volume

DIAGNOSTIC ULTRASOUND

1
volume

DIAGNOSTIC ULTRASOUND

THIRD EDITION

Carol M. Rumack, M.D.
Professor of Radiology and Pediatrics
Associate Dean for Graduate Medical Education
University of Colorado School of Medicine
University of Colorado Health Science Center
Denver, Colorado

Stephanie R. Wilson, M.D.
Professor of Medical Imaging and Obstetrics and Gynecology
University of Toronto Faculty of Medicine
Head, Section of Ultrasound
Toronto General Hospital
University Health Network
Toronto, Ontario, Canada

J. William Charboneau, M.D.
Professor of Radiology
Mayo Clinic College of Medicine
Consultant in Radiology
Mayo Clinic
Rochester, Minnesota

Associate Editor
Jo-Ann M. Johnson, M.D.
Professor, Division of Maternal Fetal Medicine
Department of Obstetrics and Gynecology
University of Calgary Faculty of Medicine
Calgary, Alberta, Canada

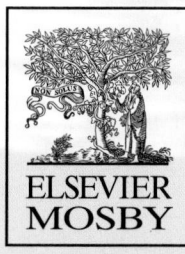

ELSEVIER
MOSBY

**ELSEVIER
MOSBY**

An Affiliate of Elsevier

11830 Westline Industrial Drive
St. Louis, Missouri 63146

DIAGNOSTIC ULTRASOUND, THIRD EDITION   0-323-02023-2

NOTICE

Radiology is an ever-changing field. Standard safety precautions must be followed, but as new research and clinical experience broaden our knowledge, changes in treatment and drug therapy may become necessary or appropriate. Readers are advised to check the most current product information provided by the manufacturer of each drug to be administered to verify the recommended dose, the method and duration of administration, and contraindications. It is the responsibility of the licensed prescriber, relying on experience and knowledge of the patient, to determine dosages and the best treatment for each individual patient. Neither the publisher nor the author assumes any liability for any injury and/or damage to persons or property arising from this publication.

Previous editions copyrighted © 1998, 1993 by Mosby, Inc.

Library of Congress Cataloging-in-Publication Data
Diagnostic ultrasound / editors, Carol M. Rumack, Stephanie R. Wilson, J. William Charboneau; associate editor, Jo-Ann M. Johnson.–3rd ed.
    p. ; cm.
Includes bibliographical references and index.
ISBN 0-323-02023-2
1. Diagnosis, Ultrasonic. I. Rumack, Carol M. II. Wilson, Stephanie R. III. Charboneau, J. William.
    [DNLM: 1. Ultrasonography. WN 208 D5357 2005]
RC78.7.U4D514 2005
616.07'543–dc22

                                                                2004050469

Acquisitions Editor: Allan Ross
Developmental Editor: Janice Gaillard
Publishing Services Manager: Tina Rebane
Project Manager: Mary Anne Folcher
Design Coordinator: Karen O'Keefe-Owens
Volume 1 9997629515
Volume 2 9997629523

Printed in China

Last digit is the print number: 9 8 7 6 5 4 3 2 1

Editors

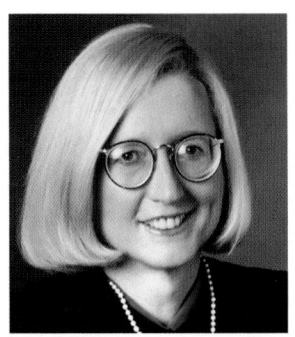

Carol M. Rumack, M.D., is Professor of Radiology and Pediatrics at the University of Colorado School of Medicine in Denver, Colorado. Her clinical practice is based at The University of Colorado Health Science Center. Her primary research has been in neonatal sonography of high-risk infants, particularly the brain. Dr. Rumack has published widely in this field and lectured frequently on pediatric ultrasound. She is an American College of Radiology Chancellor, a Chair of the American College of Radiology Commission on Ultrasound, a Fellow of both the American Institute of Ultrasound in Medicine and the Society of Radiologists in Ultrasound. She is co-editor of the most recent ACR CD-ROM Ultrasound Learning File Disk. She and her husband, Barry, have two children, Becky and Marc.

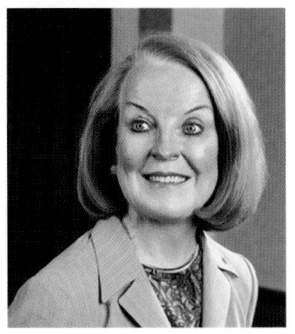

Stephanie R. Wilson, M.D., is Professor of Radiology and Obstetrics and Gynecology at the University of Toronto Faculty of Medicine and Head of the Section of Ultrasound at the Toronto General Hospital, University Health Network. Her current research endeavors, with Dr. Peter Burns, are focused on Intravascular Ultrasound Contrast Agents. Their work on the characterization and detection of focal liver masses has established them as authorities in this field. A recognized expert on ultrasound of the gastrointestinal tract and abdominal and pelvic viscera, she is the recipient of many university teaching awards and is a frequent international speaker and author. Dr. Wilson was the first woman president of the Canadian Association of Radiologists and a past vice president of the Radiological Society of North America. She was the recent recipient of the gold medal from the Canadian Association of Radiologists for recognition of her contribution to Radiology. A golf enthusiast, she and her husband, Ken, have two children, Jessica and Jordan.

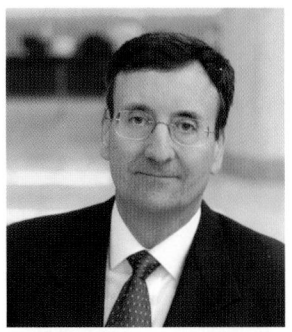

J. William Charboneau, M.D., is Professor of Radiology at the Mayo Clinic in Rochester, Minnesota. His current research interests include image-guided tumor biopsy and ablation as well as liver and small parts sonography. He is the coauthor of over 100 publications, assistant editor of the Mayo Clinic Family Health Book, and an active lecturer nationally and internationally. He and his wife, Cathy, have three children, Nick, Ben, and Laurie.

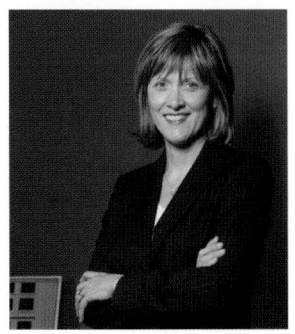

Jo-Ann M. Johnson, M.D., is Professor of Division of Maternal Fetal Medicine, Department of Obstetrics and Gynecology, University of Calgary Faculty of Medicine, Calgary, Alberta, with cross-appointment in the Department of Medical Imaging. Her main areas of clinical interest are prenatal genetic screening and diagnosis, and the ultrasound diagnosis and management of fetal anomalies. Her current research interests are in the evaluation of new ultrasound and biochemical markers for fetal abnormalities in early pregnancy. She is a frequent national and international speaker and member of the board of the International Society for Prenatal Diagnosis (ISPD). She and her husband, Patrick, have four children, Aidan, Elizabeth, Katherine, and Ciara.

Contributors

Fawaz Alkazaleh, M.D.
Assistant Professor and Consultant in Obstetrics and Gynecology; Consultant in Maternal-Fetal Medicine, Department of Obstetrics and Gynecology, Division of Maternal-Fetal Medicine, Jordan University Hospital, Amman, Jordan

Mostafa Atri, M.D., F.R.C.P.C.
Associate Professor of Radiology and Head, Abdominal Division, Department of Medical Imaging, University of Toronto Faculty of Medicine, Toronto, Ontario, Canada

Thomas D. Atwell, M.D.
Associate Professor of Radiology, Mayo Clinic College of Medicine, Consultant in Radiology, Mayo Clinic, Rochester, Minnesota

Diane S. Babcock, M.D.
Professor of Radiology and Pediatrics, University of Cincinnati College of Medicine and University Hospital, Cincinnati Children's Hospital Medical Center, Cincinnati, Ohio

Carol E. Barnewolt, M.D.
Assistant Professor of Radiology, Harvard Medical School; Pediatric Radiologist and Co-Director, Section of Fetal Imaging; Department of Radiology, Children's Hospital, Boston, Massachusetts

Carol B. Benson, M.D.
Professor of Radiology, Harvard Medical School; Director of Ultrasound and Co-Director, High-Risk Obstetrical Ultrasound, Brigham and Women's Hospital, Boston, Massachusetts

William E. Brant, M.D.
Professor of Radiology and Acting Chair, Department of Radiology, School of Medicine, University of Virginia Health System, Charlottesville, Virginia

Robert L. Bree, M.D., M.H.S.A., F.A.C.R.
Clinical Professor of Radiology, University of Washington School of Medicine, Seattle; Medical Director, Radia Medical Imaging, Everett, Washington

Dorothy I. Bulas, M.D.
Professor of Pediatrics and Radiology, George Washington University School of Medicine and Health Sciences; Director, Program in Diagnostic Imaging, Division of Diagnostic Imaging, Children's National Medical Center, Washington, DC

Peter N. Burns, Ph.D.
Professor of Medical Biophysics and Radiology, University of Toronto Faculty of Medicine; Senior Scientist, Imaging Research, Sunnybrook and Women's Health Sciences Centre, Toronto, Ontario, Canada

Barbara A. Carroll, M.D.
Professor of Radiology, Department of Radiology, Duke University Medical Center, Durham, North Carolina

J. William Charboneau, M.D.
Professor of Radiology, Mayo Clinical College of Medicine, Consultant in Radiology, Mayo Clinic, Rochester, Minnesota

David Chitayat, M.D.
Professor of Pediatrics, Obstetrics, and Gynaecology, Laboratory Medicine and Pathology, University of Toronto Faculty of Medicine, Toronto, Ontario, Canada

Simona Cicero, M.D.
Research Fellow, Harris Birthright Research Centre for Fetal Medicine, King's College Hospital, London, England

Christine H. Comstock, M.D.
Director, Division of Fetal Imaging, William Beaumont Hospital, Royal Oak; Associate Clinical Professor, Obstetrics and Gynecology, Wayne State University School of Medicine, Detroit; Clinical Professor, Obstetrics and Gynecology, University of Michigan Medical School, Ann Arbor, Michigan

Peter L. Cooperberg, M.D.C.M.
Professor and Vice Chairman of Radiology, University of British Columbia, Vancouver, British Columbia, Canada

Jeanne A. Cullinan, M.D.
Radiology Residency Program Director; Associate
Professor; Director of Women's Imaging, Department of
Radiology; Director, Comprehensive Breast Cancer
Program, James P. Wilmot Cancer Center, University of
Rochester Medical Center; Director of Women's Imaging,
Strong Health Breast Care Center at Highland Hospital,
Rochester, New York

Peter M. Doubilet, M.D., Ph.D.
Professor of Radiology, Harvard Medical School; Senior
Vice Chair of Radiology, Brigham and Women's Hospital,
Boston, Massachusetts

Dónal B. Downey, M.B.B.Ch.
Department of Diagnostic Radiology, London Health
Sciences Centre, London, Ontario, Canada

Julia A. Drose, R.D.M.S., R.D.C.S., R.V.T.
Associate Professor, Department of Radiology, University
of Colorado School of Medicine; Chief Sonographer,
Division of Ultrasound, University of Colorado Hospital,
Denver, Colorado

Beth S. Edeiken-Monroe, M.D.
Associate Professor of Radiology, University of
Texas–Houston Medical School, M. D. Anderson Cancer
Center, Houston, Texas

Sturla H. Eik-Nes, M.D., Ph.D.
Professor, Department of Obstetrics, National Center for
Fetal Medicine, Trondheim University Hospital,
Trondheim, Norway

Paul W. Finnegan, M.D.C.M.
Vice President, Alexion Pharmaceuticals, Inc, Cheshire,
Connecticut

Katherine W. Fong, M.B.
Associate Professor, Department of Medical Imaging and
Department of Obstetrics and Gynecology, University of
Toronto Faculty of Medicine; Staff Radiologist, Mount
Sinai Hospital and University Health Network, Toronto,
Ontario, Canada

Bruno D. Fornage, M.D.
Professor of Radiology and Surgical Oncology,
Department of Diagnostic Radiology, University of
Texas–Houston Medical School, M. D. Anderson Cancer
Center, Houston, Texas

J. Brian Fowlkes, Ph.D.
Associate Professor of Radiology and Biomedical
Engineering, University of Michigan Medical School,
Ann Arbor, Michigan

Margaret A. Fraser-Hill, M.D.C.M
Assistant Professor, Department of Radiology, University
of Ottawa Faculty of Medicine, Staff Radiologist,
Department of Diagnostic Imaging, Ottawa Hospital,
Ottawa, Ontario, Canada

Phyllis Glanc, M.D.
Assistant Professor, University of Toronto Faculty of
Medicine, Department of Medical Imaging, Women's
College Health Sciences Centre, Toronto, Ontario,
Canada

Charles M. Glasier, M.D.
Professor of Radiology, University of Arkansas for Medical
Sciences; Director of Magnetic Resonance Imaging,
Arkansas Children's Hospital, Little Rock, Arkansas

Brian Gorman, M.B., B.Ch., M.R.C.P.I., M.B.A.
Assistant Professor of Radiology, Mayo Clinic College of
Medicine, Consultant in Radiology, Mayo Clinic,
Rochester, Minnesota

S. Bruce Greenberg, M.D.
Associate Professor of Radiology, University of Arkansas
for Medical Sciences; Staff Radiologist, Arkansas
Children's Hospital, Little Rock, Arkansas

Leslie E. Grissom, M.D.
Associate Professor of Radiology, Jefferson Medical
College of Thomas Jefferson University, Philadelphia,
Pennsylvania; Attending Radiologist, Alfred I. duPont
Hospital for Children, Wilmington, Delaware

Anthony E. Hanbidge, M.B.B.Ch.
Assistant Professor, Department of Medical Imaging,
University of Toronto Faculty of Medicine, Division
Head, Abdominal Imaging, University Health Network
and Mount Sinai Hospital, Toronto, Ontario, Canada

H. Theodore Harcke, M.D.
Professor of Radiology and Pediatrics, Jefferson Medical
College of Thomas Jefferson University, Philadelphia,
Pennsylvania; Chief of Imaging Research, Alfred I. duPont
Hospital for Children, Wilmington, Delaware

Christopher R. Harman, M.D., F.R.C.S.
Professor and Vice-Chairman, Department of Obstetrics,
Gynecology, and Reproductive Sciences, University of
Maryland School of Medicine, Baltimore, Maryland

Ian D. Hay, M.B., Ph.D.
Professor of Medicine, Mayo Clinic College of Medicine,
Consultant of Division of Endocrinology, Metabolism,
Nutrition and Internal Medicine, Mayo Clinic, Rochester,
Minnesota

Christy K. Holland, *Ph.D.*
Associate Professor and Director of Research,
Departments of Biomedical Engineering and Radiology,
University of Cincinnati College of Medicine, Cincinnati,
Ohio

Caroline Hollingsworth, *M.D.*
Assistant Professor, Duke University Medical System,
Durham, North Carolina

Lisa K. Hornberger, *M.D.*
Associate Professor of Pediatrics and Director, Fetal
Cardiovascular Program, Departments of Pediatric
Cardiology and Surgery, University of California, San
Francisco, School of Medicine and Children's Hospital,
San Francisco, California

Bonnie J. Huppert, *M.D.*
Assistant Professor of Radiology, Mayo Clinic College of
Medicine, Consultant in Radiology, Mayo Clinic,
Rochester, Minnesota

Edgar T. Jaeggi, *M.D.*
Associate Professor of Pediatrics, University of Toronto
Faculty of Medicine; Director, Fetal Cardiovascular
Program, Division of Cardiology, Hospital for Sick
Children, Toronto, Ontario, Canada

E. Meredith James, *M.D.*
Professor of Radiology, Mayo Clinic College of Medicine,
Consultant in Radiology, Mayo Clinic, Rochester,
Minnesota

Ann Jefferies, *M.D.*
Associate Professor, Department of Pediatrics, University
of Toronto Faculty of Medicine, Staff Neonatologist,
Mount Sinai Hospital, Toronto, Ontario, Canada

Susan D. John, *M.D.*
Professor of Radiology and Pediatrics, University of
Texas–Houston Medical School; Chair, Department of
Radiology, Memorial Hermann Hospital; Chief of
Pediatric Radiology, Memorial Hermann Children's
Hospital, Houston, Texas

Jo-Ann M. Johnson, *M.D.*
Professor, Division of Maternal Fetal Medicine,
Department of Obstetrics and Gynecology, University of
Calgary Faculty of Medicine, Calgary, Alberta, Canada

Neil D. Johnson, *M.B.B.S., M.Med.*
Professor of Radiology and Pediatrics, University of
Cincinnati College of Medicine; Staff Radiologist and
Medical Director, Information Systems, Cincinnati
Children's Hospital Medical Center, Cincinnati, Ohio

Robert A. Kane, *M.D.*
Professor of Radiology, Harvard Medical School and
Brigham and Women's Hospital, Boston, Massachusetts

Korosh Khalili, *M.D., F.R.C.P.C.*
Assistant Professor, University of Toronto Faculty of
Medicine, Toronto, Ontario, Canada

John C. P. Kingdom, *M.D., M.R.C.P.*
Professor, Department of Obstetrics and Gynecology
Pathology, University of Toronto Faculty of Medicine;
Staff Obstetrician and Maternal-Fetal Medicine Director,
Mount Sinai Hospital, Toronto, Ontario, Canada

Robert A. Lee, *M.D.*
Assistant Professor of Radiology, Mayo Clinic College of
Medicine, Consultant in Radiology, Mayo Clinic,
Rochester, Minnesota

Richard E. Leithiser, Jr., *M.D., M.M.M.*
Associate Professor of Radiology, University of Arkansas
for Medical Sciences; Chief, Pediatric Radiology, Arkansas
Children's Hospital, Little Rock, Arkansas

Clifford S. Levi, *M.D.*
Professor of Radiology, University of Manitoba Faculty of
Medicine; Section Head of Diagnostic Ultrasound, Health
Sciences Centre, Winnipeg, Manitoba, Canada

Bernard J. Lewandowski, *M.D.*
Clinical Associate Professor, University of Ottawa,
Radiologist, Department of Diagnostic Imaging, Ottawa
Hospital, Ottawa, Ontario, Canada

Bradley D. Lewis, *M.D.*
Associate Professor of Radiology, Mayo Clinic College of
Medicine, Consultant in Radiology, Mayo Clinic,
Rochester, Minnesota

Edward A. Lyons, *M.D.*
Professor of Radiology, Obstetrics and Gynecology, and
Anatomy, University of Manitoba Faculty of Medicine;
Radiologist, Section of Diagnostic Ultrasound, Health
Sciences Centre, Winnipeg, Manitoba, Canada

Marie-Jocelyne Martel, *M.D.*
Clinical Associate Professor, Department of Obstetrics,
Gynecology, and Reproductive Sciences, University of
Saskatchewan College of Medicine, Saskatoon,
Saskatchewan, Canada

John R. Mathieson, *M.D., F.R.C.P.C.*
Vice Chief, Medical Imaging, Vancouver Island Health
Authority SI, Royal Jubilee Hospital, Victoria, British
Columbia, Canada

Cynthia V. Maxwell, M.D.
Assistant Professor of Obstetrics and Gynecology,
University of Toronto Faculty of Medicine; Staff,
Maternal-Fetal Medicine, Mount Sinai Hospital, Toronto,
Ontario, Canada

Fionnuala McAuliffe, M.D., M.R.C.O.G.,
M.R.C.P.I.
Senior Lecturer, Obstetrics and Gynecology, University
College Dublin, Consultant, Obstetrics and Gynecology,
National Maternity Hospital, Dublin, Ireland

John P. McGahan, M.D.
Professor of Radiology and Director, Abdominal Imaging
and Ultrasound, University of California, Davis, Medical
Center, Sacramento, California

John Mernagh, M.D., F.R.C.P.C., Ph.D.
Associate Professor, Department of Radiology, McMaster
University Faculty of Health Science, Hamilton, Ontario,
Canada

Christopher R. B. Merritt, M.D.
Professor and Vice Chair for Informatics, Department of
Radiology, Jefferson Medical College of Thomas Jefferson
University; Thomas Jefferson University Hospital,
Jefferson Ultrasound Research and Education Institute,
Philadelphia, Pennsylvania

Patrick Mohide, M.Sc., M.D.
Professor and Chair, Department of Obstetrics and
Gynecology, McMaster University Faculty of Health
Science, Hamilton, Ontario, Canada

Derek Muradali, M.D.
Assistant Professor, University of Toronto Faculty of
Medicine, Head, Division of Ultrasound, St. Michael's
Hospital, Toronto, Ontario, Canada

Khanh T. Nguyen, M.D., F.R.C.P.C.
Associate Professor, Department of Diagnostic Radiology,
Queen's University Faculty of Health Science, Kingston
General Hospital, Hotel Dieu Hospital, and St. Mary's of
the Lake Hospital, Kingston, Ontario, Canada

Kypros Nicolaides, M.B.B.S., M.R.C.O.G.
Professor of Fetal Medicine, and Consultant in Obstetrics,
Director, Harris Birthright Research Centre for Fetal
Medicine, King's College Hospital School of Medicine
and Dentistry; Director, Fetal Medicine Foundation,
London, England

Robert L. Nolan, M.D.
Professor, Department of Diagnostic Radiology, Queen's
University Faculty of Health Science, Kingston General
Hospital, Hotel Dieu Hospital, and St. Mary's of the Lake
Hospital, Kingston, Ontario, Canada

Sara M. O'Hara, M.D.
Associate Professor of Radiology and Pediatrics, University
of Cincinnati College of Medicine; Director, Ultrasound
Division, Department of Radiology, Cincinnati Children's
Hospital Medical Center, Cincinnati, Ohio

Nanette Okun, M.D.
Associate Professor, Department of Obstetrics and
Gynecology, University of Toronto Faculty of Medicine;
Staff Perinatologist, Mount Sinai Hospital, Toronto,
Ontario, Canada

Valerie Osti, M.D.
Department of Radiology, General Hospital of Saronno,
Saronno (VA), Italy

Pranav Pandya, M.D., M.B.B.S., M.R.C.O.G.
Honorary Senior Lecturer, University College London;
Consultant in Fetal Medicine and Obstetrics, University
College Hospital, London, United Kingdom

Elisabeth Peregrine, M.B.B.S., M.R.C.O.G.
Clinical Research Fellow, University College London,
London, United Kingdom

Joseph F. Polak, M.D., M.P.H.
Professor of Radiology, Tufts University Medical School;
Chief of Radiology, Lemuel Shattuck Hospital; Director
of Cardiovascular Imaging, New England Medical Center,
Boston, Massachusetts

Carl C. Reading, M.D.
Professor of Radiology, Mayo Clinic College of Medicine,
Consultant in Radiology, Mayo Clinic, Rochester,
Minnesota

Frank Reister, M.D.
Assistant Professor, Department of Obstetrics and
Gynecology and Staff Perinatologist and Consultant in
Obstetrics, University Hospital, Ulm, Germany

Henrietta Kotlus Rosenberg, M.D.
Professor of Radiology, Jefferson Ultrasound Research and
Education Institute, Jefferson Medical College of Thomas
Jefferson University, Philadelphia, Pennsylvania; Network
Section Chief of Pediatric Radiology, Generations +
Northern Manhattan Health Network, New York,
New York

Carol M. Rumack, M.D.
Professor of Radiology and Pediatrics and Associate
Dean for Graduate Medical Education, University of
Colorado School of Medicine, University of Colorado
Health Sciences Center School of Medicine, Denver,
Colorado

Greg Ryan, M.B., M.R.C.O.D.
Assistant Professor, University of Toronto Faculty of
Medicine; Director, Fetal Medicine Unit, Mount Sinai
Hospital, Toronto, Ontario, Canada

Shia Salem, M.D.
Associate Professor, Medical Imaging, University of
Toronto Faculty of Medicine, Radiologist, Medical
Imaging, Mount Sinai Hospital, Toronto, Ontario,
Canada

Kjell Å. Salvesen, M.D., Ph.D.
Professor, Department of Obstetrics, National Center for
Fetal Medicine, Trondheim University Hospital,
Trondheim, Norway

Eric E. Sauerbrei, M.Sc., M.D.
Professor of Radiology and Adjunct Professor of
Obstetrics and Gynecology, Queen's University Faculty of
Health Sciences; Director of Ultrasound and Director of
Residents' Research, Kingston General Hospital, Hotel
Dieu Hospital, Kingston, Ontario, Canada

Gareth R. Seaward, M.B.B.Ch., M.Med.
Associate Professor, Department of Obstetrics and
Gynecology, University of Toronto Faculty of Medicine;
Medical Director, Labor and Delivery, Mount Sinai
Hospital, Toronto, Ontario, Canada

Joanna J. Seibert, M.D.
Professor of Radiology and Pediatrics, University of
Arkansas for Medical Sciences; Staff Radiologist, Arkansas
Children's Hospital, Little Rock, Arkansas

Robert W. Seibert, M.D.
Professor of Otolaryngology, University of Arkansas for
Medical Sciences, Little Rock, Arkansas

Luigi Solbiati, M.D.
Director, Department of Diagnostic Imaging, General
Hospital of Busto Arsizio, Busto Arsizio (VA), Italy

A. Thomas Stavros, M.D.
Director, Ultrasound and Noninvasive Vascular Services,
Swedish Hospital, Englewood, Colorado

George A. Taylor, M.D.
John A. Kirkpatrick Professor of Radiology (Pediatrics),
Harvard Medical School; Radiologist-in-Chief, Children's
Hospital, Boston, Massachusetts

Wendy Thurston, M.D.
Assistant Professor, University of Toronto Faculty of
Medicine, Deputy Chief of Diagnostic Imaging and
Head, Division of Ultrasound, St. Joseph's Health Centre,
Toronto, Ontario, Canada

Ants Toi, M.D.
Associate Professor of Radiology, University of Toronto
Faculty of Medicine, Radiologist, Department of Medical
Imaging, University Health Network, Princess Margaret
Hospital, Toronto, Ontario, Canada

Didier H. Touche, M.D.
Staff Radiologist, Cabinet de Radiologie Buirette, Reims,
France

Jean Trines, R.N., R.D.C.S.
Educator, Echocardiography Laboratory; Coordinator,
Fetal Cardiac Outreach Program, Hospital for Sick
Children, Toronto, Ontario, Canada

Sheila Unger, M.D.
Assistant Professor of Paediatrics, Division of Clinical and
Metabolic Genetics, Hospital for Sick Children, Toronto,
Ontario, Canada

Marnix T. van Holsbeeck, M.D.
Associate Professor of Radiology, Case Western Reserve
University Medical School, Cleveland, Ohio; Division
Head, Musculoskeletal Radiology, Henry Ford Health
System, Detroit, Michigan

Sandra Viero, M.D.
Lecturer, Department of Laboratory Medicine and
Pathobiology, University of Toronto Faculty of Medicine;
Staff Pathologist, Hospital for Sick Children, Toronto
University Faculty of Medicine, Toronto, Ontario,
Canada

Patrick M. Vos, M.D.
Clinical Instructor of Radiology, University of British
Columbia Faculty of Medicine, Vancouver, British
Columbia, Canada

Stephanie R. Wilson, M.D.
Professor of Medical Imaging and Obstetrics and
Gynecology, University of Toronto Faculty of Medicine;
Head, Section of Ultrasound, Toronto General Hospital,
University Health Network, Toronto, Ontario,
Canada

Rory Windrim, M.B., M.Sc.
Associate Professor, Department of Obstetrics and
Gynecology, University of Toronto Faculty of Medicine;
Staff Perinatologist, Mount Sinai Hospital, Toronto,
Ontario, Canada

Cynthia E. Withers, M.D.
Staff Radiologist, Department of Radiology, Santa Barbara
Cottage Hospital, Santa Barbara, California

Preface

Diagnostic Ultrasound, Third Edition, builds on the strong base of the previous editions. We understand that this textbook is the most commonly used reference in ultrasound practices worldwide, and we are pleased to provide a new update of images and text with many new areas of strength. Because sonography has expanded its frontiers in the past 6 years, it was time for a major revision of *Diagnostic Ultrasound* for it to remain the definitive reference work of this specialty. In particular, greater use of color and power Doppler and harmonic images, improved high-resolution transducers, greater fields of view, and more uses for ultrasound contrast agents have required the introduction of new chapters and new authors, as well as the expansion and enhancement of the Second Edition's original material.

Great strides have been made in obstetrical sonography with fetal imaging. Growth and development of the fetus, three-dimensional imaging, and MRI correlation are bringing new areas of understanding to fetal anomalies.

Organ transplantation is now a separate chapter on key issues surrounding this intense area of interest for sonography.

Approximately 100 outstanding new and previous authors have contributed to this edition, and all are recognized experts in the field of ultrasound. There has been a substantial increase in the size of the two volumes, with the major space reallocation applied to obstetrics and gynecology. Thousands of the original images have been replaced, and new images have been added. The Third Edition now includes more than 5000 images, many in full color. The layout has been exhaustively revamped, and there are highly valuable multipart figures or key feature collages. These images all reflect the spectrum of sonographic changes that may occur in a given disease instead of the most common manifestation only.

The book's format has been redesigned to facilitate reading and review. There are again color-enhanced boxes to highlight the important or critical features of sonographic diagnoses. Key terms and concepts are emphasized in boldface type. To direct the reader to other research and literature of interest, comprehensive reference lists are organized by topic.

Diagnostic Ultrasound is again divided into two volumes. Volume I consists of Parts I to IV. Part I contains chapters on physics and biologic effects of ultrasound, as well as the latest developments in ultrasound contrast agents. Part II covers abdominal, pelvic, and thoracic sonography, including interventional procedures. There is a new chapter on organ transplantation. Part III presents intraoperative and laparoscopic sonography. Part IV contains many chapters on small-parts imaging, including carotid and peripheral artery and vein evaluation.

Volume II begins with Part V, where the greatest expansion of text and images has been on obstetric and fetal sonography. The first trimester is presented in depth in two chapters. Part VI comprehensively covers pediatric sonography.

Diagnostic Ultrasound is for practicing physicians, residents, medical students, sonographers, and others interested in understanding the vast applications of diagnostic sonography in patient care. Our goal is for *Diagnostic Ultrasound* to continue to be the most comprehensive reference book available in the sonographic literature with a highly readable style and superb images.

Preface
to the second edition

The First Edition of *Diagnostic Ultrasound*, released at the RSNA in 1991, has become the most commonly used reference textbook at ultrasound practices worldwide. Because sonography has so expanded its frontiers in the past 6 years, we believed that a major revision was required for *Diagnostic Ultrasound* to remain the definitive reference work for this specialty. In particular, greater use of color and power Doppler imaging and improved high-resolution transducers have required the introduction of new chapters and new authors, as well as the expansion and enhancement of the First Edition's original material.

Approximately 100 outstanding authors, all recognized experts in the field of ultrasound, bring you the latest state-of-the-art concepts on ultrasound performance, imaging, diagnosis, and expanded applications, including hysterosonography, laparoscopic sonography, and ultrasound-guided biopsy and drainage techniques.

There has been a 25% increase in the size of the two volumes, the major space reallocation applied to obstetrics and gynecology. Thousands of the original images have been replaced, and new images have been added. The Second Edition also includes more than 450 images in full color. The layout has been exhaustively revamped and now includes multiple-picture "Key Feature Collages." These reflect the spectrum of sonographic changes that may occur in a given disease instead of just the most common manifestation.

Many improvements in the book's format have been designed to facilitate reading and review. Color-enhanced boxes highlight the important or critical features of sonographic diagnoses. Key terms and concepts are emphasized in boldface type. To direct the reader to other research and literature of interest, the comprehensive reference lists are well organized by topic.

The book is again divided into two volumes. Volume I consists of Parts I–IV. Part I contains chapters on physics and biologic effects of ultrasound, as well as the latest developments in ultrasound contrast agents. Part II covers abdominal, pelvic, and thoracic sonography, including interventional procedures. Part III presents intraoperative and laparoscopic sonography. Part IV contains many chapters on small-parts imaging, including carotid and peripheral artery and vein evaluation. Volume II begins with Part V, a greatly expanded section on obstetric and fetal sonography. Part VI comprehensively covers pediatric sonography. Two new chapters on pediatric brain Doppler and pediatric interventional sonography have been added to Part VI.

This book is for practicing physicians, residents, medical students, sonographers, and others interested in understanding the vast applications of diagnostic sonography in patient care. As with the First Edition, *it is our goal to present to you the most comprehensive reference book available on diagnostic ultrasound.*

Acknowledgments

Our deepest appreciation and sincerest gratitude:

To all of our outstanding authors who have contributed extensive, newly updated, and authoritative text and images. We cannot thank them enough for their efforts on this project.

To Gayle Craun in Denver, Colorado, whose outstanding secretarial and communication skills with authors and editors have facilitated the review and final revision of the entire manuscript. Her enthusiastic attention to detail and accuracy helps to make this our best edition ever.

To Gordana Popovic for her beautiful new illustrations.

To Lori Kulas in Rochester, Minnesota, for her assistance in the manuscript preparation.

To Helen Robson, Research Coordinator, Division of Maternal Fetal Medicine, University of Toronto, for her special assistance to Jo-Ann Johnson.

To Janice Gaillard who has been dedicated to this project from the very beginning of the concept of the Third Edition. We also thank the enthusiastic participation of many other Elsevier Mosby staff including Allan Ross, Karen O'Keefe Owens, and Mary Anne Folcher who patiently brought the process to the final stages of development and production. It has been an intense period for everyone, and we are very proud of this superb edition of *Diagnostic Ultrasound*.

Contents

VOLUME 1

VOLUME 2

Contents xxiii

I

PHYSICS

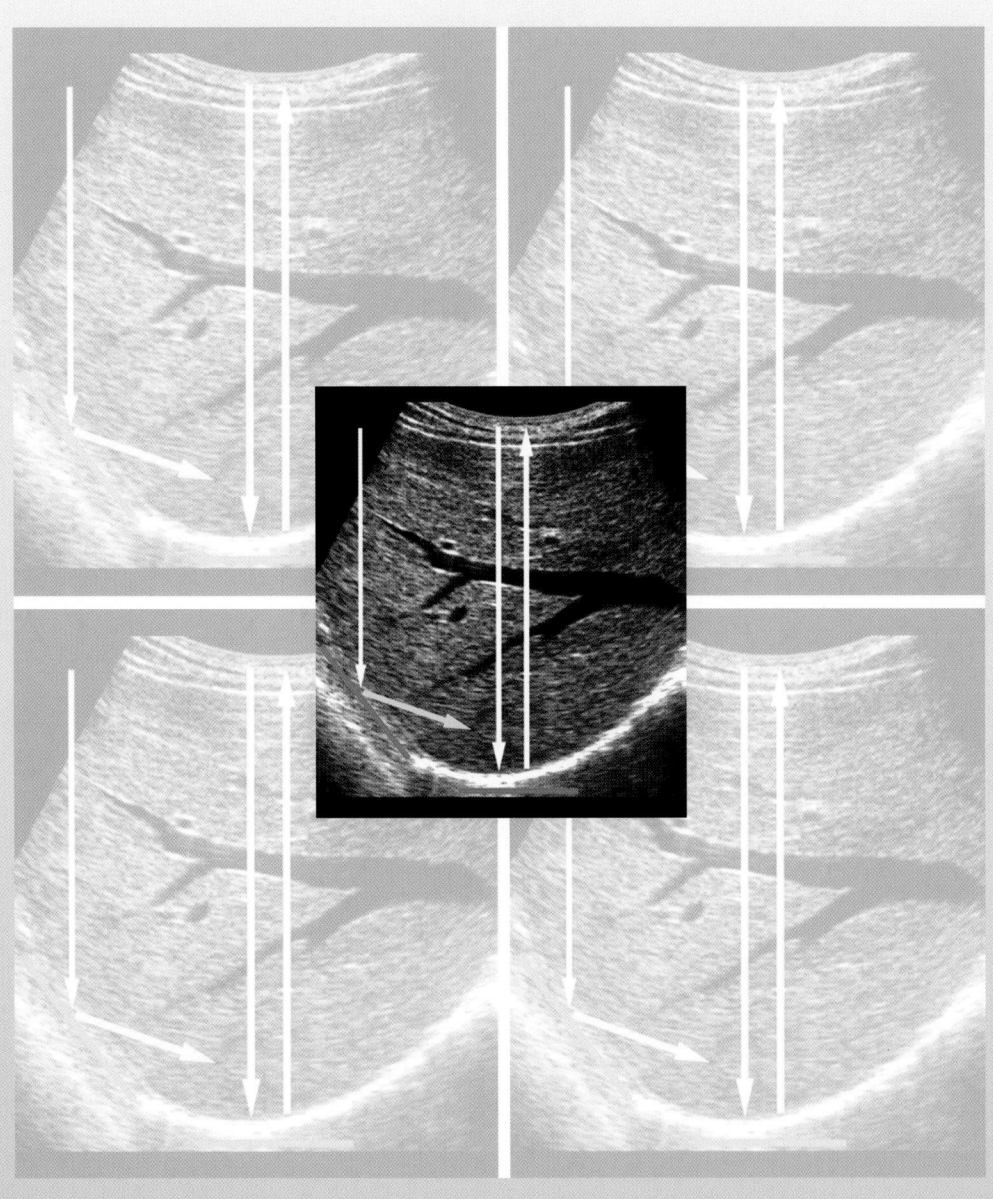

1

PHYSICS OF ULTRASOUND

Christopher R. B. Merritt

Chapter Outline

All diagnostic ultrasound applications are based on the detection and display of acoustic energy reflected from interfaces within the body. These interactions provide the information needed to generate high-resolution, gray-scale images of the body as well as display information related to blood flow. The unique imaging attributes of ultrasound have made it an important and versatile medical imaging tool. Unfortunately, the use of expensive, state-of-the-art ultrasound instrumentation does not guarantee the production of high-quality studies of diagnostic value. Gaining maximum benefit from this complex technology requires a combination of skills, including knowledge of the physical principles that empower ultrasound with its unique diagnostic capabilities. The user must understand the fundamentals of the interactions of acoustic energy with tissue and the methods and instruments used to produce and optimize the ultrasound display. With this knowledge the user can collect the maximum information from each examination, avoiding pitfalls and errors in diagnosis that may result from the omission of information or the misinterpretation of artifacts.

Ultrasound imaging and Doppler ultrasound are based on the scattering of sound energy by interfaces formed of materials of different properties through interactions governed by acoustic physics. The amplitude of reflected energy is used to generate ultrasound images, and frequency shifts in the backscattered ultrasound provide information relating to moving targets such as blood. To produce, detect, and process ultrasound data, numerous variables, many under direct user control, must be managed. To do this, the user must understand the methods used to generate ultrasound data and the theory and operation of the instruments that detect, display, and store the acoustic information generated in clinical examinations. This chapter will provide an overview of the fundamentals of acoustics, the physics of ultrasound imaging and flow detection, and ultrasound instrumentation with emphasis on points most relevant to clinical practice.

BASIC ACOUSTICS

Wavelength and Frequency

Sound is the result of mechanical energy traveling through matter as a wave producing alternating compression and rarefaction. Pressure waves are propagated by limited physical displacement of the material through which the sound is being transmitted. A plot of these

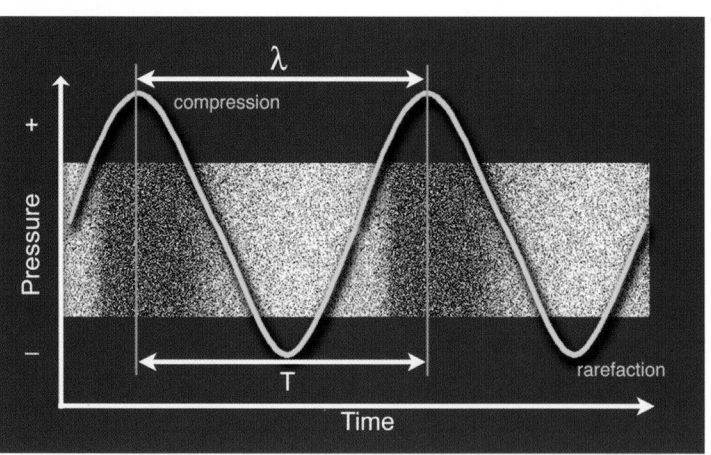

FIGURE 1-1. Sound Waves. Sound is transmitted mechanically at the molecular level. In the resting state, the pressure is uniform throughout the medium. Sound is propagated as a series of alternating pressure waves producing compression and rarefaction of the conducting medium. The time for a pressure wave to pass a given point is the period, T. The frequency of the wave is 1/T. The wavelength, λ, is the distance between corresponding points on the time-pressure curve.

changes in pressure is a sinusoidal waveform (Fig. 1-1) in which the Y axis indicates the pressure at a given point while the X axis indicates time. **Changes in pressure with time define the basic units of measurement for sound**. The distance between corresponding points on the time-pressure curve is defined as the **wavelength**, λ, and the time, T, to complete a single cycle is called the period. The number of complete cycles in a unit of time is the **frequency**, f, of the sound. Frequency and period are inversely related. If the period, T, is expressed in seconds, then $f = 1/T$ or $f = T \times sec^{-1}$. The unit of **acoustic frequency** is the **hertz** (Hz) where 1 Hz = 1 cycle per second. High frequencies are expressed in kilohertz (kHz; 1 kHz = 1000 Hz) or megahertz (MHz; 1 MHz = 1,000,000 Hz).

In nature, acoustic frequencies span a range from less than 1 Hz to more than 100,000 Hz (100 kHz). Human hearing is limited to the lower part of this range, extending from 20 to 20,000 Hz. Ultrasound differs from audible sound only in its frequency, and is 500 to 1000 times higher than the sound we normally hear. Sound frequencies used for diagnostic applications typically range from 2 to 15 MHz, although frequencies as high as 50 to 60 MHz are under investigation for certain specialized imaging applications. In general, the frequencies used for ultrasound imaging are higher than those used for Doppler. Regardless of the frequency, the same basic principles of acoustics apply.

Propagation of Sound

Most clinical applications of ultrasound use brief bursts or pulses of energy that are transmitted into the body where they are propagated through tissue. It is possible for acoustic pressure waves to travel in a direction perpendicular to the direction of the particles being displaced (transverse waves), but in tissue and fluids, sound propagation is along the direction of particle movement (longitudinal waves). The speed at which the pressure wave moves through tissue varies greatly

and is affected by the physical properties of the tissue. Propagation velocity is largely determined by the resistance of the medium to compression. This, in turn, is influenced by the density of the medium and its stiffness or elasticity. Propagation velocity is increased by increasing stiffness and reduced by increasing density. In the body, propagation velocity may be regarded as constant for a given tissue and is not affected by the frequency or wavelength of the sound. Figure 1-2 shows **typical propagation velocities** for a variety of materials. In the body, the propagation velocity of sound is assumed to be 1540 m/sec. This value is the average of measurements obtained from normal tissues.[1,2] Although this is a value representative of most soft tissues, some tissues, such as aerated lung and fat, have propagation velocities significantly less than 1540 m/sec, and others, such as bone, have greater velocities. Because a few normal tissues have propagation values significantly different from the average value assumed by the ultrasound scanner, the display of such tissues may be subject to measurement errors or artifacts (Fig. 1-3).

The propagation velocity of sound, c, is related to frequency and wavelength by the following simple equation:

$$c = f\lambda \qquad \qquad \mathbf{1}$$

Thus a frequency of 5 MHz can be shown to have a wavelength of 0.308 mm in tissue: $\lambda = c/f = 1540$ m sec^{-1}/5,000,000 sec^{-1} = 0.000308 m = 0.308 mm

Distance Measurement

Propagation velocity is a particularly important value in clinical ultrasound and is critical in determining the distance of a reflecting interface from the transducer. Much of the information used to generate an ultrasound scan is based on the precise measurement of time. If an ultrasound pulse is transmitted into the body and the time until an echo returns is measured, it is simple to calculate the depth of the interface that generated the

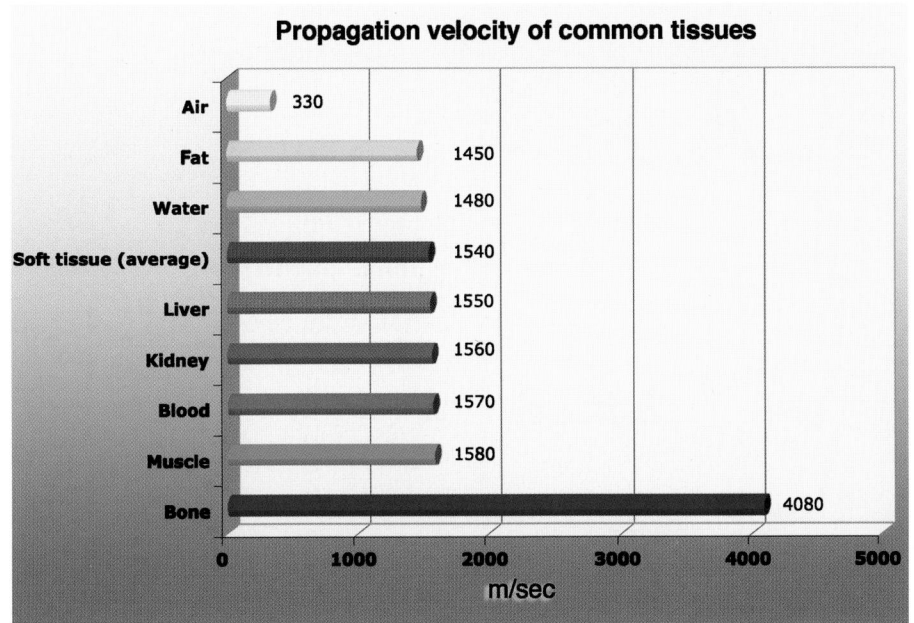

Propagation velocity of common tissues

Tissue	m/sec
Air	330
Fat	1450
Water	1480
Soft tissue (average)	1540
Liver	1550
Kidney	1560
Blood	1570
Muscle	1580
Bone	4080

m/sec

FIGURE 1-2. Propagation velocity. In the body, propagation velocity of sound is determined by the physical properties of tissue. As shown, this varies considerably. Medical ultrasound devices base their measurements on an assumed average propagation velocity of 1540 m/sec.

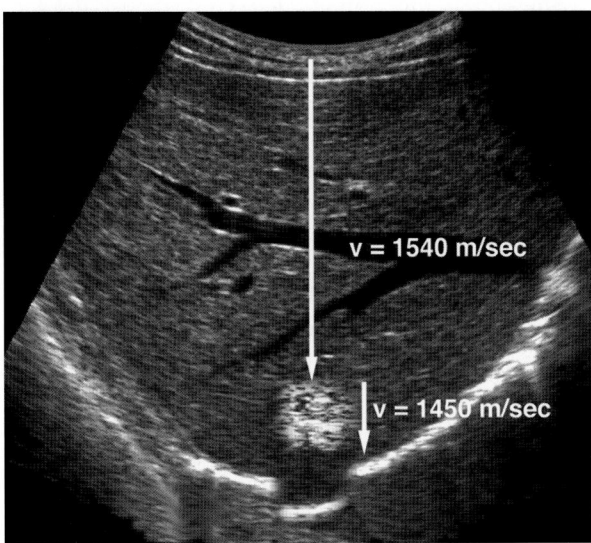

v = 1540 m/sec

v = 1450 m/sec

FIGURE 1-3. Propagation velocity artifact. When sound passes through a lesion containing fat, echo return is delayed because fat has a propagation velocity of 1450 m/sec, which is less than the liver. Because the ultrasound scanner assumes that sound is being propagated at the average velocity of 1540 m/sec, the delay in echo return is interpreted as indicating a deeper target. Therefore, the final image shows a misregistration artifact in which the diaphragm and other structures deep to the fatty lesion are shown in a deeper position than expected (simulated image).

echo, provided the propagation velocity of sound for the tissue is known. For example, if the time interval from the transmission of a pulse until the return of an echo is 0.145 ms (0.000145 sec) and the velocity of sound is 1540 m/sec, the distance that the sound has traveled must be 22.33 cm (1540 m/sec × 100 cm/m × 0.000145 sec = 22.33 cm). Because the time measured

includes the time for sound to travel to the interface and then return along the same path to the transducer, the distance from the transducer to the reflecting interface is 22.33 cm/2 = 11.165 cm (Fig. 1-4). The accuracy of this measurement is, therefore, highly influenced by how closely the presumed velocity of sound corresponds to the true velocity in the tissue being observed (see Figs. 1-2 and 1-3).

Acoustic Impedance

Current diagnostic ultrasound scanners rely on the detection and display of **reflected sound or echoes**. Imaging based on transmission of ultrasound is also possible, but is not used clinically at the present time. To produce an echo, a reflecting interface must be present. Sound passing through a **totally homogeneous medium** encounters no interfaces to reflect sound, and the medium appears anechoic or cystic. At the junction of tissues or materials with different physical properties, acoustic interfaces are present. These interfaces are responsible for the reflection of variable amounts of the incident sound energy. Thus, when ultrasound passes from one tissue to another or encounters a vessel wall or circulating blood cells, some of the incident sound energy is reflected.

The amount of reflection or backscatter is determined by the difference in the acoustic impedances of the materials forming the interface. **Acoustic impedance**, Z, is determined by product of the density, ρ, of the medium propagating the sound and the propagation velocity, c, of sound in that medium ($Z = \rho c$). Interfaces with large acoustic impedance differences, such as interfaces of tissue with air or bone, reflect almost all of the incident energy; interfaces composed of substances

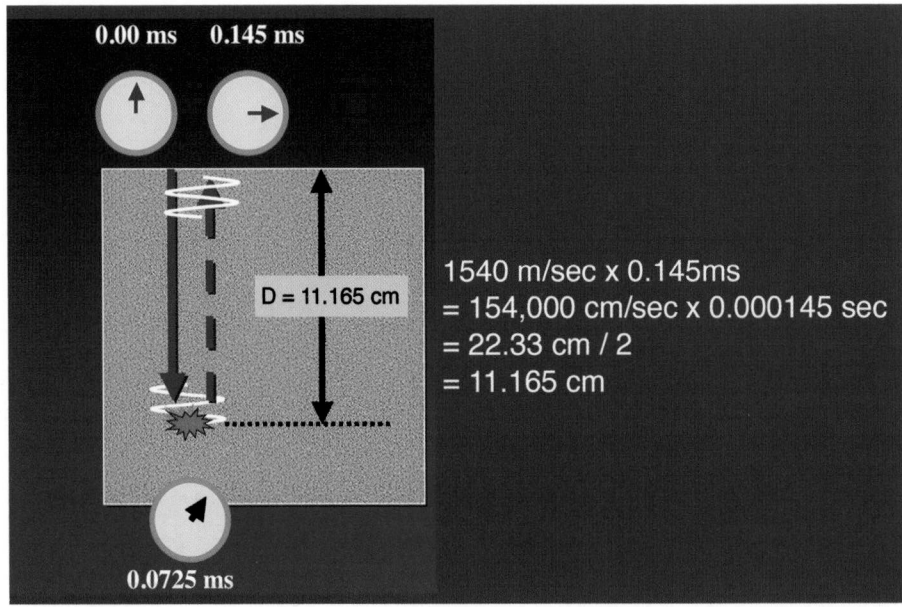

FIGURE 1-4. Ultrasound ranging. The information used to position an echo for display is based on the precise measurement of time. Here the time for an echo to travel from the transducer to the target and return to the transducer is 0.145 ms. Multiplying the velocity of sound in tissue (1540 m/sec) by the time shows that the sound returning from the target has traveled 22.33 cm. The target, therefore, lies half this distance, or 11.165 cm, from the transducer.

0.00 ms   0.145 ms

D = 11.165 cm

0.0725 ms

1540 m/sec x 0.145ms
= 154,000 cm/sec x 0.000145 sec
= 22.33 cm / 2
= 11.165 cm

SPECULAR REFLECTORS

Diaphragm
Wall of the urine-filled bladder
Endometrial stripe

with smaller differences in acoustic impedance, such as a muscle and fat interface, reflect only part of the incident energy, permitting the remainder to continue on. Like propagation velocity, acoustic impedance is determined by the properties of the tissues involved, and is independent of frequency.

Reflection

The way ultrasound is reflected when it strikes an acoustic interface is determined by the size and surface features of the interface (Fig. 1-5). If the interface is large and relatively smooth, it reflects sound much as a mirror reflects light. Such interfaces are called **specular reflectors** because they behave like mirrors for sound. Examples of specular reflectors include the diaphragm, the wall of the urine-filled bladder, and the endometrial stripe. The amount of energy reflected by an acoustic interface can be expressed as a fraction of the incident energy. This is termed the reflection coefficient, R. If a specular reflector is perpendicular to the incident sound beam, the amount of energy reflected is determined by the following relationship:

$$R = (Z_2 - Z_1)^2/(Z_2 + Z_1)^2 \qquad \textbf{2}$$

where Z_1 and Z_2 are the acoustic impedances of the media forming the interface.

Since ultrasound scanners detect only those reflections that return to the transducer, the **display of specular interfaces is highly dependent on the angle of insonation**. Specular reflectors will return echoes to the transducer only if the sound beam is perpendicular to the interface. If the interface is not at a 90-degree angle to the sound beam, it will be reflected away from the transducer, and the echo will not be detected (see Fig. 1-5A).

Most echoes in the body do not arise from specular reflectors, but come from much smaller interfaces within solid organs. In this case the acoustic interfaces involve structures with individual dimensions much smaller than the wavelength of the incident sound. The echoes from these interfaces are scattered in all directions. Such reflectors are called **diffuse reflectors** and account for the echoes that form the characteristic echo patterns seen in solid organs (see Fig. 1-5B). The constructive and destructive interference of sound scattered by diffuse reflectors results in the production of **ultrasound speckle**, a feature of tissue texture of sonograms of solid organs (Fig. 1-6). For some diagnostic applications the nature of the reflecting structures creates important conflicts. For example, most vessel walls behave as specular reflectors that require insonation at a 90-degree angle for best imaging, whereas Doppler imaging requires an angle of less than 90 degrees between the sound beam and the vessel.

Refraction

Another event that can occur when sound passes from a tissue with one acoustic propagation velocity to a tissue with a higher or lower sound velocity is a change in the direction of the sound wave. This change in direction

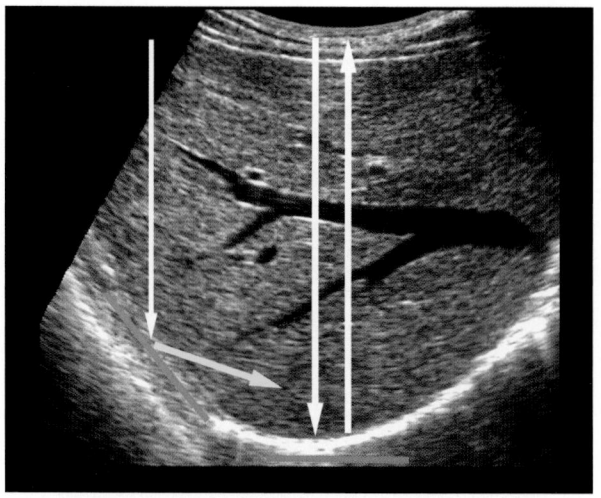
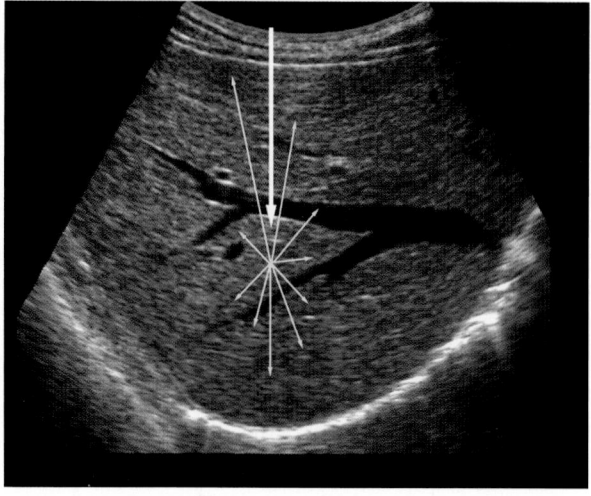

A   B

FIGURE 1-5. Specular and diffuse reflectors. Specular reflector. A, The diaphragm is a large and relatively smooth surface that reflects sound like a mirror reflects light. Thus, sound striking the diaphragm at nearly a 90-degree angle is reflected directly back to the transducer, resulting in a strong echo. Sound striking the diaphragm obliquely is reflected away from the transducer, and an echo is not displayed (*yellow arrow*). **Diffuse reflector. B,** In contrast to the diaphragm, the liver parenchyma consists of acoustic interfaces that are small in comparison to the wavelength of sound used for imaging. These interfaces scatter sound in all directions, and only a portion of the energy returns to the transducer to produce the image.

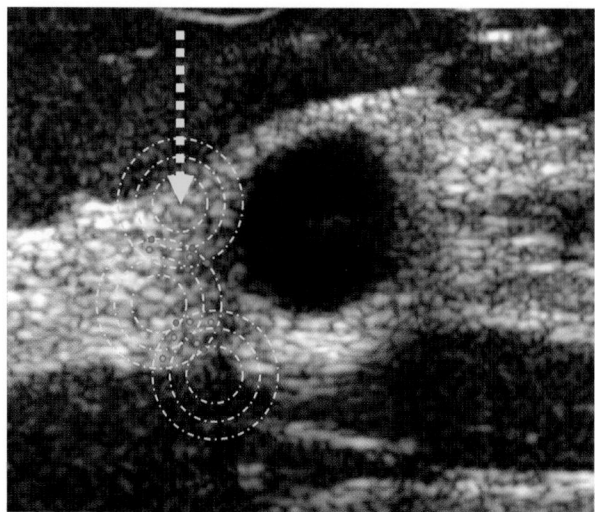

FIGURE 1-6. Speckle. Close inspection of an ultrasound image of the breast containing a small cyst reveals it to be composed of numerous areas of varying intensity (speckle). Speckle results from the constructive (*red*) and destructive (*green*) interaction of the acoustical fields (*yellow rings*) generated by the scattering of ultrasound from small tissue reflectors. This interference pattern gives ultrasound images their characteristic grainy appearance and may reduce contrast. Ultrasound speckle is the basis of the texture displayed in ultrasound images of solid tissues.

of propagation is called refraction and is governed by Snell's law:

$$\sin\theta_1/\sin\theta_2 = c_1/c_2 \qquad \mathbf{3}$$

where θ_1 is the angle of incidence of the sound approaching the interface, θ_2 is the angle of refraction,

and c_1 and c_2 are the propagation velocities of sound in the media forming the interface (Fig. 1-7). Refraction is important because it is one of the **causes of misregistration** of a structure in an ultrasound image (Fig. 1-8). When an ultrasound scanner detects an echo, it assumes that the source of the echo is along a fixed line of sight from the transducer. If the sound has been refracted, the echo detected and displayed in the image may, in fact, be coming from a different depth or location than is shown in the display. If this is suspected, **increasing the scan angle so that it is perpendicular to the interface** minimizes the artifact.

Attenuation

As the acoustic energy moves through a uniform medium, work is performed and energy is ultimately transferred to the transmitting medium as heat. The capacity to perform work is determined by the quantity of acoustic energy produced. **Acoustic power**, expressed in watts (W) or milliwatts (mW), describes the amount of acoustic energy produced in a unit of time. Although measurement of power provides an indication of the energy as it relates to time, it does not take into account the spatial distribution of the energy. **Intensity** is used to describe the spatial distribution of power. Intensity, I, is calculated by dividing the power by the area over which the power is distributed:

$$I(W/cm^2) = Power(W)/Area(cm^2) \qquad \mathbf{4}$$

The attenuation of sound energy as it passes through tissue is of great clinical importance because it influences

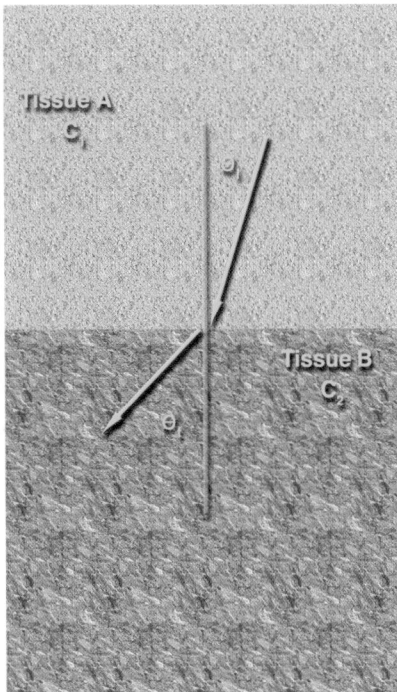

FIGURE 1-7. Refraction. When sound passes from tissue (A) with one acoustic propagation velocity (c_1) to tissue (B) which transmits sound at a different velocity (c_2) there is a change in the direction of the sound wave due to refraction. The degree of change is related to the ratio of the propagating velocities of the media forming the interface ($\sin \theta_i / \sin \theta_{tt} = c_1/c_2$).

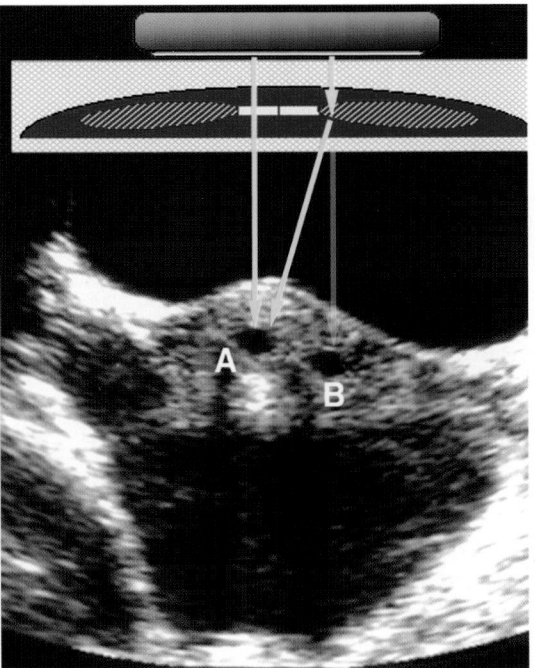

FIGURE 1-8. Refraction artifact. Axial transabdominal image of the uterus shows a small gestational sac (A) and what appears to be a second sac (B). In this case, the artifact (B) is caused by refraction at the edge of the rectus abdominis muscle. The bending of the path of the sound results in the creation of a duplicate of the image of the sac in an unexpected and misleading location (simulated image).

the depth in tissue from which useful information can be obtained. This in turn affects transducer selection and a number of operator-controlled instrument settings, including time (or depth) gain compensation, power output attenuation, and system gain levels.

Attenuation is measured in relative rather than absolute units. The decibel (dB) notation is generally used to compare different levels of ultrasound power or intensity. This value is 10 times the $\log_{10}$ of the ratio of the power or intensity values being compared. For example, if the intensity measured at one point in tissues is 10 mW/cm^2 and at a deeper point is 0.1 mW/cm^2, the difference in intensity is

$$(10)(\log_{10} 0.01/10) = (10)(\log_{10} 0.001) =$$
$$(10)(-\log_{10} 1000) = (10)(-3) = -30 \text{ dB}$$

As sound passes through tissue it loses energy, and the pressure waves decrease in amplitude as they travel farther from their source. Contributing to the attenuation of sound are the transfer of energy to tissue resulting in heating (absorption), and the removal of energy by reflection and scattering. **Attenuation** is, therefore, the result of the **combined effects of absorption, scattering, and reflection**. Attenuation depends on the insonating frequency as well as the nature of the attenuating medium. High frequencies are attenuated more rapidly

than are lower frequencies, and transducer frequency is a major determinant of the useful depth from which information can be obtained with ultrasound. Attenuation determines the efficiency with which ultrasound penetrates a specific tissue and varies considerably in normal tissues (Fig. 1-9).

INSTRUMENTATION

Ultrasound scanners are among the most complex and sophisticated imaging devices currently in use. Despite their complexity, all scanners consist of similar basic components to perform key functions—a transmitter or pulser to energize the transducer, the ultrasound transducer itself, a receiver and processor to detect and amplify the backscattered energy and manipulate the reflected signals for display, a display that presents the ultrasound image or data in a form suitable for analysis and interpretation, and a method to record or store the ultrasound image.

Transmitter

Most clinical applications use pulsed ultrasound in which brief bursts of acoustic energy are transmitted

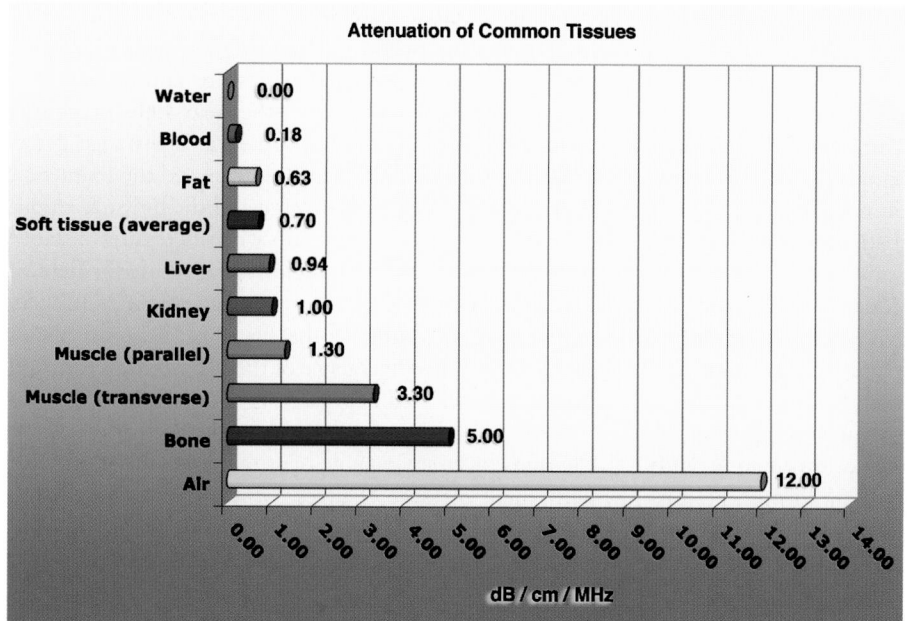

Attenuation of Common Tissues

Tissue	dB / cm / MHz
Water	0.00
Blood	0.18
Fat	0.63
Soft tissue (average)	0.70
Liver	0.94
Kidney	1.00
Muscle (parallel)	1.30
Muscle (transverse)	3.30
Bone	5.00
Air	12.00

FIGURE 1-9. Attenuation. As sound passes through tissue, it loses energy through the transfer of energy to tissue by heating, reflection, and scattering. Attenuation is determined by the insonating frequency and the nature of the attenuating medium. Attenuation values for normal tissues show considerable variation. Attenuation also increases in proportion to an increase in insonating frequency, resulting in less penetration at higher frequencies.

into the body. The ultrasound transducer that is the source of these pulses is energized by application of precisely timed, high-amplitude voltage. The maximum voltage that may be applied to the transducer is limited by federal regulations that restrict the acoustic output of diagnostic scanners. Most scanners provide a control that permits attenuation of the output voltage. Because the use of maximum output results in higher exposure of the patient to ultrasound energy, prudent use dictates use of the output attenuation controls to reduce power levels to the lowest levels consistent with the diagnostic problem.[3]

The transmitter also controls the rate of pulses emitted by the transducer or the **pulse repetition frequency (PRF).** The PRF determines the time interval between ultrasound pulses and is important in determining the depth from which unambiguous data can be obtained both in imaging and Doppler modes. The ultrasound pulses must be spaced with enough time between the pulses to permit the sound to travel to the depth of interest and return before the next pulse is sent. For imaging, PRFs from 1 to 10 kHz are used, resulting in an interval of from 0.1 to 1 ms between pulses. Thus a PRF of 5 kHz permits an echo to travel and return from a depth of 15.4 cm before the next pulse is sent.

Transducer

A transducer is any device that converts one form of energy to another. In the case of ultrasound, the transducer converts electric energy to mechanical energy and vice versa. In diagnostic ultrasound systems, the transducer serves two functions. It converts the electric energy provided by the transmitter to the **acoustic pulses**

directed into the patient. The transducer also serves as the **receiver of reflected echoes,** converting weak pressure changes into electric signals for processing. Ultrasound transducers use **piezoelectricity,** a principle discovered by Pierre Curie in 1880. Piezoelectric materials have the unique ability to respond to the action of an electric field by changing shape. They also have the property of generating electric potentials when compressed. Changing the polarity of a voltage applied to the transducer changes the thickness of the transducer, which expands and contracts as the polarity changes. This results in the generation of mechanical pressure waves that can be transmitted into the body. The piezoelectric effect also results in the generation of small potentials across the transducer when the transducer is struck by returning echoes. Positive pressures cause a small polarity to develop across the transducer; negative pressure during the rarefaction portion of the acoustic wave produces the opposite polarity across the transducer. These tiny polarity changes and the voltages associated with them are the source of all of the information processed to generate an ultrasound image or Doppler display.

When stimulated by the application of a voltage difference across its thickness, the transducer vibrates. The frequency of vibration is determined by the transducer material. When the transducer is electrically stimulated, a range or band of frequencies results. The preferential frequency produced by a transducer is determined by the propagation speed of the transducer material and its thickness. In the pulsed operating modes used for most clinical ultrasound applications, the ultrasound pulses contain additional frequencies both higher and lower than the preferential frequency. The **range of frequencies** produced by a given transducer is termed its **bandwidth**. Generally, the shorter the pulse of ultrasound produced by the transducer, the greater the bandwidth.

Most modern digital ultrasound systems employ broad bandwidth technology. Ultrasound bandwidth refers to the range of frequencies produced and detected by the ultrasound system. This is important because each tissue in the body has a characteristic response to ultrasound of a given frequency, and different tissues respond differently to different frequencies. The range of frequencies arising from a tissue exposed to ultrasound is referred to as the frequency spectrum bandwidth of the tissue or tissue signature. Broad bandwidth technology provides a means to capture the frequency spectrum of insonated tissues, preserving acoustic information and tissue signature. Broad bandwidth beam formers permit reduction of speckle artifact by a process of frequency compounding. This is possible because speckle patterns at different frequencies are independent of one another, and combining data from multiple frequency bands (i.e., compounding) results in a reduction of speckle in the final image leading to improved contrast resolution.

The length of an ultrasound pulse is determined by the number of alternating voltage changes applied to the transducer. For **continuous wave (CW) ultrasound devices**, a constant alternating current is applied to the transducer, the alternating polarity producing a continuous ultrasound wave. For imaging, a single, brief voltage change is applied to the transducer, causing it to vibrate at its preferential frequency. Because the transducer continues to vibrate or "ring" for a short time after it is stimulated by the voltage change, the ultrasound pulse will be several cycles long. The number of cycles of sound in each pulse determines the **pulse length**. For imaging, short pulse lengths are desirable because longer pulses result in poorer axial resolution. To reduce the pulse length to no more than two or three cycles, damping materials are used in the construction of the transducer. In clinical imaging applications, very short pulses are applied to the transducer, and the transducers have highly efficient damping. This results in very short pulses of ultrasound, generally consisting of only two or three cycles of sound.

The ultrasound pulse generated by a transducer must be propagated in tissue to provide clinical information. Special transducer coatings and ultrasound coupling gels are necessary to allow efficient transfer of energy from the transducer to the body. Once in the body, the ultrasound pulses are propagated, reflected, refracted, and absorbed, in accordance with the basic acoustic principles summarized earlier.

The ultrasound pulses produced by the transducer result in a series of wavefronts that form a three-dimensional beam of ultrasound. The features of this beam are influenced by constructive and destructive interference of the pressure waves, the curvature of the transducer, and acoustic lenses used to shape the beam. Interference of pressure waves results in an area near the transducer in which the pressure amplitude varies greatly. This region is termed the **near field** or Fresnel zone. Further from the transducer at a distance determined by the radius of the transducer and the frequency, the sound field begins to diverge and the pressure amplitude decreases at a steady rate with increasing distance from the transducer. This region is called the **far field** or Frauenhofer zone. In modern multielement transducer arrays, precise timing of the firing of elements allows correction of this divergence of the ultrasound beam and **focusing** at selected depths.

Only reflections of pulses that make their way back to the transducer are capable of stimulating the transducer with small pressure changes, which are converted into the voltage changes that are detected, amplified, and processed to build an image based on the echo information.

Receiver

When returning echoes strike the transducer face, minute voltages are produced across the piezoelectric elements. The receiver detects and amplifies these weak signals. The receiver also provides a means for compensating for the differences in echo strength, which result from attenuation by different tissue thickness by control of time depth compensation or **time gain compensation (TGC).**

Sound is attenuated as it passes into the body, and additional energy is removed as echoes return through tissue to the transducer. The attenuation of sound is proportional to the frequency and is constant for specific tissues. Because echoes returning from deeper tissues are weaker than those returning from more superficial structures, they must be amplified more by the receiver to produce a uniform tissue echo appearance (Fig. 1-10). This adjustment is accomplished by TGC controls that permit the user to selectively amplify the signals from deeper structures or suppress the signals from superficial tissues, compensating for tissue attenuation. Although many newer machines provide for some means of automatic TGC, the manual adjustment of this control by the user is one of the most important user controls and may have a profound effect on the quality of the ultrasound image provided for interpretation.

Another important function of the receiver is the compression of the wide range of amplitudes returning to the transducer into a range that can be displayed to the user. The ratio of the highest to the lowest amplitudes that can be displayed may be expressed in decibels and is referred to as the **dynamic range**. In a typical clinical application, the range of reflected signals may vary by a factor of as much as $1:10^{12}$, resulting in a dynamic range of up to 120 dB. Although the amplifiers

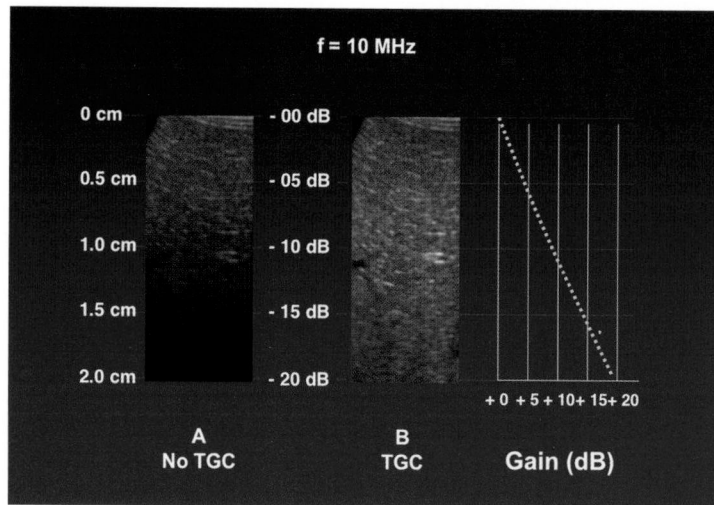

FIGURE 1-10. Time gain compensation (TGC). Without time gain compensation, tissue attenuation causes gradual loss of display of deeper tissues (**A**). In this example, tissue attenuation of 1 dB/cm/MHz is simulated for a transducer of 10 MHz. At a depth of 2 cm, the intensity is -20 dB. By applying increasing amplification or gain to the backscattered signal to compensate for this attenuation, a uniform intensity is restored to the tissue at all depths (**B**).

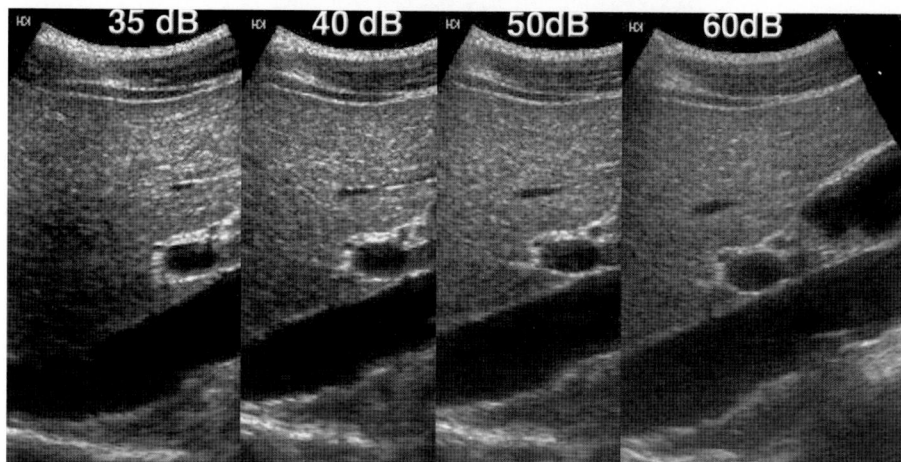

FIGURE 1-11. Dynamic range. The ultrasound receiver must compress the wide range of amplitudes returning to the transducer into a range that can be displayed to the user. Here, compression and remapping of the data to display dynamic ranges of 35 dB, 40 dB, 50 dB, and 60 dB are shown. The widest dynamic range shown (60 dB) permits the best differentiation of subtle differences in echo intensity and is preferred for most imaging applications. The narrower ranges increase conspicuity of larger echo differences.

used in ultrasound machines are capable of handling this range of voltages, gray-scale displays are limited to display a signal intensity range of only 35 to 40 dB. **Compression and remapping of the data** are required to adapt the dynamic range of the backscattered signal intensity to the dynamic range of the display (Fig. 1-11). Compression is performed in the receiver by selective amplification of weaker signals. Additional manual post-processing controls permit the user to selectively map the returning signal to the display. These controls affect the brightness of different echo levels in the image and, therefore, determine the image contrast.

Image Display

Ultrasound signals may be displayed in several ways.[4] Over the years, imaging has evolved from simple A-mode and bistable display to high-resolution, real-time, gray-scale imaging. The earliest **A-mode devices** displayed the voltage produced across the transducer by the backscattered echo as a vertical deflection on the face of an oscilloscope. The horizontal sweep of the oscilloscope was calibrated to indicate the distance from the transducer to the reflecting surface. In this form of display, the strength or amplitude of the reflected sound is indicated by the height of the vertical deflection displayed on the oscilloscope. With A-mode ultrasound, only the position and strength of a reflecting structure are recorded.

Another simple form of imaging, **M-mode ultrasound**, displays echo amplitude and shows the position of moving reflectors (Fig. 1-12). M-mode imaging uses the brightness of the display to indicate the intensity of the reflected signal. The time base of the display can be adjusted to allow for varying degrees of temporal resolution, as dictated by clinical application. M-mode ultrasound is interpreted by assessing motion patterns of specific reflectors and determining anatomic relationships from characteristic patterns of motion. Today, the major application of M-mode display is in the evaluation of the rapid motion of cardiac valves and of cardiac chamber and vessel walls. M-mode imaging may play a future role in measurement of subtle changes in vessel wall elasticity accompanying atherogenesis.

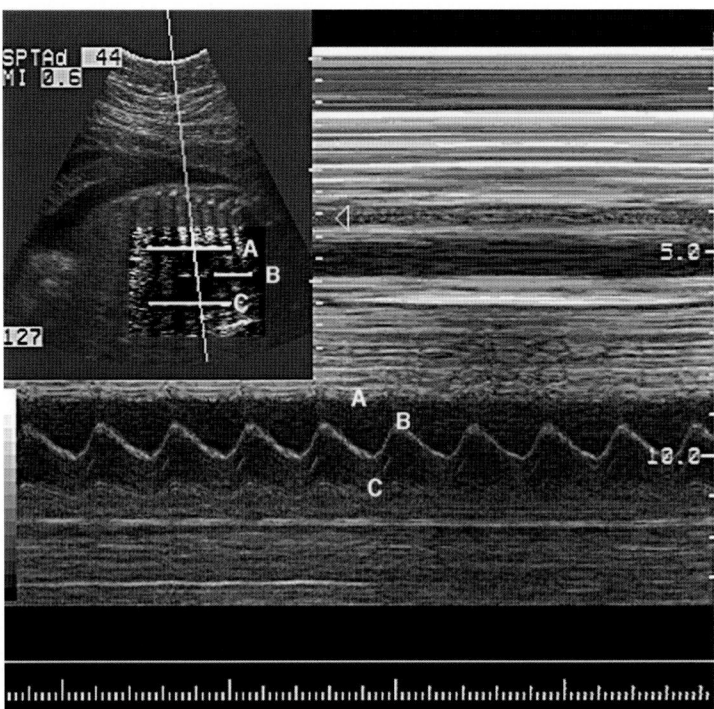

FIGURE 1-12. M-mode display. M-mode **ultrasound** displays changes of echo amplitude and position with time. Display of changes in echo position is useful in the evaluation of rapidly moving structures such as cardiac valves and chamber walls. Here, the three major moving structures in an M-mode image of the fetal heart correspond to the near ventricular wall (A), the interventricular septum (B), and the far ventricular wall (C). The baseline is a time scale, and it permits the calculation of heart rate from the M-mode data.

The mainstay of imaging with ultrasound is provided by **real-time, gray-scale, B-mode display** in which variations in display intensity or brightness are used to indicate reflected signals of differing amplitude. To generate a two-dimensional (2-D) image, multiple ultrasound pulses are sent down a series of successive scan lines (Fig. 1-13), building a 2-D representation of echoes arising from the object being scanned. When an ultrasound image is displayed on a black background, signals of greatest intensity appear as white; absence of signal is shown as black; and signals of intermediate intensity appear as shades of gray. If the ultrasound beam is moved with respect to the object being examined and the position of the reflected signal is stored, a 2-D image results, with the brightest portions of the display indicating structures reflecting more of the transmitted sound energy back to the transducer.

In most modern instruments, a digital memory of 512 × 512 or 512 × 640 pixels is used to store values that correspond to the echo intensities originating from corresponding positions in the patient. At least 2^8 or 256 shades of gray are possible for each pixel, in accord with the amplitude of the echo being represented. The image stored in memory in this fashion can then be sent to a video monitor for display. Since B-mode display relates the strength of a backscattered signal to a brightness level

on the display device (usually a video display monitor), it is important that the operator understand how the amplitude information in the ultrasound signal is translated into a brightness scale in the image display. Each ultrasound manufacturer offers several options for the way the dynamic range of the target is compressed for display, as well as the transfer function that assigns a given signal amplitude to a shade of gray. Although these technical details vary from one machine to another, the way they are used by the operator of the scanner may have a profound impact on the clinical value of the final image. In general, it is desirable to **display as wide a dynamic range as possible** in order to identify subtle differences in tissue echogenicity (see Fig. 1-9).

Real-time ultrasound produces the impression of motion by generating a series of individual 2-D images at rates from 15 to 60 frames per second. Real-time, 2-D, B-mode ultrasound is now the major method for ultrasound imaging throughout the body and is the most common form of B-mode display. Real-time ultrasound permits assessment of both anatomy and motion. When images are acquired and displayed at rates of several times per second, the effect is dynamic, and because the image reflects the state and motion of the organ at the time it is examined, the information is regarded as being shown in real time. In cardiac applications, the terms

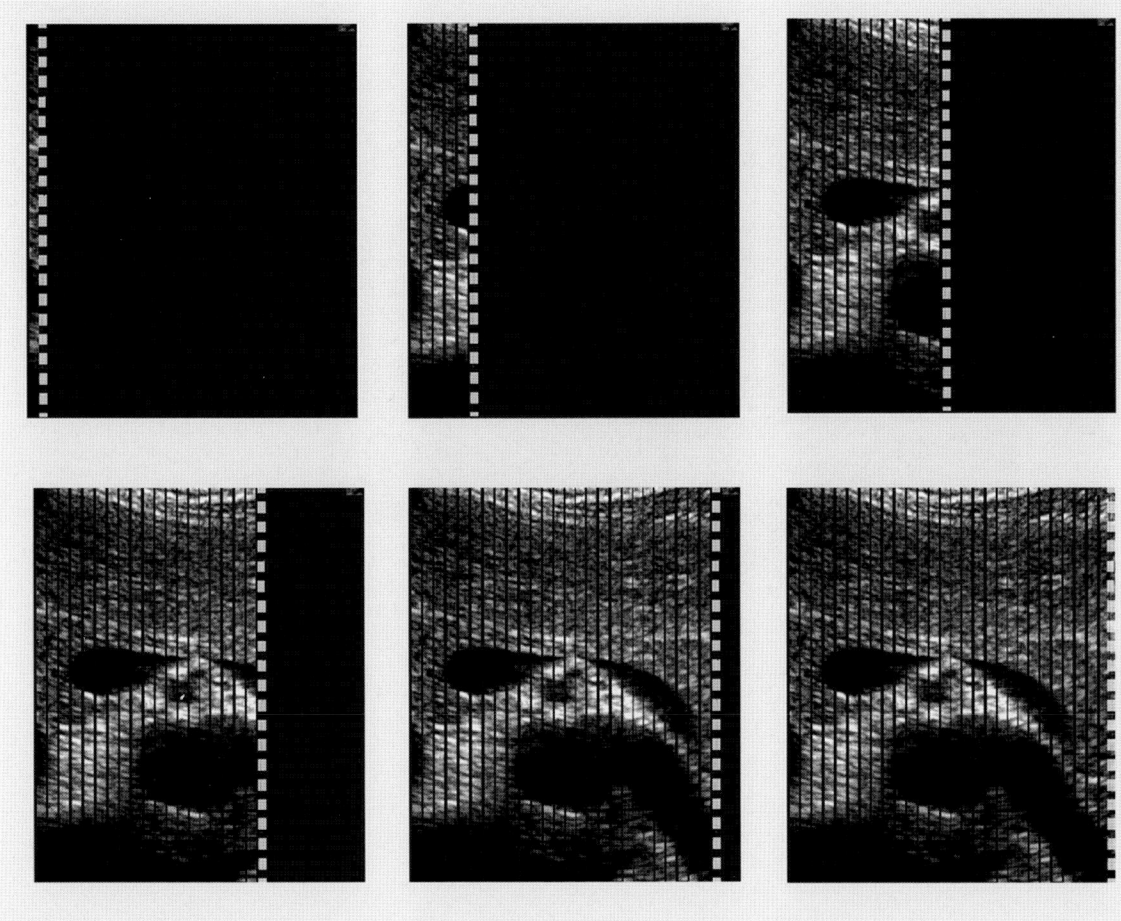

FIGURE 1-13. B-mode imaging. A 2-D, real-time image is built by ultrasound pulses sent down a series of successive scan lines. Each scan line adds to the image, building a 2-D representation of echoes from the object being scanned. In real-time imaging, an entire image is created 15 to 60 times per second.

"2-D echocardiography" and "2-D echo" are used to describe real-time, B-mode imaging; in most other applications, the term "real-time" ultrasound is used.

Transducers used for real-time imaging may be classified by the method used to steer the beam to rapidly generate each individual image, keeping in mind that as many as 30 to 60 complete images must be generated per second for real-time applications. Beam steering may be by **mechanical rotation** or **oscillation** of the transducer, or the beam may be **steered electronically** (Fig. 1-14). Electronic beam steering is used in linear array and phased array transducers and permits a variety of image display formats. Most electronically steered transducers currently in use also provide electronic focusing adjustable for depth. Mechanically steered transducers may use single-element transducers with a fixed focus or may use annular arrays of elements with electronically controlled focusing. For real-time imaging, transducers using mechanical or electronic beam steering generate display in a rectangular or pie-shaped format. For obstetric, small parts, and peripheral vascular examinations, **linear array transducers** with a rectangular image format are often used. The rectangular image display has the advantage of a larger field of view near the surface but requires a large surface area for transducer contact. **Sector scanners** with either mechanical or electronic steering require only a small surface area for contact and are better suited for examinations in which access is limited.

Mechanical Sector Scanners

Early ultrasound scanners used transducers consisting of a single piezoelectric element. To generate real-time images with these transducers, mechanical devices were required to move the transducer in a linear or circular motion. Mechanical sector scanners using one or more single-element transducers do not allow variable focusing. This problem is overcome by using annular array transducers. Although important in the early days of real-time imaging, mechanical sector scanners with fixed-focus, single-element transducers are not in common use today.

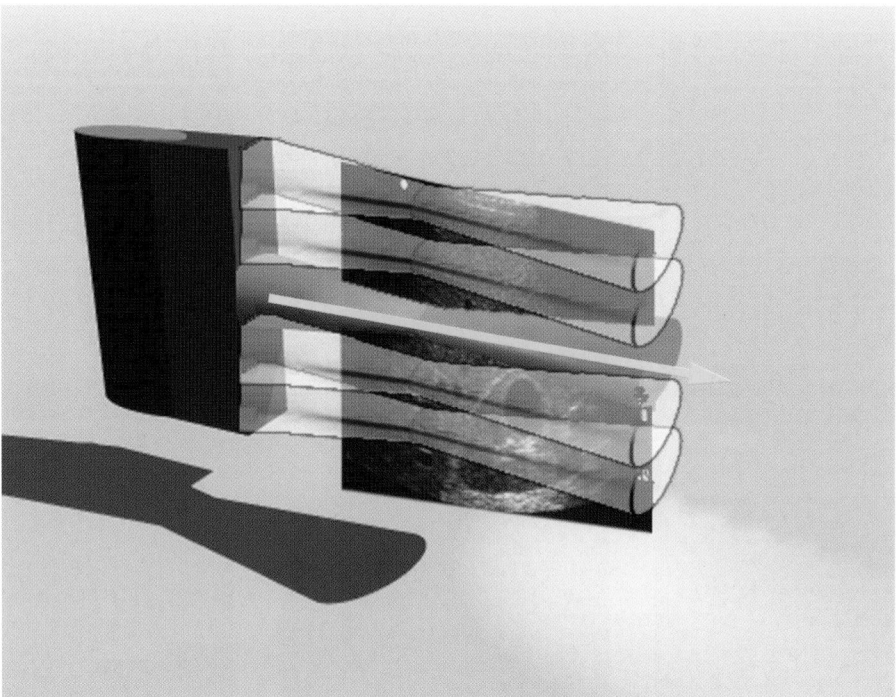

A

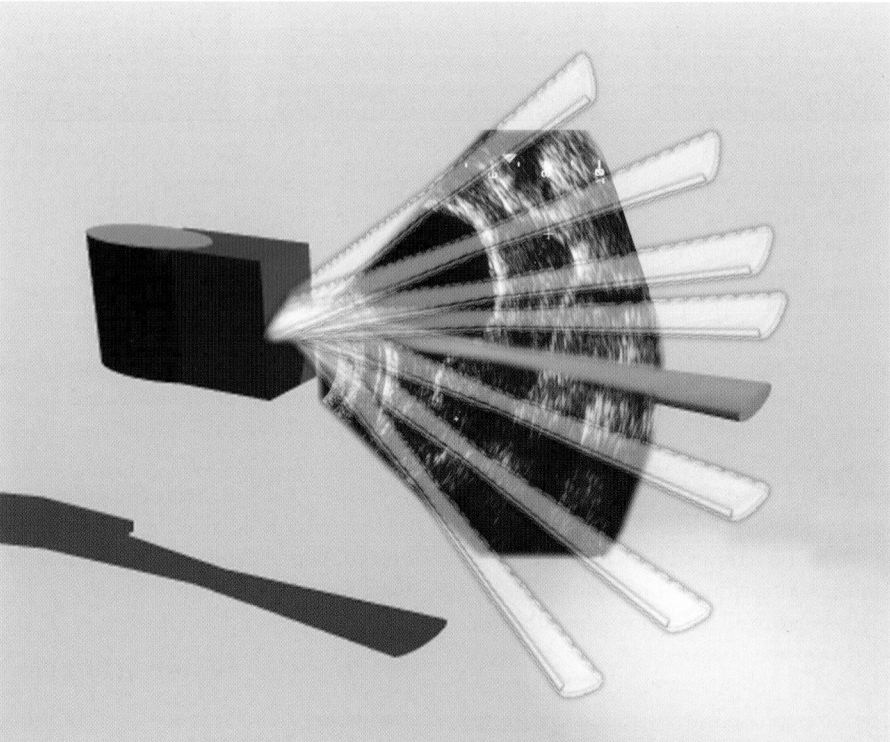

B

FIGURE 1-14. Beam steering. A, Linear array. In a linear array transducer, individual elements or groups of elements are fired in sequence. This generates a series of parallel ultrasound beams, each perpendicular to the transducer face. As these beams move across the transducer face, they generate the lines of sight that combine to form the final image. Depending on the number of transducer elements and the sequence in which they are fired, focusing at selected depths from the surface can be achieved. **B,** Phased array. A phased array transducer produces a sector field of view by firing multiple transducer elements in precise sequence to generate interference of acoustic wavefronts. The ultrasound beam that results generates a series of lines of sight at varying angles from one side of the transducer to the other, producing a sector image format.

Arrays

Current technology uses a transducer composed of multiple elements, usually produced by precise slicing of a piece of piezoelectric material into numerous small units, each with its own electrodes. Such transducer arrays may be formed in a variety of configurations. Most commonly these are linear, curved, phased, or annular arrays. High-density 2-D arrays have also been developed. By precise timing of the firing of combinations of elements in these arrays, interference of the wavefronts generated by the individual elements can be exploited to change the direction of the ultrasound beam, and this can be used to provide a steerable beam for the generation of real-time images in a linear or sector format.

Linear Arrays

Linear array transducers are commonly used for small parts, vascular, and obstetric applications because the rectangular image format produced by these transducers is well suited for these applications. In these transducers, individual elements are arranged in a linear fashion. By firing the transducer elements in sequence, either individually or in groups, a series of parallel pulses is generated, each forming a line of sight perpendicular to the transducer face. These individual lines of sight combine to form the image field of view (see Fig. 1-14A). Depending on the number of transducer elements and the sequence in which they are fired, focusing at selected depths from the surface can be achieved.

Curved Arrays

Linear arrays that have been shaped into convex curves produce an image that combines a relatively large surface field of view with a sector display format. Curved array transducers are used for a variety of applications, the larger versions serving for general abdominal, obstetric, and transabdominal pelvic scanning. Small, high-frequency, curved array scanners are often used in transvaginal and transrectal probes and for pediatric imaging.

Phased Arrays

In contrast to mechanical sector scanners, phased array scanners have no moving parts. A sector field of view is produced by multiple transducer elements fired in precise sequence under electronic control. By controlling the time and sequence in which the individual transducer elements are fired, the ultrasound wave that results can be steered in different directions as well as focused at different depths (see Fig. 1-14B). By rapidly steering the beam to generate a series of lines of sight at varying angles from one side of the transducer to the other, a sector image format is produced. This allows the fabrication of transducers of relatively small size but with large fields of view at depth. These transducers are particularly useful for intercostal scanning to evaluate the heart, liver, or spleen, and for examinations in other areas where access is limited.

Two-Dimensional Arrays

Transducer arrays can be formed by slicing a rectangular piece of transducer material perpendicular to its long axis to produce a number of small rectangular elements or by creating a series of concentric elements nested within one another in a circular piece of piezoelectric material to produce an annular array. The use of multiple elements permits precise focusing. A particular advantage of 2-D array construction is that the beam can be focused both in elevation and lateral planes, and a uniform and highly focused beam can be produced (Fig. 1-15). These arrays offer improvements in spatial resolution and contrast as well as reduction of clutter and are well-suited for the collection of data from volumes of tissue for use in 3-D processing and display. Unlike linear 2-D arrays, in which delays in the firing of the individual elements may be used to steer the beam, annular arrays do not permit beam steering, and to be used for real-time imaging they must be steered mechanically.

Transducer Selection

Practical considerations in the selection of the optimal transducer for a given application include not only the requirements for spatial resolution but the distance of the target object from the transducer because penetration of ultrasound diminishes as frequency increases. In general, the **highest ultrasound frequency permitting penetration to the depth of interest should be selected**. For superficial vessels and organs, such as the thyroid, breast, or testicle, lying within 1 to 3 cm of the surface, imaging frequencies of from 7.5 to 15 MHz are usually used. These high frequencies are also ideal for intraoperative applications. For evaluation of deeper structures in the abdomen or pelvis more than 12 to 15 cm from the surface, frequencies as low as 2.25 to 3.5 MHz may be required. When maximal resolution is needed, a high-frequency transducer with excellent lateral and elevation resolution at the depth of interest is required.

Image Display and Storage

With real-time ultrasound, user feedback is immediate and is provided by video display. The brightness and contrast of the image on this display are determined by the brightness and contrast settings of the video monitor,

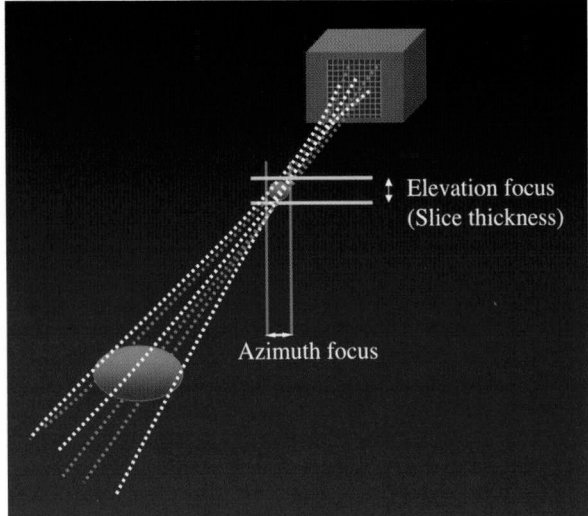

FIGURE 1-15. 2-Dimensional Array. High-density 2-dimensional arrays consist of a 2-dimensional matrix of transducer elements, permitting acquisition of data from a volume rather than a single plane of tissue. Precise electronic control of individual elements provides an opportunity for adjustable focusing on both the azimuth and elevation planes.

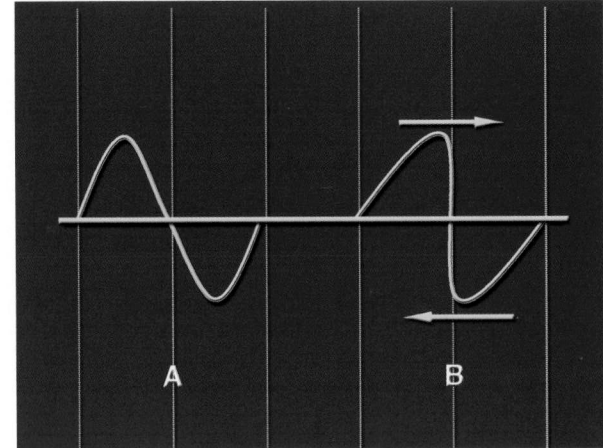

FIGURE 1-16. Harmonic generation. The transmitted waveform is shown in **A.** As the sound is propagated through tissue, the high pressure component of the wave travels more rapidly than the rarefactional component, producing distortion (**B**) of the wave and generating higher frequency components (harmonics). (From Merritt CR: Technology Update. Radiol Clin North Am 2001;39:385-397.)

by the system gain setting, and the TGC adjustment. Probably the single greatest factor affecting image quality in many ultrasound departments is improper adjustment of the video display and lack of appreciation of the relationship of the video display settings to the appearance of hard copy. Because of the importance of the real-time video display in providing feedback to the user, it is essential that the display and the lighting conditions under which the display is viewed are standardized and matched to the hard copy device.

Interpretation of images and archival storage of images may be in the form of transparencies printed on film by optical or laser cameras and printers, videotape, or through use of digital picture archiving and communications systems (PACS). Increasingly, digital storage is being used for archiving of ultrasound images.

Special Imaging Modes

Harmonic Imaging

Variation of the propagation velocity of sound in fat and other tissues near the transducer results in phase aberration that distorts the ultrasound field, producing noise and clutter in the ultrasound image. Tissue harmonic imaging provides an approach for reducing the effects of phase aberrations.[5] Nonlinear propagation of ultrasound through tissue is associated with the more rapid propagation of the high pressure component of the ultrasound pressure wave compared to its negative (rarefactional) component. This results in increasing distortion of the acoustical pulse as it travels within

the tissue, and causes the generation of multiples or harmonics of the transmitted frequency (Fig. 1-16). Tissue harmonic imaging takes advantage of the generation, at depth, of these harmonics. Because the generation of harmonics requires interaction of the transmitted field with the propagating tissue, harmonic generation is not present near the transducer/skin interface, and it only becomes important some distance from the transducer. In most cases the near and far fields of the image are affected less by harmonics than by intermediate locations. Using broad bandwidth transducers and signal filtration or coded pulses, the harmonic signals reflected from tissue interfaces can be selectively displayed. Because most imaging artifacts are caused by the interaction of the ultrasound beam with superficial structures or are due to aberrations at the edges of the beam profile, these artifacts are eliminated using harmonic imaging because the artifact-producing signals do not consist of sufficient energy to generate harmonic frequencies and are, therefore, filtered out during image formation. Images generated using tissue harmonics often exhibit reduced noise and clutter (Fig. 1-17). Because harmonic beams are narrower than the originally transmitted beams, spatial resolution is improved and side lobes are reduced.

Spatial Compounding

An important source of image degradation and loss of contrast is ultrasound speckle. Speckle results from the constructive and destructive interaction of the acoustic fields generated by the scattering of ultrasound from small tissue reflectors. This interference pattern gives

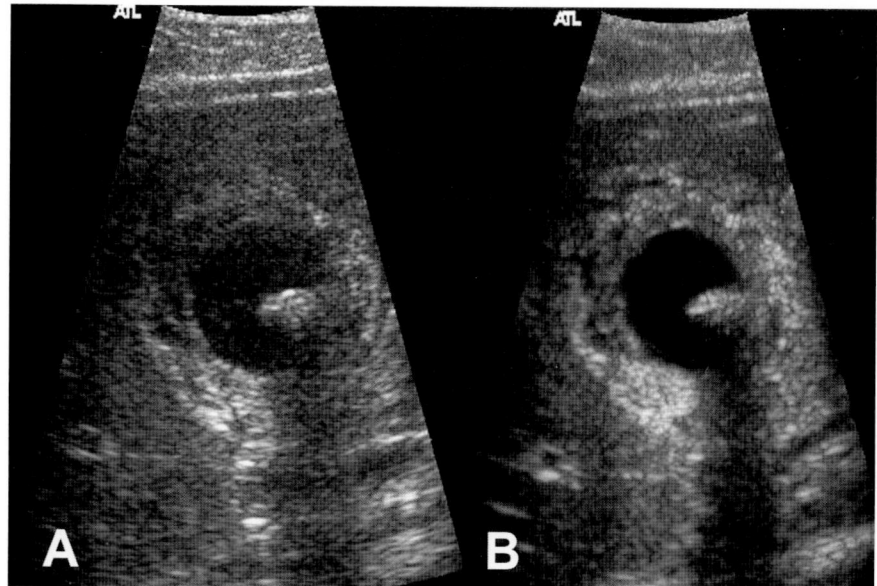

FIGURE 1-17. Tissue harmonic imaging. Conventional (**A**) and tissue harmonic (**B**) images of a gallbladder of a patient with acute cholecystitis. Note the reduction of noise and clutter in the tissue harmonic image. Because harmonic beams do not interact with superficial structures and are narrower than the originally transmitted beam, spatial resolution is improved and clutter and side lobes are reduced. (From Merritt CR: Technology Update. Radiol Clin North Am 2001;39:385-397.)

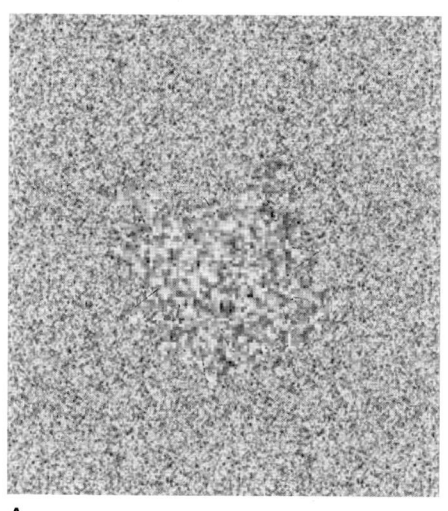
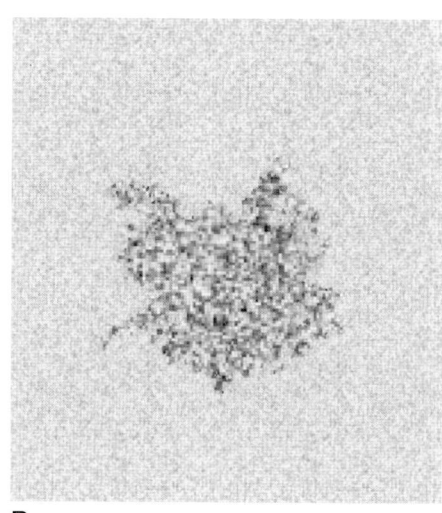

FIGURE 1-18. Speckle and contrast. The effect of speckle on contrast resolution is illustrated. Speckle noise partially obscures the simulated lesion (**A**). The speckle has been reduced (**B**), increasing the contrast between the lesion and the background. (From Merritt CR: Technology Update. Radiol Clin North Am 2001;39:385-397.)

A

B

ultrasound images their characteristic grainy appearance (see Fig. 1-6), reducing contrast (Fig. 1-18) and making the identification of subtle features more difficult. By summing images from different scanning angles through compound scanning, significant improvement in the contrast-to-noise (speckle) ratio can be achieved (Fig. 1-19). This is because speckle is random and the generation of an image by compounding will reduce speckle noise because only the signal is reinforced. In addition, spatial compounding may reduce artifacts that result when an ultrasound beam strikes a specular reflector at an angle greater or less than 90 degrees. In conventional real-time imaging, each scan line used to generate the image strikes the target at a constant fixed angle. As a result, strong reflectors that are not perpendicular to the ultrasound beam scatter sound in directions that prevent their clear detection and display. This, in turn, results in poor margin definition and

less distinct boundaries for cysts and other masses. Compounding has been found to reduce these artifacts (Fig. 1-20). Limitations of compounding are diminished visibility of shadowing and enhancement; however, these are offset by the ability to evaluate lesions, both with and without compounding, preserving shadowing and enhancement when these features are important to diagnosis.[6]

3-D Ultrasound

Dedicated 3-D scanners used for fetal, gynecologic, and cardiac scanning may employ hardware-based image registration, high density 2-D arrays, or software registration of scan planes as a tissue volume is acquired. 3-D imaging permits volume data to be viewed in multiple imaging planes and allows accurate measurement of lesion volume (Fig. 1-21).

FIGURE 1-19. Spatial compounding. Conventional imaging (**A**) is limited to a fixed angle of incidence of ultrasound scan lines to tissue interfaces, resulting in poor definition of specular reflectors that are not perpendicular to the beam. **Spatial compounding** (**B**) combines images obtained by insonating the target from multiple angles. In addition to improving detection interfaces, compounding reduces speckle noise because only the signal is reinforced, whereas speckle, being random, is not. This improves contrast.

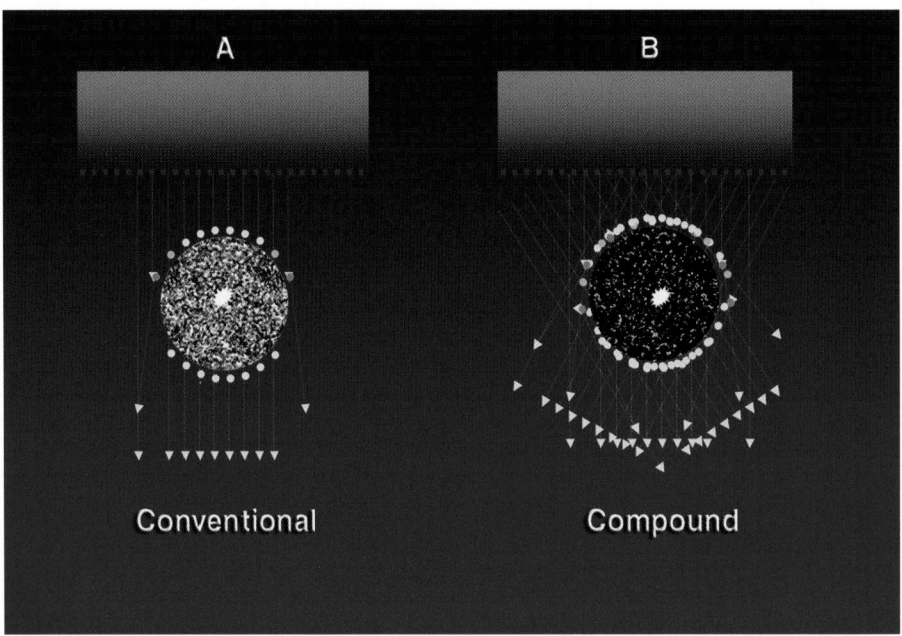

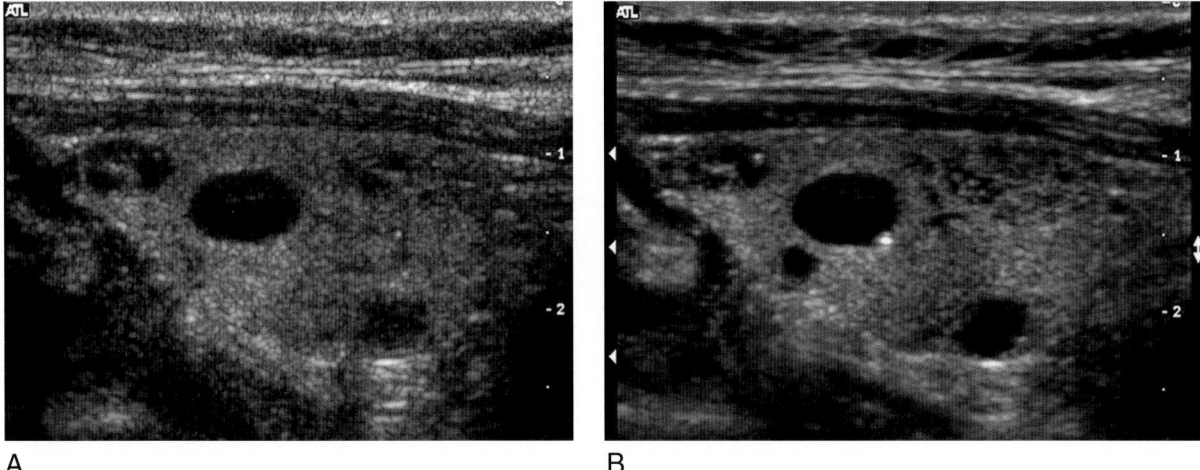

A   B

FIGURE 1-20. Spatial compounding. Conventional (**A**) and compound (**B**) images of the thyroid are compared. Note the reduced speckle as well as better definition of the margins of the solid and cystic nodules within the thyroid. Features of small cysts, calcifications, and near-field structures are shown more clearly. (From Merritt CR: Technology Update. Radiol Clin North Am 2001;39:385-397.)

IMAGE QUALITY

The key determinants of the quality of an ultrasound image include its spatial, contrast, and temporal resolution, and freedom from certain artifacts.

Spatial Resolution

The ability to differentiate two closely situated objects as distinct structures is determined by the spatial resolution of the ultrasound device. Spatial resolution must be considered in three planes, and there are different determinants of resolution in each of these. Simplest is the resolution along the axis of the ultrasound beam—**axial resolution**. With pulsed wave ultrasound, the transducer introduces a series of brief bursts of sound into the body. Each ultrasound pulse typically consists of two or three cycles of sound. The pulse length is the product of the wavelength and the number of cycles in the pulse. Axial resolution, the maximum resolution along the beam axis, is determined by the pulse length (Fig. 1-22). Because ultrasound frequency and wavelength are inversely related, the pulse length decreases as the imaging frequency increases. Because the pulse length determines the maximum resolution along the

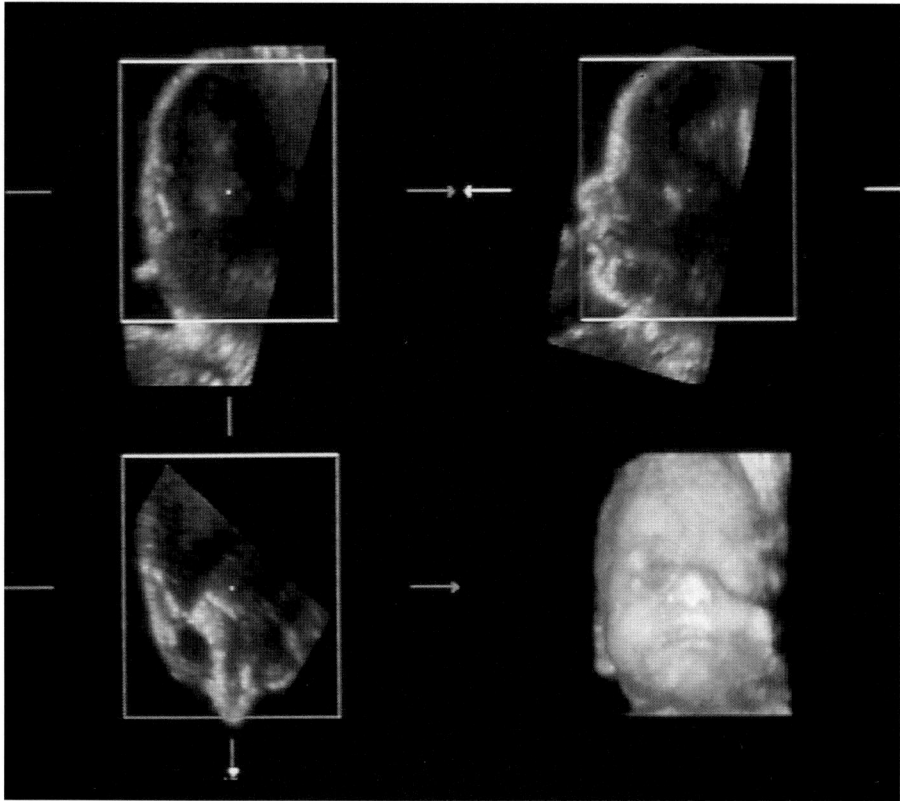

FIGURE 1-21. 3-D Ultrasound. 3-D ultrasound permits collection and review of data obtained from a volume of tissue in multiple imaging planes as well as rendering of surface features. (From Merritt CR: Technology Update. Radiol Clin North Am 2001;39:385-397.)

axis of the ultrasound beam, higher transducer frequencies provide higher image resolution. For example, a transducer operating at 5 MHz produces sound with a wavelength of 0.308 mm. If each pulse consists of three cycles of sound, the pulse length is slightly less than 1 mm, and this becomes the maximum resolution along the beam axis. If the transducer frequency is increased to 15 MHz, the pulse length is less than 0.4 mm, permitting resolution of smaller details.

In addition to axial resolution, resolution in the planes perpendicular to the beam axis must also be considered. **Lateral resolution** refers to resolution in the plane perpendicular to the beam and parallel to the transducer. **Azimuth or elevation resolution** refers to the slice thickness in the plane perpendicular to the beam and to the transducer (Fig. 1-23). Lateral resolution is determined by the width of the ultrasound beam. Ultrasound is a tomographic method of imaging that produces thin slices of information from the body, and the width and thickness of the ultrasound beam are important determinants of image quality. Excessive beam width and thickness limit the ability to delineate small features, such as the tiny cystic areas in atheromatous plaque associated with intraplaque hemorrhage. The width and thickness of the ultrasound beam determine lateral resolution and elevation resolution, respectively. Lateral and elevation resolution are significantly poorer than the axial resolution of the beam. Lateral resolution is controlled by focusing the beam, usually by electronic

phasing, to alter the beam width at a selected depth of interest. Elevation resolution is determined by the construction of the transducer and, generally, it cannot be controlled by the user.

IMAGING PITFALLS

In ultrasound, perhaps more than in any other imaging method, the quality of the information obtained is determined by the ability of the operator to recognize and avoid artifacts and pitfalls.[7] Many imaging artifacts are induced by errors in scanning technique or improper use of the instrument and are preventable. Artifacts may suggest the presence of structures that are not present, causing misdiagnosis, or they may cause important findings to be obscured. Because an understanding of artifacts is essential for correct interpretation of ultrasound examinations, several of the most important artifacts deserve discussion.

Many artifacts suggest the presence of structures not actually present. These include reverberation, refraction, and side lobes. **Reverberation artifacts** arise when the ultrasound signal reflects repeatedly between highly reflective interfaces that are usually, but not always, near the transducer (Fig. 1-24). Reverberations may also give the false impression of solid structures in areas where only fluid is present. Certain types of reverberation may be helpful because they allow the identification of a

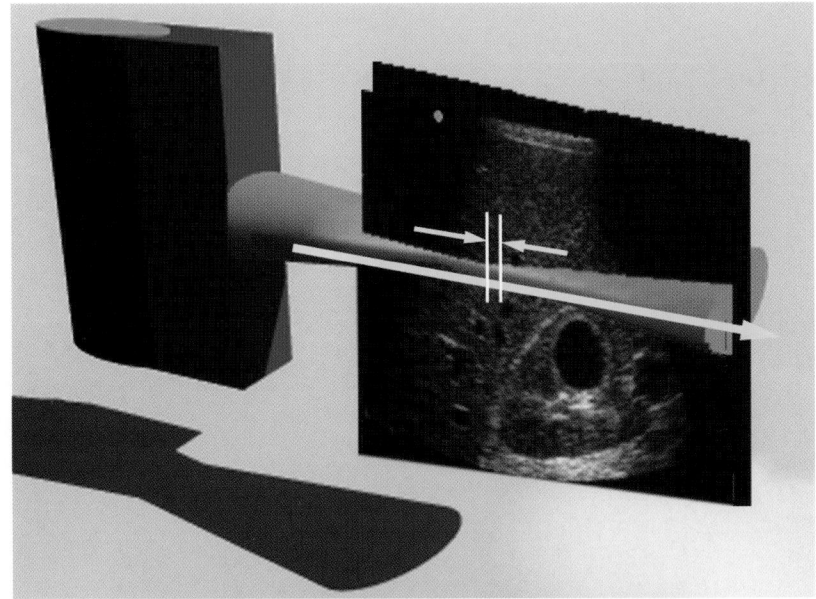

FIGURE 1-22. Axial resolution. A, Axial resolution is the resolution along the beam axis and **B** is determined by the pulse length. The pulse length is the product of the wavelength (which decreases with increasing frequency) and the number of waves (usually two to three). Because the pulse length determines axial resolution, higher transducer frequencies provide higher image resolution. For example, a transducer operating at 5 MHz produces sound with a wavelength of 0.31 mm. If each pulse consists of three cycles of sound, the pulse length is slightly less than 1 mm, and objects (A) and (B), which are 0.5 mm apart, cannot be resolved as separate structures. If the transducer frequency is increased to 15 MHz, the pulse length is less than 0.3 mm, permitting (A) and (B) to be identified as separate structures.

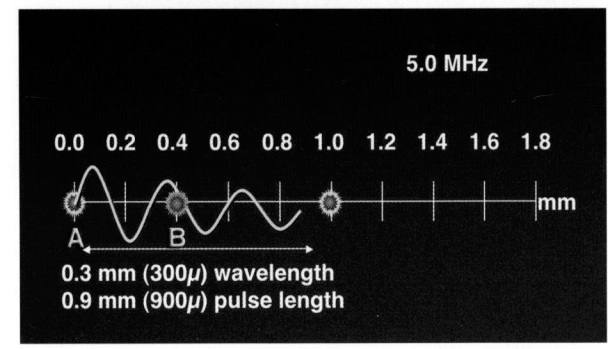

FIGURE 1-23. Lateral and elevation resolution. Resolution in the planes perpendicular to the beam axis is an important determinant of image quality. Lateral resolution (L) is resolution in the plane perpendicular to the beam and parallel to the transducer, and is determined by the width of the ultrasound beam. Lateral resolution is controlled by focusing the beam, usually by electronic phasing to alter the beam width at a selected depth of interest. Azimuth or elevation resolution (E) is determined by the slice thickness in the plane perpendicular to the beam and the transducer. Elevation resolution is controlled by the construction of the transducer. Both lateral and elevation resolution are less than the axial resolution.

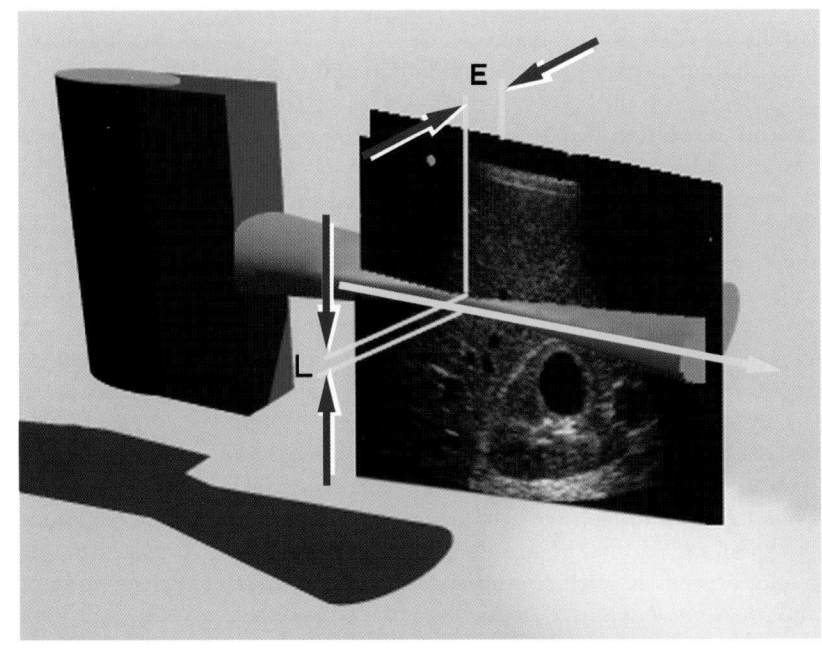

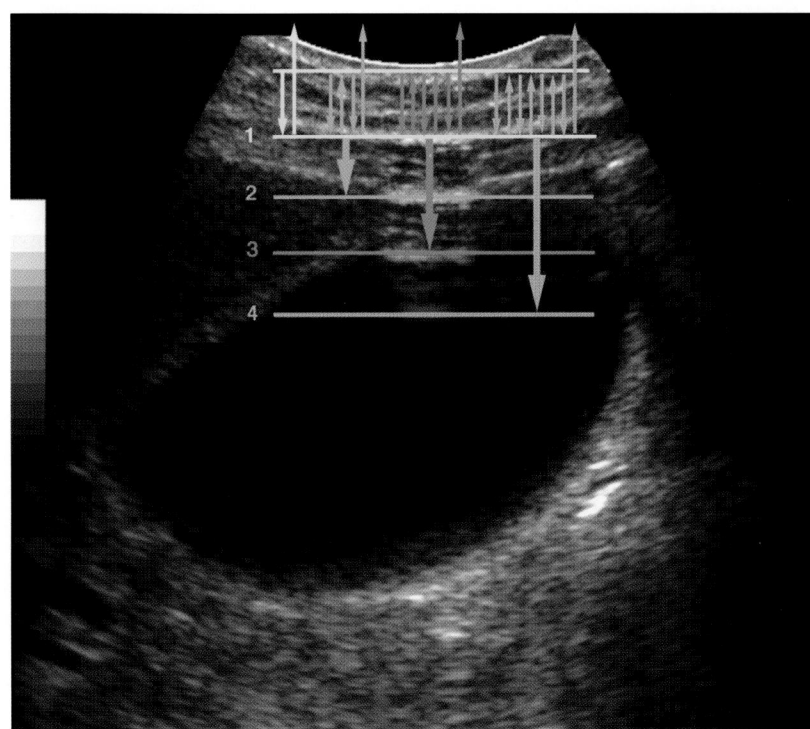

FIGURE 1-24. Reverberation artifact. Reverberation artifacts arise when the ultrasound signal reflects repeatedly between highly reflective interfaces near the transducer, resulting in delayed echo return to the transducer. This appears in the image as a series of regularly spaced echoes at increasing depth. The echo at depth 1 is produced by simple reflection from a strong interface. Echoes at levels 2 through 4 are produced by multiple reflections between this interface and the surface (simulated image).

specific type of reflector, such as a surgical clip. Reverberation artifacts can usually be reduced or eliminated by changing the scanning angle or transducer placement to avoid the parallel interfaces that contribute to the artifact.

Refraction causes bending of the sound beam so that targets not along the axis of the transducer are insonated. Their reflections are then detected and displayed in the image. This may cause structures to appear in the image that actually lie outside the volume the investigator assumes is being examined (see Fig. 1-7). Similarly, **side lobes** may produce confusing echoes that arise from sound beams that lie outside the main ultrasound beam (Fig. 1-25). These artifacts are of clinical importance because they may create the impression of structures or debris in fluid-filled structures (Fig. 1-26). Side lobes may also result in errors of measurement by reducing lateral resolution. As with most other artifacts, repositioning the transducer and its focal zone or using a different transducer will usually allow the differentiation of artifactual from true echoes.

Artifacts may also remove real echoes from the display or obscure information, and important pathology may be missed. **Shadowing** results when there is a marked reduction in the intensity of ultrasound deep to a strong reflector or attenuator. Shadowing causes partial or complete loss of information due to attenuation of the sound by superficial structures. Another common cause of loss of image information is improper adjustment of system gain and TGC settings. Many low-level echoes are near the noise levels of the equipment, and

considerable skill and experience are needed to adjust instrument settings to display the maximum information with the minimum noise. **Poor scanning angles, inadequate penetration**, and **poor resolution** may also result in loss of significant information. Careless selection of transducer frequency and lack of attention to the focal characteristics of the beam will cause loss of clinically important information from deep, low-amplitude reflectors and small targets. Ultrasound artifacts may alter the size, shape, and position of structures. For example, a **multipath artifact** is created when the path of the returning echo is not the one expected, resulting in display of the echo at an improper location in the image (Fig. 1-27).

DOPPLER SONOGRAPHY

Conventional B-mode ultrasound imaging uses pulse-echo transmission, detection, and display techniques. Brief pulses of ultrasound energy emitted by the transducer are reflected from acoustic interfaces within the body. Precise timing allows determination of the depth from which the echo originates. When pulsed wave ultrasound is reflected from an interface, the backscattered (reflected) signal contains amplitude, phase, and frequency information (Fig. 1-28). This information permits inference of the position, nature, and motion of the interface reflecting the pulse. B-mode ultrasound imaging uses only the amplitude information in the backscattered signal to generate the image, with differ-

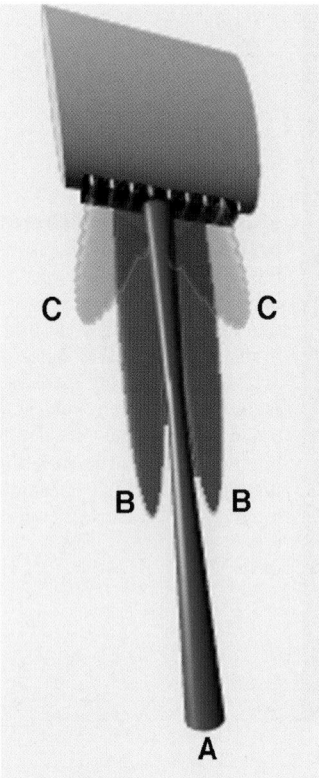

FIGURE 1-25. Side lobes. Although most of the energy generated by a transducer is emitted in a beam along the central axis of the transducer (**A**), some energy is also emitted from the sides of the primary beam (**B** and **C**). These are called side lobes and are lower in intensity than the primary beam. Side lobes may interact with strong reflectors that lie outside of the scan plane and produce artifacts that are displayed in the ultrasound image (see also Fig. 1-26).

ences in the strength of reflectors displayed in the image in varying shades of gray. Rapidly moving targets, such as red cells within the blood stream, produce echoes of low amplitude that are not commonly displayed, resulting in a relatively anechoic pattern within the lumens of large vessels.

Although gray-scale display relies on the amplitude of the backscattered ultrasound signal, additional information is present in the returning echoes that can be used to evaluate the motion of moving targets. When high-frequency sound impinges on a stationary interface, the reflected ultrasound has essentially the same frequency or wavelength as the transmitted sound (Fig. 1-29A). If, however, the reflecting interface is moving with respect to the sound beam emitted from the transducer, there is a change in the frequency of the sound scattered by the moving object (see Fig. 1-29B, C). This change in frequency is directly proportional to the velocity of the reflecting interface relative to the transducer and is a result of the Doppler effect. The relationship of the returning ultrasound frequency to the velocity of the reflector is described by the Doppler equation:

$$\Delta F = (F_R - F_T) = 2F_T \, v/c \qquad \textbf{5}$$

The Doppler frequency shift is ΔF; F_R is the frequency of sound reflected from the moving target; F_T is the frequency of sound emitted from the transducer; v is the velocity of the target toward the transducer; and c is the velocity of sound in the medium. The Doppler frequency shift ΔF, as described above, applies only if the target is moving directly toward or away from the transducer as is shown in Figure 1-30A. In most clinical

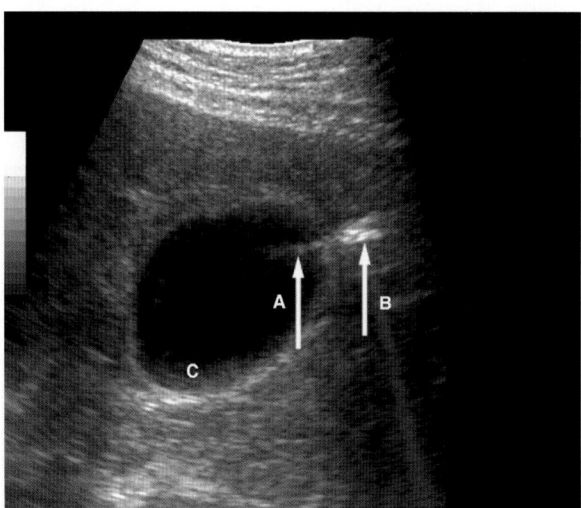

FIGURE 1-26. Side lobe artifact. Transverse image of the gallbladder reveals a bright internal echo (**A**) that suggests a band or septum within the gallbladder. This is a side lobe artifact related to the presence of a strong out-of-plane reflector (**B**) medial to the gallbladder. The low-level echoes in the dependent portion of the gallbladder (**C**) are also artifactual and are caused by the same phenomenon. Side lobe and slice thickness artifacts are of clinical importance because they may create the impression of debris in fluid-filled structures. As with most other artifacts, repositioning the transducer and its focal zone or using a different transducer will usually allow the differentiation of artifactual from true echoes.

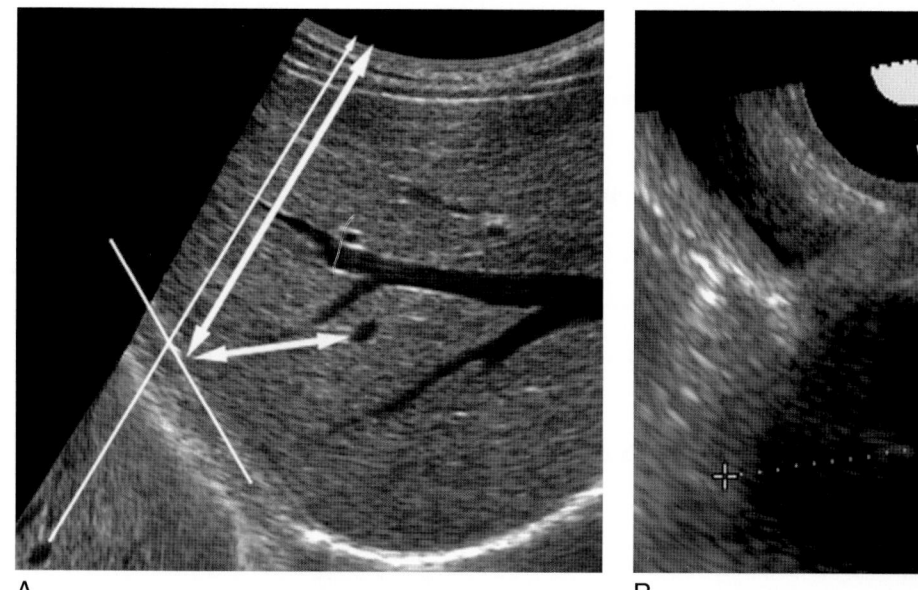

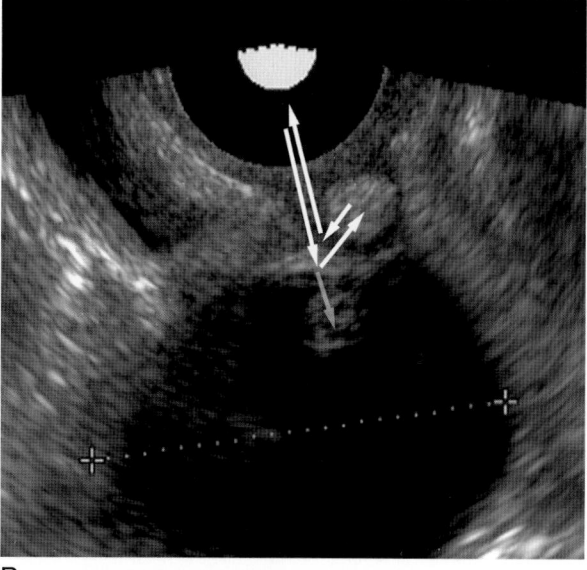

A   B

FIGURE 1-27. Multipath artifact. Echoes reflected from the **diaphragm** (**A**) and the wall of an **ovarian cyst** (**B**) create complex echo paths that delay return of echoes to the transducer. This results in the display of these echoes at a greater depth than they should normally appear. In **A**, this results in an artifactual image of the liver appearing above the diaphragm (simulated image). In **B**, the effect is more subtle and more likely to cause misdiagnosis because the artifact suggests a mural nodule in what is actually a simple ovarian cyst.

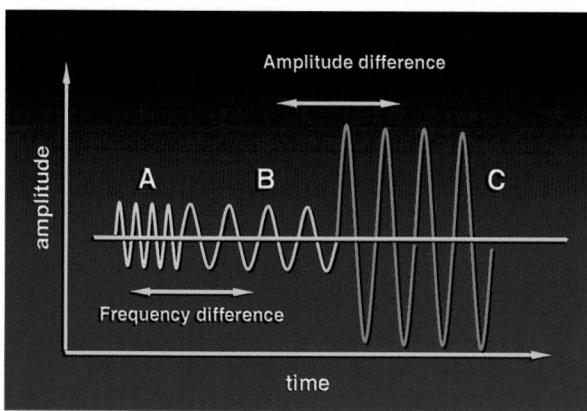

FIGURE 1-28. Backscattered information. The backscattered ultrasound signal contains amplitude, phase, and frequency information. Signals (B) and (C) differ in amplitude but have the same frequency. Amplitude differences are used to generate B-mode images. Signals (A) and (B) differ in frequency but have similar amplitudes. Such frequency differences are the basis of Doppler ultrasound.

settings, the direction of the ultrasound beam is seldom directly toward or away from the direction of flow, and the ultrasound beam usually approaches the moving target at an angle designated as the Doppler angle (Fig. 1-30B). In this case the frequency shift ΔF is reduced in proportion to the cosine of this angle. Therefore

$$\Delta F = (F_R - F_T) = (2F_T \, v/c)\cos\theta$$

where θ is the angle between the axis of flow and the incident ultrasound beam. If the Doppler angle can

be measured, estimation of flow velocity is possible. Accurate estimation of target velocity requires precise measurement of both the Doppler frequency shift and the angle of insonation to the direction of target movement. As the Doppler angle, θ, approaches 90 degrees the cosine of θ approaches 0. **At an angle of 90 degrees** there is no relative movement of the target toward or away from the transducer, and **no Doppler frequency shift is detected** (Fig. 1-31). Because the cosine of the Doppler angle changes rapidly for angles more than 60 degrees, accurate angle correction requires that Doppler measurements be made at angles of less than 60 degrees. Above 60 degrees, relatively small changes in the Doppler angle are associated with large changes in cos θ, and, therefore, a small error in estimation of the Doppler angle may result in a large error in the estimation of velocity. These considerations are important in using both duplex and color flow instruments because optimal imaging of the vessel wall is obtained when the axis of the transducer is perpendicular to the wall, whereas maximal Doppler frequency differences are obtained when the transducer axis and the direction of flow are at a relatively small angle.

In peripheral vascular applications it is highly desirable that measured Doppler frequencies be corrected for the Doppler angle to provide velocity measurement. This allows data from systems using different Doppler frequencies to be compared and eliminates error in interpretation of frequency data obtained at different Doppler angles. For abdominal applications, **angle-corrected velocity measurements**

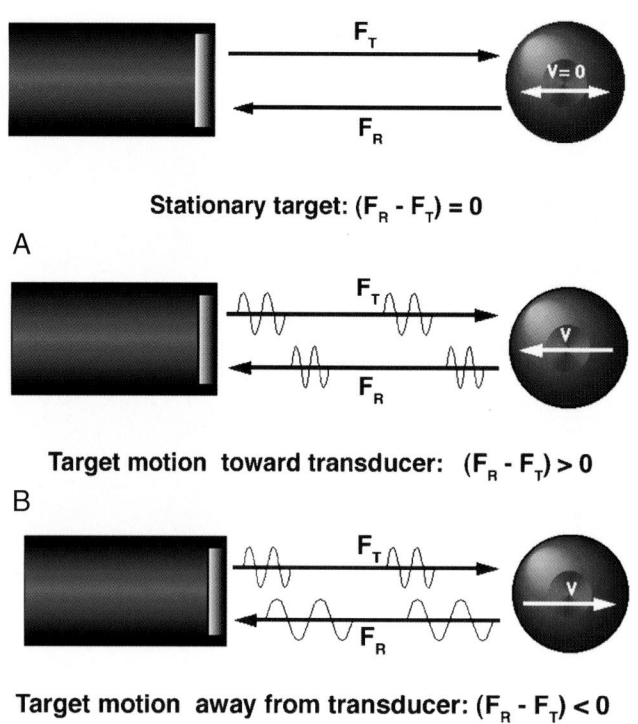

Stationary target: (F$_R$ - F$_T$) = 0

A

Target motion toward transducer: (F$_R$ - F$_T$) > 0

B

Target motion away from transducer: (F$_R$ - F$_T$) < 0

C

FIGURE 1-29. Doppler effect. A, Stationary target. If the reflecting interface is stationary, the backscattered ultrasound has the same frequency or wavelength as the transmitted sound, and there is no difference in the transmitted (F$_T$) and reflected (F$_R$) frequencies. **B and C, Moving targets**. If the reflecting interface is moving with respect to the sound beam emitted from the transducer, there is a change in the frequency of the sound scattered by the moving object. When the interface moves toward the transducer (**B**) the difference in reflected and transmitted frequencies is greater than zero. When the target is moving away from the transducer (**C**) this difference is less than zero. The Doppler equation is used to relate this change in frequency to the velocity of the moving object. (From Merritt CRB: Doppler US: The basics. Radiographics 1991;11:109-119.)

are encouraged, although qualitative assessments of flow are often made using only the Doppler frequency shift data. The interrelation of transducer frequency, F$_T$, and the Doppler angle, θ, to the Doppler frequency shift and target velocity described by the Doppler equation are important in proper clinical use of Doppler equipment.

Doppler Signal Processing and Display

Several options exist for the processing of ΔF, the Doppler frequency shift, to provide useful information regarding the direction and velocity of blood. Doppler frequency shifts encountered clinically fall in the audible range. This audible signal may be analyzed by ear and, with training, the operator can identify many flow characteristics. More commonly, the Doppler shift data are displayed in graphic form as a time-varying plot of the frequency spectrum of the returning signal. A fast Fourier transformation is used to perform the frequency analysis. The resulting Doppler frequency spectrum displays the variation with time of the Doppler frequencies present in the volume sampled, the envelope of the spectrum representing the maximum frequencies present at any given point in time, and the width of the spectrum at any point indicating the range of

frequencies present (Fig. 1-32A). In many instruments, the amplitude of each frequency component is displayed in gray scale. The presence of a large number of different frequencies at a given point in the cardiac cycle results in so-called **spectral broadening**.

In color flow Doppler imaging systems, velocity information determined from Doppler measurements is displayed as a feature of the image itself (see Fig. 1-32B). In addition to the detection of Doppler frequency shift data from each pixel in the image, these systems may also provide range-gated pulsed wave Doppler with spectral analysis for display of Doppler data.

Doppler Instrumentation

In contrast to A-mode, M-mode, and B-mode gray-scale ultrasonography, which display the information from tissue interfaces, Doppler ultrasound instruments are optimized to display flow information. The simplest Doppler devices use continuous wave rather than pulsed wave ultrasound, using two transducers that transmit and receive ultrasound continuously (**continuous wave or CW Doppler**). The transmit and receive beams overlap in a sensitive volume at some distance from the transducer face (Fig. 1-33A). Although direction of flow

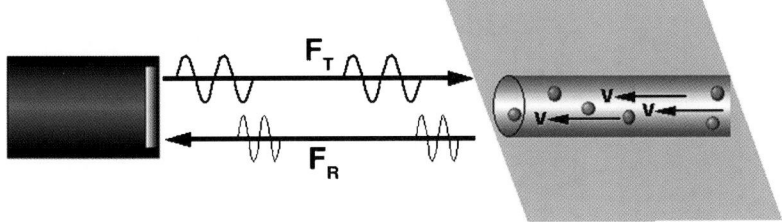

$$\Delta F = F_R - F_T = \frac{2 \cdot F_T \cdot v}{c}$$

A

FIGURE 1-30. Doppler equations. The Doppler equation describes the relationship of the Doppler frequency shift to target velocity. **A,** In its simplest form, it is assumed that the direction of the ultrasound beam is parallel to the direction of movement of the target. This situation is unusual in clinical practice. More often the ultrasound impinges on the vessel at an angle, θ. **B,** In this case the Doppler frequency shift detected is reduced in proportion to the cosine of θ. (From Merritt CRB: Doppler US: The basics. Radiographics 1991;11:109-119.)

$$\Delta F = F_R - F_T = \frac{2 \cdot F_T \cdot v \cdot \cos\varnothing}{c}$$

B

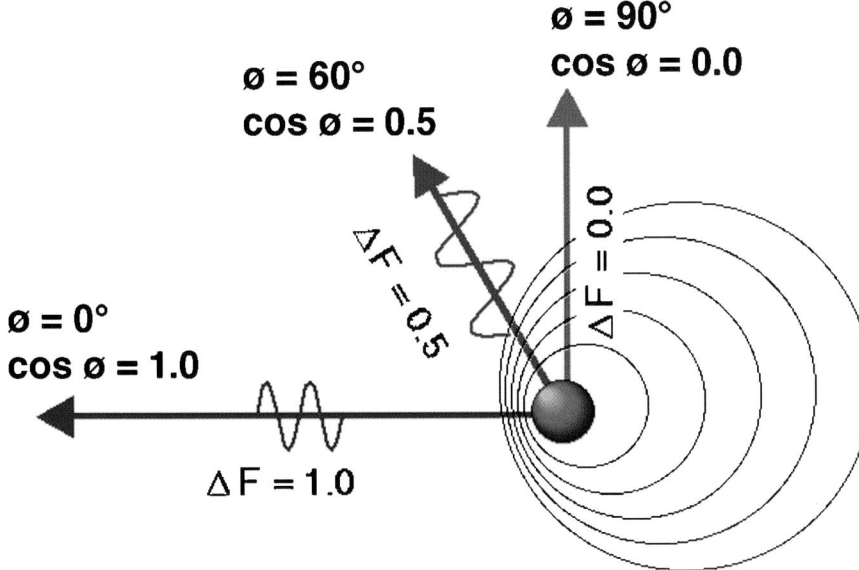

$\varnothing = 90°$
$\cos \varnothing = 0.0$

$\varnothing = 60°$
$\cos \varnothing = 0.5$

$\varnothing = 0°$
$\cos \varnothing = 1.0$

$\Delta F = 0.0$

$\Delta F = 0.5$

$\Delta F = 1.0$

FIGURE 1-31. The effect of the Doppler angle on the frequency shift detected by the transducer is illustrated. At an angle of 60 degrees, the detected frequency shift is only 50% of the shift detected at an angle of 0 degrees. At 90 degrees, there is no relative movement of the target toward or away from the transducer, and no frequency shift is detected. The detected Doppler frequency shift is reduced in proportion to the cosine of the Doppler angle. Because the cosine of the angle changes rapidly at angles above 60 degrees, the use of Doppler angles of less than 60 degrees is recommended in making velocity estimates. (From Merritt CRB: Doppler US: The basics. Radiographics 1991;11:109-119.)

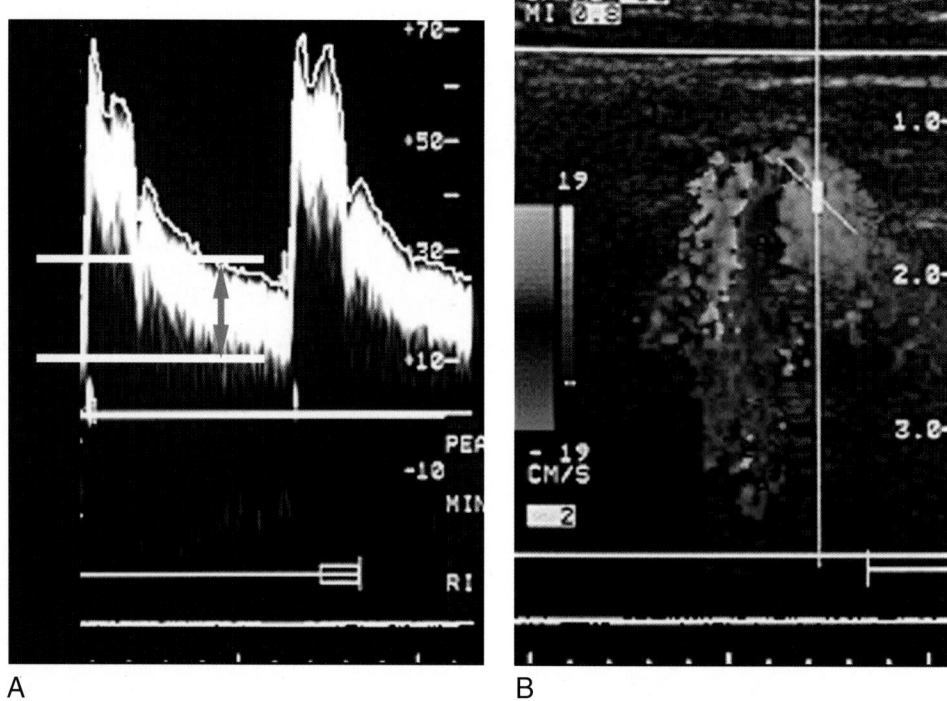

FIGURE 1-32. Doppler display. A, Doppler frequency spectrum shows changes in flow velocity and direction by vertical deflections of the waveform above and below the baseline. The width of the spectral waveform (spectral broadening) is determined by the range of frequencies present at any instant in time (*red arrow*). A brightness (gray) scale is used to indicate the amplitude of each frequency component. **B, Color flow Doppler imaging.** Amplitude data from stationary targets provide the basis for the B-mode image. Signal phase provides information about the presence and direction of motion, and changes in frequency relate to the velocity of the target. Backscattered signals from red blood cells are displayed in color as a function of their motion toward or away from the transducer, and the degree of the saturation of the color is used to indicate the frequency shift from moving red cells.

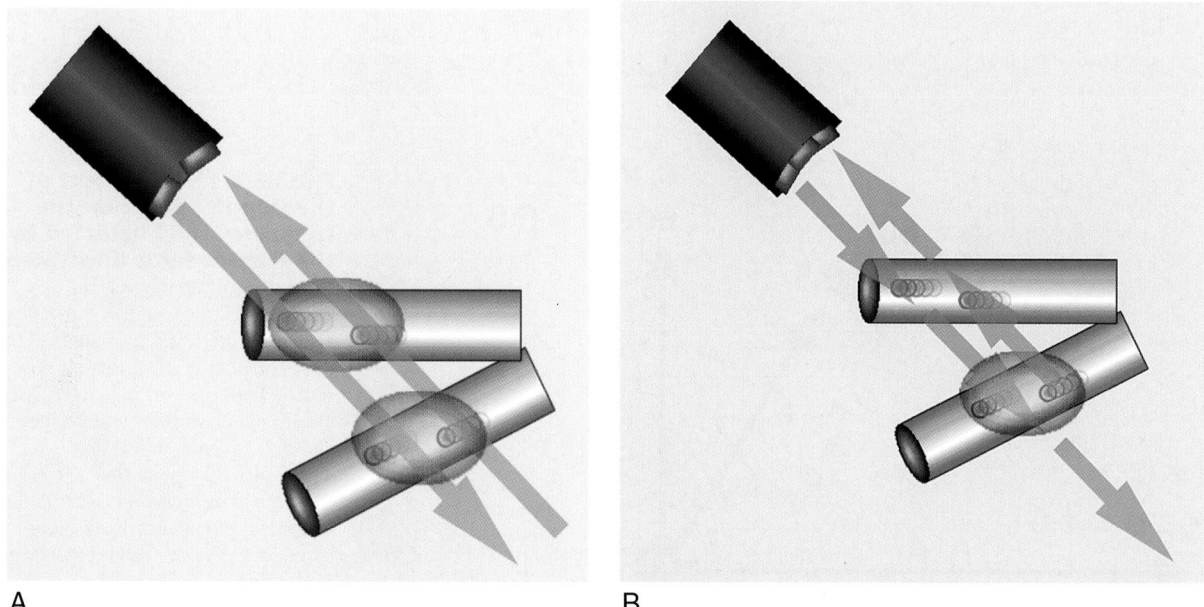

FIGURE 1-33. Continuous wave Doppler and pulsed wave Doppler. A, Continuous wave Doppler uses separate transmit and receive crystals that continuously transmit and receive ultrasound. Although able to detect the presence and direction of flow, continuous wave devices are unable to distinguish signals arising from vessels at different depths (*shaded areas*). **B, Pulsed wave Doppler** permits the sampling of flow data from selected depths by processing only the signals that return to the transducer after precisely timed intervals (*shaded area in the deeper vessel*). The operator is able to control the position of the sample volume and, in duplex systems, to view the location from which the Doppler data are obtained.

can be determined with CW Doppler, these devices do not allow discrimination of motion coming from various depths, and the source of the signal being detected is difficult, if not impossible, to ascertain with certainty. Inexpensive and portable, CW Doppler instruments are used primarily at the bedside or intraoperatively to confirm the presence of flow in superficial vessels.

Because of the limitations of CW systems, most applications use range-gated, pulsed wave Doppler. Rather than a continuous wave of ultrasound emission, pulsed wave Doppler devices emit brief pulses of ultrasound energy (see Fig. 1-33B). Using pulses of sound permits use of the time interval between the transmission of a pulse and the return of the echo as a means of determining the depth from which the Doppler shift arises. In a pulsed wave Doppler system, the sensitive volume from which flow data are sampled can be controlled in terms of shape, depth, and position. When combined with a 2-D, real-time, B-mode imager in the form of a duplex scanner, the position of the Doppler sample can be precisely controlled and monitored.

LIMITATIONS OF COLOR FLOW DOPPLER IMAGING

Angle dependence
Aliasing
Inability to display the entire Doppler spectrum in the image
Artifacts caused by noise

The most common form of Doppler ultrasound to be used for radiology applications is **color flow Doppler imaging** (Fig. 1-34A).[8] In color flow imaging systems, flow information determined from Doppler measurements is displayed as a feature of the image itself. Stationary or slowly moving targets provide the basis for the B-mode image. Signal phase provides information about the presence and direction of motion, and changes in echo signal frequency relate to the velocity of the target. Backscattered signals from red blood cells are displayed in color as a function of their motion toward or away from the transducer, and the degree of the saturation of the color is used to indicate the relative velocity of the moving red cells. Color flow Doppler imaging expands conventional duplex sonography by providing additional capabilities. The use of color saturation to display variations in Doppler shift frequency allows a **semiquantitative estimate of flow** to be made from the image alone, provided that variations in the Doppler angle are noted. The display of flow throughout the image field allows the position and orientation of the vessel of interest to be observed at all times. The display of spatial information with respect to velocity is ideal for display of small, localized areas of turbulence within a vessel, which provide clues to stenosis or irregularity of the vessel wall caused by atheroma, trauma, or other disease. Flow within the vessel is observed at all points, and **stenotic jets and focal areas of turbulence** are displayed that might be overlooked with duplex instrumentation. The contrast of flow within the vessel lumen (1) permits visualization of small vessels that are invisible when using conventional imagers and (2) enhances the visibility of wall irregularity. Color flow

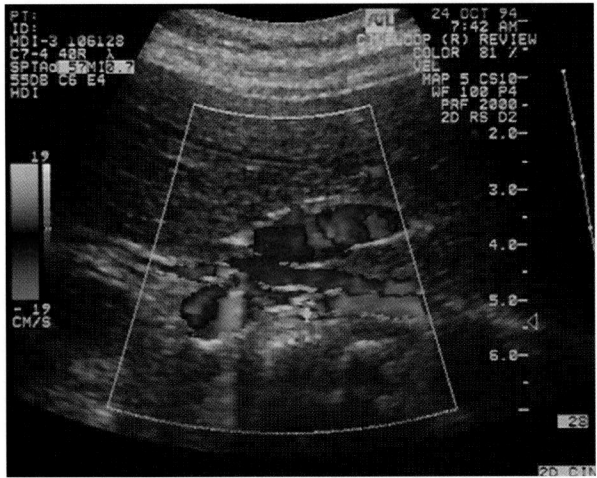
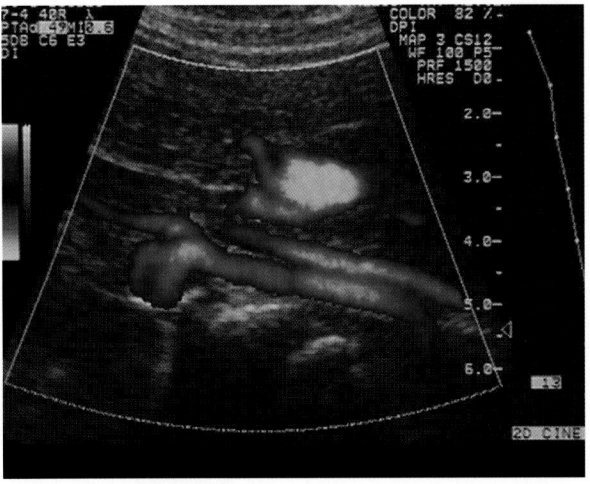

A   B

FIGURE 1-34. Color flow and power mode Doppler. **A,** Color flow Doppler imaging uses a color map to display information based on the detection of frequency shifts from moving targets. Noise in this form of display appears across the entire frequency spectrum and limits sensitivity. **B, Power mode Doppler** uses a color map to show the distribution of the power or amplitude of the Doppler signal. Flow direction and velocity information are not provided in power mode Doppler display, but noise is reduced, allowing higher gain settings and improved sensitivity for flow detection.

Doppler imaging aids in precise determination of the direction of flow and measurement of the Doppler angle. Limitations of color flow Doppler imaging include angle dependence, aliasing, inability to display the entire Doppler spectrum in the image, and artifacts caused by noise.

Power Mode Doppler

An alternative to the display of frequency information with color flow Doppler imaging is to use a color map that displays the integrated power of the Doppler signal instead of its mean frequency shift (see Fig. 1-34B).[9] Because frequency shift data are not displayed, there is no aliasing. The image does not provide any information related to flow direction or velocity, and power mode Doppler imaging is much less angle dependent than frequency-based color flow Doppler display. In contrast to color flow Doppler, where noise may appear in the image as any color, power mode Doppler permits noise to be assigned to a homogeneous background color that does not greatly interfere with the image. This results in a significant increase in the usable dynamic range of the scanner, permitting higher effective gain settings for flow detection and increased sensitivity for flow detection (Fig. 1-35).

ADVANTAGES OF POWER MODE DOPPLER

No aliasing
Much less angle dependent
Noise: a homogeneous background color
Increased sensitivity for flow detection

Interpretation of the Doppler Signal

Doppler data components that must be evaluated both in spectral display and in color flow imaging include the Doppler shift frequency and amplitude, the Doppler angle, the spatial distribution of frequencies across the vessel, and the temporal variation of the signal. Because the Doppler signal itself has no anatomic significance, the examiner must interpret the Doppler signal and then determine its relevance in the context of the image.

The detection of a Doppler frequency shift indicates movement of the target, which in most applications is related to the presence of flow. The sign of the frequency shift (positive or negative) indicates the direction of flow relative to the transducer. **Vessel stenosis** is typically associated with large Doppler frequency shifts in both

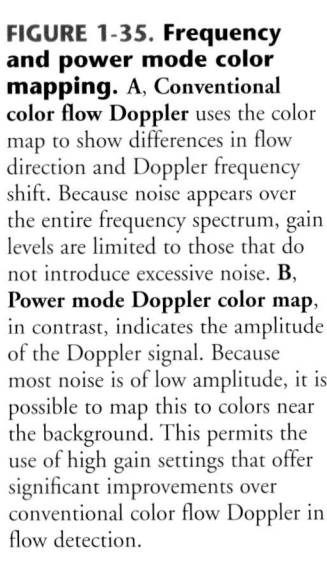
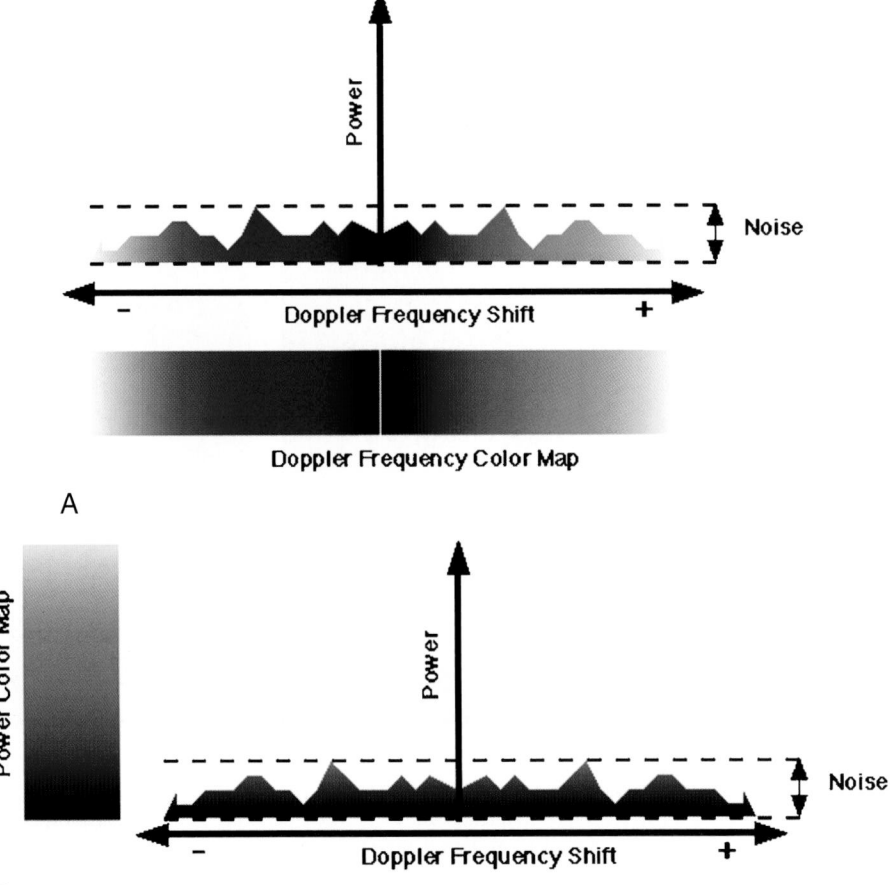

FIGURE 1-35. Frequency and power mode color mapping. A, Conventional **color flow Doppler** uses the color map to show differences in flow direction and Doppler frequency shift. Because noise appears over the entire frequency spectrum, gain levels are limited to those that do not introduce excessive noise. **B, Power mode Doppler color map,** in contrast, indicates the amplitude of the Doppler signal. Because most noise is of low amplitude, it is possible to map this to colors near the background. This permits the use of high gain settings that offer significant improvements over conventional color flow Doppler in flow detection.

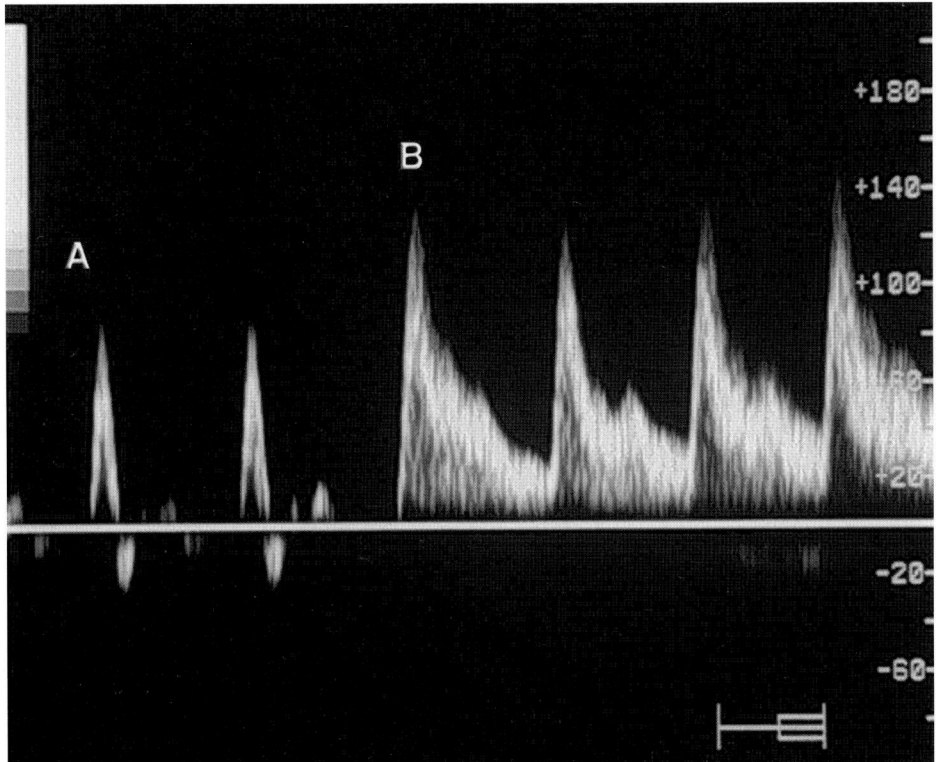

FIGURE 1-36.
Impedance. A, High-resistance waveform in the brachial artery produced by inflating blood pressure cuff applied to the forearm to a pressure above the systolic blood pressure. As a result of high peripheral resistance, there is low systolic amplitude and reversed diastolic flow. **B, Low resistance** in the peripheral vascular bed due to vasodilation stimulated by the prior ischemia. Immediately after release of 3 minutes of occluding pressure, the Doppler waveform shows increased amplitude and rapid antegrade flow throughout diastole.

systole and diastole at the site of greatest narrowing, with turbulent flow in poststenotic regions. In peripheral vessels, analysis of the Doppler changes allows accurate prediction of the degree of vessel narrowing. Information related to the resistance to flow in the distal vascular tree can be obtained by analysis of changes of blood velocity with time shown in the Doppler spectral display (Fig. 1-36), provides a graphic example of the changes in the Doppler spectral waveform resulting from physiologic changes in the resistance of the vascular bed supplied by a **normal brachial artery**. In Figure 1-36A, a blood pressure cuff has been inflated to above systolic pressure to occlude the distal branches supplied by the brachial artery. This causes reduced systolic amplitude and cessation of diastolic flow, resulting in a waveform different than that found in the normal resting state. Figure 1-36B shows the waveform in the brachial artery immediately after release of 3 minutes of occluding pressure. During the **period of ischemia** induced by pressure cuff occlusion of the forearm vessels, vasodilation has occurred. The Doppler waveform now reflects a low-resistance peripheral vascular bed with increased systolic amplitude and rapid flow throughout diastole.

Doppler indices, such as the systolic/diastolic ratio, resistive index, and pulsatility index, which compare the flow in systole and diastole, provide an indication of the resistance in the peripheral vascular bed and are used to aid in evaluation of perfusion of renal transplants, the placenta, and uterus. With Doppler ultrasound it is therefore possible to identify vessels, determine the direction of blood flow, evaluate narrowing or occlusion, and characterize flow to organs and tumors. Analysis of the Doppler shift frequency with time can be used to infer both proximal stenosis and changes in distal vascular impedance. Most work using pulsed wave Doppler imaging has emphasized the detection of stenosis, thrombosis, and flow disturbances in major peripheral arteries and veins. In these applications, measurements of peak systolic and end diastolic frequency or velocity, analysis of the Doppler spectrum, and calculation of certain frequency or velocity ratios have been the basis of analysis. Changes in the spectral waveform measured by indices comparing flow in systole and diastole provide insight into the resistance of the vascular bed supplied by the vessel and indicate changes resulting from a variety of pathologies (Fig. 1-37). Changes of these indices from normal may be important in the early identification of rejection of transplanted organs, parenchymal dysfunction, and malignancy. Although these indices are useful, it is important to keep in mind that these measurements are influenced, not only by the resistance to flow in peripheral vessels, but also by many other factors, including heart rate, blood pressure, vessel wall length and elasticity, and extrinsic organ compression. Interpretation must, therefore, always take into account all of these variables.

Although the more graphic presentation of color flow Doppler imaging suggests that interpretation is made easier, the complexity of the color flow Doppler image actually makes this a more demanding image to evaluate

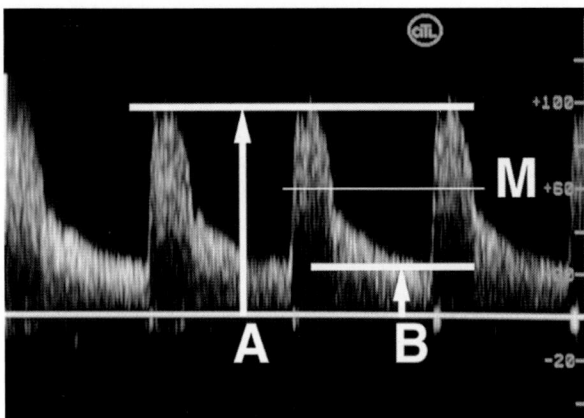

FIGURE 1-37. Doppler indices. Doppler imaging is capable of providing information about flow in both large and small vessels. Small vessel impedance is reflected in the Doppler spectral waveform of afferent vessels. Doppler flow indices used to characterize peripheral resistance are based on the **peak systolic frequency** or velocity (A), the minimum or **end diastolic frequency** or velocity (B), and the **mean frequency** or velocity (M). The most commonly used indices are the **systolic/diastolic ratio** (A/B); the **resistive index** [(A-B)/A]; and the **pulsatility index** [(A-B)/M]. In calculation of the pulsatility index, the minimum diastolic velocity or frequency is used; calculation of the systolic/diastolic ratio and resistive index use the end diastolic value.

MAJOR SOURCES OF DOPPLER IMAGING ARTIFACTS

DOPPLER FREQUENCY

Higher frequencies lead to more tissue attenuation
Wall filters
Remove signals from low-velocity blood flow

SPECTRAL BROADENING

Excessive system gain or changes in dynamic range of the gray-scale display can increase it
Excessively large sample volume increases it
Sample volume too near the vessel wall increases it

ALIASING

Decreased PRF increases aliasing
Decreasing the Doppler angle will increase aliasing
Higher Doppler frequency transducer will increase aliasing

DOPPLER ANGLE

Relatively inaccurate above 60 degrees

SAMPLE VOLUME SIZE

Increased vessel wall noise if large sample volumes

than the simple Doppler spectrum. Nevertheless, color flow Doppler imaging has important advantages over pulsed wave duplex Doppler imaging in which flow data are obtained only from a small portion of the area being imaged. To be confident that a conventional Doppler study has achieved reasonable sensitivity and specificity in detection of flow disturbances, a methodical search and sampling of multiple sites within the field of interest must be performed. Color flow Doppler imaging devices permit simultaneous sampling of multiple sites and are less susceptible to this error.

Other Technical Considerations

Although many of the problems and artifacts associated with B-mode imaging, such as shadowing, are encountered with Doppler ultrasonography, the detection and display of frequency information related to moving targets add a group of special technical considerations that are not encountered with other forms of ultrasonography. An understanding of the source of these artifacts and their influence on the interpretation of the flow measurements obtained in clinical practice is important. Major sources of Doppler artifacts are discussed subsequently.

Doppler Frequency

A primary objective of the Doppler examination is the accurate measurement of characteristics of flow within a vascular structure. The moving red blood cells that serve as the primary source of the Doppler signal act as point scatterers of ultrasound rather than specular reflectors. This interaction results in the intensity of the scattered sound varying in proportion to the fourth power of the frequency. This has an important implication with respect to the selection of the Doppler frequency to be used for a given examination. As the transducer frequency increases, Doppler sensitivity improves, but attenuation by tissue also increases, resulting in diminished penetration. Careful balancing of the requirements for sensitivity and penetration is an important responsibility of the operator during a Doppler examination. Because many abdominal vessels lie several centimeters beneath the surface, Doppler frequencies in the range of 3 to 3.5 MHz are usually required to permit adequate penetration.

Wall Filters

Doppler instruments detect motion not only from blood flow but also from adjacent structures. To eliminate these low-frequency signals from the display, most instruments use high pass filters or "wall" filters, which remove signals that fall below a given frequency limit.

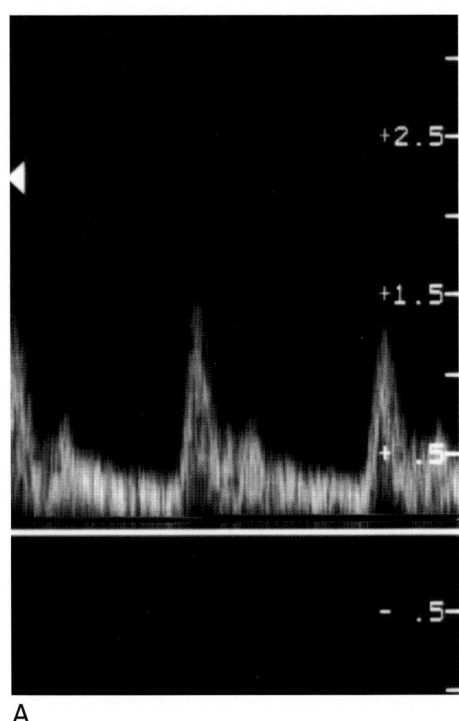

A

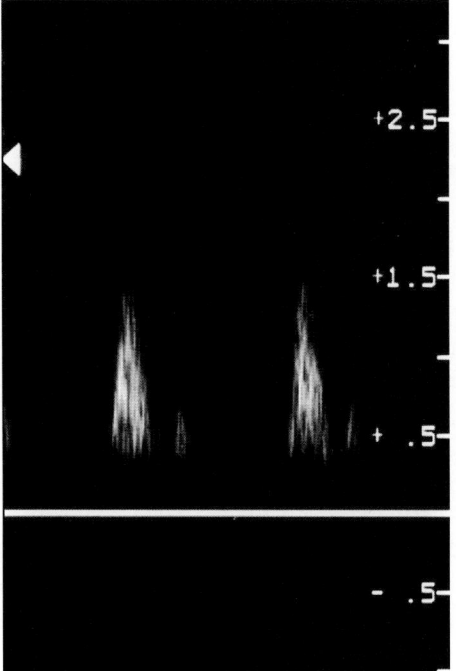

B

FIGURE 1-38. Wall filters. Wall filters are used to eliminate low-frequency noise from the Doppler display. Here the effect on the display of low-velocity flow is shown with wall filter settings of **A**, 100 Hz, and **B**, 400 Hz. High wall filter settings remove signal from low-velocity blood flow and may result in interpretation errors. In general, wall filters should be kept at the lowest practical level, usually in the range of 50 to 100 Hz.

Although effective in **eliminating low-frequency noise**, these filters may also **remove signals from low-velocity blood flow** (Fig. 1-38). In certain clinical situations, the measurement of these slower flow velocities is of clinical importance, and the improper selection of the wall filter may result in serious errors of interpretation. For example, low-velocity venous flow may not be detected if an improper filter is used, and low-velocity diastolic flow in certain arteries may also be eliminated from the display, resulting in errors in the calculation of Doppler indices, such as the systolic/diastolic ratio or resistive index. In general, the filter should be kept at the lowest practical level, usually in the range of 50 to 100 Hz.

Spectral broadening refers to the presence of a large range of flow velocities at a given point in the pulse cycle and is an important criterion of high-grade vessel narrowing. Excessive system gain or changes in the dynamic range of the gray-scale display of the Doppler spectrum may suggest spectral broadening; opposite settings may mask broadening of the Doppler spectrum, causing diagnostic inaccuracy. Spectral broadening may also be produced by the selection of an excessively large sample volume or by the placement of the sample volume too near the vessel wall where slower velocities are present (Fig. 1-39).

Aliasing

Aliasing is an artifact arising from ambiguity in the measurement of high Doppler frequency shifts. To ensure that samples originate from only a selected depth when using a pulsed wave Doppler system, it is necessary to wait for the echo from the area of interest before transmitting the next pulse. This limits the rate with which pulses can be generated, a lower PRF being required for greater depth. The PRF also determines the maximum depth from which unambiguous data can be obtained. If the PRF is less than twice the maximum frequency shift produced by movement of the target (the Nyquist limit), aliasing results. Figure 1-40 illustrates the origin of aliasing. When the PRF is less than twice the frequency shift being detected, lower frequency shifts than are actually present are displayed. Because of the need for lower PRFs to reach deep vessels, signals from deep abdominal arteries are prone to aliasing if high velocities are present. In practice, aliasing is usually readily recognized (see Fig. 1-40C, D). Aliasing can be reduced by increasing the PRF, by increasing the Doppler angle (see Fig. 1-31D)—thereby decreasing the frequency shift—or by using a lower-frequency Doppler transducer.

Doppler Angle

When making Doppler measurements, it is desirable to correct for the Doppler angle and display the measurements in terms of velocity. These measurements are independent of the Doppler frequency. The accuracy of a velocity estimate obtained with Doppler is only as great as the accuracy of the measurement of the Doppler angle. This is particularly true as the Doppler angle exceeds 60 degrees. In general, the Doppler angle is best kept at 60 degrees or less because small changes in the Doppler angle above 60 degrees result in significant

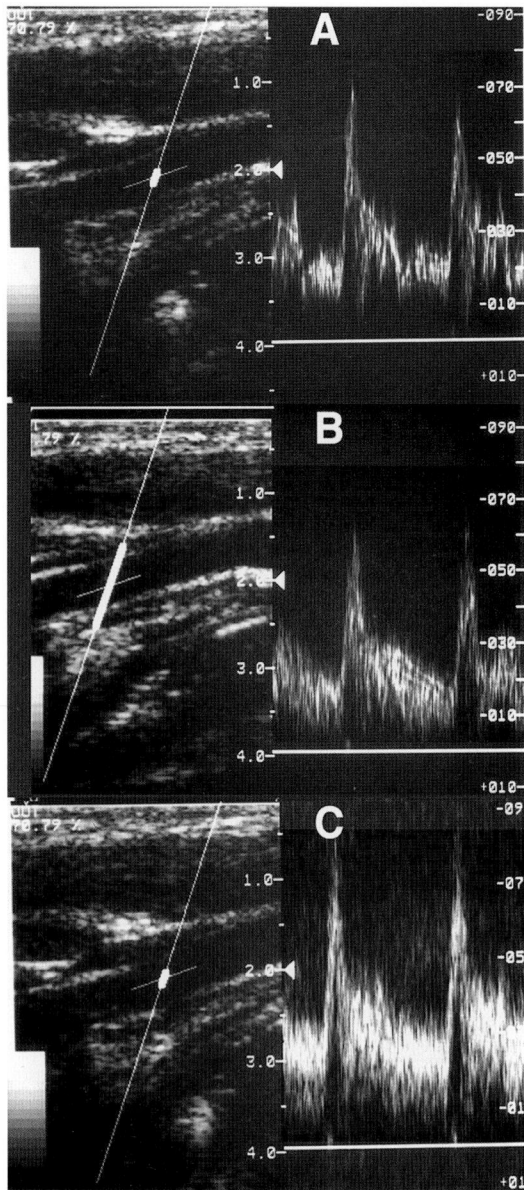

FIGURE 1-39. Spectral broadening. The range of velocities detected at a given time in the pulse cycle is reflected in the Doppler spectrum as spectral broadening. **A, Normal spectrum.** Spectral broadening may arise from turbulent flow in association with vessel stenosis. **Artifactual spectral broadening** may be produced by improper positioning of the sample volume near the vessel wall, (**B**) use of an excessively large sample volume, or (**C**) **excessive system gain**.

changes in the calculated velocity, and, therefore, measurement inaccuracies result in much greater errors in velocity estimates than do similar errors at lower Doppler angles.

Sample Volume Size

With pulsed wave Doppler systems, the length of the Doppler sample volume can be controlled by the operator, and the width is determined by the beam profile. Analysis of Doppler signals requires that the sample volume be adjusted to exclude as much of the unwanted clutter from near the vessel walls as possible.

OPERATING MODES: CLINICAL IMPLICATIONS

Ultrasound devices may operate in several modes, including real-time, color flow Doppler, spectral Doppler, and M-mode imaging. Imaging is produced in a scanned mode of operation. In scanned modes, pulses of ultrasound from the transducer are directed down lines of sight that are moved or steered in sequence to generate the image. This means that the number of ultrasound pulses arriving at a given point in the patient over a given interval of time is relatively small, and relatively little energy is deposited at any given location. In contrast, **spectral Doppler** imaging is an unscanned mode of operation in which multiple ultrasound pulses are sent in repetition along a line to collect the Doppler data. In this mode, the beam is stationary, resulting in **considerably greater potential for heating** than in imaging modes. For imaging, PRFs are usually a few thousand hertz with very short pulses. Longer pulse durations are used with Doppler than with other imaging modes. In addition, to avoid aliasing and other artifacts with Doppler imaging, it is often necessary to use higher PRFs than with other imaging applications. Longer pulse duration and higher PRF result in higher duty factors for Doppler modes of operation and increase the amount of energy introduced in scanning. Color flow Doppler, although a scanned mode, produces exposure conditions between those of real-time and Doppler imaging because color flow Doppler devices tend to send more pulses down each scan line and may use longer pulse durations than imaging devices. Clearly, every user needs to be aware that switching from an imaging to a Doppler mode changes the exposure conditions and the potential for bioeffects.

With current devices operating in imaging modes, bioeffects concerns are minimal because intensities sufficient to produce measurable heating are seldom used. With Doppler ultrasound, the potential for thermal effects is greater. Preliminary measurements on commercially available instruments suggest that at least some of these instruments are capable of producing temperature rises of greater than 1°C at soft tissue/bone interfaces, if the focal zone of the transducer is held stationary. Care is, therefore, warranted when Doppler measurements are obtained at or near soft tissue/bone interfaces as may be the case in the second and third trimester of pregnancy. In these applications, thoughtful application of the principle of ALARA (as low as reasonably achievable) is required. Under the principle of ALARA, the user should use the lowest possible

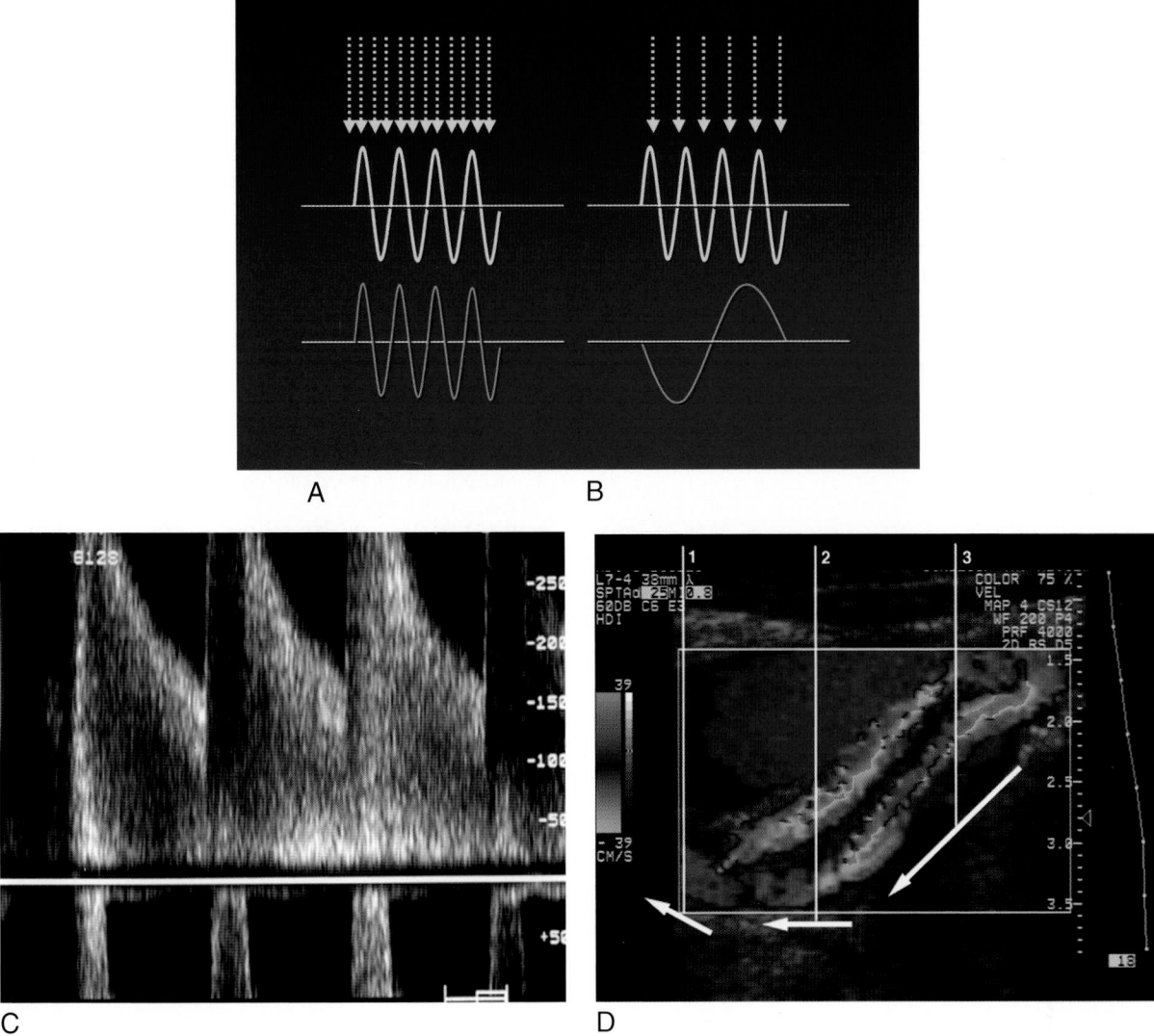

FIGURE 1-40. Aliasing. The PRF determines the sampling rate of a given Doppler frequency shift. **A,** If the PRF (*arrows*) is sufficient, the sampled waveform (*orange curve*) will **accurately** estimate the frequency being sampled (*yellow curve*). **B,** If the PRF is less than half the frequency being measured, **undersampling** will result in a lower frequency shift being displayed (*orange curve*). **C,** In a clinical setting, **aliasing** appears in the spectral display as a "wrap around" of the higher frequencies to display below the baseline. **D,** In color flow Doppler display, **aliasing** results in a wrap around of the frequency color map from one flow direction to the opposite direction, passing through a transition of unsaturated color. In **D,** the velocity throughout the vessel is constant, but **aliasing appears only in portions of the vessel.** This is because of the effect of the Doppler angle on the Doppler frequency shift. As the angle increases, the Doppler frequency shift decreases and aliasing is no longer seen.

acoustic exposure to obtain the necessary diagnostic information.

ARE BIOEFFECTS THE REAL ISSUE?

Although there is clearly a need for users of ultrasound to be aware of bioeffects concerns, it is equally important to place bioeffects concerns in perspective by considering another key element in the safe use of ultrasound—the user. The knowledge and skill of the user are major determinants of the risk-to-benefit implications of the use of ultrasound in a specific clinical situation.

For example, an unrealistic emphasis on risks may discourage an appropriate use of ultrasound, resulting in harm to the patient by preventing the acquisition of useful information or by subjecting the patient to another more hazardous examination. The skill and experience of the individual performing and interpreting the examination are likely to have a major impact on the overall benefit of the examination. In view of the rapid growth of ultrasound and its proliferation into the hands of minimally trained clinicians, it is likely that far more patients may be harmed by misdiagnosis resulting from improper indications, poor examination technique, and errors in interpretation than from biologic effects. The failure to diagnose a significant anomaly or misdiagnosis (for example, of an ectopic pregnancy) are real dangers, and poorly trained users may, in fact, turn out to be the greatest current hazard of diagnostic ultrasound.

Understanding bioeffects is essential for the prudent use of diagnostic ultrasound and is important in ensuring that the excellent risk-to-benefit performance of diagnostic ultrasound is preserved. All users of ultrasound should be prudent, understanding as fully as possible the potential risks and obvious benefits of ultrasound examinations, as well as those of alternate diagnostic methods. With this information, users can monitor exposure conditions and implement the principle of ALARA to keep patient and fetal exposure as low as possible while fulfilling diagnostic objectives.

References

Basic Acoustics
1. Chivers RC, Parry RJ: Ultrasonic velocity and attenuation in mammalian tissues. J Acoust Soc Am 1978;63:940-953.
2. Goss SA, Johnston RL, Dunn F: Comprehensive compilation of empirical properties of mammalian tissues. J Acoust Soc Am 1978;64:423-457.
3. Merritt CRB, Kremkau FW, Hobbins JC: Diagnostic Ultrasound: Bioeffects and Safety. Ultrasound Obstet Gynecol 1992;2:366-374.
4. Merritt CRB, Hykes DL, Hedrick WR, et al: Medical diagnostic ultrasound instrumentation and clinical interpretation. Topics in Radiology/Council Report. JAMA 1991;265:1155-1159.

Instrumentation
5. Krishnan S, Li P-C, O'Donnell M: Adaptive compensation of phase and magnitude aberrations. IEEE Trans Ultrasonics Fer Freq Control 1996;43:44.
6. Merritt CR: Technology Update. Radiol Clin North Am 2001;39:385-397.
7. Merritt CRB: Doppler US: The basics. RadioGraphics 1991;11:109-119.
8. Merritt CRB: Doppler color flow imaging. J Clin Ultrasound 1987;15:591-597.
9. Rubin JM, Bude RO, Carson PL, et al: Power Doppler US: A potentially useful alternative to mean frequency-based color Doppler US. Radiology 1994;190:853-856.

2

BIOLOGIC EFFECTS AND SAFETY

Christy K. Holland / J. Brian Fowlkes

Chapter Outline

OVERVIEW

Widespread Use of Ultrasound

Ultrasound has provided an incredible wealth of knowledge in diagnostic medicine. Few would be willing to deny the impact this imaging modality has had on medical practice, particularly in obstetrics. It is estimated that millions of sonographic examinations are performed each year, and ultrasound remains one of the fastest-growing imaging modalities. This growth is due to many factors, including its low cost, real-time interactions, and, to no lesser extent, its apparent lack of bioeffects. Despite the large number of sonographic examinations performed to date, there has been no causal relationship established between clinical applications of diagnostic ultrasound and biologic effects on the patient or operator.

Regulation of Ultrasound Output

At present, the U.S. Food and Drug Administration (FDA) regulates the maximal output of ultrasound devices to an established level through a marketing approval process that requires devices to be equivalent in efficacy and output to those produced prior to 1976. This historic regulation of sonography has provided a safety margin for ultrasound, while allowing clinically useful performance. The mechanism has restricted ultrasound exposure to levels that apparently produce few if any obvious bioeffects based on the epidemiologic evidence, although there has been some evidence indicating the potential for bioeffects in animal studies.

Increasing Role for Sonographers and Physicians

Proposals concerning the regulation of acoustic output from medical ultrasound systems have suggested greatly increasing the role the physician and/or sonographer play in limiting the potential for ultrasound bioeffects. Because the maximum output limit was historically set by the FDA, and because it might be diagnostically advantageous to increase this limit (e.g., patients with large amounts of subcutaneous fat are difficult to scan), ultrasound devices might produce higher outputs in the near future. As will be discussed later, for some applications the maximum acoustic output has increased through the establishment of an additional FDA market approval process, termed "Track 3," that includes additional information being reported to the operator regarding the relative potential for bioeffects. Therefore, an informed decision concerning the possible adverse effects of ultrasound in comparison to desired diagnostic information is becoming more important. Current FDA regulations that limit the maximum output are still in place, but in the future, systems might allow the discretion to increase acoustic output beyond a level that might induce a biologic response.

Although the choices made during sonographic examinations may not be equivalent to the risk versus benefit decisions associated with imaging modalities using ionizing radiation, there will be an increasing reliance on the operator to determine the amount of ultrasound exposure that is diagnostically required. For these reasons, an operator should know the potential bioeffects associated with ultrasound exposure. Patients also need to be reassured about the safety of a diagnostic ultrasound scan. The scientific community has identified some potential bioeffects from sonography, and although no causal relationship has been established, it does not mean that no effects exist, so it is important to understand the interaction of ultrasound with biologic systems.

PHYSICAL EFFECTS OF SOUND

The physical effects of sound can be divided into two principal groups: **thermal** and **nonthermal**. The thermal effects are within the common experience of most medical professionals. The effect of elevated temperature on tissue can be recognized, and the effects due to ultrasound are not substantially different from those of any other localized heat source. In this case the heating is principally due to the absorption of the sound field as it propagates through tissue. However, nonthermal mechanisms can generate heat as well.

Many nonthermal mechanisms for biologic effects exist. Acoustic fields can apply **radiation forces** (not ionizing radiation) on the structures within the body, both at the macroscopic and microscopic levels, resulting in exerted pressure and torque. The time average pressure in an acoustic field is different than the hydrostatic pressure of the fluid, and any object in the field is subject to this change in pressure. The effect is typically considered smaller than many others because it relies on less significant factors in the formulation of the acoustic field. Acoustic fields can also cause motion of fluids. Such acoustically induced flow is called **streaming**.

A topic of great interest is the effect of **acoustic cavitation**, which is the action of acoustic fields within a fluid to generate bubbles and/or cause their volume pulsation and even collapse in response to the acoustic field. The result of this activity can be heat generation and associated free radical generation, microstreaming of fluid around the bubble, radiation forces generated by the scattered acoustic field from the bubble, and mechanical actions resulting from bubble collapse. The interaction of acoustic fields with bubbles or "gas bodies" (as they are generally called) has been a significant area of bioeffects research in recent years.

THERMAL EFFECTS
Ultrasound Produces Heat

As ultrasound propagates through the body, energy is lost through **attenuation**. Attenuation causes loss in penetration and the inability to image deeper tissues. Attenuation is the result of two processes. **Scattering** of the ultrasound results from the redirection of the acoustic energy by tissue encountered during propagation. In the case of diagnostic ultrasound, some of the acoustic energy transmitted into the tissue is scattered back in the direction of the transducer (termed **backscatter**), which allows a signal to be detected and images to be made. Energy also is lost along the propagation path of the ultrasound by **absorption**. Absorption is the conversion of the ultrasound energy into heat. This heating provides a mechanism for ultrasound-induced bioeffects.

Factors Controlling Tissue Heating

The rate at which temperature will increase in tissues exposed to ultrasound depends on a number of factors. These include spatial focusing, ultrasound frequency, exposure duration, and tissue type.

Spatial Focusing

Ultrasound systems use various techniques to concentrate or focus ultrasound energy in order to improve the quality of measured signals. The analog for light is that of a magnifying glass. The glass collects all of the light striking its surface and concentrates it into a small region. In sonography and acoustics in general, the term **intensity** is used to describe the spatial distribution of ultrasonic **power** (energy per unit time) where **Intensity = Power/Area** and the area refers to the cross-sectional area of the ultrasound beam. Another beam dimension that is often quoted is the **beam width** at a specified location of the field. If the same ultrasonic power is concentrated into a smaller area, then the intensity will increase. Focusing in an ultrasound system can be used to improve the spatial resolution of the images. The side effect is an increased potential for bioeffects due to heating and cavitation. In general, the greatest heating potential will lie somewhere between the scanhead and the focus, but the exact position will depend on the focal distance, tissue properties, and heat generated within the scanhead itself.

Returning to the magnifying glass analogy, most children learn at an early age that the secret to incineration is a steady hand. Movement distributes the power of the light beam over a larger area, thereby reducing its intensity. The same is true in ultrasound imaging. Thus, imaging systems that scan a beam through tissue reduce the spatial average intensity. **Spectral Doppler** and **M-mode** imaging maintain the ultrasound beam in a stationary position (both considered **unscanned modes**) and, therefore, provide no opportunity to spatially distribute the ultrasonic power, whereas **color flow Doppler**, **power mode Doppler**, and **B-mode** (often called **gray-scale**) imaging require that the beam be moved to new locations (scanned) at a rate sufficient to produce the real-time nature of these imaging modes.

Temporal Considerations

The ultrasound power is the temporal rate at which ultrasound energy is produced; therefore, it seems reasonable that controlling how ultrasound is produced in time is a method for limiting its effects. Ultrasound can be produced in bursts rather than continuously. Ultrasound imaging systems operate on the principle of **pulse-echo** in which a burst of ultrasound is emitted followed by a quiescent period listening for echoes to return. This pulsed ultrasound is swept through the image plane numerous times during an imaging sequence. On the other hand, ultrasound may be transmitted in a **continuous wave (CW)** mode in which the ultrasound transmission is not interrupted. The **temporal peak intensity** refers to the largest intensity at any time during ultrasound exposure (Fig. 2-1). The **pulse average intensity** is the average value over the ultrasound pulse. And the **temporal average** is the average over the entire pulse repetition period (the elapsed time between the onset of ultrasound bursts). The **duty factor** is defined as the fraction of time the ultrasound field is on. Given significant time off between pulses (small duty factor), the temporal average value will be significantly smaller. For example, a duty factor of 10% will reduce the temporal average intensity by a factor of 10 compared to the pulse average. It is the time-averaged quantities that are most related to the potential for thermal bioeffects. When combined with spatial information, some common terms are produced, such as the spatial peak temporal average intensity, I_{SPTA}, or the spatial average temporal average intensity, I_{SATA}. The overall duration, or **dwell time**, of the ultrasound

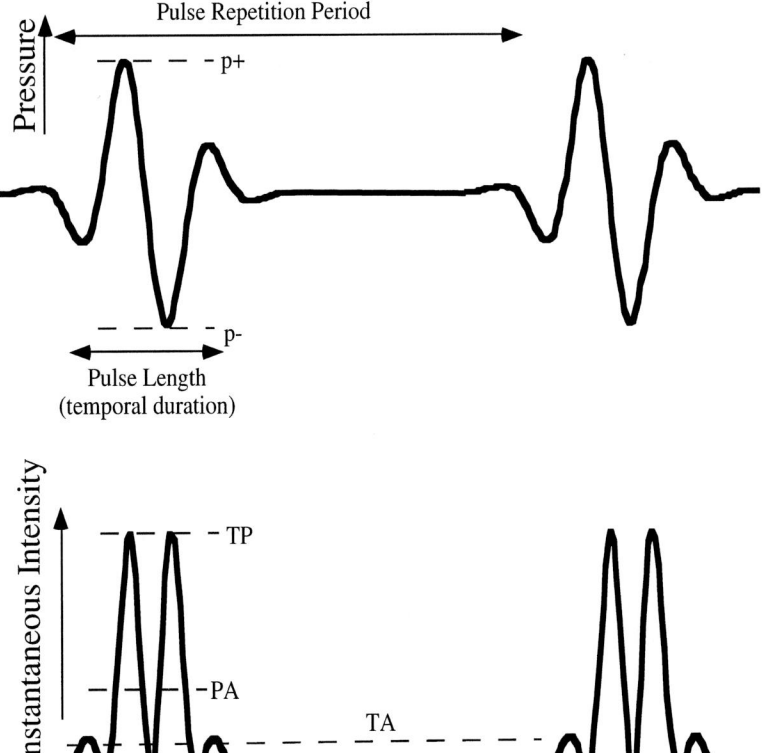

FIGURE 2-1. Pressure and intensity parameters measured in medical ultrasound. The variables are defined as follows: p+ = peak positive pressure in waveform; p- = peak negative pressure in waveform; TP = temporal peak; PA = pulse average; TA = temporal average.

TISSUE ATTENUATION

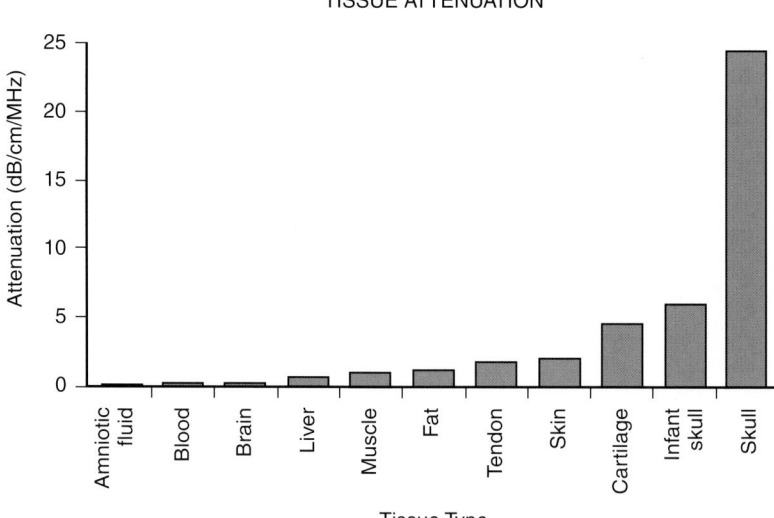

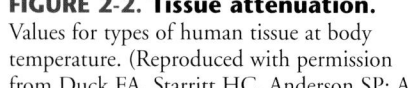

FIGURE 2-2. Tissue attenuation.
Values for types of human tissue at body temperature. (Reproduced with permission from Duck FA, Starritt HC, Anderson SP: A survey of the acoustic output of ultrasonic Doppler equipment. Clin Phys Physiol Meas 1987;8:39-49.)

exposure to a particular tissue is important because the longer the tissue is exposed, the greater the risk of bioeffects. The motion of the scanhead during an examination reduces the dwell time within a particular region of the body and minimizes the potential for bioeffects of ultrasound. Therefore, performing an efficient scan, spending only the time required for diagnosis, is a simple way to reduce exposure.

Tissue Type

Numerous physical and biologic parameters control heating of tissues. Absorption is normally the dominant contribution to attenuation in soft tissue. The attenuation coefficient is the attenuation per unit length of sound travel and is usually given in units of dB/cm-MHz. The attenuation typically increases with increasing ultrasound frequency. The attenuation ranges from a negligible amount for fluids, such as amniotic fluid, blood, and urine, to the highest value for bone with some variation among different soft tissue types (Fig. 2-2).

Another important factor is the body's ability to cool tissue via blood perfusion. Well-perfused tissue will more effectively regulate its temperature by carrying away the excess heat produced by ultrasound. The exception to this is when heat is deposited too rapidly as in thermal ablation used for therapy.[1]

From the tissue considerations noted earlier, there are two specific areas of interest based on the differences in the nature of heating phenomena. First is **bone** because of its high attenuation of incident acoustic energy. It is common in examinations during pregnancies for calcified bone to be subjected to ultrasound. A case in point is the measurement of the biparietal diameter (BPD) of the skull. Fetal bone contains increasing

degrees of mineralization as gestation progresses, thereby increasing risk of localized heating. The second is the attenuation of ultrasound by **soft tissue**. Special heating situations, which are relevant to obstetric examinations, may also occur in soft tissue where overlying structures provide little attenuation of the field, such as the fluid-filled amniotic sac.

Bone Heating

The absorption of ultrasound at bone allows for rapid deposition of energy from the field into a limited volume of tissue. The result can be a significant temperature rise. For example, Carstensen et al. combined an analytical approach and experimental measurements of the temperature rise in mouse skull exposed to continuous wave ultrasound to estimate the temperature increments in bone exposures.[2] Because bone has a large absorption coefficient, the incident ultrasonic energy is assumed to be absorbed in a thin planar sheet at the bone surface. The temperature rise of mouse skull has been studied in a 3.6-MHz focused beam with a beam width of 2.75 mm (Fig. 2-3). The temporal average intensity in the focal region was 1.5 W/cm.[2] One of two models (shown as the highest curve) in common use[3] predicts values for the temperature rise about 20% greater than that actually measured in this experiment.[1] Thus, the theoretical model is conservative in nature.

Similarly for the fetal femur, Drewniak et al.[4] indicated that the size and calcification state of the bone contributed to the *ex vivo* heating of bone (Table 2-1). To put this in perspective and to give an awareness of the role the operator can play in controlling potential heating, consider the following scenario. By reducing the output power of an ultrasound scanner by 10 dB, the predicted temperature rise would be reduced by a factor

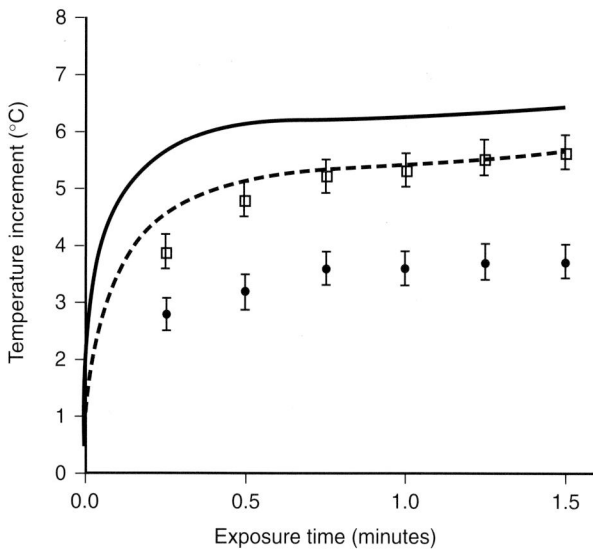

FIGURE 2-3. Heating of mouse skull in a focused sound field. For these experiments the frequency was 3.6 MHz and the temporal average focal intensity was 1.5 W/cm². Solid circles: young (<17 wks) mice (N = 7); open squares: old (>6 mo) mice (N = 4); vertical bars: two standard errors in height; top curves: theoretical estimation of the temperature increases by Nyborg. (From Carstensen EL, Child SZ, Norton S, et al: Ultrasonic heating of the skull. J Acoust Soc Am 1990;87:1310-1317; and from Nyborg WL: Solutions of the bio-heat transfer equation. Phys Med Biol 1988;33(7):785-792.)

TABLE 2-1. FETAL FEMUR TEMPERATURE INCREMENTS AT 1 W/CM²

Gestational Age (days)	Diameter (mm)	Temperature Increments (°C)
59	0.5	0.10
78	1.2	0.69
108	3.3	2.92

Temperature increments in human fetal femur exposed for 20 seconds were found to be approximately proportional to incident intensity. From Nyborg WL: Solutions of the bio-heat transfer equation. Phys Med Biol 1988;33(7):785-792.

of 10, making the 3°C rise seen by these researchers (see Table 2-1) virtually nonexistent. **This strongly suggests the use of maximum gain and reduction in output power during ultrasound examinations** (see section on controlling ultrasound output). In the case of fetal examinations, a clear attempt should be made to maximize amplifier gain because this comes at no cost to the patient in terms of exposure. Distinctions are often made between bone positioned deep to the skin at the focal plane of the transducer and bone near the skin surface, as would be the case when considering transcranial applications. This distinction is discussed later with regard to the thermal index.

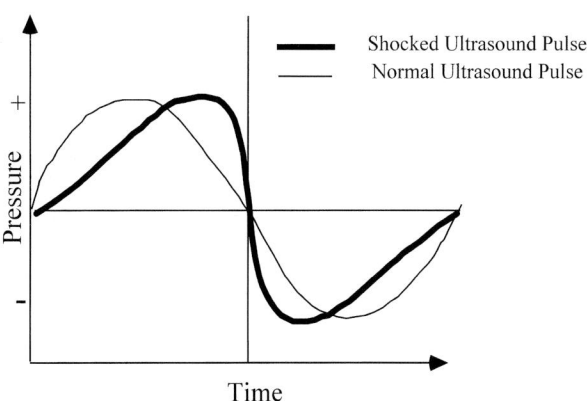

FIGURE 2-4. Effect of finite amplitude distortion on a propagating ultrasound pulse. Note the increasing steepness in the pulse, which contains higher frequency components.

Soft Tissue Heating

Two special scenarios for ultrasound exposure in soft tissue are particularly relevant to obstetric/gynecologic applications. First is the common condition of **scanning through a full bladder**. In this case, the urine is a fluid with a relatively low ultrasound attenuation coefficient. The reduced attenuation will allow larger acoustic amplitudes to be applied deeper within the body. In addition, it is possible for the propagating wave to experience **finite amplitude distortion**, resulting in energy being shifted by a nonlinear process from lower to higher frequencies. The result is a **shockwave** where a gradual wave steepening (Fig. 2-4) results in a waveform composed of higher frequency components. Because attenuation increases with increasing frequency, the absorption of a large portion of the energy in such a wave occurs over a much shorter distance, concentrating the energy deposition in the first tissue encountered, which may include the fetus. These nonlinear effects are also under extensive consideration as part of the thermal modeling for fetal exposure. Ultrasound imaging systems now include specific imaging modalities that rely on nonlinear effects. Referred to by various manufacturers as **tissue harmonic imaging**, native harmonic imaging, and other names, the image is created using the back-scatter of harmonic components induced by nonlinear propagation of the ultrasound field. This has distinct advantages in terms of reducing image artifacts and improving, especially, lateral resolution. In these nonlinear imaging modes, the acoustic output must be sufficiently high to produce the effect. So far the acoustic power used is still within the FDA limits but improvements in image quality using such modes may motivate the need to modify or relax the regulatory restrictions.

Another common situation worth noting is **transvaginal ultrasound**. This procedure is mentioned in particular because of the proximity of the transducer to sensitive tissues such as the ovaries. As will be discussed later, temperature increases near the transducer may provide a heat source at sites other than the focus of the transducer. In addition, the transducer face itself may be a significant heat source because of inefficiencies in its conversion of electrical to acoustic energy. Such considerations must be made in the estimation of potential thermal effects in transvaginal ultrasound or any other endocavitary application.

Hyperthermia and Ultrasound Safety

Our knowledge of the bioeffects for ultrasound heating is based on the experience available from other more common forms of **hyperthermia** that serve as a basis for safety criteria. There is extensive data concerning the effects of short-term and extended temperature increases, or hyperthermia. Teratologic effects due to hyperthermia have been demonstrated in birds, all the common laboratory animals, farm animals, and nonhuman primates.[5] The wide range of observed bioeffects, from subcellular chemical alterations to gross congenital abnormalities and fetal death, is an indication of the effectiveness or universality of hyperthermic conditions for perturbing living systems.[6] The National Council on Radiation Protection and Measurements (NCRP) Scientific Committee on Biological Effects of Ultrasound compiled a comprehensive list of the lowest reported thermal exposures producing teratogenic effects.[7] An examination of this data indicated a lower boundary for observed thermally induced bioeffects. This analysis of thermal effects was included in a recommendation by the NCRP, which states that a diagnostic ultrasound examination need not be withheld as long as exposure conditions do not exceed specified levels of temperature rise and duration.[7] There remain some questions as to the relevance of this analysis of hyperthermia to the application of diagnostic ultrasound.[8] Regardless, it is beneficial to provide feedback to the ultrasound operator regarding the relative potential for a temperature rise in a given acoustic field and under the current conditions associated with a particular examination. This will allow an informed decision regarding the exposure needed to obtain diagnostically relevant information.

Thermal Index

Based on analysis of hyperthermia data, a general statement was proposed by the NCRP concerning the safety of examinations in which no temperature rise greater than 1°C is expected. In an afebrile patient within this limit, it was concluded that there was no basis for expecting an adverse effect. In those cases where the temperature rise might be greater, the sonographer or physician should weigh the benefit versus the potential

risks. To assist in this decision, given the range of different imaging conditions seen in practice, a **thermal index (TI)** was approved as part of the *Standard for Real-Time Display of Thermal and Mechanical Acoustical Output Indices on Diagnostic Ultrasound Equipment*, which gives the operator an indication of the relative potential risk of heating tissue.[9]

In this standard, a series of calculations is made based on the present imaging conditions, and an on-screen display of the thermal index is provided to the operator.

The NCRP Scientific Committee on Biological Effects of Ultrasound introduced the concept of a TI.[7] The goal of the TI is to provide an indication of the relative potential for increasing tissue temperature, but it is not meant to provide the actual temperature rise. Two tissue models were recommended by the NCRP to aid in the calculation of the ultrasound power that could raise the temperature in tissue by 1° C: (1) a homogeneous model in which the attenuation coefficient is uniform throughout the region of interest and (2) a fixed-attenuation model in which the minimum attenuation along the path from transducer to a distant anatomic structure is independent of the distance because of a low-attenuation fluid path (such as amniotic fluid).[7,10,11] Because of concern for the patient, it was recommended that "reasonable worst-case" assumptions be made with respect to estimation of temperature elevations in vivo. The American Institute of Ultrasound in Medicine (AIUM), the National Electrical Manufacturers' Association (NEMA), and the FDA have adopted the TI as an output display standard. They advocate estimating the effect of attenuation in the body by reducing the acoustic power/output of the scanner (W_0) by a derating factor equal to 0.3 dB/cm-MHz for the homogeneous or soft tissue case.[9]

THE THERMAL INDEX

To more easily inform the physician of the operating conditions that could, in some cases, lead to a temperature elevation of 1°C, a thermal index is defined as

$$TI = \frac{W_0}{W_{deg}}$$

where W_{deg} is the ultrasonic source power (in watts) calculated as capable of producing a 1°C temperature elevation under specific conditions. W_0 is the ultrasonic source power (in watts) being used during the current exam.

Reproduced with permission of American Institute of Ultrasound in Medicine.

Thermal Index Models

Three tissue models were considered by the AIUM thermal index working group: a homogeneous tissue or soft tissue model; a tissue model with bone at the focus; and a tissue model with bone at the surface, or transcranial model.[9] The thermal index takes on three different forms for these tissue models.

Homogeneous Tissue Model (Soft Tissue)

The assumption of homogeneity allows for simplification in determining the effects of acoustic propagation and attenuation, as well as the heat transfer characteristics of the tissue. This is one of the most common cases for ultrasound imaging and applies to those circumstances where bone is not present and can generally be used for fetal examinations during the first trimester (low calcification in bone). Considerable effort went into the estimation of potential heating, and many assumptions and compromises had to be made in order to calculate a single quantity that would guide the operator. Calculations of the temperature rise along the axis of a focused beam are shown for a simple spherically curved single element transducer (Fig. 2-5). Note the existence of two thermal peaks. The first is in the near field (between the transducer and the focus), and the second appears close to the focal region.[12,13] The **first thermal peak** occurs in a region with low ultrasound intensity and wide beam width. When the beam width is large, cooling will occur mainly because of perfusion. In the near field, the magnitude of the local intensity will be the chief determinant of the degree of heating. The **second thermal peak** occurs at the location of high intensity (I) and narrow beam width (w) at or near the focal plane. Here the cooling will be dominated by conduction, and the total acoustic power will be the chief determinant of the degree of heating.

Given the thermal "twin peaks" dilemma, the AIUM thermal index working group compromised in creating a thermal index that included contributions from both heating domains.[9] Their rationale was based on the need to minimize the acoustic measurement load for manufacturers of ultrasound systems. In addition, adjustments had to be made to compensate for effects of the large range of potential apertures. The result is a complicated series of calculations and measurements that must be performed, and to the credit of the many manufacturers, there has been considerable effort in implementing a display standard to provide user feedback.

Tissue Model with Bone at the Focus (Fetal Applications)

Applications of ultrasound in which the acoustic beam travels through soft tissue for a fixed distance and impinges on bone occur most often in obstetric scanning during the second and third trimesters. Carson et al. have made sonographic measurements of the maternal abdominal wall thickness in various stages of pregnancy.[11] Based on their results, the NCRP recommends that the attenuation coefficients for the first, second, and third trimesters be 1.0, 0.75, and 0.5 dB/MHz, respectively.[7] These values represent "worst case" estimates. In addition, Siddiqi et al. determined the average tissue attenuation coefficient for transabdominal insonification in a patient population of nonpregnant, healthy volunteers was 2.98 dB/MHz.[14] This value

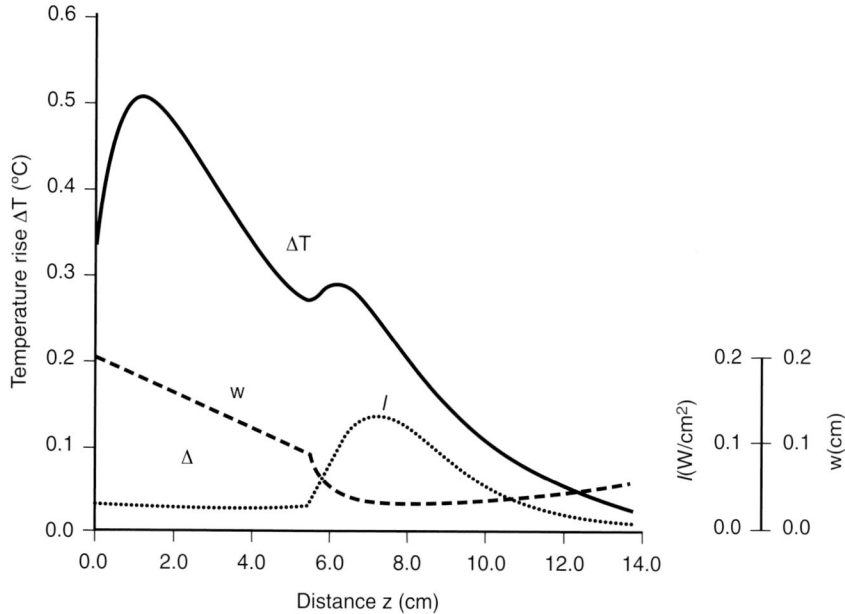

FIGURE 2-5. Thermal peaks of a single spherically focused beam. Plots of beam width (w), intensity (I), and temperature rise (ΔT) along the axis of the beam. With aperture = 2 cm, focal length = 10 cm, and center frequency = 3 MHz. The absorption coefficient and attenuation coefficient are both equal and near that of soft tissue (0.15 nepers/cm). The perfusion time is a quantity that prescribes the heat dissipation due to blood flow and was set at 1000 seconds, and the ultrasonic source power is 0.1 W. (From Scientific Committee on Biological Effects of Ultrasound. Exposure Criteria for Medical Diagnostic Ultrasound. I. Criteria based on thermal mechanisms. Bethesda, Md. National Council on Radiation Protection and Measurements, 1992. Report no. 113.)

represents an average measured value and is obviously very different from the worst case estimates listed earlier. This leads to considerable debate on how such parameters should be included in an index.

In addition, bone is a complex, hard connective tissue with a calcified collagenous intercellular substance. Its absorption coefficient for longitudinal waves is a factor of 10 greater than that for most soft tissues (see Fig. 2-2). Shear waves are also created in bone as sound waves strike bone at oblique incidence. The absorption coefficients for shear waves are even greater than those for longitudinal waves.[15-17]

Based on the data of Carstensen et al. described earlier,[2] the NCRP proposed a thermal model for bone heating. Using this model, the **thermal index for bone (TIB)** is estimated for those conditions in which the focus of the beam is at or near bone. Once again a number of assumptions and compromises had to be made to develop a functional TI for the case of bone exposure.

- For **unscanned mode** transducers (operating in a fixed position) with bone in the focal region, the location of the maximal temperature increase is at the surface of the bone. Therefore, the TIB is calculated at an axial distance that maximizes TIB, a worst case assumption.
- For **scanned modes**, the thermal index for soft tissue is used because the temperature increase at the surface is either greater than or approximately equal to the temperature increase with bone in the focus.

Tissue Model with Bone at the Surface (Transcranial Applications)

For adult cranial applications, the same model is used to estimate the temperature distribution in situ as in the focal bone case. However, because the bone is located at the surface, immediately after the acoustic beam enters the body, attenuation of the acoustic power output is not included.[9] Here, the equivalent beam diameter at the surface is used to calculate the acoustic power.

Thermal Index Estimates for Thermal Effects

There are a number of points to keep in mind when referring to the thermal index as a means of estimating the potential for thermal effects. First, the TI is not synonymous with temperature rise. A TI equal to 1 does not mean the temperature will rise 1°C. An increased potential for thermal effects can be expected as the index increases. Second, a high index does not mean that bioeffects are occurring but only that the potential exists. Several factors may reduce the actual temperature rise

generated, and these may not be taken into account by the thermal models employed for TI calculation. However, the index should be monitored during examinations and minimized when possible. Finally, there is no consideration in the TI for the duration of the scan, so minimizing the overall examination time will reduce the potential for effects.

Summary Statement on Thermal Effects

The AIUM statement concerning thermal effects[18] includes several conclusions that can be summarized as follows:

- Examinations resulting in a 2°C temperature rise or less are not expected to cause bioeffects. (Many ultrasound examinations fall within these parameters.)
- A significant number of factors control heat production by diagnostic ultrasound.
- Ossified bone is a particularly important concern for ultrasound exposure.
- A labeling standard now provides information concerning potential heating in soft tissue and bone.
- Although an FDA limit exists for fetal exposures, predicted temperature rises can exceed 2°C.
- Thermal indices are expected to track temperature increases better than any single ultrasonic field parameter.

EFFECTS OF ACOUSTIC CAVITATION
Potential Sources for Bioeffects

Our knowledge concerning the interaction of ultrasound with gas bodies (which many term "cavitation") has significantly increased recently, although our knowledge base is not as extensive as that for ultrasound thermal effects and other sources of hyperthermia. **Acoustic cavitation inception** is demarcated by a specific threshold value: the minimum acoustic pressure necessary to initiate the growth of a cavity in a fluid during the rarefaction phase of the cycle. A number of parameters affect this threshold, including initial bubble or **cavitation nucleus** size, acoustic pulse characteristics (such as center frequency, pulse repetition frequency, and pulse duration), ambient hydrostatic pressure, and host fluid parameters (such as density, viscosity, compressibility, heat conductivity, and surface tension). **Inertial cavitation** refers to bubbles that undergo large variations from their equilibrium sizes in a few acoustic cycles. Specifically during contraction, the surrounding fluid inertia controls the bubble motion.[19] Large acoustic pressures are necessary to generate inertial cavitation, and the collapse of these cavities is often violent.

The effect of **preexisting cavitation nuclei** may be

THERMAL BIOEFFECTS: CONCLUSIONS REGARDING HEAT

1. Excessive temperature increase can result in toxic effects in mammalian systems. The biological effects observed depend on many factors, such as the exposure duration, the type of tissue exposed, its cellular proliferation rate, and its potential for regeneration. These are important factors when considering fetal and neonatal safety. Temperature increases of several degrees Celsius above the normal core range can occur naturally; there have been no significant biological effects observed resulting from such temperature increases except when they were sustained for extended time periods.
   a. For exposure durations up to 50 hours, there have been no significant biological effects observed due to temperature increases less than or equal to 2°C above normal.
   b. For temperature increases greater than 2°C above normal, there have been no significant biological effects observed due to temperature increases less than or equal to

$$6 - \frac{\log_{10}(t)}{0.6}$$

   where t is the exposure duraton ranging from 1 to 250 min. For example, for temperature increases of 4°C and 6°C, the corresponding limits for the exposure duration t are 16 min. and 1. min., respectively.
   c. In general, adult tissues are more tolerant of temperature increases than fetal and neonatal tissues. Therefore, higher temperatures and/or longer exposure durations would be required for thermal damage.
2. The temperature increase during exposure of tissues to diagnostic ultrasound fields is dependent upon (a) output characteristics of the acoustical source such as frequency, source dimensions, scan rate, power, pulse repetition frequency, pulse duration, transducer self-heating, exposure time, and wave shape, and (b) tissue properties such as attenuation, absorption, speed of sound, acoustic impedance, perfusion, thermal conductivity, thermal diffusivity, anatomical structure, and nonlinear parameter.

3. For similar exposure conditions, the expected temperature increase in bone is significantly greater than in soft tissues. For this reason, conditions where an acoustic beam impinges on ossifying fetal bone deserve special attention due to its close proximity to other developing tissues.
4. Calculations of the maximum temperature increase resulting from ultrasound exposure in vivo should not be assumed to be exact because of the uncertainties and approximations associated with the thermal, acoustic, and structural characteristics of the tissues involved. However, experimental evidence shows that calculations are capable of predicting measured values within a factor of two. Thus, it appears reasonable to use calculations to obtain safety guidelines for clinical exposures where temperature measurements are not feasible. To provide a display of real-time estimates of tissue temperature increases as part of a diagnostic system, simplifying approximations are used to yield values called Thermal Indices.* Under most clinically relevant conditions, the soft-tissue thermal index, TIS, and the bone thermal index, TIB, either overestimate or closely approximate the best available estimate of the maximum temperature increase (ΔT_{max}). For example, if TIS = 2, then $\Delta T_{max} \leq 2°C$.
5. The current FDA regulatory limit for $I_{SPTA.3}$ is 720 mW/cm^2. For this, and lesser intensities, the best available estimate of the maximum temperature increase in the conceptus can exceed 2°C.
6. The TIS and the TIB are useful for estimating the temperature increase in vivo. For this purpose, these thermal indices are superior to any single ultrasonic field quantity such as the derated spatial-peak, temporal-average intensity, $I_{SPTA.3}$. That is, TIS and TIB track changes in the maximum temperature increases. $\Delta Tmax$, thus allowing for implementation of the ALARA principle, whereas $I_{SPTA.3}$ does not. For example,
   a. At a constant value of $I_{SPTA.3}$, TIS increases with increasing frequency and with increasing source diameter.
   b. At a constant value of $I_{SPTA.3}$, TIB increases with increasing focal beam diameter.

*The Thermal Indices are the nondimensional ratios of the estimated temperature increases to 1°C for specific tissue models. Reproduced with permission of American Institute of Ultrasound in Medicine.

one of the principal controlling factors in mechanical effects that result in biologic effects. The body is such an excellent filter that these nucleation sites may only be found in small numbers and only at selected sites. For instance, if water is filtered down to 2 μm, the cavitation threshold doubles.[20] Theoretically, the tensile strength of water that is devoid of cavitation nuclei is about 100 megapascal (MPa).[21] Various models have been suggested to explain bubble formation in animals,[22,23]

and these models have been used extensively in cavitation threshold determination. One model[24] is used in the prediction of SCUBA diving tables and may also have applicability to patients. It remains to be seen how well such models will predict the nucleation of bubbles from diagnostic ultrasound in the body.

A photograph of a 1-MHz therapeutic ultrasound unit generating bubbles in gas-saturated water is shown in Figure 2-6. This particular medium and ultrasound

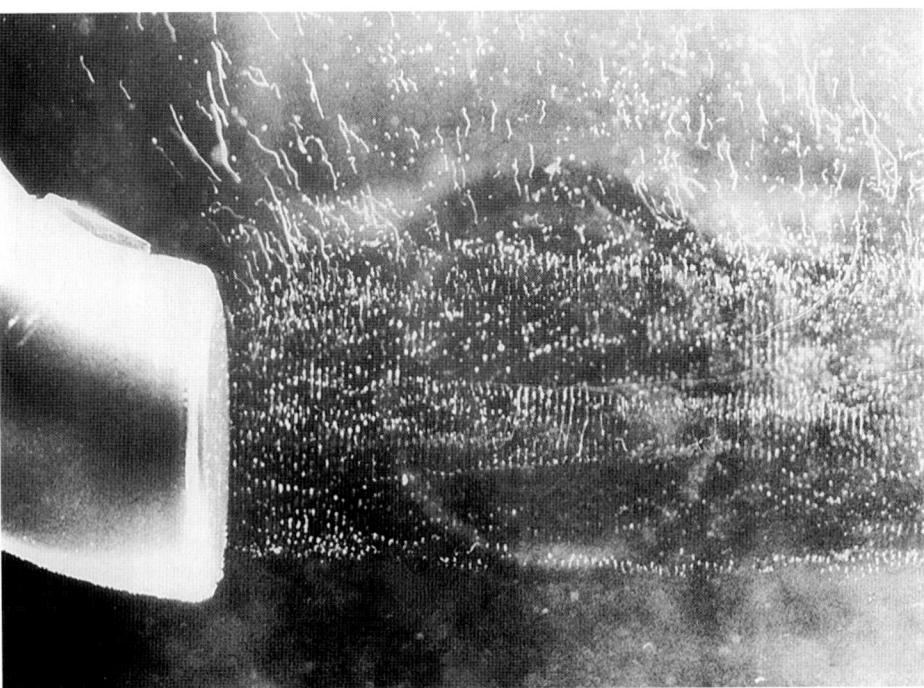

FIGURE 2-6. Acoustic cavitation bubbles. This cavitation activity is being generated in water using a common therapeutic ultrasound device. (Courtesy National Center for Physical Acoustics, University of Mississippi.)

parameters were chosen to optimize the conditions for cavitation. Using continuous wave ultrasound and plenty of preexisting gas pockets in the water set the stage for the production of cavitation. Although these acoustic pulses are longer than those typically used in diagnostic ultrasound, cavitation effects have also been observed with diagnostic pulses in fluids.[25] **Ultrasound contrast agents** composed of stabilized gas bubbles should provide a source of cavitation nuclei as will be discussed later.

Sonochemistry

Free radical generation and detection provides a means to observe cavitation and to gauge its strength and potential for damage. The sonochemistry of free radicals is the result of very high temperatures and pressures within the rapidly collapsing bubble. These conditions can even generate light, or **sonoluminescence**.[26] With the addition of the correct compounds, chemical luminescence can also be used for free radical detection.[27] **Chemiluminescence** can be generated by a therapeutic ultrasound device (Fig. 2-7). The setup is back lighted (in red) to show the bubbles and experimental apparatus. The chemiluminescence emissions are the blue bands seen through the middle of the liquid sample holder. The light emitted is sufficient to be seen by simply adapting one's eyes to darkness. Electron spin resonance can also be used with molecules that trap free radicals to detect cavitation activity capable of free radical production.[28] A number of other chemical detection schemes are presently employed to detect cavitation

from diagnostic devices in vitro.

Evidence of Cavitation from Lithotripters

It is possible to generate bubbles in vivo using short pulses with high amplitudes of an extracorporeal shockwave lithotripter (ESWL). The peak positive pressure for lithotripsy pulses can be as much as 50 MPa and the negative pressure around 20 MPa. **Finite amplitude distortion** causes high frequencies to appear in high-amplitude ultrasound fields. Although ESWL pulses have significant energy at high frequencies due to finite amplitude distortion, a large portion of the energy is actually in the 100-kHz range, much lower than frequencies in diagnostic scanners. The lower frequency makes cavitation more likely. As an example of the effect, Aymé and Carstensen have shown that the higher frequency components in nonlinearly distorted pulses contribute little to the killing of *Drosophila* larvae.[29] Interestingly enough, there is now evidence to indicate that collapsing bubbles may play a role in stone disruption.[30-32] A bubble collapsing near a surface may form a liquid jet through its center, which strikes the surface (Fig. 2-8). If a sheet of aluminum foil is placed at the focus of a lithotripter, small pinholes will be generated.[32] The impact is even sufficient to pit solid brass and aluminum plates. Clearly, lithotripsy and diagnostic ultrasound differ in the acoustic power generated and are not at all comparable in the bioeffects produced. Yet some diagnostic devices produce peak rarefactional pressures greater than 3 MPa, which is in the lower range of lithotripter outputs.[34-36] Interestingly,

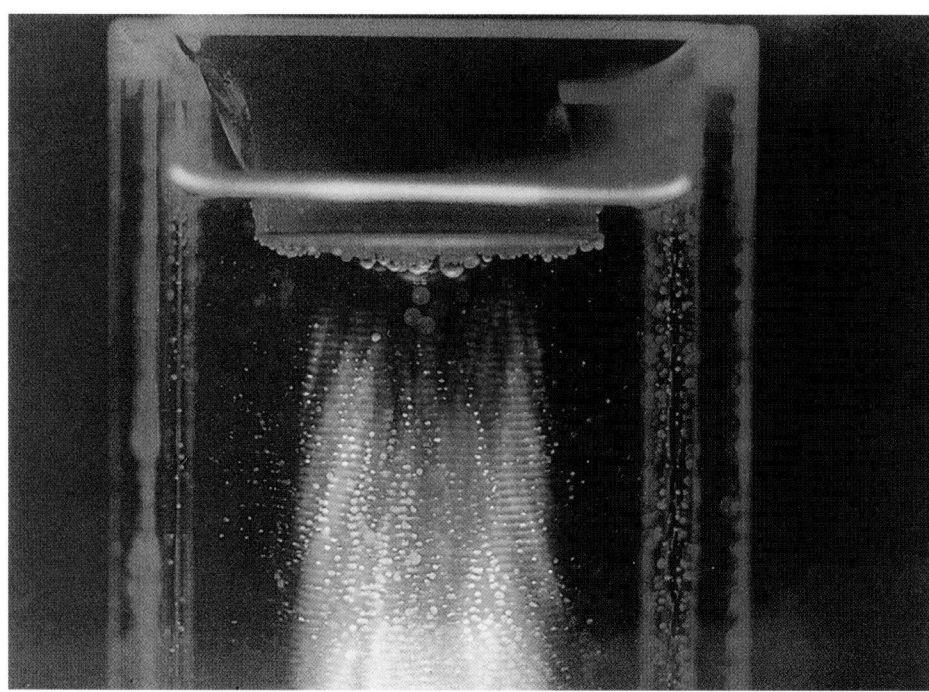

FIGURE 2-7. Chemical reaction induced by cavitation producing visible light. The reaction is the result of free radical production. (Courtesy National Center for Physical Acoustics, University of Mississippi.)

lung damage and surface petechiae have been noted as side effects of ESWL in clinical cases.[37] Inertial cavitation was suspected as the cause of this damage and has prompted several researchers to study the effects of diagnostic ultrasound exposure on the lung parenchyma.

Bioeffects in Lung

Lung tissue has proved to be an interesting location to examine for bioeffects of diagnostic ultrasound. The presence of air in the alveolar spaces constitutes a significant source of gas bodies. Child et al. measured threshold pressures for hemorrhage in mouse lung

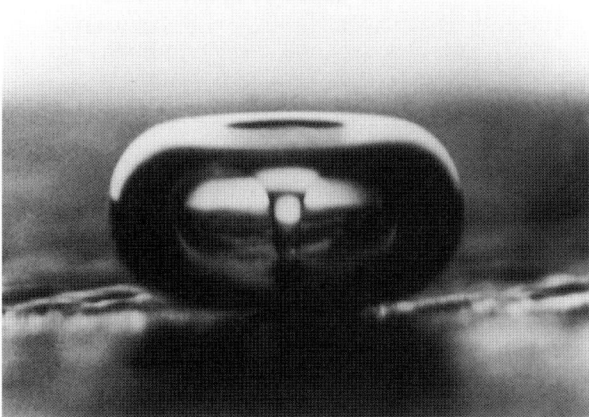

FIGURE 2-8. Collapsing bubble near a boundary. When cavitation is produced near boundaries, a liquid jet may form through the center of a bubble and strike the boundary surface. (Courtesy of Lawrence A. Crum.)

exposed to 1- to 4-MHz short-pulse diagnostic ultrasound (i.e., 10 μsec and 1 μsec pulse durations).[38] The threshold of damage in murine lung at these frequencies was established to be 1.4 MPa. Pathologic features of this damage included extravasation of blood cells into the alveolar spaces.[39] It was hypothesized that cavitation, originating from gas-filled alveoli, was responsible for the damage. Their data are the first to provide direct evidence that clinically relevant, pulsed ultrasound exposures produce deleterious effects in mammalian tissue in the absence of significant heating. Hemorrhagic foci induced by 4-MHz pulsed Doppler have also been reported in the monkey.[40] Damage in the monkey lung was of a significantly lesser degree than that in the mouse.

In these studies, it was impossible to show categorically that these effects were induced by bubbles because the cavitation-induced bubbles were themselves not observed. Kramer et al. assessed cardiopulmonary function in rats exposed to pulsed ultrasound well above the acoustic output threshold of damage (mechanical index [MI] = 9.7).[41] Measurements of cardiopulmonary function included arterial blood pressure, heart rate, respiratory rate, and arterial blood gases (PCO_2 and PO_2). If only one side of the rat lung was exposed, the cardiopulmonary measurements did not change significantly between baseline and post-exposure values because of the functional respiratory reserve in the unexposed lobes. However, when both sides of the lung had significant ultrasound-induced lesions, the rats were unable to maintain systemic arterial pressure or resting levels of arterial PO_2. Further studies are required to determine the relevance of these findings to humans.

The gross organization and cellular composition of the lung are similar in mammals, although there are significant physiologic and anatomic differences related to organization of the distal airways, alveolar morphology, and blood supply.[42] Morphologic studies demonstrate that capillaries within the alveolar septa of most mammals are arranged as a single layer separated from the air spaces by a thin cellular barrier (100 nm). Because of this anatomic configuration, Tarantal and Canfield[40] hypothesized that these regions are more susceptible to conditions where bubble oscillation and rupture may occur. They also noted that an important factor specific to the lung may be the monolayer of surfactant within the alveoli. Surfactant, the alveolar lining fluid, is responsible for modifying surface tension in order to promote lung expansion and prevent lung collapse. It is possible that, during exposure to ultrasound, small microbubbles are created within edges of the surfactant-rich alveolus. These microbubbles may oscillate and collapse, causing localized disruption of the epithelial/endothelial barrier and subsequent extravasation of red blood cells into the alveolar space. Holland and Apfel have previously shown a direct correlation between a reduction in the cavitation threshold and reduced host fluid surface tension.[43,44]

Although a proven phenomenon in vitro,[45] the occurrence of cavitation in vivo due to diagnostic ultrasound has been difficult to document in mammalian systems primarily because of the transient nature of its occurrence (i.e., μsec) and the localized character of the resultant effects (i.e., 10 microns). To explore the hypothesis of cavitation-based bioeffects from diagnostic ultrasound, research has been performed on the thresholds of damage in rat lungs exposed to 4-MHz pulsed Doppler and color Doppler ultrasound.[46] A 30-MHz active detection scheme developed by Roy et al.[47] was used to provide the first direct evidence of cavitation from diagnostic ultrasound pulses. Damage was observed with histologic features consistent with those seen in mice and monkeys because of diagnostic ultrasound exposures. However, in this limited study, bubble activity was not correlated with histologic damage.

Ultrasound Contrast Agents

The apparent absence of cavitation in many locations in the body can be due to the lack of available cavitation nuclei. Based on evidence in the lung and intestine in mammalian models described above, it is clear that in the presence of gas bodies, there is a reduction in the requisite acoustic field for producing bioeffects. Because many ultrasound contrast agents are composed of stabilized gas bubbles, they could provide readily available nuclei for potential cavitation activity. This makes the investigation of bioeffects in the presence of ultrasound contrast agents an important area of research. A review of the literature on ultrasound bioeffects associated with contrast agents is available.[48] In addition, two publications[49,50] indicated that ultrasound in the presence of contrast agents produced small vascular petechiae in mammalian systems.

As a result, the AIUM approved a safety statement related to ultrasound contrast agents. While this bioeffect may occur, there remains the issue of whether it constitutes a significant physiologic risk, which is still being researched. The safety statement is designed to make sonographers and physicians aware of the potential for bioeffects in the presence of gas contrast agents and allow them to make an informed decision based on a risk/benefit assessment.

Some research has also pointed to the production of preventricular contraction (PVC) during cardiac scanning in the presence of ultrasound contrast agents. At least one study in humans[51] indicated an increase in PVCs only when ultrasound imaging was performed with a contrast agent and not in the presence of either ultrasound imaging alone or during the injection of the agent without imaging. Other researchers are investigating this phenomenon to determine the mechanism. The importance of this bioeffect is also being debated

---

STATEMENT ON BIOEFFECTS OF DIAGNOSTIC ULTRASOUND WITH GAS BODY CONTRAST AGENTS. APPROVED MARCH, 2002

Induction of petechiae and extravasation from capillaries in mammalian tissue in vivo has been reported and independently confirmed for diagnostic ultrasound exposure with Mechanical Index above about 0.4 and gas-body contrast agent present in the circulation.

The clinical significance of these findings is presently uncertain. Only apparently minor side effects have been reported in clinical testing and use of ultrasound contrast agents. However, on the basis of these reports and a large body of data from laboratory studies in vitro and in vivo, it should be noted that the potential for any diagnostic ultrasound-induced adverse effects will depend not only on the composition, dosage, and administration of the agent, but also on operator-controlled settings of ultrasound machines, such as timing, mode, frequency, and power, as well as the anatomy scanned. Therefore, physicians and sonographers should be cognizant of the possible enhancement of nonthermal bioeffects during contrast-enhanced diagnostic ultrasound and factor this potential into risk-benefit considerations.

Reprinted with permission, AIUM.

because there is a naturally occurring rate of PVCs and a small increase may not be considered significant, particularly if there is benefit to the patient in using the agent. Additional consideration might be given to patients with specific conditions in whom additional PVCs should be avoided.

The consequences of the bioeffects reported thus far require more study. While there is the potential for a bioeffect, its scale and influence on human physiology are not clear and yet the efficacy of contrast agents for specific indications has been demonstrated. In addition, clinical trials involving many individuals receiving ultrasound and contrast agents have reported few effects. Research into the mechanism of interaction and the consequences of these effects is continuing.

Mechanical Index

Calculations for cavitation prediction have yielded a rough trade-off between peak rarefactional pressure and frequency.[52] This predicted trade-off assumes short-pulse (a few acoustic cycles) and low-duty cycle ultrasound (<1%). This relatively simple result can be used to gauge the potential for the onset of cavitation from diagnostic ultrasound. The **mechanical index**, or **MI** (see box), was adopted by the FDA, AIUM, and NEMA as a real-time output display to estimate the potential for bubble formation in vivo, in analogy to the thermal

index. As indicated before, the collapse temperature for inertial cavitation is very high. For this index, a collapse temperature of 5000 K was chosen based on the potential for free radical generation, and the frequency dependence of the pressure required to generate this thermal threshold takes a relatively simple form. The MI is a kind of "mechanical energy index" because the square of the MI is roughly proportional to mechanical work that can be performed on a bubble in the acoustic rarefaction phase.

Overview of Observed Bioeffects

A summary of results from several investigators (Fig. 2-9) indicated the MI above which bioeffects associated with cavitation have been observed in animals and insects.[18] The dotted lines are calculations for several values of the mechanical index where all of the effects appear to occur at or above an MI value of 0.3. However, it should be noted that in many of these cases stable pockets of gas (gas bodies) are known to exist in the exposed tissues. It is further suggested that other areas in the body containing gas bodies might also be particularly susceptible to ultrasound damage. These might include the intestinal lining, for example.[53] Experimentation continues, and it remains to be seen if such damage occurs in human tissue.

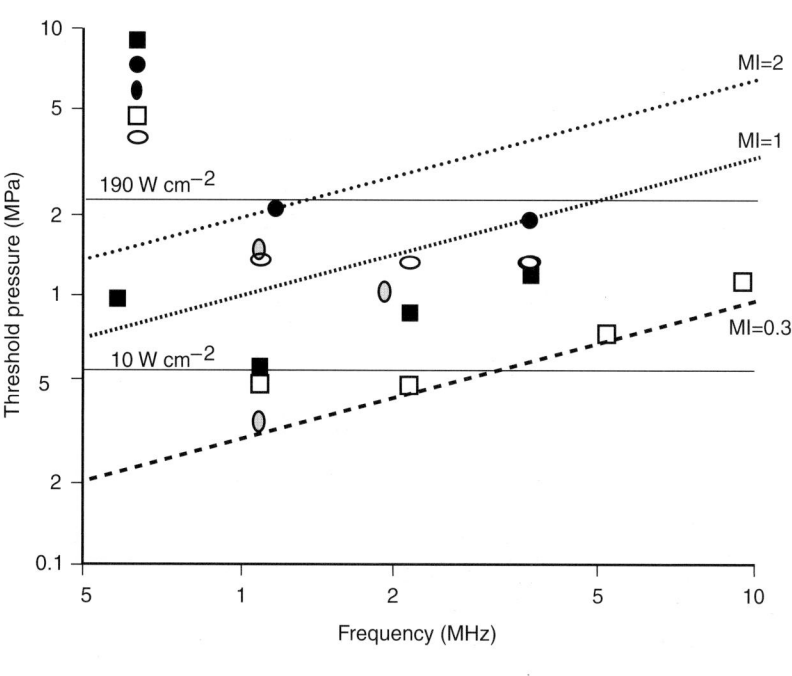

FIGURE 2-9. Threshold for bioeffects from low temporal average intensity, pulsed ultrasound. Data shown are the threshold for effects measured in peak rarefactional pressures ([p] in Fig. 2-1) as a function of ultrasound frequency used in the exposure. Pulse duration is shown in parentheses in the legend. Also shown for reference purposes are the values for the mechanical index and the local spatial peak, pulse average intensity I_{SPPA}. (From American Institute of Ultrasound in Medicine: Bioeffects and Safety of Diagnostic Ultrasound. Rockville, Md, 1993.)

■ Adult mouse lung (10 μs)
● Adult mouse lung (1μs)
◖ Neonatal mouse lung (10 μs)
□ Fruit fry larvae (10 μs)
○ Elodea leaves (5 μs)

Additional Comments on the Mechanical Index

Inherent in the formulation of the MI are the conditions only for the onset of inertial cavitation. The degree to which the threshold is exceeded, however, relates to the degree of bubble activity that may occur, and the amount of bubble activity may correlate with the probability of an undesirable bioeffect. Note that given our present knowledge, exceeding the cavitation threshold does *not* mean there will be a bioeffect. Below an MI of ~0.4, the physical conditions do not favor bubble growth, even in the presence of a broad bubble nuclei distribution in the body, which is in reasonable agreement with the results of Figure 2-9. Whereas the thermal index is a *time-averaged* measure of the interaction of ultrasound with tissue, the MI is a *peak* measure of this interaction. Thus, there is a desirable parallel between these two measures, one thermal and one mechanical, for informing the user of the extent to which the diagnostic tool can produce undesirable changes in the body.

Summary Statement on Gas Bodies Bioeffects

The AIUM statement concerning bioeffects in locations where gas bodies exist[18] (see box) includes several conclusions that can be summarized as follows:

- Current ultrasound systems can produce cavitation in vitro and in vivo and can cause blood extravasation in animal tissues.
- A mechanical index can gauge the likelihood for cavitation and apparently works better than other field parameters in predicting cavitation.
- Several interesting results have been observed concerning animal models for lung damage, which indicate a very low threshold for damage, but the implications for human exposure are not yet determined.
- In the absence of gas bodies, the threshold for damage is much higher. (This last point is significant because ultrasound examinations may be performed predominantly in tissues with no identifiable gas bodies.)

OUTPUT DISPLAY STANDARD

Several groups, including the FDA, AIUM, and NEMA, have developed the *Standard for Real-Time Display of Thermal and Mechanical Acoustical Output Indices on Diagnostic Ultrasound Equipment*, which introduces a method to provide the user with information concerning the thermal and mechanical indices. Real-time display of the MI and TI will allow a more informed decision on the potential for bioeffects during examinations. The standard requires dynamic updates of the indices as instrument output is modified and provides the opportunity for the operator to learn how controls will affect these indices. Figure 2-10 shows an example of an ultrasound system displaying the mechanical index. There are a few important things to remember about this display standard:

- It should be clearly visible on the screen and should begin to appear when the instrument exceeds an index value of 0.4. An exception is

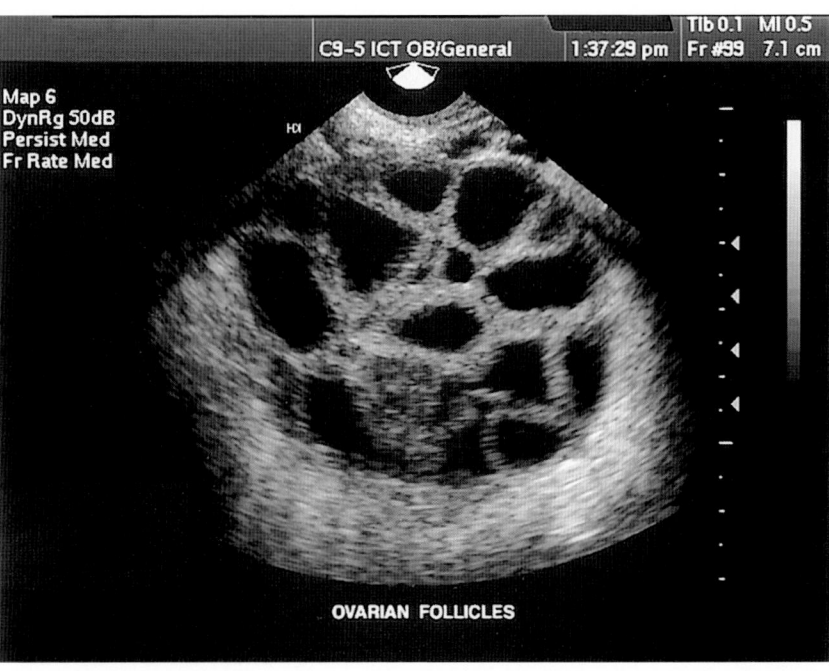

FIGURE 2-10. Display of bioeffects indices. Typical appearance of an ultrasound scanner display showing the thermal index for bone (TIB) and mechanical index (MI) (*right upper corner*) for an endocavitary transducer.

made for those instruments incapable of exceeding index values of 1. Those instruments are not required to display the bioeffects indices.

- Sometimes only one index will be displayed at a time. The choice is often based on whether a given output condition is more likely to produce an effect by either mechanism.
- The standard also requires that appropriate default output settings be in effect at power-up, new patient entry, or when changing to a fetal examination. After that time, the operator can adjust the instrument output as necessary to acquire clinically useful information while attempting to minimize the index values.
- As indicated previously, the bioeffects indices do not include any factors associated with the time taken to perform the scan. Efficient scanning is still an important component in limiting potential bioeffects.

The AIUM document entitled *Medical Ultrasound Safety*[54] suggests that the operator ask four questions to effectively use the output display.

1. Which index should be used for the examination being performed?
2. Are there factors present that might cause the reading to be too high or too low?
3. Can the index value be reduced further even when it is already low?
4. How can the ultrasound exposure be minimized without compromising the diagnostic quality of the examination?

Sonographers and physicians are being presented with real-time data on acoustic output of diagnostic scanners and are being asked not only to understand the manner in which ultrasound propagates through and interacts with tissue, but also to gauge the potential for adverse bioeffects. The output display is a tool that can be used to guide an ultrasound examination and control for potential adverse effects. The thermal and mechanical indices provide the user with more information and more responsibility in limiting outputs.

GENERAL AIUM SAFETY STATEMENTS

It is important to consider some official positions concerning the status of bioeffects resulting from ultrasound. The most important item to note is the high level of confidence in the safety of ultrasound in official statements. For example, in 1993, the AIUM reiterated its earlier statement concerning the clinical use of diagnostic ultrasound by stating that no known bioeffects have been confirmed for the use of *present diagnostic equipment* and although it remains a possibility, the patient benefits for prudent use outweigh the risks, if any, that exist. In a similar fashion, the AIUM commented on the use of diagnostic ultrasound in research by recommending that in the case of exposure for other than direct medical benefit, the person be informed concerning the exposure conditions and how these relate to normal exposures. For the most part, examinations even for research purposes are comparable to normal diagnostic examinations and pose no additional risk. In fact, many research examinations can be performed in conjunction with routine examinations.

The effects based on in vivo animal models can be summarized by the AIUM Safety Statement conclusion

---

AIUM SAFETY STATEMENTS
American Institute of Ultrasound in Medicine Official Statement on Clinical Safety. October, 1982; Revised and approved March, 1997

Diagnostic ultrasound has been in use since the late 1950s. Given its known benefits and recognized efficacy for medical diagnosis, including use during human pregnancy, the American Institute of Ultrasound in Medicine herein addresses the clinical safety of such use:

There are no confirmed biological effects on patients or instrument operators caused by exposures from present diagnostic ultrasound instruments. Although the possibility exists that such biological effects may be identified in the future, current data indicate that the benefits to patients of the prudent use of diagnostic ultrasound outweigh the risks, if any, that may be present.

American Institute of Ultrasound in Medicine Official Statement on Safety in Training and Research. Approved March, 1983; Revised and Approved March, 1997

Diagnostic ultrasound has been in use since the late 1950s. There are no confirmed adverse biological effects on patients resulting from this usage. Although no hazard has been identified that would preclude the prudent and conservative use of diagnostic ultrasound in education and research, experience from normal diagnostic practice may or may not be relevant to extended exposure times and altered exposure conditions. It is therefore considered appropriate to make the following recommendation:

In those special situations in which examinations are to be carried out for purposes other than direct medical benefit to the individual being examined, the subject should be informed of the anticipated exposure conditions, and of how these compare with conditions for normal diagnostic practice.

Reprinted with permission, AIUM.

shown in the box.[18] No independently confirmed experimental evidence indicates damage in animal models below certain prescribed levels (TI < 2 and MI < 0.3). The level for the MI is strict because tissues containing gas bodies exhibit damage at much lower levels than tissues devoid of gas bodies. Biologic effects have not been detected, even at an MI of 4 in the absence of gas bodies.

EPIDEMIOLOGY

With all of the potential causes for bioeffects, one must now examine the epidemiologic evidence that has been used, in part, to justify the apparent safety of ultrasound. Many studies of an epidemiologic nature have been conducted over the last 3 decades. Ziskin and Petitti, who reviewed these studies in 1988, concluded, "epidemiologic studies and surveys in widespread clinical usage over 25 years have yielded no evidence of any adverse effect from diagnostic ultrasound."[56]

Epidemiologic studies are difficult to conduct, and data analysis and interpretation of results are, perhaps, even more difficult. Several epidemiologic studies of fetal exposure to ultrasound have claimed to detect certain bioeffects and have also been a subject of criticism. Only one indication of an unspecified effect was reported in a general survey involving an estimated 1.2 million examinations in Canada.[57] However, this is an extremely low rate of incidence of an unspecified effect. In addition, an earlier study that included 121,000 fetal examinations reported no adverse effect.[58] Moore et al. reported an increased incidence of low birth weight.[59] However, Stark et al. examined the same data using a different statistical treatment and found no significant increase.[60] Abnormal grasp and tonic neck reflexes were noted by Scheidt et al.[61]; however, these results are difficult to interpret given the statistical treatment of the data. Increased incidence of dyslexia was detected in a study by Stark et al.,[60] yet the same children exhibited below average birth weights. As with these studies, there are a number of general problems that plague the epidemiologic studies. These include the lack of clearly stated exposure conditions and gestational age, problems in statistical sampling, which applies to both positive and negative results, and use of less than current scanning systems particularly with regard to use of fetal Doppler.

Ziskin and Petitti also provided a summary and discussion of the factors involved in the evaluation of epidemiologic evidence.[56] It is important to recognize that epidemiologic evidence can be used to identify an association between exposures and biologic effects, but this does not prove that the exposure caused that bioeffect. The strength of the association is established by the statistical significance of the relationship. Hill,[62]

Salvesen,[63] and Ziskin[64] have developed the following seven criteria for judging **causality**:

- Strength of the association
- Consistency in reproducibility and with previous related research
- Specificity to a particular bioeffect or exposure site
- Classical time relationship of cause followed by effect
- Existence of a dose response
- Plausibility of the effect
- Supporting evidence from laboratory studies

When considering these factors, there seems not to be a clear causal relationship between an adverse biologic response and ultrasound exposure of a diagnostic nature.

Recent experiments have raised the question of potential associations. The first is the study by Newnham et al., which reported the observation of higher intrauterine growth restriction during a study designed to determine the efficacy of ultrasound in reducing the number of neonatal days and prematurity rate.[65] Therefore, the study was not designed to detect an adverse bioeffect, but a statistically significant one was observed as a result of subsequent data analysis. Several other deficiencies in methodology are evident in the selection and exposure of their experimental groups, but in general, some association might be inferred from the results of this well-conducted, randomized clinical trial. In a case-control study, Campbell et al. reported a statistically significant higher rate of delayed speech in those children who were insonified *in utero*.[66] Case control studies do not provide as strong evidence of association as prospective studies, and measures of delayed speech are difficult. Follow-up prospective studies will be necessary to confirm these findings.

In 1995, the AIUM revised and approved a statement regarding the epidemiology of diagnostic ultrasound safety.[55] This statement differs only slightly from that approved in 1987 in which the statement was made that no confirmed effects associated with ultrasound exposure existed at that time. The distinction being made is that, although some effects may have been detected now, one cannot justify a conclusion of a causal relationship based on this evidence.

CONTROLLING ULTRASOUND OUTPUT: KNOBOLOGY

Perhaps the most important aspect of a discussion of potential bioeffects is what the physician or sonographer can do to minimize these effects. It is essential that operators understand the risks involved in the process, but without some ability to control the output of the ultrasound system, this knowledge has limited use. Some

OPTIMUM ULTRASOUND OUTPUT: LOWEST POWER OUTPUT THAT CREATES GOOD IMAGES

DIRECT CONTROLS

Application type: fetal, cardiac, etc.
Output intensity: power, output, transmit
Focusing: allows increasing output intensity only at the focal zone

INDIRECT CONTROLS

Ultrasound mode
  Unscanned modes (deposits heat in one area)
    Continuous wave Doppler
    Spectral or pulsed Doppler
    M-mode
  Scanned modes
    B-mode or gray-scale
    Color Doppler
    Power Doppler
Pulse repetition frequency
  Increases bursts of energy per time
Pulse length
  e.g., increasing sample volume in Doppler studies
Appropriate transducer
  High frequency will require more output for depth
  Lower frequency → less output needed at depth
Gain controls
  Time gain compensation (TGC) can increase image without more output
  Receiver gain → increases image amplitude without more output

specific methods can be used to limit ultrasound exposure while maintaining diagnostically relevant images.

Controls for the ultrasound system can be divided into two groups for the purposes of this discussion. These are **direct controls** and **indirect controls**. The direct controls are the application types and output intensity. **Application types** are those broad system controls that allow convenient selection of a particular examination type. These often come in the form of icons that are selected by the user. These default settings help to minimize the time required to optimize the imaging parameters for the myriad applications for diagnostic ultrasound. These settings should be used only as indicated; for example, do not use the cardiac settings for a fetal examination. **Output intensity** (which may be called "power," "output," or "transmit") controls the overall ultrasonic power emitted by the transducer. This control will generally affect the intensity at all points in the image to varying degrees, depending on the focusing. The lowest output intensity that produces a good image should be used to minimize the exposure intensity. **Focusing** of the system is controlled by the operator and

can be used to improve image quality in order to limit required acoustic intensity. Focusing at the correct depth can improve the image without requiring increased intensity.

The **indirect controls** are numerous but greatly affect the ultrasound exposure by dictating how the ultrasonic energy is distributed temporally and spatially. By choosing the **mode of ultrasound** used (e.g., B-mode, pulsed Doppler, color Doppler), the operator controls whether the beam is scanned. Unscanned modes deposit energy along a single path and increase the potential for heating.[67] The **pulse repetition frequency (PRF)** indicates how often the transducer is excited. Increasing the number of ultrasound bursts per second will increase the time average intensity. Control of the PRF is usually carried out by changing the maximal image depth in B-mode, or the velocity range in Doppler modes. **Burst length** (or "pulse length" or "pulse duration") controls the duration of on-time for each ultrasonic burst transmitted. Increasing the burst length while maintaining the same PRF will increase the time average intensity. The control of burst length may not be obvious. For example, in pulsed Doppler, increasing the Doppler sample volume length will increase the burst length.

The selection of the **appropriate transducer** will also limit the need for high acoustic power. Although higher frequencies provide better spatial resolution, the attenuation of tissue increases with increasing ultrasound frequency, so penetration may be lost. Perhaps most important are the **receiver gain controls**. The receiver gain control does not affect the amplitude of the acoustic output in any way. Therefore, before turning up the acoustic output intensity, try increasing receiver gain first. It should be noted that some system controls actually interact with the acoustic output intensity without direct control. Check to see whether the manufacturer provides separate controls for receiver gain, **time gain compensation (TGC),** and acoustic output intensity. The TGC can improve image quality without increasing the output.

There is really no substitute for a well-instructed operator. The indices and requirement of output display standards will help only those willing to use and understand them. Real-time display of the mechanical and thermal indices on diagnostic scanners will help clinicians evaluate and minimize potential risks in the use of such instrumentation. Physicians and sonographers are encouraged to learn more about the roles they can play in minimizing the potential effects.

ULTRASOUND ENTERTAINMENT VIDEOS

Of concern is the growing use of diagnostic ultrasound for the nonmedical scanning of pregnant women to provide a fetal "keepsake" video. Unfortunately, entertainment ultrasound is promoted most vigorously in the second and third trimesters, when bone calcification can increase thermal effects. Also, women with the economic means to schedule multiple ultrasound imaging sessions may be exposing both themselves and their fetuses to an even greater risk if ultrasound bioeffects are shown to be additive or even just by increasing the chances for a bioeffect. If there is no clinical benefit in such entertainment ultrasound, the ratio of benefit to risk is clearly zero. In addition, because oftentimes the ultrasound equipment used is identical to that used diagnostically by clinicians, the consumer may not even realize that no medical information is being generated, interpreted, or communicated to her obstetrician. The mother is asked to sign release forms, which state that there is no medical benefit. The FDA has issued a statement of concern about the nonmedical use of diagnostic ultrasound equipment as an unapproved use of a medical device.

References

Thermal Effects

1. Hynynen K: Ultrasound therapy. In Goldman LE, Fowlkes JB (eds): Medical CT and Ultrasound: Current Technology and Applications. Madison, WI, Advanced Medical Publishing, 1995, pp 249-265.
2. Carstensen EL, Child SZ, Norton S, et al: Ultrasonic heating of the skull. J Acoust Soc Am 1990;87:1310-1317.
3. Nyborg WL: Solutions of the bio-heat transfer equation. Phys Med Biol 1988;33(7):785-792.
4. Drewniak JL, Carnes KI, Dunn F: In vitro ultrasonic heating of fetal bone. J Acoust Soc Am 1989;86:1254-1258.
5. Edwards MJ: Hyperthermia as a teratogen: A review of experimental studies and their clinical significance. Teratogenesis Carcinog Mutagen 1986;6:563-582.
6. Miller MW, Ziskin MC: Biological consequences of hyperthermia. Ultrasound Med Biol 1989;15:707-722.
7. Scientific Committee on Biological Effects of Ultrasound. Exposure Criteria for Medical Diagnostic Ultrasound. I. Criteria based on thermal mechanisms. Bethesda, Md. National Council on Radiation Protection and Measurements, 1992. Report no. 113.
8. Miller MW, Nyborg WL, Dewey WC, et al: Hyperthermic teratogenicity, thermal dose and diagnostic ultrasound during pregnancy: Implications of new standards on tissue heating. Int J Hyperthermia 2002;18:361-384.
9. American Institute of Ultrasound in Medicine and National Electrical Manufacturers' Association. Standard for real-time display of thermal and mechanical acoustical output indices on diagnostic ultrasound equipment. Rockville, Md, 1992.
10. Carson PL: Medical ultrasound fields and exposure measurements. In Nonionizing Electromagnetic Radiations and Ultrasound. Bethesda, Md: National Council on Radiation Protection and Measurements, 1988, pp 287-307. NCRP Proceedings no. 8.
11. Carson PL, Rubin JM, Chiang EH: Fetal depth and ultrasound path lengths through overlying tissues. Ultrasound Med Biol 1989;15:629-663.
12. Thomenius KE: Scientific rationale for the TIS index model. Presented at the National Electrical Manufacturers' Association Output Display Standard Seminar, Rockville, Md, 1993.
13. Thomenius KE: Estimation of the potential for bioeffects. In Ziskin MC, Lewin PA (eds): Ultrasonic Exposimetry. Ann Arbor, Mich, CRC Press, 1993; pp 371–408.
14. Siddiqi T, O'Brien WD, Meyer RA, et al: In situ exposimetry: The ovarian ultrasound examination. Ultrasound Med Biol 1991;17:257-263.
15. Chan AK, Sigelman RA, Guy AW, et al: Calculation by the method of finite differences of the temperature distribution in layered tissues. IEEE Trans Biomed Eng 1973;20:86-90.
16. Chan AK, Sigelman RA, Guy AW: Calculations of therapeutic heat generated by ultrasound in fat-muscle-bone layers. IEEE Trans Biomed Eng 1974;21:280-284.
17. Frizzell LA: Ultrasonic Heating of Tissues. [Dissertation]. Rochester, NY, University of Rochester, 1975.
18. American Institute of Ultrasound in Medicine: Bioeffects and Safety of Diagnostic Ultrasound. Rockville, Md, 1993.

Effects of Acoustic Cavitation

19. Flynn HG: Cavitation dynamics. I. A mathematical formulation. J Acoust Soc Am 1975;57:1379-1396.
20. Roy RA, Atchley AA, Crum LA, et al: A precise technique for measurement of acoustic cavitation thresholds and some preliminary results. J Acoust Soc Am 1985;78(5):1799-1805.
21. Kwak H-Y, Panton RL: Tensile strength of simple liquids predicted by a model of molecular interactions. J Phys D 1985;18:647.
22. Harvey EN, Barnes DK, McElroy WD, et al: Bubble formation in animals. I. Physical factors. J Cell Compar Phys 1944;24:1-22.
23. Harvey EN, Barnes DK, McElroy WD, et al: Bubble formation in animals. II. Gas nuclei and their distribution in blood and tissues. J Cell Compar Phys 1944;24:23-34.
24. Yount DE: Skins of varying permeability: A stabilization mechanism for gas cavitation nuclei. J Acoust Soc Am 1978;65:1429-1439.
25. Holland CK, Roy RA, Apfel RE, et al: In vitro detection of cavitation induced by a diagnostic ultrasound system. IEEE Trans UFFC 1992;39:95-101.
26. Walton AJ, Reynolds GT: Sonoluminescence. Adv Physics 1984;33:595-660.

27. Crum LA, Fowlkes JB: Acoustic cavitation generated by microsecond pulses of ultrasound. Nature 1986;319(6048):52-54.

28. Carmichael AJ, Mossoba MM, Riesz P, et al: Free radical production in aqueous solutions exposed to simulated ultrasonic diagnostic conditions. IEEE Trans UFFC 33:148-155.

29. Aymé E, Carstensen EL: Occurrence of transient cavitation in pulsed sawtooth ultrasonic fields. J Acoust Soc Am 1988;84:1598-1605.

30. Coleman AJ, Saunders JE, Crum LA, et al: Acoustic cavitation generated by an extracorporeal shockwave lithotripter. Ultrasound Med Biol 1987;15:213-227.

31. Delius M, Brendel W, Heine G: A mechanism of gallstone destruction by extracorporeal shock wave. Naturwissenschaften 1988;75:200-201.

32. Williams AR, Delius M, Miller DL, et al: Investigation of cavitation in flowing media by lithotripter shock waves both in vitro and in vivo. Ultrasound Med Biol 1989; 15:53-60.

33. Coleman AJ, Saunders JE, Crum LA, et al: Acoustic cavitation generated by an extracorporeal shockwave lithotripter. Ultrasound Med Biol 1987;13(2):69-76.

34. Duck FA, Starritt HC, Aindow JD, et al: The output of pulse-echo ultrasound equipment: A survey of powers, pressures and intensities. Br J Rad 1985;58:989-1001.

35. Duck FA, Starritt HC, Anderson SP: A survey of the acoustic output of ultrasonic Doppler equipment. Clin Phys Physiol Meas 1987;8:39-49.

36. Patton CA, Harris GR, Phillips RA: Output levels and bioeffects indices from diagnostic ultrasound exposure data reported to the FDA. IEEE Trans Ultrason Ferroelec Freq Contr 1994;41:353-359.

37. Chaussy C, Schmiedt E, Jocham D, et al: Extracorporeal Shock Wave Lithotripsy. Basel, Karger, 1986.

38. Child SZ, Hartman CL, Schery LA, et al: Lung damage from exposure to pulse ultrasound. Ultrasound Med Biol 1990;16:817-825.

39. Penney DP, Schenk EA, Maltby K, et al: Morphological effects of pulsed ultrasound in the lung. Ultrasound Med Biol 1993;19:127-135.

40. Tarantal AF, Canfield DR: Ultrasound-induced lung hemorrhage in the monkey. Ultrasound Med Biol 1994;20:65-72.

41. Kramer JM, Waldrop TG, Frizzell LA, et al: Cardio-pulmonary function in rats with lung hemorrhage induced by pulsed ultrasound exposure. J Ultrasound Med 2001;20:1197-1206.

42. Tyler WS, Julian WD: Gross and subgross anatomy of lungs, pleura, connective tissue septa, distal airways, and structural units. In Parent RA (ed): Treatise on Pulmonary Toxicology. Vol. I. Comparative Biology of the Normal Lung. Boca Raton, Fla, CRC Press, 1992, pp 35-58.

43. Holland CK, Apfel RE: An improved theory for the prediction of microcavitation thresholds. IEEE Trans Ultrason Ferroelec Freq Contr 1989;36:204-208.

44. Holland CK, Apfel RE: Thresholds for transient cavitation produced by pulsed ultrasound in a controlled nuclei environment. J Acoust Soc Am 1990;88:2059-2069.

45. Holland CK, Roy RA, Apfel RE, et al: In vitro detection of cavitation induced by a diagnostic ultrasound system. IEEE Trans Ultrason Ferroelec Freq Contr 1992;39:95-101.

46. Holland CK, Deng X, Apfel RE, et al: Direct evidence of cavitation in vivo from diagnostic ultrasound. Ultrasound Med Biol 1996;22(7):939-948.

47. Roy RA, Madanshetty S, Apfel RE: An acoustic backscattering technique for the detection of transient cavitation produced by microsecond pulses of ultrasound. J Acoust Soc Am 1990;87:2451-2455.

48. Fowlkes JB, Holland CK: Mechanical bioeffects from diagnostic ultrasound: AIUM consensus statements. J Ultrasound Med 2000;19(2): 69-72.

49. Skyba DM, Price RJ, Linka AZ, et al: Direct in vivo visualization of intravascular destruction of microbubbles by ultrasound and its local effects on tissue. Circulation 1998;98:290-293.

50. Miller DL, Quddus J: Diagnostic ultrasound activation of contrast agent gas bodies induces capillary rupture in mice. Proc Natl Acad Sci USA 2000;97:10179-84.

51. Van Der Wouw PA, Brauns AC, Bailey SE, et al: Premature ventricular contractions during triggered imaging with ultrasound contrast. J Am Soc Echocardiog 2000;13:288-294.

52. Apfel RE, Holland CK: Gauging the likelihood of cavitation from short-pulse, low-duty cycle diagnostic ultrasound. Ultrasound Med Biol 1991;17:179-185.

53. Dalecki D, Raeman CH, Child SZ, et al: A test for cavitation as a mechanism for intestinal hemorrhage in mice exposed to a piezoelectric lithotripter. Ultrasound Med Biol 1996;22:493-496.

54. American Institute of Ultrasound in Medicine. Medical Ultrasound Safety. Rockville, Md, 1994.

55. American Institute of Ultrasound in Medicine. Safety Statement. Approved March 1995. Current versions are available to the public upon request or at http://www.aium.org.

Epidemiology

56. Ziskin MC, Petitti DB: Epidemiology of human exposure to ultrasound: A critical review. Ultrasound Med Biol 1988;14:91-96.

57. EDH Environment Health Directorate: Canada-Wide Survey of Nonionizing Radiation Emitting Medical Devices. II. Ultrasound Devices. 1980. Report 80-EDH-53.

58. Ziskin MC: Survey of patient exposure to diagnostic ultrasound. In Reid JM, Sikov MR (eds): Interaction of Ultrasound and Biological Tissues. 1972. U.S. Dept of Health, Education, and Welfare publication FDA 78-8008:203.

59. Moore RM Jr, Barrick KM, Hamilton TM: Ultrasound exposure during gestation and birthweight. Presented at the Meeting of the Society for Epidemiological Research, June 16-18, 1982, Cincinnati, Ohio.

60. Stark CR, Orleans M, Haverkamp AD, et al: Short- and long-term risks after exposure to diagnostic ultrasound in utero. Obstet Gynecol 1984;63:194-200.

61. Scheidt PC, Stanley F, Bryla DA: One-year follow-up of infants exposed to ultrasound in utero. Am J Obstet Gynecol 1978;131:743-748.

62. Hill AB: The environment and disease: Association or causation? Proceed Royal Soc Med 1965;58:295-300.

63. Salvesen KA, Eik-Nes SH: Is ultrasound unsound? A review of epidemiological studies of human exposure to ultrasound. Ultrasound Obstet Gynecol 1995;6(4):293-298.

64. Ziskin MC: Epidemiology of ultrasound exposure. Ultrasound Med Biol 1988;14(2):91-96.

65. Newnham B, Evans SF, Michael CA: Effects of frequent ultrasound during pregnancy: A randomized controlled trial. Lancet 1993;342:887-891.

66. Campbell S, Elford RW, Brant RF: Case-control study of prenatal ultrasonography exposure in children with delayed speech. Can Med Assoc J 1993;149:1435-1440.

67. Nyborg WL, Steele RB: Temperature elevation in a beam of ultrasound. Ultrasound Med Biol 1983;9:611-620.

68. http://www.fda.gov/cdrh/consumer/fetalvideos.html

3

MICROBUBBLE CONTRAST FOR ULTRASOUND IMAGING: WHERE, HOW, AND WHY?

Peter N. Burns

Chapter Outline

The injection of a contrast agent forms a routine part of clinical radiographs, CT, MR and radionuclide imaging in radiology. Yet in spite of the obvious significance of the vascular component of an abdominal ultrasound examination, and in spite of widespread experimentation with contrast agents for echocardiography, ultrasound imaging of the abdomen has only just begun to exploit the potential benefit of contrast enhancement. Why?

A typical response from sonographers new to contrast is that intravascular injections would detract from one of ultrasound's major attractions, that it is noninvasive. Yet, if it can be shown that the additional diagnostic information obtained with contrast enhancement will spare the patient from a more invasive procedure, it would be doing them no favor to deny them a painless intravenous injection. A more fundamental consideration appeals to the nature of the ultrasound image itself, which benefits from an intrinsically high contrast between blood and solid tissue. It could be argued that, unlike radiographic angiography, ultrasound does not need a contrast agent and an associated subtraction imaging method to *see* blood. Furthermore, if we are interested in visualizing where the blood flows, color Doppler imaging offers a powerful and effective tool, providing the additional ability to quantify hemodynamic parameters, such as the direction and velocity of flow.

It is precisely these capabilities that the new generation of ultrasound contrast agents has extended, redefining the role of ultrasound in resolving the vascular questions that were until now left to CT and MR. Contrast agents can help delineate vascular structures and enhance Doppler signals from small volumes of blood. More excitingly, contrast agents make it possible for ultrasound to achieve entirely new objectives, the most striking of which is the ability for the first time to image organ and lesion perfusion in real time. This chapter aims to provide both a tutorial and a reference for the practical use of contrast agents for these new indications.

CONTRAST AGENTS FOR ULTRASOUND

The principal requirements for an ultrasound contrast agent are that it should be easily introducible into the vascular system, be stable for the duration of the diagnostic examination, have low toxicity, and modify one or more acoustic properties of tissues which determine the ultrasound imaging process. Although it is conceivable that applications may be found for ultrasound contrast agents that will justify their injection directly into arteries, the clinical context for contrast ultrasonography requires that they be capable of administration intravenously. These constitute a demanding specification for a drug, one that only recently has been met. At the time of writing, more than 60 countries have approved the use of at least one contrast agent for abdominal ultrasound diagnosis. The technology universally adopted is that of encapsulated bubbles of gas that are smaller than red blood cells and therefore capable of circulating freely in the body. These are the so-called "blood pool" agents. Agents are also under development that are taken up by a chosen organ system or site, as are many nuclear medicine materials.

Contrast Agent Types. Contrast agents might act by their presence in the vascular system, from where they are ultimately metabolized (blood pool agents) or by their selective uptake in tissue after a vascular phase. Of the properties of tissue that influence the ultrasound image, the most important are backscatter coefficient, attenuation, and acoustic propagation velocity.[1] Most agents seek to enhance the echo by increasing the backscatter of the tissue that bears them as much as possible, while increasing the attenuation in the tissue as little as possible, thus enhancing the echo from blood.

BLOOD POOL AGENTS

Free Gas Bubbles. Gramiak and Shah first used injected bubbles to enhance the blood pool echo in 1968.[2] They injected saline into the ascending aorta during echocardiographic recording and noted strong echoes within the normally echo-free lumen of the aorta and the chambers of the heart. Subsequent work showed that these reflections were the result of free bubbles of air that

came out of solution either by agitation or by cavitation during the injection itself. In this early work, many other fluids were found to produce a contrast effect when similarly injected.[3,4] The intensity of the echoes produced varied with the type of solution used: the more viscous the solution, the more microbubbles were trapped in a bolus for a sufficient length of time to be appreciated on the image. Agitated solutions of compounds such as indocyanine green and Renografin were also used. Most of the subsequent research into the application of these bubbles as ultrasound contrast agents focused on the heart, including evaluation of valvular insufficiency,[5,6] intracardiac shunts,[7] and cavity dimensions.[8] The fundamental limitation of bubbles produced in this way is that they are large, so that they are effectively filtered by the lungs, and unstable, so that they go back into solution within a second or so. Hence this procedure was invasive and, except by direct injection, unsuitable for imaging of left-sided cardiac chambers, the coronary circulation, and the systemic arterial tree and its organs.

Encapsulated Air Bubbles. To overcome the natural instability of free gas bubbles, attempts were made to encapsulate gas within a shell so as to create a more stable particle. In 1980, Carroll et al.[9] encapsulated nitrogen bubbles in gelatin and injected them into the femoral artery of rabbits with VX2 tumors in the thigh. Ultrasound enhancement of the tumor rim was identified. However, the large size of the particles ($80\ \mu m$) precluded administration by an intravenous route. The challenge to produce a stable encapsulated microbubble of a comparable size to that of a red blood cell and which could survive passage through the heart and the pulmonary capillary network was first met by Feinstein et al. in 1984.[10] They produced microbubbles by sonication of a solution of human serum albumin and showed that it could be visualized in the left heart after a peripheral venous injection. This agent was subsequently developed commercially as Albunex (Mallinckrodt Medical, Inc., St Louis, Mo).

A burgeoning number of manufacturers have since produced forms of stabilized microbubbles that are currently being assessed for use as intravenous contrast agents for ultrasound. Several have passed through "Phase 3" clinical trials and gained regulatory approval in Europe, North America and, most recently, Japan. Levovist (Schering AG, Berlin, Germany) is a dry mixture comprising 99.9% microcrystalline galactose microparticles and 0.1% palmitic acid. On dissolution and agitation in sterile water, the galactose disaggregates into microparticles, which provide an irregular surface for the adherence of microbubbles 3 to 4 μm in size. Stabilization of the microbubbles takes place as they become coated with palmitic acid, which separates the gas—liquid interface and slows their dissolution.[11] These microbubbles are highly echogenic and are sufficiently stable for transit through the pulmonary circuit. The median bubble diameter is typical for many of the agents, approximately 2 µm with the 97th percentile at approximately 6 µm.[12] The agent is chemically related to its predecessor Echovist (SHU454, Schering AG, Berlin, Germany), a galactose agent that forms larger bubbles and that has been used principally for visualization of nonvascular ductal structures such as the fallopian tubes. Numerous studies[13,14] with Levovist demonstrate its capacity to traverse the pulmonary bed in sufficient concentrations to enhance both color and spectral Doppler signals, as well as gray-scale examinations using nonlinear imaging modes such as pulse inversion imaging. Levovist is approved for use in the European Union (EU), Canada, and Japan, but not in the United States.

Low Solubility Gas Bubbles. The "shells" which stabilize the microbubbles are extremely thin and allow a gas such as air to diffuse out and go back into solution in the blood. How fast this happens depends on a number of factors that vary, not only from agent to agent, but from patient to patient. After venous introduction, however, the effective duration of the two agents described earlier is just a few minutes. Because they are introduced as a bolus and the maximum effect of the agent is in the first pass, the useful imaging time is usually considerably less than this. Newer (sometimes referred to as second generation) agents, designed both to increase backscatter enhancement further and to last longer in the blood stream, are currently under intense development. Instead of air, many of these take advantage of low solubility gases such as perfluorocarbons, the consequent lower diffusion rate increasing the longevity of the agent in the blood. Optison (Nycomed-Amersham, Oslo, Norway) is a perfluoropropane-filled albumin shell with a size distribution similar to that of its predecessor, Albunex. The stability of the smaller bubbles in its population is the probable cause of the greater enhancement observed with this agent. It is currently approved for radiologic indications in the EU, United States, and Canada. SonoVue (Bracco, Inc., NJ) uses sulfur hexafluorane in a phospholipid shell and is available for cardiology and radiology indications in the EU. Definity (Bristol Myers-Squibb, Inc., Boston, Mass) comprises a perfluoropropane microbubble coated with a particularly flexible bilipid shell that also shows improved stability and high enhancements at low doses.[15] It is currently approved for cardiology and radiology in Canada and cardiology in the United States. Other agents are under aggressive development (Table 3-1).

Selective Uptake Agents. A perfect blood pool agent displays the same flow dynamics as blood itself and is ultimately metabolized from the blood pool. Agents can be made, however, that are capable of providing ultrasound contrast during their metabolism as well as while in the blood pool. Colloidal suspensions of liquids such as perfluorocarbons[16] and certain agents with durable shells[17] are taken up by the reticuloendothelial system from where they ultimately are excreted. There they may provide contrast from within the liver parenchyma, demarcating the distribution of Kupffer cells.[18] This application has become particularly popular for Levovist, which has been shown to provide late phase enhancement in the parenchyma of the liver and spleen after it has cleared from the vascular system.[19] It is not

TABLE 3-1. SOME ULTRASOUND CONTRAST AGENTS

Manufacturer	Name	Shell/gas	Status
Acusphere	AI-700	Polymer/perfluorocarbon	Clinical development
Alliance	Imagent	Surfactant/perfluorohexane-air	Approved in U.S. for cardiology
Bracco	SonoVue	Phospholipid/Sulfur hexafluoride	Approved in EU for radiology/cardiology
Cavcon	Filmix	Lipid/air	Preclinical development
Bristol Myers-Squibb	Definity	Liposome/perfluoropropane	Approved in U.S. for cardiology, and Canada for radiology/cardiology
Mallinckrodt/Nycomed-Amersham	Optison®	Sonicated albumin/octafluoropropane	Approved in EU and U.S. Canada, for cardiology
Mallinckrodt/Nycomed-Amersham	Albunex	Sonicated albumin/air	Approved in EU and U.S. Canada, no longer available
Nycomed-Amersham	Sonazoid	Lipid/perfluorocarbon	Clinical development
Point Biomedical	Bisphere	Polymer bilayer/air	Late clinical development (cardiology)
Porter	PESDA	Sonicated albumin/perfluorocarbon	Not commercially developed
Quadrant	Quantison	Spray-dried albumin/air	Suspended development
Schering	Echovist	Galactose matrix/air	Approved in EU, Canada
Schering	Levovist®	Lipid/air	Approved in EU, Canada, Japan. Not approved in U.S.
Schering	Sonavist®	Polymer/air	Suspended development

clear whether this is a result of phagocytosis of intact bubbles or of their adhesion to the endothelium of the hepatic sinusoids. In the future, agents with a cell-specific pathway may be used as a means both to detect and to deliver therapeutic agents to a specific site in the cardiovascular system.

The Need for Contrast or Bubble-Specific Imaging. One of the major diagnostic objectives in using an ultrasound contrast agent in an abdominal organ is to detect flow in the circulation at a level that is lower than would otherwise be possible. The echoes from blood associated with such flow—in the hepatic sinusoids, for example—exist in the midst of echoes from the surrounding solid structures of the liver parenchyma, echoes that are almost always stronger than even the contrast-enhanced blood echo. When they can be seen, blood vessels in a nonenhanced image have a low echo level, so that an **echo-enhancing agent** actually **lowers** the contrast between blood and the surrounding tissue, making the lumen of the blood vessel less visible. Thus, in order to be able to image flow in small vessels of the liver, a contrast agent is required that either enhances the blood echo to a level that is substantially higher than that of the surrounding tissue, or that can be used with a method for suppressing the echo from noncontrast-bearing structures. Radiographic angiography, which has a similar problem, deals with these "clutter" components of the image by simple subtraction of a preinjection image. What is left behind might reveal flow in individual vessels or the "blush" of perfusion at the tissue level. If, however, we subtract two consecutive ultrasound images of an abdominal organ, we are likely to get a third ultrasound image, produced by the shift or decorrelation of the speckle pattern between acquisitions. In order to show parenchymal enhancement, speckle variance must first be reduced by filtering, with an unacceptable loss of spatial or temporal resolution. Even if the speckle problem could be overcome, subtraction would still be poorly suited to the dynamic and interactive nature of ultrasound imaging.

Doppler offers an alternative method that successfully separates the echoes from blood from those of tissue. It relies on the relatively high velocity of moving blood compared to that of the surrounding tissue. Although this distinction—which allows us to use a highpass (or "wall") filter to separate the Doppler signals because of blood flow from those due to clutter—is valid for flow in large vessels, it does not work for flow at the parenchymal level, where the tissue is moving at the same speed or faster than the blood that perfuses it. In this case the Doppler shift frequency from the moving solid tissue is comparable to or higher than that of the moving blood itself. The amplitude of the solid tissue echo is typically 1000 to 10,000 times higher than that of the blood echo. Because the wall filter cannot be used without eliminating both the flow and the clutter echoes, the use of Doppler in such circumstances is defeated by the overwhelming signal from tissue movement: the **"flash" artifact** in color or the **"thump" artifact** in spectral Doppler.[20] In spite of many published claims to the contrary, true parenchymal flow cannot be imaged using conventional Doppler, with or without intravenous contrast agents (Fig. 3-1).[21]

How then might contrast agents be used to improve the visibility of small vascular structures within tissue? Clearly, a method that could identify the echo from the contrast agent and thereby suppress that from solid tissue would provide both a real time subtraction mode for contrast-enhanced B-mode imaging, and a means of suppressing Doppler clutter without the use of a velocity-dependent filter in spectral and color modes. **Contrast-specific imaging** (often referred to as **nonlinear** imaging) has provided us with such a method, and hence the means for the detection of flow in smaller vessels than has hitherto been possible.

Bubble Behavior and Incident Pressure

The key to understanding contrast imaging instruments—and the key to their successful clinical use—lies in the unique interaction between a microbubble contrast agent and the process that images them. Controlling and exploiting this interaction is central to all contrast-specific methods. Unlike tissue, microbubbles scatter

---

TABLE 3-2. THREE REGIMENS OF BUBBLE BEHAVIOR IN AN ULTRASOUND FIELD

Peak pressure (approx.)	Mechanical Index (MI) @ 1 MHz	Bubble Behavior	Acoustic Behavior	Application
<100 kPa	<0.1	Linear oscillation	Linear backscatter enhancement	Doppler signal enhancement
0.1–0.5 MPa	0.1–0.5	Nonlinear oscillation	Harmonic backscatter	Real-time (low MI) vascular imaging
>0.5 MPa	>0.5	Disruption	Transient nonlinear echoes	Interval delay (high MI) perfusion imaging

1 kPa = 1 kilopascal = 1000 Pascals; the unit of pressure.
1 MPa = 1 megapascal = 1,000,000 Pascals; the unit of pressure.

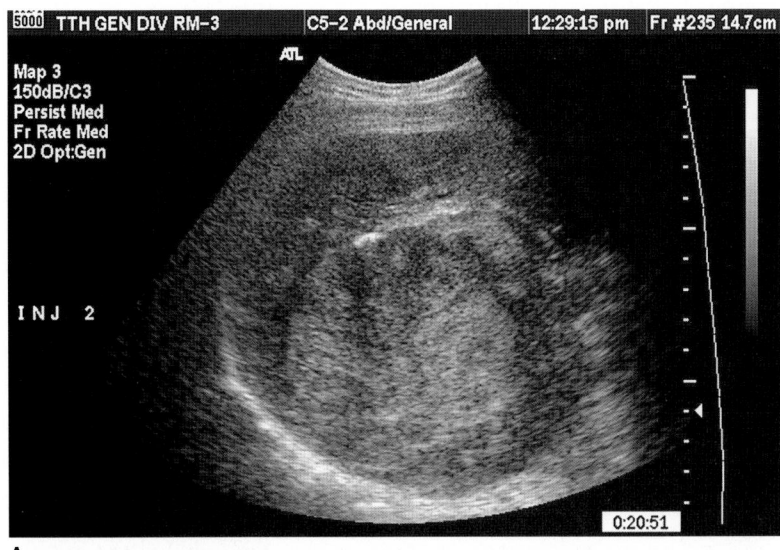

A

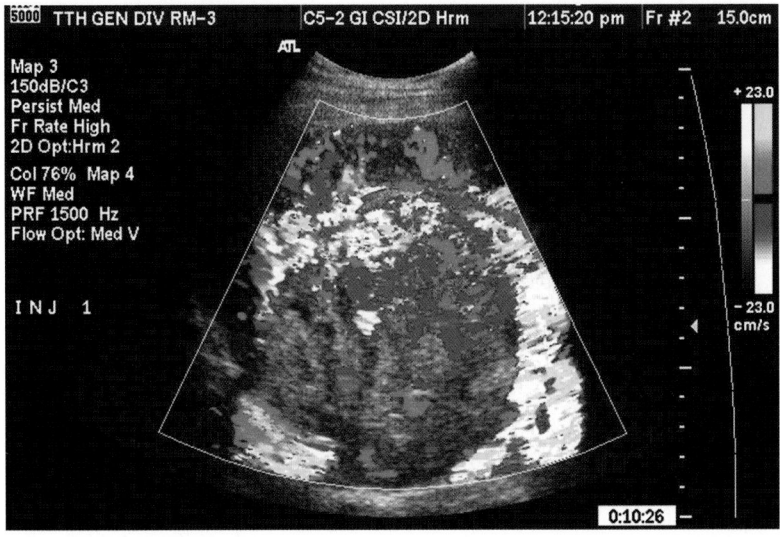

B

FIGURE 3-1. The need for contrast-specific imaging. A, Conventional image of liver containing large mass. **B**, Administration of contrast increases the echogenicity of blood but creates Doppler artifacts due to blooming and tissue motion. (From Burns PN, Wilson SR, Hope Simpson D: Pulse inversion imaging of liver blood flow: An improved method for characterization of focal masses with microbubble contrast. Invest Radiol 2000;35:58-71.)

ultrasound in a manner dependent on the amplitude of the sound to which the imaging process exposes them. The result is three broad regimens of scattering behavior, depending on the peak pressure of the incident sound field produced by the scanner. These form the basis of the contrast imaging techniques used clinically. At low incident pressures (corresponding to low transmit power of the scanner), the agents produce **linear backscatter enhancement**, resulting in an augmentation of the echo from blood. This is the behavior originally envisaged by contrast agent manufacturers for their first intended clinical indication: Doppler signal enhancement. As the transmit intensity control of the scanner is increased and the pressure incident on a bubble goes beyond about 50 to 100 kPa, which is still below the level used in most diagnostic scans, the contrast agent backscatter begins to show nonlinear characteristics, such as the **emission of harmonics**. It is the detection of these that forms the

basis of contrast specific imaging modes, such as harmonic and pulse inversion imaging and Doppler. Finally, as the peak pressure reaches nearer 100 kPa (or 1 MPa), near the maximum emitted by a typical ultrasound imaging system, many agents exhibit **transient nonlinear scattering**, resulting in their destruction. This forms the basis of triggered imaging and the most sensitive methods for detecting perfusion. It should be noted that in practice, because of the different sizes present in a realistic population of bubbles,[22] the borders between these behaviors are not sharp—nor will they be the same for different agent types, whose acoustic behavior is strongly dependent on the gas and shell properties.[23]

The Mechanical Index

For reasons unrelated to contrast imaging, ultrasound scanners marketed in the United States are required by

THE MECHANICAL INDEX (MI)

- Defined by $MI = P_{neg}/\sqrt{f}$, where P_{neg} is the peak negative ultrasound pressure, f is the ultrasound frequency
- Reflects the normalized energy to which a target (such as a bubble) is exposed in an ultrasound field
- Is defined for the focus of the ultrasound beam
- Varies with depth in the image (lessens with increasing depth)
- Varies with lateral location in the image (lessens at the sector edges)
- Varies significantly between systems from different manufacturers

the Food and Drug Administration (FDA) to carry an on-screen label of the estimated peak negative pressure to which tissue is exposed. Of course, this pressure changes according to the tissue through which the sound travels as well as the amplitude and geometry of the ultrasound beam: the higher the attenuation, the less the peak pressure in tissue will be. A scanner cannot *know* what tissue it is being used on, so the definition of an index has been formed that reflects the approximate exposure to ultrasound pressure at the focus of the beam in an average tissue. The mechanical index (MI) is defined as the peak rarefactional (that is, negative) pressure, divided by the square root of the ultrasound frequency. This quantity is related to the amount of mechanical work that can be performed on a bubble during a single negative half cycle of sound,[24] and is thought to give an indication of the propensity of the sound to cause cavitation in the medium. In clinical ultrasound systems, this index usually lies somewhere between 0.1 and 2.0. Although a single value is displayed for each image, in practice, the actual MI varies throughout the image. In the absence of attenuation, the MI is maximal at the focus of the beam. Attenuation shifts this maximum toward the transducer. Because it is a somewhat complex procedure to calculate the index, which is itself only an estimate of the actual quantity within the body, the indices displayed by different machines are not precisely comparable. For example, more bubble disruption might be observed at a displayed MI of 0.5 using one machine but at 0.6 with the same patient using another machine. For this reason, recommendations of machine settings for a specific examination are not transferable between manufacturers' instruments. Nonetheless, the MI is one of the most important machine parameters in a contrast study. It is usually controlled by means of the **output power** control of the scanner.

Nonlinear Backscatter: Harmonic Imaging

Examining the behavior of contrast-enhanced ultrasound studies reveals two important pieces of evidence. First, the size of the echo enhancement at very high dilution following a small peripheral injection (7 dB from as little as 0.01 mL/kg of Levovist, for example[25]) is much larger than would be expected from such sparse scatterers of this size in blood. Second, investigations of the acoustic characteristics of several agents[26] have demonstrated peaks in the spectra of attenuation and scattering that are dependent on both ultrasound frequency and the size of the microbubbles. This important observation suggests that the bubbles **resonate** in an ultrasound field. As the ultrasound wave—which comprises alternate compressions and rarefactions—propagates over the bubbles, the bubbles experience a periodic change in their radius in sympathy with the oscillations of the incident sound. Like vibrations in other structures, these radial oscillations have a natural—or **resonant**—frequency of oscillation at which they will both absorb and scatter ultrasound with a peculiarly high efficiency. Considering the linear oscillation of a free bubble of air in water, we can use a simple theory[1] to predict the resonant frequency of radial oscillation of a bubble of 3 μm diameter, the median diameter of a typical transpulmonary microbubble agent. As Figure 3-2 shows, it is about 3 MHz, approximately the center frequency of ultrasound used

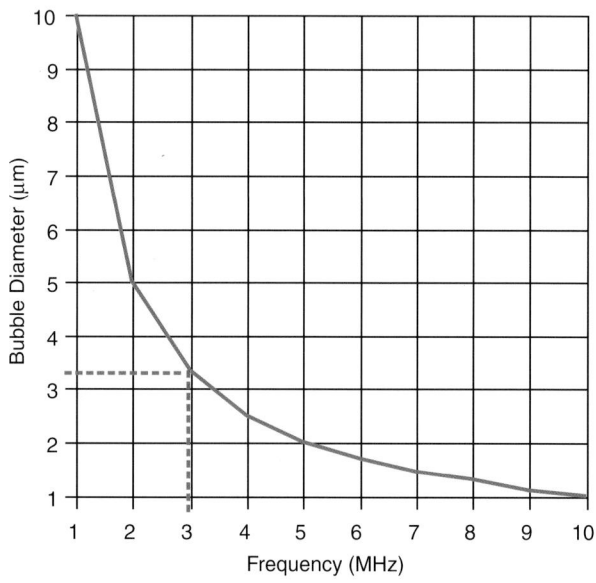

FIGURE 3-2. Microbubbles resonate in a diagnostic ultrasound field. This graph shows that the resonant—or natural—frequency of oscillation of a bubble of air in an ultrasound field depends on its size. For a 3.5 μm diameter, the size needed for an intravenously injectable contrast agent, the resonant frequency is about 3 MHz.

in a typical abdominal scan. This extraordinary—and fortunate—coincidence explains why ultrasound contrast agents are so efficient and can be administered in such small quantities. It also predicts that bubbles undergoing resonant oscillation in an ultrasound field can be induced to nonlinear motion, the basis of harmonic imaging.

It has long been recognized[27] that if bubbles are driven by an ultrasound field at sufficiently high acoustic pressures, the oscillatory excursions of the bubble reach a point where the alternate expansions and contractions of the bubble's size are not equal. Lord Rayleigh, the originator of the theoretical understanding of sound on which ultrasound imaging is based, was first led in 1917 to investigate this by his curiosity over the creaking noises that his teakettle made as the water came to a boil.[28] The consequence of such **nonlinear motion** is that the sound emitted by the bubble, and detected by the transducer, contains **harmonics**, just as the resonant strings of a musical instrument, if plucked too vigorously, will produce a harsh timbre containing overtones (the musical term for harmonics), exact octaves above the pitch of the fundamental note.

The origin of this phenomenon is the asymmetry that begins to affect bubble oscillation as the amplitude becomes large. As a bubble is compressed by the ultrasound pressure wave, it becomes stiffer and resists further reduction in its radius. Conversely, in the rarefaction phase of the ultrasound pulse, the bubble becomes less stiff and, therefore, enlarges much more (Fig. 3-3). Figure 3-4 shows the frequency spectrum of an echo produced by a microbubble contrast agent following a 3.75 MHz burst. The particular agent is Levovist, though many microbubble agents behave in a similar way. Ultrasound frequency is on the horizontal axis, with the relative amplitude on the vertical axis. A strong echo, at −13 dB with respect to the fundamental, is seen at twice the transmitted frequency, that known as the **second harmonic**. Peaks in the echo spectrum at sub- and ultra-harmonics are also seen. Here, then, is one simple method to distinguish bubbles from tissue: excite them so as to produce harmonics and detect these in preference to the fundamental echo from tissue. Key factors in the harmonic response of an agent are the incident pressure of the ultrasound field, the frequency, as well as the size distribution of the bubbles, and the mechanical properties of the bubble capsule—a stiff capsule, for example, will dampen the oscillations and attenuate its nonlinear response.

Harmonic B-Mode Imaging

An imaging and Doppler method based on this phenomenon, called **harmonic imaging**,[29] is now widely available on most modern ultrasound scanners. In harmonic mode, the system transmits normally at one

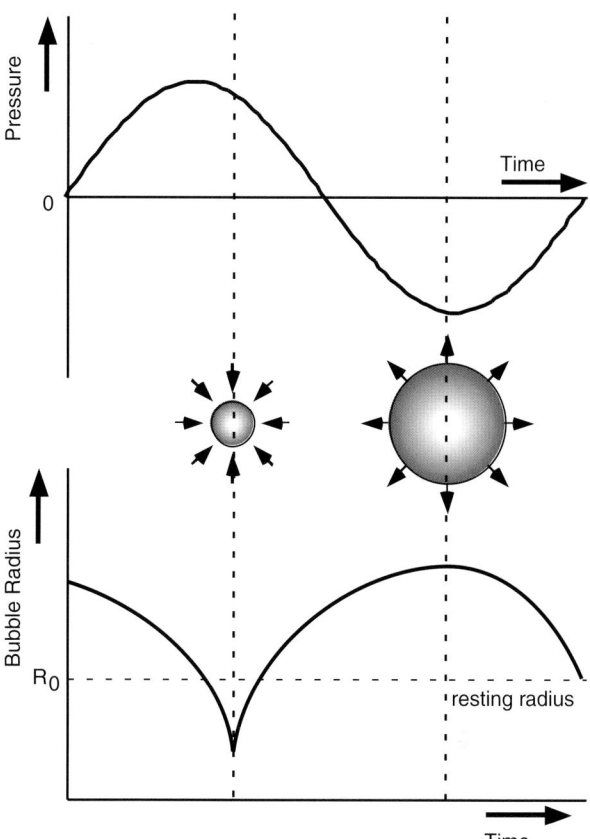

FIGURE 3-3. A microbubble in an acoustic field. Bubbles respond asymmetrically to high intensity sound waves, stiffening when compressed by sound, yielding only small changes in radius. During the low pressure portion of the sound wave, the bubble stiffness decreases and radius changes can be large. This asymmetrical response leads to the production of **harmonics** in the scattered wave.

frequency, but is tuned to receive echoes preferentially at double that frequency, where the echoes from the bubbles lie. Typically, the transmit frequency lies between 1.5 and 3 MHz and the receive frequency is selected by means of a radiofrequency bandpass filter, whose center frequency is at the second harmonic, between 3 and 6 MHz. Harmonic imaging uses the same array transducers as conventional imaging and for most of today's ultrasound systems involves only software changes. Echoes from solid tissue, as well as red blood cells themselves, are suppressed. **Real-time harmonic spectral Doppler** and **color Doppler modes** have also been implemented (sometimes experimentally) on a number of commercially available systems. Clearly, an exceptional transducer bandwidth is needed to operate over such a large range of frequencies. Fortunately much effort has been directed in recent years toward increasing the bandwidth of transducer arrays because of its significant bearing on conventional imaging performance, so harmonic imaging modes do not require the additional expense of dedicated transducers.

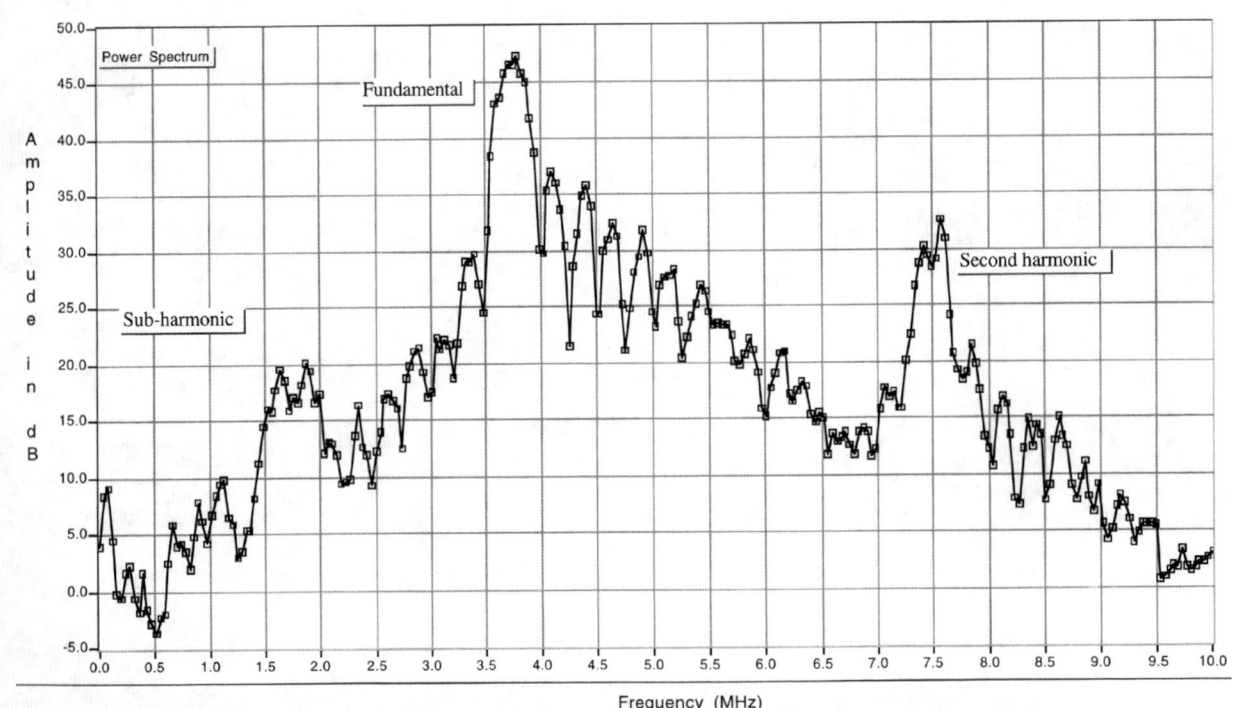

FIGURE 3-4. Harmonic emission from Levovist. A sample of a contrast agent is insonated at 3.75 MHz and the echo is analyzed for its frequency content. It is seen that most of the energy in the echo is at 3.75 MHz, but that there is a clear second peak in the spectrum at 7.5 MHz, as well as a third at 1.875 MHz. The second harmonic echo is only 13 dB less than that of the main, or fundamental, echo. Harmonic imaging and Doppler aim to separate and process this signal alone. The smaller peak is the first subharmonic. (From Becher H, Burns PN: Handbook of Contrast Echocardiography. Berlin, Springer, 2000. *http://www.sunnybrook.utoronto.ca/EchoHandbook/.*)

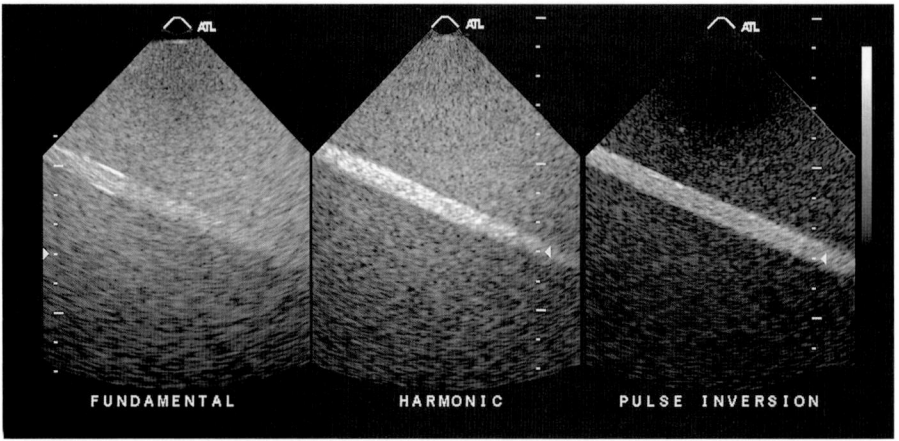

FIGURE 3-5. Comparison of conventional, harmonic, and pulse inversion imaging. In vitro images of a vessel phantom containing stationary contrast agent (Optison) surrounded by tissue equivalent material (biogel and graphite). **A,** Conventional image, MI = 0.2. **B,** Harmonic imaging, MI = 0.2, provides improved contrast between agent and tissue. **C,** Pulse inversion imaging, MI = 0.2. By suppressing linear echoes from stationary tissue, pulse inversion imaging provides better contrast between agent and tissue than conventional, fundamental, and harmonic imaging. MI, Mechanical index. (From Becher H, Burns PN: Handbook of Contrast Echocardiography. Berlin, Springer, 2000. *http://www.sunnybrook.utoronto.ca/EchoHandbook/.*)

Harmonic Doppler

In harmonic images, the echo from tissue-mimicking material is reduced—but not eliminated, reversing the contrast between the agent and its surroundings (Fig. 3-5). The value of this effect is to increase the conspicuity of the agent when it is in blood vessels normally hidden by the strong echoes from tissue. In spectral Doppler, one would expect the suppression of the tissue echo to **reduce the tissue motion thump** that is familiar to all Doppler sonographers. Figure 3-6 shows spectral Doppler applied to a region of the aorta in

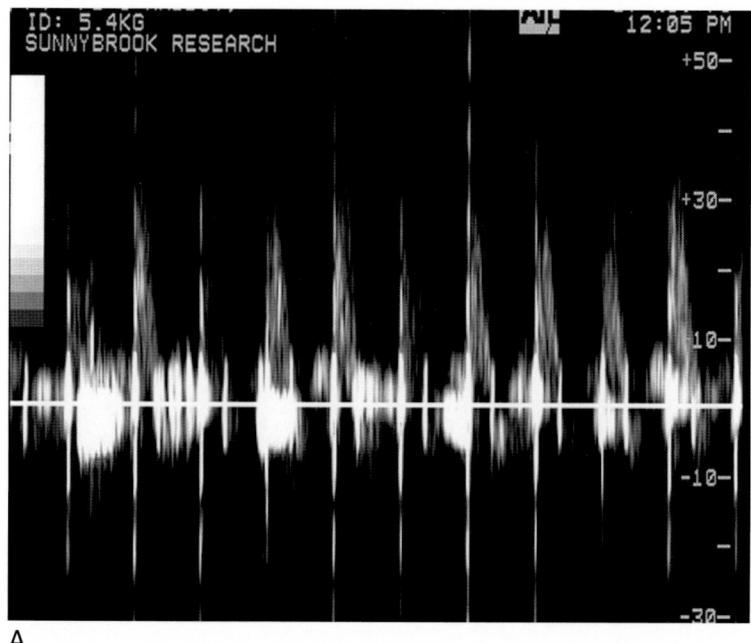

A

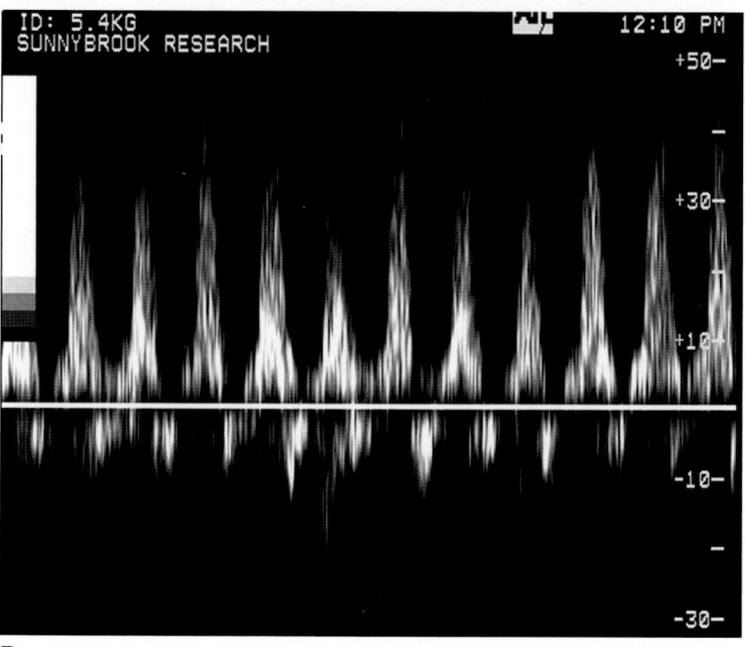

B

FIGURE 3-6. Clutter rejection with harmonic spectral Doppler. A, The abdominal aorta is examined with harmonic spectral Doppler. In conventional mode, clutter from the moving wall causes the familiar artifact that also obscures diastolic flow. **B,** In harmonic mode, the clutter is almost completely suppressed, so that flow can be resolved. The settings of the filter and other relevant instrument parameters are identical. (From Becher H, Burns PN: Handbook of Contrast Echocardiography. Berlin, Springer, 2000. *http://www.sunnybrook.utoronto.ca/EchoHandbook/*.)

which there is wall motion as well as blood flow within the sample volume. The conventional Doppler image of Figure 3-7A shows the thump artifact due to **clutter**, which is almost completely absent in the harmonic Doppler image of Figure 3-7B (all instrument settings, including the filters, are identical). In vivo measurements from spectral Doppler show that the signal-to-clutter ratio is improved by a combination of harmonic imaging and the contrast agent by as much as 35 dB.[30] Applications of this method include detection of blood flow in small vessels surrounded by tissue that is moving: the branches of the coronary arteries,[31] the myocardium,[32] and the parenchyma of the kidney[33] and liver.[34]

Harmonic Power Doppler Imaging

In color Doppler studies using a contrast agent, the effect of the arrival of the agent in a color region of interest is often to produce **blooming** of the color image, whereby signals from major vascular targets spread out to occupy the entire region. Although flow from smaller vessels might be detectable, the color images can be swamped by artifactual signals (see Fig. 3-1B). The origin of this artifact is the amplitude threshold that governs most color displays in conventional (or velocity) mode imaging. Increasing the backscattered signal power simply has the effect of displaying the velocity estimate,

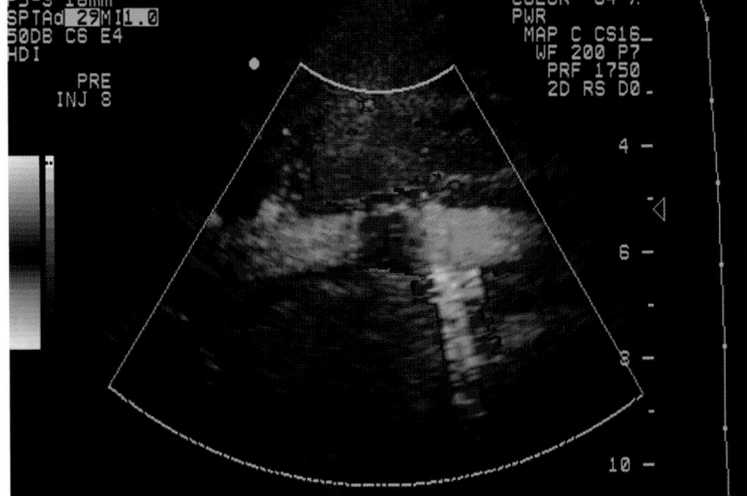

A

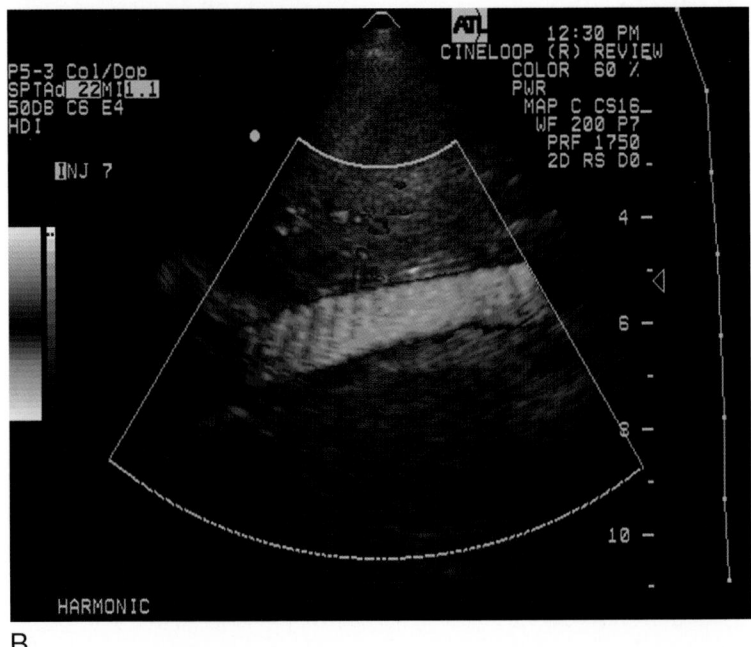

B

FIGURE 3-7. Reduction of the flash artifact in harmonic power Doppler. The harmonic contrast method helps overcome one of the principal shortcomings of power Doppler, its increased susceptibility to tissue motion. **A,** Aortic flow in power mode with flash artifact from cardiac motion of wall. **B,** In harmonic mode at the same point in the cardiac cycle, the flash is largely suppressed. All instrument settings are the same. (From Becher H, Burns PN: Handbook of Contrast Echocardiography. Berlin, Springer, 2000. *http://www.sunnybrook.utoronto.ca/EchoHandbook/.*)

at full intensity, over a wider range of pixels around the detected location. A display in which the parameter mapped to color is related directly to the backscattered signal power, however, has the advantage that such a threshold is unnecessary. Also, lower amplitude Doppler shifts, such as those that result from side lobe interference, are displayed at a lower visual amplitude, rendering them less conspicuous. Echo-enhanced flow signals, in contrast, will be displayed at a higher level. This is the basis of the **power Doppler imaging** (also known as **color power angiography**, or **color Doppler energy** mapping). Power Doppler can help eliminate

some other limitations of small vessel flow detection with color Doppler.

Low velocity detection requires lowering the Doppler pulse repetition frequency (PRF), which results in multiple aliasing and loss of directional resolution. A display method that does not use the velocity estimate is not prone to the aliasing artifact, and allows the PRF to be lowered and increases the likelihood of detection of the lower velocity flow from smaller vessels.[35] Because it maps a parameter directly related to the acoustic quantity that is enhanced by the contrast agent, the power map is a natural choice for contrast-enhanced color Doppler studies. The advantages of the power map for contrast-enhanced detection of small vessel flow are balanced by a potentially devastating shortcoming: its increased susceptibility to interference from clutter. Clutter is both detected more readily, because of the power mode's increased sensitivity, and displayed more prominently, because of the high intensity display of high amplitude signals. Frame averaging has the additional effect of sustaining and blurring the flash over the cardiac cycle, thereby exacerbating its effect on the image. This is the reason that conventional power mode, although quite popular in some organ imaging, has no application where there is tissue motion.

At the small expense of some sensitivity, amply compensated by the enhancement caused by the agent, **harmonic mode** effectively overcomes this **clutter** problem (see Fig. 3-7). Combining the harmonic method with power Doppler produces an especially effective tool for the detection of flow in the small vessels of the organs of the abdomen that may be moving with cardiac pulsation or respiration. In a study in which flow imaged on contrast-enhanced power harmonic images was compared with histologically sized arterioles in the corresponding regions of the renal cortex,[25] it was concluded that the method is capable of demonstrating flow in vessels of less than 40 μm diameter; about 10 times smaller than the corresponding imaging resolution limit, even as the organ was moving with normal respiration. Using this power mode method in the heart, flow can be imaged in the myocardium.[36,37]

Tissue Harmonic Imaging

In second harmonic imaging, an ultrasound scanner transmits at one frequency and receives at double this frequency. The resulting improved detection of the microbubble echo is due to the peculiar behavior of a gas bubble in an ultrasound field. However, any source of a received signal at the harmonic frequency that does not come from the bubble will clearly reduce the efficacy of this method. Such unwanted signals can come from nonlinearities in the transducer or its associated electronics, and these must be tackled effectively in a good harmonic imaging system. However, **tissue itself can produce harmonics** that will be received by the transducer. They are developed as a wave **propagates** through tissue. Again, this is due to an asymmetry: this time the fact that sound travels slightly faster through tissue during the compressional part of the cycle (where it is denser and hence more stiff) than during the rarefactional part. Although the effect is very small, it is sufficient to produce substantial harmonic components in the transmitted wave by the time it reaches deep tissue, so that when it is scattered by a linear target, such as the myocardium, there is a harmonic component in the echo, which is detected by the scanner along with the harmonic echo from the bubble.[38] This is the reason that solid tissue is not completely dark in a typical harmonic image. The effect is to reduce the contrast between the bubble and tissue, rendering the problem of detecting perfusion in tissue more difficult.

Tissue harmonics, though a foe to contrast imaging, are not necessarily a bad thing. In fact, an image formed from tissue harmonics without the presence of contrast agents has many properties that recommend it over conventional imaging. These come from the fact that tissue harmonics are developed as the beam penetrates tissue, in contrast to the conventional beam, which is generated at the transducer surface.[39] Artifacts, which accrue from the first few centimeters of tissue, such as reverberations, are reduced by using tissue harmonic imaging. Side lobe and other low-level interference is also suppressed, making tissue harmonic imaging the routine modality of choice in many situations, especially when visualizing fluid-filled structures.[40]

Reducing Tissue Harmonics

Nonetheless, for contrast studies, the tissue harmonics limits the visibility of bubbles within tissue and, therefore, can be considered an artifact. In considering how to reduce it, it is instructive to bear in mind differences between harmonics produced by tissue propagation and by bubble echoes. First, tissue harmonics require a high peak pressure, so are only evident at high MI. **Reducing the MI** leaves only the bubble harmonics. Second, harmonics from tissue at high MI are continuous and sustained, whereas those from bubbles at high MI are transient in nature as the bubble disrupts.

Pulse Inversion Imaging

Harmonic imaging imposes some fundamental limitations on the imaging process that restrict its clinical potential in organ imaging. To ensure that the higher frequencies are due only to harmonics emitted by the bubbles, the transmitter must be restricted to a band of frequencies around the fundamental band (Fig. 3-8A). Similarly, the received band of frequencies must be restricted to those lying around the second harmonic. If these two regions overlap (see Fig. 3-8B), the result will be that the **harmonic filter** will receive echoes from ordinary tissue, thus reducing the contrast between the agent and the tissue. However, **restricting the receive bandwidth** degrades the resolution of the resulting image, thus framing a fundamental compromise in harmonic imaging between contrast and resolution. For optimal detection of bubbles in the microvasculature, this compromise must favor contrast, so that the most sensitive harmonic images are generally of low quality. A further drawback of the filtering approach is that if the

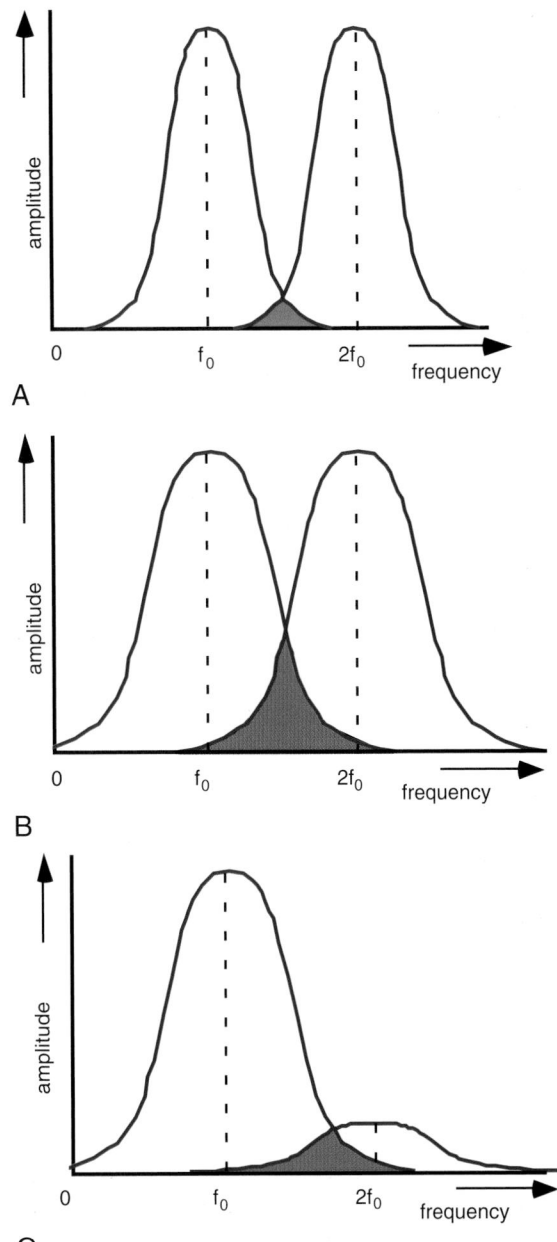

A

B

C

FIGURE 3-8. The compromises forced by harmonic imaging. A, In harmonic imaging, the transmitted frequencies must be restricted to a band around the fundamental, and the receive frequencies must be limited to a band around the second harmonic. This limits resolution. **B,** If the transmit and receive bandwidths are increased to improve resolution, some fundamental echoes from tissue will overlap the receive bandwidth and will be detected, reducing contrast between agent and tissue. **C,** When the harmonic echoes are weak, due to low agent concentration and/or low incident pulse intensity, this overlap will be especially large, and the harmonic signal may be largely composed of tissue echoes.

received echo is weak, the overlapping region between the transmit and receive frequencies becomes a larger portion of the entire received signal (see Fig. 3-8C). Thus contrast in the harmonic image is dependent on how strong the echo is from the bubbles, which is determined by the concentration of bubbles and the intensity of the incident ultrasound pulse. In practice, this forces use of a **high MI in harmonic mode**. This results in the transient and irreversible disruption of the bubbles.[41] As the bubbles enter the scan plane of a real-time ultrasound image, they provide an echo but then disappear. Thus vessels that lie within the scan plane are not visualized as continuous ducts in a typical harmonic image; but instead have a punctate appearance (Fig. 3-9A).

Principle of Pulse Inversion

Pulse inversion imaging overcomes the conflict between the requirements of contrast and resolution in harmonic imaging and provides greater sensitivity, thus allowing low incident power, nondestructive, continuous imaging of microbubbles in an organ such as the liver. The method also relies on the asymmetrical oscillation of an ultrasound bubble in an acoustic field, but detects "even" nonlinear components of the echo over the entire bandwidth of the transducer. In **pulse inversion** (also known as **phase inversion**) imaging, two pulses are sent in rapid succession into the tissue. The second pulse is a mirror image of the first (Fig. 3-10); that is, it has undergone a 180° phase change. The scanner detects the echo from these two successive pulses and forms their sum. For ordinary tissue, which behaves in a linear manner, the sum of two inverted pulses is simply zero.

For an echo with nonlinear components, such as that from a bubble, the echoes produced from these two pulses will not be simple mirror images of each other, because of the asymmetrical behavior of the bubble radius with time. The result is that the sum of these two echoes is not zero. Thus, a signal is detected from a bubble but not from tissue. It can be shown mathematically that this summed echo contains the nonlinear even harmonic components of the signal, including the second harmonic.[42] One advantage of pulse inversion over the filter approach to detect harmonics from bubbles is that it no longer suffers from the restriction of bandwidth. The full frequency range of sound emitted from the transducer can be detected in this way, providing a full bandwidth—that is high resolution—image of the echoes from bubbles.[43] Pulse inversion imaging (See Fig. 3-5C) provides better suppression of linear echoes than does harmonic imaging and is effective over the full bandwidth of the transducer, showing improvement of image resolution over harmonic mode.

Because this detection method is a more efficient means of isolating the bubble echo, weaker echoes from bubbles insonated at low, nondestructive intensities, can be detected. Figure 3-9B shows a pulse inversion image of the same liver as in Figure 3-9A, at low MI. Fourth-order branches of the portal vein are visible. It

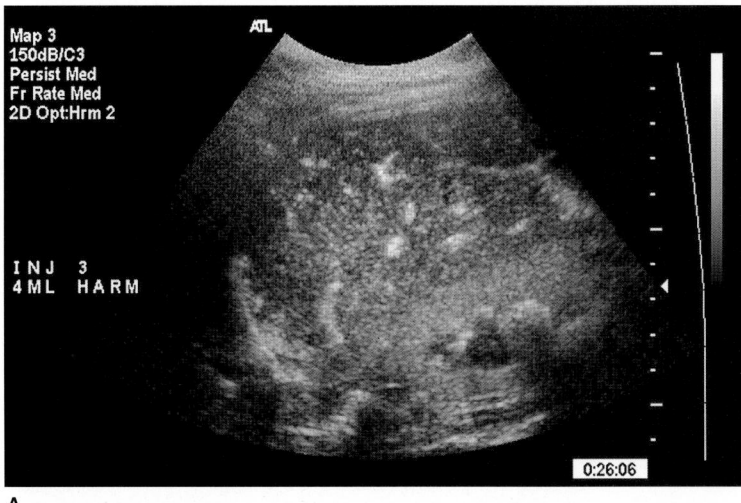

A

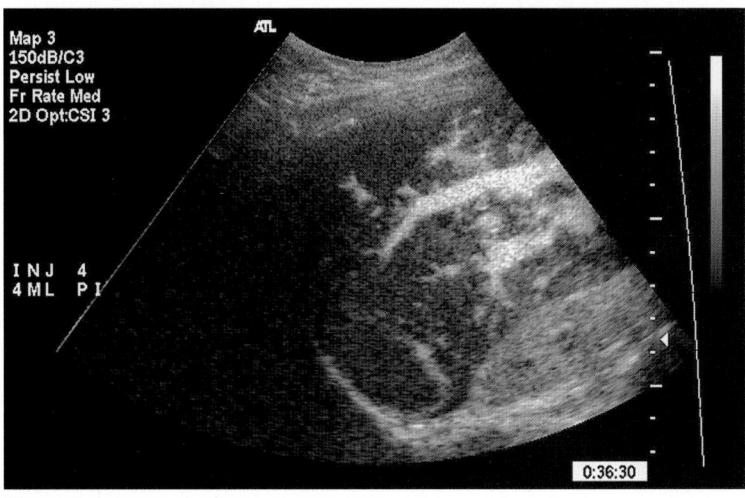

B

FIGURE 3-9. The appearance of blood vessels in harmonic and pulse inversion imaging in a study patient with an incidental hemangioma. A, In a harmonic contrast image of a liver, large vessels have a punctate appearance as the high mechanical index (MI) ultrasound disrupts the bubbles as they enter the scan plane. **B,** In the pulse inversion image of the same liver, a lower MI can be used so that continuous vessels are now seen. Improved resolution of pulse inversion imaging demonstrates 4th-order branches of the portal vein. (From Becher H, Burns PN: Handbook of Contrast Echocardiography. Berlin, Springer, 2000. *http://www.sunnybrook.utoronto.ca/EchoHandbook/.*)

should be noted, however, that as the MI increases, tissue harmonic renders the tissue brighter. Indeed, pulse inversion is now the preferred method used by many systems for tissue harmonic imaging. Optimal **pulse inversion contrast imaging** is often, then, performed at low MI. The principle of pulse inversion is the basis of many imaging modes, such as **coherent contrast imaging, ensemble harmonic imaging, phase inversion imaging**, and so on.

Pulse Inversion Doppler Imaging

In spite of the improvements offered by pulse inversion over harmonic imaging for suppressing stationary tissue, the method is somewhat sensitive to echoes from moving tissue. This is because tissue motion causes linear echoes to change slightly between pulses, so that they do not cancel perfectly. Furthermore, at high MI, nonlinear propagation also causes harmonic echoes to appear in pulse inversion images, even from linear scattering structures such as the liver parenchyma. While tissue

motion artifacts can be minimized by using a short pulse repetition interval, nonlinear tissue echoes can mask the echoes from bubbles, reducing the efficacy of microbubble contrast, especially when a high MI is used. A recent development seeks to address these problems by means of a generalization of the pulse inversion method, called pulse inversion Doppler.[42] This technique—which is also known as **power pulse inversion imaging** —combines the nonlinear detection performance of pulse inversion imaging with the motion discrimination capabilities of power Doppler. Multiple transmit pulses of alternating polarity are used and Doppler signal processing techniques are applied to distinguish between bubble echoes and echoes from moving tissue and/or tissue harmonics, as desired by the operator. This method offers potential improvements in the agent-to-tissue contrast and signal-to-noise performance, although at the cost of a somewhat reduced frame rate. The most dramatic manifestation of this method's ability to detect very weak harmonic echoes has been its first demonstration of real-time perfusion imaging of the

FIGURE 3-10. Basic principle of pulse inversion imaging. A pulse of sound is transmitted into the body and echoes are received from agent and tissue. A second pulse, which is an inverted copy of the first pulse, is then transmitted in the same direction and the two echoes are summed. Linear echoes from tissue will be inverted copies of each other and will cancel to zero. The microbubble echoes are distorted copies of each other, and the nonlinear components of these echoes will reinforce each other when summed, producing a strong harmonic signal. (From Becher H, Burns PN: Handbook of Contrast Echocardiography. Berlin, Springer, 2000. *http://www.sunnybrook.utoronto.ca /EchoHandbook/.*)

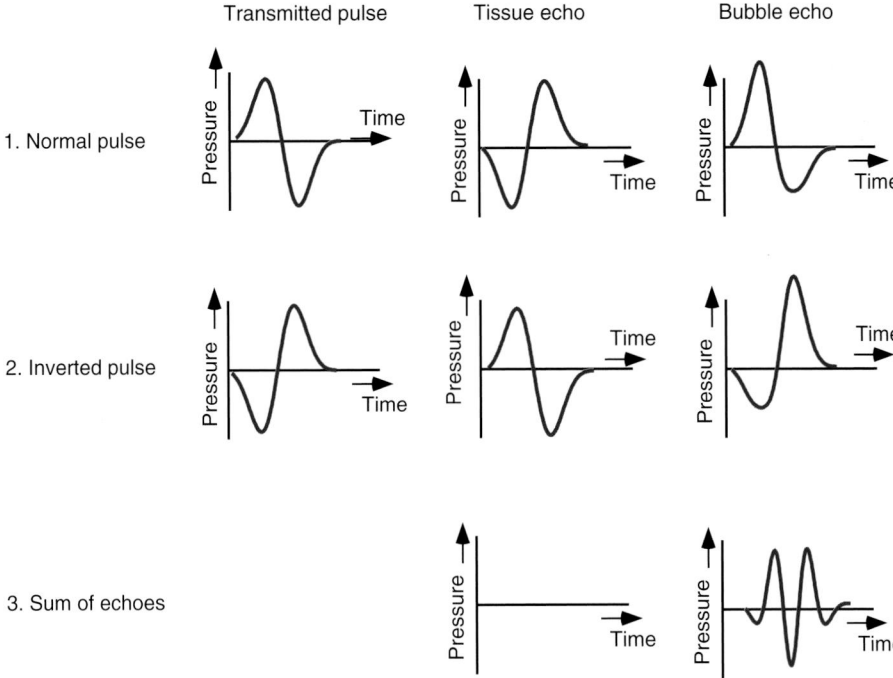

myocardium.[44] By lowering the MI to 0.1 or less, bubbles undergo stable, nonlinear oscillation, emitting continuous harmonic signals. Because of the low MI, very few bubbles are disrupted, so that imaging can take place at real-time rates. Because sustained, stable nonlinear oscillation is required for this method, perfluorocarbon gas bubbles work best.

Transient Disruption: Intermittent Imaging

As the incident pressure to which a resonating bubble is exposed increases, so its oscillation becomes more wild, with the radius increasing in some bubbles by a factor of 5 or more during the rarefaction phase of the incident sound. Just as a resonating violin string, if bowed over-zealously, will break, so a microbubble, if driven by intense ultrasound, will suffer irreversible disruption of its shell. A physical picture of precisely what happens to a disrupted bubble is only now emerging from high speed video studies (Fig. 3-11).[45] It is certain, however,

that the bubble disappears as an acoustic scatterer (not instantly, but over a period of time determined by the bubble composition), and that as it does so, it emits a strong, brief nonlinear echo. The detection of this echo is the basis of the most sensitive method to detect microbubble contrast at the perfusion level.[20]

Triggered Imaging

It was discovered during the early days of harmonic imaging that by pressing the **'freeze'** button on a scanner for a few moments, and, hence, interrupting the acquisition of ultrasound images during a contrast study, it is possible to increase the effectiveness of a contrast agent. So dramatic is this effect that it was responsible for the first ultrasound images of myocardial perfusion using harmonic imaging.[46] This is a consequence of the ability of the ultrasound field, if its peak pressure is sufficiently high, to disrupt a bubble's shell and, hence, destroy it.[41,47] As the bubble is disrupted, it releases energy, so creating a strong, transient echo, which is rich

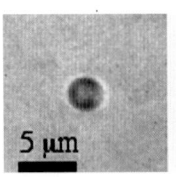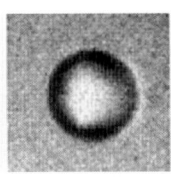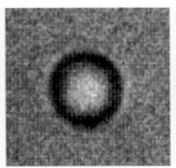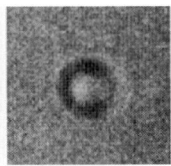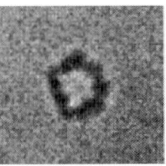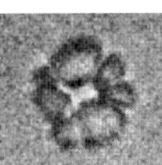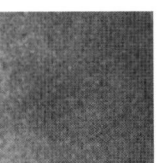

FIGURE 3-11. Fragmentation of contrast agent observed with a high-speed camera. This was done by researchers at the University of California, Davis. The frame images are captured over 50 ns. The bubble is insonated with 2.4 MHz ultrasound with a peak negative pressure of 1.1 MPa (MI ~0.7). The bubble is initially 3 μm in diameter and fragments during compression after the first expansion. Resulting bubble fragments are not seen after insonation because they are either fully dissolved or below the optical resolution. MI, Mechanical index. (From Becher H, Burns PN: Handbook of Contrast Echocardiography. Berlin, Springer, 2000. *http://www.sunnybrook.utoronto.ca/EchoHandbook/.*)

in harmonics. This process is sometimes incorrectly referred to as "stimulated acoustic emission." The fact that this echo is transient in nature can be exploited for its detection. One simple method is to subtract from a disruption image a baseline image obtained either before or (more usefully) immediately after insonation. Such a method requires offline processing of stored ultrasound images, together with software which can align the ultrasound images before subtraction, and is only useful in rare circumstances.[20]

Intermittent Harmonic Power Doppler for Perfusion Imaging

Power Doppler imaging is a technique designed to detect the motion of blood or of tissue. It works by a simple, pulse-to-pulse subtraction method,[48] in which two or more pulses are sent successively along each scan line of the image. Pairs of received echo trains are compared for each line: if they are identical, nothing is displayed, but if there is a change (due to motion of the tissue between pulses), a color is displayed whose saturation is related to the amplitude of the echo that has changed. This method, though not designed for the detection of bubble disruption, is ideally suited for high MI "destruction" imaging. The first pulse receives an echo from the bubble, the second receives none, so the comparison yields a strong signal. In a sense, power Doppler may be thought of as a line-by-line subtraction procedure on the radio frequency echo detected by the transducer. Interestingly for liver scanning, pulse inversion imaging—the most commonly used method at low MI—becomes equivalent to power Doppler if the MI is high and the bubble disrupted. Looking at Figure 3-9, one can easily see that if the echo from the second pulse is absent (because the bubble is gone), the sum of the two bubble echoes is the same as their difference, which is what is measured by power Doppler. The fact that the second transmitted pulse is inverted is immaterial for the bubble that has disappeared!

One critical question is how long one needs to wait between pulses. If the two pulses are too close together in time, the bubble's gaseous contents, which are dispersed after disruption of the shell by a process of diffusion and fragmentation, will still be able to provide an echo, so reducing the effectiveness of the detection. If the two pulses are too far apart in time, the solid tissue of the myocardium will have moved, so that the detection process will show them as well. There are two solutions. First, by using harmonic detection, some, but not all, of the moving tissue clutter can be rejected. Second, a bubble can be designed to disrupt quickly so that rapid (that is, high PRF) imaging may be used. Such a bubble will have a gas content that is highly diffusible and soluble in blood. In this respect, air is perfect. Diffusion of air after acoustic disruption is about

40 times faster than such diffusion of a perfluorocarbon gas from a similar bubble,[41] so that air-based agents such as Levovist are the most effective to image in this mode. Nonetheless, very effective imaging of perfluorocarbon bubbles throughout the liver can be made by using a sweep, a method commonly employed to map the distribution of bubbles in the postvascular phase of such agents as Levovist or SonoVue.

This, then, offers two distinct approaches to contrast imaging of the liver, which many investigators now use in combination (Fig. 3-12).[49] A **low MI**, real-time, non-destructive bubble imaging mode can be used to survey vessels in the liver. Such images show tumor vascular morphology and reveal arterialized lesions following a bolus injection of contrast (see Fig. 3-12A). The imaging modality of choice here will be **pulse inversion** (available on various systems as **phase inversion** or **coherent contrast imaging** [CCI]). Following this examination, a further injection is made and after the agent is seen to enter the hepatic arterial circulation, the scanner is set to **high MI** and frozen for an interval between 5 and 90 seconds, allowing the agent to enter the hepatic sinusoids. The scanner is unfrozen and a **flash or veil** is seen as the agent is disrupted[50] revealing the entire distribution of bubbles in the liver, including those in the parenchyma. This is a **liver perfusion image**. Depending on the delay, this can be timed to show the arterial (see Fig. 3-12B), portal (see Fig. 3-10), or postvascular phases. The preferred modes for this method are **pulse inversion**—which carries the attraction of high resolution imaging but the disadvantage of a strong tissue harmonic background—or power Doppler modes, such as **harmonic power angio** or **agent detection imaging** (ADI). Many systems now offer a low MI monitor mode that can be used to give a crude (usually fundamental) image of the liver during the interval delay which can be helpful to keep the scan plane aligned in the volume of interest. Pressing a button returns the scanner to the high MI nonlinear mode to produce the flash image of perfusion.

Summary

We have defined three regimens of behavior of bubbles in an acoustic field, which depend on the intensity of the transmitted ultrasound beam. In practice, this intensity is best monitored by means of the MI displayed by the scanner. At very low MI, the bubbles act as simple, but powerful, echo enhancers. This regimen is most useful for spectral Doppler enhancement but is rarely used in the liver. At slightly higher intensities (the bottom of the range of those used diagnostically), the bubbles emit harmonics as they undergo nonlinear oscillation. These harmonics can be detected by harmonic and pulse inversion imaging, which form the basis of real-time B-mode imaging of vascular structures in the liver. Newer

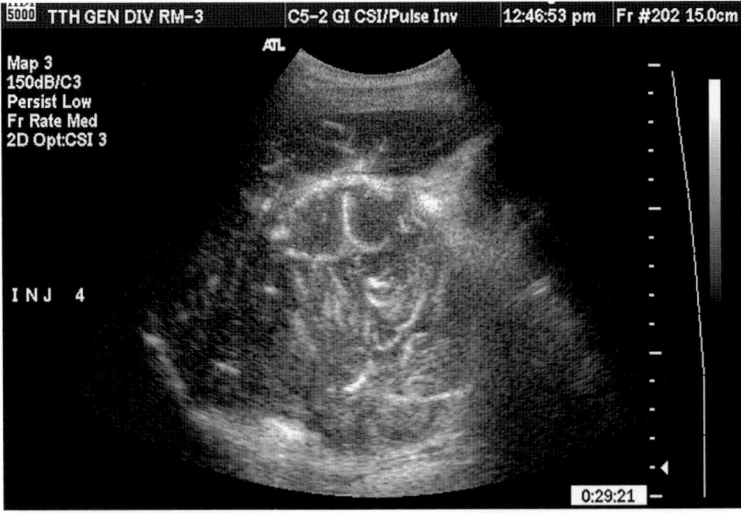

A

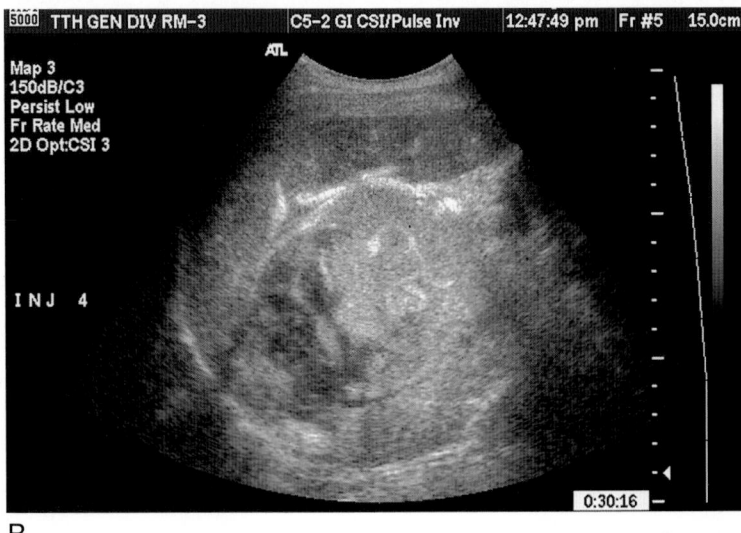

B

FIGURE 3-12. Contrast specific imaging. Using high and low MI contrast-specific imaging in the same patient as Figure 3-1. **A,** At low MI, real time pulse inversion imaging reveals the **extensive internal vasculature** of the lesion, with tortuous vessels defined with a resolution comparable to that of the conventional B-mode image. **B,** At high MI, after an 8-second interval delay, arterial perfusion is seen throughout the lesion, with the exception of an **area of necrosis**, which is well delineated. MI, Mechanical index. (From Burns PN, Wilson SR, Hope Simpson D: Pulse inversion imaging of liver blood flow: An improved method for characterization of focal masses with microbubble contrast. Invest Radiol 2000;35:58-71.)

techniques that employ many phase and/or amplitude modulated pulses, such as power pulse inversion (PPI) or contrast pulse sequence (CPS) imaging, are capable of sensitive imaging of perfusion at low MI without disrupting the bubbles. Finally, at the higher intensity setting of the machine used in routine scanning, the bubbles can be disrupted deliberately, emitting a strong, transient echo. Detecting this echo with harmonic power Doppler remains the most sensitive means we have to image bubbles in very low concentration, but it comes at the price of destroying the bubble. Because of the long reperfusion periods of hepatic flow, intermittent imaging using an interval delay in which the high MI imaging is arrested, becomes necessary.

Safety Considerations

Contrast ultrasound examinations expose patients to ultrasound in a way that is identical to that of a normal ultrasound examination. Yet the use of ultrasound pulses to disrupt bubbles that sit in microscopic vessels raises some new questions about the potential for hazard. When a bubble produces the brief echo that is associated with its disruption, it releases energy that it has stored during its exposure to the ultrasound field. Can this energy damage the surrounding tissue? At higher exposure levels, ultrasound is known to produce bioeffects in tissue, the thresholds for which have been studied extensively.[51] Do these thresholds change when bubbles are present in the vasculature? Whereas the safety of ultrasound contrast agents as drugs has been established to the satisfaction of the most stringent requirements of the regulating authorities in a number of countries, it is probably fair to say that there is much to be learned about the interaction between ultrasound and tissue when bubbles are present.

The most extreme of these interactions is known as **inertial cavitation**, which refers to the rapid formation, growth, and collapse of a gas cavity in fluid as a result of ultrasound exposure. It has been studied extensively prior to the development of microbubble contrast agents.[52] In fact, most of the mathematical models used to describe contrast microbubbles were originally developed to model cavitation.[28,53,54] When sound waves of sufficient intensity travel through a fluid, the rarefactional half-cycle of the sound wave can actually tear the fluid apart, creating spherical cavities within the fluid. The subsequent rapid collapse of these cavities during the compressional half cycle of the sound wave can focus large amounts of energy into a very small volume, raising the temperature at the center of the collapse to thousands of degrees Kelvin, forming free radicals, and even emitting electromagnetic radiation.[28,53,54]

The concern over potential cavitation-induced bioeffects in diagnostic ultrasound has led to many experimental studies. With the exception of one, which showed cavitation-induced hemorrhage in mouse lung exposed under conditions that differ substantially from those found clinically,[55] no evidence of bioeffects from clinical imaging combined with clinical contrast agent doses has been reported. Many more experiments have been made to assess whether the presence of contrast microbubbles can act as cavitation seeds, potentiating bioeffects.[56-61] While much has shown that adding contrast agents to blood increased cavitation effects (e.g., peroxide formation and acoustic emissions) and related bioeffects (e.g., hemolysis and platelet lysis), all significant bioeffects occurred with either very high agent concentration, sound pulse duration, or MI, or with a hematocrit well below the physiologic range. In experiments in which clinically relevant values of these parameters have been used (agent concentration <0.2 %, pulse duration <2 μsec, MI <1.9, hematocrit ~40% to 45%), no significant bioeffects have been reported to date.[58,62] Nonetheless, it is probably prudent to avoid the administration of lithotripter therapy within 24 hours of an ultrasound contrast examination.[63] It is also prudent to consider an extension of the ALARA (**As Low As Reasonably Achievable**) exposure principle to contrast ultrasound: The contrast ultrasound examination should expose the patient to the **lowest MI**, the **shortest total acoustic exposure time**, the **lowest contrast agent dose,** and the **highest ultrasound frequency**, consistent with obtaining adequate diagnostic information.

Conclusion

Unlike contrast agents for other imaging modalities, microbubbles are modified by the process used to image them. Understanding the behavior of bubbles when exposed to an ultrasound imaging beam is the key to performing an effective contrast ultrasound examination. The appropriate choice of a contrast-specific imaging method is based on the behavior of the agent and the requirements of the examination. MI is the major determinant of the response of contrast bubbles to ultrasound. Low MI harmonic and pulse inversion imaging offer real-time B-mode methods for liver vessel imaging. High MI harmonic power Doppler or pulse inversion can be used for intermittent imaging of liver perfusion with contrast agents, whereas pulse inversion Doppler imaging and related methods at very low MI allow real-time visualization of perfusion using perfluorocarbon agents.

References

1. Ophir J, Parker KJ: Contrast agents in diagnostic ultrasound [published erratum appears in Ultrasound Med Biol 1990;16(2):209]. Ultrasound Med Biol 1989;15:319-333.
2. Gramiak R, Shah PM: Echocardiography of the aortic root. Invest Radiol 1968;3:356-366.
3. Ziskin MC, Bonakdapour A, Weinstein DP, et al: Contrast agents for diagnostic ultrasound. Invest Radiol 1972;6:500-505.
4. Kremkau FW, Carstensen EL: Ultrasonic detection of cavitation at catheter tips. Am J Roentgenol 1968;3:159-167.
5. Kerber RE, Kioschos JM, Lauer RM: Use of an ultrasonic contrast method in the diagnosis of valvular regurgitation and intracardiac shunts. Am J Cardiol 1974;34:722-727.
6. Reid CL, Kawanishi DT, McKay CR: Accuracy of evaluation of the presence and severity of aortic and mitral regurgitation by contrast 2-dimensional echocardiography. Am J Cardiol 1983;52:519-524.
7. Sahn DJ, Valdex-Cruz LM: Ultrasonic contrast studies for the detection of cardiac shunts. J Am Coll Cardiol 1984;3:978-985.
8. Roelandt J: Contrast echocardiography. Ultrasound Med Biol 1982;8:471.
9. Carroll BA, Turner RJ, Tickner EG, et al: Gelatin encapsulated nitrogen microbubbles as ultrasonic contrast agents. Invest Radiol 1980;15:260-266.
10. Feinstein SB, Shah PM, Bing RJ, et al: Microbubble dynamics visualized in the intact capillary circulation. J Am Coll Cardiol 1984;4:595-600.
11. Schlief R: Echo enhancement: Agents and techniques—basic principles. Adv Echo-Contrast 1994;4:5-19.
12. Fritzsch T, Schartl M, Siegert J: Preclinical and clinical results with an ultrasonic contrast agent. Invest Radiol 1988;23:302-305.
13. Goldberg BB, Liu JB, Burns PN, et al: Galactose-based intravenous sonographic contrast agent: Experimental studies. J Ultrasound Med 1993;12:463-470.
14. Fobbe F, Ohnesorge O, Reichel M, et al: Transpulmonary contrast agent and color-coded duplex sonography: First clinical experience. Radiology 1992;185(P):142.
15. Unger E, Shen D, Fritz T, et al: Gas-filled lipid bilayers as ultrasound contrast agents. Invest Radiol 1994;29:134-136.
16. Mattrey RF, Scheible FW, Gosink BB, et al: Perfluorocytlbromide: A liver/spleen-specific and tumor-imaging ultrasound contrast material. Radiology 1982;145:759-762.
17. Fritzsch T, Hauff P, Heldmann F, et al: Preliminary results with a new liver specific ultrasound contrast agent. Ultrasound Med Biol 1994;20:137.
18. Mattrey RF, Leopold GR, VanSonnenberg E, et al: Perfluorochemicals as liver- and spleen-seeking ultrasound contrast agents. J Ultrasound Med 1983;2:173-176.

19. Albrecht T, Blomley M, Burns PN, et al: Improved detection of hepatic metastases with pulse inversion ultrasonography during the liver-specific phase of SHU 508A (Levovist): A multicenter study. Radiology 2003;227:361-370.

20. Becher H, Burns PN: Handbook of Contrast Echocardiography. Berlin, Springer, 2000. *http://www.sunnybrook.utoronto.ca/EchoHandbook/*.

21. Cosgrove DO, Bamber JC, Davey JB, et al: Color Doppler signals from breast tumors. Work in progress. Radiology 1990;176:175-180.

22. Chin CT, Burns PN: Predicting the acoustic response of a microbubble population for contrast imaging. In Proc, IEEE Ultrason Symp, 1997, pp 1557-1560.

23. De Jong N: Physics of Microbubble Scattering. In Nanda NC, Schlief R, Goldberg BB (eds): Advances in echo imaging using contrast enhancement. (2nd ed). Dubai Kluwer, 1997, pp 39-64.

24. Apfel RE, Holland CK: Gauging the likelihood of cavitation from short-pulse, low-duty cycle diagnostic ultrasound. Ultrasound Med and Biol 1991;17:175-185.

25. Burns PN, Powers JE, Hope Simpson D, et al: Harmonic power mode Doppler using microbubble contrast agents: An improved method for small vessel flow imaging. Proc IEEE UFFC 1994:1547-1550.

26. Bleeker H, Shung K, Barnhart J: On the application of ultrasonic contrast agents for blood flowmetry and assessment of cardiac perfusion. J Ultrasound Med 1990;9:461-471.

27. Neppiras EA, Nyborg WL, Miller PL: Nonlinear behavior and stability of trapped micron-sized cylindrical gas bubbles in an ultrasound field. Ultrasonics 1983;21:109-115.

28. Rayleigh L: On the pressure developed in a liquid during the collapse of a spherical cavity. Philosophy Magazine 1917;Series 6:94-98.

29. Burns PN, Powers JE, Fritzsch T: Harmonic imaging: A new imaging and Doppler method for contrast enhanced ultrasound. Radiology 1992;185(P):142 (Abstr).

30. Burns PN, Powers JE, Hope Simpson D, et al: Harmonic contrast enhanced Doppler as a method for the elimination of clutter—In vivo duplex and color studies. Radiology 1993;189:285.

31. Mulvagh SL, Foley DA, Aeschbacher BC, et al: Second harmonic imaging of an intravenously administered echocardiographic contrast agent: Visualization of coronary arteries and measurement of coronary blood flow. J Am Coll Cardiol 1996;27:1519-1525.

32. Porter TR, Xie F, Kricsfeld D, et al: Improved myocardial contrast with second harmonic transient ultrasound response imaging in humans using intravenous perfluorocarbon-exposed sonicated dextrose albumin. J Am Coll Cardiol 1996;27:1497-1501.

33. Mattrey RF, Steinbach G, Lee Y, et al: High-resolution harmonic gray-scale imaging of normal and abnormal vessels and tissues in animals. Acad Radiol 1998;5:S63-S65.

34. Kono Y, Moriyasu F, Yamada K, et al: Conventional and harmonic gray scale enhancement of the liver with sonication activation of a US contrast agent. Radiology 1996;201:266.

35. Rubin JM, Bude RO, Carson PL, et al: Power Doppler US: A potentially useful alternative to mean frequency-based color Doppler US. Radiology 1994;190:853-856.

36. Burns PN, Wilson SR, Muradali D, et al: Intermittent US harmonic contrast enhanced imaging and Doppler improves sensitivity and longevity of small vessel detection. Radiology 1996;201:159.

37. Becher H: Second harmonic imaging with Levovist: Initial clinical experience. In Cate FT, DeJong N (eds): Second European Symposium on Ultrasound Contrast Imaging. Book of Abstracts, Rotterdam, Erasmus Univ, 1997, p 24.

38. Hamilton MF, Blackstock DT (eds): Nonlinear Acoustics. San Diego, Academic Press, 1998.

39. Averkiou MA, Roundhill DN, Powers JE: A new imaging technique based on the nonlinear properties of tissues. In Proc IEEE Ultrason Symp, 1997, pp 1561-1566.

40. Ortega D, Wilson SR, Hope Simpson D, et al: Tissue harmonic imaging: A benefit for bile duct evaluation? Am J Roentgenol 2001;176:653-659.

41. Burns PN, Wilson SR, Muradali D, et al: Microbubble destruction is the origin of harmonic signals from FS069. Radiology 1996;201:158.

42. Hope Simpson D, Chin CT, Burns PN: Pulse inversion Doppler: A new method for detecting nonlinear echoes from microbubble contrast agents. IEEE Transactions UFFC 1999;46:372-382.

43. Burns PN, Wilson SR, Hope Simpson D: Pulse inversion imaging of liver blood flow: An improved method for characterization of focal masses with microbubble contrast. Invest Radiol 2000;35:58-71.

44. Tiemann K, Lohmeier S, Kuntz S, et al: Real-time contrast echo assessment of myocardial perfusion at low emission power: First experimental and clinical results using power pulse inversion imaging. Echocardiography 1999;16:799-809.

45. Dayton PA, Morgan KE, Klibanov AL, et al: Optical and acoustical observations of the effects of ultrasound contrast agents. IEEE Transaction on Ultrasonics, Ferroelectrics, and Frequency Control 1999;46:220-232.

46. Porter TR, Xie F: Transient myocardial contrast after initial exposure to diagnostic ultrasound pressures with minute doses of intravenously injected microbubbles: Demonstration and potential mechanisms. Circulation 1995;92:2391-2395.

47. Uhlendorf V, Scholle F-D: Imaging of spatial distribution and flow of microbubbles using nonlinear acoustic properties. Acoustical Imaging 1996;22:233-238.

48. Burns PN: Interpretation of Doppler ultrasound signals. In Burns PN, Taylor KJ, Wells PNT (eds): Clinical Applications of Doppler Ultrasound. (2nd ed). New York, Raven Press, 1996.

49. Wilson SR, Burns PN: Liver mass evaluation with ultrasound: The impact of microbubble contrast agents and pulse inversion imaging. Sem Liver Disease 2001;21:147-161.

50. Wilson SR, Burns PN, Muradali D, et al: Harmonic hepatic ultrasound with microbubble contrast agent: Initial experience showing improved characterization of hemangioma, hepatocellular carcinoma, and metastasis. Radiology 2000;215:153-161.

51. Mechanical bioeffects from diagnostic ultrasound: AIUM consensus statements. J Ultrasound Med 2000;19:120-142.

52. Brennan CE: Cavitation and Bubble Dynamics. New York, Oxford University Press, 1995.

53. Poritsky H: The collapse or growth of a spherical bubble or cavity in a viscous fluid. In Sternberg E (ed): First U.S. National Congress on Appl Mech, 1951;813-821.

54. Plesset MS: The dynamics of cavitation bubbles. J Appl Mech 1949;16:272-282.

55. Price RJ, Skyba DM, Kaul S, et al: Delivery of colloidal particles and red blood cells to tissue through microvessel ruptures created by targeted microbubble destruction with ultrasound. Circulation 1998;98:1264-1267.

56. Williams AR, Kubowicz G, Cramer E: The effects of the microbubble suspension SHU 454 (Echovist) on ultrasound-induced cell lysis in a rotating tube exposure system. Echocardiography 1991;8:423-433.

57. Miller MW, Miller DL, Brayman A: A review of in vitro bioeffects of inertial ultrasonic cavitation from a mechanistic perspective. Ultrasound Med Biol 1996;22:1131-1154.

58. Miller DL, Gies RA, Chrisler WB: Ultrasonically induced hemolysis at high cell and gas body concentrations in a thin-disk exposure chamber. Ultrasound Med Biol 1997;23:625-633.

59. Miller DL, Thomas RM: Ultrasound contrast agents nucleate inertial cavitation in vitro. Ultrasound Med Biol 1995;21:1059-1065.

60. Holland CK, Roy RA, Apfel RE, et al: In vitro detection of cavitation induced by a diagnostic ultrasound system. IEEE Trans. IEEE Transaction on Ultrasonics, Ferroelectrics, and Frequency Control 1992;29:95-101.

61. Everbach EC, Makin IRS, Francis CW, et al: Effect of acoustic cavitation on platelets in the presence of an echo-contrast agent. Ultrasound Med Biol 1998;24:129-136.

62. Uhlendorf V, Hoffmann C: Nonlinear acoustical response of coated microbubbles in diagnostic ultrasound. Proc IEEE Ultrasonics Symp 1994:1559-1562.

63. Miller DL, Gies RA: Consequences of lithotripter shockwave interaction with gas body contrast agent in mouse intestine. J Urology 1999;162:606-609.

II

*A*BDOMINAL, PELVIC, AND THORACIC SONOGRAPHY

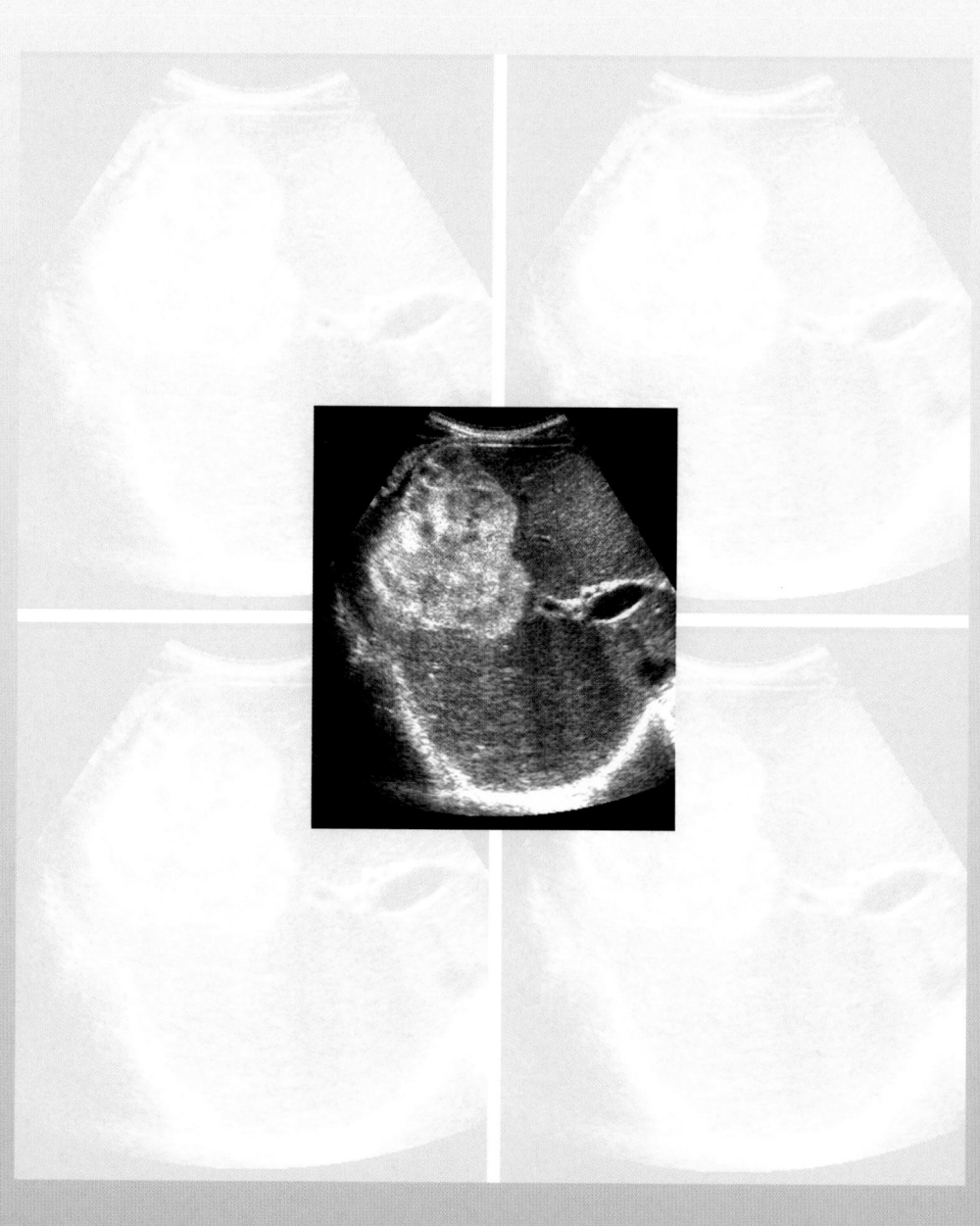

4

THE LIVER

Stephanie R. Wilson / Cynthia E. Withers

Chapter Outline

The liver is the largest organ in the human body, weighing approximately 1500 g in the adult. Because it is frequently involved in systemic and local disease, sonographic examination is often requested to assess hepatic abnormality.

TECHNIQUE

The liver is best examined with real-time sonography, ideally, following a 6-hour fast so that bowel gas is limited and the gallbladder is not contracted. Both supine and right anterior oblique views should be obtained if the patient can move or be moved. Because many patients have livers that are tucked beneath the lower right ribs, a transducer with a small scanning face, allowing an intercostal approach, is invaluable. Suspended inspiration enables examination of the dome of the liver, frequently an ultrasound *blind spot*. Sagittal, transverse, coronal, and subcostal oblique views are required for a complete survey.

NORMAL ANATOMY

The liver lies in the right upper quadrant of the abdomen, suspended from the right hemidiaphragm. Functionally, it can be divided into **three lobes**—right, left, and caudate lobes. The right lobe of the liver is separated from the left by the main lobar fissure, which passes through the gallbladder fossa to the inferior vena cava (Fig. 4-1). The **right lobe of the liver** can be further divided into anterior and posterior segments by the right intersegmental fissure. The left intersegmental

fissure divides the **left lobe** into medial and lateral segments. The **caudate lobe** is situated on the posterior aspect of the liver, having as its posterior border the inferior vena cava and as its anterior border the fissure for the ligamentum venosum (Fig. 4-2). The papillary process is the anteromedial extension of the caudate lobe, which may appear separate from the liver and mimic lymphadenopathy.

Understanding the **vascular anatomy of the liver** is essential to an appreciation of the relative positions of the hepatic segments. The major **hepatic veins** course between the lobes and segments (**interlobar and intersegmental**). They are ideal segmental boundaries but are visualized only when scanning the superior liver (Fig. 4-3). The middle hepatic vein courses within the main lobar fissure and separates the anterior segment of the right lobe from the medial segment of the left. The right hepatic vein runs within the **right intersegmental fissure** and divides the right lobe into anterior and posterior segments. In more caudal sections of the liver, the right hepatic vein is no longer identified, therefore the segmental boundary becomes a more ill-defined division between the anterior and posterior branches of the right portal vein. The major branches of the right and left **portal veins** run centrally within the segments (**intrasegmental**), with the exception of the ascending portion of the left portal vein, which runs in the left intersegmental fissure. The **left intersegmental fissure**, which separates the medial segment of the left lobe from the lateral segment, can be divided into cranial, middle, and caudal sections. The left hepatic vein forms the boundary of the cranial third, the ascending branch of the left portal vein represents the middle third, and the fissure for the ligamentum teres acts as the most caudal division of the left lobe (Table 4-1).[1]

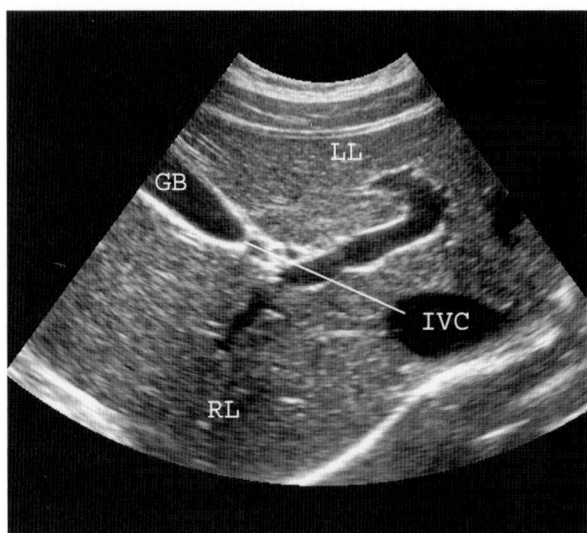

FIGURE 4-1. Normal lobar anatomy. The right lobe of the liver (RL) can be separated from the left lobe of the liver (LL) by the main lobar fissure that passes through the gallbladder fossa (GB) and the inferior vena cava (IVC).

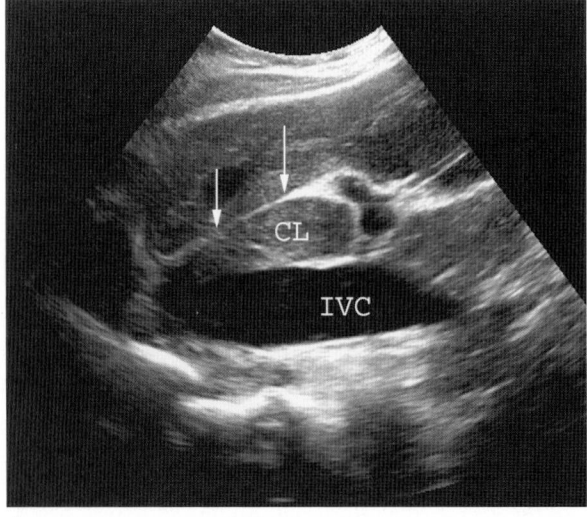

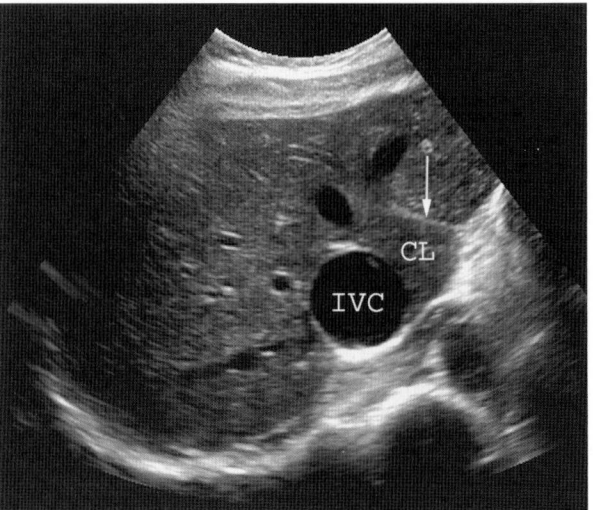

A   B

FIGURE 4-2. Caudate lobe. A, Sagittal and **B,** transverse views show the caudate lobe (CL) is separated from the left lobe by the fissure for the ligamentum venosum (*arrows*) anteriorly. Posterior is the inferior vena cava (IVC).

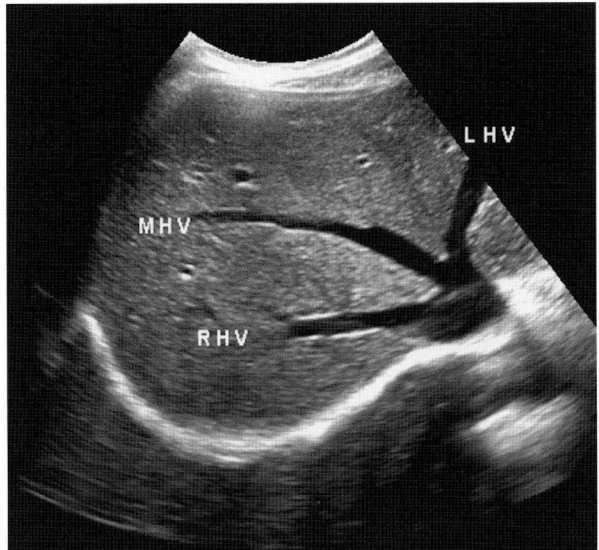

FIGURE 4-3. Hepatic venous anatomy. The three hepatic veins—right (RHV), middle (MHV), and left (LHV), are interlobar and intersegmental, separating the lobes and segments. At the level of the hepatic venous confluence with the inferior vena cava, the right hepatic vein separates the right posterior segment (segment 7) from the right anterior segment (segment 8). The left hepatic vein separates the left medial segment from the left lateral segment. The middle hepatic vein separates the right and left lobes. The hepatic veins are best seen on a subcostal oblique view as here.

Couinaud's Anatomy

Because sonography allows evaluation of liver anatomy in multiple planes, the radiologist can precisely localize a lesion to a given segment for the surgeon. Couinaud's anatomy, widely used in Europe and French Canada, is

TABLE 4-2. HEPATIC ANATOMY

Couinaud	Traditional
Segment I	Caudate lobe
Segment II	Lateral segment left lobe (superior)
Segment III	Lateral segment left lobe (inferior)
Segment IV	Medial segment left lobe
Segment V	Anterior segment right lobe (inferior)
Segment VI	Posterior segment right lobe (inferior)
Segment VII	Posterior segment right lobe (superior)
Segment VIII	Anterior segment right lobe (superior)

now becoming the universal nomenclature for hepatic lesion localization (Table 4-2).[2] This description is **based on portal segments** and is of both functional and pathologic importance. Each segment has its own blood supply (arterial, portal venous, and hepatic venous), lymphatics, and biliary drainage. Thus, the surgeon may resect a segment of a hepatic lobe, providing the vascular supply to the remaining lobe is left intact. Each segment has a branch or branches of the portal vein at its center, bounded by a hepatic vein. There are **eight segments**. The right, middle, and left hepatic veins divide the liver longitudinally into four sections. Each of these sections is further divided transversely by an imaginary plane through the right main and left main portal pedicles. Segment I is the caudate lobe, segments II and III are the left superior and inferior lateral segments, respectively, and segment IV, which is further divided into IVa and IVb, is the medial segment of the left lobe. The right lobe consists of segments V and VI, located caudal to the transverse plane, and segments VII and VIII, which are

TABLE 4-1. NORMAL HEPATIC ANATOMY: ANATOMIC STRUCTURES USEFUL FOR IDENTIFYING THE HEPATIC SEGMENTS

Structure	Location	Usefulness
RHV	Right intersegmental fissure	Divides cephalic aspect of anterior and posterior segments of right lobe
MHV	Main lobar fissure	Separates right and left lobes
LHV	Left intersegmental fissure	Divides cephalic aspect of medial and lateral segments of left lobe
RPV (anterior branch)	Intrasegmental in anterior segment of right lobe	Courses centrally in anterior segment of right lobe
RPV (posterior branch)	Intrasegmental in posterior segment of right lobe	Courses centrally in posterior segment of right lobe
LPV (horizontal segment)	Anterior to caudate lobe	Separates caudate lobe posteriorly from medial segment of left lobe anteriorly
LPV (ascending segment)	Left intersegmental fissure	Divides medial from lateral segment of left lobe
GB fossa	Main lobar fissure	Separates right and left lobes
Fissure for the ligamentum teres	Left intersegmental fissure	Divides caudal aspect of left lobe into medial and lateral segments
Fissure for the ligamentum venosum	Left anterior margin of the caudate lobe	Separates caudate lobe posteriorly from left lobe anteriorly

GB, gallbladder; LHV, left hepatic vein; LPV, left portal vein; MHV, middle hepatic vein; RHV, right hepatic vein; RPV, right portal vein.
Modified from Marks WM, Filly RA, Callen PW. Ultrasonic anatomy of the liver: A review with new applications. J Clin Ultrasound 1979; 7:137–146.

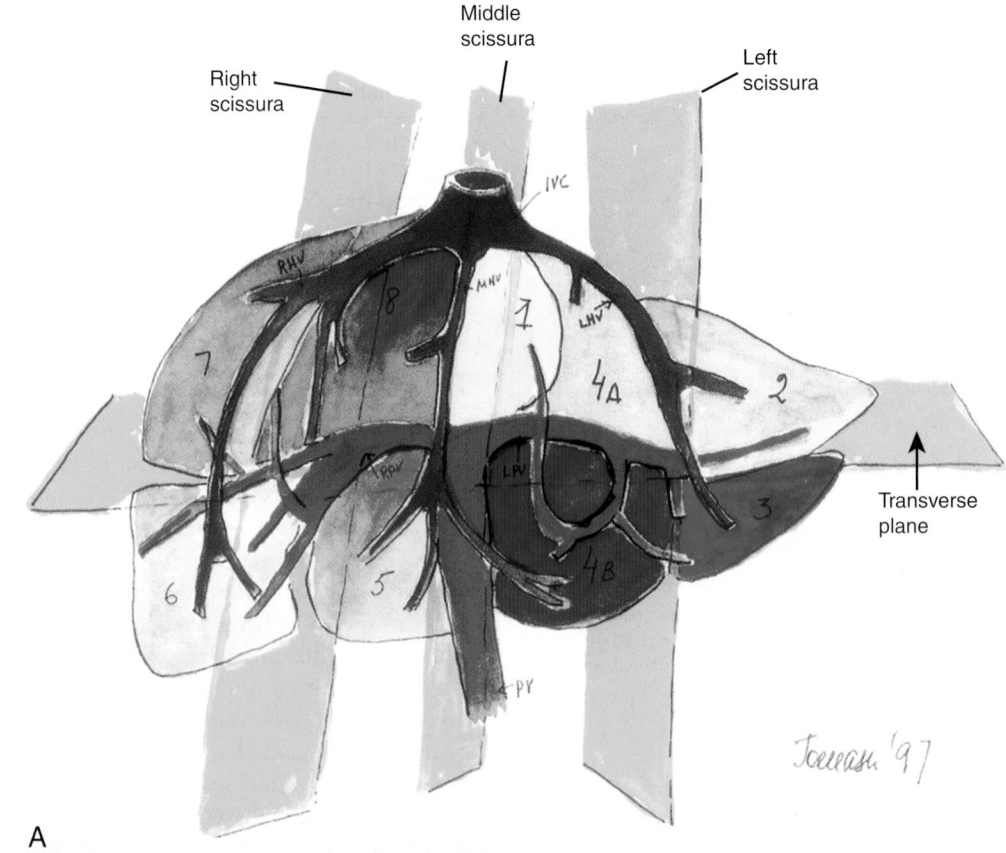

A

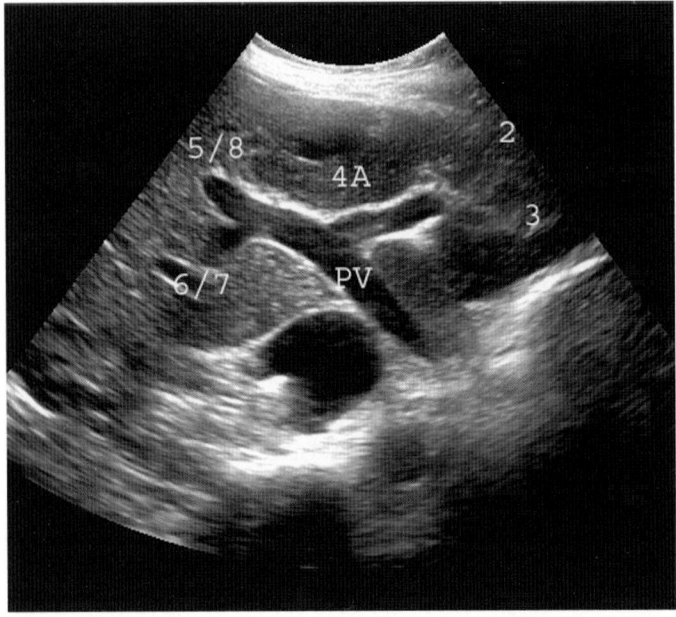

B

FIGURE 4-4. Couinaud's functional segmental anatomy. A, The liver is divided into nine segments. Yellow longitudinal boundaries (right, middle, and left scissurae) are three hepatic veins. Transverse plane is defined by right main and left main portal pedicles. Segment I, caudate lobe (*pale yellow region*), is situated posteriorly. RHV, right hepatic vein; MHV, middle hepatic vein; LHV, left hepatic vein; RPV, right portal vein; LPV, left portal vein; GB, gallbladder. **B,** Corresponding sonogram shows the main portal vein with its right and left branches. The plane through the right and left branches is the transverse separation of the liver segments. Cephalad to this level lie segments II, IVa, VII, and VIII. Caudally located are segments III, IVb, V, and VI. (From Sugarbaker PH: Toward a standard of nomenclature for surgical anatomy of the liver. Neth J Surg 1988;PO:100.)

cephalad (Fig. 4-4).[3,4,5] The caudate lobe (segment I) may receive branches of both the right and left portal veins. In contrast to the other segments, it has one or several hepatic veins which drain directly into the inferior vena cava.

The portal venous supply for the left lobe can be visualized using an oblique, cranially-angled subxiphoid view (recurrent subcostal oblique projection). A "recumbent H" is formed by the main left portal vein, the ascending branch of the left portal vein, and the branches to segments, II, III, and IV (Fig. 4-5B).[6] Segments II and III are separated from segment IV by the left hepatic vein, as well as by the ascending branch of the left portal vein and the falciform ligament. Segment IV is separated from segments V and VIII by the middle hepatic vein and the main hepatic fissure.

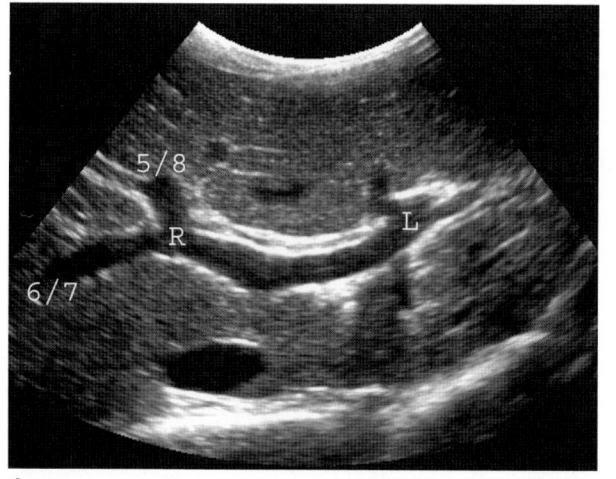
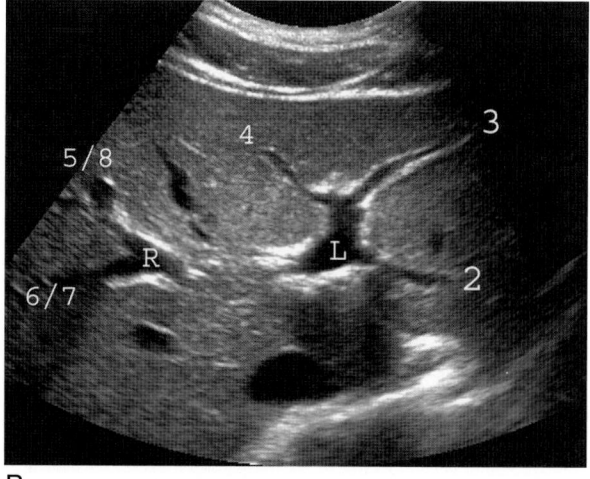

A

B

FIGURE 4-5. Portal venous anatomy in two patients. A, Best seen with a subcostal oblique view, the main portal vein is formed by the union of the right and left portal venous branches at the porta hepatis. **B,** The segmental branches of the right and left portal veins are marked. Well seen is the recumbent H shape of the left portal venous bifurcation made from the ascending and horizontal left portal vein and the segmental branches to 2, 3, and 4.

The portal venous supply to the right lobe of the liver can also be seen as a recumbent H.[6] The main right portal vein gives rise to branches that supply segments V and VI (inferiorly) and VII and VIII (superiorly). They are seen best in a sagittal or oblique-sagittal plane (Fig. 4-6).[6]

With the oblique subxiphoid view, the right portal vein is seen in cross section and enables identification of the more superiorly located segment VIII (which is closer to the confluence of hepatic veins) from segment V. Segments V and VIII are separated from segments VI and VII by the right hepatic vein.[6]

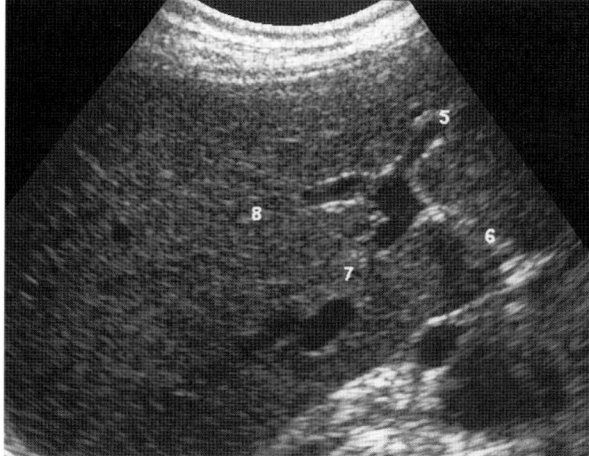

FIGURE 4-6. Recumbent H shape. Recumbent H of right portal venous bifurcation is more difficult to visualize, and is best seen with an intercostal view. Right portal venous bifurcation shows the branches to the anterior segments, 5 and 8, and the posterior segments 6 and 7.

Ligaments

The liver is covered by a thin connective tissue layer called **Glisson's capsule.** The capsule surrounds the entire liver and is thickest around the inferior vena cava and the porta hepatis. At the porta hepatis the main portal vein, the proper hepatic artery, and the common bile duct are contained within investing peritoneal folds known as the **hepatoduodenal ligament** (Fig. 4-7). The **falciform ligament** conducts the umbilical vein to the liver during fetal development (Fig. 4-8). After birth, the umbilical vein atrophies, forming the ligamentum teres. As it reaches the liver, the leaves of the falciform ligament separate. The right layer forms the upper layer of the **coronary ligament;** the left layer forms the upper layer of the **left triangular ligament.** The most lateral portion of the coronary ligament is known as the **right triangular ligament** (Fig. 4-9). The peritoneal layers that form the coronary ligament are widely separated, leaving an area of the liver not covered by peritoneum. This posterosuperior region is known as the *bare area* of the liver. The **ligamentum venosum** carries the obliterated ductus venosus, which until birth shunts blood from the umbilical vein to the inferior vena cava (Fig. 4-10).

Hepatic Circulation

Portal Veins

The liver receives a **dual blood supply** from both the portal vein and the hepatic artery. Although the portal vein carries incompletely oxygenated (80%) venous blood from the intestines and spleen, it supplies up to

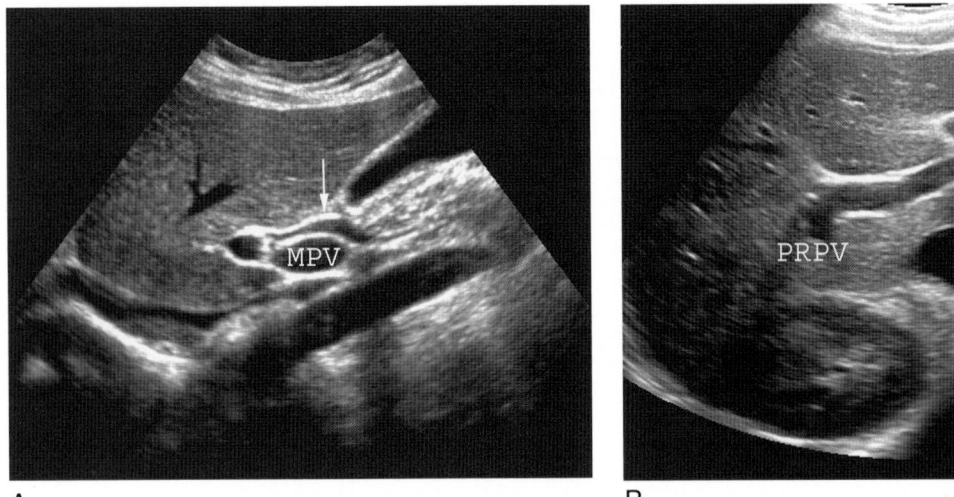

FIGURE 4-7. Porta hepatis. A, Sagittal image of the porta hepatis shows the common bile duct (*arrow*) and main portal vein (MPV), which are enclosed within the hepatoduodenal ligament. **B,** Transverse image of the porta hepatis shows the right and left portal vein branches. Posterior right portal vein (PRPV); ascending left portal vein (ALPV).

one half the oxygen requirements of the hepatocytes because of its greater flow. This dual blood supply explains the low incidence of hepatic infarction.

The **portal triad** contains a branch of the portal vein, hepatic artery, and bile duct. These are contained within a connective tissue sheath that gives the portal vein an echogenic wall on sonography and allows for its distinction from the hepatic veins, which have an almost imperceptible wall. The main portal vein divides into right and left branches. The right portal vein has an anterior branch that lies centrally within the anterior segment of the right lobe and a posterior branch that lies centrally within the posterior segment of the right lobe. The left portal vein initially courses anterior to the caudate lobe. The ascending branch of the left portal vein then travels anteriorly in the left intersegmental fissure to divide the medial and lateral segments of the left lobe.

Arterial Circulation

The branches of the hepatic artery accompany the portal veins. The terminal branches of the portal vein and their accompanying hepatic arterioles and bile ducts are known as the acinus.

Hepatic Venous System

Blood perfuses the liver parenchyma through the sinusoids and then enters the terminal hepatic venules. These terminal branches unite to form sequentially larger veins. The hepatic veins vary in number and position. However, in the general population, there are **three major veins**: the right, middle, and left hepatic veins (see Fig. 4-3). All drain into the inferior vena cava and, like the portal veins, are without valves. The **right hepatic vein** is usually single and runs in the right intersegmental fissure, separating the anterior and posterior segments of the right lobe. The **middle hepatic vein**, which courses in the main lobar fissure, forms a common trunk with the left hepatic vein in the majority of individuals. The **left hepatic vein** forms the most cephalad boundary between the medial and lateral segments of the left lobe.

Normal Liver Size and Echogenicity

The upper border of the liver lies approximately at the level of the fifth intercostal space at the midclavicular line. The lower border extends to or slightly below the costal margin. An accurate assessment of liver size is difficult with real-time ultrasound equipment because of the limited field of view. Gosink[7] proposed measuring the liver length in the midhepatic line. In 75% of patients with a liver length of greater than 15.5 cm, hepatomegaly is present. Niederau et al.[8] measured the liver in a longitudinal and anteroposterior diameter in both the midclavicular line and midline and correlated these findings with gender, age, height, weight, and body surface area. They found that organ size increases with height and body surface area and decreases with age. The mean longitudinal diameter of the liver in the midclavicular line in this study was 10.5 with 1.5 (standard deviation) cm and the mean midclavicular anteroposterior diameter was 8.1 with 1.9 (standard deviation) cm. In most patients, measurement of the liver length suffices to measure liver size. In heavy or asthenic individuals, the anteroposterior diameter should be added to avoid underestimations and over-

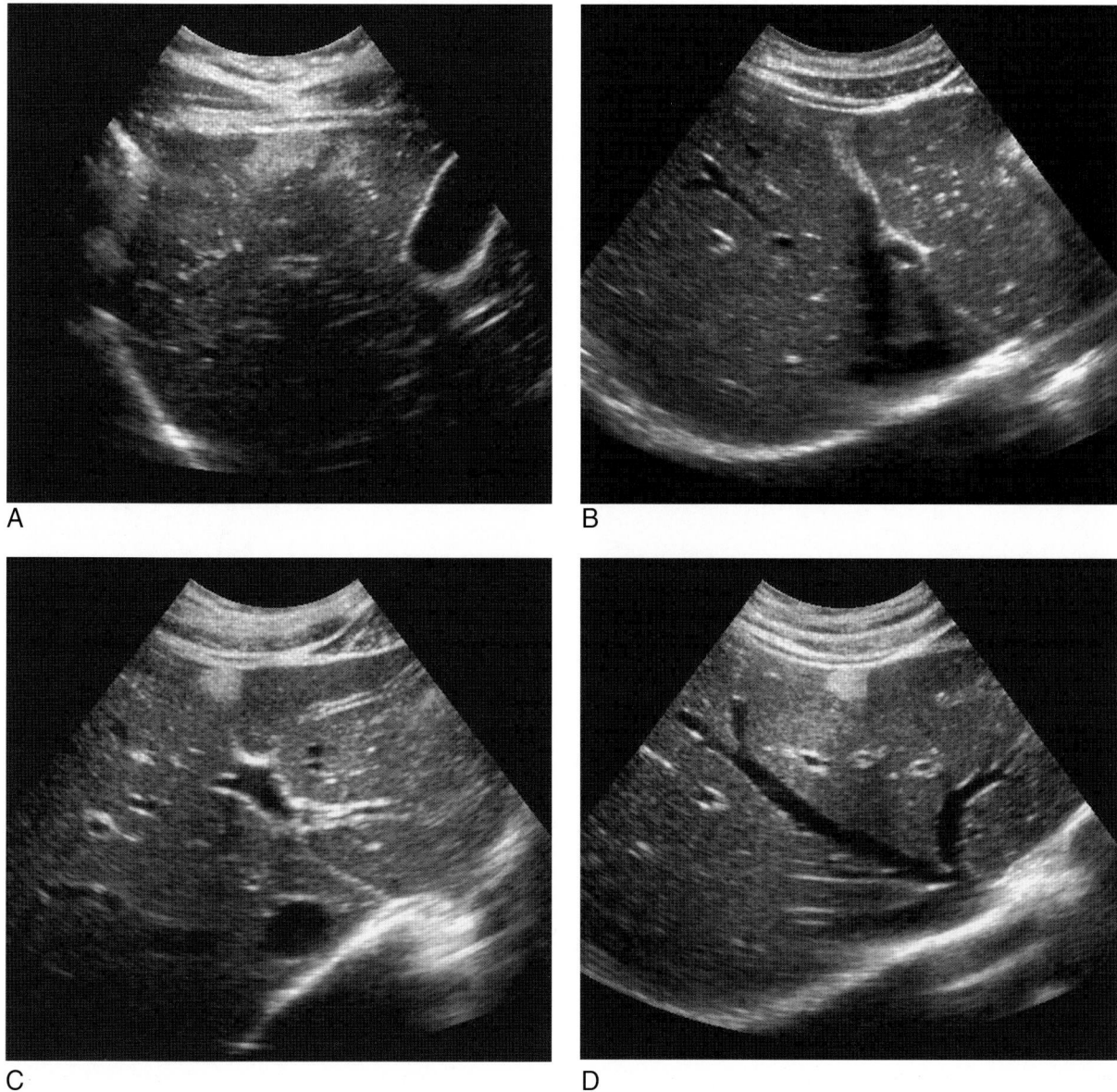

FIGURE 4-8. Falciform ligament. Contained fat helps in its localization. **A,** Sagittal image through the ligament. **B,** Subcostal oblique view of the ligament. **C,** Shows the location of the fat just anterior to the ascending branch of the left ascending portal vein branch. **D,** Shows the cephalad extent of the fat in the location of the ligament between the middle and the left hepatic veins.

estimations, respectively. Reidel's lobe is a tongue-like extension of the inferior tip of the right lobe of the liver, which is frequently found in asthenic women.

The normal liver is homogeneous, contains fine-level echoes, and is either minimally hyperechoic or isoechoic compared to the normal renal cortex (Fig. 4-11A). The liver is hypoechoic compared to the spleen. This relationship is evident when the lateral segment of the left lobe is elongated and wraps around the spleen (see Fig. 4-11B).

DEVELOPMENTAL ANOMALIES

Agenesis

Agenesis of the liver is incompatible with life. Agenesis of both the right and left lobes has been reported.[9,10] In three of five reported cases of agenesis of the right lobe, the caudate lobe was also absent.[10] Compensatory hypertrophy of the remaining lobes normally occurs, and liver function tests are normal.

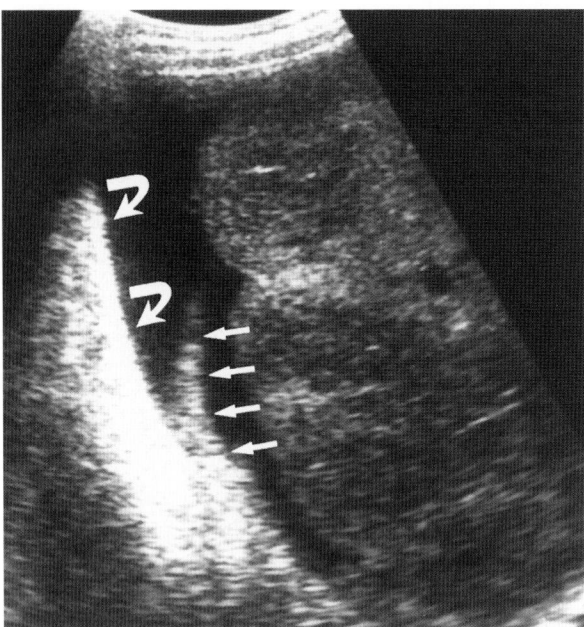

FIGURE 4-9. Right triangular ligament. Subcostal oblique scan near dome of right hemidiaphragm (*curved arrows*). Note lobulated contour and inhomogeneity of liver in this patient with cirrhosis. Right triangular ligament (*straight arrows*) is visualized because of ascites.

Anomalies of Position

In situs inversus totalis, the liver is found in the left hypochondrium. In congenital diaphragmatic hernia or omphalocele, varying amounts of liver may herniate into the thorax or outside the abdominal cavity.

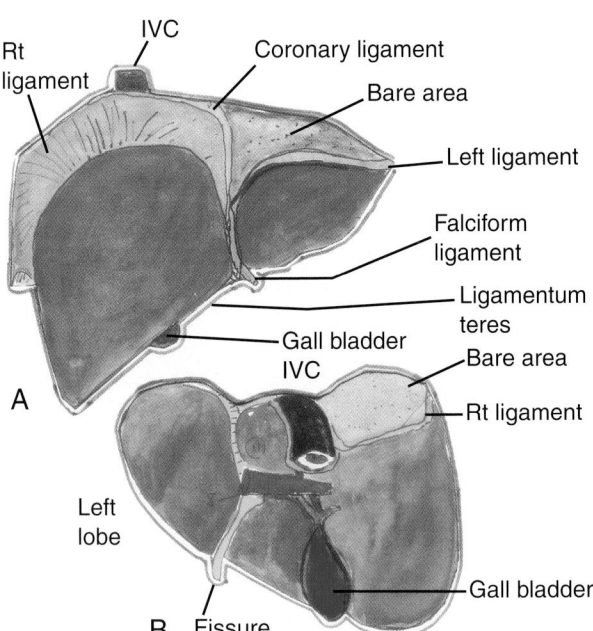

FIGURE 4-10. Hepatic ligaments. Diagram of **A**, anterior and **B**, posterior surfaces of the liver.

Accessory Fissures

Although invaginations of the dome of the diaphragm have been called accessory fissures, strictly speaking, these are not fissures but rather diaphragmatic slips. They are a cause of pseudomasses on sonography if the liver is not carefully examined in both sagittal and transverse planes (Fig. 4-12). True accessory fissures are uncommon and are caused by an infolding of perito-

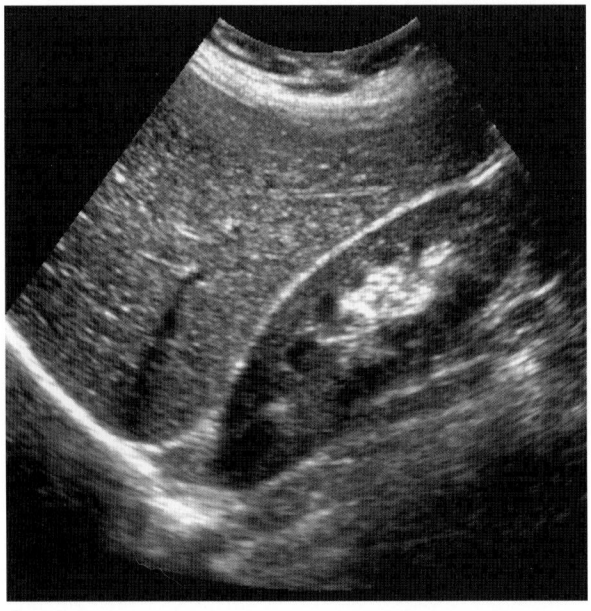

A

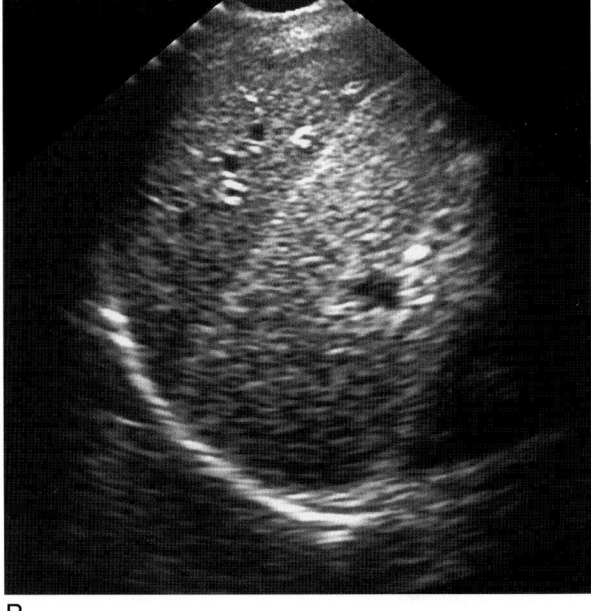

B

FIGURE 4-11. Normal liver echogenicity. A, The liver is more echogenic than the renal cortex. **B,** The liver is less echogenic than the spleen, as can be seen in many thin women, whose left lobe of the liver wraps around the spleen as seen here.

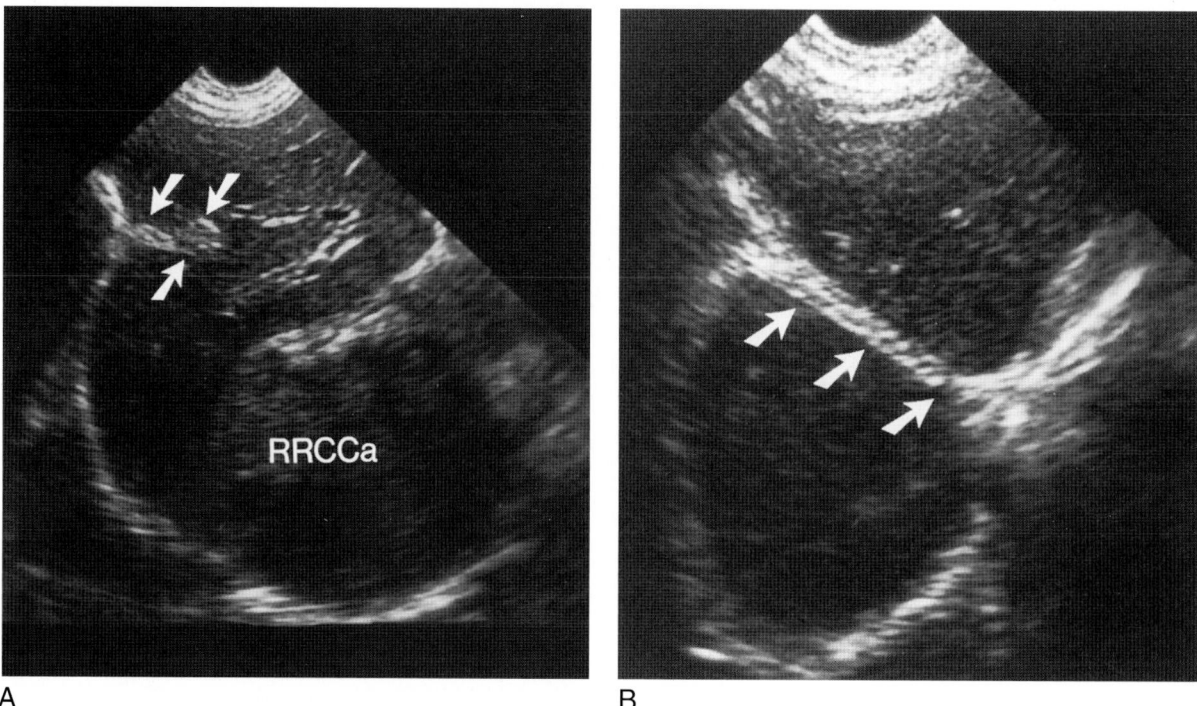

FIGURE 4-12. Diaphragmatic slip. A, Sagittal sonogram shows echogenic mass (*arrows*) adjacent to right hemidiaphragm in this patient with right renal cell carcinoma (RRCCa). **B,** Subcostal oblique image reveals mass is diaphragmatic slip (*arrows*).

neum. The inferior accessory hepatic fissure is a true accessory fissure that stretches inferiorly from the right portal vein to the inferior surface of the right lobe of the liver.[11]

Vascular Anomalies

The common hepatic artery arises from the celiac axis and divides into right and left branches at the porta hepatis. This classic textbook description of the **hepatic arterial anatomy** occurs in only 55% of the population. The remaining 45% have some **variation of this anatomy**, of which the main patterns are: (1) replaced left hepatic artery originating from the left gastric artery (10%); (2) replaced right hepatic artery originating from the superior mesenteric artery (11%); and (3) replaced common hepatic artery originating from the superior mesenteric artery (2.5%).

Congenital anomalies of the portal vein include atresias, strictures, and obstructing valves—all of which are uncommon. Sonographic variations include absence of the right portal vein with anomalies of branching from the main and left portal veins and absence of the horizontal segment of the left portal vein.[12]

In contrast, **variations in the branching of the hepatic veins** and accessory hepatic veins are relatively common. The most common accessory vein drains the superoanterior segment of the right lobe (segment VIII) and is seen in approximately one third of the population. It usually empties into the middle hepatic vein, although

occasionally it joins the right hepatic vein.[13] An inferior right hepatic vein, which drains the inferoposterior portion of the liver (segment VI), is observed in 10% of individuals. This inferior right hepatic vein drains directly into the inferior vena cava and may be as large as, or larger than, the right hepatic vein.[14] Left and right marginal veins, which drain into the left and right hepatic veins, occur in approximately 12% and 3% of individuals, respectively. Absence of the main hepatic veins is relatively less common, occurring in approximately 8% of people.[14] Awareness of the normal variations of the hepatic venous system is helpful in accurately defining the location of focal liver lesions and aids the surgeon in segmental liver resection.

CONGENITAL ABNORMALITIES

Liver Cyst

A liver cyst is defined as a fluid-filled space having an epithelial lining. Abscesses, parasitic cysts, and posttraumatic cysts are, therefore, not true cysts. The frequent presence of columnar epithelium within simple hepatic cysts suggests they have a ductal origin, although their precise cause is unclear. It is also not clear why these lesions do not appear until middle age. Although thought at one time to be relatively uncommon, ultrasound examination has shown that liver cysts occur in 2.5% of the general population, increasing to 7% in the population older than 80 years of age.[15]

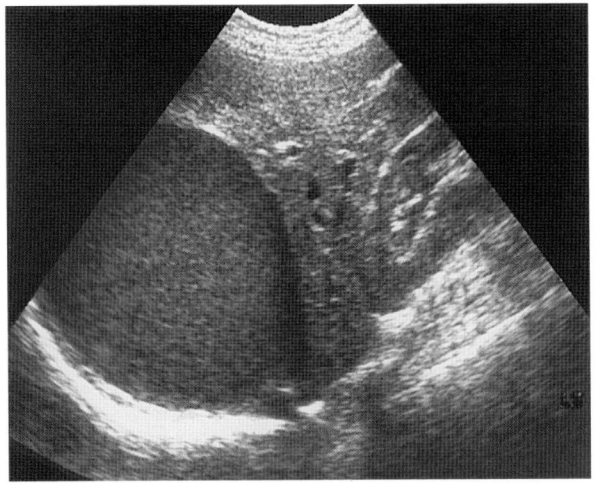

A

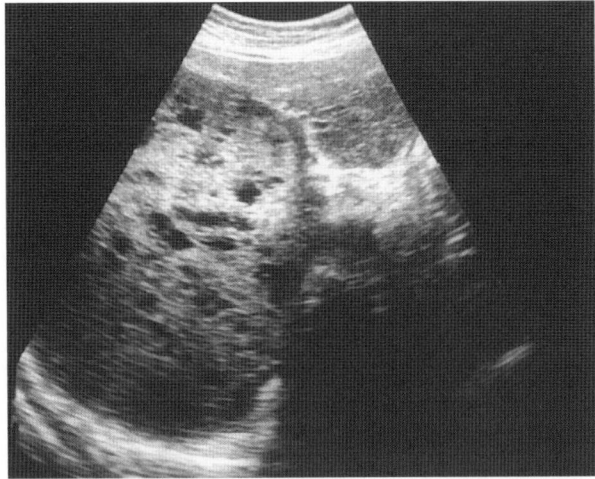

B

FIGURE 4-13. Liver cysts complicated by hemorrhage in two patients. A, Acute right upper quadrant pain in a 46-year-old woman with sagittal right lobe sonogram shows a well-defined subdiaphragmatic mass with uniform low-level internal echoes. This appearance could be misinterpreted as a solid mass. **B,** Transverse sonogram shows a large, well-defined mass with a complex but predominantly solid internal character. **C,** Enhanced computed tomography (CT) scan shows a nonenhancing low-density mass consistent with a cyst. Ultrasound is superior to CT scan at characterization of a cystic mass.

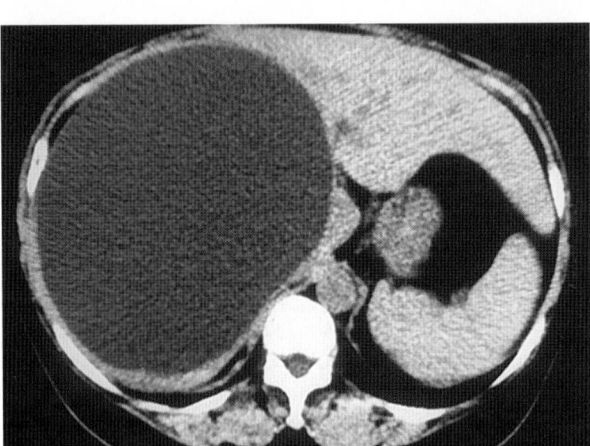

C

On **sonographic examination**, benign hepatic cysts are anechoic with a well-demarcated, thin wall and posterior acoustic enhancement. Occasionally, the patient may develop pain and fever secondary to cyst hemorrhage or infection. In this situation, the cyst may contain internal echoes (Fig. 4-13A) and septations, a thickened wall, or may appear solid (Fig. 4-13B). Active intervention is recommended only in the symptomatic patient. Although aspiration will yield fluid for evaluation, the cyst with an epithelial lining will recur. Cyst ablation with alcohol can be performed using ultrasound guidance.[16] Alternatively, surgical excision is indicated. If thick septae or nodules are seen within liver cysts, computed tomography (CT) is recommended as biliary cystadenomas and cystic metastases must be considered in the differential possibilities for complex-appearing liver cysts (Fig. 4-14).

Peribiliary Cysts

Peribiliary cysts have been described in patients with severe liver disease.[17] These cysts are small, ranging in size from 0.2 to 2.5 cm and are usually located centrally within the porta hepatis or at the junction of the main right and left hepatic ducts. They generally are asymptomatic but may rarely cause biliary obstruction.[17] Pathologically, they are believed to represent obstructed, small periductal glands. Sonographically, the peribiliary cysts may be seen as discrete, clustered cysts, or as tubular-appearing structures having thin septae, paralleling the bile ducts and portal veins.

Adult Polycystic Disease

The adult form of polycystic kidney disease is inherited in an autosomal dominant pattern. The frequency of liver cysts in association with this condition varies between 57% to 74%.[18] No correlation exists between the severity of the renal disease and the extent of liver involvement. Liver function tests are usually normal and, unlike the infantile autosomal recessive form of polycystic kidney disease, there is no association with hepatic fibrosis and portal hypertension. Indeed, if liver function tests are abnormal, complications of polycystic liver disease, such as tumor, cyst infection, or biliary obstruction, should be excluded.[18]

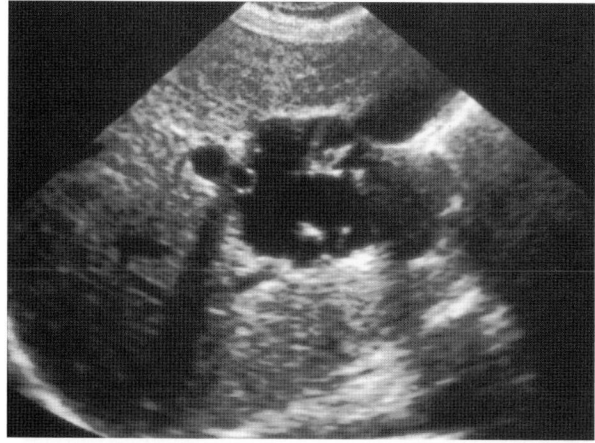

A

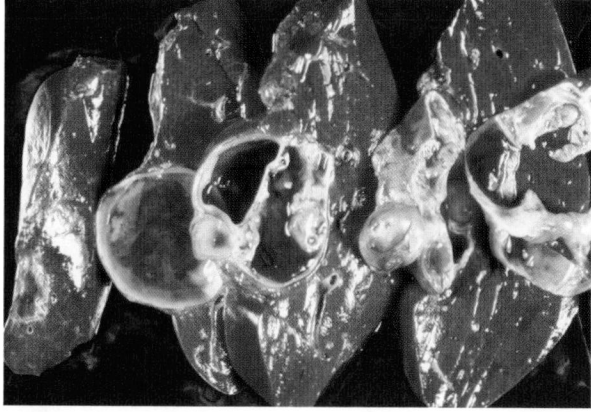

B

FIGURE 4-14. Biliary cystadenoma. A, Sagittal sonogram shows an irregular liver cyst with thick septa and mural nodules. **B,** Surgical specimen.

Biliary Hamartomas (von Meyenburg Complexes)

Bile duct hamartomas, first described by von Meyenburg in 1918,[19] are small, focal developmental lesions of the liver composed of groups of dilated intrahepatic bile ducts set within a dense collagenous stroma.[20] They are benign liver malformations that are detected incidentally in 0.6 to 5.6% of reported autopsy series.[21]

Imaging features of von Meyenburg complexes (VMC) are described in the literature in isolated case reports and a few small series including sonographic, CT, and magnetic resonance imaging (MRI) appearances.[22] VMC are often confused with metastatic cancer and reports describe single, multiple, or—most often—innumerable well-defined solid nodules usually less than 1 cm in diameter (Fig. 4-15). Nodules are usually uniformly hypoechoic[22] and less commonly hyperechoic on sonography[23,24] and hypodense on contrast-enhanced CT scan. Bright echogenic foci in the liver with distal "ringdown" artifact without obvious mass effect are also

documented on sonograms on patients with VMC (Fig. 4-16). We believe that these echogenic foci could be related to the presence of tiny cysts beyond the resolution of the ultrasound equipment. VMC are usually isolated and insignificant observations. VMC may occur with other congenital disorders such as congenital hepatic fibrosis or polycystic kidney or liver disease.[21] Association of VMC with cholangiocarcinoma has been suggested.[26]

INFECTIOUS DISEASES

Viral Hepatitis

Viral hepatitis is a common disease that occurs worldwide. It is responsible for millions of deaths secondary to acute hepatic necrosis or chronic hepatitis, which in turn may lead to portal hypertension, cirrhosis, and hepatocellular carcinoma (HCC). Recent medical advances have identified at least six distinct hepatitis viruses: hepatitis A through E and G.[27]

Hepatitis A occurs throughout the world and can be diagnosed using serosurveys with the antibody to hepatitis A (anti-HAV) as the marker. The primary mode of spread is via the fecal-oral route. In developing countries, the disease is endemic and infection occurs early in life. Hepatitis A is an acute infection leading to either complete recovery or death from acute liver failure.

Hepatitis B is transmitted parenterally, for example via blood transfusions and needle punctures as well as by nonpercutaneous exposure through sexual contact. Hepatitis B, unlike A, has a carrier state, which is esti-

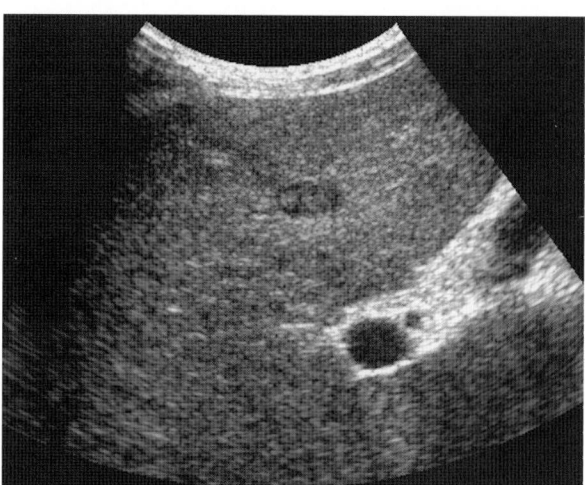

FIGURE 4-15. Von Meyenburg complex in a cancer patient. Sonogram shows a single, small, hypoechoic liver mass. Because there was no other evidence of metastatic disease, a biopsy was performed and proved the benign insignificant nature of this lesion.

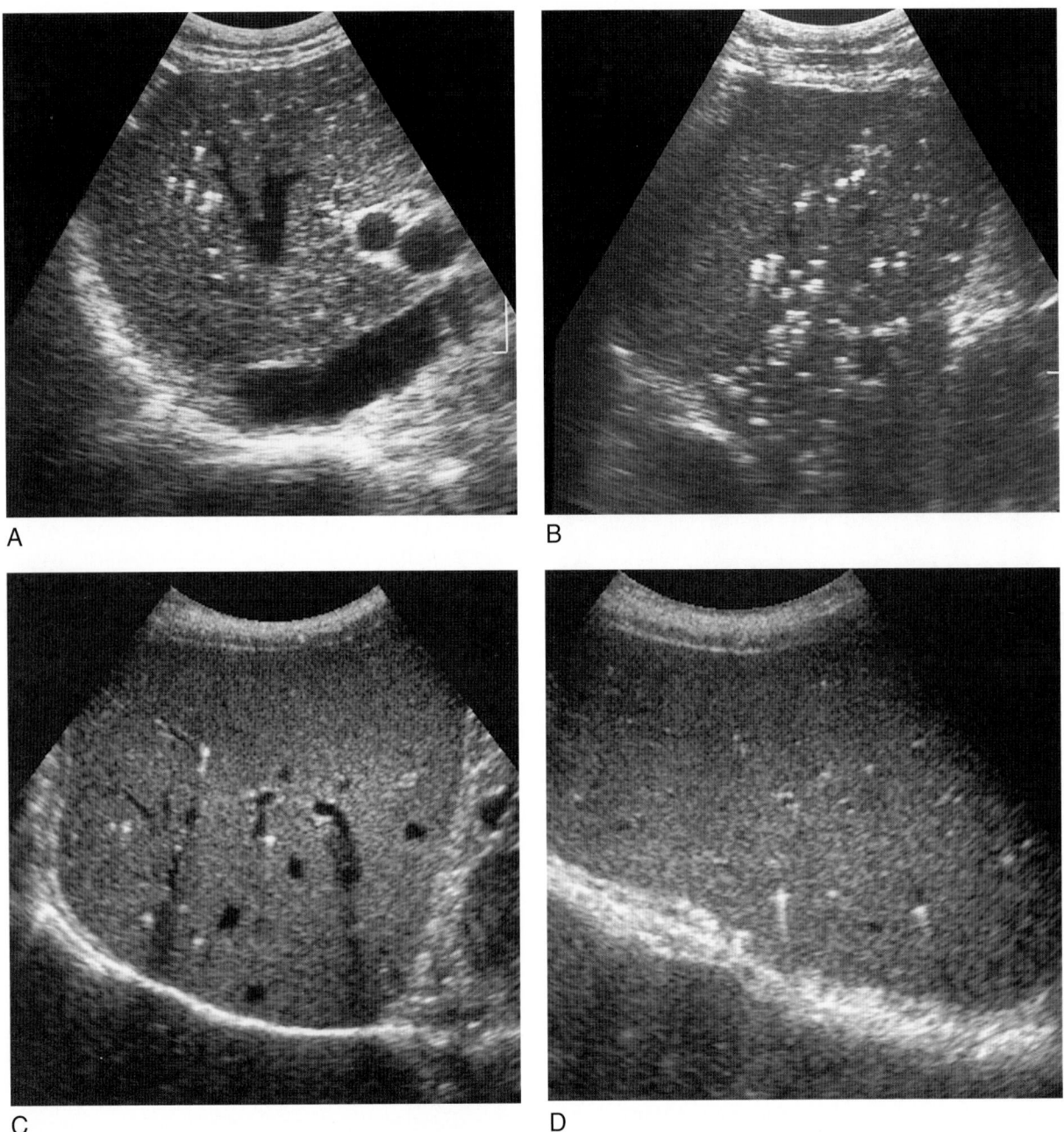

FIGURE 4-16. Bright echogenic foci with distal "ringdown" artifacts in two patients. A, Sagittal and **B,** transverse images of the left lobe of the liver show multiple, bright echogenic foci with "ringdown" artifact. Biopsy showed VMC. **C,** Sagittal and **D,** transverse images of the right lobe in an asymptomatic patient show echogenic foci with distal "ringdown" artifact.

mated worldwide at 300 million. The regions of highest carrier rates (5% to 20%) are Southeast Asia, China, sub-Saharan Africa, and Greenland. The two most useful markers for acute infection are hepatitis B surface antigen (HBsAg) and antibody to hepatitis B core antigen (anti-HBc).

Non-A, Non-B (NANB) (predominantly C) hepatitis was first recognized in 1974 to 1975. Investigators in the United States were surprised to learn that the majority of cases of post-transfusion hepatitis were not

secondary to hepatitis B but to an unknown virus or viruses. Since then, it has been realized that many cases are not the result of percutaneous transmission and that in almost 50%, no source could be identified. Acutely infected individuals have a much greater risk of chronic infection, with up to 85% progressing to chronic liver disease. Chronic hepatitis C is diagnosed by the presence in blood of the antibody to HCV (anti-HCV). Hepatitis C is a major health problem in Italy and other Mediterranean countries.

Hepatitis D or hepatitis delta virus is entirely dependent on the hepatitis B virus for its infectivity, requiring the HBsAg to provide an envelope coat for the hepatitis D virus. Its geographic distribution is, therefore, similar to that of hepatitis B. It is an uncommon infection in North America, occurring primarily in intravenous (IV) drug users.

Clinical Manifestations of Hepatitis

Uncomplicated **acute hepatitis** implies clinical recovery within 4 months. It is the outcome of 99% of cases of hepatitis A.

Subfulminant and fulminant hepatic failure occur following the onset of jaundice and include worsening jaundice, coagulopathy, and hepatic encephalopathy. Most cases are due to hepatitis B or drug toxicity. This condition is characterized by hepatic necrosis. Death occurs if the loss of hepatic parenchyma is greater than 40%.[28]

Chronic hepatitis is defined as the persistence of biochemical abnormalities beyond 6 months. It has many etiologies other than viral, i.e., metabolic (Wilson's disease, alpha-1 antitrypsin deficiency, and hemochromatosis), autoimmune, and drug induced. The prognosis and treatment of the disease depend on the specific etiology.[29]

In **acute hepatitis**, there is diffuse swelling of the hepatocytes, proliferation of Kupffer cells lining the sinusoids, and infiltration of the portal areas by lymphocytes and monocytes. The **sonographic features** parallel the histologic findings. The liver parenchyma may have a diffusely decreased echogenicity, with accentuated brightness of the portal triads, periportal cuffing (Fig. 4-17A, B and Fig. 4-18A, B). Hepatomegaly and thickening of the gallbladder wall are associated findings (see Fig. 4-17C, D and Fig. 4-18C, D). In most cases the liver appears normal.[30] Most cases of chronic hepatitis are also sonographically normal. When cirrhosis develops, sonography may demonstrate a coarsened echotexture and other morphologic changes of cirrhosis.

Bacterial Diseases

Pyogenic bacteria reach the liver by several routes, the most common being direct extension from the biliary tract in patients with suppurative cholangitis and cholecystitis. Other routes are through the portal venous system in patients with diverticulitis or appendicitis and through the hepatic artery in patients with osteomyelitis and subacute bacterial endocarditis. Pyogenic bacteria may also be present in the liver as a result of blunt or penetrating trauma. No cause can be found in approximately 50% of the cases of hepatic abscesses. Most of this latter group are caused by anaerobic infection. Diagnosis of bacterial liver infection is often delayed.

The most common presenting features of pyogenic liver abscess are fever, malaise, anorexia, and right upper quadrant pain. Jaundice may be present in approximately 25% of these patients.

Sonography has proved to be extremely helpful in the detection of abdominal abscesses. The ultrasound features of **pyogenic liver abscesses** are varied (Fig. 4-19). Frankly purulent abscesses appear cystic, with the fluid ranging from echofree to highly echogenic. Regions of early suppuration may appear solid with altered echogenicity, usually hypoechoic, related to the presence of necrotic hepatocytes.[31] Occasionally gas-producing organisms give rise to echogenic foci with a posterior reverberation artifact (see Fig. 4-19G, H, I). Fluid-fluid interfaces, internal septations, and debris have all been observed. The abscess wall can vary from well-defined to irregular and thick.

The **differential diagnosis** of pyogenic liver abscess includes amebic or echinococcal infection, simple cyst with hemorrhage, hematoma, and necrotic or cystic neoplasm. Ultrasound-guided liver aspiration is an expeditious means to confirm the diagnosis. Specimens should be sent for both aerobic and anaerobic culture. Fifty percent of abscesses in the past were considered sterile. This was almost certainly caused by failure to transport the specimen in an oxygen-free container, and, thus, anaerobic organisms were not identified.[32] Once the diagnosis of liver abscess is made by the presence of pus or a positive Gram stain and culture, the collection can be drained percutaneously using ultrasound or CT guidance.

Fungal Diseases

Candidiasis

The liver is frequently involved secondary to hematogenous spread of mycotic infections in other organs, most commonly the lungs. Patients are generally immunocompromised, although systemic candidiasis may occur in pregnancy or following hyperalimentation. The clinical characteristics include persistent fever in a neutropenic patient whose leukocyte count is returning to normal.[33]

The **ultrasound features** of hepatic candidiasis include[34]:

- "Wheel within a wheel"—Peripheral hypoechoic zone with an inner echogenic wheel and central hypoechoic nidus. The central nidus represents focal necrosis in which fungal elements are found. This is seen early in the disease.
- "Bull's eye"—1- to 4-cm lesion having a hyperechoic center and a hypoechoic rim. It is present when neutrophil counts return to normal. The echogenic center contains inflammatory cells (Fig. 4-20).

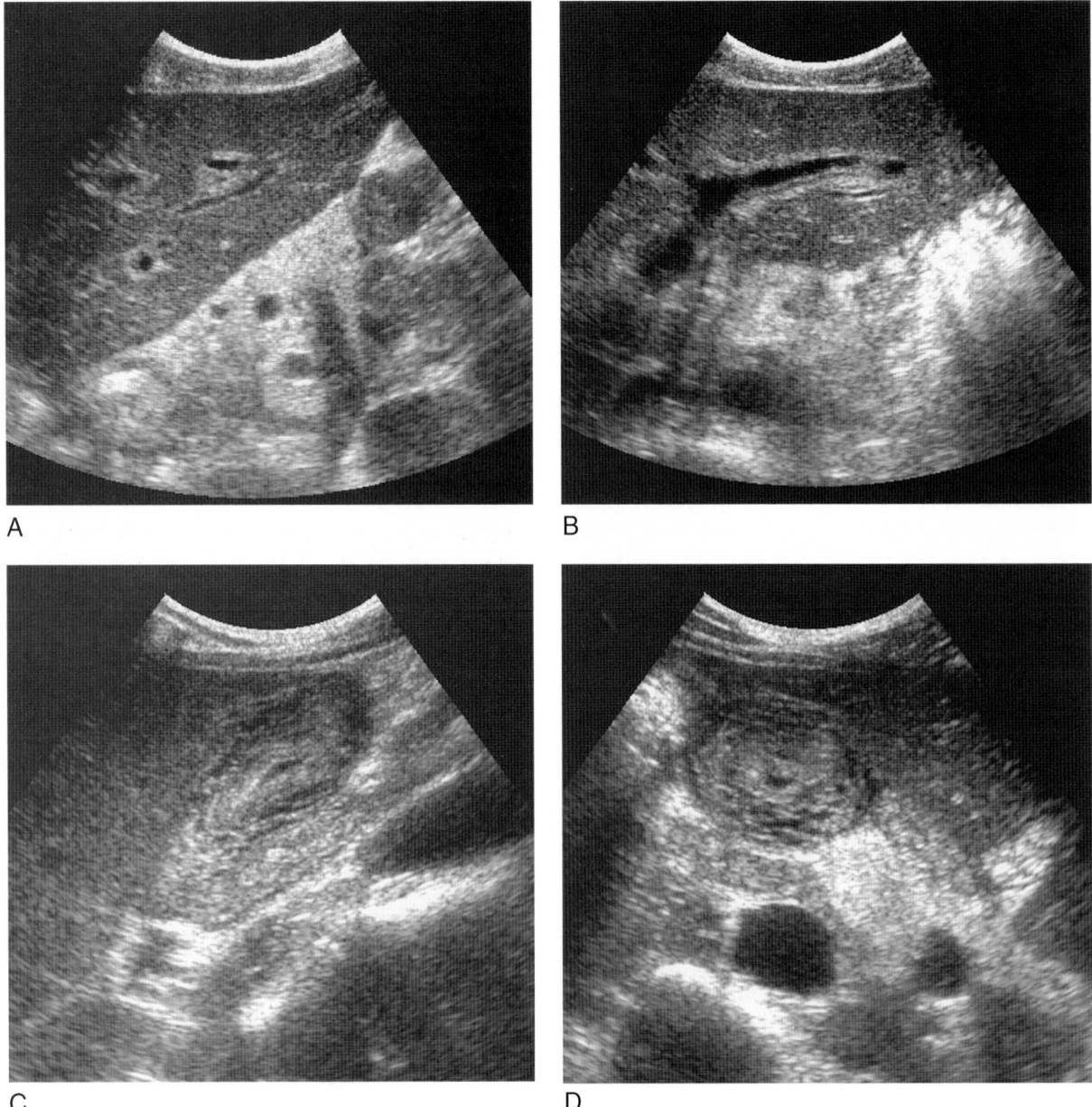

A

B

C

D

FIGURE 4-17. Acute hepatitis. A, Sagittal and **B,** transverse images of the left lobe of the liver show marked increased thickness and echogenicity of the soft tissue surrounding the portal vein branch, so called *periportal cuffing*. **C,** Sagittal and **D,** transverse views of the gallbladder show marked mural thickening, such that the lumen is virtually obliterated. The gallbladder wall shows a multilayered appearance with extensive hypoechoic pockets of edema fluid. (Reproduced with permission from ACR.)

- "Uniformly hypoechoic"—Most common. This corresponds to progressive fibrosis (Fig. 4-21A).
- "Echogenic"—Variable calcification representing scar formation (see Fig. 4-21B).

It is interesting to note that, although percutaneous liver aspiration is of great benefit in obtaining the organism in pyogenic liver abscesses, it frequently yields falsely negative results for the presence of *Candida* organisms.[34] This may be caused by failure to sample the central necrotic portion of the lesion where the pseudohyphae are found.[33]

Parasitic Diseases

Amebiasis

Hepatic infection by the parasite *Entamoeba histolytica* is the most common extraintestinal manifestation of amebiasis. Transmission is by the fecal-oral route. The protozoan reaches the liver by penetrating through the colon, invading the mesenteric venules, and entering the portal vein. However, in more than one half of patients with amebic abscesses of the liver, the colon appears normal and stool culture results are negative, thus delay-

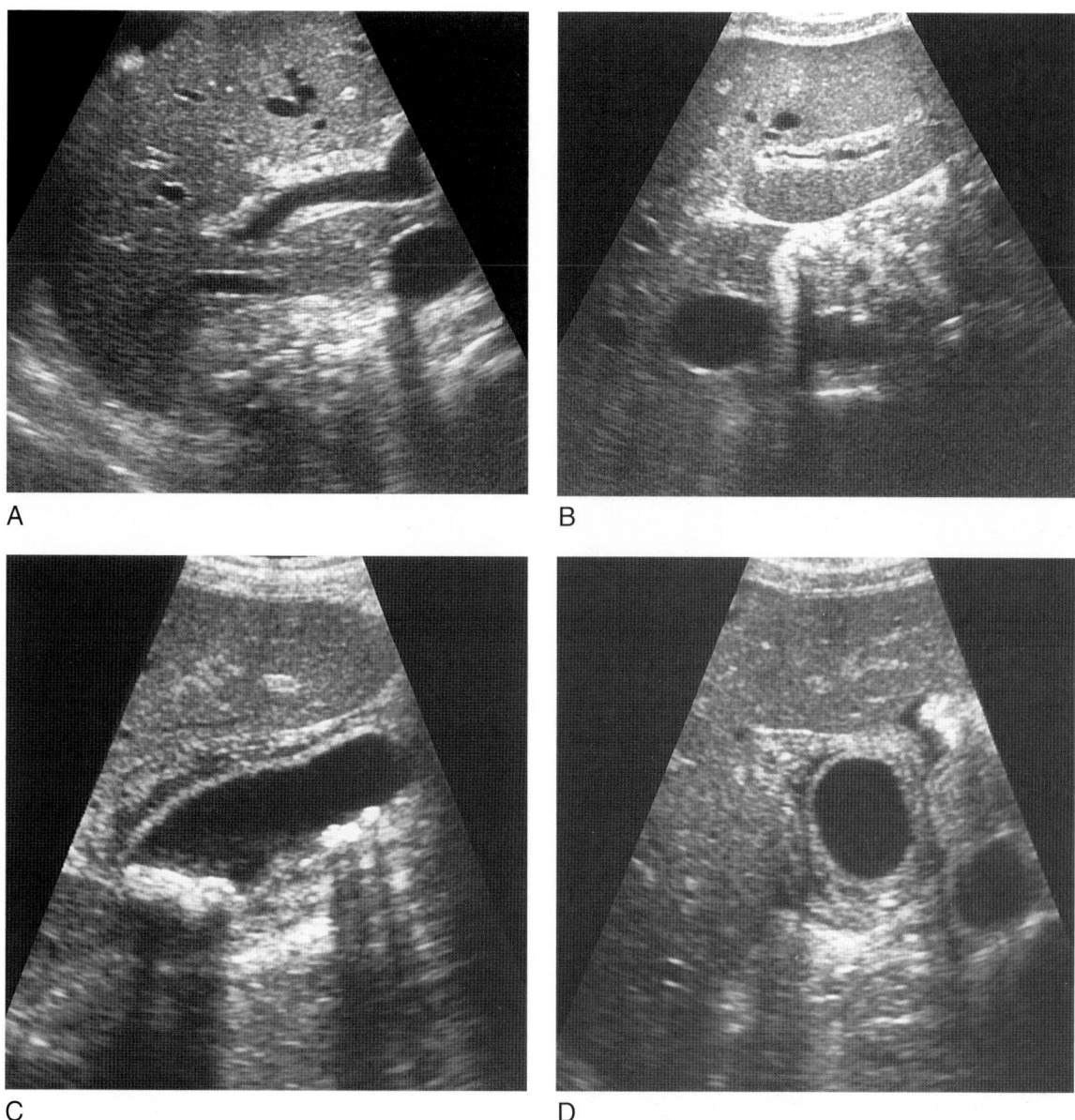

FIGURE 4-18. Acute hepatitis. Acute hepatitis in a patient with fever, abnormal liver function tests, and incidental gallstones. **A,** Transverse view of porta hepatis and **B,** transverse view of left lobe of liver both show prominent thick echogenic bands surrounding the portal veins in the portal triads, referred to as *periportal cuffing.* **C,** Sagittal and **D,** transverse views of the gallbladder show moderate edema and thickening of the gallbladder wall. The gallbladder is not large or tense and the patient does not have acute cholecystitis. Incidental cholelithiasis, as in this case, may be confusing.

ing diagnosis. The most common presenting symptom in patients with amebic abscess is pain, which occurs in 99% of patients. Approximately 15% of patients have diarrhea at the time of diagnosis.

Sonographic features include a round or oval-shaped lesion, absence of a prominent abscess wall, hypoechogenicity compared to normal liver, fine low-level internal echoes, distal sonic enhancement, and contiguity with the diaphragm (Fig. 4-22).[35,36] These features, however, can all be found in pyogenic abscesses.

In a review of 112 amebic lesions by Ralls et al., two

sonographic patterns were significantly more prevalent in amebic abscesses: (1) round or oval shapes in 82% versus 60% of pyogenic abscess and (2) hypoechoic appearance with fine internal echoes at high gain in 58% versus 36% of pyogenic abscesses.[37] Most amebic abscesses occur in the right lobe of the liver. Practically speaking, the diagnosis of amebic liver abscess is made using a combination of the clinical features, the ultrasound findings, and results of serologic testing. The indirect hemagglutination test is positive in 94% to 100% of patients.

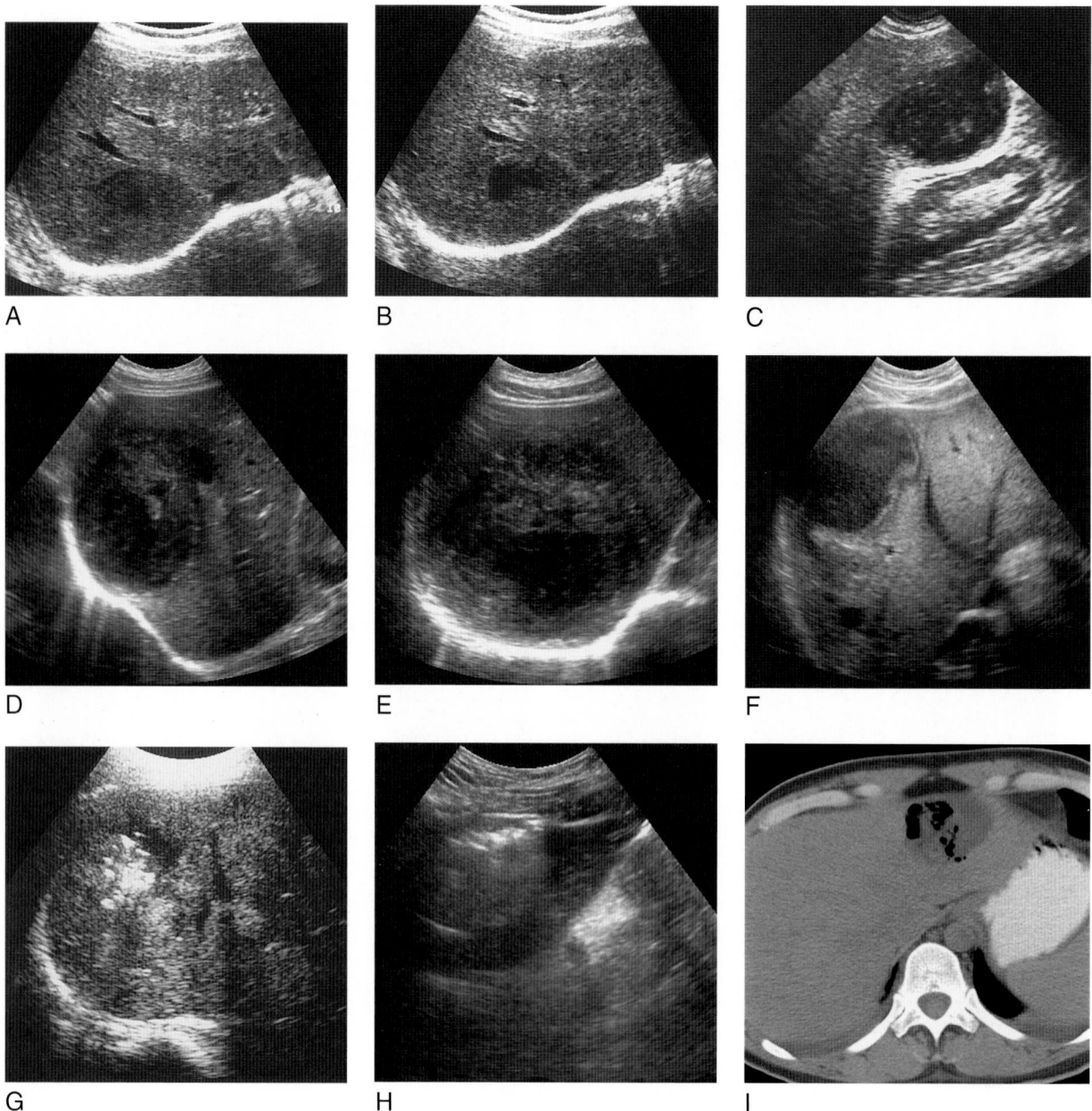

FIGURE 4-19. Pyogenic abscesses—Spectrum of appearances. Top line—early lesions. Rapid evolution from phlegmon to liquefaction is shown in **A** and **B. A,** Poorly defined mass effect or phlegmon in segment 7 of the liver. **B,** Twenty-four hours later, there is a central area of liquefaction. **C,** An early abscess is poorly marginated and bulges the liver capsule. It is difficult to characterize this mass as solid or cystic. There was no vascularity within this or other masses. **Middle line—mature abscess cavities** in three patients (**D, E,** and **F**) show a classic mature abscess as a well-defined mass with liquefaction and internal debris. **Bottom line— abscesses related to gas-forming organisms. G,** Multiple gas bubbles seen as innumerable bright echogenic foci within a poorly defined hypoechoic liver mass. **H,** Sagittal image of the left lobe of the liver and **I,** the confirmatory CT scan both show a liver mass with extensive gas content.

Amebicidal drugs are effective therapy. Patient's symptoms improve by 24 to 48 hours and most are afebrile in 4 days on medical therapy. Those who exhibit clinical deterioration may also benefit from catheter drainage; this is unusual, however. The majority of hepatic amebic abscesses disappear with adequate medical therapy.[38] The time from termination of therapy to resolution varies from 1.5 to 23 months (median 7 months).[39] A minority of patients have residual hepatic cysts and focal regions of increased or decreased echogenicity.

Hydatid Disease

The most common cause of hydatid disease in humans is infestation by the parasite *Echinococcus granulosus*. *E. granulosus* has a worldwide distribution. It is most prevalent in sheep- and cattle-raising countries, notably

ULTRASOUND FEATURES OF HEPATIC CANDIDIASIS

"Wheel within a wheel"
  Peripheral hypoechoic zone
  Inner echogenic wheel
  Central hypoechoic nidus
Bull's eye
  Hyperechoic center
  Hypoechoic rim
Uniformly hypoechoic
  Progressive fibrosis
Echogenic
  Calcification representing scar formation

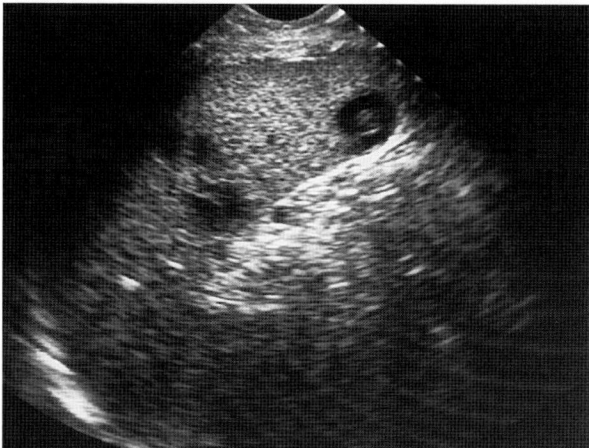

A

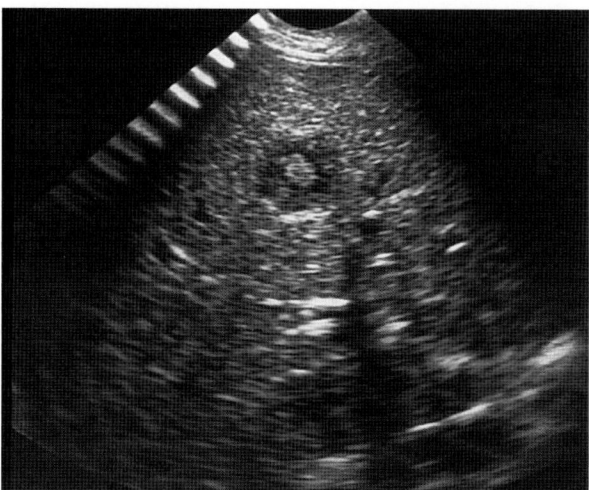

B

FIGURE 4-20. Fungal infection, bull's eye morphology, in a 24-year-old man with ALL and fever. **A,** Sagittal sonogram through the spleen shows focal hypoechoic target lesions. **B,** The liver showed multiple masses. This magnified view shows a thick, echogenic rim and a thin, hypoechoic inner rim with a dense echogenic nidus. Biopsy revealed pseudohyphae.

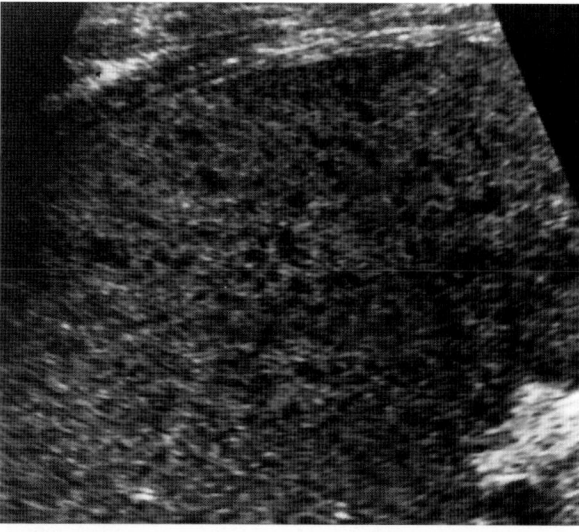

A

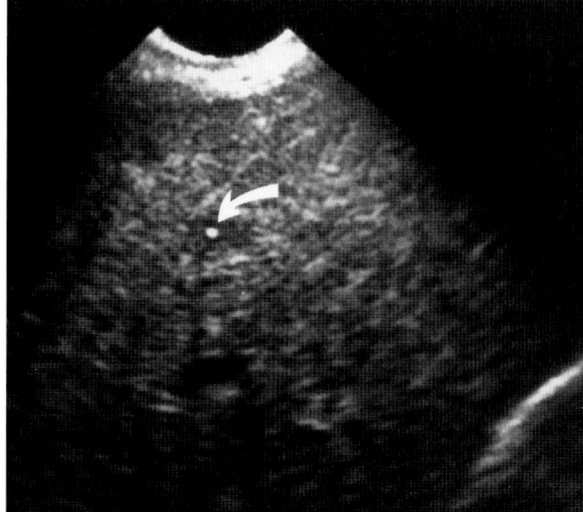

B

FIGURE 4-21. Candidiasis. A, Uniformly hypoechoic pattern. Multiple hypoechoic hepatic lesions are present in this young patient with acute myelogenous leukemia. **B,** Echogenic pattern, following medical therapy. Small calcified lesion (*arrow*) is visualized in a second immunocompromised patient.

in the Middle East, Australia, and the Mediterranean. Endemic regions are also present in the United States (the central valley in California, the lower Mississippi valley, Utah, and Arizona) and northern Canada. *E. granulosus* is a tapeworm, 3 to 6 mm in length, which lives in the intestine of the **definitive host**, usually the **dog**. Its eggs are excreted in the dog's feces and swallowed by the **intermediate hosts**—sheep, cattle, goats, or **humans**. The embryos are freed in the duodenum and pass through the mucosa to reach the liver through the portal venous system. Most of the embryos remain trapped in the liver, although the lungs, kidneys, spleen, central nervous system, and bone may become

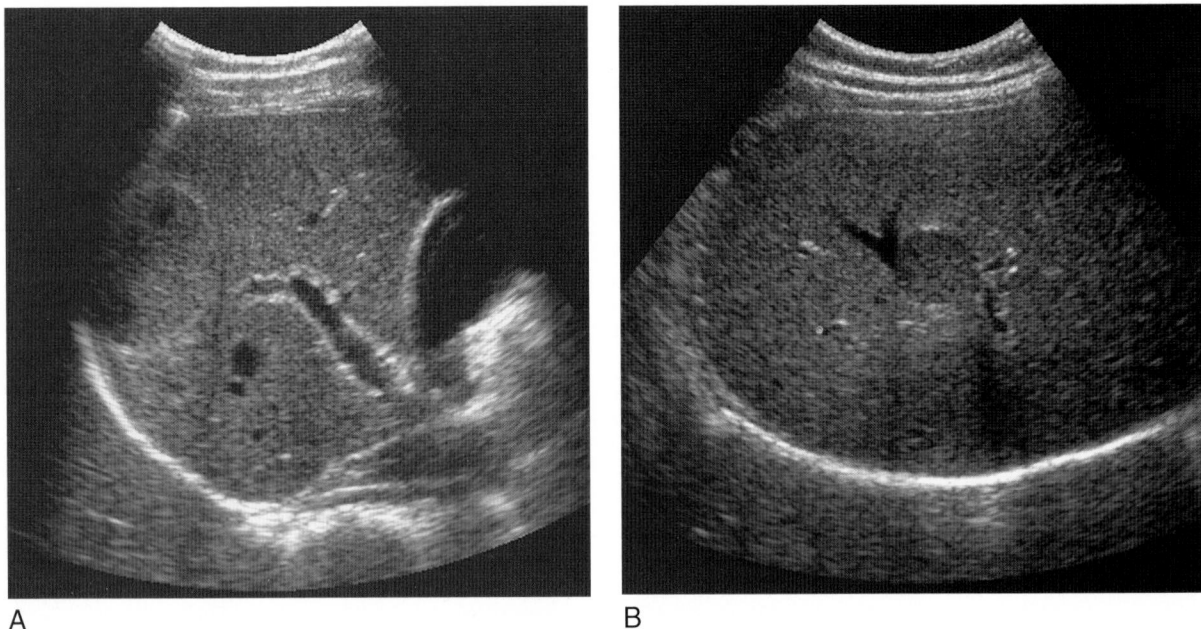

A   B

FIGURE 4-22. Amebic liver abscess—classic morphology. Transverse sonogram shows a well-defined oval subdiaphragmatic mass with increased through transmission. There are uniform low-level internal echoes and absence of a well-defined abscess wall.

secondarily involved. In the liver, the right lobe is more frequently involved. The surviving embryos form slow-growing cysts. The cyst wall consists of an external membrane that is approximately 1 mm thick, which may calcify (**the ectocyst**). The host forms a dense connective tissue capsule around the cyst (**pericyst**). The inner germinal layer (**the endocyst**) gives rise to brood capsules that enlarge to form protoscolices. The brood capsules may separate from the wall and form a fine sediment called hydatid sand. When hydatid cysts within the organs of a herbivore are eaten, the scolices attach to the intestine and grow to adult tapeworms, thus completing the life cycle.

Several reports describe the **sonographic features of hepatic hydatid disease** (Fig. 4-23 and Fig. 4-24).[40-42] Lewall proposed four groups[41]:

- Simple cysts containing no internal architecture except sand
- Cysts with detached endocyst secondary to rupture (see Fig. 4-23B)
- Cysts with daughter cysts matrix (echogenic material between the daughter cysts), or both
- Densely calcified masses

Surgery is the conventional treatment in echinococcal disease, although recent reports describe success with percutaneous drainage.[43-45] Although anaphylaxis from hydatid cyst rupture has been reported, its occurrence is rare. Ultrasound has been used to monitor the course of medical therapy in patients with abdominal hydatid disease.[46] Changes noted in the resolution of the disease

were a gradual reduction in cyst size (43%), membrane detachment (30%), progressive increase in echogenicity of the cyst cavity (12%), and wall calcification (6%). No change was identified in 26% of patients. A reappearance or persistence of fluid within the cavity may signify inadequate therapy and viability of the parasites.[47]

Hepatic alveolar echinococcus is a rare parasitic infestation by the larvae of *E. multilocularis*. The fox is the main host. The sonographic features include echogenic lesions, which may be single or multiple; necrotic, irregular lesions without a well-defined wall; clusters of calcification within lesions; and dilated bile ducts.[48]

Schistosomiasis

Schistosomiasis is one of the most common parasitic infections in humans, estimated to affect 200 million people worldwide.[49] Hepatic schistosomiasis is caused by *Schistosoma mansoni*, *S. japonicum*, *S. mekongi*, and *S. intercalatum*. Hepatic involvement by *S. mansoni* is

---

SONOGRAPHIC FEATURES OF HEPATIC HYDATID DISEASE

Simple cysts
Cysts with detached endocyst secondary to rupture
Cysts with daughter cysts
Densely calcified masses

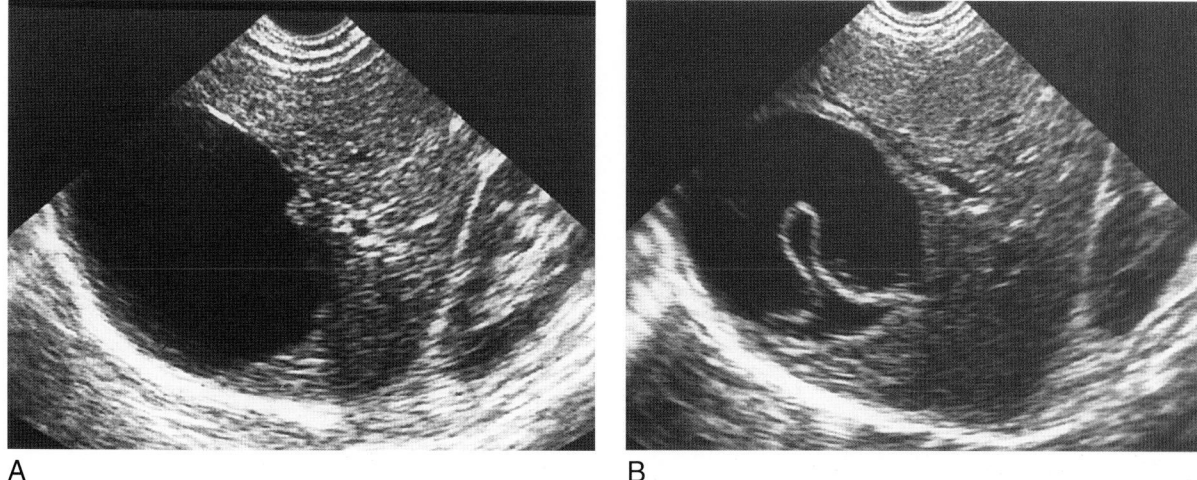

FIGURE 4-23. Hydatid cyst. A, Baseline sonogram shows a fairly simple cyst in the right lobe with a small mural nodule and a fleck of peripheral calcium anteriorly. **B,** Three weeks later, the patient presented with right upper quadrant pain and eosinophilia. The detached endocyst is floating within the lesion.

particularly severe. *S. mansoni* is prevalent in Africa, including Egypt, and South America, particularly in Venezuela and Brazil. The ova reach the liver through the portal vein and incite a chronic granulomatous reaction first described by Symmers as clay-pipestem fibrosis.[50] The terminal portal vein branches become occluded, leading to presinusoidal portal hypertension, splenomegaly, varices, and ascites.

The **sonographic features** of schistosomiasis are widened echogenic portal tracts, sometimes reaching a thickness of 2 cm.[51,52] The porta hepatis is the region most often affected. Initially the liver size is enlarged; however, as the periportal fibrosis progresses, the liver becomes contracted and the features of portal hypertension prevail.

Pneumocystis carinii

Pneumocystis carinii is the most common organism causing opportunistic infection in patients with acquired immunodeficiency syndrome (AIDS). Pneumocystis pneumonia is the most common cause of life-threatening infection in patients with human immunodeficiency virus (HIV). *Pneumocystis carinii* also affects patients undergoing bone marrow and organ transplantation, as well as those receiving corticosteroids or chemotherapy.[53] Extrapulmonic *P. carinii* infection was being reported with frequency around 1990.[54-57] It was postulated that the use of maintenance aerosolized pentamidine achieved lower systemic levels than the intravenous form, allowing subclinical pulmonary infections and systemic dissemination of the protozoa. As this treatment is no longer in frequent use by AIDS patients, disseminated infection is now rarely seen. Extrapulmonary *P. carinii* infection has been documented in the liver,

spleen, renal cortex, thyroid gland, pancreas, and lymph nodes. The **sonographic findings** of *P. carinii* involvement of the liver (Fig. 4-25) range from diffuse, tiny, nonshadowing echogenic foci to extensive replacement of the normal hepatic parenchyma by echogenic clumps representing dense calcification. A similar sonographic pattern has been identified with hepatic infection by *Mycobacterium avium-intracellulare* and cytomegalovirus.[58]

DISORDERS OF METABOLISM

Fatty Liver

Fatty liver is an acquired, reversible disorder of metabolism, resulting in an accumulation of triglycerides within the hepatocytes. Probably the most common cause of a fatty liver is obesity. Excessive alcohol intake produces a fatty liver by stimulating lipolysis, as does starvation. Other causes of fatty infiltration include poorly controlled hyperlipidemia, diabetes, excess exogenous or endogenous corticosteroids, pregnancy, total parenteral hyperalimentation, severe hepatitis, glycogen storage disease, jejunoileal bypass procedures for obesity, cystic fibrosis, congenital generalized lipodystrophy, several chemotherapeutic agents, including methotrexate, and toxins such as carbon tetrachloride and yellow phosphorus.[59] Correction of the primary abnormality will usually reverse the process, although it is now recognized that fatty infiltration of the liver is the precursor for significant chronic disease in a percentage of patients.

Sonography of fatty infiltration may be varied depending on the amount of fat and whether deposits are diffuse or focal (Fig. 4-26).[60] **Diffuse steatosis** may be:

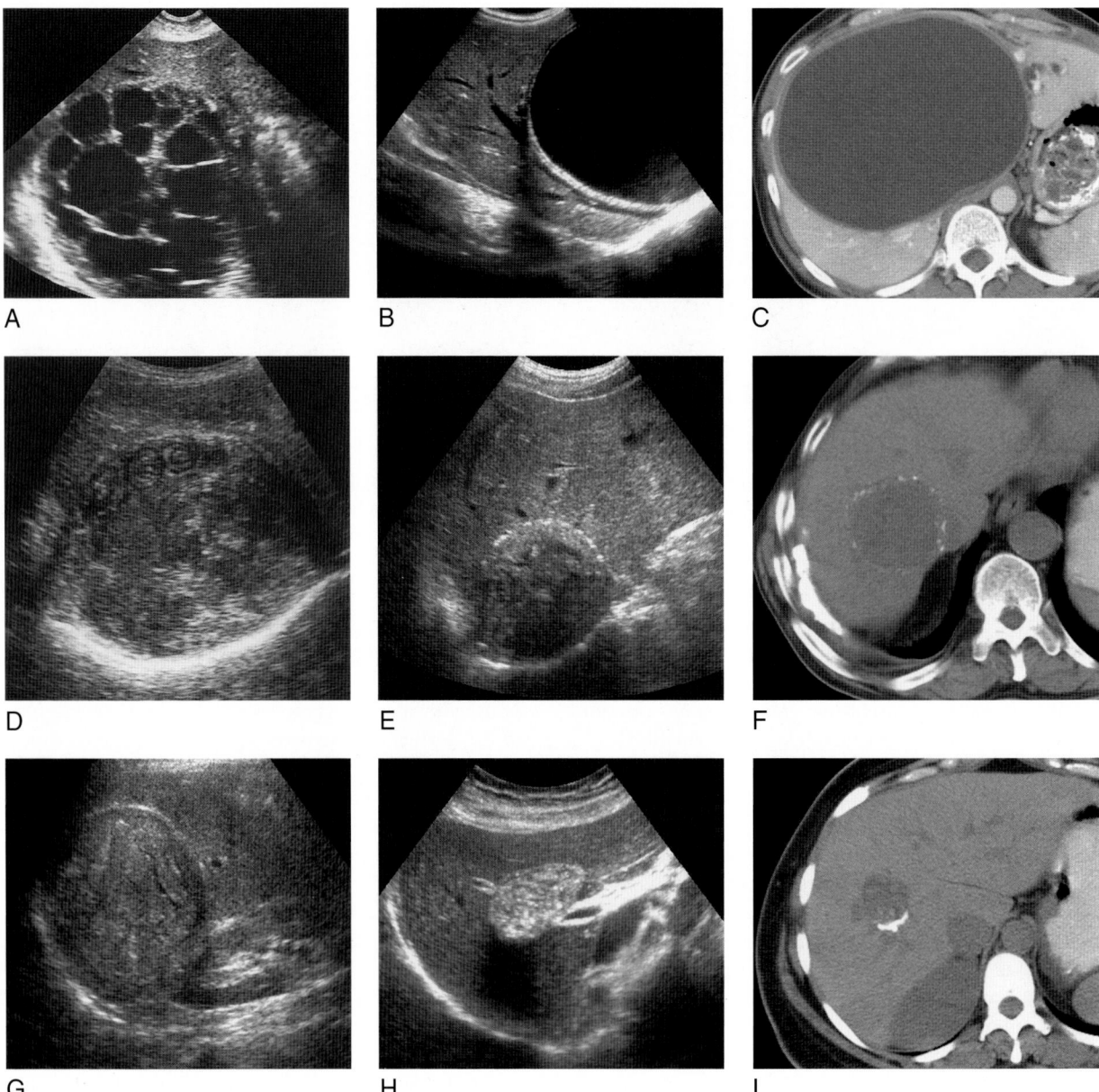

FIGURE 4-24. Hydatid liver disease—Spectrum of appearances. A, Classic appearance showing a cyst containing multiple daughter cysts. **B,** Sonogram and **C,** confirmatory CT scan show a unilocular and simple cyst, a fairly uncommon morphology for hydatid disease. **D,** Sonogram shows a complex mass. Anteriorly, there are multiple ringlike structures that raise the suspicion of hydatid disease. At surgery, the cystic mass showed thick debris and innumerable scolices. **E,** Sonogram and **F,** confirmatory CT scan show an indeterminate mass with a thin rim of calcification. **G,** Complex mass similar to that seen in **D**. There are finger-like projections within, again suggestive of hydatid disease. **H,** Sonogram and **I,** confirmatory CT scan both show a central liver mass with rim and internal punctate calcifications.

- **Mild**—Minimal diffuse increase in hepatic echogenicity; normal visualization of diaphragm and intrahepatic vessel borders.
- **Moderate**—Moderate diffuse increase in hepatic echogenicity; slightly impaired visualization of intrahepatic vessels and diaphragm.
- **Severe**—Marked increase in echogenicity; poor penetration of the posterior segment of the right

lobe of the liver and poor or nonvisualization of the hepatic vessels and diaphragm.

Focal fatty infiltration and **focal fatty sparing** may mimic neoplastic involvement.[61] In focal fatty infiltration, regions of increased echogenicity are present within a background of normal liver parenchyma. Conversely, islands of normal liver parenchyma may

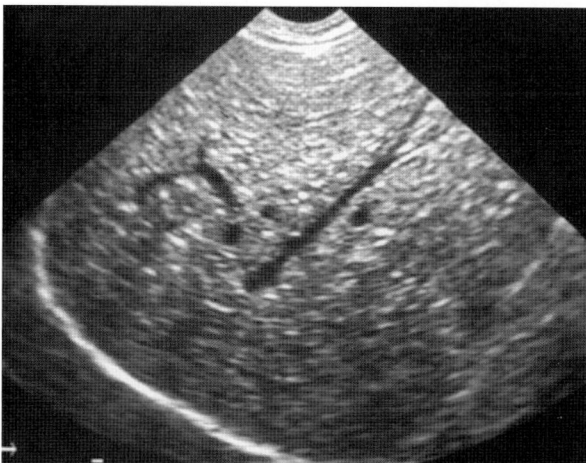

FIGURE 4-25. *Pneumocystis carinii*. Disseminated *Pneumocystis carinii* infection in an AIDS patient who had previously used a pentamidine inhaler. Sonogram shows innumerable tiny bright echogenic foci without shadowing throughout the liver parenchyma.

appear as hypoechoic masses within a dense, fatty infiltrated liver. **Features of focal fatty change** include (Fig. 4-27):

- **Focal fatty sparing** and **focal fatty liver**—both most commonly involve the periportal region of the medial segment of the left lobe (segment IV).[62,63]
- Sparing also occurs commonly by the gallbladder fossa and along the liver margins.
- Focal subcapsular fat may occur in diabetics receiving insulin in peritoneal dialysate.[64]
- **Lack of mass effect.** Hepatic vessels as a rule are not displaced. A recent report, however, has demonstrated the presence of traversing vessels in metastases.[65]
- **Geometric margins** are present, although focal fat may appear round, nodular, or interdigitated with normal tissue.[66]
- **Rapid change** with time: Fatty infiltration may resolve as early as within 6 days.
- CT scans of the liver will demonstrate corresponding regions of low attenuation.

Chemical shift MRI techniques are useful in distinguishing diffuse or focal fatty infiltration. Radionuclide liver and spleen scintigraphic examination will yield normal results, indicating adequate numbers of Kupffer cells within the fatty regions.[60] It has been postulated that these focal spared areas are caused by a regional decrease in portal blood flow as demonstrated by CT scans during arterial portographic examinations.[67] Knowledge of typical patterns and use of CT scans, MRI, or nuclear medicine scintigraphy will avoid the necessity for biopsy in the majority of cases of focal fatty alteration.

SONOGRAPHY OF DIFFUSE STEATOSIS

Mild
Minimal diffuse increase in hepatic echogenicity
Moderate
Moderate diffuse increase in hepatic echogenicity
Slightly impaired visualization of intrahepatic vessels and diaphragm
Severe
Marked increase in echogenicity
Poor penetration of the posterior liver
Poor or nonvisualization of the hepatic vessels and diaphragm

---

SONOGRAPHIC FEATURES OF FOCAL FATTY CHANGE

May show **rapid change** with time, both in appearance and resolution
Does **not** alter course or caliber of regional vessels
Does **not** produce contour abnormalities
Preferred **site for focal sparing**
　Anterior to portal vein at porta hepatis
　Gallbladder fossa
　Liver margins
Preferred **site for focal fat**
　Anterior to portal vein at porta hepatis
Geographic fat—maplike boundaries

Glycogen Storage Disease (Glycogenosis)

Recognition of glycogen storage disease (GSD) affecting the kidneys and liver was first made by von Gierke in 1929. Type 1 GSD (von Gierke's disease, glucose 6-phosphatase deficiency) is manifested in the neonatal period by hepatomegaly, nephromegaly, and hypoglycemic convulsions. Because of the enzyme deficiency, large quantities of glycogen are deposited in the hepatocytes and proximal convoluted tubules of the kidney.[68] With dietary management and supportive therapy, more patients currently are surviving to childhood and young adulthood. As a result, several patients have developed benign adenomas or, less commonly, HCC.[69] **Sonographically**, type 1 GSD appears indistinguishable from other causes of diffuse fatty infiltration. Secondary hepatic adenomas are well-demarcated, solid masses of variable echogenicity. Malignant transformation can be recognized by rapid growth of the lesions, which may become more poorly defined.[69]

CIRRHOSIS

Cirrhosis is defined by the World Health Organization (WHO) as a diffuse process characterized by fibrosis

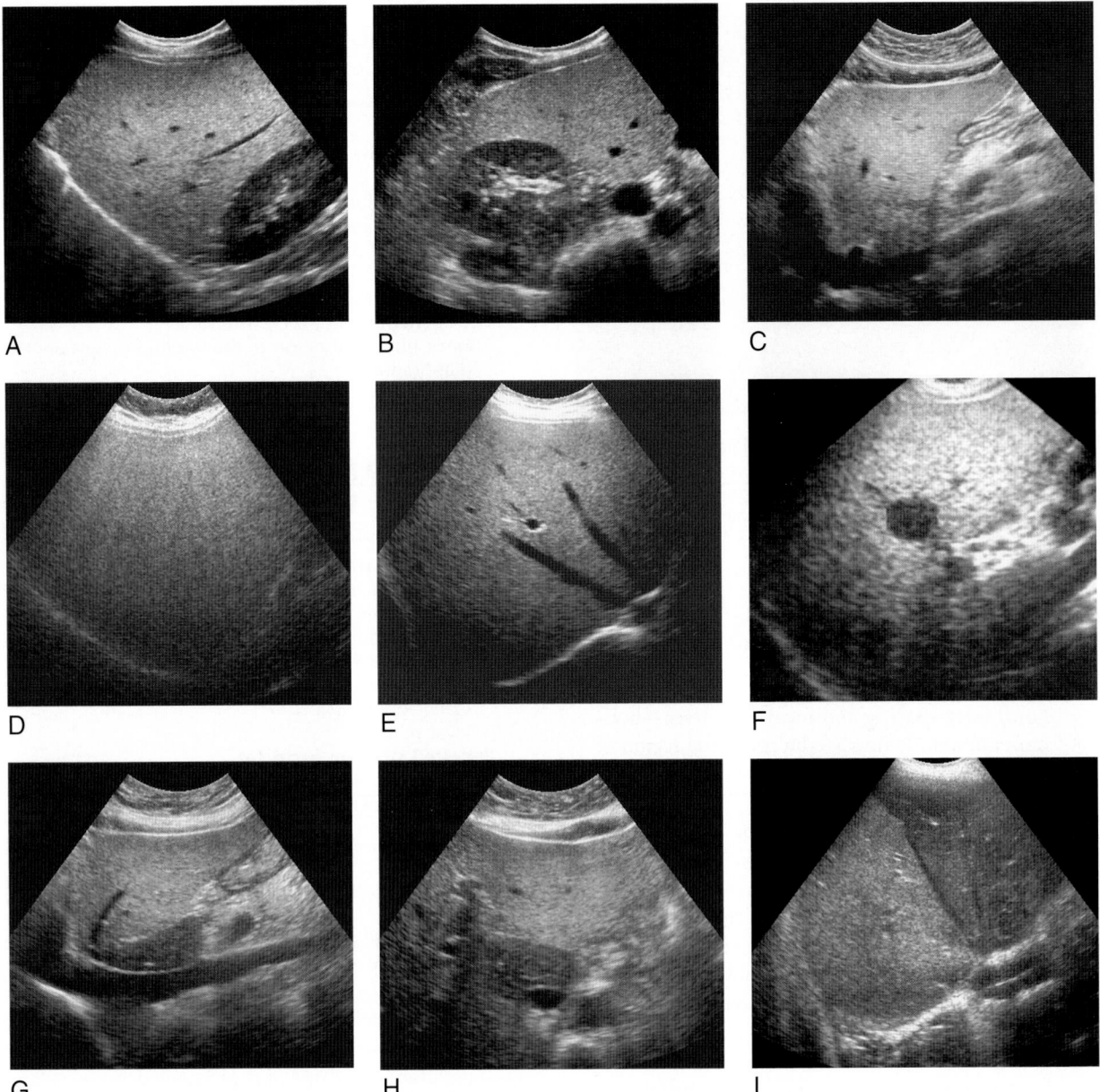

FIGURE 4-26. Diffuse fat—Spectrum of appearances. Top line—mild fatty infiltration. A, Sagittal right, **B,** transverse right and **C,** sagittal left lobe images. The liver is diffusely bright and echogenic. Sound penetration remains good. **Marked fatty infiltration** on **D,** sagittal right lobe and **E,** subcostal oblique views. The liver is enlarged and attenuating. There is poor sound penetration and the walls of the hepatic veins are not defined. **F, Focal sparing** mimicking a hypoechoic mass. Normal liver on biopsy and follow-up. **Focal fatty sparing** of the caudate lobe on **G,** sagittal and **H,** transverse images. **I, Geographic fatty sparing** of the entire left lobe marginated by the middle hepatic vein.

and the conversion of normal liver architecture into structurally abnormal nodules.[70] There are **three major pathologic mechanisms** which, in combination, create cirrhosis: cell death, fibrosis, and regeneration. Cirrhosis has been classified as **micronodular,** in which nodules are 0.1 to 1 cm in diameter, and **macronodular,** characterized by nodules of varying size, up to 5 cm in diameter. Alcohol consumption is the most common cause of micronodular cirrhosis, and chronic viral hepatitis is the most frequent cause of the macronodular

form.[71] Patients who continue to drink may go on to end-stage liver disease, which is indistinguishable from cirrhosis of other causes. Other etiologies are biliary cirrhosis (primary and secondary), Wilson's disease, primary sclerosing cholangitis, and hemochromatosis. The classic clinical presentation of cirrhosis is hepatomegaly, jaundice, and ascites. However, serious liver injury may be present without any clinical clues. In fact, only 60% of patients with cirrhosis have signs and symptoms of liver disease.

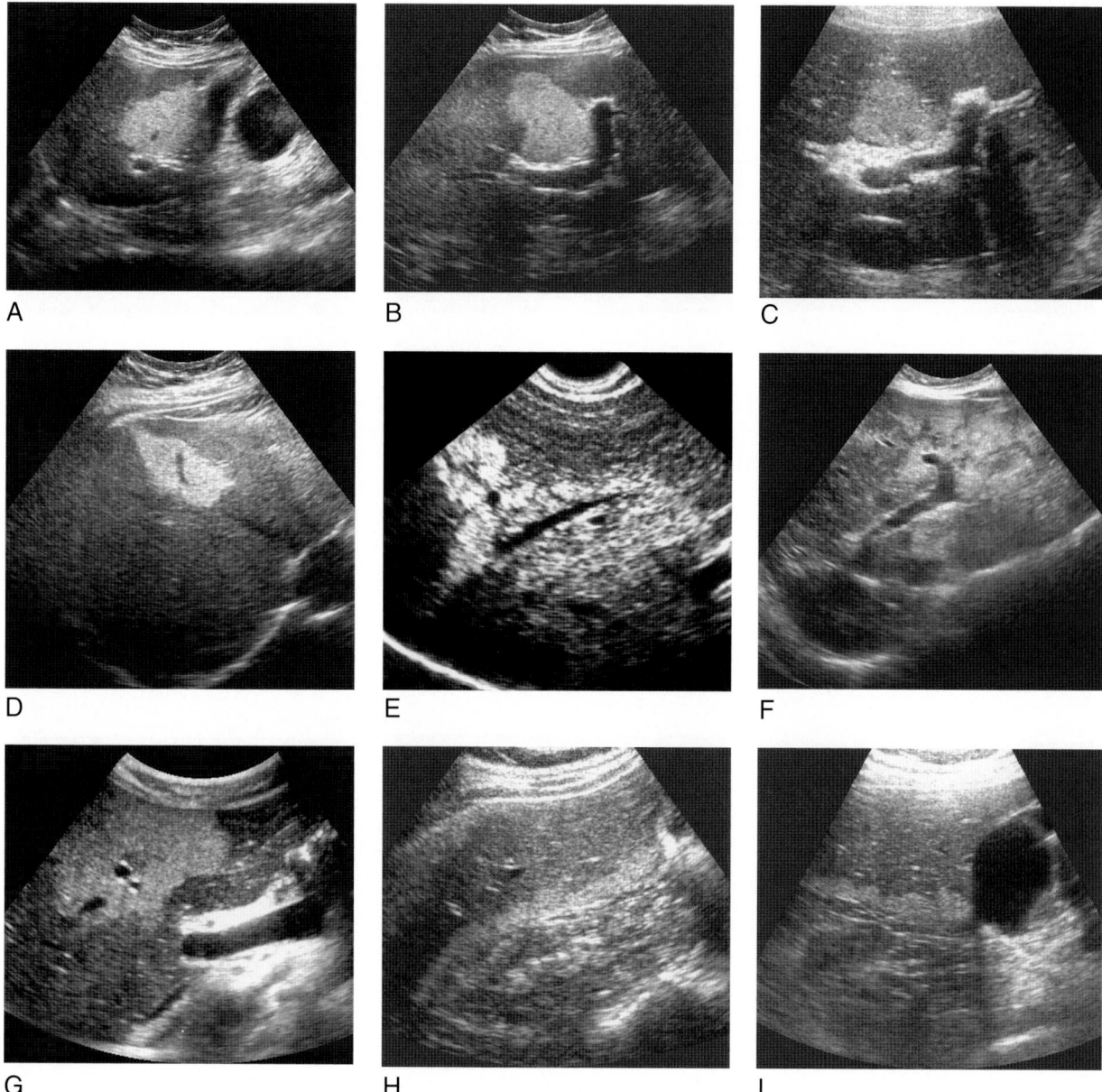

FIGURE 4-27. Focal fat—Spectrum of appearances. Classic focal fat. A, Sagittal and **B,** subcostal oblique images show the most common location for focal fat, in segment 4, anterior to the portal venous bifurcation at the porta hepatis. It may be large and masslike, as in this patient. **C,** Another patient showing a more common, milder form of the same fat deposition. **D, E, F,** and **G, Tumoral fat.** Fat deposits in all images suggest a focal liver mass. The liver vasculature is unaltered in its course at the location of the fatty masses. **E,** Focal fat of pregnancy. **H and I, Hepatic steatonecrosis** shown in views of the right lobe of the liver is a rare observation in diabetics who receive insulin in their peritoneal dialysate.

As liver biopsy is invasive, there has been great clinical interest in the ability to detect cirrhosis by noninvasive means, such as sonography. The **sonographic patterns** associated with cirrhosis include (Fig. 4-28):

- **Volume redistribution**—In the early stages of cirrhosis, the liver may be enlarged, whereas in the advanced states, the liver is often small, with relative enlargement of the caudate, left lobe, or

both, in comparison with the right lobe. Several studies have evaluated the ratio of the caudate lobe width to the right lobe width (C/RL) as an indicator of cirrhosis.[72] A C/RL value of 0.65 is considered indicative of cirrhosis. The specificity is high (100%) but the sensitivity is low (ranging from 43% to 84%), indicating that the C/RL ratio is a useful measurement if it is abnormal.[72] It should be noted, however, that there were no

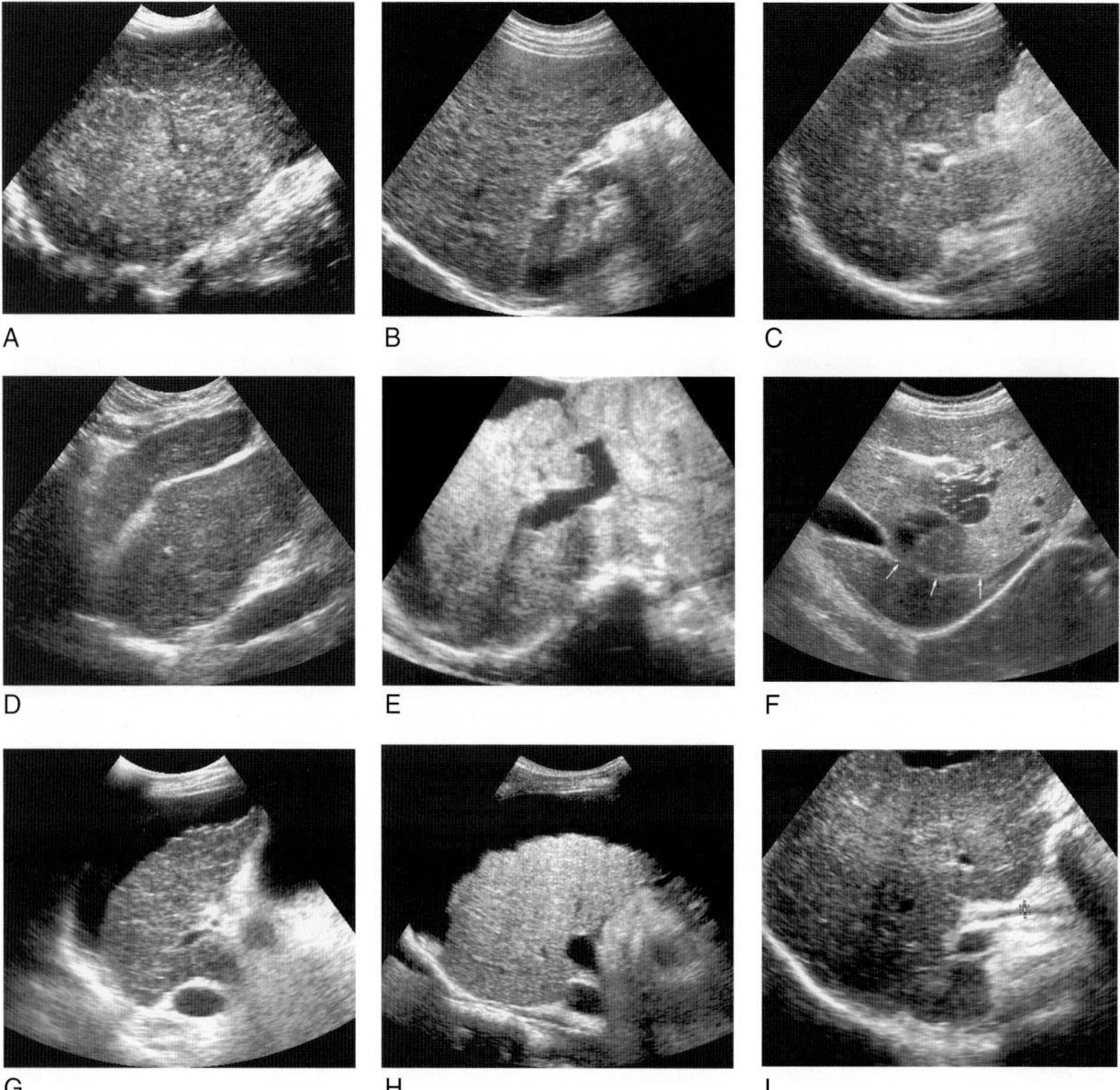

FIGURE 4-28. Cirrhosis—Spectrum of appearances. Top line—parenchymal changes (A to C). A, Coarse parenchyma and innumerable tiny, hyperechoic nodules. **B,** Coarse parenchyma and innumerable, tiny hypoechoic nodules. **C,** Coarse parenchyma and surface nodularity. **Middle line—lobar redistribution (D to F). D,** Sagittal image showing an enormous caudate lobe. **E,** Transverse sonogram shows that the right lobe is small and there is enlargement of the left lateral segment. **F,** Subcostal oblique view showing a tiny right lobe **(G to I)** of the liver, which is separated from the large left lobe by the main lobar fissure *(arrows).* **Bottom line—contour abnormality. G** and **H** show small end-stage livers with surface nodularity, best appreciated in patients with ascites, as here. **I,** There is great variation in liver contour as shown here where a large nodule protrudes from the deep liver border.

patients in these studies with Budd-Chiari syndrome, which may also cause caudate lobe enlargement.

• **Coarse echotexture**—Increased echogenicity and coarse echotexture are frequent observations in diffuse liver disease. These are subjective findings, however, and may be confounded by inappropriate time gain compensation (TGC) settings and overall gain. Liver attenuation is

correlated with the presence of fat and not fibrosis.[73] Cirrhotic livers without fatty infiltration had attenuation values similar to those of controls. This accounts for the relatively low accuracy in distinguishing diffuse liver disease[74] and for the conflicting reports regarding attenuation values in cirrhosis.

• **Nodular surface**—Irregularity of the liver surface during routine scanning has been appreciated as a

CIRRHOSIS: SONOGRAPHIC FEATURES

Volume redistribution
Coarse echotexture
Nodular surface
Nodules—regenerative and dysplastic
Portal hypertension—ascites, splenomegaly, and varices

sign of cirrhosis when the appearance is gross or when ascites is present.[75] The nodularity corresponds to the presence of regenerating nodules and fibrosis.

- **Regenerating nodules (RN)**—Regenerating nodules represent regenerating hepatocytes surrounded by a fibrotic septa. Because they have a similar architecture to the normal liver, ultrasound and CT have limited ability in their detection. RN tends to be isoechoic or hypoechoic with a thin echogenic border which corresponds to fibrofatty connective tissue.[75] MRI has a greater sensitivity than both CT and ultrasound in their detection. Because some RN contain iron, gradient echo sequences demonstrate these nodules as hypointense.[76]

- **Dysplastic nodules**—Dysplastic nodules or adenomatous hyperplastic nodules are larger than RN (diameter ≥ 10 mm) and are considered premalignant.[77] They contain well-differentiated hepatocytes, a portal venous blood supply and also atypical or frankly malignant cells. The portal venous blood supply can be detected with the use of color Doppler flow imaging and distinguished from the hepatic artery-supplied HCC.[78] In a patient with cirrhosis and a liver mass, percutaneous biopsy is often performed to exclude or diagnose HCC.

Doppler Characteristics of Cirrhosis

The normal Doppler waveform of the hepatic veins reflects the hemodynamics of the right atrium. The waveform is triphasic: two large antegrade diastolic and systolic waves and a small retrograde wave corresponding to the atrial "kick." Because the walls of the hepatic veins are thin, disease of the hepatic parenchyma may alter their compliance. In many patients with compensated cirrhosis (no portal hypertension), the Doppler waveform is abnormal. **Two abnormal patterns** have been described: decreased amplitude of phasic oscillations with loss of reversed flow; and a flattened waveform.[79,80] These abnormal patterns have also been found in patients with fatty infiltration of their livers.[80]

As cirrhosis progresses, **luminal narrowing of the hepatic veins** may be associated with flow alterations visible on color and spectral Doppler. High-velocity signals through an area of narrowing produce color aliasing and turbulence (Fig. 4-29).

The hepatic artery waveform also shows altered flow dynamics in cirrhosis and chronic liver disease. Lafortune et al.[81] found an increase in the resistive index of the hepatic artery following a meal in patients who had normal livers. The vasoconstriction of the hepatic artery occurs as a normal response to the increased portal venous flow stimulated by eating (≥20% change). In patients with cirrhosis and chronic liver disease, the normal increase in postprandial resistive index is blunted.[82]

VASCULAR ABNORMALITIES

Portal Hypertension

Normal portal vein pressure is 5 to 10 mm Hg (14 cm H_2O). Portal hypertension is defined by a wedged hepatic vein pressure or direct portal vein pressure of more than 5 mm Hg greater than inferior vena cava pressure, splenic vein pressure of greater than 15 mm Hg, or portal vein pressure (measured surgically) of greater than 30 cm H_2O. Pathophysiologically, portal hypertension can be divided into presinusoidal and intrahepatic groups, depending on whether the hepatic vein wedged pressure is normal (presinusoidal) or elevated (intrahepatic).

Presinusoidal portal hypertension can be subdivided into extrahepatic and intrahepatic forms. The causes of **extrahepatic** presinusoidal portal hypertension include thrombosis of the portal or splenic veins. This should be suspected in any patient who presents with clinical signs of portal hypertension—ascites, splenomegaly, and varices—and a normal liver biopsy. Thrombosis of the portal venous system occurs in children secondary to umbilical vein catheterization, omphalitis, and neonatal sepsis. In adults, the causes of portal vein thrombosis include trauma, sepsis, HCC, pancreatic carcinoma, pancreatitis, portacaval shunts, splenectomy, and hypercoagulable states. The **intrahepatic** presinusoidal causes of portal hypertension are results of diseases affecting the portal zones of the liver, notably schistosomiasis, primary biliary cirrhosis, congenital hepatic fibrosis, and toxic substances, such as polyvinyl chloride and methotrexate.[83]

Cirrhosis is the most common cause of **intrahepatic portal hypertension** and accounts for greater than 90% of all cases of portal hypertension in the West. In cirrhosis, most of the normal liver architecture is replaced by distorted vascular channels that provide increased resistance to portal venous blood flow and obstruction to hepatic venous outflow. Diffuse metastatic liver disease also produces portal hypertension by

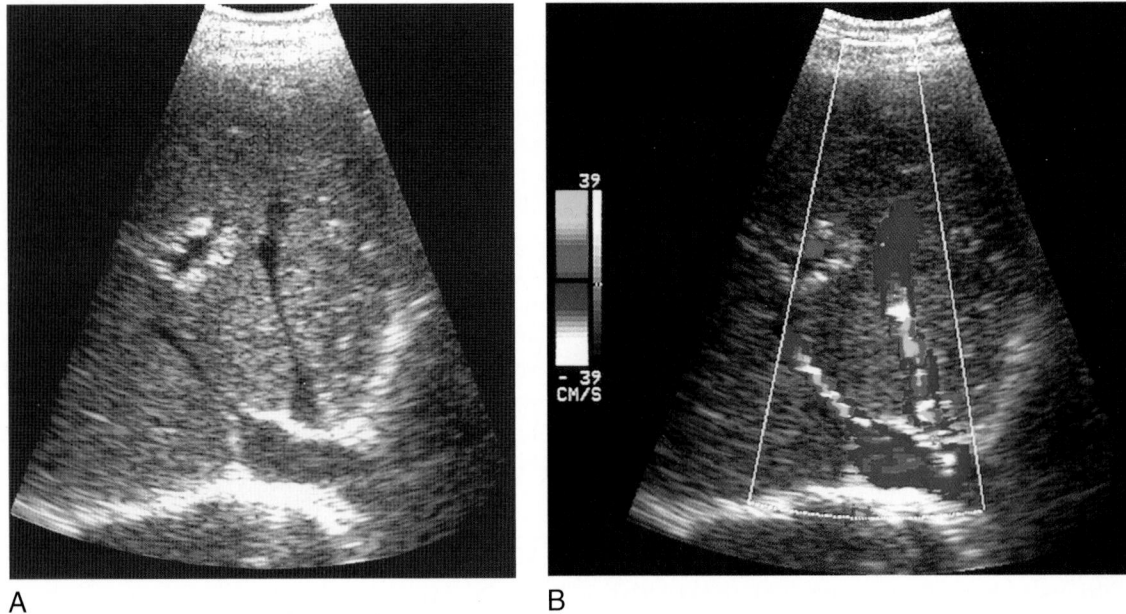

FIGURE 4-29. Hepatic vein strictures—cirrhosis. A, Gray-scale image of hepatic veins shows a tapered luminal narrowing. **B,** Color Doppler image shows appropriately directed flow toward the inferior vena cava in blue. There is color aliasing from the rapid velocity flow through the points of narrowing.

the same mechanism. Thrombotic diseases of the inferior vena cava and hepatic veins, as well as constrictive pericarditis and other causes of severe right-sided heart failure, over time, will lead to centrilobular fibrosis, hepatic regeneration, cirrhosis, and finally portal hypertension.

Sonographic findings of portal hypertension include the secondary signs of splenomegaly, ascites, and portosystemic venous collaterals (Fig. 4-30 and Fig. 4-31). When the resistance to blood flow in the portal vessels exceeds the resistance to flow in the small communicating channels between the portal and systemic circulations, portosystemic collaterals form. Thus, although the caliber of the portal vein initially may be increased (≥1.3 cm) in portal hypertension,[84] with the development of portosystemic shunts, the portal vein caliber will decrease.[85] **Five major sites of portosystemic venous collaterals** are visualized by ultrasound (see Fig. 4-30).[86-88]

- **Gastroesophageal junction**—Between the coronary and short gastric veins and the systemic esophageal veins. These varices are of particular importance because they may lead to life-threatening or fatal hemorrhage. Dilation of the coronary vein (>0.7 cm) is associated with severe portal hypertension (portohepatic gradient >10 mm Hg) (see Fig. 4-31C, D).[85]
- **Paraumbilical vein**—Runs in the falciform ligament and connects the left portal vein to the systemic epigastric veins near the umbilicus (Cruveilhier-Baumgarten syndrome) (see Fig. 4-31A).[89] Several authors have suggested

that, if the hepatofugal flow in the patent paraumbilical vein exceeds the hepatopetal flow in the portal vein, patients may be protected from developing esophageal varices.[90,91]
- **Splenorenal and gastrorenal**—Tortuous veins may be seen in the region of the splenic and left renal hilus (see Fig. 4-31E, F), which represent collaterals between the splenic, coronary, and short gastric veins and the left adrenal or renal veins.
- **Intestinal**—Regions in which the gastrointestinal tract becomes retroperitoneal so that the veins of the ascending and descending colon, duodenum, pancreas, and liver may anastomose with the renal, phrenic, and lumbar veins (systemic tributaries).
- **Hemorrhoidal**—The perianal region where the superior rectal veins, which extend from the inferior mesenteric vein, anastomose with the systemic middle and inferior rectal veins.

Duplex Doppler sonography provides additional information regarding direction of portal flow. False results may occur, however, when sampling is obtained from periportal collaterals in patients with portal vein thrombosis or hepatofugal portal flow.[92] Normal portal venous flow rates will vary in the same individual: increasing postprandially and during inspiration[82,93] and decreasing following exercise or when the patient is in the upright position.[94] An increase of less than 20% in the diameter of the portal vein with deep inspiration indicates portal hypertension with 81% sensitivity and 100% specificity.[95]

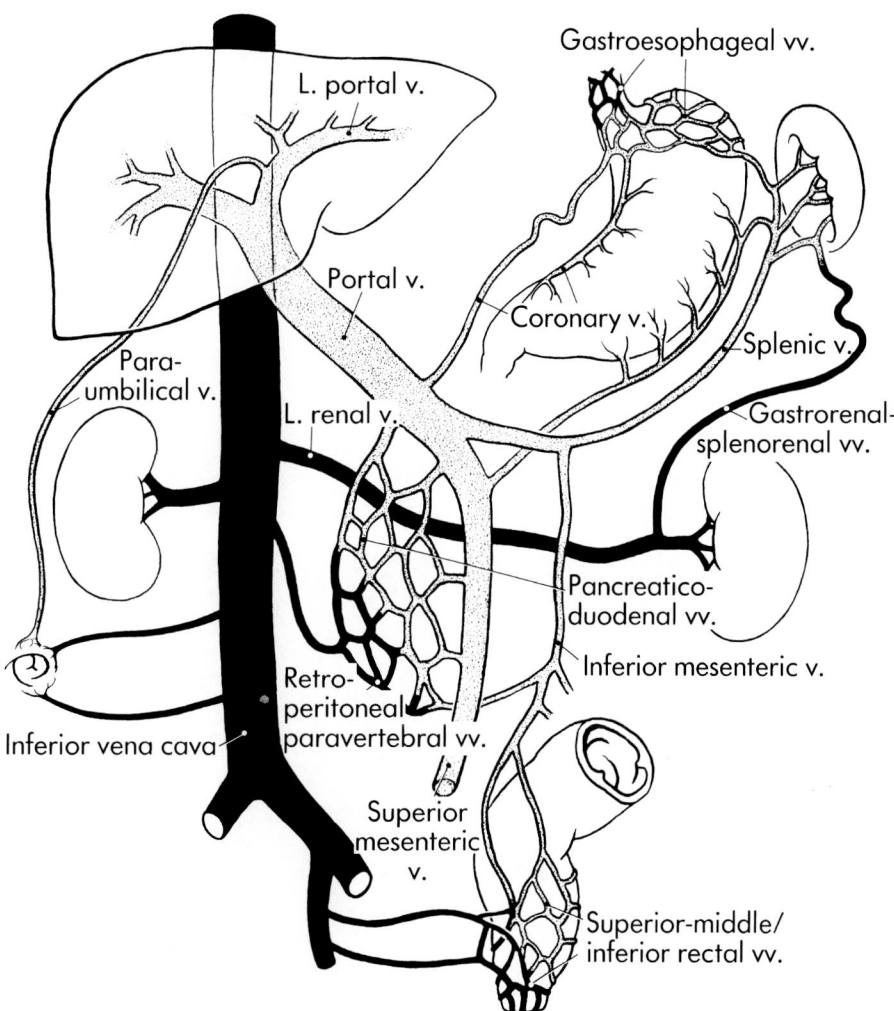

FIGURE 4-30. Portal hypertension. Major sites of portosystemic venous collaterals. (From Subramanyam BR, Balthazar EJ, Madamba MR, et al: Sonography of portosystemic venous collaterals in portal hypertension. Radiology 1983;146:161-166.)

SONOGRAPHIC IDENTIFICATION OF PORTOSYSTEMIC VENOUS COLLATERALS

Gastroesophageal junction
Paraumbilical vein in the falciform ligament
Splenorenal and gastrorenal veins
Intestinal-retroperitoneal anastomoses
Hemorrhoidal veins

The **normal portal vein** demonstrates an undulating hepatopedal (toward the liver) flow. Mean portal venous flow velocity is approximately 15 to 18 cm/sec and varies with respiration and cardiac pulsation. As portal hypertension develops, the flow in the portal vein loses its undulatory pattern and becomes monophasic. As the severity of portal hypertension increases, flow becomes biphasic and finally hepatofugal (away from the liver).

Intrahepatic arterial-portal venous shunting may also be seen.

Chronic liver disease is also associated with increased splanchnic blood flow. Recent evidence suggests that portal hypertension is, in part, caused by the hyperdynamic flow state of cirrhosis. In a study by Zweibel et al,[96] blood flow was increased in the superior mesenteric arteries and splenic arteries of patients with cirrhosis and splenomegaly, compared with normal controls. Of interest, in patients with cirrhosis and normal-sized livers, splanchnic blood flow was not increased. Patients with isolated splenomegaly and normal livers were not included in this study.

The **limitations of Doppler sonography** in the evaluation of portal hypertension include the inability to accurately determine vascular pressures and flow rates. Patients with portal hypertension are often ill, with contracted livers, abundant ascites, and floating bowel, all of which create a technical challenge. In a recent article comparing duplex Doppler with MR angiog-

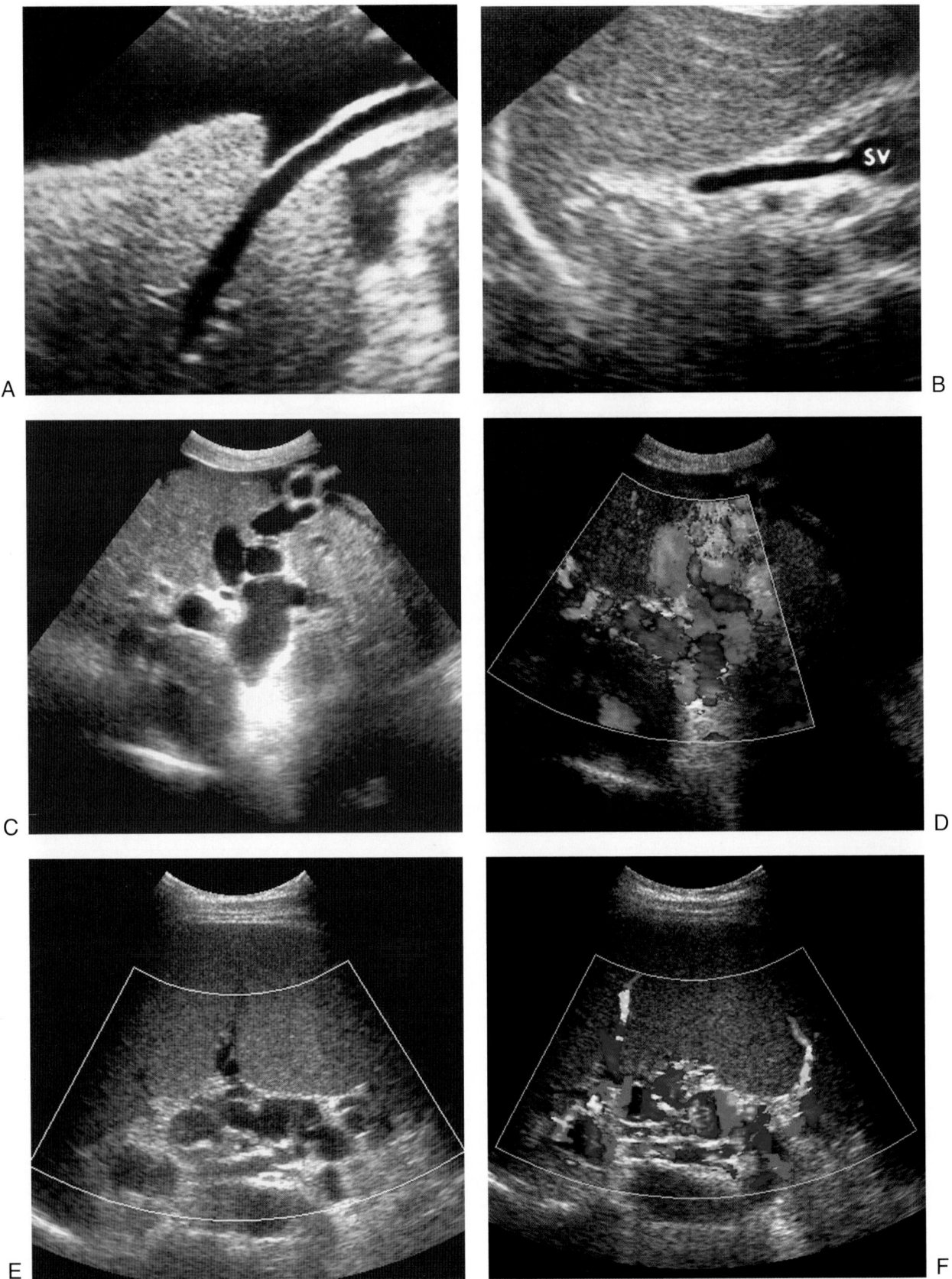

FIGURE 4-31. Portal hypertension. A, Sagittal image shows a recanalized paraumbilical vein in a patient with gross ascites. B, Enlarged coronary vein on sagittal image running cephalad from the splenic vein (SV). C and D, Gray-scale and color Doppler images showing extensive varices in the distribution of the coronary vein. E and F, Gray-scale and color Doppler images showing splenic hilar varices.

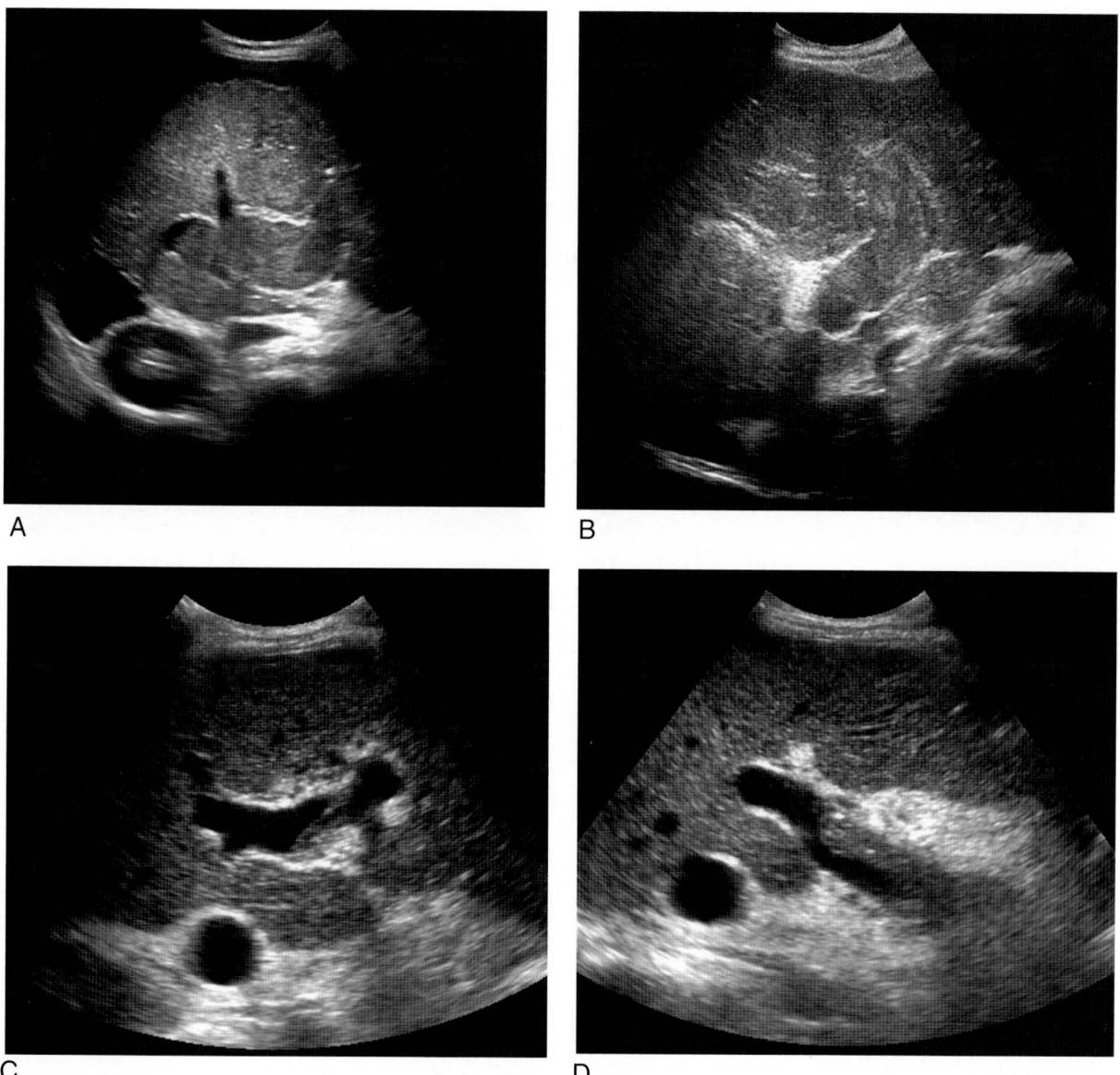

FIGURE 4-32. Portal vein thrombosis—benign and malignant. Top line—malignant thrombus (A and B).
A, Transverse view of the vein at the porta hepatis and **B,** left ascending left portal vein. Both are distended with occlusive thrombus.
Bottom line—benign thrombus (C and D). Simple bland nonocclusive thrombus in the left portal vein at the porta hepatis.
C (transverse) and **D** (sagittal) images.

raphy, MR imaging was superior in the assessment of patency of the portal vein and surgical shunts as well as in detection of varices.[97] However, when the Doppler study was technically adequate, it was accurate in the assessment of normal portal anatomy and flow direction. Duplex Doppler sonography has the added advantages of decreased cost and portability of the equipment and, therefore, should be used as the initial screening method for portal hypertension.[97]

Portal Vein Thrombosis

Portal vein thrombosis has been associated with malignancy, including HCC, metastatic liver disease,

carcinoma of the pancreas, and primary leiomyosarcoma of the portal vein[98]; as well as chronic pancreatitis; hepatitis; septicemia; trauma; splenectomy; portacaval shunts; hypercoagulable states, such as pregnancy; and in neonates, omphalitis; umbilical vein catheterization; and acute dehydration.[99]

Sonographic findings of portal vein thrombosis include echogenic thrombus within the lumen of the vein, portal vein collaterals, expansion of the caliber of the vein, and cavernous transformations (Fig. 4-32 and Fig. 4-33).[99] **Cavernous transformation of the portal vein** refers to numerous wormlike vessels at the porta hepatis, which represent periportal collateral circulation (see Fig. 4-33).[100] This pattern is observed in long-

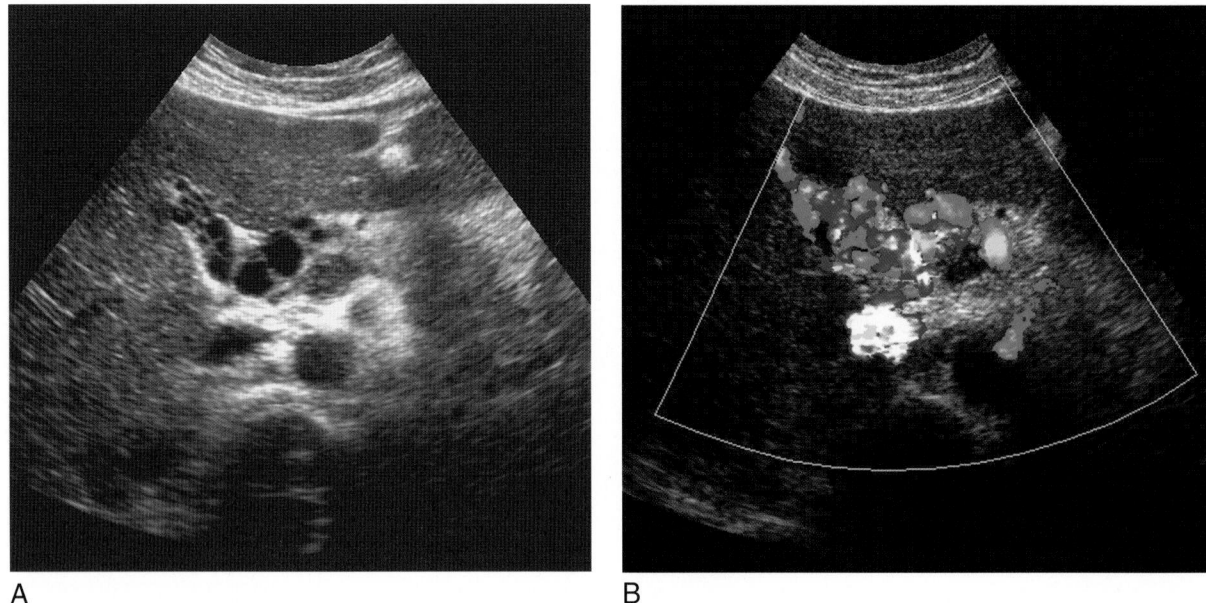

A   B

FIGURE 4-33. Cavernous transformation of portal vein. Numerous periportal collateral vessels are present.

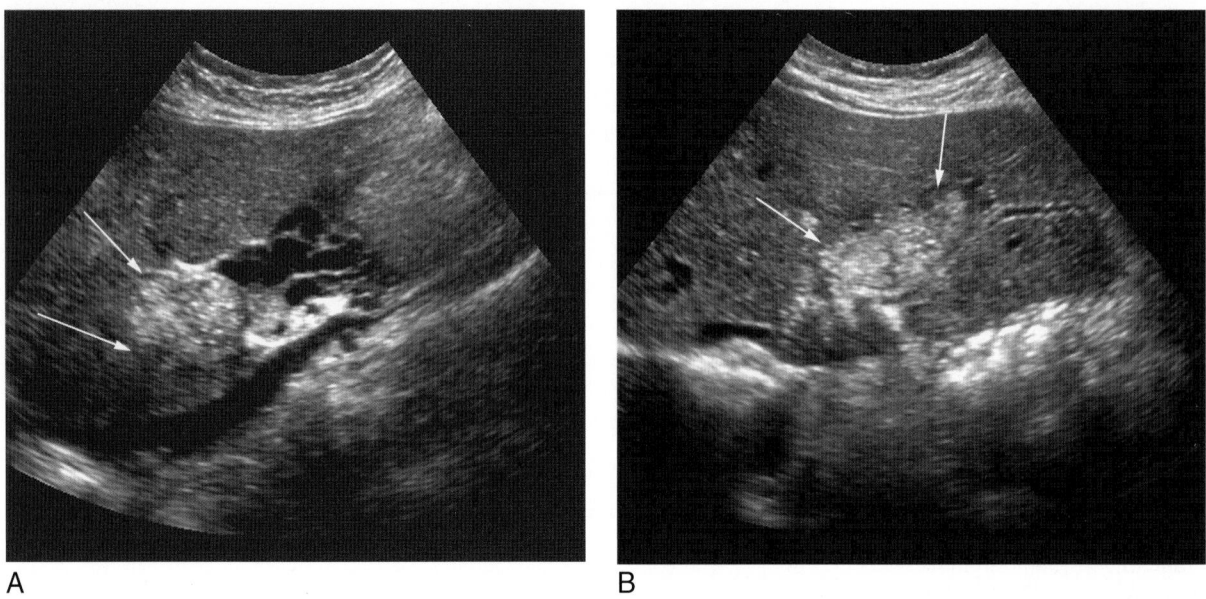

A   B

FIGURE 4-34. Metastasis to the portal vein from colon cancer. A, Sagittal view of the main portal vein at the porta hepatis and **B,** subcostal oblique sonogram of the left ascending branch of the portal vein show the portal vein is distended and highly echogenic (arrows). There is also evidence of cavernous transformation, an uncommon accompaniment of malignant portal vein occlusion.

standing thrombosis, requiring up to 12 months to occur, and thus is more likely to develop with benign disease.[101] Acute thrombus may appear relatively anechoic and, therefore, may be overlooked unless Doppler interrogation is performed. Malignant thrombosis of the portal vein has a high association with HCC and is often expansive, as is malignant occlusion from other primary or secondary disease (Fig. 4-34).

Doppler sonography is useful in distinguishing between benign and malignant portal vein thrombi in patients with cirrhosis. Both bland and malignant

thrombi may demonstrate continuous blood flow. Pulsatile flow, however, has been found to be 95% specific for the diagnosis of malignant portal vein thrombosis (see Fig. 4-32). The sensitivity was only 62% because many malignant thrombi are hypovascular.[102]

Budd-Chiari Syndrome

The Budd-Chiari syndrome is a relatively rare disorder characterized by occlusion of the lumina of the hepatic veins with or without occlusion of the lumen of the

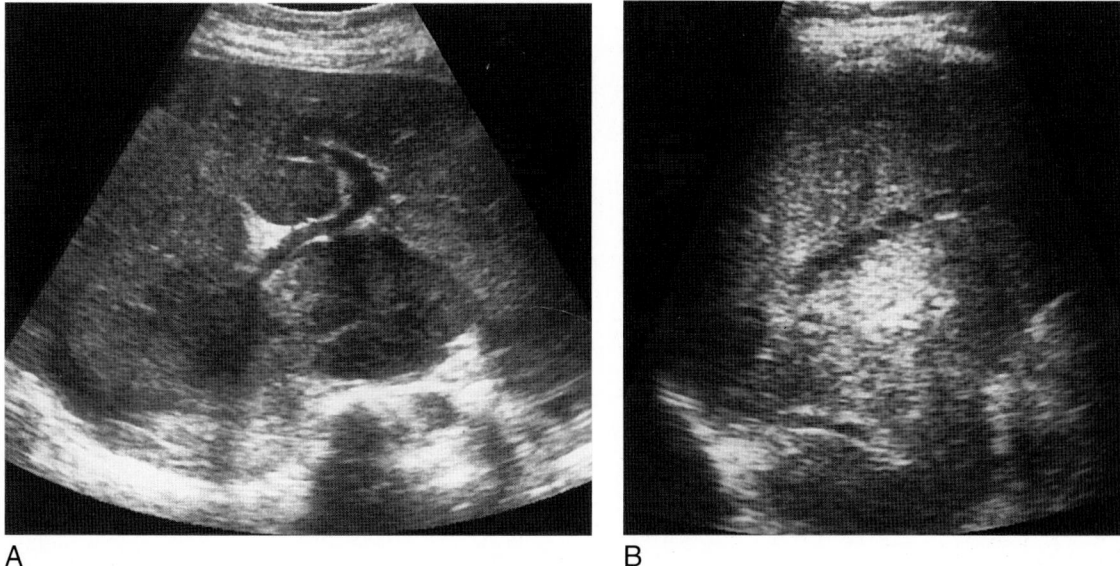

A   B

FIGURE 4-35. Acute Budd-Chiari syndrome. A, Transverse view of liver shows a large, bulbous caudate lobe. **B,** Sagittal view of right hepatic vein shows echoes within the vein lumen consistent with thrombosis, with absence of the vessel toward the inferior vena cava. Doppler showed no flow in this vessel.

inferior vena cava. The degree of occlusion and the presence of collateral circulation predicts the clinical course. Some patients die in the acute phase of liver failure. Causes of **Budd-Chiari syndrome** include coagulation abnormalities, such as polycythemia rubra vera, chronic leukemia and paroxysmal nocturnal hemoglobinuria; trauma; tumor extension from primary HCC, renal carcinoma, and adrenal cortical carcinoma; pregnancy; congenital abnormalities and obstructing membranes. The classic patient in North America is a young adult woman taking birth control pills who presents with an acute onset of ascites, right upper quadrant pain, hepatomegaly, and to a lesser extent, splenomegaly. In some cases, no etiologic factor is found. The syndrome is more common in other geographic areas including India, South Africa, and Asia.

Sonographic evaluation of the patient with Budd-Chiari syndrome includes gray-scale and Doppler features.[103-114] Ascites is an invariable observation. The liver is typically large and bulbous in the acute phase (Fig. 4-35A). Hemorrhagic infarction may produce significant altered regional echogenicity. As infarcted areas become more fibrotic, echogenicity increases.[112] The caudate lobe is often spared in Budd-Chiari syndrome because the emissary veins drain directly into the inferior vena cava at a lower level than the involved main hepatic veins. Increased blood flow through the caudate lobe leads to relative caudate enlargement.

Real-time scanning allows the radiologist to evaluate the inferior vena cava and hepatic veins noninvasively. Sonographic features include evidence of the hepatic vein occlusion (see Fig. 4-35B and Fig. 4-36) and the development of abnormal intrahepatic collaterals

(Fig. 4-37). The extent of **hepatic venous involvement** in Budd-Chiari syndrome includes partial or complete inability to see the hepatic veins, stenosis with proximal dilation, intraluminal echogenicity, thickened walls, thrombosis (Fig. 4-38 and Fig. 4-39), and extensive intrahepatic collaterals (see Fig. 4-37).[105,106] Membranous webs may be identified as echogenic or focal obliterations of the lumen.[106] Real-time ultrasonography, however, underestimates the presence of thrombosis and webs and may be inconclusive in a cirrhotic patient in whom the hepatic veins are difficult to image.[105] Intrahepatic collaterals, on gray-scale images, show as tubular vascular structures in an abnormal locale and are most commonly seen extending from a hepatic vein to the liver surface where they anastomose with systemic capsular vessels.

Duplex and color-flow Doppler imaging have considerable potential in the evaluation of patients with suspected Budd-Chiari syndrome to determine both the presence and direction of hepatic venous flow. The middle and left hepatic veins are best scanned in the transverse plane at the level of the xiphoid process. From this angle, the veins are almost parallel to the Doppler beam, allowing optimal reception of their Doppler signals. The right hepatic vein is best evaluated from a right intercostal approach.[108] The intricate pathways of blood flow out of the liver in the patient with Budd-Chiari syndrome can be mapped with documentation of hepatic venous occlusions, hepatic-systemic collaterals, hepatic venous-portal venous collaterals, and increased caliber of anomalous or accessory hepatic veins.

The normal blood flow in the inferior vena cava and hepatic veins is phasic in response to both the cardiac

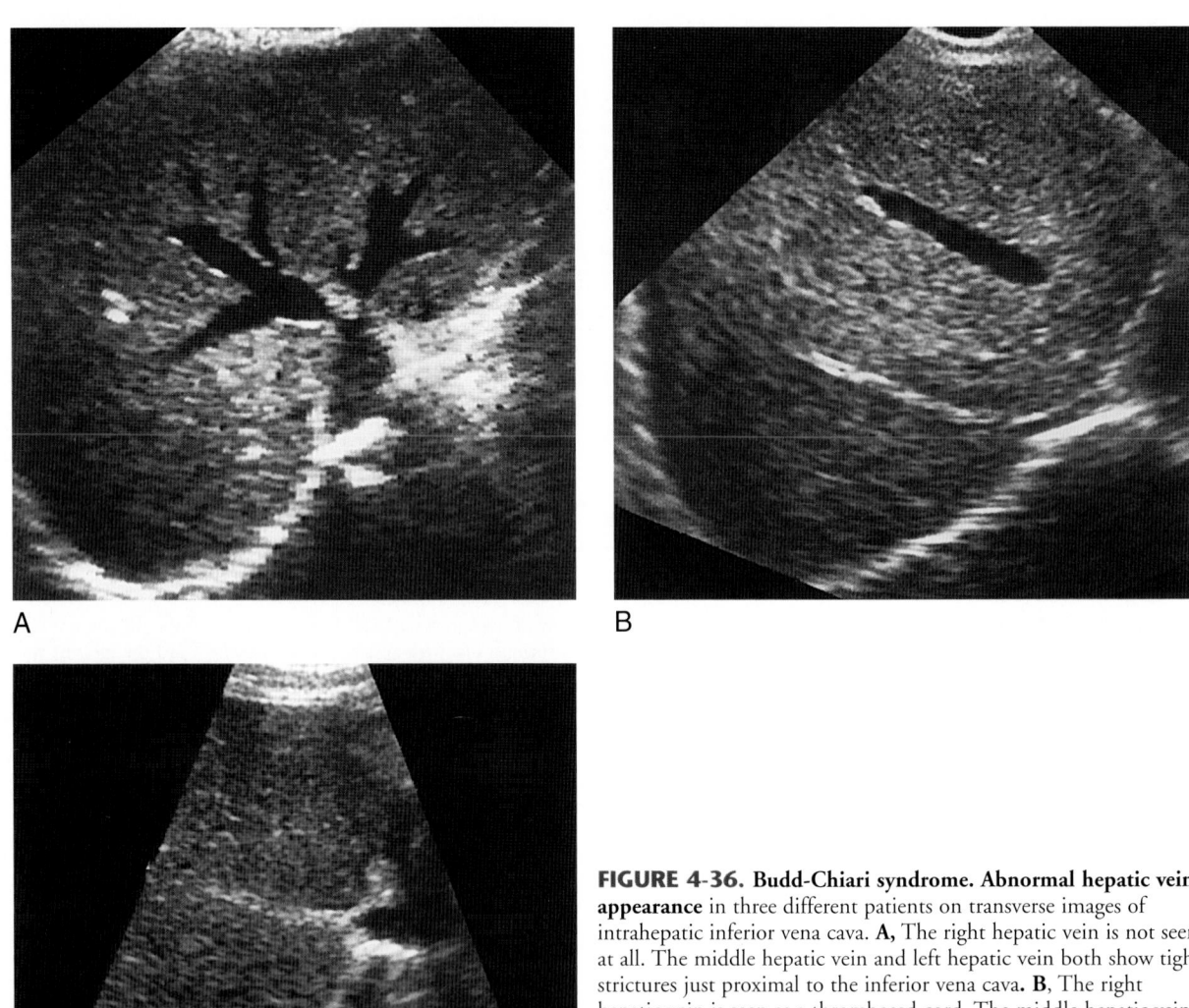

A

B

C

FIGURE 4-36. Budd-Chiari syndrome. Abnormal hepatic vein appearance in three different patients on transverse images of intrahepatic inferior vena cava. **A,** The right hepatic vein is not seen at all. The middle hepatic vein and left hepatic vein both show tight strictures just proximal to the inferior vena cava. **B,** The right hepatic vein is seen as a thrombosed cord. The middle hepatic vein does not reach the inferior vena cava. The left hepatic vein is not seen. **C,** Only a single hepatic vein, the middle hepatic vein, can be seen as a thrombosed cord.

and respiratory cycles.[115] In Budd-Chiari syndrome, flow in the inferior vena cava, hepatic veins, or both, changes from phasic to absent, reversed, turbulent, or continuous.[110,114] Continuous flow has been called the pseudoportal Doppler signal and appears to reflect either partial inferior vena cava obstruction or extrinsic inferior vena cava compression.[109] The portal blood flow also may be affected and is characteristically either slowed or reversed.[110]

The addition of Doppler to gray-scale sonography in the patient with suspect Budd-Chiari syndrome lends strong supportive evidence to the gray-scale impression of either missing, compressed, or otherwise abnormal hepatic veins and inferior vena cava.[113,114] Associated

reversal of flow in the portal vein and epigastric collaterals is also optimally assessed with this technique.[114]

Hepatic veno-occlusive disease causes progressive occlusion of the small hepatic venules. The disease is endemic in Jamaica, secondary to alkaloid toxicity from bush tea. In North America, most cases are iatrogenic, secondary to hepatic irradiation and chemotherapy used in bone marrow transplantation.[111] Patients with hepatic veno-occlusive disease are clinically indistinguishable from those with Budd-Chiari syndrome. Duplex Doppler sonography demonstrates normal caliber, patency, and phasic forward (toward the heart) flow of the main hepatic veins and inferior vena cava.[111] Flow in the portal vein, however, may be abnormal, showing either

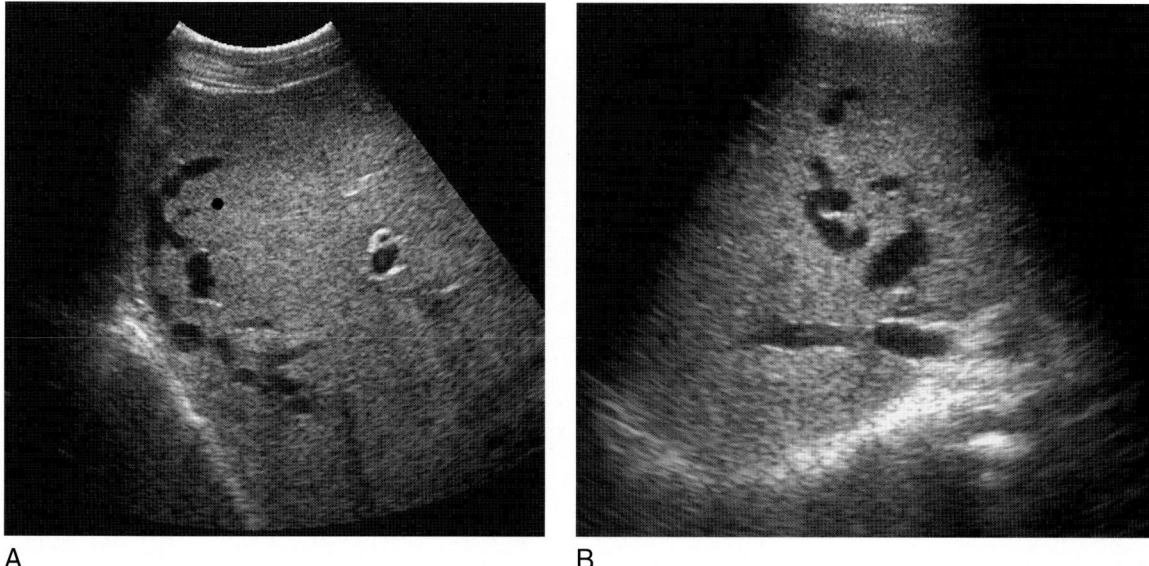

A   B

FIGURE 4-37. Budd-Chiari syndrome. Budd-Chiari with abnormal intrahepatic collaterals on gray scale in two different patients. Both images show vessels with abnormal locations and increased tortuosity as compared with the normal intrahepatic vasculature.

reversed or "to and fro" flow.[111,116] In addition, the diagnosis of hepatic veno-occlusive disease can be suggested in a patient with decreased portal blood flow (as compared with a baseline measurement performed before ablative therapy).[111]

Portal Vein Aneurysm

Aneurysms of the portal vein are rare. Their origin is believed to be either congenital or acquired secondary to portal hypertension.[117] Portal vein aneurysms have been described proximally at the junction of the superior mesenteric and splenic veins and distally involving the portal venous radicles. The sonographic appearance is that of an anechoic cystic mass, which connects with the portal venous system. Pulsed Doppler sonographic examination demonstrates turbulent venous flow.[117]

Intrahepatic Portosystemic Venous Shunts

Intrahepatic arterial-portal fistulas are well-recognized complications of large-gauge percutaneous liver biopsy and trauma. Conversely, intrahepatic portohepatic venous shunts are rare. Their cause is controversial and believed to be either congenital or related to portal hypertension.[118,119] Patients typically are middle aged and present with hepatic encephalopathy. Anatomically, portohepatic venous shunts are more common in the right lobe. Sonography demonstrates a tortuous tubular vessel or complex vascular channels, which connect a branch of the portal vein to a hepatic vein or the inferior vena cava.[118-120] The diagnosis is confirmed angiographically.

Hepatic Artery Aneurysm and Pseudoaneurysm

The hepatic artery is the fourth most common site of an intra-abdominal aneurysm, following the infrarenal aorta, iliac, and splenic arteries. Eighty percent of patients with a hepatic artery aneurysm experience catastrophic rupture into the peritoneum, biliary tree, gastrointestinal tract, or portal vein.[121] Hepatic artery pseudoaneurysm secondary to chronic pancreatitis has been described. The duplex Doppler sonographic examination revealed turbulent arterial flow within a sonolucent mass.[121] Primary dissection of the hepatic artery is rare and in most cases leads to death prior to diagnosis.[122] Sonography may show the intimal flap with the true and false channels.

Hereditary Hemorrhagic Telangiectasia

Hereditary hemorrhagic telangiectasia, or Osler-Weber-Rendu disease, is an autosomal-dominant disorder that causes arteriovenous malformations in the liver, hepatic fibrosis, and cirrhosis. Patients present with multiple telangiectasias and recurrent episodes of bleeding. Sonographic findings in hereditary hemorrhagic telangiectasia include a large feeding common hepatic artery measuring up to 10 mm, multiple dilated tubular structures representing arteriovenous malformations, and large draining hepatic veins secondary to arteriovenous shunting.[123]

Peliosis Hepatis

Peliosis hepatis is a rare liver disorder characterized by blood-filled cavities that range in size from less than a

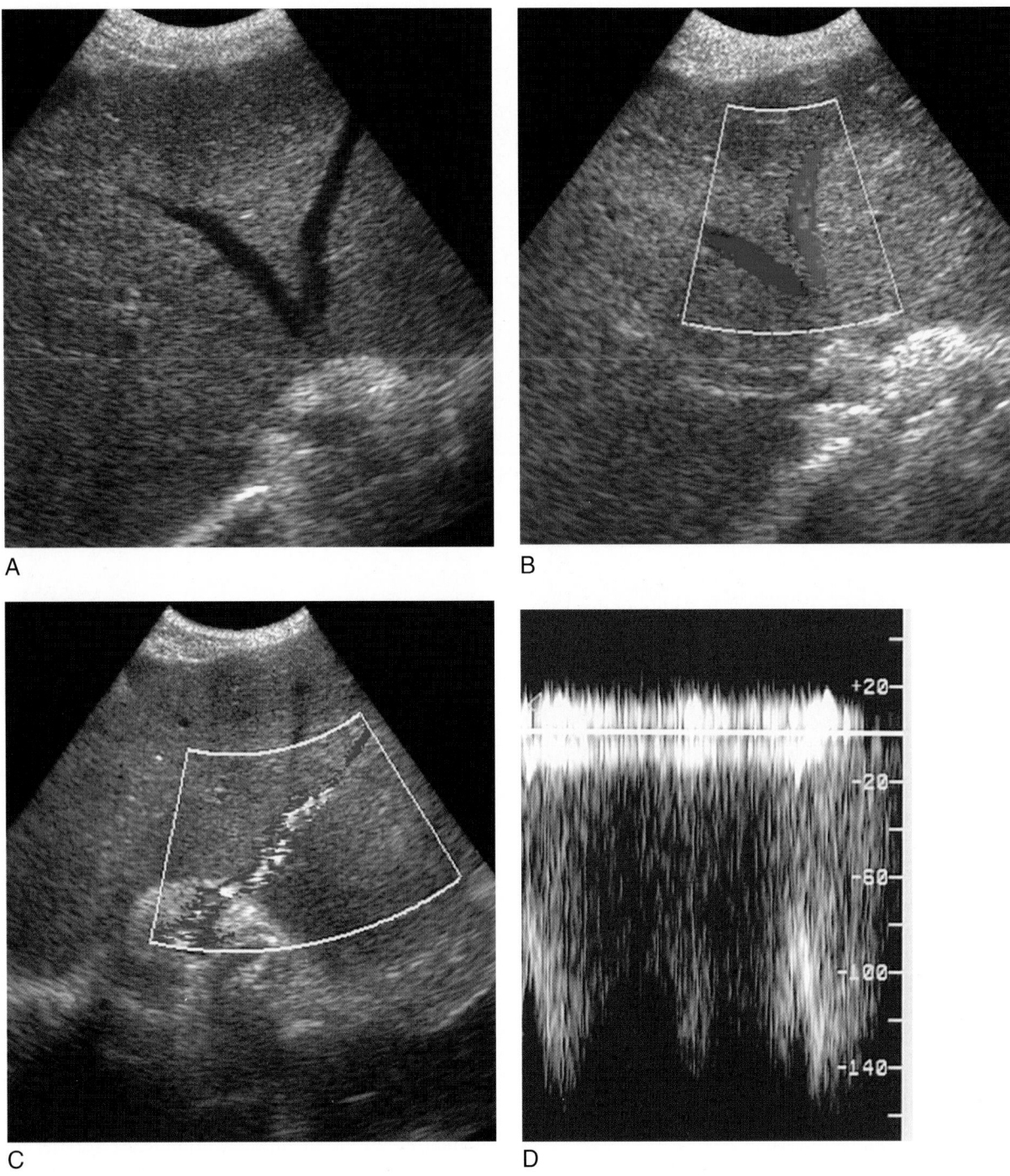

FIGURE 4-38. Budd-Chiari syndrome. A, Gray-scale transverse image of hepatic venous confluence shows complete absence of the right hepatic vein with obliteration of the lumen of a common trunk for the middle and left hepatic vein. **B,** Color Doppler shows the flow in the middle hepatic vein (*blue*) is normally directed toward the inferior vena cava. As the trunk is obliterated, all of the blood is flowing out of the left hepatic vein (*red*) that is abnormal. Other images showed anastomoses of the left hepatic vein with surface collaterals. **C,** Color Doppler image shows an anomalous left hepatic vein with flow to the inferior vena cava (normal direction) with aliasing due to a long stricture. **D,** Spectral Doppler waveform of the anomalous left hepatic vein shows a very high abnormal velocity of approximately 140 cm/sec confirming the tight stricture.

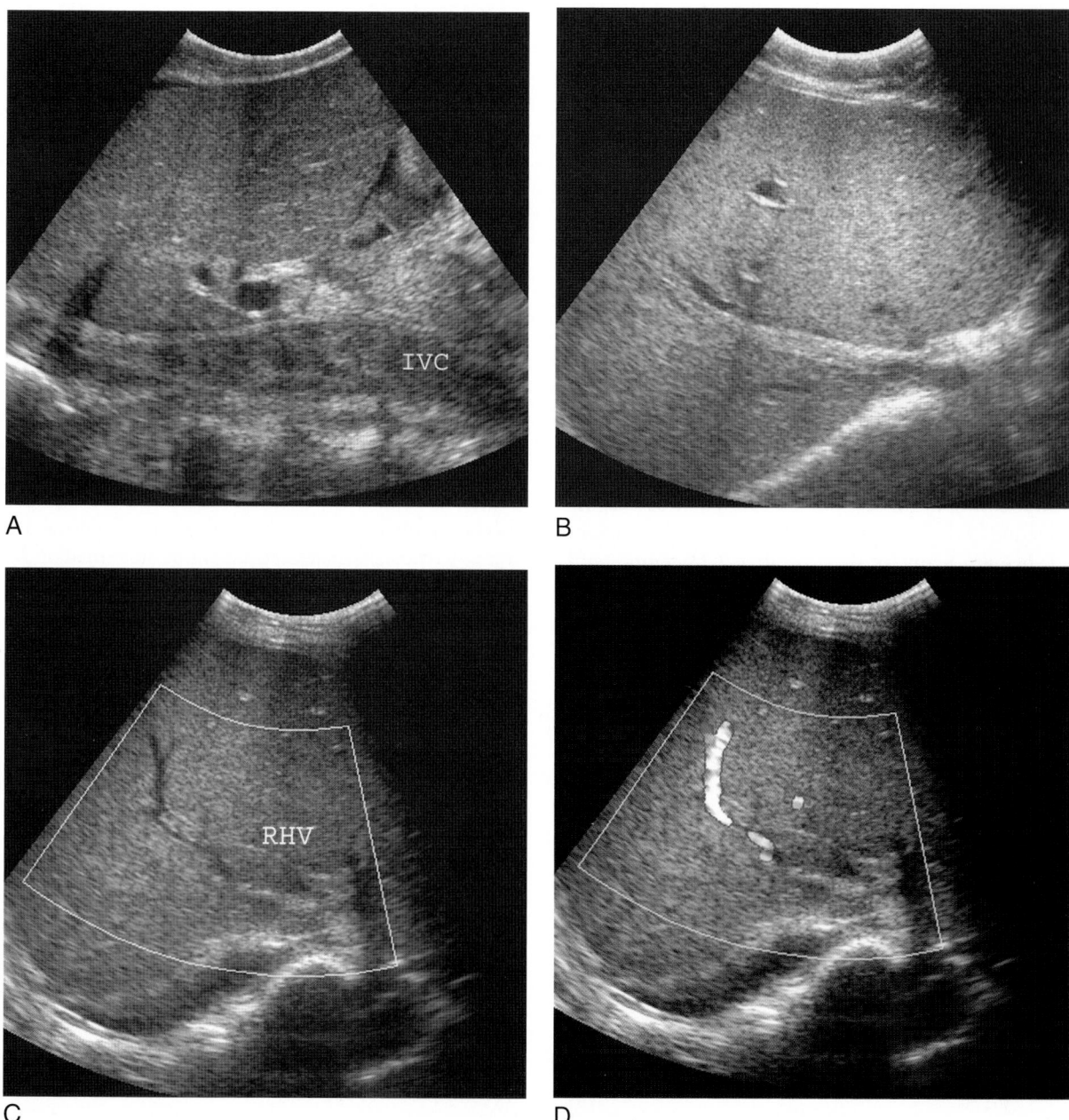

FIGURE 4-39. Budd-Chiari syndrome with extensive inferior vena cava thrombosis. A, Sagittal image of the inferior vena cava (IVC) shows that it is distended with echogenic thrombus. **B,** Middle hepatic vein as a thrombosed cord. **C,** Gray-scale right hepatic vein (RHV) and **D,** color Doppler images of an anomalous right hepatic vein show that it is distended with thrombus. There is flow in the vein proximal to the thrombus (*blue*).

millimeter to many centimeters in diameter. It can be distinguished from hemangioma by the presence of portal tracts within the fibrous stroma of the blood spaces. The **pathogenesis** of peliosis hepatis involves rupture of the reticulin fibers that support the sinusoidal walls, secondary to cell injury or nonspecific hepatocellular necrosis.[124] The diagnosis of peliosis can be made with certainty only by histologic examination. Most cases of peliosis affect the liver, although other solid internal organs and lymph nodes may be involved in the process as well.

Although early reports described incidental detection of peliosis hepatis at autopsy in patients with chronic wasting disorders, it has now been seen following renal and liver transplantation, in association with a multitude of drugs, especially anabolic steroids, and with an increased incidence in patients with HIV.[125] The latter association may occur alone or as part of bacillary angiomatosis in the spectrum of opportunistic infections of AIDS.[126] Peliosis hepatis has the potential to be aggressive and lethal.

The **imaging features** of peliosis hepatis have been described in single case reports,[127-129] although often without adequate histologic confirmation. Angiographically, the peliotic lesions have been described as accumulations of contrast detected late in the arterial phase and becoming more distinct in the parenchymal phase.[130] On sonography, described lesions are nonspecific and have shown single or multiple masses of heterogeneous echogenicity.[127,128,131] Calcifications have been reported (Fig. 4-40).[131] CT scans show low attenuation nodular lesions that may or may not enhance with contrast injection.[127,130] Peliosis hepatis is difficult to diagnose both clinically and radiologically and must be suspected in a susceptible individual with a liver mass.

MICROBUBBLE CONTRAST AGENTS FOR IMAGING FOCAL LIVER MASSES

Focal liver masses are common on pathologic or imaging evaluation of the liver and include a variety of malignant and benign neoplasms, as well as congenital and acquired masses of inflammatory and traumatic nature. Evaluation of focal liver masses is a complex issue which is often the major focus of a cross-sectional imaging study. There are two basic questions that may be posed. The first deals with characterization of a known liver lesion and answers the question—*what is it?* The second issue is that of detection and answers the question—*is it there?* The resolution of either problem requires a focused examination that is often adjusted according to the clinical situation or on the basis of information already known from previous imaging tests.

Liver Mass Characterization

Worldwide, noninvasive diagnosis of focal liver masses is achieved with contrast-enhanced CT and/or MR scan based on recognized enhancement patterns in the arterial and portal venous phases. So accurate have these techniques become that excisional and percutaneous biopsy for diagnosis of liver masses is now rarely performed.

Characterization of a liver mass on conventional sonography is based on the appearance of the mass on gray-scale imaging and vascular information derived from spectral, color, and power Doppler. Ultrasound has excellent spatial and contrast resolution. Hence, the gray-scale morphology of a mass allows for the differentiation of cystic and solid masses and, in many instances, characteristic recognized appearances may suggest the correct diagnosis without further evaluation. More often, however, definitive diagnosis is not made on the basis of gray-scale information alone, but also on vascular information that may be obtained on a conventional Doppler examination. Conventional Doppler, however, often fails in the evaluation of a focal liver mass, particularly in a large patient or on a small or deep liver lesion, or on a mass with weak Doppler signals. Motion artifact is also highly problematic for abdominal Doppler studies, and a left lobe liver mass close to the pulsation of the cardiac apex, for example, is virtually always a failure for conventional Doppler. **To remedy the problem of a failed Doppler examination** of a focal liver lesion, there are two basic approaches to improve the study. The first remedy is to inject **microbubble contrast agents** that enhance the Doppler signal from blood. The second remedy is to utilize **specialized imaging techniques,** such as pulse inversion sonography, which allow preferential detection of the signal from the contrast agent with suppression of the signal from background tissue.

Ultrasound contrast agents are composed of tiny bubbles of gas contained within a stabilizing shell. They

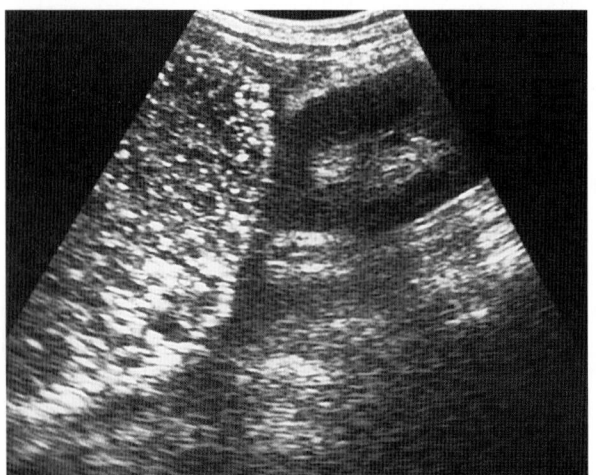
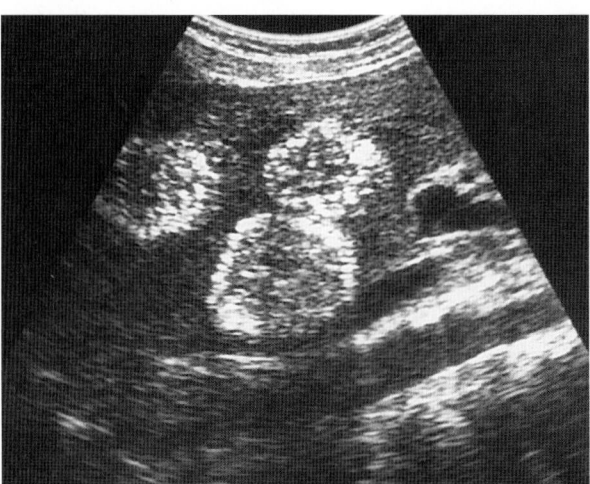

A   B

FIGURE 4-40. Peliosis hepatis. Peliosis hepatis in a 34-year-old woman with deteriorating liver function necessitating transplantation. **A,** Sagittal right lobe and **B,** sagittal left lobe scans show multiple, large liver masses with innumerable, tiny punctate calcifications. (From Muradali D, Wilson SR, Wanless IR, et al: Peliosis hepatis with intrahepatic calcifications. J Ultrasound Med 1996;16:257-260.)

are blood pool agents that do not diffuse through the vascular endothelium. This is of potential importance when imaging the liver because comparable contrast agents for CT and MR imaging may diffuse into the interstitium of a tumor. Our experience is based on the use of Levovist (Schering, Berlin, Germany),[132] a first generation air-containing microbubble agent with a lipid shell, and two perfluorocarbon agents, Definity (Bristol-Myers Squibb, Billerica, Mass.) and Optison (Mallinckrodt, St. Louis, Mo.).[133,134] The strength of imaging with Levovist is its strong liver-specific post-vascular phase, which produces bright enhancement of the liver following clearance of the microbubble from the vascular pool, when insonating with high mechanical index. By comparison, perfluorocarbon agents are ideal for the low mechanical index vascular imaging requisite for liver tumor characterization.

Microbubble contrast agents for ultrasound are unique in that they interact with the imaging process.[134] The major determinant of this interaction is the peak negative pressure of the transmitted ultrasound pulse, reflected by the **Mechanical Index (MI),** a number which is displayed on the ultrasound machine. The bubbles show stable nonlinear oscillation when exposed to an ultrasound field with a **low MI** with the production of harmonics of the transmitted frequency, including the frequency double that of the sound emitted by the transducer, the second harmonic. When the **MI is raised** sufficiently, the bubbles undergo irreversible disruption with the production of a bright, but brief, high intensity ultrasound signal. These contrast agents and their specialized imaging techniques are discussed in detail in Chapter 3, by my research colleague Peter N. Burns, and will not be discussed further in this chapter.

Liver lesion characterization with microbubble contrast agents is based on lesional vascularity and on lesional enhancement in the arterial and portal venous phase. **Lesional vascularity assessment** is dependent on continuous imaging of the agents while they are within the vascular pool. This is best performed using the perfluorocarbon agents, such as Definity, as they produce stable harmonic signals when insonated at **low MI.** We document the **presence**, **number**, **distribution**, and **morphology** of any lesional vessels (Fig. 4-41 and Fig. 4-42). A low MI is preferred as it will preserve the contrast agent population without destruction of the bubbles in the imaging field, allowing for prolonged periods of real-time observation. The morphology of the lesional vessels is discriminatory and highly helpful in diagnosis of liver lesions.

Lesional enhancement assessment is best determined by comparing the echogenicity of the lesion to the echogenicity of the liver at a similar depth on the same frame and requires some knowledge of liver blood flow for understanding. The liver has a dual blood supply from both the hepatic artery and the portal vein.

The liver derives a larger proportion of its blood from the portal vein, whereas most liver tumors derive their blood supply from the hepatic artery. At the initiation of the injection, the low MI technique will cause the entire field of view to appear virtually black, regardless of the baseline appearance of the liver and the lesion in question. In fact, a known mass may be invisible at this point (see Fig. 4-41B). As the microbubbles arrive in the field of view, first the discrete vessels in the liver and within a liver lesion will be visualized followed by a generalized increasing whiteness as the microvascular volume of each fills with the contrast agent. The liver parenchyma will appear more echogenic or whiter in the arterial phase than at baseline, and even more enhanced in the portal venous phase, as a reflection of its blood flow. Vascularity and enhancement patterns of a liver lesion, by comparison, will reflect, therefore, the actual blood flow and hemodynamics of the lesion in question, such that a hyperarterialized mass will appear white against a less white liver on an **arterial phase sequence** (see Fig. 4-41E). Conversely, a hypoperfused lesion will appear as a dark or hypoechoic region within the enhanced liver on an arterial phase sequence. In the **portal venous phase** of enhancement, malignant lesions generally are unenhanced showing as hypoechoic masses (see Fig. 4-41F). Benign lesions by comparison frequently show sustained enhancement such that their echogenicity is equal to or even greater than the liver in the portal phase.

Today, evaluation of lesional enhancement is most commonly performed with the low MI technique just described. However, lesional enhancement, as a reflection of the volume of microbubbles within the scanning plane, is most sensitively assessed using some variation of a **high MI interval delay technique.** Interruption of the imaging process for a predetermined interval allows the vascular volume to fill with the contrast agent. By freezing the mechanism on the ultrasound machine for an interval of time, followed by a brief reinsonation at high MI, bubble destruction will result in a brief and bright enhancement as the bubbles that were accumulated during the delay are disrupted in a single frame. The intensity of the brightness will be in proportion to the number of bubbles that have accumulated during the interval delay. Therefore, comparison of the changes in the echo level of the liver lesion and the adjacent liver will give a relative measurement of their vascular volumes. The timing of the interval delay, relative to the appearance of the first bubble in the imaging field, will allow for assessments in the different phases of liver enhancement—8 to 10 seconds for arterial phase imaging and 50 to 70 seconds for the portal venous phase. Longer interval delays, up to several minutes, may be appropriate for the evaluation of lesions with slow internal flow, such as hemangiomas. Although infrequently used, high MI destructive techniques remain the

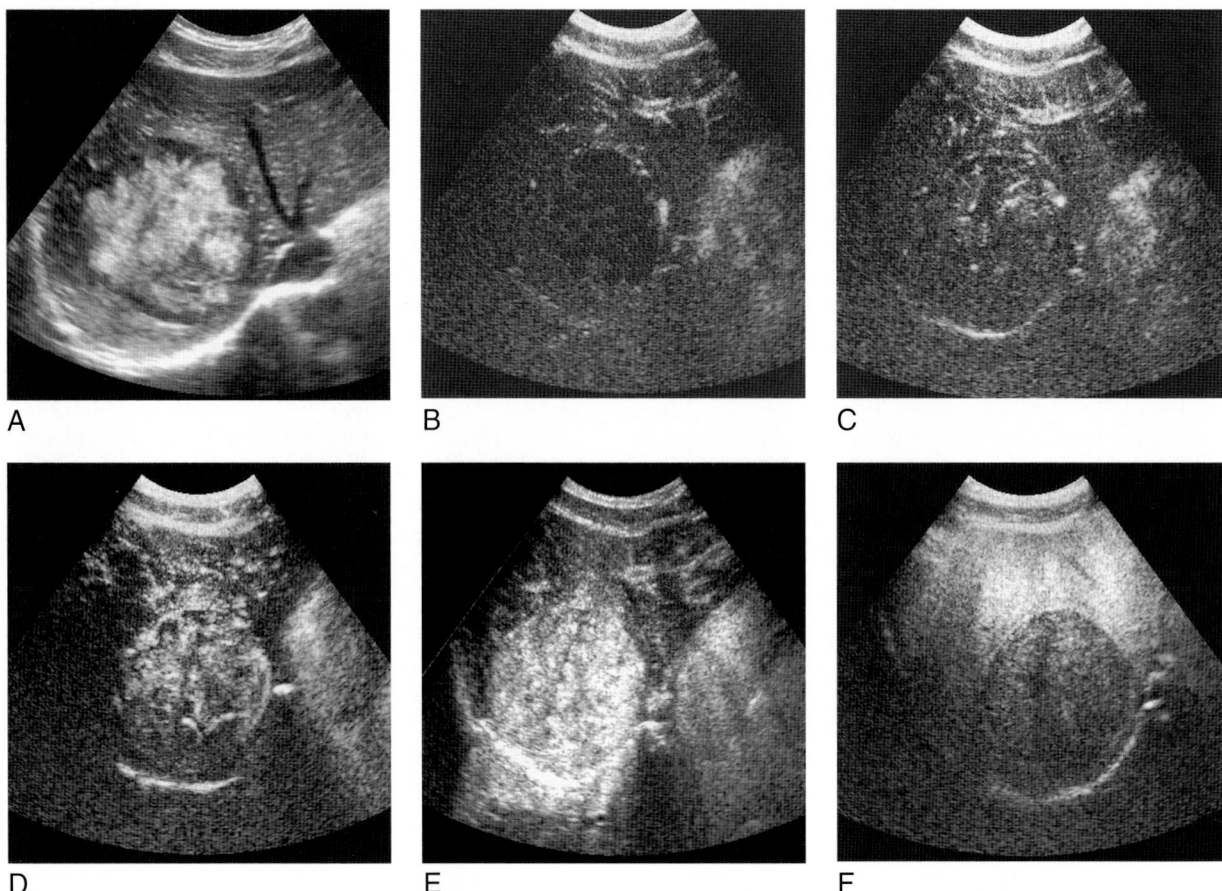

FIGURE 4-41. Characterization of a focal liver mass with microbubble contrast agents—hepatocellular carcinoma. A, Baseline gray-scale image shows a focal mass that is very echogenic with a hypoechoic rim. **B,** Taken at the same location with low MI, prior to the arrival of the microbubbles, the entire image now appears black. The lesion is barely visible and is no longer echogenic. **C** and **D,** Real-time images obtained with low MI. **C,** As the bubbles appear in the field of view, linear echogenic vessels are seen in the liver and in the lesion. **D,** Later in the arterial phase, there are more vessels in the hypervascular lesion than there are in the liver. **E,** Arterial phase interval delay image shows the enhancement of the lesion is far more than in the adjacent liver, such that the lesion is again more echogenic than the background liver. The microbubbles within the vasculature account for the echogenicity of the lesion. **F,** Portal venous phase image shows that the liver is enhanced. The lesion is less echogenic than the liver or has "washed out."

most sensitive method for evaluating lesional enhancement in difficult cases.

Where are we today? With few exceptions, incidentally discovered liver masses found on ultrasound examination are generally referred for contrast-enhanced CT or MR scan for further characterization. Using the above techniques, we have found excellent ability to diagnose focal liver masses with contrast-enhanced ultrasound. In our own clinical practice, we now try to confirm the presence of suspect benign liver masses with contrast-enhanced ultrasound without referral for further investigations. In malignant lesions, ultrasound is an integral component of patient evaluation. Based on observations in over 200 examinations, we have now established algorithms for the diagnosis of focal liver masses with ultrasound.[135] Diagnosis of benign liver masses, hemangioma, and focal nodular hyperplasia (FNH) is close to 100%. Discrimination of benign and malignant liver masses similarly has high accuracy. Algorithms are

summarized in Table 4-3 and are included in the discussions of specific lesions that follow. Knowledge obtained from these examinations forms the basis for the additions to the following sections on benign and malignant liver masses.

Liver Mass Detection

Contrary to popular belief, the excellent spatial resolution of ultrasound allows small lesions to be well seen on sonography. It is, therefore, not size but echogenicity that determines lesion conspicuity on a sonogram. That is, a tiny mass of only a few millimeters will be easily seen if it is either increased or decreased in echogenicity as compared to the adjacent liver parenchyma. As many metastases are either hypo- or hyperechoic relative to the liver, a careful examination should allow for their detection. Nonetheless, many metastatic lesions are of similar echogenicity to the background

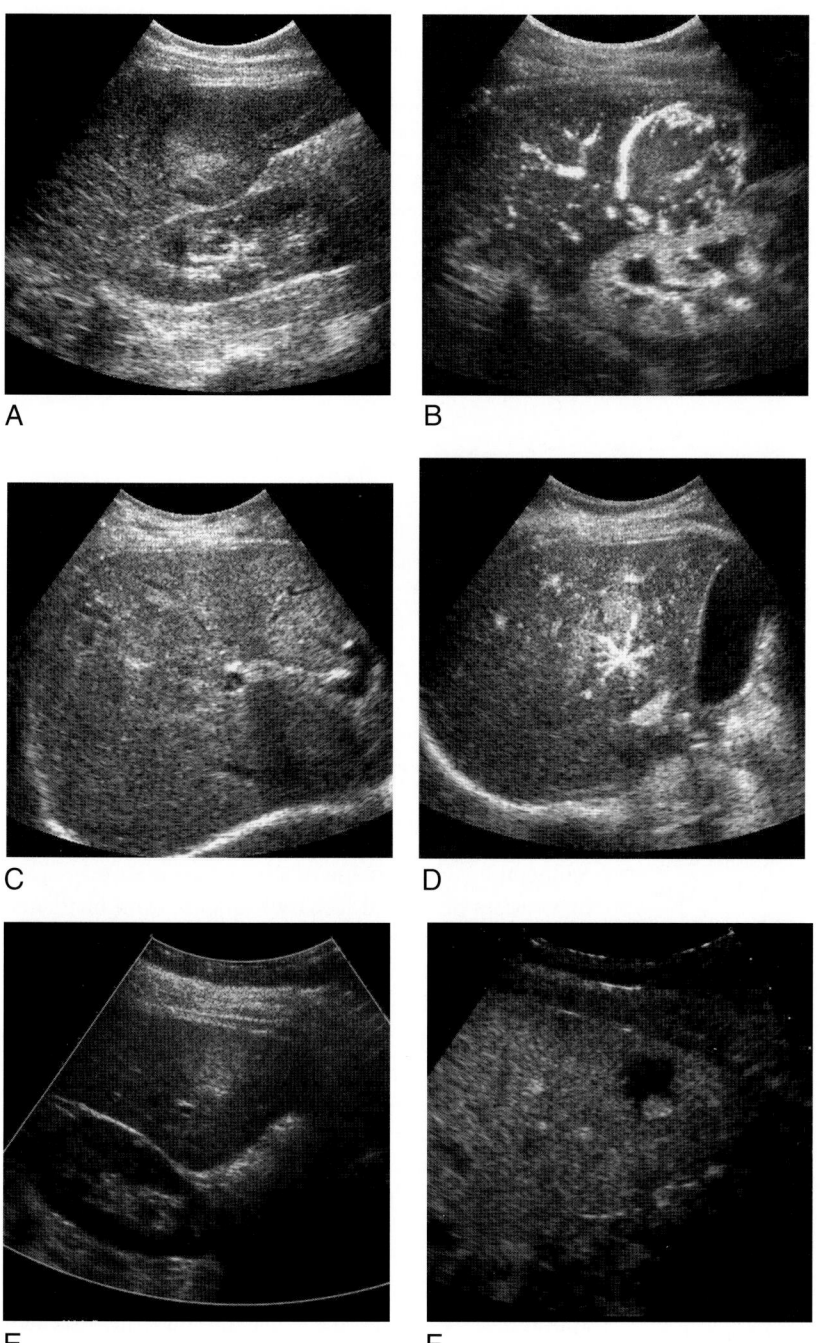

FIGURE 4-42. Discriminatory features of vascular imaging with microbubble contrast agents. Left image is a baseline image and right image is a vascular image. **Top line—hepatocellular carcinoma. A,** Baseline shows an exoplytic mass in segment 6. **B,** The vessels in the anterior part of the lesion are tortuous and dysmorphic. **Middle line—Focal nodular hyperplasia (FNH). C,** Lesion is barely visible. **D,** Stellate vessels are classic for this diagnosis. **Bottom line—hemangioma. E,** Baseline image shows the lesion is echogenic. **F,** Low MI vascular image shows brightly enhanced peripheral nodules and pools. There are no visible linear vessels. The lesion is less enhanced than the liver and appears more hypoechoic because it is hypovascular in the arterial phase. (From Brannigan M, Burns PNB, Wilson SR: Blood flow patterns in focal liver lesions at microbubble enhanced US. Radiographics 2004, in press.)

liver, making their detection difficult or impossible. This occurs when the backscatter from the lesion is virtually identical to the backscatter from the liver parenchyma. To combat this inherent problem of lack of contrast between many metastatic liver lesions and the background liver on conventional sonography, the most effective method, to date, to improve lesion visibility is to perform **contrast-enhanced liver ultrasound** (Fig. 4-43). Two methods are currently available, both of which produce enhancement of the background liver without enhancement of the metastatic lesions, thereby improving their conspicuity. Although their mechanism of action is different, in both there is microbubble

enhancement of the normal liver with no enhancement of the liver metastases. This increases the backscatter from the liver as compared with the liver lesions, thereby improving their detection.

The first method utilizes a first-generation contrast agent **Levovist** (Schering, Berlin, Germany). Following clearance of the contrast agent from the vascular pool, the microbubble persists in the liver probably within the Kupffer cells on the basis of phagocytosis. A high MI sweep through the liver will produce bright enhancement in the distribution of the bubbles. Therefore, all normal liver will enhance. Liver metastases, lacking Kupffer cells, will not enhance and, therefore, show as black or

TABLE 4-3. ALGORITHMS FOR THE DIAGNOSIS OF FOCAL LIVER MASSES ON CONTRAST-ENHANCED SONOGRAPHY

	Vascular Imaging	AP Enhancement	PVP Enhancement
Hemangioma	Marginal	Greater than liver	Equal/greater than liver
	Puddles and pools	Peripheral nodular	**Sustained enhancement**
	No linear vessel enhancement	Centripetal progression	
	(Rare—busy branching vessels that look like pools)		
FNH	Hypervascular	Greater than liver	Equal/greater than liver
	Stellate vessels		Nonenhancing scar
	Tortuous feeding artery	Diffuse	**Sustained enhancement**
		Homogeneous	
HCC	Hypervascular	Greater than liver	Less than liver
	Diffuse		**Washout over time**
	Often heterogeneous due to hemorrhage and necrosis		
Metastases	Hypovascular	Less than liver	All
	Marginal enhancement	Marginal enhancement	Less than liver
	Hypervascularity	Greater than liver	

Reproduced with permission from Brannigan M, Burns PNB, Wilson SR: Blood flow patterns in focal liver lesions of microbubble enhanced US. RadioGraphics 2004, in press.

hypoechoic holes within the enhanced parenchyma (see Fig. 4-41A, B). More and smaller lesions are seen than on baseline.[136] In a multicenter study conducted in Europe and Canada in which we participated, more lesions were seen than on baseline scan.[137] Overall, lesion detection was equivalent to CT and MR scan. The decibel difference between the lesions and the liver parenchyma is increased manifold due to increased backscatter from contrast agent within the normal liver tissue.

A second technique to improve liver lesion detection utilizes **perfluorocarbon contrast agents** with low MI scanning in both the arterial and the portal venous phases. The use of a low MI imaging technique for lesion detection has advantages in terms of scanning because the microbubble population is preserved and timing is not so critical. Virtually all metastases and HCCs will be unenhanced relative to the liver in the **portal phase** as the liver parenchyma is optimally enhanced in this phase. Therefore, all malignant lesions tend to appear hypoechoic in the portal phase allowing for improved lesion detection (see Fig. 4-41F and Fig. 4-43C, D). This observation, that malignant lesions are hypoechoic in the portal venous phase of perfluorocarbon liver enhancement, is helpful for both lesion detection and lesion characterization. Benign lesions, FNH, and hemangioma are generally enhanced equal to or more than the liver in the portal venous phase.

Detection of hypervascular liver masses, such as HCC or hypervascular metastases, is also improved by scanning with perfluorocarbon agents in the **arterial phase**. They will show as hyperechoic masses relative to the liver parenchyma in the arterial phase because they are predominantly supplied by hepatic arterial flow.

HEPATIC NEOPLASMS

An Overview

Sonographic visualization of a focal liver mass may occur in a variety of clinical scenarios ranging from incidental detection to identification in a symptomatic patient or as part of a focused search in a patient at risk for hepatic neoplasm. Hemangiomas, FNH, and adenomas are the benign neoplasms encountered regularly in the liver, whereas HCC and metastases account for the majority of malignant tumors. The role of medical imaging in the evaluation of an identified focal liver mass is to determine which masses are significant, requiring confirmation of their diagnosis, and which masses are likely to be insignificant and benign, not requiring further evaluation to confirm their nature. On a sonographic study, there is considerable overlap in the appearances of focal liver masses, but the excellent contrast and spatial resolution of state of the art ultrasound equipment allows for the development of some guidelines for the initial management of patients once a liver mass is seen.[138] These include recognition of the following features:

- A **hypoechoic halo** identified around an echogenic or isoechoic liver mass is an ominous sonographic sign necessitating definitive diagnosis.
- A **hypoechoic and solid liver mass** is highly likely to be significant and also requires definitive diagnosis.
- **Multiple solid liver masses** may be significant and raise the possibility of metastatic or

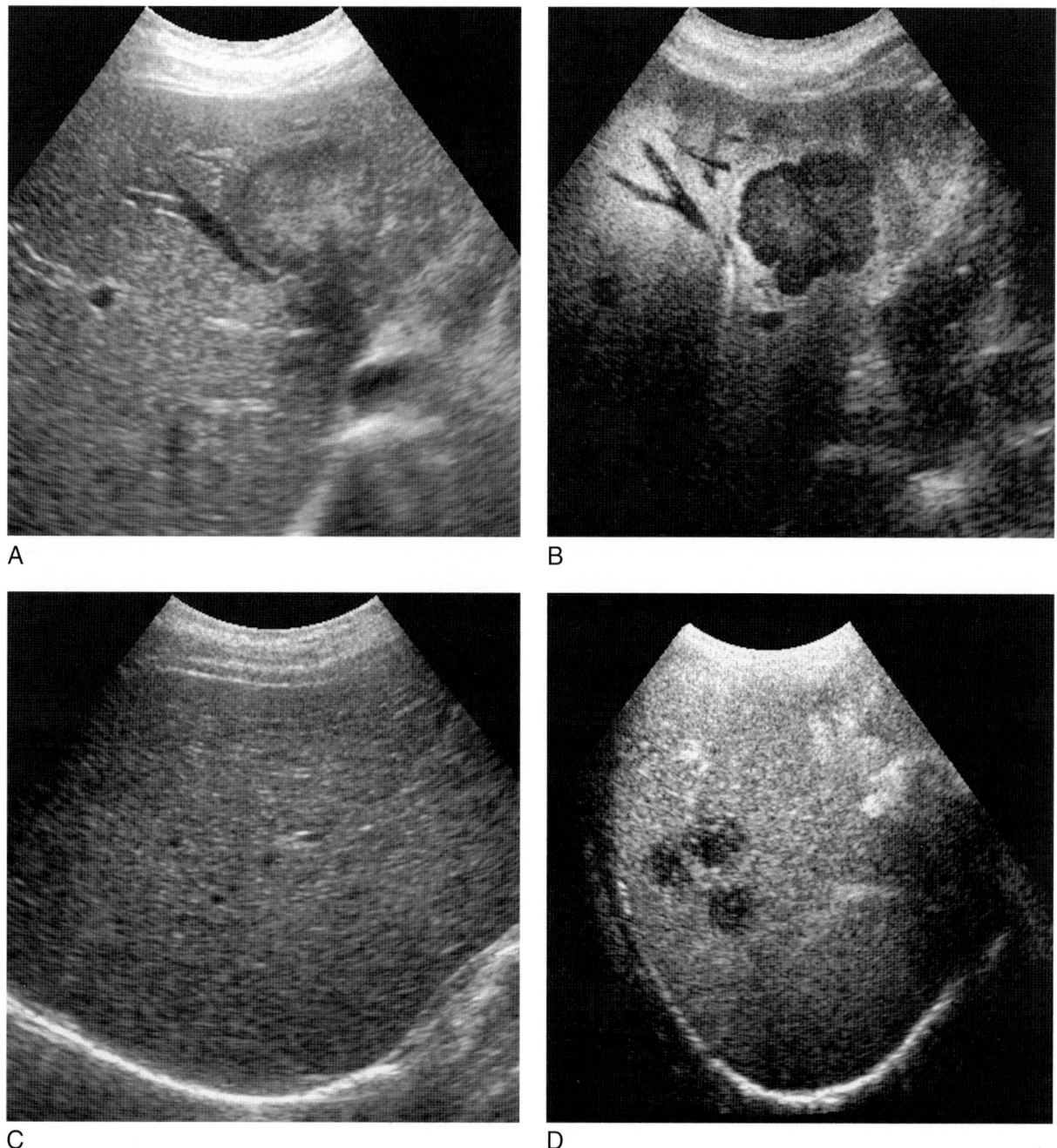

FIGURE 4-43. Improved detection of focal liver masses with two different microbubble contrast agents.
A and **B,** **Levovist** (Schering, Berlin, Germany). **A,** Baseline sonogram shows a subtle isoechoic mass with a hypoechoic halo. **B,** Postvascular Levovist image shows increased echogenicity in the liver. The lesion is strikingly hypoechoic and has increased conspicuity. **C** and **D, Definity** (Bristol-Myers Squibb, Billerica, MA). **C,** Baseline sonogram does not show any metastatic lesions in this patient with carcinoma of the lung. **D,** Portal venous phase image shows multiple focal unenhanced metastases.

multifocal malignant liver disease. Hemangiomas, however, are also frequently multiple.

- **Clinical history of malignancy**, chronic liver disease or hepatitis, and symptoms referable to the liver are requisite information for interpretation of a focal liver lesion.

Benign Hepatic Neoplasms

Cavernous Hemangioma

Cavernous hemangiomas are the **most common benign tumors** of the liver, occurring in approximately 4% of the population. They occur in all age groups but are more common in adults, particularly women. The woman to man ratio is approximately 5:1.[139] The vast majority of hemangiomas are small, asymptomatic, and discovered incidentally. Large lesions may rarely produce symptoms of acute abdominal pain caused by hemorrhage or thrombosis within the tumor. Thrombocytopenia, caused by sequestration and destruction of platelets within a large cavernous hemangioma (Kasabach-Merritt syndrome), occasionally occurs in infants and is rare in adults. Traditional teaching suggested that once hemangiomas are identified in the adult, they usually have reached a stable size and change in appearance or size is uncommon.[140,141] We now believe that this is not always true and in our own practice have documented substantial growth of some lesions over many years of follow-up. Hemangiomas may enlarge during pregnancy or with the administration of estrogens, suggesting the tumor is hormone dependent. **Histologically**, hemangiomas consist of multiple vascular channels that are lined by a single layer of endothelium and separated and supported by fibrous septa. The vascular spaces may contain thrombi.

The **sonographic appearance** of cavernous hemangioma varies (Fig. 4-44). **Typically** the lesion is small, less than 3 cm in diameter, well-defined, homogeneous and hyperechoic (see Fig. 4-44A).[142] The increased echogenicity has been related to the numerous interfaces between the walls of the cavernous sinuses and the blood within them.[143] Inconsistently seen and nonspecific, posterior acoustic enhancement has been correlated with hypervascularity on angiography (see Fig. 4-44H).[144] It is estimated that approximately 67% to 79% of hemangiomas are hyperechoic,[145,146] and of these 58% to 73% are homogeneous.[141,144] **Typical features** are also now familiar and include a nonhomogeneous central area containing hypoechoic portions, which may appear uniformly granular (see Fig. 4-44D, E, F) or lacelike in character (see Fig. 4-44D); an echogenic border, either a thin rim or a thick rind (Fig. 4-44E, F, G); and a tendency to scalloping of the margin (see Fig. 4-44B).[147] Larger lesions tend to be heterogeneous with central hypoechoic foci corresponding to fibrous collagen scars (see Fig. 4-44C), large vascular spaces, or both. A hemangioma may appear hypoechoic within the background of a fatty infiltrated liver.[148] Calcification is rare (see Fig. 4-44I).

Hemangiomas are characterized by **extremely slow blood flow** that will not routinely be detected by either color or duplex Doppler. Occasional lesions may show a low to midrange kHz shift from both peripheral and central blood vessels. The ability of power Doppler, which is more sensitive to slow flow, to detect signals within a hemangioma is still controversial.[149,150]

Cavernous hemangiomas are commonly observed on abdominal sonograms performed for any reason and confirmation of all visualized lesions has proved to be costly and unnecessary. Therefore, it is considered acceptable practice to manage some patients conservatively without confirmation of the diagnosis. When a hyperechoic lesion typical of a cavernous hemangioma is incidentally discovered, no further examination is usually necessary, or at most, a repeat ultrasound is performed in 3 to 6 months to document lack of change.

Conversely, there are potentially significant lesions that may mimic the morphology of a hemangioma on ultrasound and produce a single mass or multiple masses of uniform increased echogenicity from a colon primary or a vascular primary tumor, such as a neuroendocrine tumor; small HCCs, in particular, may show this morphology. Caturelli et al.[151] in a prospective evaluation of 1982 patients with newly diagnosed cirrhosis, found that 50% of echogenic liver lesions with a morphology suggestive of hemangioma had that ultimate diagnosis. Fifty percent, however, proved to be HCC. They also showed that in 1648 patients with known cirrhosis and new appearance of an echogenic hemangioma-like mass, all were HCC. These results emphasize the extreme necessity to prove the diagnosis of all masses with this morphology in high-risk patients. Therefore, in a patient with a known malignancy, an increased risk for hepatoma, abnormal results of liver function tests, clinical symptoms referable to the liver, or an atypical sonographic pattern, one of the following additional imaging techniques is generally recommended to confirm the suspicion of hemangioma: microbubble-enhanced sonography, computed tomography,[152,153] red blood cell scintigraphy,[154] or magnetic resonance imaging.[155]

Microbubble-enhanced sonography. On the arterial phase, hemangiomas show **peripheral puddles and pools** that are brighter than the adjacent enhanced liver parenchyma. There are no linear vessels. Over time, there is **centripetal progression** of the enhancement progressing to complete globular fill-in, with **sustained enhancement** equal to or greater than the liver in the portal venous phase, which may last for several minutes (Fig. 4-45). This enhancement may occur rapidly or may be incomplete, even in the delayed portal venous phase. In our hands, we have diagnosed close to 100% of hemangiomas including those of small size, removing the necessity for either CT, MR scan, or labeled red blood cell scintigraphy for confirmation of diagnosis, particularly in incidentally detected lesions. The best approach to the diagnosis of hemangiomas will depend on the clinical situation, the size and location of the lesion, the availability of imaging modalities, such as MRI and SPECT (single photon emission computed tomography), and the experience of the imager. In general, the combination of two confirmatory studies is diagnostic of hemangioma.[156] We are hopeful that in the future, the majority of hemangiomas seen on ultrasound will be confirmed with contrast-enhanced sonography.

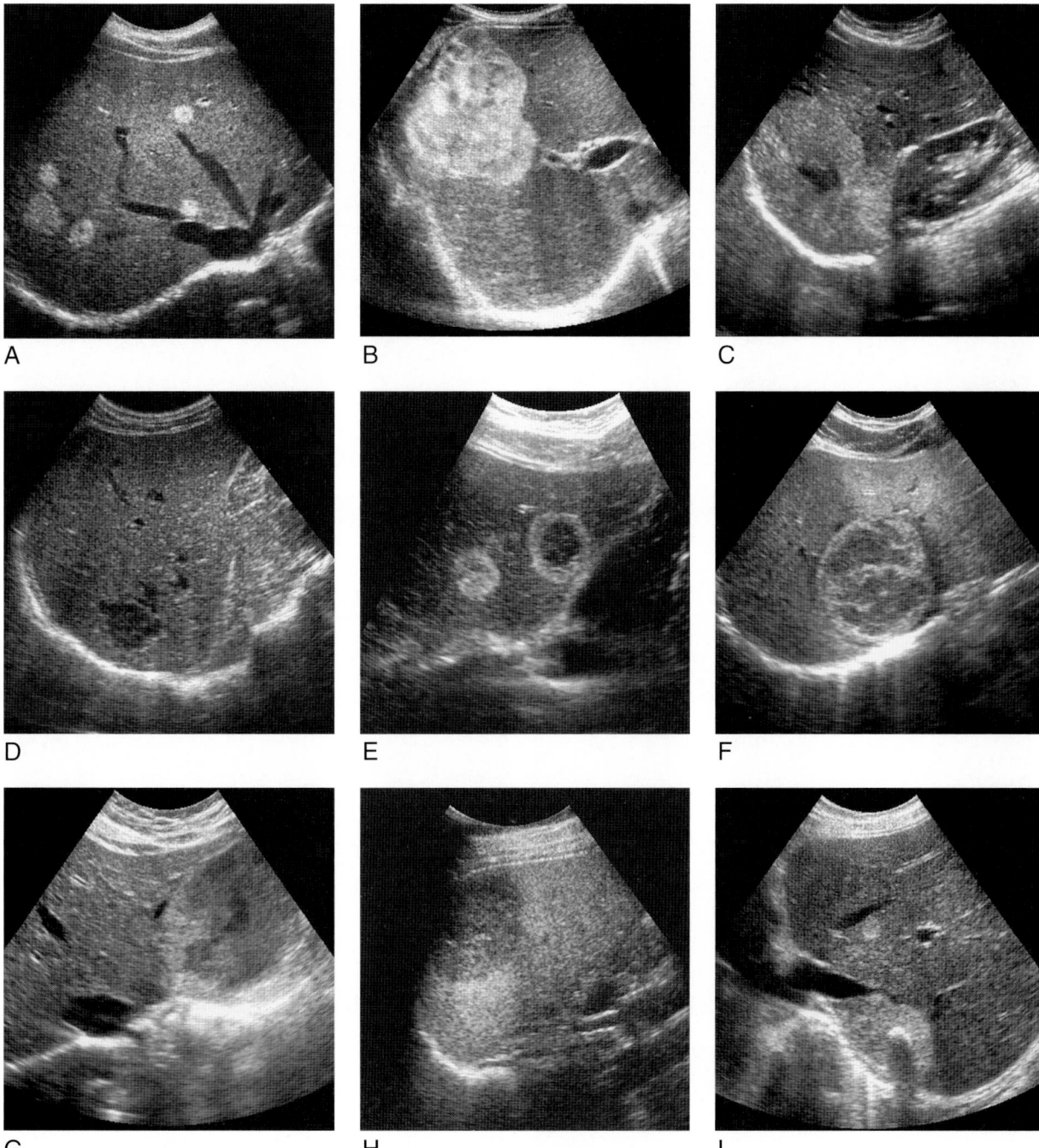

FIGURE 4-44. Hemangiomas—Spectrum of appearances. Top line—Classic morphology. A, Multiple small echogenic masses. **B,** Single, large lobulated echogenic mass. **C,** Echogenic lobulated mass with a hypoechoic area centrally, probably related to central thrombosis or scarring. **Middle line—Atypical morphology. D,** Atypical hemangioma. It is hypoechoic and has a thin echogenic border. **E,** Both classic and atypical morphologies. The atypical hemangioma has a thick, uniform echogenic border. **F,** Atypical hemangioma, which is partially hypoechoic centrally with an irregular echogenic rim. **Bottom line—infrequent observations. G,** Exophytic hemangioma bulging from the left lateral lobe of the liver. **H,** Hypoechoic mass with increased through transmission, a suggestive, but infrequently encountered, sign of hemangioma. **I,** Central calcification in a hemangioma with distal acoustic shadowing. This is a rare finding in hemangiomas.

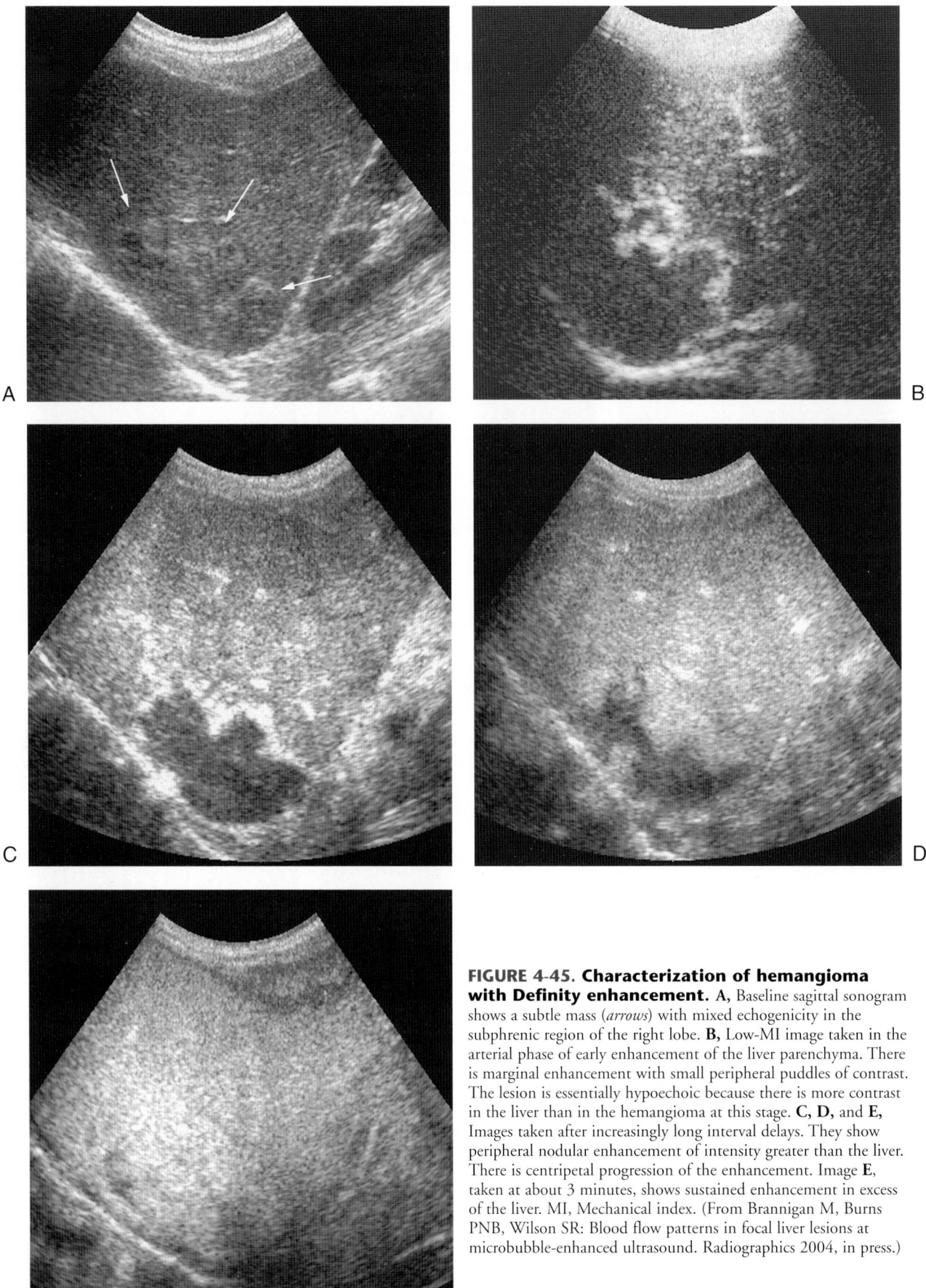

FIGURE 4-45. Characterization of hemangioma with Definity enhancement. A, Baseline sagittal sonogram shows a subtle mass (*arrows*) with mixed echogenicity in the subphrenic region of the right lobe. **B,** Low-MI image taken in the arterial phase of early enhancement of the liver parenchyma. There is marginal enhancement with small peripheral puddles of contrast. The lesion is essentially hypoechoic because there is more contrast in the liver than in the hemangioma at this stage. **C, D,** and **E,** Images taken after increasingly long interval delays. They show peripheral nodular enhancement of intensity greater than the liver. There is centripetal progression of the enhancement. Image **E,** taken at about 3 minutes, shows sustained enhancement in excess of the liver. MI, Mechanical index. (From Brannigan M, Burns PNB, Wilson SR: Blood flow patterns in focal liver lesions at microbubble-enhanced ultrasound. Radiographics 2004, in press.)

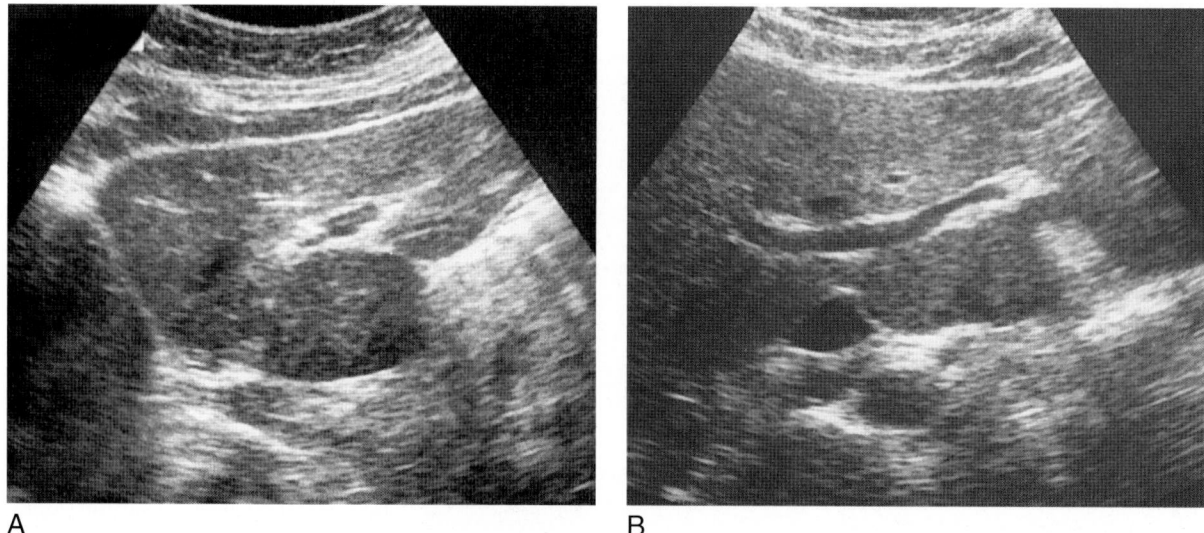

A   B

FIGURE 4-46. **Focal nodular hyperplasia. A,** Sagittal and **B,** transverse sonograms show an isoechoic, subtle caudate lobe mass. The contour variation is the key to appreciating the presence of this mass.

In a small minority of patients, imaging will not allow a definitive diagnosis of hemangioma to be made. Percutaneous biopsy of hepatic hemangiomas has been safely performed.[157,158] Cronan et al.[158] performed biopsies on 15 patients (12 of whom were outpatients) using a 20 gauge Franseen needle. In all cases, the histologic sample was diagnostic and was characterized by large spaces with an endothelial lining. It is recommended that normal liver be interposed between the abdominal wall and the hemangioma to allow hepatic tamponade of any potential bleeding.

Focal Nodular Hyperplasia

Focal nodular hyperplasia is the **second most common benign liver mass** after hemangioma.[159] These masses are believed to be developmental **hyperplastic lesions** related to an area of congenital vascular malformation, probably a preexisting arterial spider-like malformation.[162] **Hormonal influences** may be factors because FNH is more common in women than in men, particularly in the childbearing years.[161-163] Like hemangioma, FNH is invariably an incidentally detected liver mass in an asymptomatic patient.[161]

Focal nodular hyperplasia is typically a well-circumscribed and most often solitary mass that has a central scar.[161] The majority of lesions are less than 5 cm in diameter. Although usually single, cases have been reported with multiple FNH. **Microscopically,** lesions include normal hepatocytes, Kupffer cells, biliary ducts, and the components of portal triads, although no normal portal venous structures are found. As a hyperplastic lesion, there is proliferation of normal, non-neoplastic hepatocytes that are abnormally arranged. Bile ducts and thick-walled arterial vessels are prominent,

particularly in the central fibrous scar. The excellent blood supply makes hemorrhage, necrosis, and calcification rare.[161] These lesions often produce a contour abnormality to the surface of the liver or may displace the normal blood vessels within the parenchyma.

On sonography, FNH is often a subtle liver mass that is difficult to differentiate in echogenicity from the adjacent liver parenchyma. Considering the similarities in histology of FNH to normal liver, this is not a surprising fact and has led to descriptions of FNH on all imaging as a "stealth lesion" which may be extremely subtle or hide altogether.[164] Subtle contour abnormalities (Fig. 4-46 and Fig. 4-47E, F) and displacement of vascular structures should immediately raise the possibility of FNH. The central scar may be seen on gray-scale sonograms as a hypoechoic linear or stellate area within the central portion of the mass (see Fig. 4-47A).[165] On occasion, the scar may appear hyperechoic. FNH may also display a range of gray-scale appearances ranging from hypoechoic to hyperechoic on rare occasion.

Doppler features of FNH are highly suggestive, in that well-developed peripheral and central blood vessels are seen. Pathologic studies in FNH describe an anomalous arterial blood vessel larger than expected for the locale in the liver.[160] Our experience suggests that this feeding vessel is usually quite obvious on color Doppler imaging, although other vascular masses may appear to have unusually large feeding vessels as well.[166] The blood vessels can be seen to course within the central scar with either a linear or stellate configuration. Spectral interrogation usually shows predominantly arterial signals centrally with a mid-range (2 to 4 kHz) shift (see Fig. 4-55).

Similar to hemangioma, FNH is consistently diagnosed with the use of **microbubble contrast agents.** In the arterial phase, lesions are **hypervascular** and two

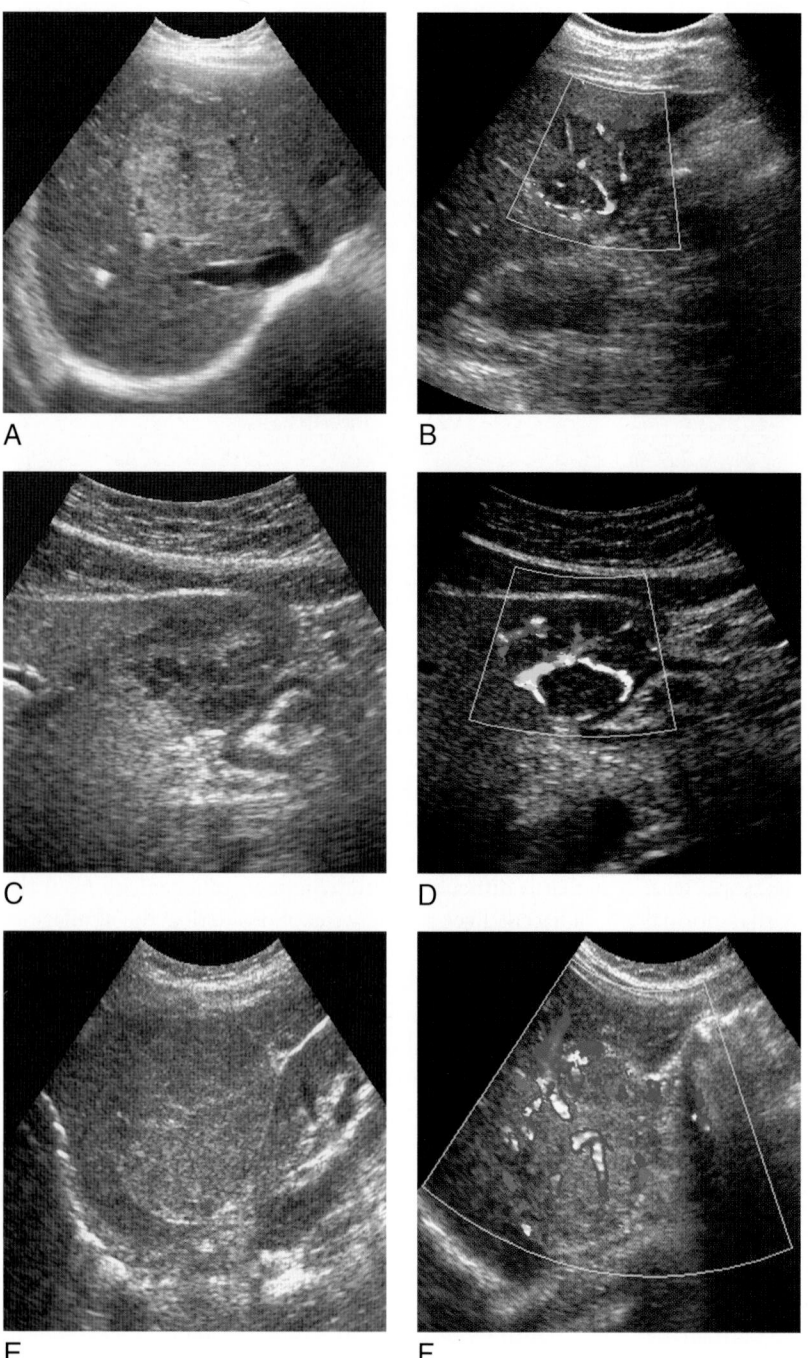

FIGURE 4-47. Focal nodular hyperplasia. Gray-scale and color Doppler features, in three patients. Left images are the gray-scale equivalents of the color Doppler images on the right. **A,** Gray-scale sonogram is virtually normal and only raises the possibility of an isoechoic and subtle mass. **B,** Doppler image, however, shows a stellate arterial pattern and confirms the authenticity of the observation. **C,** Fatty liver and a focal hypoechoic region in the tip of segment 3. Fatty sparing was considered. **D,** Doppler features, however, show a hypervascular mass with a stellate appearance. This is the classic finding in FNH. **E,** Contour-altering mass in the right lobe of the liver. **F,** Doppler again shows the central stellate vascularity suggesting FNH. This hypervascularity and stellate vasculature is usually readily observed with conventional sonography in FNH. FNH, Focal nodular hyperplasia.

highly suggestive morphologies include the presence of **stellate lesional vessels** and a **tortuous feeding artery** (Fig. 4-48). Arterial phase enhancement is homogeneous and in excess of the adjacent liver. **Portal venous enhancement is sustained** such that the lesion is enhanced equal to or more than the adjacent liver with a nonenhancing scar. An unenhanced scar may be seen in both arterial and portal phases. Ultrasound alone should be able to suggest the presence of these insignificant lesions without the necessity of referral for further imaging.

Sulfur colloid scanning is invaluable in patients with suspect FNH because 50% of lesions will take up sulfur colloid similar to the adjacent normal liver and a further 10% of lesions will be hot. Therefore, only 40% of patients with FNH will lack confirmation of their diagnosis after performing a sulfur colloid scan.[167,168] In these cases, contrast-enhanced **CT** or **MRI** scan may be performed for diagnosis.

Biopsy may be required in the minority of patients with FNH who do not have a hot or a warm lesion on sulfur colloid scanning, especially if CT or MRI features are not specific. Cytologic biopsy is not confirmatory because normal hepatocytes may be found in normal liver, adenoma, and FNH. Core liver biopsy is required

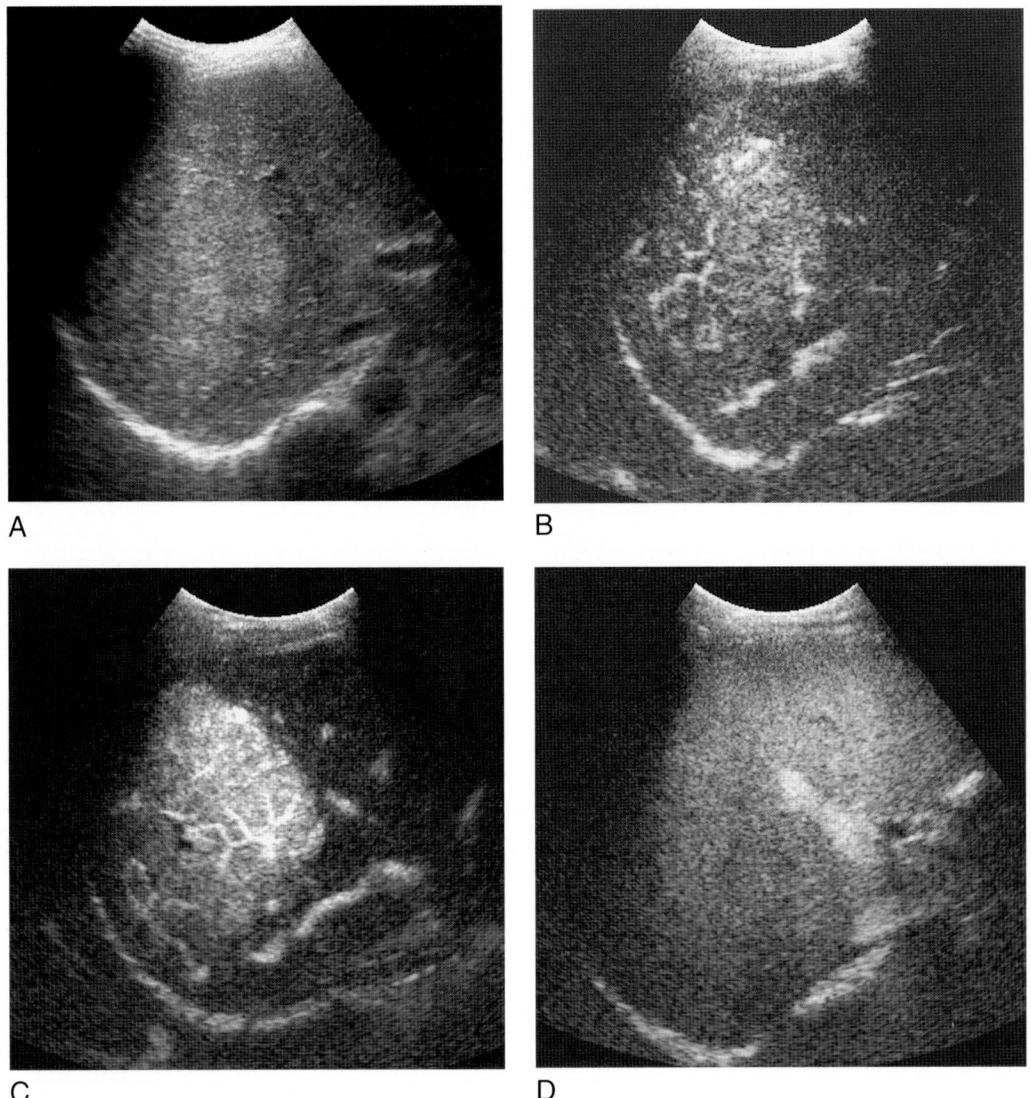

FIGURE 4-48. FNH with Definity enhancement. A, Baseline image shows a large slightly echogenic mass in the right lobe. **B,** Low-MI early arterial phase image shows linear internal vessels. **C,** Later in the arterial phase, the lesion is more enhanced than the liver. A tortuous feeding artery is also seen. **D,** Portal venous phase image shows uniform enhancement of the liver and the lesion. Enhancement of the lesion is sustained equal to the enhancement of the liver, characteristic of a benign lesion. FNH, Focal nodular hyperplasia. (From Brannigan M, Burns PNB, Wilson SR: Blood flow patterns in focal liver lesions at microbubble enhanced US. Radiographics, 2004, in press.)

to show the disorganized pattern characteristic of this pathology. Because FNH rarely leads to clinical problems and does not undergo malignant transformation, conservative management is recommended.[169]

Hepatic Adenoma

Hepatic adenomas are **less common** than FNH. Since the 1970s, however, there has been a dramatic rise in their incidence and a link clearly established to the **usage of oral contraceptive agents**. As would be expected, therefore, hepatic adenomas, similar to FNH, are more common in women. The tumor may be asymptomatic, but often the patient or the physician feels a mass in the right upper quadrant. Pain may occur as a result of bleeding or infarction within the lesion. The most alarming manifestation is shock caused by tumor rupture and hemoperitoneum. Hepatic adenomas have also been reported in association with glycogen storage disease. In particular, the frequency of adenoma for type 1 GSD (von Gierke's disease) is 40%.[170] Because of its propensity to hemorrhage and risk of malignant degeneration,[169] surgical resection is recommended.

Pathologically, the hepatic adenoma is usually solitary and well encapsulated, and ranges in size from 8 to 15 cm. Microscopically, the tumor consists of normal or slightly atypical hepatocytes. Bile ducts and Kupffer cells are either few in number or absent.[171] Hepatic

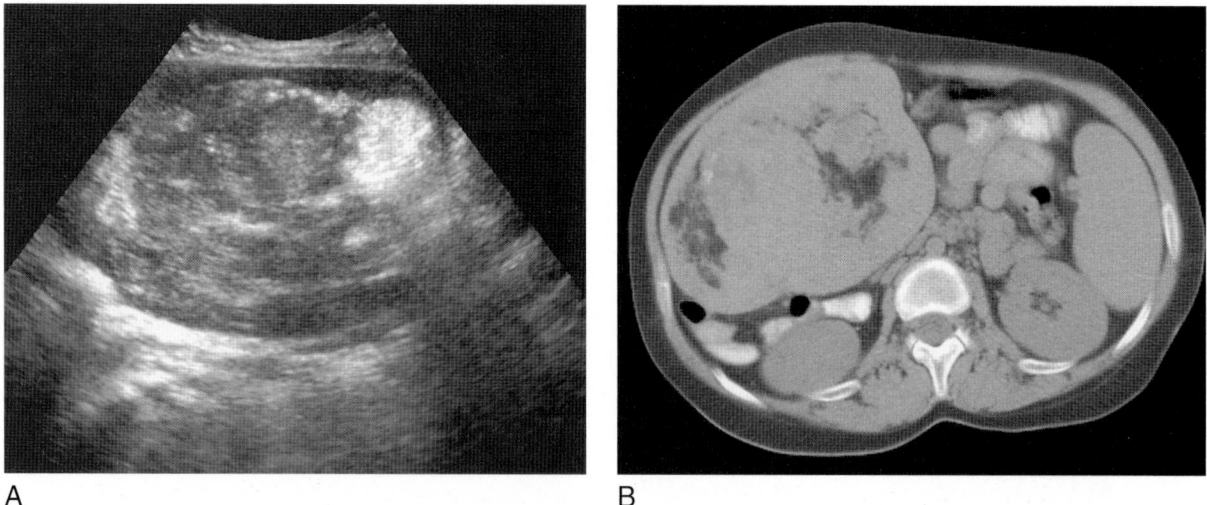

FIGURE 4-49. Hepatic adenoma. A, Sonogram and **B,** confirmatory CT scan show a large and exophytic liver mass in a young, asymptomatic woman. The mass shows highly echogenic foci, which correspond with areas of fat and calcification on the CT scan.

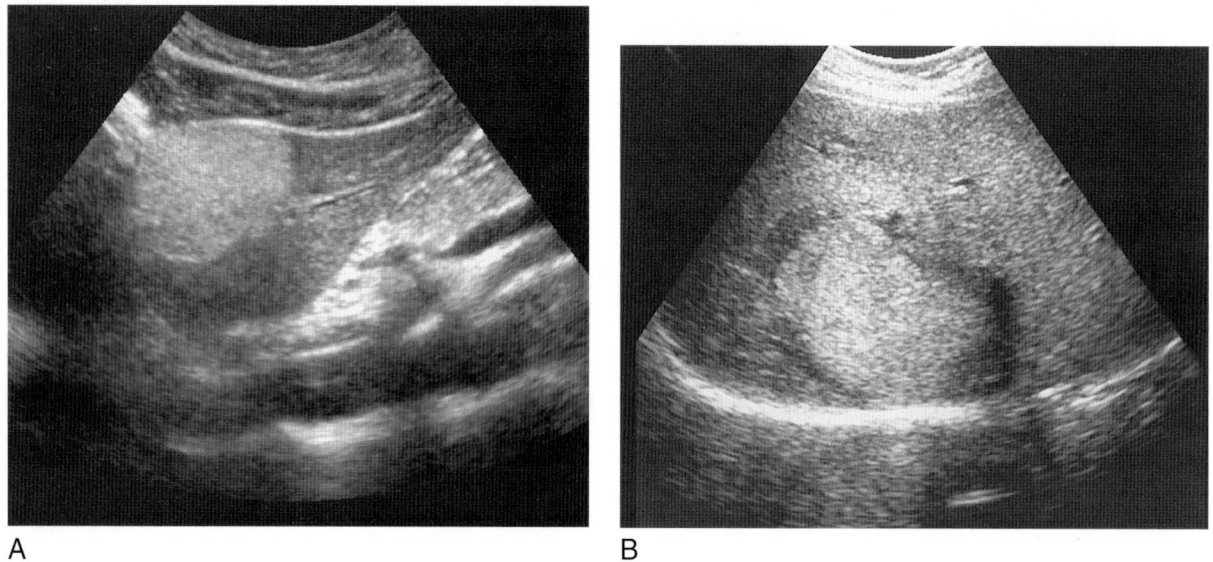

FIGURE 4-50. Hepatic adenoma—gray-scale appearances. A, Sagittal sonogram of the left lobe of the liver of an asymptomatic 35-year-old male shows a highly echogenic mass. It is unusual to see an adenoma in an otherwise normal man. **B,** Oblique sonogram of a 26-year-old Chinese woman shows a highly echogenic mass with a hypoechoic halo. The hypoechoic halo was related to a surrounding zone of liver atrophy on biopsy.

adenomas may show both calcification or fat (Fig. 4-49), both of which appear echogenic on sonography, making their gray-scale appearance suggestive in some instances.

The **sonographic appearance** of hepatic adenoma is nonspecific .The echogenicity may be hyperechoic (see Fig. 4-49 and Fig. 4-50), hypoechoic, isoechoic, or mixed.[168] With hemorrhage, a fluid component may be evident within or around the mass (Fig. 4-51) and free intraperitoneal blood may be seen. The sonographic changes with bleeding are variable, dependent on the duration and amount of hemorrhage.

It is often not possible to distinguish hepatic adenomas from FNH by their gray-scale or Doppler characteristics. Both demonstrate perilesional and intralesional well-defined blood vessels with kHz shifts in the mid-range (2 to 4 kHz). Golli et al.[166] described increased venous structures within the center of the masses and a paucity of arterial vessels. In our experience, this has not been a constant finding, although we do believe that these lesions are substantially less vascular than most FNH and certainly do not show either the intra- or perilesional vascular tortuosity that we have come to associate with FNH. The majority of adenomas are cold on ^{99}Tc-sulfur colloid imaging as a result of absent or markedly decreased numbers of Kupffer cells. Isolated cases of radiocolloid uptake by the

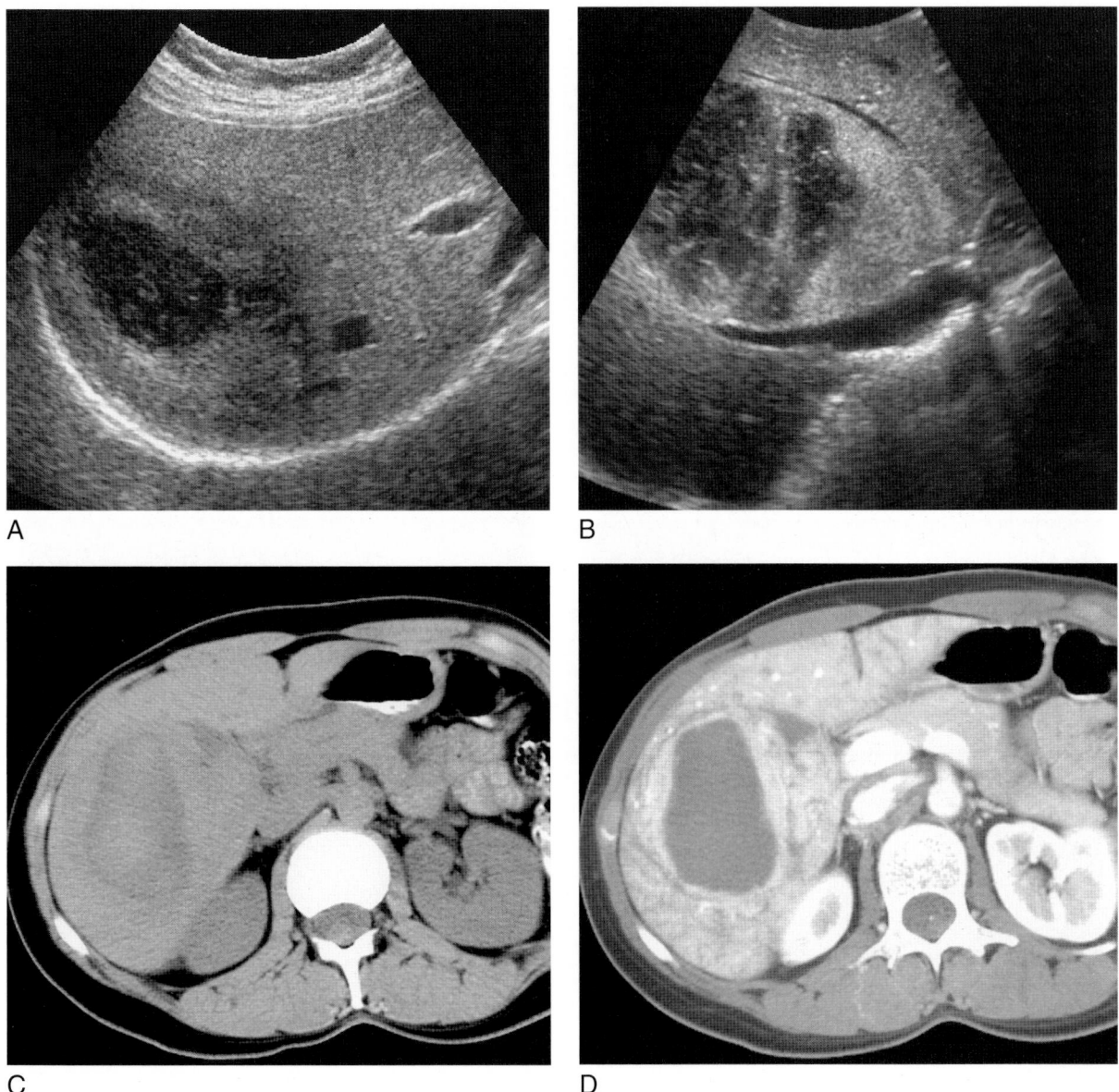

FIGURE 4-51. Bleeding adenomas. A and **B,** Sonograms of two young women presenting with acute abdominal pain from hemorrhage into hepatic adenomas. The masses are highly complex and their appearance in a patient with pain suggests hemorrhage into a preexisting lesion. **C,** Unenhanced and **D,** enhanced CT scans on the patient shown in **B,** showing the value of the unenhanced scan that confirms the high attenuation blood within the adenoma.

adenoma have been reported.[172] Hepatobiliary scans may be helpful in the diagnosis of hepatic adenomas. Because these lesions do not contain bile ducts, the tracer is not excreted and the mass persists as a photon-active region.

In a patient with right upper quadrant pain and possible hemorrhage, it is important to perform an **unenhanced CT scan** of the liver, prior to contrast injection. The hemorrhage will appear as high-density regions within the mass (see Fig. 4-51C). The lesion often demonstrates a rapid transient enhancement during the arterial phase.[173] Hepatic adenomas have a variable appearance on MRI and it is not always possible to distinguish between adenoma and HCC.

Our experience with **microbubble contrast agents** and adenomas is somewhat limited, although we have shown vascularity less than the liver in the few cases on which studies have been performed and we have not shown the marked hypervascularity of FNH.

Fatty Tumors of the Liver—Hepatic Lipomas and Angiomyolipomas

Hepatic lipomas are extremely rare, and only isolated cases have been reported in the radiologic literature.[174-176] There is an association between hepatic lipomas and renal angiomyolipomas and tuberous sclerosis. The lesions are asymptomatic. **Ultrasound** demonstrates a

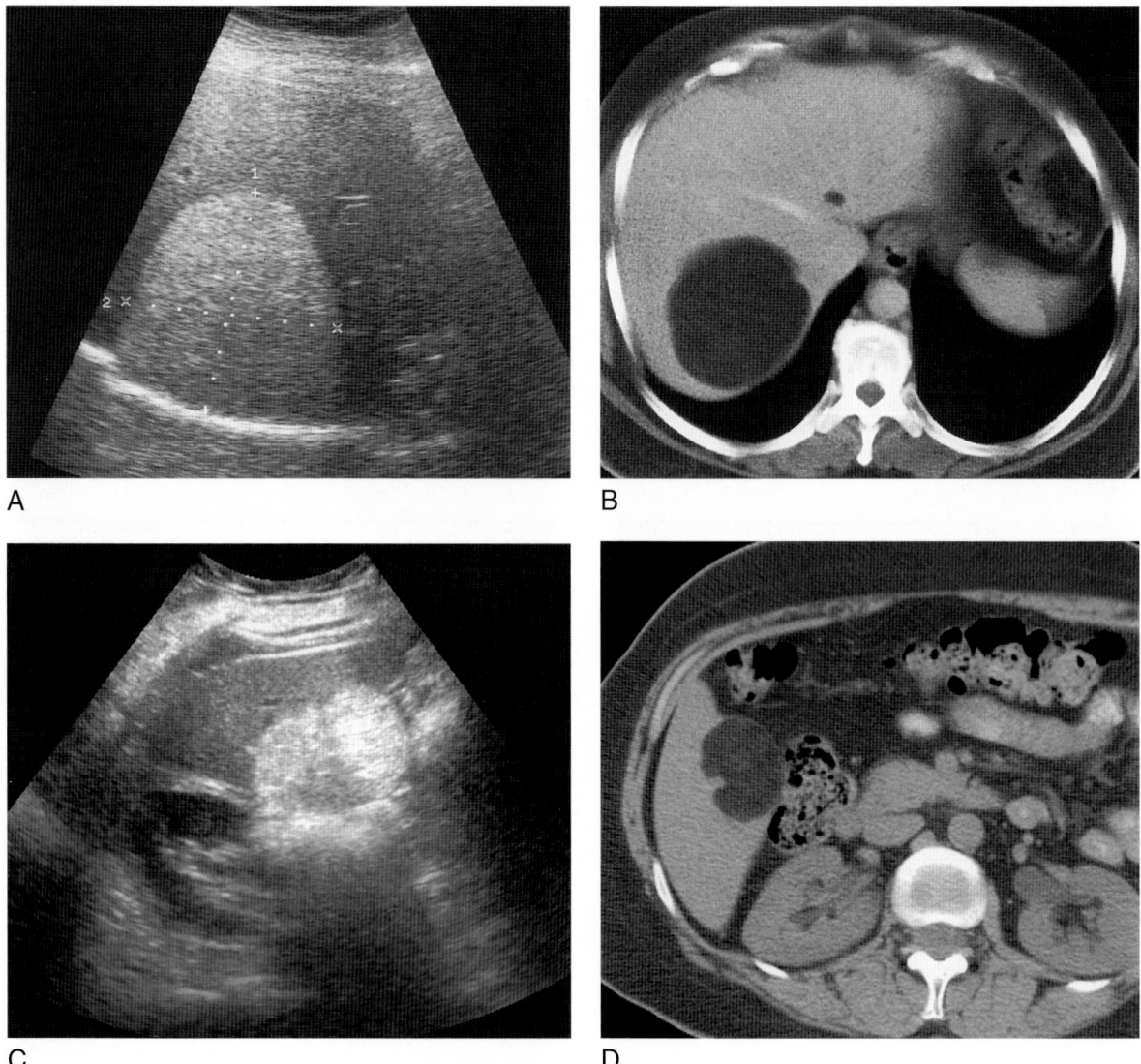

FIGURE 4-52. Fatty tumors of the liver—lipoma and angiomyolipoma. A, Sonogram shows a focal, highly echogenic, solid liver mass which initially suggests a probable hemangioma. The discontinuity of the diaphragm echo due to the altered rate of sound transmission is a clue to the correct diagnosis.[176] **B,** Confirmatory CT scan shows the fat density of the mass. A confirmed hepatic lipoma.[176] **C** and **D,** Another highly echogenic and slightly exophytic mass in the liver initially suggesting a hemangioma.[177] **E** and **F,** CT and MR scans showing the fatty nature of this angiomyolipoma. (**A** and **B** from Reinhold C, Garant M: Hepatic lipoma. C Assoc Radiol J 1996;47:140-142; **C** and **D** from Wilson SR: The Liver. Gastrointestinal Disease (Sixth Series). Test and Syllabus. American College of Radiology, Reston, Va, 2004, In press.)

well-defined echogenic mass (Fig. 4-52), indistinguishable from a hemangioma, echogenic metastasis, or focal fat—unless the mass is large and near the diaphragm—in which case differential sound transmission through the fatty mass will produce a discontinuous or broken diaphragm echo (see Fig. 4-52A).[175] The diagnosis is confirmed using CT scanning, which reveals the fatty nature of the mass by the negative Hounsfield units (-30 HU) (Fig. 4-52B).[174,177] Angiomyolipomas, by comparison, may also appear echogenic on sonography (Fig. 4-52C), although they may have insufficient fat to consistently appear of fatty attenuation on CT scan,

making confirmation of their diagnosis more difficult without biopsy.

Malignant Hepatic Neoplasms

Hepatocellular Carcinoma

Hepatocellular carcinoma is one of the most common malignant tumors, particularly in Southeast Asia, sub-Saharan Africa, Japan, Greece, and Italy. It occurs predominantly in men, with a sex ratio of approximately 5:1.[171] **Etiologic factors** contributing to the development of HCC depend on the geographic distribution. Although alcoholic cirrhosis remains a common predisposing cause for hepatoma in the West, both hepatitis C and hepatitis B are now of worldwide significance. In addition to their growing importance in Western countries, these viral infections also account for the high incidence of HCC in sub-Saharan Africa, Southeast Asia, China, Japan, and in the Mediterranean. Aflatoxins, which are toxic metabolites produced by fungi in certain foods, have also been implicated in the pathogenesis of hepatomas in developing countries.[171] The clinical presentation is often delayed until the tumor reaches an advanced stage. Symptoms include right upper-quadrant pain, weight loss, and abdominal swelling when ascites is present.

Pathologically, HCC occurs in three forms:

- Solitary tumor
- Multiple nodules
- Diffuse infiltration

There is a propensity toward **venous invasion**. The portal vein is involved more commonly than the hepatic venous system, occurring in 30% to 60% of cases (see Fig. 4-53G).[178-180]

The **sonographic appearance** of HCC is variable (Fig. 4-53). The masses may be hypoechoic, complex, or echogenic. Most small (<5 cm) HCCs are hypoechoic, (see Fig. 4-53A), corresponding histologically to a solid tumor without necrosis.[181,182] A thin, peripheral hypoechoic halo, which corresponds to a fibrous capsule, is seen most often in small HCCs.[183] With time and increasing size, the masses tend to become more complex and inhomogeneous as a result of necrosis and fibrosis (see Fig. 4-53E). Calcification is uncommon but has been reported.[184] Small tumors may appear diffusely hyperechoic, secondary to fatty metamorphosis or sinusoidal dilation (see Fig. 4-53C), making them indistinguishable from focal fatty infiltration, cavernous hemangiomas, and lipomas.[181,182,185] Intratumoral fat also occurs in larger masses. Because it tends to be focal, it is unlikely to cause confusion in diagnosis. Patients with rare surface lesions may present with spontaneous rupture and hemoperitoneum (see Fig. 4-53I).

Studies evaluating focal liver lesions with **duplex and color flow Doppler** ultrasound suggest HCC has characteristic high-velocity signals.[186-188] Doppler is excellent for detecting neovascularity within tumor thrombi within the portal veins, diagnostic of HCC even without demonstration of the parenchymal lesion (Fig. 4-54).

Highly superior to conventional Doppler for **characterization of HCC** in the cirrhotic liver, **microbubble-enhanced sonography** is much more sensitive in the detection of lesional vascularity (see Fig. 4-41). Lesions are **hypervascular,** often showing dysmorphic vessels (see Fig. 4-42B). Enhancement in the arterial phase is in excess of the adjacent liver, frequently showing non-enhanced regions representing either necrosis or scarring. In the portal venous phase, lesions show **washout,** such that they are less enhanced than the adjacent liver (see Fig. 4-41F). Lesions appear, therefore, hypoechoic relative to the enhanced liver. Regenerative nodules, by comparison, show similar arterial phase and portal venous phase vascularity and enhancement in the remainder of the cirrhotic liver.

Microbubble-enhanced sonography is, as yet, untested in terms of its role in the **detection** of HCC. Sweeps of the liver in the arterial phase have the potential to detect hypervascular foci potentially representing HCC. Sweeps in the portal venous phase, by comparison, show HCC as hypoechoic regions, again allowing for the detection of unsuspected lesions. The arterialized liver of cirrhosis, however, is problematic for several reasons. First, it shows dysmorphology of all liver vessels, in general, and the appreciation of focal increased vascularity in a small nodule is more difficult. Portal venous-phase imaging is also weakened when the liver receives a greater proportion of its blood supply from the hepatic artery. Therefore washout of a specific nodule may not be as evident as in a normal liver. This area remains of high interest to us and investigations are ongoing in terms of evaluation of chronically diseased livers. **CT scanning**[189] and **MRI**[190] are both frequently performed to screen for and to evaluate HCC.

Fibrolamellar carcinoma is a histologic subtype of HCC that is found in younger patients (adolescents and young adults) without coexisting liver disease. The serum alpha-fetoprotein levels are usually normal. The tumors are usually well-differentiated, often encapsulated by fibrous tissue, and solitary. The size ranges from 6 to 22 cm.[191-193] The prognosis is generally better for fibrolamellar carcinoma compared with HCC with 5-year survival rates approximately 25% to 30%.[194,195] Most patients, however, demonstrate advanced disease at the time of diagnosis. Aggressive surgical resection of tumor is recommended at the time of presentation as well as for recurrent disease.[193] The echogenicity of fibrolamellar carcinoma is variable. Punctate calcification and a central echogenic scar—features that are distinctly unusual in hepatomas—are more common in the fibrolamellar subtype.

Hemangiosarcoma (Angiosarcoma)

Hepatic hemangiosarcoma is an extremely rare malignant tumor. It occurs almost exclusively in adults, reaching its peak incidence in the sixth and seventh decades of life. Hemangiosarcoma is of particular interest because of its association with specific carcinogens—Thorotrast, arsenic, and polyvinyl chloride.[171] Only a few cases of hepatic hemangiosarcoma have been reported in the

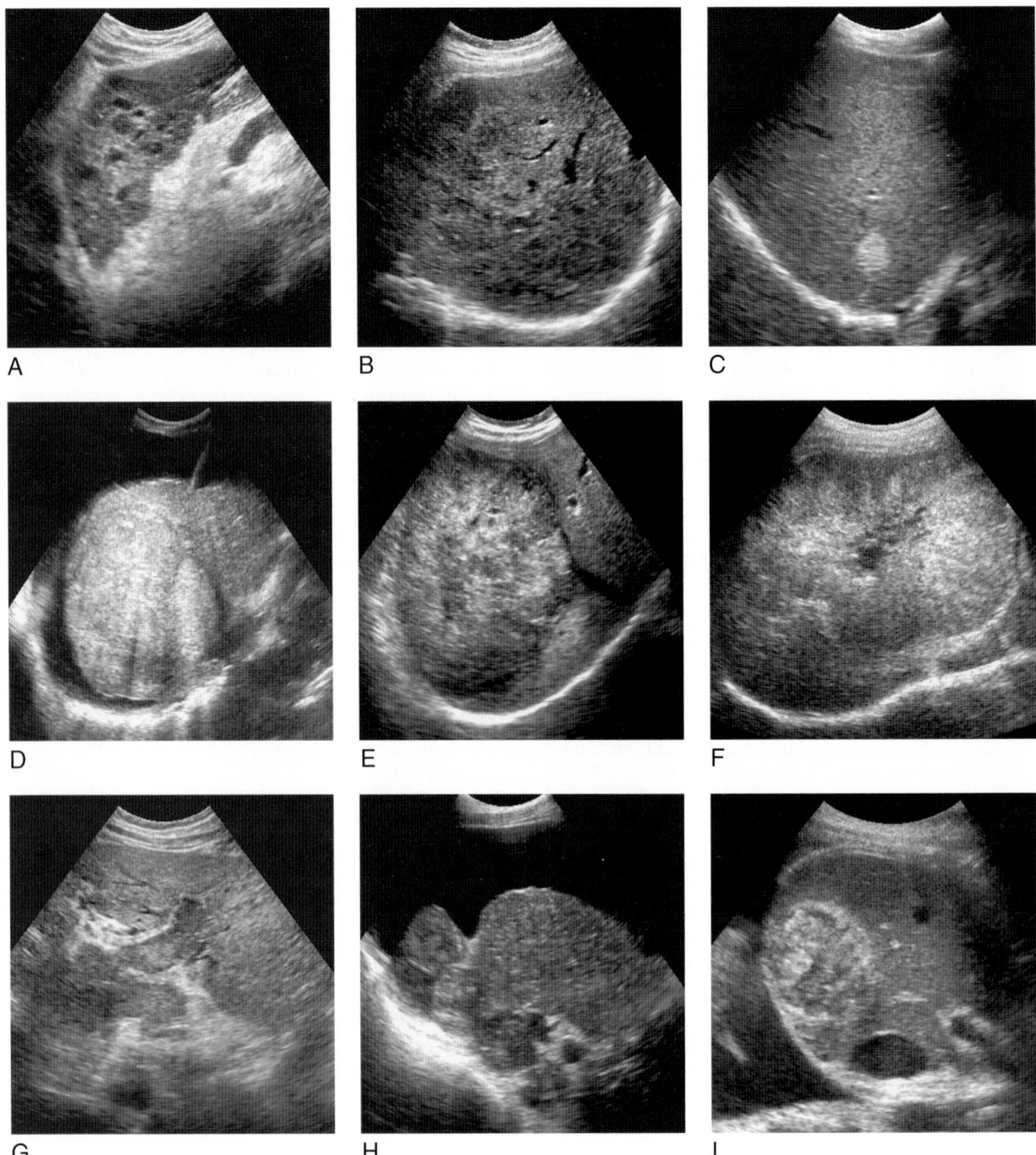

FIGURE 4-53. Hepatocellular carcinoma—Spectrum of appearances. A, Small focal hypoechoic nodules. **B,** Multifocal hypoechoic nodules, which may be difficult to differentiate from the background cirrhotic nodules. **C,** Focal echogenic nodule mimicking hemangioma, **D,** Large echogenic nodule in a cirrhotic liver. **E,** Large mixed echogenic mass. Hypoechoic regions corresponded at pathology with areas of necrosis. **F,** Large lobulated mass with central hypoechoic region suggesting a scar. **G,** Expansive tumor filling the portal vein as the only observation seen on the sonogram. **H,** Small cirrhotic liver showing exophytic tumors. **I,** Superficial mass of mixed echogenicity in a young hepatitis B patient presenting with spontaneous liver rupture.

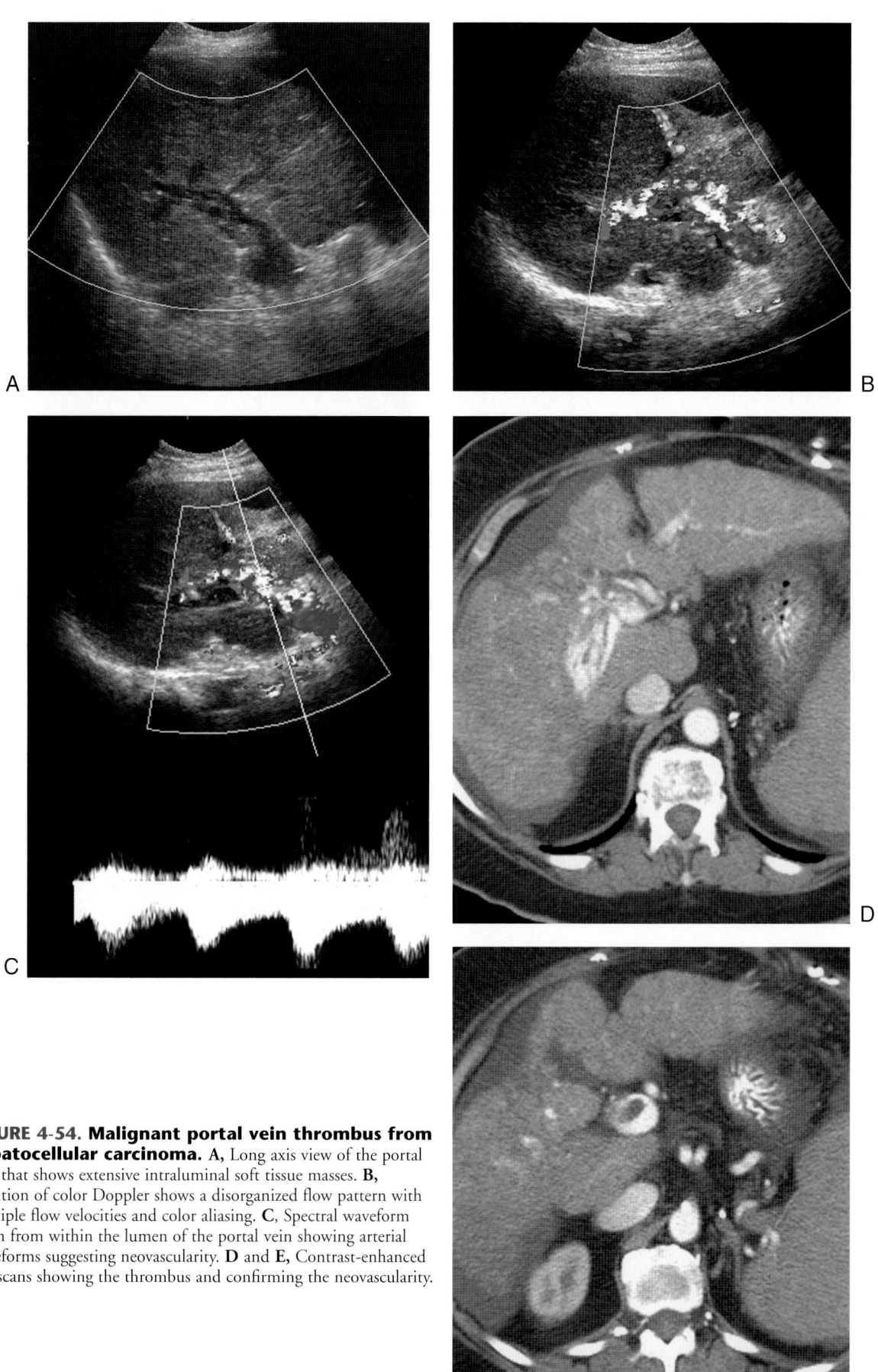

FIGURE 4-54. Malignant portal vein thrombus from hepatocellular carcinoma. A, Long axis view of the portal vein that shows extensive intraluminal soft tissue masses. **B,** Addition of color Doppler shows a disorganized flow pattern with multiple flow velocities and color aliasing. **C,** Spectral waveform taken from within the lumen of the portal vein showing arterial waveforms suggesting neovascularity. **D** and **E,** Contrast-enhanced CT scans showing the thrombus and confirming the neovascularity.

radiologic literature. The sonographic appearance is that of a large mass of mixed echogenicity.[196,197]

Hepatic Epithelioid Hemangioendothelioma

Epithelioid hemangioendothelioma (EHE) is a rare malignant tumor of vascular origin that occurs in adults. Soft tissues, lung, and liver are affected. The prognosis is variable. Many patients survive longer than 5 years with or without treatment.[198] Hepatic EHE begins as multiple hypoechoic nodules. Over time, the nodules grow and coalesce, forming larger confluent hypoechoic masses, which tend to involve the periphery of the liver. Foci of calcification may be present.[198,199] The hepatic capsule overlying the lesions of EHE may be retracted inward, secondary to fibrosis incited by the tumor. This is an unusual feature that is highly suggestive of this diagnosis. One should keep in mind that peripheral postchemotherapy metastases and tumors causing biliary obstruction may result in segmental atrophy and have a similar appearance.[200] The diagnosis is made by percutaneous liver biopsy, providing immunohisto-chemical staining is performed.

COMMON PATTERNS FOR METASTATIC LIVER DISEASE

Echogenic metastases
  Gastrointestinal tract
  Hepatocellular carcinoma
  Vascular primaries
  Islet cell carcinoma
  Carcinoid
  Choriocarcinoma
  Renal cell carcinoma
Hypoechoic metastases
  Breast cancer
  Lung cancer
  Lymphoma
  Esophagus, stomach, and pancreas
Bull's eye or target pattern
  Lung cancer
Calcified metastases
  Frequently—mucinous adenocarcinoma
  Less frequently—osteogenic sarcoma
  Chondrosarcoma
  Teratocarcinoma
  Neuroblastoma
Cystic metastases
  Necrosis—sarcomas
  Cystic growth patterns—cystadenocarcinoma of
    ovary and pancreas
  Mucinous carcinoma of colon
Infiltrative patterns
  Breast cancer
  Lung cancer
  Malignant melanoma

Metastatic Disease

In the United States, metastatic liver disease is 18 to 20 times more common than HCC. Its detection greatly alters the patient's prognosis and quite often the management.

The **incidence** of hepatic metastases depends on the type of tumor and its stage at initial detection. At autopsy, 25% to 50% of patients dying from cancer have liver metastases. Patients with short survival rates (<1 year) after initial detection of liver metastases are those with HCC and carcinomas of the pancreas, stomach, and esophagus. Patients with a more prolonged survival are those with head and neck carcinomas and carcinoma of the colon. Most patients with melanoma have an extremely low incidence of hepatic metastases at diagnosis. Liver involvement at autopsy, however, may be as high as 70%.

The **most common primary tumor sites** resulting in liver metastases in decreasing order of frequency are: gallbladder, colon, stomach, pancreas, breast, and lung. Most metastases to the liver are blood-borne via the hepatic artery or portal vein, but lymphatic spread of tumors from stomach, pancreas, ovary, or uterus may also occur. The portal vein provides direct access to the liver for tumor cells originating from the gastrointestinal tract and probably accounts for the high frequency of liver metastases from organs that drain into the portal circulation.

Advantages of ultrasound as a screening test for metastatic liver disease include its relative accuracy, speed, lack of ionizing radiation, and availability. Further, the multiplanar capability of ultrasound allows for excellent segmental localization of masses with the ability to detect proximity to or involvement of the vital vascular structures. Although isolated reports describe detection of metastases on sonography in skilled hands, competitive with CT and MR scan,[201] sonography is not uniformly used as the first line investigative technique to search for metastatic disease worldwide where CT has filled that role. Our experience and that of others suggests that US without microbubble-contrast agents does not compete with triphasic CT scan for metastases detection.[137] Although greatly improved with the addition of contrast agents as described earlier in the chapter, we doubt that this will ever be widely utilized in routine clinical practice for the large numbers of patients who have scans to search for metastatic disease. Nonetheless, on a case-by-case basis, and as a problem-solving modality, contrast-enhanced ultrasound may play a contributory role in the evaluation of the patient with metastatic liver disease.

On **conventional gray-scale sonography**, patients with metastatic liver disease may present as with a single liver lesion (Fig. 4-55A) although more commonly they present with multiple focal liver masses. All metastatic

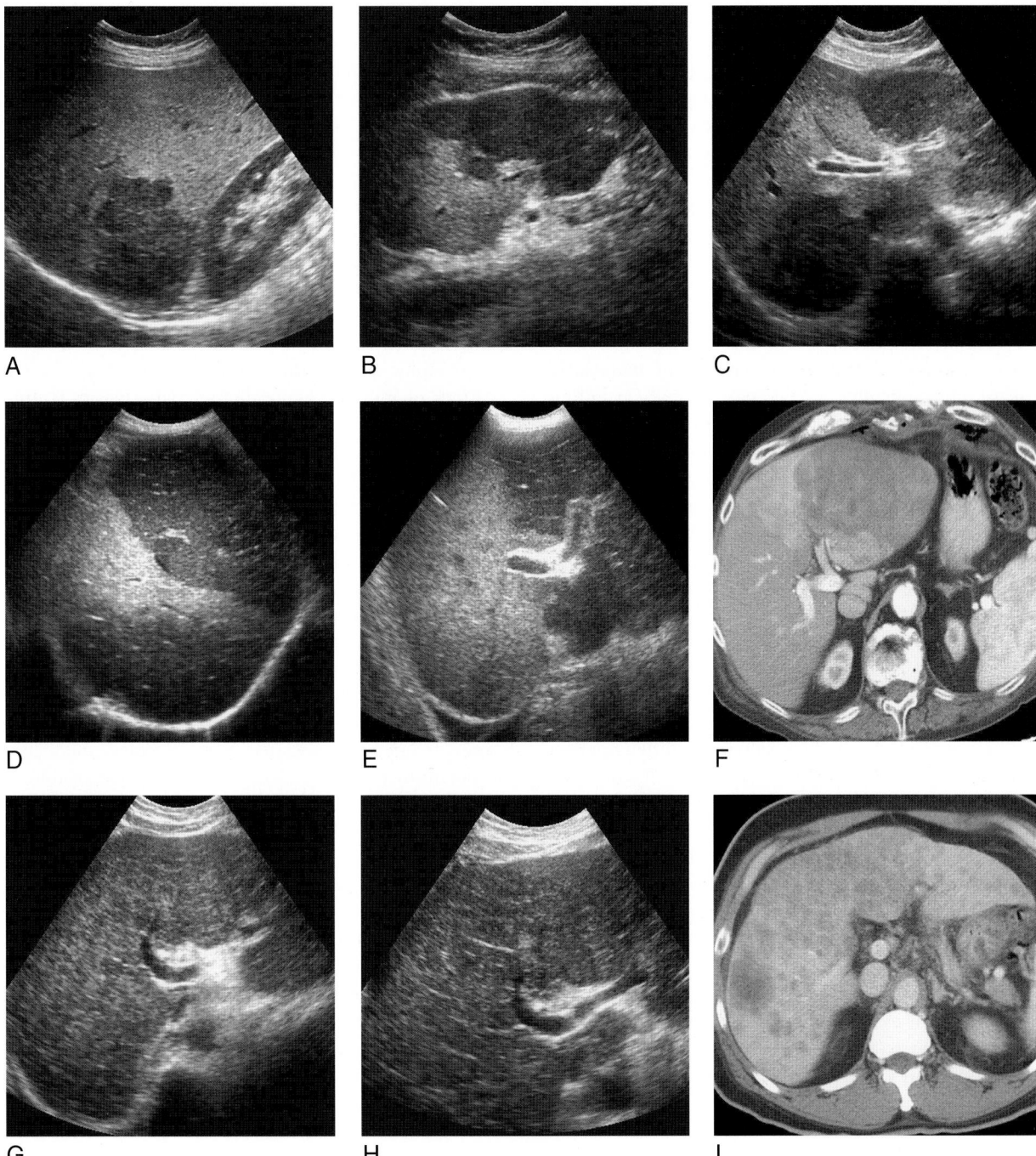

FIGURE 4-55. Liver involvement with metastases in three patients. Top line—most common variety and easiest to appreciate—focal liver mass(es). **A,** Sagittal image of the right lobe shows a well-defined and lobulated hypoechoic mass. **B,** Sagittal image of the left lobe shows confluent masses in segment 3. **C,** Transverse image shows the two focal hypoechoic masses separated by normal liver. **Middle line—rare geographic pattern of metastases. D** and **E,** Subcostal views showing the right and left lobes of the liver. A sharp geographic or maplike border separates the normal echogenic liver from the hypoechoic tumor. The distribution and echogenicity variation both suggest possible fatty change or perfusion abnormality. **F,** Confirmatory CT scan. **Bottom line—diffuse tumor involvement.** Often the most difficult to appreciate on ultrasound as here. **G,** Transverse sonogram and **H,** similar view with greater magnification. Both images show a coarse liver parenchyma. It is more suggestive of cirrhosis than the extensive tumor that is shown on the CT scan in **I.**

lesions in a given liver may have identical sonographic morphology; however, biopsy-confirmed lesions of differing appearances may have the same underlying histology. Of importance, metastases may also be present in a liver that already has an underlying diffuse or focal abnormality, most commonly hemangioma. Metastatic involvement of the liver may take on different forms, showing diffuse liver involvement and, rarely, geographic infiltration (Fig. 4-55C-F).

Knowledge of a prior or concomitant malignancy and features of disseminated malignancy at the time of a sonogram are helpful in correct interpretation of a sonographically detected liver mass(es). Although there are no absolutely confirmatory **features of metastatic disease** on sonography, several are suggestive, including the presence of **multiple solid lesions** of varying size and the presence of a **hypoechoic halo** surrounding a liver mass. A halo around the periphery of a liver mass on sonography has been regarded as an ominous sign with a high association with malignancy, particularly metastatic disease, but also HCC.

In our own investigation of 214 consecutive patients with focal liver lesions, 66 patients had lesions that showed a hypoechoic halo; 13 HCCs (Fig. 4-56A, B); 43 metastases (see Fig. 4-56C-F); 4 focal nodular hyperplasia; and 2 adenomas (see Fig. 4-50). Four lesions were unconfirmed. In 1992, Wernecke et al.[202] described the importance of the hypoechoic halo in the differentiation of malignant from benign focal hepatic lesions. Its identification has a positive and negative predictive value of 86% and 88%, respectively. Therefore, we conclude that although a halo is not absolutely indicative of malignancy, it is seen with lesions that require further investigation and confirmation of their nature, regardless of the patient's presentation or status. Radiologic-histologic correlation of a hypoechoic halo surrounding a liver mass has revealed that, in the majority of cases, the hypoechoic rim corresponds to normal liver parenchyma, which is compressed by the rapidly expanding tumor. Less commonly, the hypoechoic rim represents proliferating malignant cells, tumor fibrosis or vascularization, or a fibrotic rim.[203-205]

The following **sonographic appearances** of **metastatic liver disease** have been described (Fig. 4-57): echogenic, hypoechoic, target, calcified, cystic, and diffuse. Although the ultrasound appearance is not specific for determining the origin of the metastasis, certain generalities apply.

Echogenic metastases tend to arise from a gastrointestinal origin or from HCC (see Fig. 4-57I). The more vascular the tumor, the more likely the lesion is to be echogenic.[187,206] Therefore, metastases from renal cell carcinoma, carcinoid, choriocarcinoma, and islet cell carcinoma tend to be hyperechoic (see Fig. 4-57I). It is this particular group of tumors that may potentially mimic a hemangioma on sonography.

Hypoechoic metastases are generally hypovascular and may be mono- and hypercellular without interstitial stroma. They are the typical pattern seen in untreated metastatic breast or lung cancer (see Fig. 4-56 and Fig. 4-57), as well as gastric, pancreatic, and esophageal tumors. Lymphomatous involvement of the liver may also manifest as hypoechoic masses (Fig. 4-58). The uniform cellularity of lymphoma without significant background stroma is thought to be related to its hypoechoic appearance on sonography. Although at autopsy the liver is often a secondary site of involvement by Hodgkin's and non-Hodgkin's lymphoma, the disease tends to be diffusely infiltrative and undetected by sonographic examination and CT scanning.[207] The pattern of multiple hypoechoic hepatic masses is more typical of primary non-Hodgkin's lymphoma of the liver or lymphoma associated with AIDS.[207,208] The lymphomatous masses may appear anechoic and septated, mimicking hepatic abscesses.

The **bull's eye or target pattern** is characterized by a peripheral hypoechoic zone (see Fig. 4-56). The appearance is nonspecific and common, although it is frequently identified in metastases from bronchogenic carcinoma.[209]

Calcified metastases are distinctive by virtue of their marked echogenicity and distal acoustic shadowing (see Fig. 4-57B). Mucinous adenocarcinoma of the colon is most frequently associated with calcified metastases. Calcium may appear as large, echogenic, and shadowing foci or, more often, shows innumerable tiny punctate echogenicities without clear shadowing. Other primary malignancies that give rise to calcified metastases are endocrine pancreatic tumors, leiomyosarcoma, adenocarcinoma of the stomach, neuroblastoma, osteogenic sarcoma, chondrosarcoma, and ovarian cystadenocarcinoma and teratocarcinoma.[210]

Cystic metastases are fortunately uncommon and generally exhibit features that enable them to be distinguished from the ubiquitous benign hepatic cyst—for example, mural nodules, thick walls, fluid-fluid levels, and internal septations.[211,212] Primary neoplasms having a cystic component, such as cystadenocarcinoma of the ovary and pancreas and mucinous carcinoma of the colon, may produce cystic secondary lesions, although uncommonly. More often, cystic neoplasms occur secondary to extensive necrosis, seen most commonly in metastatic sarcomas, which typically have low-level echoes and a shaggy, thickened wall (see Fig. 4-57H). Metastatic neuroendocrine and carcinoid tumors are typically highly echogenic and often show secondary cystic change (see Fig. 5-57I). Large colorectal metastases may also rarely be necrotic, producing a predominantly cystic liver mass.

Diffuse disorganization of the hepatic parenchyma reflects an infiltrative form of metastatic disease and is the most difficult to appreciate on sonography, probably

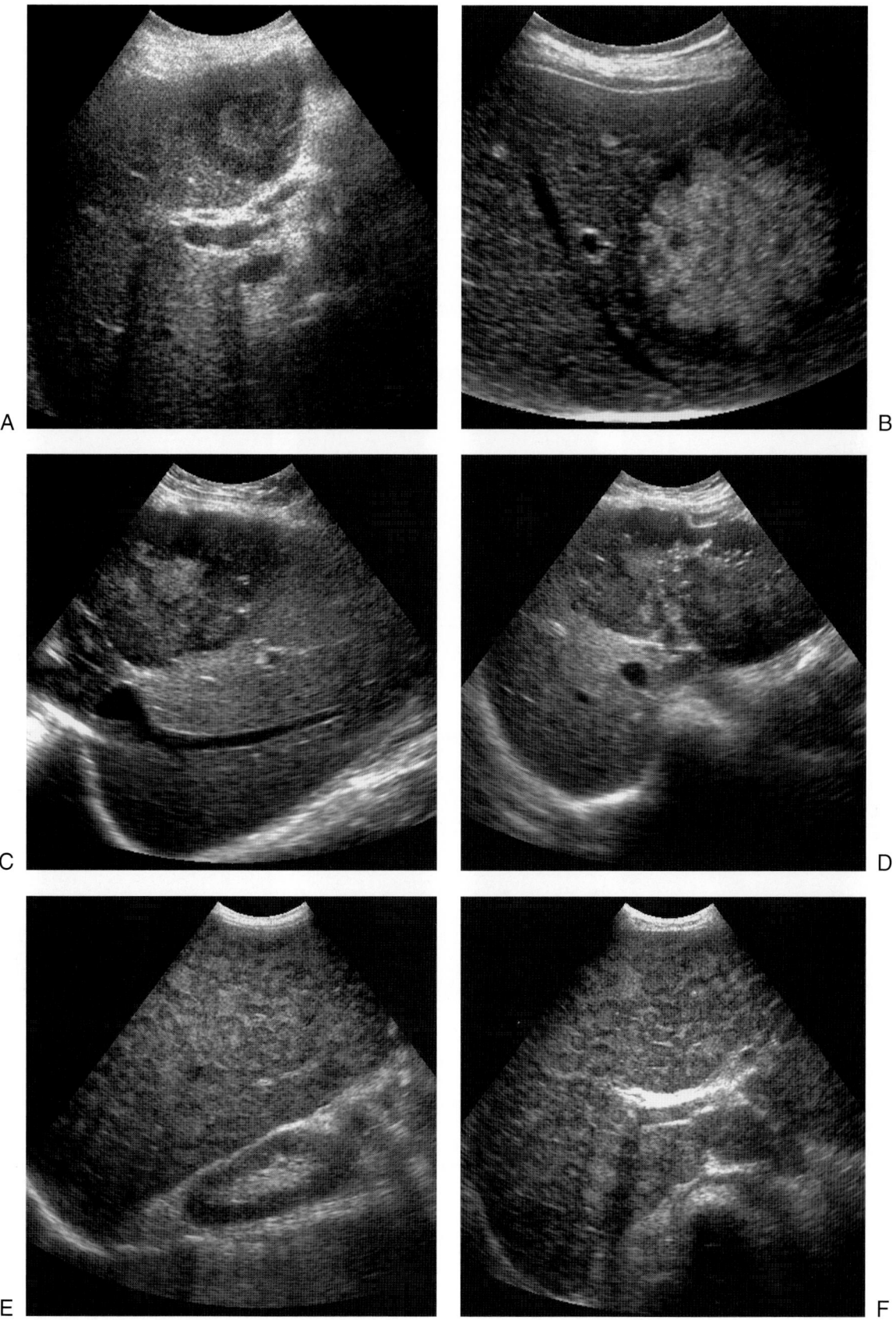

FIGURE 4-56. Hypoechoic Halo. A and **B,** Hepatocellular carcinoma showing as echogenic masses with a surrounding halo. **C** and **D,** Sagittal and transverse images of a large solitary breast metastasis. **E** and **F,** Large liver full of small masses with hypoechoic halos from small cell carcinoma of the lung.

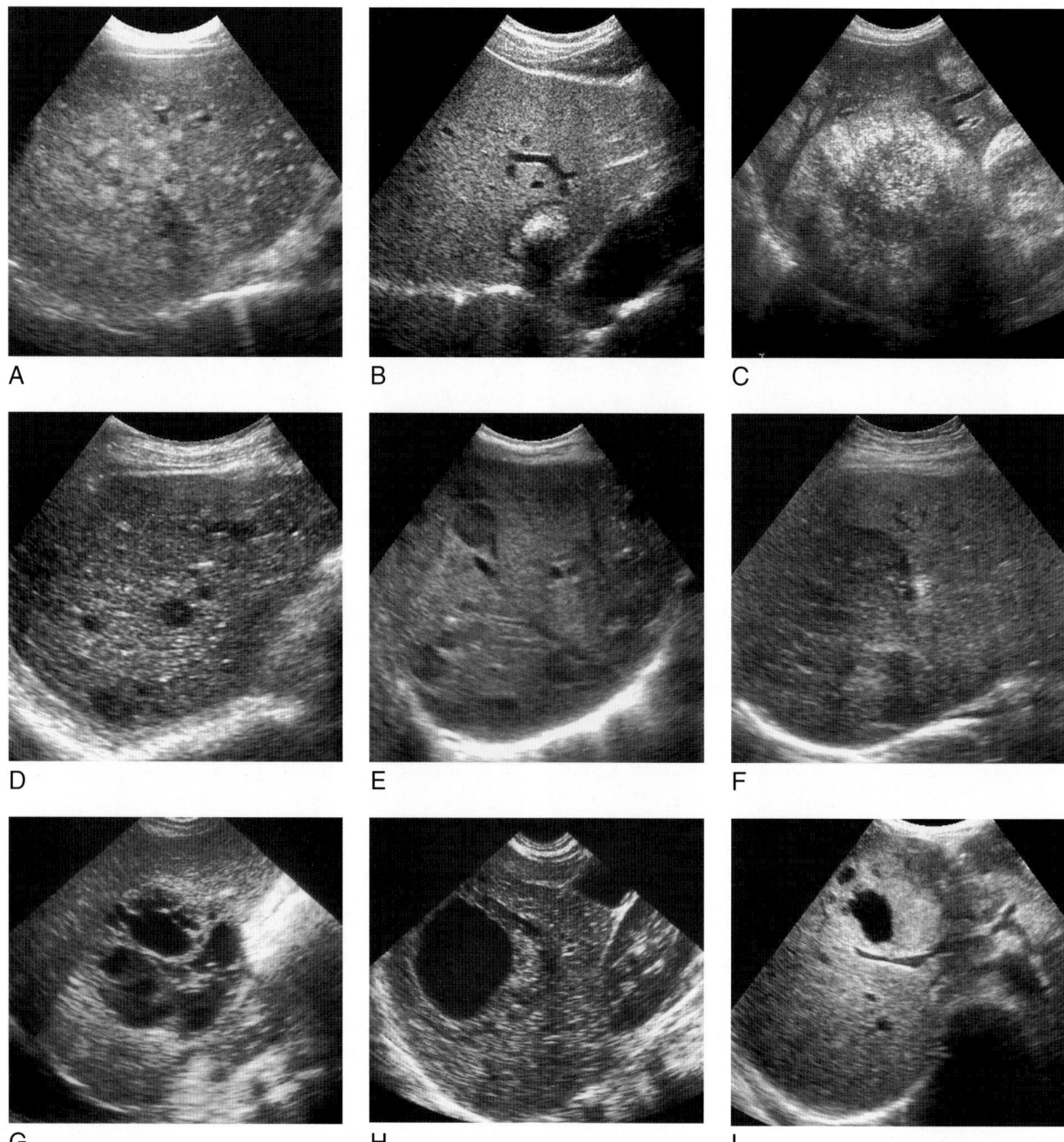

FIGURE 4-57. Patterns of metastatic liver disease. Top line—echogenic lesions. A, Multiple, tiny echogenic metastases from choriocarcinoma. **B,** Colon metastasis with clump of calcium with distal acoustic shadowing. **C,** Large, metastatic, poorly differentiated adenocarcinoma with tiny punctate echogenicities suggesting microcalcification. **Middle line—hypoechoic lesions of increasing size from D,** pancreas, **E,** lung, and **F,** adenocarcinoma from unknown primaries. **Bottom line—cystic metastases. G,** Rare metastatic liposarcoma from the thigh. Metastasis has a cystic growth pattern. **H,** Metastatic sarcoma from the small bowel with necrosis and **I,** highly echogenic metastasis with a well-defined cystic component highly suggestive of metastatic carcinoid or neuroendocrine tumor.

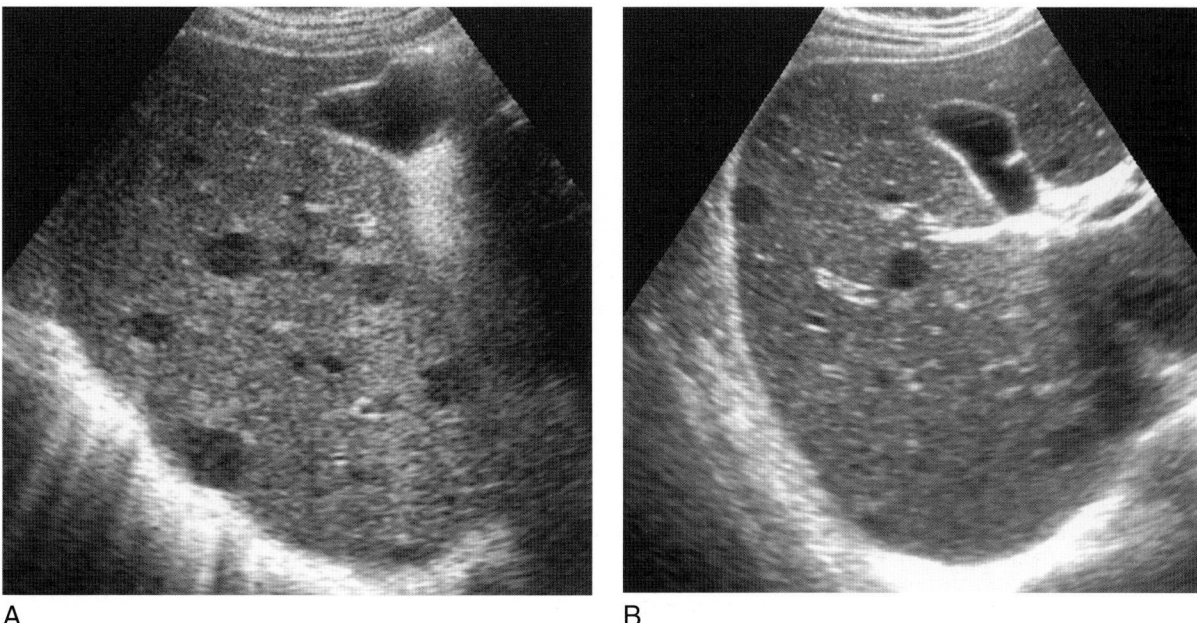

A   B

FIGURE 4-58. Lymphoma of the liver. A, Sagittal and **B,** transverse sonograms show small focal hypoechoic nodules throughout the liver. Lymphoma may also involve the liver diffusely without producing a focal sonographic abnormality.

as a loss of the reference normal liver for comparison (see Fig. 4-55G-I). In our experience, breast and lung carcinomas, as well as malignant melanomas, are the most common primary tumors to give this pattern. The diagnosis can be even more difficult if the patient has a fatty liver from chemotherapy. In these patients, CT scanning or MRI may be helpful. Segmental and lobar tumor infiltration by secondary tumor may also be difficult to detect because it may mimic other and benign conditions, such as fatty infiltration (see Fig. 4-55D-F).

Cholangiocarcinoma extending to involve the liver parenchyma may also be difficult to appreciate on sonograms. Both subtle parenchymal infiltration and invasion of the portal triads are recognized. Hepatic involvement by **Kaposi's sarcoma**, although frequent in patients with AIDS at autopsy, is rarely diagnosed by imaging studies.[213] Sonography has demonstrated periportal infiltration and multiple, small, peripheral hyperechoic nodules.[214,215] Because of the nonspecific appearance of metastatic liver disease, ultrasound-guided biopsy is widely used to establish a primary tissue diagnosis. In addition, ultrasound is an excellent means to monitor the response to chemotherapy in oncology patients.

HEPATIC TRAUMA

The approach to the management of **blunt hepatic injury** is becoming increasingly more conservative. Operative exploration is indicated for patients in shock or for those who are hemodynamically unstable.[216] In the hemodynamically stable patient, many institutions

initially perform abdominal CT scans to assess the extent of liver trauma. Ultrasound may be used to serially monitor the pattern of healing.

The predominant site of **hepatic injury** in blunt trauma is the right lobe—in particular, the posterior segment.[217] In the study series by Foley et al.[218] the most common type of injury was a perivascular laceration paralleling branches of the right and middle hepatic veins and the anterior and posterior branches of the right portal vein. Other findings were subcapsular, pericapsular, or isolated hematomas, liver fracture (which was defined as a laceration extending between two visceral surfaces), lacerations involving the left lobe, and hemoperitoneum (Fig. 4-59).[218] Hepatic infarcts are rarely identified following blunt abdominal trauma because of the dual blood supply of the liver.

Van Sonnenberg et al.[219] evaluated the sonographic findings of acute trauma to the liver (<24 hours following injury or transhepatic cholangiogram) and determined that fresh hemorrhage was echogenic (see Fig. 4-59C, D).[221] Within the first week, the hepatic laceration becomes more hypoechoic and distinct as a result of resorption of devitalized tissue and ingress of interstitial fluid. At 2 to 3 weeks later, the laceration becomes increasingly indistinct as a result of resorption of the fluid and filling of the spaces with granulation tissue.[220]

PORTOSYSTEMIC SHUNTS
Surgical Tips

Surgical portosystemic shunts are performed to decompress the portal system in patients with portal

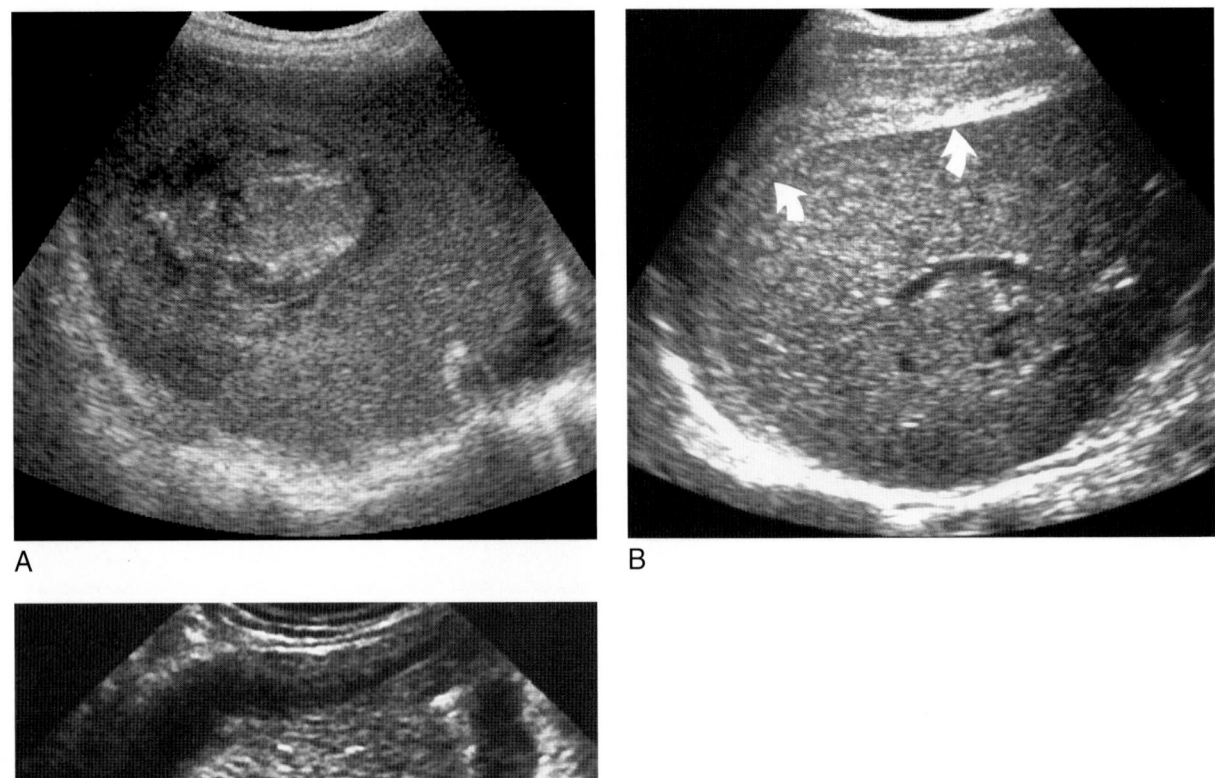

FIGURE 4-59. Liver trauma. A, An acute intrahepatic bleed and **B,** an acute perihepatic hematoma (*arrows*) between the liver surface and the overlying abdominal wall show increased echogenicity. **C,** An older hematoma surrounds the tip of the right lobe of the liver, appearing as a fluid collection with strands.

hypertension. The most commonly created surgical shunts include mesocaval, distal splenorenal (Warren), mesoatrial, and portacaval. Duplex Doppler sonography and color Doppler imaging appear to be reliable noninvasive methods of assessing shunt patency or thrombosis.[220-223] Both modalities are effective in assessing portacaval, mesoatrial, and mesocaval shunts.[222] Shunt patency is confirmed by demonstrating flow at the anastomotic site. If the anastomosis cannot be visualized, hepatofugal portal flow is an indirect sign of patency.[220,221]

Distal splenorenal communications are particularly difficult to examine with duplex Doppler sonography because overlying bowel gas and fat hinder accurate placement of the Doppler cursor.[222,224] Color Doppler imaging more readily locates the splenic and renal limbs of Warren shunts. The splenic limb is best imaged from a left subcostal approach, whereas the left renal vein is

optimally scanned through the left flank. In the study by Grant et al.,[222] color Doppler sonography correctly inferred patency or thrombosis in all 14 splenorenal communications by evaluating the flow in both limbs of the shunt.

Transjugular Intrahepatic Portosystemic Shunts

Transjugular intrahepatic portosystemic shunts (TIPS) are the most recently developed and now most popular technique for relief of symptomatic portal hypertension, specifically varices with gastrointestinal bleeding, and less often, refractory ascites. Performed percutaneously with insertion of an expandable metal stent, TIPS have less morbidity and mortality than surgical shunt procedures.[225]

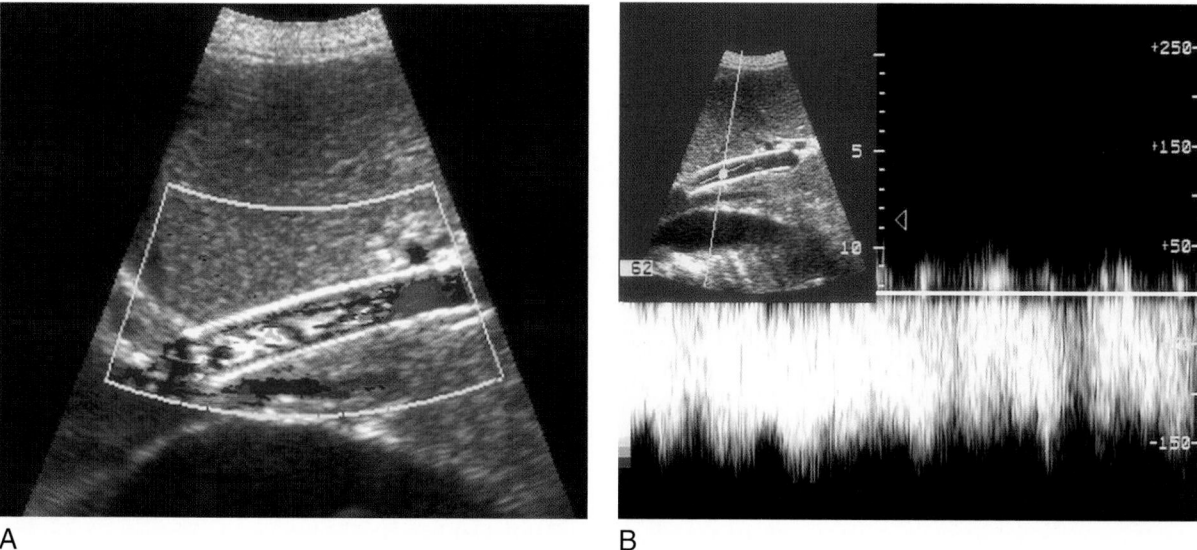

A   B

FIGURE 4-60. TIPS. A, Color Doppler image of TIPS shunt shows flow throughout the shunt appropriately directed toward the heart with a turbulent pattern. **B,** Angle corrected mid-shunt velocity is normal at 150 cm/sec. TIPS, Transjugular intrahepatic portosystemic shunts.

The **technique of performing TIPS** requires transjugular access to the infrahepatic inferior vena cava with selection of the optimal hepatic vein on the basis of its angle and diameter, most often the right hepatic vein. After targeting the portal vein with either fluoroscopy or Doppler sonography, a transjugular puncture needle is passed from the hepatic vein to the intrahepatic portal vein and a shunt is created. The tract is dilated to an approximate diameter of 10 mm with monitoring of the portal pressure gradient and filling of varices on portal venography. A bridging stent is left in place.[226]

In addition to acute problems directly attributed to the procedure itself, TIPS may be complicated by stenosis or occlusions of the stent caused by hyperplasia of the pseudointimal lining. At 1 year, primary patency rates vary from 25% to 66% with a primary assisted patency of approximately 83%.[227,228] Sonography with Doppler provides a noninvasive method for monitoring of TIPS patients following their procedure because malfunction of the graft may be silent in its early phase. Scans should be performed immediately postprocedure, at three monthly intervals, and/or as indicated clinically.

Normal postprocedure Doppler findings include high-velocity, turbulent blood flow (mean peak systolic velocity, 135 to 200 cm/sec)[229] throughout the stent and hepatofugal flow in the intrahepatic portal venous branches as the liver parenchyma drains through the shunt into the systemic circulation. Increased hepatic artery peak systolic velocity is also a normal observation, as is increased velocity in the main portal vein, as the stent serves as a low resistance conduit, bypassing the high-resistance hepatic circulation. The reported mean **main portal vein velocity** in patients with patent shunts ranged from 37 to 47 cm/second.[230-232] **Hepatic**

artery velocities increase from 79 cm/second preshunt to 131 cm/second following the procedure.[229]

The **technique of sonographic evaluation** should include measurement of angle corrected stent velocities at three points along the stent and in the main portal vein as well as evaluation of the direction of flow in the intrahepatic portal vein and in the involved hepatic vein (Fig. 4-60 and Fig. 4-61).

Sonographic detected complications include:

- Stent occlusion;
- Stent stenosis; and
- Hepatic venous stenosis.

PERCUTANEOUS LIVER BIOPSY

Percutaneous biopsy of malignant disease involving the liver has a sensitivity greater than 90% in most study series.[237,238] **Relative contraindications** to percutaneous biopsy are an uncorrectable bleeding diathesis, an unsafe access route, and a patient who cannot adequately cooperate. **Ultrasound guidance** allows real-time observation of the needle tip as it is advanced into the lesion. Several biopsy attachments have been developed that allow continuous observation of the needle as it follows a predetermined path. Alternatively, many experienced radiologists prefer a "free-hand" technique. Even small masses (2.5 cm) can undergo successful biopsy using sonographic guidance.[249] Ultrasound guidance may also be used in percutaneous aspiration and drainage of complicated fluid collections in the liver. Ultrasound-guided percutaneous ethanol injection has been used in the treatment of HCC and hepatic metastases.[239,240]

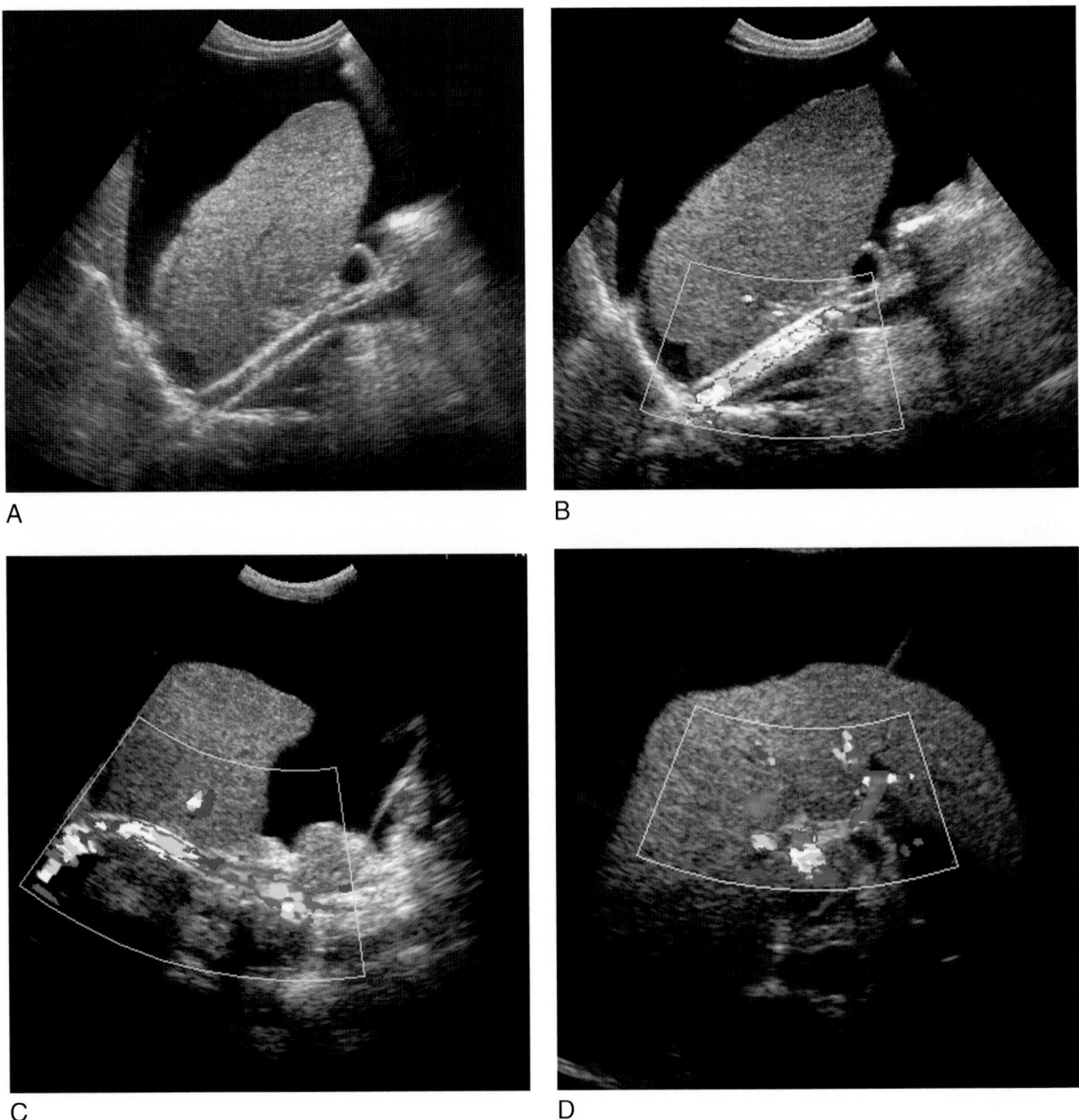

FIGURE 4-61. Secondary signs of a functional shunt. All images show gross ascites, which raises the possibility of a dysfunctional shunt. **A**, Gray-scale and **B**, color Doppler images show a patent TIPS shunt. Velocities throughout the shunt were about 130 cm per second, which is normal. **C,** Sagittal image shows flow in the main portal vein is appropriately directed toward the shunt, appearing *red*. **D**, Transverse image of the porta hepatis shows the ascending left portal venous branch is *blue*, flowing toward the shunt. This is also the correct direction. Therefore, in spite of the ascites, the ultrasound evaluation does not show a dysfunctional shunt.

MALFUNCTION OF TIPS: SONOGRAPHIC SIGNS[235-236]

DIRECT SIGNS

no flow, consistent with shunt thrombosis or occlusion;

peak shunt velocity of <90 cm/second or >190 cm/second

a **change** in the **peak shunt velocity**—decrease of >40 cm/second or an increase of >60 cm/second

main portal vein velocity <30 cm/second

reversal of flow in the **hepatic vein** away from the inferior vena cava suggesting hepatic vein stenosis

hepatopedal intrahepatic **portal venous flow**

SECONDARY SIGNS

Reaccumulation of ascites
Reappearance of varices
Reappearance of recanalized paraumbilical vein

INTRAOPERATIVE ULTRASOUND

Intraoperative ultrasound is now an established application of ultrasound technology. The exposed liver is scanned with a sterile 7.5 MHz transducer, or one covered by a sterile sheath. Intraoperative ultrasound has been found to change the operative strategy in 31% to 49% of patients undergoing hepatic resection, either by allowing more precise resection or by indicating inoperability because of unsuspected masses or venous invasion.[241,242]

References

Normal Anatomy

1. Marks WM, Filly RA, Callen PW: Ultrasonic anatomy of the liver: A review with new applications. J Clin Ultrasound 1979;7:137-146.
2. Couinaud C. Le foie. In Etudes Anatomiques et Chirugicales, Paris, 1957, Masson et Cie.
3. Sugarbaker PH: Toward a standard of nomenclature for surgical anatomy of the liver. Neth J Surg 1988;PO:100.
4. Nelson RC, Chezmar JL, Sugarbaker PH, et al: Preoperative localization of focal liver lesions to specific liver segments: Utility of CT during arterial portography. Radiology 1990;176:89-94.
5. Soyer P, Bluemke DA, Bliss DF, et al: Surgical segmental anatomy of the liver: Demonstration with spiral CT during arterial portography and multiplanar reconstruction. AJR 1994;163:99-103.
6. Lafortune M, Madore F, Patriquin HB, et al: Segmental anatomy of the liver: A sonographic approach to Couinaud nomenclature. Radiology 1991;181:443-448.
7. Gosink BB, Leymaster CE: Ultrasonic determination of hepatomegaly. J Clin Ultrasound 1981;9:37-44.
8. Niederau C, Sonnenberg A, Muller JE, et al: Sonographic measurements of the normal liver, spleen, pancreas, and portal vein. Radiology 1983;149:537-540.

Developmental Anomalies

9. Belton R, Van Zandt TF: Congenital absence of the left lobe of the liver: A radiologic diagnosis. Radiology 1983;147:184.
10. Radin DR, Colletti PM, Ralls PW, et al: Agenesis of the right lobe of the liver. Radiology 1987;164:639-642.
11. Lim JH, Ko YT, Han MC, et al: The inferior accessory hepatic fissure: Sonographic appearance. AJR 1987;149:495-497.
12. Fraser-Hill MA, Atri M, Bret PM, et al: Intrahepatic portal venous system: Variations demonstrated with duplex and color Doppler US. Radiology 1990;177:523-526.
13. Cosgrove DO, Arger PH, Coleman BG: Ultrasonic anatomy of hepatic veins. J Clin Ultrasound 1987;15:231-235.
14. Makuuchi M, Hasegawa H, Yamazaki S, et al: The inferior right hepatic vein: Ultrasonic demonstration. Radiology 1983;148:213-217.

Congenital Abnormalities

15. Gaines PA, Sampson MA: The prevalence and characterization of simple hepatic cysts by ultrasound examination. Br J Radiol 1989;62:335-337.
16. Bean WJ, Rodan BA: Hepatic cysts: Treatment with alcohol. AJR 1985;144:237-241.
17. Baron RL, Campbell WL, Dodd GD 3rd: Peribiliary cysts associated with severe liver disease: Imaging-pathologic correlation. AJR 1994;162:631-636.
18. Levine E, Cook LT, Grantham JJ: Liver cysts in autosomal-dominant polycystic kidney disease: Clinical and computed tomographic study. AJR 1985;145:229-233.
19. von Meyenburg H: Uber die Cystenliber. Beitr Pathol Anat 1918;64:477-532.
20. Chung ED: Multiple bile duct hamartomas. Cancer 1970;26:287.
21. Redston MS, Wanless IR: The hepatic von Meyenburg complex: Prevalence and association with hepatic and renal cysts among 2843 autopsies. Mod Pathol 1996;9:233-237.
22. Lev-Toaff AS, Bach AM, Wechsler RJ, et al: The radiologic and pathologic spectrum of biliary hamartomas. AJR 1995;165:309-313.
23. Salo J, Bru C, Vilella A, et al: Bile duct hamartomas presenting as multiple focal lesions on hepatic ultrasonography. Am J Gastroenterol 1992;87:221-223.
24. Tan A, Shen J, Hecht A: Sonogram of multiple bile duct hamartomas. Clin Ultrasound 1989;17:667-669.
25. Burns CD, Huhns JG, Wieman TJ: Cholangiocarcinoma in association with multiple biliary microhamartomas. Arch Pathol Lab Med 1990;114:1287-1289.

Infectious Diseases

26. Wilson SR: The Gallbladder. In Gastrointestinal Disease (Sixth Series). Test and Syllabus. American College of Radiology. Reston, VA. In press.
27. Seeft LB. Acute Viral Hepatitis. In: Kaplowitz N, ed. Liver and Biliary Disease, 2nd ed. Baltimore; Williams & Wilkins, 1996, pp 289-316.
28. Douglas DD, Rakela J: Fulminant hepatitis. In Kaplowitz N (ed): Liver and Biliary Disease, 2nd ed. Baltimore, Williams & Wilkins, 1996, pp 317-326.
29. Davis GL: Chronic hepatitis. In Kaplowitz N (ed): Liver and Biliary Disease, 2nd ed. Baltimore, Williams & Wilkins, 1996, pp 327-337.
30. Zweibel WJ: Sonographic diagnosis of diffuse liver disease. Semin US, CT, MRI 1995;16:8-15.
31. Wilson SR, Arenson AM: Sonographic evaluation of hepatic abscesses. J Can Assoc Radiol 1984;35:174-177.
32. Sabbaj J, Sutter VL, Finegold SM: Anaerobic pyogenic liver abscess. Ann Intern Med 1972;77:629-638.
33. Lawrence PH, Holt SC, Levi CS, et al: Ultrasound case of the day. Hepatosplenic candidiasis. Radiographics 1994;14:1147-1149.
34. Pastakia B, Shawker TH, Thaler M, et al: Hepatosplenic candidiasis: Wheels within wheels. Radiology 1988;166:417-421.
35. Ralls PW, Colletti PM, Quinn MF, et al: Sonographic findings in hepatic amebic abscess. Radiology 1982;145:123-126.
36. Berry M, Bazaz R, Bhargava S: Amebic liver abscess: Sonographic diagnosis and management. J Clin Ultrasound 1986;14:239-242.
37. Ralls PW, Barnes PF, Radin DR: Sonographic features of amebic and pyogenic liver abscesses: A blinded comparison. AJR 1987;149:499-501.
38. Ralls PW, Barnes PF, Johnson MB, et al: Medical treatment of hepatic amebic abscess: Rare need for percutaneous drainage. Radiology 1987;165:805-807.
39. Ralls PW, Quinn MF, Boswell WD, et al: Patterns of resolution in successfully treated hepatic amebic abscess: Sonographic evaluation. Radiology 1983;149:541-543.

40. Gharbi HA, Hassine W, Brauner MW, et al: Ultrasound examination of the hydatic liver. Radiology 1981;139:459-463.

41. Lewall DB, McCorkell SJ: Hepatic echinococcal cysts: Sonographic appearance and classification. Radiology 1985;155:773-775.

42. Beggs I: Radiology of hydatid disease. AJR 1985;145:639-648.

43. Mueller PR, Dawson SL, Ferrucci JT, Jr, et al: Hepatic echinococcal cyst: Successful percutaneous drainage. Radiology 1985;155:627-628.

44. Bret PM, Fond A, Bretagnolle M, et al: Percutaneous aspiration and drainage of hydatid disease of the liver. Radiology 1988;168:617-620.

45. Akhan O, Ozmen MN, Dincer A, et al: Liver hydatid disease: Long-term results of percutaneous treatment. Radiology 1996;198:259-264.

46. Bezzi M, Teggi A, De Rosa F, et al: Abdominal hydatid disease: Ultrasound findings during medical treatment. Radiology 1987;162:91-95.

47. Jha R, Lyons EA, Levi CS: Ultrasound case of the day. Hydatid cyst (*Echinococcus granulosus*) in the right lobe of the liver. Radiographics 1994;14:455-458.

48. Didier D, Weiler S, Rohmer P, et al: Hepatic alveolar echinococcus: Correlative ultrasound and computed tomography study. Radiology 1985;154:179-186.

49. McCully RM, Barron CM, Cheever AW: Schistosomiasis. In Binford CH, Connor DH (eds): Pathology of Tropical and Extraordinary Disease. Washington, DC. Armed Forces Institute of Pathology; 1976, pp 482-508.

50. Symmers W St C. Note on a new form of liver cirrhosis due to the presence of the ova of *Bilharzia hematobilia*. J Pathol 1904;9:237-239.

51. Cerri GG, Alves VAF, Magalhaes A. Hepatosplenic schistosomiasis mansoni: Ultrasound manifestations. Radiology 1984;153:777-780.

52. Fataar S, Bassiony H, Satyanath S, et al: Characteristic sonographic features of schistosomal periportal fibrosis. AJR 1984;143:69-71.

53. Kuhman JE: Pneumocystic infections: The radiologist's perspective. Radiology 1996;198:623-635.

54. Radin DR, Baker EL, Klatt EC, et al: Visceral and nodal calcification in patients with AIDS-related *Pneumocystis carinii* infection. AJR 1990;154:27-31.

55. Spouge AR, Wilson SR, Gopinath N, et al: Extrapulmonary *Pneumocystis carinii* in a patient with AIDS: Sonographic findings. AJR 1990;155:76-78.

56. Telzak EE, Cote RJ, Gold JWM, et al: Extrapulmonary *Pneumocystis carinii* infections. Rev Infect Dis 1990;12:380-386.

57. Lubat E, Megibow AJ, Balthazar EJ, et al: Extrapulmonary *Pneumocystis carinii* infection in AIDS: Computed tomography findings. Radiology 1990;174:157-160.

58. Towers MJ, Withers CE, Hamilton PA, et al: Visceral calcification in AIDS may not be always due to *Pneumocystis carinii*. AJR 1991;156:745-747.

Disorders of Metabolism

59. Zakim D: Metabolism of glucose and fatty acids by the liver. In Zakim D, Boyer TD (eds): Hepatology: A Textbook of Liver Disease, Philadelphia; WB Saunders, 1982, pp 76-109.

60. Wilson SR, Rosen IE, Chin-Sang HB, et al: Fatty infiltration of the liver: An imaging challenge. J Can Assoc Radiol 1982;33:227-232.

61. Yates CK, Streight RA: Focal fatty infiltration of the liver simulating metastatic disease. Radiology 1986;159:83-84.

62. Sauerbrei EE, Lopez M: Pseudotumor of the quadrate lobe in hepatic sonography: A sign of generalized fatty infiltration. AJR 1986;147:923-927.

63. White EM, Simeone JF, Mueller PR, et al: Focal periportal sparing in hepatic fatty infiltration: A cause of hepatic pseudomass on ultrasound. Radiology 1987;162:57-59.

64. Wanless IR, Bargman JM, Oreopoulos DG, et al: Subcapsular steatonecrosis in response to peritoneal insulin delivery: A clue to the pathogenesis of steatonecrosis in obesity. Mod Pathol 1989;2:69-74.

65. Apicella PL, Mirowitz SA, Weinreb JC: Extension of vessels through hepatic neoplasms: MR and CT findings. Radiology 1994;191:135-136.

66. Quinn SF, Gosink BB: Characteristic sonographic signs of hepatic fatty infiltration. AJR 1985;145:753-755.

67. Arai K, Matsui O, Takashima T, et al: Focal spared areas in fatty liver caused by regional decreased blood flow. AJR 1988;151:300-302.

68. Ishak KG, Sharp HL: Metabolic errors and liver disease. In: MacSween RNM, Anthony PP, Scheuer PJ (eds): Pathology of the Liver, 2nd ed, New York; Churchill Livingstone, 1987, pp 99-180.

69. Grossman H, Ram PC, Coleman RA, et al: Hepatic ultrasonography in type 1 glycogen storage disease (von Gierke disease). Radiology 1981;141:753-756.

Cirrhosis

70. Anthony PP: The morphology of cirrhosis: Definition, nomenclature, and classification. Bull WHO 1977; 55:521.

71. Millward-Sadler GH: Cirrhosis. In MacSween RNM, Anthony PP, Scheuer PJ (eds): Pathology of the Liver, 2nd ed. New York, Churchill Livingstone, 1987, pp 342-363.

72. Giorgio A, Amoroso P, Lettiri G, et al: Cirrhosis: Value of caudate to right lobe ratio in diagnosis with ultrasound. Radiology 1986;161:443-445.

73. Taylor KJW, Riely CA, Hammers L, et al: Quantitative ultrasound attenuation in normal liver and in patients with diffuse liver disease: Importance of fat. Radiology 1986;160:65-71.

74. Sandford N, Walsh P, Matis C, et al: Is ultrasonography useful in the assessment of diffuse parenchymal liver disease? Gastroenterology 1985;89:186-191.

75. Freeman MP, Vick CW, Taylor KJW, et al: Regenerating nodules in cirrhosis: Sonographic appearance with anatomic correlation. AJR 1986;146:533-536.

76. Murakami T, Nakamura H, Hori S, et al: Regenerating nodules in hepatic cirrhosis. MR findings with pathologic correlation. AJR 1990;155:1227-1231.

77. Theise ND: Macroregenerative (dysplastic) nodules and hepatocarcinogenesis: Theoretical and clinical considerations. Semin Liver Dis 1995;15:360-371.

78. Tanaka S, Kitamra T, Fujita M, et al: Small hepatocellular carcinoma: Differentiation from adenomatous hyperplastic nodule with color Doppler flow imaging. Radiology 1997;182:161-165.

79. Bolondi L, Bassi S, Gaiani S, et al: Liver cirrhosis: Changes of Doppler waveform of hepatic veins. Radiology 1991;178:513-516.

80. Colli A, Cocciolo M, Riva C, et al: Abnormalities of Doppler waveform of the hepatic veins in patients with chronic liver disease: Correlation with histologic findings. AJR 1994;162:833-837.

81. Lafortune M, Dauzat M, Pomier-Layrargues E, et al: Hepatic artery: Effect of a meal in healthy persons and transplant recipients. Radiology 1993;187:391-394.

82. Joynt LK, Platt JF, Rubin JM, et al: Hepatic artery resistance before and after standard meal in subjects with diseased and healthy livers. Radiology 1995;196:489-492.

Vascular Abnormalities

83. Boyer TD: Portal Hypertension and its Complications. In Zakim D, Boyer TD (eds): Hepatology: A Textbook of Liver Disease, Philadelphia, WB Saunders, 1982, pp 464-499.

84. Bolondi L, Gandolfi L, Arienti V, et al: Ultrasonography in the diagnosis of portal hypertension: Diminished response of portal vessels to respiration. Radiology 1982;142:167-172.

85. Lafortune M, Marleau D, Breton G, et al: Portal venous system measurements in portal hypertension. Radiology 1984;151:27-30.

86. Juttner H-U, Jenney JM, Ralls PW, et al: Ultrasound demonstration of portosystemic collaterals in cirrhosis and portal hypertension. Radiology 1982;142:459-463.

87. Subramanyam BR, Balthazar EJ, Madamba MR, et al: Sonography of portosystemic venous collaterals in portal hypertension. Radiology 1983;146:161-166.

88. Patriquin H, Lafortune M, Burns PN, et al: Duplex Doppler examination in portal hypertension. AJR 1987;149:71-76.

89. Lafortune M, Constantin A, Breton G, et al: The recanalized umbilical vein in portal hypertension: A myth. AJR 1985;144:549-553.

90. DiCandio G, Campatelli A, Mosca F, et al: Ultrasound detection of unusual spontaneous portosystemic shunts associated with uncomplicated portal hypertension. J Ultrasound Med 1985;4:297-305.

91. Mostbeck GH, Wittich GR, Herold C, et al: Hemodynamic significance of the paraumbilical vein in portal hypertension: Assessment with duplex ultrasound. Radiology 1989;170:339-342.

92. Nelson RC, Lovett KE, Chezmar JL, et al: Comparison of pulsed Doppler sonography and angiography in patients with portal hypertension. AJR 1987;149:77-81.

93. Bellamy EA, Bossi MC, Cosgrove DO: Ultrasound demonstration of changes in the normal portal venous system following a meal. Br J Radiol 1984;57:147-149.

94. Ohnishi K, Saito M, Nakayama T, et al: Portal venous hemodynamics in chronic liver disease: Effects of posture change and exercise. Radiology 1985;155:757-761.

95. Bolondi L, Maziotti A, Arienti V, et al: Ultrasonography in the diagnosis of portal hypertension and after portosystemic shunt operations. Surgery 1984;95:261-269.

96. Zweibel WJ, Mountford RA, Halliwell MJ, et al: Splanchnic blood flow in patients with cirrhosis and portal hypertension: Investigation with duplex Doppler US. Radiology 1995;194:807-812.

97. Finn JP, Kane RA, Edelman RR, et al: Imaging of the portal venous system in patients with cirrhosis: MR angiography vs. duplex Doppler sonography. AJR 1993;161:989-994.

98. Wilson SR, Hine AL: Leiomyosarcoma of the portal vein. AJR 1987;149:183-184.

99. Van Gansbeke D, Avni EF, Delcour C, et al: Sonographic features of portal vein thrombosis. AJR 1985;144:749-752.

100. Kauzlaric D, Petrovic M, Barmeir E: Sonography of cavernous transformation of the portal vein. AJR 1984;142:383-384.

101. Aldrete JS, Slaughter RL, Han SY: Portal vein thrombosis resulting in portal hypertension in adults. Am J Gastroenterol 1976;65:3-11.

102. Dodd GD, Memel OS, Baron RL, et al: Portal vein thrombosis in patients with cirrhosis. Does sonographic detection of intrathrombus flow allow differentiation of benign and malignant thrombus? AJR 1995;165:573-577.

103. Stanley P: Budd-Chiari syndrome. Radiology 1989;170:625-627.

104. Makuuchi M, Hasegawa H, Yamazaki S, et al: Primary Budd-Chiari syndrome: Ultrasonic demonstration. Radiology 1984;152:775-779.

105. Menu Y, Alison D, Lorphelin J-M, et al: Budd-Chiari syndrome: Ultrasound evaluation. Radiology 1985;157:761-764.

106. Park JH, Lee JB, Han MC, et al: Sonographic evaluation of inferior vena caval obstruction: Correlative study with vena cavography. AJR 1985;145:757-762.

107. Murphy FB, Steinberg HV, Shires GT, et al: The Budd-Chiari syndrome: A review. AJR 1986;147:9-15.

108. Grant EG, Perrella R, Tessler FN, et al: Budd-Chiari syndrome: the results of duplex and color Doppler imaging. AJR 1989;152:377-381.

109. Keller MS, Taylor KJW, Riely CA: Pseudoportal Doppler signal in the partially obstructed inferior vena cava. Radiology 1989;170:475-477.

110. Hosoki T, Kuroda C, Tokunaga K, et al: Hepatic venous outflow obstruction: Evaluation with pulsed Duplex sonography. Radiology 1989;170:733-737.

111. Brown BP, Abu-Youssef M, Farner R, et al: Doppler sonography: A non-invasive method for evaluation of hepatic veno-occlusive disease. AJR 1990;154:721-724.

112. Becker CD, Scheidegger J, Marincek B: Hepatic vein occlusion: Morphologic features on computed tomography and ultrasonography. Gastrointest Radiol 1986;11:305-311.

113. Ralls PW, Johnson MB, Radin RD, et al: Budd-Chiari syndrome: Detection with color Doppler sonography. AJR 1992;159:113-116.

114. Millener P, Grant EG, Rose S, et al: Color Doppler imaging findings in patients with Budd-Chiari syndrome: Correlation with venographic findings. AJR 1993;161:307-312.

115. Taylor KJW, Burns PN, Woodcock JP, et al: Blood flow in deep abdominal and pelvic vessels: Ultrasonic pulsed Doppler analysis. Radiology 1985;154:487-493.

116. Kriegshauser SJ, Charboneau JW, Letendre L: Hepatic venocclusive disease after bone marrow transplantation: Diagnosis with duplex sonography. AJR 1988;150:289-290.

117. Vine HS, Sequira JC, Widrich WC, et al: Portal vein aneurysm. AJR 1979;132:557-560.

118. Chagnon SF, Vallee CA, Barge J, et al: Aneurysmal portohepatic venous fistula: Report of two cases. Radiology 1986;159:693-695.

119. Mori H, Hayashi K, Fukuda T, et al: Intrahepatic portosystemic venous shunt: Occurrence in patients with and without liver cirrhosis. AJR 1987;149:711-714.

120. Park JH, Cha SH, Han JK, et al: Intrahepatic portosystemic venous shunt. AJR 1990;155:527-528.

121. Falkoff GE, Taylor KJW, Morse S: Hepatic artery pseudo-aneurysm: Diagnosis with real-time and pulsed Doppler ultrasound. Radiology 1986;158:55-56.

122. Garcia P, Garcia-Giannoli H, Meyron S, et al: Primary dissecting aneurysm of the hepatic artery: Sonographic, CT and angiographic findings. AJR 1996;166:1316-1318.

123. Cloogman HM, DiCapo RD: Hereditary hemorrhagic telangiectasia: Sonographic findings in the liver. Radiology 1984;150:521-522.

124. Wanless IR: Vascular Disorders. In MacSween RNM, Anthony PP, Scheuer PJ, et al (eds): Pathology of the Liver, 3rd ed. Edinburgh, Churchill Livingstone, 1994, p 535.

125. Czapar CA, Weldon-Linne CM, Moore DM, et al: Peliosis hepatis in the acquired immunodeficiency syndrome. Arch Pathol Lab Med 1986;110:611.

126. Leong SS, Cazen RA, Yu GSM, et al: Abdominal visceral peliosis associated with bacillary angiomatosis. Ultrasound evidence of endothelial destruction by bacilli. Arch Pathol Lab Med 1992;116:866.

127. Jamadar DA, D'Souza SP, Thomas EA, et al: Radiological appearances in peliosis hepatis. Br J Radiol 1994; 67:102.

128. Toyoda S, Takeda K, Nakagawa T, et al: Magnetic resonance imaging of peliosis hepatis: A case report. Eur J Radiol 1993;16:207.

129. Lloyd RL, Lyons EA, Levi CS, et al: The sonographic appearance of peliosis hepatis. J Ultrasound Med 1982;1:293.

130. Tsukamoto Y, Nakata H, Kimoto T, et al: CT and angiography of peliosis hepatis. AJR 1984;142:539.

131. Muradali D, Wilson SR, Wanless IR, et al: Peliosis hepatis with intrahepatic calcifications. J Ultrasound Med 1996;16:257-260.

Microbubble Contrast Agents

132. Dill-Macky MJ, Burns PN, Khalili K, et al: Focal hepatic masses: Enhancement patterns with SH U 508A and pulse-inversion US. Radiology 2002;222:95-102.

133. Wilson SR, Burns PN, Muradali D, et al: Harmonic hepatic ultrasound with microbubble contrast agent: Initial experience showing improved characterization of hemangioma, hepatocellular carcinoma, and metastasis. Radiology 2000;215:153-161.

134. Burns PN, Wilson SR, Simpson DH: Pulse inversion imaging of liver blood flow: Improved method for characterizing focal masses with microbubble contrast. Invest Radiol 2000;35:58-71.

135. Brannigan M, Burns PNB, Wilson SR: Blood flow patterns in focal liver lesions at microbubble enhanced ultrasound. Radiographics 2004, in press.

136. Blomley MJK, Albrecht T, Cosgrove DO, et al: Improved imaging of liver metastases with stimulated acoustic emission in the late phase of enhancement with the US contrast agent SHU 508A: Early experience. Radiology 1999;210:409-416.

137. Albrecht T, Blomley MJK, Burns PN, et al: Improved detection of hepatic metastases with pulse-inversion US during the liver-specific phase of SHU 508A: Multicentre Study. Radiology 2003;227(2):361-370.

Hepatic Neoplasms

138. Charboneau JW: There is a hyperechoic mass in the liver: What does that mean? 2002 Categorical Course in Diagnostic Radiology: Findings at US—What do they mean? PL Cooperberg (ed): RSNA, 73-78.

139. Edmondson HA: Tumors of the liver and intrahepatic bile ducts. In Atlas of Tumor Pathology, Washington, DC; Armed Forces Institute of Pathology, 1958, p 113.

140. Gibney RG, Hendin AP, Cooperberg PL: Sonographically detected hemangiomas: Absence of change over time. AJR 1987;149:953-957.

141. Mungovan JA, Cranon JJ, Vacarro J: Hepatic cavernous hemangiomas: Lack of enlargement over time. Radiology 1994;191:111-113.

142. Bree RL, Schwab RE, Neiman HL: Solitary echogenic spot in the liver: Is it diagnostic of a hemangioma? AJR 1983;140:41-45.

143. McCardle CR: Ultrasonic appearances of a hepatic hemangioma. J Clin Ultrasound 1978;6:122-123.

144. Taboury J, Porcel A, Tubiana J-M, et al: Cavernous hemangiomas of the liver studied by ultrasound. Radiology 1983;149:781-785.

145. Itai Y, Ohnishi S, Ohtomo K, et al: Hepatic cavernous hemangioma in patients at high risk for liver cancer. Acta Radiol 1987;28:697-701.

146. Itai Y, Ohtomo K, Araki T, et al: Computed tomography and sonography of cavernous hemangioma of the liver. AJR 1983;141:315-320.

147. Moody AR, Wilson SR: Atypical hemangioma: A suggestive sonographic morphology. Radiology 1993; 188:413-417.

148. Marsh JI, Gibney RG, Li DKB: Hepatic hemangioma in the presence of fatty infiltration: An atypical sonographic appearance. Gastrointest Radiol 1989;14:262-264.

149. Choi BI, Kim TK, Han JK, et al: Power versus conventional color Doppler sonography: Comparison in depiction of vasculature in liver tumors. Radiology 1996;200:55-58.

150. Porzio ME, Pellerito JS, D'Agostino CA, et al: Improved characterization of hepatic hemangioma with color power angiography. In RSNA Scientific Program 1995, Supplement to Radiology 1995,197(P), pp 401-402.

151. Caturelli E, Pompili M, Bartolucci F, et al: Hemangioma-like lesions in chronic liver disease: Diagnostic evaluation in patients. Radiology 2001;220(2):337-342.

152. Freeny PC, Marks WM: Hepatic hemangioma: Dynamic bolus computed tomography. AJR 1986;147:711-719.

153. Scatarige JC, Kenny JM, Fishman EK, et al: Computed tomography of hepatic cavernous hemangioma. J Comput Assist Tomogr 1987;11:455-460.

154. Brunetti JC, Van Heertum RL, Yudd AP: SPECT in the diagnosis of hepatic hemangioma (Abstract). J Nucl Med 1985;26:8.

155. Birnbaum BA, Weinreb JC, Megibow AJ, et al: Definitive diagnosis of hepatic hemangiomas: Magnetic resonance imaging versus Tc-99m-labeled red blood cell SPECT. Radiology 1990;176:95-101.

156. Nelson RC, Chezmar JL: Diagnostic approach to hepatic hemangiomas. Radiology; 1990;176:11-13.

157. Solbiati L, Livraghi T, DePra L, et al: Fine-needle biopsy of hepatic hemangioma with sonographic guidance. AJR 1985;144:471-474.

158. Cronan JJ, Esparza AR, Dorfman GS, et al: Cavernous hemangioma of the liver: Role of percutaneous biopsy. Radiology 1988;166:135-138.

159. Craig JR, Peters RL, Edmondson HA: Tumors of the liver and intrahepatic bile ducts. Fasc 26, 2nd ser, Washington, DC, 1989, Armed Forces Institute of Pathology.

160. Wanless IR, Mawdsley C, Adams R: On the pathogenesis of focal nodular hyperplasia of the liver. Hepatology 1985;5:1194-1200.

161. Saul SH: Masses of the liver. In Sternberg SS (ed): Diagnostic Surgical Pathology, 2nd ed. New York, Raven, 1994, pp 1517-1580.

162. Knowles DM 2nd, Casarella WJ, Johnson PM, et al: The clinical, radiologic and pathologic characterization of benign hepatic neoplasms: Alleged association with oral contraceptives. Medicine 1978;57:223-237.

163. Ross D, Pina J, Mirza M, et al: Regression of focal nodular

hyperplasia after discontinuation of oral contraceptives. Ann Intern Med 1976;85:203-204.

164. Buetow PC, Pantongrag-Brown L, Buck JL, et al: Focal nodular hyperplasia of the liver: Radiologic-pathologic correlation. Radiographics 1996;16:369-388.

165. Scatarige JC, Fishman EK, Sanders RC: The sonographic "scar sign" in focal nodular hyperplasia of the liver. J Ultrasound Med 1982;1:275-278.

166. Golli M, Van Nhieu JT, Mathieu D, et al: Hepatocellular adenoma: Color Doppler US and pathologic correlations. Radiology 1994;190:741-744.

167. Drane WE, Krasicky GA, Johnson DA: Radionuclide imaging of primary liver tumors and tumor-like conditions of the liver. Clin Nucl Med 1987;12:569.

168. Welch TJ, Sheedy PF, Johnson CM, et al: Focal nodular hyperplasia and hepatic adenoma: Comparison of angiography, CT, US and scintigraphy. Radiology 1985;156:593.

169. Kerlin P, Davis GL, McGill DB, et al: Hepatic adenoma and focal nodular hyperplasia: Clinical, pathologic and radiologic features. Gastroenterology 1983; 84:994-1002.

170. Brunelle R, Tammam S, Odievre M, et al: Liver adenomas in glycogen storage disease in children: Ultrasound and angiographic study. Pediatr Radiol 1984;14:94-101.

171. Kew MC: Tumors of the liver. In Zakim D, Boyer TD (eds): Hepatology: A Textbook of Liver Disease. Philadelphia, WB Saunders, 1982, pp 1048-1084.

172. Lubbers PR, Ros PR, Goodman ZD, et al: Accumulation of technetium-99m sulfur colloid by hepatocellular adenoma: Scintigraphic-pathologic correlation. AJR 1987;148:1105-1108.

173. Katsuyoshi I, Kazumitsu H, Fujita T, et al: Liver neoplasms: Diagnostic pitfalls in cross sectional imaging. Radiographics 1996;16:273-293.

174. Roberts JL, Fishman E, Hartman DS, et al: Lipomatous tumors of the liver: Evaluation with computed tomography and ultrasound. Radiology 1986; 158:613-617.

175. Marti-Bonmati L, Menor F, Vizcaino I, et al: Lipoma of the liver: Ultrasound, computed tomography and magnetic resonance imaging appearance. Gastrointest Radiol 1989;14: 155-157.

176. Reinhold C, Garant M: Hepatic lipoma. Can Assoc Radiol J 1996;47:140-142.

177. Wilson SR: The Liver. Gastrointestinal Disease (Sixth Series). Test and Syllabus. American College of Radiology, Reston, VA, 2004, In press.

178. Jackson VP, Martin-Simmerman P, Becker GJ, et al: Real-time ultrasonographic demonstration of vascular invasion by hepatocellular carcinoma. J Ultrasound Med 1983;2:277-280.

179. Subramanyam BR, Balthazar EJ, Hilton S, et al: Hepatocellular carcinoma with venous invasion: Sonographic-angiographic correlation. Radiology 1984;150:793-796.

180. LaBerge JM, Laing FC, Federle MP, et al: Hepatocellular carcinoma: Assessment of resectability by computed tomography and ultrasound. Radiology 1984;152:485-490.

181. Sheu J-C, Chen D-S, Sung J-L, et al: Hepatocellular carcinoma: Ultrasound evaluation in the early stage. Radiology 1985;155:463-467.

182. Tanaka S, Kitamura T, Imaoka S, et al: Hepatocellular carcinoma: Sonographic and histologic correlation. AJR 1983;140:701-707.

183. Choi BI, Takayasu K, Han MC: Small hepatocellular carcinomas associated with nodular lesions of the liver: Pathology, pathogenesis and imaging findings. AJR 1993;160:1177-1188.

184. Teefey SA, Stephens DH, Weiland LH: Calcification in hepatocellular carcinoma: Not always an indicator of fibrolamellar histology, AJR 1987;149:1173-1174.

185. Yoshikawa J, Matsui O, Takashima T, et al: Fatty metamorphosis in hepatocellular carcinoma: Radiologic features in 10 cases. AJR 1988;151:717-720.

186. Taylor KJW, Ramos I, Morse SS, et al: Focal liver masses: Differential diagnosis with pulsed Doppler ultrasound. Radiology 1987;164:643-647.

187. Tanaka S, Kitamura T, Fujita M, et al: Color Doppler flow imaging of liver tumors. AJR 1990;154:509-514.

188. Reinhold C, Hammers L, Taylor CR, et al: Characterization of focal hepatic lesions with duplex sonography: Findings in 198 patients. AJR 1995;164:1131-1135.

189. Baron RL, Oliver JH 3rd, Dodd GD 3rd, et al: Hepatocellular carcinoma: Evaluation with biphasic, contrast-enhanced, helical CT. Radiology 1996;199:505-511.

190. Johnson CD: Imaging of hepatocellular carcinoma. In Freeny PC (ed): Radiology of the Liver, Biliary Tract and Pancreas. San Diego, ARRS Categorical Course Syllabus 1996, 96th Annual Meeting, pp 41-46.

191. Friedman AC, Lichtenstein JE, Goodman Z, et al: Fibrolamellar hepatocellular carcinoma. Radiology 1985;157:583-587.

192. Brandt DJ, Johnson CD, Stephens DH, et al: Imaging of fibrolamellar hepatocellular carcinoma. AJR 1988;151:295-299.

193. Stevens WR, Johnson CD, Stephens DH, et al: Fibrolamellar hepatocellular carcinoma: Stage at presentation and results of aggressive surgical management. AJR 1995;164:1153-1158.

194. Kanai T, Hirohashi S, Upton MP, et al: Pathology of small hepatocellular carcinoma: A proposal for new gross classification. Cancer 1987;60:810-819.

195. Okuda K, Musha H, Nakajuma Y, et al: Clinicopathologic features of encapsulated hepatocellular carcinoma: A study of 26 cases. Cancer 1977;40:1240-1245.

196. Mahony B, Jeffrey RB, Federle MP: Spontaneous rupture of hepatic and splenic angiosarcoma demonstrated by computed tomography. AJR 1982;138:965-966.

197. Fitzgerald EJ, Griffiths TM: Computed tomography of vinyl-chloride-induced angiosarcoma of liver, Br J Radiol 1987;60:593-595.

198. Furui S, Itai Y, Ohtomo D, et al: Hepatic epithelioid hemangioendothelioma: Report of five cases. Radiology 1989;171:63-68.

199. Radin R, Craig JR, Colletti PM, et al: Hepatic epithelioid hemangioendothelioma. Radiology 1988;169:145-148.

200. Oliver JH 3rd: Malignant hepatic neoplasms, excluding hepatocellular carcinoma and cholangiocarcinoma. In Freeny PC (ed): Radiology of the Liver, Biliary Tract and Pancreas. San Diego; ARRS Categorical Course Syllabus; 1996, pp 27-32.

201. Kane RA, Longmaid HE, Costello P, et al: Noninvasive imaging in patients with hepatic masses: A prospective comparison of ultrasound. CT and MR Imaging (abstract). RSNA Scientific Program, 1993.

202. Wernecke K, Vassallo P, Bick U, et al: The distinction between benign and malignant liver tumors on

sonography: Value of a hypoechoic halo. AJR1992; 159:1005-1009.

203. Marchal GJ, Pylyser K, Tshibwabwa-Tumba EA: Anechoic halo in solid liver tumors: Sonographic, microangiographic, and histologic correlation. Radiology 1985; 156:479-483.

204. Wernecke K, Henke L, Vassallo P, et al: Pathologic explanation for hypoechoic halo seen on sonograms of malignant liver tumors: An in vitro correlative study. AJR 1992;159:1011-1016.

205. Kruskal JB, Thomas P, Nasser I, et al: Hepatic colon cancer metastases in mice: Dynamic in vivo correlation with hypoechoic rims visible at US. Radiology 2000;215:852-857.

206. Rubaltelli L, Del Mashio A, Candiani F, et al: The role of vascularization in the formation of echographic patterns of hepatic metastases: Microangiographic and echographic study. Br J Radiol 1980;53:1166-1168.

207. Sanders LM, Botet JF, Straus DJ, et al: Computed tomography of primary lymphoma of the liver. AJR 1989;152:973-976.

208. Townsend RR, Laing FC, Jeffrey RB, et al: Abdominal lymphoma in AIDS: Evaluation with ultrasound. Radiology 1989;171:719-724.

209. Yoshida T, Matsue H, Okazaki N, et al: Ultrasonographic differentiation of hepatocellular carcinoma from metastatic liver cancer. J Clin Ultrasound 1987; 15:431-437.

210. Bruneton JN, Ladree D, Caramella E, et al: Ultrasonographic study of calcified hepatic metastases: A report of 13 cases. Gastrointest Radiol 1982;7:61-63.

211. Wooten WB, Green B, Goldstein HM: Ultrasonography of necrotic hepatic metastases. Radiology 1978; 128:447-450.

212. Federle MP, Filly RA, Moss AA: Cystic hepatic neoplasms: Complementary roles of computed tomography and sonography. AJR 1981;136:345-348.

213. Nyberg DA, Federle MP: AIDS-related Kaposi sarcoma and lymphomas. Semin Roentgenol 1987;22(1):54-65.

214. Luburich P, Bru C, Ayuso MC, et al: Hepatic Kaposi sarcoma in AIDS: Ultrasound and computed tomography findings. Radiology 1990;175:172-174.

215. Towers MJ, Withers CE, Rachlis AR, et al: Ultrasound diagnosis of hepatic Kaposi sarcoma. J Ultrasound Med 1991;10:701.

Hepatic Trauma

216. Anderson CB, Ballinger WF: Abdominal injuries. In Zuidema GD, Rutherford RB, Ballinger WF (eds): The Management of Trauma, 4th ed. Philadelphia, WB Saunders, 1985, pp 449-504.

217. Moon KL, Federle MP: Computed tomography in hepatic trauma. AJR 1983;141:309-314.

218. Foley WD, Cates JD, Kellman GM, et al: Treatment of blunt hepatic injuries: Role of computed tomography. Radiology 1987;164:635-638.

219. van Sonnenberg E, Simeone JF, Mueller PR, et al: Sonographic appearance of hematoma in the liver, spleen, and kidney: A clinical, pathologic, and animal study. Radiology 1983;147:507-510.

Portosystemic Shunts

220. Lafortune M, Patriquin H, Pomier G, et al: Hemodynamic changes in portal circulation after portosystemic shunts: Use of duplex sonography in 43 patients. AJR 1987;149:701-706.

221. Chezmar JL, Bernardino ME: Mesoatrial shunt for the treatment of Budd-Chiari syndrome: Radiologic evaluation in eight patients. AJR 1987;149:707-710.

222. Grant EG, Tessler FN, Gomes AS, et al: Color Doppler imaging of portosystemic shunts. AJR 1990;154:393-397.

223. Ralls PW, Lee KP, Mayekawa DS, et al: Color Doppler sonography of portocaval shunts. J Clin Ultrasound 1990;18:379-381.

224. Foley WD, Gleysteen JJ, Lawson TL, et al: Dynamic computed tomography and pulsed Doppler sonography in the evaluation of splenorenal shunt patency. J Comput Assist Tomogr 1983;7:106-112.

225. Freedman AM, Sanyal AJ, Tisnado J, et al: Complications of transjugular intrahepatic portosystemic shunt: A comprehensive review. Radiographics 1993; 13:1185-1210.

226. Kerlan RK, Jr, LaBerge JM, Gordon RL, et al: Transjugular intrahepatic portosystemic shunts: Current status. AJR 1995;164:1059-1066.

227. LaBerge JM, Ring EJ, Gordon RL, et al: Creation of transjugular intrahepatic portosystemic shunts with the Wallstent endoprosthesis: Results in 100 patients. Radiology 1993;187:413-420.

228. Haskal ZJ, Pentecost MJ, Soulen MC, et al: Transjugular intrahepatic portosystemic shunt stenosis and revision. AJR 1994;163:439-444.

229. Foshager MC, Ferral H, Nazarian GK, et al: Duplex sonography after transjugular intrahepatic portosystemic shunts (TIPS): Normal hemodynamic findings and efficacy in predicting shunt patency and stenosis. AJR 1995;165:1-7.

230. Haskal ZJ, Carrol JW, Jacobs JE, et al: Sonography of transjugular intrahepatic portosystemic shunts: Detection of elevated portosystemic gradients and loss of shunt function. JVIR 1997;8:549-556.

231. Murphy TP, Beecham RP, Kim HM, et al: Long-term follow-up after TIPS: Use of Doppler velocity criteria for detecting elevation of the portosystemic gradient. JVIR 1998;9:275-281.

232. Surratt RS, Middleton WD, Darcy MD, et al: Morphologic and hemodynamic findings at sonography before and after creation of a transjugular intrahepatic portosystemic shunt. AJR 1993;160:627-630.

233. Chong WK, Malisch TA, Mazar MJ, et al: Transjugular intrahepatic portosystemic shunts: US assessment with maximum flow velocity. Radiology 1993; 189:789-793.

234. Dodd GD 3rd, Zajko AB, Orons PD, et al: Detection of transjugular intrahepatic portosystemic shunt dysfunction: Value of duplex Doppler sonography. AJR 1995;164:1119-1124.

235. Feldstein VA, LaBerge JM: Hepatic vein flow reversal at duplex sonography: A sign of transjugular intrahepatic portosystemic shunt dysfunction, AJR 1994;162:839-841.

236. Kanterman RY, Darcy MD, Middleton WD, et al: Doppler sonography findings associated with transjugular intrahepatic portosystemic shunt malfunction. AJR 1997;168:467-472.

Percutaneous Liver Biopsy

237. Charboneau JW, Reading CC, Welch TJ. CT and sonographically guided needle biopsy: Current techniques and new innovations. AJR 1990;154:1-10.

238. Downey DB, Wilson SR: Ultrasonographically guided

biopsy of small intra-abdominal masses. Can Assoc Radiol J 1993;44:350-353.

239. Livragi T, Festi D, Monti F, et al: US-guided percutaneous alcohol injection of small hepatic and abdominal tumors. Radiology 1986;161:309-312.

240. Shiina S, Yasuda H, Muto H, et al: Percutaneous ethanol injection in the treatment of liver neoplasms. AJR 1987;149:949-952.

Intraoperative Ultrasound

241. Rifkin MD, Rosato FE, Mitchell Branch H, et al: Intraoperative ultrasound of the liver: An important adjunctive tool for decision making in the operating room. Ann Surg 1987;205:466-471.

242. Parker GA, Lawrence J, Jr, Horsley JS, et al: Intraoperative ultrasound of the liver affects operative decision making, Ann Surg 1989;209:569-577.

5

THE SPLEEN

Patrick M. Vos / John R. Mathieson / Peter L. Cooperberg

Chapter Outline

*J*n patients with palpable splenomegaly or left upper quadrant trauma, sectional imaging techniques are indispensable to diagnose or rule out splenic abnormalities. Although in many centers computed tomography is the technique of choice for evaluation of the spleen and surrounding structures, ultrasound can be particularly useful in the first stage of the investigation and also in the follow-up of suspected or confirmed abnormalities. In general the spleen and other structures in the left upper quadrant can easily be examined without the patient's having to be moved. If necessary, examination can be carried out using a portable ultrasound machine.

Because the normal spleen is uniform in echogenicity, abnormalities stand out clearly. Similarly, perisplenic fluid collections and other abnormalities are usually identified easily. Inadequate sonographic assessment of the spleen and surrounding structures is rare. Occasionally, because the spleen is located high in the left upper quadrant, difficulties can be encountered. Shadowing from ribs, overlying bowel gas, and overlying lung in the costophrenic angle can obscure visualization of the deeper structures. Expertise and persistence may be required to overcome these obstacles.

EMBRYOLOGY AND ANATOMY

Embryologically, the spleen arises from a mass of mesenchymal cells located between the layers of the dorsal mesentery, which connects the stomach to the posterior peritoneal surface over the aorta (Fig. 5-1A). These mesenchymal cells differentiate to form the splenic pulp, the supporting connective tissue structures, and the capsule of the spleen. The splenic artery penetrates the primitive spleen, and arterioles branch through the connective tissue into the splenic sinusoids.

As the embryonic stomach rotates 90° on its longitudinal axis, the spleen and dorsal mesentery are carried to the left along with the greater curvature of the stomach (see Fig. 5-1B). The base of the dorsal mesentery fuses with the posterior peritoneum over the left kidney, giving rise to the splenorenal ligament. This explains why, although the spleen is intraperitoneal, the splenic artery enters from the retroperitoneum via the splenorenal ligament (see Fig. 5-1C). In most adults, a portion of the splenic capsule is firmly adherent to the fused dorsal mesentery anterior to the upper left kidney, giving rise to the so-called bare area of the spleen. The size of

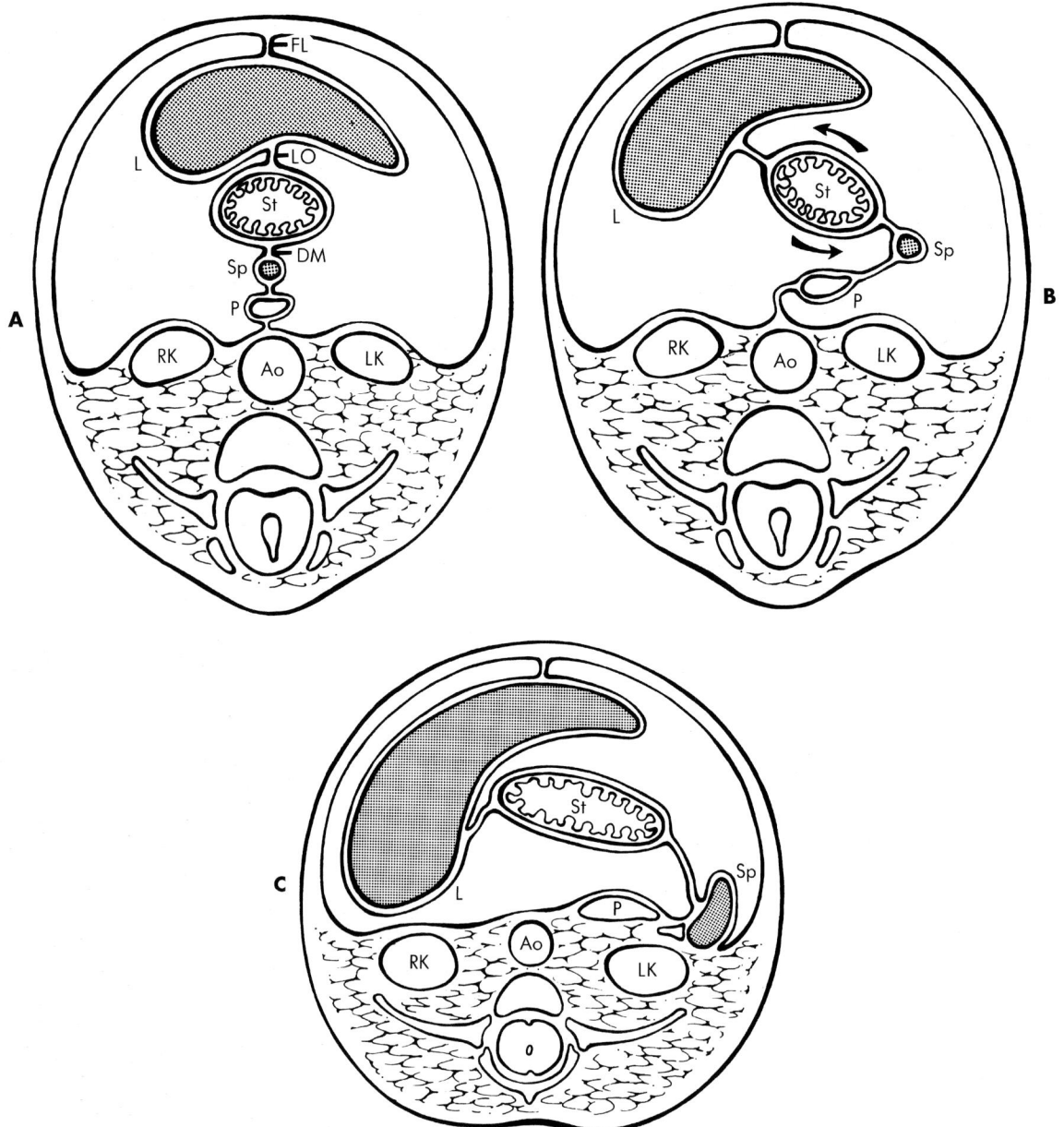

FIGURE 5-1. Schematic axial drawings of the upper abdomen showing the embryologic development of splenic anatomy. **A,** Embryo of 4 to 5 weeks. The mesentery anterior to the stomach (ST) is the ventral mesentery. Posterior to the stomach is the dorsal mesentery (DM). Note the spleen and pancreas developing within the dorsal mesentery. The dorsal mesentery is divided into two portions by the spleen: the splenogastric ligament anteriorly and the splenorenal ligament posteriorly. The pancreas (P) has not yet become retroperitoneal and remains within the dorsal mesentery. The ventral mesentery is divided into the falciform ligament (FL) anteriorly and the gastrohepatic ligament, or lesser omentum (LO), posteriorly by the liver (L). **B,** 8-week embryo. The stomach rotates counterclockwise, displacing the liver to the right and the spleen to the left. The portion of the dorsal mesentery containing the pancreas, the splenic vessels, and the spleen begins to fuse to the anterior retroperitoneal surface, giving rise to the splenogastric ligament and the "bare area" of the spleen. If fusion is incomplete, the spleen will be attached to the retroperitoneum only by a long mesentery, giving rise to a mobile or "wandering" spleen. **C,** Newborn baby. Fusion of the dorsal mesentery is now complete. The pancreas is now completely retroperitoneal, and a portion of the spleen has fused with the retroperitoneum. Note the close relation of the tail of the pancreas to the splenic hilum. Ao, aorta; FL, falciform ligament; L, liver; LK, left kidney; LO, lesser omentum or gastrohepatic ligament; P, pancreas; RK, right kidney; SP, spleen; ST, stomach.

the splenic bare area is variable, but it usually involves less than half of the posterior splenic surface (Fig. 5-2). This anatomic feature is analogous to the bare area of the liver and, similarly, can be helpful in distinguishing intraperitoneal from pleural fluid collections.[1]

The normal adult spleen is convex superolaterally, concave inferomedially, and has a very homogeneous echo pattern. The spleen lies between the fundus of the stomach and the diaphragm, with its long axis in the line of the left tenth rib. The diaphragmatic surface is convex

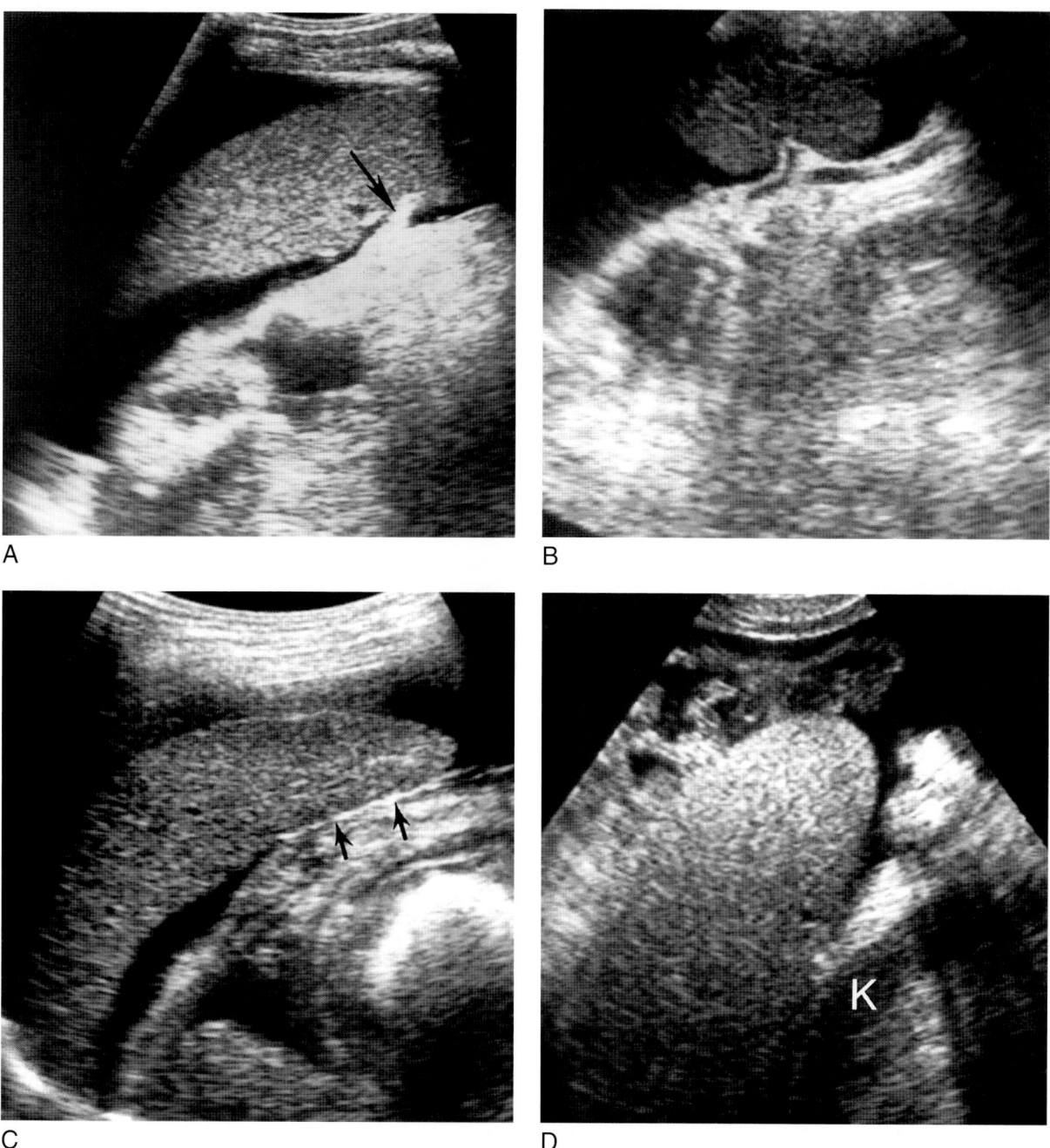

FIGURE 5-2. Variability in the relation of the spleen to the anterior retroperitoneal surface. All of these patients have gross ascites, which clearly demonstrates the extent of the splenic "bare area." **A,** This patient has no bare area. The splenorenal ligament (arrow) is outlined on both sides by ascitic fluid. **B,** Part of the lower pole of the spleen is fused posteriorly. **C,** The lower pole of the spleen is fused to the retroperitoneum (arrows). **D,** A large proportion of this patient's spleen is fused posteriorly. Note the close relation of the spleen to the left kidney (K).

and is usually situated between the ninth and eleventh ribs. The visceral or inferomedial surface has gentle indentations where it comes into contact with the stomach, left kidney, pancreas, and splenic flexure. The spleen is suspended by the splenorenal ligament, which is in contact with the posterior peritoneal wall, the phrenicocolic ligament and the gastrosplenic ligament.

The gastrosplenic ligament is composed of the two layers of the dorsal mesentery that separate the lesser sac posteriorly from the greater sac anteriorly.

The average adult spleen measures 12 cm in length, 7 cm in breadth, and 3 to 4 cm in thickness and has an average weight of 150 g, varying between 80 and 300 g. A normal spleen decreases in size and weight with advancing age. It also increases slightly during digestion and can vary in size in accordance with the nutritional status of the body.

Splenic functions include phagocytosis, fetal hematopoiesis, adult lymphopoiesis, immune response, and erythrocyte storage. Under a variety of conditions, including surgical misadventure, the spleen may be removed. It is common for a person to live successfully without a spleen. However, particularly in childhood, the immune response may be impaired, particularly to encapsulated bacteria. Recently, the surgical trend is toward splenic preservation whenever possible.

EXAMINATION TECHNIQUE

All routine abdominal sonographic examinations, regardless of the indications, should include at least one coronal view of the spleen and the upper pole of the left kidney. This view is easy to obtain with real-time scanning, particularly by using the sector format. The most common approach to visualizing the spleen is to maintain the patient in the supine position and place the transducer in the coronal plane of section posteriorly in one of the lower left intercostal spaces. The patient can then be examined in various degrees of inspiration to maximize the window to the spleen. Excessive inspiration introduces air into the lung in the lateral costophrenic angle and may obscure visualization. A modest inspiration depresses the central portion of the left hemidiaphragm and spleen inferiorly so that they can be visualized (Fig. 5-3). The plane of section should then be swept posteriorly and anteriorly to view the entire volume of the spleen. We generally find that a thorough examination in the coronal plane of section is highly accurate for ruling out any lesion within or around the spleen and for documenting approximate splenic size. If an abnormality is discovered within or around the spleen, other planes of section can be used. An oblique plane of section along the intercostal space can avoid rib shadowing (Fig. 5-4). Because the long axis of the spleen lies obliquely, this oblique plane of section is also convenient with the upper pole located posterior to the lower pole. A transverse plane from a lateral, usually intercostal, approach may help to localize a lesion within the spleen anteriorly and posteriorly. In this regard, especially for beginners, it must be emphasized that the apex of the sector image is always placed at the top of the screen. However, on a left lateral intercostal transverse image, the top of the screen—the apex of the sector—is actually to the patient's left; the right side of the sector image is posterior, and the left side of the image is anterior. To look at the image appropriately, one would have to rotate it 90° in a clockwise direction or turn one's head in a 90° counterclockwise direction.

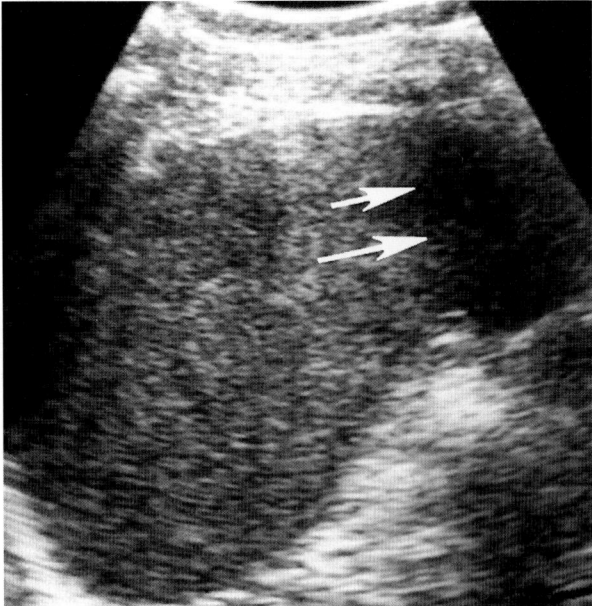

FIGURE 5-3. Coronal scan of a normal spleen. The lower pole is partially obscured by a rib shadow (*arrows*). Note the homogeneous echo texture.

If the spleen is not enlarged and is not surrounded by a large mass, scanning from an anterior position—as one would for imaging the liver—is not helpful because of the interposition of gas within the stomach and the splenic flexure of the colon.[2] However, if the patient has a relatively large liver, one may be able to see the spleen through the left lobe of the liver and the collapsed stomach, analogous to the image seen on the transverse CT scan of the upper abdomen. Also, if the spleen is enlarged or if there is a mass in the left upper quadrant, the spleen may be visualized from an anterior approach (Fig. 5-5). If there is free intraperitoneal fluid around the spleen or if there is a left pleural effusion, the spleen may be better visualized from an anterolateral approach. Often, it is beneficial to have the patient roll onto his or her right side as much as 45°, or even 90°, so that a more posterior approach can be used to visualize the spleen. We no longer use the prone position.

Generally, the same technical settings for gain, time-gain compensation, and power are used for examination of the spleen as for examination of the other organs in the upper abdomen. We normally use 2-5 MHz curvilinear transducers; if necessary, linear array transducers can be used for more detail. There is a slight disadvantage in intercostal scanning with the larger transducer face, but the image quality is significantly improved with these transducers. It is important to appreciate that the ribs can often be broader and flatter than expected and may encroach on the intercostal spaces, making them particularly narrow. This can severely impair the quality of the image seen from an intercostal space.

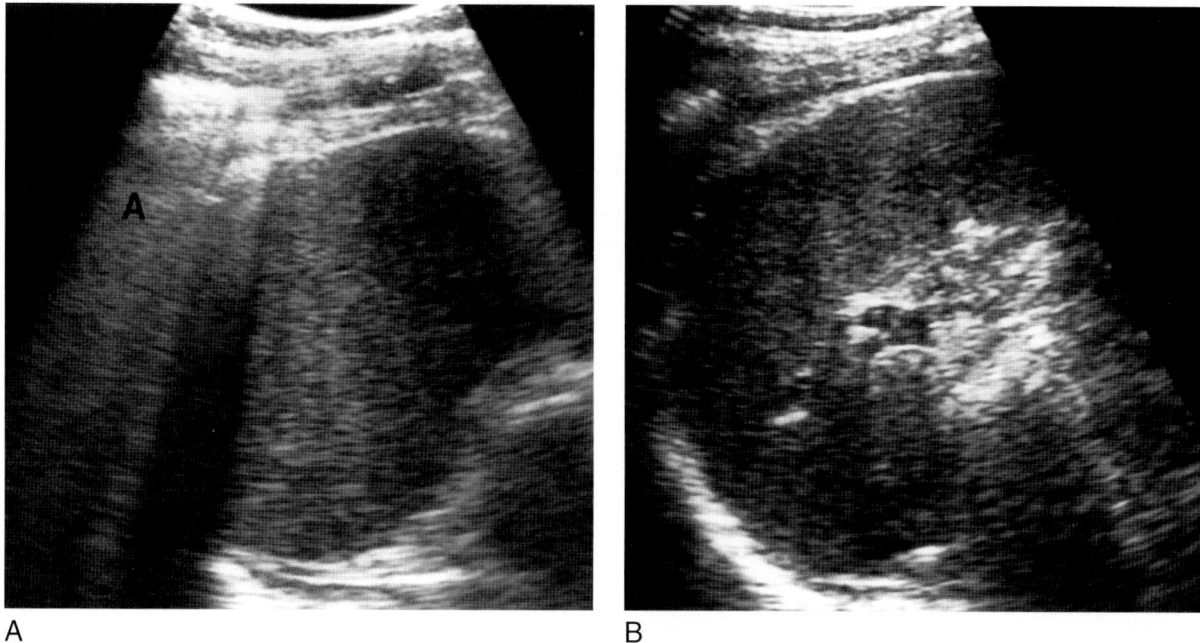

A   B

FIGURE 5-4. Importance of scan plane. A, Coronal scan showing partial obscuration of the spleen by air in the lung (A) and by a rib shadow. **B,** Oblique coronal scan, aligned with the 10th interspace, shows improved visualization of the spleen.

SONOGRAPHY OF THE SPLEEN

The shape of the normal spleen is variable. The spleen consists of two components joined at the hilum: a supero-medial component and an inferolateral component. More superiorly, on transverse scanning, the spleen has a typical fat "inverted comma" shape with a thin component extending anteriorly and another component extending medially, either superior to or adjacent to the upper pole of the kidney. This is the component that can be seen to indent the gastric fundus on plain films of the abdomen or in barium studies. As one moves the scan plane inferiorly, only the inferior component of the spleen is seen. This component can be outlined by a thin rim of fat above the splenic flexure as can be seen on a plain film of the abdomen. It may extend inferiorly to the costal margin and present clinically as a palpable spleen. However, either component can enlarge independently without the enlargement of the other component.

It is important to recognize the normal structures that are anatomically related to the spleen. The diaphragm cradles the spleen posteriorly, superiorly, and laterally. If the left liver lobe is large, it may extend into the left upper quadrant superior to the spleen (Fig. 5-6). The fundus of the stomach and lesser sac are medial and anterior to the splenic hilum. It is important to appreciate that the fundus may contain gas or fluid. The tail of the pancreas lies posterior to the stomach and lesser sac. It approaches the hilum of the spleen, closely related to the splenic artery and vein. Consequently, the spleen

can be used as a window to evaluate the pancreatic tail area. The left kidney generally lies inferior and medial to the spleen. A useful landmark in identifying the spleen and splenic hilum is the splenic vein, which generally can be demonstrated without difficulty.

The splenic parenchyma is extremely homogeneous, and therefore the spleen has a uniform mid- to low-level echogenicity. It is generally considered that the liver is more echogenic than the spleen but, in fact, the echogenicity of the parenchyma is higher in the spleen than in the liver. Using a dual image setting, one may compare the echogenicity of these two organs. The impression that the liver has greater echogenicity occurs because of its large number of reflective vessels. When the spleen enlarges, it can become more echogenic. Unfortunately, one cannot differentiate between the different types of enlargement on the basis of the degree of echogenicity.

PATHOLOGIC CONDITIONS OF THE SPLEEN

Splenomegaly

Frequently, sonography is performed to determine the presence or absence of splenomegaly. If there is gross enlargement of the spleen, confirmation of splenomegaly is easy. However, if there is only mild enlargement, it can be difficult to make the decision based on a sonographic study. Techniques have been developed to measure serial sections of the spleen by planimetry and then compute the volume of the spleen by adding the values for each

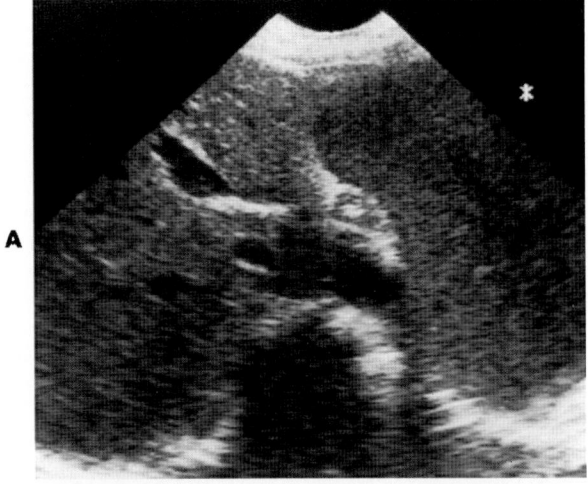

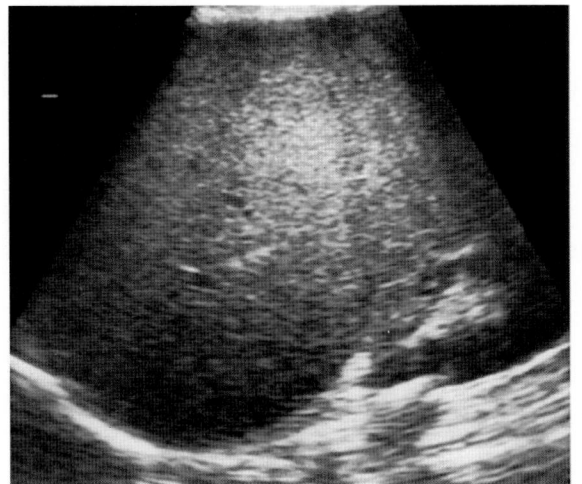

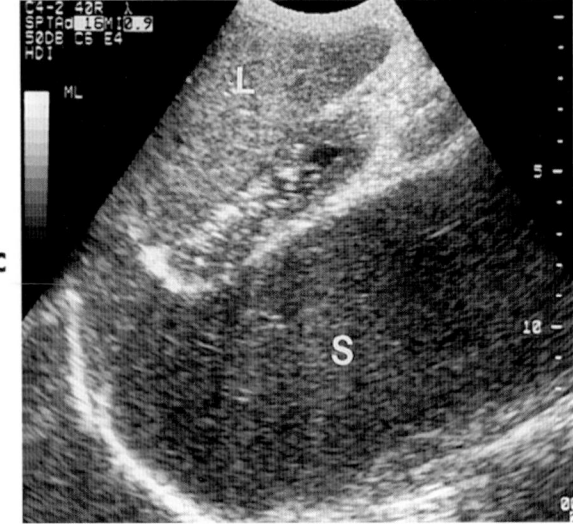

FIGURE 5-5. Splenomegaly. A, Transverse scan in the upper abdomen showing the liver apparently continuous with the large spleen across the inferior aspect of the abdomen. **B,** Coronal scan showing only the midportion of the spleen, with the superior and inferior aspects beyond the sector format. **C,** Sagittal scan through the left lobe of the liver (L), with the markedly enlarged spleen (S) posterior to the stomach and liver.

section.[3] However, these techniques are cumbersome and not popular. The most commonly used method is the "eyeball" technique: if it looks big, it is (see Figs. 5-5 and 5-7).

Unfortunately, this method of assessment requires considerably more experience than is necessary for other imaging techniques. Furthermore, it is relatively inaccurate. As in measuring all other structures in the body, it is helpful to have measurements that establish the upper limits of normal. The wide range of what is considered to be a normal-sized adult spleen, combined with its complex three-dimensional shape, makes it particularly difficult to establish a normal range of sonographic measurements. Nonetheless, a study of almost 800 normal adults found that in 95% of patients, the length of the spleen was less than 12 cm, the breadth less than 7 cm, and the thickness less than 5 cm.[4] These measurements may be useful for borderline cases. According to a recent study from Lamb et al., who correlated spleen measured by ultrasound with the splenic volume measured by helical CT, measurement of splenic length correlates well with splenic volume,

particularly when performed with the patient in the right lateral decubitus (RLD) position.[5] The spleen is capable of growing to an enormous size. It may extend inferiorly into the left iliac fossa. It can cross the midline and appear as a mass inferior to the left lobe of the liver on longitudinal section.

The differential diagnosis of splenomegaly is exceedingly long. It includes infection, neoplasia, infiltration, trauma, blood dyscrasias, storage disorders, and portal hypertension. Sonography is not usually helpful in the specific diagnosis of splenomegaly. However, the degree of splenomegaly can help to narrow the differential diagnosis. Mild-to-moderate splenomegaly is usually caused by **infection**, **portal hypertension**, or **AIDS**. More marked splenomegaly is usually the result of hematologic disorders, including **leukemia** and **lymphoma,** as well as **infectious mononucleosis.** Massive splenomegaly can be seen in **myelofibrosis**. In addition, focal lesions within the spleen may suggest **lymphomatous involvement, metastatic disease, cysts,** or **hematomas.** Nonsplenic abnormalities such as lymph node enlargement or liver involvement may suggest lymphoma,

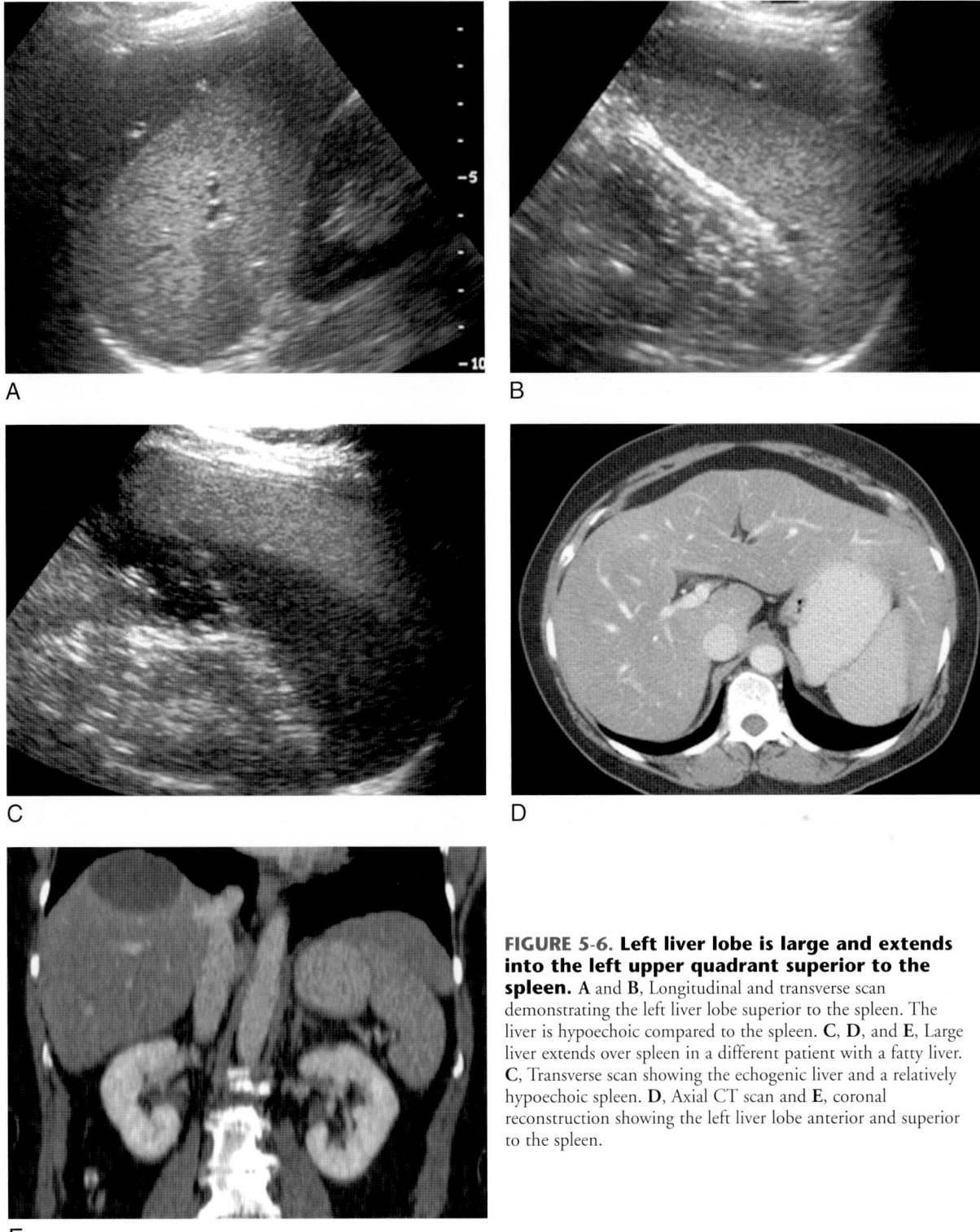

FIGURE 5-6. Left liver lobe is large and extends into the left upper quadrant superior to the spleen. A and B, Longitudinal and transverse scan demonstrating the left liver lobe superior to the spleen. The liver is hypoechoic compared to the spleen. C, D, and E, Large liver extends over spleen in a different patient with a fatty liver. C, Transverse scan showing the echogenic liver and a relatively hypoechoic spleen. D, Axial CT scan and E, coronal reconstruction showing the left liver lobe anterior and superior to the spleen.

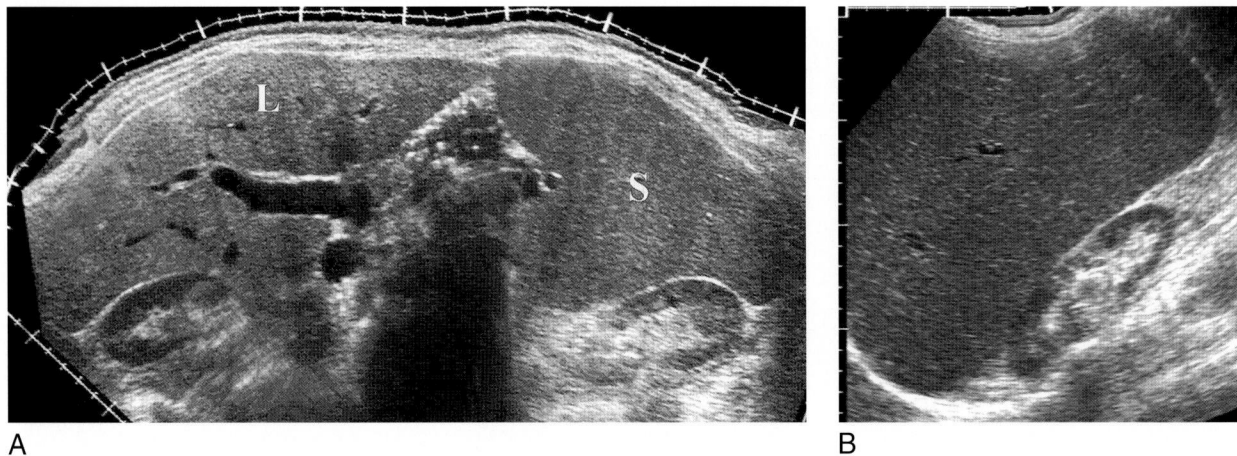

FIGURE 5-7. Splenomegaly. A, Transverse and **B,** longitudinal Siescape images show marked splenic (S) enlargement. L, liver.

whereas recanalization of the umbilical vein or other evidence of portal systemic collaterals, such as lienorenal shunts, splenic vein varices, or ascites, can establish **portal hypertension** as the cause of splenomegaly (Fig. 5-8). In most cases, however, splenomegaly may be the sole finding or only one of several nonspecific sonographic findings.

Several investigators have attempted to quantify the degree of diffuse splenic fibrosis or tumor infiltration by analyzing various parameters of the reflected ultrasound signal. Speed and attenuation measurements have been studied, but to date, such parameters are not regarded as clinically useful.[6-8]

Focal Abnormalities

Cysts

Splenic cysts, like cysts located elsewhere in the body, characteristically appear as echo-free areas with smooth, sharp borders and enhancement of the echoes deep into the lesions. When small, they may be located within the splenic parenchyma. Occasionally, these cysts can grow very large and become mainly exophytic. It may then be difficult to appreciate their intrasplenic origin (Fig. 5-9).

Infectious cysts may be caused by **echinococcus**. The spleen is one of the least common sites for the development of hydatid cysts, however. Calcification may be identified in the wall of the cyst (Fig. 5-10).

The diagnosis is made with a combination of appropriate history, geographic background, serologic testing, and ultrasound appearance.[9,10] Percutaneous fine-needle aspiration can be diagnostic, provided the pathologist has been alerted to search for the scoleces.

Posttraumatic cysts have no cellular lining and are also called **pseudocysts**.[11] The walls of these cysts, like echinococcal cysts, may become calcified. These cysts may contain low-level echoes that can be cholesterol crystals or debris.[12] Hemorrhage into any cyst can also give rise to echogenic fluid (Fig. 5-11).[13] **Primary congenital cysts**, also called **epidermoid cysts**, can be differentiated from posttraumatic cysts by the presence of an epithelial or endothelial lining. Congenital cysts are thought to arise from embryonal rests of primitive mesothelial cells within the spleen. Intracystic fluid may have increased echogenicity owing to cholesterol crystals, inflammatory debris, or hemorrhage. Reliable differentiation between true cysts and pseudocysts is usually not possible with ultrasound (Fig. 5-12). Endothelial-lined cysts are rare; they include lymphangiomas and, very rarely, cystic hemangiomas.[14]

Pancreatic pseudocysts extending into the spleen can be diagnosed by the associated features of pancreatitis. **Splenic abscesses** may have an appearance similar to that of simple cysts, but the diagnosis can easily be made in conjunction with the clinical findings. There may be gas within an abscess cavity in the spleen, which should point to an infectious cause. Gas can cause a confusing picture if only a small area of increased echogenicity is seen in the spleen (Fig. 5-13).

However, there may be acoustic shadowing and/or

CAUSES OF MILD-TO-MODERATE SPLENOMEGALY

Portal hypertension
Infection
AIDS

CAUSES OF MARKED SPLENOMEGALY

Leukemia
Lymphoma
Myelofibrosis

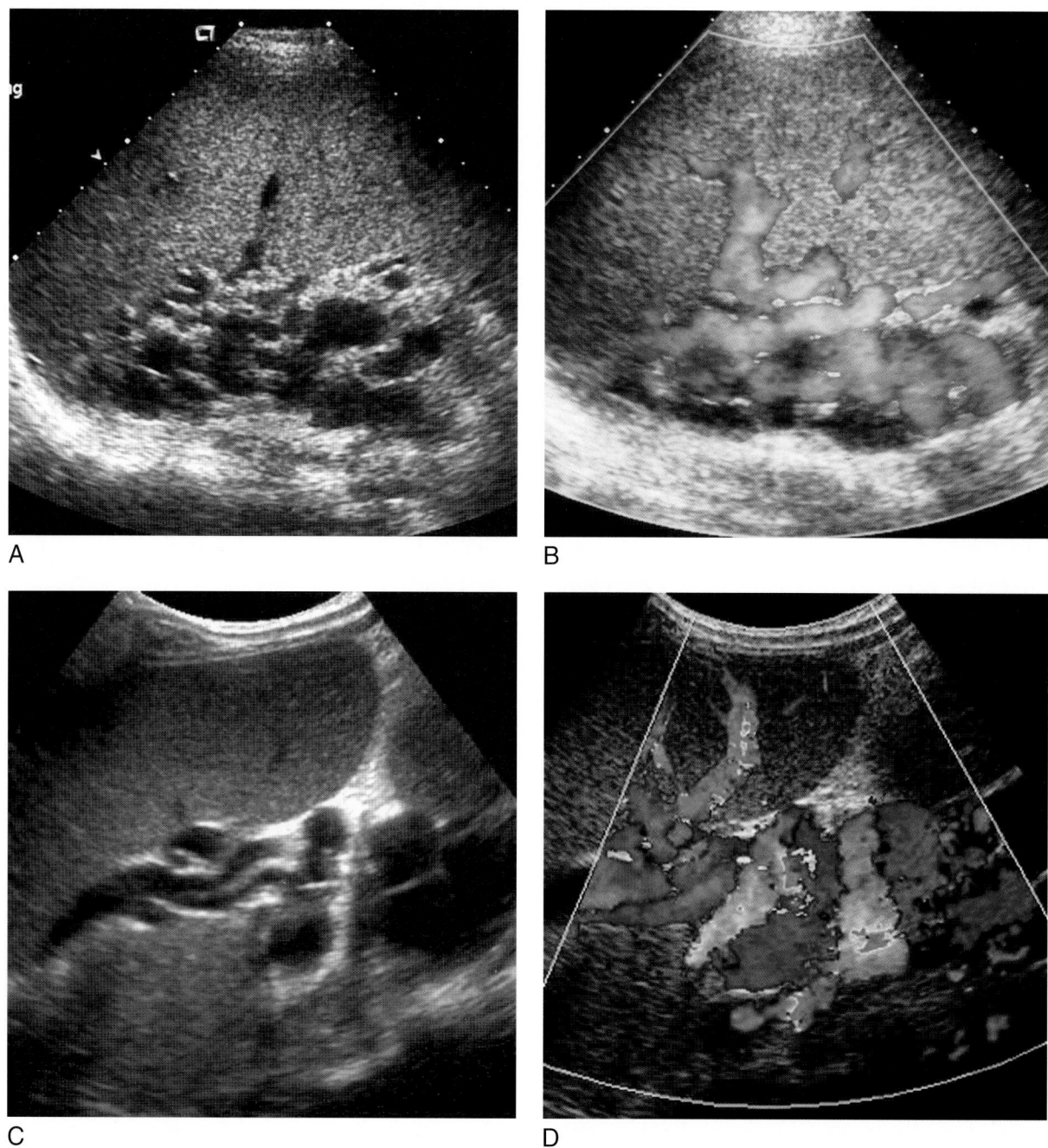

FIGURE 5-8. Varices. A and **B**, Longitudinal and power Doppler images show splenomegaly and tortuous varices medial to the spleen. **C** and **D**, Longitudinal and color Doppler images show varices medial and inferior to the spleen representing a splenorenal shunt.

CATEGORIES OF CYSTIC LESIONS OF THE SPLEEN

Infectious cysts
Posttraumatic cysts
Primary congenital cysts
Intrasplenic pancreatic pseudocysts

a ring-down artifact. The sonographic findings can be variable and in questionable cases, aspiration can be useful for diagnosis.[15,16] Catheter drainage, guided by sonography, can be safely and successfully performed.[17]

Solid Masses

Solid focal lesions in the spleen are uncommon, but they can be caused by a large number of diseases. The most common focal lesions result from previous granuloma-

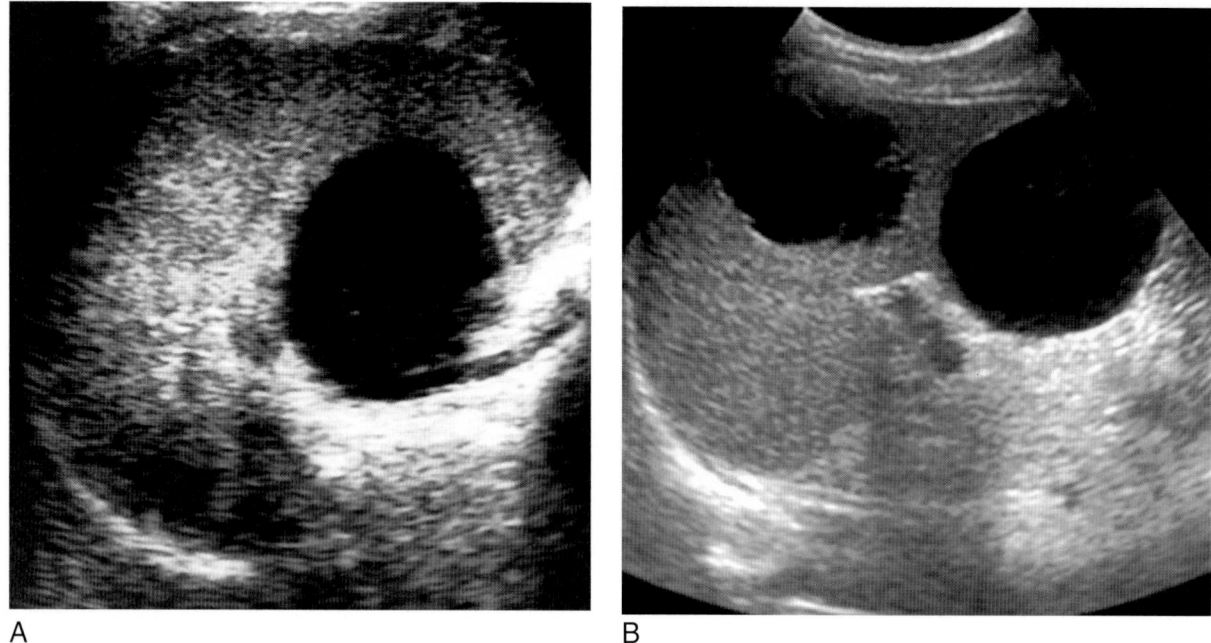

FIGURE 5-9. Splenic cyst. A, Coronal scan of the spleen showing a cyst 5 cm in diameter in the hilar region of the spleen adjacent to the splenic vein from trauma to the left upper quadrant several years earlier. **B,** Longitudinal scan of the spleen in an asymptomatic female showing two cysts. One central 5 cm cyst with somewhat irregular borders and a 6 cm cyst at the inferior portion of the spleen.

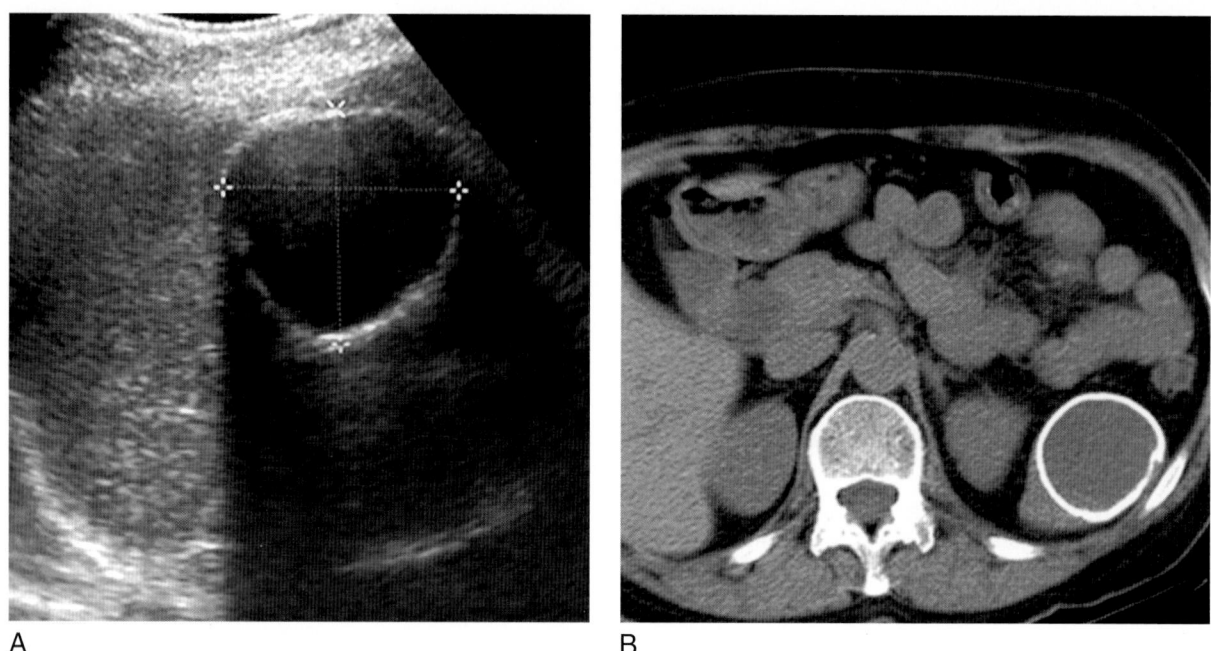

FIGURE 5-10. Calcified splenic cysts. A, Longitudinal scan. Note the shadowing from the near side of the splenic cyst. **B,** Noncontrast CT demonstrating the wall calcification. Both "burned out" hydatid cysts and posttraumatic cysts can look like this.

Continued

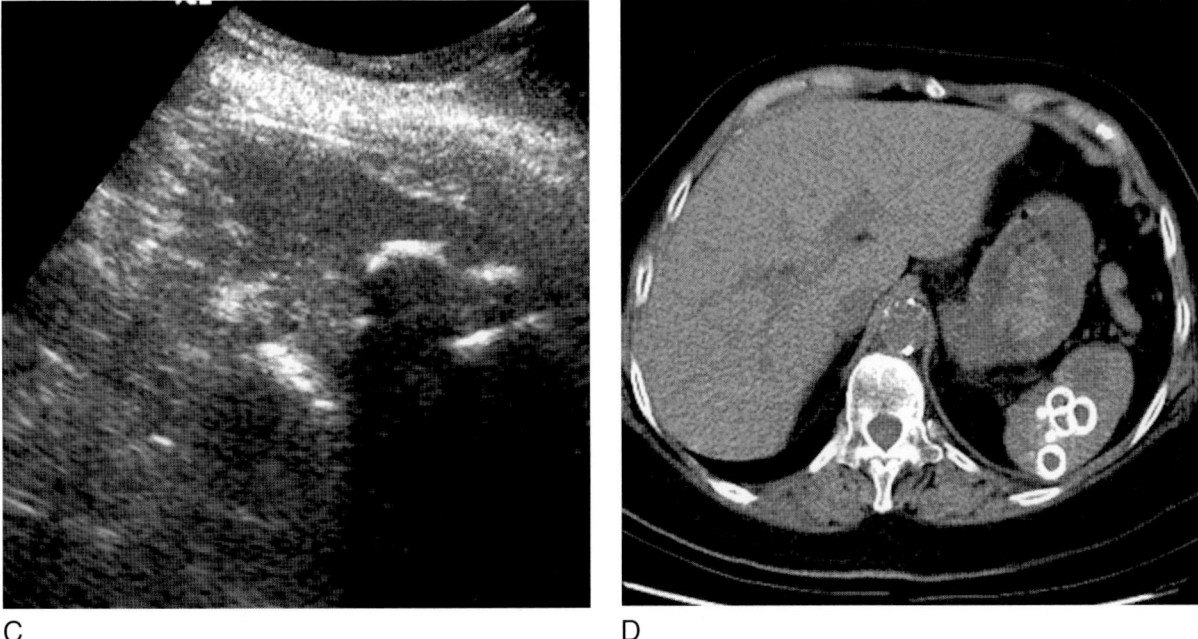

C   D

FIGURE 5-10, *cont'd.* **Calcified splenic cysts. C,** Coronal scan and **D,** noncontrast CT of the spleen in a patient with a history of hydatid disease. Dense calcification in the near wall causes extensive shadowing. **D,** Small, well-defined, rounded wall calcifications compatible with calcified cysts.

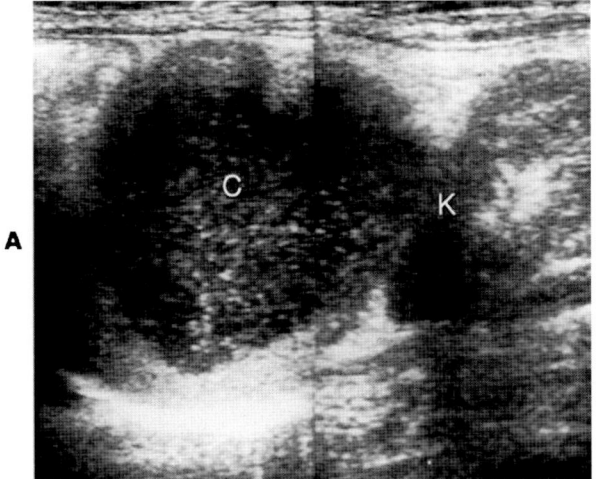

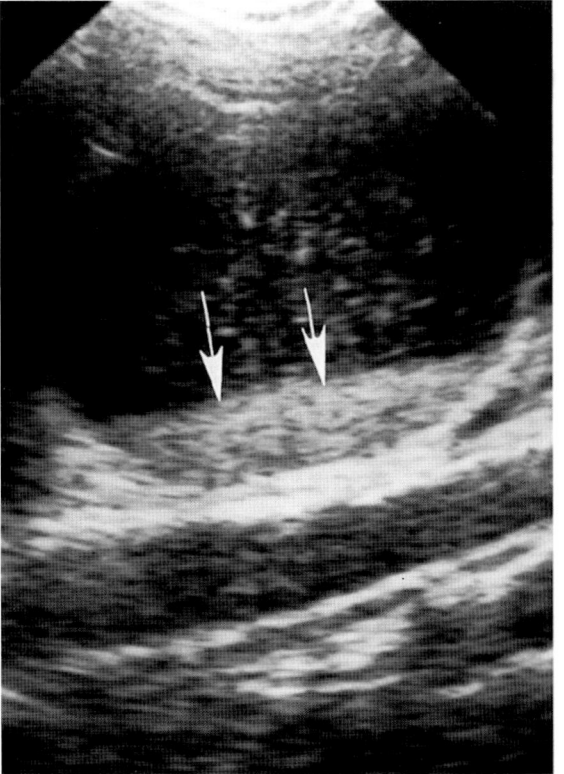

FIGURE 5-11. Splenic cyst. A, Composite linear array images. Note the 8 cm splenic cyst (C). Only a small rim of spleen noted superiorly and medially that displaces the left kidney (K) inferiorly toward the right of the image. The echoes from the cholesterol crystals and debris within the cyst mimic a solid lesion. **B,** Sector image shows a more echogenic, dependent layer (*arrows*).

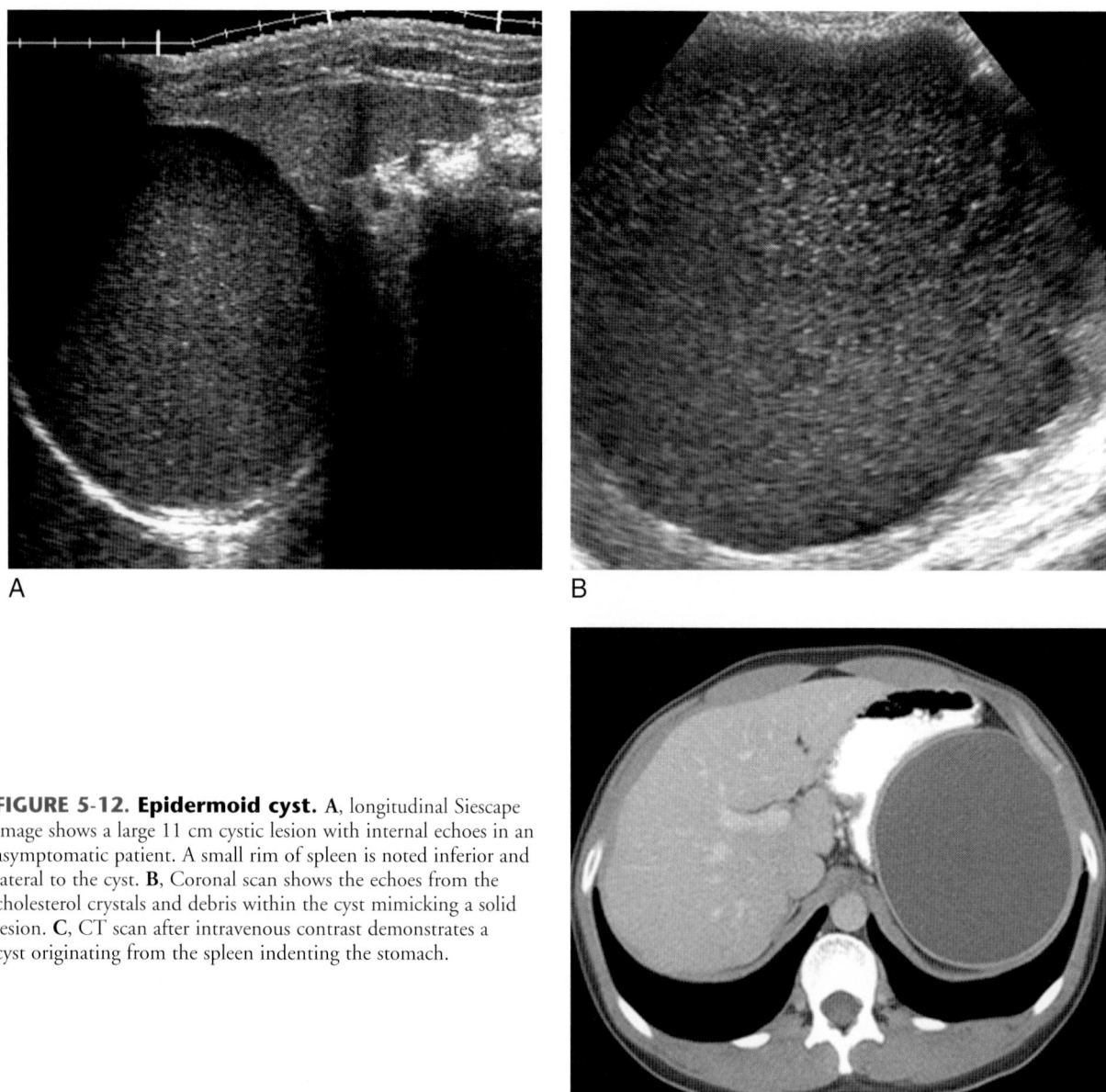

FIGURE 5-12. Epidermoid cyst. A, longitudinal Siescape image shows a large 11 cm cystic lesion with internal echoes in an asymptomatic patient. A small rim of spleen is noted inferior and lateral to the cyst. **B,** Coronal scan shows the echoes from the cholesterol crystals and debris within the cyst mimicking a solid lesion. **C,** CT scan after intravenous contrast demonstrates a cyst originating from the spleen indenting the stomach.

tous infections, typically seen as focal, bright, echogenic lesions with or without shadowing. **Histoplasmosis** and **tuberculosis** are the most common causes, although granulomas may occur in the spleen in patients with **sarcoidosis** (Fig. 5-14).[18,19] Calcification in the splenic artery is common and should not be confused with calcification in a lesion (Fig. 5-15). Primary malignancies of the spleen are extremely rare, but primary lymphoma and angiosarcoma have been reported (Fig. 5-16).[20,21]

Metastatic involvement of the spleen generally occurs as a late phenomenon rather than as a presenting feature. Splenic **metastases** occur most commonly in **malignant melanoma**, **lymphoma**, and **leukemia**, but they can also occur in **carcinoma of the ovary**, **breast**, **lung**, and

stomach (Fig. 5-17).[22] Metastases are usually hypoechoic but may be echogenic or of mixed echogenicity.[23]

Hemangiomas of the spleen have been reported in up to 14% of patients undergoing autopsy,[24,25] but the typical appearance of hemangioma is seen far less frequently in the spleen than in the liver. Hemangiomas are usually isolated phenomena but they may occur in association with other stigmata of the Klippel-Trenaunay-Weber syndrome.[26] The sonographic appearance of hemangiomas is variable. The lesions may have a well-defined echogenic appearance that is similar to the typical appearance of hemangiomas in the liver (Figs. 5-18 and 5-19).

However, lesions of mixed echogenicity with cystic spaces of variable sizes have been reported. Occasionally, foci of calcification have been found.[26-28] Lymph-

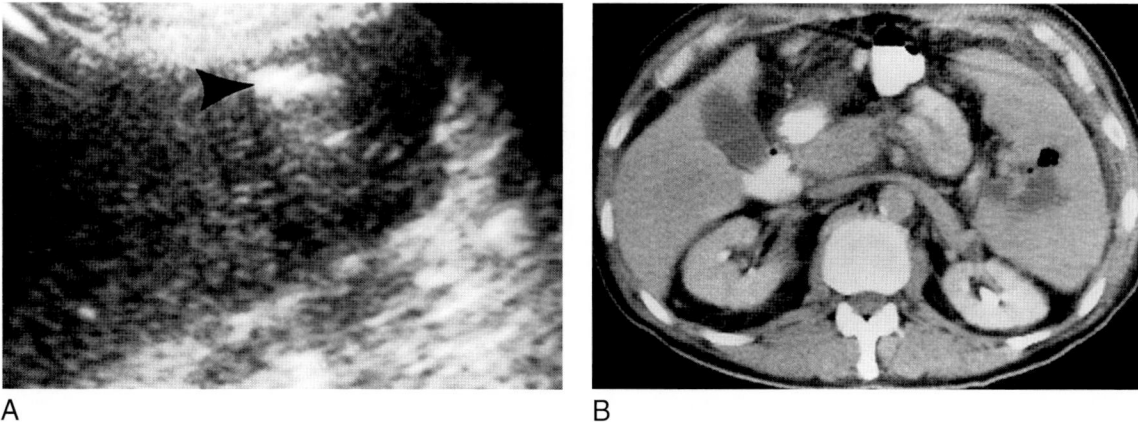

FIGURE 5-13. Splenic abscess. A, Coronal scan shows a gas collection with "dirty shadowing" (*arrowhead*). **B**, CT scan confirms the presence of gas and fluid within the spleen.

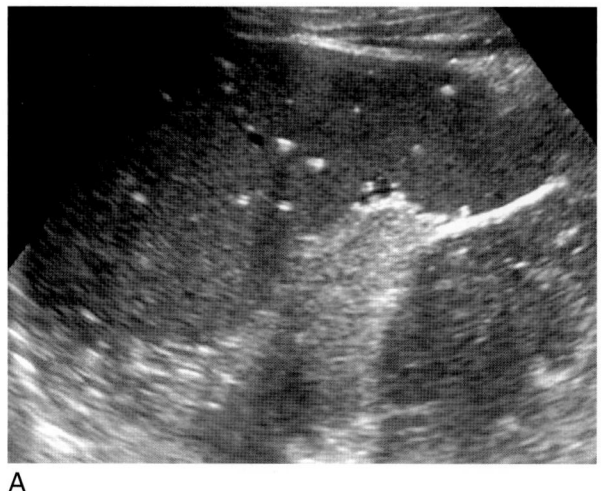

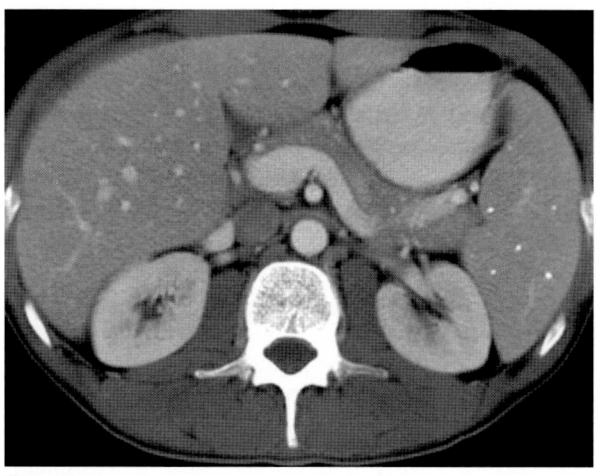

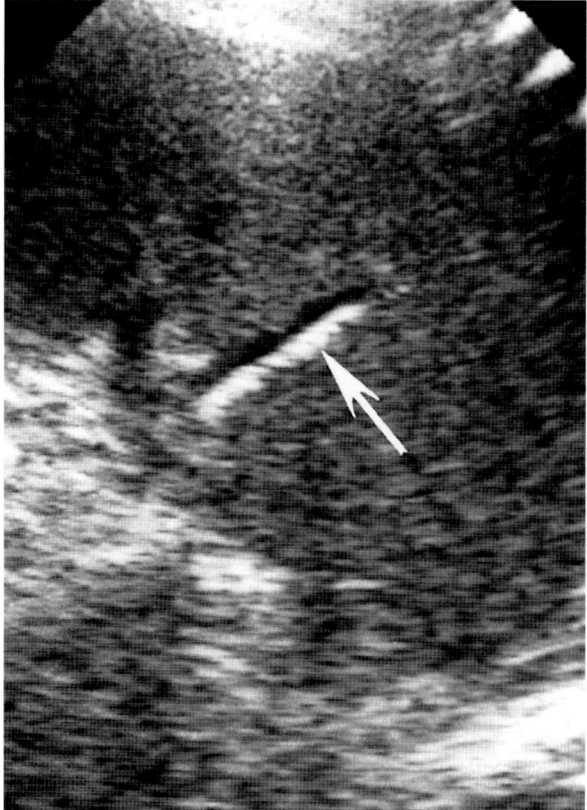

FIGURE 5-15. Calcified splenic artery. Transverse scan of the spleen showing calcification of the splenic artery coursing parallel to the splenic vein.

FIGURE 5-14. Granulomatous disease of the spleen: sarcoidosis. A, Longitudinal scan showing tiny bright echoes measuring 2 to 3 mm throughout the spleen, some demonstrating shadowing. **B**, CT scan after IV contrast showing multiple well-defined, small parenchymal calcifications throughout the spleen.

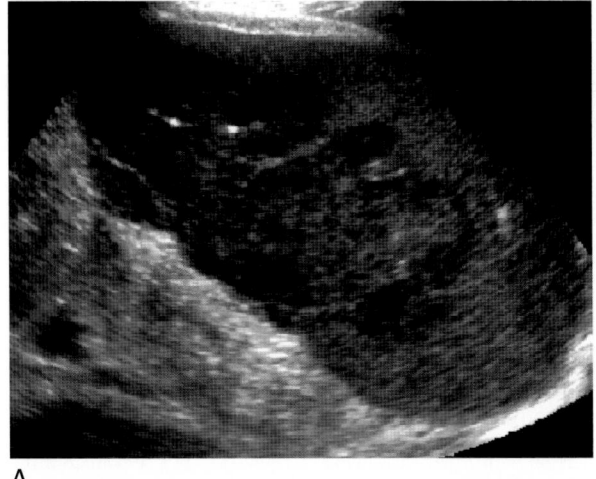

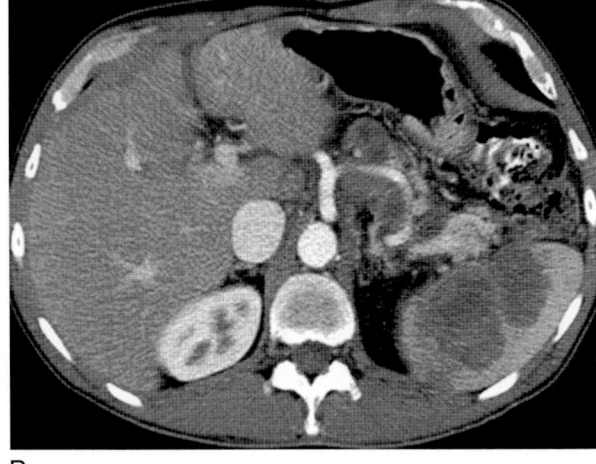

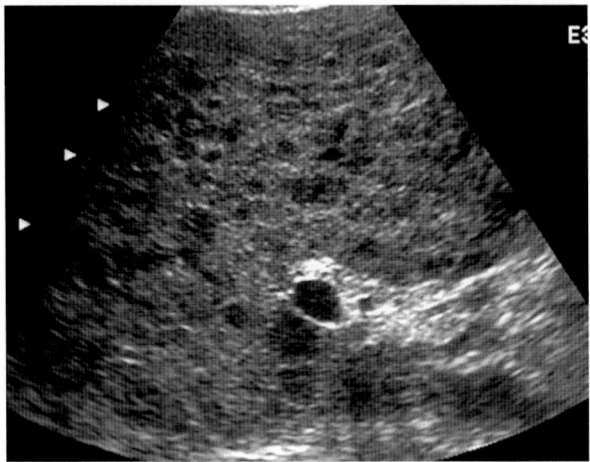

FIGURE 5-16. Primary malignancies. A, Lymphoma. Transverse scan of the spleen showing multiple ill-defined hypoechoic lesions throughout the spleen. **B,** CT scan after IV contrast demonstrating the hypodense areas and extensive lymphadenopathy. **C,** Angiosarcoma of the liver and the spleen. Transverse scan of the spleen demonstrating multiple ill-defined hypoechoic lesions throughout the spleen.

angiomas may also occur in the spleen and may have an appearance similar to that of hemangiomas.[29] It remains to be shown whether MRI will be as helpful for confirming the diagnosis of hemangioma in the spleen as it is in the liver.[30]

Splenic infarction is one of the more common causes of focal splenic lesions. If a typical peripheral, wedge-shaped, hypoechoic lesion is noted, splenic infarction should be the first diagnostic consideration (Figs. 5-20 and 5-21).

However, splenic infarctions do not always have this typical appearance but may have a nodular appearance or, as fibrosis progresses, a hyperechoic appearance. The temporal evolution of the ultrasonic appearance of splenic infarctions has been studied and has shown that the echogenicity of the lesion is related to the age of the infarction. Infarctions are hypoechoic, or echo-free, in early stages, and they progress to hyperechoic lesions over time.[32,33]

Several relatively rare diseases have a high frequency of associated splenic abnormalities. For example, in **Gaucher's disease**, splenomegaly occurs almost univer-

sally, and approximately one third of patients have multiple splenic nodules. These nodules are frequently well-defined hypoechoic lesions, but they may also be irregular, hyperechoic, or of mixed echogenicity.[34-36] Pathologically, these nodules represent focal areas of Gaucher cells associated with fibrosis and infarction. Rarely, the entire spleen may be involved, with ultrasound showing diffuse inhomogeneity.[34] In patients with **schistosomiasis**, splenomegaly is found universally, and focal hyperechoic nodules are seen in 5% to 10% of patients.[37]

Multiple nodules may also be found in patients with splenic infections, particularly in immunocompromised patients. The so-called wheels-within-wheels appearance has been described in patients with hepatosplenic **candidiasis**. The outer "wheel" is thought to represent a ring of fibrosis surrounding the inner echogenic "wheel" of inflammatory cells and a central hypoechoic, necrotic area. This appearance is not universally seen in splenic candidiasis; nodules in some patients may have a bull's-eye appearance or may be hypoechoic or hyperechoic (Fig. 5-22).[38]

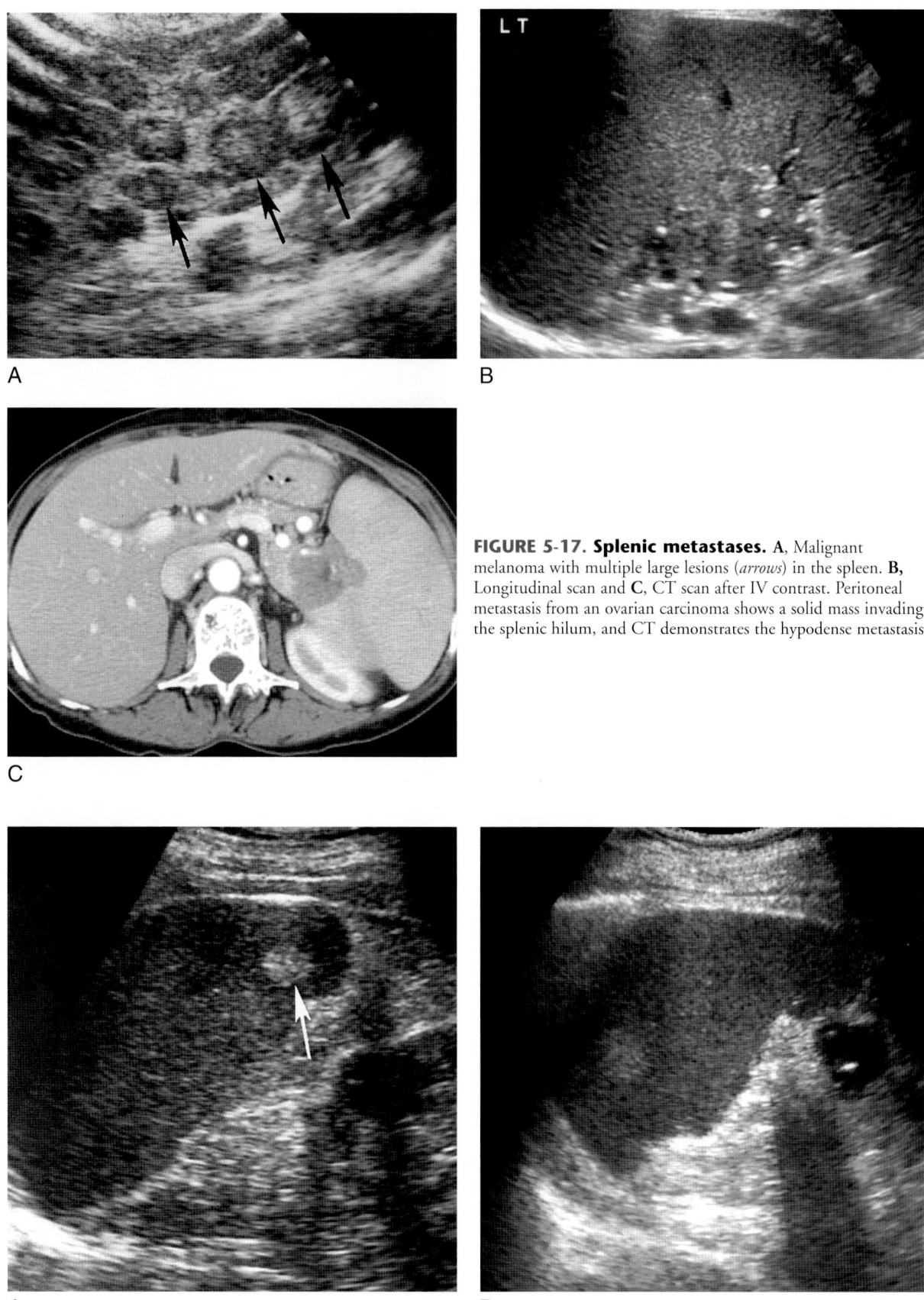

FIGURE 5-17. Splenic metastases. A, Malignant melanoma with multiple large lesions (*arrows*) in the spleen. **B,** Longitudinal scan and **C,** CT scan after IV contrast. Peritoneal metastasis from an ovarian carcinoma shows a solid mass invading the splenic hilum, and CT demonstrates the hypodense metastasis.

FIGURE 5-18. Splenic hemangioma. A, Note the small (1.4 cm), well-defined, rounded, echogenic lesion (*arrow*). This is similar to the typical appearance of hemangiomas in the liver. **B,** Different patient with a 2 cm hemangioma.

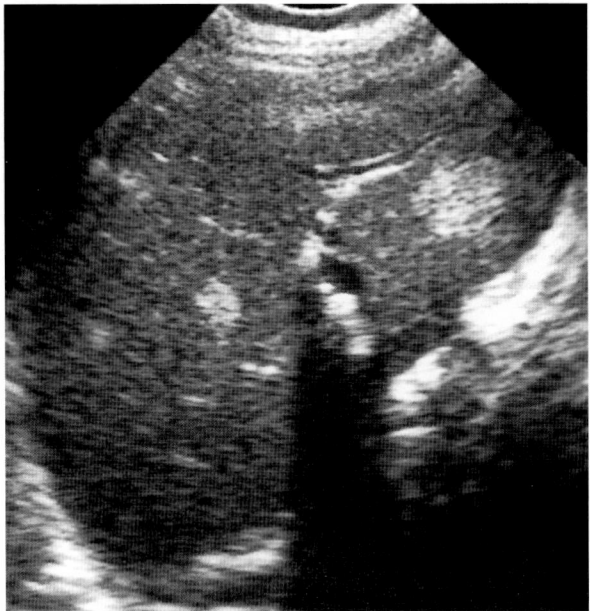

FIGURE 5-19. Multiple splenic hemangiomas. The coronal scan shows multiple echogenic lesions of different sizes in the spleen. Note the calcified splenic artery adjacent to the vein in the splenic hilum.

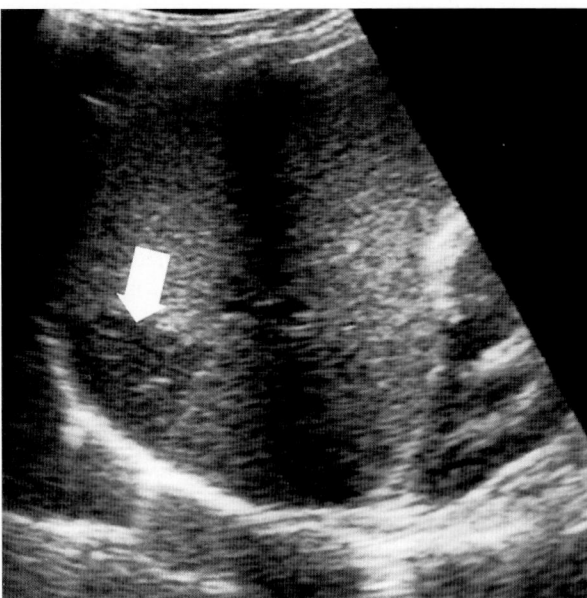

FIGURE 5-20. Splenic infarct. The triangular hypoechoic, wedge-shaped infarct (*arrow*) in the superior aspect of the spleen extends to the splenic capsule, analogous to the pleural wedge-shaped density seen in pulmonary infarction.

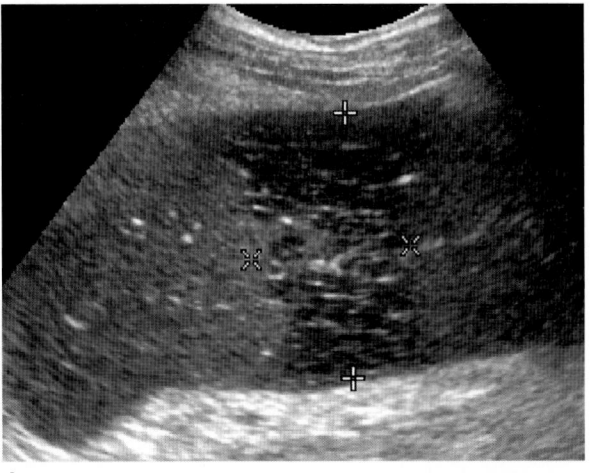

A

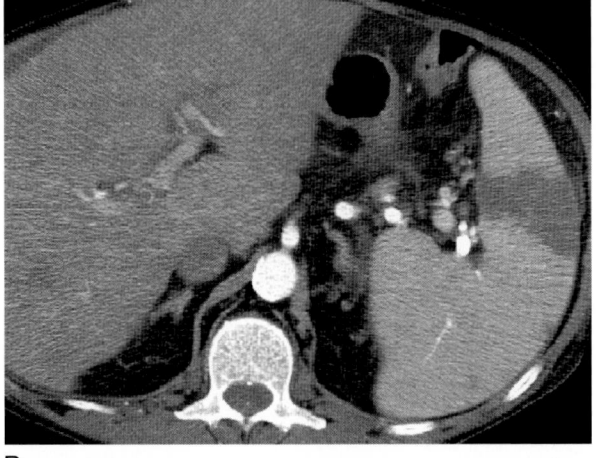

B

FIGURE 5-21. Splenic infarct. A, Coronal longitudinal scan showing a hypoechoic, well-defined central area reaching the splenic capsule medial and lateral in a patient with splenomegaly on peritoneal dialysis. **B**, CT scan after IV contrast with a wedge-shaped nonenhancing area.

Miliary tuberculosis can occur with both typical and **atypical mycobacterial infection** and is more commonly seen in immunocompromised patients. Innumerable tiny, echogenic foci can be seen diffusely throughout the spleen (Fig. 5-23). In active tuberculosis, echo-poor or cystic lesions representing tuberculous abscesses may be seen (Fig. 5-24).

Although ultrasound is very helpful in finding focal splenic lesions, there is so much overlap in the appearance of the different pathologies that it is rarely possible to make a specific diagnosis. Splenic biopsy and even fine-needle biopsy is considered a greater risk than a similar biopsy of the liver because of potential hemorrhage. Therefore, splenic biopsies are not often performed in clinical practice, and most splenic lesions remain unproved and even undiagnosed. If a typical appearance of splenic infarction is found, serial observations may be used to confirm the diagnosis. If a very well defined echogenic lesion is found in an asymptomatic patient, the lack of change on serial ultrasound examina-

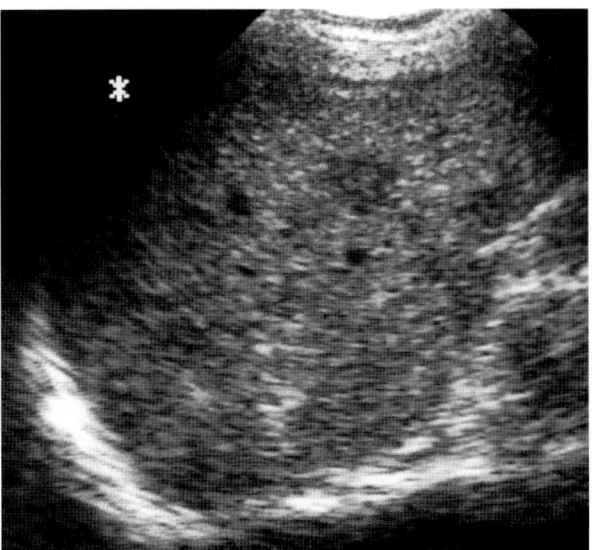

FIGURE 5-22. *Candida* **abscesses of the spleen in an AIDS patient.** Note the lesion in the middle has an echogenic center characteristic of *Candida*.

tions may be used to confirm the diagnosis of hemangioma. Calcified lesions in the spleen may be safely followed with serial ultrasound scanning because they are unlikely to represent any condition requiring treatment.

Splenic Trauma

Ultrasound can be very useful and highly accurate in the diagnosis of subcapsular and pericapsular hematomas of the spleen. Nonetheless, this is one area in which CT has proved particularly useful because more upper abdominal pathology can be identified in one examination.[39,40] However, splenic trauma from blunt, nonpenetrating injuries to the left upper quadrant is not always an emergency, and ultrasound can be useful.[41] Advantages of US are that it is fast, portable, and easily integrated into the resuscitation of patients with trauma without a delay of therapeutic measures.[42] In addition, if the patient is in extreme distress, the CT scanner often cannot be made available quickly enough, so ultrasound can play an important role in that circumstance as well. Furthermore, now that nonoperative management is preferred, ultrasound is preferable for numerous follow-up examinations. If the spleen is involved in blunt abdominal trauma, two outcomes are possible. If the capsule remains intact, the outcome may be an intraparenchymal or subcapsular hematoma (Figs. 5-25 and 5-26).

If the capsule ruptures, a focal or free intraperitoneal hematoma may result. With capsular rupture, it might be possible to demonstrate fluid surrounding the spleen in the left upper quadrant. Although blood may spread within the peritoneal cavity and be found in the flanks or in Morison's pouch, on most occasions it

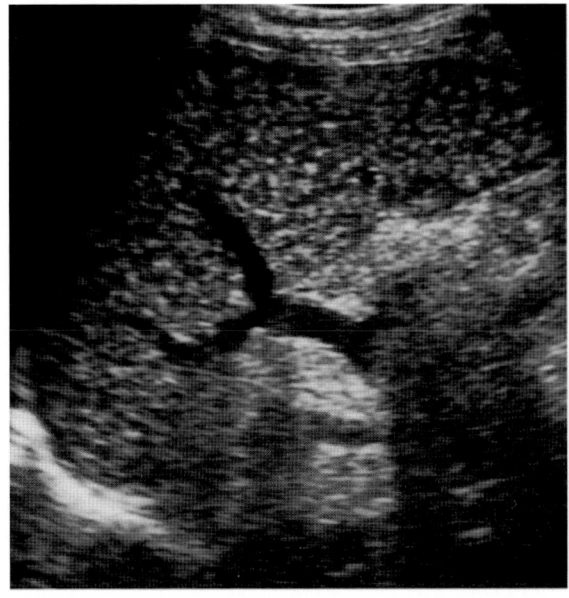

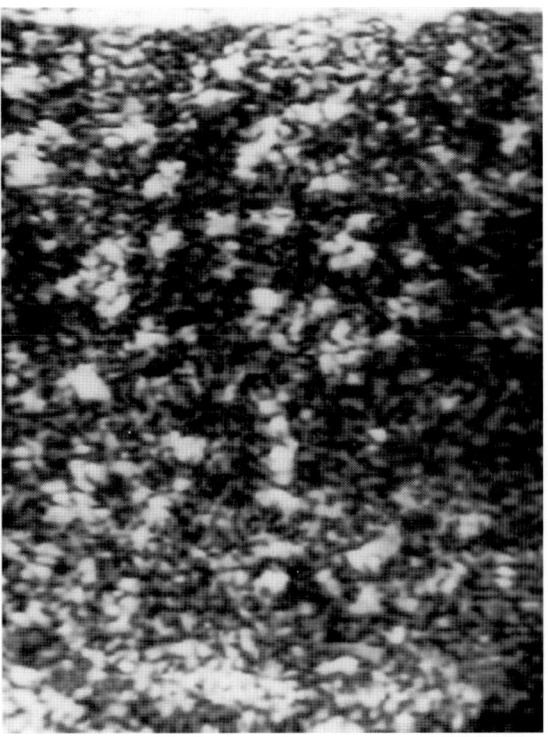

FIGURE 5-23. Miliary tuberculosis of the spleen. A, Coronal and **B,** high-resolution linear array images showing multiple tiny echogenic foci of tuberculous granulomata. This was active tuberculosis.

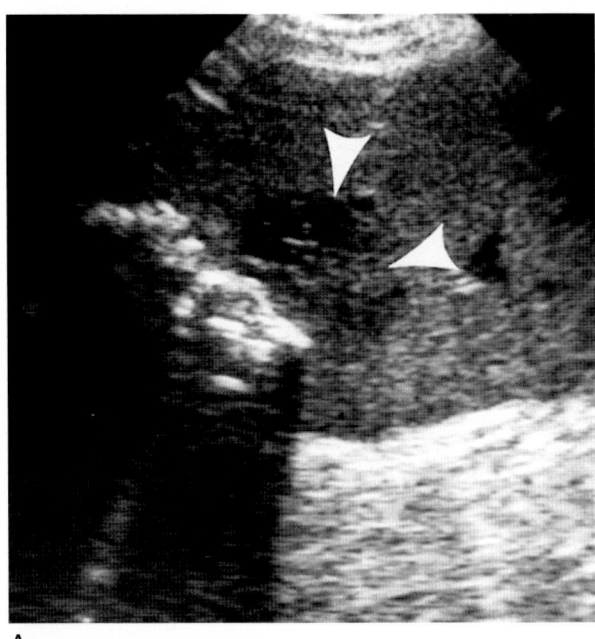

FIGURE 5-24. Old and active tuberculosis in the spleen. A, Longitudinal, coronal image shows old calcified granulomas with shadowing in the superior aspect of the spleen, and echo-poor lesions (*arrowheads*) in the midportion resulting from reactivated tuberculosis. **B** and **C**, Transverse and longitudinal Siescape images in a young AIDS patient with active miliary tuberculosis. Note the numerous, tiny, hypoechoic foci throughout the enlarged spleen.

A

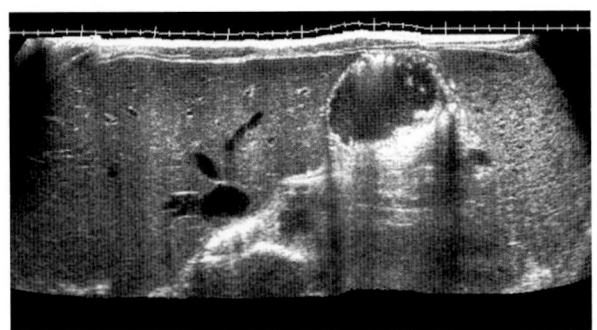

B

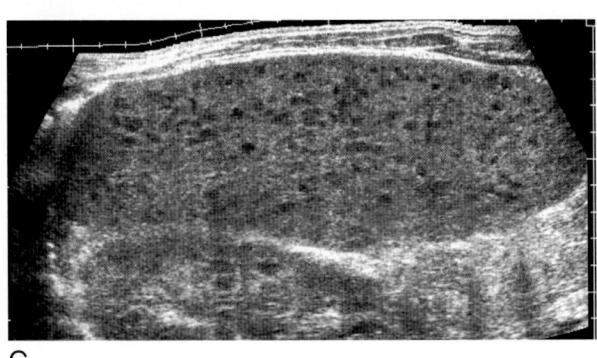

C

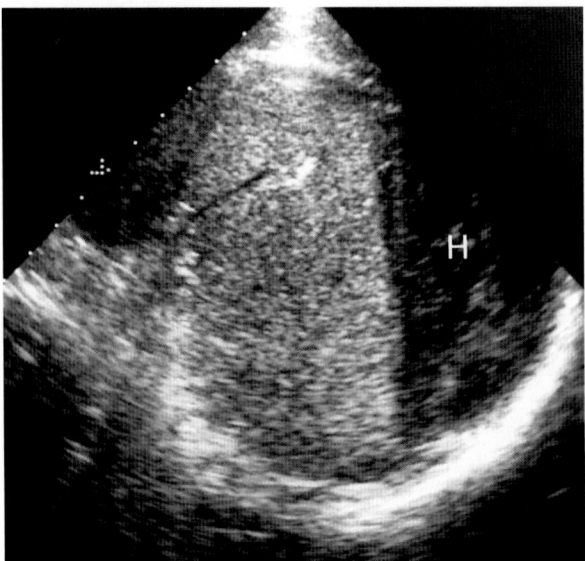

FIGURE 5-25. Subcapsular hematoma of the spleen. Transverse scan showing a fluid- and debris-filled crescentic hematoma (H) in the lateral aspect of the spleen.

becomes walled off in the left upper quadrant (Figs. 5-27 and 5-28).

It is important to consider the timing of the sonographic examination relative to the trauma. Immediately after the traumatic incident, the hematoma is liquid and can easily be differentiated from splenic parenchyma. However, after the blood clots, and for the subsequent 24 to 48 hours, the echogenicity of the perisplenic clot may closely resemble the echogenicity of normal splenic parenchyma. The appearance may mimic that of an enlarged spleen. Subsequently, the blood reliquefies and the diagnosis becomes easy again. Usually, by the time the patient has been admitted and has settled down, one sees only an irregularly marginated, echogenic mass that is larger than one would expect for a normal spleen. There are often focal areas of inhomogeneity within the spleen to indicate that there is an abnormality. Because current therapy for stable patients with suspected splenic trauma consists of nonintervention and temporization, a follow-up sonogram is suggested in 2 or 3 days to demonstrate reliquefaction of the hematoma. With time,

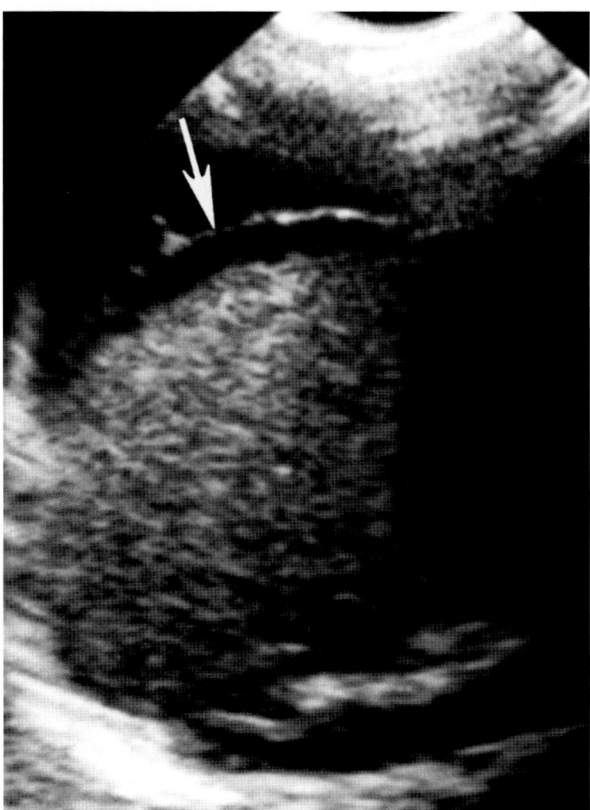

FIGURE 5-26. Subcapsular and perisplenic hematomas. The thin, brightly echogenic crescentic line (*arrow*) represents the splenic capsule.

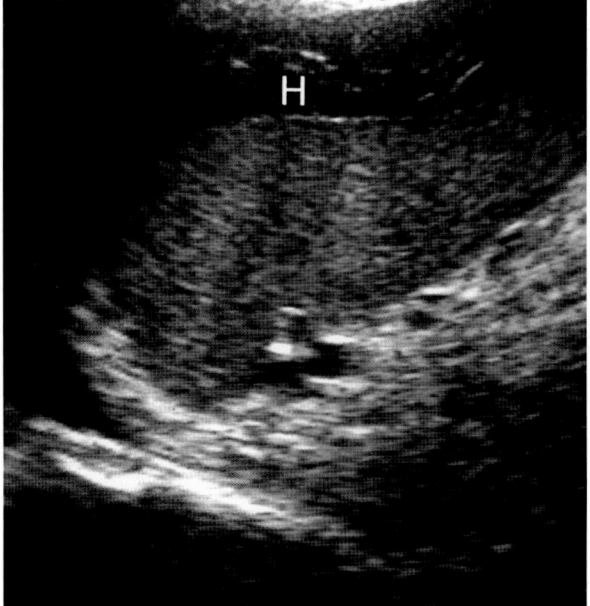

FIGURE 5-27. Posttraumatic perisplenic hematoma. Coronal scan showing hematoma (H) around the lateral aspect of the spleen. There is also a left pleural effusion.

one may clearly see the subcapsular hematoma differentiated from the pericapsular, walled-off hematoma by the capsule itself.[41] The splenic capsule is very thin and is frequently not visualized separately from adjacent fluid. In these cases, the shape of the fluid collection can provide an important clue to the location of the hematoma. If the collection is crescentic and conforms to the contour of the spleen, the hematoma should be assumed to be subcapsular. More irregularly shaped collections are seen with perisplenic hematomas.

Perisplenic fluid may persist for weeks or even months following the trauma. Although there may actually be a condition of delayed rupture of the spleen, it is possible that all ruptures of the spleen occurred at the time of injury and were walled off initially. Delayed rupture may only be the extension of a perisplenic hematoma into the peritoneal cavity.

Aside from splenic capsule rupture, there may be internal damage to the spleen with an intact splenic capsule. This can result in intraparenchymal or subcapsular hematoma of the spleen, which initially appears only as an inhomogeneous area in the otherwise uniform splenic parenchyma. Subsequently, the hematoma may resolve, and repeat scans can show the cyst at the site of the original injury.

Sonographically, a perisplenic hematoma can closely mimic a perisplenic abscess. The hematoma can easily become infected and transform into a left subphrenic abscess.[43] Generally, the distinction can be made clinically. If it is not clinically obvious, fine-needle aspiration can differentiate quickly between hematoma and abscess. Catheter drainage for definitive therapy can then be performed under ultrasound or CT guidance.

Acquired Immune Deficiency Syndrome

The most common splenic ultrasound finding in patients with acquired immune deficiency syndrome (AIDS) is moderate splenomegaly, reported in 50% to 70% of patients referred for abdominal ultrasound.[44,45] Splenomegaly has been noted more frequently in patients with sexually transmitted HIV infection than in patients who acquired the disease through intravenous drug use. Focal lesions can occur in patients with AIDS. They may be caused by opportunistic infections such as *Candida* (see Fig. 5-22), *Pneumocystis carinii*, or *Mycobacterium avium*. There have been reports of disseminated pneumocystis appearing as tiny focal echoes throughout the liver, spleen, and kidneys.[46] We have seen an identical case caused by atypical mycobacteria (Fig. 5-29). The spleen may also be involved in Kaposi's sarcoma or lymphoma.

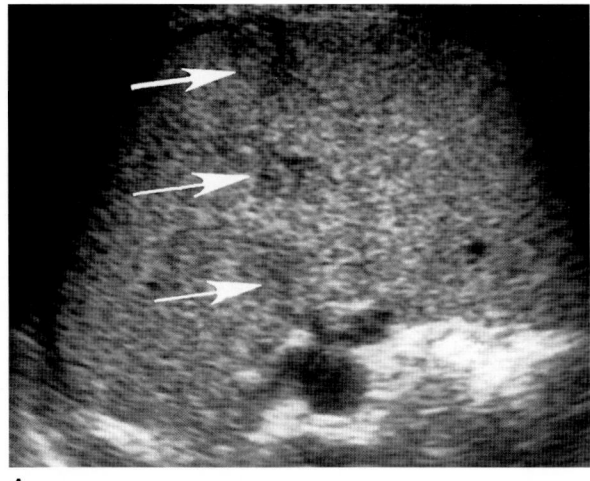

A

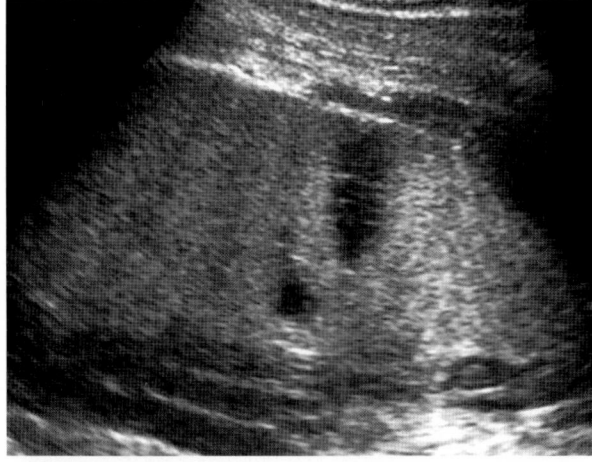

B

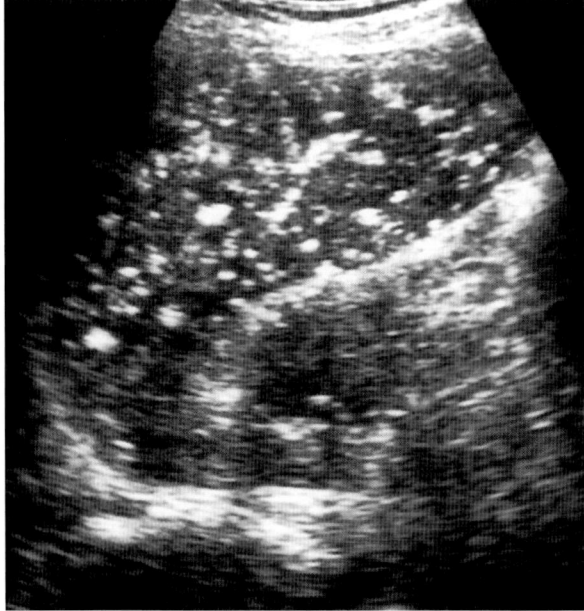

C

FIGURE 5-28. Splenic laceration. A, Coronal scan showing irregular subtle, hypoechoic areas (*arrows*). There is a small amount of blood (anechoic) around the spleen. **B** and **C,** Different patient. **B,** Longitudinal scan showing ovoid hypoechoic areas. **C,** Coronal reconstructed CT scan, after IV contrast, demonstrating the splenic lacerations and a large perisplenic hematoma.

FIGURE 5-29. Atypical tuberculosis of the spleen in an AIDS patient. Tiny calcifications throughout the spleen were also present throughout the liver, and isolated foci were identified in the kidney. Several core biopsies through the liver confirmed these to be *Mycobacterium avium intracellulare* granulomas. Disseminated *Pneumocystis carinii* can also look like this.

CONGENITAL ANOMALIES

Accessory spleens are common normal variants found in up to 30% of autopsies. They are also referred to as **splenunculi.** They may be confused with enlarged lymph nodes around the spleen or with masses in the tail of the pancreas (Fig. 5-30). When the spleen enlarges, the accessory spleens may also enlarge. Ectopic accessory spleens may be confused with abnormal masses or may rarely undergo torsion and cause acute abdominal pain.[47-50] The vast majority of accessory spleens, however, are easy to recognize sonographically as small rounded masses, less than 5 cm in diameter (Fig. 5-31). They are located near the splenic hilum and have echogenicity identical to that of the adjacent spleen. A CT scan or scintigraphy with Tc[99m] heat-damaged red blood cells can confirm the diagnosis.

The spleen may have a long, mobile mesentery if the dorsal mesentery fails to fuse with the posterior peritoneum. The "wandering" spleen can be found in unusual locations and may be mistaken for a mass. It

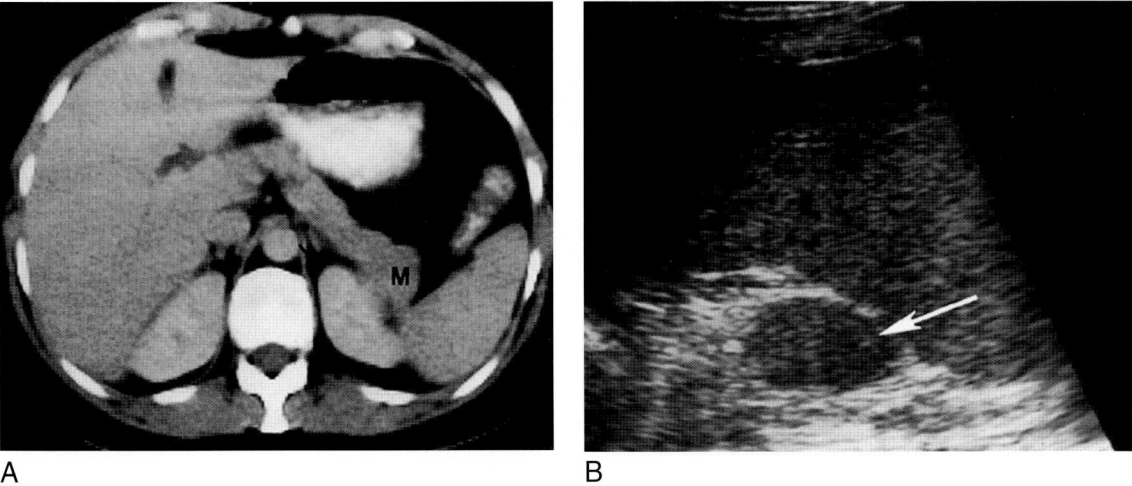

FIGURE 5-30. Accessory spleen appearing as possible mass (M) in the tail of the pancreas. A, CT scan was done first and the patient was referred for an ultrasound-guided biopsy of the pancreatic tail. **B**, Coronal sonogram shows that the apparently enlarged pancreatic tail is actually an accessory spleen (*arrow*) lying adjacent to the tail of the pancreas.

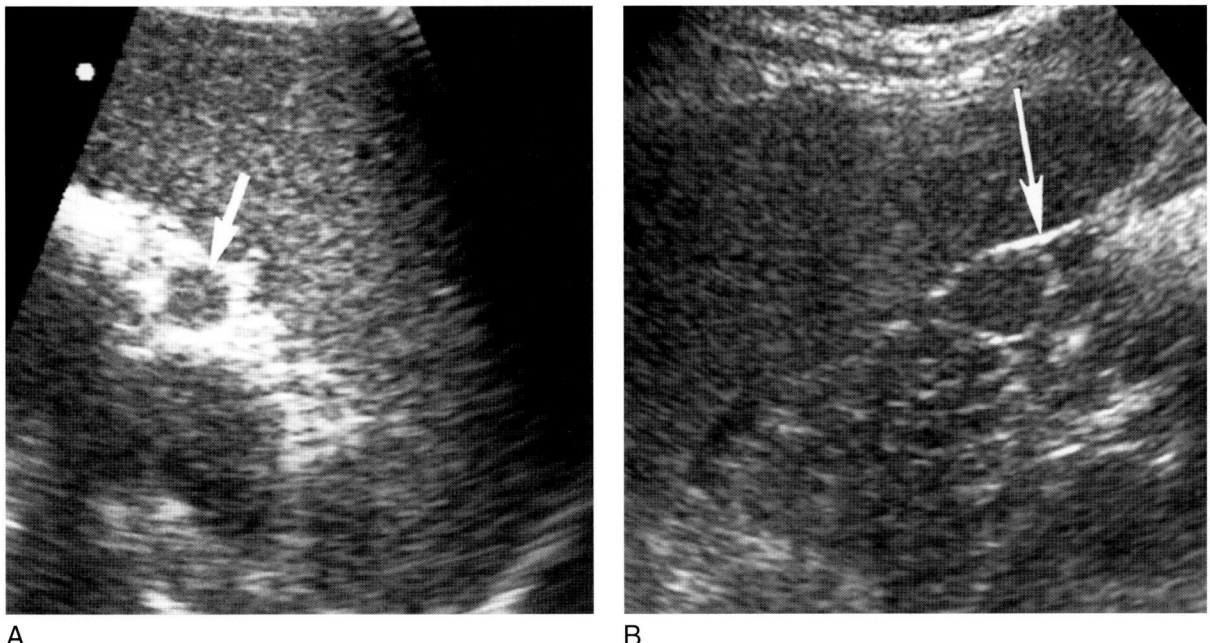

FIGURE 5-31. Accessory spleen. A, Coronal scan showing an accessory spleen (*arrow*) (splenunculus) in the splenic hilum, with homogeneous echogenicity identical to that of the remainder of the spleen. **B**, Longitudinal scan in a different patient showing a medial accessory spleen.

may undergo torsion and result in acute or chronic abdominal pain.[51-53] If the diagnosis of a wandering spleen is made in a patient with acute abdominal pain, the diagnosis of torsion may be supported by a color flow Doppler examination showing absence of blood flow.

The other two major congenital splenic anomalies are the **asplenia** and **polysplenia syndromes**. These conditions are best understood if viewed as part of the spectrum of anomalies known as visceral heterotaxy. A normal arrangement of asymmetric body parts is known as *situs solitus*. The mirror image condition is called *situs inversus*. In between these two extremes is a wide spectrum of abnormalities called *situs ambiguous*. Splenic abnormalities in patients with visceral heterotaxy consist of polysplenia and asplenia. Interestingly, patients with **polysplenia** have bilateral left-sidedness, or a dominance of left-sided over right-sided body structures. They may have two morphologically left lungs, left-sided azygous continuation of an interrupted inferior vena cava, biliary atresia, absence of the gallbladder, gastrointestinal malrotation, and, frequently, cardiovascular abnormalities. Conversely, patients with asplenia may have bilateral right-sidedness. They may have two morphologically right lungs, midline location of the liver, reversed position of the abdominal aorta and inferior vena cava, anomalous pulmonary venous return, and horseshoe kidneys. The wide variety of possible anomalies obviously accounts for the wide variety of presenting symptoms, but absence of the spleen per se causes impairment of the immune response, and such patients can present with serious infections, such as bacterial meningitis.

Polysplenia must be differentiated from posttraumatic splenosis. Following splenic rupture, splenic cells may implant throughout the peritoneal cavity and increase in size, resulting in multiple ectopic splenic rests.[54-56] Nuclear studies with technetium-labeled, heat-damaged red blood cells are the most sensitive studies for both posttraumatic splenosis and congenital polysplenia. Accessory spleens as small as 1 cm can be demonstrated by this method.[57-59]

INTERVENTIONAL PROCEDURES

Despite the fact that ultrasound-guided fine-needle aspiration biopsy and catheter drainage have been established as safe and successful techniques for most areas of the abdomen, many interventional radiologists have been reluctant to apply these techniques to the spleen. The main concern has been fear of bleeding caused by the highly vascular nature of the organ. Reluctance also exists because of the frequent necessity to transgress the pleural space or colon to reach the spleen. In recent years, however, a number of reports have appeared that describe ultrasound-guided interventional procedures in the spleen and demonstrate safety and success records similar to those obtained elsewhere in the abdomen.[15,60,61] Fine- and core-cutting-needle biopsies have been performed for the diagnosis of focal lesions, including abscesses, sarcoidosis, primary splenic malignancies, metastases, and lymphoma.[62-67] Successful catheter drainage of abscesses, cysts, hematomas, and infected necrotic tumors has been reported. However, only very small numbers of cases have been reported, and further experience will be needed to verify the safety and efficacy of these procedures.

PITFALLS

Several sonographic pitfalls exist, and one must be wary of them when scanning the left upper quadrant and spleen. The first pitfall is the crescentic, echo-poor area superior to the spleen, which can be caused by the **left lobe of the liver** in thin individuals (see Fig. 5-6 A,B).[68-71]

It can mimic the appearance of a subcapsular hematoma or a subphrenic abscess. The correct interpretation can be made by noting the hypoechoic liver sliding over the more echogenic spleen during quiet respiration. It would be desirable to follow the liver from the anterior axillary line in the midline over to the posterior axillary line in the coronal plane, but this is usually not possible because of the presence of gas in the stomach. Hepatic and/or portal veins may help to identify this structure as the liver.

The **tail of the pancreas** may look large and may simulate a mass adjacent to the hilum of the spleen. This is particularly true if the plane of section is aimed along the long axis of the tail of the pancreas. Identifying the splenic artery and vein may be helpful in confirming it as the normal tail of the pancreas.

Similarly, the **fundus of the stomach** may nestle in the hilum of the spleen. A particular oblique plane of section may pass through the spleen and include the hilum, with an echogenic portion of the stomach simulating an intrasplenic lesion. Sometimes this is just the fat around the stomach. Occasionally, fluid in the fundus of the stomach can simulate an intrasplenic fluid collection or an abscess in the hilum of the spleen. This can usually be resolved by scanning transversely and, if necessary, giving the patient water to drink.

An occasional anatomic variant can occur if the inferior portion of the spleen lies posterolateral to the upper pole of the left kidney. This variant has been called the **retrorenal spleen**. Awareness of its existence can prevent the misdiagnosis of an abnormal mass. If it is visualized sonographically, it should be avoided in any interventional procedure performed on the left kidney.[72]

It can be very difficult to determine the site of origin of large, left upper quadrant masses arising from the spleen, left adrenal gland, left kidney, tail of the pancreas, stomach, or retroperitoneum. Differential motion observed during shallow respiration can sometimes be helpful. Additionally, the identification of the splenic vein entering the splenic hilum can be definitive. CT or MRI can usually solve difficult cases.

References

Embryology and Anatomy
1. Vibhakar SD, Bellon EM: The bare area of the spleen: A constant computed tomography feature of the ascitic abdomen. AJR 1984;141(5):953-955.

Examination Technique
2. Hicken P, Sauerbrei EE, Cooperberg PL: Ultrasonic coronal, scanning of left upper quadrant. J Can Assoc Radiol 1981;32:107-110.

Pathologic Conditions of the Spleen

3. Breiman RS, Beck JW, Korobkin M, et al: Volume determinations using computed tomography. AJR 1982;138(2):329-333.

4. Frank K, Linhart P, Kortsik C, et al: Sonographic determination of spleen size: Normal dimensions in adults with a healthy spleen. Ultraschall Med 1986;7(3):134-137.

5. Lamb PM, Lund A, Kanagasabay RR, et al: Spleen size: How well do linear ultrasound measurements correlate with three-dimensional CT volume assessments? Br J Radiol 2002;75(895):573-577.

6. Manoharan A, Chen CF, Wilson LS, et al: Ultrasonic characterization of splenic tissue in myelofibrosis: Further evidence for reversal of fibrosis with chemotherapy. Eur J Haematol 1988;40(2):149-154.

7. Wilson LS, Robinson DE, Griffiths KA, et al: Evaluation of ultrasonic attenuation in diffuse diseases of spleen and liver. Ultrasound Imaging 1987;9(4):236-247.

8. Rubinson DE, Gill RW, Kossoff G: Quantitative sonography. Ultrasound Med Biol 1986;12(7):555-565.

9. Franquet T, Montes M, Lecumberri FJ, et al: Hydatid disease of the spleen: Imaging findings in nine patients. AJR 1990;154(3):525-528.

10. Al-Moyaya S, Al-Awami M, Vaidya MP, et al: Hydatid cyst of the spleen. Am J Trop Med Hyg 1986;35(5):995-999.

11. Bhimji SD, Cooperberg PL, Naiman S: Ultrasound diagnosis of splenic cysts. Radiology 1977;122:787-789.

12. Thurber LA, Cooperberg PL, Clemente JG, et al: Echogenic fluid: A pitfall in the ultrasonographic diagnosis of cystic lesions. JCU 1979;7:273-278.

13. Propper RA, Weinstein BJ, Skolnick ML, et al: Ultrasonography of hemorrhagic splenic cysts. JCU 1979;7:18-20.

14. Duddy MJ, Calder CJ: Cystic hemangioma of the spleen: Findings on ultrasound and computed tomography. Br J Radiol 1989;62(734):180-182.

15. Quinn SF, Van Sonnenberg E, Casola G, et al: Interventional radiology in the spleen. Radiology 1986;161:289–291.

16. Changchien CS: Sonographic patterns of splenic abscess: An analysis of 34 proven cases. Abdom Imaging 2002;27(6):739-745.

17. Learner RM, Spataro RF: Splenic abscess: Percutaneous drainage. Radiology 1994;153:643-645.

18. Kessler A, Mitchell DG, Israel L, et al: Hepatic and splenic sarcoidosis: Ultrasound and MR imaging. Abdom Imag 1993;18:159-183.

19. Schaeffer A, Vasile N: Computed tomography of sarcoidosis (case report). J Comput Assist Tomogr 1986;10(4):679-680.

20. Iwasaki M, Hiyama Y, Myojo S, et al: Primary malignant lymphoma of the spleen: Report of a case. Rinsho Hoshasen 1988;33(3):405-408.

21. Neuhauser TS, Derringer GA, Thompson LD, et al: Splenic angiosarcoma: A clinicopathologic and immunophenotypic study of 28 cases. Mod Pathol 2000;13(9):978-987.

22. Costello P, Kane RA, Oster J, et al: Focal splenic disease demonstrated by ultrasound and computed tomography. J Can Assoc Radiol 1985;36:22-28.

23. Goerg C, Schwerk WB, Goerg K: Sonography of focal lesions of the spleen. AJR 1991;156(5):949-953.

24. Manor A, Starinsky R, Gorfinkel D, et al: Ultrasound features of a symptomatic splenic hemangioma. J Clin Ultrasound 1984;12:95-97.

25. Ross PR, Moser RP, Dackman AH, et al: Hemangioma of the spleen: Radiologic-pathologic correlation in ten cases. AJR 1987;162:73-77.

26. Pakter RL, Fishman EK, Nussbaum A, et al: Computed tomography findings in splenic hemangiomas in the Klippel-Trenaunay-Weber syndrome. J Comput Assist Tomogr 1987;11(1):88-91.

27. Moss CN, Van Dyke JA, Koehler RE, et al: Multiple cavernous hemangiomas of the spleen: Computed tomography findings. J Comput Assist Tomogr 1986;10(2):338-340.

28. Kagalwala TY, Vaidya VU, Bharucha BA, et al: Cavernous hemangiomas of the liver and spleen. Indian Pediatr 1987;24(5):427-430.

29. Pistoia F, Markowitz SK: Splenic lymphangiomatosis: Computed tomography diagnosis. AJR 1988;150:121-122.

30. Soyer P, Dufresne AC, Somveille E, et al: Hepatic cavernous hemangioma: Appearance on T2-weighted fast spin-echo MR imaging with and without fat suppression. AJR 1997;168(2):461-465.

31. Maresca G, Mirk P, DeGaetano AM, et al: Sonographic patterns in splenic infarction. J Clin Ultrasound 1986;14:23-28.

32. Goerg C, Schwerk WB: Splenic infarction: Sonographic patterns, diagnosis, follow-up, and complications. Radiology 1990;174(3 Pt 1):803-807.

33. Balcar I, Seltzer SE, Davis S, et al: Computed tomography patterns of splenic infarction: A clinical and experimental study. Radiology 1984;151:723-729.

34. Hill SC, Reinig JW, Barranger JA, et al: Gaucher's disease: Sonographic appearance of spleen. Radiology 1986;160:631-634.

35. Stevens PG, Kumari-Subaiya SS, Kahn LB: Splenic involvement in Gaucher's disease: Sonographic findings. J Clin Ultrasound 1987;15:397-400.

36. Patlas M, Hadas-Halpern I, Abrahamov A, et al: Spectrum of abdominal sonographic findings in 103 pediatric patients with Gaucher disease. Eur Radiol 2002;12(2):397-400.

37. Cerri GG, Alvis VAF, Magalhaes A: Hepatosplenic schistosomiasis mansoni: Ultrasound manifestations. Radiology 1984;153:777-780.

38. Pastakia B, Shawker TH, Thalar M, et al: Hepatosplenic candidiasis: Wheels within wheels. Radiology 1988;166:417-421.

39. Jeffrey RB, Laing FC, Federle MP, et al: Computed tomography of splenic trauma. Radiology 1981;141:729-732.

40. Lawson DE, Jacobson JA, Spizarny DL, et al: Splenic trauma: Value of follow-up CT. Radiology 1995;194:97-100.

41. Siniluoto TM, Paivansalo MJ, Lanning FP, et al: Ultrasonography in traumatic splenic rupture. Clin Radiol 1992;46(6):391-396.

42. Brown MA, Casola G, Sirlin CB, et al: Blunt abdominal trauma: Screening US in 2,693 patients. Radiology 2001;218(2):352-358.

43. Epstein NB, Omar GM: Infective complications of splenic trauma. Clin Radiol 1983;34:91-94.

44. Langer R, Langer M, Schutze B, et al: Ultrasound findings in patients with AIDS. Digitale Bilddiagn 1988;8(2):93-96.

45. Yee JM, Raghavendra BN, Horii SC, et al: Abdominal sonography in AIDS: A review. J Ultrasound Med 1989;8(12):705-714.

46. Spouge AR, Wilson SR, Gopinath N, et al: Extrapulmonary pneumocystis carinii in a patient with AIDS: Sonographic findings. AJR 1990;155(1):76-78.

47. Hansen S, Jarhult J: Accessory spleen imaging: Radionuclide, ultrasound and computed tomography investigations in a patient with thrombocytopenia 25 years after splenectomy for ITP. Scand J Haematol 1986;37(1):74-77.

48. Mostbeck G, Sommer G, Haller J, et al: Accessory spleen: Presentation as a large abdominal mass in an asymptomatic young woman. Gastrointest Radiol 1987;12:337-339.

49. Muller H, Schneider H, Ruchauer K, et al: Accessory spleen torsion: Clinical picture, sonographic diagnosis and differential diagnosis. Klin Pediatr 1988;200(5):419-421.

50. Nino-Murcia M, Friedland GW, Gross DL: Imaging the effects of an ectopic spleen on the urinary tract. Urol Radiol 1988;10(4):195-197.

51. Plaja Ramon P, Aso Puertolas C, Sanchis Solera L: Wandering spleen: Discussion apropos of a case. An Esp Pediatr 1987;26(1):69-70.

52. Scicolone G, Contin I, Bano A, et al: Wandering spleen: Preoperative diagnosis by echotomography of the abdomen. Chir Ital 1986;38(1):72-79.

53. Azoulay D, Gossot D, Sarfati E, et al: Volvulus of a mobile spleen: Apropos of a case diagnosed in the preoperative period by ultrasonography. J CLIR 1987;124(10):520-522.

54. Maillard JC, Menu Y, Scherrer A, et al: Intraperitoneal splenosis: Diagnosis by ultrasound and computed tomography. Gastrointest Radiol 1989;(2):179-180.

55. Delamarre J, Capron JP, Drouard F, et al: Splenosis: Ultrasound and computed tomography findings in a case complicated by an intraperitoneal implant traumatic hematoma. Gastrointest Radiol 1988;13(3):275-278.

56. Turk CO, Lipson SB, Brandt TD: Splenosis mimicking a renal mass. Urology 1988;31(3):248-250.

57. Nishitani H, Hayashi T, Onitsuka H, et al: Computed tomography of accessory spleens. Radiat Med 1984;2(4):222.

58. Nielsen JL, Ellegaard J, Marqversen J, et al: Detection of splenosis and ectopic spleens with 99mTc-labelled heat damaged autologous erythrocytes in 90 splenectomized patients. Scand J Haematol 1981;27(1):51-56.

59. Normand JP, Rioux M, Dumont M, et al: Ultrasonographic features of abdominal ectopic splenic tissue. Can Assoc Radiol J 1993;44(3):179-184

Interventional Procedures

60. Lucey BC, Boland GW, Maher MM, et al: Percutaneous nonvascular splenic intervention: A 10-year review, AJR 2002;179(6):1591-1657.

61. Vyborny CJ, Merrill TN, Reda J, et al: Subacute subcapsular hematoma of the spleen complicating pancreatitis: Successful percutaneous drainage. Radiology 1989;169:161-162.

62. Suzuki T, Shibuya H, Yoshimatsu S, et al: Ultrasonically guided staging splenic tissue core biopsy in patients with non-Hodgkin's lymphoma. Cancer 1987;60:879-882.

63. Cavanna L, Civardi G, Fornari F, et al: Ultrasonically guided percutaneous splenic tissue core biopsy in patients with malignant lymphomas. Cancer 1992;15;69(12): 2932-2936.

64. Silverman JF, Geisinger KR, Raab SS, et al: Fine needle aspiration biopsy of the spleen in the evaluation of neoplastic disorders. Acta Cytol 1993;37(2):158-162.

65. Zeppa P, Vetrani A, Luciano L, et al: Fine needle aspiration biopsy of the spleen. A useful procedure in the diagnosis of splenomegaly. Acta Cytol 1994;38(3):299-309.

66. Keogan MT, Freed KS, Paulson EK, et al: Imaging-guided percutaneous biopsy of focal splenic lesions: Update on safety and effectiveness. AJR 1999;172(4):933-937.

67. Venkataramu NK, Gupta S, Sood BP, et al: Ultrasound guided fine needle aspiration biopsy of splenic lesions. Br J Radiol 1999;72(862):953-956.

Pitfalls

68. Rao MG: Enlarged left lobe of the liver mistaken for a mass in the splenic region. Clin Nucl Med 1989;14(2):134.

69. Li DK, Cooperberg PL, Graham MF, et al: Pseudo peri-splenic "fluid collections" a clue to normal liver and spleen echogenic texture. J Ultrasound Med 1986;5(7):397-400.

70. Crivello MS, Peterson IM, Austin RM: Left lobe of the liver mimicking perisplenic collections. JCU 14(9):697-701.

71. Arenson AM, McKee JD: Left upper quadrant pseudolesion secondary to normal variants in liver and spleen. JCU 1986;14(7):558-561.

72. Dodds WJ, Darweesh RMA, Lawson TL, et al: The retroperitoneal spaces revisited. AJR 1986;174:1155-1161.

6

THE BILIARY TREE AND GALLBLADDER

Korosh Khalili / Stephanie R. Wilson

Chapter Outline

$\mathcal{S}$onographic evaluation of the biliary tract is one of the most appropriate and efficacious uses of the ultrasound examination. The cystic nature of both the gallbladder and the bile ducts, particularly when dilated, provides an inherently high contrast resolution in comparison to the adjacent tissues. This factor, the excellent spatial resolution of sonography, and the acoustic window provided by the liver allow for a high-quality examination in the majority of patients. Today, sonography remains the **modality of choice** for the detection of gallstones, assessment of acute right upper quadrant pain, and for the initial evaluation of the patient with jaundice or elevated liver function tests. In conjunction with MRI/MRCP and contrast enhanced CT scan, sonography also plays a key role in the **multimodality evaluation** of more complex biliary problems, such as the diagnosis and staging of hilar cholangiocarcinoma. The recent development of contrast-enhanced sonog-

raphy for detection of hepatic masses further broadens this role. From the smallest of ultrasound departments operating in remote geographic areas to the largest of tertiary institutions, there is no other anatomic location in the body that is better studied with sonography than the biliary tract.

THE BILIARY TREE

Anatomy of the Biliary Tree and Normal Variants

An understanding of the normal location of the bile ducts and common anatomic variations is quite important in staging of malignancies and directing intervention. In biliary terminology, **proximal** denotes the portion of the biliary tree that is in relative proximity to the liver and hepatocytes, whereas **distal** refers to the

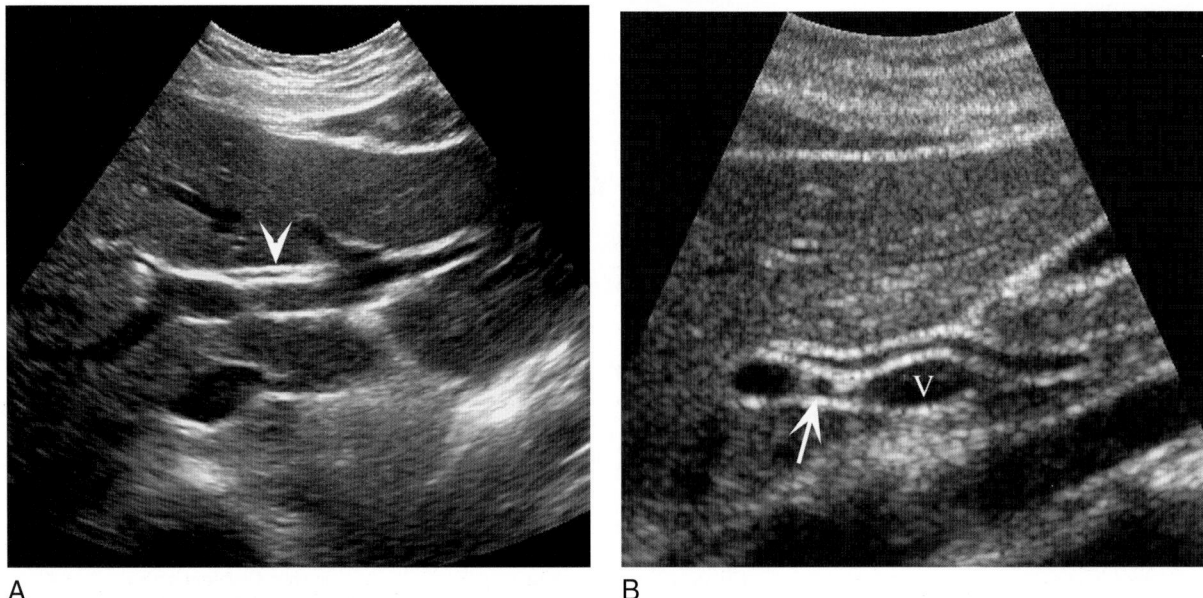

A   B

FIGURE 6-1. Normal bile ducts. A, Right and left hepatic ducts (*arrowhead*) are commonly seen in normal studies lying anteriorly to the portal veins. **B, Common hepatic/common bile ducts** of normal caliber in sagittal view lying in the typical position anterior to the portal vein (V) and hepatic artery (*arrow*).

caudal end closer to the bowel. The term **"branching order"** applies to the level of division of the bile ducts starting from the common hepatic duct (CHD), with first order branches being the right and left hepatic ducts, second order branches, their respective divisions (also known as secondary biliary radicals), and so on. **Central** specifies proximity to the porta hepatis, whereas **peripheral** refers to the higher order branches of the intrahepatic biliary tree extending well into the hepatic parenchyma. Knowledge of **Couinaud's functional anatomy of the liver** is also vital in description of the intrahepatic biliary abnormalities (see Hepatic Anatomy in Chapter 4).

The **intrahepatic ducts** are not in a fixed relation to the portal veins within the portal triads, and can be anterior or posterior to the vein or even tortuous about the vein.[1] The right and left hepatic ducts, that is, the first order branches of the CHD, are routinely seen on sonography, and it is not uncommon to visualize normal second order branches (Fig. 6-1).[2] The use of spectral and color Doppler is often needed to distinguish hepatic arteries from ducts. In our experience, visualization of third or higher order branches is often an abnormal finding and requires a search for the cause of dilation. Most of the right and left hepatic ducts are extrahepatic and, along with the CHD, form the hilar or central portion of the biliary tree at the porta hepatis. This is the most common location for cholangiocarcinoma. The **normal diameter** of the first and higher order branches of the CHD has been suggested to be 2 mm or less, and no more than 40% of the diameter of the adjacent portal vein.[2]

The most common **branching pattern of the biliary tree** occurs in 56% to 58% of the population (Figs. 6-2 and 6-3).[3,4] On the right side, the right hepatic duct forms from the right anterior and posterior branches, draining the anterior (segments 5 and 8) and posterior segments (segments 6 and 7) of the right lobe, respectively. On the left side, segment 2 and 3 branches join to the left of the falciform ligament to form the left hepatic duct. This duct becomes extrahepatic in location as it extends to the right of the falciform ligament, where it is joined by segment 4 and 1 ducts.

The key to understanding the common **normal variants of biliary branching** lies in the variability of the site of insertion of the **right posterior (segment 6 and 7) duct (RPD).** This duct often extends centrally toward the porta hepatis in a cranial direction. It passes superior and posterior to the right anterior duct (RAD) and then turns caudally, joining the RAD to form the short right hepatic duct (see Fig. 6-2). There are three other common sites of insertion of the RPD, which account for the majority of the anatomic variations. If the RPD extends more to the left than usual, it can join the junction of the right and left hepatic ducts (the so called trifurcation pattern, ~8% of normals) or the left hepatic duct (~13% of normals). If the RPD extends in a caudal-medial direction instead, it can join the CHD or CBD directly (~5%). Anomalous drainage of various segmental hepatic ducts directly into the common hepatic ducts is less common.

The **normal caliber of the common hepatic/bile duct** in patients without history of biliary disease has been quoted as up to 6 mm by most studies (see Fig. 6-1).[5]

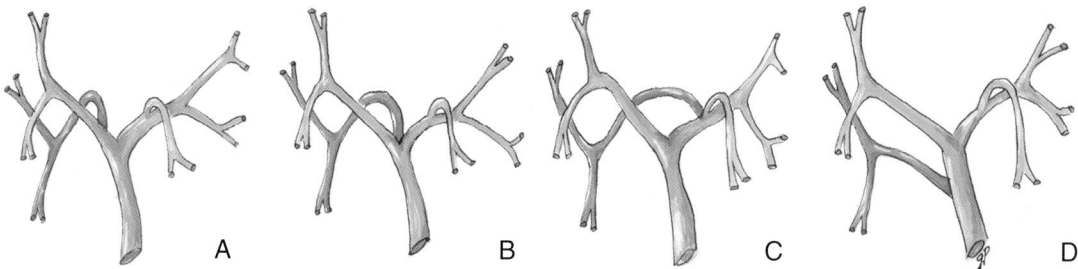

FIGURE 6-2. Common variants of bile duct branching. Right posterior duct (RPD) is in red. **A,** RPD joins the right anterior duct in 56% to 58% of population. **B,** Trifurcation pattern, 8%. **C,** RPD joins the left hepatic duct, 13%. **D,** RPD joins the common hepatic or common bile duct directly, 5%.

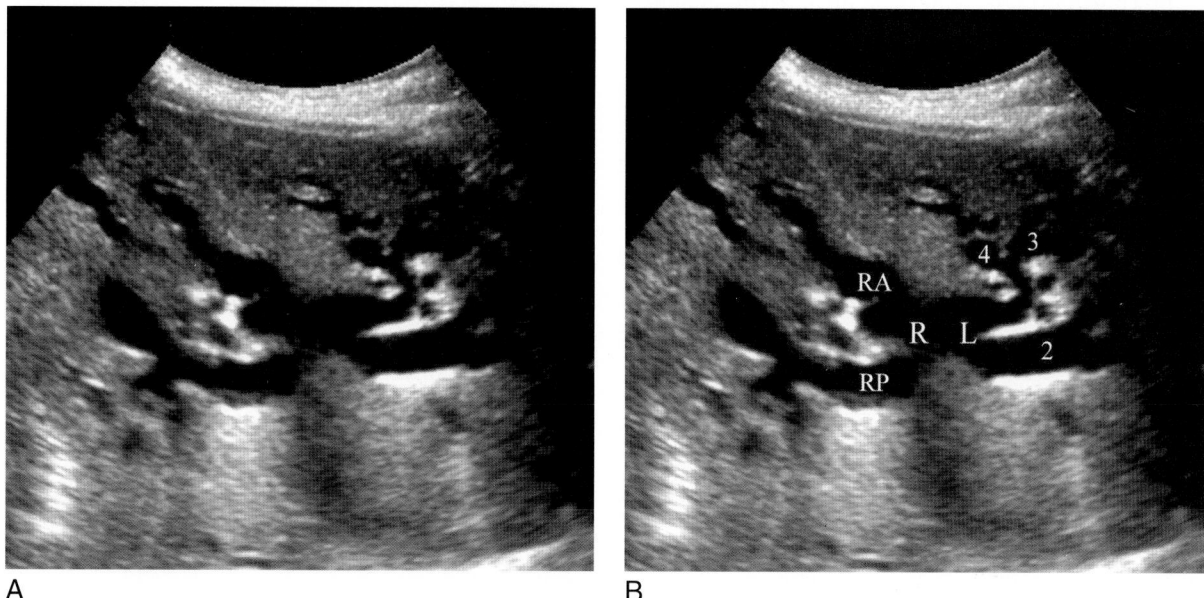

FIGURE 6-3. Typical ductal branching order. A and B, Intrahepatic biliary tree is dilated due to an obstructed common bile duct (*not shown*). This subcostal oblique view foreshortens the right (R) and left (L) hepatic ducts. RA, right anterior duct; RP, right posterior duct; 2, segment 2 duct; 3, segment 3 duct; 4, segment 4 duct.

There is controversy about whether there is a normal widening of the duct with increasing age.[6] Similarly, the literature is inconclusive with regard to an association between cholecystectomy and a large caliber common bile duct. Although diameters of up to 10 mm have been recorded in an asymptomatic normal population, the great majority of the diameters lie under 7 mm. Therefore, a ductal diameter of 7 mm or greater should prompt further investigations, such as correlation with serum levels of cholestatic liver parameters.

The site of insertion of the **cystic duct** into the bile duct is quite variable. The cystic duct may join the bile duct along its lateral, posterior, or medial border. It may also run a parallel course to the duct and insert into the lower one third of the duct, close to the ampulla of Vater.[7] The **common bile duct (CBD)** extends caudally within the hepatoduodenal ligament, lying anterior to the portal vein, and to the right of the hepatic artery.

It then passes posterior to the first portion of the duodenum and the head of the pancreas, sometimes embedded in the latter. It ends in the ampulla of Vater, which is rarely identified on transabdominal ultrasound.

Ultrasound Technique

Our technique for assessment of the **intrahepatic ducts** includes a routine scan as would be performed for evaluation of the liver, including both **sagittal and transverse scans**. In addition, we perform a focused scan to assess the porta hepatis, recognizing that its orientation requires an oblique plane to show the length of the right and left hepatic ducts in a single image. For this we utilize a **subcostal oblique view** with the left edge of the transducer more cephalad than the right edge. The face of the transducer is directed toward the right shoulder. With a full suspended inspiration, a sweep of the transducer, directed from the shoulder to the umbilical region, will show the middle hepatic vein and then the long axis of the right and left hepatic ducts at the porta hepatis, followed by the common duct in cross section. By rotating the transducer 90 degrees to this plane, a second suspended inspiration will allow for a long axis view of the common hepatic and common bile duct at the porta hepatis. **Harmonic imaging** allows for improved contrast between the ducts and adjacent tissues, leading to improved visualization of the duct, its luminal contents and wall (Fig. 6-4). We advocate routine use of harmonic imaging in the assessment of the biliary tree. Specific scanning techniques for assessment of choledocholithiasis and cholangiocarcinoma are discussed in the appropriate sections.

Choledochal Cysts

Choledochal cysts represent a heterogeneous group of diseases that may manifest as congenital, focal, or diffuse cystic dilation of the biliary tree. These cysts occur most commonly in the East Asian populations; the incidence in Japan is 1 in 13,000 as compared to 1 in 100,000 in Western populations.[8,9] There is a 3-4 to 1 female-to-male predominance.

Although most patients present early in life, about 20% of choledochal cysts are encountered in adulthood, when sonography is performed for symptoms of gallstone disease.[10] The most widely used classification system divides choledochal cysts into five types (Fig. 6-5).[11] **Type I choledochal cysts**, a **fusiform dilation of the**

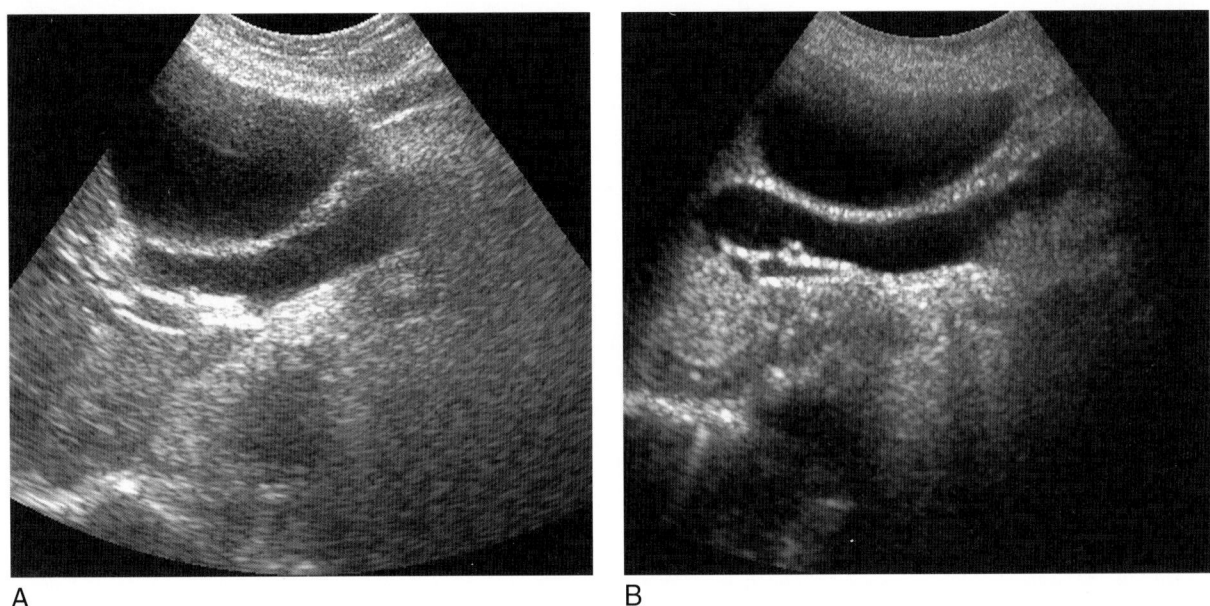

A   B

FIGURE 6-4. Harmonic imaging of biliary tree. A, Longitudinal view of the common bile duct with **fundamental frequencies** and **B, with harmonic imaging.** There is increased contrast to noise with harmonic imaging, effectively clearing the artifactual, low-level echoes over the fluid-filled duct. (From Ortega D, Burns PN, Hope Simpson D, Wilson SR: Tissue harmonic imaging: Is it a benefit for bile duct sonography? AJR 2001;176(3):653-659.)

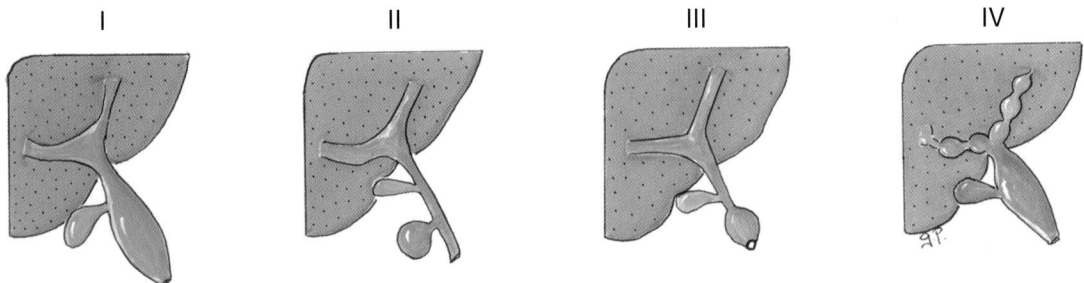

FIGURE 6-5. Choledochal cysts. Todani Classification System. Type I cyst, diffuse dilation of the extrahepatic bile duct; this is the most common type (80%). **Type II cyst,** true diverticulum of the bile duct; very rare. **Type III cyst,** also called choledochocele, diffuse dilation of the very distal (intraduodenal) CBD. **Type IV cyst,** multifocal dilations of the intra- and extrahepatic bile ducts. **Type V cyst,** which is Caroli's disease, is omitted because it is not a true choledochal cyst. (From Todani T, Watanabe Y, Narusue M, et al: Congenital bile duct cysts, classification, operative procedures, and review of thirty-seven cases including cancer arising from choledochal cyst. Am J Surg 1977;134:263-269.)

CBD, are the most common (80%) and, along with **type IVa,** are associated with an abnormally long common channel (>20 mm) between the distal bile duct and the pancreatic duct. It has been suggested that this long common channel allows for reflux of pancreatic juices into the CBD, causing dilation, but this remains controversial.[8,12] **Type II cysts** are **true diverticuli** of the bile ducts and are very rare. **Type III cysts,** the so-called **choledochoceles,** are confined to the intraduodenal portion of the CBD. **Type IVa cysts** are **multiple intra- and extrahepatic biliary dilations,** whereas **type IVb**

cysts are confined to the extrahepatic biliary tree. Caroli's disease has been classified as **type V** cysts, but is of a different embryonic origin and, therefore, is not a true choledochal cyst.[9]

On sonography, a cystic structure is identified which may contain internal sludge, stones, or even solid neoplasm (Fig. 6-6). In some cases, the cyst is large enough that its connection to the bile duct is not immediately recognized. Use of various scanning windows and angles allows for demonstration of the relationship of the lesion to the biliary tract, differentiating it from pancreatic

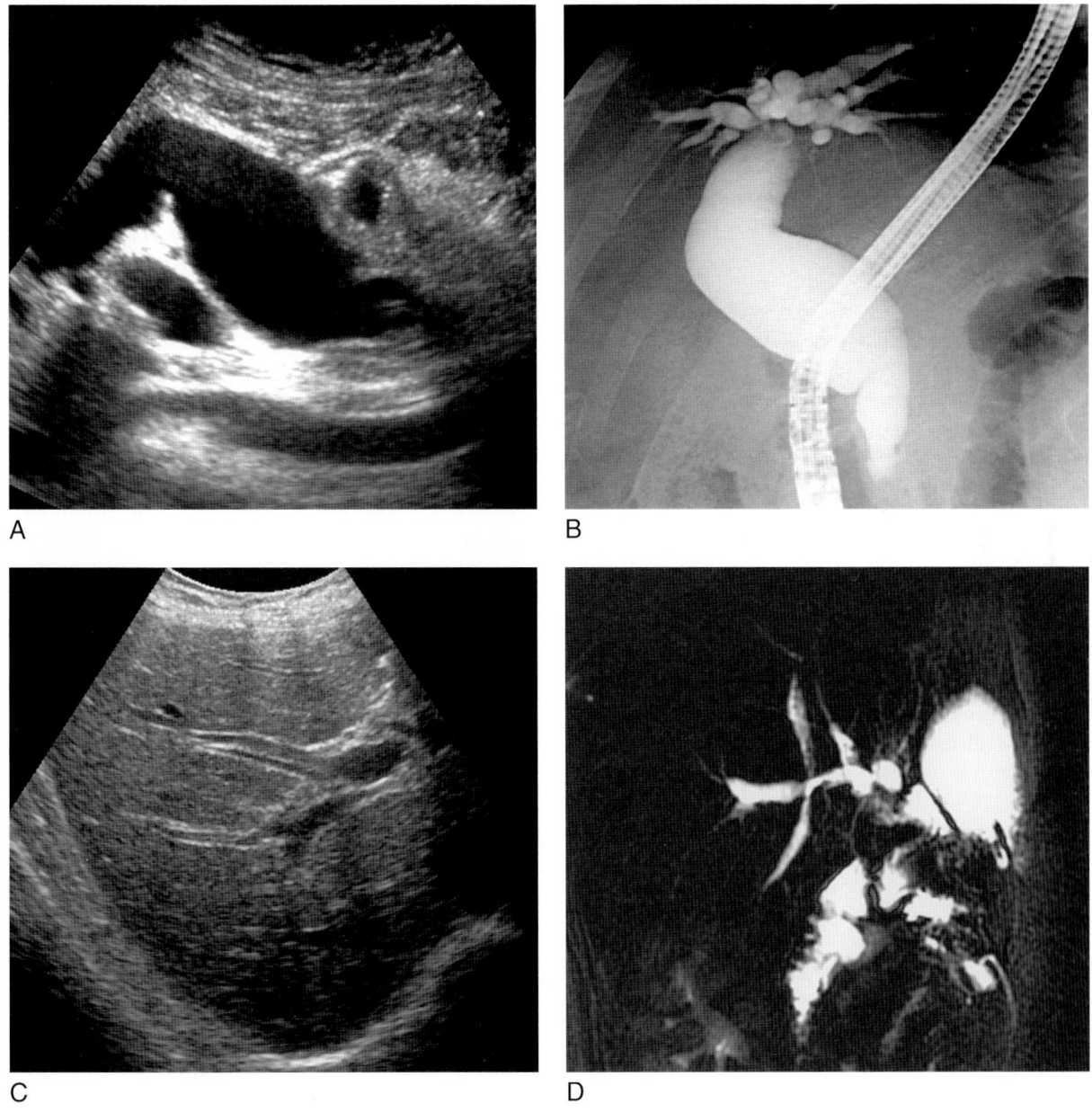

A

B

C

D

FIGURE 6-6. Choledochal cysts. A and **B, Type I.** Fusiform dilation of the **common bile duct** is seen, but no obstructive lesion is noted. This is the most common type of choledochal cyst. An **ERCP** is obligatory to ensure that an ampullary tumor does not exist. **C,** Sonogram and **D, MRCP, Type IV.** There is tubular dilation of the more central intrahepatic biliary tree. The dilated extrahepatic ducts have been previously resected.

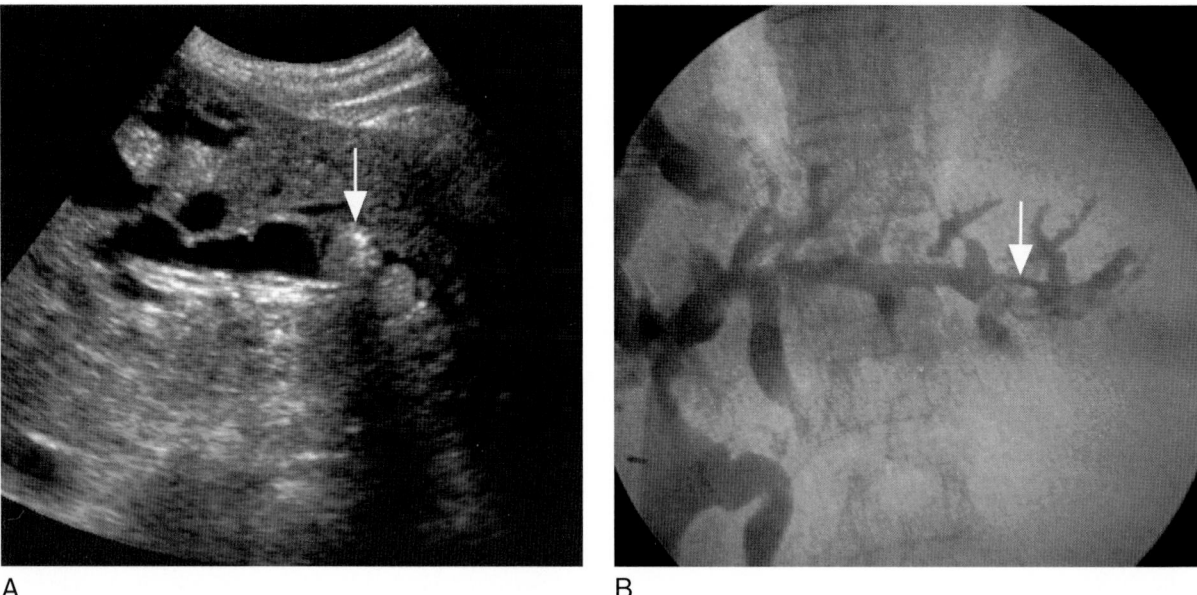

FIGURE 6-7. Caroli's disease. A, Transverse image through the left lobe of the liver demonstrates a dilated duct with sacculations typical of Caroli's disease. Mildly shadowing stones (*arrow*) are seen in the proximal duct. **B,** Corresponding **cholangiogram** shows the stones (*arrow*) as filling defects.

pseudocysts or enteric duplication cysts. Biliary scintigraphy, MRCP, and ERCP have all been used to further delineate the structure of choledochal cysts. ERCP is necessary to ensure that the dilation is not a result of distal neoplasm, especially in the case of type I choledochal cysts (see Fig. 6-6). Because there is a proven risk of cholangiocarcinoma with all choledochal cysts, surgical resection is advocated.

Caroli's Disease

Caroli's disease is a rare congenital disease of the **intrahepatic biliary tree** that forms as a result of malformation of the ductal plates, the primordial cells that give rise to the intrahepatic bile ducts. There are two types of **Caroli's disease**, the simple, classic form, and the second, more common form, which occurs with periportal hepatic fibrosis.[13] This latter form has also been called **Caroli's syndrome**. The disease has associated cystic renal disease, most commonly renal tubular ectasia (medullary sponge kidneys). However, both forms may also be seen in patients with autosomal-recessive polycystic kidney disease. The disease affects men and women equally, and more than 80% of patients present before the age of 30 years.[14]

Caroli's disease leads to saccular or, less often, fusiform dilation of the intrahepatic biliary tree resulting in biliary stasis, stone formation, and bouts of **cholangitis and sepsis** (Fig. 6-7). The disease most often diffusely affects the intrahepatic biliary tree, but it may be focal. The dilated ducts contain stones and sludge. In distinction to recurrent pyogenic cholangitis, the ductal

contents do not form a cast of the dilated system and thus are more easily identified as ductal contents.[15] As well, small portal vein branches surrounded by dilated bile ducts and bridging echogenic septa traversing the dilated ducts have been described on ultrasound. These correspond to persistent embryonic ductal structures.[16] If associated with congenital hepatic fibrosis, finding of cirrhosis and portal hypertension is also present. **Cholangiocarcinoma** develops in 7% of patients with Caroli's disease.[14]

Obstruction of the Biliary Tree

Elevation of cholestatic liver parameters, which may appear clinically as jaundice, is a frequent indication for sonographic examination of the abdomen. The major objective in performing these scans is to determine if the patient has obstruction of the bile ducts, as opposed to a hepatocellular or biliary ductule diseases. Sonography is highly sensitive in the **detection of dilation of the biliary tree** and is, therefore, an excellent modality for initiation of the imaging investigation (Fig. 6-8). These scans should be performed with knowledge of the **patient's clinical condition**, most particularly as to whether the patient has **painless** or **painful jaundice**. The latter is seen with acute obstruction and/or infection affecting the biliary tree.

Performance of the ultrasound examination should be focused on answering several **key questions** as follows:

- Are the bile ducts or gallbladder dilated?
- If yes, to what level?

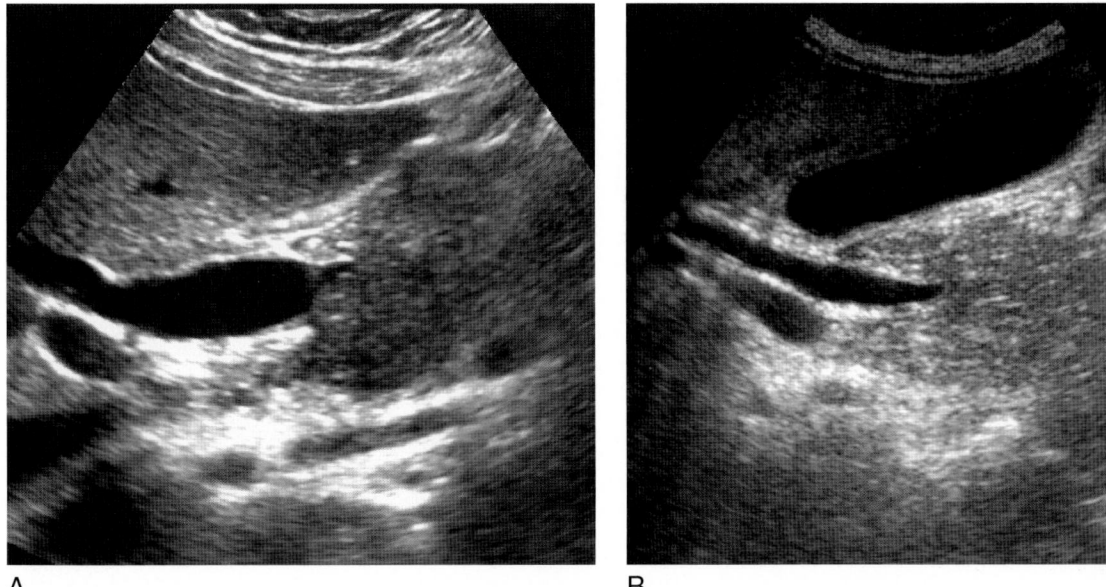

A   B

FIGURE 6-8. CBD obstruction due to extrinsic causes. A, Pancreatic adenocarcinoma. Short transition zone with shouldering, large duct caliber, along with an obstructive mass are typical findings in malignant obstruction. **B, Pancreatitis.** Elongated tapering of the duct suggests a benign cause. Note mild sympathetic gallbladder wall thickening due to adjacent inflammation.

- If yes, what is the cause?
  Causes of biliary obstruction are listed in Table 6-1.

Choledocholithiasis

Choledocholithiasis may be classified into primary and secondary forms. Primary choledocholithiasis denotes *de novo* formation of stones, often made of calcium bilirubinate (pigment stones) within the ducts. The **etiologic factors** are often related to diseases causing strictures or dilation of the bile ducts, leading to stasis, as follows:

- Sclerosing cholangitis
- Caroli's disease
- Parasitic infections of the liver (*Clonorchis, Fasciola,* and *Ascaris*)[17]
- Chronic hemolytic diseases, such as sickle cell disease
- Prior biliary surgery, such as biliary-enteric anastomoses

Migration of stones from the gallbladder into the common bile duct constitutes secondary choledocholithiasis. Whereas primary choledocholithiasis is relatively rare outside endemic regions (East Asia), secondary choledocholithiasis is quite common, representing the worldwide distribution of gallstone disease. Bile duct stones are found in 8% to 18% of patients with symptomatic gallstones.[18]

TABLE 6-1. CAUSES OF BILIARY OBSTRUCTION

Choledocholithiasis*
  Hemobilia*

Congenital Biliary Diseases
  Caroli's disease*
  Choledochal cysts

Cholangitis
  Infectious
    Acute pyogenic cholangitis*
    Biliary parasites*
    Recurrent pyogenic cholangitis*
    HIV cholangiopathy
  Sclerosing cholangitis

Neoplastic
  Cholangiocarcinoma
  Gallbladder carcinoma
  Locally invasive tumors (esp. pancreatic adenocarcinoma)
  Ampullary tumors
  Metastases

Extrinsic Compression
  Mirizzi's syndrome*
  Pancreatitis

Denotes causes of painful jaundice.

Intrahepatic Stones

With the recent advent of harmonic and compound imaging, the ability to find small stones within the intrahepatic bile ducts has improved, especially in the setting of dilated ducts. Our own experience suggests that sonography competes well with, and occasionally surpasses, other biliary imaging methods, including MRCP. The current sensitivity of sonography in detecting intrahepatic stones is unknown, however.

The **appearance** of stones depends on their size and texture (Fig. 6-9). Most stones are highly echogenic with posterior acoustic shadowing. Small (<5 mm) or soft pigment stones in the setting of recurrent pyogenic cholangitis may not shadow (see Fig. 6-17D). When the affected ducts are filled with stones, the individual stones may not be appreciated; instead, a bright echogenic linear structure with posterior shadowing is seen. Stones should always be suspect if discrete or linear echogenicities with or without shadowing are seen in the

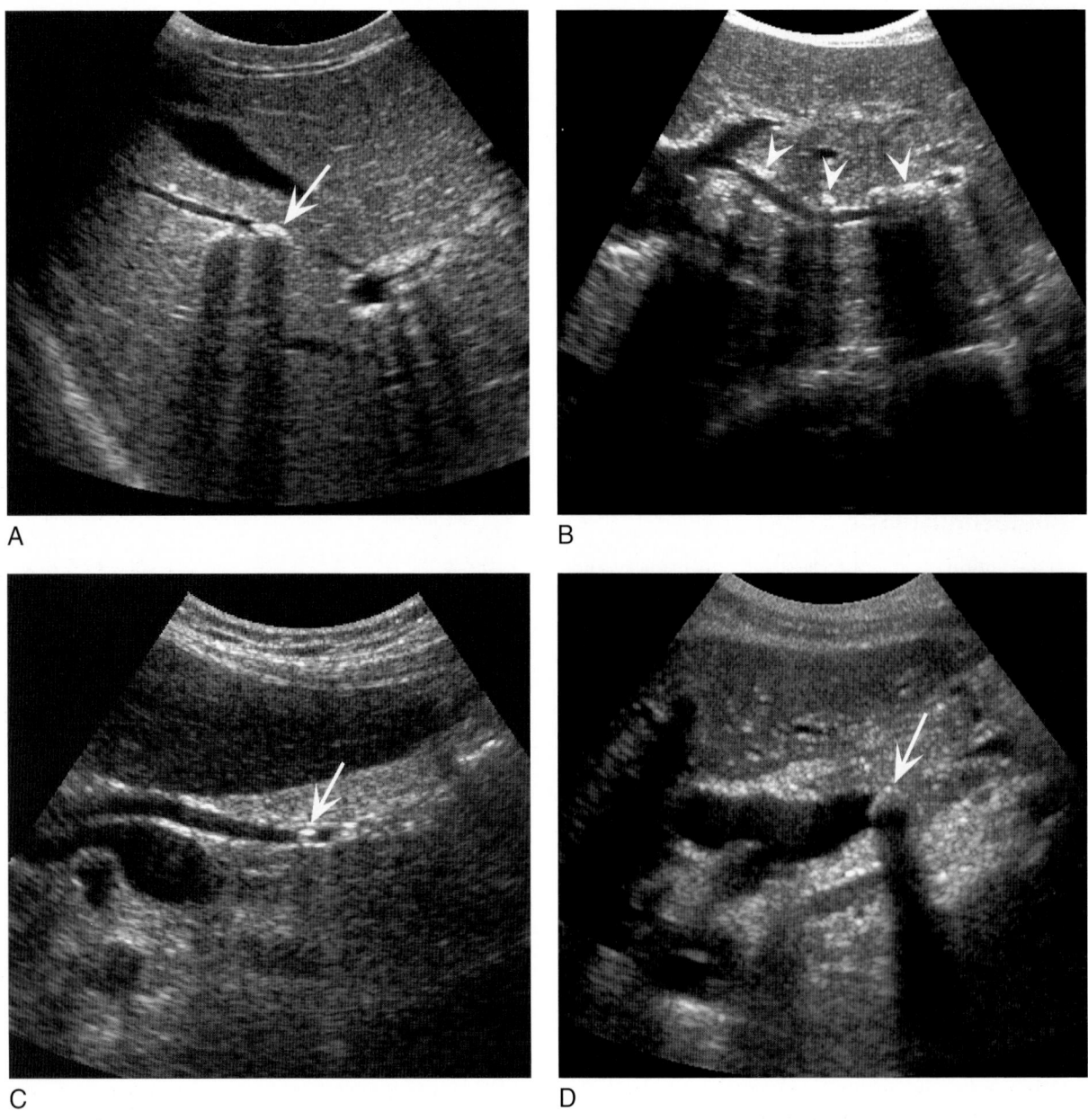

FIGURE 6-9. Choledocholithiasis. A, Intrahepatic stones. Small stones (*arrow*) are seen in the right lobe causing acoustic shadowing. Note the dilated duct proximal to the larger stone. **B,** Multiple stone clusters (*arrowheads*) in the left lobe appearing as echogenic linear structures with shadowing. Both patients **A** and **B** had cystic fibrosis. **Common bile duct stones. C, Small stone** (*arrow*) may not shadow, whereas **D, large stone** (*arrow*) has classic findings within a dilated CBD. (**C** and **D** from Ortega D, Burns PN, Hope Simpson D, Wilson SR: Tissue harmonic imaging: Is it a benefit for bile duct sonography? AJR 2001;176(3):653-659.)

region of the portal triads paralleling the course of the portal veins within the liver. Harmonic imaging improves both the contrast resolution and detection of the acoustic shadow and is, therefore, recommended for routine assessment of the biliary tree.[19]

Common Bile Duct Stones

The majority of stones in the CBD will be in the distal duct right at the ampulla of Vater. Therefore, sonographic evaluation should include assessment of the entire duct with detailed effort focused on the peri-ampullary region. Regrettably, this exact area is often the most difficult to see as it may be hidden by bowel gas, making detection of distal CBD stones most difficult. **Optimal technical factors** to improve assessment include:

- **Changes in patient position.** The CBD may be examined in supine, left lateral decubitus, and standing positions. The change in the relative position of adjacent organs and bowel gas may allow significantly improved visualization of the distal duct.
- **Choice of sonographic window.** The subcostal view is most useful for the assessment of the porta hepatis and proximal CBD. An epigastric view is best for the distal CBD.
- **Use of compression sonography.** Physically compressing the epigastrium may collapse the superficial bowel and displace the bowel gas blocking the view.
- **Detailed assessment of the distal CBD.** The distal intrapancreatic CBD is often best visualized with the probe focused on the pancreatic head in the transverse plane. Once the dilated CBD is identified, a slight rocking of the transducer to just "peek" at the point of caliber change will often allow a glimpse of a stone impacted in the distal duct, which is otherwise hidden from sonographic view. Similarly, a sagittal view focused on the pancreatic head should show the dilated CBD on the dorsal aspect of the head. Again, slight manipulation of the transducer focusing on the point of caliber change is best to see a solitary stone impacted in the distal duct.

The classic **appearance** of CBD stones is that of a rounded echogenic lesion with posterior acoustic shadowing (see Fig. 6-9). It should be recognized that there will not be a fluid rim around an impacted distal CBD stone because it is compressed against the duct wall. The lateral margins of the stone are, therefore, not seen, decreasing the conspicuity of the stone versus a stone seen in the gallbladder or proximal duct, where it is likely to be surrounded by bile. **Small stones** may lack good acoustic shadows and appear only as a **reproducible, bright linear echogenicity**, either straight or curved. Awareness of this subtle appearance of CBD stones definitely improves their detection.

Pitfalls in the diagnosis of choledocholithiasis include blood clot (hemobilia), papillary tumors, and occasionally biliary sludge; none of these will shadow. Surgical clips in the porta hepatis, mostly due to previous cholecystectomy, appear as linear echogenic foci with shadowing.[20] The short length, relative high degree of echogenicity, lack of ductal dilation, and absence of the gallbladder should allow differentiation of surgical clips from stones.

Mirizzi Syndrome

Mirizzi syndrome describes a **clinical syndrome** of jaundice with pain and fever resulting from obstruction of the common hepatic duct by a stone impacted in the cystic duct. It occurs most commonly when the cystic duct and common hepatic ducts run a parallel course. The stone is often impacted in the distal cystic duct, and the accompanying inflammation and edema result in the obstruction of the adjacent common hepatic duct. The obstruction of the cystic duct results in recurrent bouts of cholecystitis, and the impacted stone may erode into the common hepatic duct, resulting in a cholecysto-choledochal fistula and biliary obstruction.[22] Identification of this complication (called Mirizzi type II) is important because the treatment requires surgical repair of the fistula. Acute cholecystitis, cholangitis, and even pancreatitis may occur.[21]

Mirizzi syndrome should be considered on **sonography** when biliary obstruction with dilation of the biliary ducts to the level of the common hepatic duct is seen in conjunction with a picture of acute or chronic cholecystitis. Thus, the gallbladder has features of acute cholecystitis, but may or may not be distended.[2] A stone impacted in the cystic duct with surrounding edema at the level of the obstruction is confirmatory (Fig. 6-10).

Hemobilia

Iatrogenic biliary trauma, mostly due to percutaneous biliary procedures or liver biopsies, accounts for approximately 65% of all causes of hemobilia reported in the recent literature. Other etiologies include cholangitis/cholecystitis (10%), vascular malformations/aneurysms (7%), abdominal trauma (6%), and malignancies, especially hepatocellular carcinoma and cholangiocarcinoma (7%).[23] Pain, bleeding, and biochemical jaundice are the usual complaints at presentation. Apart from the blood loss, which occasionally is severe, complications are rare; they include cholecystitis, cholangitis, and pancreatitis.[23]

The appearance of blood within the biliary tree is not unlike blood clots encountered elsewhere (Fig. 6-11).

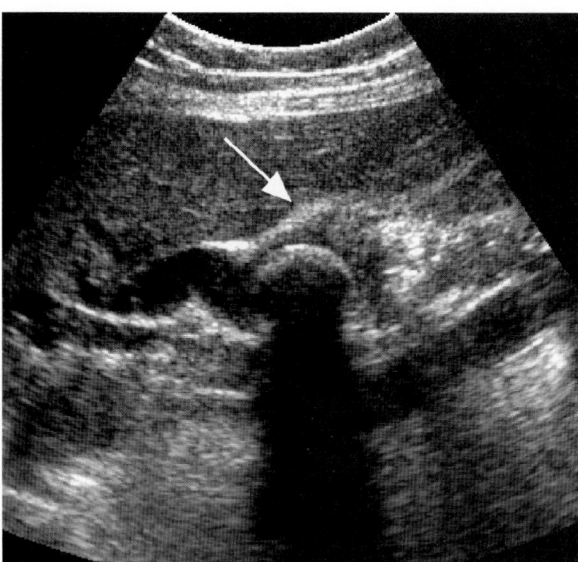

FIGURE 6-10. Mirizzi's syndrome. Mirizzi's syndrome in a patient with abdominal pain and jaundice. Sagittal sonogram shows a dilated common bile duct obstructed by a large stone impacted in the distal cystic duct. This appearance may be mistaken for a common bile duct stone. There is thickening of the wall of the cystic duct (*arrow*).

Most often, the clot is echogenic or of mixed echogenicity, and retractile, conforming to the shape of the duct. Occasionally it may appear tubular with a central hypoechoic area. Acute hemorrhage will appear as fluid with low-level internal echoes. Blood clots may be mobile. Extension into the gallbladder is common. The clinical history is often very useful in assisting with the diagnosis.

Pneumobilia

Air within the biliary tree is most commonly seen as a result of previous biliary intervention, biliary-enteric anastomoses, or common bile duct stents. In the **acute abdomen**, pneumobilia may be caused primarily by three entities. **Emphysematous cholecystitis** may lead to pneumobilia; its risk factors and findings are discussed under Acute Cholecystitis. Inflammation caused by an impacted stone in the common bile duct may cause erosion of the duct wall leading to a **choledocho-duodenal fistula**. The third entity, **prolonged acute cholecystitis,** may lead to erosion into an adjacent loop of bowel, most commonly the duodenum or transverse colon, called **cholecysto-enteric fistula**. Stones may then pass from the gallbladder into the bowel and can cause bowel obstruction called **gallstone ileus.**

Air in the bile ducts has a characteristic appearance. **Bright, echogenic linear structures** following the portal triads are seen, more commonly in a nondependent position (Fig. 6-12). Posterior dirty shadowing and reverberation artifact (ringdown) are seen with large quantities of air. **Movement** of the air bubbles, best seen just after changing the patient's position, is diagnostic. Extensive arterial calcifications, seen especially in diabetics, can mimic pneumobilia.

Acute (Bacterial) Cholangitis

Antecedent biliary obstruction is an essential component of bacterial cholangitis, associated in 85% of cases with common bile duct stones.[24] Other causes of obstruction include biliary stricture as a result of trauma or surgery, congenital abnormalities, such as choledochal cysts, and partially obstructive tumors. Intrinsic or extrinsic neoplasms causing complete biliary obstruction rarely cause pyogenic cholangitis prior to biliary intervention.[25] The **clinical presentation** is usually that of fever (~90%), right upper quadrant pain (~70%), and jaundice (~60%), the classic Charcot's triad. There is leukocytosis, or at least a left shift, and elevation of serum alkaline phosphatase and bilirubin in the great majority of patients. Often mild serum transaminitis is present, but occasional levels above 1000 are seen early in the disease due to sudden increase in intrabiliary pressures.[25] The bile is most commonly infected by gram-negative enteric bacteria, which are often retrieved in blood cultures.

Acute cholangitis is a medical emergency. **Sonography** is advocated as the first imaging modality to determine **the cause** and **level** of obstruction, and to **exclude other diseases,** such as cholecystitis, acute hepatitis, or Mirizzi's syndrome. Sonography is more accurate than CT and more practical than MR, endoscopic ultrasound, and ERCP in the initial assessment of patients with potential acute biliary disease.[26]

The **sonographic findings** of bacterial cholangitis are shown in Figure 6-13 and include the following:

- Dilation of the biliary tree
- Choledocholithiasis and possibly sludge
- Bile duct **wall thickening**
- Hepatic abscesses

Dilation of the biliary tree, when present, can be well diagnosed by sonography. A diameter of common bile duct greater than 6 mm is considered abnormal in most patients. Subtle dilation of the intrahepatic biliary tree is a finding that is frequently overlooked, and should be specifically sought. This includes use of subcostal oblique scanning of the porta hepatis to assess the caliber of the right and left hepatic ducts and evaluation of the CBD, which may measure normal but still show a somewhat tense or distended morphology. Dilation of the biliary tree is seen in 75% of patients. The obstructive stone is usually lodged in the distal common bile duct, but may be mobile causing intermittent obstruction. It is rare to see air within the ducts; its presence suggests a **choledochoenteric fistula** in the absence of previous

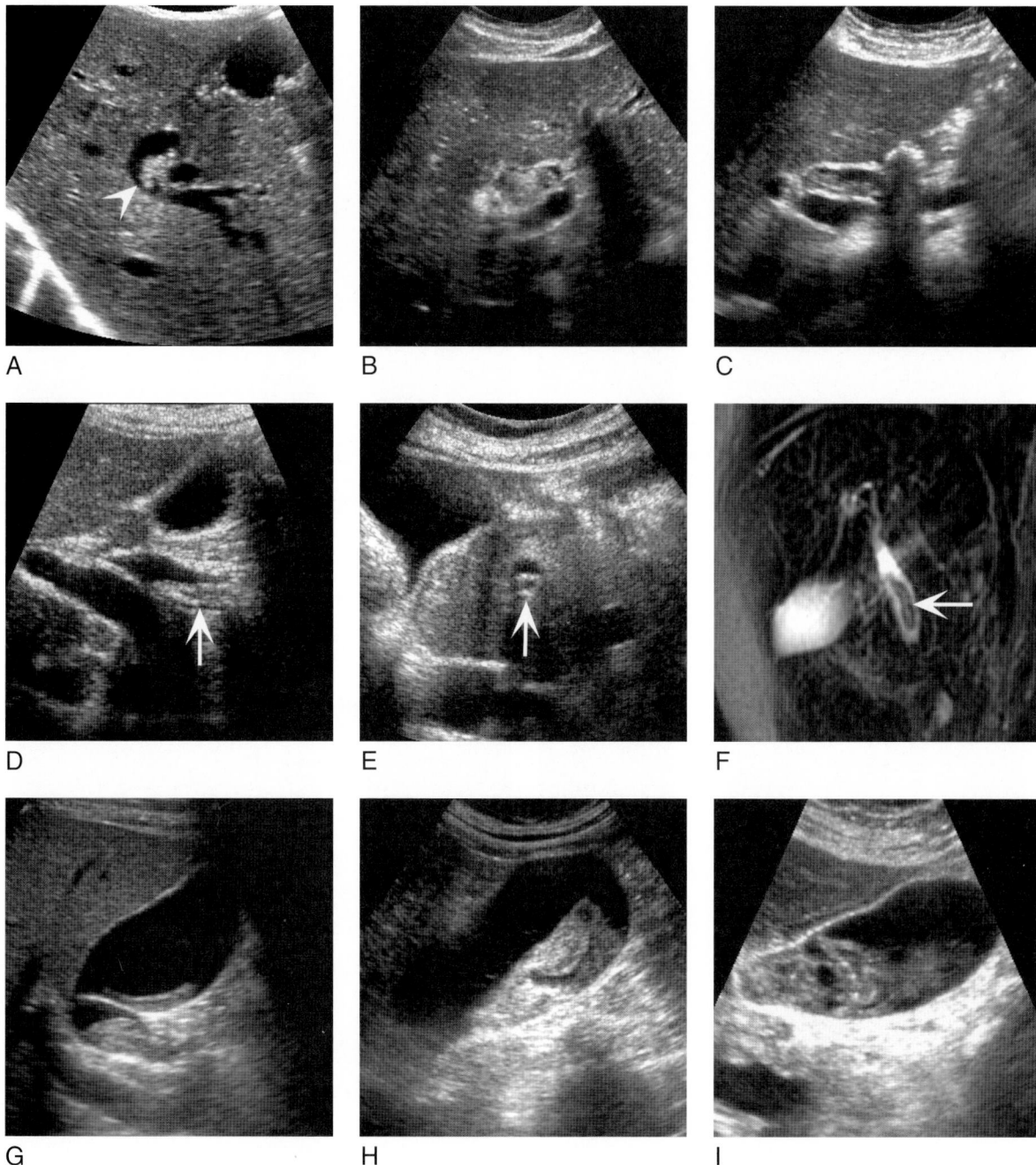

FIGURE 6-11. Hemobilia—spectrum on sonography. A, Echogenic blood clot (*arrowhead*) within a dilated duct, after insertion of biliary drainage catheter. Biliary obstruction was due to pancreatic tumor. **B** and **C,** Echogenic clot in the common hepatic duct in two patients after liver biopsy. **D** and **E,** Spontaneous hemobilia in patient on anticoagulation therapy. Note the tubular appearance of the clot (*arrow*) with central anechoic lumen. **F,** Corresponding **MRCP image** depicts the same. **G, H,** and **I, Blood in gallbladder** in three different patients. All patients developed pain after liver biopsy. Note the angled edges of the clot in **G,** quite typical of blood clots.

biliary manipulation. Circumferential thickening of the bile duct wall, similar to other causes of cholangitis, may be present, and may extend to the gallbladder. Multiple, small hepatic abscesses—sometimes grouped in a lobe or segment of the liver—are not uncommon but tend to become visible on sonography when they have undergone liquefaction and are a late finding.

Recurrent Pyogenic Cholangitis

Recurrent pyogenic cholangitis has been known by other names including **hepatolithiasis** and **oriental cholangiohepatitis**. It is a disease characterized by chronic biliary obstruction, stasis, and stone formation, leading to recurrent episodes of acute pyogenic cholangitis. Its

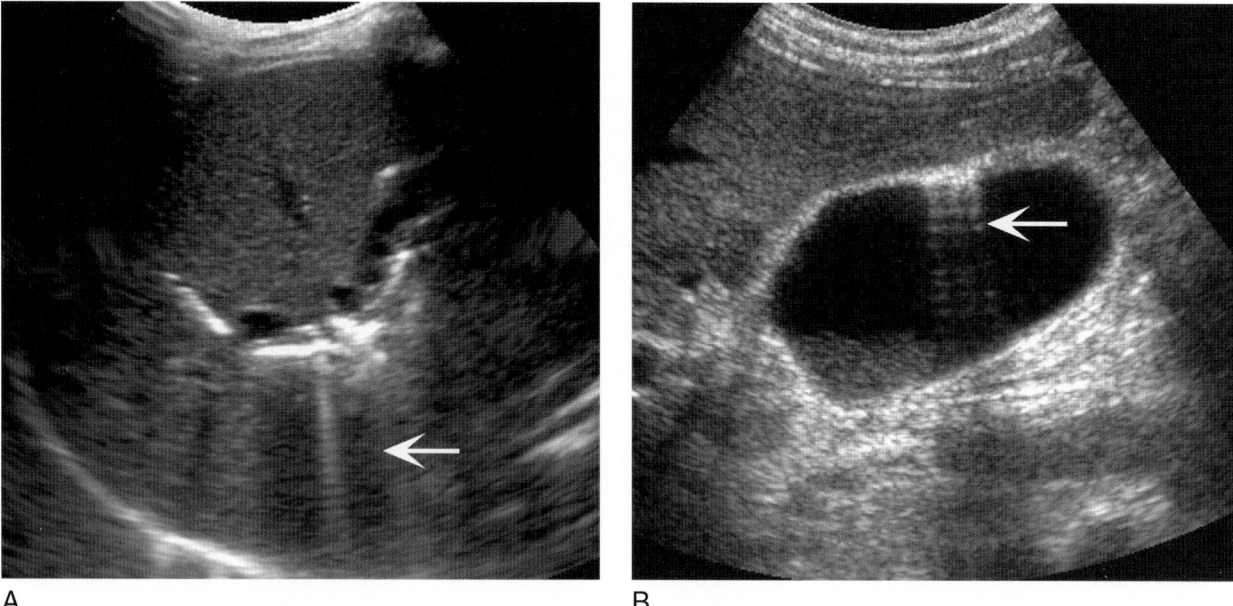

A   B

FIGURE 6-12. Pneumobilia. A, Extensive air within the central ducts manifests as linear echogenic structures paralleling the portal veins. Note the dirty shadowing (*arrow*) and reverberation artifact. **B, Air in the gallbladder.** Pneumobilia often extends into the gallbladder. Note the reverberation artifact (*arrow*).

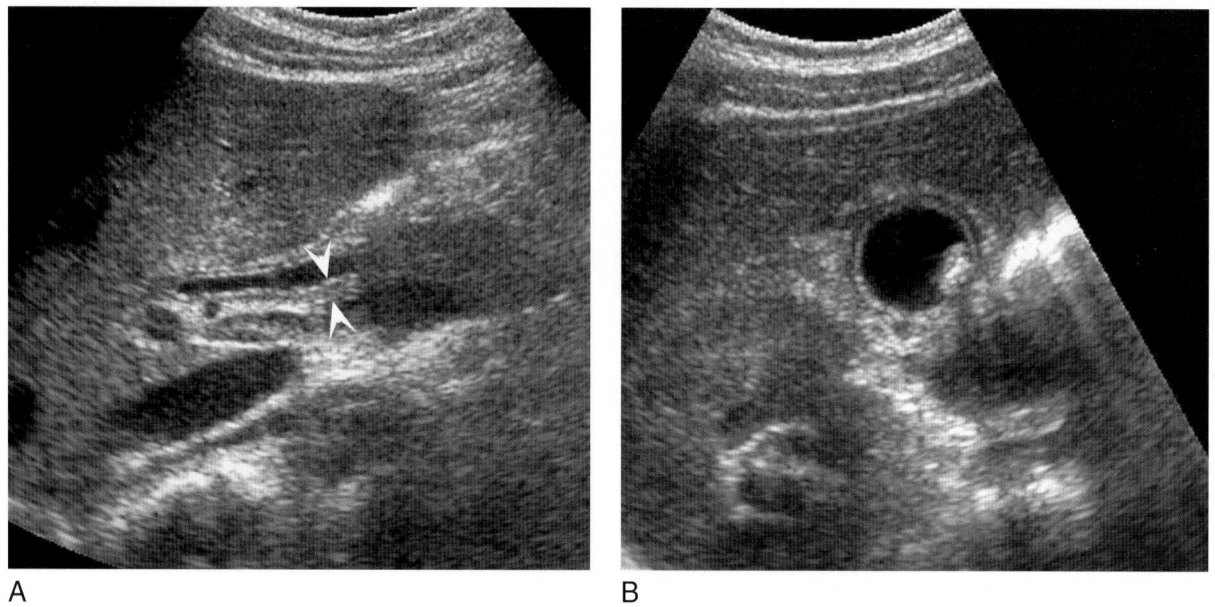

A   B

FIGURE 6-13. Acute bacterial cholangitis in a 22-year-old female. A, Bile duct wall thickening (*arrowheads*) and **B, gallbladder wall thickening**. Presence of gallbladder wall thickening helps to differentiate from primary sclerosing cholangitis, where the gallbladder is affected in only 10% to 15% of cases. Note gallstone in the gallbladder.

incidence is highest in people of Southeast and East Asian descent; it is rare and sporadic in other populations. Although liver fluke infections (especially *Clonorchis sinensis*), malnutrition, and portal bacteremia have all been implicated, the etiology of the disease remains unknown.[27] Any segment of the liver may be affected, but the lateral segment of the left lobe is most often involved. **Acute complications** of the disease, namely sepsis, may be fatal and may need urgent percutaneous biliary decompression or surgery. The chronic stasis and inflammation eventually leads to severe atrophy of the affected segment; biliary cirrhosis and cholangiocarcinoma are long-term complications. The **treatment** of the disease lies in repeated biliary dilation and stone removal.[28]

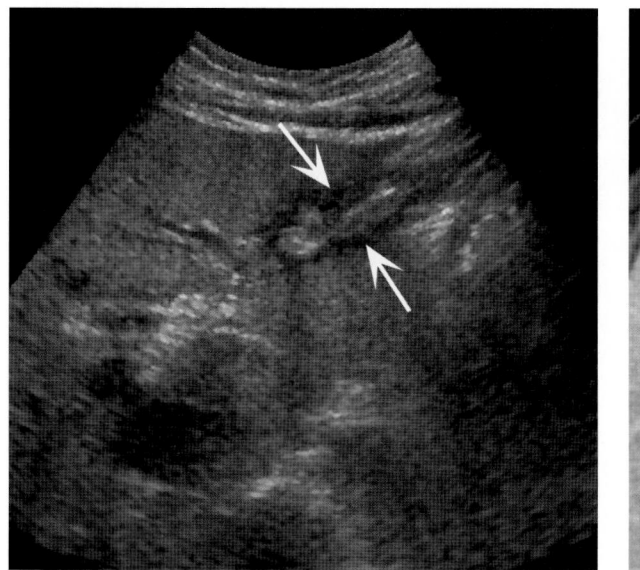
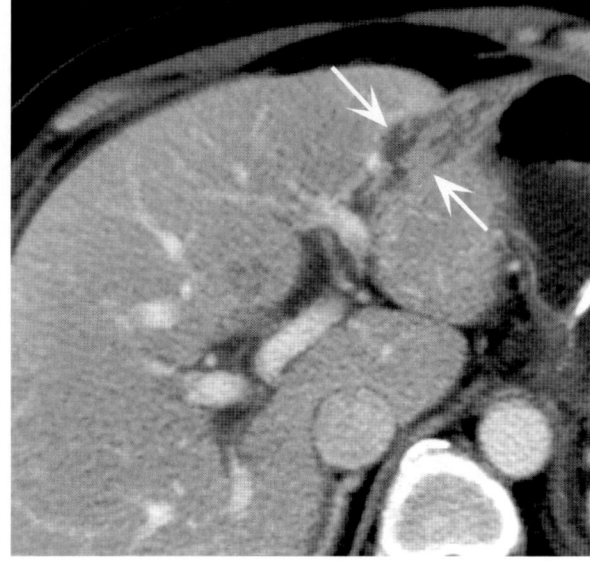

A   B

FIGURE 6-14. Segmental recurrent pyogenic cholangitis. A, Transverse sonogram and **B, CT scan** depict severe atrophy of segment 3 (*arrows*) about abnormal, stone-filled ducts.

Ultrasound is commonly used for both disease screening and monitoring.[25] The common appearance on sonography is that of dilated ducts filled with sludge and stones, confined to one or more segments of the liver (Figs. 6-14 and 6-15). Patients may also present with multiple echogenic masses in the liver, and recognizing that these, in fact, lie within markedly dilated ducts requires care. When dilated ducts are identified, their contents may be hypoechoic or echogenic and the stones need not shadow. With severe atrophy of the affected segment, very little liver parenchyma may be present, and the crowded, stone-filled ducts may appear as a single heterogeneous mass.

Ascariasis

Ascaris lumbricoides is a parasitic roundworm which has been estimated to infect up to one quarter of the world's population. It uses a fecal-oral route of transmission and is most common in children, presumably due to their lower hygiene levels.[29] The worm is generally 20 to 30 cm long and up to 6 mm in diameter. It is active within the small bowel and may enter the biliary tree retrogradely through the ampulla of Vater, causing acute biliary obstruction. Generally, infected patients are asymptomatic but may present with biliary colic, cholangitis, acalculous cholecystitis, or pancreatitis.

The **appearance** of biliary ascariasis on sonography depends on the number of worms within the bile ducts at the time of the study. Most commonly, a single worm is identified, which appears as a tube or as parallel echogenic lines within the bile ducts. The appearance is quite similar to a biliary stent, which should be excluded on clinical history. On the transverse view, the rounded worm surrounded by the duct wall gives a target appearance. The worm may be folded unto itself or occupy any portion of the ductal system, including far out into the liver parenchyma, close to the capsule, or within the gallbladder. Movement of the worm during the scan facilitates the diagnosis. When infestation is heavy, multiple worms may lie adjacent to each other within a distended duct, giving a spaghetti like appearance. Occasionally, the worms may appear as an amorphous, echogenic filling defect, making the diagnosis more difficult.[29]

HIV Cholangiopathy

HIV cholangiopathy, also known as **AIDS cholangitis**, is an inflammatory process affecting the biliary tree in the advanced stages of HIV infection. It is most commonly due to an opportunistic infection and, therefore, occurs in patients with CD4 counts of less than 100. Patients present with severe right upper quadrant or epigastric pain, a nonicteric cholestatic picture; and markedly elevated serum alkaline phosphatase with a normal bilirubin level. In most patients, a pathogen is recovered, most commonly *Cryptosporidium* or, less commonly, cytomegalovirus.[30]

Sonography has been advocated as the first imaging test for assessment of HIV cholangiopathy (Fig. 6-16). A negative scan effectively rules out the disease. The findings include the following:

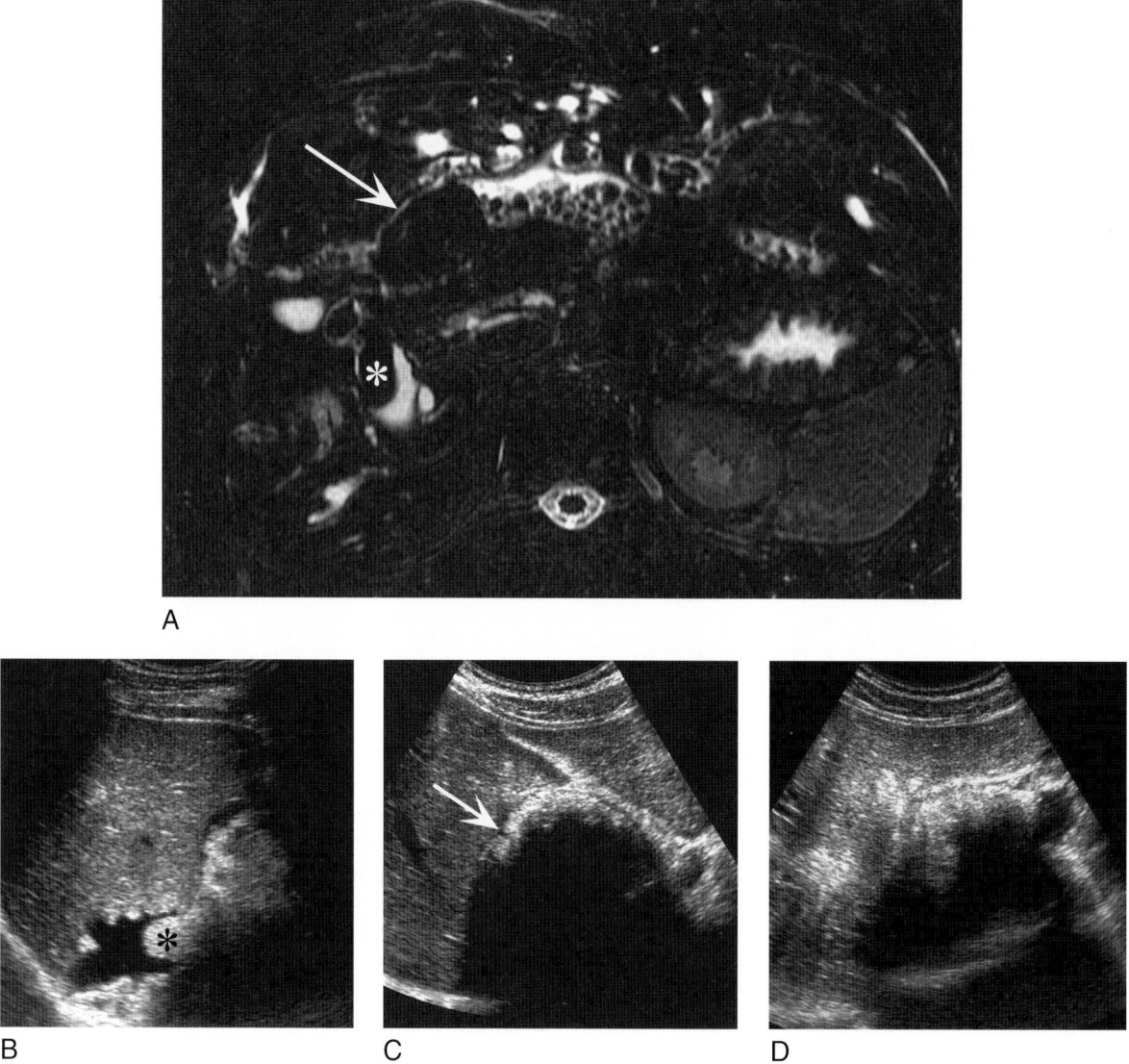

FIGURE 6-15. Recurrent pyogenic cholangitis. A, Axial MRCP view through the liver demonstrates markedly dilated biliary tree filled with stones. **B, Transverse image of the right lobe** shows a large stone (*) in the dilated right posterior duct, corresponding to abnormality (*) on the MRCP. **C, Huge stone in the central duct** (*arrow*) with marked posterior acoustic shadowing. **D, Multiple small stones in the left lobe** which appear as masslike, echogenic conglomerate on the sonogram. This, especially when accompanied by atrophy of the hepatic parenchyma, is the most common appearance of recurrent pyogenic cholangitis.

- Bile duct **wall thickening** of the intra- and extrahepatic biliary tree
- Focal **strictures and dilations** identical to primary sclerosing cholangitis
- Dilation of the common bile duct due to an inflamed and stenosed papilla of Vater (**papillary stenosis**). The inflamed papilla itself may be seen as an echogenic nodule protruding into the distal duct.[31]
- Diffuse gallbladder wall thickening, seen much more commonly than in primary sclerosing cholangitis.[32]

Autoimmune Cholangiopathy

Autoimmune cholangiopathy may affect small or large ducts. Diseases involving the small ductules, such as primary biliary cirrhosis and autoimmune cholangitis, affect ducts that are too small to resolve by imaging; only gross changes in the liver architecture, such as lobar redistribution and cirrhosis, are detected. Primary sclerosing cholangitis affects larger caliber ducts and, thus, has typical abnormal ductal features seen on sonography.

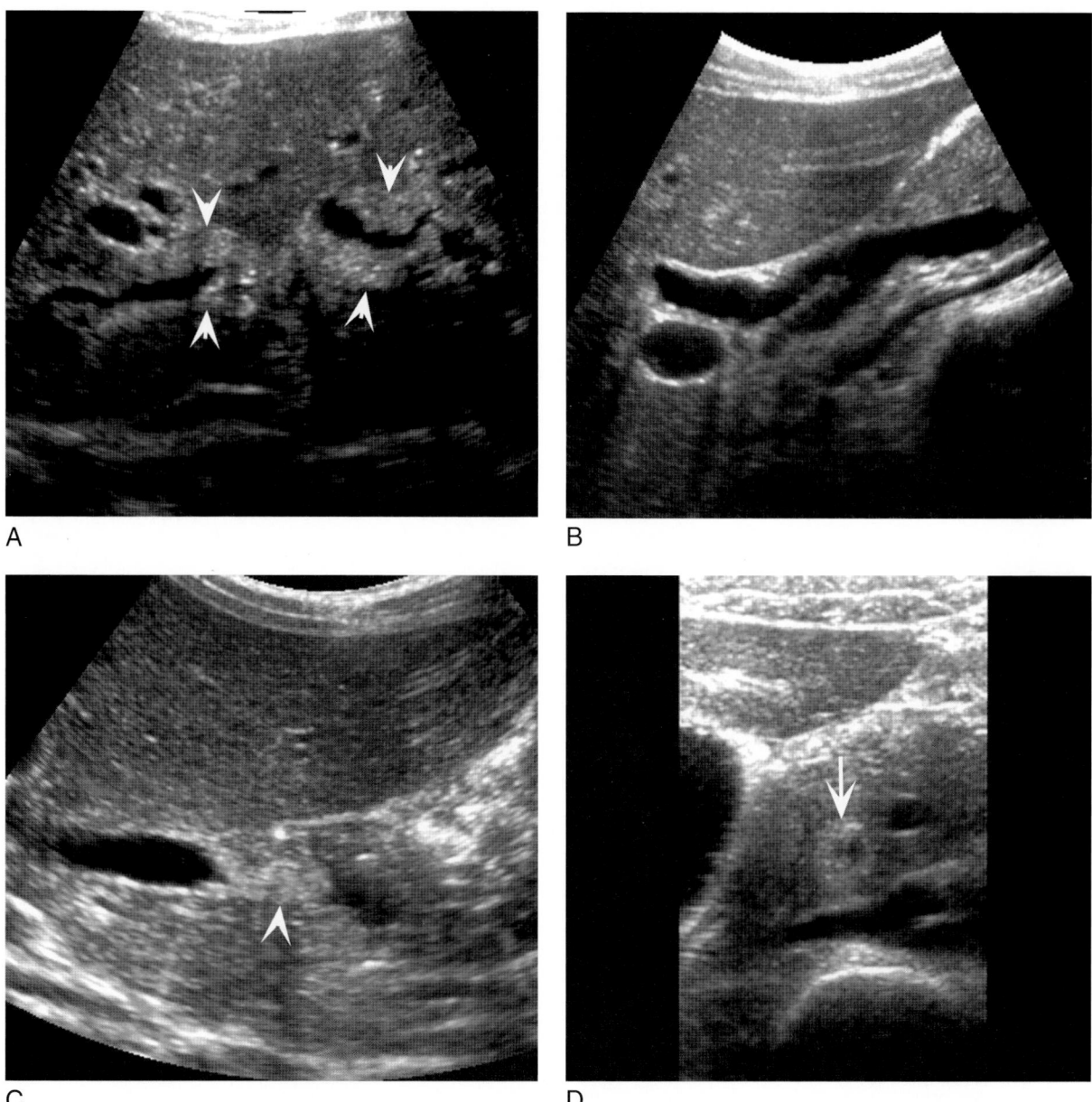

FIGURE 6-16. HIV cholangiopathy. A, Intrahepatic biliary tree. Note the thick rind of echogenic tissue (*arrowheads*) surrounding the central portal triads and causing irregular narrowing of the bile ducts. **B, Common bile duct** (CBD) is dilated and its wall is minimally irregular. **C, Papillary stenosis.** The dilated CBD abruptly tapers in an echogenic, inflamed ampulla (*arrowhead*). **D, Transverse view of ampulla** (*arrow*), which is enlarged and echogenic, viewed in the caudal aspect of pancreatic head.

Primary Sclerosing Cholangitis

Sclerosing cholangitis (SC) is a chronic inflammatory disease process affecting the biliary tree. If the etiology of the disease is unknown, the term primary sclerosing cholangitis is used; the causes of secondary SC are listed in Table 6-2.

Primary sclerosing cholangitis is a chronic disease affecting the entire biliary tree. The process involves a **fibrosing inflammation** of the small and large bile ducts leading to **biliary strictures and cholestasis**, and eventually to biliary cirrhosis, portal hypertension, and

hepatic failure.[33,34] It occurs more frequently in men, with median age of 39 years at diagnosis.[35] About 80% of the patients have concomitant inflammatory bowel disease, typically **ulcerative colitis**, but this association occurs less often in a non-Western population. It may also occur in conjunction with other autoimmune disorders or systemic sclerosing conditions (such as retroperitoneal fibrosis).[27]

Most patients diagnosed with primary sclerosing cholangitis are asymptomatic. **Sonographic findings** include irregular, circumferential bile duct wall thickening of varying degree, encroaching on and narrowing

TABLE 6-2. CAUSES OF SECONDARY SCLEROSING CHOLANGITIS

AIDS cholangiopathy
Bile duct neoplasm (PSC previously not established)
Biliary tract surgery, trauma
Choledocholithiasis
Congenital abnormalities of the biliary tract
Ischemic stricturing of bile ducts
Toxic strictures related to intra-arterial infusion of
    floxuridine
Post-treatment for hydatid cyst

PSC, Primary sclerosing cholangitis. From Narayanan Menon KV, Wiesner RH: Etiology and natural history of primary sclerosing cholangitis. J Hepatobiliary Pancreat Surg 1999;6(14):343-351.

the lumen (Fig. 6-17). **Focal strictures and dilations** of the bile ducts ensue. The extrahepatic disease is more easily visible. A high degree of suspicion and careful examination of the portal triads in all hepatic segments is required to detect intrahepatic ductal involvement. An earlier study suggested false normal appearance of the intrahepatic bile ducts in 25% of patients.[36] The gallbladder and cystic duct are involved in 15% to 20% of patients.[37] Choledocholithiasis, once thought to exclude the disease, is now recognized as a complication and is more frequently seen in symptomatic patients.[38] In more advanced cases, findings of cirrhosis are also present.

Cholangiocarcinoma develops in 7% to 30% of patients with primary sclerosing cholangitis and is particularly a difficult diagnosis to make in this setting.[34] Rapid progression of the disease or development of a visible mass is a clue to this complication. Hepatic

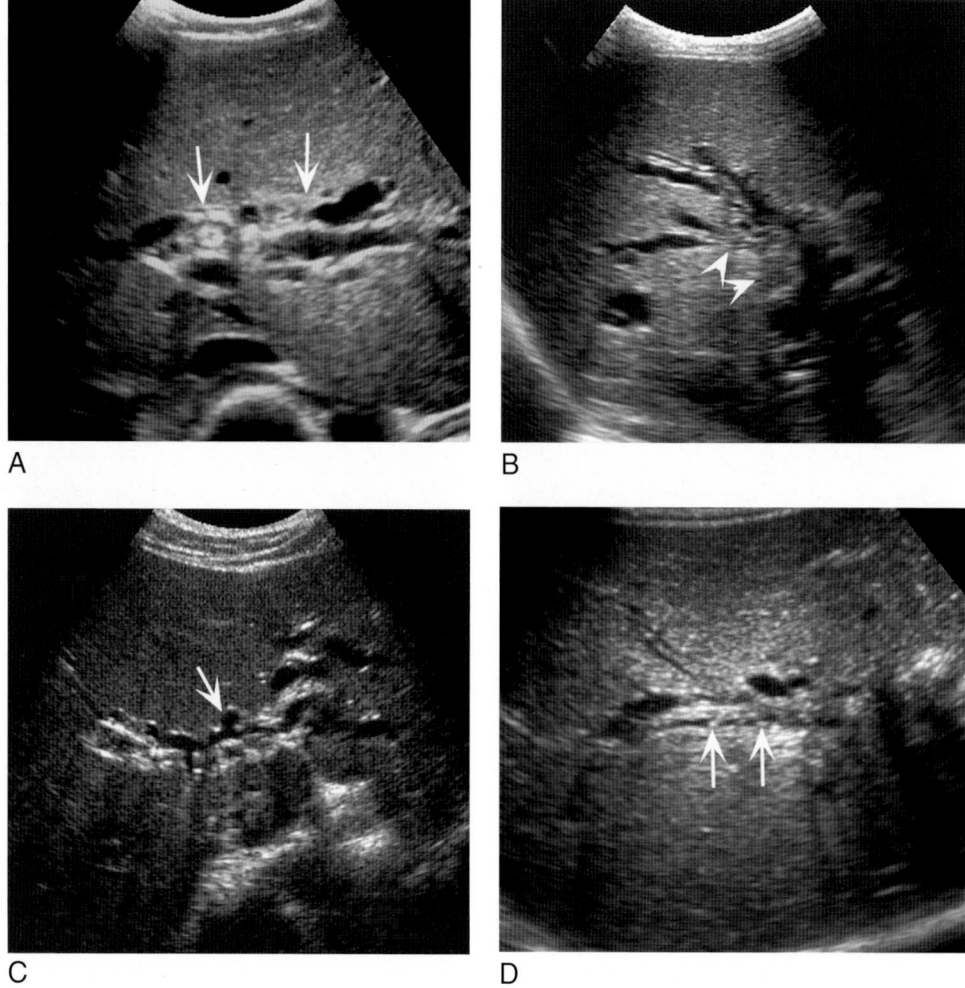

A

B

C

D

FIGURE 6-17. Primary sclerosing cholangitis. A, Isoechoic inflammatory tissue causing obliteration of the right and left hepatic ducts (*arrows*) with proximal dilation. **B, Dilated intrahepatic ducts** "rat-tail" as they extend centrally toward the hepatic hilum. Note the hypoechoic ductal/periductal tissue obstructing the central ducts (*arrowheads*). **C, Saccular diverticuli** (*arrow*) of the duct are occasionally seen. Note the variable caliber of the dilated ducts. **D, Minute intraductal stones** (*arrows*) are seen in irregular, mildly dilated ducts.

Continued

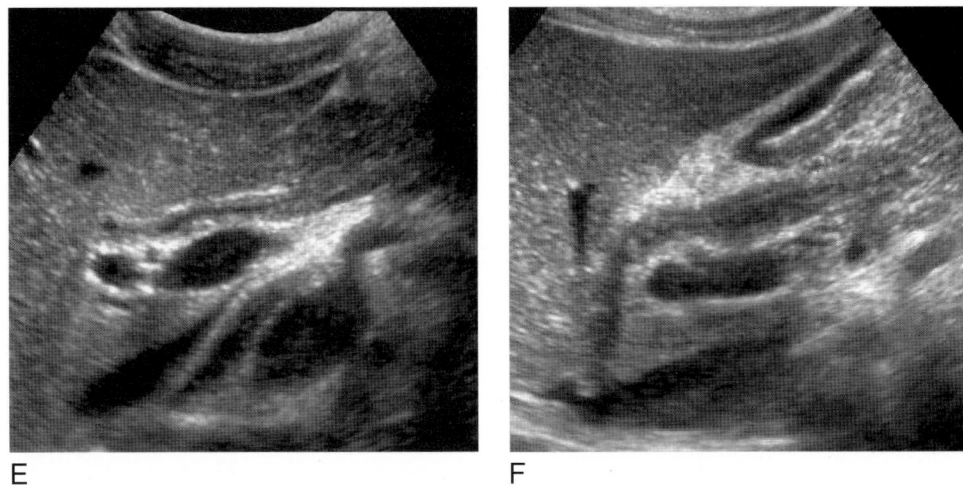

E   F

FIGURE 6-17, *cont'd*. Primary sclerosing cholangitis. E and F, **CBD wall thickening** of moderate and severe degrees, respectively. Note the markedly narrowed anechoic central lumen.

transplantation is required in the latter stages of the disease. Unfortunately, the disease may recur in the transplanted organ in 1% to 20% of patients.[39]

Cholangiocarcinoma

Cholangiocarcinoma is an uncommon neoplasm that may arise from any portion of the biliary tree. Its incidence varies geographically, being highest in populations harboring known risk factors. Overall incidence, per 100,000 population, ranges between 1 to 2 in the United States, 2 to 6 in other Western countries, 5.5 in Japan, and up to 80 to 130 in northeastern Thailand, where the liver fluke *Opisthorchis viverrini* is endemic.[40,41] The frequency of cholangiocarcinomas increases with age, with the peak incidence in the 8th decade of life. The majority of cholangiocarcinomas are **sporadic**; however, there are a number of risk factors, most of which are related to chronic biliary stasis and inflammation (see Table 6-1). Primary sclerosing cholangitis is the most common risk factor in the Western world; the lifetime risk of developing a clinically detectable cholangiocarcinoma in patients with PSC is approximately 10%.[42] The most common risk factors in other populations are recurrent biliary infections and stone disease.

Cholangiocarcinomas are **classified based on the anatomic location** as follows: **intrahepatic**, also called peripheral (~10%); **hilar**, also called **Klatskin's** (~60%); and **distal** (~30%).[43] Approximately 90% of cholangiocarcinomas are adenocarcinomas, with squamous carcinomas being the next most common subtype.[44] **Macroscopically**, they are divided into three subtypes: sclerosing, nodular, and papillary. Because the first two subtypes frequently occur together, the term **nodular-sclerosing** has been used to describe them. Nodular-sclerosing tumors, the most common subtype, appear as a firm mass surrounding and narrowing the affected duct, with a nodular intraductal component. Most hilar cholangiocarcinomas are of the nodular-sclerosing variety. These tumors incite a prominent desmoplastic reaction and demonstrate a periductal, perineural, and lymphatic pattern of spread along the ducts, as well as subendothelial spread within the ducts. Papillary tumors represent approximately 10% of all cholangiocarcinomas and are most common in the distal CBD. Patients present with an intraductal polypoid mass that expands, rather than constricts, the duct.[43,45,46] The overall **prognosis** for cholangiocarcinoma is dismal. In one single-center, large series, the 5-year survival rates for patients with intrahepatic, hilar, and distal cholangiocarcinoma have been reported to be 23%, 6%, and 24%, respectively, and improve to only 44%, 11%, and 28%, respectively, in patients who underwent resection.[47]

Intrahepatic Cholangiocarcinoma

Intrahepatic cholangiocarcinomas are the least common location for cholangiocarcinomas, but they represent the second most common primary malignancy of the liver. They arise from the second or higher order branches of the biliary tree within the liver parenchyma, and their histologic origin is different than that of extrahepatic ducts. The incidence of intrahepatic cholangiocarcinomas has been dramatically rising in the past 2 decades, due in part to the increase in numbers of patients with liver cirrhosis and long-term hepatitis C infection.[48,49] These tumors are associated with a poor prognosis because the mass is often unresectable.[50,51]

The most common manifestation of intrahepatic cholangiocarcinoma is that of a large hepatic mass. The sonographic appearance is often that of a hypovascular solid mass with heterogeneous echotexture, and it may appear hypo-, iso- or hyperechoic (Fig. 6-18). A clue to

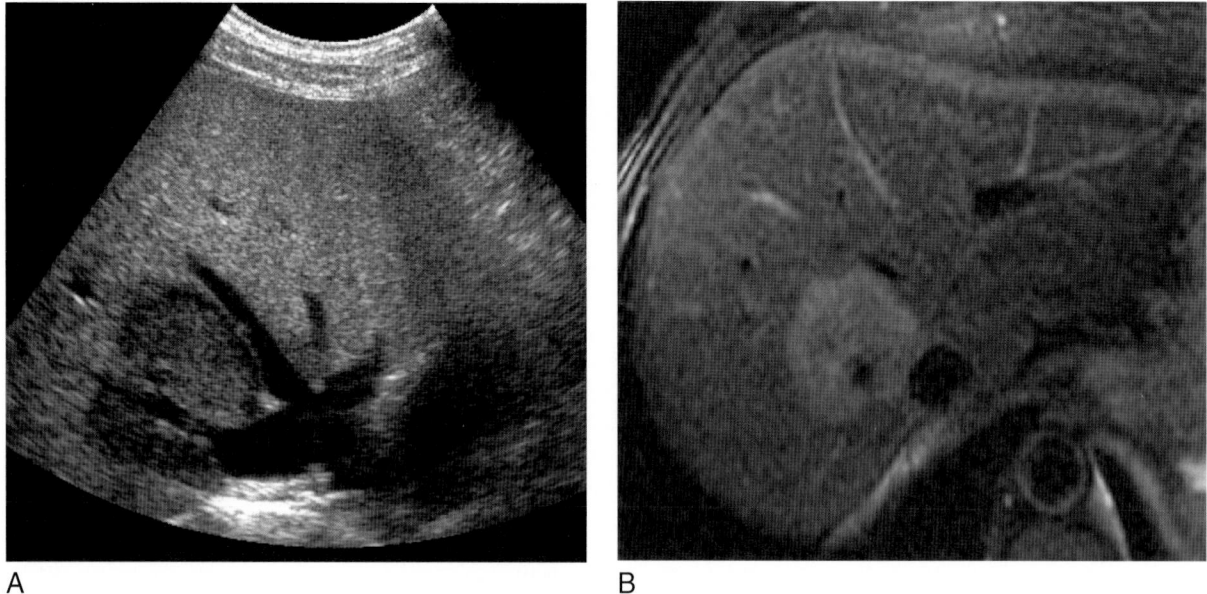

A   B

FIGURE 6-18. Peripheral cholangiocarcinoma. A, Ultrasound and B, T2W MRI depict a solid mass encasing the right hepatic vein. Differentiation from a metastasis is not possible by imaging.

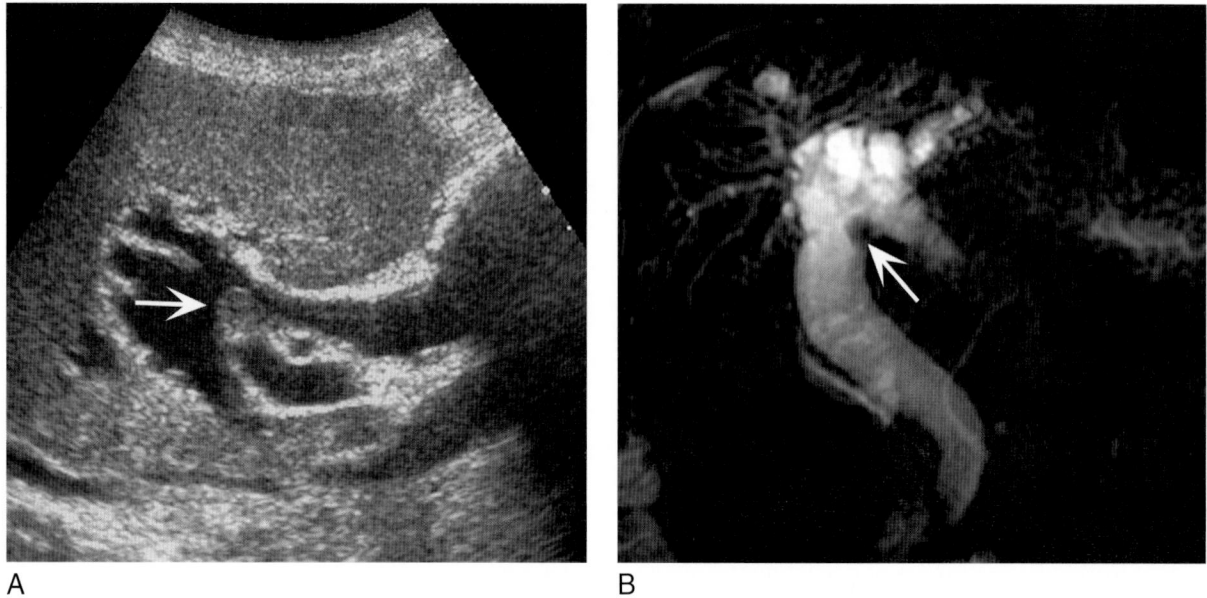

A   B

FIGURE 6-19. Intraductal papillary mucin-producing tumor of bile ducts. A, Ultrasound and B, MRCP show papillary tumor arising from the common hepatic duct (*arrow*) and causing diffuse ductal dilation due to excessive mucin production.

the differentiation from hepatocellular carcinoma (HCC) is a much higher incidence of ductal obstruction, reportedly occurring in 31% of intrahepatic cholangiocarcinomas and only 2% of HCC.[52,53] However, metastasis to the liver not uncommonly may cause intrahepatic ductal obstruction and, therefore, may be indistinguishable.[54]

A more unusual manifestation of intrahepatic cholangiocarcinoma is that of a purely intraductal mass. These are polypoid masses distending the affected ducts, often third or fourth order branches, spreading within

the duct and filling it with mucin. These tumors have a much better prognosis and are thought to be histologically separate from other intrahepatic cholangiocarcinomas, resembling papillary tumors of the extrahepatic bile ducts.[51,55]

The most common appearance of the intraductal intrahepatic cholangiocarcinoma is one or more polypoid masses confined to the bile ducts. Abundant mucin production can markedly distend the affected lobar and distal ducts (Fig. 6-19). A less common form may present as a solid mass within a cystic

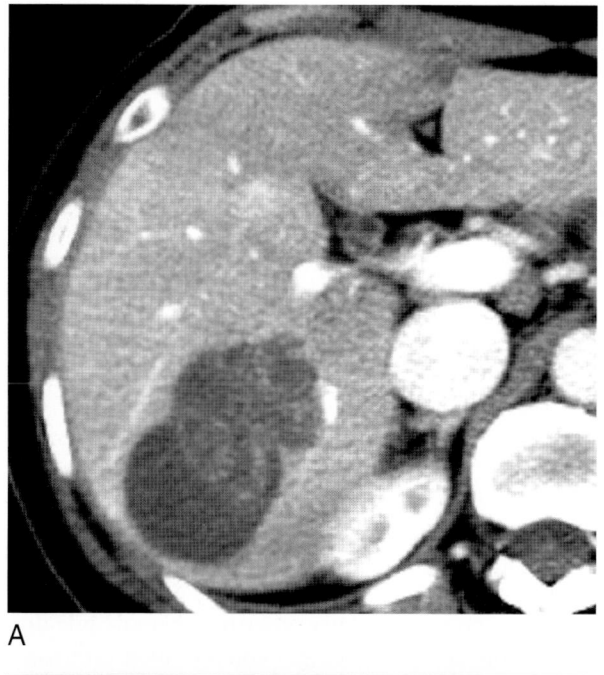

A

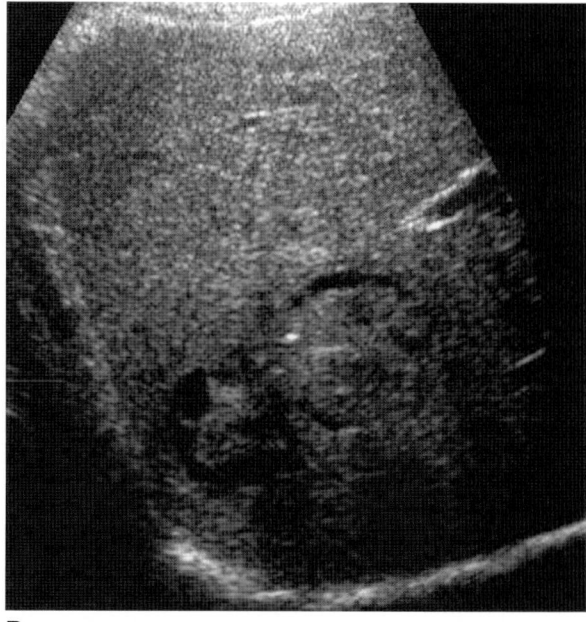

B

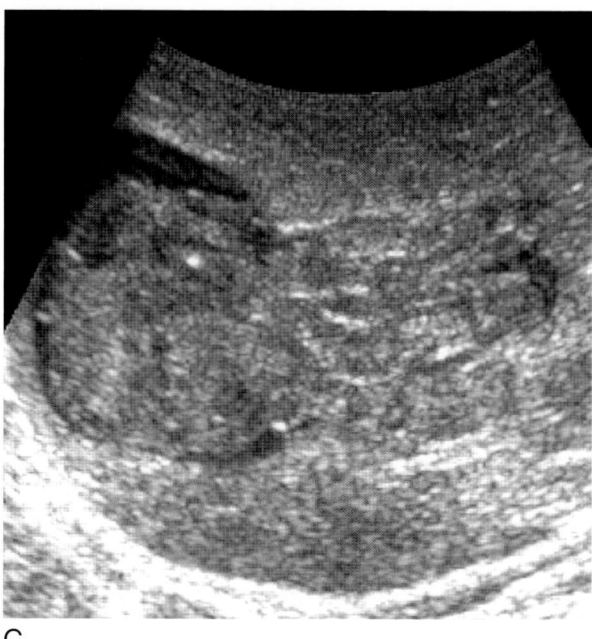

C

FIGURE 6-20. Intraductal intrahepatic cholangiocarcinoma. A, CT and **B, ultrasound** show a solid and cystic mass in the right lobe of the liver. **C, Intraoperative ultrasound** demonstrates the mass to lie entirely within a markedly dilated duct. Low-grade cholangiocarcinoma was found at pathologic examination.

structure, representing tumor within a markedly distended duct that does not communicate with the biliary tree (Fig. 6-20).

Hilar Cholangiocarcinoma

The correct identification and staging of hilar cholangiocarcinoma is challenging with all imaging modalities. This is due to the desmoplastic nature of the tumor, its peribiliary and subendothelial patterns of growth, and the complex anatomy of the porta hepatis with structures lying just outside the liver and surrounded by connective tissue. Ultrasound plays an important role in

both detection and staging of hilar cholangiocarcinomas because it is often the first modality used in assessment of these tumors. Furthermore, ultrasound is often performed prior to any biliary manipulation and stent placement. As biliary intervention often significantly obscures the intraductal disease and causes secondary bile duct thickening, sonography may be the only cross-sectional modality to assess the unmanipulated ducts. Most patients with hilar cholangiocarcinoma present for a sonographic evaluation with jaundice, pruritus, and elevated cholestatic liver parameters, or with vague symptoms and elevated serum alkaline phosphatase or gamma glutamyltranspeptidase levels.

Patterns of Tumor Growth and Staging. Hilar cholangiocarcinomas often begin in either the right or left bile ducts and extend both proximally into higher order branches and distally into the common hepatic duct and contralateral bile ducts. The spread of tumor may be subendothelial, or within the peribiliary connective tissue, leading to obstruction or irregular ductal narrowing. The tumors also extend outside of the ducts to involve adjacent portal vein and arteries. Chronic obstruction, especially if accompanied with portal vein involvement, leads to atrophy of the involved lobe. Nodal disease often begins in the porta hepatis and within the hepatoduodenal ligaments (local nodes) and extending to celiac, superior mesenteric, peripancreatic, and posterior pancreatoduodenal stations (distant nodes).[56] **Metastases** are usually to the liver and peritoneal surfaces.

Curative treatment of cholangiocarcinoma requires surgical resection; the vast majority of patients with unresectable disease die within 12 months of diagnosis.[43] The current **surgical approach** to patients with hilar cholangiocarcinoma is resection of the involved lobe with extensive hilar dissection to remove tumor extending to the contralateral lobe (an extended lobectomy). A biliary-enteric anastomosis is created to allow bile drainage. There are currently no widely used staging systems that accurately stratify patients based on surgical resectability. Jarnagin et al. have recently proposed a new system, however, which allows for preoperative staging of hilar cholangiocarcinoma.[56] Because a lobectomy is performed, the remaining liver parenchyma, its portal vein, hepatic artery, and at least some proximal length of its lobar bile duct (first order branch of the common hepatic duct) should be free of disease. The main portal vein and proper hepatic artery should also be disease free. The remaining liver should not have undergone significant atrophy because it may not be able to maintain hepatic function. Although regional nodes may be removed *en-bloc* with the tumor, distant nodal disease precludes resection. The criteria of nonresectability are listed in Table 6-3.

Assessment by Conventional Gray-Scale and Doppler Sonography. An accurate assessment of hilar cholangiocarcinoma requires a patient and diligent, hands-on involvement by the responsible physician. The use of various views and patient positions as well as familiarity with biliary anatomy and common variants significantly improves sonographic performance. Once dilated intrahepatic ducts have been detected, the following parameters should be assessed:

- The level of the obstruction
- The presence of a mass
- Lobar atrophy
- Patency of main, right, and left portal veins
- Encasement of hepatic artery

TABLE 6-3. CRITERIA FOR UNRESECTABLE HILAR CHOLANGIOCARCINOMA*

Hepatic duct involvement up to secondary biliary radicles bilaterally
Encasement or occlusion of the main portal vein proximal to its bifurcation
Atrophy of one hepatic lobe with encasement of contralateral portal vein branch
Atrophy of one hepatic lobe with contralateral involvement of secondary biliary radicles
Distant metastases (peritoneum, liver, and lung)

From Jarnagin WR: Cholangiocarcinoma of the extrahepatic bile ducts. Semin Surg Oncol 2000;19:156-176.

- Local and distant adenopathy
- Presence of metastases

Dilation of the higher order intrahepatic bile ducts with non-union of the right and left ducts is the classic appearance of hilar cholangiocarcinomas (Fig. 6-21).[54] When dilated ducts are encountered, they should be followed centrally toward the hepatic hilum to determine which order branching (segmental ducts and higher or right/left hepatic ducts) is involved with tumor. Tumor extension into segmental ducts bilaterally precludes resection.

The obstructing tumor is not always visualized by sonography. Various studies have reported rates of mass detection from 21% to 87%, with more recent studies showing higher rates.[57,58,59] When a mass is not directly visualized, its presence can be inferred based on the level of obstruction, though this often underestimates the tumor extent.[60] **Lobar atrophy** (Fig. 6-22) leads to crowding of the dilated bile ducts and, if longstanding, a shift in the axis of the liver due to hypertrophy of the contralateral side. The atrophy of the lobe is often accompanied by obliteration of its portal vein, and precludes its resection. **Differences in lobar echogenicity**, due to the varying degree of ductal and vascular obstruction between the two lobes, is an uncommon finding (see Fig. 6-22).

The main, right, and left portal veins should all be examined with both gray-scale and color Doppler sonography. **Narrowing of the right or left portal veins leads to compensatory increased flow in the accompanying hepatic artery**; when prominent arterial signal is noted on color Doppler, the portal venous flow should be carefully examined (see Fig. 6-22). Tumor encasing, narrowing, or obliterating the main portal vein or the proper hepatic artery renders the tumor unresectable. The detection of the extrahepatic tumor infiltration and early peritoneal metastases is difficult with sonography, and CT or MRI scan is recommended as an adjunct study for preoperative assessment.

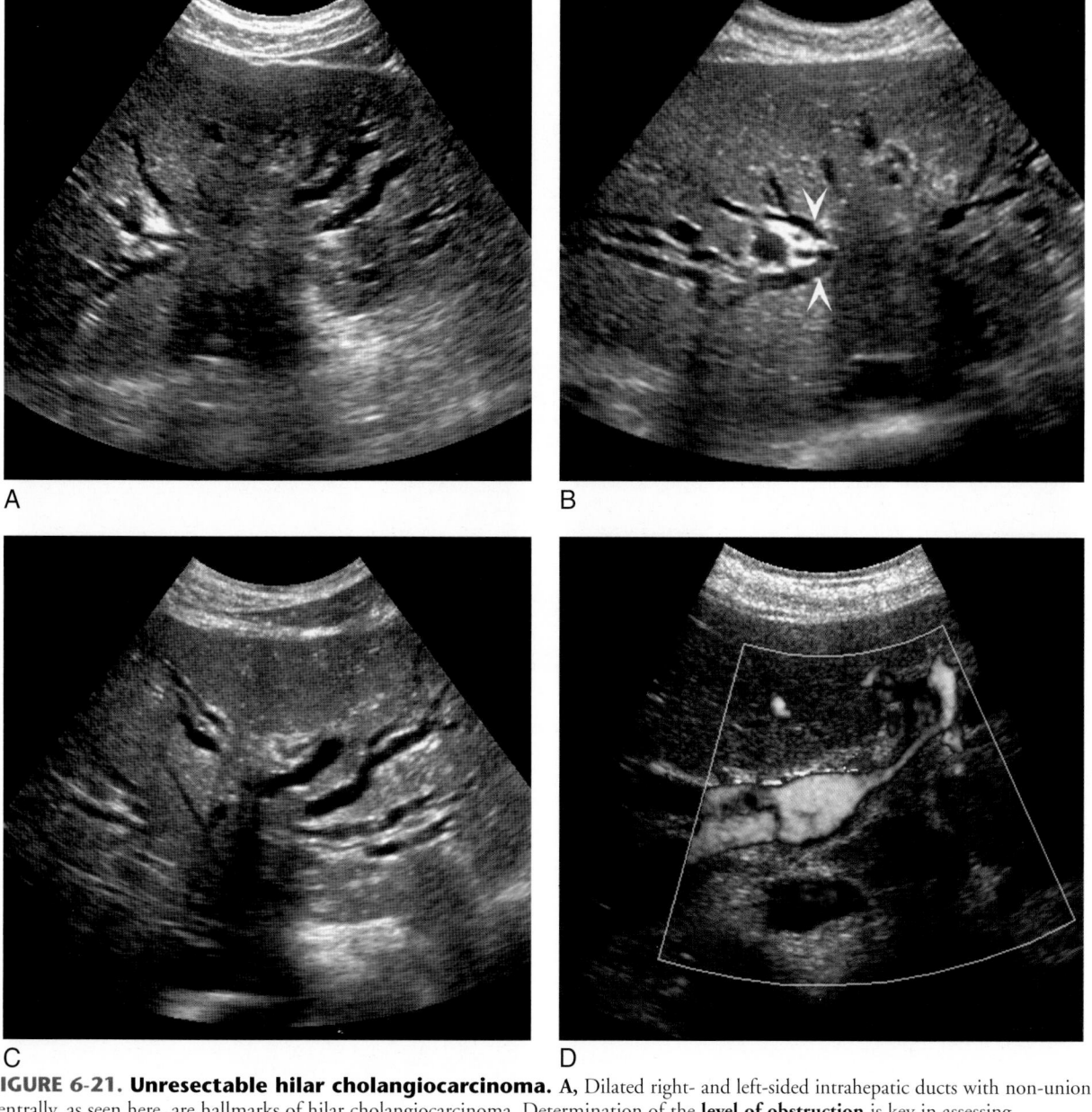

FIGURE 6-21. Unresectable hilar cholangiocarcinoma. A, Dilated right- and left-sided intrahepatic ducts with non-union centrally, as seen here, are hallmarks of hilar cholangiocarcinoma. Determination of the **level of obstruction** is key in assessing resectability. **B, Right lobe,** the right anterior and posterior ducts (*arrowheads*) approach each other, but never join to form the right hepatic duct. **C, Left lobe,** second and third order branches end abruptly because they are blocked by tumor. Because the tumor completely involves the first order branches (right and left hepatic ducts) bilaterally, it is unresectable. **D,** The tumor also encases and narrows the **left portal vein.**

Assessment by Contrast Enhanced Sonography. Some ultrasound contrast agents persist in the liver parenchyma after a brief intravascular phase. This **postvascular**, liver-specific phase of enhancement significantly increases the contrast difference between the liver parenchyma and invasive tumors that do not enhance. Therefore, the invasive component of cholangiocarcinoma—not seen in a significant minority of patients—becomes visible in most, if not all, cases (Fig. 6-23).[60] The ability to directly visualize the invasive tumor also allows for improved performance of sono-

graphy in the staging of hilar cholangiocarcinomas.[60] Currently, Levovist is the most widely used agent with this postvascular, liver-specific phase of enhancement, although some second-generation ultrasound contrast agents under development also have the same property.

Distal Cholangiocarcinoma

Distal cholangiocarcinomas are clinically indistinguishable from the hilar forms, with progressive jaundice seen in 75% to 90% of patients.[43] Although the nodular

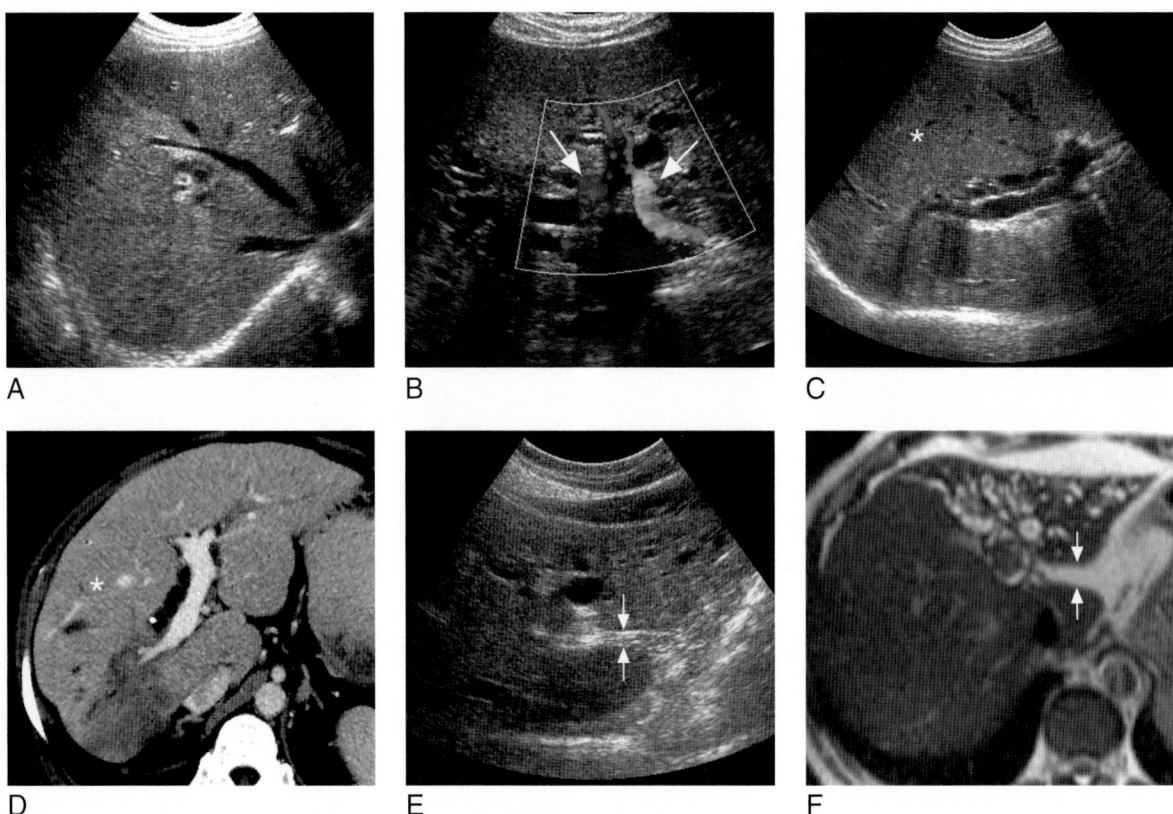

FIGURE 6-22. Secondary findings in hilar cholangiocarcinoma. A, Difference in lobar echogenicity. The right lobe of the liver is demarcated from the left by its increased echogenicity. The right biliary system was obstructed by tumor centrally. **B, Compensatory increased flow in hepatic arteries.** Enlarged hepatic arterial branches (*arrows*) on either side of the ascending branch of the left portal vein are clearly seen, whereas no flow is noted in the portal vein. This finding suggests severe stenosis or obstruction of the portal vein. **C and D, Lobar atrophy.** There is marked atrophy of the right lobe with compensatory hypertrophy of the left. Enlarged medial segment of the left lobe (*asterisk*). **E and F, Lobar atrophy.** There is marked atrophy of the left lobe of the liver. Apart from the small size, widening of the fissure for ligamentum venosum (*arrows*) and concave liver margins are secondary clues. **F,** Axial SSFSE T2W MR image shows the same.

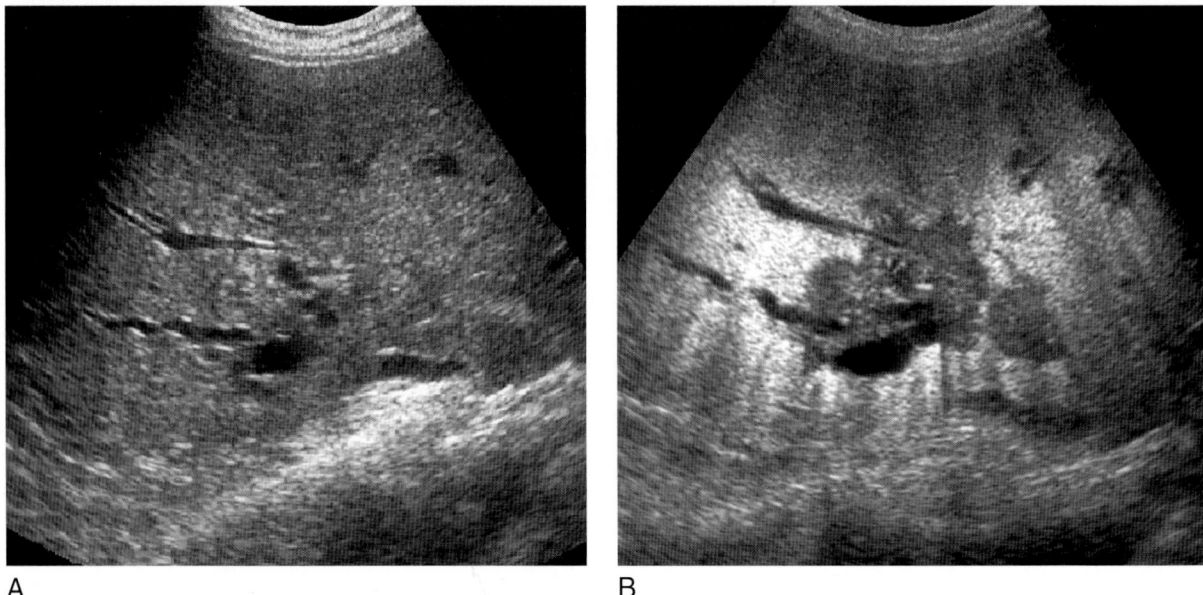

FIGURE 6-23. Cholangiocarcinoma. Evaluation with ultrasound contrast. **A,** Routine gray-scale image demonstrates dilated ducts terminating abruptly. The tumor is not visible. **B,** Levovist-enhanced image obtained in the postvascular phase clearly depicts the margins of the nonenhancing tumor.

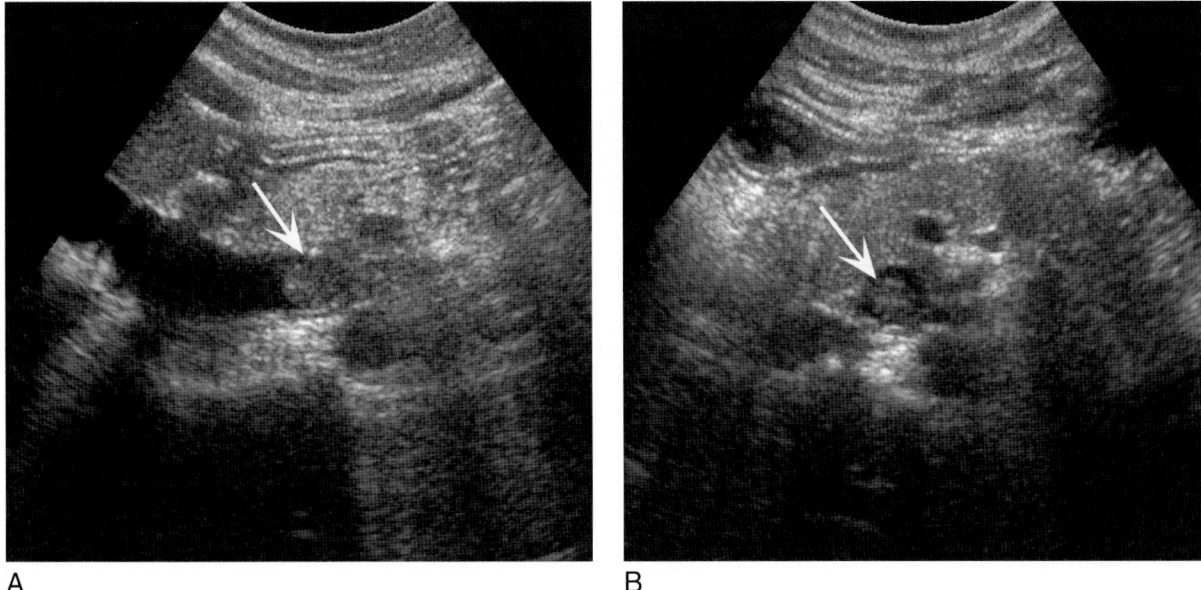

A   B

FIGURE 6-24. Distal cholangiocarcinoma. A and **B,** Polypoid solid intraductal mass (*arrows*) within the distal common bile duct causing ductal obstruction.

sclerosing type still predominates, polypoid masses are seen more frequently. Surgical resection is the most effective therapy; therefore, a careful search for spread that would preclude resection is vital. The tumor may locally extend cranially within the ducts, even involving the cystic and right and left hepatic ducts. Therefore, the superior extent of the tumor must be clearly defined. The tumor may also extend beyond the duct walls. Patients may present with a distal obstructive mass with identical appearance to pancreatic adenocarcinoma. The status of the adjacent vascular structures, including the portal and superior mesenteric veins and the common hepatic artery, must be determined. Spread to lymph nodes adjacent to the tumor is common. Spread to more distant nodes, such as celiac, superior mesenteric, and periportal regions may preclude resection.[43] Surgical approach to a **distal cholangiocarcinoma** is a pancreaticoduodenectomy.

On **sonography**, the **distal cholangiocarcinoma** may have several appearances. A polypoid tumor appears as a duct-expanding, well-defined intraductal mass often with no internal vascularity (Fig. 6-24). The nodular-sclerosing subtype causes focal irregular ductal constriction and duct wall thickening. In more advanced disease, the tumor appears as a hypoechoic, hypovascular mass with poorly defined margins invading adjacent structures.

Metastases to the Biliary Tree

Metastases to the biliary tree mimic the different appearances of cholangiocarcinoma, affecting both the intra- and extrahepatic ducts (Fig. 6-25). The history of past or concurrent malignancy, along with multiplicity, should raise the possibility of metastases. Breast, colon, and melanoma constitute the majority of primary sites of malignancy in our experience.

THE GALLBLADDER

The Anatomy of the Gallbladder and Normal Variants

The gallbladder is a pear-shaped organ lying in the inferior margin of the liver, between the right and left lobes (Fig. 6-26). The middle hepatic vein lies in the same anatomic plane and may be used to help find the gallbladder fossa. The **interlobar fissure**, the third structure separating the two hepatic lobes, extends from the origin of the right portal vein to the gallbladder fossa. It has been seen in up to 70% of hepatic ultrasounds[61] and may also be used as a landmark for the **gallbladder fossa**. The **gallbladder** is divided into the fundus, body, and neck, with the fundus being the most anterior, and often inferior, segment. In the region of the neck, there may be an infundibulum, called **Hartmann's Pouch**, which is a common location for impaction of gallstones.[10]

Consumption of food, particularly of a fatty nature, stimulates gallbladder contraction. The contracted gallbladder appears thick walled and may obscure luminal or wall abnormalities. Therefore, examination of the gallbladder should be performed after a minimum of 4 hours of fasting.

The gallbladder derives as an outpouching from the embryonic biliary tree. The proximal portion of the

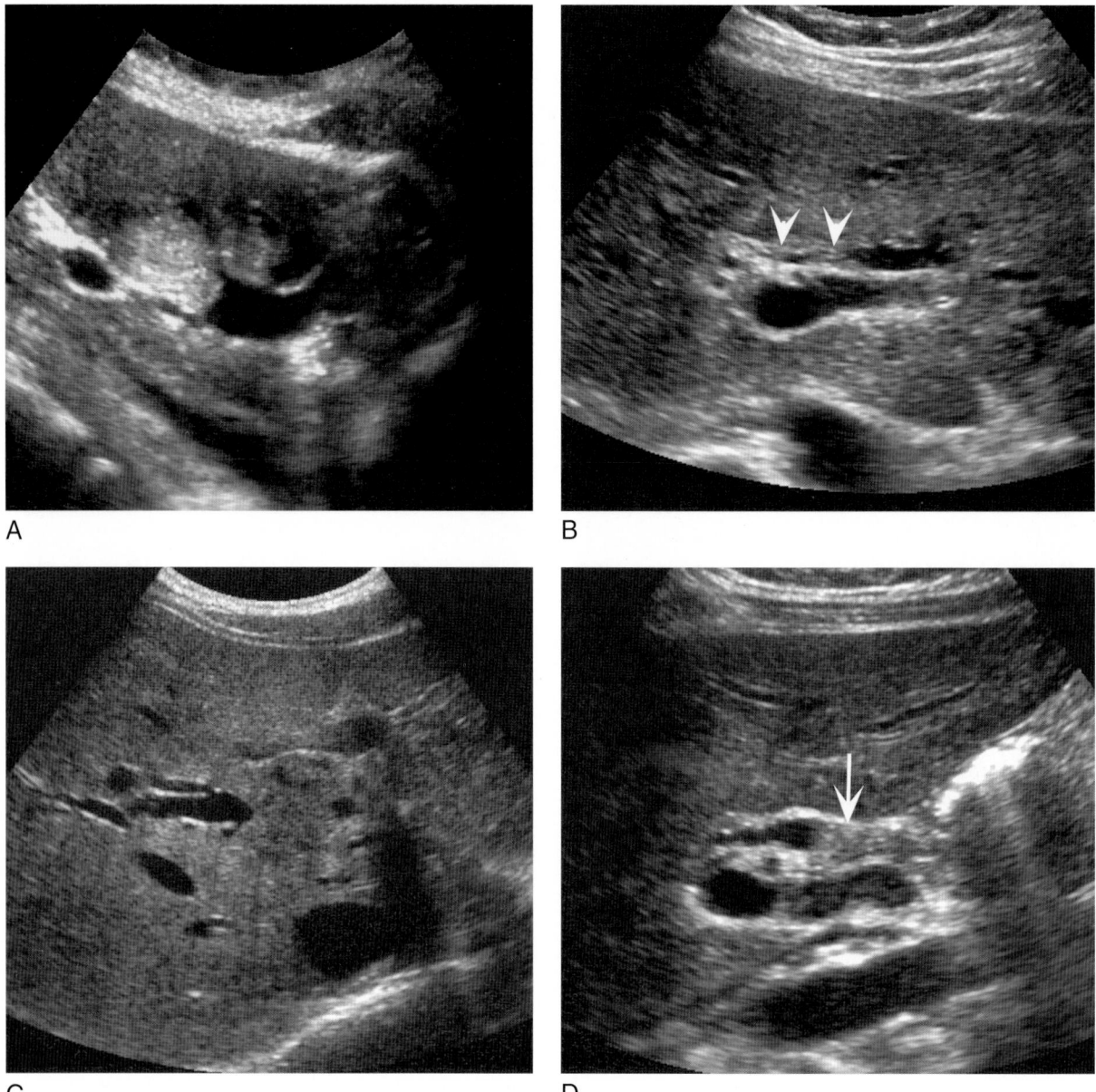

FIGURE 6-25. Metastases to the biliary tree—spectrum of appearances. A, Entirely intraductal echogenic mass obstructing left lobe of liver. **B,** Periductal/duct wall infiltration (*arrowheads*) with obliteration of the left hepatic duct. **C,** Poorly defined hilar tumor with ductal obstruction. **D,** Echogenic intraductal tumor (*arrow*) within the extrahepatic ducts. In all cases, tumor mimics cholangiocarcinoma. The diagnosis in all four images was metastatic breast carcinoma.

pouch forms the cystic duct, the distal portion forming the gallbladder. Within the cystic duct and sometimes the gallbladder neck, small mucosal folds exist called the **spiral valves of Heister**; these are occasionally identified on sonography. During its initial development, the gallbladder lies in an intrahepatic position, but as it migrates to the surface of the liver, it acquires a peritoneal covering (part of the liver capsule) over 50% to 70% of its surface.[10] The remainder of the gallbladder surface is covered with adventitial tissue that merges with connective tissue in contiguity with the liver. In generalized edematous processes or local inflammation, this potential space between the gallbladder and liver is a common

area for edema to collect. Failure to migrate may lead to an intrahepatic, or partially **intrahepatic, gallbladder,** a rare but significant finding that may preclude laparoscopic surgery.[62] Conversely, the gallbladder may become fully enveloped in visceral peritoneum, hanging from a mesentery that extends from the liver. This leads to increased mobility of the gallbladder and appears to be a risk factor in the rare development of torsion (volvulus) of the gallbladder.[63]

Failure to identify the gallbladder on sonographic examination is most often due to a previous cholecystectomy. Occasionally, chronic cholecystitis leading to a collapsed and fibrosed gallbladder makes its detection

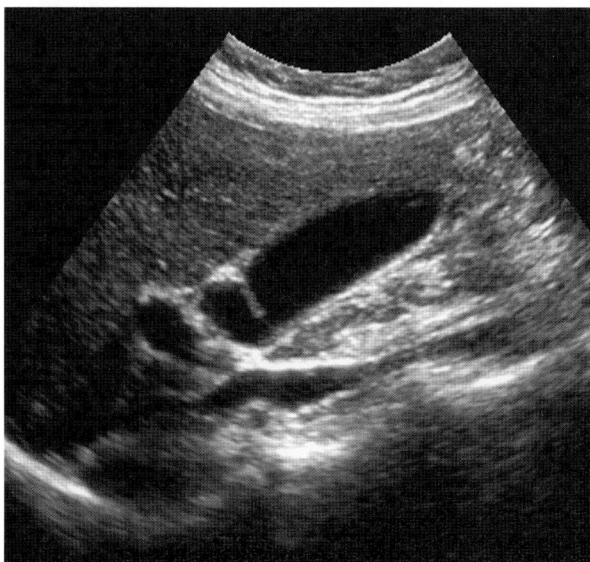

FIGURE 6-26. Normal gallbladder. Normal gallbladder showing a thin fold.

difficult. **Agenesis of the gallbladder** is rare, occurring in up to 0.09% of the population.[64] Although most often incidental, dilation of the bile duct and choledocholithiasis may occur with gallbladder agenesis, leading to attempted cholecystectomies in some patients.[10] In the majority of the cases, the cystic duct is also absent. The lack of visualization of the gallbladder on sonography in symptomatic patients should lead to MRCP or ERCP to avoid an unnecessary surgical procedure. The gallbladder may also lie in **ectopic** positions, including suprahepatic, suprarenal, within the anterior abdominal wall, or in the falciform ligament.[10]

The gallbladder may fold unto itself the body onto the neck, or the fundus onto the body. The latter is called a **Phrygian cap** and has no clinical significance. A **septate gallbladder** is composed of two or more intercommunicating compartments divided by thin septa.[10] This is distinguished from the hourglass gallbladder (see adenomyomatosis) which has thick septa separating the components. **Duplication of the gallbladder** often occurs with duplication of the cystic duct and may be diagnosed prenatally. Variations of the cystic duct are discussed under the anatomy of the biliary tree.

The gallbladder derives its **blood supply** from the cystic artery, which arises from the right hepatic artery, or less commonly, from the gastroduodenal artery. In acute cholecystitis, an enlarged prominent cystic artery may be identified on sonography.

Sonographic Technique

Evaluation of the gallbladder is usually easily performed with routine sagittal and transverse sonograms. If the gallbladder is not visualized, however, maneuvers to evaluate the gallbladder fossa are essential to avoid missing gallbladder pathology. This is done primarily with subcostal oblique sonograms, performed with the left edge of the transducer more cephalad than the right edge. The face of the transducer is directed toward the right shoulder. A sweep from cephalad to caudad will show the middle hepatic vein superiorly and the gallbladder fossa inferiorly in a single plane as they form the anatomic boundary separating the right and left liver lobes. The fossa runs from the anterior surface of the right portal vein obliquely to the surface of the liver. It may have variable appearances largely influenced by the state of the gallbladder, and following its removal shows as an echogenic line related to the remaining connective tissues.

Ingestion of food, particularly of a fatty nature, stimulates the gallbladder to contract. The contracted gallbladder appears thick walled and may obscure luminal or wall abnormalities. Therefore, the examination of the gallbladder should be performed after a minimum of 4 hours of fasting.

Gallstone Disease

Gallstone disease is common worldwide. The prevalence of gallstones is highest in the European and North American populations (~10%) and lowest in the East Asian (~4%) and sub-Saharan African populations (2% to 5%).[65] Common risk factors are increasing age, female sex (not in the Asian populations), fecundity, obesity, diabetes, and pregnancy. Although most patients are asymptomatic, approximately one in five develops a complication, most usually biliary colic. The risk of acute cholecystitis or other serious complications of gallstones in patients with a history of biliary colic is about 1% to 2% per year.[66]

Sonography is highly sensitive in the detection of stones within the gallbladder. The variable size and number of stones within the gallbladder give them several different appearances on sonography (Fig. 6-27). The large difference in the acoustic impedance of stones and adjacent bile makes them highly reflective; this results in an echogenic appearance with strong posterior acoustic shadowing. Small stones (<5 mm) may not shadow, but will still appear echogenic. Mobility is a key feature of stones, allowing differentiation from polyps or other entities. Various maneuvers may be used to demonstrate mobility of a stone: scanning with the patient in the right or left lateral decubitus or upright standing positions may allow the stone to roll within the gallbladder.

Multiple stones may appear as one large stone, producing uniform acoustic shadowing. When the gallbladder is filled with small stones, or with a single giant stone, the gallbladder fossa will appear as an echogenic line with posterior shadowing. This can be

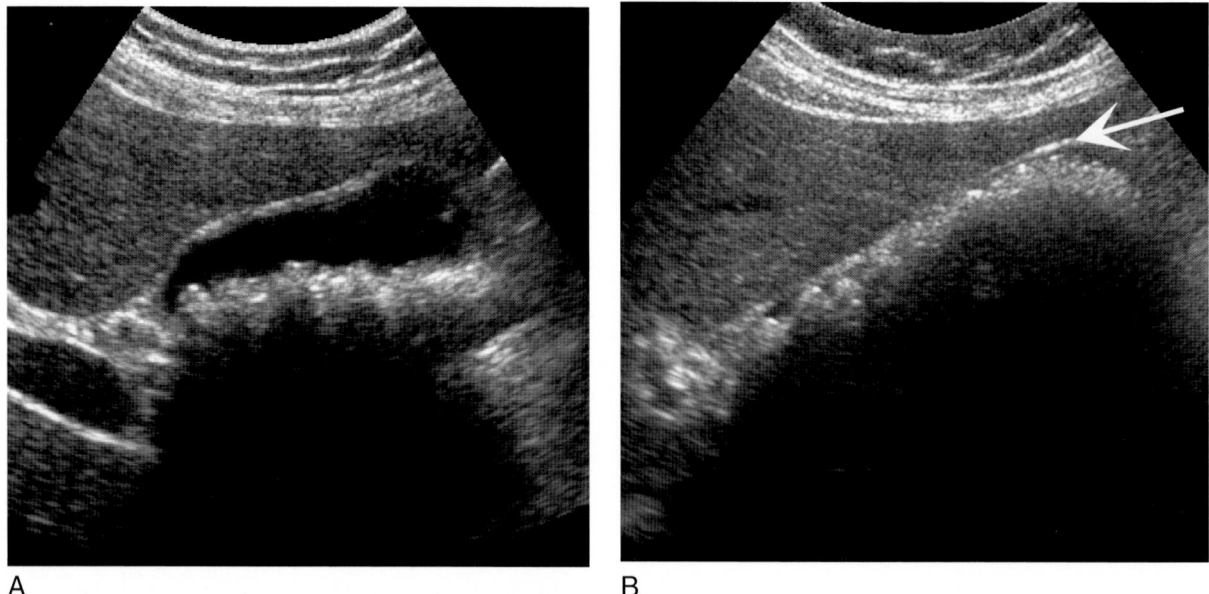

FIGURE 6-27. Gallbladder stones. A, Sagittal images show multiple dependent stones appearing as echogenic foci with posterior acoustic shadowing. **B, "Wall-echo-shadow complex"** in a gallbladder filled with stones. Gallbladder wall (*arrow*) is thin.

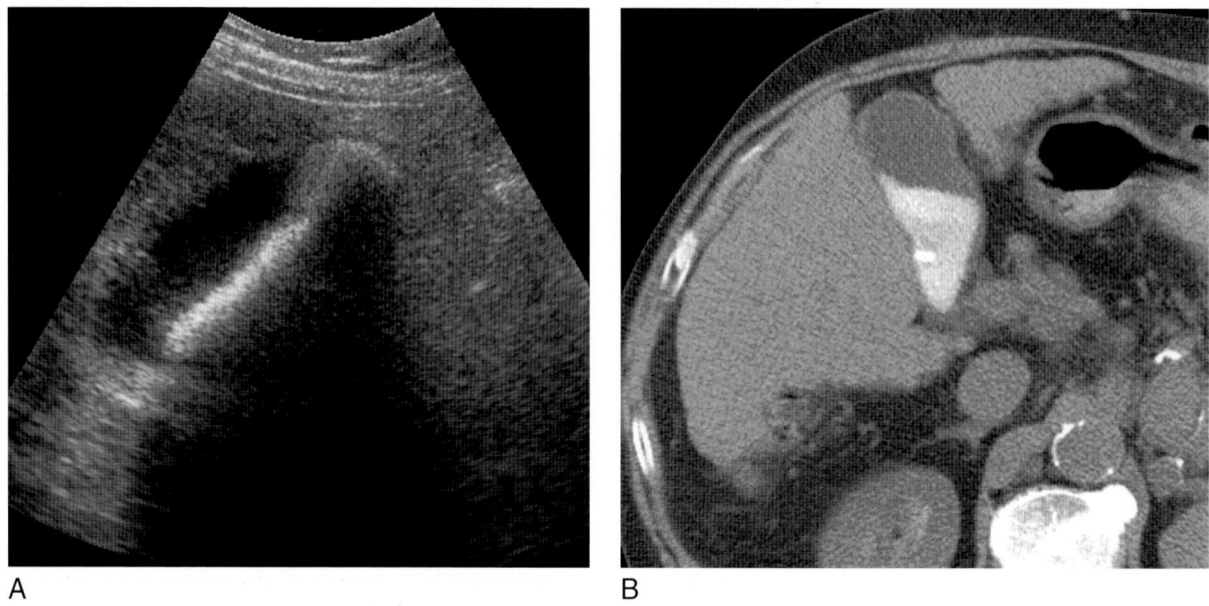

FIGURE 6-28. Milk of calcium bile. A, Sonogram and **B,** corresponding CT scan show a bile calcium level.

differentiated from air or calcification in the gallbladder wall by analysis of the echoes. In case of stones, the gallbladder wall is first visualized in the near field, followed by the bright echo of the stone, followed by the acoustic shadowing, the so-called, wall-echo-shadow or WES complex (see Fig. 6-27). When air or calcification is present, the normal gallbladder wall is not seen; only the bright echo and the posterior shadowing are seen.

Milk of calcium bile, also known as limey bile, is a rare condition in which the gallbladder becomes filled with a pasty semi-solid substance made mostly of calcium carbonate.[67] It is often associated with gall-

bladder stasis and rarely may cause acute cholecystitis or migrate into the bile ducts. The appearance on sonography is that of highly echogenic material with posterior acoustic shadowing, forming a level on various patient positions (Fig. 6-28).

Biliary Sludge

Biliary sludge, also known as *biliary sand* or *microlithiasis*, is defined as a mixture of particulate matter and bile that occurs when solutes in bile precipitate.[68] It was first recognized with the advent of sonography. The exact prevalence of sludge is unknown in the general population because most studies have examined high-risk populations. The predisposing factors in development of sludge are pregnancy, rapid weight loss, prolonged fasting, critical illness, long-term total parenteral nutrition (TPN), ceftriaxone or prolonged octreotide therapy, and bone marrow transplantation.[68] It has been suggested that over a 3-year period, approximately 50% of cases resolve spontaneously; approximately 20% persist asymptomatically; approximately 5% to 15% develop gallstones; and 10% to 15% become symptomatic.[68] The complications of biliary sludge are stone formation, biliary colic, acalculous cholecystitis, and pancreatitis.

The sonographic appearance of sludge is that of amorphous, low-level echoes within the gallbladder in a dependent position, with no acoustic shadowing (Fig. 6-29). With a change in the position of the patient, sludge may slowly resettle in the most dependent location. In fasting, critically ill patients, sludge may be present in large quantities and completely fill the gallbladder. Sludge may mimic polypoid tumors, so called **"tumefactive sludge."** Lack of internal vascularity, potential mobility of the sludge, and a normal gallbladder wall are all clues to the presence of sludge. When doubts persist, lack of contrast enhancement on CT or MRI allows conservative management. Occasionally, sludge has the same echotexture as the liver, leading to camouflage of the gallbladder. This has been called **"hepatization"** of the gallbladder and may be easily recognized by identifying the normal gallbladder wall (see Fig. 6-29).

Acute Cholecystitis

Acute cholecystitis is a relatively common disease, accounting for 5% of the patients presenting to the emergency department with abdominal pain, and 3% to 9% of hospital admissions.[69] It is caused by gallstones in more than 90% of cases.[70] Impaction of the stones in the cystic duct or the gallbladder neck results in obstruction with luminal distention, ischemia, superinfection, and eventually, necrosis of the gallbladder. Women have a three times higher incidence of acute cholecystitis than do men younger than 50 years of age, but similar incidence at higher age groups.[66] Clinically, patients present with a prolonged, constant right upper quadrant or epigastric pain associated with right upper quadrant tenderness. Fever, leukocytosis, and increased serum bilirubin and alkaline phosphatase levels all may be present.

Sonography is currently the most practical and accurate method of diagnosis of acute cholecystitis. The sensitivity and specificity of sonography, when adjusted for verification bias, is approximately 88% and 80%, respectively.[71] Cholescintigraphy uses ionizing radiation, cannot be performed at the bedside, and also has a significant false-positive rate. CT scanning has been found to be less accurate than sonography in the diagnosis of acute cholecystitis, although it may be useful for depiction of its complications.[72]

Sonographic findings include (Figures 6-30,[73] 6-31 and Table 6-4):

SONOGRAPHIC NONVISUALIZATION OF GALLBLADDER

CONSIDER

Previous cholecystectomy
Physiologic contraction
Fibrosed gallbladder duct—chronic cholecystitis
Air-filled gallbladder or emphysematous
  cholecystitis
Tumefacient sludge
Agenesis of gallbladder
Ectopic location

TABLE 6-4. ACUTE CALCULOUS CHOLECYSTITIS

Pathophysiology	Sonographic Appearance
Obstruction of the cystic duct or neck of the gallbladder	Stones in gallbladder, possibly in the neck or cystic duct
Continued secretions	Gallbladder distention
Inflammatory cell infiltration	Thickening of the gallbladder wall
AND	Often striated with pockets of edema fluid
Gallbladder wall edema	Positive sonographic Murphy's sign (>90%)
Hypervascularity	Hyperemia of the gallbladder wall
Gallbladder stasis with bacterial overgrowth by 72 hrs ⇒	Biliary sludge
Empyema of gallbladder	Heterogeneous luminal contents of variable echogenicity with layering
Increased pressure in the gallbladder lumen and wall ⇒	Sloughed membranes, hypovascularity,
Gangrene	Loss of Murphy's sign
Perforation	Loss of gourd-shaped collection in or adjacent to gallbladder fossa

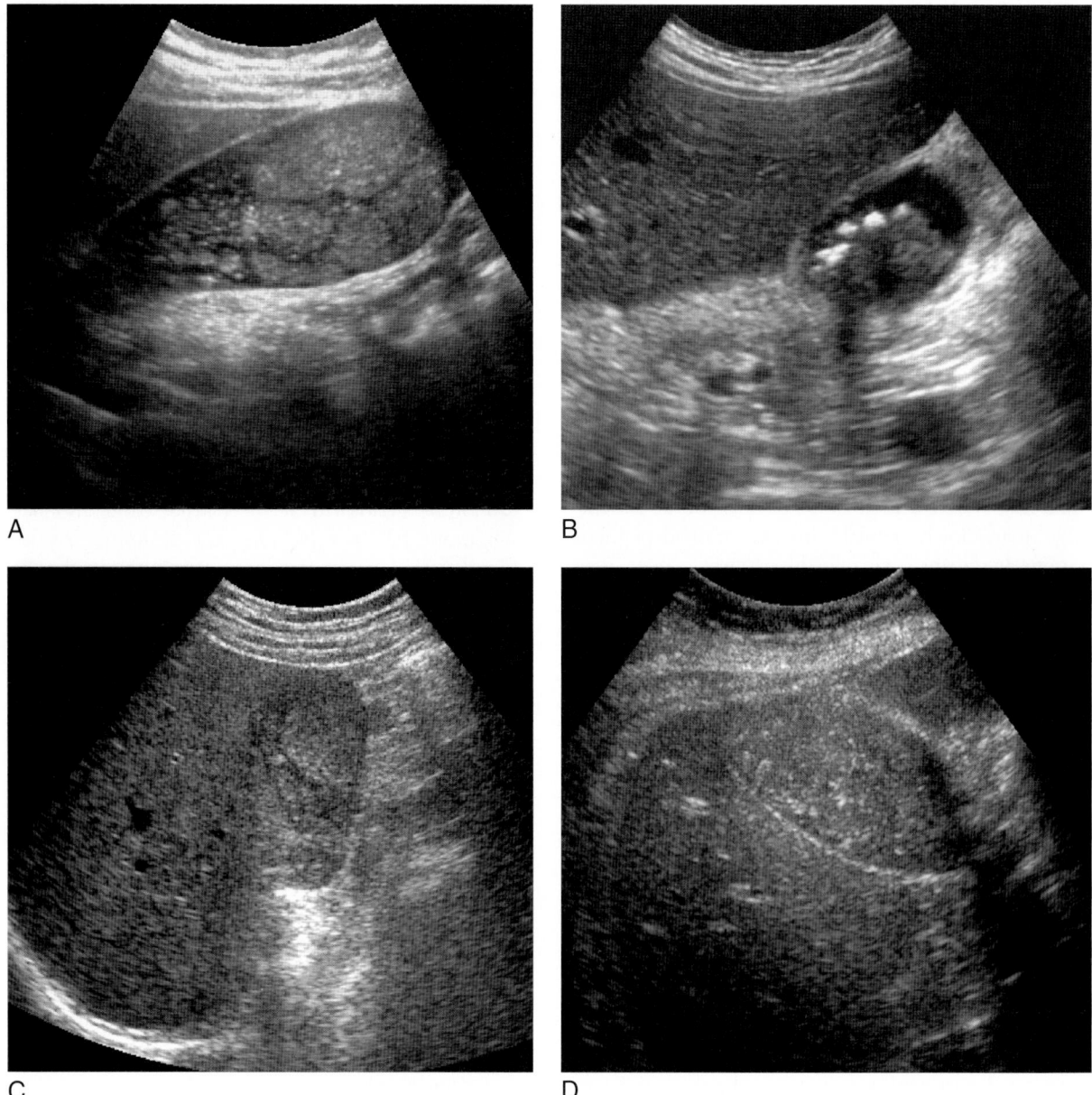

FIGURE 6-29. Tumefactive sludge in three patients. A, Sagittal sonogram shows gallbladder filled with tumor-like sludge. **B,** Transverse image shows a polypoid appearance of sludge on the dependent gallbladder wall with stones along its margin. **C,** Sagittal and **D,** subcostal oblique sonograms of the same patient show "hepatization" of the gallbladder with internal echoes mimicking the normal liver parenchyma. In all three patients, the gallbladder wall was normal. There was no vascularity detected from the tumefacient sludge.

- Thickening of the gallbladder wall (>3 mm)
- Distention of the gallbladder lumen (diameter >4 cm)
- Gallstones
- Impacted stone in cystic duct or gallbladder neck
- Pericholecystic fluid collections
- Positive sonographic Murphy's sign
- Hyperemic gallbladder wall on Doppler interrogation

There are many causes for **gallbladder wall thickening** (Table 6-5). The appearance of the gallbladder wall in acute cholecystitis is nonspecific, but marked thickening of the wall with visible stratification, as seen in generalized edematous states, tends not to be present (Fig. 6-32). Multiple focal noncontiguous hypoechoic pockets of edema fluid within the thickened wall are observed commonly. The inflamed gallbladder is very often significantly distended unless there is perforation of its walls. Gallstones, including the obstructing stone, and sludge are commonly identified. A thin rim of fluid, representing edema, is often seen about much of the organ.

A **sonographic Murphy's sign** is maximal tenderness over the gallbladder when the probe is used to compress

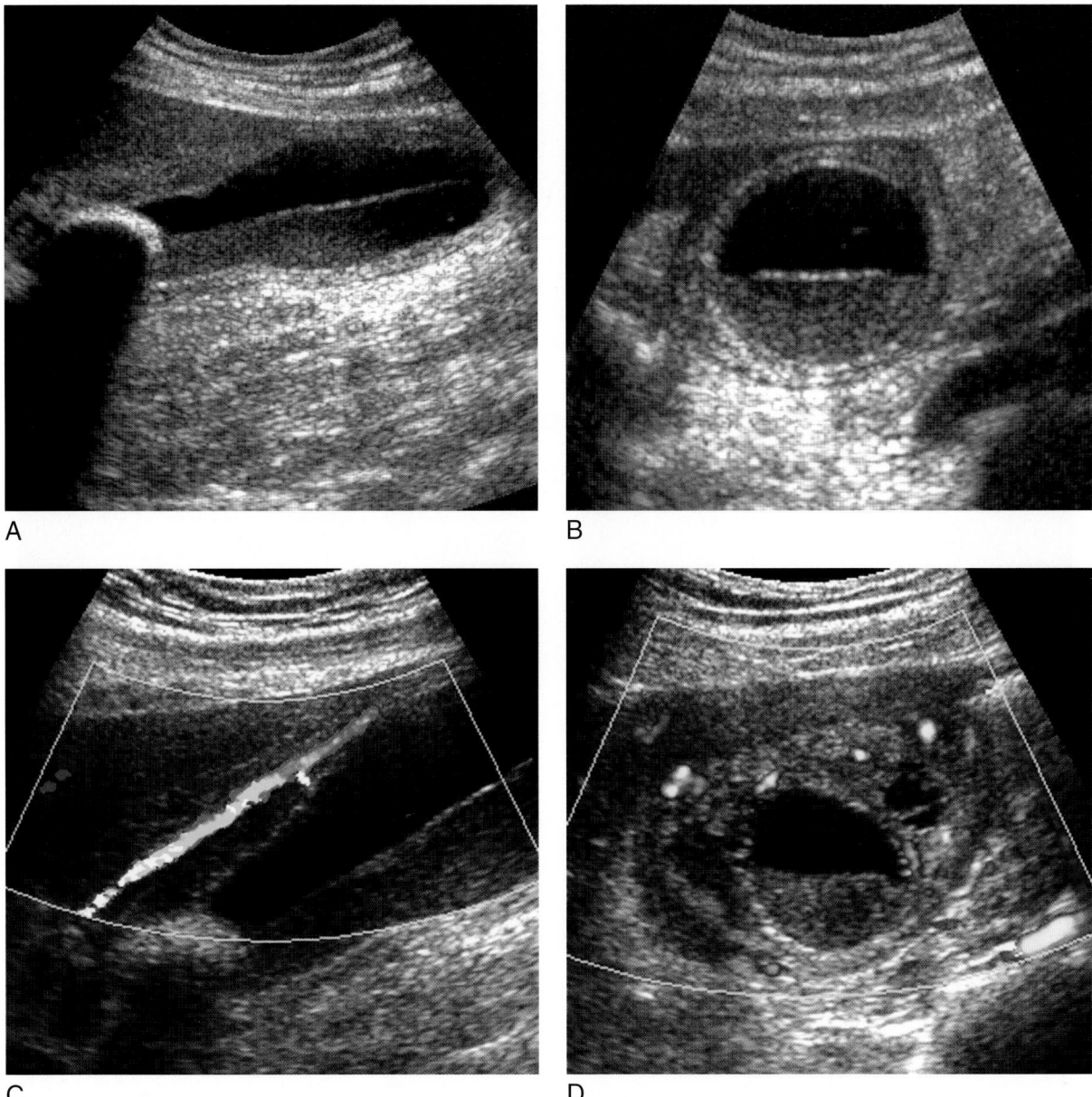

FIGURE 6-30. Classic acute cholecystitis in a young woman with a negative Murphy's sign who had received narcotic analgesics. A, Sagittal and **B,** transverse images show a tense gallbladder, wall thickening, fluid-debris level, and an obstructing stone in the gallbladder neck. **C, Color Doppler** image shows a large cystic artery. **D, Transverse power Doppler** image shows pockets of edema fluid within the thickened, hyperemic wall. (From Wilson SR: Gastrointestinal Disease (Sixth Series) test and syllabus. American College of Radiology, Reston, Va. In press.)

the right upper quadrant. It is often better elicited with deep inspiration which displaces the gallbladder fundus below the costal margin, allowing for more direct compression. **Sonographic Murphy's sign may be absent** in elderly patients, when analgesics have been administered prior to the study, or when prolonged inflammation has led to gangrenous cholecystitis. Hyperemia detected in the gallbladder wall and the presence of a prominent cystic artery have been shown to be relatively specific findings in acute cholecystitis (see Fig. 6-30); power Doppler has been shown to be superior to color

Doppler in detecting such hyperemia.[74] Hyperemia is only qualitatively assessed, however, and motion artifact somewhat limits the utility of power Doppler. Despite the reported usefulness of Doppler interrogation of the gallbladder wall, we have not found this to be consistently helpful in equivocal cases. In fact, we rely heavily on the morphologic changes in the gallbladder for the diagnosis of acute cholecystitis in our own practice and use Doppler only as a supportive test.

Although none of the signs described above are pathognomonic of acute cholecystitis, the combination

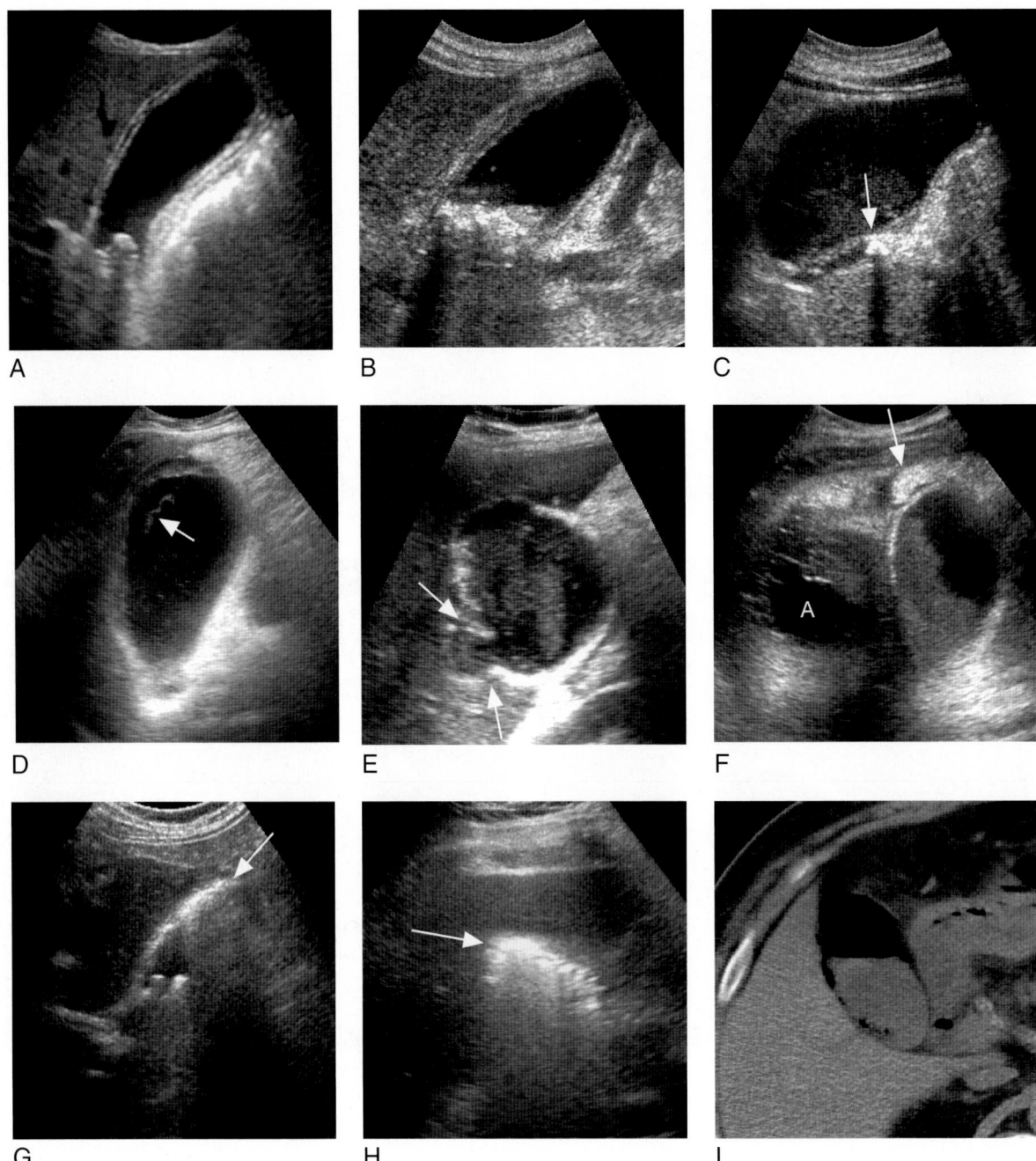

FIGURE 6-31. Acute cholecystitis—spectrum of appearances. Uncomplicated acute cholecystitis. **A,** Classic appearance with gallbladder distention, mild wall thickening, and gallstones. **B, Acute cholecystitis.** More advanced classic changes with a thicker wall and a larger lumen. There are multiple dependent stones. **C,** Distended gallbladder filled with sludge. After careful scrutiny, a stone (*arrow*) was detected in the cystic duct. **Gangrenous cholecystitis. D,** Sloughed membrane (*arrow*) appearing as a linear intraluminal echo. **E,** Perforation shown as disruption of the gallbladder wall (*arrows*). **F,** Pericholecystic inflammatory change. There is echogenic inflamed fat (*arrow*) and an abscess (A). The gallbladder remains large and tense. **Emphysematous cholecystitis. G,** Sagittal sonogram of the gallbladder with a focus of intraluminal air appearing as a bright echogenic focus (*arrow*) with dirty shadowing. **H,** Gallbladder that is filled with air (*arrow*). The gallbladder is not actually visualized, and knowledge of the location of the gallbladder fossa is essential to avoid mistaking this for bowel gas. **I,** Corresponding CT scan shows air in the gallbladder wall and lumen. (**F,** Courtesy of Dr. A.E. Hanbidge, University of Toronto.)

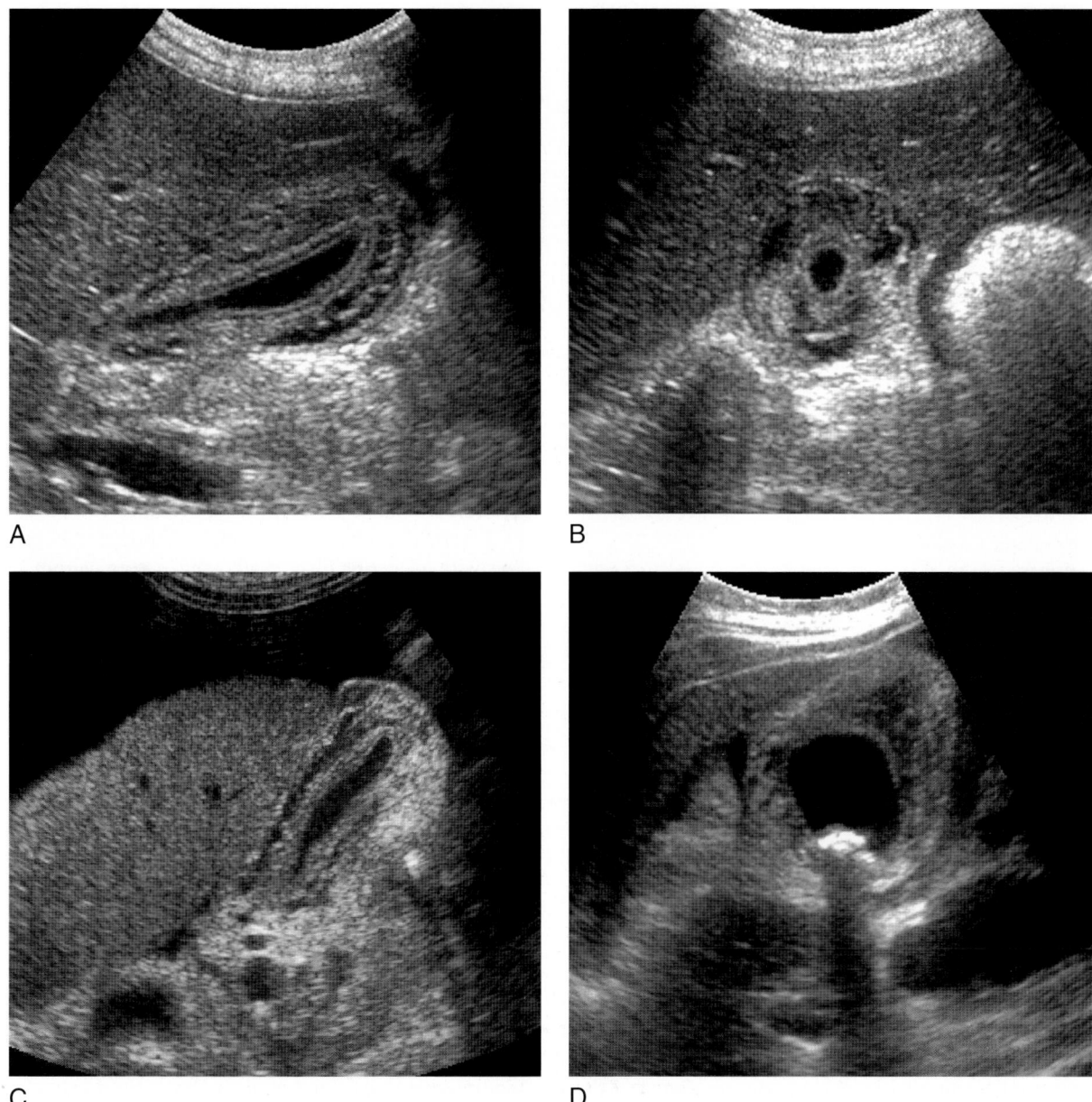

FIGURE 6-32. Systemic causes of gallbladder wall edema. A, Sagittal and **B,** transverse images of **hypoalbuminemia** show marked thickening of the gallbladder wall with a small lumen. **C,** Sagittal image of the gallbladder in a patient with **cirrhosis** demonstrating similar changes to those in **A** and **B. D,** Patient with **congestive heart failure.** There is marked wall thickening. There are incidental gallstones in this patient with no pain and a negative Murphy's sign.

of multiple findings should make the correct diagnosis. It is our experience that in some patients, acute cholecystitis may not show classic findings and so can be quite challenging. This occurs in patients with mild inflammation; but it occurs more so in those hospitalized and ill for other reasons, not on an oral diet, and unable to communicate symptoms. A high index of suspicion should be present when a distended gallbladder is encountered in these patients, and careful scanning of the right upper quadrant is recommended. Perforated duodenal ulcer, acute hepatitis, colitis or diverticulitis, and even pyelonephritis can demonstrate a Murphy's sign

and sympathetic gallbladder wall thickening (Fig. 6-33). Absence of a distended gallbladder and gallstones is often a clue to the nonbiliary origin of the process.

Complications of Acute Cholecystitis

Gangrenous Cholecystitis. When acute cholecystitis is especially severe, prolonged, or infected, the gallbladder may undergo necrosis. Sonographic findings of gangrenous cholecystitis include bands of nonlayering, echogenic tissue within the lumen representing sloughed membranes and blood (see Fig. 6-31). The gallbladder

TABLE 6-5. CAUSES OF GALLBLADDER WALL THICKENING

Generalized edematous states
Congestive heart failure
Renal failure
End-stage cirrhosis
Hypoalbuminemia

Inflammatory Conditions
Primary
  Acute cholecystitis
  Cholangitis
  Chronic cholecystitis
Secondary
  Acute hepatitis
  Perforated duodenal ulcer
  Pancreatitis
  Diverticulitis/colitis

Neoplastic Conditions
Gallbladder adenocarcinoma
Metastases

Miscellaneous
Adenomyomatosis
Mural varicosities

wall also becomes quite irregular with small collections within the wall, which may represent abscesses or hemorrhage.[66] Murphy's sign is absent in two thirds of patients,[75] presumably due to necrosis of the nervous supply to the gallbladder. **Hemorrhagic cholecystitis** represents a rare gangrenous process in which bleeding within the gallbladder wall and lumen predominates. The clinical symptoms are indistinguishable, and only occasionally does the patient experience a gastrointestinal bleed.

Perforated Cholecystitis. Perforation occurs in 5% to 10% of patients, generally in cases of prolonged inflammation.[66] The focus of perforation, seen as a small defect or rent in the wall of the gallbladder, is often, but not always, visible (see Fig. 6-31). Clues to perforation are the deflation of the gallbladder with loss of its normal gourdlike shape, and a pericholecystic fluid collection. The latter is often a small fluid collection about the wall defect, in distinction to the thin rim of fluid about the entire organ present in uncomplicated cholecystitis.[76] The collection may have internal strands typical of abscesses elsewhere (see Fig. 6-31). Perforation of the gallbladder **may extend into the adjacent liver parenchyma**, forming an abscess collection. The presence of a cystic liver lesion about the gallbladder fossa should raise the possibility of a pericholecystic abscess.

Emphysematous Cholecystitis. Emphysematous cholecystitis represents fewer than 1% of all cases of acute cholecystitis, but it is rapidly progressive and fatal in approximately 15% of patients. Emphysematous cholecystitis differs from acute cholecystitis in several ways: it is 3 to 7 times more common in men than in women, approximately one half of the patients are diabetic, and one third to one half of the patients have no gallstones.[66,77] The gas is produced by gas-forming bacteria, presumably after an ischemic event affecting the gallbladder.[77] There is a much higher incidence of perforation than in the usual acute cholecystitis, and urgent surgical management is advocated for all patients.

The **appearance** of emphysematous cholecystitis on sonography depends on the amount of gas present (see Fig. 6-31). The gas is often both within the lumen and the wall of the gallbladder. Small amounts of gas appear as echogenic lines with posterior dirty shadowing or reverberation artifact (ringdown). Large amounts of gas can be more difficult to appreciate; the absence of a normal gallbladder is a clue. A bright echogenic line with posterior dirty shadowing is seen within the entire gallbladder fossa. Movement of gas bubbles is a helpful finding, and compression of the gallbladder fossa may precipitate this sign. Pneumobilia is not uncommon.[77]

Acalculous Cholecystitis

Acalculous cholecystitis may occur in patients with no risk factors, but is more commonly seen in critically ill patients, thereby having a worse prognosis. **Risk factors** include major surgery, severe trauma, sepsis, total parenteral nutrition, diabetes, atherosclerotic disease, and HIV infection.[70] In nonhospitalized patients, it is more common in elderly male patients with atherosclerotic disease,[78] with a much better prognosis.

The **diagnosis of acalculous cholecystitis** can be difficult to make as gallbladder distention, wall thickening, internal sludge, and pericholecystic fluid may all be present in critically ill patients without cholecystitis.[79] The patients may be obtunded or receiving analgesics, reducing the sensitivity of Murphy's sign. It is the combination of the findings that suggests the diagnosis; the more signs present, the more the likelihood of cholecystitis.[80] Nevertheless, cholescintigraphy or percutaneous sampling of the luminal contents should be used more liberally to aid in establishing the diagnosis.

Torsion (Volvulus) of the Gallbladder

Gallbladder torsion is a rare, acute entity. Patients present with symptoms of acute cholecystitis. It is often seen in elderly females and may be related to a mobile gallbladder with a long suspensory mesentery. The hallmarks on imaging are a massively distended and inflamed gallbladder lying in an unusual **horizontal** position, with its long axis oriented in a left to right

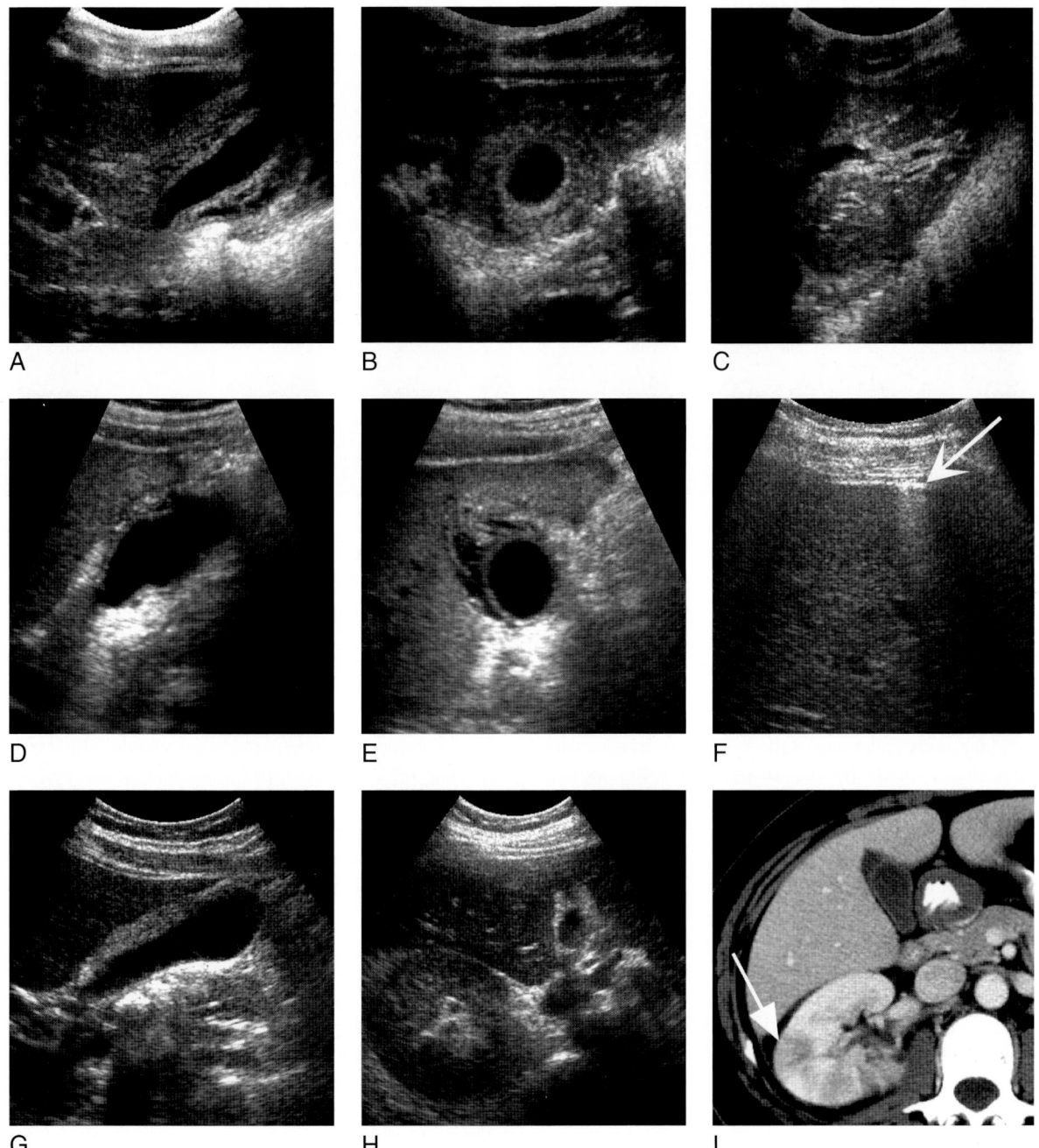

FIGURE 6-33. Sympathetic thickening of the gallbladder wall. Sympathetic thickening of the gallbladder wall in three patients with positive sonographic Murphy's sign. **Acute hepatitis. A** and **B,** Views of the gallbladder show marked circumferential thickening of the gallbladder wall. The lumen is not distended. **C,** Left lobe of the liver shows periportal cuffing. **Perforation of a duodenal ulcer. D** and **E,** Demonstrate asymmetrical marked thickening of the gallbladder wall. **F,** Free intraperitoneal air. The peritoneal line in the epigastrium (*arrow*) marks a focus of increased brightness (enhancement) with posterior dirty shadowing. **Acute pyelonephritis. G** and **H,** Asymmetrical thickening of the gallbladder wall. **I,** CT scan shows striated nephrogram (*arrow*). (**D, E,** and **F** Courtesy of Dr. A.E. Hanbidge, University of Toronto.)

direction. A twist of the cystic artery and the cystic duct may be visible. If the torsion is greater than 180 degrees, gangrene of the gallbladder ensues, otherwise obstruction of the cystic duct and acute cholecystitis occur. In either case, treatment is usually surgical.[81]

Chronic Cholecystitis

Chronic cholecystitis is associated with the mere presence of gallstones; therefore, it is most commonly asymptomatic and mild in degree. It has the same incidence and risk factors as gallstone disease. In more

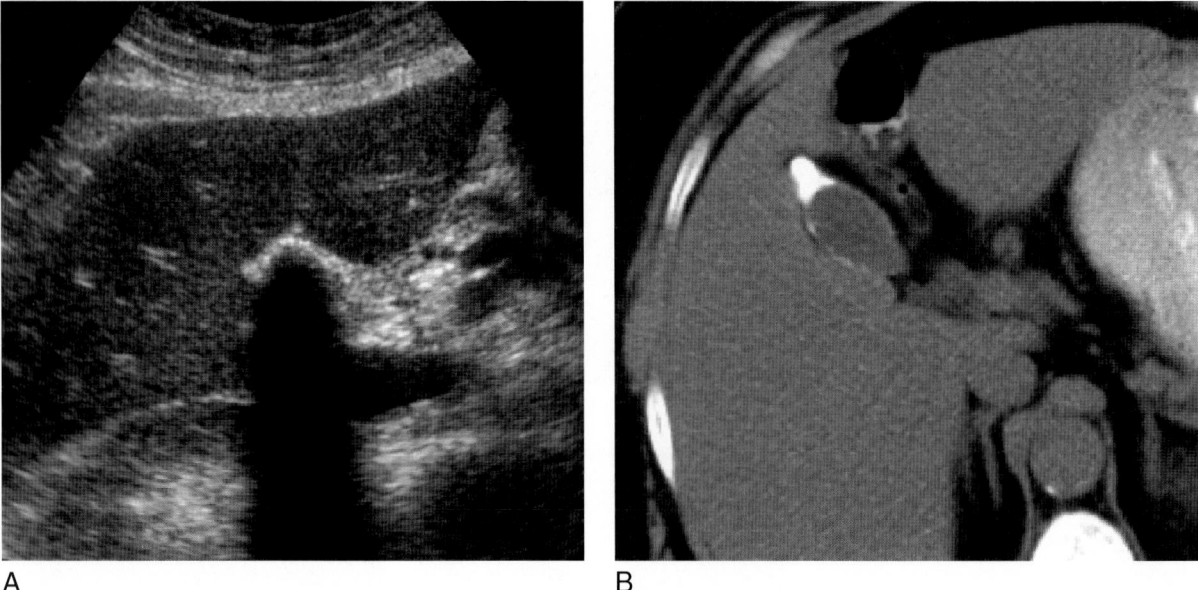

FIGURE 6-34. Porcelain gallbladder. A, Sonogram and **B, corresponding CT.** On ultrasound, this appearance could be mistaken for a stone within the gallbladder lumen. There is, however, no gallbladder wall superficial to the echogenic focus.

advanced cases, it leads to thickening and fibrosis of the gallbladder wall. In such cases, chronic cholecystitis appears on **sonographic examination** as a thick-walled gallbladder with gallstones. Differentiation from acute cholecystitis is made by the **absence of other signs**, namely gallbladder distention, Murphy's sign, and hyperemia in the wall.[82] Bouts of acute cholecystitis may complicate chronic cholecystitis.

Xanthogranulomatous cholecystitis is a rare form of chronic cholecystitis, in which collections of lipid-laden macrophages occur within grayish-yellow nodules or streaks within the gallbladder wall. Apart from gall-stones, hypoechoic nodules or bands within the thickened wall, representing the lipid-laden xantho-granulomatous nodules, may be seen suggesting the diagnosis.[83]

Porcelain Gallbladder

Calcification of the gallbladder wall is termed **porcelain gallbladder**. Its cause is unknown, but occurs in association with gallstone disease and may represent a form of chronic cholecystitis. It is a rare entity, occurring in up to 0.8% of cholecystectomy specimens. There is a female predominance, most commonly found in the sixth decade of life.[84] Two recent large studies have disputed a **high incidence of gallbladder carcinoma** in porcelain gallbladder, suggesting a coincidence of the two entities in 0% to 7% of patients.[85,86] Nevertheless, prophylactic resection is advised.[84]

The degree and pattern of calcification determines the **sonographic appearance** (Fig. 6-34). When the entire gallbladder wall is thickly calcified, a hyperechoic

semilunar line with dense posterior acoustic shadowing is noted. Mild calcification appear as an echogenic line with variable degrees of posterior acoustic shadowing. The luminal contents may be visible. Interrupted clumps of calcium appears as echogenic foci with posterior shadowing.[66] **Differential diagnosis** includes gallstones and emphysematous cholecystitis. Because the calcifications occur in the wall of the gallbladder, the WES complex is absent (see section on gallstone disease).

Adenomyomatosis (Adenomatous Hyperplasia)

Gallbladder adenomyomatosis is a benign condition caused by exaggeration of the normal invaginations of the luminal epithelium (Rokitansky-Aschoff sinuses) with associated smooth muscle proliferation (Fig. 6-35). The affected areas demonstrate thickening of the gallbladder wall with internal cystic spaces that are the key to the radiologic diagnosis. The great majority of adenomyomatoses are asymptomatic.[87]

Adenomyomatosis may be focal or diffuse. The most common appearance on sonography is that of tiny echogenic foci in the gallbladder wall that create comet-tail artifacts, presumably caused by either the cystic space itself or the internal debris (Fig. 6-36). Prominent mass-like focal areas of adenomyomatosis, called **adenomyomas**, are the next most common manifestation. Careful evaluation of the adenomyoma, sometimes requiring higher frequency or linear probes, can show several features that are diagnostic of the entity and allow for differentiation from neoplasm. The most telling finding is the presence of cystic spaces; however, this is not the

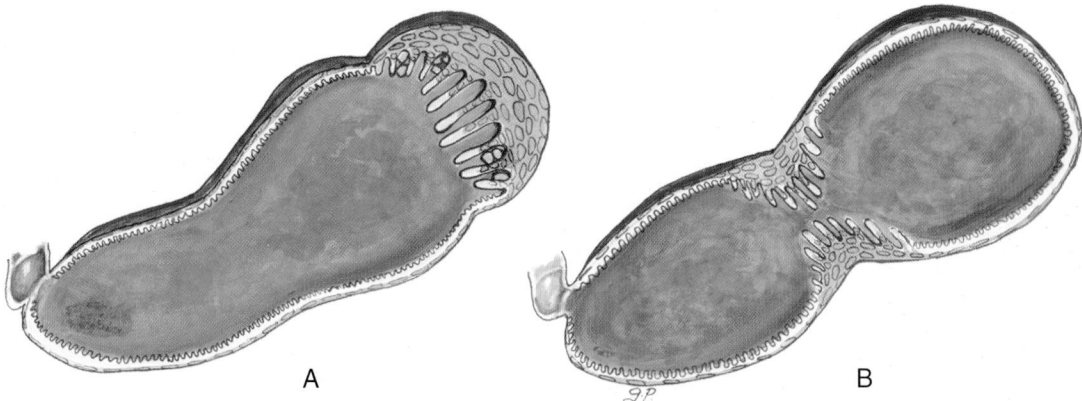

FIGURE 6-35. Segmental adenomyomatosis. A, Fundal adenomyoma. B, Hourglass adenomyomatosis. In both cases, note the constricted contour of the gallbladder and thickening of the wall with hypertrophy of the smooth muscle. On sonography, the exaggerated Rokitansky-Aschoff sinuses may appear as cystic spaces or as echogenic foci with comet-tail artifact, possibly due to cholesterol crystals (depicted here as yellow particles) lodged in them.

most common. Echogenic foci with ringdown or with twinkling artifact on Doppler examination are also typical. Focal adenomyomatosis is most common in the gallbladder fundus, but may less commonly affect the midportion of the gallbladder to create a narrowing of the midportion of the organ, called **hourglass gallbladder** (Fig. 6-37). Fundal adenomyomas are often folded onto the body of the gallbladder and can occasionally be mistaken for a pericholecystic or even a hepatic mass. The entire gland wall may be involved, causing collapse of the lumen. The absence of the cystic spaces, echogenic foci, or twinkling artifact, or the presence of internal vascularity should prompt further investigation to differentiate from neoplasm. MRI/MRCP allows for improved specificity, the diagnosis being made by the presence of cystic spaces within the thickened wall.[88]

Polypoid Masses of the Gallbladder

Polypoid masses of the gallbladder are listed in Table 6-6. Differentiation of benign and malignant polyps is

TABLE 6-6. COMMON POLYPOID MASSES OF THE GALLBLADDER

Cholesterol polyps*—50-60%
Inflammatory polyps*—5-10%
Adenoma*—<5%
Focal adenomyomatosis
Gallbladder adenocarcinoma
Metastases (esp. melanoma)

*Data from Bilhartz LE: Acalculous cholecystitis, cholesterolosis, adenomyomatosis, and polyps of the gallbladder. In Feldman M, et al: (eds): Sleisenger & Fordtran's Gastrointestinal and Liver Disease, 7th ed. Elsevier Science, 2002, pp 1116-1130.

very important because the former are very common, and the latter require early intervention to improve outcome. Multiplicity and size of up to 10 mm are the most frequently used criteria for benignity. Lesions measuring less than 10 mm are most often benign when resected, and do not change in size when followed.[89] Malignancy has been documented in 37% to 88% of resected polyps greater than 10 mm.[90] Other factors that increase the risk of malignancy are age older than 60 years, singularity, gallstone disease, rapid change in size on follow-up sonography, and a sessile morphology.[91] There is overlap of Doppler features of benign and malignant masses; however, a blood velocity of greater than 20 cm/sec and resistive index of less than 0.65 are more suggestive of malignancy.[92]

Cholesterol Polyps

Approximately one half of all polypoid gallbladder lesions are cholesterol polyps. These represent the focal form of gallbladder **cholesterolosis**, a common non-neoplastic condition of unknown etiology. Cholesterolosis results in accumulation of lipids within macrophages. The diffuse form, commonly known as **strawberry gallbladder**, is not visible on imaging. Cholesterolosis has the same risk factors as gallstone disease, but the two conditions rarely coexist.[93] Cholesterol polyps are often between 2 and 10 mm, although lesions up to 20 mm have been described.[90] On pathologic series, one fifth are solitary but the mean number of polyps is eight.[93]

The sonographic appearance of **cholesterol polyps** is that of multiple, nonshadowing, oval lesions attached to the gallbladder wall (Fig. 6-38). In distinction to small nonshadowing stones, polyps are not mobile. Larger lesions may contain a fine pattern of echogenic foci within them.[94]

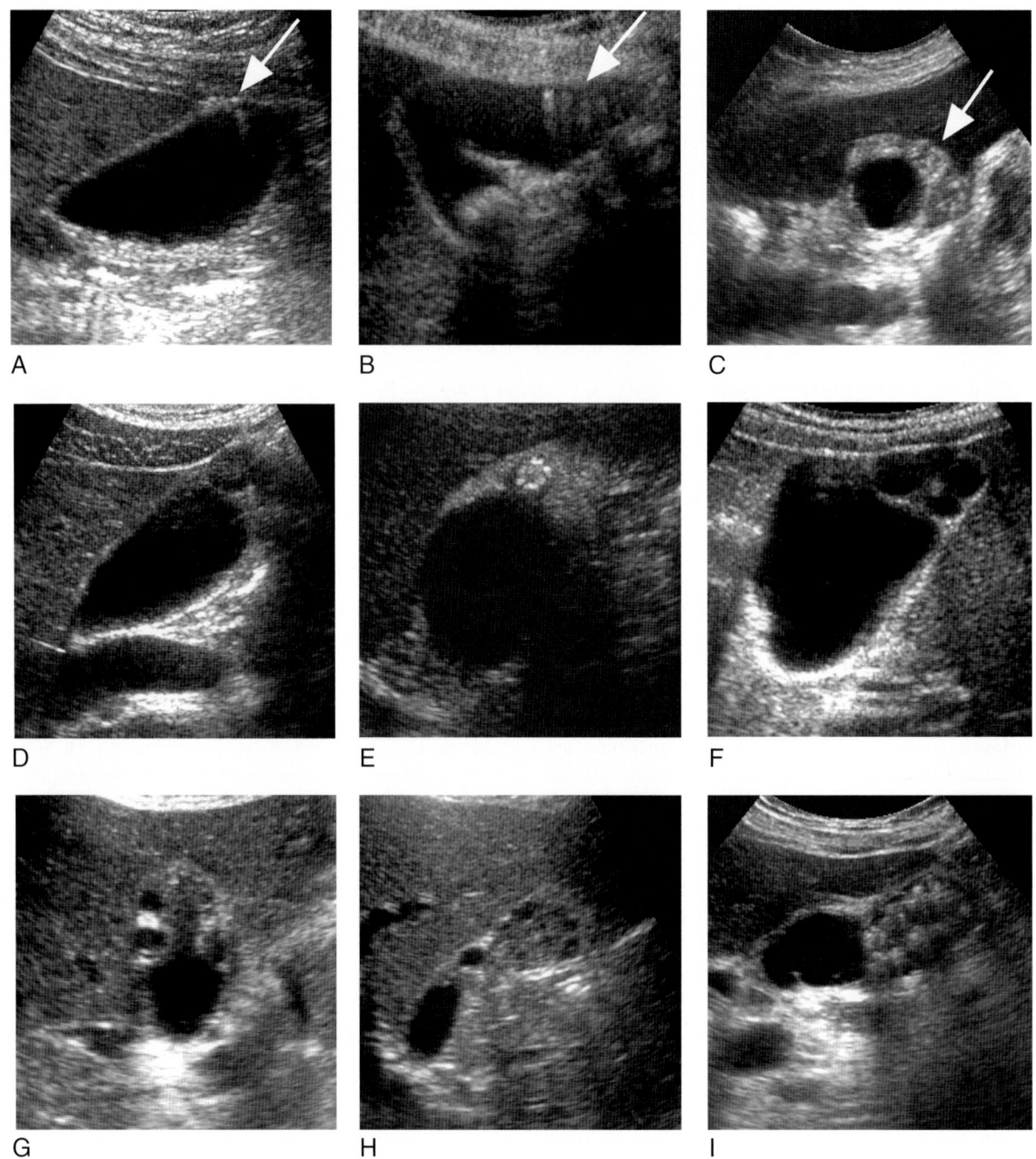

FIGURE 6-36. Adenomyomatosis—spectrum of appearances. Focal adenomyomatosis, the most common manifestation. **A,** Small focal area of thickening of the anterior fundal wall (*arrow*) with a bright echogenic focus with a distal comet-tail artifact. **B,** Multiple bright foci (*arrow*) with distal artifacts. **C,** Highly echogenic focal thickening of the gallbladder wall (*arrow*). Increased echogenicity is unusual for a malignant tumor that is more likely to appear hypoechoic. **Fundal adenomyomas. D,** Appears hypoechoic and masslike. **E,** Caplike area with multiple tiny highly echogenic foci that suggest multiple crystals in the Rokitansky-Aschoff sinuses. **F,** Multiple cystic spaces within the adenomyoma. **Segmental adenomyomatosis. G** and **H,** Masslike areas obliterating the gallbladder lumen. Multiple cystic spaces suggest the correct diagnosis. **I,** Shows multiple echogenic foci suggestive of crystals in the Rokitansky-Aschoff sinuses.

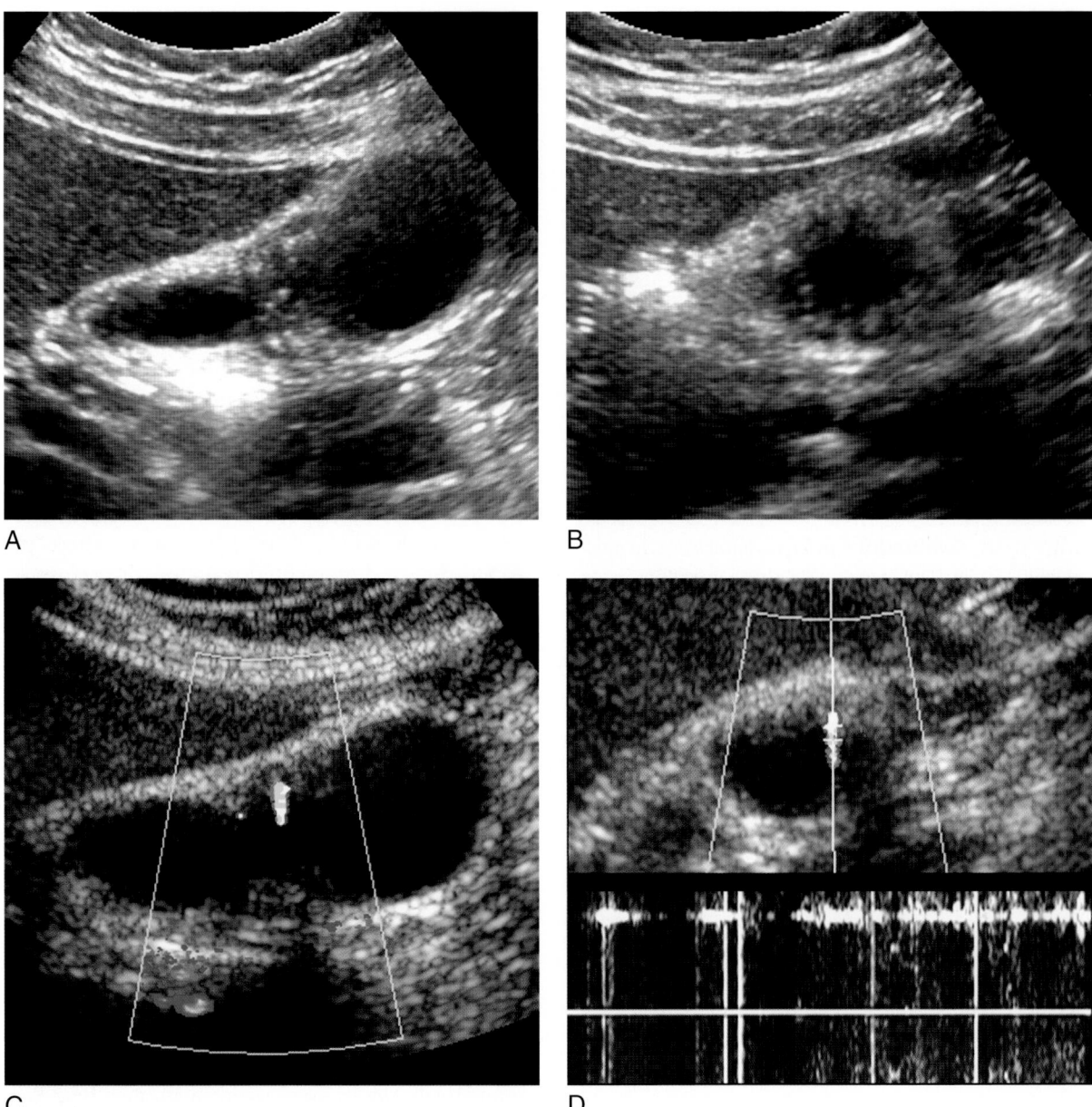

FIGURE 6-37. Hourglass adenomyoma. A, Sagittal and **B,** transverse sonograms show thickening of the gallbladder wall creating an hourglass configuration. At the point of wall thickening there are innumerable bright echogenic foci with ringdown artifact suggesting cholesterol crystals in Rokitansky-Aschoff sinuses. **C** and **D, Color and spectral Doppler** show a twinkle artifact without real vascularity, supportive of the correct diagnosis.

Adenomas, Adenomyomas, and Inflammatory Polyps

Adenomas are true benign neoplasms of the gallbladder with a premalignant potential much lower than colonic adenomas. They represent less than 5% of gallbladder polyps and occur as a solitary lesion. Adenomas are usually pedunculated and larger lesions may contain foci of malignant transformation.[93] Adenomas tend to be homogeneously hyperechoic, but become more heterogeneous as they increase in size.[90] Thickening of the gallbladder wall adjacent to an adenoma should raise the possibility of malignancy. On occasion, an adenomyoma may appear as a sessile polypoid gallbladder lesion. Imaging features, described under the adenomyomatosis section, should allow differentiation. Inflammatory polyps of the gallbladder comprise 5% to 10% of gallbladder polyps, and are multiple in half the cases.[93] They tend to occur in the background of gallstone disease and chronic cholecystitis.[95] The sonographic appearance of these lesions has not been systematically studied.

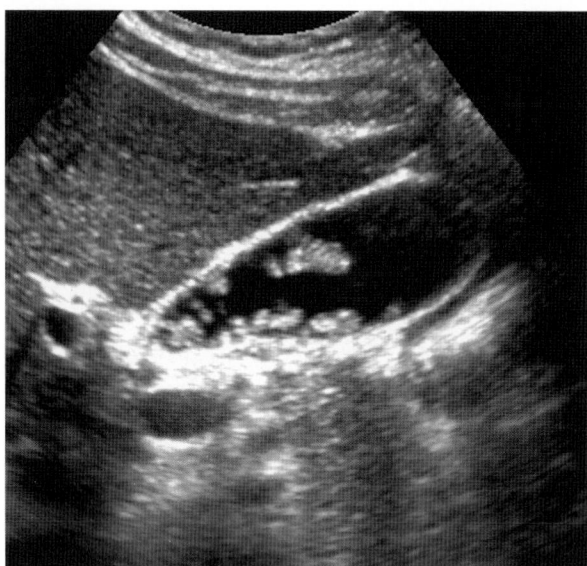

FIGURE 6-38. Gallbladder polyps. Small size (≤10 mm) and multiplicity are features most suggestive of benignity.

Malignancies

Primary gallbladder adenocarcinomas may appear as a polypoid mass; their appearance is discussed subsequently. Melanoma is the cause of 50% to 60% of metastases to the gallbladder. These appear as hyperechoic, broad-based polypoid lesions, which may be multiple. They are often >10 mm in diameter.[96] Other adenocarcinomas can rarely metastasize to the gallbladder. Advanced hepatocellular carcinoma can directly invade the gallbladder fossa and extend through the gallbladder wall to appear as a luminal mass. The large hepatic component of the mass, along with its hypervascular nature, should be helpful in the diagnosis.

Gallbladder Carcinoma

Gallbladder carcinoma is an uncommon malignancy occurring mainly in the elderly population, with a 3:1 female to male predominance. In a majority of cases, it is associated with gallstones; chronic gallstones disease and resultant dysplasia have been cited as a causative factor.[97] About 98% of gallbladder carcinomas are adenocarcinomas, with squamous cell carcinoma and metastases accounting for the rest.

The following three **patterns of disease** have been described:

- Mass arising in the gallbladder fossa, obliterating the gallbladder and invading the adjacent liver. This is the most common.
- Focal or diffuse, irregular wall thickening
- Intraluminal polypoid mass

Patterns of Tumor Spread

Because the wall of the gallbladder is quite thin and little connective tissue separates it from the liver parenchyma, **contiguous hepatic invasion** is the most common pattern of spread. Gallbladder tumors also extend along the cystic duct into the **porta hepatis**, where they mimic hilar cholangiocarcinomas. Tumor extension into bile ducts or encasement of the portal vein or hepatic artery may ensue. Direct invasion into adjacent loops of bowel, especially the duodenum or colon, is not unusual. A resultant cholecystoenteric fistula and inflammation may be mistaken for a benign abscess collection. Metastases to the peritoneum are a common finding.

Lymphatic spread is also a common feature of the disease and may occur in the absence of invasion of adjacent organs.[98] The first nodes to be affected are in the hilar region. Adenopathy then may either extend down the hepatoduodenal ligament to affect peripancreatic and mesenteric nodes or across the gastrohepatic ligament to celiac nodal stations.

Surgical resection is the only chance of cure; however, reported resection rates range between 10% to 30%.[98] If the tumor is not confined to the mucosa, an extended cholecystectomy involving resection of 3 to 5 cm rim of liver adjacent to the gallbladder fossa, cystic and common bile ducts, and regional lymph node dissection is required. The presence of noncontiguous hepatic or peritoneal metastases, celiac or peripancreatic nodal disease, or encasement of the main portal vein or hepatic artery renders the patient unresectable and should be carefully sought.

Sonographic Appearance

The appearance on sonography varies depending on the pattern of disease (Fig. 6-39). Masses replacing the normal gallbladder fossa, when small, may be difficult to appreciate because they may blend into the liver. The **absence of a normal-appearing gallbladder** with no history of cholecystectomy should raise suspicion. A clue to the diagnosis is the common presence of an immobile stone that is engrossed by the tumor, the so-called **"trapped stone."** On Doppler interrogation, the mass may demonstrate internal arterial and venous flow. **Diffuse malignant thickening** of the wall differs from other causes in that the wall is irregular with loss of the normal mural layers. **Polypoid intraluminal masses** are differentiated from non-neoplastic abnormalities by immobility of the mass, larger size (>1 cm), and prominent internal vascularity. Gallbladder carcinomas may produce large quantities of mucin, which distends the gallbladder.

Sonography performs very well in locally staging gallbladder carcinoma. Bach et al. have reported a 94% sensitivity and a 63% accuracy for prediction of

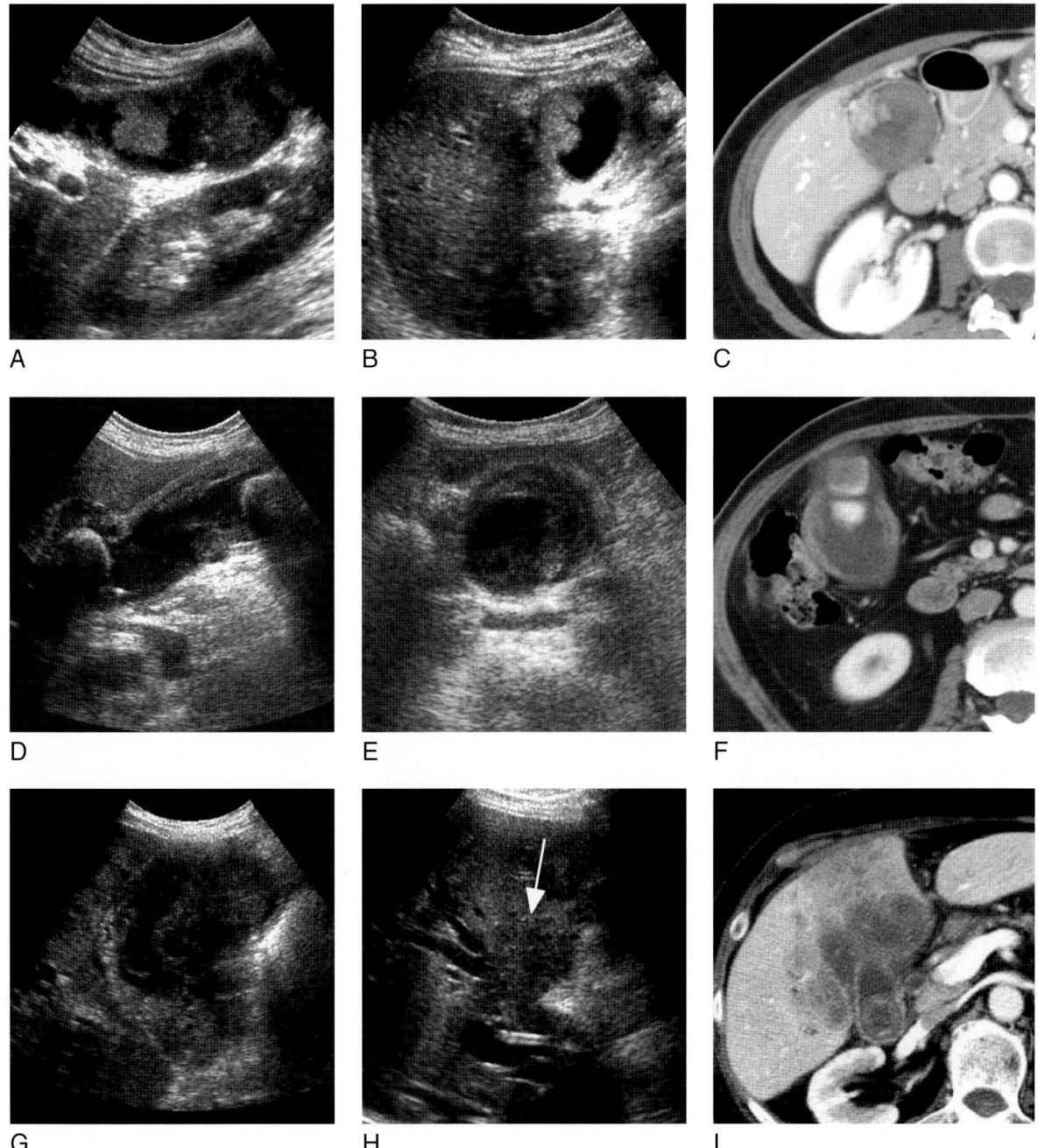

FIGURE 6-39. Gallbladder cancer—spectrum of appearances. Polypoid masses. A and **B,** Large intraluminal polypoid masses. **C,** Corresponding CT scan shows enhancing polyps. **Wall thickening. D** and **E,** Extensive asymmetrical heterogeneous wall thickening. **F,** Corresponding CT scan. **Invasive gallbladder cancer. G** and **H,** Huge mass replacing the gallbladder fossa and invading the liver. **H,** Biliary obstruction due to the invasive mass (*arrow*). **I,** Corresponding CT scan.

resectability when compared to operative findings.[99] However, sonography is often difficult in patients with unresectable disease due to limited detection of noncontiguous hepatic, lymph node, and, particularly, peritoneal metastases. A CT scan is recommended to improve detection of metastatic disease.

References

1. Bret PM, De Stempel JV, Atri M, et al: Intrahepatic bile duct and portal vein anatomy revisited. Radiology 1988;169(2):405-407.
2. Bressler EL, Rubin JM, McCracken S: Sonographic parallel channel sign: A reappraisal. Radiology 1987;164(2):343-346.

3. Puente SG, Bannura GC: Radiological anatomy of the biliary tract: Variations and congenital abnormalities. World J Surg 1983;7(2):271-276.

4. Russell E, Yrizzary JM, Montalvo BM, et al: Left hepatic duct anatomy: Implications Radiology 1990;174:353-356.

5. Bowie JD: What is the upper limit of normal for the common bile duct on ultrasound: How much do you want it to be? Am J Gastroenterol 2000;95(4):897-900.

6. Horrow MM, Horrow JC, Niakosari A, et al: Is age associated with size of adult extrahepatic bile duct: Sonographic study. Radiology 2001;221(2):411-414.

7. Lamah M, Karanjia ND, Dickson GH: Anatomical variations of the extrahepatic biliary tree: Review of the world literature. Clin Anat 2001;14(3):167-172.

8. Sato M, Ishida H, Konno K, et al: Choledochal cyst due to anomalous pancreatobiliary junction in the adult: Sonographic findings. Abdom Imaging 2001;26:395-400.

9. De Vries JS, De Vries DC, Aronson DK, et al: Choledochal cysts: Age of presentation, symptoms, and late complications related to Todani's classification. J Pediatr Surg 2002;37:1568-1573.

10. Adkins RB Jr, Chapman WC, Reddy VS: Embryology, anatomy, and surgical applications of the extrahepatic biliary system. Surg Clin North Am 2000;80(1):363-379.

11. Todani T, Watanabe Y, Narusue M, et al: Congenital bile duct cysts, classification, operative procedures, and review of thirty-seven cases including cancer arising from choledochal cyst. Am J Surg 1977;134:263-269.

12. Matsumoto Y, Fujii H, Itakura J, et al: Recent advances in pancreaticobiliary maljunction. J Hepatobiliary Pancreat Surg 2002;9:45-54.

13. Parada LA, Hallén M, Hägerstrand I, et al: Clonal chromosomal abnormalities in congenital bile duct dilatation (Caroli's disease). Gut 1999;45:780-782.

14. Suchy FJ: Anatomy, histology, embryology, developmental anomalies, and pediatric disorders of the biliary tract. In Feldmen M, et al (eds): Sleisenger & Fordtran's Gastrointestinal and Liver Disease, 7th ed. Elsevier Science, 2002, p 1033.

15. Fulcher AS, Turner MA, Sanyal AJ: Case 38: Caroli disease and renal tubular ectasia. Radiology 2001;220:720-723.

16. Marchal GJ, Desmet VJ, Proesmans WC, et al: Caroli disease: High-frequency US and pathologic findings. Radiology 1986;158:507-511.

17. Greenberger NJ, Paumgartner G: Diseases of the gallbladder and bile ducts. In Braunwald E, et al (eds): Harrison's Principles of Internal Medicine, 15th ed. New York, McGraw-Hill, 2001.

18. Ko CW, Lee SP: Epidemiology and natural history of common bile duct stones and prediction of disease. Gastrointest Endosc 2002;56 (Supp 6):165-169.

19. Ortega D, Burns PN, Hope Simpson D, Wilson SR: Tissue harmonic imaging: Is it a benefit for bile duct sonography? AJR 2001;176(3):653-659.

20. Baron RL, Tublin ME, Peterson MS: Imaging the spectrum of biliary tract disease. Radiol Clin North Am 2002;40(6):1325-1354.

21. Abou-Saif A, Al-Kawas FH: Complications of gallstone disease: Mirizzi syndrome, cholecystocholedochal fistula, and gallstone ileus. Am J Gastroenterol 2002;97(2):249-254.

22. Turner MA, Fulcher AS: The cystic duct: Normal anatomy and disease processes. Radiographics 2001;21:3-22.

23. Green MH, Duell RM, Johnson CD, Jamieson NV: Haemobilia. Br J Surg 2001;88(6):773-786.

24. Horton JD, Bilhartz LE: Gallstone disease and its complications. Clinical manifestations of gallstone disease. In Feldman M, et al (eds): Sleisenger & Fordtran's Gastrointestinal and Liver Disease, 7th ed. Elsevier Science, 2002; pp 1065-1087.

25. Hanau LH, Steigbigel NH: Infections of the liver: Acute (ascending) cholangitis. Infect Dis Clin North Am 2000;14(3):521-546.

26. Harvey RT, Miller WT, Jr: Acute biliary disease: Initial CT and follow-up US versus initial US and follow-up CT. Radiology 1999;213:831-836.

27. Mahadevan U, Bass NM: Sclerosing cholangitis and recurrent pyogenic cholangitis. In Feldman M, et al: (eds): Sleisenger & Fordtran's Gastrointestinal and Liver Disease, 7th ed. Elsevier Science, 2002, pp 1131-1152.

28. Cosenza CA, Durazo F, Stain SC, et al: Current management of recurrent pyogenic cholangitis. Am Surg 1999;65(10):939-943.

29. Schulman A: Ultrasound appearances of intra- and extrahepatic biliary ascariasis. Abdom Imaging 1998;23:60-66.

30. Mahajani RV, Uzer MF: Cholangiopathy in HIV-infected patients. Clin Liver Dis 1999;3(3):669-684.

31. Da Silva F, Boudghene F, Lecomte I, et al: Sonography in AIDS-related cholangitis: Prevalence and cause of an echogenic nodule in the distal end of the common bile duct AJR 1993;160(6):1205-1207.

32. Defalque D, Menu Y, Girard PM, et al: Sonographic diagnosis of cholangitis in AIDS patients. Gastrointest Radiol 1989;14(2):143-147.

33. MacCarty RL: Noncalculous inflammatory disorders of the biliary tract. In Gore RM, Levine MS, Laufer I (eds): Textbook of Gastrointestinal Radiology. Philadelphia, WB Saunders, 1994, pp 1727-1745.

34. Narayanan Menon KV, Wiesner RH: Etiology and natural history of primary sclerosing cholangitis. J Hepatobiliary Pancreat Surg 1999;6(14):343-351.

35. Olsson R, Danielsson A, Jarnerot G, et al: Prevalence of primary sclerosing cholangitis in patients with ulcerative colitis. Gastroenterology 1991;100 (5 Pt 1):1319-1323.

36. Majoie CB, Smits NJ, Phoa SS, et al: Primary sclerosing cholangitis: Sonographic findings. Abdom Imaging 1995;20(2):109-112.

37. Stockbrugger RW, Olsson R, Jaup B, et al: Forty-six patients with primary sclerosing cholangitis: Radiological bile duct changes in relationship to clinical course and concomitant inflammatory bowel disease. Hepatogastroenterology 1988;35:289-294.

38. Pokorny CS, McCaughan GW, Gallagher ND, et al: Sclerosing cholangitis and biliary tract calculi—primary or secondary? Gut 1992;33(10):1376-1380.

39. Graziadei IW, Wiesner RH, Batts KP, et al: Recurrence of primary sclerosing cholangitis following liver transplantation. Hepatology 1999;29:1050-1056.

40. Kennedy A: Emedicine article *http://www.emedicine.com/med/topic343.htm*.

41. Watanapa P, Watanapa WB: Liver fluke-associated cholangiocarcinoma. Br J Surg 2002;89(8):962-970.

42. De Groen PC, Gores GJ, Larusso NF, et al: Biliary tract cancers. N Engl J Med 1999;341(18):1368-1378.

43. Jarnagin WR: Cholangiocarcinoma of the extrahepatic bile ducts. Semin Surg Oncol 2000;19:156-176.

44. Sohn TA, Lillemoe KD: Tumors of the gallbladder, bile ducts, and ampulla. In Feldman M, et al (eds): Sleisenger & Fordtran's Gastrointestinal and Liver Disease, 7th ed. Elsevier Science, 2002, pp 1153-1165.

45. Colombari R, Tsui WM: Biliary tumors of the liver. Semin Liver Dis 1995;15:402-413.

46. Gihara S, Kojiro M: Pathology of cholangiocarcinoma. In

Okuda K, Ishak KG, (eds): Neoplasms of the Liver. Tokyo, Springer Verlag, 1987, pp 236 -301.

47. Nakeeb A, Pitt HA, Sohn TA, et al: Cholangiocarcinoma. A spectrum of intrahepatic, perihilar and distal tumors. Ann Surg 1996;224:463-475.

48. Patel T: Worldwide trends in mortality from biliary tract malignancies. BMC Cancer 2002;2(1):10.

49. Patel T: Increasing incidence and mortality of primary intrahepatic cholangiocarcinoma in the United States. Hepatology 2001;33(6):1353-1357.

50. Maetani Y, Itoh K, Watanabe C, et al: MR imaging of intrahepatic cholangiocarcinoma with pathologic correlation. AJR 2001;176:1499-1507.

51. Sano T, Kamiya J, Nagino M, et al: Macroscopic classification and preoperative diagnosis of intrahepatic cholangiocarcinoma in Japan. J Hepatobiliary Pancreat Surg 1999;6(2):101-107.

52. Wibulpolprasert B, Dhiensiri T: Peripheral cholangiocarcinoma: Sonographic evaluation. J Clin Ultrasound 1992;20:303-314.

53. Lee NW, Wong KP, Siu KF, et al: Cholangiography in hepatocellular carcinoma with obstructive jaundice. Clin Radiol 1984;35:119-123.

54. Bloom CM, Langer B, Wilson SR: Role of US in the detection, characterization, and staging of cholangiocarcinoma. Radiographics 1999;19(5):1199-1218.

55. Lee JW, Han JK, Kim TK: CT Features of intraductal intrahepatic cholangiocarcinoma. AJR 2000;175:721-725.

56. Jarnagin WR, Fong Y, DeMatteo RP, et al: Staging, resectability, and outcome in 225 patients with hilar cholangiocarcinoma. Ann Surg 2001;234(4):507-517.

57. Robledo R, Muro A, Prieto ML: Extrahepatic bile duct carcinoma: US characteristics and accuracy in demonstration of tumors. Radiology 2000;198:869-873.

58. Hann LE, Greatrex KV, Bach AM, et al: Cholangiocarcinoma at the hepatic hilus: Sonographic findings. AJR 1997;168:985-989.

59. Choi BI, Lee JH, Han MC, et al: Hilar cholangiocarcinoma: Comparative study with sonography and CT. Radiology 1989;172:689-692.

60. Khalili K, Metser U, Wilson SR: Hilar biliary obstruction: Preliminary results with Levovist-enhanced sonography. AJR 2003;180(3):687-693.

61. Fried AM, Kreel L, Cosgrove DO: The hepatic interlobar fissure: Combined in vitro and in vivo study. AJR 1984;143(3):561-564.

62. Martin DF, Laasch HL: The biliary tract. In Grainger RG, Allison DJ (eds): Diagnostic Radiology: A Textbook of Medical Imaging, 4th ed. Churchill Livingstone, 2001, p 1277.

63. Stieber AC, Bauer JJ: Volvulus of the gallbladder. Am J Gastroenterol 1983;78:96-98.

64. Waisberg J, Pinto Junior PE, Gusson PR, et al: Agenesis of the gallbladder and cystic duct. Sao Paulo Med J 2002;120(6):192-194.

65. Kratzer W, Mason RA, Kachele V: Prevalence of gallstones in sonographic surveys worldwide. J Clin Ultrasound 1999;27(1):1-7.

66. Gore RM, Yaghmai V, Newmark GM, et al: Imaging benign and malignant disease of the gallbladder. Radiol Clin North Am 2002;40(6):1307-1323.

67. Naryshkin S, Trotman BW, Raffensperger EC: Milk of calcium bile. Evidence that gallbladder stasis is a key factor. Dig Dis Sci 1987;32(9):1051-1055.

68. Ko CW, Sekijima JH, Lee SP: Biliary sludge. Ann Intern Med 1999;130:301-311.

69. Trowbridge RL, Rutkowski NK, Shojania KG: Does this patient have acute cholecystitis? JAMA 2003;1;289(1):80-86.

70. Indar AA, Beckingham IJ: Acute cholecystitis. BMJ 2002;21;325(7365):639-643.

71. Shea JA, Berlin JA, Escarce JJ, et al: Revised estimates of diagnostic test sensitivity and specificity in suspected biliary tract disease. Arch Intern Med 1994;154:2573-2581.

72. Fidler J, Paulson EK, Layfield L: CT evaluation of acute cholecystitis: Findings and usefulness in diagnosis. AJR 1996;166:1085-1088.

73. Wilson SR: Gastrointestinal Disease (Sixth Series) test and syllabus. American College of Radiology, Reston, Va. In press.

74. Uggowitzer M, Kugler C, Schramayer G, et al: Sonography of acute cholecystitis: Comparison of color and power Doppler sonography in detecting a hypervascularized gallbladder wall. AJR 1997;168(3):707-712.

75. Simeone JF, Brink JA, Mueller PR, et al: The sonographic diagnosis of acute gangrenous cholecystitis: Importance of the Murphy sign. AJR 1989;152:289-290.

76. Sood BP, Kalra N, Gupta S, et al: Role of sonography in the diagnosis of gallbladder perforation. J Clin Ultrasound 2002;30(5):270-274.

77. Konno K, Ishida H, Naganuma H, et al: Emphysematous cholecystitis: Sonographic findings. Abdom Imaging 2002;27(2):191-195.

78. Ryu JK, Ryu KH, Kim KH: Clinical features of acute acalculous cholecystitis. J Clin Gastroenterol 2003;36(2):166-169.

79. Boland GW, Slater G, Lu DS, et al: Prevalence and significance of gallbladder abnormalities seen on sonography in intensive care unit patients. AJR 2000;174(4):973-977.

80. Helbich TH, Mallek R, Madl C, et al: Sonomorphology of the gallbladder in critically ill patients. Value of a scoring system and follow-up examinations. Acta Radiol 1997;38(1):129-134.

81. Ikematsu Y, Yamanouchi K, Nishiwaki Y, et al: Gallbladder volvulus: Experience of six consecutive cases at an institute. J Hepatobiliary Pancreat Surg 2000;7(6):606-609.

82. Schiller VL, Turner RR, Sarti DA: Color Doppler imaging of the gallbladder wall in acute cholecystitis: Sonographic-pathologic correlation. Abdom Imaging 1996;21:233-237.

83. Parra JA, Acinas O, Bueno J, et al: Xanthogranulomatous cholecystitis: Clinical, sonographic, and CT findings in 26 patients. AJR 2000;174:979-983.

84. Opatrny L: Porcelain gallbladder. AMAJ 2002;166(7):933.

85. Towfigh S, McFadden DW, Cortina GR, et al: Porcelain gallbladder is not associated with gallbladder carcinoma. Am Surg 2001;67:7-10.

86. Stephen AE, Berger DL: Carcinoma in the porcelain gallbladder: A relationship revisited. Surgery 2001;129(6):699-703.

87. Bilhartz LE: Acalculous cholecystitis, cholesterolosis, adenomyomatosis, and polyps of the gallbladder. In Feldman M, et al (eds): Sleisenger & Fordtran's Gastrointestinal and Liver Disease, 7th ed. Elsevier Science, 2002, pp 1123-1125.

88. Yoshimitsu K, Honda H, Aibe H, et al: Radiologic diagnosis of adenomyomatosis of the gallbladder: Comparative study among MRI, helical CT, and transabdominal US. J Comput Assist Tomogr 2001;25(6):843-850.

89. Csendes A, Burgos AM, Csendes P, et al: Late follow-up of polypoid lesions of the gallbladder smaller than 10 mm. Ann Surg 2001;234(5):657-660.

90. Levy AD, Murakata LA, Abbott RM, et al: From the archives of the AFIP. Benign tumors and tumorlike lesions

of the gallbladder and extrahepatic bile ducts: Radiologic-pathologic correlation. Armed Forces Institute of Pathology. Radiographics 2002;22(2):387-413.

91. Mainprize KS, Gould SW, Gilbert JM: Surgical management of polypoid lesions of the gallbladder. Br J Surg 2000;87(4):414-417.

92. Hirooka Y, Naitoh Y, Goto H, et al: Differential diagnosis of gallbladder masses using colour Doppler ultrasonography. J Gastroenterol Hepatol 1996;11(9):840-846.

93. Bilhartz LE: Acalculous cholecystitis, cholesterolosis, adenomyomatosis, and polyps of the gallbladder. *In Feldman M, et al: (eds): Sleisenger & Fordtran's Gastrointestinal and Liver Disease, 7th ed. Elsevier Science, 2002, pp 1116-1130.

94. Sugiyama M, Atomi Y, Kuroda A, et al: Large cholesterol polyps of the gallbladder: Diagnosis by means of US and endoscopic US. Radiology 1995;196(2):493-497.

95. Maeyama R, Yamaguchi K, Noshiro H, et al: A large inflammatory polyp of the gallbladder masquerading as gallbladder carcinoma. J Gastroenterol 1998;33(5):770-774.

96. Holloway BJ, King DM: Ultrasound diagnosis of metastatic melanoma of the gallbladder. Br J Radiol 1997;70(839):1122-1125.

97. Levy AD, Murakata LA, Rohrmann CA, Jr: Gallbladder carcinoma: Radiologic-pathologic correlation. Radiographics 2001;21:295-314.

98. Curley SA: The Gallbladder. In Abeloff MD (ed): Clinical Oncology, 2nd ed. Churchill Livingstone, 2000, pp 1415-1420.

99. Bach AM, Loring LA, Hann LE, et al: Gallbladder cancer: Can ultrasonography evaluate extent of disease? J Ultrasound Med 1998;17:303-309.

7

THE PANCREAS

Mostafa Atri / Paul W. Finnegan

Chapter Outline

*B*efore 1970, imaging of the pancreas was limited to the assessment of its surrounding structures or its vascular tree by angiography. With the advent of sonography, visualization of the pancreas itself became a reality. Since then, other imaging modalities such as computed tomography (CT) and magnetic resonance imaging (MRI) have become available to examine the pancreatic parenchyma. The development of fiberoptic technology has allowed physicians to examine the pancreatic duct with endoscopic retrograde cholangiopancreatography (ERCP) and, more recently, has allowed the examiner to apply high-resolution sonography with the use of endoscopic sonography (EUS). Although CT has played a major role, ultrasound remains the most widely available and least expensive means of visualizing the pancreas.

Although a spectrum of pathologic processes affects the pancreas, the major tasks of the imager are to distinguish a normal from an abnormal pancreas and to differentiate pancreatitis from malignancies. With the development of ultrasound-guided percutaneous fine-needle aspiration (PFNA) biopsy, accuracy in differentiating pancreatitis from carcinoma has significantly improved. Ultrasound guidance has also helped to promote the percutaneous interventional procedure as an alternative to surgical treatment for a number of pathologic processes related to the pancreas.

EMBRYOLOGY

The primitive pancreas consists of a dorsal and a ventral bud.[1] The dorsal bud arises as a diverticulum of the dorsal aspect of the duodenum, whereas the ventral bud originates as a common diverticulum with the primitive common bile duct (Fig. 7-1A). At 6 weeks' gestation, the ventral bud rotates 270 degrees to lie posteroinferior to the dorsal bud (see Fig. 7-1B). Fusion of these two buds

213

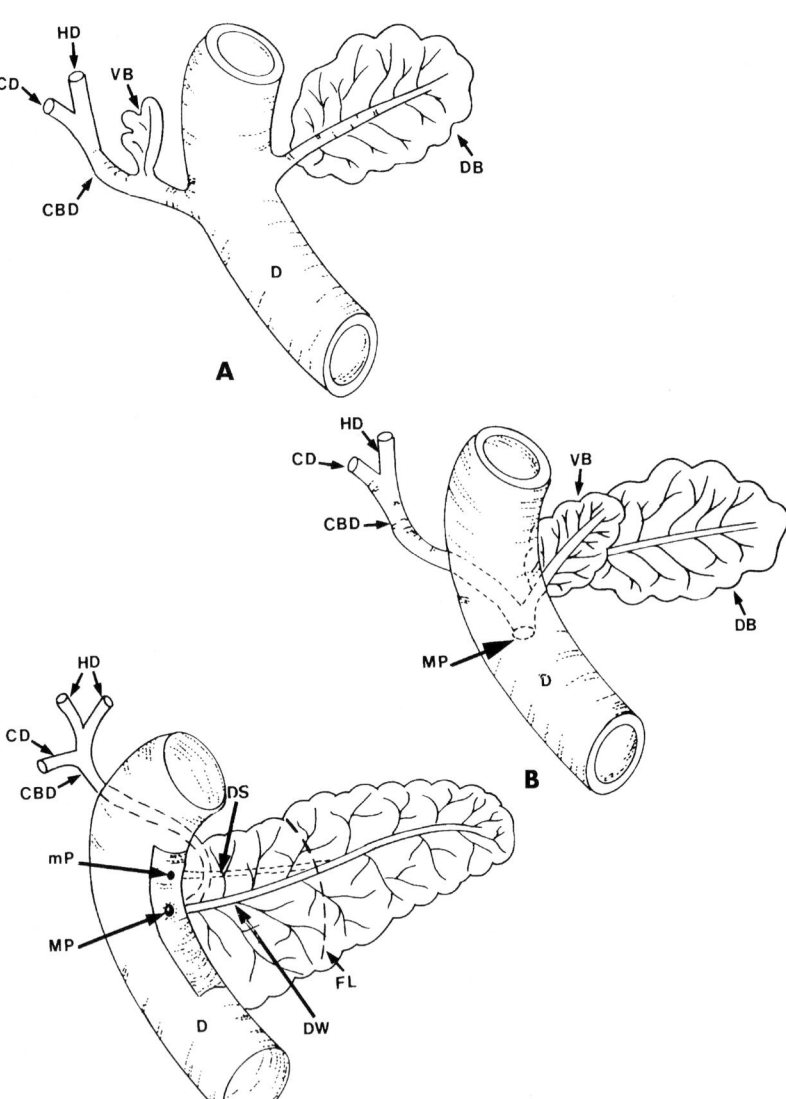

FIGURE 7-1. Stages in development of pancreas. A, Original pancreatic buds: ventral and dorsal. **B,** Rotation of ventral bud 270 degrees. **C,** Fusion of two buds and formation of final pancreatic duct. CBD, Common bile duct; CD, cystic duct; D, duodenum; DB, dorsal bud; DS, duct of Santorini; DW, duct of Wirsung; FL, fusion line; HD, hepatic duct; MP, major papilla; mP, minor papilla; VB, ventral bud.

forms the final pancreas. The dorsal bud develops into the cephalad aspect of the head, neck, body, and tail, whereas the caudal aspect of the head and the uncinate process originates from the ventral bud (see Fig. 7-1C). Initially, each pancreatic bud has its own duct, which drains separately into the duodenum at two different openings, the major and minor papillae. After fusion of the two buds, the ventral duct in the head anastomoses with the proximal part of the dorsal duct in the body and tail to form the final main pancreatic duct **(duct of Wirsung),** which drains most of the pancreas (see Fig. 7-1C). This main duct empties into the duodenum through the major papilla together with the common bile duct. The remaining portion of the dorsal pancreatic duct, called the accessory pancreatic duct **(duct of Santorini),** opens into the duodenum at the minor papilla. Various degrees of regression affecting the terminal part of the dorsal pancreatic duct result in multiple anatomic variants of the pancreatic duct (Fig. 7-2).[2]

ANATOMY

The pancreas can be localized with ultrasound by identifying its parenchymal architecture and the surrounding anatomic landmarks. The level of the pancreas is known to change slightly, depending on the phase of respiration. With maximal inspiration and expiration, the organ has been shown to shift 2 to 8 cm in the craniocaudad axis.[3] These respiratory migrations should be taken into consideration when imaging the pancreas and especially during ultrasound-guided biopsy.

The pancreas is a nonencapsulated, retroperitoneal structure that lies in the anterior pararenal space between the duodenal loop and the splenic hilum over a length of 12.5 to 15 cm.[1] The head, uncinate process, neck, body, and tail constitute the different parts of the pancreas (Fig. 7-3). The superior mesenteric vessels course posterior to the neck of the pancreas, separating the head

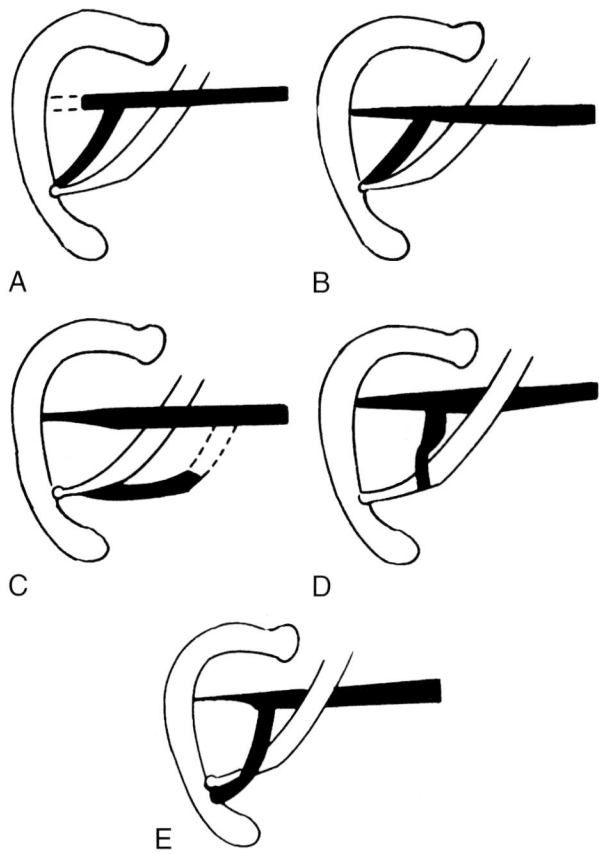

FIGURE 7-2. Variations, pancreatic duct anatomy. A, Complete regression of duct of Santorini (40% to 50%). **B,** Persistence of the duct of Santorini (35%). **C,** Persistence of both Santorini and Wirsung ducts without communication (5% to 10%). **D,** Communication of Santorini and Wirsung ducts, with duct of Wirsung entering common bile duct proximal to ampulla (5% to 10%). **E,** Separate entrance of duct of Wirsung and common bile duct with variable persistence of duct of Santorini (5%). (From Berman LG, Prior JT, Abramow SM, et al: A study of the pancreatic duct system in man by the use of vinyl acetate cases of postmortem preparations. Surg Gynecol Obstet 1960;110:391-403.)

from the body. The uncinate process represents the medial extension of the head and lies behind the superior mesenteric vessels. No anatomic landmark separates the body from the tail.

The pancreas comprises exocrine and endocrine tissues. The exocrine pancreas constitutes 80% of the pancreatic tissue and is composed of ductal and acinar cells. The endocrine islet cells of Langerhans form only 2% of the pancreatic substance. The remaining 18% consists of fibrous stroma that contains blood vessels, nerves, and lymphatics.[4]

Surrounding Structures

Gastrointestinal Tract, Ligaments, and Peritoneal Spaces

The antrum of the stomach lies transversely across the midline, usually anterior to the pancreas, with the gastric

body located anterior to the pancreatic tail. However, depending on the patient's body habitus, which alters the shape and orientation of the stomach, the pancreas may occupy a position cephalad or caudad to the stomach. The **duodenal loop,** except for the first segment, is retroperitoneal and encircles the pancreatic head.

The **transverse mesocolon** attaches posteriorly to the anterior aspect of the head, body, and proximal tail of the pancreas and anteriorly to the greater omentum. At the level of the head of the pancreas, the mesocolon joins midway between the superior and the inferior borders; at the level of the body, it suspends from the inferior border of the pancreas, dividing the organ into supramesocolic and inframesocolic portions. The stomach, omentum, and lesser sac lie anterior to the pancreas in the **supramesocolic portion.**[1]

The **lesser omentum,** which is a double layer of peritoneum, bridges the abdominal part of the esophagus, lesser curvature of the stomach, and first portion of the duodenum to the fissure for the ligamentum venosum of the liver. The **greater omentum,** which is also double-layered, hangs down from the greater curvature of the stomach and attaches to the transverse colon after looping back on itself. The lesser sac is a potential space situated between the lesser omentum, greater omentum, and the stomach anteriorly and the parietal peritoneum posteriorly. Depending on the position of the stomach, different parts of the lesser and greater omentum, stomach, and lesser sac are related to the pancreas anteriorly.[1] The **lesser sac** is often partially or completely obliterated by adhesions, and, therefore, the stomach and greater and lesser omentum come in close contact with the anterior surface of the pancreas. The jejunal loops, duodenojejunal junction, and splenic flexure of the colon lie anterior to the pancreas in the **inframesocolic space.**[1] The tip of the tail of the pancreas is intraperitoneal because it is ensheathed in the lienorenal ligament.[1]

Vessels

Arteries. The **abdominal aorta** runs posterior to the body of the pancreas. The **celiac axis** arises from the abdominal aorta at the superior border of the pancreas and divides into the left gastric, common hepatic, and splenic arteries. The common hepatic artery proceeds anteriorly to the right, cephalad to the head, of the pancreas. At the inferior border of the epiploic foramen, the common hepatic artery divides into its two terminal branches: the hepatic proper and the gastroduodenal arteries. The hepatic artery proper travels superiorly toward the liver along the free edge of the lesser omentum anterior to the portal vein and to the left of the bile duct. A common normal variant, present in 25% of the population, consists of a completely or incompletely

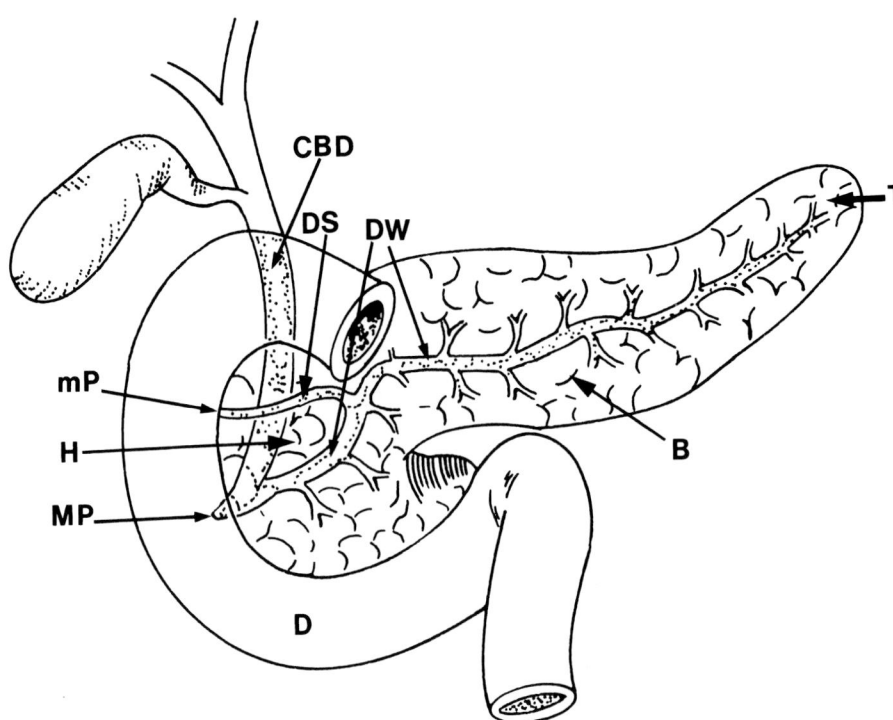

FIGURE 7-3. Schematic drawing of pancreas, duodenum, and bile duct. B, Body of pancreas; CBD, common bile duct; DS, duct of Santorini; DW, duct of Wirsung; H, head of pancreas; mP, minor papilla; MP, major papilla; T, tail of pancreas.

replaced hepatic artery, which arises from the right lateral aspect of the superior mesenteric artery. This accessory (or replaced hepatic artery) usually courses between the portal vein and the inferior vena cava as opposed to the normal hepatic artery that runs anterior to the portal vein. The gastroduodenal artery travels a short distance posterior to the junction of the pylorus and the first portion of the duodenum within a groove on the superior border of the pancreas lateral to the neck. Then, passing anterior to the head of the pancreas, it divides into its terminal branches, the right gastro-epiploic and the superior pancreaticoduodenal arteries.[1] The splenic artery follows a tortuous course along the superior border of the body and the tail of the pancreas. The **superior mesenteric artery** arises from the abdominal aorta just caudad to the inferior border of the pancreas, descending anterior to the uncinate process of the pancreas and the third portion of the duodenum to enter the mesentery.

Veins. The **inferior vena cava** lies posterior to the head of the pancreas. Depending on the level at which the renal veins drain into the inferior vena cava, the left renal vein may travel posterior to the head of the pancreas, although it is usually more caudad.

The **splenic vein** runs from its origin in the splenic hilum along the posteroinferior aspect of the pancreas to join the **superior mesenteric vein.** The superior mesenteric vein travels to the right of the superior mesenteric artery and ascends anterior to the third portion of the duodenum and the uncinate process of the pancreas. The superior mesenteric vein and the splenic vein join posterior to the neck of the pancreas to form the portal vein. The **portal vein** ascends toward the porta hepatis cephalad to the head of the pancreas.[1]

Common Bile Duct

The common bile duct passes inferiorly in the free edge of the lesser omentum to the level of the duodenum. It then travels posterior to the first portion of the duodenum and the head of the pancreas to lie to the right of the main pancreatic duct. The common bile duct then opens into the duodenum at the hepaticopancreatic ampulla on the summit of the major papilla after forming a common trunk with the pancreatic duct (80%). In 20% of people, the common bile duct has its own separate ampulla but still enters the duodenum at the major papilla.[5] In its course behind the head of the pancreas, it lies in a groove on the posterior aspect of the pancreas or is embedded in its substance.

PANCREATIC SONOGRAPHY

Head

Transverse Plane

The pancreatic head may be quite long, extending over several centimeters. The sonographic appearance varies from the most cephalad to the most caudal image. **Cephalad to the pancreatic head,** the hepatic artery and bile duct are seen anterior to the portal vein. The air- or fluid-filled pylorus and the first portion of the duodenum may also be seen at this level. In the **superior**

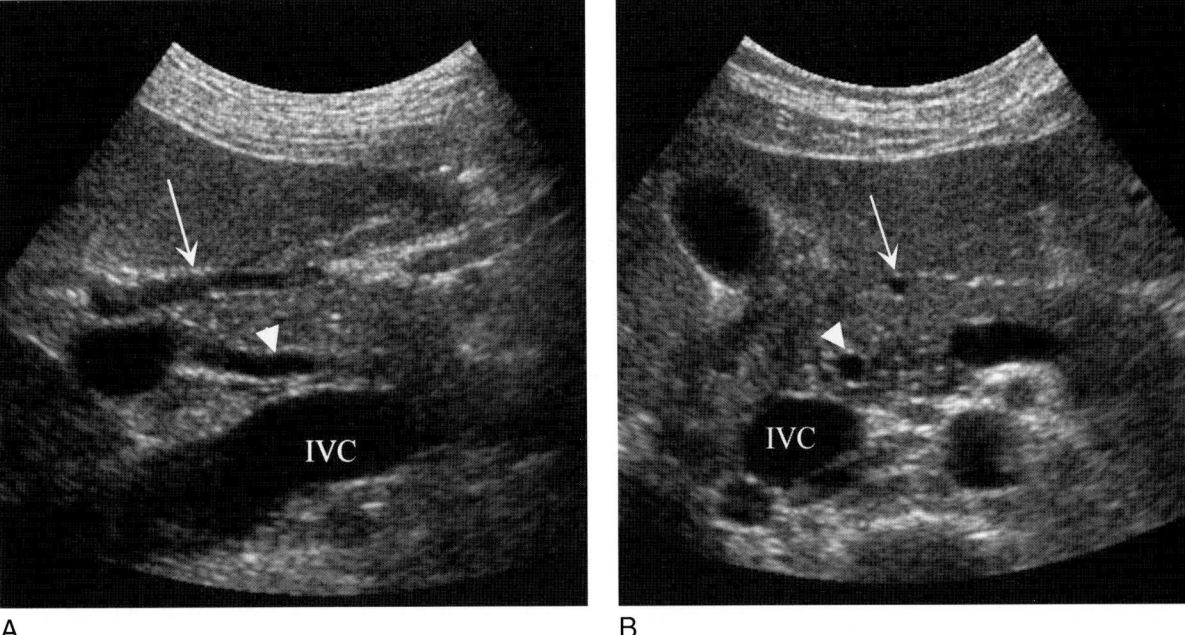

A   B

FIGURE 7-4. Normal pancreatic head. A, Sagittal and **B,** transverse images show the pancreas anterior to the inferior vena cava (IVC). Two tubular structures related to the pancreatic head are the gastroduodenal artery *(arrow)*, which is on the right anterolateral margin, and the common bile duct *(arrowhead)*, which is on the right posterolateral boundary. (Courtesy of Stephanie Wilson, M.D., University of Toronto, Toronto, Ontario.)

aspect of the head, two circular structures can be identified on the right lateral aspect of the head that represent a cross-sectional view of the **gastroduodenal artery** anteriorly and the **common bile duct** posteriorly (Fig. 7-4). The latter structures demarcate the lateral aspect of the pancreatic head, allowing for separation of the head of the pancreas from the more laterally placed duodenum. However, in some individuals, the lateral extent of the head may extend beyond a line drawn between the gastroduodenal artery and common bile duct.[6] At this level, the medial extent of the head merges with the neck of the pancreas. The inferior vena cava lies posterior to the head. However, the relation of the pancreas to the inferior vena cava and aorta is variable and can occasionally be off center to the left of the major vessels, especially in thin patients and in patients lying in the left decubitus position. The main pancreatic duct and its branches may be seen extending obliquely between the neck of the pancreas more superiorly and to the second portion of the duodenum more inferiorly, where it may or may not join the common bile duct before entering the duodenum. In its most **inferior aspect,** the medial portion of the pancreatic head tapers to form the **uncinate process.** At this level in cross section, the superior mesenteric vein is seen to the right and the superior mesenteric artery to the left between the uncinate process and the neck of the pancreas. A replaced hepatic artery is commonly shown by sonographic examination,[7] arising from the right lateral aspect of the superior mesenteric artery and running

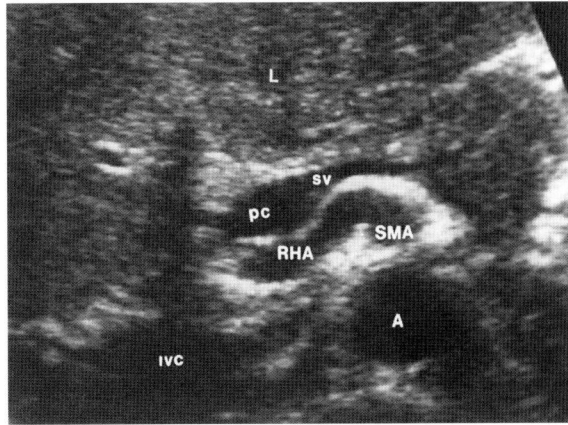

FIGURE 7-5. Replaced hepatic artery (RHA). Transverse scan shows RHA running between portal confluence (PC) and inferior vena cava (IVC). A, aorta; L, liver; SMA, superior mesenteric artery; SV, splenic vein.

toward the liver between the portal vein and inferior vena cava (Fig. 7-5). **Caudad to the head,** the third portion of the duodenum may be seen running transversely from right to left.

Sagittal Plane

On the right and lateral to the head, the second portion of the duodenum projects in a cephalocaudal direction. In the lateral aspect of the head in some patients, the gastroduodenal artery may be seen coursing in a cephalocaudal direction anterior to the pancreas with the common bile duct running parallel but more posteriorly (Fig. 7-4A). The latter may lie posterior to the pancreas or be embedded in its posterior aspect. The third portion of the duodenum is seen in cross-sectional views caudad to the pancreas. More medially, the longest cephalocaudal dimension of the head is displayed. A longitudinal view of the main portal vein projects superior to the head of the pancreas at this level.

Neck, Body, and Tail

The pancreatic neck lies between the head and body anterior to the portal venous confluence. There is no anatomic landmark separating the body and the tail of the pancreas, but the left lateral border of the vertebral column is considered the arbitrary plane demarcating these two segments. The level of the tail in relation to the body of the pancreas on the horizontal plane varies depending on the body habitus. It may be located cephalad, at the same level, or (rarely) lower than the body.

Transverse Plane

The celiac axis is seen **cephalad** to the body of the pancreas at this level, dividing similar to a "Y" into the hepatic and splenic arteries (see Fig. 7-6B). At the **level of the neck,** the confluence of the splenic and superior mesenteric veins is seen posterior to the pancreas. More laterally, the splenic vein runs posterior to the body and the tail. The abdominal aorta lies posterior to the proximal body of the pancreas. The left renal vein courses between the superior mesenteric artery and the aorta and posterior to the pancreas to drain into the inferior vena cava. The upper pole of the left kidney and the left renal vessels may also be seen posterior to the tail of the pancreas. Depending on the location of the stomach, its posterior wall may be visualized anterior to the pancreas. **Caudad** to the pancreas lie the third and fourth portions of the duodenum. Caution should be exercised not to mistake a jejunal branch draining into the superior mesenteric vein for a splenic vein. In the presence of splenic vein thrombosis, this jejunal branch may be mistaken for a patent splenic vein.

Sagittal Plane

At the level of the neck, the superior mesenteric vein is seen posterior to the pancreas (Fig. 7-7A). The uncinate process of the head is seen posterior to the superior mesenteric vein. A longitudinal view of the aorta is identified with the **body** of the pancreas situated between the celiac axis and the superior mesenteric artery (see Fig. 7-7B). At the levels of the body and the tail, the stomach lies anteriorly (see Fig. 7-7C). A cross

section of the splenic vein is seen posteriorly, whereas a cross section of the splenic artery appears cephalad. The third portion of the duodenum projects inferiorly. By using the spleen as an acoustic window, the **tail** of the pancreas is occasionally seen medial to that organ on both transverse and coronal planes (see Fig. 7-7D). When the pancreas is echogenic, a distinct echogenic structure representing the tail may be seen through the spleen.

Pancreatic Duct

The normal pancreatic duct is seen at least partially in 86% of patients.[8] On the transverse plane, it is optimally visualized in the central portion of the body where the duct is perpendicular to the ultrasound beam. Based on the resolution of the ultrasound system, the patient's body habitus, and the angle of insonation, the pancreatic duct is seen as a single linear structure (Fig. 7-8A) or as double-parallel lines (see Fig. 7-8B). The mean internal diameter on sonographic examination has been reported to measure 3 mm in the head, 2.1 mm in the body, and 1.6 mm in the tail.[9] The dimensions of the pancreatic duct obtained sonographically are smaller than the corresponding ERCP measurements as a result primarily of x-ray magnification and overdistention of the duct.[10] Its diameter increases with age, probably because of parenchymal atrophy. Although a 2- to 2.5-mm diameter has been reported as the upper limit of normal,[8,10] for practical purposes the pancreatic duct is probably normal as long as the walls maintain their parallel course and the duct can be followed along its whole length to the duodenum. It has been shown that the diameter of pancreatic duct may vary with respiration, increasing at end inspiration.[11] When the pancreatic duct becomes dilated, its side branches may also be seen and may be mistaken for pancreatic cysts. Occasionally, the accessory duct of Santorini and some normal branches of the main pancreatic duct can be identified in the pancreatic head. The normal pancreatic duct can change caliber during the examination (see Fig. 7-8C and D).

Pancreatic Echotexture

The normal pancreas is usually homogeneous. The echogenicity, when compared with the normal liver, is either isoechoic or, more commonly, hyperechoic (Fig. 7-9). Sometimes a mottled appearance may be seen. The contour of the pancreas is distinct when its echogenicity is less than the surrounding retroperitoneal fat. The gland usually appears smoothly contoured, although a lobulated contour is occasionally discerned. With aging and obesity, the pancreas becomes more echogenic as a result of the presence of **fatty infiltration** and in up to 35% of cases may be as echogenic as the

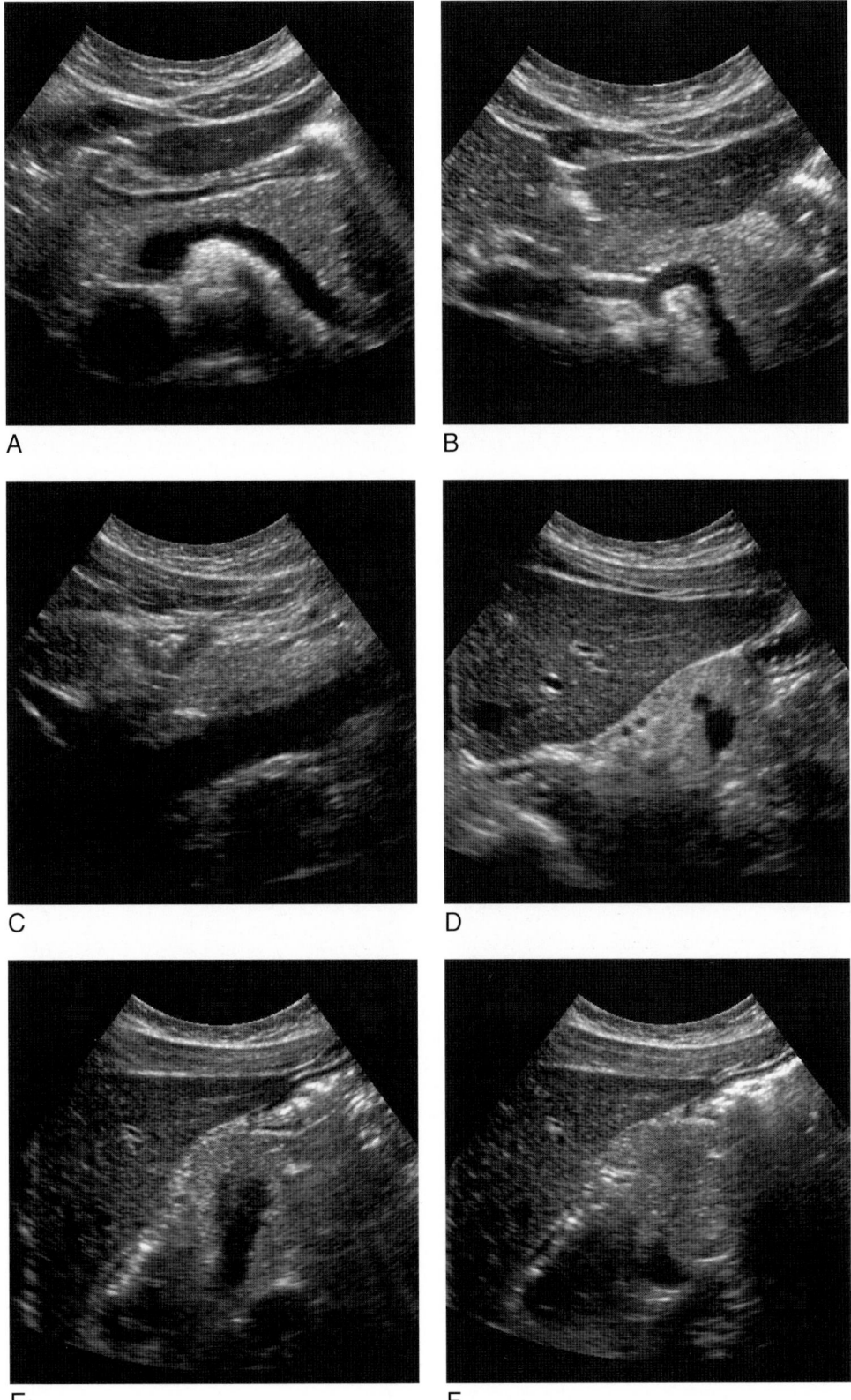

FIGURE 7-6. Normal pancreas sonogram. A, Transverse image showing the pancreas and the most consistent vascular landmark—the splenic vein and portal venous confluence. **B,** Body of the pancreas anterior to the branches of the celiac axis, which limits the pancreas on its cephalad margin. **C,** Longitudinal right paramedian scan showing the inferior vena cava. The head of the pancreas lies on the IVC. **D, E,** and **F,** Left paramedian images taken in sequence beginning in the midline and progressively angling to the left. **D,** Splenic artery and splenic vein in cross section. **E,** Splenic vein in long axis. **F,** The pancreatic tail.

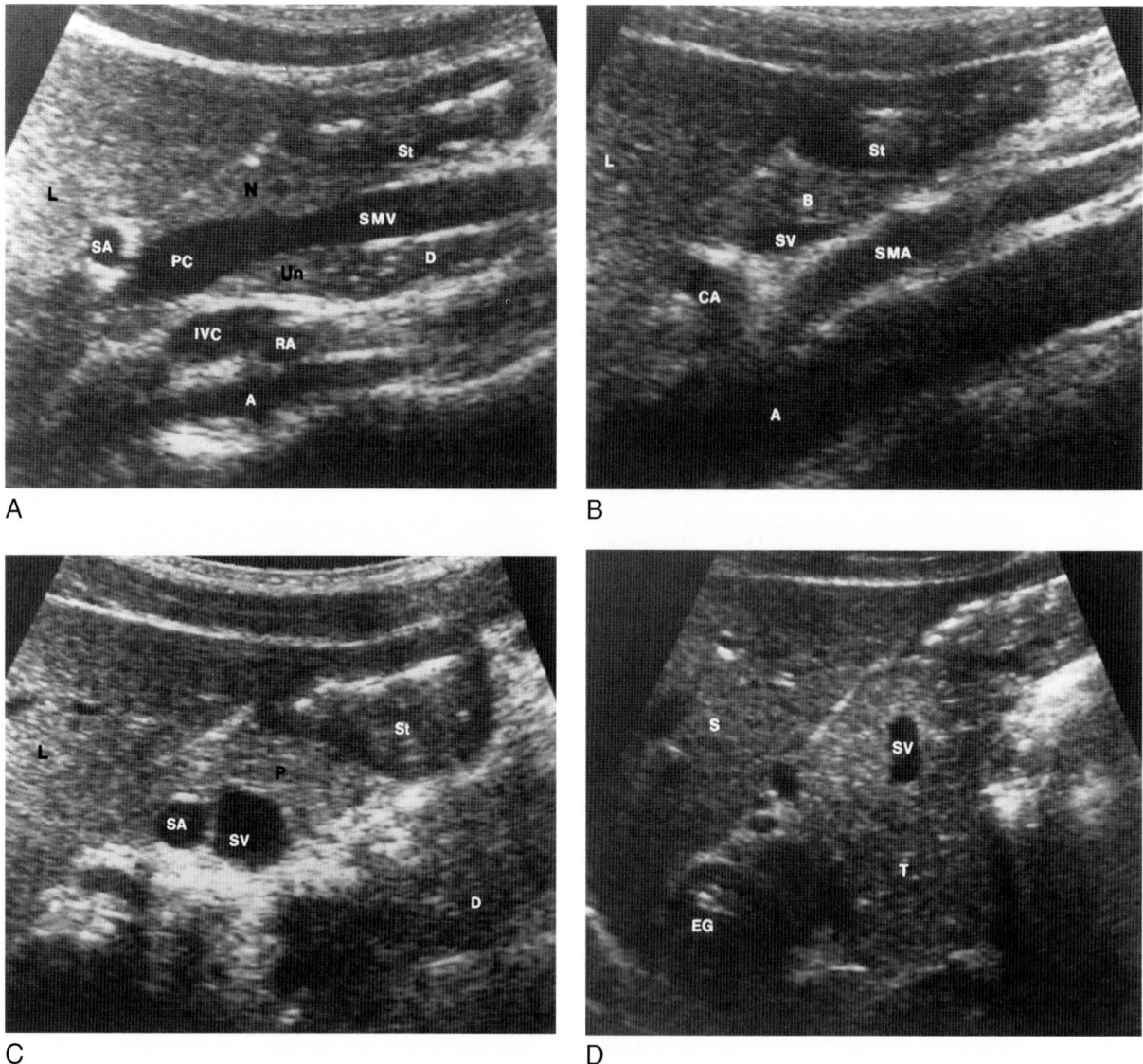

FIGURE 7-7. Neck, body, and tail of pancreas, sagittal view. A, Level of neck. **B,** Slightly to left of neck. **C,** Level of body. **D,** Level of tail on coronal plane through spleen. Projection of splenic vein (SV) in middle of tail of pancreas is due to averaging. A, aorta; B, body of stomach; CA, celiac artery; D, third portion of duodenum; EG, esophagogastric junction; IVC, inferior vena cava; L, liver; N, neck of pancreas; P, body of pancreas; PC, portal confluence; RA, right renal artery; S, spleen; SA, splenic artery; SMA, superior mesenteric artery; SMV, superior mesenteric vein; St, stomach; SV, splenic vein; T, tail of pancreas; Un, uncinate process.

adjacent retroperitoneal fat.[12] The increased echogenicity resulting from excessive body fat is reversible.[12] Hyperechogenicity may account for difficulty in visualizing the pancreas as it blends with the adjacent retroperitoneal fat, making its contour and true size impossible to identify. In such patients, the gland can be assessed only by describing the pancreatic fossa using the vascular anatomy as landmarks. Because the size of the pancreas cannot be evaluated in these patients, pancreatic atrophy resulting in pancreatic insufficiency should not be excluded.[13] Also, retroperitoneal fat in the bed of a congenitally absent or atrophic body and tail of the pancreas may mimic pancreatic tissue on ultrasound. CT scans are indicated in these patients. **Causes of fatty**

infiltration of the pancreas include aging, obesity, chronic pancreatitis, dietary deficiency, viral infection, corticosteroid therapy, cystic fibrosis, diabetes mellitus, hereditary pancreatitis, and obstruction caused by a stone or pancreatic carcinoma.[13] In lipomatous pseudohypertrophy, the pancreas is massively enlarged as a result of fatty replacement.[14]

Dimensions

The normal head of the pancreas generally has the largest dimensions, with the neck having the smallest.[15] The body and most of the tail are slightly smaller than the head. In one study,[16] the anteroposterior dimension of

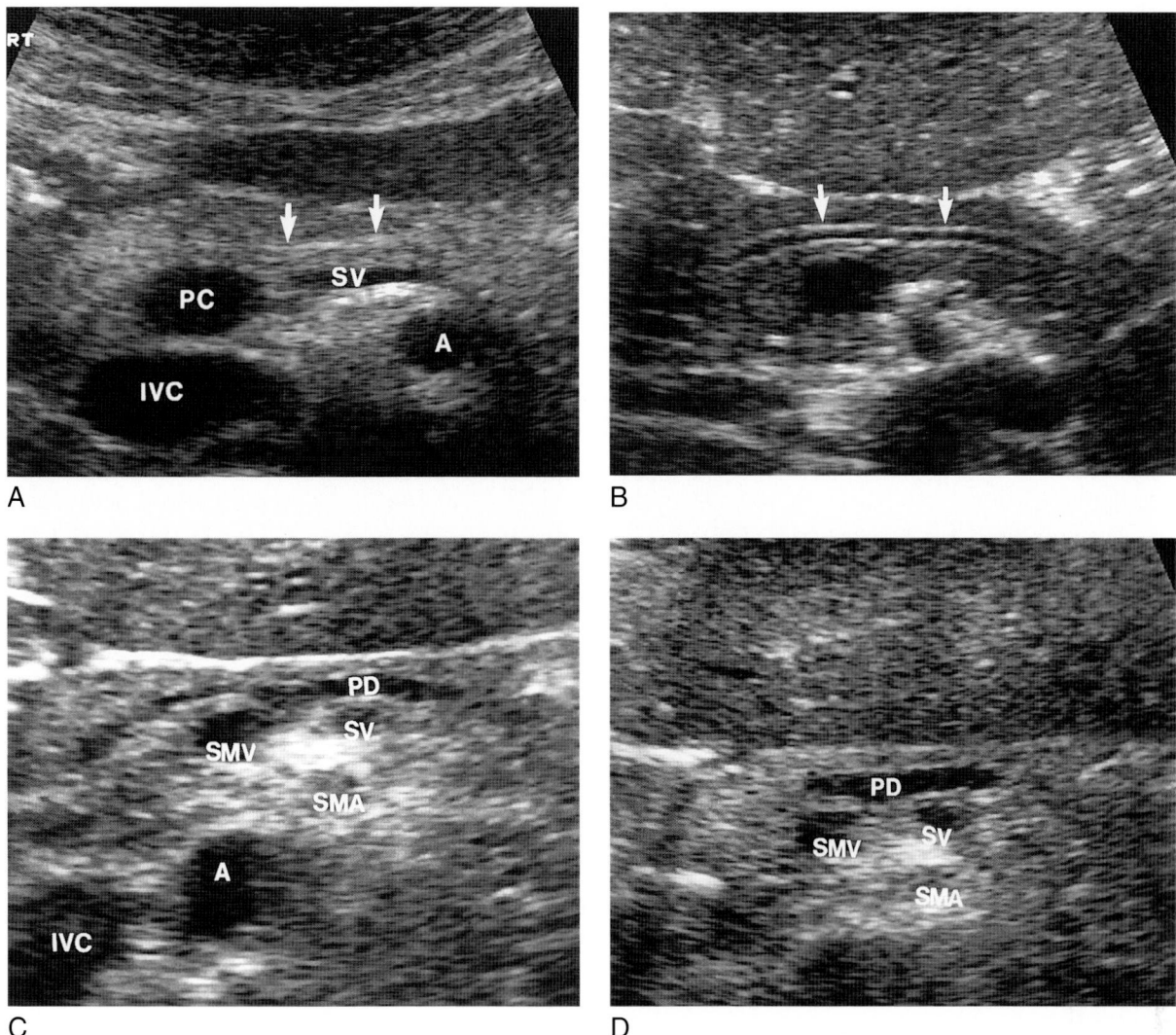

FIGURE 7-8. Pancreatic duct, transverse scan. A, Single line pancreatic duct *(arrows).* **B,** Double-line pancreatic duct *(arrows).* **C,** Small caliber pancreatic duct (PD). **D,** Changing to a larger caliber during the same examination. A, aorta; IVC, inferior vena cava; PC, portal confluence; SMA, superior mesenteric artery; SMV, superior mesenteric vein; SV, splenic vein.

the normal head measured 2.2 to 0.3 cm, with the body measuring 1.8 to 0.3 cm. The cephalocaudal dimension of the head has been reported as 2.01 to 0.39 cm and that of the body as 1.18 to 0.36 cm.[15] The pancreas may appear larger in obese patients, because it blends with the excessive retroperitoneal fat. The size of the pancreas diminishes with age.[17]

Pitfalls and Normal Variants

Pancreas

Structures that may be mistaken for the pancreas or a pancreatic pathologic process include the following:

- The **posterior part (segment 2)** of the lateral segment of the left lobe of the liver, when it is less echogenic than the anterior part (segment 3) because of sound attenuation by perivascular fat

- The **papillary process of the caudate lobe,** when it is completely separated from the liver
- The **third part of the duodenum,** when it is collapsed or filled with echogenic fluid (bowel wall layers and peristalsis differentiate)
- **Retroperitoneal fibrosis,** when seen as a midline band (it usually occurs inferior to the pancreas between the aorta and the mesenteric vessels)
- **Horseshoe kidney,** which is usually inferior and posterior to the mesenteric vessels, continuous with kidneys, and reniform
- **Lymph nodes,** which can simulate a bandlike pancreas (associated aortocaval, retrocaval, or retroaortic lymphadenopathy helps to differentiate them from the pancreas)
- **Intrapancreatic collateral veins** secondary to portal vein thrombosis, which may mimic intrapancreatic cystic lesions (Fig. 7-10)

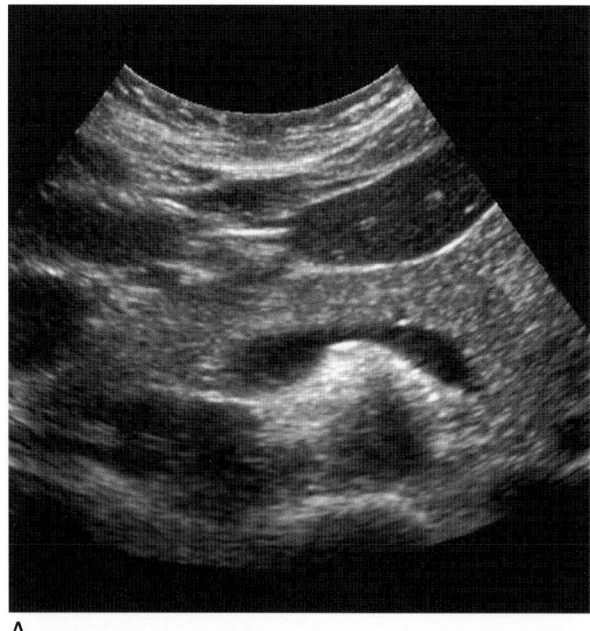

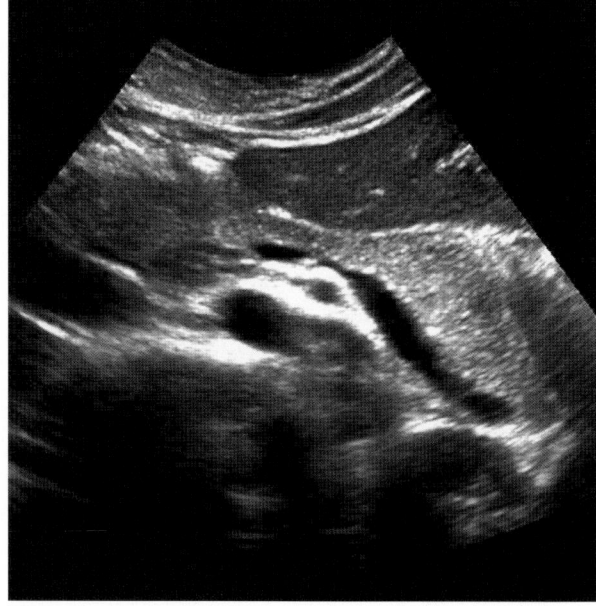

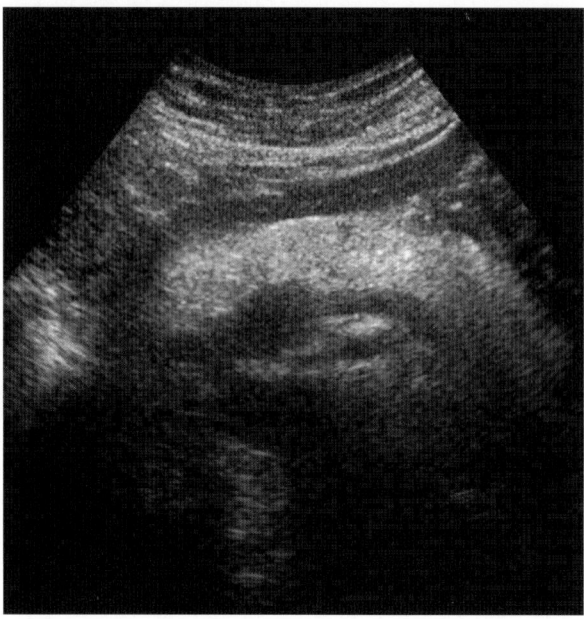

FIGURE 7-9. Normal variation of the echogenicity of the pancreas. The pancreas is generally more echogenic than the spleen and liver, and the degree of echogenicity is variable. Different degrees of hyperechogenicity of the pancreas are shown in **A** to **C**.

The embryologic **ventral aspect of the head and uncinate process of the pancreas** may be hypoechoic relative to the rest of the pancreas in some individuals (Fig. 7-11).[18-20] The distribution of the hypoechogenicity and geographic appearance, sharp demarcation from the rest of the pancreas, and the identification of the normal pancreatic duct and common bile duct within this zone help to distinguish it from a pathologic process.

We have shown on correlation of ultrasound and pathology in vitro that this area of hypoechogenicity corresponds to less fatty infiltration of the embryologic ventral pancreas.[20] The corresponding finding on CT is higher attenuation of the ventral pancreas. In our series,

the prevalence of this finding was 54% on the pancreas autopsy specimens and 22% on the CT scan. In vivo prevalence of this finding on ultrasound was 28.1% in the series of Donald and colleagues.[18] CT may or may not show an area of high density corresponding to the hypoechogenicity on ultrasound, presumably depending on the discrepancy in fat content. Areas of focal fatty infiltration are occasionally seen in the pancreas, presenting as hyperechoic or hypoechoic nodules.

Pancreatic Duct

Structures that are confused with the pancreatic duct and errors of interpretation include the layers of the

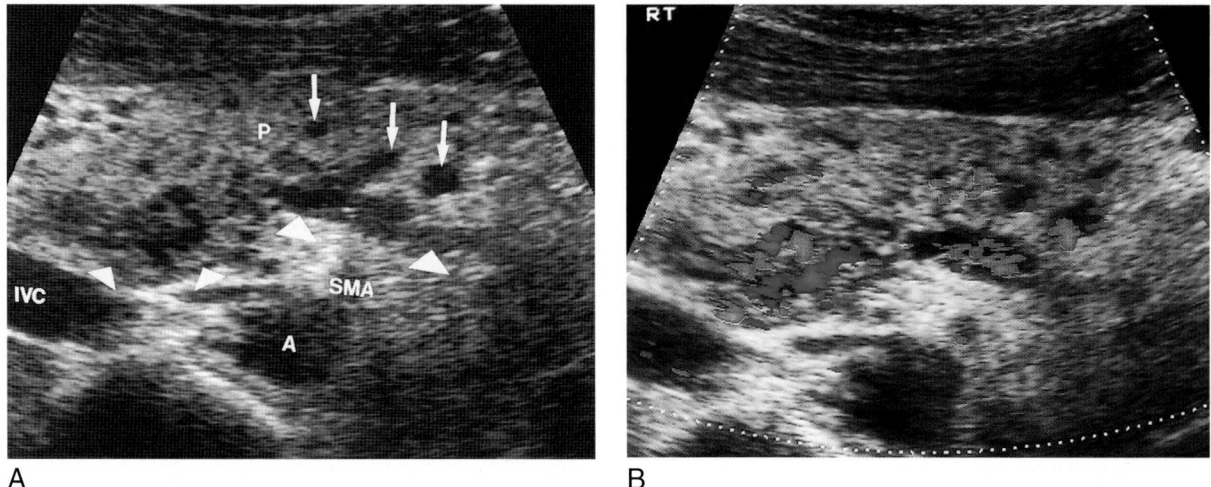

FIGURE 7-10. Pitfalls and normal variants of pancreas. Thrombosis of the splenoportal circulation in a patient with pancreatic carcinoma. Transverse views. **A,** Splenoportal vein thrombosis *(arrowheads)*. Collateral veins *(arrows)* in pancreas (P). A, aorta; SMA, superior mesenteric artery; IVC, inferior vena cava. **B,** Color Doppler examination of the same patient demonstrating color flow in the vascular spaces of the pancreas.

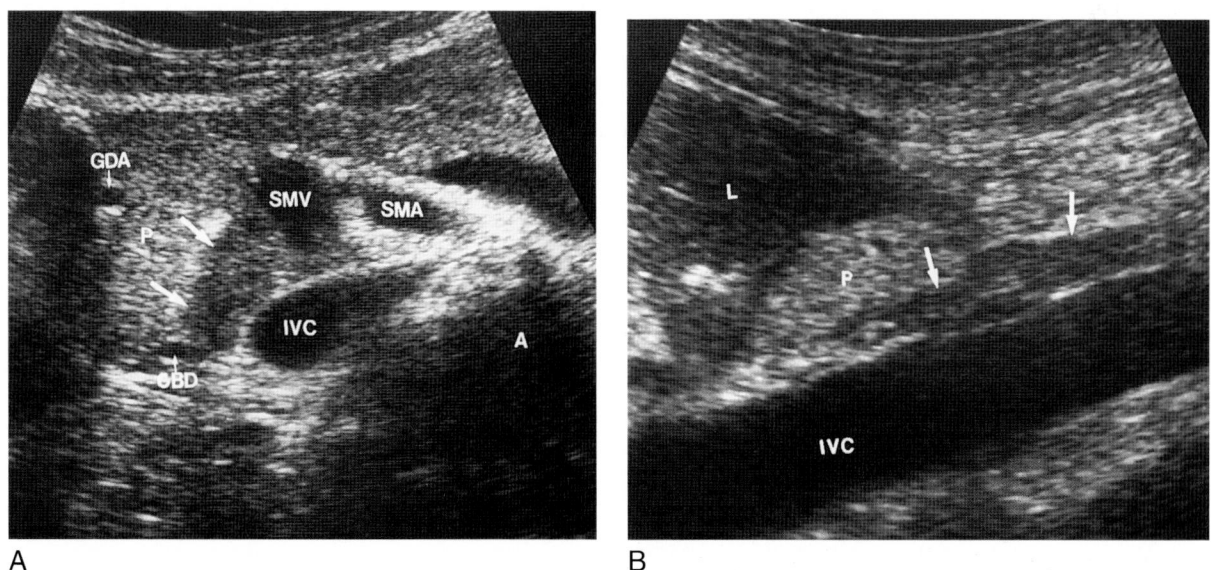

FIGURE 7-11. Hypoechoic ventral aspect of head of pancreas. Transverse (**A**) and sagittal (**B**) views show well-defined hypoechogenicity of embryologic ventral aspect of head of pancreas *(arrows)*. Notice the undisturbed common bile duct (CBD). A, aorta; GDA, gastroduodenal artery; IVC, inferior vena cava; L, liver; P, pancreas; SMA, superior mesenteric artery; SMV, superior mesenteric vein.

posterior wall of the stomach and the outline of the splenic vein. No pancreatic parenchyma surrounds them, they are not located in the middle of an apparent pancreas, and their course is not toward the second portion of the duodenum. A jejunal branch of the superior mesenteric vein may have an appearance and orientation similar to that of the pancreatic duct because it may be surrounded by retroperitoneal fat that can simulate pancreatic tissue on a sonogram. Following the vessel to its junction with the superior mesenteric vein and Doppler interrogation help to differentiate a vascular structure from the pancreatic duct. Artifacts

inherent to the ultrasound technology, such as beam width, can cause averaging of a tortuous splenic artery within the pancreas and may simulate a dilated pancreatic duct. With significant pancreatic atrophy caused by obstruction, no pancreatic tissue is seen around the dilated duct, creating the potential for an erroneous interpretation of a vascular structure. This is more likely to happen when the pancreas is very anterior as a result of significant emaciation caused by pancreatic carcinoma. On rare occasions, venous branches draining into the portal vein are seen in the head of the pancreas, which can be mistaken for the pancreatic duct. Intra-

STRUCTURES THAT MAY BE MISTAKEN FOR THE PANCREAS OR A PANCREATIC PATHOLOGIC PROCESS

Posterior part of the lateral segment of the left lobe of the liver because of sound attenuation by perivascular fat

Papillary process of the caudate lobe when it is completely separated from the liver

Third part of the duodenum collapsed or filled with echogenic fluid

Retroperitoneal fibrosis when seen as a midline band inferior to the pancreas between the aorta and the mesenteric vessels

Horseshoe kidney usually inferior and posterior to the mesenteric vessels

Lymph nodes simulate a bandlike pancreas

Intrapancreatic collateral veins secondary to portal vein thrombosis may mimic intrapancreatic cystic lesions (see Fig. 7-10).

Ventral aspect of the head and uncinate process may be hypoechoic relative to the rest of the pancreas (see Fig. 7-11).

STRUCTURES THAT ARE CONFUSED WITH THE PANCREATIC DUCT

Layers of the posterior wall of the stomach and the splenic vein

Jejunal branch of the superior mesenteric vein may be surrounded by retroperitoneal fat that can simulate pancreatic tissue

Averaging of a tortuous splenic artery within the pancreas

Significant pancreatic atrophy Erroneous interpretation of a vascular structure

Venous branches draining into the portal vein

Intrapancreatic collateral veins

Air in the pancreatic duct Mistaken for ductal calculi

pancreatic collaterals in the presence of portal vein thrombosis may be mistaken for a pancreatic duct. The course of these structures and documentation of flow on Doppler help differentiation. Air in the pancreatic duct, usually secondary to pancreaticoenterostomy, may be mistaken for ductal calculi.

Intrapancreatic Common Bile Duct

A normal posterior-superior pancreaticoduodenal vein is occasionally seen running in the cephalocaudal dimension in the head of the pancreas to insert on the caudal aspect of the portal vein (Fig. 7-12). This vein is reported to parallel the common bile duct posteriorly in 98% and anteriorly in 2% in one series.[21] It can potentially be mistaken for the common bile duct.

Technical Aspects

Patient Preparation

Evaluation of the pancreas is usually performed as part of the ultrasound examination of the upper abdomen and especially in conjunction with assessment of the biliary system. Because optimal gallbladder distention requires fasting, ultrasound examination of the pancreas has been traditionally performed after a minimum fast of 6 hours. Theoretically, fasting also diminishes gaseous distention of the upper gastrointestinal tract, which can interfere with the visualization of the pancreas. However, in some patients, evaluating the pancreas alone appears to be feasible in the postfasting state.[22]

Considerations of Technique

There are two major factors preventing optimal visualization of the pancreas: fat and interfering gastrointestinal gas. Because the pancreas is retroperitoneal, it is a deep structure in larger patients and a particular technical challenge because it is covered by the gas-filled gastrointestinal tract. Scanning principles used for the examination of the pancreas include the following:

- Place the area of interest within the focal zone of the transducer.
- Alter the patient's position to include erect, supine, both oblique views, both decubitus views, and even prone positions, to displace the gas-containing structures or transfer the gas into another part of the gastrointestinal tract. The erect position displaces the gas-filled stomach or colon away from the pancreas and causes the liver to move down over the pancreas, becoming an acoustic window. The erect position appears to be most effective if used in the beginning of the examination because aerophagia caused by deep inspirations during the examination may fill the stomach with gas.
- Furthermore, breathing mechanisms, including suspended inspiration or expiration, and a Valsalva maneuver may be helpful. Differentiation of a pancreatic mass from a lesion arising from surrounding structures may be helped by evaluating the mobility of the mass relative to these structures during respiration. The mobility of the pancreas is not as great as the intraperitoneal structures.[3]
- Lastly, increasing stomach distention with fluid when there is a large amount of interfering gas and when the upright position has failed to demonstrate the pancreas may allow pancreatic visualization.

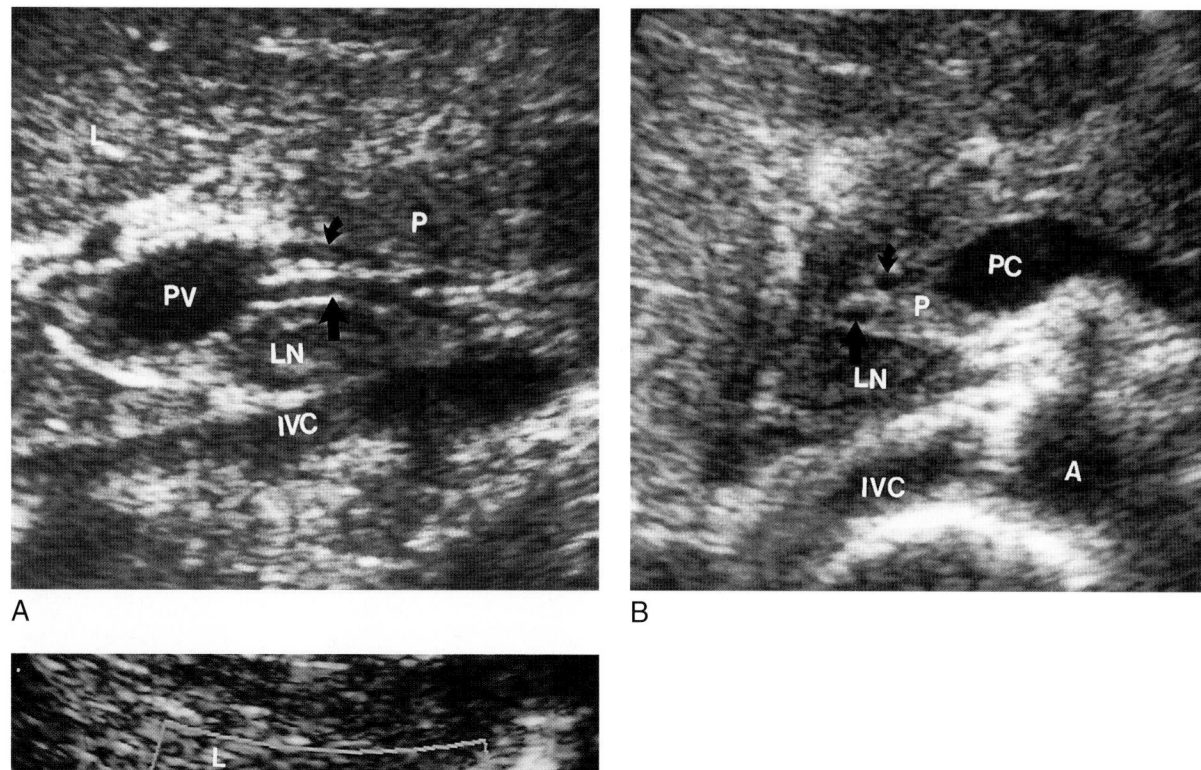

A

B

C

FIGURE 7-12. Normal posterior superior pancreaticoduodenal vein (PSPDV). A, Sagittal view of head of pancreas (P) shows parallel course of PSPDV *(straight arrow)* posterior to common bile duct *(curved arrow).* **B,** Transverse plane of head of pancreas demonstrates PSPDV *(straight arrow)* posterior to common bile duct *(curved arrow).* **C,** Color Doppler view showing PSPDV *(straight arrow)* entering caudal aspect of portal vein *(curved arrow).* A, aorta; IVC, inferior vena cava; L, liver; LN, lymph node; P, pancreas; PC, portal confluence; PV, portal vein. (Courtesy of R. H. Wachsberg, MD, New Jersey Medical Center, Newark, NJ.)

Ultrasonic oral contrast agents are also being developed to reduce artifacts from a gas-filled gastrointestinal tract, which may help visualization of the pancreas.[23] The fluid-filled stomach provides an acoustic window, causes movement of the intragastric gas, and acts as a balloon, displacing the gas-filled colon and small bowel loops inferiorly. Ingestion of deionized water through a straw minimizes air swallowing. Some investigators have advocated the use of tubeless hypotonic duodenography with glucagon to facilitate visualization of the head of the pancreas.[24] Alternatively, some authors have shown that using agents such as metoclopramide, which increases gastric and duodenal contractility, can improve visualization of the pancreas.[25] However, in practice, ingestion of water alone is adequate for most patients and no additional medication is required. Visualization

of the pancreatic tail has been shown to improve with the use of simethicone as the oral contrast agent.[26] In patients who have had barium studies of the upper gastrointestinal tract, ultrasound evaluation of the pancreas with a water-filled stomach 1 hour after the upper gastrointestinal study has been shown to provide better results than an ultrasound examination performed immediately after or 1 hour after the barium examination without a fluid-filled stomach.[27]

Sonographic Examination of the Pancreas

Sonographic examination of the pancreas should begin with the patient in the erect position. Transverse scans in the midline below the xiphoid are made using the related vascular landmarks to identify the region of the pancreas.

The probe may need to be oblique to visualize the gland in its entirety. Angling the transducer cephalad and caudad from the level of the longitudinal view of the splenic vein appears to be adequate in most patients to scan through the entire gland.

Sagittal scanning of the pancreas is initiated with the transducer in the midline below the xiphoid. The level of the pancreas is easily localized by identification of the portal splenic confluence. There should be minimal movement of the transducer to the left or right of the midline, and, in practice, side-tilting of the probe has proved more effective than a lateral-sliding displacement.

By using the left kidney as an acoustic window the tail of the pancreas may be visualized anterior to its upper pole with a left coronal view. In some thin patients, the tail of the pancreas can also be seen through the spleen from the left lateral intercostal approach using a coronal plane. The head can occasionally be seen through the right lateral approach on a coronal plane.

CONGENITAL ANOMALIES

Agenesis

Congenital absence of the body and tail of pancreas has been reported.[28] The remaining pancreatic head may show compensatory hypertrophy. This condition should be differentiated from acquired atrophy by CT scan.

Congenital Cysts

Epithelium-lined true cysts of the pancreas are believed to be congenital in origin, representing anomalous development of the pancreatic ducts.[29] Multiple congenital cysts, ranging from microscopic to 3 to 5 cm,[29] are associated with cystic disease of the pancreas, liver, spleen, and kidneys as part of the broad spectrum of adult type polycystic kidney disease. The von Hippel-Lindau syndrome is another entity associated with multiple true pancreatic cysts.[29] Solitary congenital pancreatic cysts are rare and usually seen in infancy and childhood.[30]

Cystic Fibrosis

Cystic fibrosis is characterized by viscous secretions and dysfunction of multiple glands, including the pancreas. It can lead to pancreatic insufficiency, with the majority of patients showing evidence of exocrine pancreas dysfunction. When severely affected, the pancreas is shrunken with marked fibrosis, fatty replacement, and cysts secondary to the obstruction of small ducts.[31]

The most common **sonographic manifestation** is increased echogenicity caused by fibrosis or fatty replacement resulting from glandular atrophy (Fig. 7-13).[32,33]

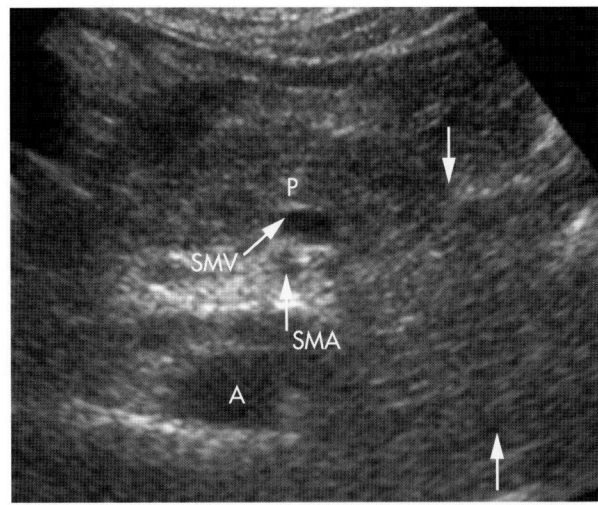

A

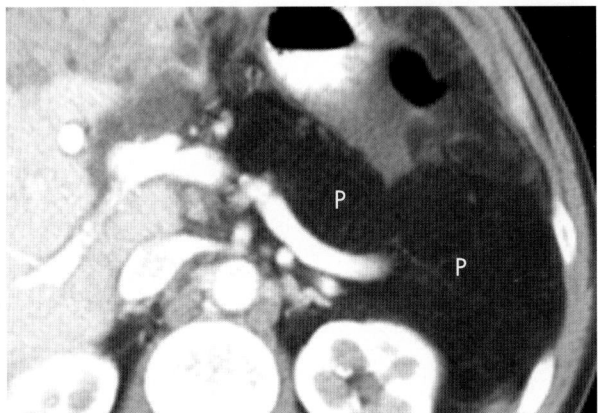

B

FIGURE 7-13. Cystic fibrosis of the pancreas. A, Transverse ultrasounds. **B,** Axial enhanced CT show echogenic poorly defined enlargement of the tail of pancreas (P) *(arrows)* on ultrasound corresponding to complete fatty replacement on CT. A, aorta; SMA, superior mesenteric artery; SMV, superior mesenteric vein.

In one series, all patients demonstrated abnormal pancreatic echo patterns when compared with an age- and gender-matched normal population.[34] The pancreas may be small,[34] but this can only be appreciated in cases in which the pancreas is less echogenic than the adjacent retroperitoneal fat. If the pancreas is enlarged, it indicates the presence of complicating pancreatitis, and it is usually associated with a hypoechoic parenchyma.[34] The pancreatic duct is less often visualized in patients with cystic fibrosis than in the normal population.[35] Small cysts of 1 to 3 mm are seen on pathologic examination of the pancreas but are uncommonly seen on sonography.[34] Individual larger cysts, less than 5 cm in diameter, have been reported on ultrasound examinations.[33] Rarely, pancreatic cystosis or multiple cysts can completely replace the pancreatic parenchyma. A high amylase content has been shown on aspiration biopsy of these cysts.[36]

Pancreas Divisum

Pancreas divisum, caused by the lack of fusion of the dorsal and ventral pancreatic buds, occurs in 10% of the population on anatomic studies.[37,38] Drainage of the entire dorsal pancreas is through the minor papilla, with only the ventral part draining through the major papilla. There is controversy regarding the predisposition of patients with pancreas divisum to pancreatitis, which may be related to the drainage of most of the pancreatic secretions through the relatively small orifice of the minor papilla. In a group of patients with recurrent idiopathic pancreatitis, Cotton[38] reported an incidence of 25.6% with associated pancreas divisum. Involvement of the pancreas with acute pancreatitis is usually limited to the dorsal part of the gland.[38] However, isolated ventral pancreatitis has also been documented.[39] A persistent dorsal pancreatic duct in the head may be identified on ultrasound, but the presence or absence of communication with the ventral duct is difficult to ascertain. Increased prominence of the ventral pancreas, suggesting preservation of this part of pancreas from chronic pancreatitis, has been reported as an indication of pancreas divisum.[17]

Von Hippel-Lindau Syndrome

Pancreatic cysts are common in von Hippel-Lindau syndrome and are described in 72% of autopsy results[38] and 25% of patients on sonographic examination.[40] Other associated lesions include apudomas, microcystic adenomas, ductal cell adenocarcinomas, ampullary cell carcinomas, and hemangioblastomas.[41]

INFLAMMATORY PROCESSES

Acute Pancreatitis

The diagnosis of acute pancreatitis is usually based on clinical and laboratory findings, with clinical severity best determined by Ranson's criteria[42] or Acute Physiology and Chronic Health Evaluation (APACHE) II criteria.[43] Radiologic examinations are helpful for patients with a confusing history or clinical findings. The role of ultrasound lies in the detection of gallstones or common bile duct calculi, a survey of possible complications such as peripancreatic fluid, follow-up of complications arising from acute pancreatitis, and guidance of interventional procedures. Ultrasound is limited in its usefulness as part of the early investigation of acute pancreatitis or traumatic pancreatic injury,[44] whereas CT has been shown to be useful in helping to predict the outcome of acute pancreatic inflammation and to detect necrosis and fracture of the pancreas.[45,46]

Pathologic changes in acute pancreatitis depend on the severity of the disease. Mild forms consist of interstitial edema limited to the gland with no or slight peripancreatic inflammation. Although parenchymal necrosis is not visible grossly, small foci of acinar cell necrosis occasionally may be found. Necrosis of intrapancreatic and peripancreatic adipose tissue is common. Inflammation is associated with extravasation of enzymes into the surrounding tissues. More severe cases show fat necrosis, parenchymal necrosis, and necrosis of blood vessels, with subsequent hemorrhage and more severe peripancreatic inflammatory changes appearing in 1 to 2 days.[47] If the patient survives, the necrotic tissue is replaced by diffuse or focal parenchymal or stromal fibrosis, calcifications, and irregular ductal dilations. Pseudocysts may form by the accumulation of enzyme-rich fluid and necrotic debris confined by a nonepithelialized capsule of connective tissue.[29]

Acute pancreatitis has numerous causes; however, the precise pathophysiologic factors are yet to be elucidated. Congenital causes include hereditary pancreatitis and compression from a congenital choledochal cyst. The role of pancreas divisum as a predisposing factor to pancreatitis is controversial, with some studies showing increased[38] and others showing similar[48] incidence of acute pancreatitis in these patients. Acquired conditions such as alcohol abuse and biliary calculi account for the majority of the cases of acute pancreatitis. Trauma and other less common entities can induce acute pancreatitis.[49]

CAUSES OF ACUTE PANCREATITIS

Biliary tract disease
Ethyl alcohol abuse
Peptic ulcer
Trauma, surgery (cardiopulmonary bypass surgery), hypotensive shock
Pregnancy
Hyperlipoproteinemias (types I, IV, and V)
Hypercalcemia (primary and secondary, hyperparathyroidism, multiple myeloma)
Drugs (azathioprine, estrogens, corticosteroids, and thiazides)
Hereditary pancreatitis, idiopathic fibrosing pancreatitis
Infectious agents (mumps, *Ascaris, Campylobacter,* and *Mycoplasma* infections, and hydatid)
Methyl alcohol, L-asparaginase
Scorpion bites
Carcinoma of pancreas (primary and metastatic); ductal obstruction by tumor
Endoscopic retrograde cholangiopancreatography, upper gastrointestinal endoscopy, percutaneous transhepatic biliary tract drainage
Post-transplantation
Legionnaires' disease

Modified with permission from Goekas MC: Etiology and pathogenesis of acute pancreatic inflammation: Acute pancreatitis. Ann Intern Med 1985;103:86-100.

Because the natural history of acute pancreatitis is variable, serial examination by ultrasound plays an important role in monitoring the inflammatory process of the pancreas after an initial attack. The process can take several directions: resolution, pseudocyst formation, or chronic pancreatitis. Cases of mild pancreatitis, or self-limiting disease, often revert to normal organ echotexture and size. More severe disease may result in increased echogenicity of the pancreas. This increase may be homogeneous and accompanied by scattered, random, bright reflections representing minute calcifications (often without acoustic shadowing) or inhomogeneous and mottled in appearance. These changes reflect the healing of the pancreas by fibrosis accompanied by calcifications deposited along the main pancreatic duct or in the branches within the parenchyma.

Pseudocyst formation is an attempt by the body to wall off the pancreatic secretions to prevent further autodigestion of the peripancreatic tissue or other structures. In many instances patients feel better at the time of pseudocyst formation because it acts as a cordon, enclosing the active inflammation.

Chronic pancreatitis usually results from repeated bouts of acute pancreatitis. This condition is progressive, with indolent destruction and fibrosis of the organ leading to functional exocrine and endocrine glandular failure.

Sonography

Sonographic findings of acute pancreatitis can be classified by distribution (focal or diffuse) and by severity (mild, moderate, and severe).[50] Ultrasound findings may be negative in the milder forms of acute pancreatitis. The examination may, however, find the cause of pancreatitis, such as choledocholithiasis, or an alternative diagnosis in questionable cases. Mild pancreatitis is a self-limiting disease responding to conservative treatment. In more severe cases, CT is the primary modality of choice to identify necrotic parenchyma and extraparenchymal involvement because the associated ileus limits sonographic visualization.[51] The technical success of the ultrasound examination improves 48 hours after the acute episode, as the paralytic ileus resolves.[50] Complications may be found, such as **inflammatory mass, hemorrhage, intrapancreatic and extrapancreatic fluid collections,** and **pseudocyst formation.** Sonograms may differentiate between inflammatory masses and fluid collections and can also be used to guide needle aspiration that would help to differentiate between infected and noninfected inflammatory masses and pseudocysts.

Focal pancreatitis, presenting as focal isoechoic or hypoechoic enlargement of the pancreas without extrapancreatic manifestations, poses a dilemma to the imager. This presentation generally occurs in the pancreatic head (Fig. 7-14).[52] These patients usually are alcohol abusers and have a previous history of pancreatitis or pain. This suggests that focal pancreatitis tends to occur in the background of chronic pancreatitis.[52] Differentiation from neoplasm may be difficult because both conditions create a focal hypoechoic mass on sonograms. If the serum amylase level is normal and the patient is asymptomatic, the mass is likely to represent a neoplasm. If the patient's symptoms and signs are severe, the focal hypoechogenicity is more likely to be caused by pancreatitis than by a tumor. The presence of calcification within the mass and abnormal ductal changes outside the focal enlargement on ERCP (suggestive of chronic pancreatitis) also favor an inflammatory mass.[52] Identification of a gradually tapering common bile duct or pancreatic duct on imaging is also suggestive of focal pancreatitis. In addition, serial sonographic examination while the patient is undergoing treatment may differentiate focal pancreatitis from tumor. EUS may provide better resolution of the pancreas and reveal parenchymal features suggestive of chronic pancreatitis other than a mass.[53-54] CT can be helpful by showing peripancreatic soft tissue inflammation (see Fig. 7-14C). Percutaneous biopsy should be performed on patients whose diagnoses remain questionable, keeping in mind that a negative biopsy finding does not exclude malignancy. Focal pancreatitis may also be caused by an adjacent inflammatory process, such as a penetrating peptic ulcer (Fig. 7-15).

In **diffuse pancreatitis** the pancreas becomes increasingly hypoechogenic relative to the normal liver and increases in size (Fig. 7-16). The assessment of relative pancreatic echogenicity may be difficult because of the alcohol-induced fatty liver present in a large number of these patients. Therefore, comparison of the echogenicity of the pancreas with the liver may be of little practical value. In mild acute pancreatitis, sonograms show a normal pancreas with abnormal clinical and laboratory findings. As the condition worsens, decreased echogenicity and increased size are more evident as a result of the increased fluid content in the interstitium secondary to inflammation. The pancreas may also appear inhomogeneous (Fig. 7-17). The pancreatic duct may be compressed or dilated. Ductal dilation is usually caused by a focal pancreatic inflammation located upstream from the dilated pancreatic duct. Rarely, another cause of duct obstruction such as a calculus, tumor, or ascariasis can be detected by transcutaneous or endoscopic sonography.[55]

Differentiation cannot be made between necrotic and non-necrotic pancreatitis by ultrasound but is evident on CT (Fig. 7-18). Focal hemorrhage is detected as a focal echogenic mass. When acute inflammation of the pancreas becomes masslike and is accompanied by severe symptoms and clinical findings, the term *inflammatory mass* can be employed (see Fig. 7-17). Conservative

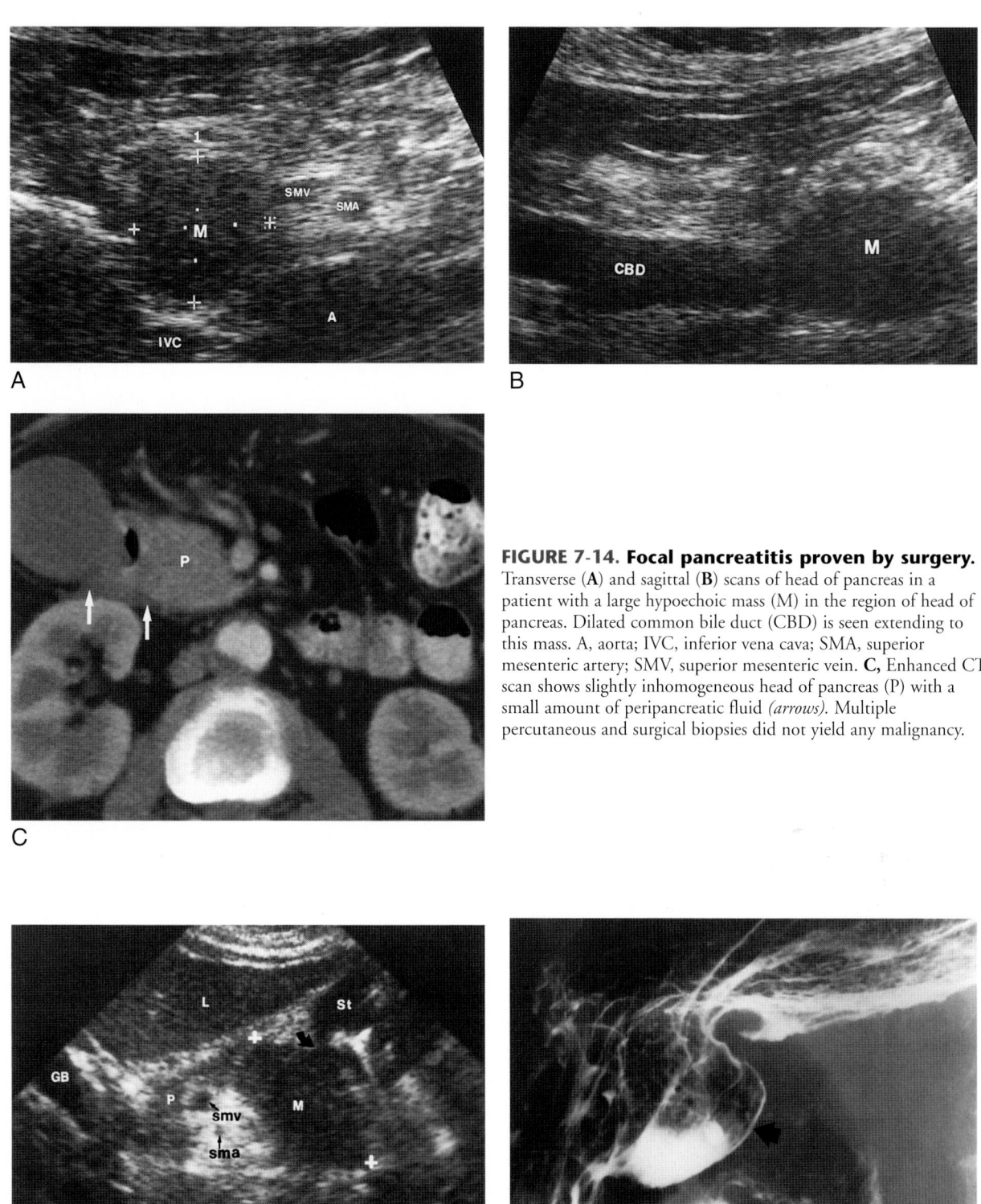

FIGURE 7-14. Focal pancreatitis proven by surgery.
Transverse (**A**) and sagittal (**B**) scans of head of pancreas in a patient with a large hypoechoic mass (M) in the region of head of pancreas. Dilated common bile duct (CBD) is seen extending to this mass. A, aorta; IVC, inferior vena cava; SMA, superior mesenteric artery; SMV, superior mesenteric vein. **C,** Enhanced CT scan shows slightly inhomogeneous head of pancreas (P) with a small amount of peripancreatic fluid *(arrows)*. Multiple percutaneous and surgical biopsies did not yield any malignancy.

FIGURE 7-15. Focal pancreatitis caused by penetrating benign gastric ulcer. A, Transverse scan of pancreas shows hypoechoic masslike enlargement (M) of body and tail. No fat plane is present between this mass and adjacent stomach (St). A, aorta; GB, gallbladder; IVC, inferior vena cava; L, liver; P, pancreas; sma, superior mesenteric artery; smv, superior mesenteric vein. **B,** Large ulcer of posterior wall of body of stomach *(arrows on A and B).*

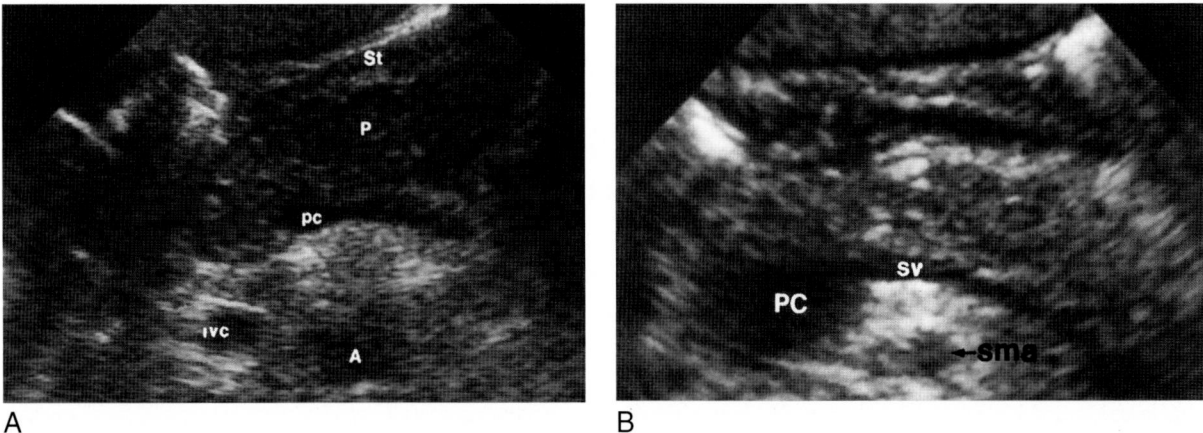

FIGURE 7-16. Acute pancreatitis with resolution. A, Transverse scan of enlarged hypoechoic pancreas (P). **B,** Same patient after resolution. Pancreas has returned to normal size and echogenicity. A, aorta; IVC, inferior vena cava; PC, portal confluence; sma, superior mesenteric artery; St, stomach; sv, splenic vein.

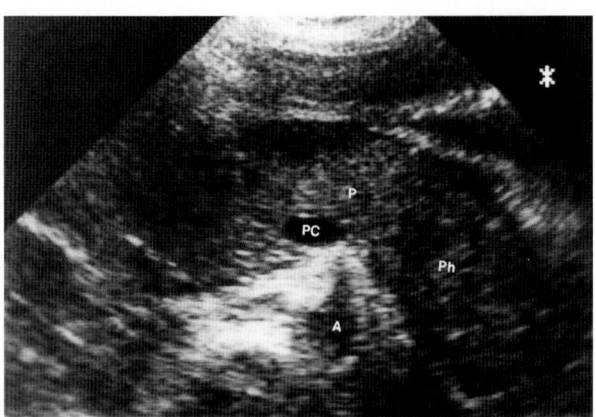

FIGURE 7-17. Severe acute pancreatitis. Transverse scan shows large pancreas (P) with inhomogeneous, hypoechoic area in tail, which represents phlegmon (Ph) or an inflammatory mass. A, aorta; PC, portal confluence.

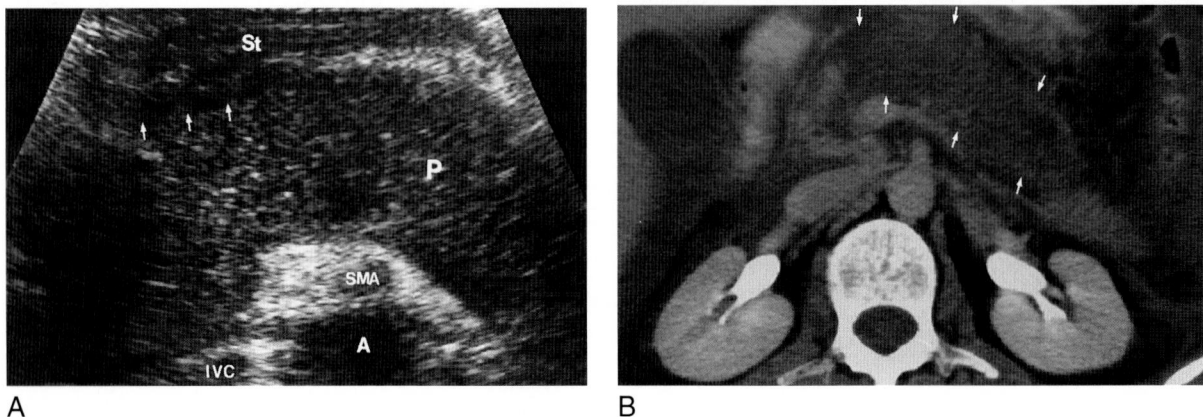

FIGURE 7-18. Acute pancreatitis with pancreatic necrosis. A, Transverse ultrasonic view. Enlarged hypoechoic inhomogeneous pancreas (P) surrounded by a small amount of fluid anteriorly *(arrows)*. **B,** Corresponding CT scan shows lack of enhancement of body and most of tail of pancreas *(arrows)*. A, aorta; IVC, inferior vena cava; SMA, superior mesenteric artery; St, stomach.

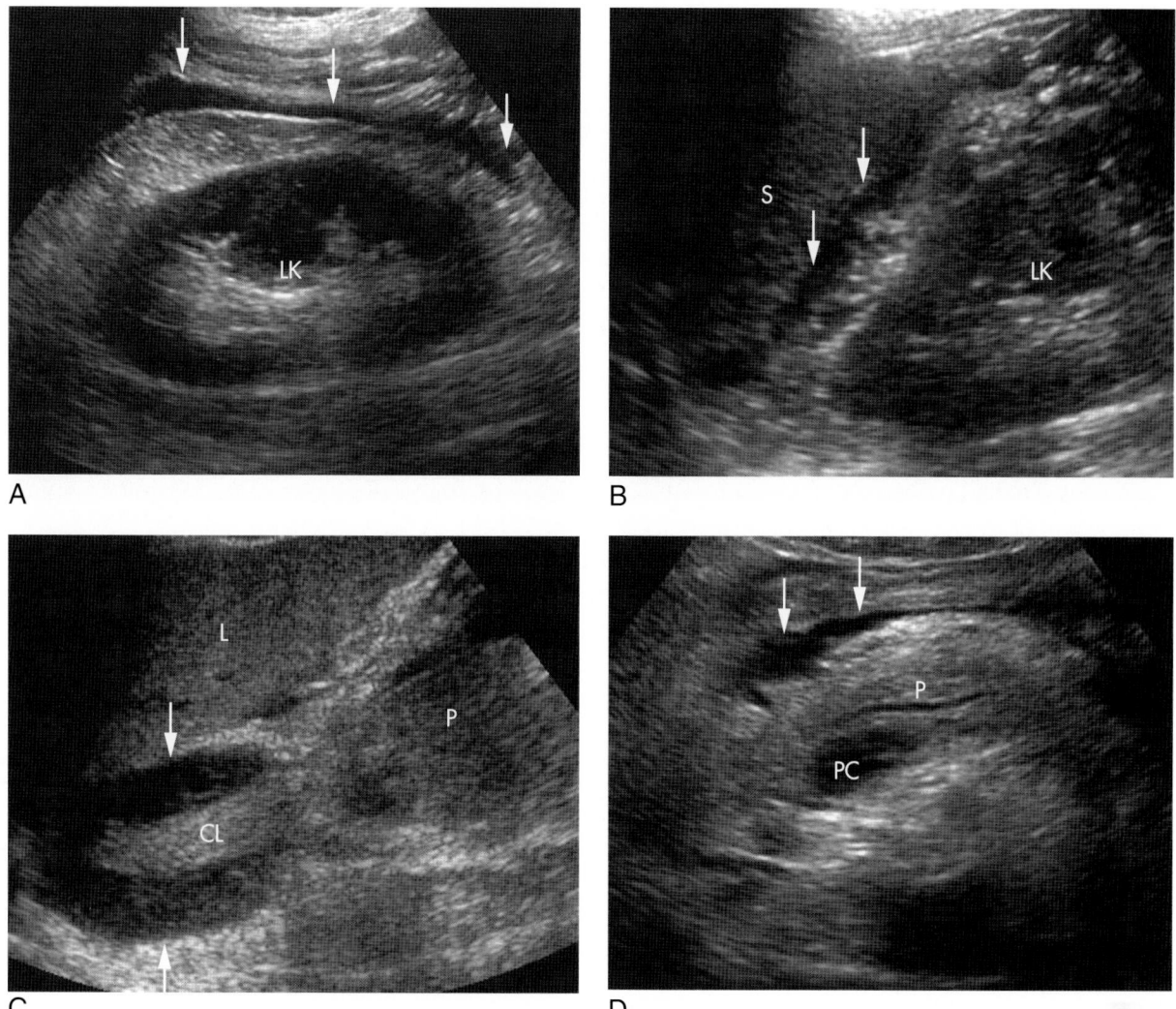

FIGURE 7-19. Acute pancreatitis, fluid collection in the spaces in the vicinity of the pancreas. A, Sagittal view shows fluid in the anterior pararenal space *(arrows).* **B,** Sagittal view demonstrates fluid *(arrows)* in the hilum of the spleen (S). **C,** Sagittal view shows fluid *(arrows)* surrounding the caudate lobe (CL). **D,** Fluid *(arrows)* anterior to the pancreas (P) in the lesser sac. A, aorta; PC, portal confluence.

management with serial sonographic imaging is advised because most inflammatory masses resolve without intervention.[56]

Extrapancreatic manifestations in patients with acute pancreatitis are important and should be sought because intrapancreatic changes tend to be subjective.[51] They consist of **fluid collections** and **edema** along the different soft tissue planes and are generally seen in severe cases. The common spaces for the extrapancreatic fluid to collect include the lesser sac, anterior pararenal spaces, mesocolon, perirenal spaces, and peripancreatic soft tissues.[51] Lesser sac fluid located between the pancreas and the stomach is the easiest to visualize with sonography (Fig. 7-19). If the fluid is located in the superior recess of the lesser sac, it tends to surround the caudate lobe (see Fig. 7-19C).[51] The free edge of the gastrohepatic ligament may be visualized with a combination of lesser sac and greater sac fluid. Perirenal

fluid is also readily demonstrated (see Fig. 7-19B). However, edema or fluid in the anterior pararenal space is more difficult to see and may require coronal scanning; a hypoechoic band separated from the kidney by the echogenic perirenal fat would represent fluid in the pararenal space (see Fig. 7-19A and B).[51] Fluid collections in the mesocolon are the most difficult to identify by sonographic examination. They present in the midline just caudad to the pancreas. Peripancreatic soft tissue changes are seen as hypoechoic bands adjacent to the pancreas or surrounding the portal venous system (Fig. 7-20).[51] In less severe cases, the only finding may be a small amount of fluid (Fig. 7-21) or hypoechoic linear edema (see Fig. 7-21) in the retroperitoneal fat immediately surrounding the pancreas anteriorly or posteriorly. The presence of fluid between the pancreas and the splenic vein has been reported as the only indication of pancreatic injury on CT scan in trauma patients.[57]

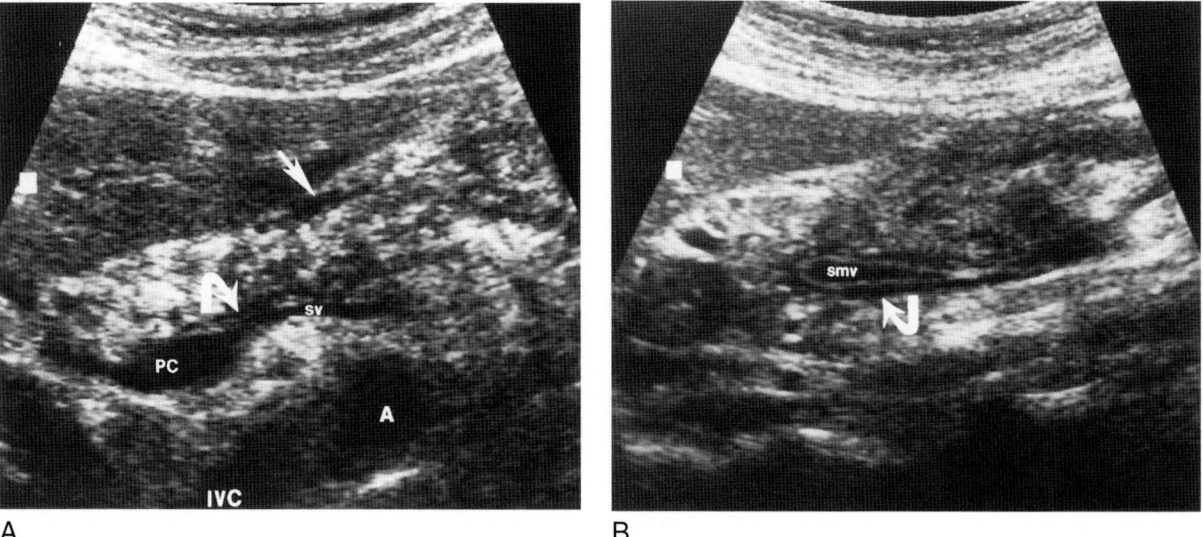

FIGURE 7-20. Acute pancreatitis, extrapancreatic soft tissue edema. A, Transverse scan. **B,** Longitudinal scan. Pancreas echotexture is inhomogeneous. Peripancreatic edema *(straight arrow)* and periportal system edema *(curved arrow)* are present. A, aorta; IVC, inferior vena cava; PC, portal confluence; smv, superior mesenteric vein; SV, splenic vein.

Fluid or edema may also be visualized around the ligamentum teres.

Pancreatic fluid is either clear or septated as a result of associated hemorrhage or infection. Retroperitoneal or intraperitoneal fluid collections may be inhomogeneous and solid looking as a result of the inflammatory nature of the edematous retroperitoneal tissues (Fig. 7-22). Extrapancreatic fluid collections occur within 4 weeks from the onset of an acute attack and have a high incidence of spontaneous regression; therefore, they can be treated conservatively in conjunction with serial sonographic scanning.[58] The term *pseudocyst* is used when a pancreatic fluid collection has developed into a well-defined, walled-off fluid structure that persists on serial imaging examinations for an interval of at least 4 weeks from the onset of acute inflammation.[59]

Other extrapancreatic findings include **ascites, thickening of the adjacent gastrointestinal tract** (stomach, duodenum, and colon), and a **thickened gall-bladder wall** with or without pericholecystic fluid, which may simulate acute cholecystitis (see Fig. 7-22D).[60]

Complications

Pancreatic Pseudocysts. A pancreatic pseudocyst is a fluid collection that has developed a well-defined non-epithelialized wall in response to extravasated enzymes.[61] It is generally spherical and distinct from other structures. Four to 6 weeks are necessary for a fluid collection to enclose itself by forming a wall composed of collagen and vascular granulation tissue.[62] Pseudocysts occur in 10% to 20% of patients who have had acute pancreatitis.[63] Most commonly, pseudocyst formation is associated with an alcoholic or biliary etiology. However,

COMPLICATIONS OF PANCREATITIS

Pancreatic pseudocyst
Obstruction of the stomach, small bowel, colon, or the bile ducts
Pseudocysts dissect into adjacent organs
Gastrointestinal hemorrhage
    From direct erosion
    From variceal bleeding
Acute peritonitis
Chronic pancreatitis

it may also occur after blunt trauma or secondary to pancreatic malignancy (Fig. 7-23). Persistent pain and elevation of amylase levels suggest the diagnosis; however, it can be confirmed by imaging. Classically, a pseudocyst is seen on sonographic examination as a well-defined, smooth-walled, anechoic structure with acoustic enhancement. Occasionally, it may also appear solid or complex, especially during formation.[61,64] As a pseudocyst matures, serial scanning will generally reveal gradual clearing of the internal echoes. Debris within a pseudocyst may occur with complications such as hemorrhage or infection (Fig. 7-24).[61] A pseudocyst may also remain multiloculated without complications and may develop calcifications within its walls (see Fig. 7-24). A heavily calcified pseudocyst may be difficult to see on sonograms because of the presence of shadowing. Pseudocysts can migrate outside the abdomen and have been reported to occur in the mediastinum and the thigh.[65,66]

Complications have been reported in 30% to 50% of the patients with a pancreatic pseudocyst.[67] These lesions

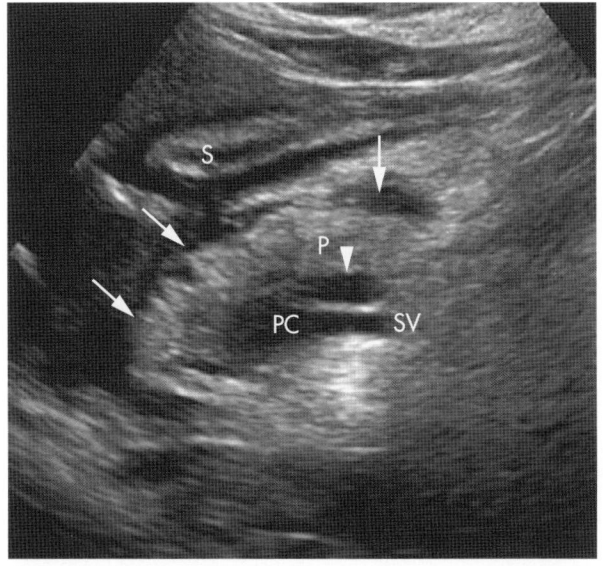

A

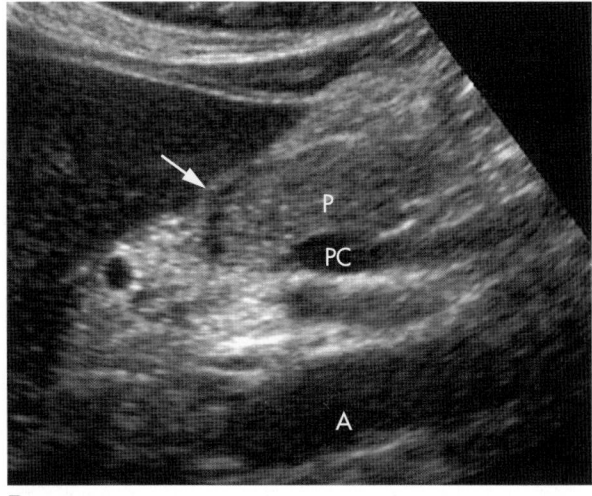

B

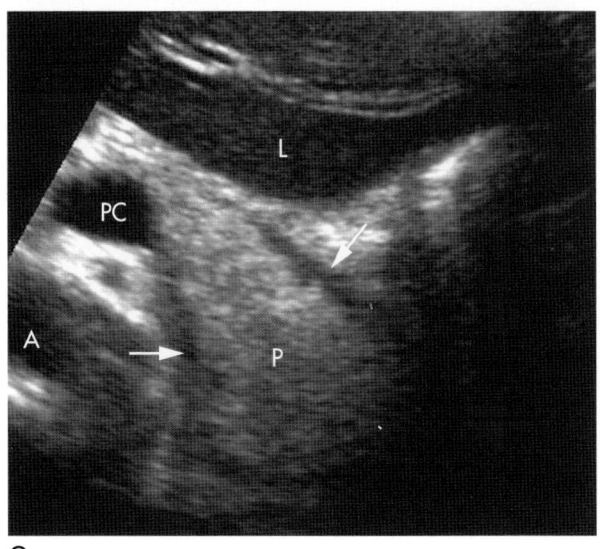

C

FIGURE 7-21. Subtle peripancreatic changes in acute pancreatitis. Transverse (**A**) and sagittal (**B**) views. Small amount of fluid is seen anterior, superior, and lateral *(arrows)* to the head and body of pancreas (P). Fluid is present *(arrowhead)* anterior to splenic vein (SV). **C,** Transverse view of another patient with proven pancreatitis demonstrates fluid *(arrows)* anterior and posterior to the tail of the pancreas (P). A, aorta; PC, portal confluence; S, stomach; SV, splenic vein.

may become large or may be strategically placed and cause obstruction of the stomach, small bowel (especially duodenum), colon, or bile ducts.[68] The latter may progress from obstructive jaundice to obstructive cholangitis. Bowel obstruction occurs by extrinsic compression or by intramural extension of the pseudocyst between the serosa and muscularis or between the muscularis and mucosa (Fig. 7-25).[69] Pseudocysts can also **dissect** into the parenchyma of the adjacent organs such as the liver, spleen, and kidney (Fig. 7-26).[70]

Gastrointestinal hemorrhage may occur from direct erosion of the pseudocyst into the stomach or from variceal bleeding secondary to local portal hypertension caused by portosplenic venous compression or thrombosis.[67,71] A pseudocyst or pancreatic secretion alone may erode into an adjacent visceral artery, most commonly the splenic, with resultant intracystic hemorrhage or

formation of a pseudoaneurysm. Hemorrhage may also occur with a pancreatic abscess and severe necrotizing pancreatitis without pseudocyst formation.[72,73] Hemorrhage can be suspected by identifying areas of increased echogenicity. With the addition of Doppler insonation, the presence of a **pseudoaneurysm** and **portosplenic thrombosis** can be revealed.[74] If thrombosis becomes chronic, cavernous transformation of the portal venous system may follow.

Acute peritonitis can ensue with rupture of a pseudocyst into the peritoneal cavity. This serious complication should be differentiated clinically from pancreatic ascites, which is caused by a slow leakage of fluid into the peritoneal cavity, unassociated with peritonitis.

A pseudocyst that forms during acute necrotizing pancreatitis has a high propensity toward spontaneous

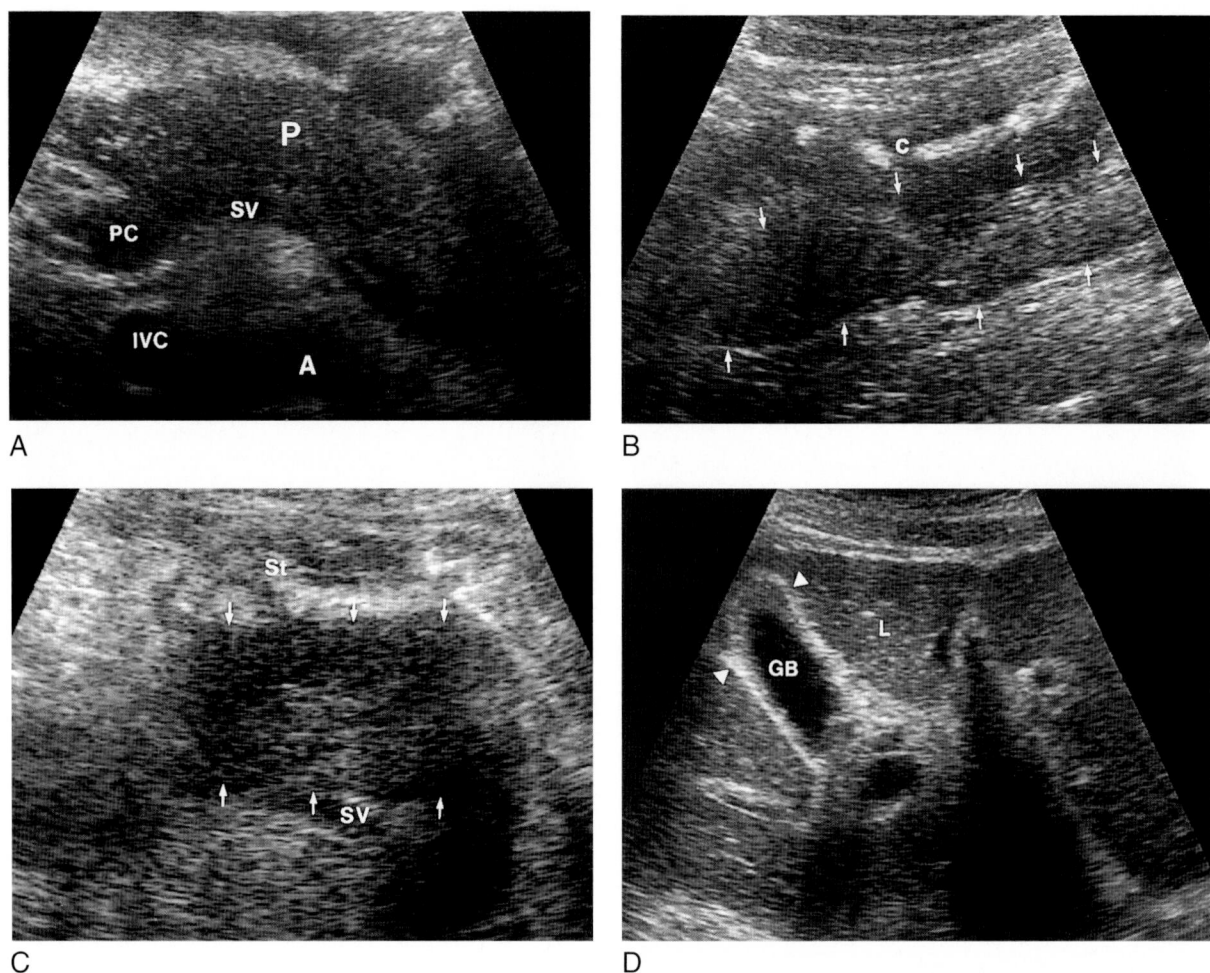

FIGURE 7-22. Acute pancreatitis with solid-looking extrapancreatic inflammation (*arrows*). A, Transverse view of inflamed pancreas (P). **B,** Sagittal view of left flank. **C,** Transverse view of lesser sac. **D,** Transverse view of gallbladder (GB) with thickening of gallbladder wall *(arrowheads)*. A, aorta; C, colon; GB, gallbladder; IVC, inferior vena cava; L, liver; P, pancreas; PC, portal confluence; St, stomach; SV, splenic vein.

regression, whereas a pseudocyst that forms as a result of chronic pancreatitis does not generally resolve on its own, especially when calcifications occur within the walls.[75] Spontaneous decompression of the pseudocyst may occur by rupturing into the pancreatic duct, the adjacent portion of the gastrointestinal tract (usually the stomach), or the common bile duct.[76] In general, pseudocysts that persist beyond 6 weeks require decompression, and the risk of complications rises significantly.[61] A pseudocyst will persist as long as disruption of the pancreatic ducts exists; on healing of this disruption, spontaneous resorption will occur.[76] The **criteria for decompression** of a pancreatic pseudocyst include (1) persistence greater than 6 weeks; (2) size larger than 5 cm in diameter without evidence of ongoing regression on follow-up sonographic or CT examination; (3) smaller pseudocysts causing symptoms; and (4) presence of complications such as infection, internal hemorrhage, or intra-abdominal perforation.

Nonsurgical decompression is becoming more popular, with more favorable results obtained in the past few years.[74] There remains controversy over the choice of approach; some large series advocate the transgastric approach as the primary route,[77] whereas others initially prefer the direct approach and reserve the transgastric, transduodenal, or transhepatic approaches for inaccessible locations.[77] Single aspiration has been abandoned because of a high recurrence rate.[77] Percutaneous transgastric pseudocyst drainage is a combined technique of percutaneous gastrostomy with cystogastrostomy using a Mitty-Pollack needle (Cook, Bloomingdale, IN) performed under fluoroscopy and ultrasound guidance. There is a minimal chance of pseudocyst recurrence because of internal drainage to the stomach. In one study series using this technique, a success rate of 67% was observed with a recurrence rate of 12.5%.[78] This approach is considered the route of choice in pseudocysts associated with obstruction of the pancreatic duct.

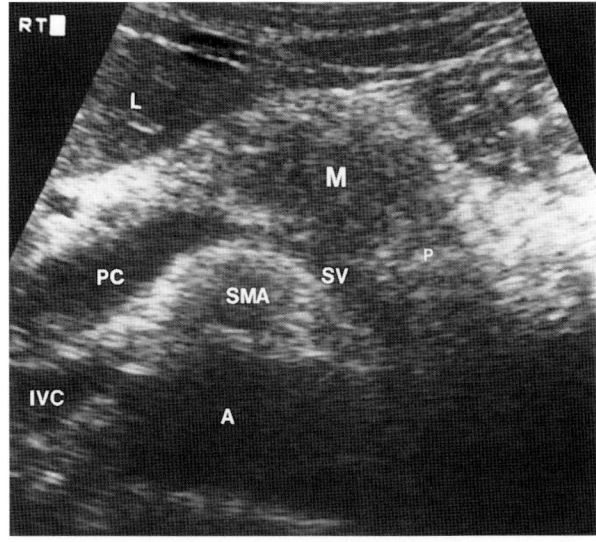

A

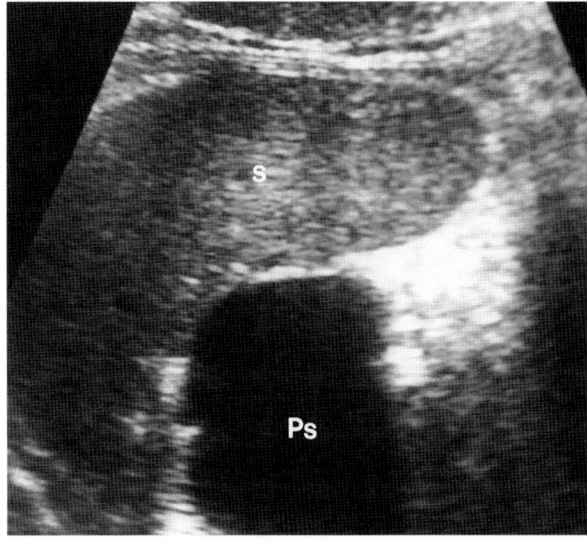

B

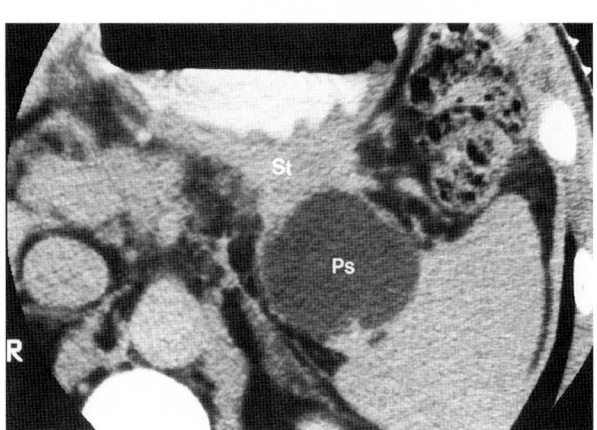

C

FIGURE 7-23. Pseudocyst of pancreas tail from pancreatic body carcinoma. A, Transverse view of pancreas (P) shows a poorly defined hypoechoic mass in the body (M). **B,** Coronal view of spleen (S) demonstrates a pseudocyst (Ps) in the splenic hilum. **C,** Enhanced CT scan shows the pseudocyst (Ps) and inflammatory changes in the adjacent stomach wall (St). A, aorta; IVC, inferior vena cava; L, liver; PC, portal confluence; SMA, superior mesenteric artery; SV, splenic vein.

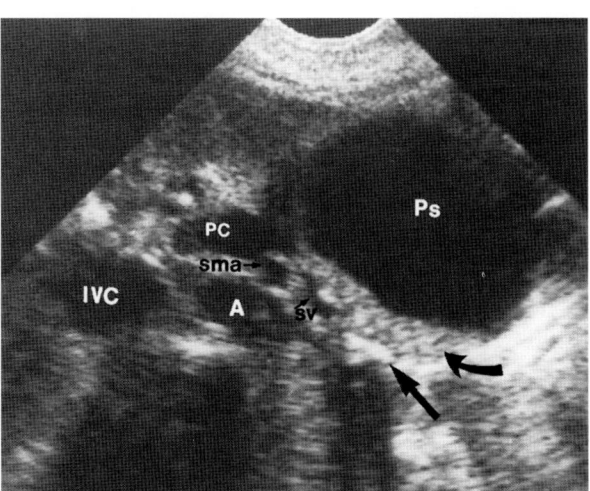

FIGURE 7-24. Complicated pseudocyst. Transverse scan of partially calcified *(straight arrow)* pseudocyst (Ps) containing debris *(curved arrow)* in tail of pancreas. A, aorta; IVC, inferior vena cava; PC, portal confluence; sma, superior mesenteric artery; SV, splenic vein.

The direct approach is performed using the usual percutaneous technique. The reported success rate for the combined approach (with the majority being drained directly) is 86%.[77] The catheter is left in place until drainage ceases, the pseudocyst resolves, and there is no communication with the pancreatic duct.[77] The drainage period is generally longer than an uncomplicated abscess and closer to abscesses associated with fistula to the gastrointestinal tract.[79] Recently, the systemic administration of octreotide acetate, to reduce pancreatic exocrine function, is suggested to improve the success rate of percutaneous drainage of pseudocyst.[77]

Endoscopic cystogastrostomy or duodenostomy is an alternative approach; however, it may be more time consuming than the radiologically guided percutaneous approach.[80] If the just-described techniques are unavailable, the anatomy precludes their usage, or a pseudocyst is extensively multiloculated, a surgical decompression should be used.

Infected Pancreatic Lesions. The uncircumscribed infected pancreatic focus consists of secondarily infected

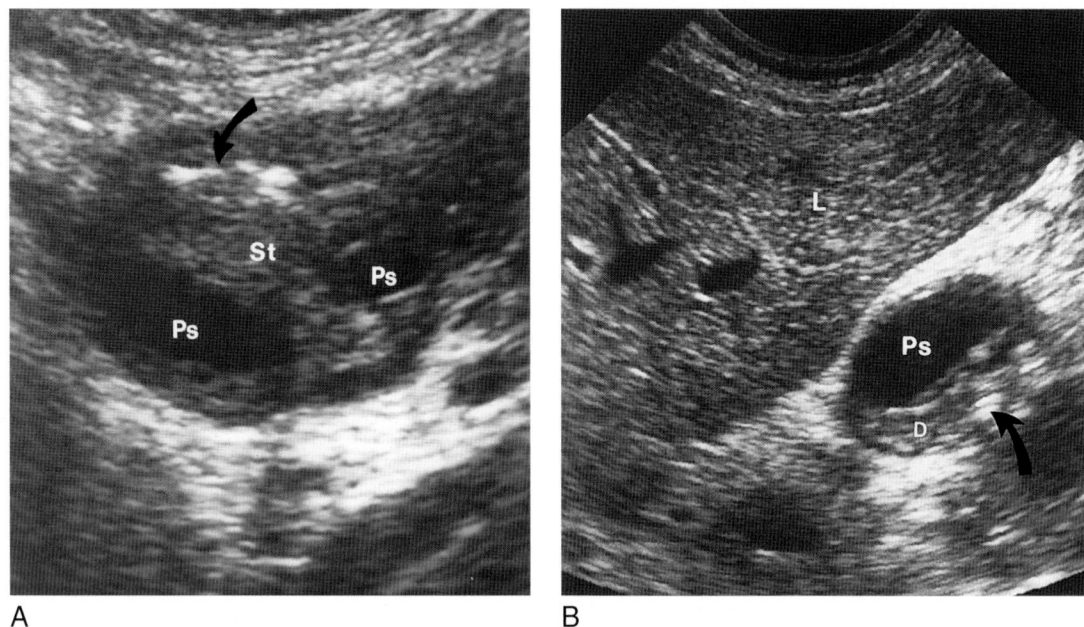

A   B

FIGURE 7-25. Pseudocyst in the wall of gut. A, Intramural pseudocyst in the wall of stomach (St). Transverse view of antrum showing multiple pseudocysts (Ps) in thickened wall. **B,** Intramural pseudocyst (Ps) in the wall of duodenum in a different patient. D, duodenum; L, liver. Notice gas *(curved arrow)* in lumen.

CRITERIA FOR DECOMPRESSION OF A PANCREATIC PSEUDOCYST

Persistence greater than 6 weeks
Larger than 5 cm in diameter without evidence of
    ongoing regression
Smaller pseudocysts causing symptoms
Complications such as infection, internal
    hemorrhage, or intra-abdominal perforation

entities that are not delimited by a wall, such as pancreatic necrosis, pancreatic fluid collections, and pancreatic hemorrhage. Bacterial contamination of necrotic pancreatic tissue and fluid rises to a significant rate (71.4%) after 2 weeks of acute necrotic pancreatitis.[81] Sonographically, a sterile, uncircumscribed focus cannot be distinguished from an infected one. Therefore, a high index of suspicion is necessary to detect these lesions, and an ultrasound-guided (or CT-guided) needle aspiration with Gram stain and culture of the aspirate should be performed to confirm the presence of infection. An uncircumscribed infected pancreatic focus is best treated by surgical débridement.[82] Percutaneous catheter drainage is reserved for cases in which the patient is in refractory shock or cannot withstand immediate surgery.[83]

Sonographically, an **infected pancreatic pseudocyst** cannot be distinguished from a sterile pseudocyst with certainty. Clinically, the patient may appear well with stable vital signs, except for an elevated temperature.

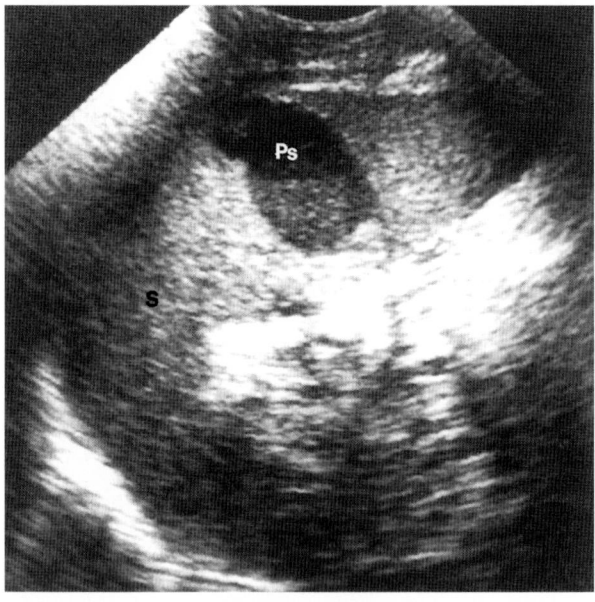

FIGURE 7-26. Pseudocyst of spleen. Sagittal view of spleen (s) shows cyst (Ps) containing a fluid level.

Therefore, a high degree of suspicion is again necessary and a percutaneous ultrasound-guided aspiration with Gram stain and culture should be employed whenever the question of infection arises. An infected pseudocyst is best treated (94% reported success) by percutaneous image-guided catheter drainage.[77,78]

A **pancreatic abscess** is distinguished from an infected pseudocyst by its greater risk of mortality (near 100% mortality if left untreated) and its need for surgical débridement when associated with pancreatic

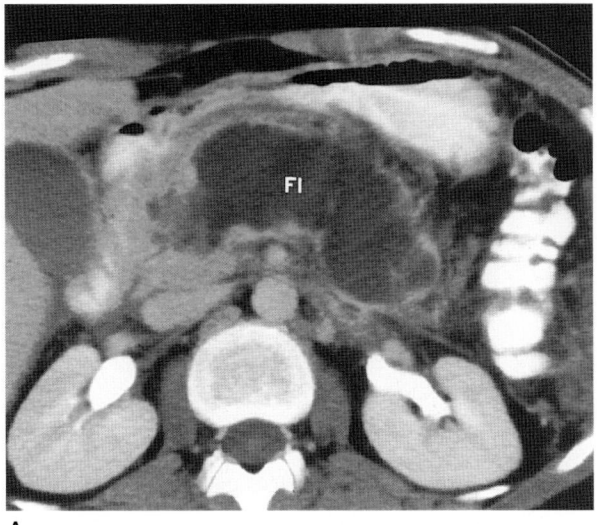
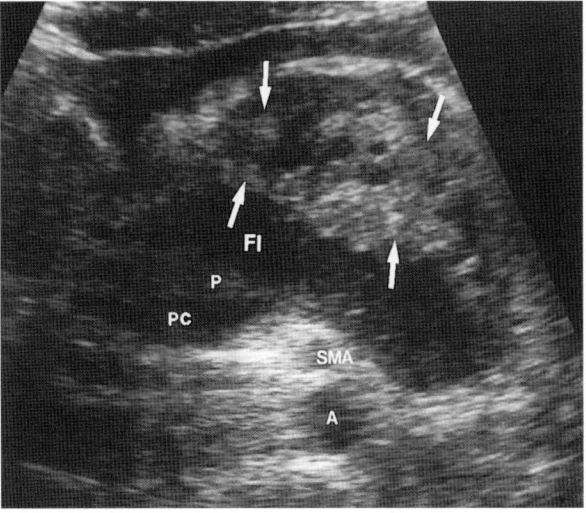

A   B

FIGURE 7-27. Value of ultrasound to determine the nature of pancreatic fluid collection following pancreatic necrosis. Some patient as in Fig. 7-21, 15 days later. **A**, Enhanced computed tomography scan shows a walled-off homogeneous fluid collection (FI). **B**, Transverse ultrasound confirms fluid nature of the posterior aspect of this mass (FI) but the anterior aspect is solid (arrows). Residual pancreatic tissue is seen posteriorly (P). A, aorta; PC, portal confluence; SMA, superior mesentric artery.

necrosis (versus percutaneous catheter drainage).[82,84] The organisms obtained are usually gram-negative enteric bacteria, and approximately half of the cultures are polymicrobial.[85] Pancreatic abscesses occur more frequently in postoperative patients than in those with alcohol or biliary pancreatitis.[86]

On sonography, one sees a thick-walled, mostly anechoic mass containing debris with bright echoes from gas bubbles. However, gas collections can also arise from uninfected fistulous communications with the gastro-intestinal tract.[87] Whether one sees gas bubbles, the absence of gas, or a cystic, complex, or a solid structure, suspicious areas must be aspirated with a fine needle (22 gauge) under ultrasound or CT guidance to obtain specimens for Gram stain, culture, and sensitivity tests. Pancreatic abscesses require surgical débridement. CT scan is required to evaluate the extent of the disease before catheter placement or surgical intervention. The information obtained from the CT scan may help to predict the success of draining a pancreatic abscess with a radiologic catheter.[88] However, ultrasound and, more recently, MRI are superior to CT for determining the nature of fluid and thus its ability to be drained by a percutaneous image-guided catheter (Fig. 7-27). An uncomplicated clear pancreatic abscess without necrotic tissue is likely to respond to percutaneous drainage.[77] Residual collections left after surgery can also have a percutaneous catheter placed radiologically to help affect a complete cure.[88]

Vascular Complications. Vascular complications may be related to the pancreatitis or may occur secondary to the pseudocyst formation. They include venous or arterial thrombosis with splenic infarct as a rare complication of vascular involvement (Fig. 7-28)[89] or pseudoaneurysm formation.[90] A high degree of suspicion is crucial to diagnose a pseudoaneurysm because of the potential to mistake it for a much more common complication of this condition (e.g., a pseudocyst). The presence of an echogenic crescent in the periphery of a cystic mass is highly suggestive of an aneurysm. Doppler imaging should be used to confirm the existence of these vascular complications.

Pancreatic Ascites and Pleural Effusion. Pancreatic ascites results from slow leakage of pancreatic enzymes into the peritoneal cavity from a disruption of the main pancreatic duct or a poorly walled pseudocyst.[91] Anterior enzyme leakage enters the lesser sac and the peritoneal cavity, causing ascites. Posterior enzyme leakage moves cephalad into the mediastinum and the pleural space, resulting in pancreatic pleural effusion (classically, left sided).[92] A "leaky" diaphragm or a pleural-subdiaphragmatic fistula may also allow ascites to become a pleural effusion. Pancreatic ascites is asymptomatic, causing an enlarging abdomen. ERCP can detect the location of pancreatic duct disruption.

Chronic Pancreatitis

Chronic pancreatitis is a progressive, irreversible destruction of the pancreas by repeated bouts of mild or subclinical pancreatitis resulting from high alcohol intake or biliary tract disease. In chronic alcoholic pancreatitis, the chronic alcohol intake causes increased pancreatic protein secretion with subsequent obstruction of the ducts by the protein-rich plugs, resulting in the more common type, namely, **chronic calcifying**

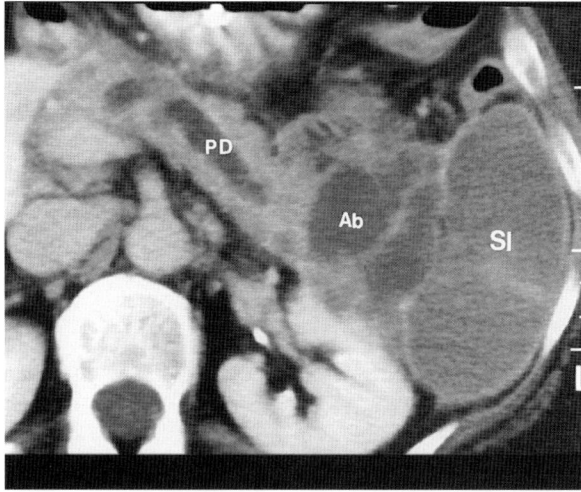
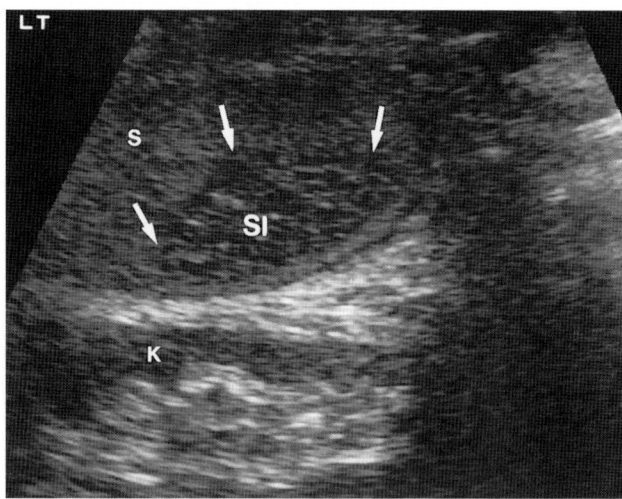

A

B

FIGURE 7-28. Vascular complications of acute pancreatitis. Splenic infarct (SI), dilatation of pancreatic duct (PD), and an abscess (Ab) in the tail of pancreas are shown. Enhanced CT scan (**A**) and ultrasound (**B**) show a wedge-shaped area of hypoechogenicity with multiple interfaces *(arrows)* in the spleen (S) diagnostic of infarct. K, Kidney.

pancreatitis.[29] The fibrous connective tissue proliferates around ducts and between parenchymal lobules, causing interstitial scarring accompanied by loss of acini.[93] This process eventually leads to an irregular, nodular appearance of the surface of the pancreas and pancreatic calculi.[29,93] The less common type is **chronic obstructive pancreatitis** with a nonlobular distribution, less ductal epithelial damage, and rare calcified stones. This is usually caused by stenosis of the sphincter of Oddi by cholelithiasis or pancreatic carcinoma.[29]

Sonographic findings of chronic pancreatitis consist of changes in the size and echotexture of the pancreas, focal mass lesions, calcifications, pancreatic duct dilation, and pseudocyst formation (Fig. 7-29). Bile duct dilation and portal vein thrombosis are other associated findings.[17] The echotexture of the pancreas is usually a mixture of patches of hypoechoic and hyperechoic foci. The hyperechoic foci are probably caused by a combination of fibrosis and calcification. Hypoechoic areas are likely due to the associated inflammation.[17,94] The echotexture changes are relatively sensitive but nonspecific.[17] The size of the pancreas depends on the degree of associated inflammation. In the absence of significant acute inflammation, the pancreas tends to be atrophied.

A **focal mass** or enlargement is found in approximately 40% of patients.[94,95] These changes result from progressive, mostly perilobular scarring in the interstitium accompanied by chronic edema and inflammatory infiltration. The presence of calcification helps to differentiate these focal enlargements from neoplasms. However, in some cases differentiation is not possible (see Fig. 7-14). Irregular **dilation of the pancreatic duct** occurs in chronic pancreatitis. In advanced cases, the duct becomes very tortuous. The differential diagnosis

between chronic pancreatitis and pancreatic carcinoma in a patient with duct dilation can be difficult. However, as a general rule, chronic pancreatitis is more highly suspected when the duct contains calcification and no obstructing mass lesion is seen, whereas carcinoma is suggested when a parenchymal mass lesion is identified at the site of obstruction of the pancreatic duct.[96] In normal subjects, it has been shown that variable degrees of pancreatic duct dilation occur after a standard meal or secretin stimulation.[17] An absent or diminished response has been shown in patients with chronic pancreatitis.[17]

Pancreatic calcifications are mostly intraductal in location and result from deposition of calcium carbonate on intraductal protein plugs.[97] They may (see Fig. 7-29) or may not (Fig. 7-30) be obstructive. The presence of these calcifications has been used diagnostically and as a basis for treatment of chronic pancreatitis because they were believed to be associated with clinical pancreatic insufficiency. However, contrary to previous opinion, one study showed a poor correlation between exocrine function and pancreatic calcification.[98] Moreover, the degree and pattern of pancreatic calcification have been shown to change with time.[99] Three phases were identified: (1) increasing calcifications; (2) stationary calcifications; and (3) decreasing calcifications. The third phase, not previously recognized, occurred to a significant degree in one third of the patients studied; some of this loss resulted from drainage procedures, whereas others occurred spontaneously with continued loss of exocrine function.

Pancreatic pseudocysts are reported in 25% to 40% of patients with chronic pancreatitis.[17] They are better walled-off in chronic pancreatitis than in the acute stage and tend not to resolve spontaneously.

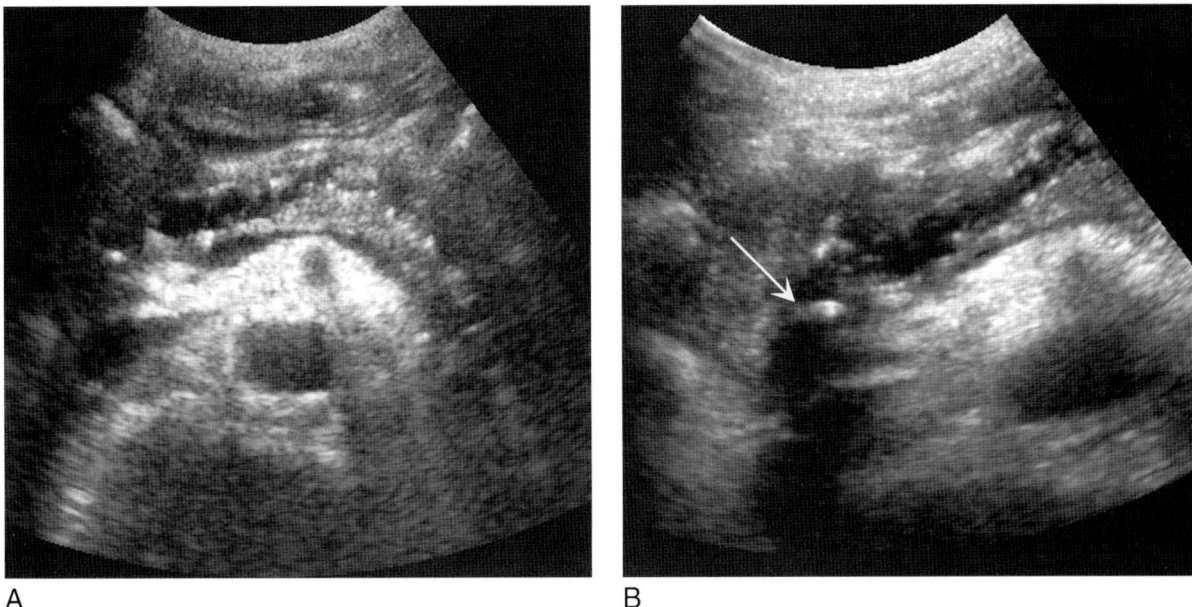

A   B

FIGURE 7-29. Chronic calcific pancreatitis. A, Transverse image of the pancreas shows a dilated and irregular duct. **B,** Transverse image of the pancreatic head shows the dilated duct. There is a bright focus with shadowing within the duct consistent with a calculus *(arrow).* (Courtesy of Stephanie Wilson, M.D., University of Toronto, Toronto, Ontario.)

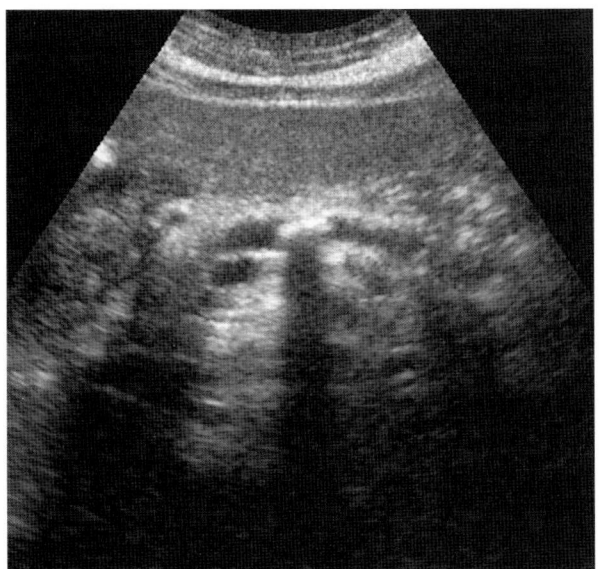

FIGURE 7-30. Pancreatic duct calculus. Transverse image of the pancreas shows a dilated duct. A bright echogenic focus with shadowing is consistent with a calculus. (Courtesy of Stephanie Wilson, M.D., University of Toronto, Toronto, Ontario.)

Dilation of the common bile duct is present in 5% to 10% of the patients with chronic pancreatitis and characteristically causes smooth gradual tapering, although abrupt tapering is rarely seen.[17]

Portosplenic vein thrombosis may occur as a complication of chronic pancreatitis and was recently reported as occurring in 5.1% of patients.[100] Because of the chronic nature of the disease, cavernous transformation may be present.

There is relatively good functional and morphologic correlation in advanced pancreatic disease but poor correlation for mild-to-moderate disease. In chronic pancreatitis, bicarbonate secretion seems to correlate best with ductal imaging (i.e., ERCP), whereas enzyme secretion correlates with gland imaging (i.e., ultrasound and CT).[101] However, a revised "Cambridge" classification of chronic pancreatitis has been proposed and preliminary studies indicate good correlations based on findings of ERCP and ultrasound (Table 7-1). Ductal abnormalities of more than three side branches are diagnostic of the early stages of chronic pancreatitis, whereas abnormality of the main duct indicates at least moderate disease.[102] The finding of intraductal calculi constitutes sufficient evidence for grading as advanced chronic pancreatitis.[103] Therefore, correlation of ultrasound findings with that of ERCP has become part of the basis of treatment of chronic pancreatitis.

NEOPLASMS

Adenocarcinoma

Pancreatic carcinoma is the fourth leading cause of death from cancer in the United States, preceded by cancer of the lung, colon, and breast. The incidence of this neoplasm has increased threefold in the past 40 years. Carcinoma of the pancreas is extremely rare before 40 years of age, and two thirds of patients present after age 60 years.[104] The prognosis is particularly poor, with a median survival time of 2 to 3 months and a 1-year survival of 8%. **Clinical symptoms** depend on the

TABLE 7-1. REVISED "CAMBRIDGE" CLASSIFICATION OF CHRONIC PANCREATITIS

Class*	Ultrasound
Normal	Visualization of entire gland and demonstration and measurement of main pancreatic duct
Equivocal	Less than two abnormal signs
	Main duct enlarged (less than 4 mm)
	Gland enlarged (up to twice normal)
	Cavities (less than 10 mm)
	Irregular ducts
Mild	Focal reduction in parenchymal echogenicity
Moderate	Two or more abnormal signs
	Echogenic foci in parenchyma
	Increased or irregular echogenicity of wall of main duct
	Irregular contour to gland, particularly focal enlargement
Marked	Large cavities (greater than 10 mm)
	Calculi
	Duct obstruction (greater than 4 mm)
	Major duct irregularity
	Gross enlargement (greater than 4 mm)
	Contiguous organ invasion

If pathologic changes are limited to one third of the gland or less, they are classified as focal.
Modified with permission from Jones SN, Lees WR, Frost RA: Diagnosis and grading of chronic pancreatitis by morphological criteria derived by ultrasound and pancreatography. Clin Radiol 1988;39:43-48.

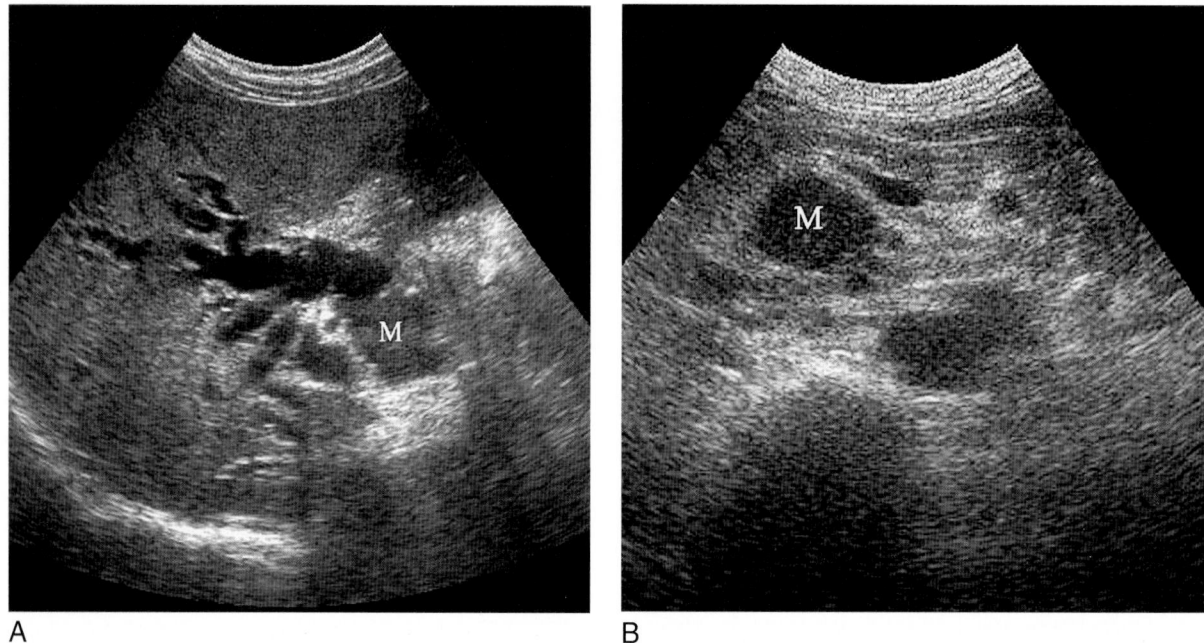

FIGURE 7-31. Pancreatic head cancer presenting as painless jaundice. A, Sagittal sonogram through the porta hepatis shows markedly dilated biliary duct. The common bile duct terminates in a solid mass (M) in the pancreatic head. **B,** Transverse image of the caudal aspect of the pancreatic head shows the hypoechoic mass (M). (Courtesy of Stephanie Wilson, M.D., University of Toronto, Toronto, Ontario.)

location. Tumors arising in the pancreatic head present earlier because of associated bile duct obstruction (Fig. 7-31). A palpable, nontender gallbladder accompanied by jaundice (Courvoisier's sign) is present in approximately 25% of patients.[4] Tumors in the body and tail present later with less specific symptoms, most commonly weight loss, pain, jaundice, and vomiting

when the gastrointestinal tract is invaded by the tumor. Diabetes and malabsorption are late findings.

Pathologically, almost all adenocarcinomas originate in the ductal epithelium, with less than 1% arising in the acini. They may be either mucinous or nonmucinous.[29] Approximately 70% of the pancreatic cancers arise in the region of the head, 15% to 20% in the body, and 5% in

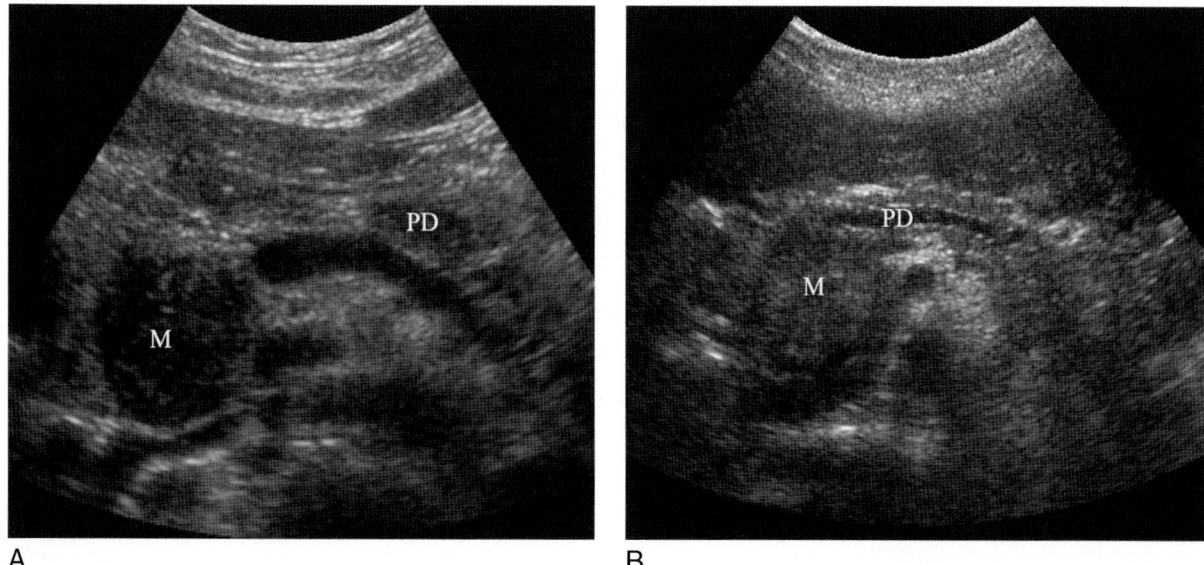

FIGURE 7-32. Pancreatic head cancer in two patients. Transverse sonograms of the pancreas each show a mass in the head. **A,** The most common appearance is a poorly defined and very hypoechoic mass. A dilated pancreatic duct (PD) is incompletely seen on this view. **B,** A subtle, slightly echogenic mass is most evident as the dilated pancreatic duct can be traced to its margin. (Courtesy of Stephanie Wilson, M.D., University of Toronto, Toronto, Ontario.)

the tail. In 20% of cases, the tumor is distributed diffusely throughout the gland.[29]

Because pancreatic head tumors present earlier, they can be fairly small and cause little or moderate expansion of the head. They may be unapparent on external examination and only create an impression of abnormal consistency or nodularity. On cut cross section, they are poorly defined and present an irregular margin with few, if any, foci of hemorrhage.[29] Carcinomas of the body and tail of the pancreas are, on the average, larger than those of the head and tend to invade adjacent organs, including the stomach, transverse colon, spleen, and adrenal gland. Carcinomas in the region of the body and tail are more likely to present as metastases, probably as a result of late presentation.[104] Massive hepatic metastases are characteristic. Metastases occur most frequently in the regional lymph nodes, liver, lungs, peritoneum, and adrenal glands. Peripancreatic, gastric, mesenteric, omental, and portohepatic nodes are frequent sites of spread.

Sonography

Direct Signs. The most common sonographic finding in pancreatic carcinoma is a **poorly defined, homogeneous or inhomogeneous hypoechoic mass** in the pancreas or pancreatic fossa (Fig. 7-32).[105] This may or may not be associated with expansion of the pancreas or compression of the adjacent structures. In patients whose pancreas shows increased echogenicity, the tumor will be better visualized as the contrast between the neoplasm and the normal pancreatic echotexture is accentuated. When an isoechoic mass is identified,

attention should be given to the size of the pancreas and nodularity of its contour. In the uncinate process, the presence of a mass changes its pointed contour to a rounded appearance. Necrosis, seen as a cystic area within the mass, is a rare manifestation of pancreatic carcinoma (Fig. 7-33).[106] However, pseudocysts caused by associated pancreatitis may be seen adjacent to the carcinoma (see Fig. 7-23). The less common diffuse tumors can be mistaken for acute pancreatitis. The lobulated appearance of the pancreatic mass and clinical presentation help in differentiation. At the time of diagnosis by sonography, pancreatic carcinomas usually measure more than 2 cm. The tumor size is usually larger at surgery or autopsy than on the sonograms. This may be caused by the presence of microscopic infiltration of the tissues surrounding the tumor itself, which is undetected by ultrasound. **Lesional vascularity is uncommonly shown with conventional Doppler imaging** (Fig. 7-34).

Indirect Signs. Dilation of the pancreatic duct proximal to a pancreatic mass is a common finding. A normal pancreatic duct usually measures less than 2 to 3 mm and has parallel walls and a straight course. When obstructed, it loses its parallel nature, becomes tortuous, and ends or tapers abruptly. The pancreatic duct distends with aging, but it maintains its parallel straight course and can be followed to its entrance into the duodenum. Recognition of a dilated pancreatic duct is an important observation, because it can lead to detection of small pancreatic carcinoma (Fig. 7-35). However, in the absence of a mass, the appearances of the pancreatic duct in both pancreatic carcinoma and pancreatitis may overlap.

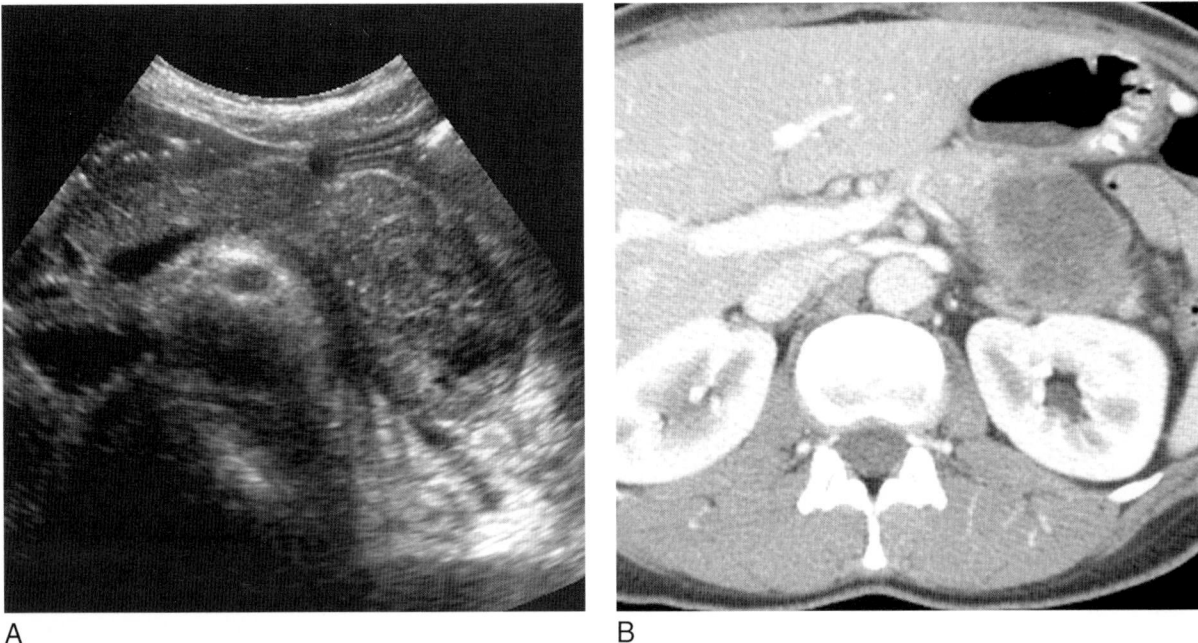

FIGURE 7-33. Pancreatic tail adenocarcinoma. In a 41-year-old woman showing infrequent small cystic areas related to necrosis. **A,** Sonogram and **B,** CT scan both show a large and bulky mass in the pancreatic tail.

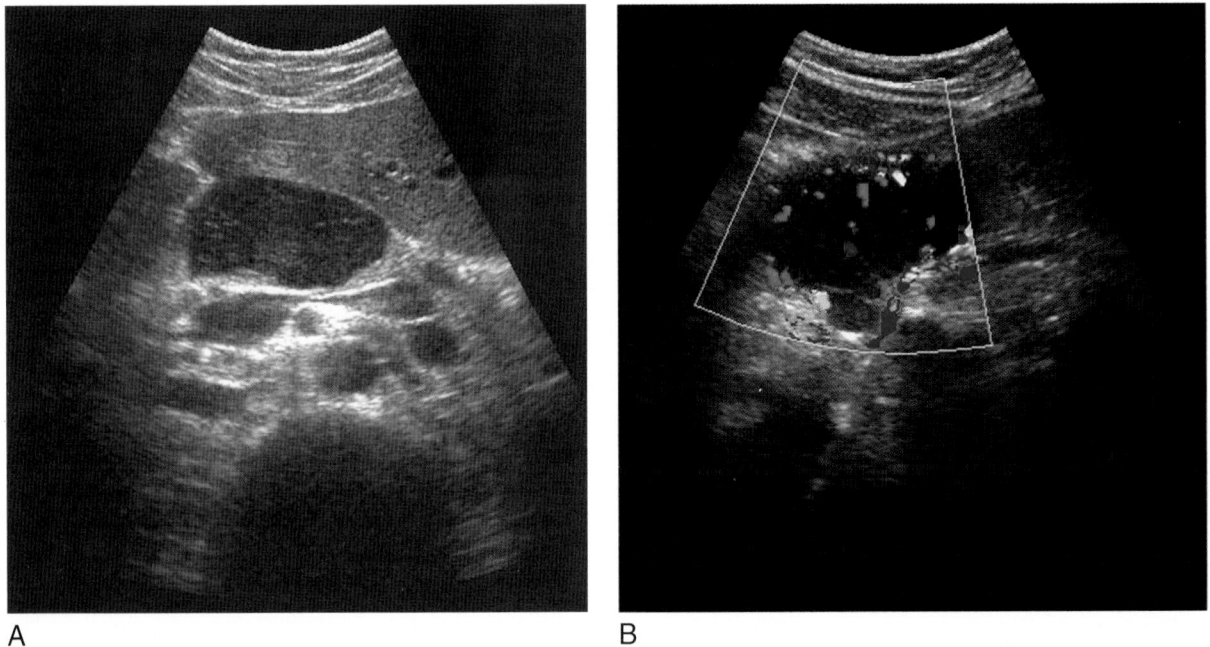

FIGURE 7-34. Unusual appearance of pancreatic ductal adenocarcinoma showing an exophytic and well-defined mass with vascularity. A, Transverse sonogram shows a very well-defined exophytic solid hypoechoic mass in the pancreatic neck/body. **B,** Color Doppler shows lesional vascularity. Both the well-defined margin and the vascularity are not commonly seen in pancreatic cancer.

Bile duct dilation is commonly seen with lesions in the head of the pancreas (see Fig. 7-31). The gallbladder and cystic duct may or may not be dilated. The level of obstruction may be in the head, above the head, or in the porta hepatis, depending on the extent of the lesion or associated lymphadenopathy. Abrupt termination of the dilated bile duct is strongly suggestive of malignancy. Thick, echogenic sludge in the common bile duct proximal to a tumor should not be mistaken for the tumor itself. These patients also often have thick sludge in the gallbladder. Uncommonly, the mass itself extends inside the bile duct. Dilation of the common bile duct,

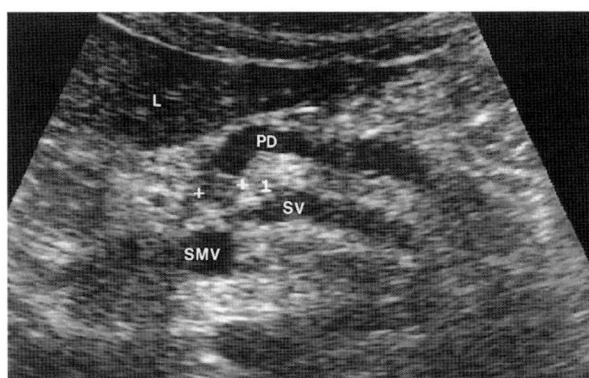

FIGURE 7-35. Small pancreatic carcinoma.
Transverse ultrasound. Detection of this small slightly
hypoechoic mass *(between cursors)* was facilitated by following
the dilated pancreatic duct (PD). This mass was not evident on
CT scan. L, liver; PD, pancreatic duct; SMV, superior
mesenteric vein; SV, splenic vein.

pancreatic duct (see Fig. 7-35), or both, may occasionally be the only sonographic finding. Although the
double-duct sign (combined dilation of the pancreatic
and common bile duct) is also seen with chronic pancreatitis, it usually indicates the presence of pancreatic
adenocarcinoma (Fig. 7-36).

Displacement and involvement of adjacent vascular
structures may occur (Fig. 7-37). Compression of the
inferior vena cava by the head of the pancreas has been
reported as an indication of a mass lesion.[107] Pancreatic
cancer may originate from the pancreas in an exophytic
fashion (Fig. 7-38).

Associated pancreatitis proximal to the mass may
obscure the underlying primary tumor because of the
similar echogenicity. This is especially true when
pseudocyst formation from pancreatitis distorts the
gland and the underlying tumor. In these cases, sonographic differentiation may be difficult (see Fig. 7-23).

Atrophy of the gland proximal to an obstructing mass
in the head may occur and may appear hypoechoic or
hyperechoic. In the presence of a hypoechoic body and
tail, disproportionate size of the head may be the only
clue to the presence of a mass.

Some patients presenting with carcinoma of the
pancreas are very cachectic. In these circumstances,
because the pancreas is situated anteriorly and close to
the abdominal wall, a 7.5-MHz transducer or a transducer with a good near field should be used. Occasionally, when there is occlusion of the pancreatic duct,
the dilated duct may be the only structure left in the
atrophied pancreas and the entire pathologic state can be
overlooked if the duct is mistaken for a blood vessel.
When dilation of the pancreatic duct or common bile
duct or both are present, meticulous scanning should be
performed in the region where one or both dilated ducts
terminate, to identify the mass.

Doppler Findings. Pancreatic carcinoma appears to
have Doppler features similar to other malignant lesions
(increased velocity and diminished flow impedance).[108]
Taylor and coworkers[108] have reported a velocity greater
than 3 kHz and a systolic/diastolic ratio of less than 3
in pancreatic carcinomas. These results are similar to
those reported for primary liver, kidney, and adrenal
neoplasms. The increased velocity is attributed to
arteriovenous shunting and the diminished impedance
to vascular spaces that lack muscular walls.[108] However,
Doppler has not proven effective in differentiating
benign from malignant pancreatic masses.

Color and pulsed Doppler can be used to evaluate
venous and arterial structures for the presence or absence
of encasement, occlusion, or thrombosis. Increased focal
arterial or venous flow velocity indicates the presence of
compression or encasement of a vessel.

Staging of Pancreatic Carcinomas. The role of ultrasound is important not only in diagnosing pancreatic
carcinomas but also in assessing tumor resectability.
Surgery is still the treatment of choice in carcinomas that
are considered resectable. However, surgery still carries a
high rate of mortality and morbidity and provides poor
results. Therefore, every attempt should be made to
preoperatively confirm the diagnosis and properly stage
the disease to prevent unnecessary surgery.

Extension of pancreatic carcinomas beyond the
pancreatic parenchyma—including venous invasion,
involvement of the retroperitoneal fat and adjacent
organs, lymphadenopathy, and liver metastasis—
precludes the feasibility of surgery. Some surgeons also
consider arterial involvement a contraindication to
surgery. It is generally difficult to differentiate between
compression and **invasion** of the **venous structures.**
Occlusion or thrombosis of the splenic vein is suggested
with interruption of the vein, splenomegaly, and
collateral formation in the peripancreatic and periportal
region and along the stomach wall. Intrapancreatic
collaterals are rarely seen (see Fig. 7-10). Enlargement of
the gastrocolic vein draining into the superior mesenteric
vein providing a collateral pathway via the gastroepiploic
vein may be seen when there is involvement of the
splenic vein or superior mesenteric portal vein confluence above the gastrocolic trunk. A gastrocolic vein
greater than 5 mm is reported to be suggestive of occlusion of the splenic vein or superior mesenteric portal
vein confluence above gastrocolic trunk on CT examination.[109] Also, lack of visualization of the splenic vein
should be regarded as suspicious for its invasion.
Involvement of the superior mesenteric and portal veins
may also result in collateral formation in the mesentery.
Although cavernous transformation is rare because of
the short duration of portal thrombosis in these patients,
it can occur. **Encasement** of the celiac axis or superior
mesenteric artery as a result of lymphatic involvement is
more easily recognizable and may be the only indication
of the presence of the disease (Figs. 7-39 and 7-40; see
also Fig. 7-37).

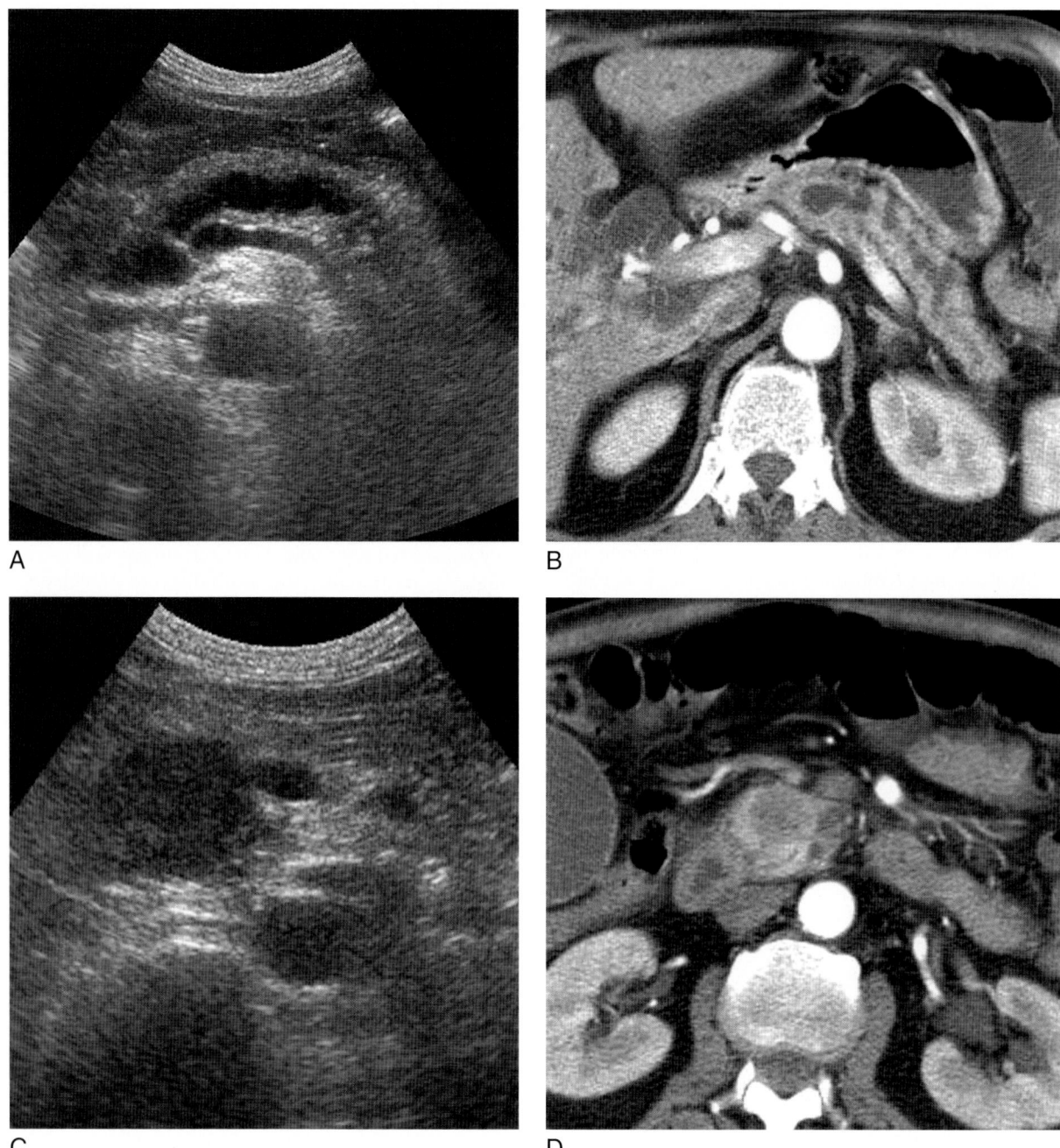

FIGURE 7-36. Double-duct sign. Pancreatic and common bile duct dilation as manifestation of pancreatic head cancer. A, Sonogram and **B,** CT scan show a dilated pancreatic duct and a dilated CBD, that is suspect for pancreatic head cancer shown on other views. **C,** Sonogram and **D,** CT scans taken at the caudal aspect of the pancreatic head show the head cancer. (Courtesy of Stephanie Wilson, M.D., University of Toronto, Toronto, Ontario.)

Vascular structures should be evaluated with the help of the Doppler examination (Figs. 7-41 and 7-42). Ascites is seen in more advanced cases. Involvement of the duodenum may be appreciated on ultrasound.

Comparative Imaging

There is controversy concerning the role of ultrasound and CT in the detection of pancreatic carcinoma.[110-113] The superiority of ultrasound over CT for tissue charac-

terization is generally accepted. Because sonography relies more on tissue characterization, which is a more objective sign than pancreatic enlargement for the diagnosis of pancreatic carcinoma, sonography should be more accurate than CT when the pancreas is optimally seen. Because CT relies more on indirect signs, such as enlargement of the pancreas, it has a lower specificity than ultrasound.[110] In one study, 59% of the CT results falsely suggested a pancreatic mass solely on the basis of apparent localized enlargement of the pancreas without

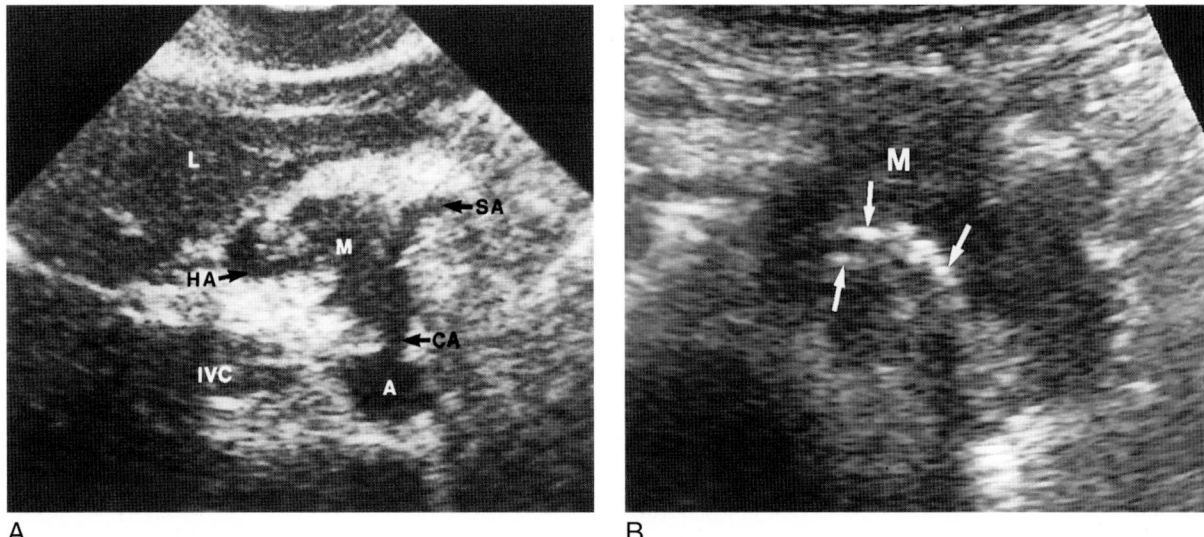

FIGURE 7-37. Pancreatic cancer involving adjacent vascular structures in two patients. Transverse (**A**) and sagittal (**B**) views showing encasement of celiac artery (CA) and splenic artery (*arrows*). A, aorta; HA, hepatic artery; IVC, inferior vena cava; L, liver; M, mass; SA, splenic artery.

any other findings. All proved to be normal on the sonographic examination.[110] In another series comparing CT and ultrasound for the detection of pancreatic carcinoma, ultrasound showed the tumor itself in 86% as compared with 69% with CT. Ultrasound identified secondary signs but not the tumor in 11% of patients compared with 25% for CT, and the findings were normal in 3% as compared with 6% for CT.[112] However, with the advent of helical CT and the possibility of visualizing the normal pancreas at its peak enhancement, which occurs early, the increased contrast between the very vascular normal parenchyma and the hypovascular adenocarcinoma of the pancreas has improved the sensitivity and specificity of CT for diagnosing pancreatic carcinoma.[114] The sensitivity of ultrasound for the detection of pancreatic carcinoma is more operator dependent and is related to the time spent in visualizing the entire pancreas. In general, if the pancreas is optimally seen in its entirety and is normal, pancreatic carcinoma can be excluded with a high degree of certainty, considering the reported 98% sensitivity of ultrasound for detection of pancreatic carcinoma.[110] However, if the whole length of the pancreas is not seen, pancreatic carcinoma cannot be excluded.

CT should be performed after the sonographic diagnosis of pancreatic carcinoma to assess resectability. CT appears to be more sensitive when assessing local extension with regard to involvement of the adjacent retroperitoneal fat, although assessment of vascular involvement has improved with advances in color Doppler imaging, including power Doppler. In a recent cost-effectiveness study of different imaging modalities to assess for resectability of pancreatic cancer, a strategy of CT, laparoscopy, and laparoscopic ultrasound

consistently resulted in significantly lower costs than other imaging tests under a wide range of scenarios.[115]

However, if ultrasound confirms nonresectability, no additional information is gained by performing CT.[110] Angiography is useful for the assessment of vascular invasion. ERCP should only be used in conjunction with ultrasound or CT, when there is a question of differentiation of malignant from inflammatory masses.[116] ERCP has no role if the malignant nature of a pancreatic mass is confirmed on ultrasound or CT.

Differential Diagnosis

The main differential diagnosis of pancreatic carcinoma is focal pancreatitis, or a focal mass associated with chronic pancreatitis. If the findings are localized to the pancreas and limited to a hypoechoic area with or without mass effect, pancreatic carcinoma cannot be differentiated from focal pancreatitis unless the area has foci of calcification. With pancreatitis, CT may show more diffuse involvement of the pancreas or soft tissue changes in the adjacent fat (see Fig. 7-14C). Cross-sectional imaging and ERCP may show smooth tapering of the ducts at the site of the mass and associated changes of pancreatitis, especially upstream to the mass.[116]

Peripancreatic lymphadenopathy can usually be differentiated from pancreatic cancer by the identification of echogenic septa between individual nodes. The absence of jaundice when a large pancreatic head mass is present close to the distal common bile duct favors lymphadenopathy.

Ampullary adenocarcinomas should be differentiated from pancreatic adenocarcinomas because the former has a better prognosis. For the three gross patterns

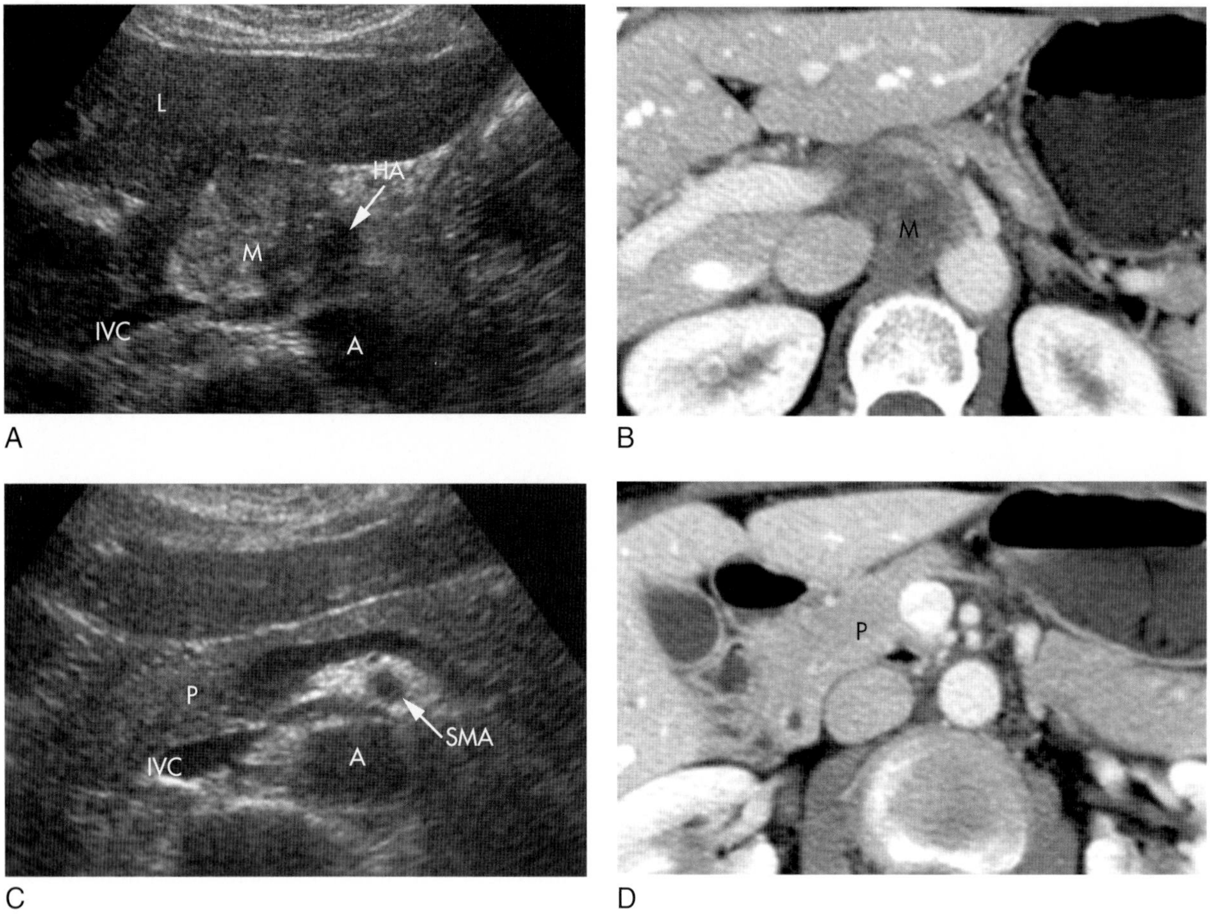

A

B

C

D

FIGURE 7-38. Exophytic pancreatic mass. Transverse ultrasound (**A**) and axial CT scan (**B**) show a mass (M) arising from the superior aspect of pancreas invading the hepatic artery (HA). Transverse ultrasound (**C**) and axial CT scan (**D**) show normal inferior aspect of head of pancreas (P). A, aorta; IVC, inferior vena cava; L, liver; SMA, superior mesenteric artery.

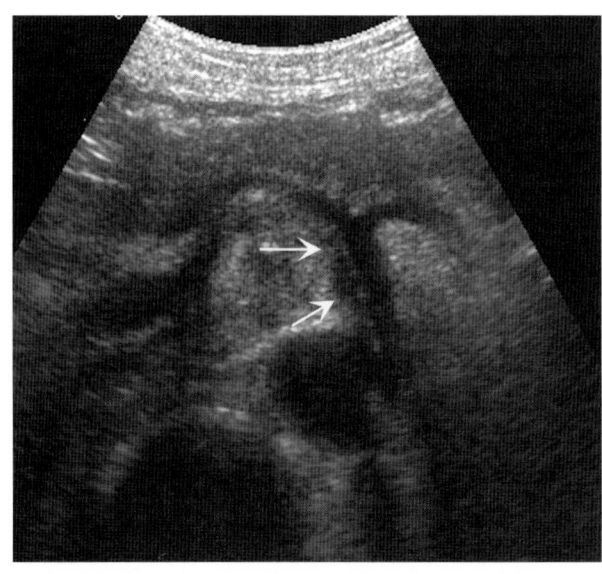

FIGURE 7-39. Soft tissue cuff around the celiac axis. Transverse sonogram shows the celiac axis arising from the ventral aspect of the aorta. A hypoechoic soft tissue cuff (arrows) is seen along the right lateral wall of the vessel. This may be seen with inflammatory or neoplastic infiltration, as in this patient with pancreatic cancer.

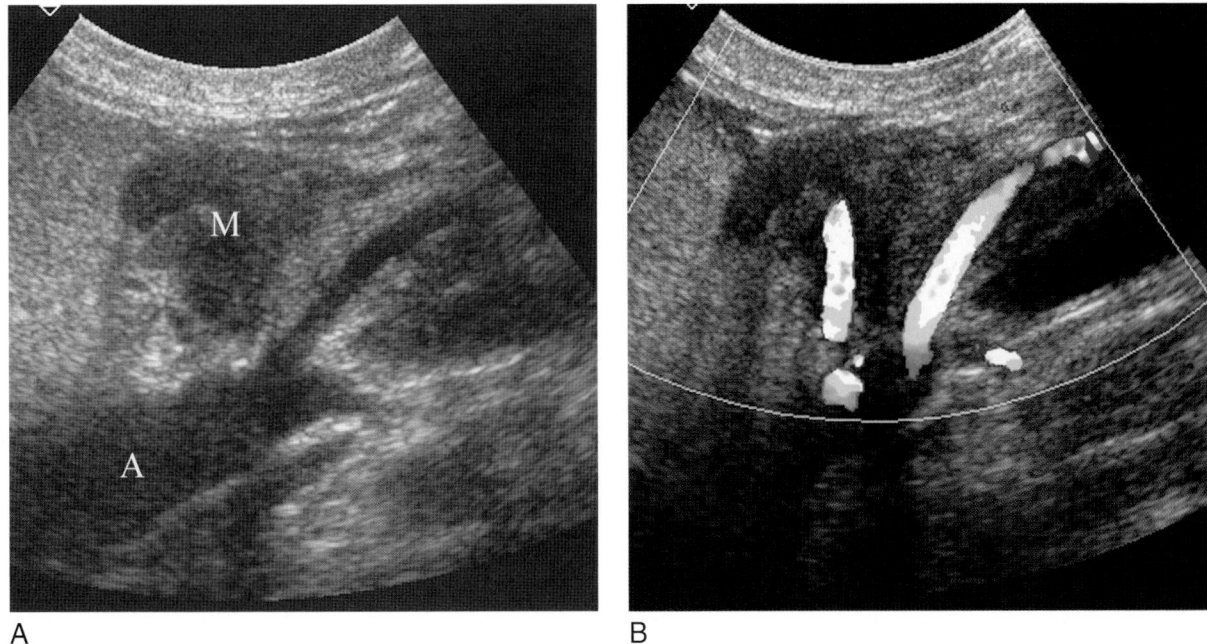

FIGURE 7-40. Vascular encasement from locally invasive pancreatic cancer. A, Sagittal midline image shows the aorta (A) and the superior mesenteric artery. There is a hypoechoic mass (M) anterior to the aorta. **B,** Color Doppler image at the same level shows flow in the SMA and also within the celiac axis (CA) that is not shown on the grayscale image. The CA lies within the soft tissue mass. (Courtesy of Stephanie Wilson, M.D., University of Toronto, Toronto, Ontario.)

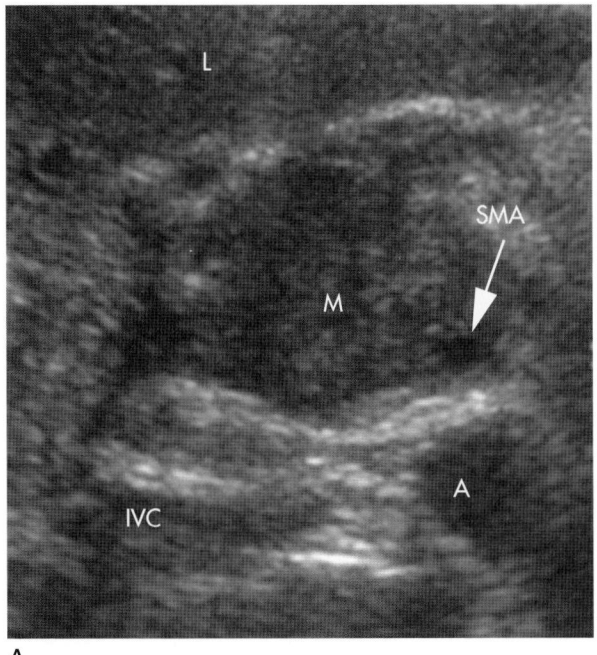

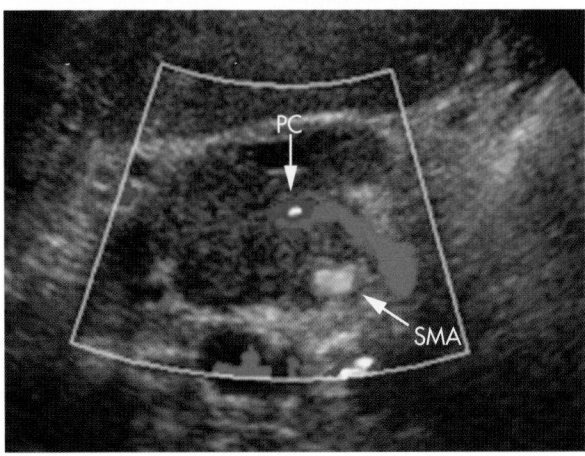

FIGURE 7-41. Contribution of Doppler imaging to staging of pancreatic carcinoma. Transverse gray-scale (**A**) and transverse color Doppler (**B**) views demonstrate a mass (M) in the head of pancreas encasing portal confluence (PC) and superior mesenteric artery (SMA), better appreciated on color Doppler. A, aorta; IVC, inferior vena cava; L, liver.

of ampullary adenocarcinoma—intra-ampullary, peri-ampullary, and mixed—the prognosis diminishes respectively. Masses larger than 2 cm have a similar prognosis to that of pancreatic carcinoma.[117] Most patients present with dilation of both the common bile duct and the pancreatic duct. However, the bile duct may be the only involved duct (Fig. 7-43). Occasionally, an intraluminal mass is seen at the distal end of a dilated bile duct.[118] EUS has improved the accuracy of ultrasound for diagnosing ampullary carcinoma, allowing its differentiation from pancreatic carcinoma and the staging of ampullary carcinoma (see the section on EUS).

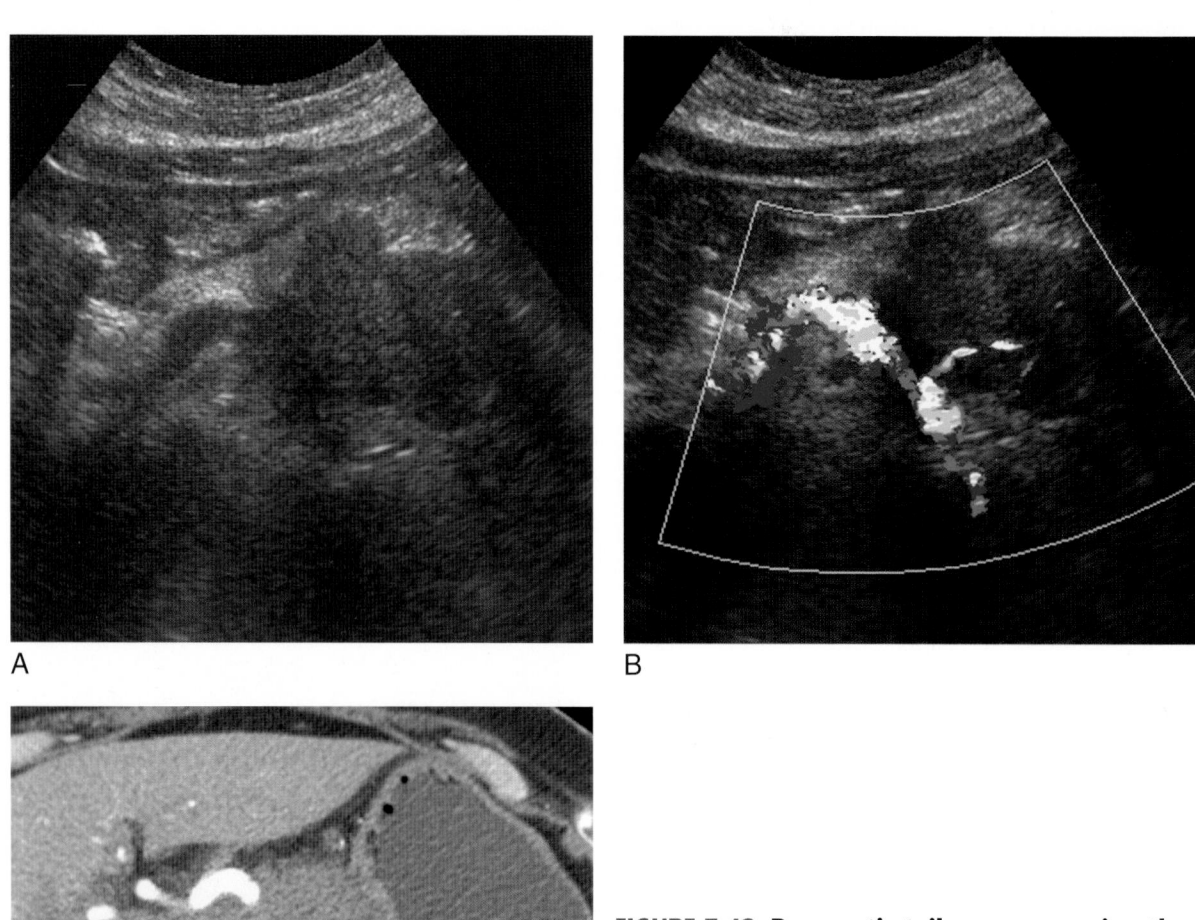

FIGURE 7-42. Pancreatic tail cancer encasing the branches of the celiac axis. A, Transverse sonogram shows a lobulated pancreatic tail mass. The hepatic artery is seen but not the remainder of the celiac axis. **B,** The addition of color Doppler shows the celiac axis. The splenic artery is narrowed and totally encased within the tumor. The hepatic artery is involved to a lesser extent. **C,** confirmary CT scan shows the mass and the encased arteries.

Cystic Neoplasms

Cystic neoplasms of the pancreas represent 10% to 15% of all pancreatic cysts and 1% of all pancreatic cancers. There are two main categories of cystic neoplasms: microcystic or serous type and macrocystic or mucinous type. Both types of cystic neoplasms have a female-to-male preponderance that is 3:2 for the microcystic and 6:1 for the macrocystic group.[119,120] Microcystic neoplasms are usually seen in patients older than 60 years of age, whereas macrocystic tumors occur in both middle and old age.[120] Patients present with nonspecific abdominal symptoms, weight loss, abdominal mass, or jaundice. Tumors may be found incidentally at surgery or autopsy.[121] Microcystic neoplasms constitute a high percentage of cysts seen in patients with von Hippel-Lindau syndrome.[119]

Microcystic or serous cystadenoma is a moderately well-circumscribed, multilocular mass, without a true capsule, often containing a central stellate scar with occasional calcification within this scar. Microcystic neoplasms are always benign and therefore do not require surgery, especially because they usually present in older patients. The cysts vary in size from less than 1 mm to 2 cm and are more numerous peripherally. The cysts are lined with glycogen-containing cells.[119] In one study

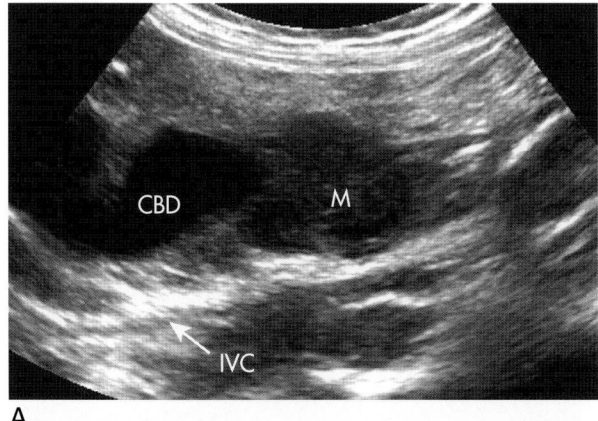

A

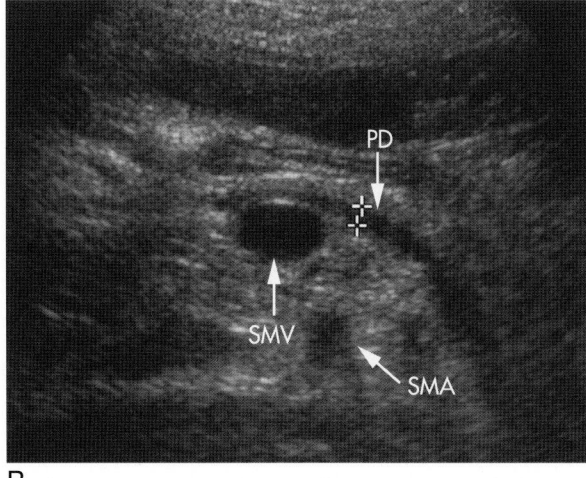

B

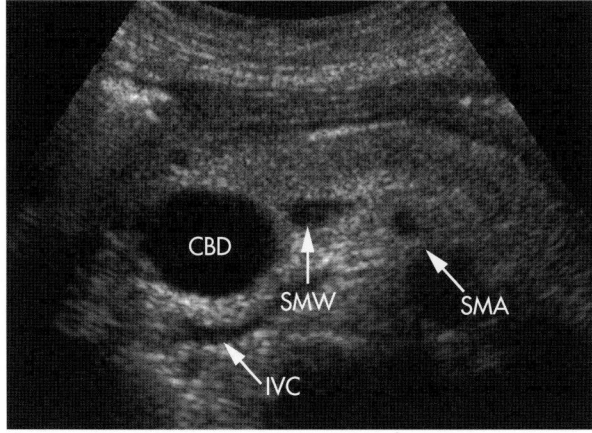

C

FIGURE 7-43. Large ampullary carcinomas. Sagittal (**A**) and transverse (**B** and **C**) views. A hypoechoic mass is seen in the region of the head of the pancreas (M) obstructing the common bile duct (CBD). There is minimal dilatation of the pancreatic duct *(cursors)*. IVC, inferior vena cava; SMA, superior mesenteric artery; SMV, superior mesenteric vein.

series, almost 30% of these cysts were located in the pancreatic head, with the rest distributed between the body and the tail.[119]

Macrocystic or mucinous cystadenoma and cystadenocarcinoma are unilocular or multilocular smooth-surfaced cystic masses with occasional papillary projections or calcification. The cysts usually measure more than 2 cm and are lined with cells containing mucinous material.[120] These tumors are malignant or potentially malignant. Differentiation of benign and malignant forms is difficult (except when there are obvious papillary projections) even at surgery, and tumors presumed to be benign can present a few years later with metastasis. However, even the malignant macrocystic tumors have a better prognosis than adenocarcinomas. Therefore, these tumors should be surgically removed if possible.

Sonography

Microcystic adenomas are relatively well-defined tumors with external lobulation. Depending on the size of the individual cysts, the ultrasound appearance may vary from a well-defined, slightly echogenic, solid-appearing mass (Fig. 7-44) (because the smaller cysts are

only depicted as interfaces) to a partly solid-looking mass with cystic areas, more commonly peripherally to a multicystic mass (Figs. 7-45 and 7-46). Individual cysts range from 1 to 20 mm. The scar that is present in some of these lesions is depicted at the sonographic examination as a central, stellate-shaped echogenic area. Calcifications may be present within this scar.[121] The scar is present in up to 20% of cases.[121,122] The pseudocapsule and septa of these tumors tend to be very vascular. This increased vascularity may be detected on Doppler imaging. Although pancreatic and common bile duct dilatation is uncommonly seen, these tumors tend not to obstruct these ducts, presumably because of their soft nature.

Macrocystic neoplasms commonly manifest sonographically as well-circumscribed, smooth-surfaced, thin- or thick-walled, unilocular, or multilocular cystic lesions of variable sizes, usually more than 2 cm in diameter and fewer than six in number (Figs. 7-47 and 7-48).[121-123] The appearances of these cysts have been classified into four types:[124]

- Clear cysts
- Echogenic cysts containing debris
- Cysts with solid mural vegetations
- Completely filled or solid-looking cysts

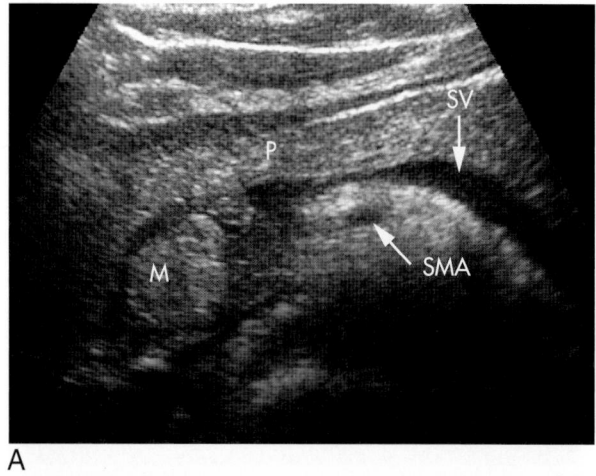

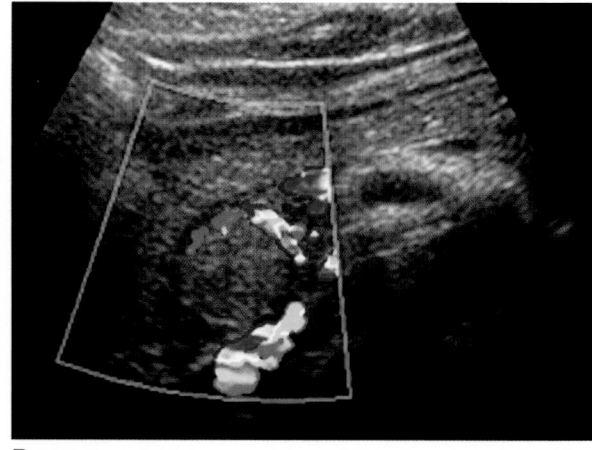

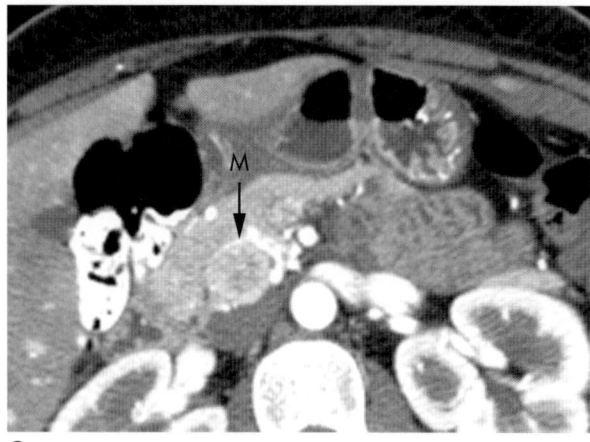

FIGURE 7-44. Microcystic neoplasm. Transverse (**A**), transverse color Doppler (**B**), and axial enhanced CT scans (**C**) demonstrate a homogeneously echogenic, vascular, solid mass (M) in the head of pancreas. P, pancreas; SMA, superior mesenteric artery; SV, splenic vein.

The presence of a solid component in a predominantly cystic mass is diagnostic of this condition. Cysts with multiple thick septa as well as multicystic masses with dominant cysts larger than 2 cm are also very suggestive of a macrocystic tumor. In fact, these tumors have gross features similar to those of an ovarian surface epithelial tumor. The first two types must be differentiated from a pseudocyst. The cysts may show peripheral or mural calcifications.[123] Although it is not possible to definitely differentiate between benign and malignant types, the lesions demonstrating more solid components or papillary projections are usually malignant.[121,123]

It has been shown that the internal architecture of cystic neoplasms is better appreciated on EUS.[125] Although most microcystic neoplasms can be differentiated from macrocystic tumor, there is overlap between the imaging features of these two entities.[126]

Intraductal papillary mucinous tumor (IPMT) is a form of mucinous cystic neoplasm that has been reported under different terms: mucinous ductal ectasia, papillary adenocarcinoma, ductectatic tumor, intraductal mucin-hypersecreting neoplasm, and mucin villous adenomatosis. However, in 1997, the unified IPMT was adopted.[127] Ductal tumors originate from the main pancreatic duct (MPD) or its branches and demonstrate four main patterns at imaging.[128] Both are seen with equal frequency in male and female patients. The peak age at occurrence is in the sixth decade but at a slightly higher age for the branch type.[128] The histology of these tumors ranges from benign to frankly malignant. The most common presentation is recurrent pancreatitis that occurs more frequently in the MPD type.[129] The MPD type presents as segmental or diffuse dilatation of the MPD with or without side branch dilatation (Fig. 7-49). The branch type manifests as a single or multicystic mass with a microcystic or macrocystic appearance. Differentiation from other cystic neoplasms is made by identifying communication with the pancreatic duct.[129] This is best achieved by ERCP but may be evident on cross-sectional imaging.[129] The presence of vascular nodules and a thick wall differentiate benign from malignant lesions. Although MR and CT are more accurate than transabdominal ultrasound to assess the internal architecture of these lesions, endoscopic and intraductal ultrasound appear to be most accurate.[130] These tumors tend to secrete mucinous material that may present as nonvascular nodules within the dilated ducts. ERCP is the gold standard to diagnose

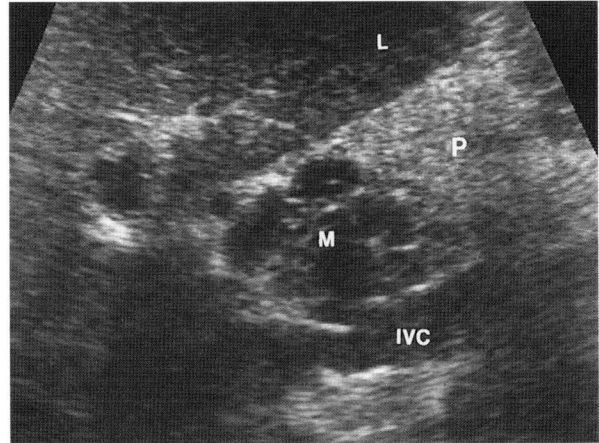

A

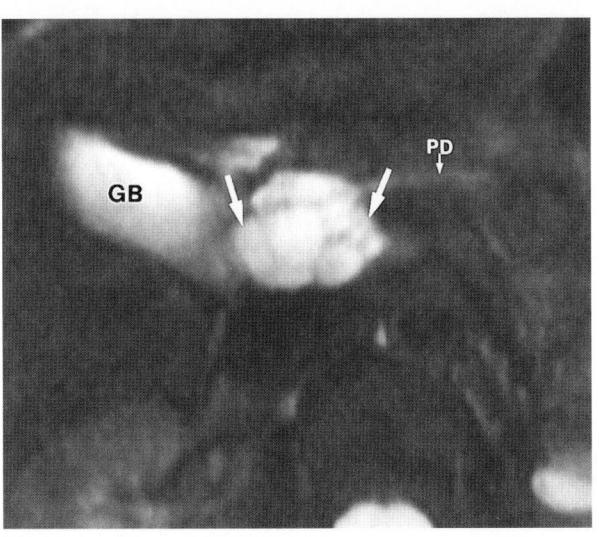

B

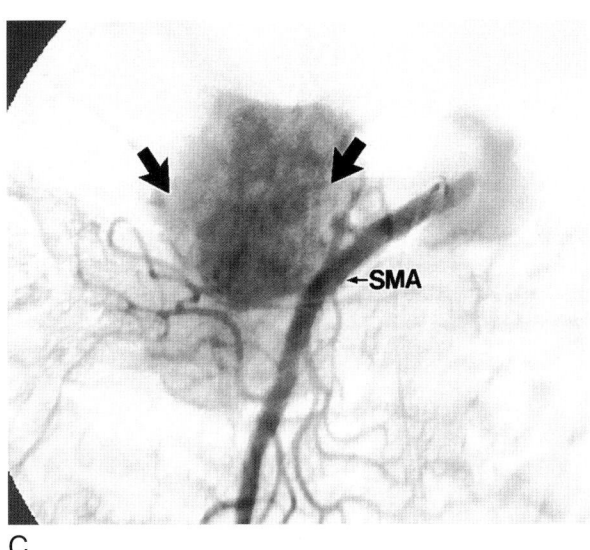

C

FIGURE 7-45. Cystic-appearing microcystic neoplasm. A, Sagittal ultrasound shows multicystic mass (M) in head of pancreas (P) containing multiple small cysts. **B,** Confirmatory heavily T2-weighted axial MRI with fat saturation confirms the multicystic mass *(arrows)* and no solid component. **C,** Superior mesenteric angiogram demonstrates an intensely vascular mass *(arrows)*. GB, gallbladder; IVC, inferior vena cava; L, liver; M, mass; P, pancreas; PD, pancreatic duct; SMA, superior mesenteric artery.

these tumors by observing mucinous material exuding from the ampulla if the cysts are communicating with the pancreatic duct, presence of filling defects in the duct, and communication of the cystic masses with the pancreatic duct. However, ERCP may underestimate the extent of disease because of obstructing mucin plug and solid components.

It is recommended that masses less than 3 cm that do not contain mural nodularity, especially in the branch type tumors, are in general benign and can be followed up.[131]

Comparative Imaging

Small cysts and mural nodules are better recognized on sonographic examinations than CT scans, whereas calcification is more evident on CT scan. Also, CT may show septal or mural enhancement.[121] Angiography shows significant vascularity of the microcystic tumors (see Fig. 7-45C). MRI, particularly heavily T2-weighted sequences, helps resolve these cysts irrespective of their size (see Fig. 7-45B).[132] The combination of an apparent, solid, echogenic mass on ultrasound that appears cystic on MRI is very suggestive of a microcystic tumor. ERCP rarely shows communication with the pancreatic duct in macrocystic neoplasms.[133]

Differential Diagnosis

The microcystic type can be differentiated from an **adenocarcinoma** by its well-circumscribed nature and if tiny cysts are visualized on ultrasound or the multicystic nature of an apparently solid mass on ultrasound is confirmed on MRI. Multilocularity with solid components and multiple septa are more in keeping with a mucinous cystic tumor than a serous type. Communication with the pancreatic duct and parenchymal changes of pancreatitis on ERCP and lack of multilocularity or septa on ultrasound favor the diagnosis of a pseudocyst. Uncommonly, necrotic or cystic islet cell and solid and papillary neoplasms can mimic mucinous tumors.[132] **Choledochal cysts** may present as a cystic mass in the

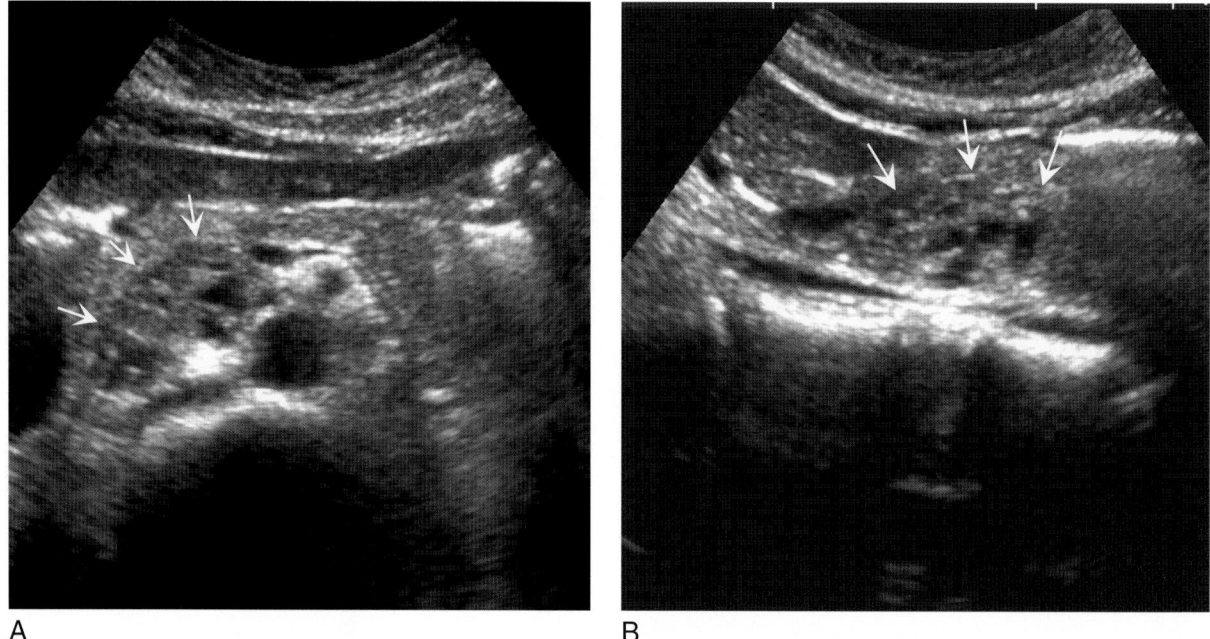

FIGURE 7-46. Microcystic neoplasm of the pancreatic head. A focal hypoechoic mass *(arrows)* is shown with small cystic components measuring less than 2 cm in diameter on **A,** transverse and **B,** sagittal sonograms.

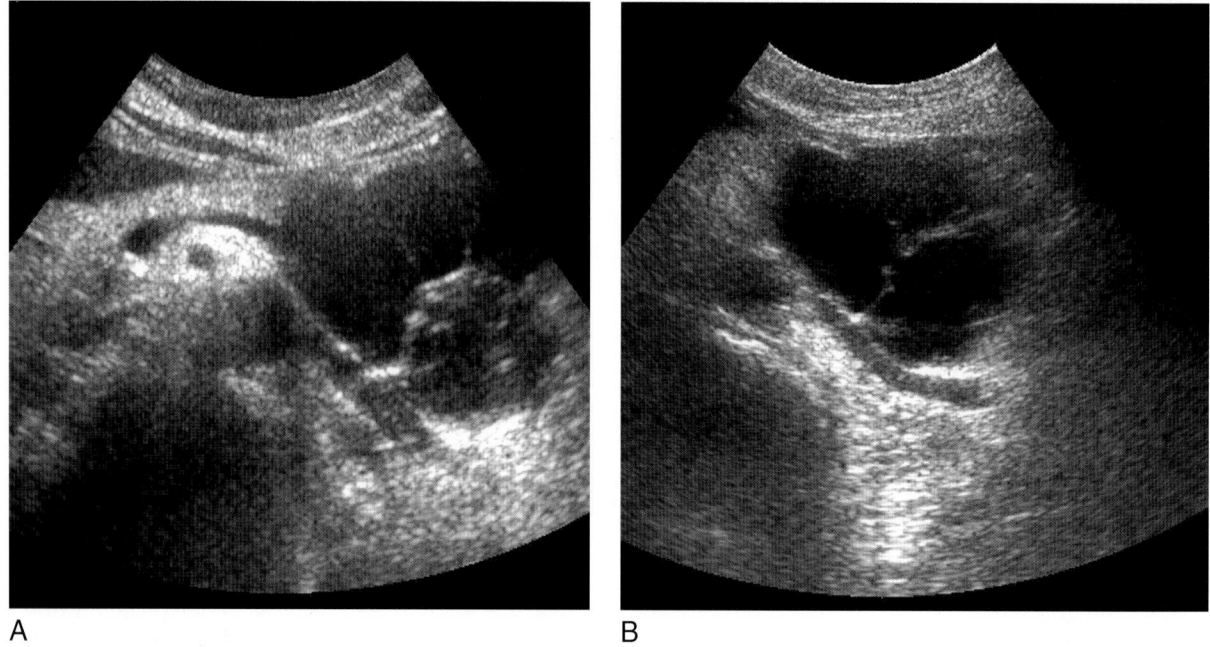

FIGURE 7-47. Macrocystic neoplasm of pancreatic tail. A, Transverse and **B,** sagittal sonograms show a big mass in the tail. The mass is complex, predominantly cystic, with thick septations. Cystic components are greater than 2 cm.

region of the head of the pancreas, but their communication with the common bile duct on cholangiography or direct opacification helps to differentiate them from the cystic neoplasms.[134]

Percutaneous fine-needle aspiration (PFNA) has been used to differentiate between pancreatic cystic masses. Despite the findings of recent reports,[135-138] experience with cyst fluid analysis is still limited. Some authors have

shown a high accuracy for aspiration cytology by identifying inflammatory cells in pseudocysts, hypocellular material with rare strips of cuboidal cells, positive stain for glycogen in microcystic tumors, and moderately cellular material with columnar cells containing mucin in macrocystic tumors.[137,138] Other experts question the diagnosis of pseudocyst made on the basis of the presence of an inflammatory smear.[135] Also, some smears

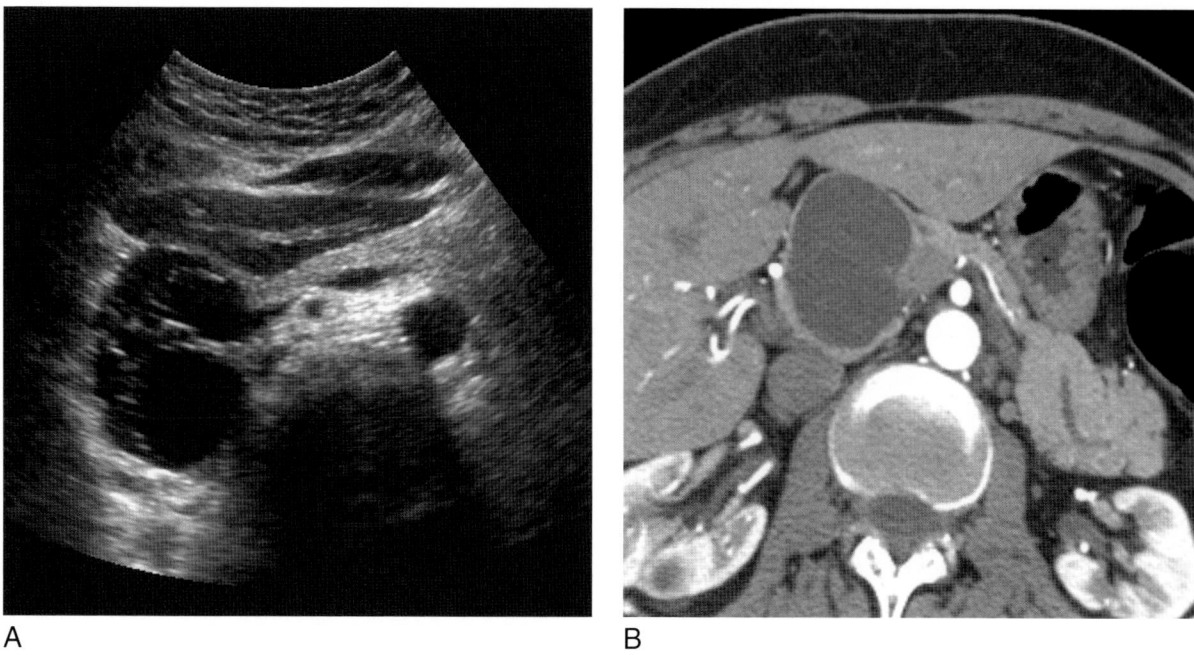

A   B

FIGURE 7-48. Macrocystic pancreatic neoplasm of the pancreatic head. A, sonogram and **B,** contrast-enhanced CT scan.

from cystic tumors lack epithelial cells.[135] The amylase content of pseudocysts is almost always high, whereas the level in neoplastic cysts is generally low.[136] However, cystic tumors of all types may exhibit elevated amylase levels.[135] Some tumor markers, especially carcino-embryonic antigen (CEA), are high in mucinous tumors and low in pseudocysts and microcystic tumors.[135] High viscosity of the cyst content has been shown to be highly specific for mucinous tumors.[135]

Islet-Cell Tumors

Islet-cell tumors of the pancreas appear to arise from multipotential stem cells in ductal epithelium, referred to as the **amine precursor uptake** and **decarboxylation (APUD) system.** Islet-cell tumors can be part of the multiple endocrine neoplasia (MEN) syndrome, in which multiple tumors can secrete different poly-peptides.[139] Although each specific tumor secretes multiple peptides, the clinical picture depends on the dominant hormone. Each of the syndromes may be caused by diffuse hyperplasia, benign adenoma, and malignant neoplasm.

Islet-cell tumors are equally distributed throughout the gland.[29] Electron microscopy and immunoassay techniques are required for specific marking of the tumor.[29] Necrosis, hemorrhage, and calcification are more prominent in larger, malignant types, but malignancy cannot be differentiated microscopically and only dissemination provides indisputable evidence of malignancy. Even malignant tumors are slow growing, and spread beyond regional lymph nodes and liver is

rare. Islet-cell tumors are classified as functioning or nonfunctioning (silent). Silent tumors secrete a bio-logically inactive polypeptide hormone, or target cells are unresponsive or have blocked receptors.[140]

Functioning Tumors

B-Cell Tumors (Insulinomas). Insulinomas are the most common type of islet-cell tumors. They are usually benign, presenting in the fourth through sixth decades of life with hypoglycemic symptoms. B-cell tumors are most commonly found in the body or tail of the pancreas.[29] They are usually well encapsulated and do not differ from normal islet cells on microscopic exam-ination. Of these lesions, 70% are solitary adenomas, 10% are multiple adenomas, and 10% are malignant. The remaining 10% are diffuse hyperplasia or extra-pancreatic. Tumors range in size from minute lesions, difficult to locate on the dissecting table, to huge masses over 1500 g (90% < 2 cm in diameter).[141] Ten to 27 percent of patients with biochemical and clinical indication of insulinomas have no tumor discovered at the time of the initial operation, in which case a blind distal pancreatectomy may be performed.[142]

G-Cell Tumors (Gastrinomas). Gastrinomas, which produce Zollinger-Ellison syndrome, are the second most common islet-cell tumors after insulinomas. The presenting symptoms include diarrhea and peptic ulcer disease with a patient mean age of 50 at presentation.[143] Most gastrinomas are in the pancreas, with 10% to 15% arising in the duodenum.[29] Of those located in the pancreas, only 25% are solitary. Earlier reported

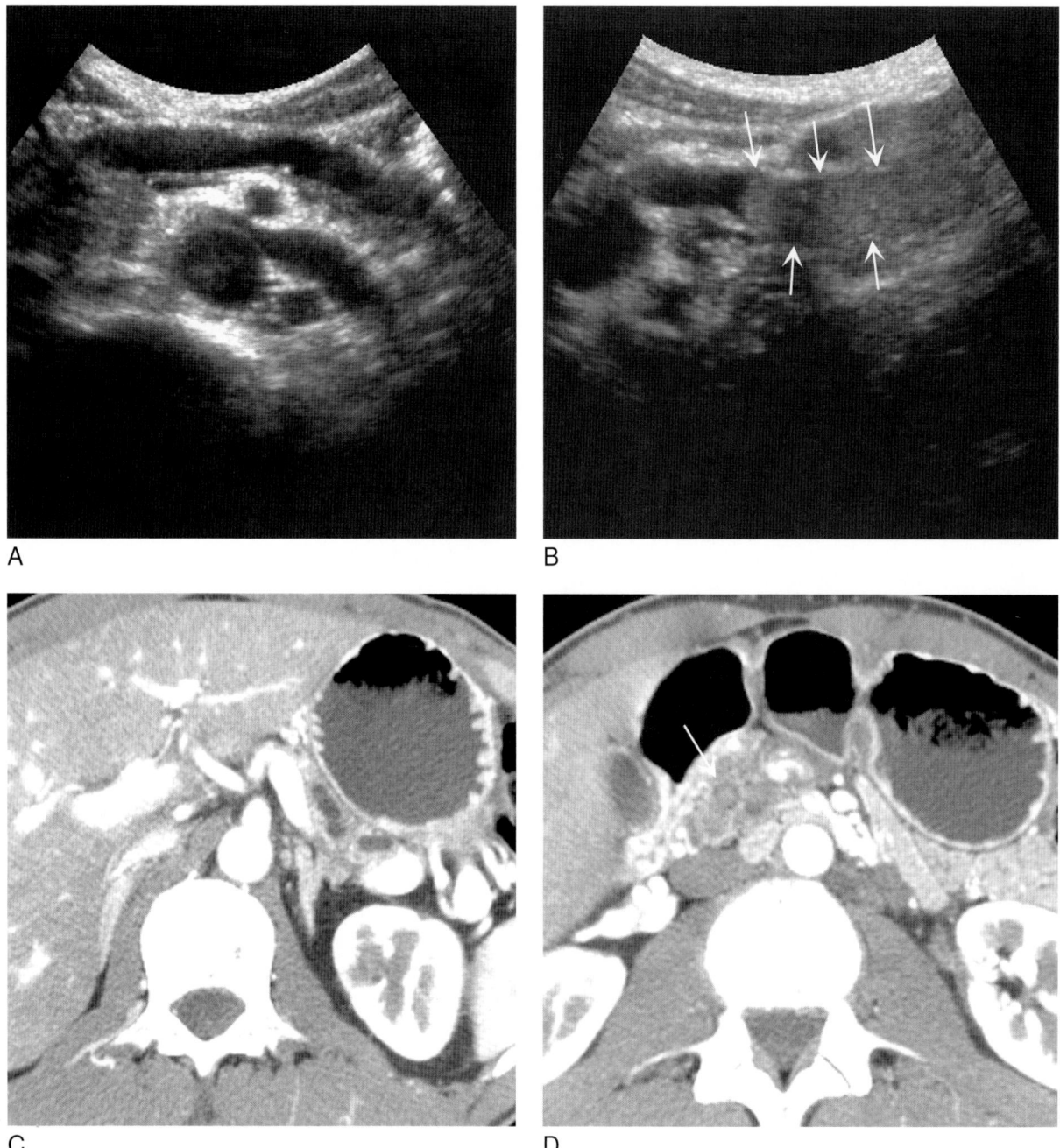

FIGURE 7-49. Intraductal papillary mucinous tumor (IPMT) of the pancreas. A, Transverse sonogram of the pancreas shows marked ductal dilatation with parenchymal atrophy. **B,** Sagittal sonogram of the pancreatic head shows that the dilated pancreatic duct is filled with a papillary soft tissue mass *(arrows)*. **C** and **D** are confirmatory CT images of the pancreatic duct dilatation, the atrophy of the parenchyma, and the soft tissue mass within the dilated duct in the pancreatic head *(arrow)*.

malignancy rates were as high as 60% at presentation,[144] but recent studies confirm a decline in malignant cases, probably as a result of earlier detection because of radio-immunoassay tests for plasma gastrin levels.[145] However, all lesions are potentially malignant. Current management consists of medical treatment of the symptoms. Surgical intervention is limited to patients whose lesions are accurately localized.[145]

Rare Islet-Cell Tumors. Glucagonoma (Fig. 7-50), vipoma, somatostatinoma, and carcinoid (Fig. 7-51) and multihormonal tumors constitute rare functioning islet-cell tumors. There is a high incidence of malignancy in glucagonomas and vipomas.[146] Vipomas are also associated with dilation of the gallbladder (caused by its paralysis as it fills with diluted bile), fluid-filled distended bowel loops (caused by inhibition of bowel

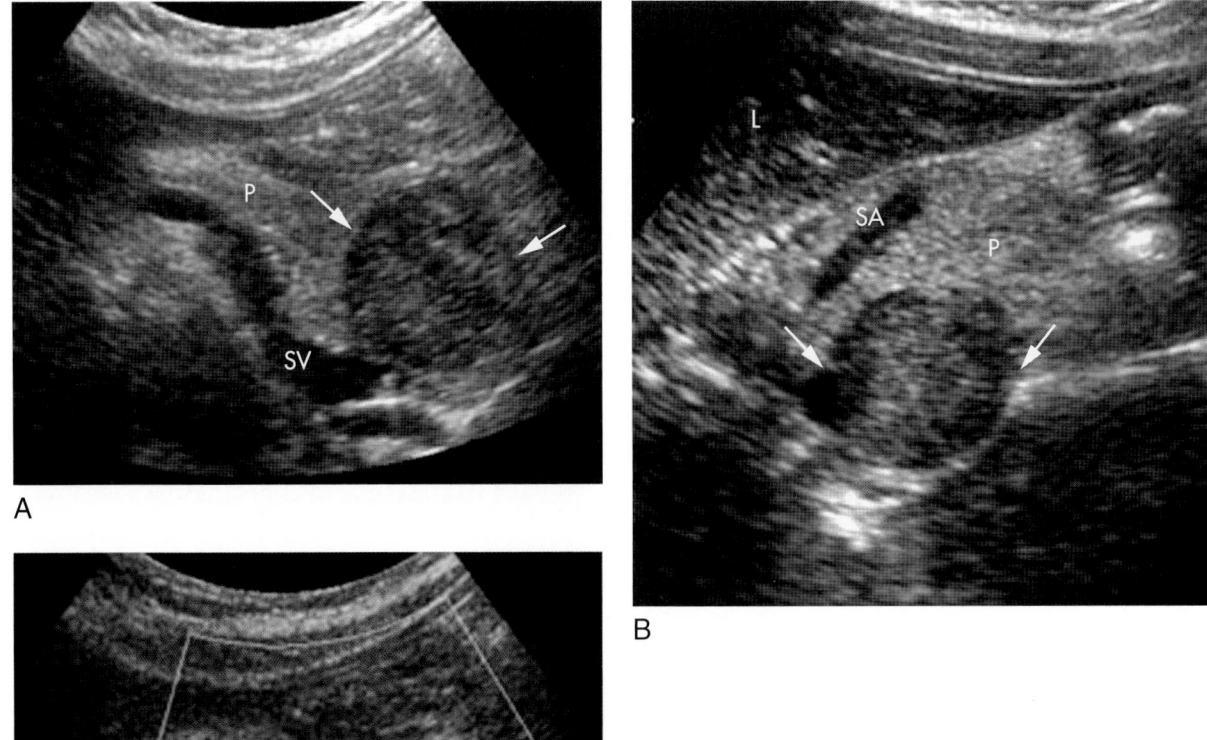

FIGURE 7-50. Glucagonoma. Transverse (**A**), sagittal (**B**), and transverse color Doppler (**C**) views demonstrate a well-defined vascular hypoechoic mass *(arrows)* in the tail of the pancreas (P). L, liver; SA, splenic artery; SV, splenic vein.

motility), and excessive secretion of fluid and electrolytes. The gastric wall may also be thickened.[147]

Nonfunctioning islet-cell tumors constitute one third of all islet-cell neoplasms and have a tendency to present as large tumors with a high incidence of malignancy (Fig. 7-52). They are usually located in the head of the pancreas.[143]

Sonography

Preoperative sonographic examination for the detection of islet-cell tumors is generally difficult, with identification varying from 25% to 60%.[146,147] This difficulty is the small size of these tumors in patients who are generally obese because of overeating for fear of hypoglycemic episodes. Gastrinomas are even smaller, with an average detection rate of 20%.[148] However, recent experience with EUS has allowed more reliable detection of these intrapancreatic endocrine neoplasms, increasing the detection rate to a level of 80%.[149] The usual small

islet-cell tumors are hypoechoic and well defined without calcifications or necrosis. However, these lesions can be isoechoic and only detectable by contour changes.[150] Larger tumors can be hypoechoic or echogenic and irregular and may contain calcifications or areas of necrosis (see Fig. 7-52). The latter findings are usually associated with malignancy.[151] Metastatic lesions tend to be echogenic.[151]

One of the most important contributions of **intraoperative ultrasound** (IOUS) is in the detection of islet-cell tumors (Fig. 7-53).[148,149] IOUS has improved the sensitivity of sonographic detection from 61% to 84%,[148] and, combined with palpation, it has a reported sensitivity of 100%.[142] In another series, 86% of insulinomas and 83% of gastrinomas were detected by IOUS and intrapancreatic lesions were identified in 100% of cases.[152] IOUS can also outline the relation of the neoplasm to the pancreatic or common bile duct.[148] Although more sensitive than both CT and preoperative sonography, IOUS is less accurate for the detection of

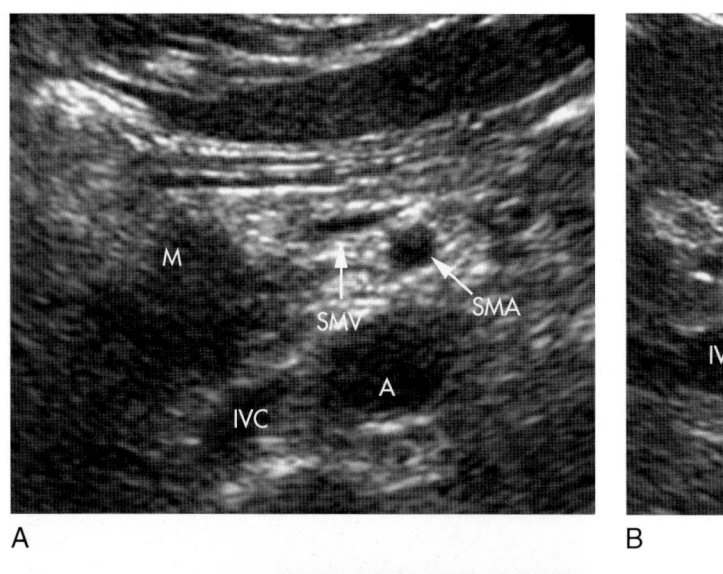

A

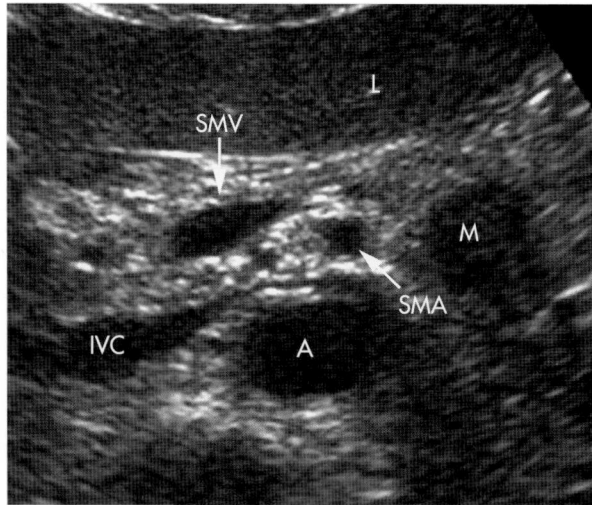

B

C

FIGURE 7-51. Carcinoid. A and **B,** Transverse views show two well-defined hypoechoic masses (M) in the head and tail of pancreas. **C,** Axial enhanced CT scan demonstrates a subtle corresponding mass *(arrows)* similar to the adjacent pancreas. A, aorta; IVC, inferior vena cava; L, liver; SMA, superior mesenteric artery; SMV, superior mesenteric vein.

multiple adenomas, with a sensitivity of 36% because of the small size of the tumors.[146]

Comparative Imaging

Preoperative localization of islet-cell tumors remains extremely difficult because of the small size and rare occurrence, which limits the experience of individual institutions.[152-155] Preoperative sonographic, CT, and angiographic examinations appear to be comparable in the detection of islet-cell tumors that are larger than 2 cm. For smaller tumors, the accuracy of various modalities for the investigation of islet-cell tumors depends on the specific expertise available in different institutions.

The reported sensitivity of CT for the detection of insulinomas is 40% to 66%,[153] whereas angiographic sensitivity varies from 29% to 90%.[152,153] Success rates of as high as 97% have been reported with venous sampling.[154] The advent of helical CT appears to have improved the ability of islet cell tumors to be detected by

CT. Considering that these tumors are generally vascular, the addition of early arterial (parenchymal) phase helical CT with thin slices enhances the detection of these tumors. Van Hoe and coworkers[155] detected 9 of 11 islet-cell tumors including a 4-mm gastrinoma using both arterial- and venous-phase helical CT. Also, combinations of fat-suppressed T1-weighted spin-echo, T2-weighted spin-echo, dynamic gadolinium DTPA gradient recalled echo, and gadolinium-enhanced fat-suppressed T1-weighted images appear to be superior to conventional CT and ultrasound.[156-158] Further studies are required to compare the performance of multi-detector helical CT and MRI. Currently, intraoperative ultrasound is considered the most accurate test to localize functioning islet cell tumors.[159]

Non–Islet-Cell Tumors

The rare non–islet-cell tumors of the pancreas include giant cell tumors, adenosquamous carcinomas, mucinous adenocarcinomas, anaplastic carcinomas, solid and

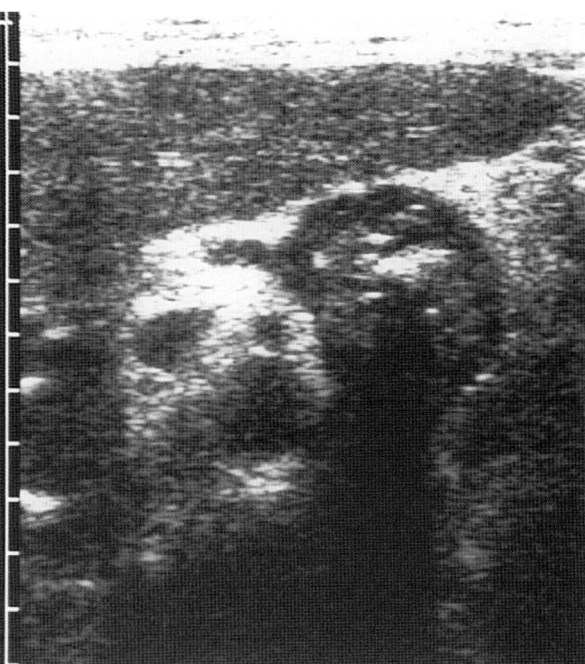

FIGURE 7-52. Islet-cell carcinoma of the body of the pancreas. Transverse sonogram shows a sharply marginated focal hypoechoic mass with internal calcifications that cast an acoustic shadow. (Courtesy of J. William Charboneau, MD, Mayo Clinic, Rochester, MN.)

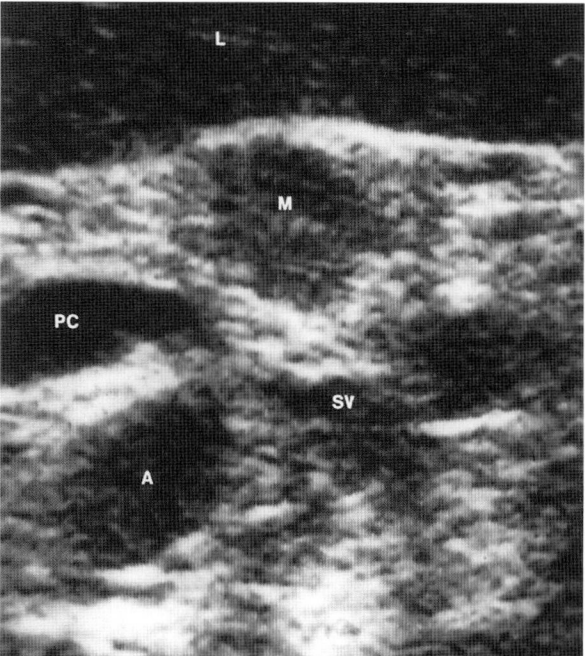

FIGURE 7-53. Islet-cell tumor. Intraoperative scan shows hypoechoic mass (M) in body of pancreas. A, aorta; L, liver; PC, portal confluence; SV, splenic vein.

papillary epithelial neoplasms, acinar cell carcinomas, pancreaticoblastomas, connective tissue tumors, metastases, lymphomas, and plasmacytomas.[160] There is no reported sonographic description for most of these tumors.

Solid and papillary tumors are usually seen in young women as large, well-defined, encapsulated tumors that may contain thick-walled cystic areas as a result of hemorrhage and necrosis. They have a predilection for the pancreatic tail and have a better prognosis and a tendency for long patient survival because of their local invasion and lack of metastases.[161]

Pancreatic metastasis is not common and usually occurs as direct extensions from adjacent structures, such as the stomach, or contiguous lymphadenopathy. On autopsy, only 3% of all patients with a proven malignancy had metastasis to the pancreas.[162] **Metastasis to the pancreas occurs in 8.4% of patients with lung cancer,[163] 19% of those with breast cancer,[164] and 37.5% of those with malignant melanomas.[165] Pancreas is one of the sites for early or late metastasis from renal cell carcinoma (Fig. 7-54). Pancreatic metastasis[166] is usually hypoechoic and small, so the contour of the pancreas is not always affected. Larger lesions, especially from the ovary and melanoma, may show cystic changes. Single lesions may be mistaken for primary adenocarcinomas and multiple ones for acute pancreatitis, diffuse adenocarcinoma, or lymphoma.[166]

Non-Hodgkin's lymphoma, especially the histiocytic type, tends to involve the extra lymph node organs. This extranodal involvement is usually associated with concomitant intra-abdominal lymphadenopathy. Involvement of the pancreas may be either solitary or diffuse,[167] with multiple discrete nodules (Fig. 7-55A and B) or diffuse involvement (see Fig. 7-55C and D). In some cases, the pancreas is embedded in massive peripancreatic lymphadenopathy, in which case it is not possible to know if the pancreas is involved or merely compressed.

ULTRASOUND-GUIDED PANCREATIC INTERVENTION

Biopsy

A percutaneous biopsy of pancreatic masses is in general performed to differentiate an inflammatory process from pancreatic carcinoma. Although the sensitivity of PFNA biopsy for the diagnosis of pancreatic malignancy (50% to 86%)[168,169] is not as high as for the diagnosis of liver malignancy, its reported specificity is as high as 100%.[168-170] Lower sensitivity results, both percutaneous and at surgery, are due to several factors[170]:

- Presence of necrosis that is not visible on sonograms
- Tendency for the neoplasm to produce significant desmoplastic fibrous reaction, causing a negative biopsy result

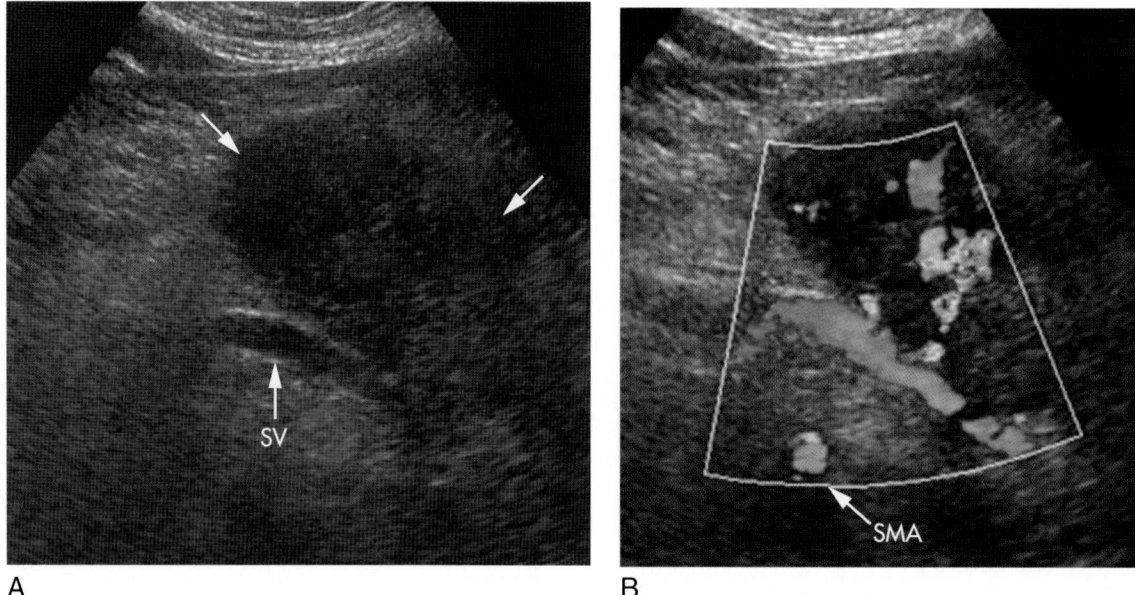

FIGURE 7-54. Renal cell carcinoma. Transverse gray-scale (**A**) and transverse color Doppler (**B**) views show a well-defined hypoechoic vascular mass *(arrows)* in the body of the pancreas. SV, splenic vein; SMA, superior mesenteric artery.

- Associated pancreatitis that may complicate localization of the tumor
- Well-differentiated tumors that can be difficult to diagnose on cytologic examinations

However, more recent reports using larger cutting needles to obtain core biopsy samples have shown better results, with sensitivities of 92% and 94% without increase in complication rate.[171,172] It is most efficacious to obtain biopsy specimens in the region where the pancreatic duct tapers. Endosonographically guided biopsy of pancreatic masses and peripancreatic lymph nodes, when available, can improve accuracy of tissue diagnosis of pancreatic masses and cancer staging.[173-174] A positive biopsy result prevents unnecessary surgery when unresectability is confirmed by prior imaging.

The main complication of PFNA of the pancreas is the induction of pancreatitis, and a few deaths have been reported from fulminant pancreatitis.[175-177] This usually occurs when a normal pancreas has undergone biopsy. There have also been isolated reports of seeding of pancreatic cancer along the path of the biopsy needle.[175,178]

Percutaneous Pancreatography

Although performing percutaneous pancreatography is feasible in a nondilated system (considering the fact that the pancreatic duct is almost always seen under ultrasound guidance), the opacification of a nondilated pancreatic duct should be left to ERCP. In patients with a dilated duct, a plain radiograph is obtained to document calcifications. The pancreatic duct is then punctured under ultrasound guidance using a 22 gauge

needle. A small amount of pancreatic juice is aspirated for cytologic assessment, and water-soluble contrast medium is injected at a low pressure using fluoroscopy.[179] The amount of contrast agent injected varies with visualization of the pancreatic duct or, in cases of occlusion, the amount of pressure needed to opacify the duct and the patient's response to the injection. Excessive injection should be avoided, and the contrast medium should be aspirated at the end of the procedure.[179] A success rate of 89% has been obtained in the largest study series reported.[179] No complications are reported, except for one case of bile leakage as a result of transgression of a dilated intrahepatic bile duct.[179]

Indications for percutaneous pancreatography include:

- Technical difficulty with ERCP, either as a result of failure of the procedure or modified anatomy from previous surgery (e.g., prior gastrectomy, pancreaticojejunostomy, or a Whipple procedure)[179]
- Lack of ERCP visualization of the pancreatic duct in spite of opacification of the common bile duct
- Poor or nonopacification of the proximal pancreatic duct caused by significant narrowing or occlusion of the distal pancreatic duct
- Determination of the presence of stones and creation of a surgical map before pancreatic surgery
- A dilated pancreatic duct but no demonstrable mass on sonographic or CT examinations (a pancreatogram can precisely localize a lesion for biopsy) (Fig. 7-56).

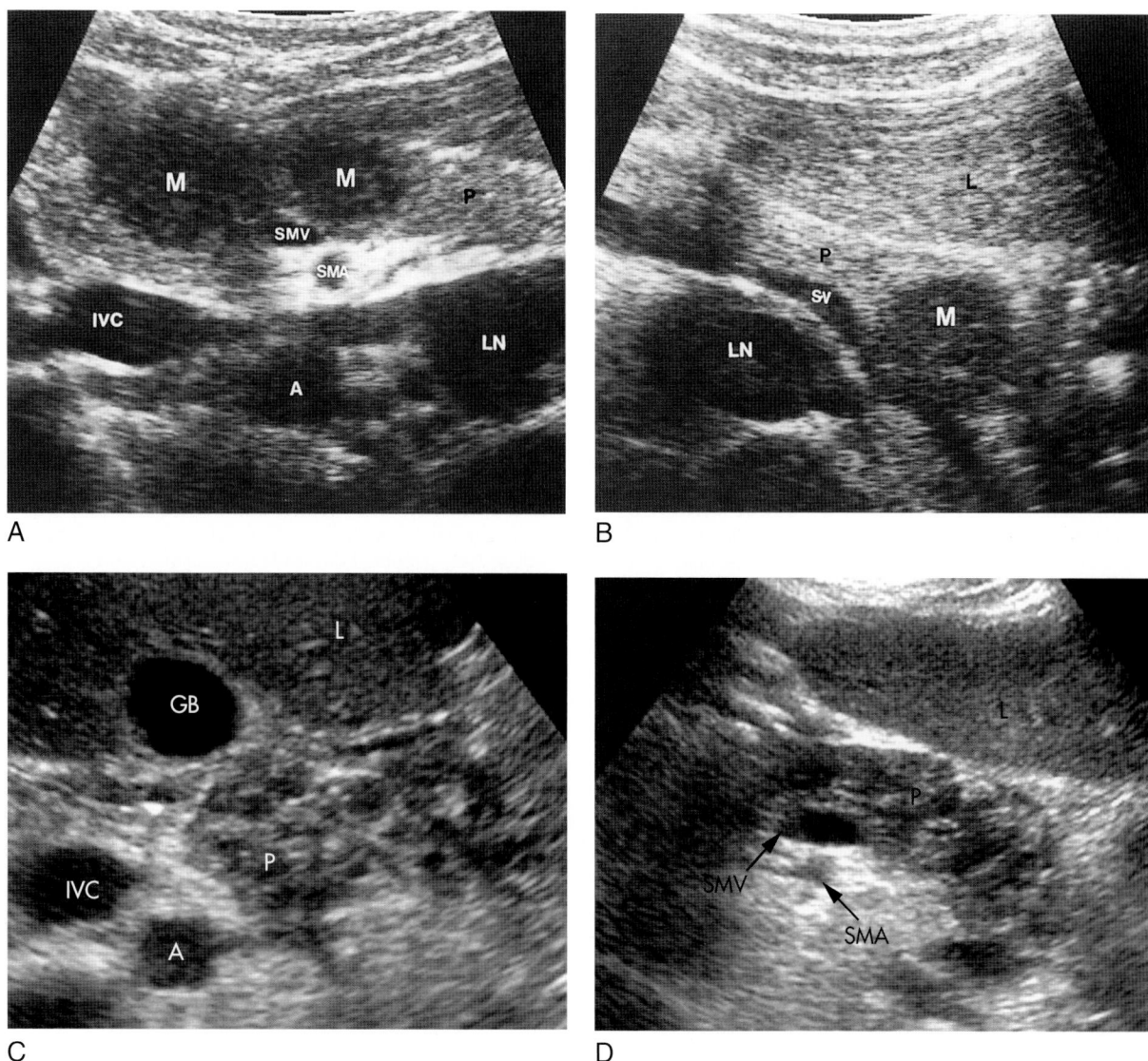

FIGURE 7-55. Non-Hodgkin's lymphoma. A and **B,** Transverse ultrasound of head, body, and tail of pancreas demonstrate multiple well-defined hypoechoic masses (M) throughout pancreas (P). **C,** Transverse view of head of pancreas. **D,** Transverse view of body of pancreas in another patient shows diffuse nodular heterogeneity of pancreas (P). A, aorta; IVC, inferior vena cava; L, liver; LN, lymph node; SMA, superior mesenteric artery; SMV, superior mesenteric vein; SV, splenic vein.

The introduction of magnetic resonance cholangio-pancreatography (MRCP) may obviate the need for percutaneous pancreatography in some cases of failed or inadequate ERCP because it provides noninvasive visualization of the pancreatic duct.[180]

ENDOSCOPIC SONOGRAPHY

EUS is a technique that combines endoscopy with high-resolution sonography. High-resolution sonograms of the pancreas can be obtained because of the proximity to the pancreas provided by the intragastrointestinal position of the endoscopic probe. EUS can overcome factors that limit transabdominal sonography, such as overlying bowel gas, morbid obesity, or the patient's

inability to cooperate with respiratory instructions.[181] As in all forms of sonography, this procedure is highly operator dependent. In addition, it is available in only a few institutions. With increased expertise, the rate of technical failure has decreased from 25% to a level below 5% in the hands of experienced endoscopists.[182] The few remaining failures relate to the inability to pass the endoscope into the third portion of the duodenum in cases where a detailed view of the uncinate and head of pancreas is needed.

Two types of endosonographic scopes are commercially available. The radial type uses a high-frequency (7.5 and 12 MHz) radial scanner capable of producing 360-degree cross-sectional images. This type of scope is useful for surveying the gastrointestinal tract and the surrounding organs. The orientation within the scan

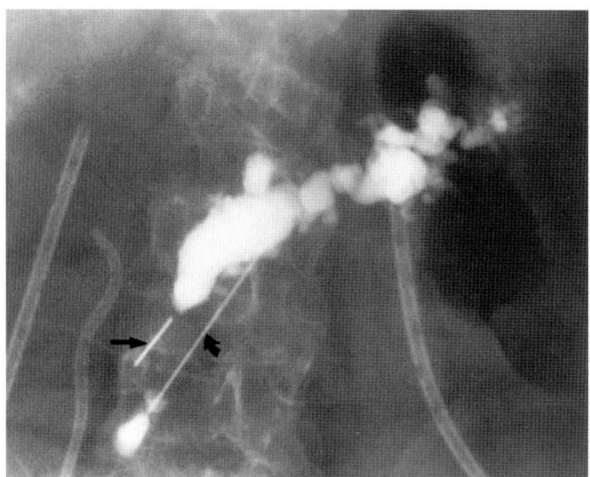

FIGURE 7-56. Percutaneous pancreatogram performed under ultrasound guidance using 22 gauge needle (*curved arrow*). Biopsy of site of occlusion using 22 gauge needle (*straight arrow*) under fluoroscopic guidance.

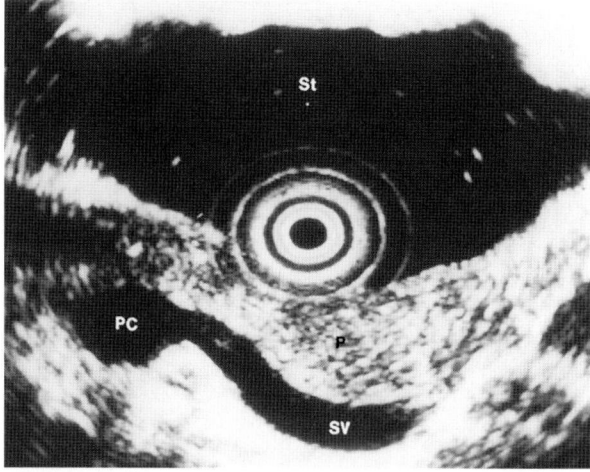

FIGURE 7-57. Transgastric endosonography, body and tail of normal pancreas. P, pancreas; PC, portal confluence; St, stomach; SV, splenic vein. (Courtesy of P. J. Valette, MD, Hôpital Edouard Herriot, Lyon, France.)

plane is relatively straightforward. The commercially available unit does not have color Doppler capability and has relatively limited scanning depth. Biopsy capability is not yet commercially available. The commercially available sector-type scanner employs a lower-frequency (5 and 7.5 MHz) transducer. At this level of transducer frequency, detection of small intrapancreatic lesions is still excellent. Color Doppler and biopsy capabilities are available with the sector units, although endosonographic-guided biopsies have not currently matured as a widely employed technique. The lower transducer frequencies permit deeper tissue penetration, which is useful in identifying deep lesions, such as intrapancreatic endocrine tumors. However, the smaller field of view can make it difficult to maintain scan orientation.

Transverse and coronal oblique views of the pancreatic head can be obtained from the duodenal bulb or the second part of the duodenum. The body and tail of the pancreas can be visualized through the greater curvature of the stomach. High-resolution images of the entire pancreas, as well as the portal venous confluence, the common bile duct, the pancreatic duct, and the superior mesenteric vessels, can be obtained (Fig. 7-57).[183] Two methods of contact are employed to provide adequate interface between the gut wall and the transducer. The first is the balloon method, which is preferred when examining the pancreas and uses a water-filled balloon at the tip of the scope surrounding the transducer. The second is the water-filled stomach method, which consists of placing an uncovered transducer in the stomach filled with 300 to 800 mL of de-aerated water.[184] The complete examination lasts 15 to 30 minutes.[185]

EUS is highly accurate in identifying the presence of a pancreatic abnormality. The sensitivity of EUS in detecting **pancreatic lesions** has been reported to be 98% to 100%. In comparison, the sensitivities of trans-abdominal ultrasound (TA-US), CT scan, and ERCP are 67% to 72%, 71% to 78%, and 88% to 94%, respectively.[182,186,187] EUS is especially useful in detecting pancreatic lesions that are less than 3 cm. In one study, the EUS detection rate was 100% versus 50% for TA-US, 55% for CT, and 90% for ERCP.[187]

Indications for EUS include detection and staging of pancreatic adenocarcinoma (especially tumors <3 cm), evaluation for pancreatic neuroendocrine tumors, assessment of the pancreas in morbidly obese patients, and high-resolution anatomic assessment of the pancreatic head and the ampulla.[181,182] EUS is showing promise in the assessment of patients with abdominal pain who are suspected of having chronic pancreatitis.[188]

EUS appears to be the single most accurate technique in both localizing pancreatic lesions and assessing resectability of a pancreatic malignancy (Fig. 7-58). Accuracies of EUS, TA-US, CT, and MRI for detecting pancreatic cancers are reported to be 91% to 96%, 64% to 88%, 66% to 88%, and 83%, respectively.[189-192] EUS has also been shown to be accurate both in localizing and staging the ampullary tumors and differentiating them from pancreatic cancer (Fig. 7-59).[193,194] The sonographic appearance of pancreatic carcinoma on EUS is similar to that of conventional ultrasound; however, EUS affords better characterization of the mass in regard to tumor margin, shape, echogenicity, and echotexture. Although most pancreatic carcinomas are described as being hypoechoic with irregular margins and mottled echotexture, substantial overlap exists with the features seen in chronic pancreatitis.[182,191] Moreover, examination of a pancreatic mass greater than 5 cm greatly hampers the ability of EUS because of the limited field

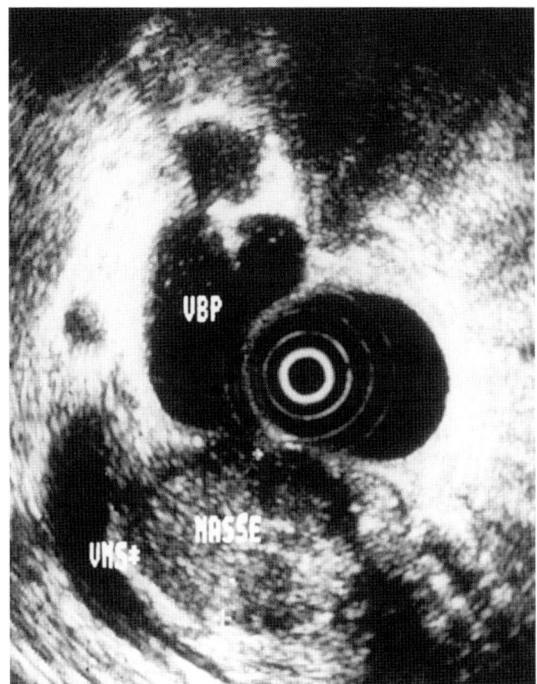

FIGURE 7-58. Transduodenal endosonography of pancreatic carcinoma. MASSE, pancreatic mass; VBP, common bile duct; VMS, superior mesenteric vein. (Courtesy of P. Taourel, MD, Hôpital St. Eloi, Montpellier, France.)

EUS shortcomings include the difficulty in performing EUS-guided needle biopsy with currently available instrumentation and its inability to accurately detect the liver, peritoneal, and omental metastases. At present, there seems to be no substitute for laparoscopy in detecting these metastases when they are small, which is crucial in determining the resectability status for a patient with pancreatic carcinoma.[196]

EUS is an important nonsurgical localization study in patients with insulinomas and gastrinomas. In patients with sporadic insulinomas, EUS provides a detection rate of 80% to 90%.[188] If an insulinoma is identified by EUS, no other study is required. Pancreatic angiography and arterial stimulation study are performed only if EUS is negative in a patient suspected of having sporadic insulinomas. IOUS as a stand-alone diagnostic procedure has disadvantages, such as extended intraoperative time. IOUS is therefore recommended as an image-guidance adjunct to insulinoma enucleation or as a second-line diagnostic modality when all other studies fail.

In patients with hyperinsulinoma secondary to multiple endocrine neoplasia type I syndrome, EUS is used to evaluate only the head and uncinate process because a distal pancreatectomy is performed regardless of other findings. In patients with a clinical diagnosis of Zollinger-Ellison syndrome, EUS can detect virtually all intrapancreatic gastrinomas. Sensitivity of a negative EUS of the pancreas predicting extrapancreatic gastrinoma is 100%.[188] A negative EUS in combination with a negative CT scan in a patient with Zollinger-Ellison syndrome strongly suggests the probability that a small submucosal gastrinoma will be found in the duodenum.

The superior resolution of EUS over TA-US can help to characterize cystic neoplasms. The cystic nature of serous cystadenomas can be better appreciated on EUS by identification of small cysts in an apparent solid mass on TA-US (Fig. 7-60).

of view and acoustic penetration (a function of the high-frequency transducer). In determining resectability of a pancreatic carcinoma, EUS has been found to be particularly useful in evaluating the presence or absence of invasion into the portal, splenic, and superior mesenteric veins, the duodenal wall, or the ampulla.[195] Clinical utility of EUS in determining the presence of lymph node metastasis as well as invasion of the celiac and superior mesenteric arteries is not convincing at this time when compared with other imaging modalities.

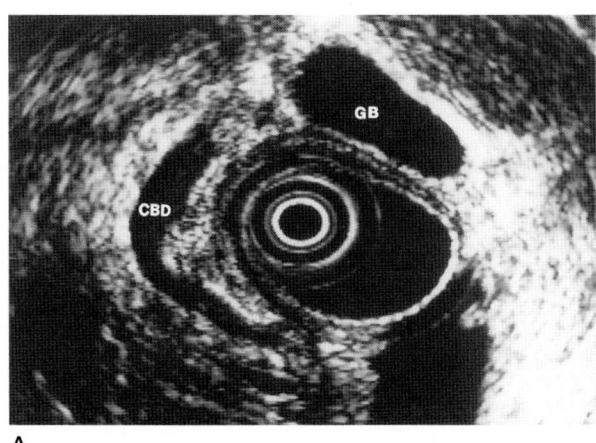

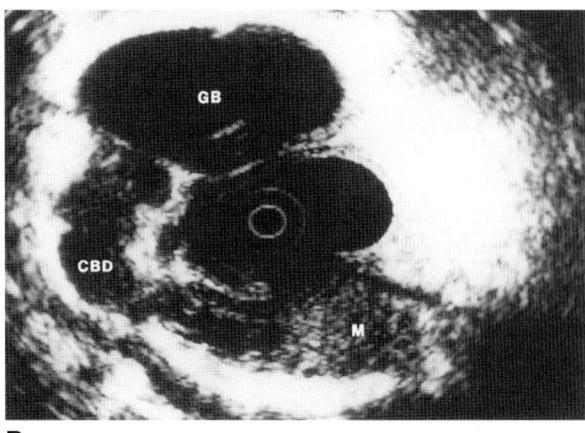

A   B

FIGURE 7-59. Transduodenal endosonography, common bile duct (CBD) and gallbladder (GB). A, Normal common bile duct. **B,** Solid intraluminal mass (M) in distal dilated common bile duct is ampullary carcinoma. Gallbladder is distended (Courtesy of P. J. Valette, MD, Hôpital Edouard Herriot, Lyon, France.)

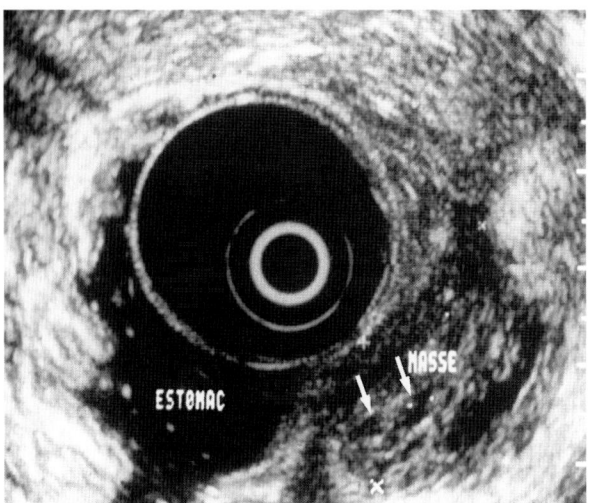

FIGURE 7-60. Transgastric endosonography of solid-appearing pancreatic serous cystadenoma on transabdominal ultrasound examination.
Endoscopic ultrasound shows multiple small cysts *(arrows)* that were not seen by transabdominal ultrasound. Estomac, stomach; Masse, mass. (Courtesy of P. Taourel, M.D., Hôpital St. Eloi, Montpellier, France.)

EUS is sensitive to parenchymal changes associated with chronic pancreatitis. Eight EUS features have been described: (1) inhomogeneous echogenicities; (2) accentuation of parenchymal lobulations; (3) irregular margin of the pancreas; (4) increased thickness or echogenicity of the main pancreatic ductal wall; (5) dilatation of the main pancreatic duct and side branches; (6) echogenic foci within the gland; (7) intraductal calcifications; and (8) pancreatic or peripancreatic cystic structures.[197,198] Specificity and accuracy of EUS in the diagnosis of chronic pancreatitis is reported to be in the range of 80% to 86%.[204] However, no major double-blinded or histologically confirmed study has been published. Therefore, the observed EUS features in patients suspected of having chronic pancreatitis with a normal ERCP result may represent either greater sensitivity of EUS to early chronic pancreatic changes or false-positive results. Nevertheless, in doubtful cases where chronic pancreatitis is clinically suspected but cannot be confirmed by TA-US or CT scan, EUS is recommended (prior to ERCP), because it has been shown to be sensitive to parenchymal changes and also does not carry the risk of procedure-related acute pancreatitis.

EUS is still a developing sonographic modality, although its use outside the university teaching centers is beginning to be accepted. It requires the combined expertise of an endoscopist and a sonologist. EUS-guided biopsy capability is yet to be refined to the level of consistent reliability. Development of the anticipated EUS biopsy guide and needle system would make EUS an even more powerful investigative modality. Finally, high-frequency mini-probes (daughter scopes introduced through the interventional channel of a mother scope) with 20- to 30-MHz scan heads are being developed for examination of the pancreatic duct, which may prove to be useful in the search of an intraductal papillary carcinoma.[172]

Acknowledgment

The author would like to thank Mrs. Carole Leduc for her assistance in the preparation of this chapter.

References

Embryology

1. Clemente CD: The digestive system. In Gray's Anatomy, 30th ed. Philadelphia, Lea & Febiger, 1985, pp 1502-1507.
2. Berman LG, Prior JT, Abramow SM, et al: A study of the pancreatic duct system in man by the use of vinyl acetate casts of postmortem preparations. Surg Gynecol Obstet 1960;110:391-403.

Anatomy

3. Suramo I, Peivensalo M, Myllyle V: Cranio-caudal movements of the liver, pancreas and kidneys in respiration. Acta Radiol 1984;25:129-131.
4. Valenzvela JE: Pancreas. In Gitnick G, Hollander D, Samloff IM (eds): Principles and Practice of Gastroenterology and Hepatology. New York, Elsevier Science, 1988.
5. Newman BM, Lebenthal E: In Vay Liang WG, Gardner JD, Brooks FP, et al (eds): Congenital Anomalies of the Exocrine Pancreas. New York, Raven, 1986.
6. Ross BA, Jeffrey RB Jr, Mindelzun RE: Normal variations in the lateral contour of the head and neck of the pancreas mimicking neoplasm: Evaluation with dual-phase helical CT. AJR Am J Roentgenol 1996;166:799-801.

Pancreatic Sonography

7. Bret PM, Reinhold C, Herba M, et al: Replaced or right accessory hepatic artery: Can ultrasound replace angiography? J Clin Ultrasound 1988;16:245-249.
8. Bryan PJ: Appearance of normal pancreatic duct: A study using real-time ultrasound. J Clin Ultrasound 1982;10:63-66.
9. Hadidi A: Pancreatic duct diameter: Sonographic measurement in normal subjects. J Clin Ultrasound 1983;11:17-22.
10. Didier D, Deschamps JP, Rohmer P, et al: Evaluation of the pancreatic duct: A reappraisal based on a retrospective correlative study by sonography and pancreatography in 117 normal and pathologic subjects. Ultrasound Med Biol 1983;9:509-518.
11. Wachsberg RH: Respiratory variation of the diameter of the pancreatic duct on sonography. AJR Am J Roentgenol 2000;175:1459-1461.
12. So CB, Cooperberg PL, Gibney RG, et al: Sonographic findings in pancreatic lipomatosis. AJR Am J Roentgenol 1987;149:67-68.
13. Patel S, Bellon EM, Haaga J, et al: Fat replacement of the exocrine pancreas. AJR Am J Roentgenol 1980;135:843-845.
14. Nakamura M, Katada N, Sakakibara, et al: Huge lipomatous pseudohypertrophy of the pancreas. Am J Gastroenterol 1979;72:171-174.

15. de Graaff CS, Taylor KJW, Simonds BD, et al: Gray-scale echography of the pancreas: Re-evaluation of normal size. Radiology 1978;129:157-161.

16. Niederau C, Sonnenberg A, Muller JE, et al: Sonographic measurements of the normal liver, spleen, pancreas, and portal vein. Radiology 1983;149:537-540.

17. Bolondi L, Bassi SL, Gaiani S: Sonography of chronic pancreatitis. Radiol Clin North Am 1989;27:815-833.

18. Donald JJ, Shorvon PJ, Lees WR: A hypoechoic area within the head of the pancreas: A normal variant. Clin Radiol 1990;41:337-338.

19. Marchal G, Verbeken E, Van Steenbergen W, et al: Uneven lipomatosis: A pitfall in pancreatic sonography. Gastrointest Radiol 1989;14:233-237.

20. Atri M, Nazarnia S, Mehio A, et al: Hypoechogenic embryologic ventral aspect of the head and uncinate process of the pancreas: *In vitro* correlation of US with histopathologic findings. Radiology 1994;190:441-444.

21. Wachsberg RH: Posterior superior pancreaticoduodenal vein: Mimic of distal common bile duct at sonography. AJR Am J Roentgenol 1993;160:1033-1037.

22. Tszekessy D, Pochhammer KF: Diurnal sonographic imaging of the pancreas. Ultraschall Med 1985; 6:134-136.

23. Muradali D, Wilson SR, Hope-Simpson D, et al: Oral contrast agents for sonography: Improved visualization of the abdomen and gut. Radiol Soc North Am 1995;197:611.

24. Op den Orth JO: Tubeless hypotonic duodenography with water: A simple aid in sonography of the pancreatic head. Radiology 1985;154:826.

25. duCret RP, Jackson VP, Rees C, et al: Pancreatic sonography: Enhancement by metoclopramide. AJR Am J Roentgenol 1986;146:341-343.

26. Abu-Yousef MM, El-Zein Y: Improved US visualization of the pancreatic tail with simethicone, water, and patient rotation. Radiology 2000;217:780-785.

27. Rauch RF, Bowie JD, Rosenberg ER, et al: Can ultrasonic examination of the pancreas and gallbladder follow a barium UGI series on the same day? Invest Radiol 1983;18:523-525.

Congenital Anomalies

28. Gold RP: Agenesis and pseudo-agenesis of the dorsal pancreas. Abd Imaging 1993;18:141-144.

29. Cotran RC, Kumar V, Robbins SL: The Pancreas: Robins' Pathologic Basis of Disease, 4th ed. Philadelphia, WB Saunders, 1989.

30. Mares AJ, Hirsch M: Congenital cysts of the head of the pancreas. J Pediatr Surg 1977;12:547-552.

31. Oppenheimer EH, Esterly JR: Pathology of cystic fibrosis review of the literature and comparison with 146 autopsied cases. Perspect Pediatr Pathol 1975;2:241-278.

32. Swobodnik W, Wolf A, Wechsler JG, et al: Ultrasound characteristics of the pancreas in children with cystic fibrosis. J Clin Ultrasound 1985;13:469-474.

33. Dobson RL, Johnson MA, Henning RC, et al: Sonography of the gallbladder, biliary tree, and pancreas in adults with cystic fibrosis. Can Assoc Radiol J 1988;39:257-259.

34. Daneman A, Gaskin K, Martin DJ, et al: Pancreatic changes in cystic fibrosis: Computed tomography and sonographic appearances. AJR Am J Roentgenol 1983;141:653-655.

35. Graham N, Manhire AR, Stead RJ, et al: Cystic fibrosis: Sonographic findings in the pancreas and hepatobiliary system correlated with clinical data and pathology. Clin Radiol 1985;36:199-203.

36. Hernanz-Schulman M, Teele RL, Perez-Atayde A, et al: Pancreatic cytosis in cystic fibrosis. Radiology 1986;158:629-631.

37. Cooperman M, Ferrara JJ, Fromkes JJ, et al: Surgical management of pancreas divisum. Am J Surg 1982;143:107-112.

38. Cotton PB: Congenital anomaly of pancreas divisum as cause of obstructive pain and pancreatitis. Gut 1980;21:105-114.

39. Brinberg DE, Carr MF Jr, Premkumar A, et al: Isolated ventral pancreatitis in an alcoholic with pancreas divisum. Gastrointest Radiol 1988;13:323-326.

40. Jennings CM, Gaines PA: The abdominal manifestation of von Hippel-Lindau disease and a radiological screening protocol for an affected family. Clin Radiol 1988; 39:363-367.

41. Levine E, Collins DL, Horton WA, et al: Computed tomography screening of the abdomen in von Hippel-Lindau disease. AJR Am J Roentgenol 1982;139:505-510.

Inflammatory Processes

42. Ranson JHC, Rifkind KM, Turner JW: Prognostic signs and nonoperative peritoneal lavage in acute pancreatitis. Surg Gynecol Obstet 1976;143:209-219.

43. Knaus W, Draper E, Wagner D, et al: APACHE II: A severity of disease classification system. Crit Care Med 1985;13:818-829.

44. Jeffrey RB, Laing FC, Wing VW: Ultrasound in acute pancreatic trauma. Gastrointest Radiol 1986;11:44-48.

45. Jeffrey RB Jr, Federle MP, Crass RA: Computed tomography of pancreatic trauma. Radiology 1983;147:491-494.

46. Balthazar EJ, Robinson DL, Megibow AJ, et al: Acute pancreatitis: Value of CT in establishing prognosis. Radiology 1990;174:331-336.

47. Gyr KE, Singer MV, Sarles H: Pancreatitis: Concepts and Classification. International Congress Series 1985, p 642.

48. Delhaye M, Engelholm L, Cremer M: Pancreas divisum: Congenital anatomic variant or anomaly? Contribution of endoscopic retrograde dorsal pancreatography. Gastroenterology 1985;89:951-958.

49. Goekas MC: Etiology and pathogenesis of acute pancreatic inflammation: Acute pancreatitis. Ann Intern Med 1985;103:86-100.

50. Freeny PC: Classification of pancreatitis. Radiol Clin North Am 1989;27:1-3.

51. Jeffrey RB, Laing FC, Wing VW: Extrapancreatic spread of acute pancreatitis: New observations with real-time ultrasound. Radiology 1986;159:707-711.

52. Neff CC, Simeone JF, Wittenberg J, et al: Inflammatory pancreatic masses: Problems in differentiating focal pancreatitis from carcinoma. Radiology 1984;150:35-40.

53. Zuccaro G Jr, Sivak MV Jr: Endoscopic sonography in the diagnosis of chronic pancreatitis. Endoscopy 1992; 24:347-349.

54. Nattermann D, Goldschmidt AJ, Dancygier H: Endosonography in chronic pancreatitis—a comparison between ERCP and EUS. Endoscopy 1993;25:565-570.

55. Price J, Leung JWC: Ultrasound diagnosis of *Ascaris lumbricoides* in the pancreatic duct: The "four-lines" sign. Br J Radiol 1988;61:411-413.

56. Warshaw AL: Inflammatory masses following acute pancreatitis. Surg Clin North Am 1974;54:621-636.

57. Lane MJ, Mindelzun RE, Sandhu JS, et al: CT diagnosis of blunt pancreatic trauma: Importance of detecting fluid between the pancreas and the splenic vein. AJR Am J Roentgenol 1994;163:833.

58. Bradley EL III, Clements JL Jr, Gonzalez AC: The natural history of pancreatic pseudocysts: A unified concept of management. Am J Surg 1979;137:135-141.

59. Donovan PJ, Sanders RC, Siegelman SS: Collections of fluid after pancreatitis: Evaluation of computed tomography and sonography. Radiol Clin North Am 1982;20:653-665.

60. Nyberg DA, Laing F: Sonographic findings in peptic ulcer disease and pancreatitis that simulate primary gallbladder disease. J Ultrasound Med 1983;2:303-307.

61. Lee CM, Chang-Chien CS, Lim DY, et al: Real-time sonography of pancreatic pseudocyst: Comparison of infected and uninfected pseudocysts. J Clin Ultrasound 1988;16:393-397.

62. Bradley EL III: Pancreatic pseudocyst. In Bradley EL III (ed): Complications of Pancreatitis: Medical and Surgical. Philadelphia, WB Saunders, 1982.

63. Rattner DW, Warshaw AL: Surgical intervention in acute pancreatitis. Crit Care Med 1988;16:85-95.

64. Laing FC, Gooding GAW, Brown T, et al: Atypical pseudocysts of the pancreas: An ultrasonographic evaluation. J Clin Ultrasound 1979;7:27-33.

65. Maier W, Roscher R, Malfertheinar P, et al: Pancreatic pseudocyst of the mediastinum: Evaluation by computed tomography. Eur J Radiol 1986;6:70-72.

66. Lye DJ, Stark RH, Cullen GM, et al: Ruptured pancreatic pseudocysts: Extension into the thigh. AJR Am J Roentgenol 1987;49:937-938.

67. Grace RR, Jordan PH Jr: Unresolved problems of pancreatic pseudocysts. Ann Surg 1976;184:16-21.

68. Rheingold OJ, Wilbar JA, Barkin JS: Gastric outlet obstruction due to pancreatic pseudocyst: A report of two cases. Am J Gastroenterol 1978;69:92-96.

69. Bellon EM, George CR, Schreiber H, et al: Pancreatic pseudocysts of the duodenum. AJR Am J Roentgenol 1979;133:827-831.

70. Vick CW, Simeone JF, Ferrucci JT, et al: Pancreatitis associated fluid collection involving the spleen: Sonographic and computed tomographic appearance. Gastrointest Radiol 1981;6:247-250.

71. Stanley JL, Frey CF, Miller TA, et al: Major arterial hemorrhage: A complication of pancreatic pseudocyst and chronic pancreatitis. Arch Surg 1976;111:435-440.

72. Frey CF, Lindenaver SM, Miller TA: Pancreatic abscess. Surg Gynecol Obstet 1979;149:722-726.

73. White AF, Barum S, Buranasiri S: Aneurysms secondary to pancreatitis. AJR Am J Roentgenol 1976;127:393-396.

74. Falkoff GE, Taylor KJW, Morse SS: Hepatic artery pseudoaneurysm: Diagnosis with real-time and pulsed Doppler ultrasound. Radiology 1986;58:55-56.

75. Crass RA, Way LW: Acute and chronic pancreatic pseudocysts are different. Am J Surg 1981;142:660-663.

76. Sarti DA: Rapid development and spontaneous regression of pancreatic pseudocysts documented by ultrasound. Radiology 1977;125:789-793.

77. van Sonnenberg E, Wittich GR, Casola G, et al: Percutaneous drainage of infected and noninfected pancreatic pseudocysts: Experience in 101 cases. Radiology 1989;170:757-761.

78. Matzinger FRK, Ho CS, Yee AC, et al: Pancreatic pseudocysts drained through a percutaneous transgastric approach: Further experience. Radiology 1988; 167:431-434.

79. D'Agostino HB, vanSonnenberg E, Sanchez RB, et al: Treatment of pancreatic pseudocyst with percutaneous drainage and octreotide: Work in progress. Radiology 1993;187:685-688.

80. Cremer M: Endoscopic cystoduodenostomy. Endoscopy 1981;2:29-30.

81. Beger HG, Bittner R, Block S, et al: Bacterial contamination of pancreatic necrosis: A prospective clinical study. Gastroenterology 1986;91:433-438.

82. Doglietto GB, Gui D, Pacelli F, et al: Open vs. closed treatment of secondary pancreatic infection: Review of 42 cases. Arch Surg 1994;129:689-693.

83. van Sonnenberg E, Wittich GR, Casola G, et al: Complicated pancreatic inflammatory disease: Diagnostic and therapeutic role of interventional radiology. Radiology 1985;155:340-355.

84. Banks PA: Clinical manifestations and treatment of pancreatitis. Ann Intern Med 1985;103:91-95.

85. Seiler JG, Polk HC: Factors contributing to fatal outcome after treatment of pancreatic abscess. Ann Surg 986;203:605-612.

86. Ranson JHC, Spencer FC: Prevention, diagnosis and treatment of pancreatic abscess. Surgery 1977; 82:99-105.

87. Federle MP, Jeffrey RB, Crass RA, et al: Computed tomography of pancreatic abscess. AJR Am J Roentgenol 1981;136:879-882.

88. Vernacchia FS, Jeffrey RB Jr, Federle MP, et al: Pancreatic abscess: Predictive value of early abdominal computed tomography. Radiology 1987;162:435-438.

89. Fishman EK, Soyer P, Bliss DF, et al: Splenic involvement in pancreatitis: Spectrum of CT findings. AJR Am J Roentgenol 1995;164:631-635.

90. Kahn LA, Kamen C, McNamara MP Jr: Variable color Doppler appearance of pseudoaneurysm in pancreatitis. AJR Am J Roentgenol 1994;162:187-188.

91. Sankaran S, Walt A: Pancreatic ascites: Recognition and management. Arch Surg 1976;430-434.

92. Belfar HL, Radecki PD, Friedman AC, et al: Pancreatitis presenting as pleural effusions: Computed tomography demonstration of pleural extension of pancreatic exudate. Comput Tomogr 1987;11:184-186.

93. Howard JM, Nedurich A: Correlation of the histologic observations and operative findings in patients with chronic pancreatitis. Surg Gynecol Obstet 1971; 132:387-395.

94. Alpern MB, Sandler MA, Kellman GM, et al: Chronic pancreatitis: Ultrasonic features. Radiology 1985; 155:215-219.

95. Ferrucci J Jr, Wittenberg J, Black EB, et al: Computed body tomography in chronic pancreatitis. Radiology 1979;130:175-182.

96. Fishman EK, Siegelman SS: Pancreatitis and its complications. In Tavares JM, Ferrucci JT (eds): Radiology: Diagnosis, Imaging, Intervention. Philadelphia, JB Lippincott, 1986.

97. Weinstein BJ, Weinstein DP, Brodmeckel GJ Jr: Ultrasonography of pancreatic lithiasis. Radiology 134:185-189, 1980.

98. Lankish PG, Otto J, Erkelenz I, et al: Pancreatic calcifications: No indicator of severe exocrine pancreatic insufficiency. Gastroenterology 1986;90:617-621.

99. Ammann RW, Meunch R, Otto R, et al: Evolution and regression of pancreatic calcification in chronic pancreatitis. Gastroenterology 1988;95:1018-1028.

100. Rosch N, Lux G, Rieman JF, et al: Chronic pancreatitis and the neighboring organs. Fortschr Med 1981; 99:1118-1125.

101. Malfertheiner P, Buchler M: Correlation of imaging and function in chronic pancreatitis. Radiol Clin North Am 1989;27:51-64.

102. Ason ATA: Endoscopic retrograde cholangiopancreatography in chronic pancreatitis: Cambridge classification. Radiol Clin North Am 1989;27:39-50.

103. Jones SN, Lees WR, Frost RA: Diagnosis and grading of chronic pancreatitis by morphological criteria derived by ultrasound and pancreatography. Clin Radiol 1988; 39:43-48.

Neoplasms

104. Kissane JM: Anderson's Pathology, 9th ed. St Louis, Mosby–Year Book, 1990.

105. Weinstein DP, Weinstein BJ: Pancreas. In Goldberg BB (ed): Clinics in Diagnostic Ultrasound: Ultrasound in Cancer. New York, Churchill Livingstone, 1981.

106. Kaplan JO, Isikoff MB, Barkin J, et al: Necrotic carcinoma of the pancreas. "The pseudo-pseudocyst." J Comput Assist Tomogr 1980;4:166-167.

107. Walls WJ, Templeton AW: The ultrasonic demonstration of inferior vena caval compression: A guide to pancreatic head enlargement with emphasis on neoplasm. Radiology 1977;123:165-167.

108. Taylor KJW, Ramos I, Carter D: Correlation of Doppler US tumor signals with neovascular morphologic features. Radiology 1988;166:57-62.

109. Mori H, McGrath FP, Malone DE, et al: The gastrocolic trunk and its tributaries: CT evaluation. Radiology 1992;182:871-877.

110. Campbell JP, Wilson S: Pancreatic neoplasms: How useful is evaluation with ultrasound? Radiology 1988;167:341-344.

111. Kaneko T, Kimata H, Sugimoto H, et al: Power Doppler ultrasonography for the assessment of vascular invasion by pancreatic cancer. Pancreatology 2002;2:61-68.

112. Peivensalo M, Lehde S: Sonography and computed tomography in pancreatic malignancy. Acta Radiol 1988;29:343-344.

113. Kamin PD, Bernardino ME, Wallace S, et al: Comparison of ultrasound and computed tomography in the detection of pancreatic malignancy. Cancer 1980;46:2410-2412.

114. Bluemke DA, Cameron JL, Hruban RH, et al: Potentially resectable pancreatic adenocarcinoma: Spiral CT assessment with surgical and pathologic correlation. Radiology 1995;197:381-385.

115. McMahon PM, Halpern EF, Fernandez-del Castillo C, et al: Pancreatic cancer: Cost-effectiveness of imaging technologies for assessing resectability. Radiology 2001;221:93-106.

116. Hildell J, Aspelin P, Wehlin L: Grayscale ultrasound and endoscopic ductography in the diagnosis of pancreatic disease. Acta Chir Scand 1979;145:239-245.

117. Cubilla AL, Fitzgerald PJ: Surgical pathology aspects of cancer of the ampulla-head-of-pancreas region. Monogr Pathol 1980;21:67-81.

118. Robledo R, Prieto ML, Perez M, et al: Carcinoma of the hepaticopancreatic ampullar region: role of ultrasound. Radiology 1988;166:409-412.

119. Compagno J, Oertel JE: Microcystic adenomas of the pancreas (glycogen-rich cystadenomas): A clinicopathologic study of 34 cases. Am J Clin Pathol 1978;69:289-298.

120. Compagno J, Oertel JE: Mucinous cystic neoplasms of the pancreas with overt and latent malignancy (cystadenocarcinoma and cystadenoma): A clinicopathologic study of 41 cases. Am J Clin Pathol 1978;69:573-580.

121. Friedman AC, Lichtenstein JE, Dachman AH: Cystic neoplasms of the pancreas: Radiological-pathological correlation. Radiology 1983;149:45-50.

122. Johnson CD, Stephens DH, Charboneau JW, et al: Cystic pancreatic tumors: Computed tomography and sonographic assessment. AJR Am J Roentgenol 1988;151:1133-1138.

123. Bastid C, Sahel J, Sastre B, et al: Mucinous cystadenocarcinoma of the pancreas: Sonographic findings in 5 cases. Acta Radiol 1989;30:45-47.

124. Busilacchi P, Rizzatto G, Bazzocchi M, et al: Pancreatic cystadenocarcinoma: Diagnostic problems. Br J Radiol 1982;55:558-561.

125. Brugge WR: Role of endoscopic ultrasound in the diagnosis of cystic lesions of the pancreas. Pancreatology 2001;1:637-640.

126. Yeh HC, Stancato-Pasik A, Shapiro RS: Microcystic features at US: A nonspecific sign for microcystic adenomas of the pancreas. Radiographics 2001; 21:1455-1461.

127. Solcia E, Capella C, Klöppel G: Tumors of the pancreas. In Atlas of tumor Pathology, fascicle 20, series 3. Washington, DC, Armed Forces Institute of Pathology, 1997, pp 53-64.

128. Procacci C, Megibow AJ, Carbognin G, et al: Intraductal papillary mucinous tumor of the pancreas: A pictorial essay. Radiographics 1999;19:1447-1463.

129. Barbe L, Ponsot P, Vilgrain V, et al: Intraductal papillary mucinous tumors of the pancreas: Clinical and morphological aspects in 30 patients. (French). Gastroenterol Clin Biol 1997;21:278-286.

130. Yamao K, Ohashi K, Nakamura T, et al: Evaluation of various imaging methods in the differential diagnosis of intraductal papillary-mucinous tumor (IPMT) of the pancreas. Hepatogastroenterology 2001;48:962-966.

131. Wakabayashi T, Kawaura Y, Morimoto H, et al: Clinical management of intraductal papillary mucinous tumors of the pancreas based on imaging findings. Pancreas 2001;22:370-377.

132. Ros PR, Hamrick-Turner JE, Chiechi MV, et al: Cystic masses of pancreas. Radiographics 1992;12:673-686.

133. Herrera L, Glassman CI, Komins JI: Mucinous cystic neoplasm of the pancreas demonstrated by ultrasound and endoscopic retrograde pancreatography. Am J Gastroenterol 1980;73:512-515.

134. Markle BM, Friedman AC, Sachs L: Anomalies and congenital disorders. In Friedman AC (ed): Radiology of the Liver, Biliary Tree, Pancreas, and Spleen. Baltimore, Williams & Wilkins, 1987.

135. Lewandrowski K, Lee J, Southern J, et al: Cyst fluid analysis in the differential diagnosis of pancreatic cysts: A new approach to the preoperative assessment of pancreatic cystic lesions. AJR Am J Roentgenol 1995;164:815-819.

136. Hammel P, Levy P, Voitot H, et al: Preoperative cyst fluid analysis is useful for the differential diagnosis of cystic lesions of the pancreas. Gastroenterology 1995; 108:1230-1235.

137. Laucirica R, Schwartz MR, Ramzy I: Fine needle aspiration of pancreatic cystic epithelial neoplasms. Acta Cytol 1992;36:881-886.

138. Jorda M, Essenfeld H, Garcia E, et al: The value of fine-needle aspiration cytology in the diagnosis of inflammatory pancreatic masses. Diagn Cytopathol 1992;8:65-67.

139. Friesen SR: Tumors of the endocrine pancreas. N Engl J Med 1982;306:580-590.

140. Toledo-Pereyra LH: The Pancreas: Principles of Medical and Surgical Practice. New York, Wiley Medical, 1985.

141. van Heerden JA, Edis AJ, Service FJ: The surgical aspects of insulinomas. Ann Surg 1979;189:677-682.

142. Grant CS, van Heerden J, Charboneau JW, et al: Insulinoma: The value of intraoperative sonography. Arch Surg 1988;123:843-848.

143. Rossi P, Allison DJ, Bezzi M, et al: Endocrine tumors of the pancreas. Radiol Clin North Am 1989;27:129-161.

144. Jensen RT, Gardner JD, Raufman JP, et al: Zollinger-Ellison syndrome: Current concepts and management. Ann Intern Med 1983;98:59-75.

145. Stadil F: Gastrinomas: Clinical syndromes. Acta Oncol 1989;28:379-381.

146. Galiber AK, Reading CC, Charboneau JW, et al: Localization of pancreatic insulinoma: Comparison of pre- and intraoperative ultrasound with computed tomography and angiography. Radiology 1988;166:405-408.

147. Gorman B, Charboneau JW, James EM, et al: Benign pancreatic insulinoma: Preoperative and intraoperative sonographic localization. AJR Am J Roentgenol 1986;147:929-934.

148. Kuhn FP, Gunther R, Ruckert K, et al: Ultrasonic demonstration of small pancreatic islet cell tumors. J Clin Ultrasound 1982;10:173-175.

149. Norton JA, Cromack DT, Shawker TH: Intraoperative sonographic localization of islet cell tumors. Ann Surg 1988;207:160-168.

150. Katz LB, Aufses AH, Rayfield E, et al: Preoperative localization and intraoperative glucose monitoring in the management of patients with pancreatic insulinoma. Surg Gynecol Obstet 1986;163:509-512.

151. Rossi P, Baert A, Passariello R, et al: Computed tomography of functioning tumors of the pancreas. AJR Am J Roentgenol 1985;144:57-60.

152. Montenegro-Rodas F, Samaan NA: Glucagonoma tumors and syndrome. Curr Prob Cancer 1981;6:1-54.

153. Roche A, Raisonnier A, Gillon-Savouret MC: Pancreatic venous sampling and arteriography in localizing insulinomas and gastrinomas: Procedure and results in 55 cases. Radiology 1982;145:621-627.

154. Tjon A, Tham RT, Jansen JB, et al: Magnetic resonance, computed tomography, and ultrasound findings of metastatic vipoma in pancreas. J Comput Assist Tomogr 1989;13:142-144.

155. Van Hoe L, Gryspeerdt S, Marchal G, et al: Helical CT for the preoperative localization of islet cell tumors of the pancreas: Value of arterial and parenchymal phase images. AJR Am J Roentgenol 1995;165:1437-1439.

156. Moore NR, Rogers CE, Britton BJ: Magnetic resonance imaging of endocrine tumours of the pancreas. Br J Radiol 1995;68:341-347.

157. Aspestrand F, Kolmannskog F, Jacobsen M: CT, MR imaging and angiography in pancreatic apudomas. Acta Radiol 1993;34:468-473.

158. Semelka RC, Cumming MJ, Shoenut JP, et al: Islet cell tumors: Comparison of dynamic contrast-enhanced CT and MR imaging with dynamic gadolinium enhancement and fat suppression. Radiology 1993;186:799-802.

159. Hiramoto JS, Feldstein VA, LaBerge J, et al: Intraoperative ultrasound and preoperative localization detects all occult insulinomas. Arch Surg 2001;136:1020-1025.

160. Rice NT, Woodring JH, Mostowycz L, et al: Pancreatic plasmacytoma: Sonographic and computerized tomographic findings. J Clin Ultrasound 1981; 9:46-48.

161. Lin JT, Wang TH, Wei TC, et al: Sonographic features of solid papillary neoplasm of the pancreas. J Clin Ultrasound 1985;13:339-342.

162. Willis RA: The Spread of Tumors in the Human Body. New York, Butterworths, 1975.

163. Budinger JM: Untreated bronchogenic carcinoma: A clinicopathological study of 250 autopsied cases. Cancer 1958;11:106-116.

164. de la Monte SM, Hutchins GM, Moore GW: Endocrine organ metastases from breast carcinoma. Am J Pathol 1984;114:131-136.

165. Patel JK, Didolkar MS, Pickren JW, et al: Metastatic pattern of malignant melanoma: A study of 216 autopsy cases. Am J Surg 1978;135:807-810.

166. Wernecke K, Peters PE, Galanski M: Pancreatic metastases: Ultrasound evaluation. Radiology 1986;160:339-402.

167. Glazer HS, Lee JKT, Balfe DM, et al: Non-Hodgkin lymphoma: Computed tomographic demonstration of unusual extranodal involvement. Radiology 1983; 149:211-217.

Ultrasound-Guided Pancreatic Intervention

168. Pilotti S, Rilke F, Claren R, et al: Conclusive diagnosis of hepatic and pancreatic malignancies by fine needle aspiration. Acta Cytol 1988;32:27-38.

169. Ekberg O, Bergenfeldt M, Aspelin P, et al: Reliability of ultrasound-guided fine-needle biopsy of pancreatic masses. Acta Radiol 1988;29:535-539.

170. Yamamoto R, Tatsuta M, Noguchi S, et al: Histocytologic diagnosis of pancreatic cancer by percutaneous aspiration biopsy under ultrasonic guidance. Am J Clin Pathol 1985;83:409-414.

171. Brandt KR, Charboneau JW, Stephens DH, et al: CT- and US-guided biopsy of the pancreas. Radiology 1993; 187:99-104.

172. Elvin A, Andersson T, Scheibenpflug L, et al: Biopsy of the pancreas with a biopsy gun. Radiology 1990;176:677-679.

173. Mallery JS, Centeno BA, Hahn PF, et al: Pancreatic tissue sampling guided by EUS, CT/US, and surgery: A comparison of sensitivity and specificity. Gastrointest Endosc 2002;56:218-224.

174. Shin HJ, Lahoti S, Sneige N: Endoscopic ultrasound-guided fine-needle aspiration in 179 cases: The M. D. Anderson Cancer Center experience. Cancer 2002;96:174-180.

175. Hancke S, Holm HH, Koch F: Ultrasonically guided puncture of solid pancreatic mass lesions. Ultrasound Med Biol 1984;10:613-615.

176. Evans WK, Ho CS, McLoughlin MJ, et al: Fatal necrotizing pancreatitis following fine-needle aspiration biopsy of the pancreas. Radiology 1981;141:61-62.

177. Levin DP, Bret PM: Percutaneous fine-needle aspiration biopsy of the pancreas resulting in death. Gastrointest Radiol 1991;16:67-69.

178. Caturelli E, Rapacci GL, Anti M, et al: Malignant seeding after fine-needle aspiration biopsy of the pancreas. Diagn Imaging Clin Med 1985;54:88-91.

179. Matter D, Bret PM, Bretagnolle M, et al: Pancreatic duct: Ultrasound guided percutaneous opacification. Radiology 1987;163:635-636.

180. Soto JA, Barish MA, Yucel EK, et al: MR cholangio-pancreatography with a three-dimensional fast spin-echo technique. Radiology 1995;196:459-464.

Endoscopic Sonography

181. Kaplan DS, Heisig DG, Roy AK, et al: Endoscopic ultrasound in the morbidly obese patient: A new indication. Am J Gastroenterol 1993;88:593-594.

182. Kelsey PJ, Warshaw AL: EUS: An added test or a replacement for several? Endoscopy 1993;25:179-181.

183. Zerbey AL, Lee MJ, Brugge WR, et al: Endoscopic sonography of the upper gastrointestinal tract and pancreas. AJR Am J Roentgenol 1996;166:45-50.

184. Boyce GA, Sivak MV Jr: Endoscopic sonography in the diagnosis of pancreatic tumors. Gastrointest Endosc 1990;36:S28-S32.

185. Kaufman AR, Sivak MV Jr: Endoscopic sonography in the differential diagnosis of pancreatic disease. Gastrointest Endosc 1989;35:214-219.

186. Rosch T, Lorenz R, Braig C, et al: Endoscopic ultrasound in pancreatic tumor diagnosis. Gastrointest Endosc 1991;37:347-352.

187. Snady H, Cooperman A, Siegel J: Endoscopic sonography compared with computed tomography and ERCP in patients with obstructive jaundice or small peripancreatic mass. Gastrointest Endosc 1992;38:27-34.

188. Thompson NW, Czako PF, Fritts LL, et al: Role of endoscopic sonography in the localization of insulinomas and gastrinomas. Surgery 1994;116:1131-1138.

189. Palazzo L, Roseau G, Gayet B, et al: Endoscopic sonography in the diagnosis and staging of pancreatic adenocarcinoma: Results of a prospective study with comparison to sonography and CT scan. Endoscopy 1993;25:143-150.

190. Nakaizumi A, Uehara H, Iishi H, et al: Endoscopic sonography in diagnosis and staging of pancreatic cancer. Digest Dis Sci 1995;40:696-700.

191. Yasuda K, Mukai H, Fujimoto S, et al: The diagnosis of pancreatic cancer by endoscopic sonography. Gastrointest Endosc 1988;34:1-8.

192. Ahmad NA, Lewis JD, Ginsberg GG, et al: EUS in preoperative staging of pancreatic cancer. Gastrointest Endosc 2000;52:463-468.

193. Tio TL, Tytgat GN, Cikot RJ, et al: Ampullopancreatic carcinoma: Preoperative TNM classification with endosonography. Radiology 1990;175:455-461.

194. Tomazic A, Pegan V: Preoperative staging of periampullar cancer with US, CT, EUS and CA 19-9. Hepatogastroenterology 2000;47:1135-1137.

195. Snady H, Bruckner H, Siegel J, et al: Endoscopic sonographic criteria of vascular invasion by potentially resectable pancreatic tumors. Gastrointest Endosc 1994;40:326-333.

196. Cuesta MA, Meijer S, Borgstein PJ, et al: Laparoscopic sonography for hepatobiliary and pancreatic malignancy. Br J Surg 1993;12:1571-1574.

197. Wiersema MJ, Hawes RH, Lehman GA, et al: Prospective evaluation of endoscopic sonography and endoscopic retrograde cholangiopancreatography in patients with chronic abdominal pain of suspected pancreatic origin. Endoscopy 1993;25:555-564.

198. Rosch T: Endoscopic sonography-more questions than answers? Endoscopy 1993;25:600-602.

8

THE GASTROINTESTINAL TRACT

Stephanie R. Wilson

Chapter Outline

BASIC PRINCIPLES

Gastrointestinal tract sonography is frequently frustrating and always challenging. Gas content within the gut lumen can make visibility difficult and even impossible, intraluminal fluid may mimic cystic masses, and fecal material may create a variety of artifacts and pseudo-tumors. Nevertheless, normal gut has a reproducible pattern or **gut signature,** and a variety of gut pathologies create recognizable sonographic abnormalities. In addition, in a few conditions—such as acute appendicitis and acute diverticulitis—sonography may play a major primary investigative role. Further, endosonography, performed with high-frequency transducers in the lumen of the gut, is an increasingly popular technique for assessing the esophagus, stomach, and rectum.

The Gut Signature

The gut is a continuous hollow tube with **four concentric layers** (Fig. 8-1). From the lumen outward, they are: (1) mucosa, which consists of an epithelial lining, loose connective tissue or lamina propria, and muscularis mucosa; (2) submucosa; (3) muscularis propria, with inner circular and outer longitudinal fibers; and (4) serosa or adventitia. These histologic layers correspond with the sonographic appearance as depicted in Figure 8-2[1-3] and referred to as the **gut signature**, where up to **five layers** may be visualized (Fig. 8-3). The sonographic layers appear alternately echogenic and hypoechoic: the first, third, and fifth layers are echogenic; and the second and fourth layers are hypoechoic. This relationship of the histologic layering with the sonographic layering is best remembered by recognition that the muscular compo-

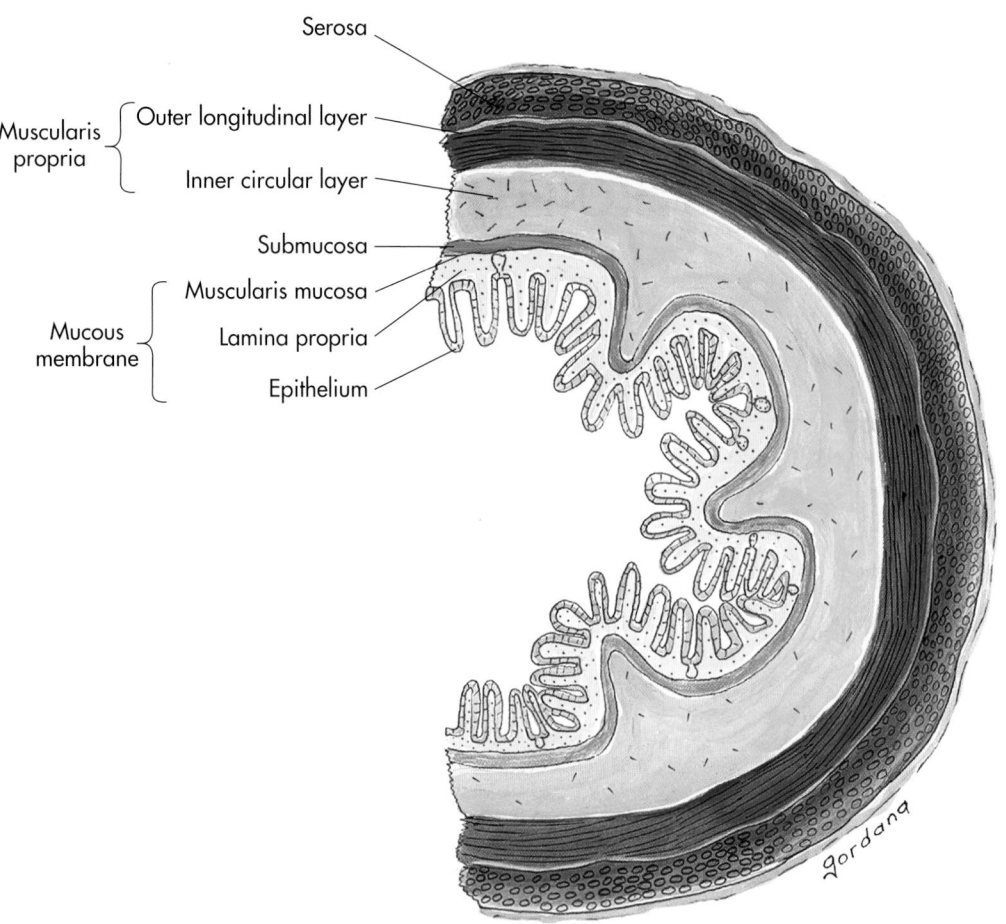

FIGURE 8-1. Schematic depiction of the histologic layers of the gut wall.

nents of the gut wall, the muscularis mucosa and the muscularis propria, constitute the hypoechoic layers on sonography.

On routine sonograms, the gut signature may vary from a bull's eye in cross-section, with an echogenic central area and a hypoechoic rim, to full depiction of the five sonographic layers. The quality of the scan and the resolution of the transducer determine the degree of layer differentiation. The normal gut wall is uniform and compliant, with an average thickness of 3 mm if distended and 5 mm if not. In addition to recognition of the gut signature, there are other morphologic features that allow recognition of specific portions of the gut, including the gastric rugae (Fig. 8-4A, B), the valvulae conniventes (see Fig. 8-4C, D), and the colonic haustrations.

The **content** and **diameter** of the gastrointestinal lumen and the **motor activity** of the gut are also assessed. Hypersecretion, mechanical obstruction, and ileus are implicated when gut fluid is excessive. Peristalsis is normally seen in the small bowel and stomach. Activity may be increased with mechanical obstruction and inflammatory enteritides. Decreased activity is seen with paralytic ileus and in the end stages of mechanical bowel obstruction.

Gut Wall Pathology

Evaluation of **thickened gut** on sonography is far superior to the evaluation of normal gut for two important reasons. Thick gut, particularly if associated with abnormality of the perienteric soft tissues, creates a *mass effect*, which is easily seen on sonography. In addition, thickened gut is frequently relatively gasless, improving its sonographic evaluation.[6] Gut wall pathology creates characteristic sonographic patterns (Fig. 8-5). The most familiar, the **target pattern** (see Fig. 8-5 middle), was first described by Lutz and Petzoldt[4] in 1976 and later by Bluth et al.,[5] who referred to the pattern as a **"pseudo-kidney"** (see Fig. 8-5), noting that a pathologically significant lesion was found in more than 90% of patients with this pattern. In both descriptions, the hypoechoic external rim corresponds to thickened gut wall, whereas the echogenic center relates to residual gut lumen or

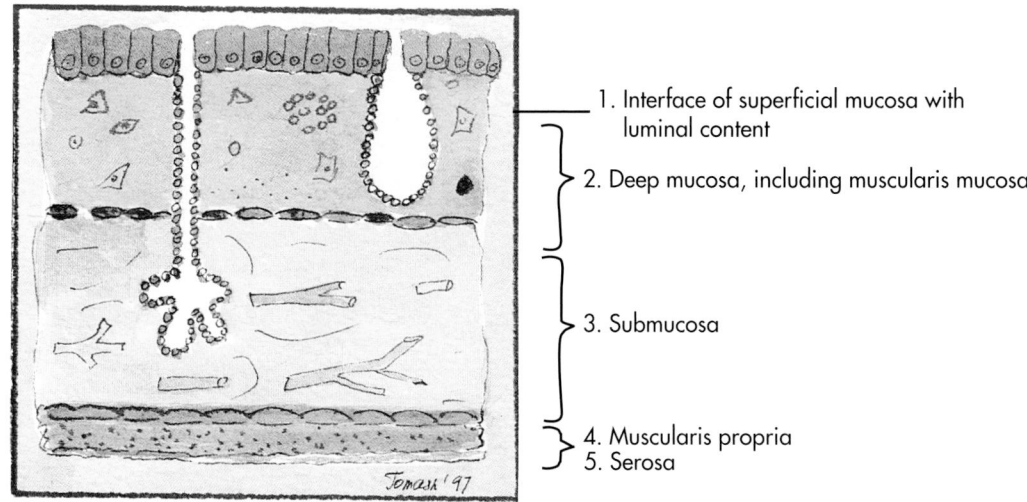

1. Interface of superficial mucosa with luminal content

2. Deep mucosa, including muscularis mucosa

3. Submucosa

4. Muscularis propria
5. Serosa

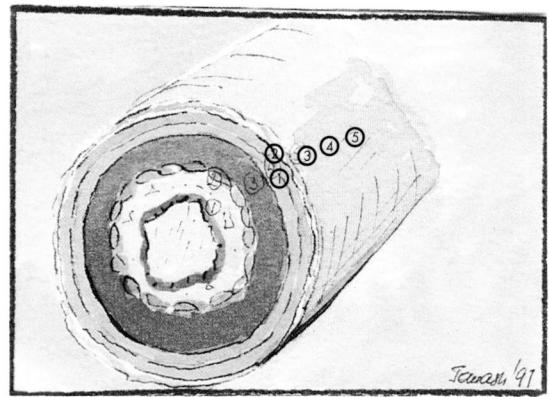

Sonographic appearance from the lumen ontward

1. Echogenic

2. Hypoechoic

3. Echogenic

4. Hypoechoic

5. Echogenic

FIGURE 8-2. Correlation of sonographic and histologic layers of the gut wall. Top schematic shows histologic layers of the gut wall. Bottom schematic shows gut in cross section with documented layer echogenicity as it relates to the histologic image shown above.

FOUR HISTOLOGIC LAYERS OF THE GUT

MUCOSA

Consists of an epithelial lining, loose connective tissue or lamina propria, and muscularis mucosa

SUBMUCOSA

MUSCULARIS PROPRIA

Consists of inner circular and outer longitudinal fibers

SEROSA OR ADVENTITIA

mucosal ulceration. The target and pseudokidney are the abnormal equivalents of the gut signature created by normal gut.

Identification of **thickened gut on sonography** may be related to a variety of pathologies.[6] Diagnostic possibilities are predicted by determining the extent and location of disease, the preservation or destruction of wall layering, and the concentricity or eccentricity of wall involvement. **Benignancy** is favored by long segment involvement with concentric thickening and wall layer preservation. The classic benign pathology showing gut wall thickening is Crohn's disease. **Malignancy** is favored by short segment involvement with eccentric disease and wall layer destruction. The classic malignant pathology showing gut wall thickening is adenocarcinoma of the stomach or colon. The foregoing are guidelines rather than hard and fast rules because chronically

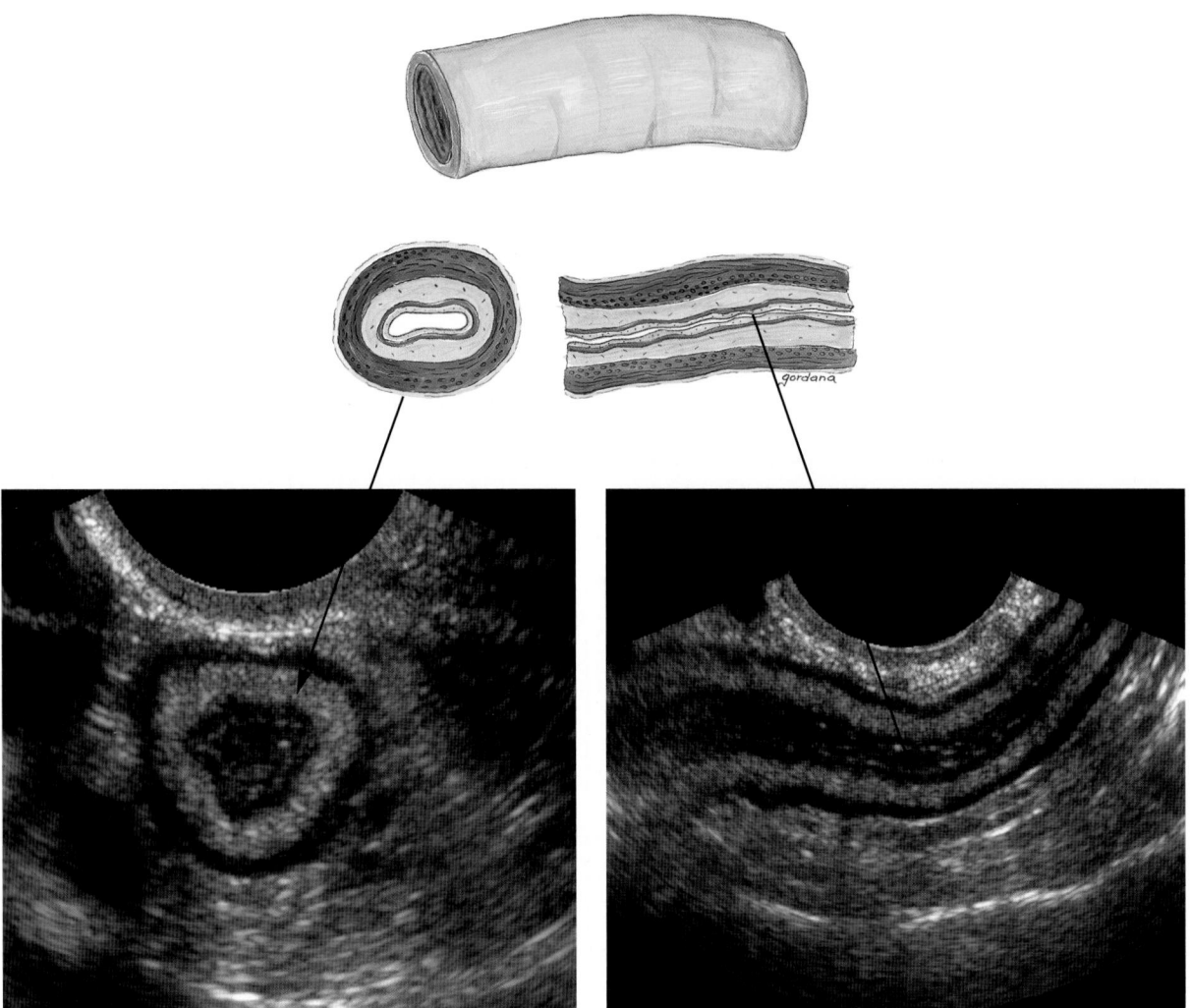

FIGURE 8-3. Gut signature. *Top,* schematic and *bottom,* corresponding ultrasound in a patient with mild gut thickening from Crohn's disease. *Blue layers,* representing the muscle, are black or hypoechoic on the sonogram. *Yellow layers,* representing the submucosa and the superficial mucosa, are hyperechoic. There is a small amount of fluid and air in the gut lumen on the sonogram.

thickened gut in Crohn's disease may show layer destruction related to fibrotic change and infiltrative adenocarcinoma may show some wall layer preservation. Lymphadenopathy and hyperemia of the thickened gut wall are seen in association with both malignant and benign gut wall thickening.

Gut wall masses, as distinct from thickened gut wall, may be intraluminal, mural, or exophytic, all with or without ulceration (see Fig. 8-5). Intraluminal gut masses and mucosal masses may have a variable appearance on sonography but are frequently hidden by gas or luminal content. In contrast, gut pathology creating an exophytic mass without or with mucosal involvement or ulceration may form masses that are more readily visualized. They may be difficult to assign to a gastrointestinal tract origin if typical gut signatures, targets, or pseudokidneys are not seen on sonography. Conse-

quently, intraperitoneal masses of varying morphology, which do not clearly arise from the solid abdominal viscera or the lymph nodes, should be considered to have a potential gut origin.

Technique

Routine sonograms are best performed when the patient has fasted. A real-time survey of the entire abdomen is performed with a 3.5- and/or a 5-MHz transducer and any obvious masses or gut signatures are observed. The pelvis is scanned before and after the bladder is emptied because the full bladder facilitates visualization of pathologic conditions in some patients and displaces abdominal bowel loops in others. Areas of interest then receive detailed analysis, including **compression sonography** (Fig. 8-6).[7] Although this technique was initially

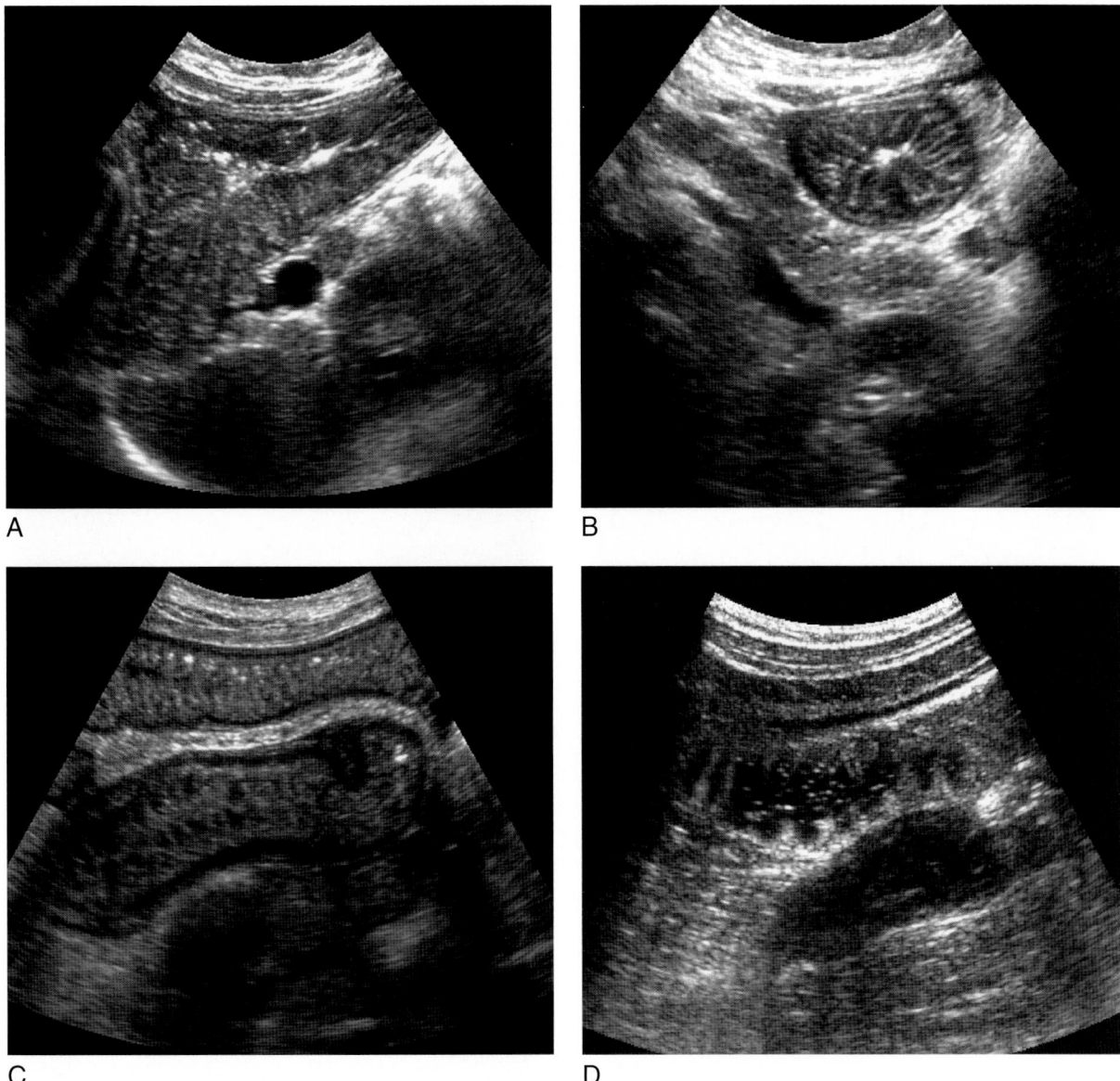

FIGURE 8-4. GUT recognition. A, Sagittal and **B,** cross-sectional views of the stomach show normal **gastric rugae.** The collapsed stomach shows variable wall thickness. **C** and **D** show **valvulae conniventes** of the small bowel. These are more easily seen when there is fluid in the lumen of the bowel as in **C,** or if the valvulae are edematous as in **D.**

described using high-frequency linear probes, 5-MHz convex linear and some sector probes work extremely well.[8] The critical factor is a transducer with a short focal zone allowing optimal resolution of structures close to the skin. Slow, graded pressure is applied. Normal gut will be compressed, and gas pockets displaced away from the region of interest. In contrast, thickened abnormal loops of bowel and/or obstructed noncompressible loops will remain unchanged. Patients with peritoneal irritation or local tenderness will usually tolerate the slow gentle increase in pressure of compression sonography, whereas they show a marked painful response if rapid, uneven scanning is performed. In women, **transvaginal sonography** is invaluable for evaluation of the portions of the gut within the true pelvis, most particularly the rectum and sigmoid colon. On occasion, oral fluid or a fluid enema may be helpful aids to sonography. This is true if one is attempting to determine the origin of a documented fluid collection. Further, oral fluid and a Fleet enema may improve localization and diagnosis of intraluminal or intramural gastric and rectal masses respectively.

Doppler Evaluation of the Gut Wall

Normal gut shows little signal on conventional color Doppler because interrogation is difficult in a normal and mobile bowel loop. Both neoplasia and inflammatory disease show increased vascularity when compared with the normal gut wall (Fig. 8-7), whereas ischemic

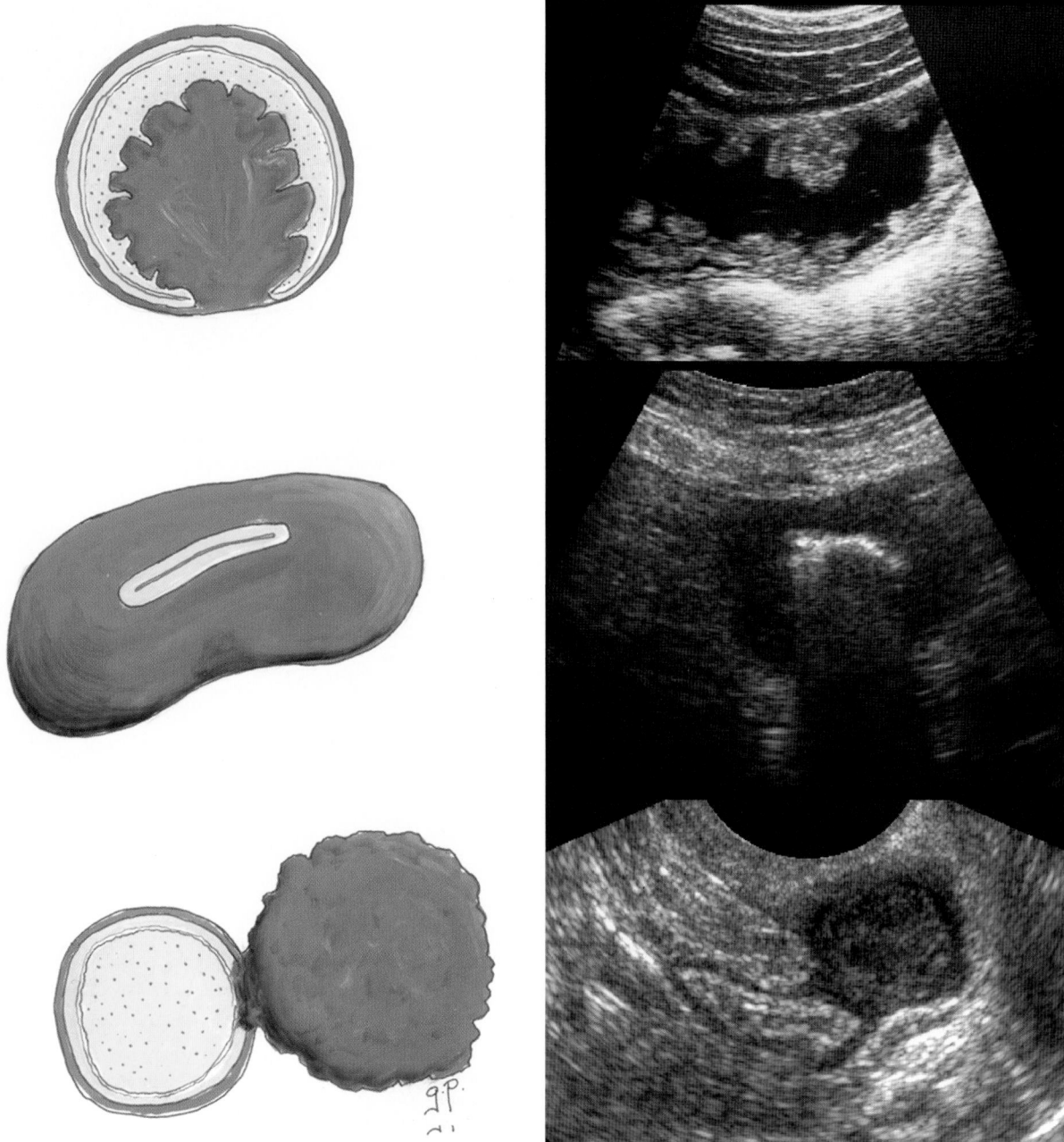

FIGURE 8-5. Gut wall pathology. Schematic of sonographic appearances with sonographic equivalents.
Top—Intraluminal mass. Inflammatory pseudopolyp on sonogram.[22] *Middle*—Pseudokidney sign with symmetrical wall thickening and wall layer destruction. Carcinoma of the colon on sonogram. *Bottom*—Exophytic mass. Serosal seed on visceral peritoneum of the gut on sonogram. (From Wilson SR: The bowel wall looks thickened: What does that mean? Categorical course in diagnostic radiology: Findings at US—what do they mean? Radiological Society of North America. 2002, 219-228.)

and edematous gut tend to be relatively hypovascular. The addition of color and spectral Doppler evaluation to the study of the gut wall allows for supportive evidence that gut wall thickening is due to either ischemic or inflammatory change in the patient with acute abdominal pain. Teefey et al.[9] examined 35 patients and found absent or barely visible blood flow on

color Doppler and absence of arterial signal to be suggestive of ischemia. In contrast, readily detected color Doppler flow and a resistance index less than 0.6 were consistent with inflammation. In our own experience, we have found color Doppler to be of great value in confirming our suspicion of an inflammatory gut process.

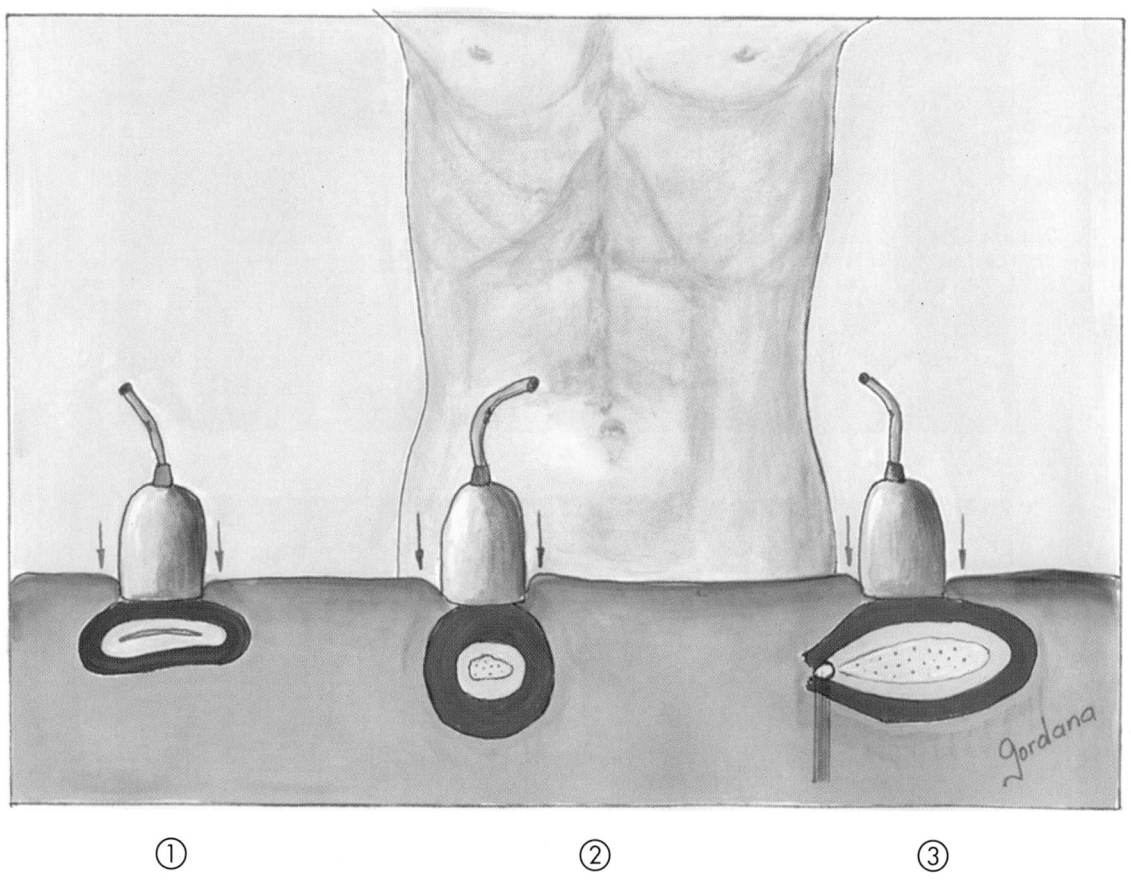

① ② ③

FIGURE 8-6. Compression sonography, schematic depiction. *Left*—Normal gut is compressed. *Middle*—Abnormally thickened gut or, *right*—an obstructed loop, such as that seen in acute appendicitis, will be noncompressible. (From Puylaert JBCM: Acute appendicitis: Ultrasound evaluation using graded compression. Radiology 1986;158:355-360.)

GASTROINTESTINAL TRACT NEOPLASMS

The role of sonography in the evaluation of gastrointestinal tract neoplasms is similar to that of computed tomography (CT) scan. Visualization is rarely obtained in early mucosal lesions or with small intramural nodules, whereas tumors growing to produce an exophytic mass, a thickened segment of gut with or without ulceration (Fig. 8-8), or a sizable intraluminal mass (Fig. 8-9) may all be seen. Sonograms are frequently performed early in the diagnostic work-up of patients with gastrointestinal tract tumors, often before their initial identification. Vague abdominal symptomatology, abdominal pain, a palpable abdominal mass, and anemia are common indications for these scans. Appreciation of the typical morphologies associated with gastrointestinal tract neoplasia may lead to accurate recognition, localization, and even staging of disease with the opportunity for directing appropriate further investigation, including sonography-guided aspiration biopsy.

Adenocarcinoma

Pathology. Adenocarcinoma is the most common malignant tumor of the gastrointestinal tract. It accounts for 80% of all malignant gastric neoplasms. These tumors arise most commonly in the prepyloric region, the antrum, and the lesser curve, which are the most optimally assessed portions of the stomach on sonography. Grossly it has variable growth patterns including infiltrative (see Fig. 8-8), polypoid (see Fig. 8-9), fungating, and ulcerated tumors. Infiltration may be superficial or transmural, the latter creating a **linitis plastica** or a **"leather bottle" stomach**.

Adenocarcinoma is much less frequent in the **small bowel** than in either the stomach or the large bowel. It accounts for approximately 50% of the tumors found in this region, 90% of them arising in either the proximal jejunum (Fig. 8-10) or the duodenum.[10] **Crohn's disease** is associated with a significantly increased incidence of adenocarcinoma that usually develops in the ileum. Small bowel adenocarcinomas are generally annular in gross morphology, frequently with ulceration.

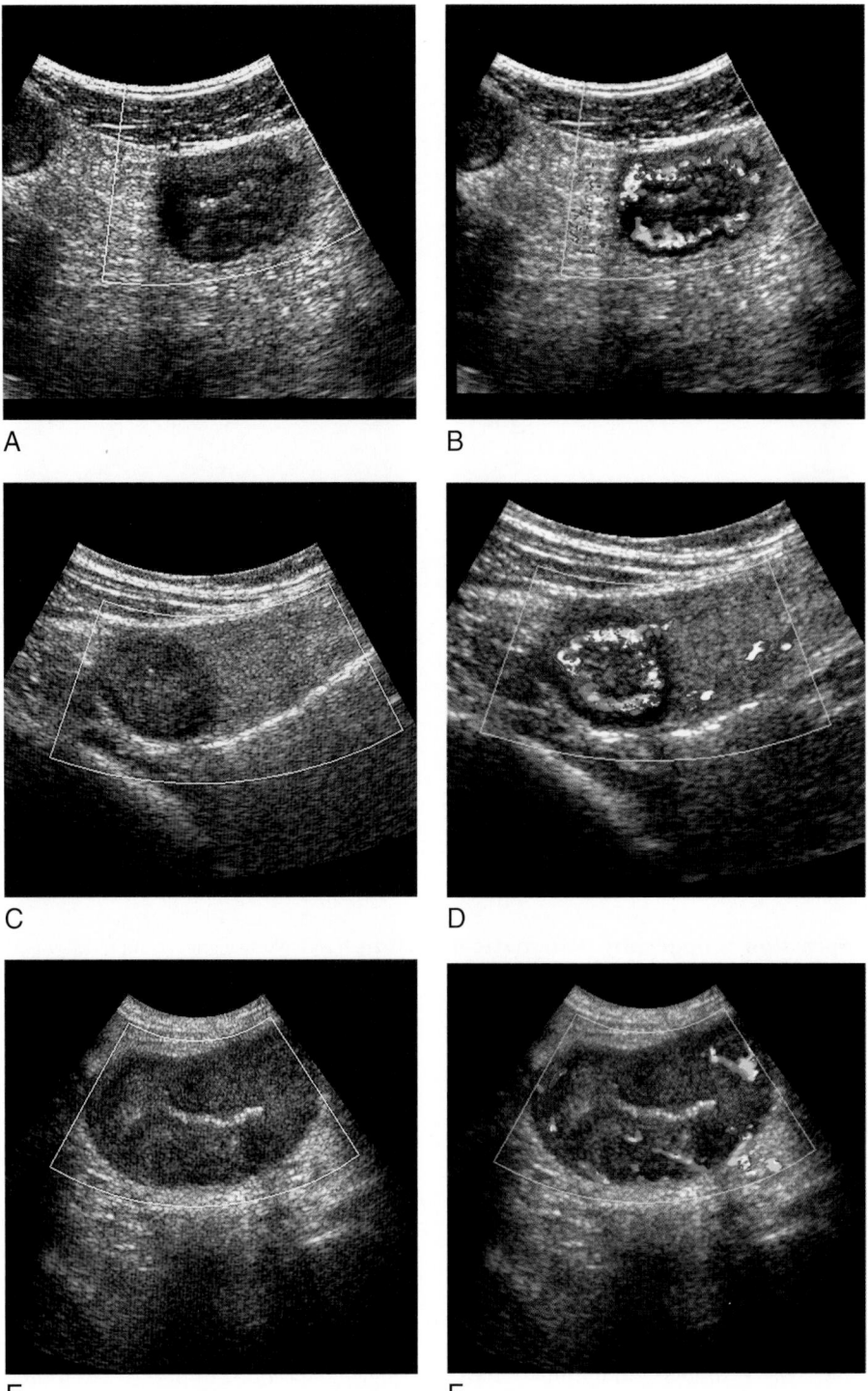

FIGURE 8-7. Contribution of Doppler to gut assessment in three patients. **A** and **B,** Cross-sectional views of the terminal ileum in a patient with Crohn's disease show marked symmetrical thickening of the gut wall. Color Doppler image shows marked hyperemia of the gut wall and surrounding actively inflamed fat. **C** and **D,** Featureless loop of gut with eccentric fat in the small bowel mesentery. Hyperemia of the fat and the gut wall reflect the active inflammation. **E** and **F,** Transverse images of the ascending colon show wall thickening with total layer destruction related to invasive colon carcinoma. Neoplastic tumors of the gut invariably show vascularity as here.

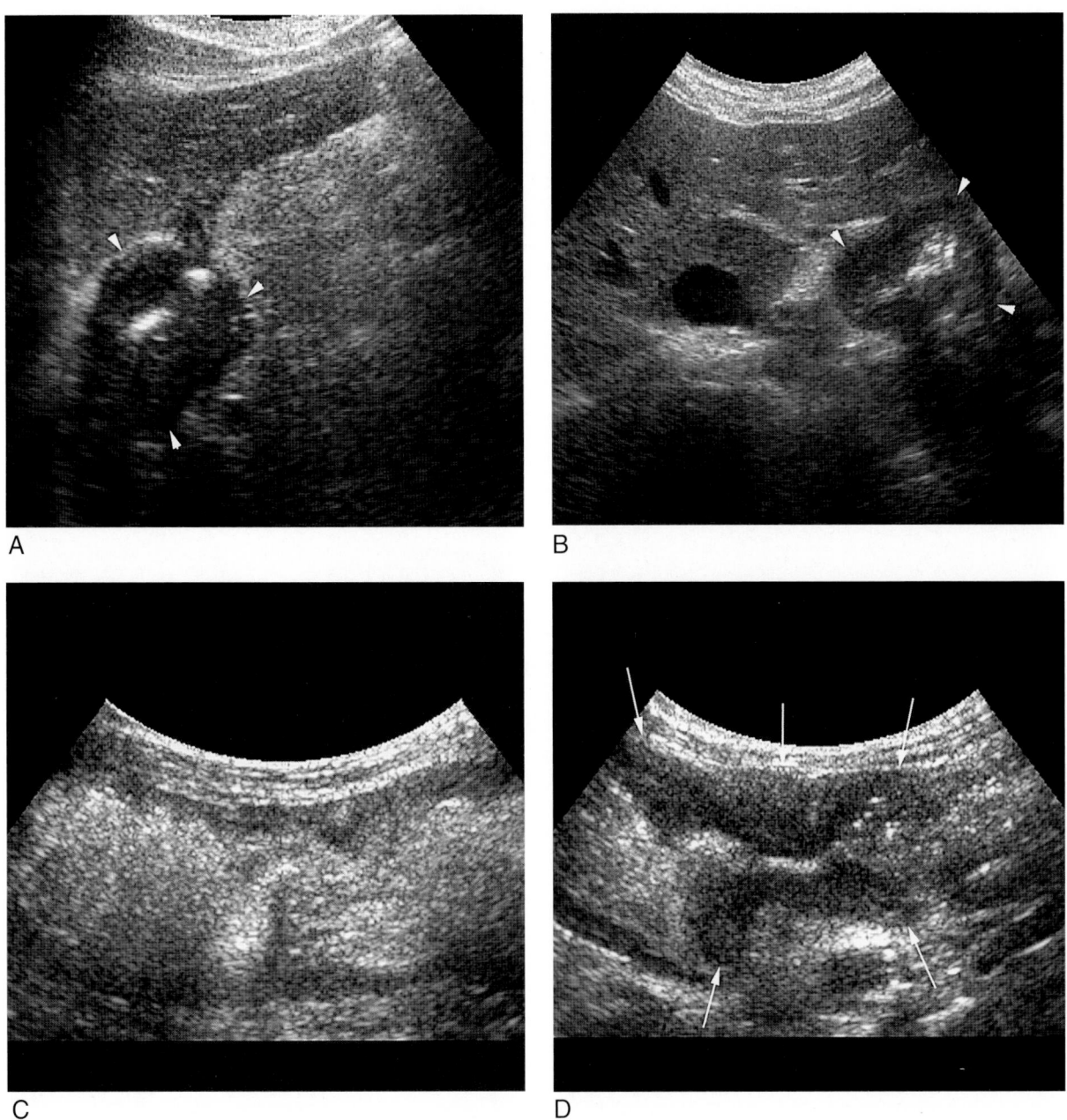

FIGURE 8-8. Adenocarcinoma of the gut in two patients. A, Sagittal and **B,** transverse sonograms of the upper abdomen show a pseudokidney (*arrowheads*) adjacent to the left lobe of the liver, representing a carcinoma at the gastroesophageal junction. **C,** Long axis sonogram of the proximal transverse colon shows a fluid-filled dilated lumen of the colon. **D,** More distally, a segment of thickened gut (*arrows*) shows wall layer destruction and a narrow central lumen from an annular carcinoma of the colon.

Colon carcinoma is very common, its incidence surpassed only by lung and breast cancer. Colon carcinoma accounts for virtually all malignant colorectal neoplasms. Colorectal adenocarcinoma grows with two major gross morphologic patterns: polypoid intraluminal tumors, which are most prevalent in the cecum and ascending colon; and annular constricting lesions (see Fig. 8-8H, I), which are most common in the descend-ing and sigmoid colon. Rarely, infiltrative tumors similar to those seen in the stomach may occur in the colon (Fig. 8-11).

Sonography. Most gastrointestinal tract mucosal cancers are not visualized on sonography; however, large masses, either intraluminal (see Fig. 8-9) or exophytic, and annular tumors (see Fig. 8-8H, I) create sonographic abnormalities.[11,12] Tumors of variable length may

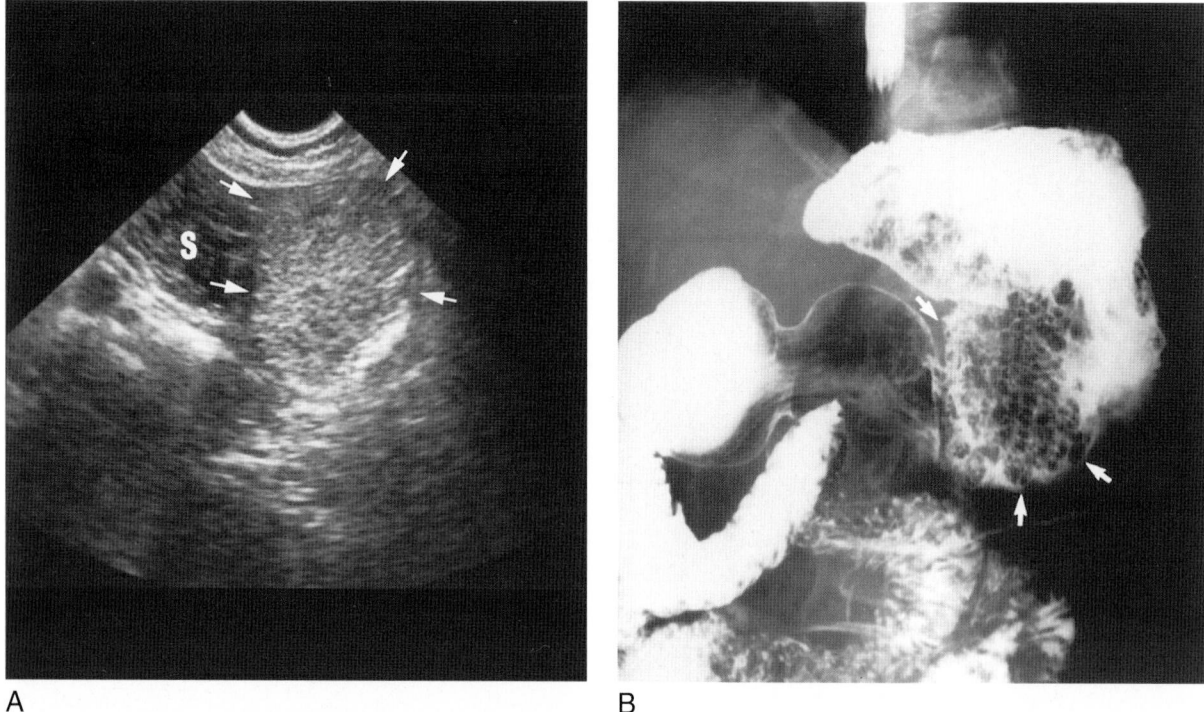

FIGURE 8-9. Intraluminal villous adenocarcinoma of the stomach. A, Transverse sonogram following oral fluid ingestion shows a relatively well-defined, nonhomogeneous, echogenic mass (*arrows*) within the body of the stomach. Fluid is in the stomach lumen (S). **B,** Confirmatory barium swallow shows the villous tumor (*arrows*).

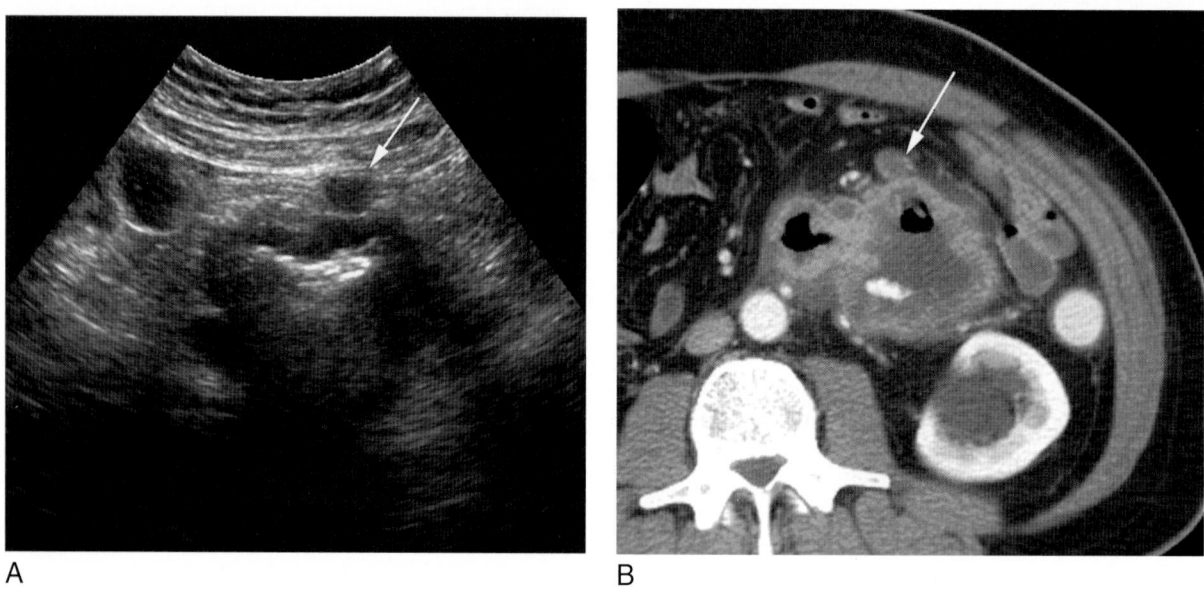

FIGURE 8-10. Adenocarcinoma of the jejunum. A, Sonogram and **B,** CT scan both show a large and necrotic left upper quadrant mass with enlargement of the perienteric lymph nodes (*arrow*) in a 60-year-old man who presented with abdominal discomfort and blood loss.

thicken the gut wall in either a concentric symmetrical or an asymmetrical pattern. A target or pseudokidney (see Fig. 8-5) morphology may be created. Air in mucosal ulcerations typically produces linear echogenic foci, often with "ringdown" artifact, within the bulk of the mass. Tumors are usually, but not invariably, hypoechoic.

Annular lesions may produce gut obstruction with dilation, hyperperistalsis, and increased luminal fluid of the gut proximal to the tumor site (see Fig. 8-8H, I).[12] Evidence of direct invasion, regional lymph node enlargement (see Fig. 8-8C), and liver metastases should be specifically sought in all cases.

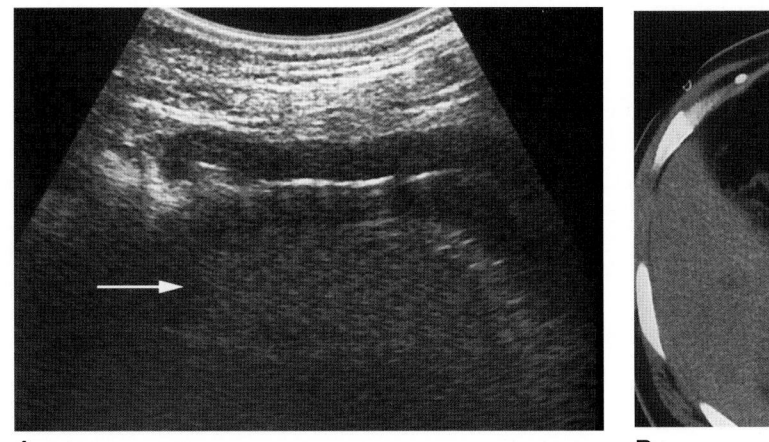
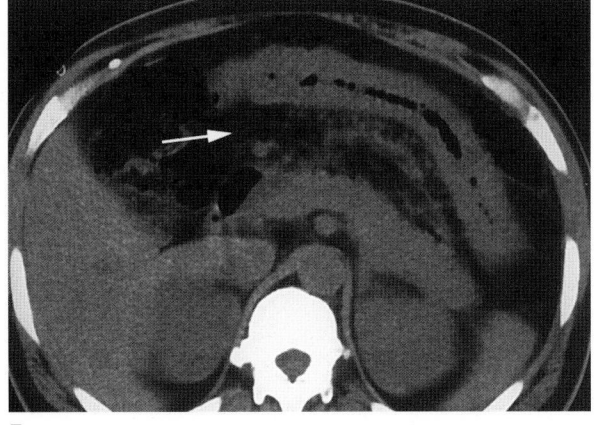

A   B

FIGURE 8-11. Infiltrative carcinoma of the transverse colon. A 42-year-old black man presented to the emergency department with acute abdominal pain. **A,** Transverse view of the epigastrium shows a featureless segment of thick gut with total loss of wall layering in the location of the transverse colon. Deep to the gut is a diffuse echogenic mass effect (*arrow*) suggesting infiltrated or inflamed fat. **B,** Confirmatory computed tomography scan. Neoplasia was not suspected on the basis of either imaging test or at surgery.

Gastrointestinal Stromal Tumors (GIST)

Pathology. Of the mesenchymal tumors affecting the gut, those of smooth muscle origin are the most common and account for about 1% of all gastrointestinal tract neoplasms. They are found most often in the stomach and the small bowel. Colonic tumors are the least frequent and occur most often in the rectum. Although they may be found as an incidental observation at surgery, sonography, or autopsy, these vascular tumors frequently become very large and may undergo ulceration, degeneration, necrosis, and hemorrhage.[13]

Sonography. Smooth muscle tumors typically produce round mass lesions of varying size and echogenicity (Fig. 8-12), often with central cystic areas (Fig. 8-13)[14] related to either hemorrhage or necrosis. Their gut origin is not always easily determined but if ulceration is present, pockets of gas in an ulcer crater may suggest their origin. Smooth muscle tumors of gut origin should be considered in the differential diagnosis of incidentally noted, indeterminate abdominal masses in asymptomatic patients, particularly if they show central cystic or necrotic change (see Fig. 8-13). These tumors are very amenable to sonographic-guided aspiration biopsy.

Lymphoma

Pathology. The gut may be involved with lymphoma in two basic forms: as widespread dissemination in stage III or IV lymphoma of any cell type or, more commonly, as primary lymphoma of the GI tract, which is virtually always a non-Hodgkin's lymphoma. Primary tumors constitute only 2% to 4% of all gastrointestinal tract malignant tumors[15] but account for 20% of those found in the small bowel. **Three predominant growth patterns** are observed: nodular or polypoid, carcinoma-

GROWTH PATTERNS OF LYMPHOMA

Nodular or polypoid
Carcinoma-like ulcerative lesions
Infiltrating tumor masses
Invade the adjacent mesentery and lymph nodes

like ulcerative lesions, and infiltrating tumor masses that frequently invade the adjacent mesentery and lymph nodes.[10]

Sonography. Small submucosal nodules may be easily overlooked on sonography. However, many affected patients have large, very hypoechoic, ulcerated masses in the stomach or small bowel (Fig. 8-14).[16,17] Long, linear, high-amplitude echoes with "ringdown" artifacts, indicating gas in the residual lumen or ulcerations, are frequently seen. This particular pathology has been recognized as one of the more frequent presentations of patients with **AIDS-related lymphoma** as compared with other lymphoma populations. Regional lymph node enlargement may be visualized, although generalized lymph node abnormality is uncommon.

Metastases

Pathology. Malignant melanoma and primary tumors of the **lung** and **breast** are the tumors most likely to have secondary involvement of the gastrointestinal tract.[18] In order of frequency, the stomach, small bowel, and colon are involved. Secondary neoplasm affecting the omentum and peritoneum may cause ascites, tiny or confluent superficial secondary nodules on the gut surface (see Fig. 8-21), or extensive omental cakes that virtually engulf the involved gut loops.[19,20] Metastases to the

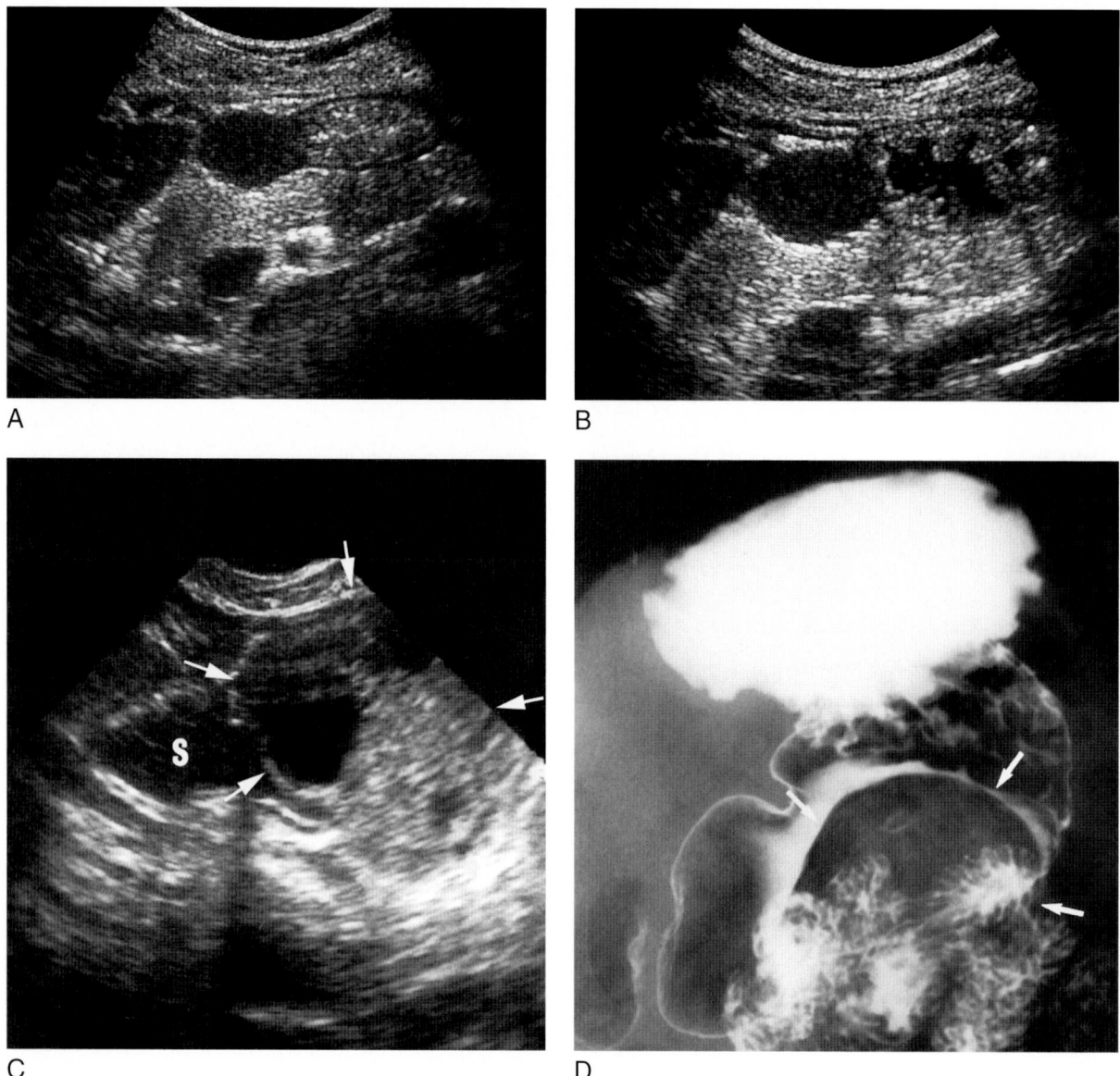

FIGURE 8-12. Gastrointestinal stromal tumors (GIST) in two patients. A and B, Exophytic gut mass, a gastric leiomyoma, analogous to the bottom schematic and image from Figure 8-5. **A,** Transverse sonogram of epigastrium shows the normal gastric gut signature and the focal exophytic mass. **B,** Following water ingestion, the lumen contains fluid that appears black. The solid mass is now clearly seen. **C** and **D,** Gastric leiomyosarcoma. **C,** Transverse sonogram following oral ingestion of fluid shows a complex smooth intramural mass (*arrows*) projecting into the fluid-filled stomach lumen (S). **D,** Confirmatory barium swallow shows the intramural tumor (*arrows*).

peritoneum most commonly arise from primary tumors in the **ovary** or the **gut** (see Fig. 8-16).

Sonography. Small submucosal nodules, with a tendency to ulcerate, are rarely seen on sonography, whereas large, diffusely infiltrative tumors with large ulcerations are common, particularly in the small bowel (Fig. 8-15), where they create hypoechoic, well-defined masses that often have bright, specular echoes with "ringdown" artifacts in areas of ulceration. Particulate ascites, omental thickening, and visceral and parietal peritoneal nodules and plaques (see Figs. 8-5, bottom and 8-22) should all raise the suspicion of metastatic disease.

INFLAMMATORY BOWEL DISEASE (CROHN'S DISEASE)

Inflammatory bowel disease includes Crohn's disease and ulcerative colitis. The latter is a mucosal inflammation and shows little in the way of sonographic change even with acute disease. Crohn's disease, a transmural process, therefore, constitutes the majority of patients scanned with inflammatory bowel disease.

Pathology. Crohn's disease, a chronic inflammatory disorder of the gastrointestinal tract of unknown patho-

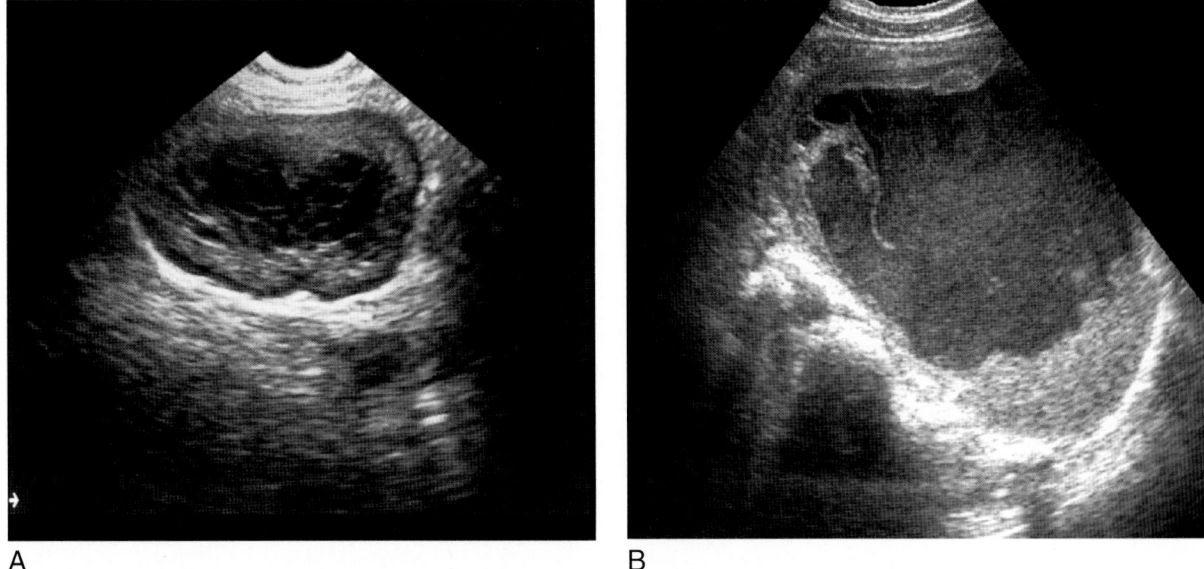

FIGURE 8-13. Leiomyosarcoma with suggestive morphology for GIST in two patients. A, Left flank sonogram shows a well-defined mass with a solid rim and nonuniform cystic center suggestive of necrosis. Proven leiomyosarcoma of the jejunum. **B,** Large necrotic leiomyosarcoma of the stomach showing as an enormous highly complex left upper quadrant mass. Its appearance raises the possibility of a GIST. The gut origin of this mass could not be shown on sonography. The complex nature of the mass, however, correctly suggested its nature although not its precise origin. GIST, Gastrointestinal stromal tumor.

genesis and etiology, most commonly affects the terminal ileum and the colon—although any portion of the gut may be involved. It is a transmural, granulomatous inflammatory process affecting all layers of the gut wall. Grossly, the gut wall is typically very thick and rigid with secondary luminal narrowing. Discrete or continuous ulcers and deep fissures are characteristic, frequently leading to fistula formation. Mesenteric lymph node enlargement and matting of involved loops are common. The mesentery may be markedly thickened and fatty, creeping over the edges of the gut to the antimesenteric border. Recurrence after surgery and perianal disease is a classic clinical feature.

Although barium study and endoscopy remain the major tools to evaluate mucosal and luminal abnormality, sonography, like CT, may offer valuable additional information about the gut wall, the lymph nodes, the mesentery, and the regional soft tissues.[21] The chronic nature of inflammatory bowel disease, characterized by multiple remissions and exacerbations, is well assessed by a noninvasive, sensitive modality, such as sonography. The degree of thickening of the gut wall and the frequent association of extraluminal disease make Crohn's disease the most optimally studied disorder. Baseline examination with follow-up predicts complications, such as abscess, fistula, or obstruction; detects postoperative recurrence; and identifies patients who require more invasive imaging techniques.[22] Radiation exposure is significant in the young population frequently affected with Crohn's disease if a CT scan is performed with each exacerbation of disease. Sonography is, therefore,

our routine evaluation technique for patients with this diagnosis.

Sonography. The objectives of a sonogram on a patient with known or suspected inflammatory bowel disease include the documentation of the **classic features:** gut wall thickening, creeping fat, hyperemia, mesenteric lymphadenopathy, strictures, and mucosal abnormalities. The distribution and extent of disease should also be documented. Sonography may also detect the **complications** of disease including: inflammatory masses (phlegmon or abscess), fistulae, obstruction, perforation, and appendicitis.[22]

Classic Features of Crohn's Disease

Gut Wall Thickening

This is the most frequently observed abnormality in patients with Crohn's disease. Sonography may be appropriate for initial detection, for detection of recurrence,[23] for determining the extent of disease, and in the assessment of response to treatment. Gut wall thickening is most frequently concentric and may be quite marked.[24,25] Wall echogenicity varies depending on the degree of inflammatory infiltration and fibrosis. Stratification with retention of the gut layers is typical (see Figs. 8-3B, 8-17A, B, and 8-18), or a target or pseudokidney appearance is possible with long-standing fibrotic disease as the gut wall layering is progressively lost (see Fig. 8-17C, D). Long-standing and often burnt out disease may also show subtle wall thickening with fat

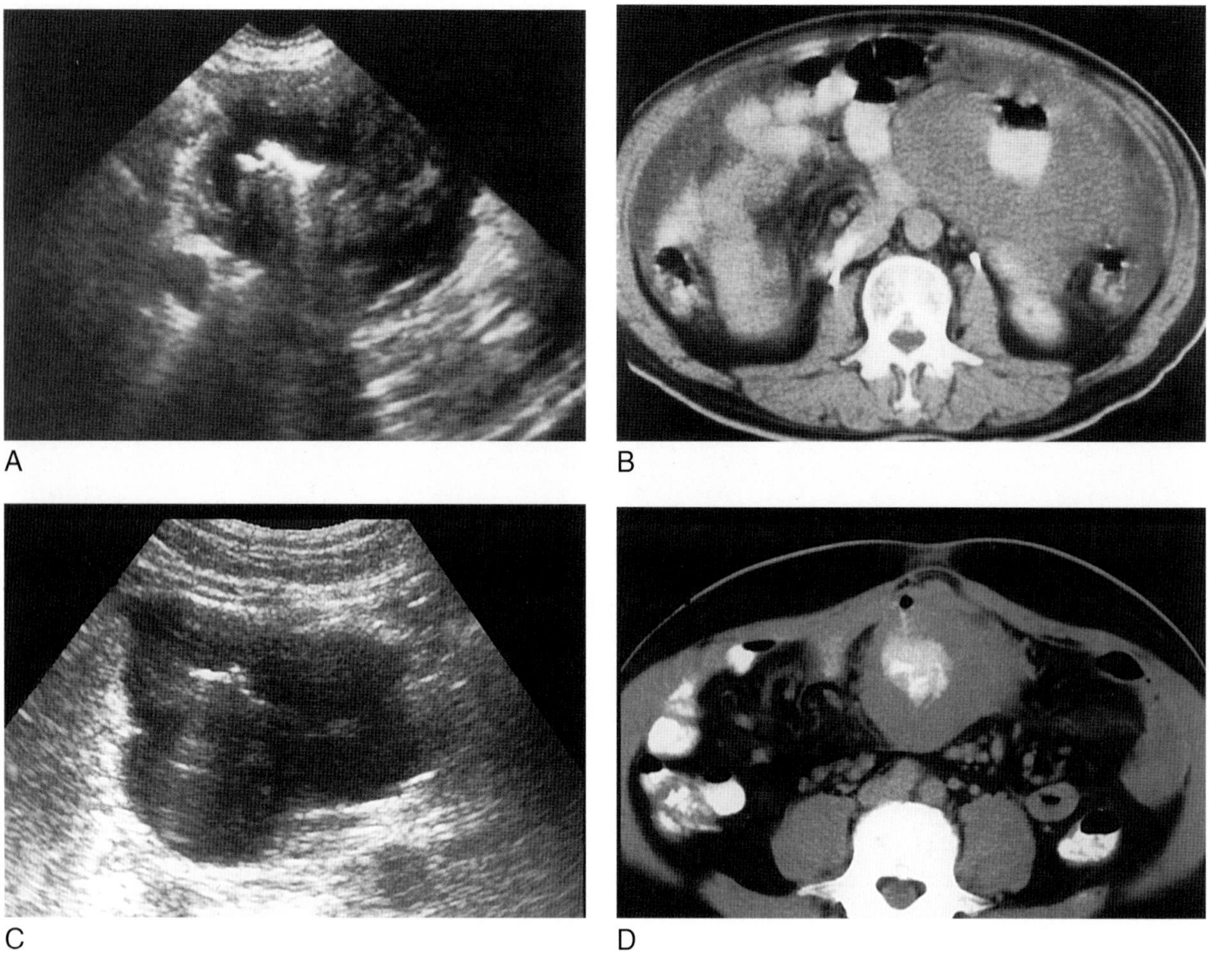

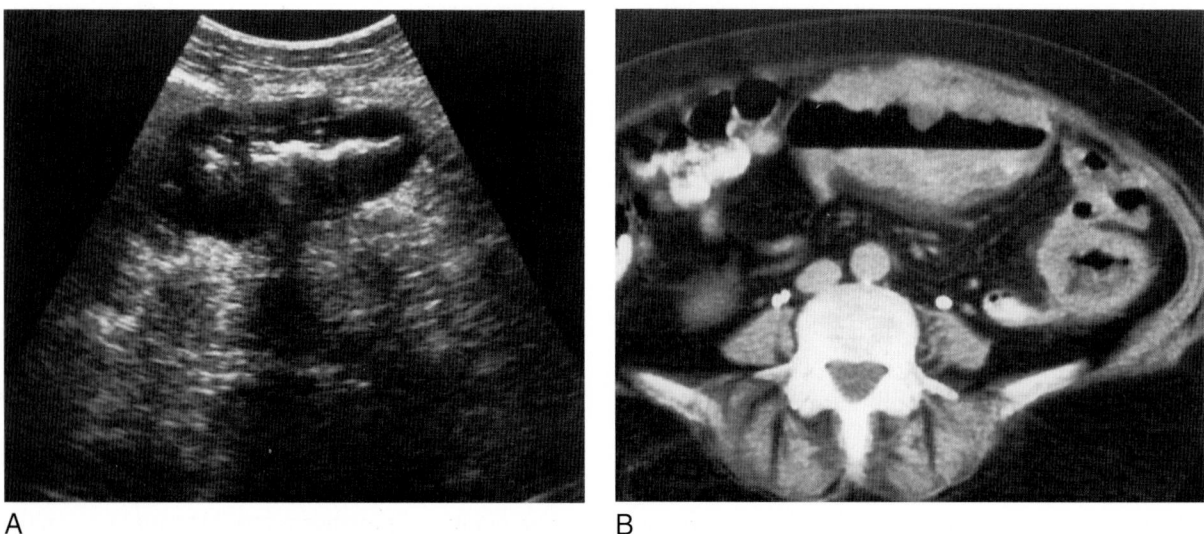

FIGURE 8-14. Small bowel lymphoma in two patients. A, Transverse left paramedian sonogram shows a hypoechoic round mass lesion. Central echogenicity with ringdown gas artifact suggests its gut origin. **B,** Confirmatory CT scan shows large, soft tissue mass with corresponding residual gut lumen. **C** and **D,** AIDS patient. **C,** Sonogram shows a focal midabdominal, very hypoechoic (*black*) mass with no wall layer definition, which is classic for gut lymphoma. The luminal gas appears as central bright echogenicity with dirty shadowing. **D,** Confirmatory CT scan.

FIGURE 8-15. Metastatic malignant melanoma to small bowel. A, Transverse paraumbilical sonogram shows well-defined, hypoechoic mass with central irregular echogenicity with gas artifact suggesting, correctly, its gut origin. **B,** Confirmatory CT scan.

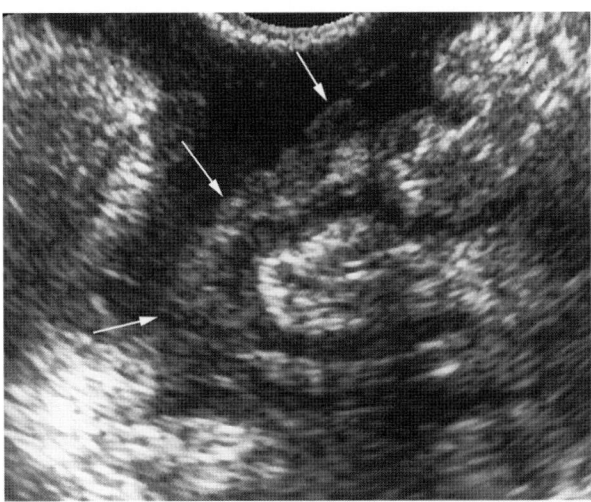

FIGURE 8-16. Visceral peritoneal plaque on small bowel surface—metastatic ovarian cancer. Transvaginal image shows ascites. A plaque of soft tissue (*arrows*) is seen on the surface of the small bowel loop.

SONOGRAPHIC FEATURES OF CROHN'S DISEASE

CLASSIC FEATURES

Gut wall thickening
Strictures
Creeping fat
Hyperemia
Mesenteric lymphadenopathy
Mucosal abnormalities

COMPLICATIONS

Inflammatory masses
Fistula
Obstruction
Perforation
Appendicitis

deposition in the submucosa, which shows as increased echogenicity of this layer (see Fig. 8-17E, F). Actively involved gut typically appears rigid and fixed with decreased or absent peristalsis. Skip areas are frequent. Involved segments vary in length from a few millimeters to many centimeters. Activity of inflammatory change correlates with hyperemia as seen on color Doppler evaluation.

Edema and Fibrosis of the Adjacent Mesentery

These are characteristic features of Crohn's disease and produce a mass in the mesentery adjacent to the diseased gut which may creep over the border of the abnormal gut or completely engulf it. Fat creeping onto the margins of the involved gut creates a uniform **echogenic halo** around the mesenteric border of the gut with a thyroid-like appearance in cross-section (Fig. 8-19). It may become more heterogeneous and even hypoechoic in long-standing disease. **Creeping fat** is the most common cause to explain gut loop separation as seen on contrast gastrointestinal studies (see Fig. 8-19).[22] It is also the most striking and easy to detect abnormality on sonography of patients with perienteric inflammatory processes (Fig. 8-20). Its detection should provoke the examiner to perform a detailed evaluation of the regional gut.

Lymphadenopathy

This is seen in virtually all patients in the active phase of inflammation with Crohn's disease. It is not nearly as commonly observed in the inactive phase. Perienteric nodes and nodes in the mesentery (Fig. 8-21) are involved and show as focal hypoechoic masses circumferentially surrounding the gut and in the expected location of the mesenteric attachment. Nodes are frequently quite round and typically lose the normal linear echogenic streak from the nodal hilum. The lymph nodes show hyperemia similar to the gut as a reflection of their inflammation. Nodes are usually of moderate size and are tender. Larger nodes, over 3 cm in diameter, raise the possibility of a malignant complication of Crohn's disease.

Hyperemia

This is a reflection of the activity of the inflammatory process. Although subjective, the addition of color Doppler to gray-scale sonography is valuable supportive evidence of inflammatory change in the gut and adjacent inflamed fat (see Fig. 8-7A-D).[22] Evaluation of blood flow is a useful tool to monitor inflammatory activity in response to therapy.

Strictures

These are due to rigid narrowing of the gut lumen and fixed angulations are common observations in Crohn's disease. The luminal surfaces of involved segments of gut most often appear to be in apposition, with the lumen appearing as a linear echogenic central area within a thickened gut loop (Fig. 8-22). This is in contrast to thickened sections, where the luminal diameter may be maintained (Fig. 8-23). Incomplete mechanical obstruction may be inferred if dilated, hyperperistaltic segments are seen proximal to a stricture. Peristaltic waves from the obstructed gut, proximal to a narrowed segment, may produce visible movement through the strictured segment. Less often, involved segments of gut may show **luminal dilation** (see Fig. 8-23) with sacculation, as well as narrowing, and the retained lumen may be of variable

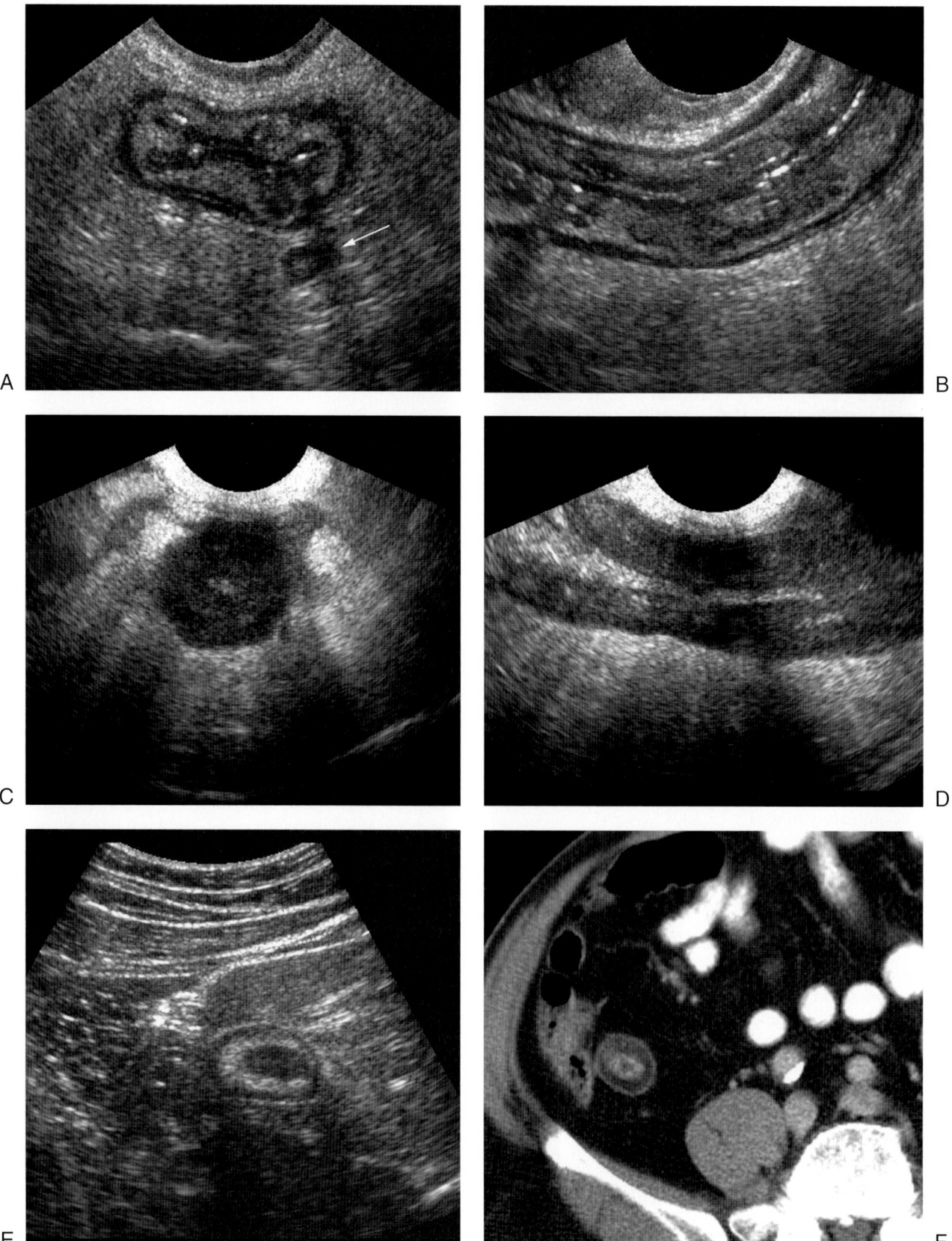

FIGURE 8-17. Crohn's disease—classic feature, gut wall thickening in three patients. A and **B,** Sagittal and cross-sectional views showing the typical thickening in active disease with wall layer retention. *Arrow,* lymph node. **C** and **D** are sagittal and cross-sectional views showing complete loss of wall layering.[6] This is seen uncommonly in patients who often have long-standing but active disease as in this case. **E** and **F,** Corresponding sonogram and CT images of the terminal ileum in a patient with burnt out disease with fatty deposition in the submucosa. This appears echogenic on the sonogram. (**C** and **D,** From Wilson SR: The bowel wall looks thickened: What does that mean? Categorical course in diagnostic radiology: Findings at US—what do they mean? Radiological Society of North America. 2002, 219-228.)

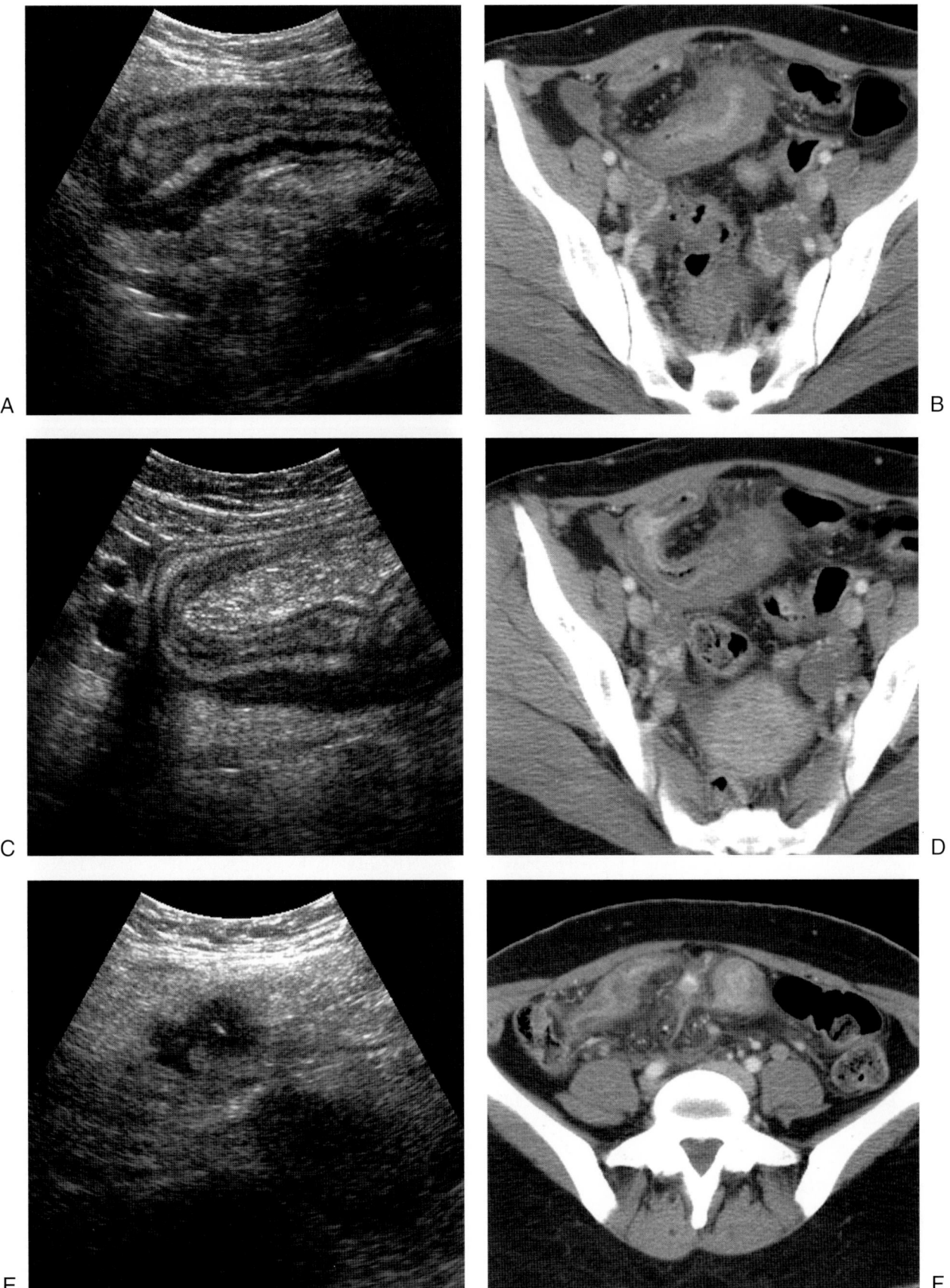

FIGURE 8-18. Crohn's disease—classic feature, gut wall thickening in active disease. A, Sonogram shows the ileum in long axis. The wall is very thick and wall layering is preserved. **B,** Confirmatory CT scan shows the thickened wall but does not resolve the wall layers. **C,** Sonogram and **D,** CT scan show another loop of ileum with acute angulation and less wall thickening. **E** and **F,** Sonogram and confirmatory CT show a central inflammatory mass made of inflamed fat. The hypoechoic zone with ill-defined borders on the sonogram suggests phlegmonous change.

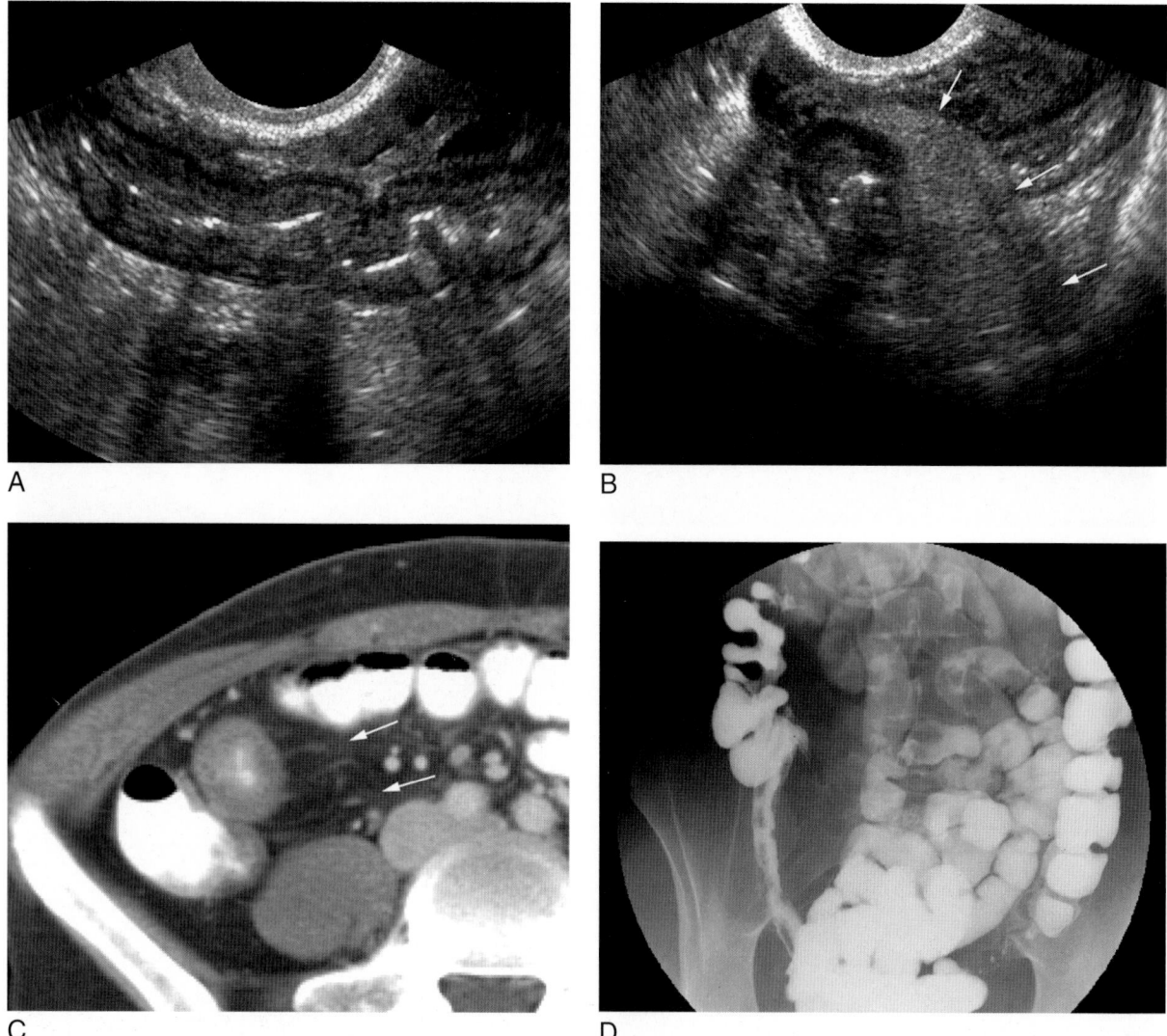

FIGURE 8-19. Crohn's disease—classic feature, creeping fat. A, Long axis view of a thickened terminal ileum (TI). Wall layering is preserved. **B,** TI in cross section. A hyperechoic mass effect (*arrows*) is seen along the medial border of the gut and represents creeping fat. **C,** Confirmatory CT scan showing both the thick wall of the TI and the streaky fat (*arrows*). **D,** Subsequent barium study showing separation of loops of small bowel in the same location. Creeping fat is the most common explanation for this bowel separation.

caliber. **Concretions** and **bezoars** (Fig. 8-24) may develop in gut between strictured segments. Parente et al. have recently shown that bowel ultrasound is an accurate technique for detecting small bowel strictures, especially in very severe cases that are candidates for surgery.[26]

Conglomerate Masses

These may be related to clumps of matted bowel, inflamed edematous mesentery, increased fat deposition in the mesentery, and uncommonly mesenteric lymphadenopathy. Involved loops may demonstrate angulation and fixation resulting from retraction of the thickened fibrotic mesentery.

Complications of Crohn's Disease

Inflammatory Masses

These involving the fibrofatty mesentery are the most common complication of Crohn's disease, although the development of abscesses with drainable pus occurs infrequently. Prior to the stage of liquefaction, **phlegmonous change** may be noted as ill-defined hypoechoic zones without fluid content within areas of inflamed fat (Fig. 8-25). **Abscess formation** shows as a complex or fluid-filled mass (see Fig. 8-25). Gas content within an abscess is both helpful in raising suspicion of an abscess (see Fig. 8-25) and also a potential source of sonographic error, particularly if large quantities are

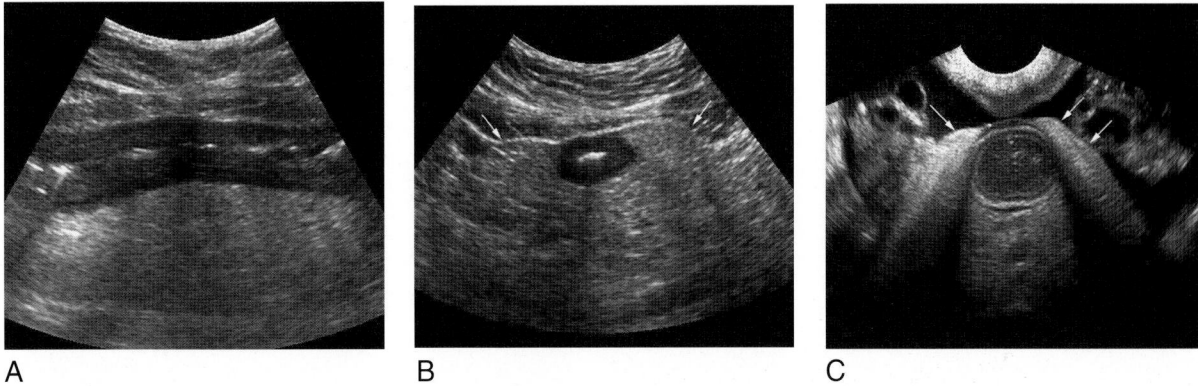

FIGURE 8-20. Spectrum of appearances of inflamed fat in two patients. A, Long axis and **B,** cross-sectional images of the sigmoid colon in a patient with Crohn's disease show the gut wall is thickened. Inflamed fat in the sigmoid mesentery shows an echogenic mass effect mainly on the deep border of the abnormal gut in long axis. In cross section the fat (*arrows*) creeps around the margins of the gut loop. **C,** Rectosigmoid colon on a transvaginal scan in a patient with generalized edema and ascites. The perienteric fat (*arrows*) is thick and echogenic. The gut loop shows a fluid-filled lumen and mild gut wall thickening.

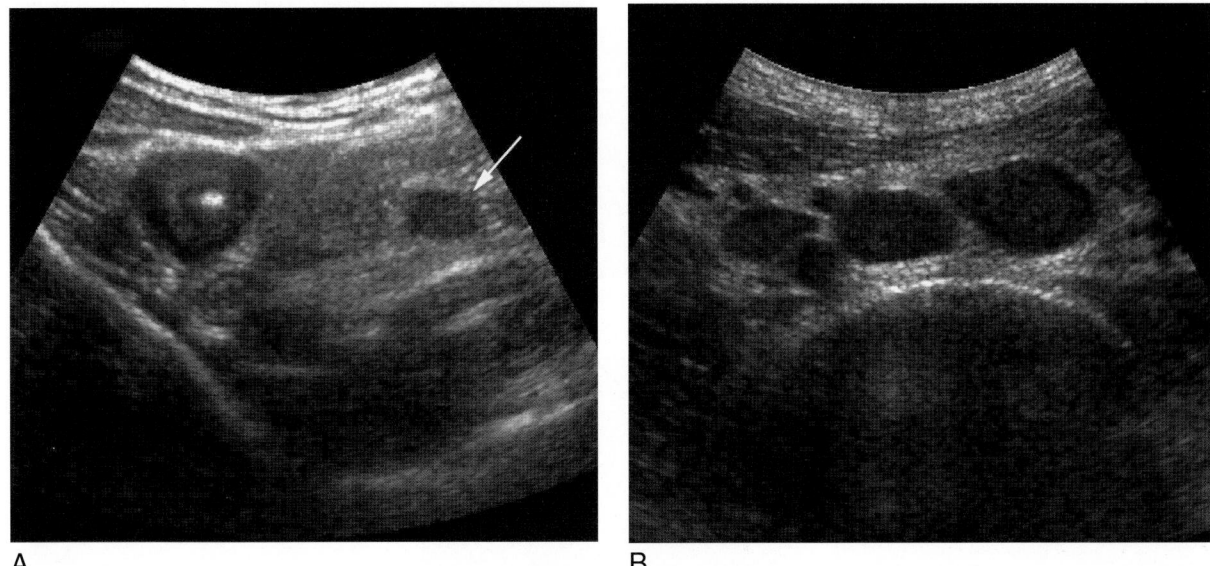

FIGURE 8-21. Crohn's disease—classic feature, lymphadenopathy in two patients. A, Transverse image in the right lower quadrant shows a thick terminal ileum in cross section. There is inflamed fat in the location of the mesentery. A mesenteric node (*arrow*) shows as a small, solid hypoechoic mass within the fat. **B,** Multiple mesenteric nodes of varying size show as hypoechoic soft tissue masses within the mesentery, optimally shown in an oblique plane between the region of the ileocecal valve and the aortic bifurcation.

present. Abscesses may be intraperitoneal or extraperitoneal (see Fig. 8-25) or may be in remote locations such as the liver or the psoas muscles.

Fistula Formation

This is a characteristic complication of Crohn's disease and occurs most commonly at the proximal end of a thickened and strictured segment of bowel. Although mucosal ulcerations are not well assessed on sonography, deep fissures in the gut wall appear as echogenic linear areas penetrating deeply into the wall beyond the margin of the gut lumen (Fig. 8-26). With fistula formation,

linear bands of varying echogenicity can be seen extending from segments of abnormal gut to the skin (see Fig. 8-26C), bladder (see Fig. 8-26A), or to other abnormal loops. If there is gas or movement in the fistula during sonographic study, the fistula will usually appear bright or echogenic, with or without "ringdown" artifact related to the presence of air in the tract (see Figs. 8-26A and D) Conversely, if the tract is empty or partially closed, it may appear as a black or hypoechoic tract (see Figs. 8-26B and C). Palpation of the abdomen during the examination may produce movement of fluid or air through the fistula, thereby increasing its identification.

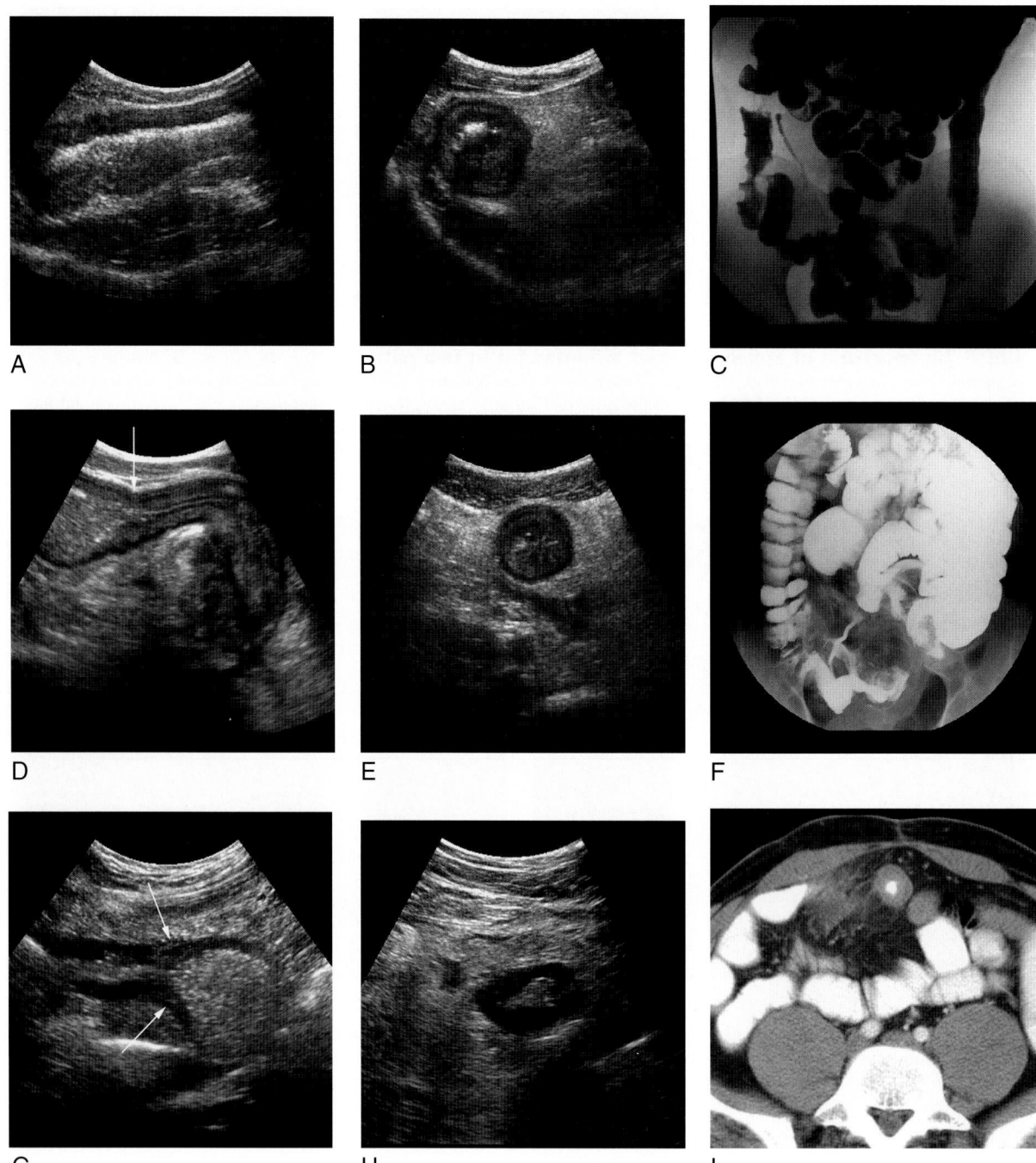

FIGURE 8-22. Crohn's disease—classic feature. Strictures in three different patients, one per line. **A,** Long axis, and **B,** short axis sonograms show a diffusely thickened loop of gut, the ileum proximal to the ileocecal valve, with narrowing of the central echogenic lumen. There is inflammation of the mesenteric fat. **C,** Confirmatory small bowel enema shows the long and tight stricture in the ileum. **D,** Long axis, and **E,** short axis sonograms of the terminal ileum show an abrupt transition in the caliber of the gut (*arrow*). The gut proximal to the arrow is dilated and fluid filled. The distal gut has a stricture, confirmed on **F,** the small bowel enema. **G,** Long axis image of the neoterminal ileum shows a thickened and featureless wall with a caliber alteration (*arrows*). **H,** Short axis image through the stricture shows the thickened wall and surrounding inflamed fat. **I,** Confirmatory CT scan.

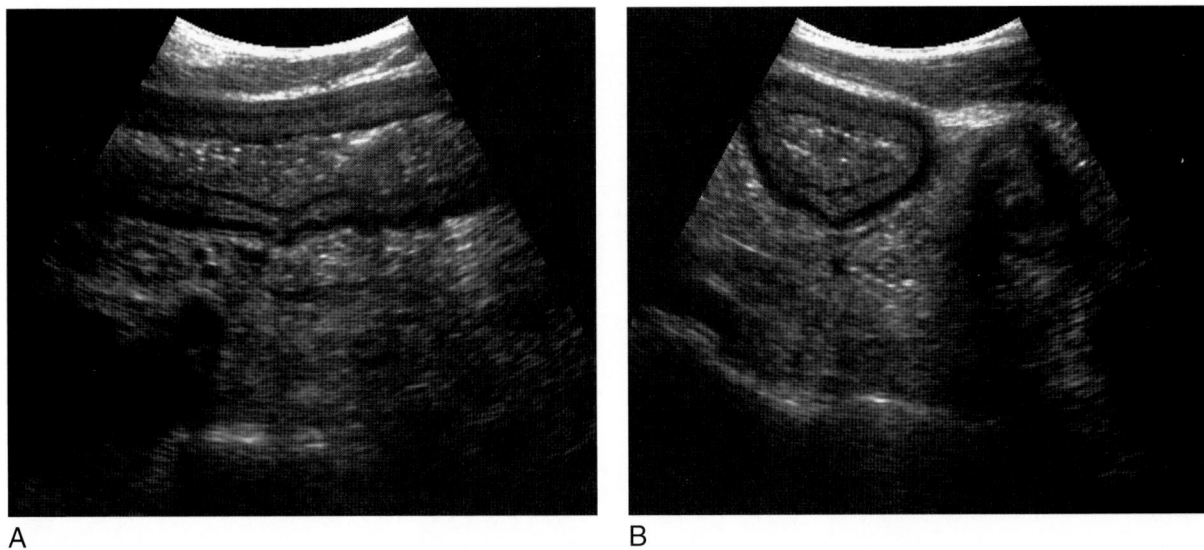

FIGURE 8-23. Crohn's disease—segment of involved gut proximal to a strictured segment. A, Long axis and **B,** cross-sectional images show thickening of the gut wall with layer preservation. The lumen is fluid filled and substantial in caliber.

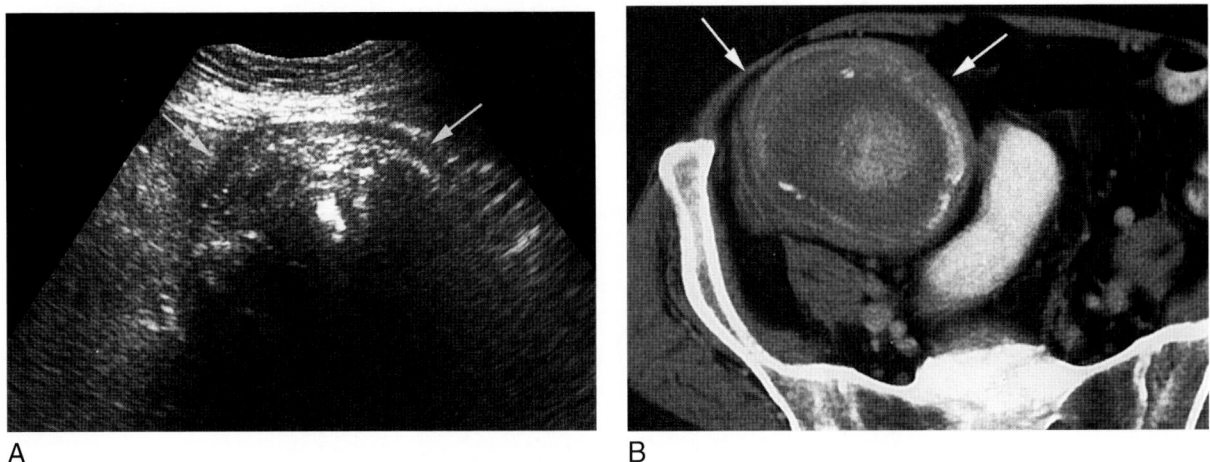

FIGURE 8-24. Small bowel bezoar in a patient with Crohn's disease with strictures. A, Sonogram of right lower quadrant shows a highly attenuating intraluminal mass. **B,** Confirmatory CT scan.

Perianal Inflammatory Problems

These are a frequent and debilitating complication of Crohn's disease. Highly complex transsphincteric tracts, which may extend to involve the deep tissues of the buttocks, the perineum, the scrotum in men, and the labia and vagina in women, are documented. Unlike commonly encountered perianal fistulae based on the crypto-glandular theory, fistulae in Crohn's disease have no predilection for the location of the internal openings and are highly complex. Transrectal ultrasound (TRUS) is frequently ordered in patients with rectal Crohn's disease or perianal pathology and may successfully show abscesses and fistulous tracts. However, we have not had uniform success with this procedure, which is often painful and noncontributory in this particular population. In contrast, in patients of either gender, we have found transperineal scanning to be a more comfortable and often more informative technique used alone or in combination with transrectal ultrasound.[27] Further, in women, we have found transvaginal scan to contribute greatly to our assessment of rectal and perirectal disease. It is also ideal for showing **enterovesical** (see Fig. 8-26A, B), **enterovaginal,** and **rectovaginal fistulae** (see Fig. 8-26D).[28] If bladder symptoms are present, we recommend that transvaginal sonography be performed with a partially full bladder. Further, the probe should be fully inserted and slowly withdrawn while elevating the examining hand to allow for evaluation of the entire rectum and anal canal in both sagittal and transverse planes. Rectal involvement in Crohn's disease is characterized by thickening of the rectal wall with wall layer preservation, inflammation of the perirectal fat, and enlargement of the perirectal lymph nodes (Fig. 8-27).

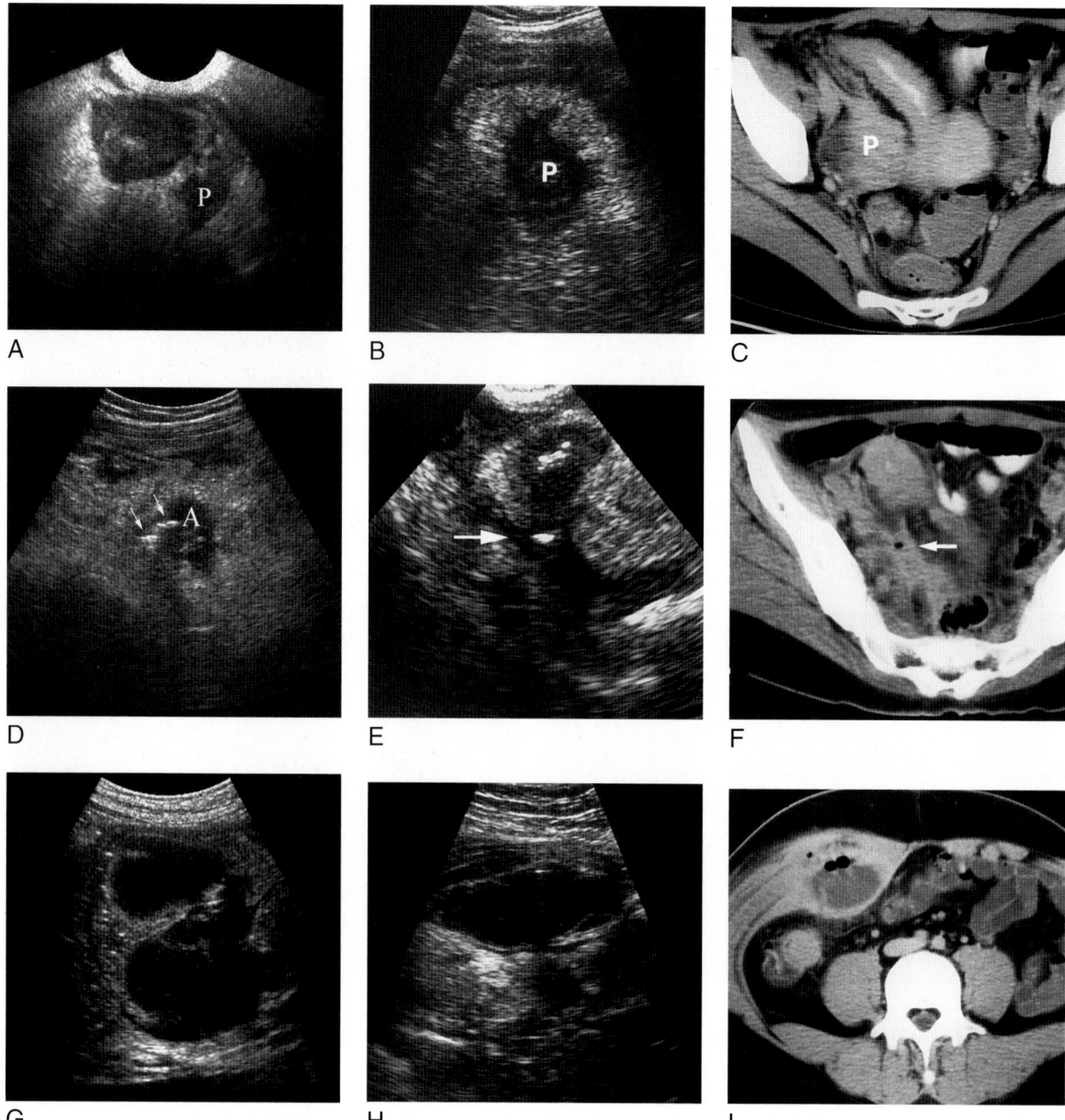

FIGURE 8-25. Crohn's complication—inflammatory masses. *Top line*—**phlegmons** (P). **A,** Loop of thick sigmoid colon is seen in cross section. Adjacent to the margin is a poorly defined, hypoechoic zone within extensive inflamed fat. **B,** Transverse sonogram in the right lower quadrant showing a thick terminal ileum superficially. There is extensive inflamed fat within which there is a poorly defined, hypoechoic zone representing the phlegmon (P). **B**—*Middle line*—**inflammatory masses with air but no drainable pus. C,** Confirmatory CT scan for image. **D,** Transverse image of the right lower quadrant. There is abundant inflamed fat. Centrally, there is a small fluid collection or abscess (A) with small echogenic shadowing foci (*arrows*) due to air bubbles. **E,** Cross-sectional sonogram through the terminal ileum shows thickening of the gut, echogenic, inflamed fat, and a poorly defined, focal hypoechoic area deep to the gut. Bubbles of gas outside of the gut are seen as bright echogenic foci (*arrow*) on sonography. **F,** Confirmatory CT scan for image. *Bottom line*—**drainable abscesses. G,** Large interloop fluid collection. **H,** Ultrasound and **I,** confirmatory CT scan, show a superficial fluid collection, with small gas bubbles, within the anterior abdominal wall. (**B, E, F, H, I,** From Sarrazin J, Wilson SR: Manifestations of Crohn disease at US. Radiographics 1996;16:499-520.)

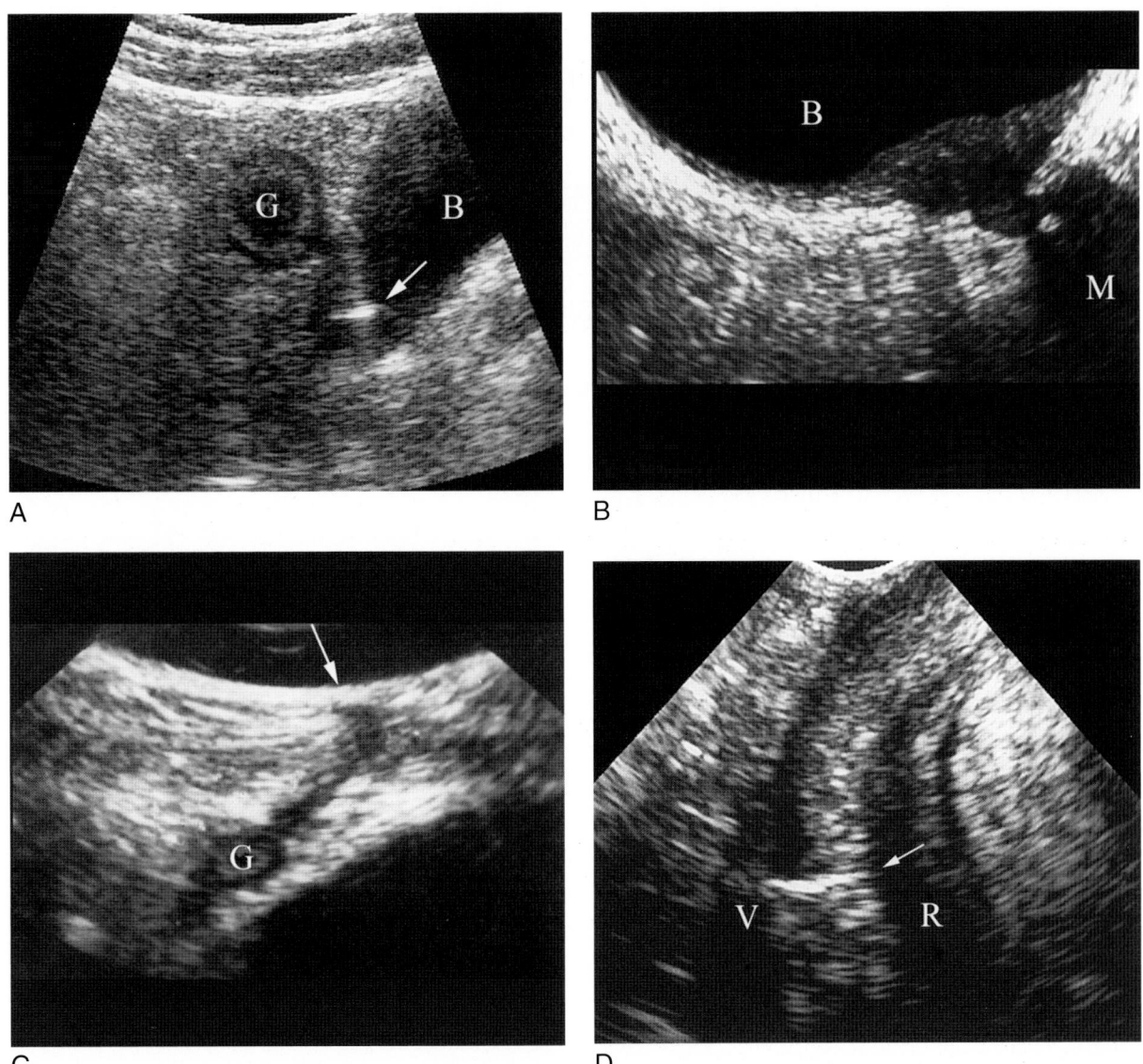

FIGURE 8-26. Crohn's complication—fistulae. A, Enterovesical fistula. There is a tract between the abnormal gut (G) and the bladder (B). An air bubble within shows as a bright echogenic focus (*arrow*). **B,** Enterovesical fistula. A hypoechoic tract connects an inflammatory mass (M) to the bladder (B). **C,** Enterocutaneous fistula. A hypoechoic tract runs from a loop of abnormal gut (G) to the skin surface (*arrow*). **D,** Rectovaginal fistula seen on transvaginal sonogram shows as an air-containing bright tract (*arrow*) which runs from the rectum (R) to the vagina (V).

The principles of interpretation of perianal inflammatory disease are discussed later in the section on endosonography.

ACUTE ABDOMEN

Sonography is a valuable imaging tool in patients who may have specific gastrointestinal disease, such as acute appendicitis or acute diverticulitis[29]; however, its contribution to the assessment of patients with possible GI tract disease is less certain. Seibert et al.[30] emphasized its great value in assessing the patient with a distended and gasless abdomen, in detecting ascites, unsuspected masses, and abnormally dilated fluid-filled loops of small bowel. In my experience, sonography has been helpful, not only in the gasless abdomen, but also in a wide variety of other situations. Sonography may add greatly to diagnostic acumen if used in conjunction with plain film radiography, CT, and other imaging modalities. The real-time aspect of sonographic study allows for direct interaction of the sonographer/physician with the patient with confirmation of palpable masses and/or focal points of tenderness. The doctrine **"scan where it hurts"** is invaluable and has led sonographers to describe the value of the sonographic equivalent to clinical examination with such descriptors as a *sonographic Murphy* or *sonographic McBurney* sign. Similar to the radiographic

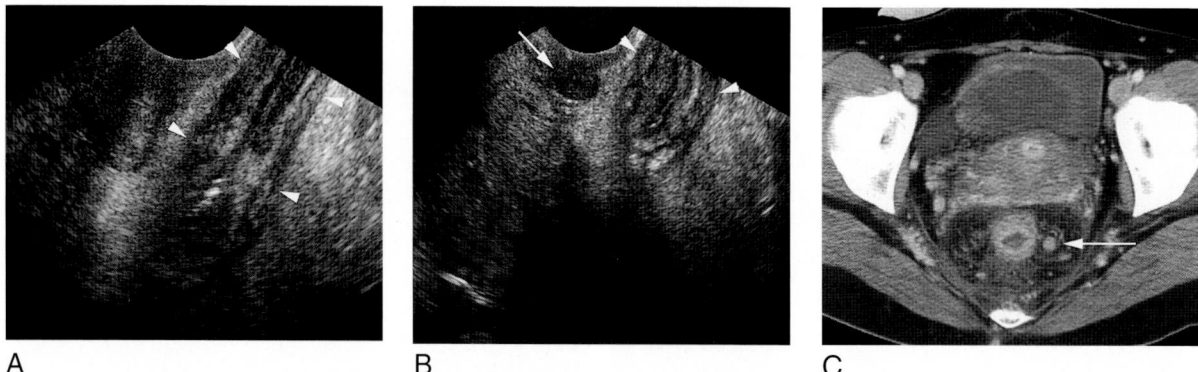

FIGURE 8-27. Crohn's complication—perianal inflammatory disease. A, Long axis view of the rectum taken with the probe in the vagina shows a thick rectum with wall layer preservation (*arrowheads*). Each wall measures 1.4 cm. Surrounding the rectum is an echogenic mass effect related to inflamed fat. **B,** Oblique view showing the thick-walled rectum (*arrowheads*), the echogenic, inflamed fat, and a hypoechoic, solid mass (*arrow*) representing an enlarged perirectal lymph node. **C,** Confirmatory CT scan shows the thick rectum, the inflamed fat, and the lymph nodes (*arrow*).

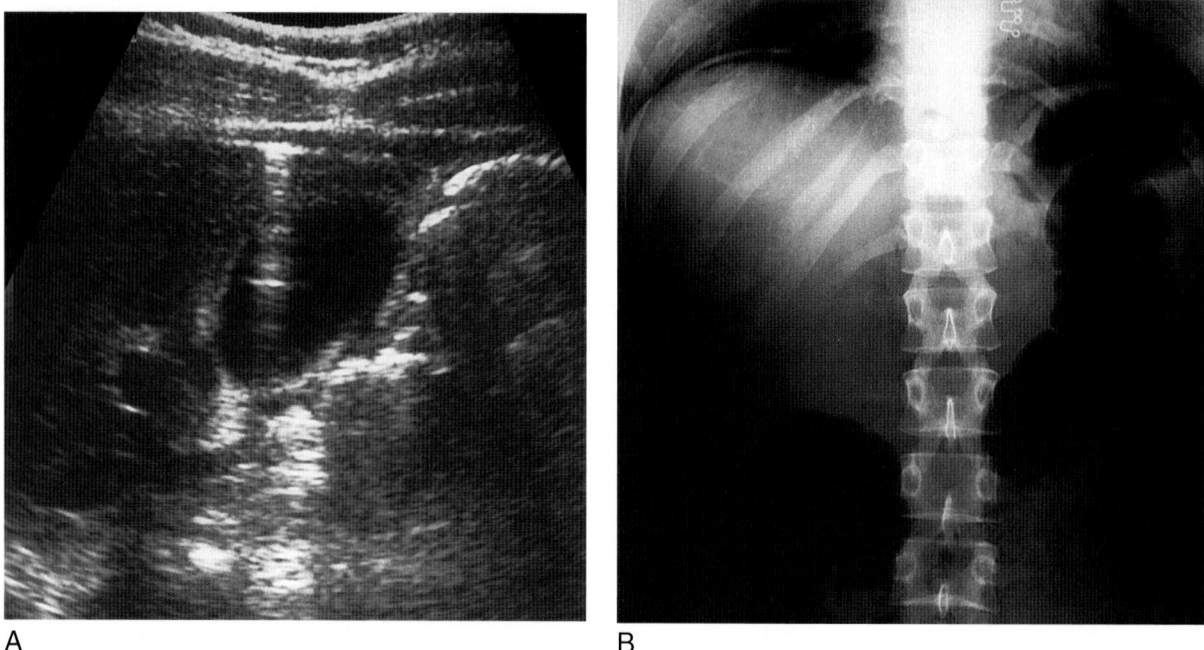

FIGURE 8-28. Gas—pneumoperitoneum. A, Sonogram shows a bright, echogenic focus representing free air between the abdominal wall and liver. Also shown is enhancement of the peritoneal stripe. **B,** Confirmatory plain film. (From Muradali D, Wilson S, Burn PN, et al: A specific sign of pneumoperitoneum on sonography: Enhancement of the peritoneal stripe. AJR 1999; 17(5):1257-1262.)

approach to plain film interpretation, a **systematic approach** is essential in the sonographic assessment of the abdomen in a patient with an acute abdomen of uncertain etiology.

This should include evaluation of visible **gas** and **fluid** to determine their luminal or extraluminal location, evaluation of the **perienteric soft tissues**, and the evaluation of the **gastrointestinal tract** itself. Identification of gas in a location where it is not usually found is a clue to many important diagnoses. The gas itself may appear as a bright echogenic focus, but it is the identification of the artifacts associated with the gas pockets that usually

leads to their detection. These include both "ringdown" artifacts and so-called *dirty shadowing*. Extraluminal gas may be intraperitoneal or retroperitoneal and its presence should raise the possibility of either hollow viscus perforation (Fig. 8-28) or infection with gas-forming organisms (Fig. 8-29).[31] Nonluminal gas may be easily overlooked, particularly if the collection is large. Gas in the wall of the gastrointestinal tract, pneumatosis intestinalis, with or without gas in the portal veins, raises the possibility of ischemic gut. Gas in the biliary ducts or gallbladder may be seen with spontaneous biliary enteric anastomosis or emphysematous cholecystitis.

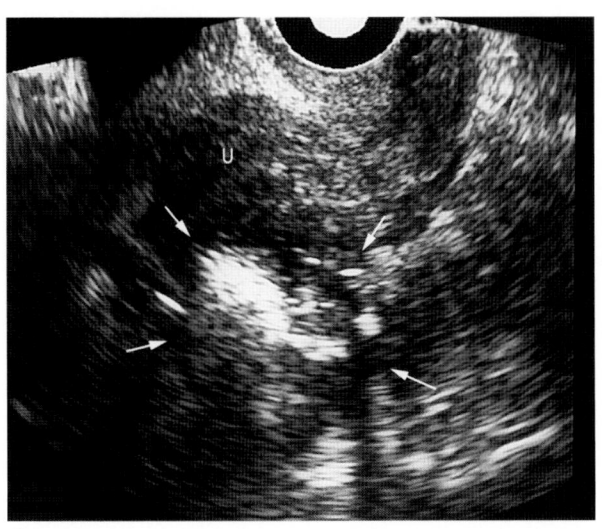
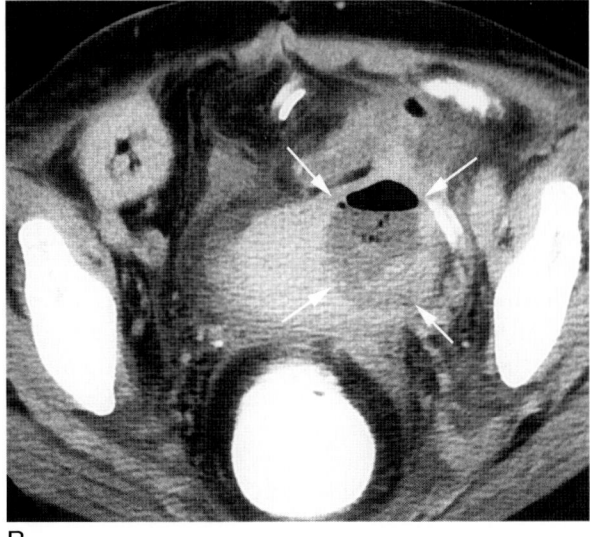

A   B

FIGURE 8-29. Gas-containing abscess. Unsuspected gas-containing abscess secondary to acute diverticulitis in a renal transplant recipient. **A,** Transvaginal image shows a large gas-containing mass (*arrows*) posterior to the uterus. **B,** CT scan confirms gas-containing abscess. This type of abscess may be very difficult to appreciate on suprapubic scan.

SONOGRAPHIC APPROACH TO THE PATIENT WITH AN ACUTE ABDOMEN

Gas	Intraluminal
	Extraluminal
	Intraperitoneal
	Retroperitoneal
	Gut wall
	Gallbladder/biliary ducts
	Portal veins
Fluid	Intraluminal
	Normal caliber gut
	Dilated gut
	Extraluminal
	Free
	Loculated

Masses
  Neoplastic
  Inflammatory
Perienteric soft tissues
  Inflamed fat
  Lymph nodes
Gut
  Wall
  Caliber
  Peristalsis
Clinical interaction
  Palpable mass
  Maximal tenderness
  Sonographic
    Murphy sign
  Sonographic
    McBurney sign

Free intraperitoneal gas may be difficult to detect on sonography and suspicion of its presence should prompt recommendation for further imaging. The potential for large artifacts from gas to obscure visualization of part or all of a sonographic image leads many to avoid the challenge of ultrasound interpretation with a preference for CT scan. However, there are valuable clues to the presence of intraperitoneal gas on sonography.

The likelihood of gas artifacts between the abdominal wall and the underlying liver to be related to free intra-peritoneal gas was nicely described by Lee et al.[31] In our own work, we have found that the peritoneal stripe appears as a bright, continuous echogenic line and that air adjacent to the peritoneal stripe produces enhancement of this layer because the gas has a higher acoustic impedance to sound waves than does the peritoneum itself (see Fig. 8-28). Careful peritoneal assessment is best done with a 5- or even 7.5-mHz probe with the focal zone set at the expected level of the peritoneum. In a clinical situation, **enhancement of the peritoneal stripe** is a highly specific but insensitive sign to detect pneumoperitoneum.[32]

Loculated fluid collections can mimic portions of the gastrointestinal tract. Left upper quadrant and pelvic collections suggestive of the stomach and rectum may be clarified by adding fluid orally and rectally. Assessing peristaltic activity and wall morphology also helps in distinguishing luminal from extraluminal collections. Interloop and flank collections are aperistaltic and tend to correspond in contour to the adjacent abdominal wall or intestinal loops, frequently forming acute angles, which are rarely seen with intraluminal fluid.

The appearance of the **perienteric soft tissues** is frequently the first and most obvious clue to abdominal pathology on abdominal sonograms. **Inflammation of the perienteric fat** shows as a hyperechoic mass effect (see Fig. 8-20) often with absence of the usual appearance created by normal gut with its contained small pockets of gas. Neoplastic infiltration of the perienteric fat is often indistinguishable from inflammatory infiltration on ultrasound (see Fig. 8-11).

Mesenteric adenopathy is another manifestation of both inflammatory and neoplastic processes of the gut, which should be specifically sought when performing abdominal sonography. As elsewhere, lymph nodes tend to change in size and shape when they are replaced by abnormal tissue. A normal oval or flattened lymph node with a normal linear hilar echo becomes increasingly round and hypoechoic with either inflammatory or neoplastic replacement. In contrast to the sonographic appearance of loops of gut, mesenteric lymph nodes typically appear as focal, discrete hypoechoic masses of varying size (Figs. 8-8C and 8-21). Their identification on sonography suggests enlargement because they are not normally seen on routine examinations. Abnormal masses related to or causing gastrointestinal tract abnormality should also be sought. These are most commonly neoplastic or inflammatory in origin.

Right Lower Quadrant Pain

Acute Appendicitis

Acute appendicitis is the most common explanation for the so-called acute abdomen presentation to an emergency department. Patients typically have right lower quadrant pain, tenderness, and leucocytosis. A mass may also be palpable. With a classic presentation, the patient is often treated with surgery for appendectomy without preoperative imaging. This is often complicated by surgical removal of a normal appendix in a patient for whom there is another explanation for their symptomatology. Furthermore, surgery may be delayed in some patients with acute appendicitis if the presentation is atypical. This may lead to perforation prior to the surgery, making it a complicated and difficult procedure, often followed by abscess formation. In the clinical literature, laparotomy resulting in removal of normal, noninflamed appendices is reported in 16% to 47% of cases, mean 26%.[33-35] Equally distressing, perforation may occur in up to 35%.[36] It is a balance between this *negative laparotomy rate* and the *perforation rate at surgery* that motivates cross-sectional imaging prior to initiating treatment for the patient who presents with acute right lower quadrant pain. In performing a sonogram on a patient with suspected appendicitis, the objectives are: **to identify the patient with acute appendicitis, to identify the patient without acute appendicitis**, and in this latter population, **to identify an alternate explanation for their right lower quadrant pain**.

There is a well-recognized overlap of symptomatology of appendicitis with a variety of other gastrointestinal conditions, including **acute typhlitis**, **acute mesenteric adenitis**, **variations of Crohn's disease**, **right-sided diverticulitis**, and **acute segmental infarction of the omentum**. In women, this list is expanded to include acute gynecologic conditions.[37] It is important to recognize that not only can other conditions suggest acute appendicitis but that acute appendicitis may also suggest other diagnoses, particularly acute pelvic inflammatory disease. This occurs most often when the appendix is located in the true pelvis, in which case acute inflammatory change may implicate the uterine cervix and ovaries on clinical examination. The appendix is most commonly located caudal to the base of the cecum. It may also be retrocecal and retroileal. In a minority of patients, the appendix may be located in the true pelvis. It is in this situation that confusion in diagnosis occurs, most often in terms of mistaken diagnosis with gynecologic disease.

From a retrospective review of 462 patients with suspected appendicitis who underwent appendectomy, Bendeck et al. found that women, in particular, benefit most from preoperative imaging, with a statistically significant lower negative appendectomy rate than that in women who undergo no preoperative imaging.[38] In their study, they found no similar improvement in the negative appendectomy rate for girls, boys, or men. CT and ultrasound both provide sensitive and accurate diagnosis of appendicitis. The choice of imaging modality is motivated to some extent on local expertise.[39] Some institutions also screen patients on the basis of their weight, sending thin patients for ultrasound and

---

SONOGRAPHIC DIAGNOSIS OF ACUTE APPENDICITIS

Patient with right lower-quadrant pain/elevated white blood cell count

IDENTIFY APPENDIX

Blind ended
Noncompressible
Aperistaltic tube
Gut signature
Arising from base of cecum
Diameter greater than 6 mm

SUPPORTIVE FEATURES

Inflamed perienteric fat
Pericecal collections
Appendicolith

reserving CT for larger patients. These considerations aside, we recommend sonographic evaluation of all women—with the addition of transvaginal scan in all patients on whom the explanation for the pain is not evident on completion of a traditional suprapubic pelvic sonogram.

The **pathophysiology** in the development of acute appendicitis is believed to be obstruction of the appendiceal lumen, 35% of cases demonstrating a fecalith.[40] Mucosal secretions continue, increasing the intraluminal pressure and compromising venous return. The mucosa becomes hypoxic and ulcerates. Bacterial infection ensues with ultimate gangrene and perforation. Walled-off abscess is more common than free peritoneal contamination.

Acute appendicitis begins with transient, visceral, or referred crampy pain in the periumbilical area associated with nausea and vomiting. Coincident with inflammation of the serosa of the appendix, the pain shifts to the right lower quadrant and may be associated with physical signs of peritoneal irritation. Both clinical and experimental data support the belief that some patients have repeated attacks of appendicitis.[41,42] Surgical specimens have shown chronic inflammatory infiltrate in patients with recurrent attacks of right lower-quadrant pain before appendectomy.

In 1986, Julien Puylaert described the value of **graded compression sonography** in the evaluation of 60 consecutive patients suspected of having acute appendicitis.[7] Since then, other investigators have improved the sonographic criteria for diagnosis, firmly establishing the value of sonography in assessing patients with equivocal evidence of this disease. The accuracy afforded by sonography should keep negative laparotomy rates at approximately 10%,[43] clearly an improvement over the rate achieved by instinct alone.

Puylaert's[7] initial reports of success in diagnosing acute appendicitis with compression sonography depended solely on visualization of the appendix: a blind-ended, noncompressible, aperistaltic tube, arising from the tip of the cecum with a gut signature (Figs. 8-30 and 8-31). However, other investigators have reported seeing normal appendices on a sonogram (Fig. 8-32).[44,45] The normal appendix is compressible with wall thickness of less than or equal to 3 mm.[46] Jeffrey and colleagues[43] concluded that the size of an appendix can differentiate the normal from the acutely inflamed. Threshold levels for the diameter of the appendix, above which acute appendicitis is highly likely to be present, have been set at either 6 or 7 mm, with resultant change of sensitivity and specificity. Sonographic visualization of an appendix with an appendicolith, regardless of appendiceal diameter, should also be regarded as a positive test (see Fig. 8-30). Rettenbacher et al.[47] have recently described the additional value of assessment of appendiceal morphology in confirming suspicion of

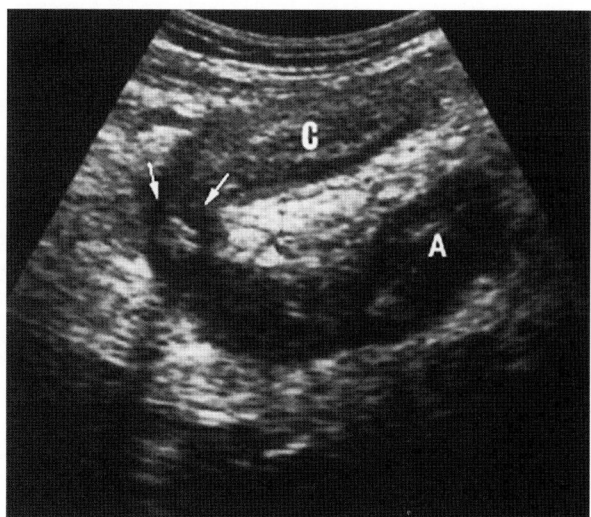

FIGURE 8-30. Acute appendicitis. The inflamed appendix (A) is seen as a blind-ended, aperistaltic, noncompressible tubular structure, arising from the cecum (C). A faintly shadowing appendicolith (*arrows*) is seen.

appendicitis. A round or partly round appendix had a high correlation with acute appendicitis as compared with an ovoid appendix, which did not (see Fig. 8-31). Color Doppler is also contributory, showing hyperemia in the appendiceal wall in the acutely inflamed appendix.

Recently Lee et al.[48] described graded compression sonography with adjuvant use of a **posterior manual compression technique** for the sonographic diagnosis of acute appendicitis. With graded compression sonography alone, they achieved visualization of the vermiform appendix in 485 (85%) of 570 patients. After the adjuvant use of a posterior manual compression technique, the vermiform appendix was found in an additional 57 of 85 patients, with the number of identified vermiform appendices increasing to 542 (95%) of 570 patients.

Inflammation of the **appendix that is positioned in the true pelvis** may show subtle evidence of this on a suprapubic scan because the pathology may be deep in the pelvic cavity. In our experience, this occurs most often in women, possibly related to a more capacious pelvis, and the clinical presentation is frequently that of pelvic inflammatory disease. This particular pathology is optimally studied with transvaginal placement of

SONOGRAPHY OF APPENDICEAL PERFORATION

Loculated pericecal fluid
  Phlegmon
  Abscess
Prominent pericecal fat
Circumferential loss of the submucosal layer

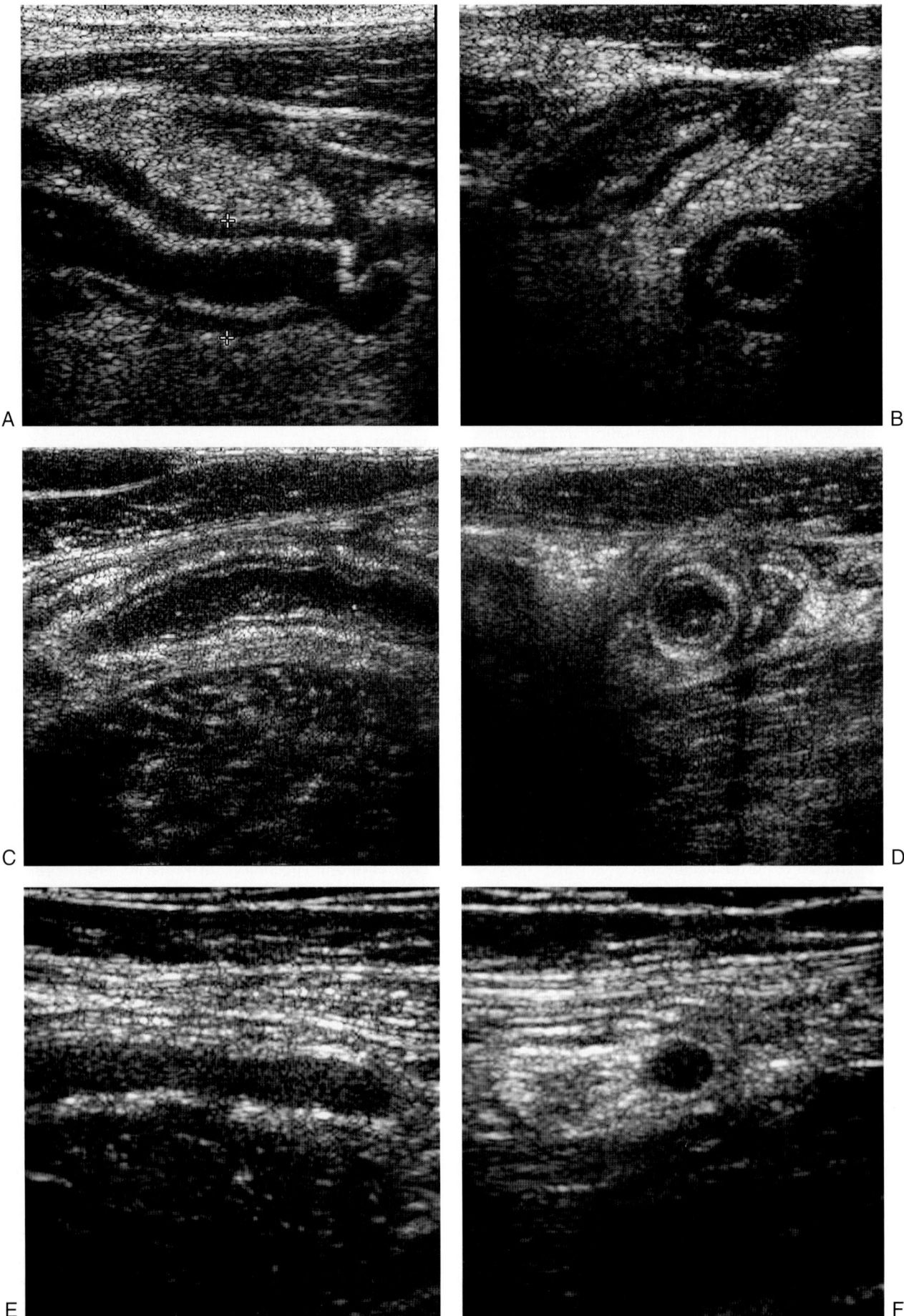

FIGURE 8-31. Acute appendicitis in three patients—spectrum of appearances. A, C, and **E** are long axis views and show the blind-ended tip of the appendix. In **C,** the tip is directed to the left of the image as the appendix ascends cephalad from its origin from the cecum. **B, D, and F** are corresponding cross-sectional views. The appendix looks round in short axis on all cases and the lumen is distended with fluid. The appendix is surrounded with inflamed fat. The gut signature is preserved in the top two cases. The bottom case shows loss of definition of the wall layers, suggestive of gangrenous change.

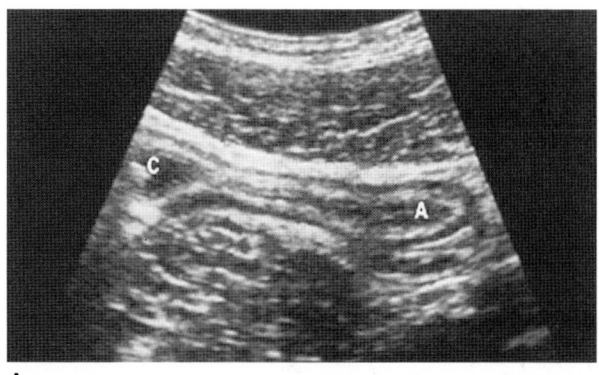
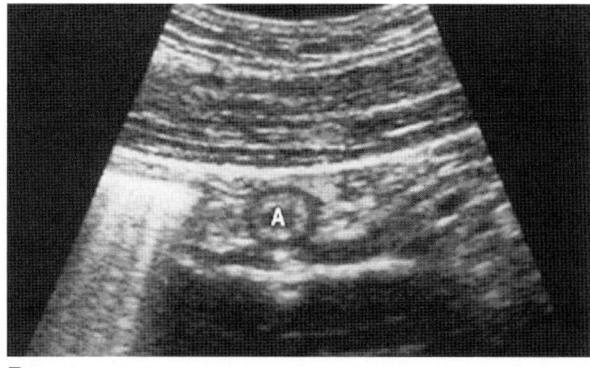

A   B

FIGURE 8-32. Normal appendix. A, Long axis and **B,** cross-sectional images show the normal appendix (A) arising from the base of the cecum (C). The appendix shows a gut signature, a blind end, and measures 6 mm or less in diameter.

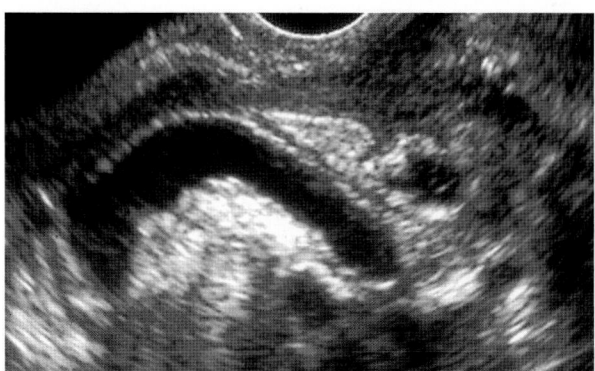

FIGURE 8-33. Acute appendicitis of a pelvic appendix seen on transvaginal sonogram only.
Sonogram shows the blind-ended tip of the fluid-distended appendix.

the ultrasound probe because the appendix is often intimately related to either the uterus and/or the ovaries. The sonographic features required for diagnosis are identical, although the origin of such an appendix from the base of the cecum may be impossible to determine on transvaginal sonography, and compression with the ultrasound probe is often not feasible. Nonetheless, the identification of the blind-ended tip of the appendix with an increased diameter, luminal distention, and inflammation of the surrounding fat is obvious (Fig. 8-33). If rupture of a pelvic appendix has occurred prior to the sonogram, the identification of a pelvic abscess without identification of the appendix itself may produce an equivocal result as to the source of the pelvic inflammatory problem.

Although the sensitivity of sonography for the diagnosis of appendicitis decreases with **perforation**, features statistically associated with its occurrence include loculated pericecal fluid, phlegmon or abscess, prominent pericecal or periappendiceal fat, and circumferential loss of the submucosal layer of the appendix (Fig. 8-34).[49] False-positive diagnosis for acute appendicitis may occur if a normal appendix or a thickened

terminal ileum is mistaken for an inflamed appendix. Awareness of the diagnostic criteria stated previously, particularly related to appendiceal diameter and morphology, should minimize these errors.

Clinical misdiagnosis of appendicitis occurs most frequently in young women with gynecologic conditions, especially **acute pelvic inflammatory disease, rupture or torsion of ovarian cysts,** and **postpartum ovarian vein thrombosis.** Bendeck et al.[38] have recently confirmed that women suspected of having appendicitis benefit the most from preoperative CT or ultrasound, with a statistically significant lower negative appendectomy rate than women who undergo no preoperative imaging. They concluded that preoperative imaging should be part of the routine evaluation of women suspected of having acute appendicitis.

Other diseases than those of gynecologic origin may also be misdiagnosed as acute appendicitis. Gastrointestinal illnesses include acute terminal ileitis with **mesenteric adenitis,**[50] **acute typhlitis, acute diverticulitis,** especially of a cecal tip diverticulum, and **Crohn's disease** in the ileocecal area or involving the appendix itself.[52] Urologic disease, especially **stone-related** and **right-sided segmental omental infarction,** may also mimic acute appendicitis. The value of sonography in establishing an **alternative diagnosis** in patients with suspected acute appendicitis was addressed by Gaensler et al.,[51] who found that 70% of patients with another diagnosis had abnormalities visualized on the sonogram.

Crohn's Appendicitis

Patients with Crohn's disease may present with acute appendicitis due to inflammatory bowel involvement of the appendix as distinct from acute suppurative appendicitis. The **wall of the appendix** is typically **markedly thickened** and hyperemic with wall layer preservation, and the **luminal surfaces are often in apposition** (Fig. 8-35).[52] This is in sharp contrast with the appearances in suppurative appendicitis, where luminal

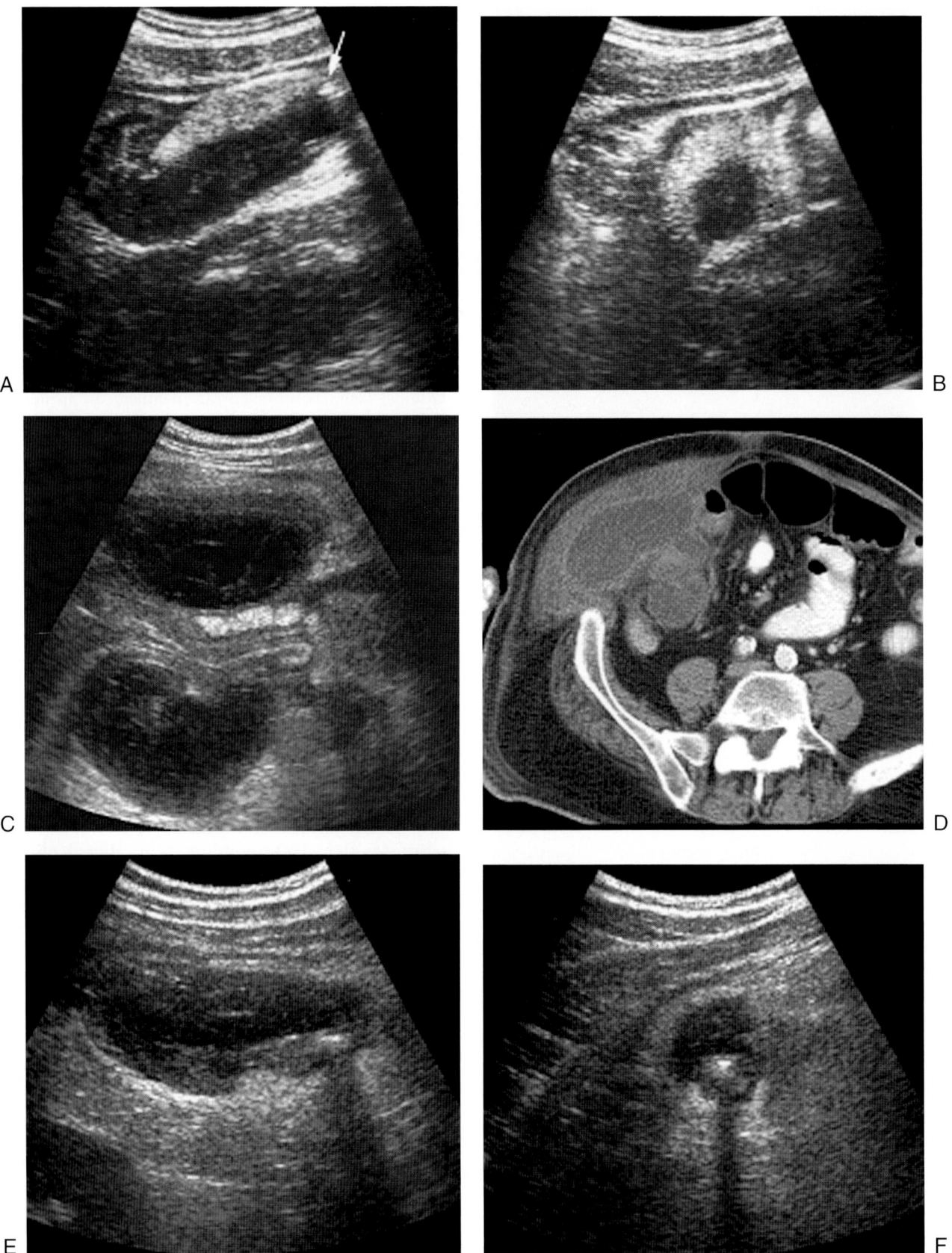

FIGURE 8-34. Perforation of the appendix in three patients—spectrum of appearances. **A,** Long axis and **B,** cross-sectional images show the blind-ended appendix. There is loss of definition of the wall layers and the appendix is surrounded by an echogenic mass effect representing inflamed fat in the mesoappendix. The *arrow* points to a bubble of extraluminal gas at the tip of the appendix. Confirmed tip perforation at surgery. **C,** Sonogram and **D,** CT scan show a periappendiceal fluid collection or abscess.[39] The decompressed appendix is seen centrally on the sonogram. **E** and **F,** Long axis and transverse images in the right lower quadrant showing an abscess with an escaped appendicolith with acoustic shadowing. The appendix is no longer visible. (**C,** From Birnbaum BA, Wilson SR: Appendicitis at the millennium. Radiology 2000;215(2):337-348.)

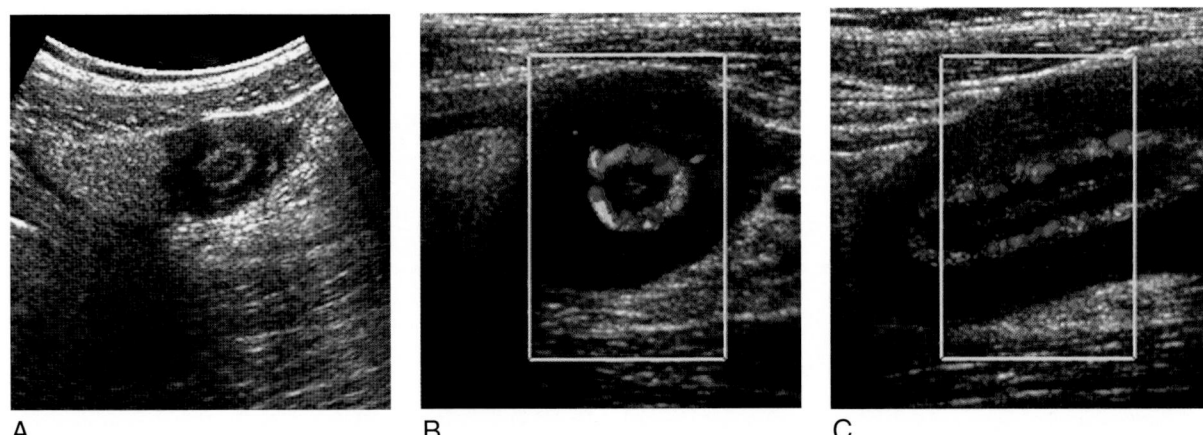

A   B   C

FIGURE 8-35. Crohn's appendicitis. A, Transverse sonogram in the right lower quadrant shows a very thick-walled loop of gut surrounded by inflamed fat. High frequency linear images of this loop of gut. **B,** Cross section and **C,** long axis show that it is blind ended. There is massive mural thickening and hyperemia. The luminal surfaces are in apposition. All changes resolved completely with conservative management. (From Wilson SR: The bowel wall looks thickened: What does that mean? Categorical course in diagnostic radiology: Findings at US—what do they mean? Radiological Society of North America. 2002, 219-228.)

distention is the expectation and wall thickening is usually moderate at most.

Crohn's appendicitis is a self-limited process[53,54] and **treatment** may be conservative if the appropriate diagnosis can be established with noninvasive techniques. In a small number of patients on whom we have suggested this diagnosis, follow-up sonograms have shown resolution of the sonographic findings with no progression of their disease. Patients with Crohn's disease who present with Crohn's appendicitis account for about 10% of total presentations. This patient population typically has a more benign course. If the appendix is removed surgically in the mistaken belief that the patient has acute suppurative appendicitis, recurrence or progression of Crohn's disease is rare.

Right-sided Diverticulitis

Acute inflammation of a right-sided diverticulum is distinct from the more common diverticulitis that is encountered in the left hemicolon. These diverticula occur more often in women than in men and have a predilection for Asian populations. Most affected patients are young adults. Right-sided diverticula are usually solitary and are congenital in origin. They are **true diverticula** and have, therefore, all layers of the gut wall. Their inflammation is associated with right lower quadrant pain, tenderness, and leukocytosis with a mistaken diagnosis of appendicitis in virtually all cases.

On sonography, acute diverticulitis is associated with inflammation of the pericolonic fat. The diverticula may be located in the cecum or the adjacent ascending colon. When inflamed, they may have one of two appearances.[55] Most commonly, the diverticulum may show as a **pouch or saclike structure** arising from the colonic wall (Fig. 8-36).[56] Wall layers are continued into the wall of the congenital diverticulum. Hyperemia of the diverticulum and the inflamed fat is typical. If a **fecalith** is present within the diverticulum, it may show as a **bright echogenic focus** located within or beyond a segment of thickened colonic wall. On occasion, the culprit diverticulum may not be evident and the only observations may be the inflamed fat and the focal thickening of the colonic wall (see Fig. 8-36). In the appropriate clinical milieu, this is highly suspicious for acute diverticulitis.

Treatment of acute diverticulitis is conservative and not surgical, emphasizing the importance of preoperative imaging in patients with right lower quadrant pain attributed to this condition.

Acute Typhlitis

Immunocompromised patients are most often affected, with AIDS patients accounting for the overwhelming majority of cases of acute typhlitis seen since 1990. Cytomegalovirus (CMV) and *Cryptosporidium* are the pathogens isolated most often in patients with typhlitis and colitis, although other organisms have been implicated. Sonographic study most commonly shows striking **concentric, uniform thickening of the colon wall**, usually localized to the cecum and the adjacent ascending colon (Fig. 8-37).[57] The colon wall may be several times normal in thickness, reflecting inflammatory infiltration throughout the gut wall.[58,59] Acute abdominal catastrophe in patients with AIDS is usually a complication of CMV colitis with deep ulceration and may result in hemorrhage, perforation, and peritonitis.[60] Tuberculous colitis may similarly affect the right colon and is frequently associated with lymphadenopathy

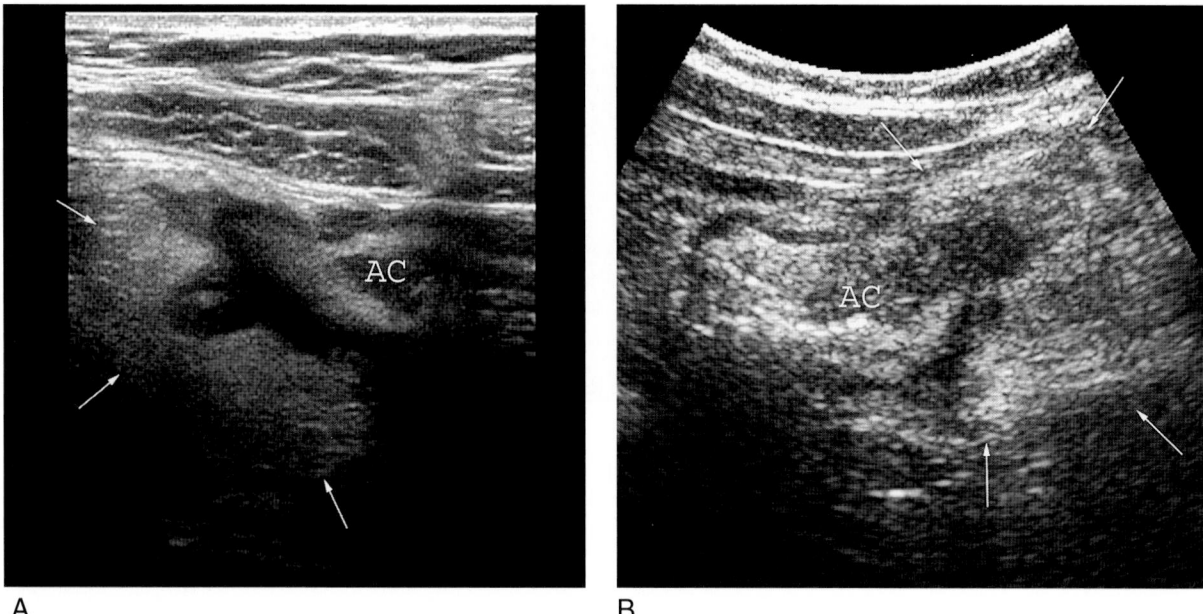

FIGURE 8-36. Right sided diverticulitis in two patients. Transverse sonograms through the ascending colon (AC) show a hypoechoic pouch-like projection, representing the inflamed diverticulum, which arises from the lateral wall of the gut in **A** and from the medial border of the gut in **B**. Both are surrounded by inflamed fat (*arrows*).

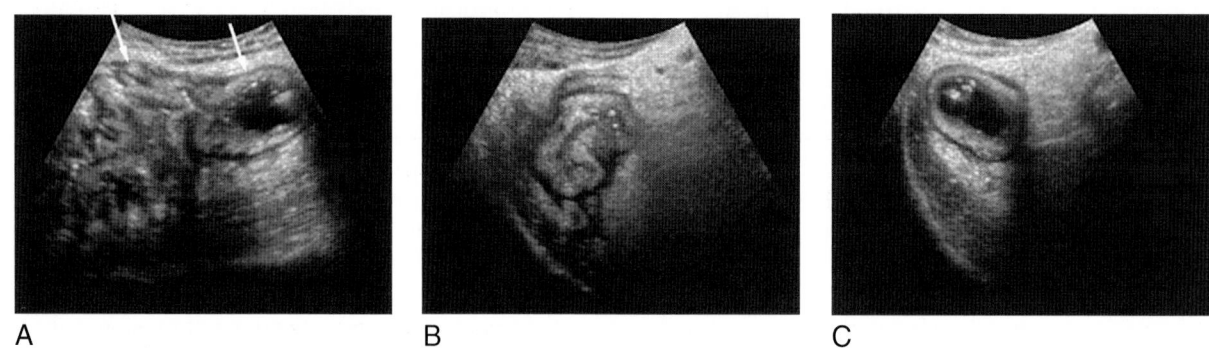

FIGURE 8-37. Acute typhlitis. A, Long axis view of the ascending colon shows marked mural thickening of the cecum and the wall of the ascending colon. Wall layer preservation is noted. **B,** At the level of the *left arrow* in **A** is a cross-sectional view of the thickened colon, with luminal surfaces in apposition. **C,** At the level of the *right arrow* in **A** is a cross-sectional view of the cecum, which is thick walled and shows a fluid-filled lumen. (From Wilson SR: The bowel wall looks thickened: What does that mean? Categorical course in diagnostic radiology: Findings at US—what do they mean? Radiological Society of North America. 2002, 219-228.)

(particularly involving the mesenteric and omental nodes), splenomegaly, intrasplenic masses, ascites, and peritoneal masses, all of which may be assessed using sonography.

Mesenteric Adenitis and Acute Terminal Ileitis

Mesenteric adenitis, in association with acute terminal ileitis, is the most frequent gastrointestinal cause of misdiagnosis of acute appendicitis. Patients typically have right lower-quadrant pain and tenderness. On the **sonographic examination**, **enlarged mesenteric lymph nodes** and **mural thickening of the terminal ileum** are noted. *Yersinia enterocolitica* and *Campylobacter jejuni* are the most common causative agents.[50,61]

Right-sided Segmental Omental Infarction

Right-sided segmental infarction of the omentum is a rare condition that is virtually always mistaken clinically for acute appendicitis.[62] Of unknown etiology, it is postulated to occur with an anomalous and fragile blood supply to the right lower omentum, making it susceptible to painful infarction.[63] Patients present with right lower-quadrant pain and tenderness and are invariably thought to have acute appendicitis clinically. On sonography, **a plaque or cake-like area of increased echogenicity** suggesting inflamed or infiltrated fat is seen superficially in the right flank with adherence to the peritoneum (Fig. 8-38).[62] No underlying gut abnormality is shown. As segmental infarction is a self-limited process, its correct diagnosis will prevent unnecessary

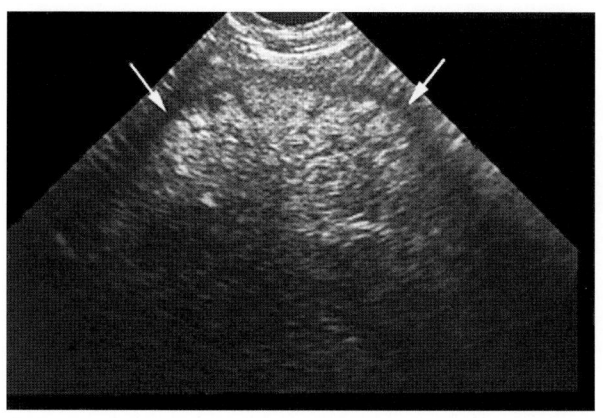
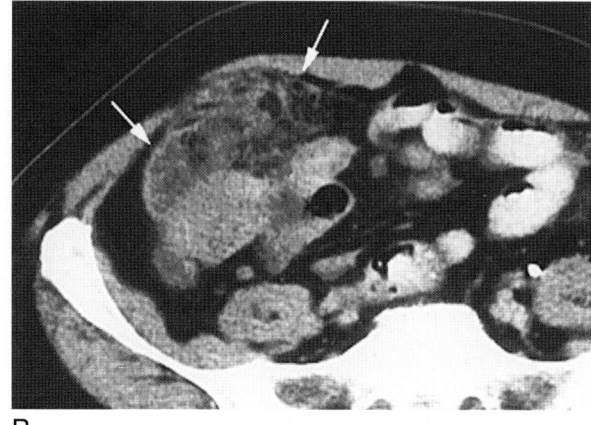

A   B

FIGURE 8-38. Acute omental infarction in an elderly man with acute right lower-quadrant pain. A, Sonogram shows a large, tender mass in the right lower quadrant (*arrows*). The mass is uniformly echogenic and attenuating, with an ultrasound appearance suggesting inflamed fat. **B,** Confirmatory CT scan.

SONOGRAPHY OF DIVERTICULITIS

Segmental concentric thickening of gut wall
   Hypoechoic reflecting muscular hypertrophy
Inflamed diverticula
   Echogenic foci within or beyond gut wall
   Acoustic shadowing or "ringdown" artifact
Inflammation of pericolonic fat
   Hyperechoic mass effect
Abscess formation
   Loculated fluid collection
   Often with gas component
Intramural sinus tracts
   High-amplitude linear echoes within gut wall
   Fistulae
   Linear tracts from gut to bladder, vagina, or
     adjacent loops
   Hypo- or hyperechoic
Thickening of the mesentery

surgery. CT scan is confirmatory, showing streaky fat in a masslike configuration in the right side of the omentum.

Left Lower Quadrant Pain

The sonographic evaluation of the patient with left lower quadrant pain is less problematic than the evaluation of the patient with pain on the right side. The wide differential possibilities for right lower-quadrant pain are not present and acute diverticulitis is the explanation for the overwhelming majority of cases for which a valid explanation for the pain is found. The diagnostic features of acute diverticulitis are also less variable than those for acute appendicitis, making a suspicion of diverticulitis a very good indication for the use of sonographic examination.

Acute Diverticulitis

Diverticula of the colon are usually acquired deformities and are found most frequently in western urban civilizations.[64] The incidence of diverticula increases with age,[65] affecting approximately one half the population by the ninth decade. Muscular dysfunction and hypertrophy are constant associated features. Diverticula are usually multiple: their most common location is the sigmoid and left colon. Acute diverticulitis and spastic diverticulosis may both be associated with a classic triad of presentation: left lower-quadrant pain, fever, and leukocytosis. Diverticula may also be found singly and in the right colon, where no association with muscular hypertrophy and dysfunction has been established.

Inspissated fecal material is believed to incite the initial inflammation in the apex of the diverticulum leading to acute diverticulitis.[66] Spread to the peridiverticular tissues and microperforation or macroperforation may follow. Localized abscess formation occurs more commonly than does peritonitis. Fistula formation, with communication to the bladder, vagina, skin, or other bowel loops, is present in the minority of cases. Surgical specimens demonstrate shortening and thickening of the involved segment of colon, associated with muscular hypertrophy. The peridiverticular inflammatory response may be minimal or very extensive.

Sonography appears to be of value in early assessment of patients thought to have acute diverticulitis.[67,68] Classic features include segmental thickened gut and inflamed diverticula and inflamed perienteric fat. A negative scan combined with a low clinical suspicion is usually a good indication to stop investigation. However, a negative scan in a patient with a highly suggestive clinical picture justifies a CT scan. Similarly, demonstration of extensive pericolonic inflammatory changes on the sonogram may be appropriately followed by

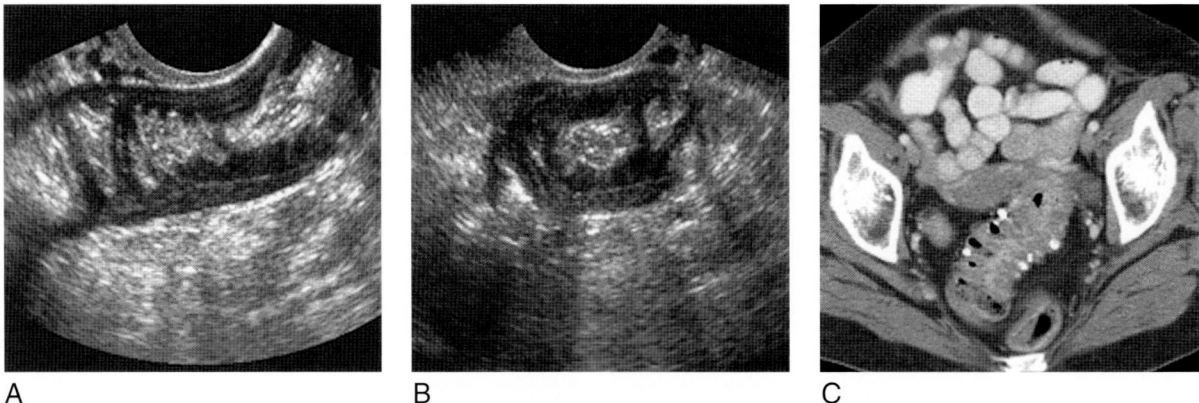

A   B   C

FIGURE 8-39. Muscular hypertrophy from diverticular disease of the colon. A, Long axis sonogram of the sigmoid colon shows prominence of the outer muscular layer, the muscularis propria, which appears hypoechoic. The outer longitudinal muscle fibers are slightly more echogenic than the inner circular muscle fibers. **B,** Cross-sectional view. **C,** Characteristic CT scan showing the effects of the smooth-muscle hypertrophy.

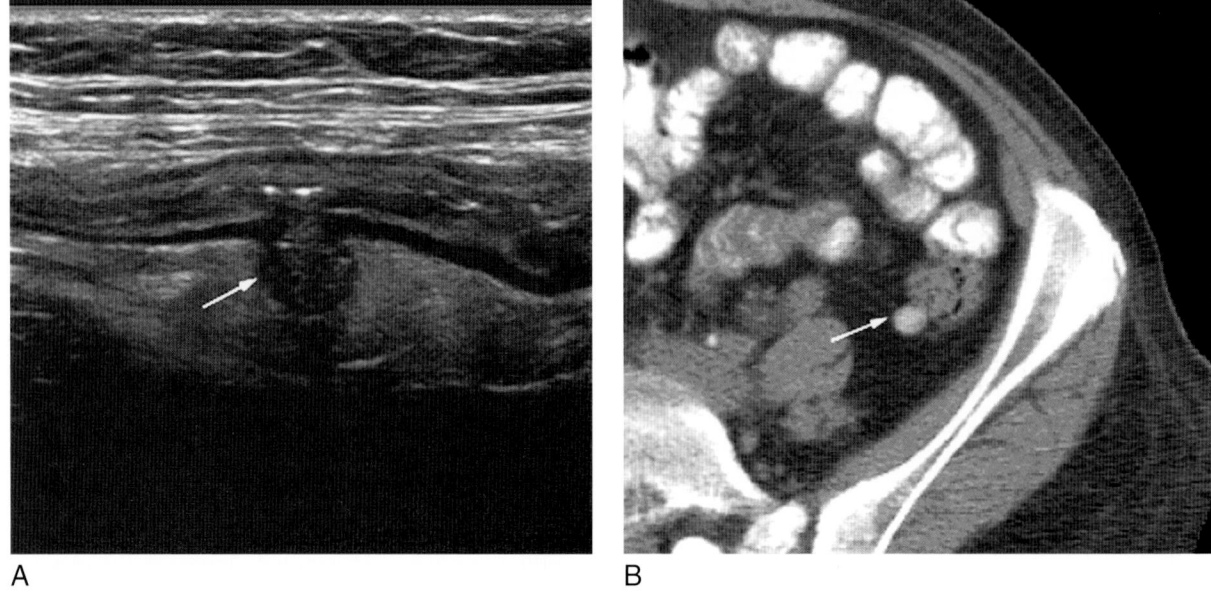

A   B

FIGURE 8-40. Diverticulum of the colon. A, Long axis sonogram and **B,** correlative CT scan both show a small pouch (*arrow*) arising from the wall of the descending colon. There is mild inflammatory change in the perienteric fat.

CT scan to better define the nature and extent of the pericolonic disease before surgery or other intervention.

Because diverticula and smooth muscle hypertrophy of the colon are so prevalent, it seems likely that they would be commonly seen on routine sonography, but this is not the usual experience. However, with the development of acute diverticulitis, both the inflamed diverticulum and the thickened colon become evident. Presumably the impacted fecalith, with or without microabscess formation, accentuates the diverticulum, whereas smooth muscle spasm, inflammation, and edema accentuate the gut wall thickening. Identification of diverticula on the sonogram strongly indicates diverticulitis.[69]

Diverticula are arranged in parallel rows along the margins of the teniae coli; therefore careful technique is required to make their identification. Following demonstration of a thickened loop of gut (Fig. 8-39), the long axis of the loop should be determined. Slight tilting of the transducer to the margins of the loop will increase visualization of the diverticula because they may be on the lateral and medial edges of the loop rather than directly anterior or posterior. Cross-sectional views are then obtained running along the entire length of the thickened gut. Abnormalities must be confirmed on both views. Errors related to overlapping gut loops, in particular, can be virtually eliminated with this careful technique. Identification of diverticula on sonography is correlated highly with inflammation, because it is unusual to show the diverticula in the absence of inflammation (Fig. 8-40).

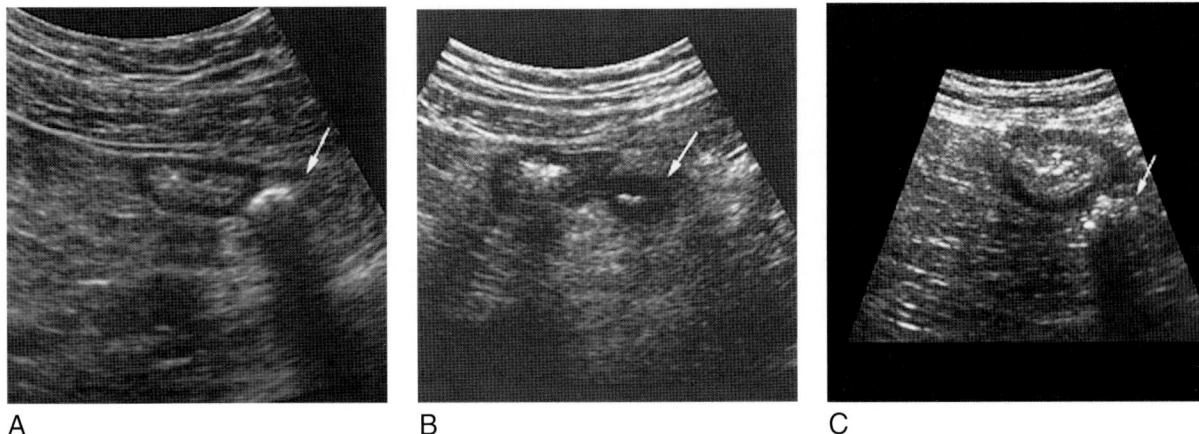

FIGURE 8-41. Acute diverticulitis of the sigmoid colon in three patients. A, B, and **C,** Cross sectional views of part of the left colon. **A,** Mild prominence of the muscular layer. The diverticulum (*arrow*) shows as a bright, echogenic shadowing focus possibly related to a fecalith within. The wall of the diverticulum is not evident. There is little inflamed fat. **B,** Diverticulum (*arrow*) has a thick and hypoechoic wall. There is a small, bright focus centrally but no shadowing. **C,** Larger focus of echogenicity and shadowing related to the abscess that forms at the base of the inflamed diverticulum (*arrow*). Diverticula frequently show optimally on the cross-sectional images.

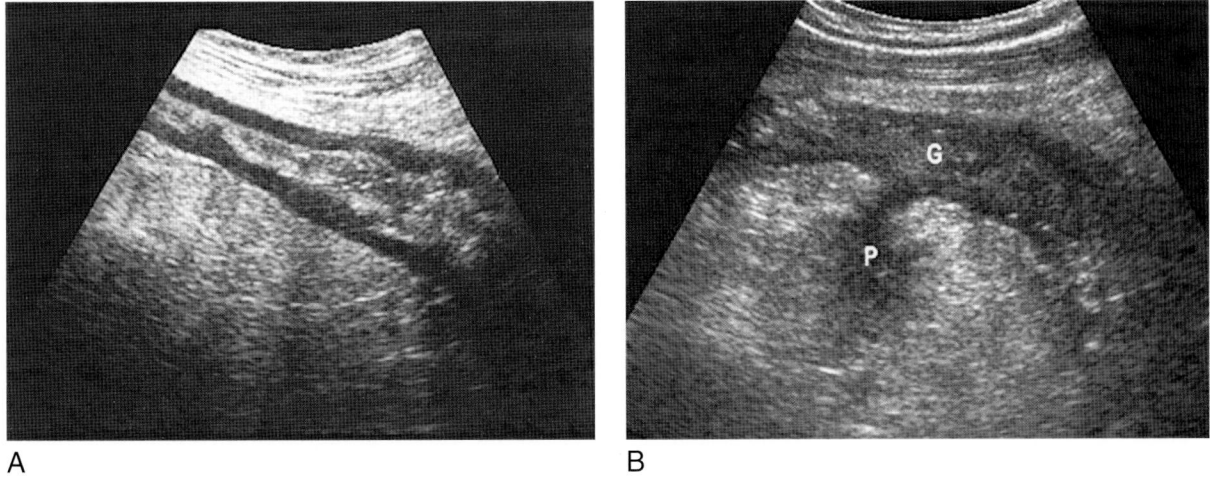

FIGURE 8-42. Pericolonic changes with diverticulitis in two patients. A, Long axis view of descending colon shows a long segment of thickened gut with prominent muscularis propria. Edema of the perienteric fat is striking and shows as a homogeneous echogenic mass effect deep to the gut. **B,** Similar inflamed fat. Phlegmonous change (P) shows as a hypoechoic zone centrally within the fat. G, Gut.

Failure to identify gas-containing abscesses and inter-loop abscesses are the major potential sources of error when using sonography to evaluate patients thought to have diverticulitis. The meticulous technique of following involved thickened segments of colon in long axis and transverse section will help detect even small amounts of extraluminal gas.

Sonographic features of diverticulitis include: segmental concentric **thickening of the gut wall** that is frequently strikingly hypoechoic, reflecting the predominant thickening in the muscular layer (see Fig. 8-39); **inflamed diverticula**, seen as bright echogenic foci with acoustic shadowing or "ringdown" artifact within or beyond the thickened gut wall (Fig. 8-41); acute **inflammatory changes in the pericolonic fat**, seen as

poorly defined hyperechoic zones without obvious gas or fluid content (Fig. 8-42); and **abscess formation**, seen as loculated fluid collections in an intramural, pericolonic, or remote location. With the development of extraluminal inflammatory masses, the diverticulum may no longer be identified on sonography, presumably being incorporated into the inflammatory process. Therefore, demonstration of a thickened segment of colon with an adjacent inflammatory mass may be consistent with diverticulitis but also with neoplastic or other inflammatory disease. **Intramural sinus tracts** appear as high-amplitude, linear echoes, often with "ringdown" artifact, within the gut wall. Typically they are deep, between the muscularis propria and the serosa. **Fistulae** appear as linear tracts that extend from the

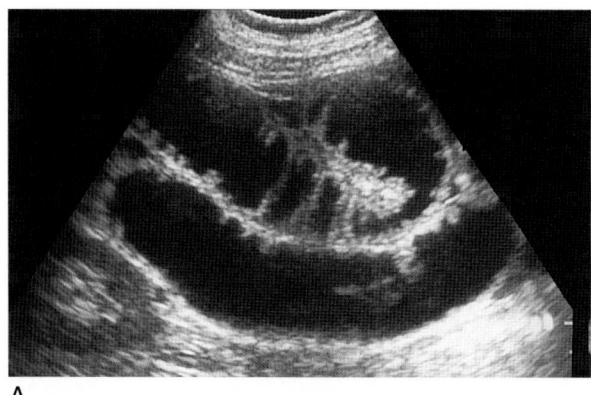
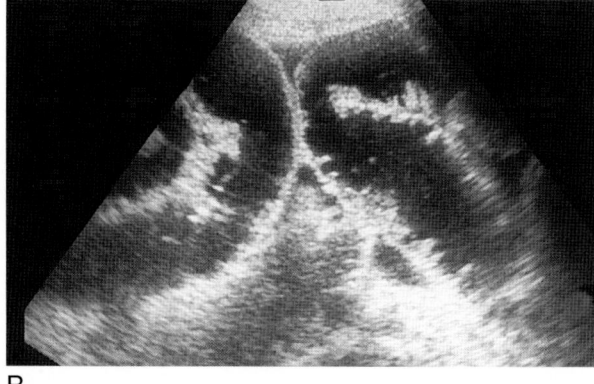

A   B

FIGURE 8-43. Mechanical small bowel obstruction. A, Sagittal image of right flank shows multiple, adjacent, long loops of dilated, fluid-filled small bowel with the classic morphology for a distal mechanical small bowel obstruction. **B,** Transverse image in the left lower quadrant confirms the multiplicity of dilated loops involved in the process. A small amount of ascites is seen between the dilated loops.

involved segment of gut to the bladder, vagina, or adjacent loops. Their echogenicity depends on their content, usually gas or fluid. Thickening of the mesentery and inflamed mesenteric fat (see Fig. 8-42) may also be seen.

The sonographic and clinical features of diverticulitis are more specific than those of acute appendicitis and errors of diagnosis occur less often. However, **torsion of appendices epiploicae** may produce a sonographic appearance so closely resembling acute diverticulitis that differentiation may be difficult.[69] The inflamed/infarcted fat of the appendix shows as a **shadowing area of increased echogenicity** related to the margin of the colon, mimicking an inflamed diverticulum. Regional perienteric inflammatory change, however, is usually minimal and systemic symptoms are fewer. The non-inflamed colonic appendices epiploicae are not visible—except with ascites, where they are seen as uniformly spaced echogenic foci along the margins of the colon.

MISCELLANEOUS GASTROINTESTINAL TRACT ABNORMALITIES

Mechanical Bowel Obstruction

Occlusion of the gastrointestinal tract lumen producing obstruction may be mechanical—where an actual physical impediment to the progression of the luminal content exists, or it may be functional—where paralysis of the intestinal musculature impedes progression (paralytic ileus).[70]

Mechanical bowel obstruction (MBO) is characterized by dilation of the intestinal tract proximal to the site of luminal occlusion, accumulation of large quantities of fluid and/or gas, and hyperperistalsis as the gut attempts to pass the luminal content beyond the obstruction. If the process is prolonged, exhaustion and over-distention of the bowel loops may occur

with secondary decrease in the peristaltic activity. There are **three broad categories** of mechanical obstruction: **obturation obstruction**, related to blockage of the lumen by material in the lumen; **intrinsic abnormalities** of the gut wall associated with luminal narrowing; and **extrinsic bowel lesions, including adhesions. Strangulation obstruction** develops when the circulation of the obstructed intestinal loop becomes impaired.

Sonography in patients suspected to have mechanical obstruction is usually not helpful. This is easily appreciated if one remembers that adhesions, the most common cause of intestinal obstruction, are not visible on the sonogram. Also, the presence of abundant gas in the intestinal tract, characteristic of most patients with obstruction, frequently produces sonograms of non-diagnostic quality. However, in the minority of patients with mechanical obstruction who do not have significant gaseous distention, sonography may be very helpful. In a prospective study of 48 patients, Meiser et al.[71] found that ultrasound was positive in 25% of the patients when the plain film was considered normal. Ultrasound alone allowed complete diagnosis of the cause of obstruction in six patients[12] in a retrospective study of sonography on 26 patients with known colonic obstruction, correctly predicted the location of colonic obstruction in 22 cases (85%), and the etiology of the obstruction in 21 cases (81%). Of 13 patients ultimately proven to have adenocarcinoma, five had a mass on sonography, five had segmental thickening, and 11 others showed a target sign of intussusception.

Sonographic study of potential bowel obstruction should include assessment of:

- Gastrointestinal tract **caliber** from the stomach to the rectum, noting any point at which the caliber alters (Fig. 8-43).
- **Content** of any dilated loops, with special

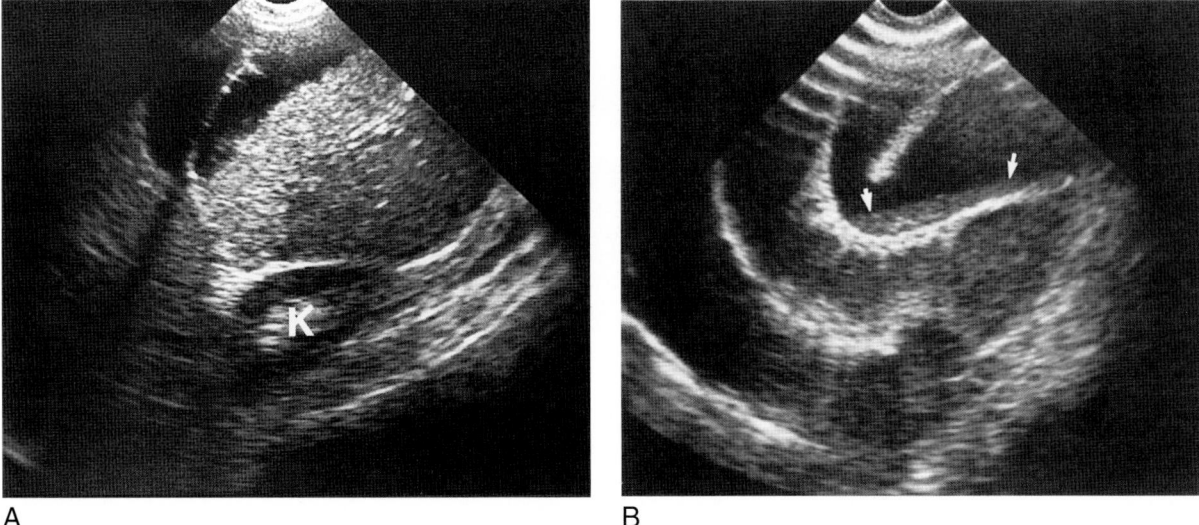

FIGURE 8-44. Dilated hypoperistaltic segments. A, Sagittal sonogram in the right flank shows gross dilation of the ascending colon. There is a long fluid-sediment level seen as a reflection of the hypoperistalsis of this segment of obstructed gut in a patient with a Crohn's stricture. Kidney (k). **B,** Sagittal sonogram in a patient with paralytic ileus shows extensive small bowel dilation. Loops are fluid filled and quiet with fluid-fluid level (*arrows*). (**A,** From Sarrazin J, Wilson SR: Manifestations of Crohn disease at US. Radiographics 1996;16:499-520.)

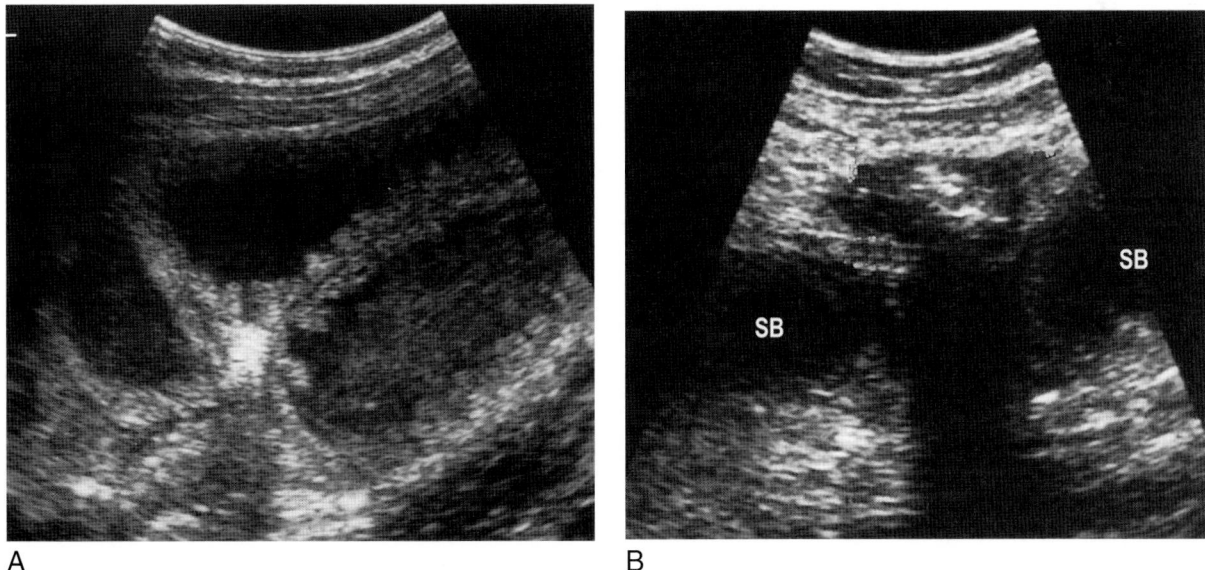

FIGURE 8-45. Mechanical small bowel obstruction—ventral hernia. A, Sonogram shows dilated fluid-filled loops of small bowel with edematous valvulae conniventes. **B,** Transverse paraumbilical sonogram shows normal caliber gut lying in abnormal superficial location between two dilated loops of small bowel (SB).

attention to their fluid and/or gaseous nature (Fig. 8-44).

- **Peristaltic activity** within the dilated loops, which is typically markedly exaggerated and abnormal, frequently producing a to-and-fro motion of the luminal content. With strangulation, peristalsis may decrease or cease.
- **Site of obstruction** for luminal (large gallstones, bezoars,[72] foreign bodies, intussusception, and occasional polypoid tumors); intrinsic (segmental gut wall thickening and stricture formation from Crohn's disease and annular carcinomas); and extrinsic (abscesses and endometriomas) abnormality as a cause of the obstruction.
- **Location of gut loops,** noting any abnormal position. Obstruction associated with external hernias is ideal for sonographic detection in that dilated loops of gut may be traced to a portion of the gut with normal caliber but abnormal location (Fig. 8-45). Spigelian and inguinal hernias are the disorders most commonly seen on sonograms.

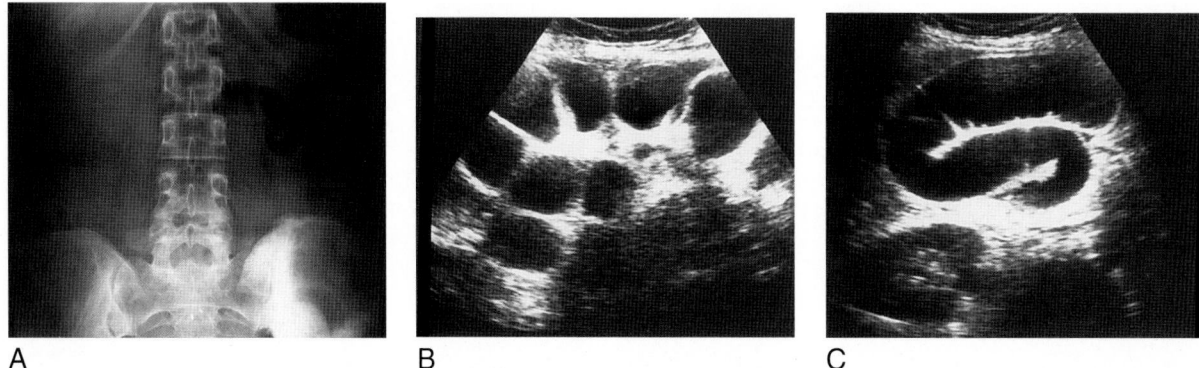

FIGURE 8-46. Closed loop obstruction. A, Plain film is unremarkable. **B,** Sonogram shows grossly dilated, gasless, fluid-filled, small bowel loops. **C,** Single loop shows a suggestive C- or U-shape.

Unique sonographic features are seen in the following:

Closed loop obstruction occurs if the bowel lumen is occluded at two points along its length, a serious condition that facilitates strangulation and necrosis. As the obstructed loop is closed off from the more proximal portion of the gastrointestinal tract, little or no gas is present within the obstructed segments, which may become very dilated and fluid filled. Consequently, the abdominal radiograph may be quite unremarkable (Fig. 8-46A) and sonography may be most helpful by showing the dilated involved segments (see Fig. 8-46B) and often the normal caliber bowel distal to the point of obstruction. The CT features of closed loop obstruction are well described and include dilated small bowel, a C- or U-shaped bowel loop (see Fig. 8-46C), a whirl sign, and two adjacent collapsed loops.[73,74] The latter important specific observation is very difficult to observe on ultrasound, in contrast to CT scan. However, we have correctly suspected closed loop obstruction in many patients on the basis of virtually normal plain films, small bowel dilation and a **U- or C-shaped bowel loop** (see Fig. 8-46), especially if there is gut wall thickening and/or pneumatosis intestinalis suggesting gut infarction.

Afferent loop obstruction is an uncommon complication of subtotal gastrectomy, with Billroth II gastrojejunostomy, that may occur by twisting at the anastomotic site, internal hernias, or with anastomotic stricture. Again, a gasless, dilated loop may be readily recognized on sonography in a location consistent with the enteroenteric anastomosis running from the right upper quadrant across the midline. Its detection, location, and shape should allow for correct sonographic diagnosis of this condition.[75]

Intussusception, invagination of a bowel segment (the intussusceptum) into the next distal segment (the intussuscipiens), is a relatively infrequent cause of mechanical obstruction in the adult in whom it is usually associated with a tumor as a lead point. In our experience, this is frequently a lipoma that appears as a highly echogenic intraluminal mass related to its fat content. A **sonographic appearance** of **multiple concentric rings**, related to the invaginating layers of the telescoped bowel, seen in cross-section is virtually pathognomonic (Fig. 8-47A).[76] Occasionally, only a target appearance may be seen.[77] The longitudinal appearance suggesting a "**hay fork**"[78] is not as reliably detected. In both projections, the mesenteric fat invaginating with the intussusceptum will show as an eccentric area of increased echogenicity. A lipoma, as a lead point, similarly shows as a focus of increased echogenicity (see Fig. 8-47B, C).

Midgut malrotation predisposes to bowel obstruction and infarction. It is infrequently encountered in adults. Sonographic abnormality related to the superior mesenteric vessels is suggestive of malrotation.[79] On transverse sonograms, the superior mesenteric vein is seen on the left ventral aspect of the superior mesenteric artery, a reversal of the normal relationship.

Paralytic Ileus

Paralytic ileus is a type of bowel obstruction related to adynamic function of the bowel wall. Paralysis of the intestinal musculature, in response to general or local insult, may impede the progression of luminal content. Although the lumen remains patent, no progression occurs. Sonography is usually of little value because these patients characteristically have poor-quality sonograms resulting from large quantities of gas in the intestinal tract. However, on rare occasions, the sonogram may demonstrate dilated, fluid-filled, very quiet, or aperistaltic loops of intestine. A fluid-fluid level in a dilated loop is characteristic of paralytic ileus, reflecting lack of movement of the intestinal contents (see Fig. 8-44B).

Gut Edema

Patients with acute vasculitis of various association may present with acute abdominal pain and ascites with

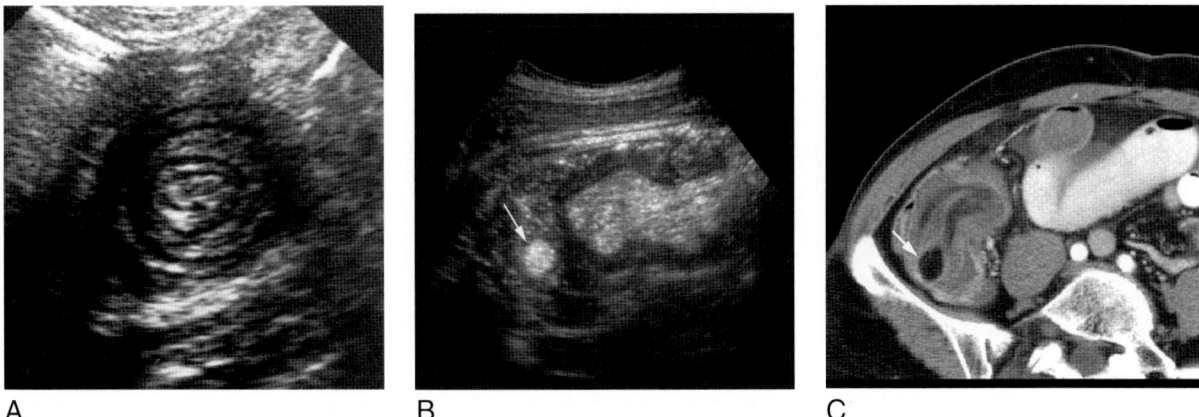

A   B   C

FIGURE 8-47. Intussusception in two patients. A, Sonogram shows multiple concentric rings representative of the invaginating intussuscipiens and the intussusceptum. Submucosal metastatic nodule as lead point. **B,** Sonogram of the right lower quadrant shows a highly echogenic lead point related to a lipoma (*arrow*). The invaginating fat in the mesentery is also echogenic. **C,** Confirmatory CT scan for image B. (**B** and **C,** From Wilson SR: The bowel wall looks thickened: What does that mean? Categorical course in diagnostic radiology: Findings at US—what do they mean? Radiological Society of North America. 2002, 219-228.)

massive edema of the small bowel wall seen as the major abnormality on imaging. Hypoalbuminemia, congestive heart failure, and spontaneous venous thrombosis may also show diffuse edema of the gut wall. Prominent thickened hypoechoic valvulae conniventes (Fig. 8-48)[80] and gastric rugae are relatively easy to recognize on the sonographic study, which should also include Doppler evaluation of the mesenteric and portal veins.

Gastrointestinal Tract Infections

Although fluid-filled, actively peristaltic gut may be seen with infectious viral or bacterial gastroenteritis, most affected patients do not demonstrate a sonographic abnormality. However, some pathogens, notably *Yersinia enterocolitica*, *Mycobacterium tuberculosis*, and *Campylobacter jejuni*, produce highly suggestive sonographic abnormalities in the ileocecal area that are partially described earlier in the section on right lower quadrant pain. Certain high-risk populations, such as those with AIDS and neutropenia,[57] appear to be susceptible to acute typhlitis and colitis, which also have a highly suggestive sonographic appearance.

The AIDS Population

AIDS patients are at increased risk for development of both gastrointestinal tract neoplasia, especially lymphoma (Fig. 8-14C, D), and unusual opportunistic infections, most commonly *Candida* esophagitis and CMV colitis.[58,59] The relative incidence of infection compared with neoplasia is about 4 or 5 to 1. Acute typhlitis (see Fig. 8-37) is described above in the section on right lower quadrant pain. The frequent symptom of watery diarrhea, associated with a variety of small bowel pathogens, often shows nothing on sonography apart from active and fluid-filled small bowel of normal thickness.

Pseudomembranous Colitis

Pseudomembranous colitis is a necrotizing inflammatory bowel condition that may occur as a response to a heterogeneous group of insults. Today, antibiotic therapy with effects from the toxin of *Clostridium difficile*, a normal inhabitant of the gastrointestinal tract, is most commonly implicated.[81] Watery diarrhea is the most common symptom and usually occurs during antibiotic therapy but may be quite remotely associated, occurring up to 6 weeks later. Endoscopic demonstration of pseudomembranous exudative plaques on the mucosal surface of the gut and culture of the enterotoxin of *C. difficile* are diagnostic. Superficial ulceration of the mucosa is associated with inflammatory infiltration of the lamina propria and the submucosa, which may be thickened to many times normal size.[82]

Sonography is frequently performed before pseudomembranous colitis is diagnosed, often based on a history of fever, abdominal pain, and watery diarrhea. **Sonographic features** have only rarely been described[83,84] but are suggestive of pseudomembranous colitis. Usually the entire colon is involved in a process that may produce **striking thickening of the colon wall**. Exaggerated haustral markings and a nonhomogeneous thickened submucosa, with virtual **apposition of the mucosal surfaces** of the thickened walls, are characteristic (Fig. 8-49).[56] Pseudomembranous colitis should be suspected in any patient with diffuse colonic wall thickening without a previous history of inflammatory bowel disease. Because the history of concurrent or prior antibiotic therapy is not always given, direct questioning of the patient is frequently helpful.

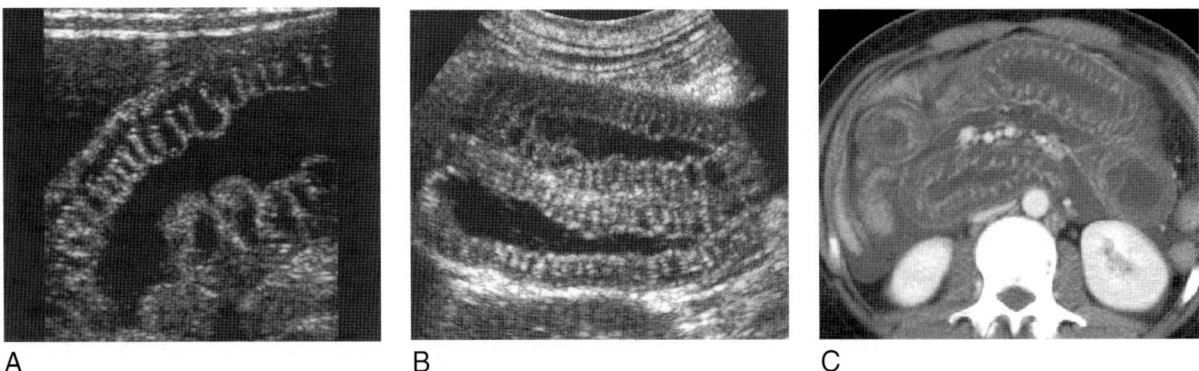

FIGURE 8-48. Small bowel edema secondary to vasculitis. A and **B,** Sonograms show marked edema of the valvulae conniventes of the entire small bowel. **C,** Confirmatory CT scan. (From Wilson SR: Evaluation of the small intestine by ultrasonography. In Gourtsoyiannis NC [ed]: Radiological Imaging of the Small Intestine. Heidelberg, Germany, Springer-Verlag, 2002, pp 73-86.)

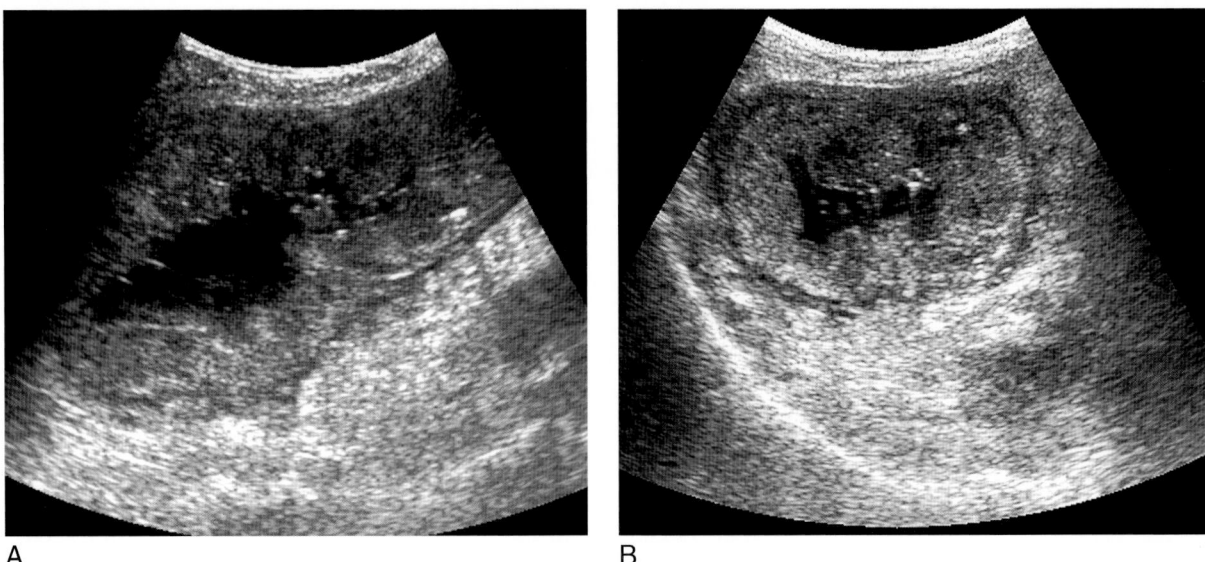

FIGURE 8-49. Pseudomembranous colitis. A, Long axis and **B,** cross-sectional views of the ascending colon show striking mural thickening of the gut wall. (From O'Malley ME, Wilson SR: US of gastrointestinal tract abnormalities with CT correlation. Radiographics 2003;23:59-72.)

Congenital Abnormalities of the Gastrointestinal Tract

Duplication cysts, characterized by the presence of the normal layers of the gut wall, may occur in any portion of the gastrointestinal tract. These cysts may be visualized on sonogram, either routine or endoscopic, and should be considered as diagnostic possibilities whenever unexplained abdominal cysts are seen (Fig. 8-50A, B). Tail-gut cysts are variants of abdominal cysts that are seen in the presacral region and are related to the rectum (Fig. 8-50C, D).

Ischemic Bowel Disease

Ischemic bowel disease most commonly affects the colon and is most prevalent in elderly persons who have arteriosclerosis. In younger patients, it may complicate cardiac arrhythmia, vasculitis, coagulopathy, embolism, shock, or sepsis.[85] Sonographic features have been poorly described, although gut wall thickening may be encountered. Pneumatosis intestinalis may complicate gut ischemia with a characteristic sonographic appearance.

Pneumatosis Intestinalis

Pneumatosis intestinalis is a relatively rare condition in which intramural pockets of gas are found throughout the GI tract. It has been associated with a wide variety of underlying conditions including **obstructive pulmonary disease**, **collagen vascular disease**, **inflammatory bowel disease**, **traumatic endoscopy**, and **postjejunoileal bypass**. In many situations, affected patients are

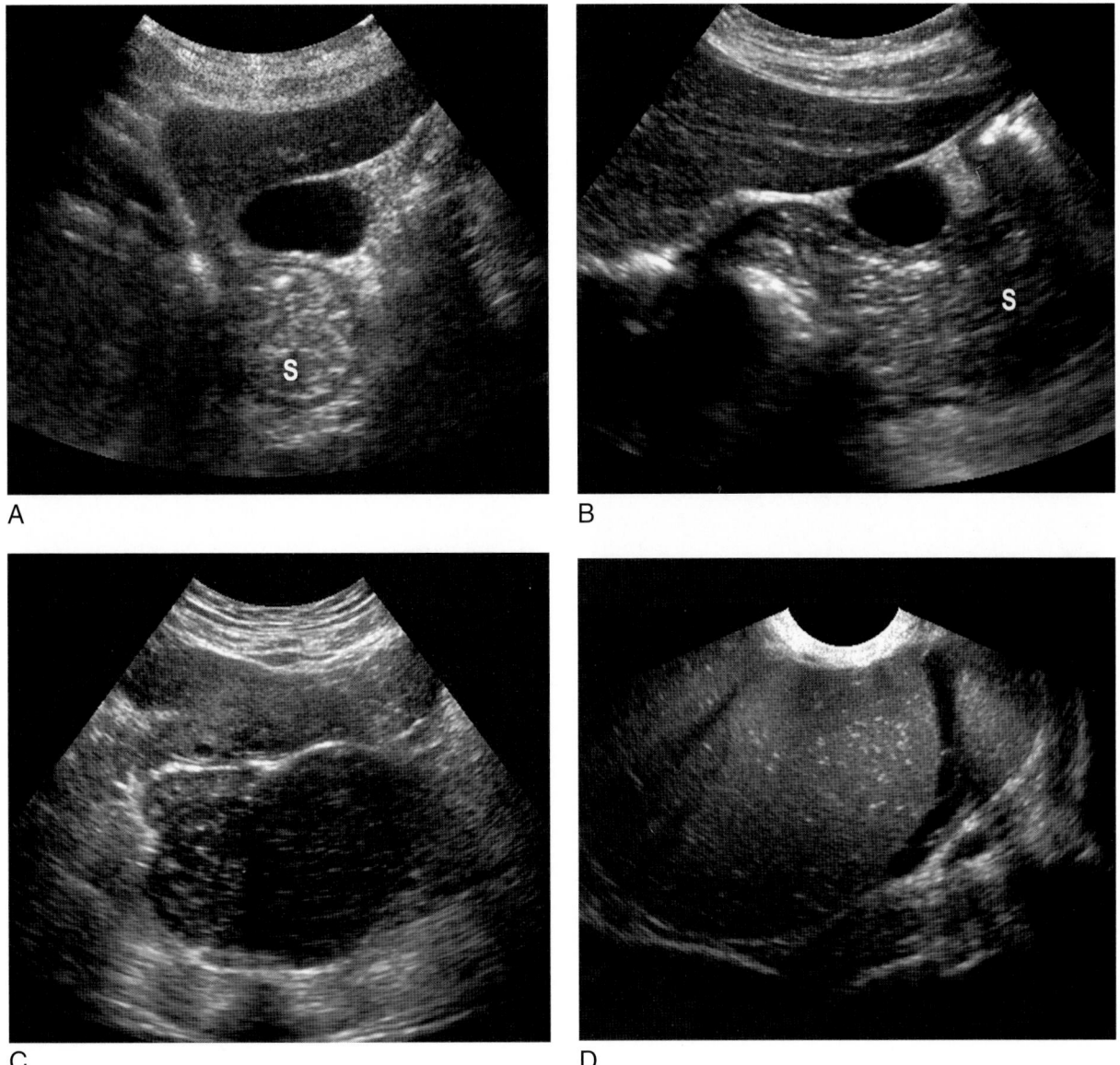

FIGURE 8-50. Congenital cysts. A, Sagittal and **B,** transverse sonograms in the epigastrium show an incidental gastric duplication cyst adjacent to the lesser curve of the stomach(s). **C,** Suprapubic and **D,** transvaginal pelvic scans show a complex, presacral pelvic mass, an incidental tail-gut cyst.

asymptomatic and the observation is incidental. However, its demonstration is of great clinical significance when **necrotizing enterocolitis** or **ischemic bowel disease** is present. Both conditions are associated with mucosal necrosis in which gas from the lumen passes to the gut wall.

Sonographic description is limited to isolated case reports. **High-amplitude echoes** may be demonstrated in the gut wall with **typical air artifact** or shadowing (Fig. 8-51).[86,87] Gut wall thickening may be noted if the pneumatosis is associated with underlying inflammatory bowel disease. If gut ischemia is suspected, careful evaluation of the liver is recommended to look for evidence of portal venous air.

Mucocele of the Appendix

Mucocele of the appendix is relatively uncommon, occurring in about 0.25% of 43,000 appendectomy specimens in one series.[88] Many patients with this condition are asymptomatic. A mass may be palpated in approximately 50% of cases. Both benign and malignant varieties occur in a ratio of approximately 10:1.[89] In the benign form, the appendiceal lumen is obstructed by either inflammatory scarring or fecaliths. The glandular mucosa in the isolated segment continues to secrete sterile mucus. The neoplastic variety of mucocele is associated with primary mucous cystadenoma or cystadenocarcinoma of the appendix. Although the gross

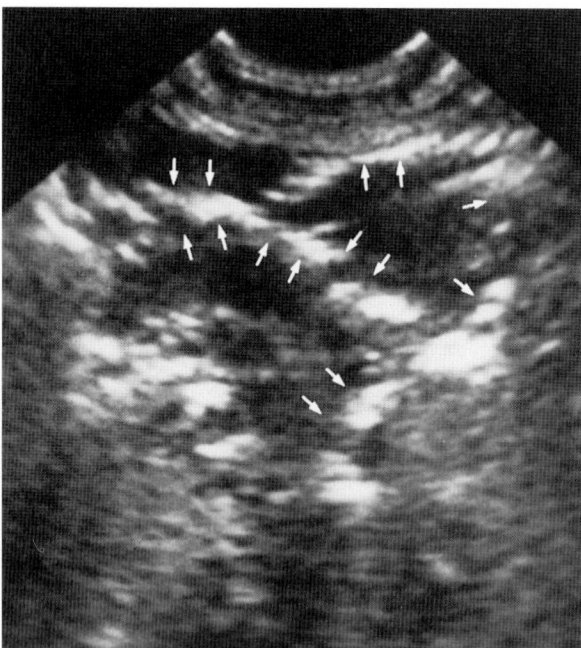

FIGURE 8-51. Pneumatosis intestinalis. Sonogram shows three loops of gut with bright, high-amplitude echoes (*arrows*) originating within the gut wall.

morphology of the appendix may be similar in the benign and malignant varieties, the malignant form is often associated with pseudomyxoma peritonei if rupture occurs.[90]

On sonography, mucoceles typically produce large, hypoechoic, well-defined **right lower-quadrant cystic masses** with variable internal echogenicity, wall thickness, and wall calcification (Fig. 8-52). The internal contents often show a laminated or whorled appearance. These masses are frequently retrocecal and may be

mobile. Although their sonographic appearance is not always specific, this diagnostic possibility should be considered when an elongated oval cystic mass is found in the right lower quadrant in any patient with an appendix.[91]

Gastrointestinal Tract Hematoma

Blunt abdominal trauma, complicated by duodenal hematoma and rectal trauma, either sexual or iatrogenic following rectal biopsy, are the major causes of local hematomas seen on sonography. Hematoma is usually localized to the submucosa. Larger or more diffuse hematomas may complicate anticoagulation therapy or bleeding disorders associated with leukemia. If hematomas are large, diffuse gut wall thickening may be seen on sonograms.

Peptic Ulcer

Peptic ulcer, a defect in the epithelium to the depth of the submucosa, may be seen in either gastric or duodenal locations. Although rarely visualized, peptic ulcer has a fairly characteristic sonographic appearance. A gas-filled ulcer crater is seen as a **bright echogenic focus** with **"ringdown" artifact**, either in a focal area of wall thickening or beyond the wall, depending on the depth of penetration (Fig. 8-53). Edema in the acute phase and fibrosis in the chronic phase may produce localized wall thickening and deformity.

Bezoars

Bezoars are masses of foreign material or food, typically found in the stomach after surgery for peptic ulcer

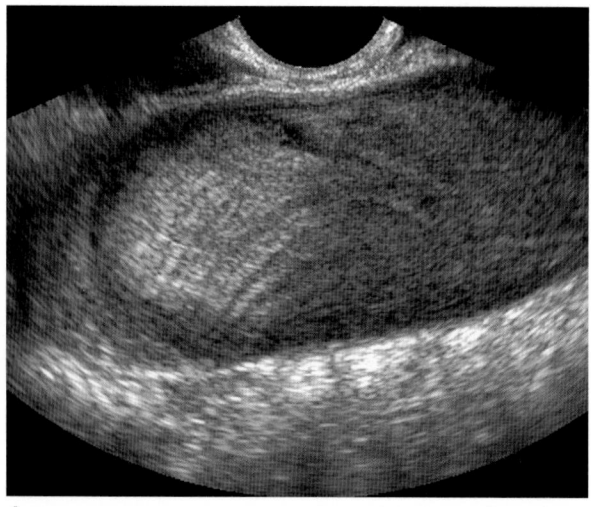

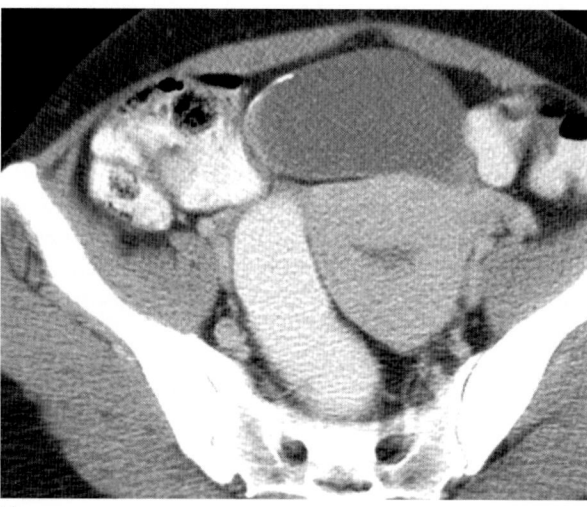

A   B

FIGURE 8-52. Mucocele of the appendix. A, Sonogram and **B,** CT scan show a large mucus-filled appendix as an incidental observation. The whorled appearance on the sonogram is characteristic. There is a fleck of calcification in the wall on the CT scan.

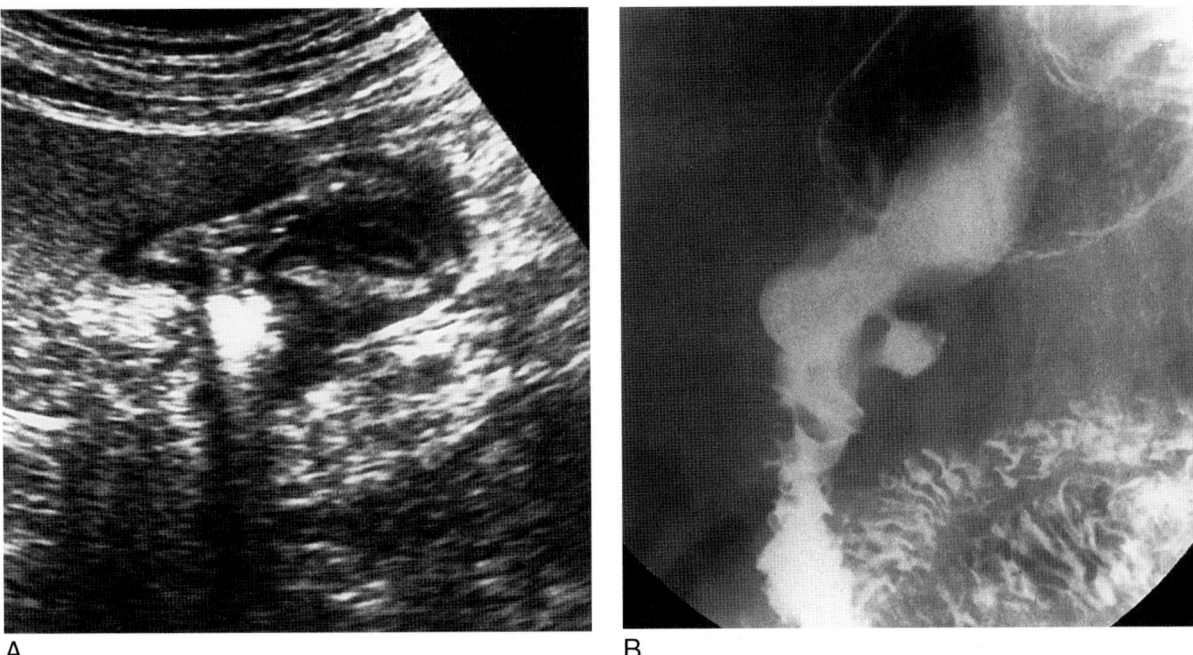

A   B

FIGURE 8-53. Peptic ulcer. A, Cross-sectional sonogram of the stomach shows a hypoechoic eccentric mass with a bright, central echogenic focus representing air in the ulcer crater. **B,** Confirmatory barium swallow.

disease (*phytobezoars*) or after ingestion of indigestible organic substances such as hair (*trichobezoars*). These masses may produce **shadowing intraluminal densities** on the sonogram and have been documented as a rare cause of small bowel obstruction.[72] They may also form in the small bowel in association with chronic stasis.

Intraluminal Foreign Bodies

Large foreign bodies, including bottles, candles, sexual vibrators, contraband, tools, and food, may be identified, particularly in the rectum and sigmoid colon where they produce fairly sharp, distinct specular echoes with sharp, acoustic shadows. Their recognition is enhanced by suspicion of their presence.

Celiac Disease

Undiagnosed adult patients with celiac disease are encountered infrequently in general ultrasound departments. Nonetheless, we have, on occasion, seen patients where sonography is the first to suggest the correct diagnosis. Sonographic observations include abnormal fluid-filled small intestine with moderate dilation of the involved loops. Alteration of the morphology from normal is observed and described by Dietrich et al. as reduction of Kerckring's plicae circulares with loss of density and uniformity.[92] Peristalsis is increased above normal. An increase in the caliber of the superior mesenteric artery and portal vein may also be seen.[93] We have also observed frequent intermittent intussusception in this patient population.

Cystic Fibrosis

Aggressive treatment of the pulmonary problems of cystic fibrosis increases the likelihood of encountering adult patients in a general ultrasound department performing abdominal sonography. Thickening of the wall of particularly the right hemicolon, and to a lesser extent also the left colon and the small bowel, may be seen in association with infiltration of both the pericolonic and the mesenteric fat (Fig. 8-54).[94] These may often be incidental observations without significant associated symptomatology. In its advanced stage, a fibrosing colonopathy with stricture may be seen.[95,96] The culture of *C. difficile* is also documented in some patients with cystic fibrosis and colon-wall thickening without the accompanying symptoms of abdominal pain and diarrhea.[97] Positive stool culture, however, is not the rule in cystic fibrosis patients with detectable colon wall thickening.

ENDOSONOGRAPHY

Endosonography, performed with high-frequency transducers in the lumen of the gut, allows for detection of mucosal abnormality, delineation of the layers of the gut wall, and definition of the surrounding soft tissues to a depth of 8 to 10 cm from the transducer crystal. Thus, tumors hidden below normal mucosa, tumor penetration into the layers of the gut wall, and tumor involvement of surrounding vital structures or lymph nodes may be well evaluated. Staging of previously iden-

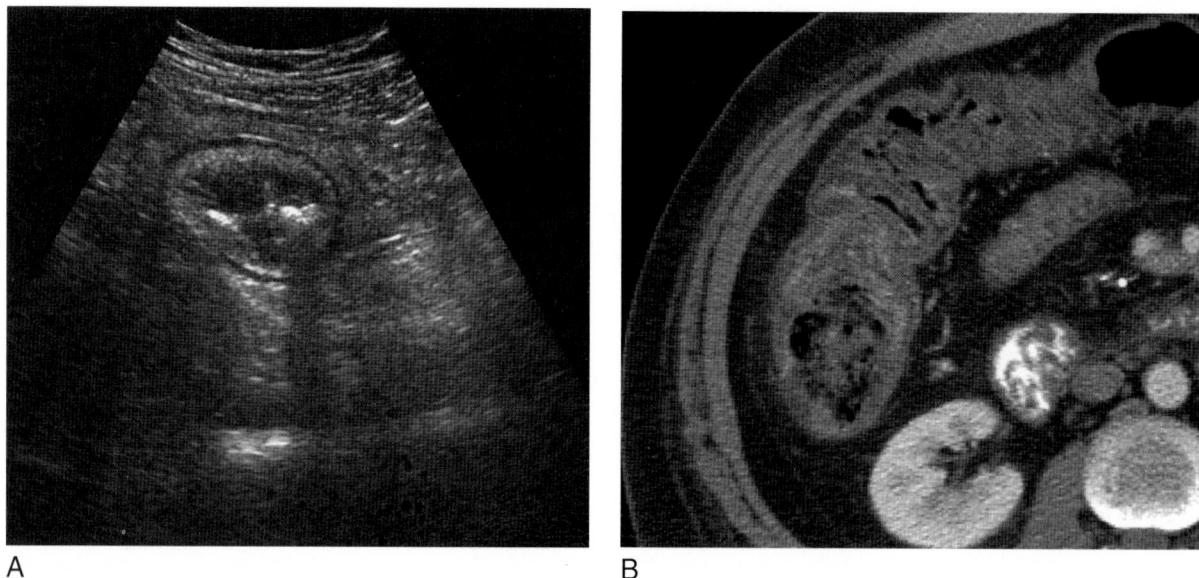

A   B

FIGURE 8-54. Cystic fibrosis. A, Cross-sectional sonogram of the ascending colon shows moderate wall thickening with layer preservation. **B,** Confirmatory CT scan.

tified mucosal tumors is one of the major applications of this technique.

Upper Gastrointestinal Tract

Rotating high-frequency transducers, using 7.5-MHz crystals fitted into a fiberoptic endoscope, are most suitable for endosonography of the esophagus, stomach, and duodenum. Light sedation of the patient is usually required. The patient is placed in the left lateral decubitus position, and the endoscope is inserted to the desired location. Intraluminal gas is aspirated, and a balloon covering the transducer crystal is inflated with deaerated water. Localization is determined from the distance of insertion from the teeth and identification of anatomic landmarks, such as the spleen, liver, pancreas, and gallbladder. Rotation and deflection of the transducer tip allow scanning of visualized lesions in different planes.[98]

Identification, localization, and characterization of **benign masses** are possible with endoscopic sonography. **Varices** are seen as compressible hypoechoic or cystic masses deep to the submucosa or in the outer layers of the esophagus, gastroesophageal junction, or gastric fundus.[99] **Benign tumors**, such as fibromas or leiomyomas, are well-defined, solid masses without mucosal involvement that can be localized to the layer of the wall from which they arise, usually the submucosa and the muscularis propria, respectively. **Peptic ulcer** typically produces marked thickening of all layers of the gastric wall with a demonstrated ulcer crater. **Ménétrier's disease** produces thickening of the mucosal folds.

Staging of **esophageal carcinoma** involves assessment of depth of tumor invasion and evaluation of involvement of the local lymph nodes and adjacent vital

structures.[100] Constricting lesions that do not allow passage of the endoscope may produce technically unsatisfactory or incomplete examinations.

Gastric lymphoma is typically very hypoechoic, its invasion is along the gastric wall or horizontal, and involvement of extramural structures and lymph nodes is less than with gastric carcinoma. Thus, localized mucosal ulceration with extensive infiltration of the deeper layers suggests lymphoma that may also grow with a polypoid pattern or as a diffuse infiltration without ulceration.[101] **Gastric carcinoma**, in contrast, arises from the gastric mucosa, is usually more echogenic, tends to invade vertically or through the gastric wall, and frequently involves the perigastric lymph nodes by the time of diagnosis.

The Rectum

Tumor Staging of Rectal Carcinoma

Although a variety of pathologic conditions may be assessed with endorectal sonography, the staging of previously detected rectal carcinoma is its major role. Patients are scanned in the left lateral decubitus position following a cleansing enema. Both axial and sagittal images are obtained. A variety of rigid intrarectal probes are now commercially available using a range of transducer technologies with phased array, mechanical sector, and rotating crystals. A sterile condom covers an inner balloon, which is inflated with 35 to 70 mL of deaerated water. The probe is moved to allow for visualization of the tumor within the focal zone of the transducer. Axial images demonstrate the rectum as a multilayered circle (Fig. 8-55).

Recently, we have been evaluating women with rectal carcinoma using a transvaginal probe placed in the vagina

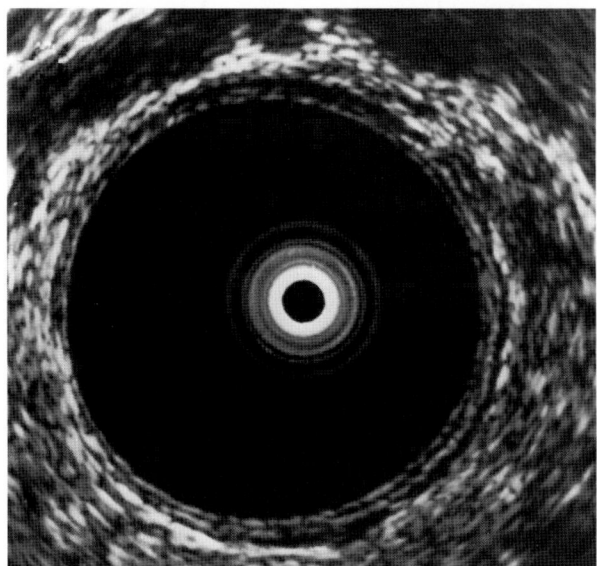

FIGURE 8-55. Normal rectal endosonogram. Axial view shows the probe centrally within the rectal lumen. The five layers of the gut wall are most optimally seen between the 3 o'clock and 7 o'clock positions.

following Fleet enema. This technique is excellent, especially for larger tumors because the rectovaginal septum, the tumor, and the lymph nodes in the mesorectum are more optimally seen.

Tumors are staged according to the Astler-Coller modification of the Dukes' classification[102] or, more simply, with the primary tumor (T) component of the Union Internationale Contre le Cancer (UICC) TNM classification[103]—where T represents the primary tumor, N the nodal involvement, and M the distant metastases (Fig. 8-56).

Rectal carcinoma arises from the mucosal surface of the gut. Tumors appear as relatively hypoechoic masses that may distort the rectal lumen. Invasion of the deeper layers, the submucosa, the muscularis propria, and the perirectal fat produces discontinuity of these layers on the sonogram. Superficial ulceration or crevices that allow small bubbles of gas to be trapped deep to the inflated balloon may demonstrate "ringdown" artifact and shadowing, with loss of layer definition deep to the ulceration. Lymph nodes appear as round or oval, hypoechoic masses in the perirectal fat. Sonographically, many visible nodes may be reactive rather than neoplastic, and normal-sized nodes may have microscopic invasion. Therefore, definitive staging requires pathologic assessment of both the tumor and the regional nodes.

Wang et al.[104] studied 6 normal and 16 neoplastic colorectal specimens in vitro with an 8.5-MHz ultrasound transducer. They accurately demonstrated invasion of the submucosa in 92.5% and invasion of the muscularis propria in 77%. Invasive tumors with extension

beyond the muscularis propria were accurately predicted 90% of the time. In vivo studies support this excellent result.[105,106] Comparing preoperative transrectal ultrasound and CT staging in 102 consecutive patients, Rifkin et al.[107] found transrectal sonography superior to CT in assessment of tumor extent and in the detection of lymph node involvement.

Limitations of rectal sonography include:

- Inability to identify microscopic tumor invasion
- Inability to image stenotic tumors
- Inability to image tumors greater than 15 cm from the anal verge
- Inability to distinguish nodes involved with tumor from those with reactive change
- Inability to identify normal-sized nodes with microscopic tumor invasion

Despite these limitations, endorectal ultrasound appears to be an excellent imaging tool for preoperative staging of accessible rectal cancers.

Recurrent rectal cancer after local resection is usually extraluminal, involving the resection margin secondarily. Serial transrectal sonography may be used in conjunction with serum chorioembryonic antigen levels to detect these recurrences. A pericolic hypoechoic mass or local thickening of the rectal wall, in either deep or superficial layers, is taken as evidence of recurrence. **Previous radiation treatment** may produce a diffuse thickening of the entire rectal wall, usually of moderate or high echogenicity with an appearance that is usually easily differentiated from the focal hypoechoic appearance of recurrent cancer. Sonographic-guided biopsy of a detected abnormality facilitates histologic differentiation of recurrence from postoperative, inflammatory, or postradiation change.

Prostatic carcinoma may invade the rectum directly, or more remote tumors may involve the rectum, usually as a result of seeding to the posterior peritoneal pouch. Because these tumors initially involve the deeper layers of the rectal wall with mucosal involvement occurring as the disease progresses, their sonographic appearance is distinct from that of primary rectal carcinoma (see Fig. 8-56D).

Benign mesenchymal tumors, especially of smooth muscle origin, are uncommon in the rectum. When seen, their sonographic features are the same as elsewhere. **Mucous retention cysts,** caused by the obstruction of mucous glands, produce cystic masses of varying size that are located deep in the rectal wall.

The Anal Canal

Fecal Incontinence

Anal endosonography, performed with the addition of a hard cone attachment to a radial 7.5-MHz probe, allows accurate assessment of the anal canal, including the

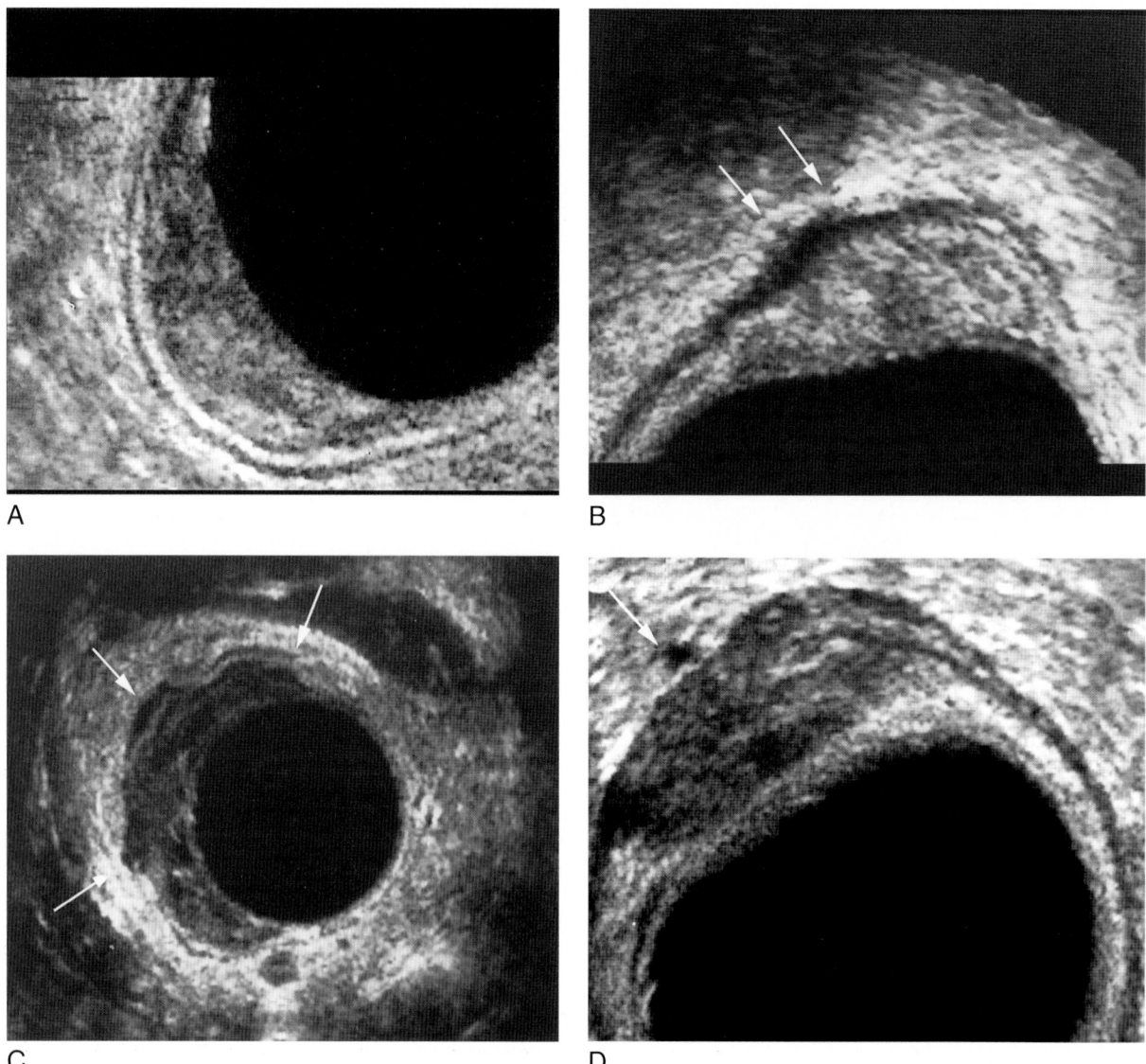

FIGURE 8-56. Rectal tumors seen at transrectal sonography. A, Rectal carcinoma—T$_1$. A hypoechoic mass between the 6 o'clock and 8 o'clock positions is noted. The submucosa—the echogenic line—and the muscularis propria—the external hypoechoic line—are intact. **B,** Rectal carcinoma—T$_2$. A tumor is seen anteriorly. The muscularis propria (*arrows*) is the hypoechoic line that is thickened and nodular, consistent with tumor involvement. **C,** Rectal carcinoma—T$_3$. A large tumor involves the entire right lateral wall of the rectum. Invasion of the perirectal fat (*arrows*) is noted in several locations. A large node is seen at the 6 o'clock position; smaller nodes are seen at the 5 o'clock and 8 o'clock positions. **D,** Metastatic carcinoma to rectal wall. A hypoechoic mass is seen between the 10 o'clock and 1 o'clock positions. It involves the deep layers of the rectal wall and not the rectal mucosa. There is a small lymph node (*arrow*).

internal and external sphincters.[108] Performed primarily for assessment of fecal incontinence, this test shows the integrity of the sphincters with documentation of the degree and size of muscle defects.

Young women, following traumatic obstetric delivery, are most often afflicted with fecal incontinence. We, and others, have found transvaginal assessment of the anal sphincter—performed with a side-firing transvaginal probe close to the introitus—to be equally as effective as a transanal approach.[28,109,110]

The **internal anal sphincter,** in continuity with the muscularis propria of the rectum above, is seen as a circular hypoechoic or black ring just deep to the convoluted mucosal echoes (Fig. 8-57). The **external anal sphincter,** in contrast, is less well defined and more echogenic, appearing gray on the ultrasound examination, and in continuity with fibers from the puborectalis sling. Traumatic disruption of the muscle layers will show as defects in the continuity of the normal muscle texture most commonly anterior (Fig. 8-58). Posttraumatic scarring may be associated with a change of shape of the anal canal from round to oval (see Fig. 8-58).

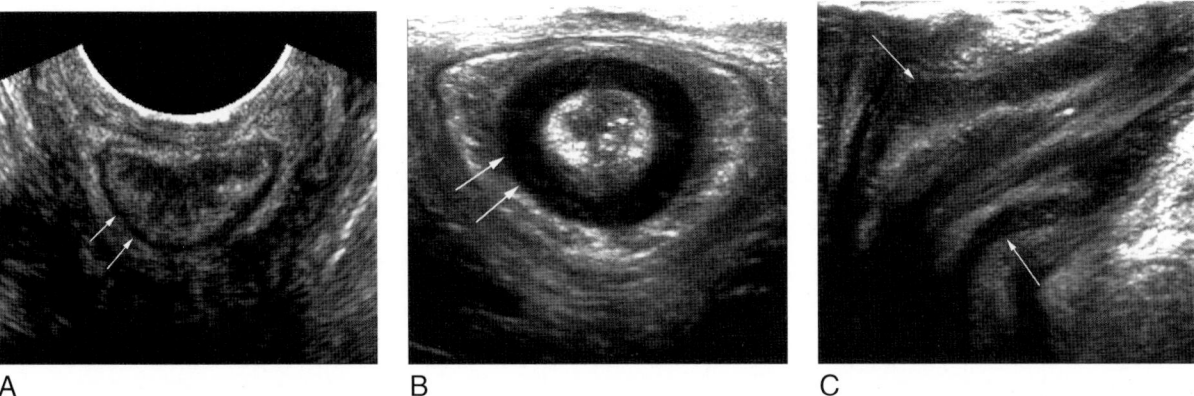

A   B   C

FIGURE 8-57. Normal rectum and anal canal. **A,** Transvaginal and, **B** and **C,** transperineal approach. **A,** Cross-sectional image of rectum taken with vaginal probe showing the normal convoluted rectal mucosa, prominent submucosa (*white*) and the muscularis propria as a black thin rim (*arrows*). The rectum is usually oval, as shown here. **B,** Anal canal shows the thick, well-defined, internal anal sphincter (*arrows*) as a continuous black ring that is in continuity with the muscularis propria of the rectal wall above. The external anal sphincter is less well defined and echogenic. **C,** Rotation of the probe by 90 degrees shows the anal canal in long axis. Internal anal sphincter (*arrows*).

A

B

C

D

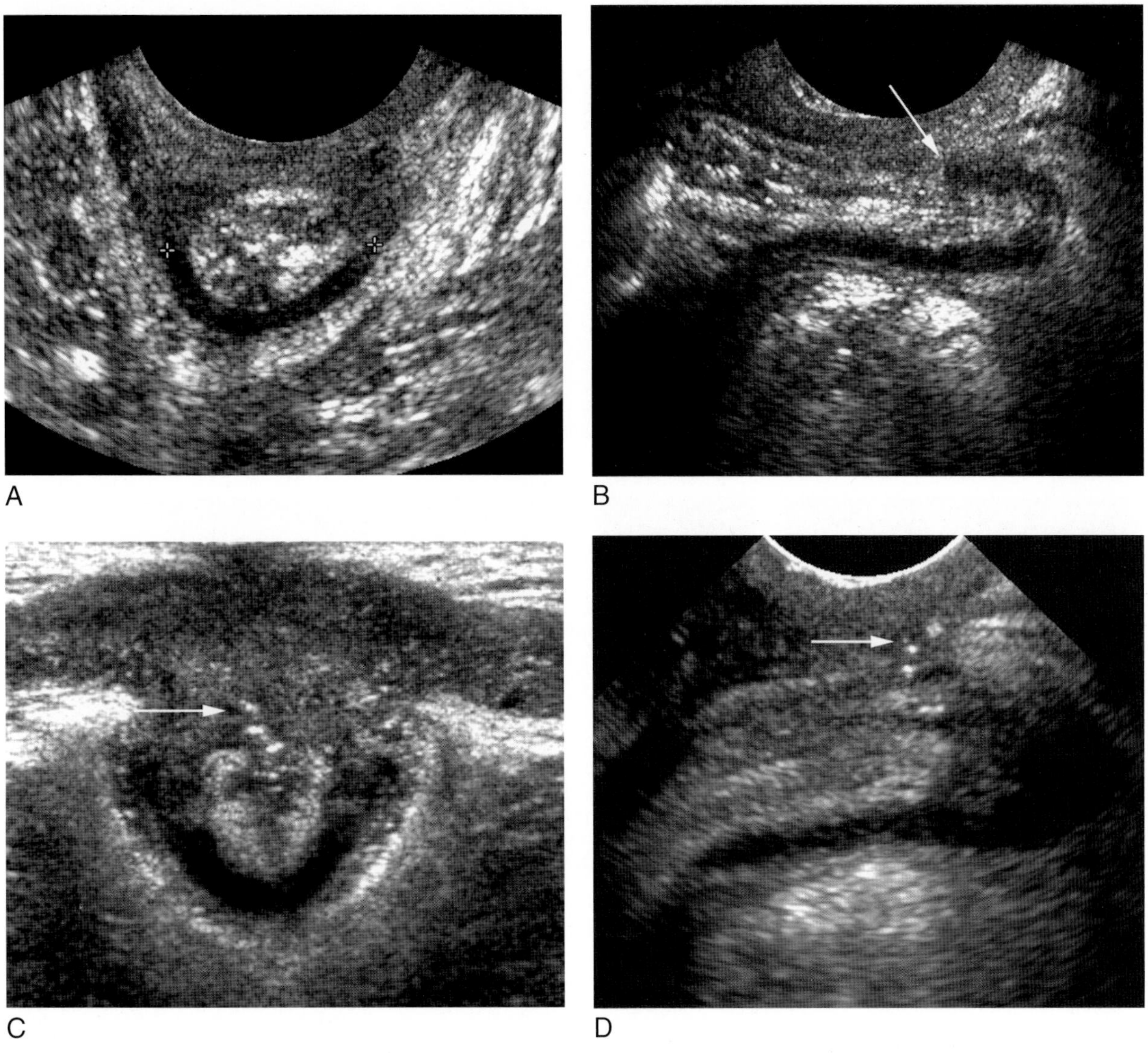

FIGURE 8-58. Traumatic disruption of the anal sphincter in two patients. **A,** Cross-sectional and **B,** long-axis views of the anal canal taken from a transvaginal approach show disruption of the sphincter anteriorly from 9 to 3 o'clock. The arrow on the sagittal image shows the cephalad extent of the internal anal sphincter. **C,** Cross-sectional and **D,** long-axis views of the anal canal show full thickness disruption of the anterior anal canal between 11 and 1 o'clock. The *arrow* in each image shows air bubbles within an anovaginal fistula.

Perianal Inflammatory Disease

Perianal inflammatory disease is seen in two distinct populations, those with Crohn's disease who develop perianal inflammation as part of their disease, and patients who develop a perianal abscess or fistula as a spontaneous event. The former is described earlier in the section on Crohn's disease. In other patients, perianal infection arises in small intersphincteric anal glands predominantly located at the dentate line. This occurs most frequently in young adult males. Documentation of fluid collections and the relationship of inflammatory

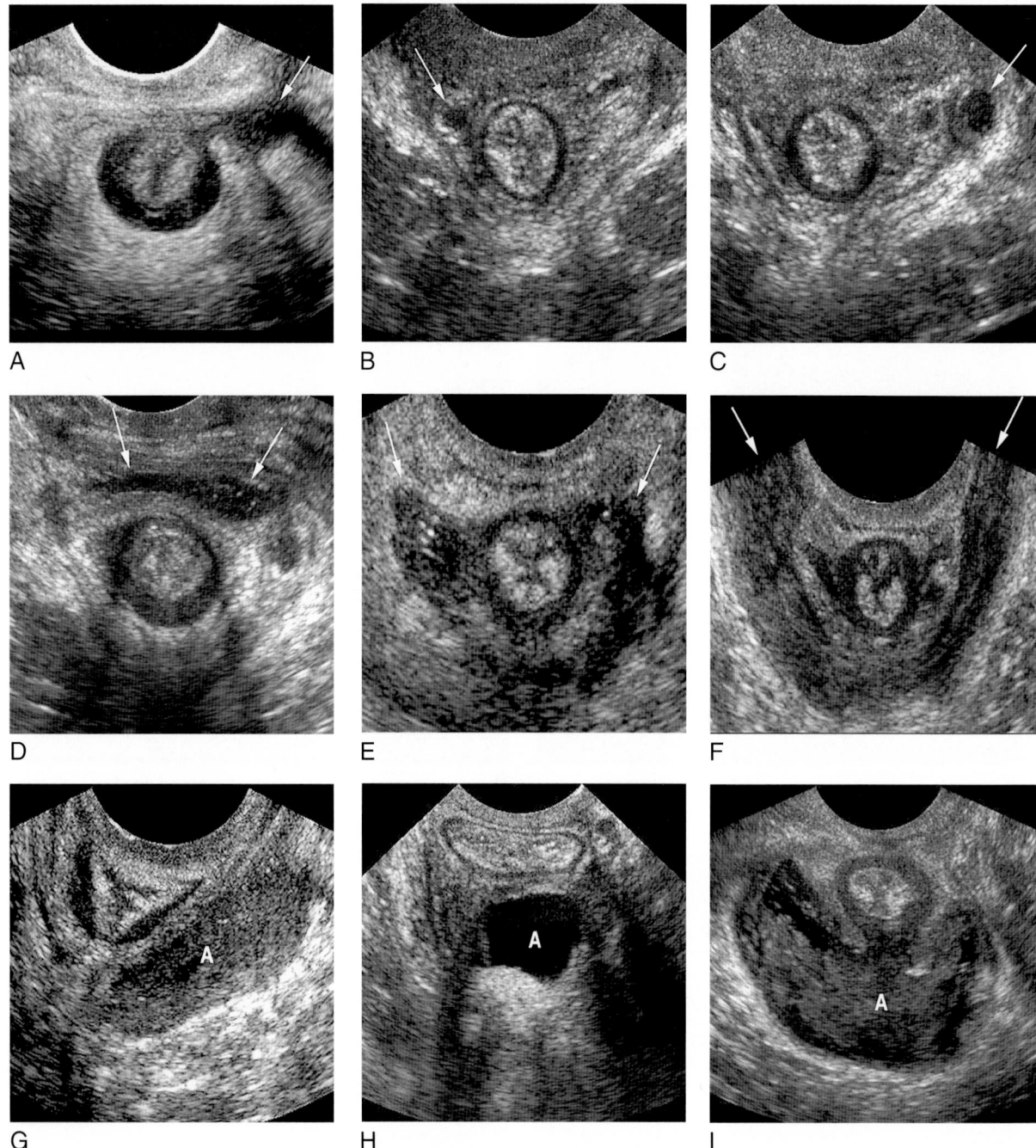

FIGURE 8-59. Perianal inflammatory disease in nine patients. *Top line*—Simple inflammatory openings and tracts (*arrows*). **A,** Cross-sectional images of the anal canal show internal opening at 1 o'clock with a transsphincteric tract running to a small collection. **B,** Intersphincteric tract and **C,** larger extrasphincteric tract. *Middle line*—**More complex tracts** (*arrows*). **D,** Anterior extrasphincteric tract shows fluid within. **E,** Bilateral, complex, intersphincteric tracts and collections show bright, echogenic foci representing extraluminal air. **F,** Boomerang, or horseshoe tract, surrounds the anal canal posteriorly and laterally. There are internal openings at 2, 4, and 9 o'clock. *Bottom line*—**Perianal abscesses** (A). **G,** Abscess on left posterolateral aspect of the anal canal is particle filled. **H,** Large, posterior abscess is complex with a dependent debris level, and **I,** large posterior abscess shows a large internal opening posteriorly at 6 o'clock.

tracts to the sphincter mechanism are important for surgical treatment.

Transanal sonography for assessment of perianal inflammatory disease is limited because placement of the rigid probe into the anal canal does not allow assessment of disease in the perineal region. We prefer transvaginal sonography in conjunction with transperineal sonography in women and transperineal sonography in men for evaluation of this problem.

Scans are performed with curved and high frequency linear probes placed firmly on the skin of the perineum between the introitus and the anal canal in women and between the scrotum and the anal canal in men. Firm pressure on the transducer is required to afford good visualization of the anal canal. We begin the procedure with the transducer in the transverse plane relative to the body. The transducer should be directed cephalad and anterior to the plane of the anal canal and then angled slowly through the plane of the anal canal, which will show it in cross section from the anorectal junction to the external anal opening. Rotation of the transducer by 90 degrees will allow for imaging in the longitudinal plane. Tracts and collections in the perineum, buttocks, scrotum, and labia can also all be assessed and followed in a retrograde direction to their connection with the anal canal.

Perianal inflammatory tracts and masses are classified according to the classification of Parks.[111] His classification provides an anatomic description of fistulous tracts, which acts as a guide to operative treatment. According to this classification, there are four main subtypes: intersphincteric (between the internal and external sphincter), transsphincteric (crossing both the internal and external anal sphincter into the ischiorectal or ischioanal fossa), suprasphincteric, and extrasphincteric. In each patient, we document also the internal opening and the external openings as possible. Tracts show on the ultrasound scan as hypoechoic linear areas or fluid-containing tubular areas depending on their size and activity (Fig. 8-59). As with fistulas elsewhere, air bubbles within the tract show as bright echogenic foci that may move during the scan, helping with their identification. In our initial experience with 54 patients with perianal inflammatory masses, sonographic findings were confirmed in 22 (85%) of 26 patients who underwent surgical treatment for their disease.[27]

Acknowledgments

The author would like to acknowledge Gordana Popovich and Jenny Tomashpolskaya for their artwork.

References

Basic Principles

1. Heyder N, Kaarmann H, Giedl J: Experimental investigations into the possibility of differentiating early from invasive carcinoma of the stomach by means of ultrasound. Endoscopy 1987;19:228-232.
2. Bolondi L, Caletti G, Casanova P, et al: Problems and variations in the interpretation of the ultrasound feature of the normal upper and lower gastrointestinal tract wall. Scand J Gastroenterol 1986;21:16-26.
3. Kimmey MB, Martin RW, Haggitt RC, et al: Histologic correlates of gastrointestinal ultrasound images. Gastroenterology 1989;96:433-441.
4. Lutz H, Petzoldt R: Ultrasonic patterns of space occupying lesions of the stomach and the intestine. Ultrasound Med Biol 1976;2:129-131.
5. Bluth EI, Merritt CRB, Sullivan MA: Ultrasonic evaluation of the stomach, small bowel, and colon. Radiology 1979;133:677-680.
6. Wilson SR: The bowel wall looks thickened: What does that mean? Categorical course in diagnostic radiology: Findings at US—what do they mean? Radiological Society of North America. 2002, 219-228.
7. Puylaert JBCM: Acute appendicitis: Ultrasound evaluation using graded compression. Radiology 1986;158:355-360.
8. Wilson SR: Gastrointestinal sonography. Abdom Imaging 1996;21:1-8.
9. Teefey SA, Roarke MC, Brink JA, et al: Bowel wall thickening: Differentiation of inflammation from ischemia with color Doppler and duplex US. Radiology 1996;198:547-551.

Gastrointestinal Tract Neoplasms

10. Winawer SJ, Sherlock P: Malignant neoplasms of the small and large intestine. In Sleisenger MH, Fordtran JS (eds): Gastrointestinal Disease: Pathophysiology Diagnosis Management, 3rd ed. Philadelphia, 1983, WB Saunders.
11. Lim JH: Colorectal cancer: Sonographic findings. AJR 1996;167:45-47.
12. Lim JH, Ko YT, Lee DH, et al: Determining the site and causes of colonic obstruction with sonography. AJR 1994;163:1113-1117.
13. Fenoglio-Preiser CM, Lantz PE, Listrom MB, et al (eds): Gastrointestinal Pathology: An Atlas and Text, 2nd ed. New York, Raven Press, 1998, pp 1169-1215.
14. Kaftori JK, Aharon M, Kleinhaus U: Sonographic features of gastrointestinal leiomyosarcoma. J Clin Ultrasound 1981;9:11-15.
15. Fenoglio-Preiser CM, Lantz PE, Listrom MB, et al (eds): Gastrointestinal Pathology: An Atlas and Text, 2nd ed. New York, Raven Press, 1998, pp 1129-1168.
16. Salem S, Hiltz CW: Ultrasonographic appearance of gastric lymphosarcoma. J Clin Ultrasound 1978; 6:429-430.
17. Derchi LE, Bandereali A, Bossi MC, et al: Sonographic appearance of gastric lymphoma. J Ultrasound Med 1984;3:251-256.
18. Telerman A, Gerend B, Van der Heul B, et al: Gastrointestinal metastases from extraabdominal tumors. Endoscopy 1985;17:99.
19. Rubesin SE, Levine MS: Omental cakes: Colonic involvement by omental metastases. Radiology 1985;54:593-596.
20. Yeh H-C: Ultrasonography of peritoneal tumors. Radiology 1979;133:419-424.

Inflammatory Bowel Disease (Crohn's Disease)

21. Seitz K, Rettenmaier G: Inflammatory bowel disease. Sonographic Diagnostics. Dr. Falk Pharmac, West Germany, GmbH, 1988.

22. Sarrazin J, Wilson SR: Manifestations of Crohn disease at US. Radiographics 1996;16:499-520.

23. DiCandio G, Mosca F, Campatelli A, et al: Sonographic detection of postsurgical recurrence of Crohn's disease. AJR 1986;146:523-526.

24. Worlicek H, Lutz H, Heyder N, et al: Ultrasound findings in Crohn's disease and ulcerative colitis: A prospective study. J Clin Ultrasound 1987;15:153-163.

25. Dubbins PA: Ultrasound demonstration of bowel wall thickness in inflammatory bowel disease. Clin Radiol 1984;35:227-231.

26. Parente F, Maconi G, Bollani SL, et al: Bowel ultrasound in assessment of Crohn's disease and detection of related small bowel strictures: A prospective comparative study versus x ray and intraoperative findings. Gut 2002; 50:490-495.

27. Stewart LK, McGee J, Wilson SR: Transperineal and transvaginal sonography of perianal inflammatory disease. AJR 2001;177(3):627-632.

28. Damani N, Wilson SR: Nongynecologic findings of transvaginal sonography. Radiographics 1999;19: S179-200.

Acute Abdomen

29. Puylaert JB: Ultrasound of acute GI tract conditions. Eur Radiol 2001;11:1867-1877.

30. Seibert JJ, Williamson SL, Golladay ES, et al: The distended gasless abdomen: A fertile field for ultrasound. J Ultrasound Med 1986;5:301-308.

31. Lee DH, Lim JH, Ko YT, et al: Sonographic detection of pneumoperitoneum in patients with acute abdomen. AJR 1990;154:107-199.

32. Muradali D, Wilson S, Burn PN, et al: A specific sign of pneumoperitoneum on sonography: Enhancement of the peritoneal stripe. AJR 1999;17(5):1257-1262.

33. Kazarian KK, Roeder W, Mersheiner WL: Decreasing mortality and increasing morbidity from acute appendicitis. Am J Surg 1970;119:681-685.

34. Pieper R, Forsell P, Kager L: Perforating appendicitis: A nine-year survey of treatment and results. Acta Chir Scand 1986;530:51-57.

35. Go PMNYH, Luyendijk R, Murting JDK: Metnonidazo-protylaxe bij appendectomie. Med Tijdschr Geneejk 1986;130:775-778.

36. Van Way CW III, Murphy JR, Dunn EL, et al: A feasibility study in computer-aided diagnosis in appendicitis. Surg Gynecol Obstet 1982;155:685-688.

37. Berry J Jr, Malt RA: Appendicitis near its centenary. Ann Surg 1984;200(5):567-575.

38. Bendeck SE, Nino-Murcia NM, Berry GJ, Jeffrey RB: Imaging for suspected appendicitis: Negative appendectomy and perforation rates. Radiology 2002;225:131-136.

39. Birnbaum BA, Wilson SR: Appendicitis at the millennium. Radiology 2000;215(2):337-348.

40. Shaw RE: Appendix calculi and acute appendicitis. Br J Surg 1965;52:452-459.

41. Savrin RA, Clauren K, Martin EW, Jr, et al: Chronic and recurrent appendicitis. Am J Surg 1979;137:355-357.

42. Dachman AH, Nichols JB, Patrick DH, et al: Natural history of the obstructed rabbit appendix: Observations with radiography, sonography, and computed tomography. AJR 1987;148:281-284.

43. Jeffrey RB, Jr, Laing FC, Lewis FR: Acute appendicitis: High-resolution real-time ultrasound findings. Radiology 1987;163:11-14.

44. Abu-Yousef MM, Bleicher JJ, Maher JW, et al: High-resolution sonography of acute appendicitis. AJR 1987;149:53-58.

45. Jeffrey RB, Jr, Laing FC, Townsend RR: Acute appendicitis: Sonographic criteria based on 250 cases. Radiology 1988;67:327-329.

46. Rioux M: Sonographic detection of the normal and abnormal appendix. AJR 1992;158:773-778.

47. Rettenbacher T, Hollerweger A, Macheiner P, et al: Ovoid shape of the vermiform appendix: A criterion to exclude acute appendicitis—evaluation with US. Radiology 2003;226:95-100.

48. Lee JH, Jeong YK, Hwang JC, et al: Graded compression sonography with adjuvant use of a posterior manual compression technique in the sonographic diagnosis of acute appendicitis. AJR 2002;178(4):863-868.

49. Borushok KF, Jeffrey RB, Jr, Laing FC, et al: Sonographic diagnosis of perforation in patients with acute appendicitis. AJR 1990;154:275-278.

50. Puylaert JB, Lalisang RI, van der Werf SD, et al: Campylobacter ileocolitis mimicking acute appendicitis: Differentiation with graded-compression ultrasound. Radiology 1988;166:737-740.

51. Gaensler EHL, Jeffrey RB, Jr, Laing FC, et al: Sonography in patients with suspected acute appendicitis: Value in establishing alternative diagnoses. AJR 1989;152:49.

52. Agha FP, Ghahremani GG, Panella JS, et al: Appendicitis as the initial manifestation of Crohn's disease: Radiologic features and prognosis. AJR 1987;149:515-518.

53. Roth T, Zimmer G, Tschantz P. Crohn's disease of the appendix. Ann Chir 2000;125(7):665-667.

54. Higgins MJ, Walsh M, Kennedy SM, et al: Granulomatous appendicitis revisited: Report of a case. Dig Surg 2001;18(3):245-248.

55. Chou YH, Chiou HJ, Tiu CM, et al: Sonography of acute right side colonic diverticulitis. Am J Surg 2001 Feb;181(2):122-127.

56. O'Malley ME, Wilson SR: US of gastrointestinal tract abnormalities with CT correlation. Radiographics 2003;23:59-72.

57. Teefey SA, Montana MA, Goldfogel, et al: Sonographic diagnosis of neutropenic typhlitis. AJR 1987;149:731-733.

58. Frager DH, Frager JD, Brandt LJ, et al: Gastrointestinal complications of AIDS: Radiologic features. Radiology 1986;158:597-603.

59. Balthazar EJ, Megibow AJ, Fazzini E, et al: Cytomegalovirus colitis in AIDS: Radiographic findings in 11 patients. Radiology 1985;155:585-589.

60. Teixidor HS, Honig CL, Norsoph E, et al: Cytomegalo-virus infection of the alimentary canal: Radiologic findings with pathologic correlation. Radiology 1987; 163:317-323.

61. Puylaert JB: Mesenteric adenitis and acute terminal ileitis: US evaluation using graded compression. Radiology 1986;161:691-695.

62. Puylaert JB: Right-sided segmental infarction of the omentum: Clinical, US, and CT findings. Radiology 1992;185:169-172.

63. Bender MD, Ockner RK: Diseases of the peritoneum, mesentery and diaphragm. In Sleisenger MH, Fordtran JS (eds): Gastrointestinal Disease, 5th ed, vol. 2. Philadelphia, WB Saunders, 1993, pp 2004-2011.

Left Lower Quadrant Pain

64. Painter NS, Burkitt DP: Diverticular disease of the colon, a 20th century problem. Clin Gastroenterol 1975;4:3.

65. Parks TG: Natural history of diverticular disease of the colon. Clin Gastroenterol 1975;4:53.

66. Ming SC, Fleischner FG: Diverticulitis of the sigmoid colon: Reappraisal of pathology and pathogenesis. Surgery 1965;58:627.

67. Wilson SR, Toi A: The value of sonography in the diagnosis of acute diverticulitis of the colon. AJR 1990;154:1199-1202.

68. Parulekar SG: Sonography of colonic diverticulitis. J Ultrasound Med 1985;4:659-666.

69. Derchi LE, Reggiani L, Rebaudi F, et al: Appendices epiploicae of the large bowel. Sonographic appearance and differentiation from peritoneal seeding. J Ultrasound Med 1988;7:11-14.

Miscellaneous Abnormalities

70. Jones RS: Intestinal obstruction, pseudo-obstruction, and ileus. In Sleisenger MH, Fordtran JS (eds): Gastrointestinal Disease: Pathophysiology Diagnosis Management, 5th ed, vol 1. Philadelphia, WB Saunders, 1993, pp 898-903.

71. Meiser G, Meissner K: Sonographic differential diagnosis of intestinal obstruction—results of a prospective study of 48 patients. Ultraschall Med 1985;6:39-45.

72. Tennenhouse JE, Wilson SR: Sonographic detection of a small bowel bezoar. J Ultrasound Med 1990;9:603-605.

73. Siewert B, Raptopoulos V: CT of the acute abdomen: Findings and impact on diagnosis and treatment. AJR 1994;163:1317-1324.

74. Balthazar EJ: CT of small-bowel obstruction. AJR 1994;162: 255-261.

75. Lee DH, Lim JH, Ko YT: Afferent loop syndrome: Sonographic findings in seven cases. AJR 1991; 157:41-43.

76. Parienty RA, Lepreux JF, Gruson B: Sonographic and computed tomography features of ileocolic intussusception. AJR 1981;136:608-610.

77. Weissberg DL, Scheible W, Leopold GR: Ultrasonographic appearance of adult intussusception. Radiology 1977;124:791-792.

78. Alessi V, Salerno G: The "hay-fork" sign in the ultrasonographic diagnosis of intussusception. Gastrointest Radiol 1985;10:177-179.

79. Gaines PA, Saunders AJS, Drake D: Midgut malrotation diagnosed by ultrasound. Clin Radiol 1987;38:51-53.

80. Wilson SR: Evaluation of the small intestine by ultrasonography. In Gourtsoyiannis NC (ed): Radiological Imaging of the Small Intestine. Heidelberg, Germany: Springer-Verlag, 2002, pp 73-86.

81. Bartlett JG: The pseudomembranous enterocolitides. In Sleisenger MH, Fordtran JS (eds): Gastrointestinal Disease: Pathophysiology Diagnosis Management, 5th ed, vol. 2. Philadelphia, WB Saunders, 1993, pp 1174-1189.

82. Totten MA, Gregg JA, Fremont-Smith P, et al: Clinical and pathological spectrum of antibiotic-associated colitis. Am J Gastroenterol 1978;69:311-319.

83. Bolondi L, Ferrentino M, Trevisani F, et al: Sonographic appearance of pseudomembranous colitis. J Ultrasound Med 1985;4:489-492.

84. Downey DB, Wilson SR: The role of sonography in pseudomembranous colitis. Radiology 1991;180:61-64.

85. Fenoglio-Preiser CM, Lantz PE, Listrom MB, et al (eds): Gastrointestinal Pathology: An Atlas and Text, 2nd ed. New York, 1998, Raven Press, pp 763-908.

86. Sigel B, Machi J, Ramos JR, et al: Ultrasonic features of pneumatosis intestinalis. J Clin Ultrasound 1985; 13:675-678.

87. Vernacchia FS, Jeffrey RB, Laing FC, et al: Sonographic recognition of pneumatosis intestinalis. AJR 1985; 145:51-52.

88. Woodruff R, McDonald JR: Benign and malignant cystic tumors of the appendix. Surg Gynecol Obstet 1940;71:750-755.

89. The gastrointestinal tract. In Robbins SL, Cotran RS, Kumar V (eds): Pathologic Basis of Disease, 5th ed. Philadelphia, WB Saunders, 1994, pp 755–830.

90. Young RH, Gilks CB, Scully RE: Mucinous tumors of the appendix associated with mucinous tumors of the ovary and pseudomyxoma peritonei. A clinicopathological analysis of 22 cases supporting an origin in the appendix. Am J Surg Pathol 1991;15(5):415-429.

91. Horgan JG, Chow PP, Richter JO, et al: Computed tomography and sonography in the recognition of mucoceles of the appendix. AJR 1984;143:959.

92. Dietrich CF, Brunner V, Seifert H, et al: Intestinal B-mode sonography in patients with endemic sprue. Intestinal sonography in endemic sprue. Ultraschall Med 1999;20(6):242-247.

93. Rettenbacher T, Hollerweger A, Macheiner P, et al: Adult celiac disease: US signs. Radiology 1999;211(2):389-394.

94. Pickhardt PJ, Yagan N, Siegel MJ, et al: Cystic fibrosis: CT findings of colonic disease. Radiology 1998 Mar;206(3):725-730

95. Haber HP, Benda N, Fitzke G, et al: Colonic wall thickness measured by ultrasound: Striking differences in patients with cystic fibrosis versus healthy controls. Gut 1997;40(3):406-411.

96. Connett GJ, Lucas JS, Atchley JT, et al: Colonic wall thickening is related to age and not dose of high strength pancreatin microspheres in children with cystic fibrosis. Eur J Gastroenterol Hepatol 1999;11(2):181-183.

97. Welkon CJ, Long SS, Thompson CM Jr, et al: Clostridium difficile in patients with cystic fibrosis. Am J Dis Child 1985 Aug;139(8):805-808.

Endosonography

98. Shorvon PJ, Lees WR, Frost RA, et al: Upper gastrointestinal endoscopic ultrasonography in gastroenterology. Br J Radiol 1987;60:429-438.

99. Strohm WD, Classen M: Benign lesions of the upper GI tract by means of endoscopic ultrasonography. Scand J Gastroenterol 1986;21(123):41-46.

100. Takemoto T, Ito T, Aibe T, et al: Endoscopic ultrasonography in the diagnosis of esophageal carcinoma, with particular regard to staging it for operability. Endoscopy 1986;18(3):22-25.

101. Bolondi L, Casanova P, Caletti GC, et al: Primary gastric lymphoma versus gastric carcinoma: Endoscopic ultrasound evaluation. Radiology 1987;165:821-826.

102. Astler VB, Coller FA: The prognostic significance of direct extension of carcinoma of the colon and rectum. Ann Surg 1954;139:816.

103. Spiessel B, Schiebe O, Wagner G: Union International Contre le Cancer (UICC) TNM Atlas, New York, 1982, Springer Verlag.

104. Wang KY, Kimmey MB, Nyberg DA, et al: Colorectal neoplasms: Accuracy of ultrasound in demonstrating the depth of invasion. Radiology 1987;165:827-829.

105. Yamashita Y, Machi J, Shirouzu K, et al: Evaluation of endorectal ultrasound for the assessment of wall invasion of rectal cancer: Report of a case. Dis Colon Rectum 1988;31(8):617-623.

106. Hildebrandt U, Feifel G: Preoperative staging of rectal cancer by intrarectal ultrasound. Dis Colon Rectum 1985;28(1):42-46.

107. Rifkin MD, Ehrlich SM, Marks G: Staging of rectal carcinoma: Prospective comparison of endorectal

ultrasound and computed tomography. Radiology 1989;170:319-322.

108. Law PJ, Bartman CI: Anal endosonography: Technique and normal anatomy, Gastrointest Radiol 1989; 14:349-353.

109. Stewart LK, Wilson SR: Transvaginal sonography of the anal sphincter: Reliable or not? AJR 1999;173:179-185.

110. Sudakoff GS, Quiroz F, Foley WD: Sonography of anorectal, rectal, and perirectal abnormalities. AJR 2002;179:131-136.

111. Parks AG, Gordon PH, Hardcastle JE: A classification of fistula-in-ano. Br J Surg 1976;63:1-12.

9

THE URINARY TRACT

Wendy Thurston / Stephanie R. Wilson

Chapter Outline

Chapter Outline—cont'd

$\mathcal{T}$he prime function of the kidney is excretion of metabolic waste product. The kidneys do this by converting more than 1700 liters of blood per day into 1 liter of highly concentrated urine.[1] The kidney is an endocrine organ secreting many hormones including erythropoietin, renin, and prostaglandins. The kidneys also function to maintain homeostasis by regulating water/salt and acid/base balance. The renal collecting system, ureters, and urethra function as conduits and the bladder serves as a reservoir for urinary excretion.

EMBRYOLOGY

Development of the Kidneys and Ureter

Three sets of kidneys develop in human embryos: the pronephros, mesonephros, and metanephros (the permanent kidney).[2] The **pronephros** appear early in the fourth embryologic week and are rudimentary and nonfunctioning. The **mesonephros** form late in the fourth week and function as interim kidneys until the metanephros develop (fifth week) and begin to function (ninth week).

The **metanephros** (permanent kidneys) develop from two sources: (1) the **ureteric bud** and (2) the **metanephrogenic blastema**.[2] The ureteric bud, which forms the ureter, renal pelvis, calices, and collecting ducts, interacts with and penetrates the blastema. This interaction is necessary to initiate ureteric bud branching and differentiation of nephrons within the metanephrogenic blastema (Fig. 9-1). Initially, the permanent kidneys are found in the pelvis. With fetal growth, the kidneys come to lie in the upper retroperitoneum. With ascent, the kidneys rotate medially 90 degrees so that the renal pelvis is directed anteromedially. The kidneys are in their adult location and position by the ninth gestational week. As the kidneys ascend, they derive their blood supply from nearby vessels. Their adult blood supply is from the abdominal aorta.

Development of the Bladder

In the seventh gestational week the urorectal septum fuses with the cloacal membrane, dividing it into a **ventral urogenital sinus** and a **dorsal rectum**. The bladder develops from the urogenital sinus. Initially, the bladder is continuous with the allantois, which eventually becomes a fibrous cord called the **urachus** (known as the median umbilical ligament in the adult). As the bladder enlarges, the distal portion of the mesonephric ducts is incorporated as connective tissue into the bladder trigone.[2] At the same time, the ureters come to open separately into the bladder.[2] In infants and children, the bladder is an abdominal organ and it is not until after puberty that it becomes a true pelvic structure (Fig. 9-2).[2]

Development of the Urethra

The epithelium of most of the male urethra and the entire female urethra is derived from the endoderm of the urogenital sinus.[2] The urethral connective tissue and smooth muscle form from adjacent splanchnic mesenchyme.[2]

ANATOMY

Kidney

In the adult, each kidney is about 11 cm long, 2.5 cm thick, 5 cm wide, and weighs between 120 and 170 grams.[3] Emamian et al.[4] demonstrated, using 665 volunteers, that parenchymal volume of the right kidney is smaller than the left. Possible explanations for this include (1) the spleen is smaller than the liver and there is more space for left kidney growth, and (2) the left renal artery is shorter than the right and, therefore, increased blood flow on the left results in increased renal volume. They also demonstrated that renal length correlates best with body height and renal size decreases with advancing age because of parenchymal reduction.

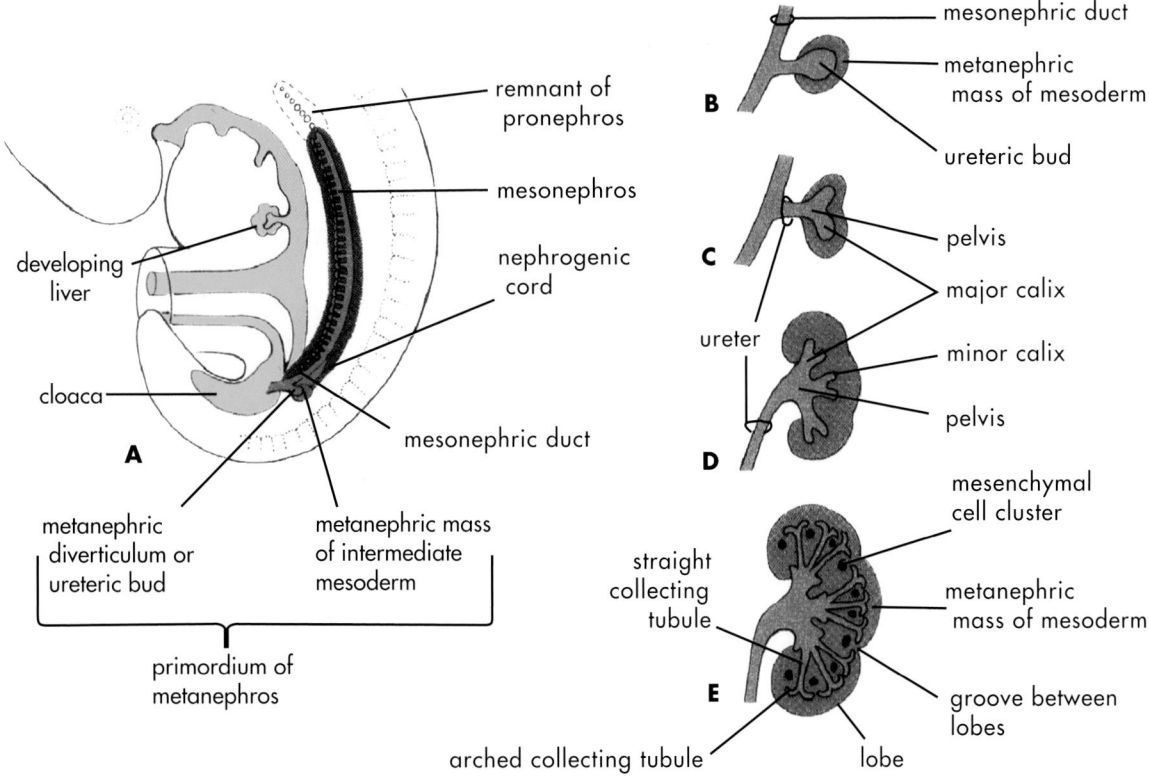

FIGURE 9-1. Embryology of the kidney and ureter. A, Lateral view of a 5-week embryo showing the three embryologic kidneys that develop. **B** through **E,** Successive stages of development of the ureteric bud (fifth to eighth week) into the ureter, pelvis, calices, and collecting tubules. (From The urogenital system. In Moore KL, Persaud TVN (eds): The Developing Human. 5th ed. Philadelphia, WB Saunders, 1993, pp 265-303.)

The left kidney usually lies 1 to 2 cm higher than the right.[3] The kidneys are mobile and will move depending on body position. In the supine position, the superior pole of the left kidney is at the level of the twelfth thoracic vertebrae and the inferior pole at the level of the third lumbar vertebrae.

The normal adult kidney is bean shaped with a smooth convex contour anteriorly, posteriorly, and laterally. Medially, the surface is concave and known as the **renal hilum**. The renal hilum is continuous with a central cavity called the **renal sinus**. Within the renal sinus are the major branches of the renal artery, major tributaries of the renal vein, and the collecting system.[3] The remainder of the renal sinus is packed with fat. The collecting system (renal pelvis) lies posterior to the renal vessels in the renal hilum (Fig. 9-3).

The **renal parenchyma** is composed of **cortex** and **medullary pyramids**. The renal medullary pyramids are hypoechoic relative to the renal cortex and can be identified in most normal adults (Fig. 9-4). The normal renal cortex has classically been described as being less echogenic than adjacent liver and spleen. Platt et al.[5] evaluated 153 patients and found that 72% of patients with renal cortical echogenicity equal to that of the liver had normal renal function. If renal echogenicity greater than the liver were used as the criterion, both specificity

and positive predictive value for abnormal renal function rose to 96% and 67%, respectively. However, sensitivity is poor—only 20%.[5]

During normal development, there is partial fusion of two parenchymal masses called *renunculi*. **Parenchymal junctional defects** occur at the site of fusion and must not be confused with pathologic processes such as renal scars and angiomyolipoma. The junctional parenchymal defect is most typically located anteriorly and superiorly and can be traced medially and inferiorly into the renal sinus. Usually, it is oriented more horizontally than vertically; therefore, it is best appreciated on sagittal

SONOGRAPHIC CRITERIA FOR HYPERTROPHIED COLUMN OF BERTIN

Indentation of the renal sinus laterally
Bordered by a junctional parenchymal defect
Location at the junction of the upper and middle thirds
Continuous with adjacent renal cortex
Contains renal pyramids
Less than 3 cm in size

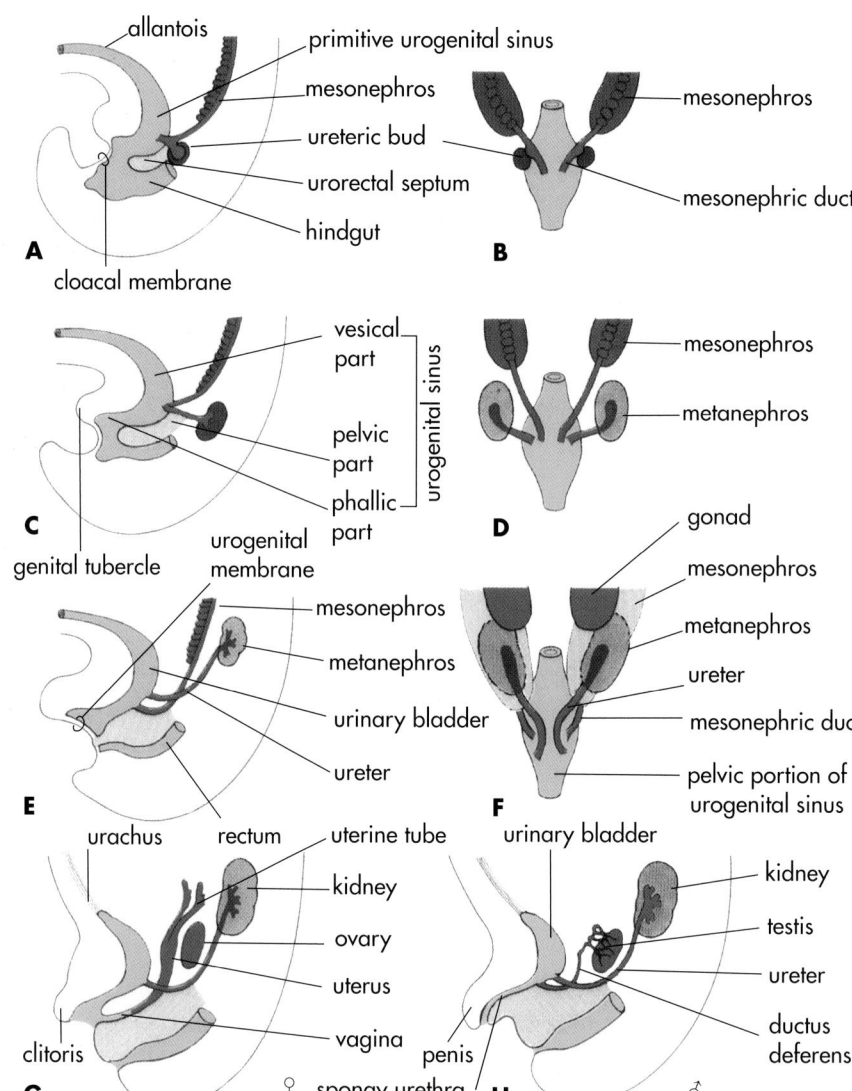

FIGURE 9-2. Embryology of the bladder and urethra. Diagrams showing division of the cloaca into the urogenital sinus and rectum; absorption of the mesonephric ducts; development of the urinary bladder, urethra and urachus; and change in location of the ureters. **A** and **B**, 5-week embryo. **C** through **H**, 7- to 12-week embryo. (From The urogenital system. In Moore KL, Persaud TVN (eds): The Developing Human. 5th ed. Philadelphia, WB Saunders, 1993, pp 265-303.)

scans (Fig. 9-5).[6] It is seen more often on the right; however, when a good acoustic window is present (splenomegaly), it can also be seen on the left.

Hypertrophied column of Bertin (HCB) is a normal variant and represents unresorbed polar parenchyma from one or both of the two subkidneys that fuse to form the normal kidney.[7] Sonographic criteria used to allow diagnosis of HCB include indentation of the renal sinus laterally, bordered by a junctional parenchymal line and defect. It is usually at the junction of the upper and middle thirds of the kidney and contains renal cortex that is continuous with the adjacent renal cortex of the same subkidney. HCB contains renal pyramids. The largest dimension is less than 3 cm (Fig. 9-6).[7,8]

Echogenicity of the HCB and renal cortex depends on the scan plane in relation to the tissue structures. The differences in tissue orientation produce different acoustic reflectivity.[7] The echoes of the HCB are brighter than those of adjacent renal cortex when seen *en face* (see

Fig. 9-6).[7] It may be difficult to differentiate a small avascular tumor from an HCB; however, demonstration of arcuate arteries by color Doppler indicates HCB rather than tumor. Occasionally, intravenous pyelography (IVP), computed tomography (CT), or renal scintigraphy will be required to make the differentiation.

Renal duplication artifact can occur as a result of sound beam refraction between the lower portion of the spleen or liver and adjacent fat.[9] Middleton et al.[9] analyzed duplication artifact in 20 patients and found that it mimicked duplication of the collecting system, suprarenal mass, and upper-pole renal cortical thickening. This artifact is seen most commonly on the left and in obese patients. Changing the transducer position or using deep inspiration so that the liver and spleen are interposed as an acoustic window will eliminate the false impression.

The kidney has a thin, fibrous true capsule. Outside this capsule is the **perirenal fat**. The fat is encased

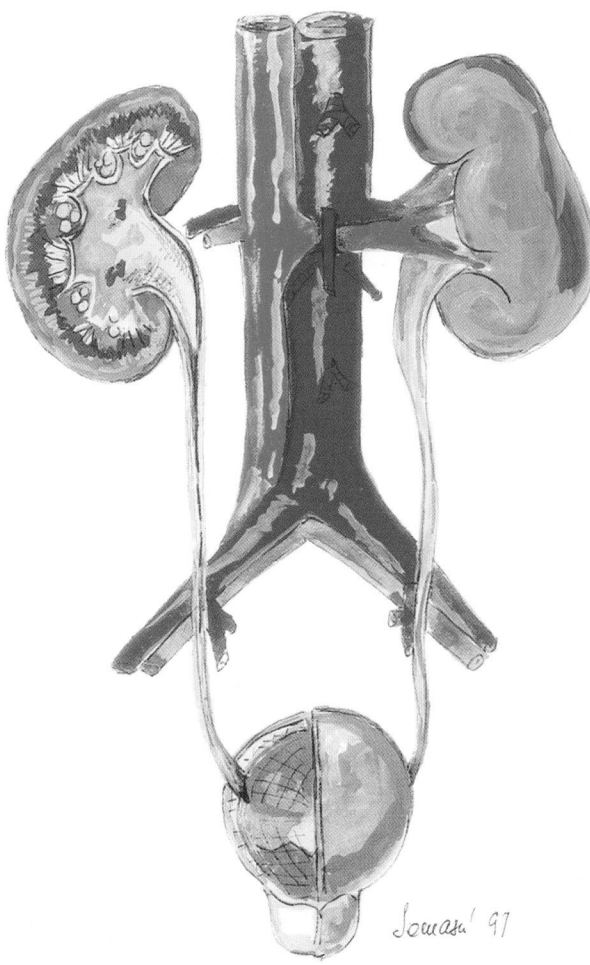

FIGURE 9-3. Anatomy of the kidney, ureter, and bladder.

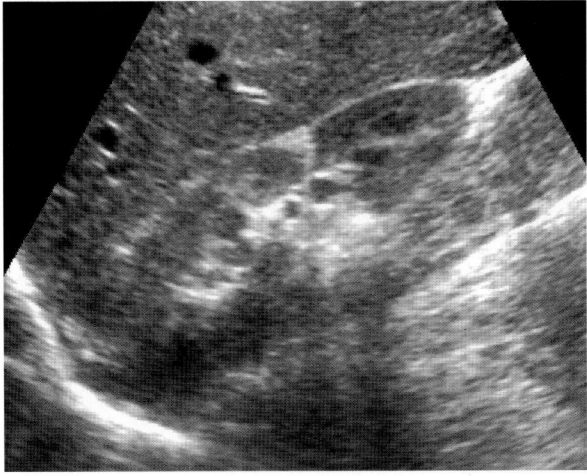

FIGURE 9-5. Anterior junction line. Sagittal sonogram demonstrating the echogenic line that extends from the renal sinus to the perinephric fat, most commonly located at the junction of the upper and middle thirds of the kidney.

anteriorly by the **fibrous fascia of Gerota** and posteriorly by the **fibrous fascia of Zuckerkandl**.[10] The perirenal space is open superiorly on the right to the bare area of the liver, allowing communication between the retroperitoneum and intraperitoneal space.[11] The perirenal spaces communicate with one another at the level of the third to fifth lumbar vertebrae.[11]

Ureter

The ureter is a long (30 to 34 cm)[3] mucosal-lined conduit that delivers urine from the renal pelvis to the bladder. Each ureter varies in diameter from 2 to 8 mm.[3] As the ureter enters the pelvis, it passes anterior to the common, or external, iliac artery. The ureter has an oblique course through the bladder wall (see Fig. 9-3).

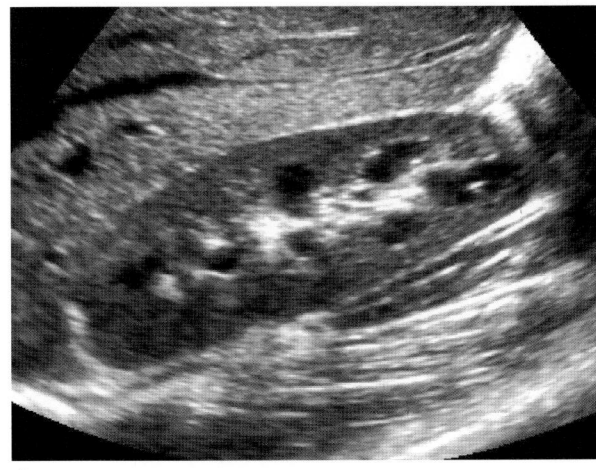

A

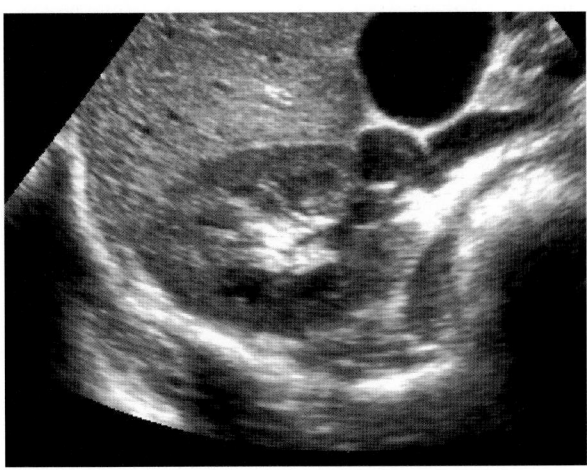

B

FIGURE 9-4. Normal kidney. A, Sagittal and **B,** transverse sonograms demonstrating normal anatomy with corticomedullary differentiation.

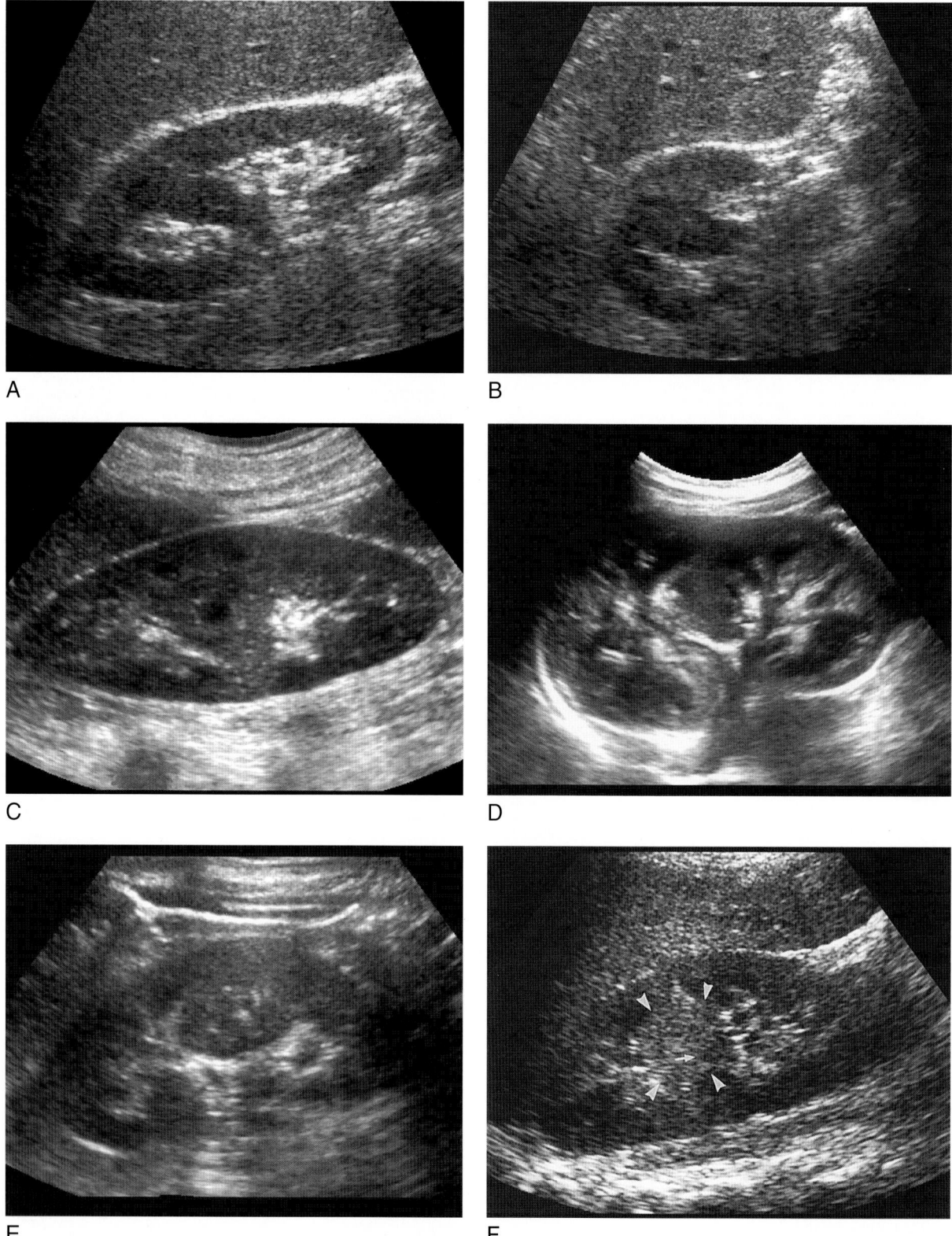

FIGURE 9-6. Appearances of hypertrophied column of Bertin. **A**, Sagittal and **B**, transverse sonograms show classic appearance of the column. **C**, Medullary pyramids can be seen within the hypertrophied column of Bertin. **D**, **E** and **F** show variations of echogenicity and shape. In **F**, the *arrowheads* outline the hypertrophied column.

Bladder

The bladder is in the pelvis inferior and anterior to the peritoneal cavity and posterior to the pubic bones.[3] Superiorly, the peritoneum is reflected over the anterior aspect of the bladder. Within the bladder the ureteric and urethral orifices demarcate an area known as the **trigone**. The urethral orifice marks the area known as the bladder neck. The bladder neck and trigone remain constant in shape and position; however, the remainder of the bladder will change shape and position depending on the volume of urine within it. Deep to the peritoneum covering the bladder lies a loose, connective tissue layer of subserosa, which forms the adventitial layer of the bladder wall. Adjacent to the adventitia are three muscular layers that include (1) outer or longitudinal muscle layer; (2) middle or circular muscle layer; and (3) internal longitudinal muscle layer. Adjacent to the muscle, the innermost layer of the bladder is composed of mucosa. The bladder wall should be smooth and of uniform thickness. The wall thickness depends on the degree of bladder distention.

GENITOURINARY TRACT SONOGRAPHY

Technical Aspects

Ability to visualize organs of the genitourinary tract sonographically is multifactorial related to (1) body habitus; (2) operator experience; and (3) type of equipment. The patient should fast a minimum of 6 hours before the examination in an attempt to limit bowel gas. High-resolution, real-time sector scanners should be used. Harmonic imaging should be routinely used in the evaluation of genitourinary tract stones.

Scanning Technique

Kidney. The kidneys should be assessed in the transverse and coronal plane. Patient position should include the supine, oblique, lateral decubitus, and, occasionally, prone position. Usually, a combination of subcostal and intercostal approaches is necessary to fully evaluate the kidneys, particularly the upper pole of the left kidney.

Ureter. The proximal ureter is best visualized using a coronal-oblique view with the kidney as an acoustic window. An attempt is made to follow the ureter to the bladder maintaining the same approach. A nondilated ureter may be impossible to visualize because of overlying bowel gas. Transverse scanning of the retroperitoneum will often demonstrate a dilated ureter, which can then be followed caudally with both transverse and sagittal imaging. In women, a dilated distal ureter can be well seen with transvaginal scanning if visualization through the abdominal wall is poor because of intervening bowel gas or if the bladder is empty.

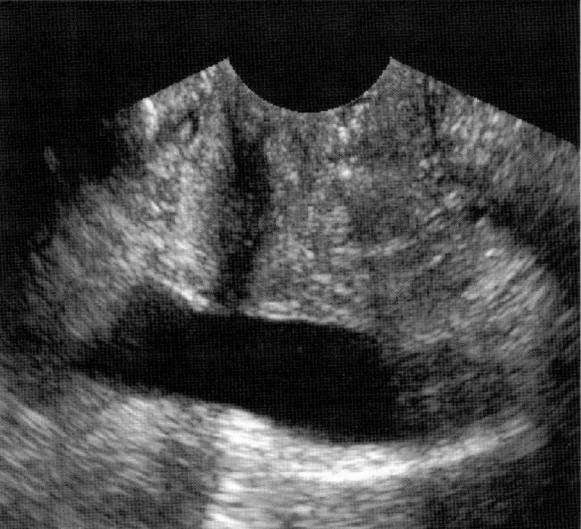

FIGURE 9-7. Translabial ultrasound of the female urethra. Sagittal sonogram shows the tubular hypoechoic urethra extending from the bladder to the skin surface.

Bladder. The bladder is best evaluated when it is moderately filled. When overfilled, patient discomfort occurs. The bladder should be scanned in the transverse and sagittal plane and occasionally in a decubitus position. To better visualize the bladder wall in women, transvaginal scanning can be helpful. If the nature of a large fluid-filled mass in the pelvis is uncertain, either voiding or insertion of a Foley catheter will clarify the location and appearance of the bladder relative to the fluid-filled mass.

Urethra. The urethra in a woman can be scanned with transvaginal, transperineal or translabial sonography (Fig. 9-7).[12] The posterior or prostatic urethra in men is best visualized with endorectal probes (Fig. 9-8).

CONGENITAL ANOMALIES OF THE GENITOURINARY TRACT

Anomalies Related to Renal Growth

Hypoplasia. Renal hypoplasia represents a renal parenchymal anomaly in which there are too few nephrons. Renal function is normal in proportion to the mass of the kidney. True hypoplasia is a rare anomaly. Many patients with unilateral hypoplasia are asymptomatic and the condition is detected as an incidental finding. Patients with bilateral hypoplasia often have evidence of renal insufficiency. Hypoplasia is believed to result from the ureteral bud making contact with the caudal-most portion of the metanephrogenic blastema. This can occur with delayed development of the ureteric bud or from delayed contact of the bud with the cranially migrating blastema. Morphologically, the diagnosis is established by the finding of fewer renal lobules which

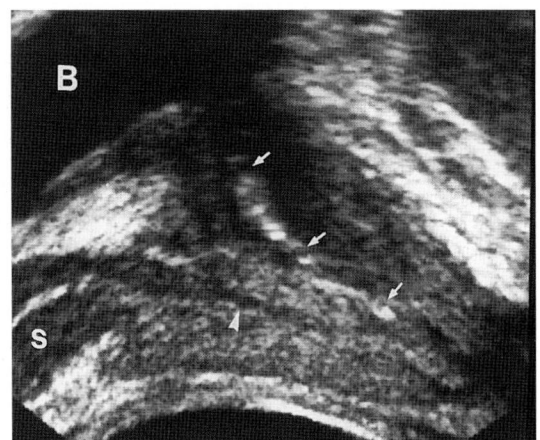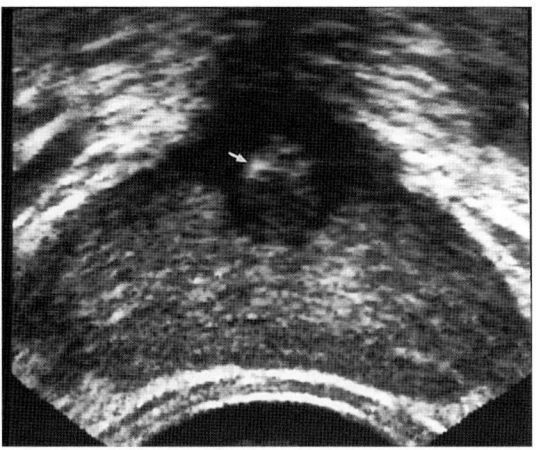

FIGURE 9-8. Transrectal ultrasound of the male urethra. **A,** Sagittal and **B,** transverse sonograms show the urethra with calcifications in the urethral glands (*arrows*) surrounded by the echo-poor muscle of the internal urethral sphincter. Bladder (B), ejaculatory duct (*arrow*), seminal vesicles (S). (Courtesy of Ants Toi, M.D., The Toronto Hospital.)

otherwise have a normal microscopic appearance.[13] **Sonographically,** the kidney is small but otherwise normal. Sometimes the kidney may be difficult to identify, particularly on the left side.

Fetal Lobulation. Fetal lobulation is usually present until 4 or 5 years of age; however, persistent lobulation is seen in 51% of adult kidneys.[14] There is infolding of the cortex without loss of cortical parenchyma. On **sonography,** sharp clefts are seen overlying the septa of Bertin.[15]

Compensatory Hypertrophy. Compensatory hypertrophy may be diffuse or focal and occurs when existing healthy nephrons enlarge to allow the healthy renal parenchyma to perform more work. The diffuse form is seen with **nephrectomy, renal agenesis, renal hypoplasia, renal atrophy,** or **renal dysplasia.** The focal form is seen when **residual islands of normal tissue** enlarge in an otherwise diseased kidney (**reflux nephropathy**). On **sonography,** diffuse compensatory hypertrophy reveals an enlarged but otherwise normal kidney. In nodular compensatory hypertrophy, large areas of nodular normal renal tissue are seen between scars and may mimic a solid renal mass.[5]

Anomalies Related to Ascent of the Kidney

Ectopia. Failure of the kidney to ascend during embryologic development results in a **pelvic kidney** that is estimated to occur in 1 in 724 pediatric autopsies.[15] These kidneys are often small and abnormally rotated. Fifty percent of pelvic kidneys have decreased function.[15] The ureters are often short. These kidneys are prone to poor drainage and may develop dilation of the collecting system with susceptibility to infection and stone formation. The blood supply is derived from the regional vessels, usually the common or internal iliac artery, and

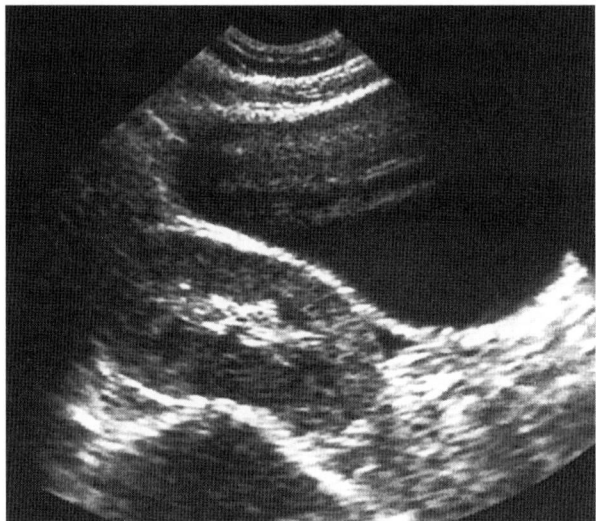

FIGURE 9-9. Pelvic kidney. Sagittal sonogram demonstrates a kidney posterior to the bladder.

is often multiple. If the kidney ascends too high, it may pass through the foramen of Bochdalek and become a true **thoracic kidney.** This is usually of no clinical significance. On **sonography,** the kidney location can usually be ascertained if not found in its normal location (Fig. 9-9). Particularly with kidneys that have ascended too high, ultrasound is helpful to determine whether or not the diaphragm is intact.

Crossed Renal Ectopia. In crossed renal ectopia, both kidneys are found on the same side. In 85% to 90% of cases, the ectopic kidney will be fused to the other kidney. The upper pole of the ectopic kidney is usually fused to the lower pole of the other kidney, although fusion may occur anywhere. The incidence at autopsy is one in 1000 to 1500.[14] Embryologically, there is fusion of the metanephrogenic blastema, which does not allow proper rotation or ascent; therefore, both kidneys are

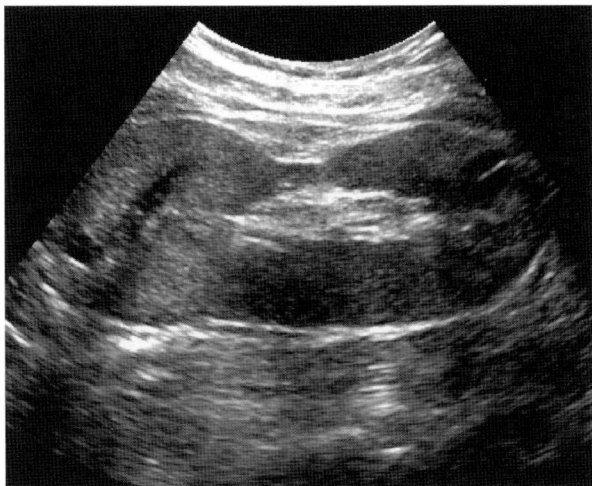

FIGURE 9-10. Cross-fused ectopia. Sagittal sonogram demonstrates two kidneys fused to each other.

more caudally located. The ureterovesical junctions will be located in their normal position. On **sonography**, both kidneys will be on the same side with the majority demonstrating fusion (Fig. 9-10). In patients with renal colic, the knowledge that the ureterovesical junctions are normally located is particularly important.

Horseshoe Kidney. Horseshoe kidney occurs with an incidence of 0.01% to 0.25%. These kidneys fail to rotate properly and often demonstrate ureteropelvic junction obstruction, which leads to an increased incidence of infection and stone formation. The horseshoe kidney sits anterior to the abdominal great vessels and derives its blood supply from the aorta and other regional vessels such as inferior mesenteric, common iliac, internal iliac, and external iliac arteries. Fusion of the metanephrogenic blastema, usually at the lower poles (95%), prior to ascent will result in a horseshoe kidney. Usually, the isthmus is composed of functioning renal tissue, although sometimes it may be a fibrous connection. Associated anomalies include ureteropelvic junction obstruction, vesicoureteral reflux, collecting system duplication, renal dysplasia, retrocaval ureter, supernumerary kidney, anorectal malformation, esophageal atresia, rectovaginal fistula, omphalocele, and cardiovascular and skeletal abnormalities. On **sonography**, the kidneys are usually lower than normal with the lower poles projecting medially. Transverse imaging of the retroperitoneum will demonstrate the renal isthmus crossing the midline anterior to the abdominal great vessels (Fig. 9-11). Pelvicaliectasis and collecting system stones may be evident.

Anomalies Related to the Ureteral Bud

Renal Agenesis. Renal agenesis may be unilateral or bilateral. Bilateral renal agenesis is a rare anomaly, incompatible with life and found in 0.04% of autopsies with a 3:1 male predominance.[14] Unilateral renal agenesis is usually an incidental finding with the remaining kidney demonstrating compensatory hypertrophy. Renal agenesis will occur when there is (1) absence of the metanephrogenic blastema; (2) absence of ureteral bud development; or (3) absence of interaction and penetration of the ureteral bud with the metanephrogenic blastema. Renal agenesis is associated with genital tract anomalies, which are often cystic pelvic masses in both men and women. Other associated anomalies include skeletal abnormalities, anorectal malformations, and cryptorchism. On **sonography**, the kidney is absent; however, a normal adrenal gland is usually found. The adrenal gland will be absent in 8% to 17%.[15] It may be difficult to differentiate between renal agenesis and a small hypoplastic or dysplastic kidney. The other kidney will demonstrate compensatory hypertrophy with all these conditions. Usually, the colon falls into the empty

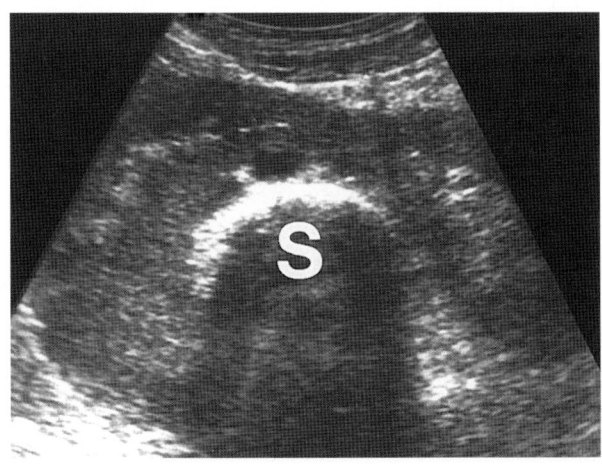

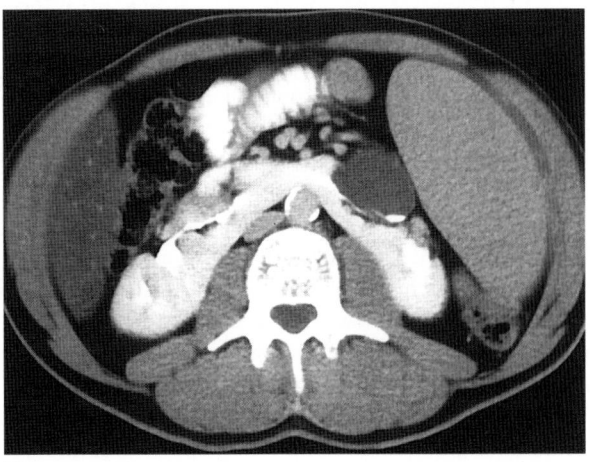

A   B

FIGURE 9-11. Horseshoe kidney. A, Transverse sonogram shows the isthmus crossing anterior to the retroperitoneal great vessels with the renal parenchyma of each limb of the horseshoe draping over the spine (S). **B,** Confirmatory computed tomography.

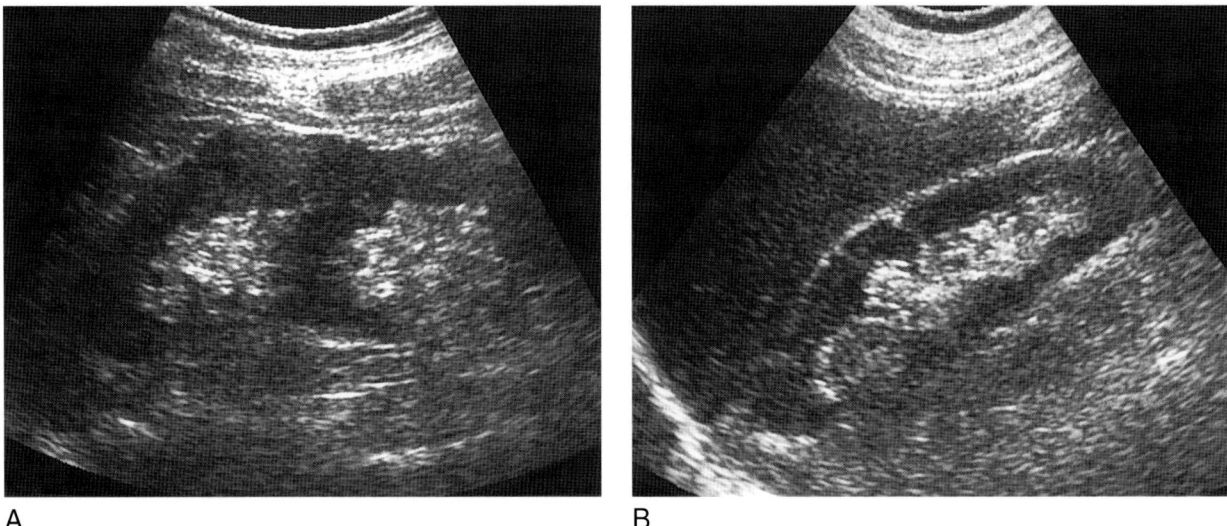

A   B

FIGURE 9-12. Supernumerary kidney. Sagittal sonograms demonstrate **A**, two fused kidneys on the left and **B**, normal right kidney.

renal bed and care should be taken not to confuse a loop of gut with a normal kidney.

Supernumerary Kidney. Supernumerary kidneys are an exceedingly rare anomaly. The supernumerary kidney is usually smaller than normal and can be found above, below, in front of, or behind the normal kidney. The supernumerary kidney often has only a few calices and a single infundibulum. The formation of a supernumerary kidney is likely caused by the same mechanism as that which gives rise to a duplex collecting system.[14] Two ureteric buds reach the metanephrogenic blastema, which then divides, or there are two blastema initially present. On **sonography**, an extra kidney will be found (Fig. 9-12).

Duplex Collecting System and Ureterocele. Duplex collecting system is the most common congenital anomaly of the urinary tract with a reported incidence of 0.5% to 10% of all live births.[14] The degree of duplication is variable. Duplication is **complete** when there are two separate collecting systems and two separate ureters, each with their own ureteral orifice. Duplication is **incomplete** when the ureters join and enter the bladder through a single ureteral orifice. Ureteropelvic duplication arises when two ureteral buds form and join with the metanephrogenic blastema or when there is division of a single ureteral bud early in embryogenesis. Normally during embryologic development, the ureteral orifice migrates superiorly and laterally to become part of the bladder trigone. With complete duplication, the ureter from the lower pole of the kidney migrates to assume its normal location, whereas the ureter draining the superior pole of the kidney doesn't migrate normally, resulting in a more medial and inferior located ureteral orifice. There is an increased incidence of ureteropelvic junction obstruction and uterus didelphys.[15]

In complete duplication, the ureter draining the lower pole has a more perpendicular course through the bladder wall making it more prone to **reflux**. The ectopic ureter from the upper pole is prone to obstruction, reflux, or both. If obstruction is present, it can result in cystic dilation of the intramural portion of the ureter, giving rise to a **ureterocele**. Ureteroceles may be unilateral or bilateral and may occur in normal, duplicated, or ectopic ureters. Clinically, ureteroceles may produce obstruction and give rise to recurrent or persistent urinary tract infections. If large, they may block the contralateral ureteral orifice and/or the urethral orifice at the bladder neck. Ureterocele treatment is surgical. Ureteroceles are a common observation at sonography in asymptomatic patients. They are often transient, incidental, and insignificant.

On **sonography**, a duplex collecting system is seen as two central echogenic renal sinuses with intervening bridging renal parenchyma. Unfortunately, this sign is insensitive and only seen in 17% of duplex kidneys.[16] Hydronephrosis of the upper pole moiety and visualization of two distinct collecting systems and ureters are diagnostic (Fig. 9-13). The bladder should always be carefully evaluated for the presence of a ureterocele. A ureterocele will appear as a round, cystlike structure within the bladder (see Fig. 9-13). Occasionally, it may be large enough to occupy the entire bladder with obstruction of the bladder neck. In female patients, transvaginal sonography can be helpful to identify small ureteroceles (Fig. 9-14).[17] These ureteroceles may be transient. Madeb et al.[18] demonstrated that transvaginal sonography with color Doppler and spectral analysis could provide additional information about flow dynamics, thereby eliminating the need for invasive procedures.

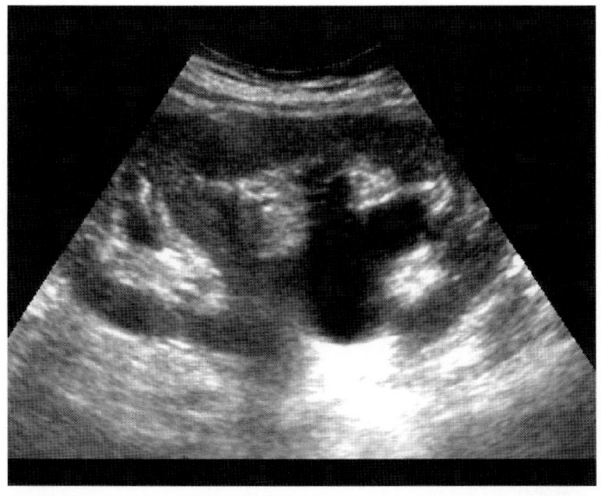

A

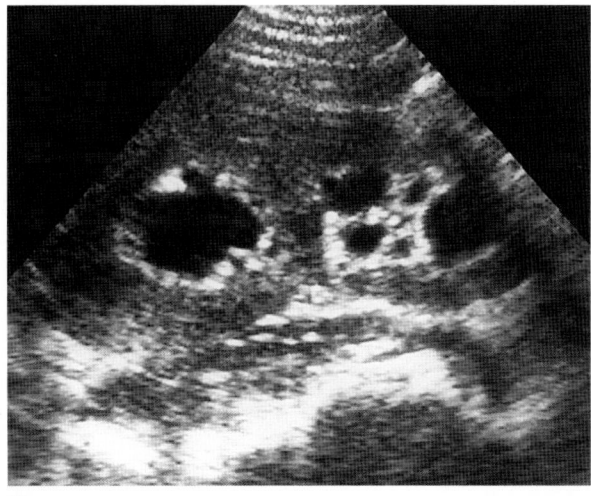

B

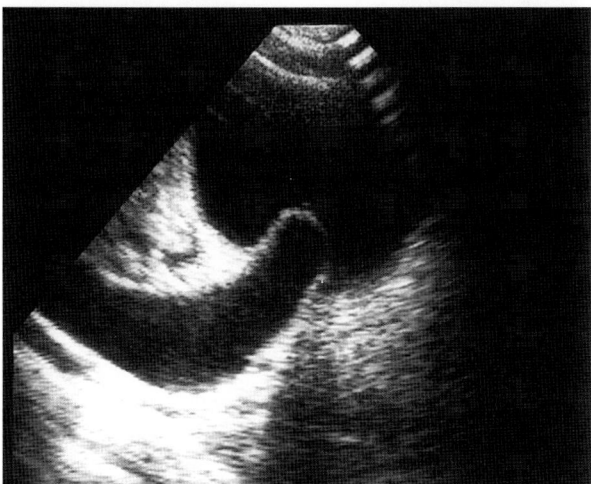

C

FIGURE 9-13. Duplex collecting system. A, Sagittal sonogram shows dilation of the lower pole moiety likely related to reflux. **B,** Sagittal sonogram shows central parenchyma separating the upper and lower-pole moieties. There is moderate dilation of both moieties. **C,** Sagittal sonogram of the bladder and distal ureter of the patient in **B**. There is dilation of the ureter from the upper pole moiety with a large ureterocele.

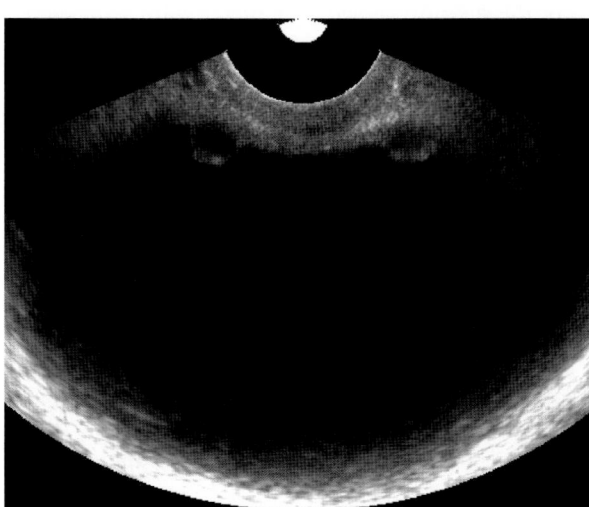

FIGURE 9-14. Bilateral small ureteroceles. Transverse transvaginal sonogram demonstrates two small cystic structures related to the bladder wall. With the probe in the vagina the bladder trigone and the ureteric orifices show as depicted in the image.

Ureteropelvic Junction Obstruction. Ureteropelvic junction (UPJ) obstruction is a common anomaly and is found in men with a 2:1 predominance. The left kidney is affected twice as frequently as the right. It is bilateral in 10% to 30%.[19] Most adult patients will present with chronic, vague back or flank pain. Symptomatic patients or patients with complications, including superimposed infection, stones, or impairment of renal function, should be treated. There is an increased incidence of contralateral multicystic dysplastic kidney and renal agenesis. It is believed that most idiopathic UPJ obstructions are functional rather than anatomic.[19] Histologic evaluation of affected resected specimens has demonstrated excessive collagen between muscle bundles, deficient or absent muscle, and excessive longitudinal muscle.[19] Occasionally, intrinsic valves, true luminal stenosis, and aberrant arteries are the cause of obstruction. On **sonography,** pelvicaliectasis is present to the level of the UPJ (Fig. 9-15). Often marked ballooning of the renal pelvis is present, and if long-standing, there will be associated renal parenchymal atrophy. The ureter is of

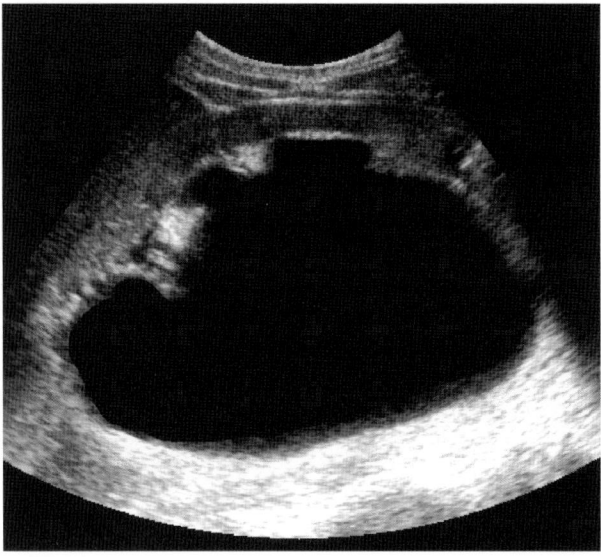
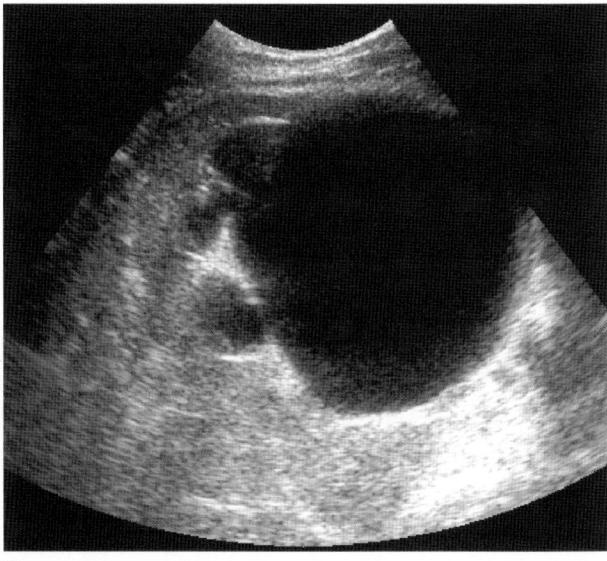

A

B

FIGURE 9-15. Ureteropelvic junction obstruction. A, Sagittal and **B,** transverse sonograms demonstrate marked ballooning of the renal pelvis with associated proximal caliectasis.

normal caliber. Careful evaluation of the contralateral kidney should be performed to assess for the presence of associated anomalies.

Congenital Megacalices. Congenital megacalices is an entity producing nonobstructive enlargement of the calices, which is usually unilateral. It is nonprogressive and patients have normal renal function and parenchyma. There is an increased incidence of infection and stone formation because of caliceal enlargement. The exact pathogenesis is speculative. The most common association is with primary megaureter.[20] On **sonography**, enlarged clubbed calices are seen which are usually increased in number. Papillary impressions are absent. Cortical thickness is maintained.

Congenital Megaureter. Congenital megaureter results in functional ureteric obstruction. The distal-most segment of ureter is aperistaltic giving rise to a wide spectrum of findings, ranging from insignificant distal ureterectasis to progressive hydronephroureterosis. Men are more commonly affected as is the left side.[19] Bilateral involvement has been demonstrated in 8% to 50% of patients. On **sonography**, fusiform dilation of the distal third of the ureter is classic (Fig. 9-16). Depending on the severity, associated pelvicaliectasis may or may not be present. The ureter will demonstrate normal or increased peristalsis with the waves disappearing at the distal aperistaltic segment. Calculi may form just proximal to the adynamic segment.

Anomalies Related to Vascular Development

Aberrant Vessels. As the kidney ascends during embryologic development, it derives its blood supply from the aorta at successively higher levels with regression of the lower level vessels. If the lower level vessels persist, aberrant renal arteries will be present. Aberrant vessels can compress the ureter anywhere along its course, giving rise to obstruction. With color Doppler, aberrant vessels may be seen crossing the ureter at the level of ureteric obstruction.

Retrocaval Ureter. Retrocaval ureter is a rare but well-recognized congenital anomaly. There is a 3:1 predominance in men, with most patients presenting with pain in the second to fourth decade of life. Normally, the infrarenal inferior vena cava (IVC) develops from the supracardinal vein. If this portion of the cava develops from the subcardinal vein, the ureter will pass posterior to the IVC. The ureter then passes medially and anteriorly between the aorta and IVC to cross the right iliac vessels. It then enters the pelvis and bladder in a normal fashion. On **sonography**, there will be pelvicaliectasis and proximal hydroureter to the level where the ureter turns medial to pass posterior to the IVC.

Anomalies Related to Bladder Development

Agenesis. Bladder agenesis is a rare anomaly. Most infants with bladder agenesis are stillborn with virtually all surviving infants being female.[21] Often, many associated anomalies are present. Sonographically, the bladder is absent.

Duplication. Bladder duplication has been divided into three types:

- **Type 1**—A peritoneal fold, which may be complete or incomplete, separates the two bladders.

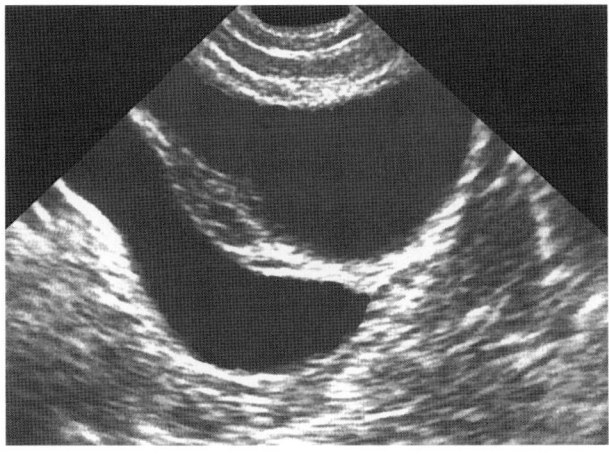
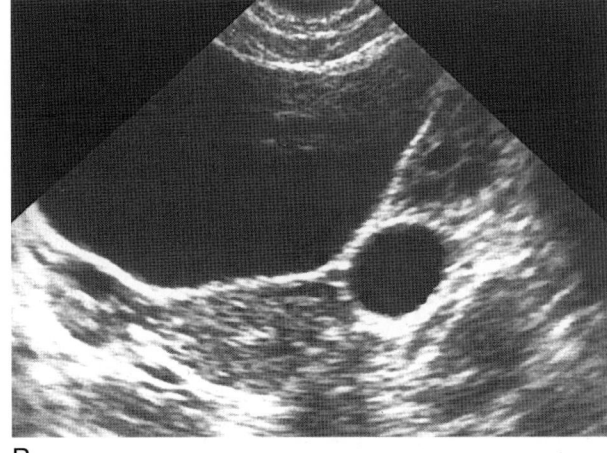

A   B

FIGURE 9-16. Congenital megaureter. A, Sagittal and **B,** transverse sonograms show fusiform dilation of the distal ureter. Associated pelvicaliectasis may or may not be present.

- **Type 2**—An internal septum is present, dividing the bladder. The septum may be complete or incomplete and may be oriented in a sagittal or coronal plane. There may be multiple septa.
- **Type 3**—There is a transverse band of muscle dividing the bladder into two unequal cavities.[15]

Exstrophy. Bladder exstrophy occurs in 1 in 30,000 live births.[15] There is a 2:1 predominance in males.[15] Failure in development of the mesoderm below the umbilicus leads to absence of the lower abdominal and anterior bladder wall. There is a high incidence of associated musculoskeletal, gastrointestinal, and genital tract anomalies. These patients have an increased incidence of **bladder carcinoma** (200×) which is adenocarcinoma in 90% of cases.[15]

Urachal Anomalies. Normally, the urachus closes in the last half of fetal life.[15] There are four types of congenital urachal anomalies.[15,22,23]

- patent urachus (50%)
- urachal cyst (30%)
- urachal sinus (15%)
- urachal diverticulum (5%) (Fig. 9-17)

There is a 2:1 predominance in males. A **patent urachus** is usually associated with urethral obstruction and serves as a protective mechanism to allow normal fetal development. A **urachal cyst** forms if the urachus closes at the umbilical and bladder ends but remains patent in between. The cyst is usually situated in the lower one third of the urachus. There is an increased incidence of **adenocarcinoma**. On **sonography**, a cyst with or without internal echoes is seen superior to the bladder, near the midline. A **urachal sinus** forms when the urachus closes at the bladder end but remains patent at the umbilicus. A **urachal diverticulum** forms if the urachus closes at the umbilical end but remains patent at

the bladder. They are usually incidentally found. There is, however, an increased incidence of **carcinoma** and **stone formation**.

Anomalies Related to Urethral Development

Diverticulum. The majority of **urethral diverticula** are acquired through injury or infection, although some are congenital developmental anomalies. Most urethral diverticula in women form as a result of infection of the periurethral glands. Some may be related to childbirth. Most are found in the midurethra and are bilateral. Often, a fluctuant anterior vaginal mass is felt. Stones may develop because of urinary stasis. **Transvaginal** or **translabial** scanning may demonstrate a simple or complex cystic structure communicating with the urethra through a thin neck (Fig. 9-18).

INFECTIONS OF THE GENITOURINARY TRACT

Pyelonephritis

Acute Pyelonephritis. Acute pyelonephritis is a tubulointerstitial inflammation of the kidney. Two routes may give rise to inflammation and these are: (1) **ascending infection** (*Escherichia coli*) 85% and (2) **hematogenous seeding** (*Staphylococcus aureus*) 15%. Women 15 to 35 years of age are most commonly affected.[24] Two percent of pregnant women will develop acute pyelonephritis.[25] Most adults present with flank pain and fever and can be diagnosed clinically with the aid of laboratory studies (bacteriuria, pyuria, and leukocytosis). Treatment with appropriate antibiotics results in rapid improvement in both clinical and laboratory findings. Imaging is only necessary to rule out potential

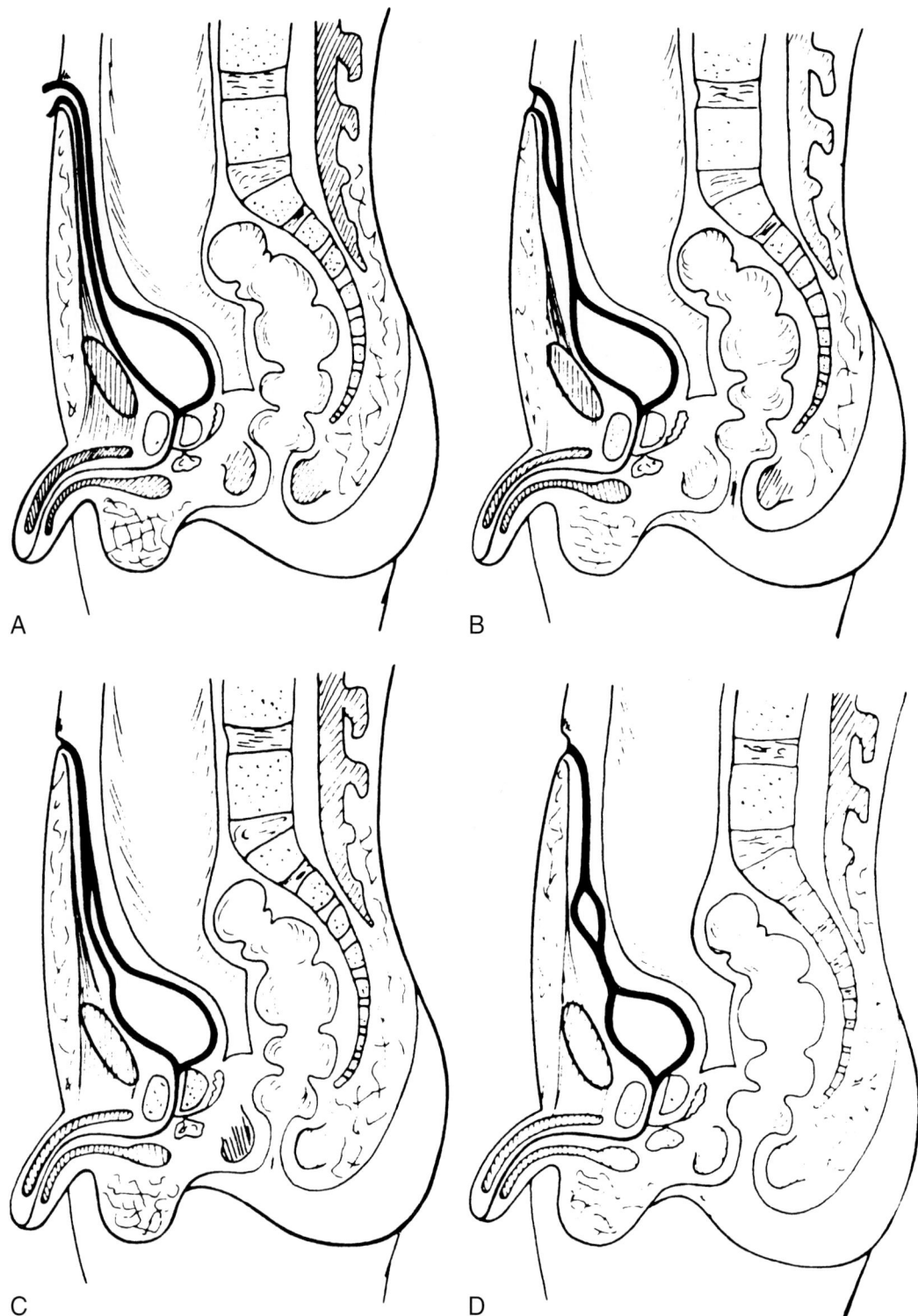

FIGURE 9-17. Congenital urachal anomalies. A, Patent urachus. **B**, Urachal sinus. **C**, Urachal diverticulum. **D**, Urachal cyst. (From Schnyder PA, Candarjia G: Vesicourachal diverticulum. CT diagnosis in two adults. AJR 1981;137:1063-1065. Modified with permission.)

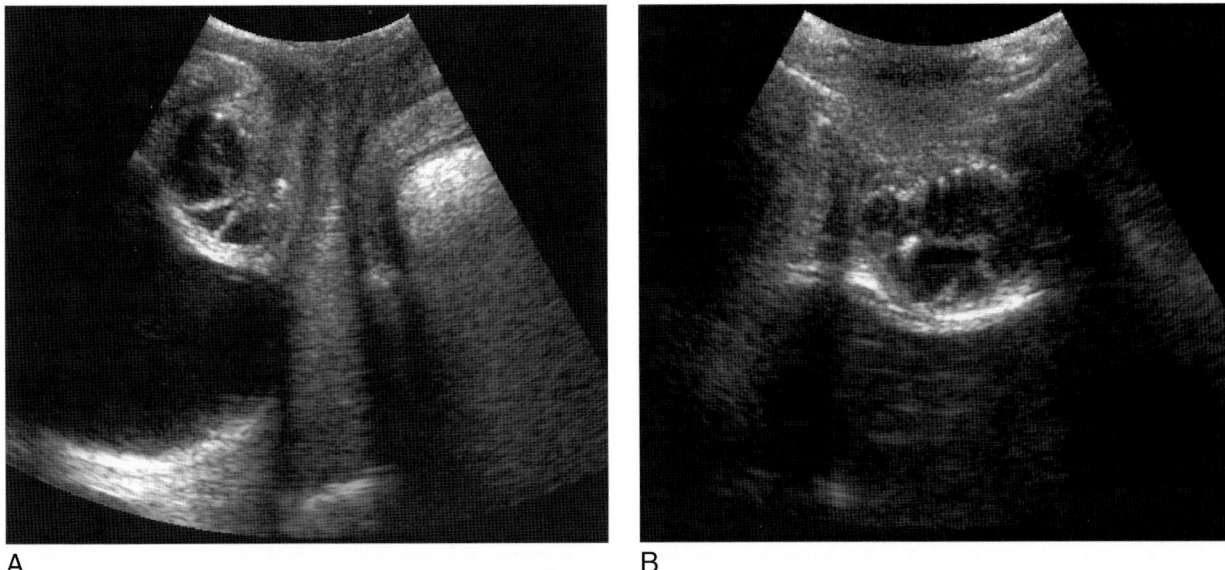

A   B

FIGURE 9-18. Urethral diverticulum in a young woman with a palpable vaginal mass. **A**, Sagittal and **B**, transverse sonograms show a complex cystic mass adjacent to the anterior urethra.

complications (such as renal or perirenal abscess development) when symptoms and laboratory abnormalities persist. The Society of Uroradiology has proposed a simplified terminology describing acutely infected kidneys.[26] The term **acute pyelonephritis** should be used, thus eliminating the need for terms such as **bacterial nephritis, lobar nephronia, renal cellulitis, lobar nephritis, renal phlegmon,** and **renal carbuncle.**[26]

On **sonography**, the majority of kidneys with acute pyelonephritis appear normal. If abnormality is present, the following can be seen (Fig. 9-19):

- renal enlargement
- compression of the renal sinus
- alteration of the echotexture, which may be hypoechoic (edema) or hyperechoic (hemorrhage)
- loss of corticomedullary differentiation
- poorly marginated mass(es)
- gas within the renal parenchyma.[25,26]
- focal or diffuse absence of perfusion corresponding to the swollen inflamed areas

If the pyelonephritis is focal, the poorly marginated masses may be echogenic, hypoechoic, or of mixed echogenicity. Echogenic masses may be the most common appearance of focal pyelonephritis.[27]

Sonography, including power Doppler, is less sensitive than CT, MRI, or Tc-99m DMSA SPECT cortical scintigraphy for demonstrating changes of acute pyelonephritis but is more accessible and less expensive and, therefore, an excellent screening modality for the development and follow-up of complications.[28] Ultrasound also is an excellent modality in the assessment of

pregnant patients with acute pyelonephritis because of its lack of ionizing radiation.[25,26]

Another new entity known as **alkaline-encrusted pyelitis** has been described in renal transplants and native kidneys of debilitated and immunocompromised patients.[29] This entity is most frequently caused by *Corynebacterium urealyticum*, a urea-splitting microorganism. There is stone encrustation in the wall of the urinary tract, and usually in the kidney and the bladder. If the kidney is affected, the patient may present with hematuria, stone passage, or an ammonium odor to the urine. Dysuria and suprapubic pain are the most common clinical signs if the bladder is involved. Treatment is with antibiotics and local acidification of the urine. On **sonography**, the appearance of alkaline-encrusted pyelitis is calcification of a thickened urothelial wall rather than the calcification lying free within the collecting system.[29] The calcification can be thin and smooth or thick and irregular.[29]

Renal and Perinephric Abscess. Untreated or inadequately treated acute pyelonephritis may lead to parenchymal necrosis with abscess formation. Patients

---

ACUTE PYELONEPHRITIS ON SONOGRAPHY

Renal enlargement
Compression of the renal sinus
Abnormal echotexture
Loss of corticomedullary differentiation
Poorly marginated mass(es)
Gas within the renal parenchyma

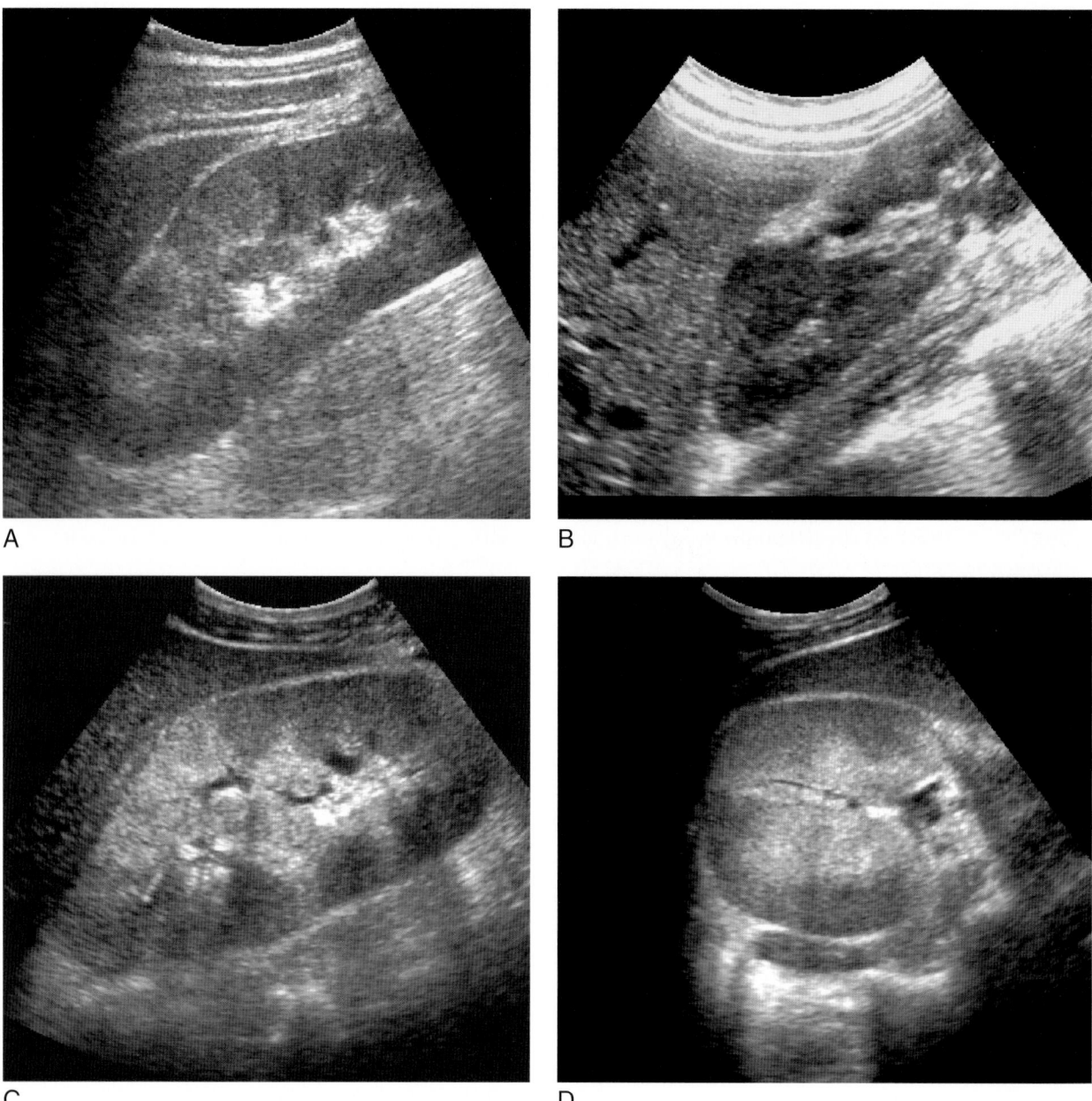

FIGURE 9-19. Acute pyelonephritis. A, Subtle focal increased echogenic areas are seen in the anterior cortex of the right kidney. **B**, A single focal hypoechoic area is seen in the upper pole of the kidney. **C**, Sagittal and **D**, transverse sonograms on the same patient show a swollen and edematous kidney with focal altered echogenicity and loss of corticomedullary differentiation. The renal sinus fat is attenuated by the swollen parenchyma.

at increased risk for abscess development include those with diabetes, urinary tract obstruction, infected renal stones, immune compromise, IV drug abuse, or chronic debilitating disease.[25,30] **Renal abscesses** tend to be solitary and may spontaneously decompress into the collecting system or perinephric space. **Perinephric abscess** may also result from a ruptured pyonephrosis, direct extension of peritoneal or retroperitoneal infection, or following intervention, such as surgery, endoscopy, or percutaneous procedures.[23] Small abscesses may be treated conservatively with antibiotics, whereas larger ones will

require percutaneous drainage and, if unsuccessful, surgery.

On **sonography**, a renal abscess will appear as a round, thick-walled, hypoechoic complex mass often with some through transmission (Fig. 9-20). Internal mobile debris may be seen. Occasionally, gas with dirty shadowing may be noted within the abscess. Septations may be present. The differential diagnosis includes (1) hemorrhagic or infected cysts; (2) parasitic cysts; (3) multiloculated cysts; and (4) cystic neoplasm. Sonography is not as accurate as CT in determining the presence and extent of peri-

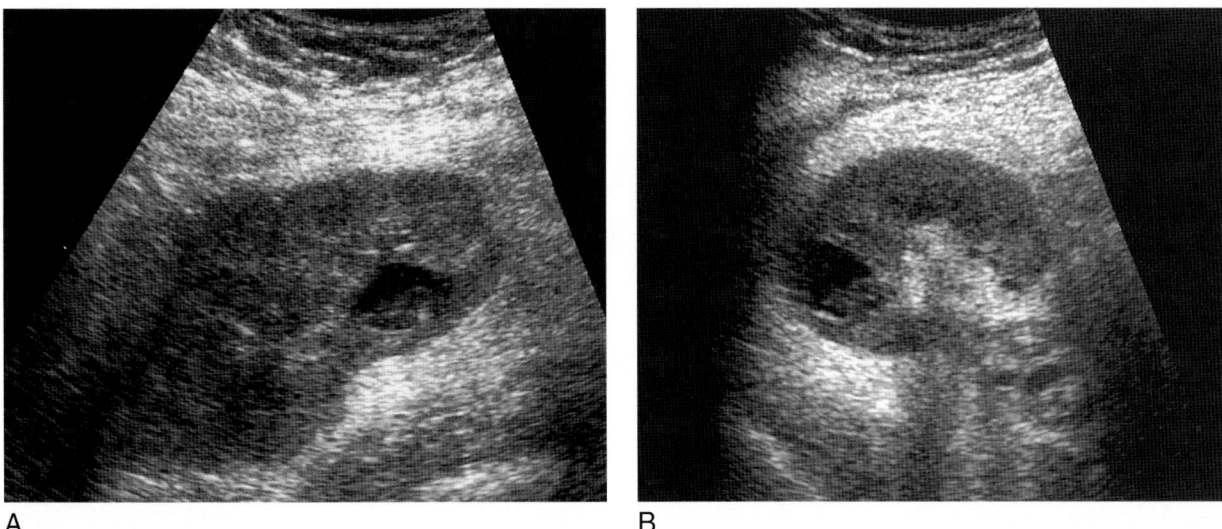

A   B

FIGURE 9-20. Renal abscess. A, Sagittal and **B**, transverse sonograms show a complex cystic mass in the lower pole of the kidney containing internal debris.

nephric abscess extension.[25] Sonography is, however, an excellent modality for following patients with abscesses that are being treated conservatively to document resolution.

Pyonephrosis. Pyonephrosis implies purulent material in an obstructed collecting system. Depending on the level of obstruction, any portion of the collecting system, including the ureter, can be affected. Early diagnosis and treatment are crucial to prevent development of bacteremia and life-threatening septic shock. The mortality rate of bacteremia and septic shock is 25% and 50%, respectively.[31] Fifteen percent of patients will be asymptomatic at presentation.[32] In the young adult, ureteropelvic junction obstruction and stones are the most frequent cause of pyonephrosis development, whereas malignant ureteral obstruction is usually the cause in the elderly.[25] On **sonography**, hydronephrosis, with or without hydroureter, will be seen. Mobile collecting system debris—with or without a fluid-debris level—collecting system gas, and stones can be seen (Fig. 9-21). **Emphysematous Pyelonephritis.** This is an uncommon, life-threatening infection of the renal parenchyma characterized by gas formation.[33] Most patients are women (2:1) and diabetic (90%) with a mean age of 55 years. Twenty percent of diabetic patients with emphysematous pyelonephritis (EPN) will have urinary obstruction compared with nondiabetic patients, in whom urinary tract obstruction is present in 75%. Bilateral disease occurs in 5% to 10%. *Escherichia coli* is the offending organism in 62% to 70%, *Klebsiella* 9%, *Pseudomonas* 2%, with *Proteus*, *Aerobacter*, and *Candida* occasionally involved.[25,30] At presentation most patients are extremely ill with fever, flank pain, hyperglycemia, acidosis, dehydration, and electrolyte imbalance.[34] Eighteen percent of patients will present only with fever of unknown origin.[35]

Wan et al.[36] retrospectively studied 38 patients with EPN and identified two types of disease. **EPN1** was characterized by parenchymal destruction with presence of streaky or mottled gas. **EPN2** was characterized as either renal or perirenal fluid collections with bubbly or loculated gas or gas in the collecting system. They found the mortality rate for EPN1 and for EPN2 was 69% and 18%, respectively. They postulate that the difference between EPN1 and EPN2 is related to the severity of immune compromise of the patient, as well as to the vascular insufficiency of the affected kidney. Emergency nephrectomy is the treatment of choice of EPN1, whereas percutaneous drainage is recommended for patients with EPN2. CT is the preferred method to image patients with EPN to determine the location and extent of renal and perirenal gas. **Sonographic evaluation** can be difficult, because gas will produce echogenic foci with **distal dirty shadowing** obscuring visualization of deeper structures. The gas could potentially be misinterpreted as bowel gas or renal calculi. (Figs. 9-22 and 9-23).[37]
Emphysematous Pyelitis. This entity refers to abnormal air within the urinary collecting system only.[33] This disease is seen most often in women with diabetes or obstructing stone disease and carries a mortality rate of 20%. It is important to exclude iatrogenic causes of air within the collecting system. On **sonography**, nondependent linear echogenic lines with dirty distal posterior acoustic shadowing, indicative of air, are seen within the collecting system. CT is often required because the dirty acoustic shadow from air on ultrasound may obscure the exact extent of renal and perirenal disease.
Chronic Pyelonephritis. Chronic pyelonephritis is an interstitial nephritis often associated with vesicoureteric reflux. Reflux nephropathy is believed to cause 10% to 30% of all cases of end-stage renal disease.[38] Chronic

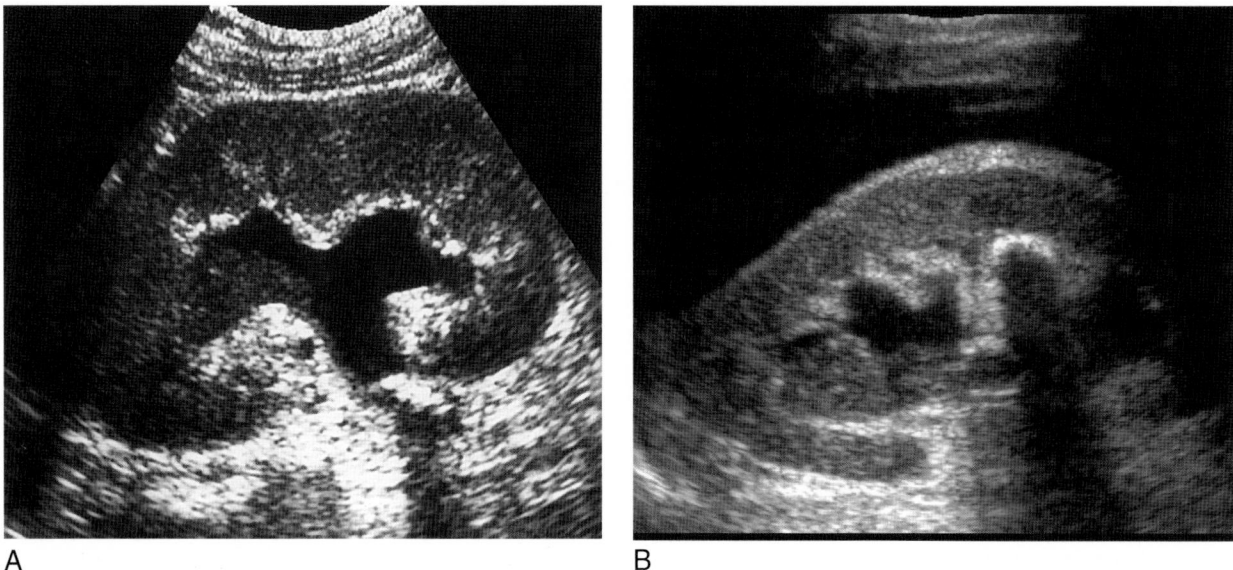

A   B

FIGURE 9-21. Pyonephrosis. A and **B,** sagittal sonograms in two different patients showing dilated collecting systems with dependent internal debris. **A,** Shows a stone in the ureteropelvic junction. **B,** Shows a nonobstruting caliceal stone.

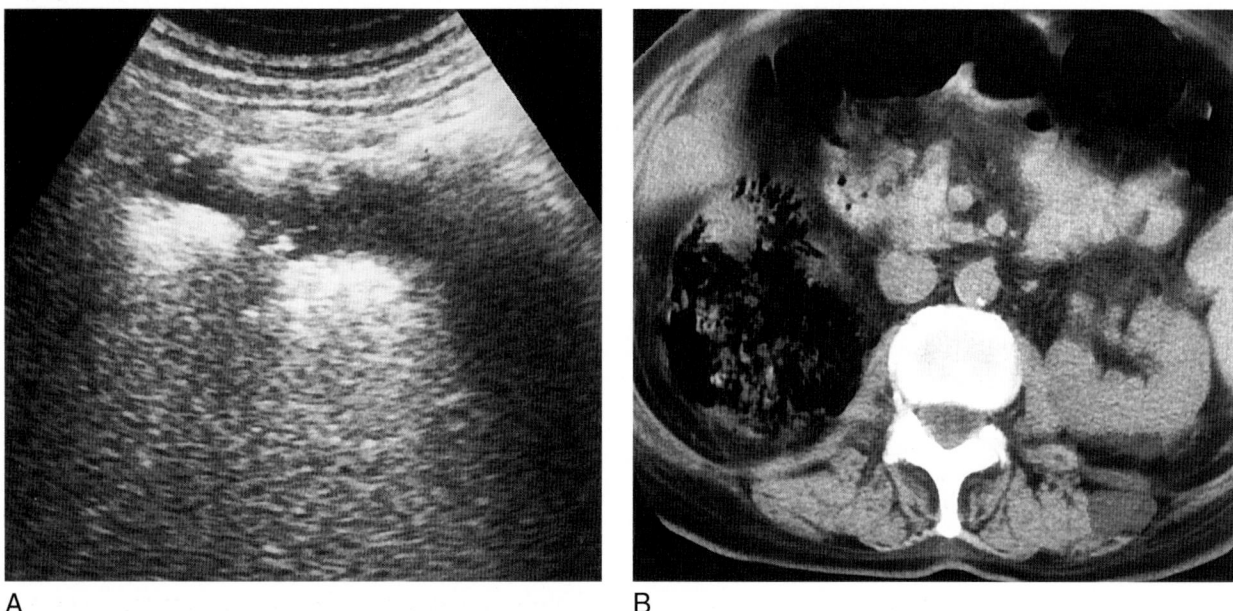

A   B

FIGURE 9-22. Emphysematous pyelonephritis (type 1). A, Sagittal sonogram of right renal bed reveals extensive air obscuring visualization of the kidney. **B,** Computed tomography demonstrates diffuse parenchymal destruction of the right kidney with extensive mottled gas. Caution must be exercised to avoid missing this diagnosis altogether on ultrasound. Failure to see a kidney in a septic patient warrants computed tomography scan.

pyelonephritis usually begins in childhood and is more common in women. The renal changes may be unilateral or bilateral but usually are asymmetrical. Reflux into the collecting tubules occurs when the papillary duct orifices are incompetent. This occurs more often in compound papillae which are typically found at the poles of the kidneys. Cortical scarring, therefore, tends to be predominantly polar overlying the involved calix. There is associated papillary retraction with caliceal clubbing. On **sonography,** a dilated blunt calix is seen that is associated with an overlying cortical scar or cortical atrophy (Fig. 9-24).[39] These changes may be multicentric and bilateral. If the disease is unilateral, there may be compensatory hypertrophy of the contralateral kidney. If the disease is multicentric, compensatory hypertrophy of normal intervening parenchyma may create islands of normal tissue simulating a tumor.

Xanthogranulomatous Pyelonephritis. Xanthogranulomatous pyelonephritis (XGP) is a chronic, suppurative renal infection causing destruction of renal parenchyma

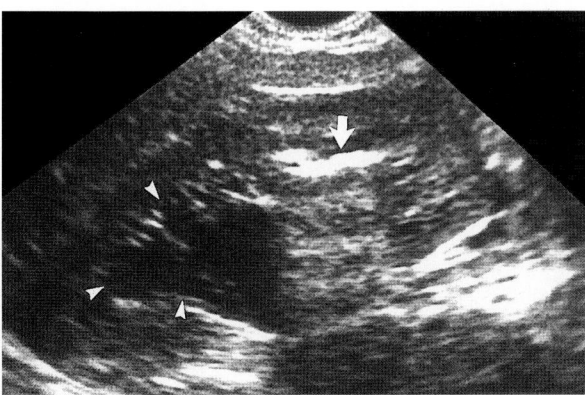

FIGURE 9-23. Emphysematous pyelonephritis (type 2). Sagittal sonogram shows a dilated collecting system (*arrowheads*) containing air (*arrow*) which appears as a bright, nondependent echogenic line with dirty shadowing.

and replacement of it with lipid-laden macrophages. The disease is usually unilateral and may be **diffuse**, **segmental**, or **focal**. XGP is usually associated with nephrolithiasis (70%) and obstructive nephropathy.[40-42] The disease is found most commonly in middle-aged women and diabetics.[42] Presenting signs are nonspecific and include pain, mass, weight loss, and urinary tract infection (*Proteus* or *E. coli*).[40] In the diffuse variety, the kidney is usually nonfunctioning. On **sonography**, the **diffuse variety** will show renal enlargement with maintenance of the reniform shape and lack of corticomedullary differentiation. Multiple hypoechoic areas are seen corresponding to dilated calices or inflammatory parenchymal masses.[40] Through transmission is variable depending on the degree of liquefaction of the parenchymal masses. The central renal sinus may be extremely echogenic with shadowing corresponding to a large staghorn calculus (Fig. 9-25). Perinephric extension may be present and is often best appreciated with CT. Occasionally, in the diffuse variety, the kidney demonstrates large complex cystic masses with irregular thick walls and fluid levels mimicking pyonephrosis. Diffuse XGP does not have any specific sonographic features but is suggested when parenchymal thinning, hydronephrosis, stones, debris in a dilated collecting system, and perinephric fluid collections are present.[43] **Segmental XGP** will be seen as one or more hypoechoic masses often associated with a single calix.[40,44] An obstructing calculus may be seen near the papilla.[40] **Focal XGP** arises in the renal cortex and does not communicate with the renal pelvis. It cannot be distinguished sonographically from tumor or abscess.[40]

Papillary Necrosis

Many causative factors are implicated in the ischemia leading to the development of papillary necrosis and these include (1) **analgesic abuse**, (2) **diabetes**, (3)

SONOGRAPHIC FINDINGS OF PAPILLARY NECROSIS

Swollen pyramids
Papillary cavitation
Adjacent clubbed calix
Sloughed papilla in the collecting system that can calcify and simulate a stone
Sloughed papilla may cause obstruction

urinary tract infection, (4) **renal vein thrombosis**, (5) **prolonged hypotension**; (6) **urinary tract obstruction**; (7) **dehydration**, (8) **sickle cell anemia**, and (9) **hemophilia**.[45] Initially, the papilla swells and then a communication with the caliceal system occurs. Central papillary cavitation then occurs and the papilla may slough. Occasionally, a necrotic papilla may calcify. The **sonographic findings** parallel the pathologic changes. Swollen pyramids may be seen but can be difficult to recognize sonographically (Fig. 9-26). With papillary cavitation, cystic collections within the medullary pyramids will be noted. If the papilla sloughs, the affected adjacent calix will be clubbed. The sloughed papilla can be seen in the collecting system as an echogenic nonshadowing structure. If the sloughed papilla calcifies, distal acoustic shadowing simulating a stone will be seen.[46] If the sloughed papilla passes into the ureter, obstruction may occur with development of hydronephrosis.

Tuberculosis

Urinary tract tuberculosis (TB) occurs with hematogenous seeding of the kidney by *Mycobacterium tuberculosis* from an extraurinary source, most commonly the lung. Urinary tract TB will usually manifest in 5 to 10 years following the initial pulmonary infection.[47] Chest radiographs can be normal (35% to 50%) or demonstrate active (10%) or inactive healed TB (40% to 55%).[47] Most patients present with lower urinary tract signs and symptoms that include frequency, dysuria, nocturia, urgency, and gross (25%) or microscopic (75%) hematuria. Approximately 10% to 20% of patients will be asymptomatic.[47] Urinalysis demonstrating sterile pyuria, microscopic hematuria, and acid pH suggests urinary tract TB. Definitive diagnosis is demonstration of acid-fast bacilli in the urine; however, this usually requires 6 to 8 weeks for growth.

Although both kidneys are seeded initially, clinical manifestations are usually unilateral. The **early or acute changes** include development of bilateral multiple small tuberculomas. Das et al.[48] reviewed the **sonographic features** of genitourinary TB in 20 patients. They found the most frequently encountered abnormality was focal renal lesions. Small focal lesions (5 to 15 mm) were

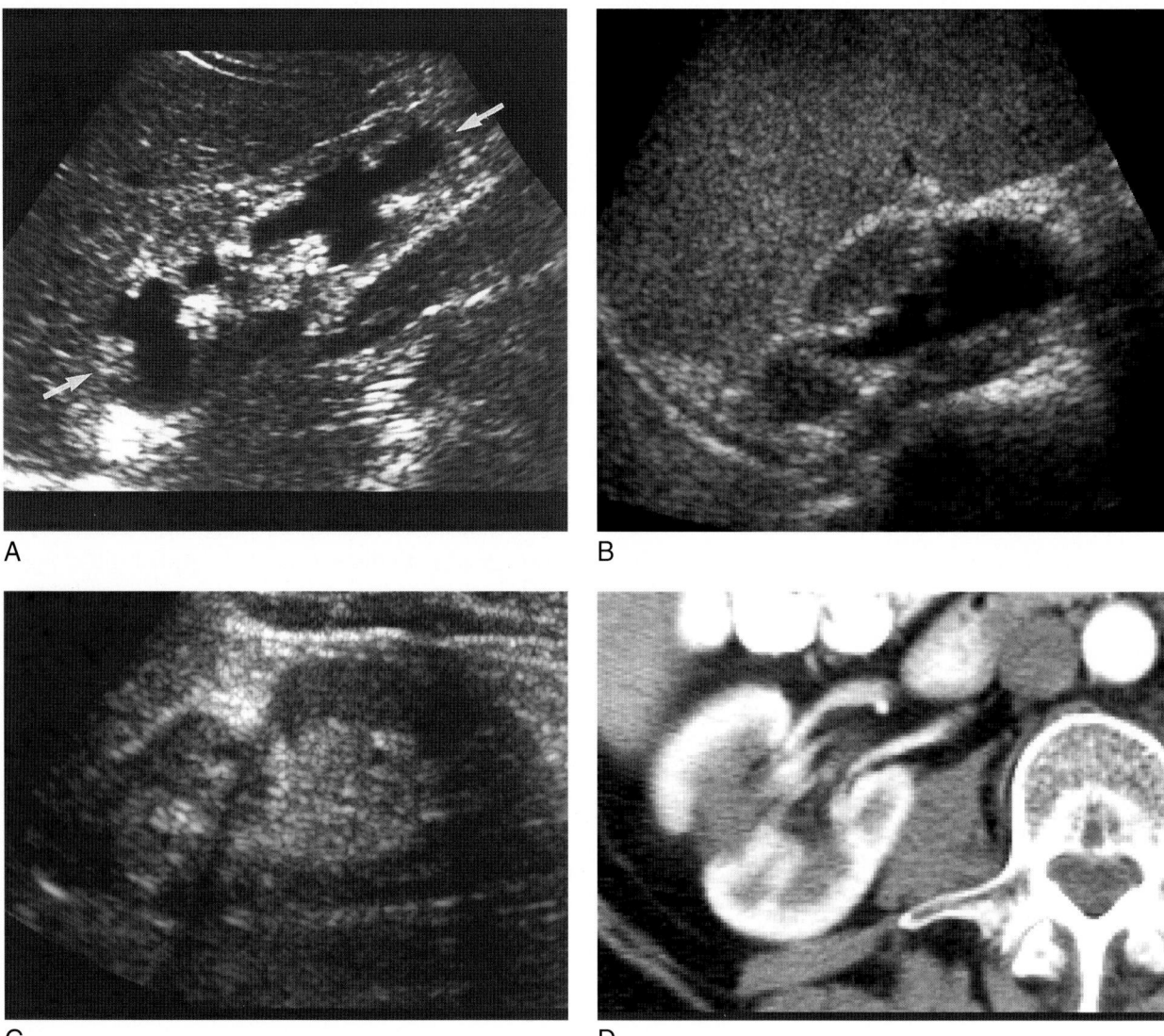

FIGURE 9-24. Chronic pyelonephritis. A, Sagittal sonogram demonstrates echogenic parenchyma with atrophy most marked at the renal poles (*arrows*). Dilation of the collecting system is from chronic vesicoureteric reflux. **B,** Sagittal sonogram shows an atrophic kidney with scarring and dilation of the collecting system due to reflux. **C,** Sagittal sonogram showing an echogenic wedge shaped scar in the mid-pole of the kidney and **D,** a confirmatory CT scan.

echogenic or were hypoechoic with an echogenic rim. Larger focal lesions (>15 mm) were of mixed echogenicity with poorly defined borders. Bilateral disease was noted in 30% of their patients. Most will heal spontaneously or following antituberculous therapy. At some later date (perhaps years later), one or more of the tubercles may enlarge. With enlargement, cavitation and communication with the collecting system will occur with changes resembling papillary necrosis. Papillary involvement is noted when a sonolucent linear tract is seen extending from the involved calix into the papilla. Soft tissue caliceal masses representing sloughed papilla can be seen. Following rupture into the collecting system, *M. tuberculosis* bacilluria develops and allows the spread of the renal infection to other parts of the urinary tract. Spasm or edema in the region of the ureterovesical junction (UVJ) may occur, giving rise to pelvicaliectasis and hydroureter. Ureteric linear ulcers may also occur, most commonly in the distal portion. Involvement of the bladder is frequent and is responsible for the initial clinical symptoms of dysuria and frequency. The early bladder manifestations include mucosal edema and ulceration. If edema occurs at the bladder trigone, ureteric obstruction may occur. Bladder involvement will be seen in 33% of patients with genitourinary tract TB.[48] Bladder wall tuberculomas may be single or multiple and can be quite large (Fig. 9-27).

The later or more **chronic** changes of genitourinary tract TB include **fibrotic strictures, extensive cavitation, calcification, mass lesions, perinephric abscess,**

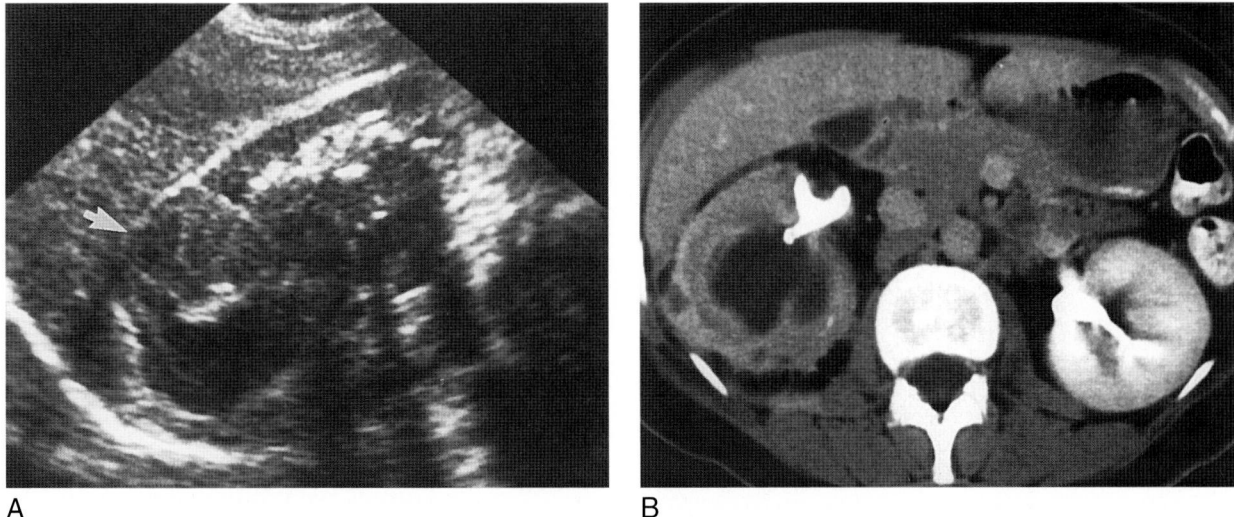

FIGURE 9-25. Xanthogranulomatous pyelonephritis. A, Sagittal sonogram demonstrates a large central mass with calcification. Caliceal dilation with purulent debris is noted (*arrow*). **B,** Confirmatory computed tomography shows a large staghorn calculus with proximal hydronephrosis and multiple intrarenal abscesses.

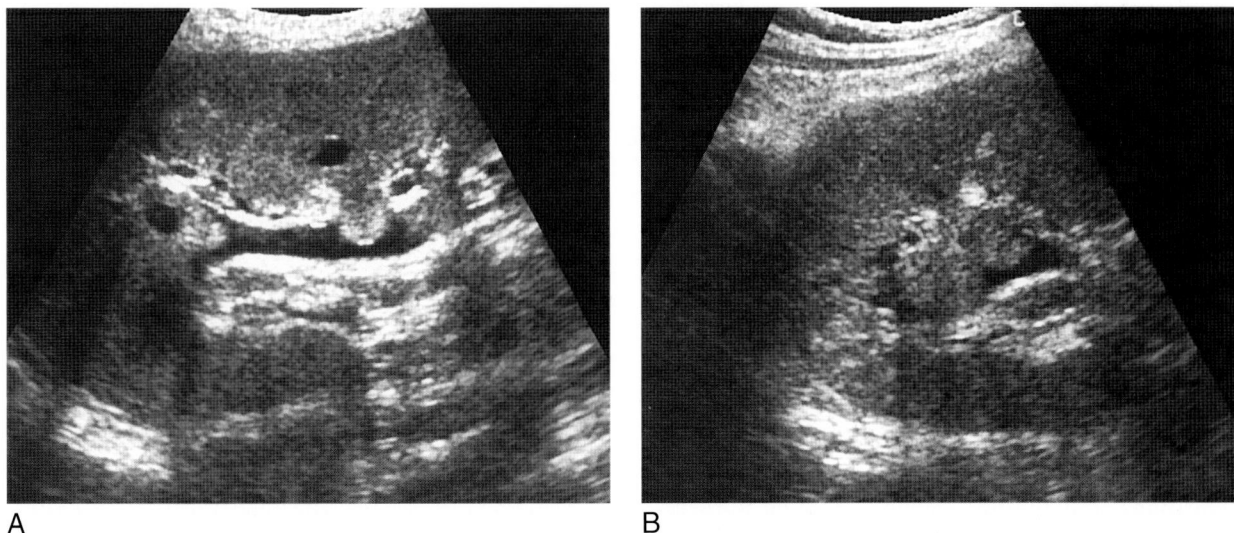

FIGURE 9-26. Papillary necrosis. A, Sagittal and **B,** transverse sonograms show swollen bulbous papillae.

and **fistula**.[47] The chronic changes, in particular those related to fibrotic strictures, result in significant renal damage. Strictures may occur anywhere in the intrarenal collecting system and ureter. The obstruction then results in proximal collecting system dilation and pressure atrophy of the renal parenchyma (Fig. 9-28). With time, calcification in the areas of caseation or sloughed papilla may occur. If renal infection ruptures into the perinephric space, an abscess may develop. If the perinephric abscess extends to involve adjacent viscera, fistula formation can occur. Eventually, the kidney will become nonfunctioning, small, and totally calcified (**autonephrectomy or putty kidney**). In the bladder, chronic fibrotic healing results in a thick-walled, small, symmetric bladder.[47] Speckled or curvilinear calcification of the bladder wall may occur but is rare.[49]

Most cases of genitourinary tract TB can be diagnosed with a combination of IVP, retrograde pyelography, ultrasound, and CT.[50] Premkumar et al.[50] demonstrated in 14 patients with advanced urinary tract TB that detailed morphologic information and functional renal status are best assessed with CT and urography. Das et al.[51] demonstrated that ultrasound-guided, fine-needle aspiration is useful in making the diagnosis of renal TB in patients with negative urine cultures and in defining the nature of obvious sonographic lesions in patients with positive urine cultures.

Unusual Infections

Fungal. Patients with diabetes mellitus, indwelling catheters, malignancy, hematopoietic disorders, chronic

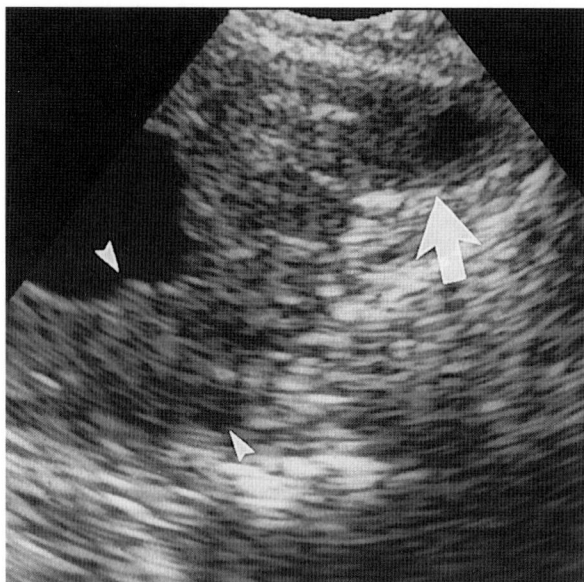

FIGURE 9-27. Acute urinary bladder tuberculosis. Transverse transvaginal sonogram shows marked urothelial thickening of left bladder wall (*arrowheads*) and of the distal left ureter at the ureterovesical junction (*arrow*).

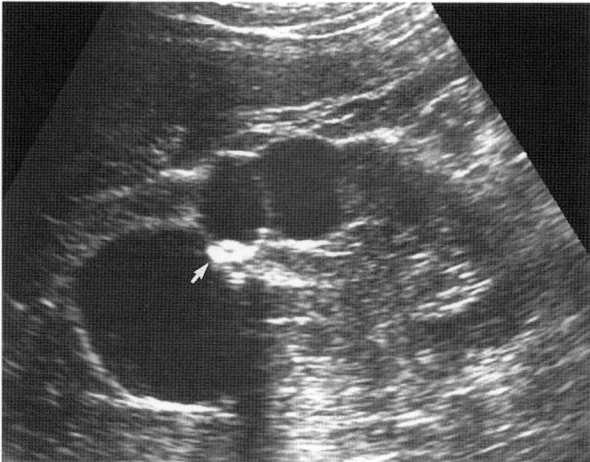

FIGURE 9-28. Chronic renal tuberculosis. Sagittal sonogram shows upper and mid-pole caliceal clubbing with marked overlying parenchymal atrophy. A focal area of calcification (*arrow*) in the region of the upper-pole infundibulum is noted.

antibiotic or steroid therapy, transplant, and IV drug abuse are at increased risk for developing fungal infections of the urinary tract.[52]

Candida albicans. Candida albicans is the most common fungal agent that affects the urinary tract. Renal parenchymal involvement usually occurs with diffuse systemic involvement. Multiple small, focal parenchymal abscesses occur that may calcify with time.[53] Extension into the perinephric space is possible. Invasion of the collecting system may occur, ultimately resulting in formation of **fungal balls** that need to be differentiated from **blood clot**, **radiolucent stones**, **transitional cell tumors**, **sloughed papilla**, **fibroepithelial polyps**, **cholesteatomas**, and **leukoplakia**.[54,55] On **sonography**, the microabscesses appear similar to bacterial abscesses and are small hypoechoic parenchymal masses. Fungus balls appear as echogenic nonshadowing soft tissue masses within the collecting system.[56] Fungus balls are mobile and may cause obstruction that leads to development of hydronephrosis.

Parasitic. In developing countries, parasitic infections are common. For all practical purposes, there are three parasitic infections of the urinary tract that need to be considered: (1) **schistosomiasis**, (2) **echinococcus (hydatid disease)**, and (3) **filariasis**.

Schistosomiasis. *Schistosoma haematobium* is the most common agent to affect the urinary tract. The worms enter the human host by penetrating the skin. They are then carried via the portal venous system to the liver, where they mature into their adult form. *S. haematobium* likely enters the perivesical venous plexus from the hemorrhoidal plexus.[57] The female worm then deposits

eggs into the venules of the bladder wall and ureter. Granuloma formation and obliterative endarteritis occur. Serologic tests demonstrating ova allow diagnosis. Hematuria is the most frequent complaint.[57] On **sonography**, the kidneys are normal until late in the disease. **Pseudotubercles** develop in the ureter and bladder and the urothelium becomes thickened (Fig. 9-29). With time, the pseudotubercles will calcify. The calcification may be fine and granular, fine and linear, or thick and irregular.[58] If repeated infections occur, the bladder will become small and fibrosed. There is an increased incidence of ureteral and bladder calculi.[57] With chronic disease, there is also an increased incidence of squamous cell carcinoma.[57]

Echinococcus (Hydatid Disease). Two major types of hydatid disease exist that affect the urinary tract: *Echinococcus multilocularis* and *Echinococcus granulosus*. The latter is the more common offending organism. Renal hydatid disease is found in 2% to 5% of patients with hydatid disease[57] and is usually solitary, involving the renal poles.[59] Hydatid cysts may occur along the ureter or in the bladder. Each hydatid cyst consists of (1) the **pericyst**; (2) the **ectocyst**; and (3) the **endocyst**. The disease is often silent until the cyst has grown large enough to either rupture or cause pressure on adjacent structures. On **sonography**, early in its development, an anechoic cyst is seen that may have a perceptible wall. Mural nodularity suggests scolices. When daughter cysts are present, a multiloculated cystic mass will be seen. The membranes from the endocyst may detach and precipitate to the bottom of the hydatid fluid to become "**hydatid sand**."[60] Calcification is variable in its appearance, ranging from eggshell to dense reticular. Ring-shaped calcifications inside a larger calcified lesion suggests calcified daughter cysts.[57,60]

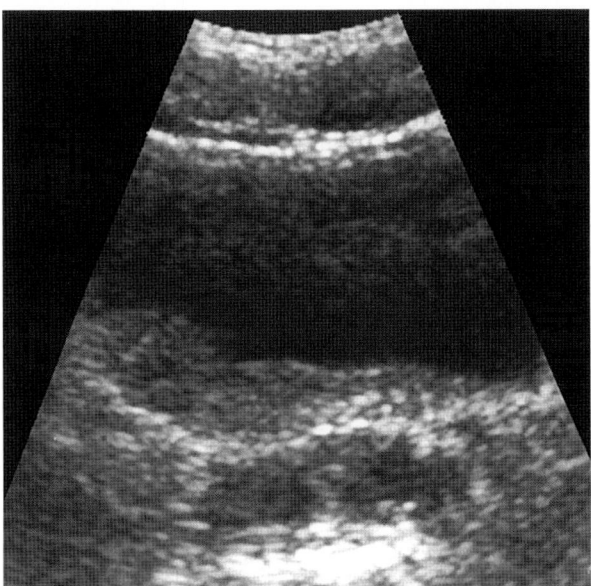

FIGURE 9-29. Bladder schistosomiasis. Sagittal sonogram reveals asymmetrical bladder wall thickening.

Filariasis. Most people with **filariasis** (*Wuchereria bancrofti*) are infected between 10 and 12 years of age, although the signs and symptoms of elephantiasis, chyluria, and chylous ascites usually do not develop for many years (5 to 20 years).[57] Filariasis is transmitted to humans by mosquitoes, and the worms migrate into the lymphatics.[57] A granulomatous inflammatory reaction occurs. Obstruction of the retroperitoneal lymphatics occurs leading to dilation, proliferation, and subsequent rupture of these lymphatics into the pelvicaliceal system. Diagnosis is usually made by lymphangiography.[61] **Sonography** is not helpful.

AIDS. Many renal abnormalities have been described in AIDS patients including: **acute tubular necrosis, nephrocalcinosis,** and **interstitial nephritis.**[62] Pathologic changes in the kidney include focal and segmental glomerulosclerosis and tubular abnormalities.[62] These changes lead to increased renal parenchymal echogenicity on ultrasound.[62,63] There is also an increased incidence of **opportunistic infection** (cytomegalovirus, *Candida albicans, Cryptococcus, Pneumocystis carinii, Mycobacterium avium-intracellulare* and mucormycosis[64]) and **tumor** (lymphoma and Kaposi's sarcoma). Pyelonephritis, renal abscess, and cystitis may occur. Diffuse visceral calcifications, including renal, may be seen with disseminated *P. carinii,* cytomegalovirus and *M. avium-intracellulare* infections (Fig. 9-30).[65-67] With the advent of improved medical therapy for patients with AIDS, these complications are seen with much less frequency today.

Cystitis

Infectious. Cystitis is a disease found predominantly in women and involves colonization of the urethra by rectal flora. In men, it is associated with bladder outlet obstruction or prostatitis. The most common offending pathogen is *E. coli.*[68] Mucosal edema and decreased bladder capacity are common. Findings may be more prominent at the trigone and bladder neck. Patients will present with bladder irritability and hematuria. On

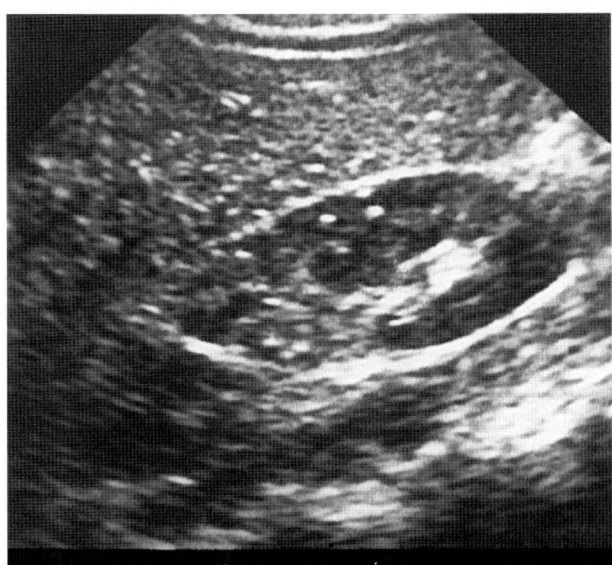

A

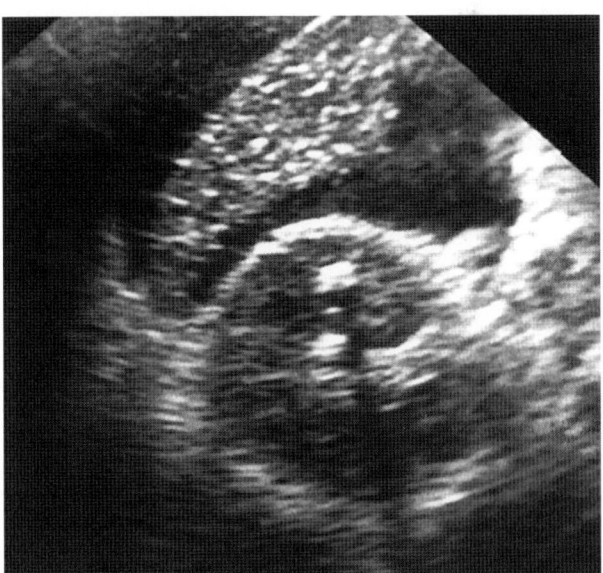

B

FIGURE 9-30. Proven pneumocystis nephropathy in an AIDS patient. A, Sagittal and **B,** transverse sonograms show multiple scattered echogenic foci within the renal parenchyma. Some foci demonstrate the distal acoustic shadowing of calcification. Similar findings are seen in the liver. (From Spouge AR, Wilson S, Gopinath N, et al: Extrapulmonary Pneumocystis carinii in a patient with AIDS. Sonographic findings. AJR 1990;155:76-78.)

CAUSES OF BLADDER WALL THICKENING

FOCAL

Neoplasm

Transitional cell
  carcinoma
Squamous cell
  carcinoma
Adenocarcinoma
Lymphoma
Metastases

**Infectious/
Inflammatory**

Tuberculosis (acute)
Schistosomiasis (acute)
Cystitis
Malakoplakia
Cystitis cystica
Cystitis glandularis
Fistula

Medical Diseases

Endometriosis
Amyloidosis

Trauma

Hematoma

DIFFUSE

Neoplasm

Transitional cell
  carcinoma
Squamous cell carcinoma
Adenocarcinoma

**Infectious/
Inflammatory**

Cystitis
Tuberculosis (chronic)
Schistosomiasis (chronic)

Medical Diseases

Interstitial cystitis
Amyloidosis

Neurogenic Bladder

Detrusor hyperreflexia

Bladder outlet

**Obstruction with
Muscular Hypertrophy**

sonography, the most typical finding is that of diffuse bladder wall thickening. If cystitis is focal, pseudopolyps may form which are impossible to differentiate from tumor (Fig. 9-31).[69]

Malakoplakia. Malakoplakia is a rare granulomatous infection with a predilection for the urinary bladder. The remainder of the urothelium can be affected. The disease is seen more commonly in women (4:1) with a peak incidence in the sixth decade.[70] Pathogenesis is not known; however, its increased association in patients with diabetes mellitus, alcoholic liver disease, mycobacterial infections, sarcoidosis, and following transplantation suggests an altered immune response.[71] Patients may present with hematuria and symptoms of bladder irritability.[70] On **sonography**, single or multiple mucosal-based mass(es) ranging from 0.5 to 3.0 cm are seen most commonly at the bladder base. The disease may be locally invasive (see Fig. 9-31).[70]

Emphysematous Cystitis. Emphysematous cystitis occurs most commonly in female patients and those with diabetes. Patients present with symptoms of cystitis and occasionally have pneumaturia.[68] The most common offending organism is *E. coli*. Both intraluminal and intramural gas is present. Frank gangrene of the bladder

rarely occurs. In these severely ill patients, the urothelium is ulcerated, necrotic, and may slough completely. The **sonographic identification** of this entity depends on the demonstration of echogenic foci with ringdown or dirty shadowing (air) within the bladder wall (Fig. 9-32).[73] Air is often seen in the lumen as well. The bladder wall is usually thickened and demonstrates increased echogenicity.[33]

Chronic Cystitis. Chronic inflammation of the bladder causes predictable histologic change. Brunn's nests are solid nests of urothelium in the lamina propria.[74] If the central portion of a Brunn's nest degenerates, a cyst results (**cystitis cystica**). If chronic irritation persists, the Brunn's nests may develop into glandular structures (**cystitis glandularis**) and may be a precursor of adenocarcinoma.[68] **Sonographically**, these chronic inflammatory changes may be visible. Cysts or solid papillary masses may be seen (see Fig. 9-31). Differentiation from malignancy is impossible with imaging, and cystoscopy with biopsy is necessary for diagnostic confirmation.

Bladder Fistula. Bladder fistula may be congenital or acquired. When acquired, etiologies include **trauma**, **inflammation**, **radiation**, and **neoplasm**. Fistula formation may occur with the vagina, the gut, the skin, the uterus, and the ureter. **Vesicovaginal fistulas** are most commonly related to gynecologic or urologic surgery, bladder carcinoma, and carcinoma of the cervix. **Vesicoenteric fistulas** are most commonly related to diverticulitis and Crohn's disease. **Vesicocutaneous fistulas** occur following surgery or trauma. **Vesicouterine fistulas** occur most commonly following cesarean section. **Vesicoureteral fistulas** are rare and usually occur following hysterectomy.[75] On **sonography**, fistulas are difficult to diagnose, because they are often thin, short communications. Occasionally, linear bands of varying echogenicity[76,77] are seen extending from the bladder to the organ with which fistulous communication exists. If the bladder communicates with gut, vagina, or skin, an abnormal collection of air may be seen in the bladder lumen as a nondependent linear echogenic focus with distal dirty shadowing. Palpation of the abdomen during scanning may cause gas to percolate through the fistula, thereby enhancing its detection (Fig. 9-32).[77] The use of ultrasound contrast agents and color Doppler may be helpful in diagnosing vesicovaginal fistulas with the identification of a jet phenomenon into the vagina as bubbles are introduced into the bladder.[78]

GENITOURINARY TRACT STONES AND CALCIFICATION

Stones

Renal stones are very common, affecting 12% of the population at some time in their life.[79] Stone disease

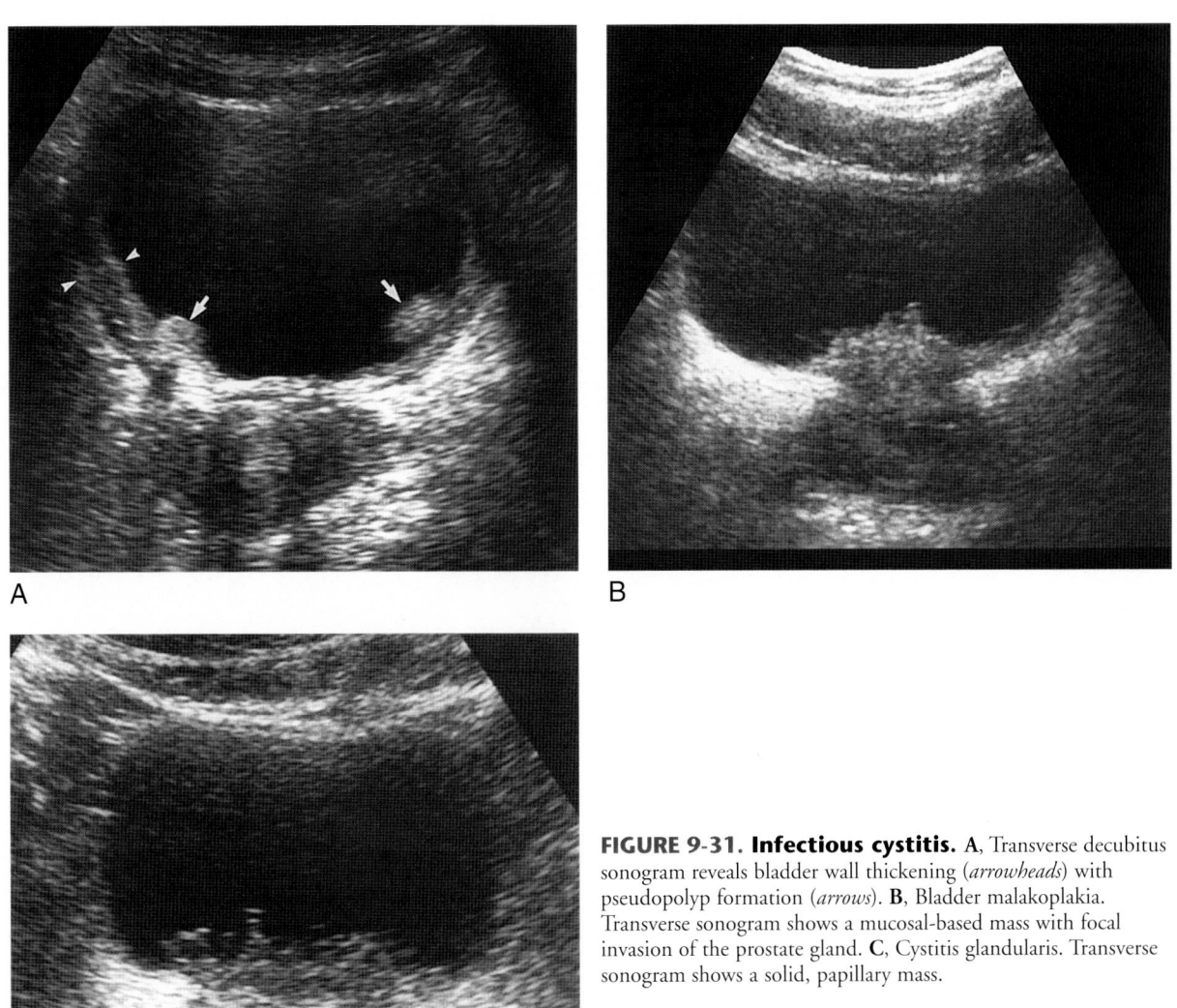

FIGURE 9-31. Infectious cystitis. A, Transverse decubitus sonogram reveals bladder wall thickening (*arrowheads*) with pseudopolyp formation (*arrows*). **B,** Bladder malakoplakia. Transverse sonogram shows a mucosal-based mass with focal invasion of the prostate gland. **C,** Cystitis glandularis. Transverse sonogram shows a solid, papillary mass.

increases with advancing age, and white men are most commonly affected. The most common type of stone is calcium oxalate (60% to 80%).[80] The etiology of stone formation is largely unknown, although it is believed to be multifactorial. Caliceal stones that are nonobstructing are usually asymptomatic, although patients may have hematuria (gross or microscopic) or pain. If a stone moves and causes infundibular or UPJ obstruction, clinical signs and symptoms of flank pain and infection often occur. If a stone passes into the ureter, there are **three areas of ureteric narrowing** where the stone may lodge: (1) just past the UPJ; (2) where the ureter crosses the iliac vessels; and (3) at the UVJ. The majority of stones will lodge at the UVJ (75% to 80%), where the ureter has its smallest diameter of 1 to 5 mm.[80]

Approximately 80% of stones smaller than 5 mm will pass spontaneously.

Renal calculi can be detected using many different imaging modalities, including plain films, tomography, ultrasound, and CT. Many studies have been undertaken evaluating the sensitivity for stone detection utilizing these various imaging modalities. Middleton et al.[81] demonstrated that sonography has a 96% sensitivity for renal stone detection, which was slightly inferior to a combination of plain radiography with tomography. They also found that stones greater than 5 mm in size were detected with 100% sensitivity sonographically. On **sonography,** renal calculi are seen as echogenic foci with sharp distal acoustic shadowing (Fig. 9-33). Small stones in the urinary tract may be hard to find if they have

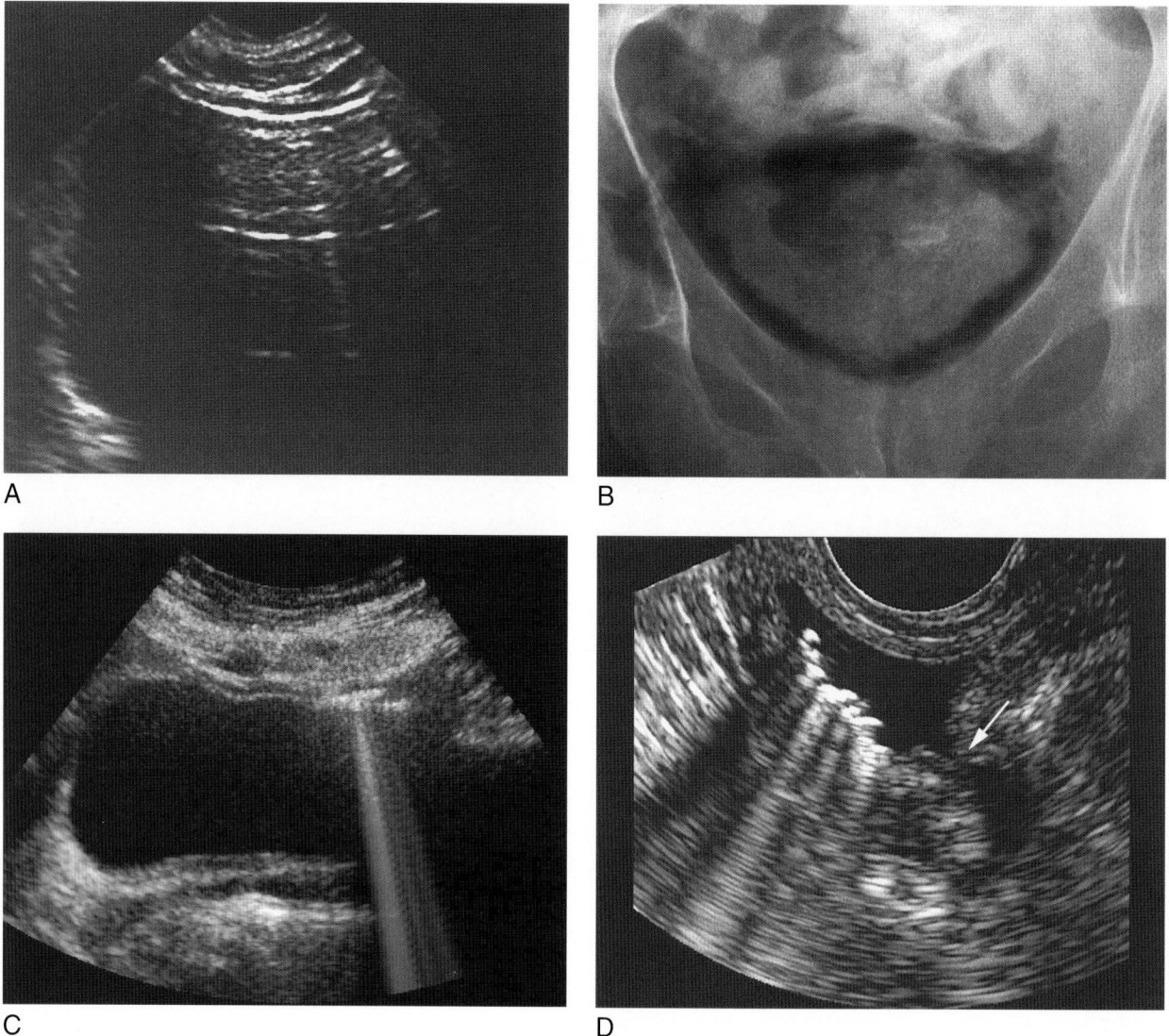

FIGURE 9-32. Air in the bladder. Emphysematous cystitis. A, Transverse sonogram shows an anterior linear echogenic line with dirty shadowing and a multiple reflection artifact distally in the bladder that represents air. **B**, Confirmatory plain film demonstrates extensive air in the bladder wall. **C**, Iatrogenic air introduced at cystoscopy shows as a nondependent bright echogenic focus with multiple reflection artifact. **D**, Enterovesical fistula (*arrow*) showing air in the bladder as multiple bright echogenic foci on a transvaginal sonogram. (From Damani N, Wilson S: Nongynecologic applications of transvaginal US. RadioGraphics 1999;19:S179-S200. Reproduced with permission.)

a weak posterior acoustic shadow. Lee et al.[82] have demonstrated that most urinary tract stones (83%) show color and power Doppler twinkling artifacts. In equivocal cases, this appears to be a helpful ancillary finding (Fig. 9-34). Smith et al.[83] have demonstrated that annular array transducers are able to demonstrate stone shadowing to better advantage than mechanical sector transducers. Harmonic imaging may also help, and this technique should be employed when assessing for the presence or absence of urinary tract stones. Certain entities may **mimic renal calculi** sonographically including (1) intrarenal gas; (2) renal artery calcification; (3) calcified sloughed papilla; (4) calcified transitional cell tumor; (5) alkaline-encrusted pyelitis;

and (6) encrusted calcification of the ends of a ureteric stent.

For patients presenting with **acute renal colic**, the role of imaging is to confirm the diagnosis, define stone size, stone location, stone number, and to assess for associated complications. Normally, this is accomplished by plain renal tomography followed by intravenous pyelography (IVP). The ability of urography to provide information regarding anatomy and function still makes it a widely performed test. Alternatively, a plain film of the abdomen combined with renal sonography has been advocated as a replacement.[84-87] This approach has not gained universal acceptance.[88,89] There are many sonographic pitfalls for this approach including (1)

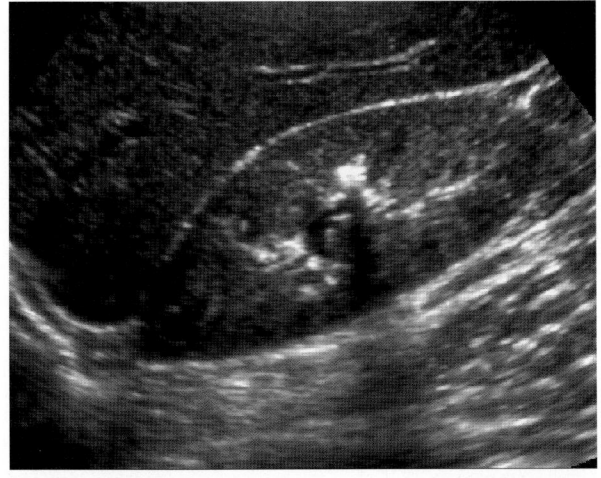

A

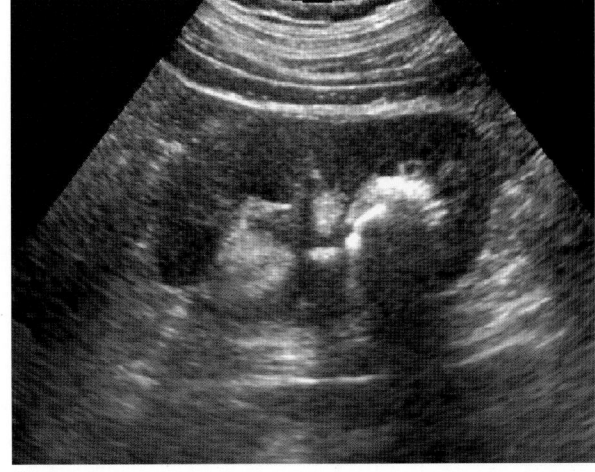

B

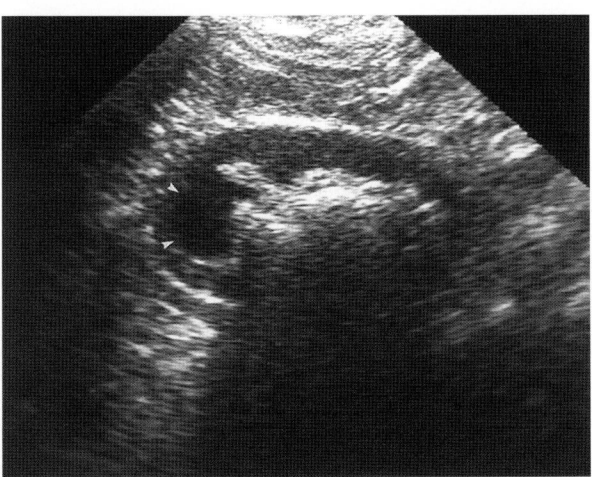

C

FIGURE 9-33. Renal stones. Sagittal sonograms show **A**, a small mid-pole echogenic focus with shadowing representing a nonobstructing stone. **B**, Multiple lower pole and renal pelvic stones with associated mild hydronephrosis. **C**, A large staghorn calculus with severe upper pole caliectasis (*arrowheads*).

ENTITIES THAT MIMIC RENAL CALCULI

Intrarenal gas
Renal artery calcification
Calcified sloughed papilla
Calcified transitional cell tumor
Alkaline-encrusted pyelitis
Encrusted calcification of a ureteric stent

evaluation before hydronephrosis develops, leading to a false-negative result; and (2) mistaking parapelvic cysts and nonobstructive pelvicaliectasis as hydronephrosis.[89]

One study by Patlas et al.[90] suggested a 93% sensitivity and 95% specificity for the sonographic diagnosis of ureteral stones. They suggest that because of lack of ionizing radiation and lower cost, this test should be employed initially before CT. If sonography is unavailable or is nondiagnostic, then CT could be performed. On **sonography**, the search for **ureteral calculi** can be difficult because of overlying bowel gas and the deep retroperitoneal location of the ureter (Fig. 9-35). However, transvaginal or transperineal scanning may be an optimal way to detect and demonstrate distal ureteral calculi that are not seen with a transabdominal suprapubic approach.[77,91,92] When the ureter is dilated, the distal 3 cm will be seen as a tubular hypoechoic structure entering the bladder obliquely. A stone will be identified as an echogenic focus with distal sharp acoustic shadowing within the ureteric lumen (Fig. 9-36). There may be associated mucosal edema at the bladder trigone. Transabdominal evaluation of the ureteral orifices for **jets** is helpful to assess for obstruction.[93] On gray scale, a stream of low-level echoes can be seen entering the bladder from the ureteral orifice. It is believed that density differences between the jet and bladder urine allow its sonographic visualization.[94] Good hydration prior to the study is important. In addition, patients should not be allowed to completely empty the bladder following hydration, prior to the study, so that concentrated urine remains in the bladder. This will then cause a density difference between the ureteric and bladder urine, allowing a jet to be seen.[95]

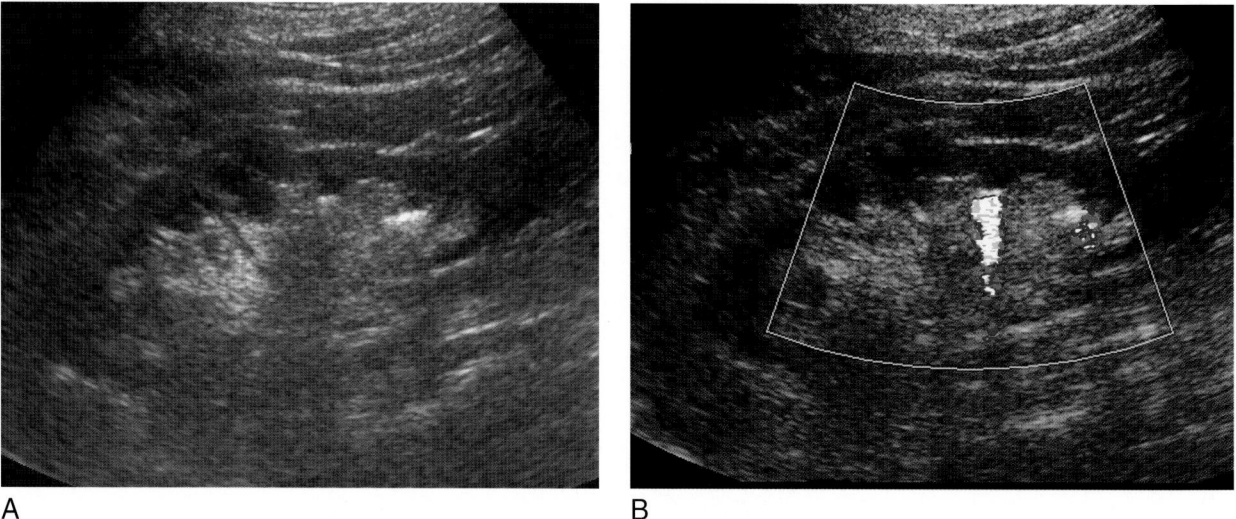

A   B

FIGURE 9-34. Twinkle artifacts indicating renal calculi. A, Sagittal sonogram shows two subtle echogenic foci in the lower pole of the kidney. **B,** The addition of color Doppler showing a twinkle artifact confirms their nature.

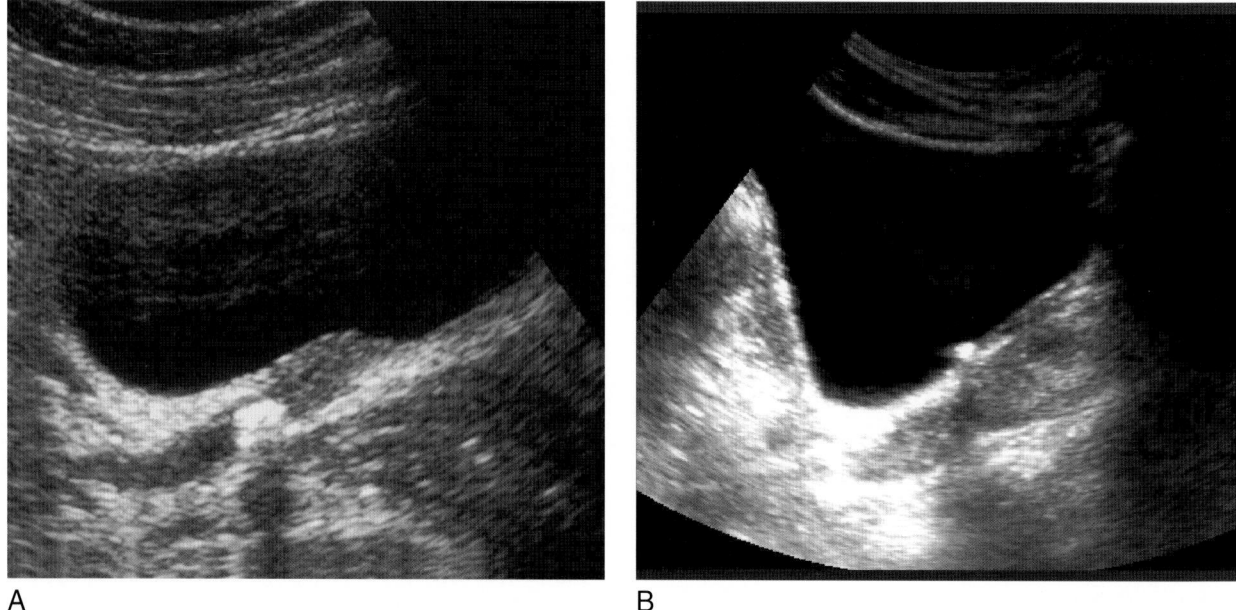

A   B

FIGURE 9-35. Distal ureteric stones. Sagittal sonograms of the distal ureters in two different patients show a stone in **A,** 1 cm from the ureterovesical junction with extensive edema of the distal ureteric mucosa and **B,** a tiny stone at the ureterovesical junction with no obvious edema. Both stones show distal acoustic shadowing.

In addition to gray-scale evaluation, Doppler improves detection of ureteric jets. The use of color Doppler over duplex Doppler has the advantage of being less prone to sampling error and also of allowing simultaneous visualization of both ureteral orifices (Fig. 9-37).[93] Depending on the state of hydration, jet frequency may vary from less than 1 per minute to continuous flow; however, both sides should be symmetrical in a healthy individual. Patients with high-grade ureteric obstruction will have asymmetrical jets on color Doppler imaging, which will be detected as either complete absence of the jet on the affected side, or as continuous, low-level flow

from the symptomatic side. Patients with low-grade obstruction may or may not have asymmetry of their jets.[93] The use of color Doppler should be adjunctive in assessing for ureteric obstruction and possibility of spontaneous ureteral stone passage. Geavlete et al.[96] found if there was an intravesical ureteric jet on the renal colic side associated with resistive index (RI) values less than or equal to 0.7 and delta RI less than or equal to 0.06, spontaneous passage of the stone occurred 71% of the time.

Recently, it has been suggested that the addition of **duplex renal Doppler** to the gray-scale examination may allow diagnosis of both **acute and chronic urinary**

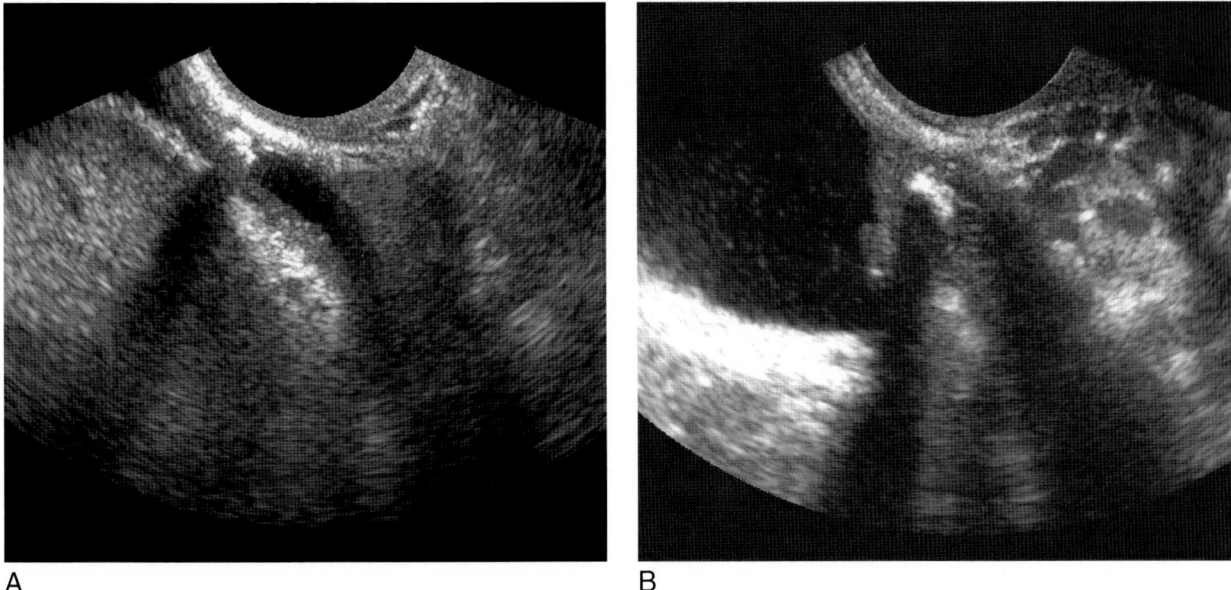

FIGURE 9-36. Ureterovesical stone. Transvaginal sonograms in two different patients show the value of this technique. **A,** A small stone obstructing a mildly dilated ureter at the ureterovesical junction. **B,** A larger stone with extensive surrounding ureteric edema.

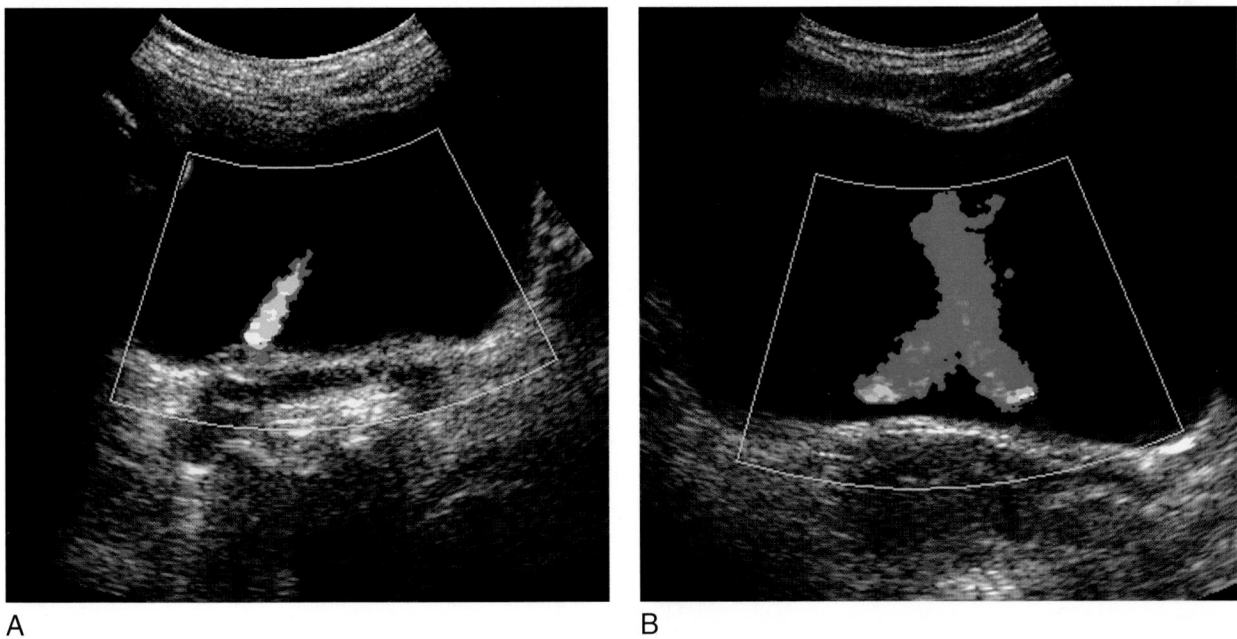

FIGURE 9-37. Color Doppler evaluation. Value of color Doppler evaluation of ureteric jets to discriminate degree of urinary tract obstruction. Transverse sonograms in two different patients show **A,** a single right jet and **B,** bilateral jets.

tract obstruction.[97] It is believed that with obstruction, the renal pelvic wall tension increases, resulting in elevation of prostaglandins that initially causes vasodilation.[98] With prolonged obstruction, many hormones, including renin-angiotensin, kallikrein-kinin, and prostaglandin-thromboxane, reduce vasodilation and produce diffuse vasoconstriction. Platt et al.[97] used a threshold resistance index (RI) of greater than 0.70 to indicate obstruction. They also noted a difference in RI of 0.08 to 0.1 when comparing the patients' obstructed and nonobstructed kidneys. Others have not had the same success using duplex Doppler.[89,98] Some of the potential problems include (1) there is no elevation of RI with partial obstruction; (2) the use of nonsteroidal anti-inflammatory medication for pain control appears to alter the RI by interfering with vasodilation and vasoconstriction; and (3) antecedent IVP causes vasoconstriction, altering the RI.[89,98]

IVP or unenhanced helical CT is most accepted as the initial imaging test in patients with acute renal colic, with the exception of pregnant patients in whom sonography should be used to eliminate radiation exposure.[89,99-101] Helical CT can be performed rapidly and with no patient preparation required. There is no risk of contrast reaction, and the associated findings of hydronephrosis, hydroureter, perinephric stranding, and ureteric edema are easily assessed, although at a higher cost than with ultrasound.[99] In addition, extraurinary tract causes of acute flank pain may be noted with helical CT.

Bladder calculi occur most commonly as a result of either migration from the kidney or urinary stasis in the bladder. Urinary stasis is usually related to bladder outlet obstruction, cystocele, neurogenic bladder, or a foreign body in the bladder. Bladder calculi may be asymptomatic. If symptomatic, patients will complain of bladder pain or foul smelling urine with or without hematuria. On **sonography**, a mobile, echogenic focus with distal acoustic shadowing will be seen in the bladder (Fig. 9-38). If the stone is large, edema of the ureteral orifices and thickening of the bladder wall may be seen. Occasionally, stones can adhere to the bladder wall because of adjacent inflammation, and these are known as **"hanging" bladder stones**.

Nephrocalcinosis

Nephrocalcinosis refers to renal parenchymal calcification. The calcification may be dystrophic or metastatic. With **dystrophic calcification**, there is deposition of calcium in devitalized tissue, usually resulting from

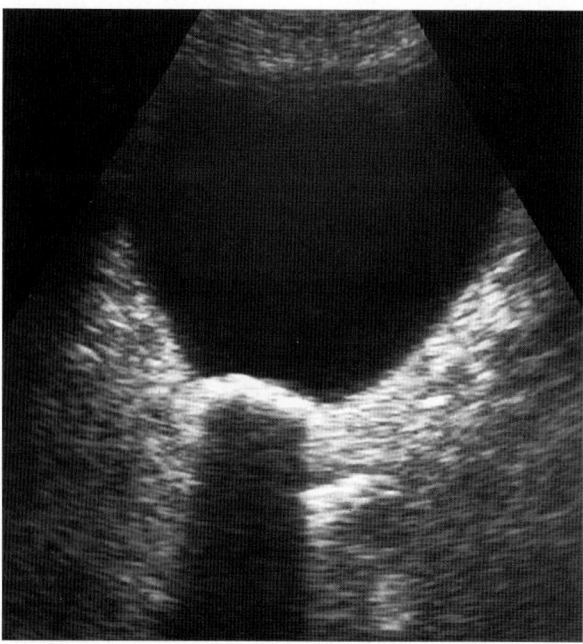

FIGURE 9-38. Bladder stone. Transverse sonogram shows a dependent echogenic focus with distal sharp acoustic shadowing.

ischemia or necrosis.[102] This type occurs in tumors, abscesses, and hematomas. **Metastatic nephrocalcinosis** occurs most commonly with hypercalcemic states caused by hyperparathyroidism, renal tubular acidosis, and renal failure. Metastatic nephrocalcinosis can be further categorized by the location of the calcium deposits into **cortical** or **medullary nephrocalcinosis**. Causes of **cortical nephrocalcinosis** include acute cortical necrosis, chronic glomerulonephritis, chronic hypercalcemic states, ethylene glycol poisoning, sickle cell disease, and rejected renal transplants. Causes of **medullary nephrocalcinosis** include hyperparathyroidism (40%), renal tubular acidosis (20%), medullary sponge kidney, bone metastases, chronic pyelonephritis, Cushing's syndrome, hyperthyroidism, malignancy, renal papillary necrosis, sarcoidosis, sickle cell disease, vitamin D excess, and Wilson's disease.[102]

The **Anderson-Carr-Randall theory of stone progression** postulates that the concentration of calcium is high in the fluid around the renal tubules. The calcium is removed by lymphatics and if the amount exceeds lymphatic capacity, deposits of calcium in the fornical tips and margins of the medulla will occur, producing a striking appearance on sonography with nonshadowing echogenic rims surrounding all medullary pyramids (Fig. 9-39). Plaques form that may perforate the calix and form a nidus for further stone growth.[103]

Sonographically, cortical nephrocalcinosis is seen as increased cortical echogenicity, which may produce acoustic shadowing. **Medullary nephrocalcinosis** is apparent when the medullary pyramids become more echogenic than the adjacent cortex. With time, further calcium deposition and stone formation occur with acoustic shadowing becoming apparent (see Fig. 9-39).

TUMORS OF THE GENITOURINARY TRACT

Renal Cell Carcinoma

Renal cell carcinoma (RCC) accounts for approximately 3% of all adult malignancies and 86% of all primary malignant renal parenchymal tumors.[104] There is a 2:1 predominance in men. Peak age is between 50 and 70 years. The etiology is unknown, although a moderate association with smoking,[105] chemical exposure, asbestosis, obesity and hypertension has been shown. Although most RCCs occur sporadically, a **familial variety** does occur.[106,107] It is estimated that about 4% of renal cancers are hereditary.[107] This variety occurs at an earlier age, is multifocal and bilateral, and affects men and women equally.[106] There is also an association with **von Hippel-Lindau disease**, in which 24% to 45% of affected patients develop RCC.[108] Seventy-five percent of these patients will have multicentric and bilateral tumors.[109] There is also an increased incidence of RCC

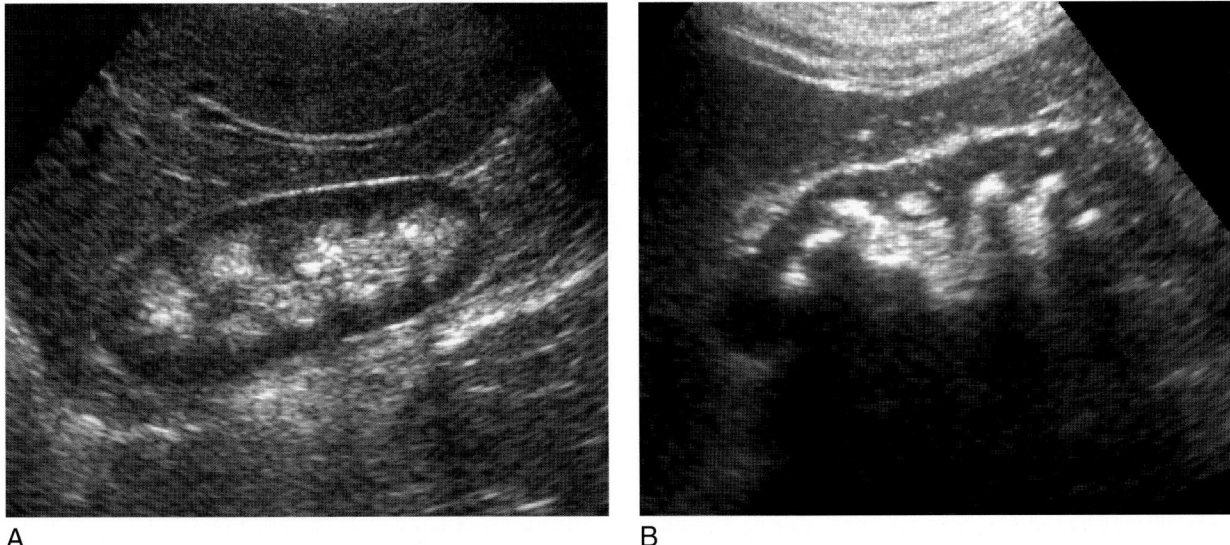

FIGURE 9-39. Medullary nephrocalcinosis in two different patients. A, Anderson-Carr kidney. Sagittal sonogram demonstrates increased echogenicity in a rimlike pattern around all medullary pyramids. **B,** Sagittal sonogram shows extensive medullary calcification.

in patients with **tuberous sclerosis**. Other syndromes associated with hereditary renal cancers include **hereditary papillary renal cancer, Birt-Hogg-Dubé syndrome, hereditary leiomyoma, renal cell carcinoma, familial renal oncocytoma, hereditary nonpolyposis colon cancer,** and **medullary carcinoma of the kidney.** Many other syndromes associated with hereditary renal cancers are also under investigation.[107] Patients with chronic renal failure, who have been on long-term hemodialysis or peritoneal dialysis, develop **acquired cystic kidney disease (ACKD)** and have an increased incidence of RCC. RCC associated with ACKD is often small and hypovascular.[110,111]

There are many different **histologic subtypes of RCC.** These include clear cell (70% to 75%); papillary (15%); chromophobe (5%); oncocytoma (2% to 3%); and collecting duct or medullary tumors (<1%). Patients with papillary, chromophobic, and oncocytic tumors have a much better prognosis than those with clear cell and collecting duct tumors. There have been attempts to differentiate subtypes on the basis of imaging, predominantly CT. Enhancement patterns seem to be the most helpful, although much work remains to be done. Lack of necrosis and presence of calcification appear to be associated with a better prognosis (papillary and chromophobe subtypes).[112] Necrosis and calcification can be seen sonographically.

The **classic diagnostic triad** of flank pain, gross hematuria, and palpable renal mass is seen in 4% to 9% of patients at presentation.[113] Systemic symptoms, such as anorexia and weight loss, are common. Many manifestations secondary to hormone production occur, including erythrocytosis (erythropoietin); hypercalcemia (parathormone, vitamin D metabolites, and prostaglan-

dins); hypokalemia (ACTH); galactorrhea (prolactin); hypertension (renin); and gynecomastia (gonadotropin). RCC has been described as having metastases to virtually every organ in the body. Spontaneous regression of the primary tumor may occur, although the mechanism for this is unclear.[114]

With the rapidly changing and improved superior technology of current cross-sectional imaging techniques, we are able to detect smaller renal masses. The prevalence rate of incidentally discovered occult renal cell carcinoma on CT is 0.3%.[115] Before the advent of CT, renal tumors less than 3 cm represented 5% of lesions, whereas now these small lesions represent 9% to 38% of all renal tumors.[116] Warshauer et al.[117] demonstrated the relative insensitivity of excretory urography/linear tomography for renal masses less than 3 cm in diameter and of ultrasound for masses less than 2 cm. Jamis-Dow et al.[118] found that CT was more sensitive than ultrasound for the detection of small renal masses (<1.5 cm) and that both ultrasound and CT were equally able to characterize a mass larger than 1 cm. They also demonstrated that a combination of ultrasound and CT allowed accurate characterization of a lesion larger than 1.0 cm 95% of the time. Neither method was able to accurately characterize lesions less than 1 cm in diameter. Therefore, a combination of both ultrasound and CT is superior to either one alone. With the advent of helical CT, respiratory misregistration and partial volume averaging can be eliminated. Many authors[119-122] have demonstrated that nephrographic phase helical CT scans enable better lesion detection and characterization. With the combined use of ultrasound and helical CT, there is usually no need for other imaging in the evaluation of renal masses.

Magnetic resonance imaging (MRI) for renal mass characterization has improved significantly with the development of phased-array multicoils, fast breath-hold imaging, and gadopentetate dimeglumine contrast enhancement. This method is assuming an increasingly important role in the detection and characterization of some renal masses.[123,124] This is particularly so in patients with allergy to iodinated contrast, renal failure, pregnancy, and when indeterminate renal masses or extent of vascular involvement cannot be adequately determined with a combination of ultrasound and CT.

With the detection of small (<3 cm) renal masses, the controversy now is how to manage them. The choice is either watchful waiting or surgery (radical nephrectomy, partial nephrectomy, enucleation , cryotherapy, or radio-frequency ablation). As a result of preliminary experience, Bosniak et al.[125] suggest watchful waiting in some elderly patients and in those patients at risk for surgery, who have small, incidentally discovered lesions. Gervais et al.[126] have found that radiofrequency ablation of exophytic RCC (up to 5 cm in size) can be performed successfully. Tumors that have a component in the renal sinus are more difficult to treat.

On **sonography**, most tumors are solid with no predilection for either kidney and no predilection for the upper, mid-, or lower pole. Tumors may be hypoechoic, isoechoic, or hyperechoic (Fig. 9-40). Charboneau et al.[127] demonstrated that the majority (86%) are iso-echoic, whereas the minority were hypoechoic (10%) or echogenic (4%). More recently, it has been demonstrated that small renal tumors (<3 cm) tend to be echogenic when compared with normal renal parenchyma. Forman et al.[128] found that 77% of their small RCCs (<3 cm) and Yamashita et al.[129,130] found 61% of their small RCCs were more echogenic than renal parenchyma. In comparing hyperechoic RCCs and angiomyolipomas (AMLs), Yamashita et al.[129,130] found considerable overlap in the echogenicity of these two tumors. They demonstrated a **hypoechoic rim** sonographically, which represented a pseudocapsule histologically, in 84% of the RCCs and in none of the AMLs. As well, **intratumoral cystic spaces** were noted in their hyperechoic RCCs and not in any of the AMLs (see Fig. 9-40). The exact pathologic basis for the hyper-echoic appearance of RCC is not understood, but in their study this appearance was seen in RCCs with papillary, tubular, or microcystic architecture or in tumors with minute calcification, necrosis, cystic degeneration, or fibrosis.[116] RCC will demonstrate **calcification** in 8% to 18% of cases. This calcification may be punctate, curvilinear, diffuse (rare), central, or peripheral.[131-135] Daniels et al.[134] demonstrated that central calcification was associated with a malignant tumor 87% of the time. Rim or diffuse calcification of a renal mass may obscure adequate sonographic visualization, and CT is advised to look for features of malignancy, including the presence of a soft tissue mass extending beyond the calcification.[136]

Fifteen percent of RCCs will be of a **papillary variety**.[112,137] This type of tumor is characterized by slower growth, lower stage at presentation, and better prognosis.[138] These tumors tend to be hypoechoic or isoechoic, although no consistent sonographic pattern exists because some may also be hyperechoic.[137] Five percent to 7% of all RCCs will be of a **cystic variety**.[139] **Four histologic growth patterns** have been described: (1) multilocular; (2) unilocular; (3) cystic necrosis; and (4) tumors originating in a simple cyst (Fig. 9-41).[140] Yamashita et al.[139] believe that recognition of subtypes may have clinical significance because the multilocular and unilocular subtypes seem to be less aggressive. On sonography, **multilocular cystic RCC** will demonstrate a cystic mass with internal septations. These septations may be thick (>2 mm), nodular, and contain calcification (see Fig. 9-40). **Unilocular cystic RCC** will demonstrate a debris-filled cystic mass with thick, irregular walls which may be calcified. **Necrotic RCCs** show various sonographic findings depending on the degree of necrosis. **Tumors originating in a simple cyst** are rare and a mural tumor nodule will be found at the base of a simple cyst. Helical-enhanced CT in conjunction with ultrasound will usually allow accurate characterization of the internal nature of a cystic renal lesion.[141] Silverman et al.[142] demonstrated that spiral CT alone can underestimate the number of septations in small (≤3 cm) cystic renal lesions. The majority of cystic RCCs will demonstrate features of malignancy in 88% of cases.

The use of **Doppler ultrasound** for detection of tumor vascularity has shown high sensitivity for malignant lesions in the liver, kidneys, adrenal glands, and pancreas. Most malignant renal tumors (70% to 83%) will have Doppler shift frequency of 2.5 kHz.[143-147] Similar changes may be noted with inflammatory masses; however, patients with renal infection should be clinically apparent. Absence of high-frequency Doppler shift does not exclude malignancy.[145] Confirmation of blood flow within malignant solid and cystic renal tumors has also recently been performed with micro-bubble contrast agents and pulse inversion sonography. Initial investigations suggest that characteristics of indeterminate cystic masses as seen on CT scan may have the most significant impact on patient management in the future (Fig. 9-42).

Tumor stage at diagnosis is important for patient prognosis. **Robson staging** classification is:

- **I**—tumor confined within the renal capsule;
- **II**—tumor invasion of perinephric fat;
- **III**—tumor involvement of regional lymph nodes or venous structures;
- **IV**—invasion of adjacent organs or distant metastases.

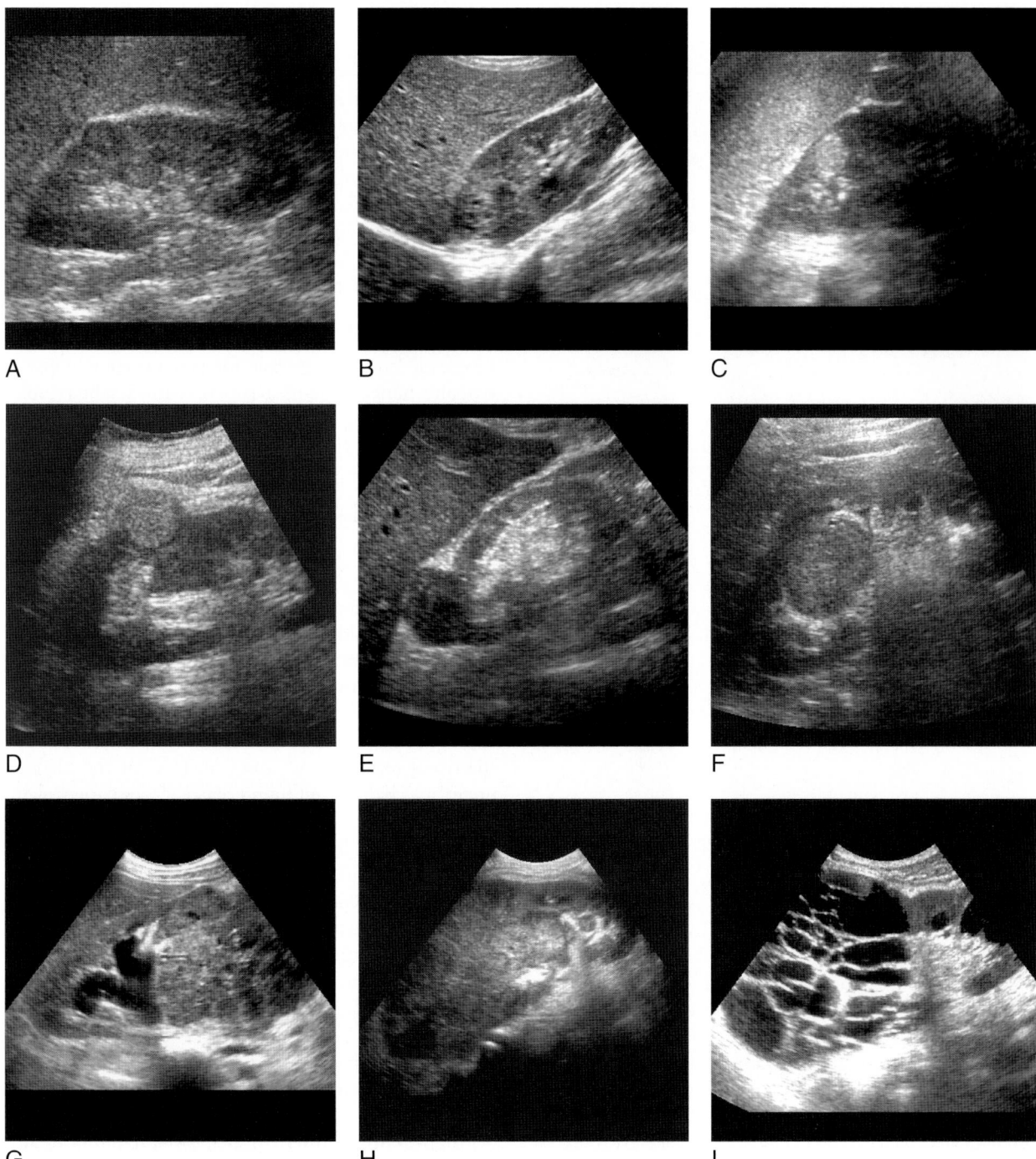

FIGURE 9-40. Sonographic appearances of renal cell carcinoma on sagittal sonograms. A, Tiny incidental hypoechoic tumor. **B,** Small echogenic tumor with central cystic spaces. **C,** Small echogenic nodule, simulating an angiomyolipoma. **D,** Exophytic echogenic mid-pole renal mass. **E,** Exophytic hypoechoic upper pole renal mass. **F,** Large central renal sinus mass with no associated caliectasis. **G,** Large solid heterogeneous mass in the lower pole of the kidney compressing the renal pelvis with upper pole caliectasis. **H,** Large infiltrative renal mass with maintenance of the reniform shape. **I,** Large upper pole cystic mass showing numerous thick internal septations.

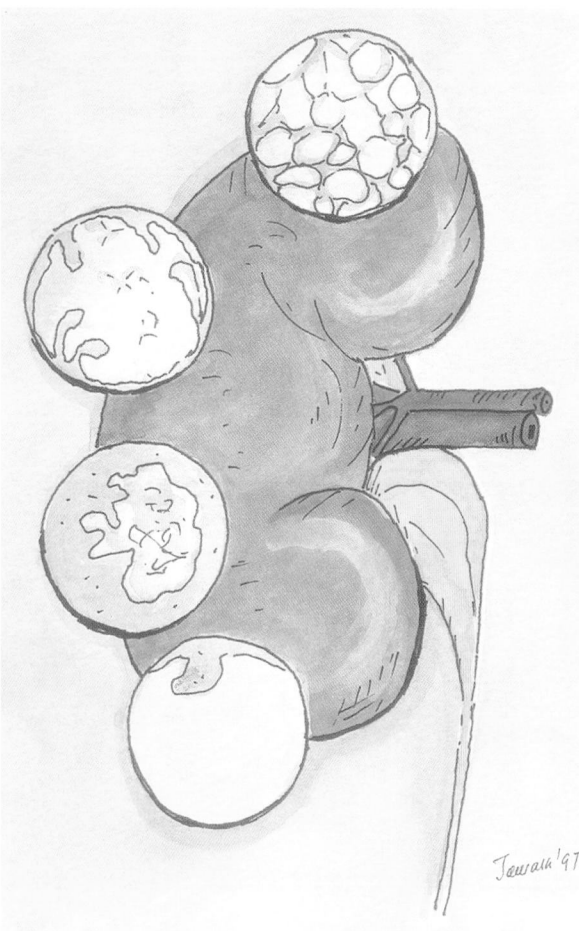

FIGURE 9-41. Cystic growth patterns of renal cell carcinoma. Upper pole, multilocular; upper lateral, unilocular; lower lateral, cystic necrosis; lower pole, origin in the wall of a simple cyst. (From Yamashita Y, Watanabe O, Miyazaki H, et al: Cystic renal cell carcinoma. Acta Radiologica 1994;35(1):19-24.)

Five-year survival rates for Robson stage I, II, III, and IV are 67%, 51%, 33.5%, and 13.5%, respectively.[148] Patients with stage I and II disease are treated surgically (partial or radical nephrectomy). Patients with stage III disease, with extensive metastatic lymphadenopathy, are often treated palliatively. Patients with stage III disease and with tumor thrombus are treated with radical nephrectomy and thrombectomy. Patients with stage IV disease usually receive palliative treatment only.[149] Ultrasound is inferior to CT and MRI for staging RCC. Unfortunately, obese patients and overlying bowel gas make it difficult to assess for lymphadenopathy and/or vascular involvement.

In thin patients and in those with minimal bowel gas, the renal veins and retroperitoneum can be well assessed with ultrasound and an attempt should be made to do so in all patients with a renal mass (Fig. 9-43). Sonography is excellent for assessment of the intrahepatic IVC and determination of the cephalad extent of venous tumor

thrombus (Fig. 9-44). Habboub et al.[150] found the accuracy of detecting renal vein and IVC involvement on sonography was 64% and 93%, respectively. They also demonstrated that addition of color Doppler improved accuracy for diagnosing both renal vein and IVC thrombus to 87% and 100%, respectively. It is crucial to determine the location and extent of vascular tumor thrombus to plan the surgical approach. Many staging limitations, however, are shared by ultrasound, CT, and MRI. These include (1) microscopic tumor invasion of the renal capsule; (2) detection of metastatic tumor deposits in normal-sized lymph nodes; and (3) differentiation of inflammatory hyperplastic nodes from neoplastic ones.[151] The role for percutaneous biopsy is virtually nonexistent in a patient with a solitary solid renal mass and no other known malignancy. Good radiologic imaging is virtually diagnostic in all cases.[152-154]

Transitional Cell Carcinoma

Transitional cell carcinoma (TCC) of the renal pelvis accounts for 7% of all primary renal tumors.[155] They are two to three times more common than ureteral neoplasms. Bladder TCC, because of its large surface area, is 50 times more common than renal pelvic TCC.[156] The multifocal and bilateral nature of this disease requires accurate diagnosis and staging to allow appropriate surgical planning. Yousem et al.[157] retrospectively reviewed 645 cases of TCC of the bladder, ureter, and kidney and found that 3.9% of patients with bladder cancer developed an upper tract lesion (mean = within 61 months). Thirteen percent of patients with ureteral TCC and 11% of patients with renal TCC developed metachronous tumors (mean = within 28 and 22 months, respectively). Synchronous TCC was present in 2.3% of patients with bladder TCC, 39% with ureteral TCC, and 24% with renal TCC. Surveillance with IVP, retrograde pyelography, and cystoscopy is recommended. Some patients at increased risk for development of TCC may require closer surveillance and include those with (1) **Balkan nephritis**; (2) **vesicoureteric reflux**; (3) **multifocal recurrent bladder** TCC; (4) **high-grade bladder tumors**; (5) **carcinoma in situ** of the distal ureters following cystectomy; (6) **analgesic abuse**; (7) **heavy smoking**; (8) **exposure to carcinogens**; and (9) **treatment with cyclophosphamide**.[157]

TCC may be **papillary** or **nonpapillary**. Papillary forms are exophytic polypoid lesions attached to the mucosa by a stalk. This type tends to be low grade, slow to infiltrate, late to metastasize, and follows a more benign course. Nonpapillary tumors present as nodular or flat tumors demonstrating mucosal thickening. These tumors are usually high grade and infiltrating.[156]

Kidney. Transitional cell tumors of the kidney are more common in men than in women (4:1) with a mean age at diagnosis of 65 years.[156] Seventy-five percent

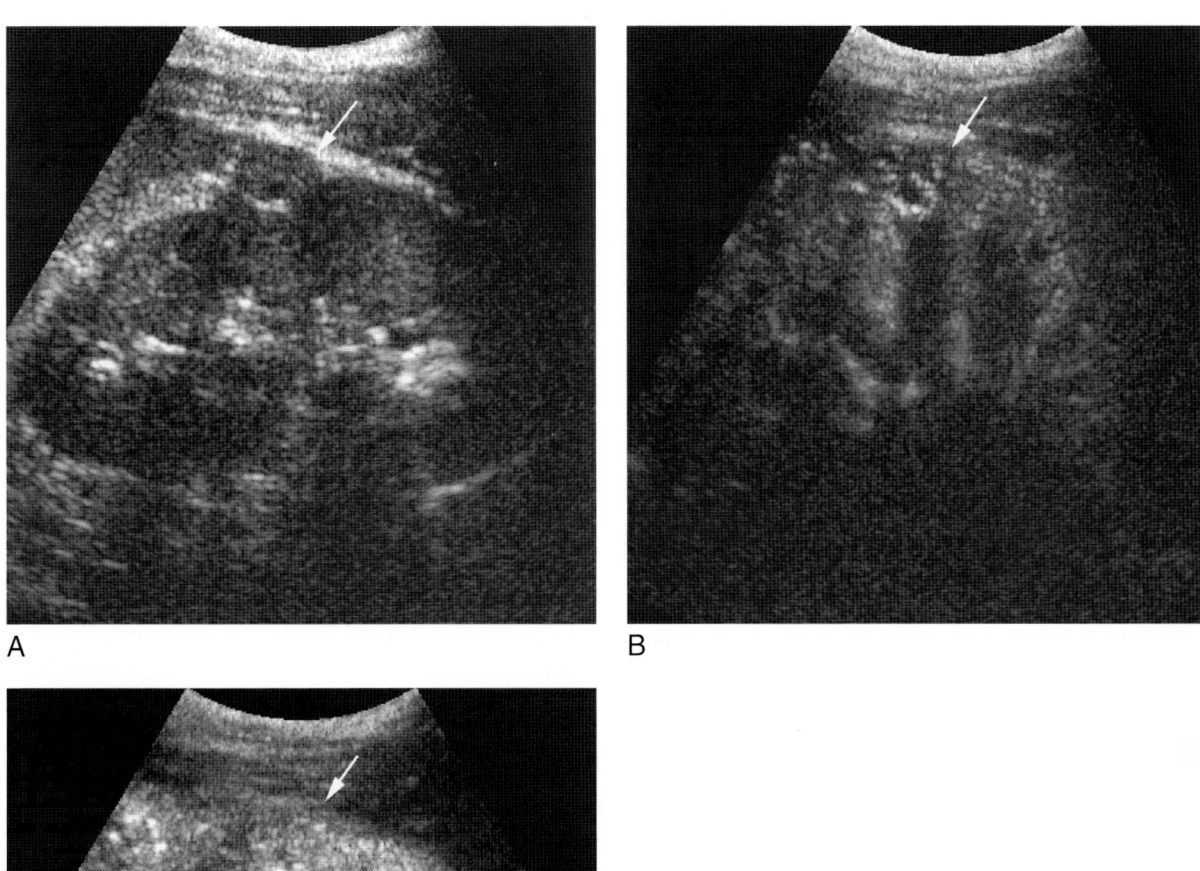

A

B

C

FIGURE 9-42. Value of microbubble enhanced sonography for determining the vascularity of a renal mass. **A**, Sagittal sonogram shows a small exophytic isoechoic solid mid-pole renal mass (*arrow*). **B**, Immediately following bolus injection of Definity (Bristol-Myers Squibb, Billerica, MA). There are small linear vessels in the mass (*arrow*). **C**, Arterial phase image shows that the renal parenchyma and the renal mass are both enhanced relative to the presence of microbubbles in the vasculature (*arrow*).

of patients with renal pelvic tumors will present with gross or microscopic hematuria. Twenty-five percent of patients will have flank pain. Incidental tumor discovery occurs in less than 5%.[156]

Sonographic assessment of the **renal sinus** poses unique problems and is a challenge to evaluate for pathologic processes because of its variable morphologic appearance. The presence of fat within the renal sinus can appear as a hypoechoic mass simulating a solid TCC (Fig. 9-45). In uncertain cases, confirmation with IVP is recommended to rule out neoplasm, particularly in patients with hematuria.

The **sonographic appearance** of renal TCC is quite variable and depends on tumor morphology (papillary,

nonpapillary, or infiltrative), location, size, and presence or absence of hydronephrosis (Fig. 9-46). Small, non-obstructing tumors may be impossible to visualize. With growth, papillary tumors will be seen as discrete, solid, central, hypoechoic renal sinus masses with or without associated proximal caliectasis (Fig. 9-47). The differential diagnosis includes **blood clots**, **sloughed papilla**, and **fungus ball**.

The tumor may demonstrate peripelvic or paren-chymal extension. Tumor growth may be in a diffusely infiltrative pattern. These destructive tumors distort and enlarge the renal architecture with maintenance of reniform shape (see Fig. 9-47). Flat tumors are difficult to see, although the associated pelvicaliectasis may be

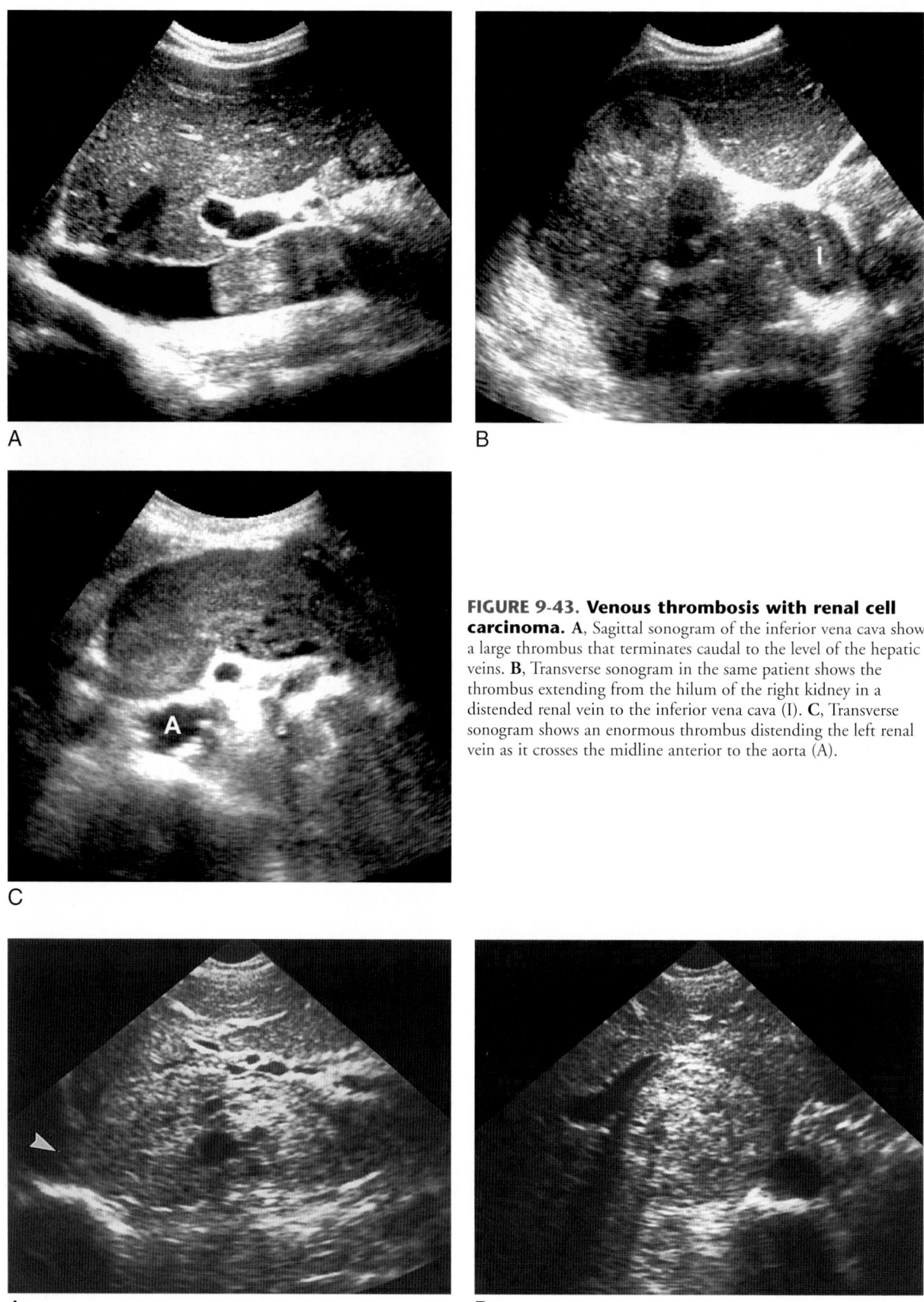

FIGURE 9-43. Venous thrombosis with renal cell carcinoma. A, Sagittal sonogram of the inferior vena cava shows a large thrombus that terminates caudal to the level of the hepatic veins. **B**, Transverse sonogram in the same patient shows the thrombus extending from the hilum of the right kidney in a distended renal vein to the inferior vena cava (I). **C**, Transverse sonogram shows an enormous thrombus distending the left renal vein as it crosses the midline anterior to the aorta (A).

FIGURE 9-44. Tumor thrombus in inferior vena cava. A, Sagittal and **B**, transverse sonograms demonstrate a large, expansile tumor thrombus extending cephalad to the diaphragm (*arrowhead*) in **A**.

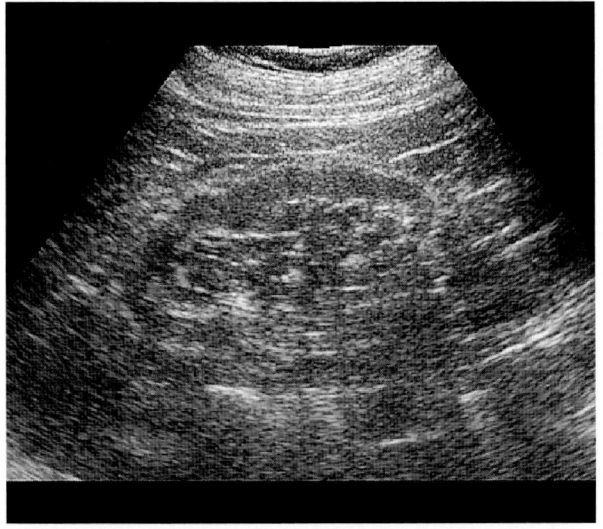
A

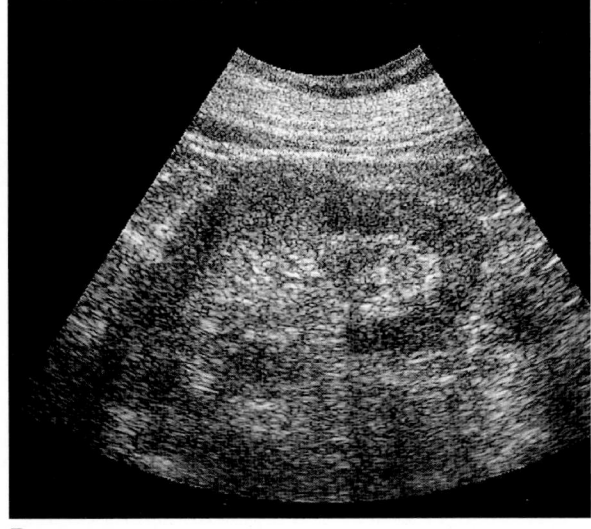
B

C

FIGURE 9-45. Renal sinus fat mimicking transitional cell carcinoma on sagittal sonograms in two different patients. A, An atrophic kidney shows small size and thin cortex. The renal sinus shows increased deposition of fat. **B,** A small focal area of hypoechogenicity is seen within the more echogenic sinus fat in the lower pole. **C,** Color Doppler image at the same level as in **B** shows normal vessels running through this area, confirming insignificant fat rather than tumor.

visualized sonographically. Both sessile and papillary TCCs may demonstrate dystrophic calcification creating difficulty in the differentiation of tumor from stones or sloughed calcified papilla.[158] TCC may invade the renal vein in 7% of cases.[159] This is usually a late finding.

Ureter. Transitional cell carcinoma (TCC) of the ureter is rare, accounting for only 1% to 6% of all upper urinary tract cancers.[156,160] Men are more commonly affected (3:1), with peak prevalence between the fifth and seventh decade.[156] The tumors are usually found in the lower third of the ureter (70% to 75%).[156,160] Sixty percent of the tumors are **papillary** and 40% are **non-papillary**.[156] The most frequent symptoms are hematuria, frequency, dysuria, and pain.[160] The imaging modalities of choice for evaluation include retrograde pyelography for direct ureteral visualization and CT for evaluation of extraureteral tumor extent. On **sonography,** hydronephrosis and hydroureter will be seen and occasionally a solid ureteral mass will be depicted.[160]

Bladder. Transitional cell carcinoma (TCC) of the bladder is a common malignant tumor. These tumors occur more commonly in men (3:1), with a peak incidence in the sixth and seventh decades. They occur most frequently at the trigone and along the lateral and posterior walls of the bladder. Approximately 70% of bladder cancers are superficial, whereas the remaining 30% are invasive. Patients most commonly present with hematuria. Frequency, dysuria, and suprapubic pain may also be present. **Sonographic detection** of bladder tumors is excellent and is greater than or equal to 95%.[161] The appearance is that of a focal nonmobile mass or of urothelial thickening (Fig. 9-48). The appearances, however, are nonspecific and the **differential diagnosis** is extensive and includes **cystitis, wall thickening** due to bladder outlet obstruction, **postradiation change, postoperative change, adherent blood clot, invasive prostate carcinoma, lymphoma, metastases, endometriosis,** and **neurofibromatosis.** Some papillary

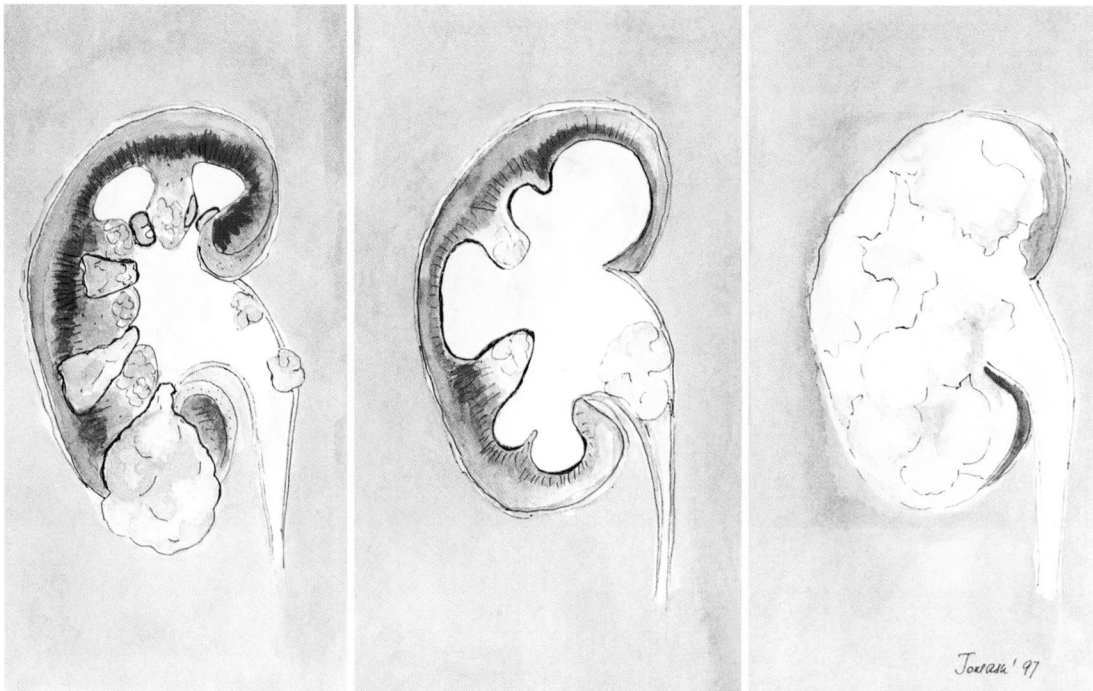

FIGURE 9-46. Morphologic growth patterns of renal transitional cell carcinoma.

bladder tumors may demonstrate focal areas of calcification (Fig. 9-49). Cystoscopy and biopsy are necessary for diagnosis. Both transvaginal and transrectal ultrasound may be used to assess a bladder wall mass if suprapubic visualization is poor (see Fig. 9-48). Transitional tumors may also arise within urinary bladder diverticula. Many diverticula have narrow necks, making them inaccessible for cystoscopic examination, and imaging plays an important role in the detection of these tumors. The periureteric and posterolateral wall locations of most bladder diverticula allow for adequate sonographic visualization.[162] Diverticular tumors are seen as a moderately echogenic nonshadowing mass. Although ultrasound is good for tumor detection, staging is still best performed clinically in combination with CT or contrast-enhanced MRI.[163]

Squamous Cell Carcinoma

Squamous cell carcinoma (SCC) is rare but is the second most common malignant tumor arising from urothelium after TCC. It represents 6% to 15% of renal pelvic tumors and 5% to 8% of all bladder tumors.[164,165] Chronic infection, irritation, and stones lead to squamous metaplasia and leukoplakia of the urothelium. Leukoplakia is felt to be premalignant. SCC tends to be solid, flat, and infiltrative with extensive ulceration and very rarely is exophytic and fungating. Distant metastases are usually present at the time of diagnosis. On **sonography**, **renal SCC** is seen as a diffusely enlarged kidney which has maintained its reniform shape. The normal renal echotexture is destroyed and often a stone (47% to 58%)[164] will be present. It may be impossible to differentiate this from xanthogranulomatous pyelonephritis. Often, perinephric tumor extension and metastases are present. **Ureteral SCC** is rare and hydronephroureterectasis proximal to the tumor mass will be apparent. Occasionally, the tumor mass is seen as a poorly defined, irregular, solid mass. Associated stones are often present. **Bladder SCCs** tend to be large, solid, and infiltrating. Ultrasound is an effective modality for detection but is less reliable in its ability to stage these tumors. Staging is best done with CT or MRI.

Adenocarcinoma

Adenocarcinoma of the renal pelvis, ureter, and bladder is rare. Almost all patients with adenocarcinoma of the renal pelvis will have urinary tract infection[166] and two thirds will have a stone, usually a staghorn calculus. Most will have hematuria. One must be careful to differentiate adenocarcinoma of the bladder from adenocarcinoma of the rectum, uterus, or prostate that has invaded the bladder. The prognosis of this tumor is poor. On **sonography**, a renal pelvic, ureteric, or bladder mass will be seen occasionally with calcification. An associated stone will often be present.

Oncocytoma

Oncocytes are large epithelial cells with granular eosinophilic cytoplasm caused by extensive cytoplasmic mito-

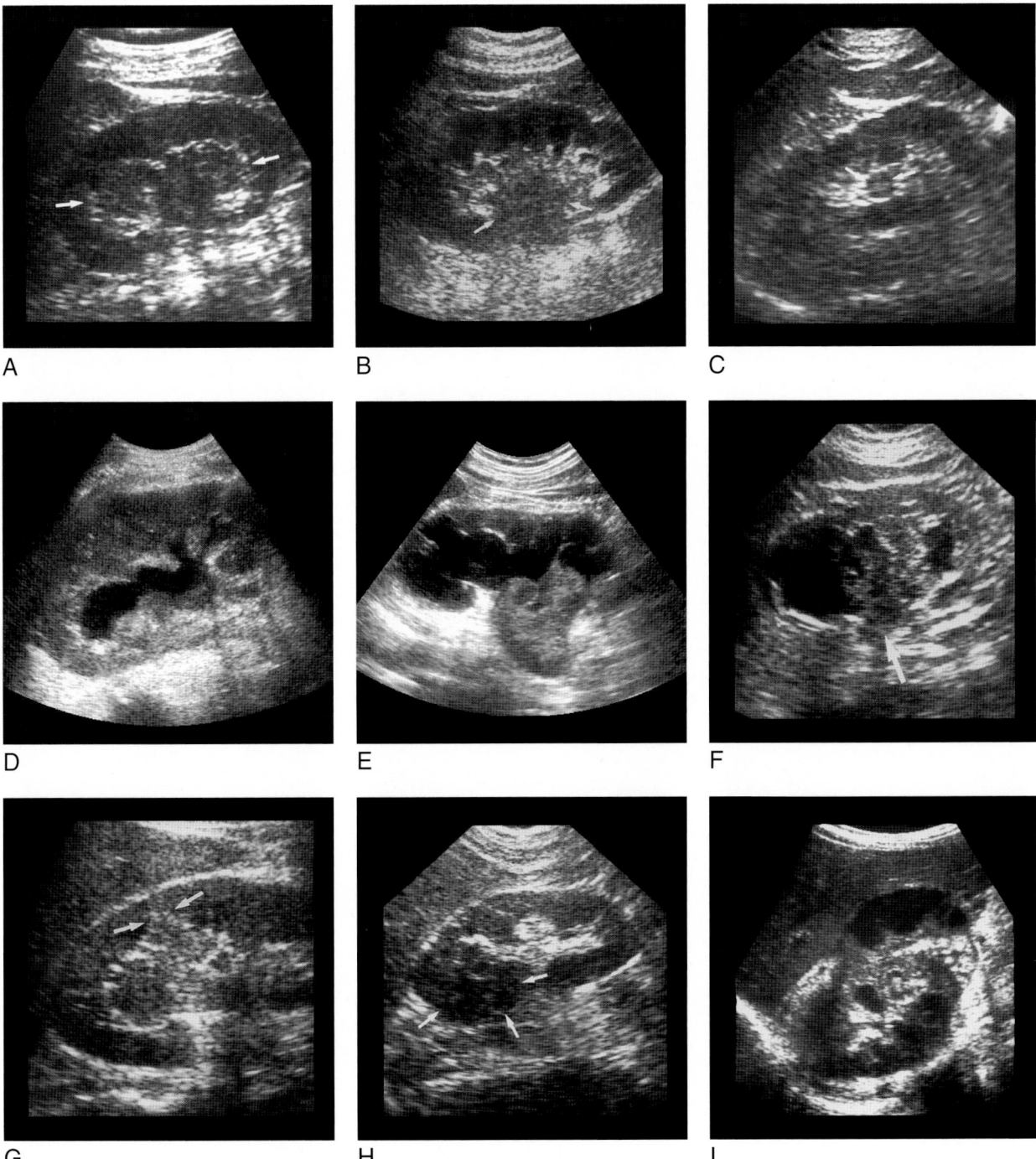

FIGURE 9-47. Transitional cell carcinoma of the kidney. **A** and **B**, Sagittal sonograms in two patients show normal and fat-filled renal sinuses (*arrows*) that appear hypoechoic, mimicking transitional cell carcinoma. **C**, Small, central nonobstructing hypoechoic mass (*arrow*). **D**, **E**, and **F**, Sagittal sonograms in three different patients showing hydronephrosis related to large central solid pelvic tumors (*arrow* in **F**). **G**, Infiltrative transitional cell carcinoma in the upper pole extends from the calix into the renal parenchyma (*arrows*). **H**, Large, lobulated solid parenchymal infiltrative mass (*arrows*) with no associated caliectasis. **I**, Perirenal tumor extension.

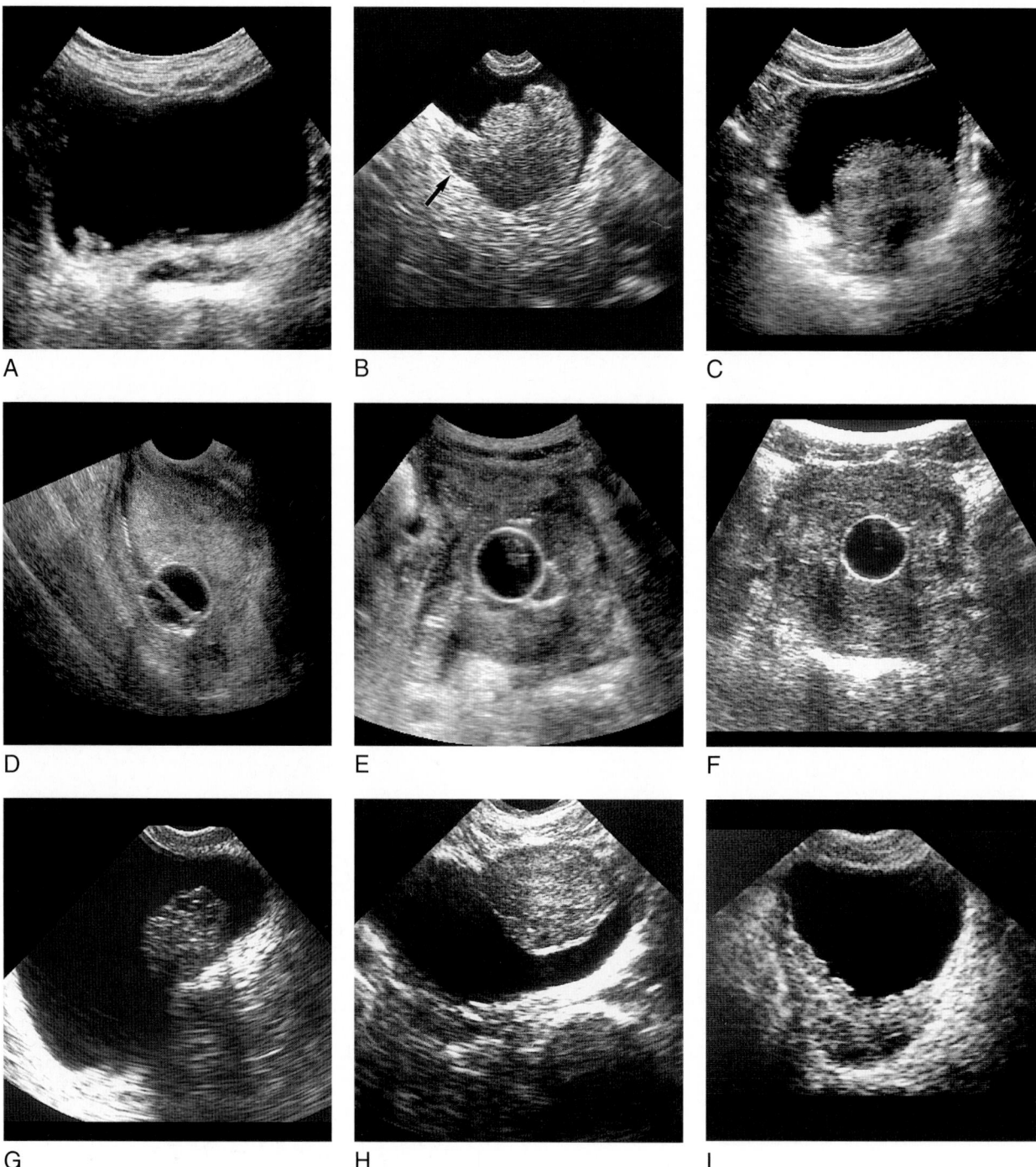

FIGURE 9-48. Appearances of bladder masses. A, Small polypoid transitional cell carcinoma. **B,** Invasive transitional cell carcinoma involving the perivesical fat (*arrow*).[77] **C,** Benign prostatic hypertrophy simulating a large invasive bladder wall mass. **D,** Diffuse transitional cell carcinoma on a transvaginal sagittal image. A Foley catheter is in place. **E,** Diffuse invasive transitional cell carcinoma on suprapubic scan. **F,** Interstitial cystitis closely simulates diffuse tumor. **G,** An endometrioma shows a solid mass with small cystic spaces. **H,** Pheochromocytoma appears as an anterior wall submucosal mass. **I,** Lymphoma of the posterior bladder wall.[77]

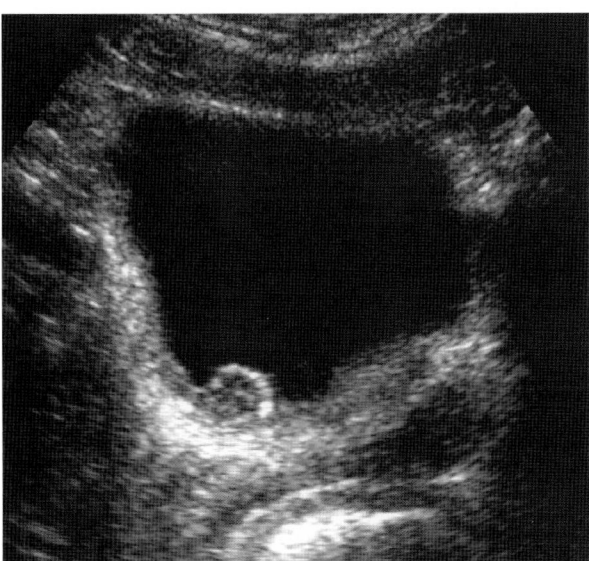

FIGURE 9-49. Calcified bladder transitional cell carcinoma. Sagittal sonogram demonstrates a polypoid solid mass with superficial echogenic foci representing calcification.

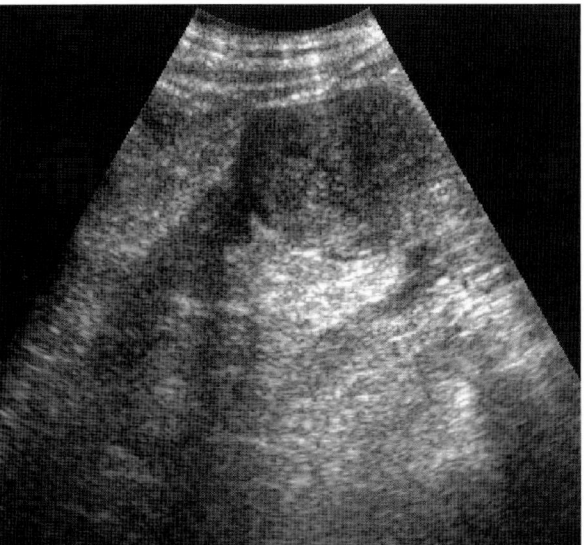

FIGURE 9-50. Renal oncocytoma. Sagittal sonogram shows a large isoechoic tumor at the lower pole of the kidney. It cannot be differentiated from renal cell carcinoma.

chondria. **Oncocytomas** may occur in the parathyroid glands, the thyroid gland, the adrenal glands, the salivary glands, and the kidneys. They represent 3.1% to 6.6% of all renal tumors.[167,168] They occur most commonly in men (1.7:1), with a peak incidence in the sixth and seventh decades.[169] Most patients are asymptomatic.[167] Oncocytomas may be small or extremely large (mean = 3 to 8 cm). On cut surface, they have a mahogany color. Hemorrhage and calcification are uncommon. These tumors histologically may have a benign or more malignant appearance. Patients with benign-appearing tumors clinically do well. Pathologically these tumors are multicentric and bilateral in 5% to 10% and 3%, respectively.[168]

On the basis of imaging, oncocytoma and renal cell adenocarcinoma cannot be differentiated. Davidson et al.[170] demonstrated that CT homogeneity, lack of homogeneity, and a central stellate "scar" are poor predictors in differentiating oncocytomas from RCCs. Oncocytomas represent about 5% of all tumors originally diagnosed as RCC on imaging.[171] On **sonography,** oncocytomas are variable in appearance and may be isoechoic, hypoechoic, or hyperechoic. These tumors may be homogeneous or heterogeneous with a well- or poorly demarcated wall depending on its size (Fig. 9-50).[172] A central scar, central necrosis, or calcification may be seen. These features may also be seen with RCC. If a solid mass is found in the kidney on sonography, CT is required for both staging and to look for the presence of fat. Most nonfat-containing solid renal mass(es) are either RCC or oncocytoma.[170] With a large oncocytoma, perinephric engulfment of fat may occur.[173] In these cases, care must be taken not to mistakenly diagnose angiomyolipoma.

In certain patients, partial nephrectomy and laparoscopic surgical techniques can be used.[174]

Angiomyolipoma

Angiomyolipomas (AML) are benign renal tumors composed of varying proportions of adipose tissue, smooth muscle cells, and blood vessels. Angiomyolipomas may occur sporadically or be found in patients with **tuberous sclerosis**. Tumors in patients, without stigmata of tuberous sclerosis, most commonly are unilateral and demonstrate a middle-aged predominance in women. Up to 50% of patients with AML will have stigmata of tuberous sclerosis (mental retardation, epilepsy, and sebaceous adenomas of the face) and up to 80% of patients with tuberous sclerosis will have one or more AMLs.[175] AMLs associated with tuberous sclerosis are usually small, multiple, and bilateral with no sex predilection. Sporadic tumors are histologically identical to those associated with tuberous sclerosis. It is unusual for small tumors (<4 cm)[176] to be symptomatic; however, with growth, these tumors may hemorrhage, giving rise to signs and symptoms of hematuria, flank pain, or palpable flank mass.

On **sonography,** the echopattern of the AML depends on the proportion of fat, smooth muscle, vascular elements, and hemorrhage. Classically, AMLs are markedly hyperechoic relative to renal parenchyma (Fig. 9-51). The tumors may be within the parenchyma or exophytic (see Fig. 9-51). If muscle, vascular elements, or hemorrhage predominate, the tumor may be hypoechoic (see Fig. 9-51). Small (<3 cm) renal cell carcinomas (RCC) are also hyperechoic and may sim-

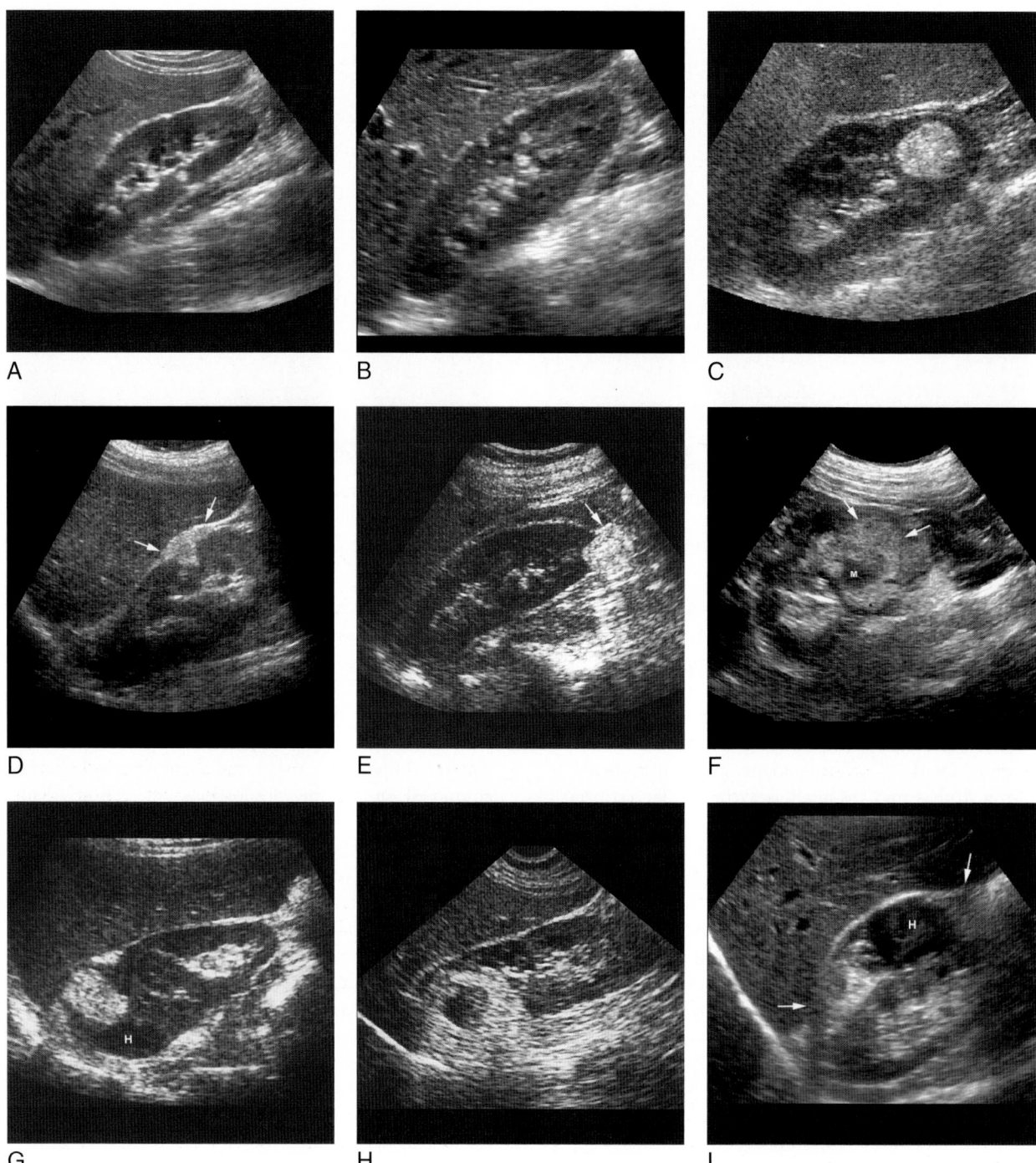

FIGURE 9-51. Spectrum of appearances of angiomyolipoma (AML). A, A classic small hyperechoic intraparenchymal tumor. **B,** Multiple small echogenic foci in the anterior cortex of the mid-pole. **C,** A solitary, large, highly echogenic mass in the lower pole. **D,** An exophytic echogenic mass involves the cortex and the perirenal space (*arrows*). The flat appearance suggests a compliant soft tumor. **E,** A large exophytic lower pole echogenic mass (*arrow*). The echogenicity of the mass may be very similar to the perirenal fat. **F,** A large complex intrarenal mass (*arrows*) is mildly echogenic and has a hypoechoic component representing myomatous elements (M). **G, H,** and **I** are hemorrhagic AML. **G,** An exophytic ruptured upper pole AML with a perirenal hematoma (H). **H,** An echogenic mass with a central hypoechoic hemorrhage. **I,** A large predominantly exophytic AML. The kidney appears quite normal. The mass (*arrows*) shows increased echogenicity from the fat in the AML and a large hypoechoic hemorrhage (H).

ulate AML up to 33% of the time (see Fig. 9-40).[128,129] Therefore, CT imaging is necessary to demonstrate the presence of fat, and helical CT is superior to conventional CT.[177] Yamashita et al.[130] demonstrated that intratumoral cystic spaces and a peripheral hypoechoic rim in an echogenic solid lesion suggest RCC rather than AML. Siegel et al.[178] have also shown that the multiple fat and nonfat interfaces in an AML, along with the large acoustic impedance differences at these interfaces, cause scattering and attenuation of the sound waves, giving rise to an echogenic lesion with detectable shadowing (Fig. 9-52). Shadowing was seen in 33% of their AMLs and in none of their RCCs. Involvement of regional lymph nodes and extension of tumor into the inferior vena cava have been described.[179] If an AML is large and exophytic, it might be difficult to differentiate from a large retroperitoneal liposarcoma. Some helpful features that may allow differentiation include defect in the renal parenchyma where the tumor originates and presence of enlarged vessels and other associated AMLs.[180] The blood vessels in an AML lack normal elastic tissue and are prone to aneurysm formation and hemorrhage.[181] Color flow Doppler appears to be the best imaging modality to detect an intratumoral pseudoaneurysm in a hemorrhagic AML.[182]

Small, asymptomatic AMLs may be followed for growth. If they are large, symptomatic, or have hemorrhaged, surgery is often performed. If possible, renal-sparing surgery is preferable, particularly because these tumors are benign or may be multiple. Embolization may also be used to treat actively bleeding AMLs.[183]

Lymphoma

Kidney. The kidney does not contain lymphoid tissue, and lymphomatous involvement of the kidney occurs

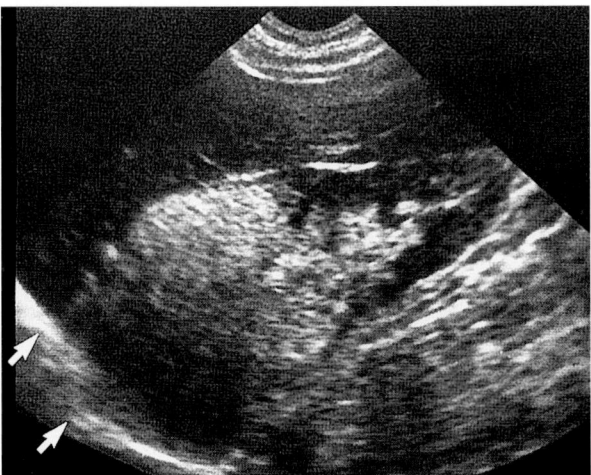

FIGURE 9-52. Exophytic angiomyolipoma. Sagittal sonogram shows a large exophytic tumor with shadowing. Diaphragmatic interruption (*arrows*) indicates fatty nature of the mass.

SONOGRAPHIC APPEARANCE OF RENAL LYMPHOMA

Focal parenchymal involvement
Diffuse infiltration
Invasion from a retroperitoneal mass
Perirenal involvement

---

from either hematogenous dissemination or contiguous extension of retroperitoneal disease. Renal disease is more commonly **non-Hodgkin's lymphoma** than **Hodgkin's lymphoma**. By the time renal disease is evident, there is usually apparent disseminated disease. Urinary tract symptoms are uncommon. Occasionally flank pain, flank mass, or hematuria may occur. At autopsy, renal involvement will be found in one third of lymphoma patients[184] and bilateral renal disease is more common than unilateral disease. Isolated renal disease may be seen in patients undergoing treatment.

The **sonographic appearance** of **renal lymphoma** is variable depending on the pattern of involvement. Four patterns are recognized and include focal parenchymal involvement, diffuse infiltration, invasion from a retroperitoneal mass, and perirenal involvement.

Focal parenchymal involvement may manifest as solitary or multiple nodules. These masses appear homogeneous and hypoechoic or anechoic (Fig. 9-53). They may simulate cysts; however, appropriate through transmission for the size of the lesion is not apparent.[185,186] **Diffuse infiltration** is seen as complete disruption of the normal renal architecture with maintenance of the reniform shape. The kidney may be enlarged (Fig. 9-54). The tumor may invade the renal sinus and destroy the echogenic central echo complex.[187] **Direct invasion** of the kidney by large retroperitoneal lymph node masses may occur with associated vascular and ureteral encasement. Large retroperitoneal hypoechoic lymph node masses will be seen extending into the kidney, causing hydronephrosis. Rarely, **perirenal involvement** is noted as a surrounding hypoechoic perirenal mass/rind which may be confused with hematoma or extramedullary hematopoiesis (Fig. 9-55).[188,189]

Ureter. Lymphomatous involvement of the ureter occurs with either displacement or encasement. Displacement is more common with encasement, representing 1% to 16%. Of these cases, actual invasion of the ureter wall occurs in only one third.[160] The result is usually dilation of the intrarenal collecting system and ureter to the level of the retroperitoneal mass. This is usually easily appreciated on sonography.

Bladder. Primary bladder lymphoma arises from lymph follicles in the submucosa and usually does not infiltrate the other layers of the bladder wall.[190] Most patients are between 40 to 60 years of age, with women

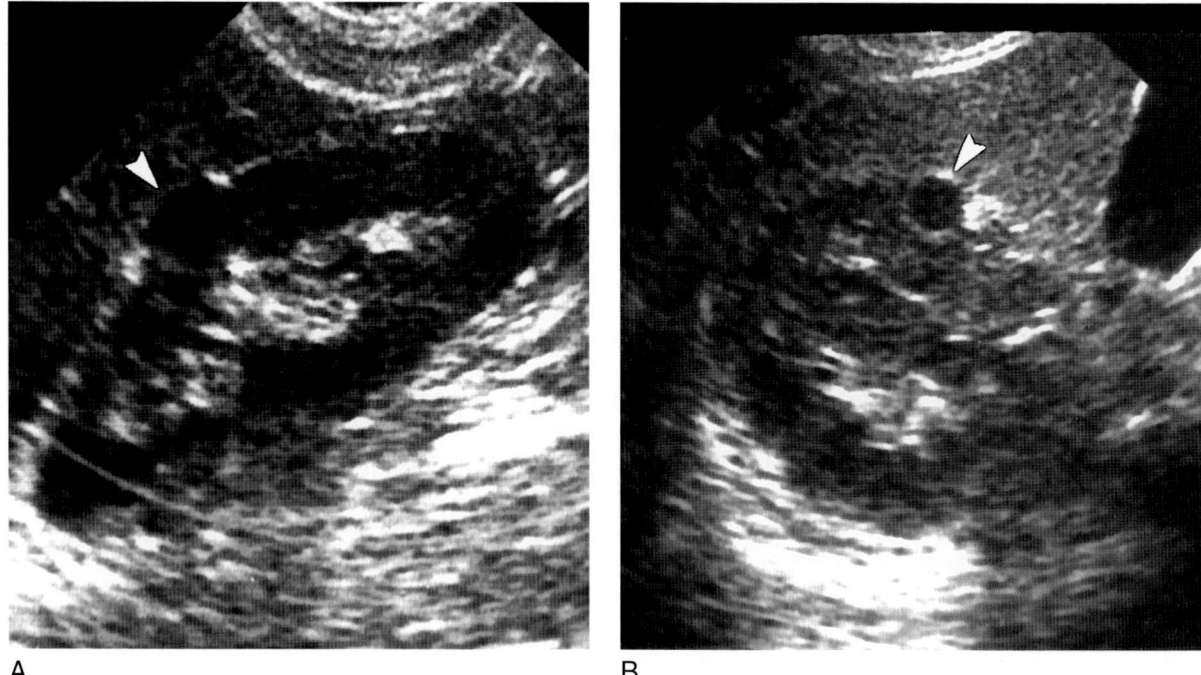

A   B

FIGURE 9-53. Renal lymphoma. A, Sagittal and **B,** transverse sonograms demonstrate a small hypoechoic renal mass (*arrowhead*) simulating a cyst. Through transmission is not seen, indicating a solid lesion.

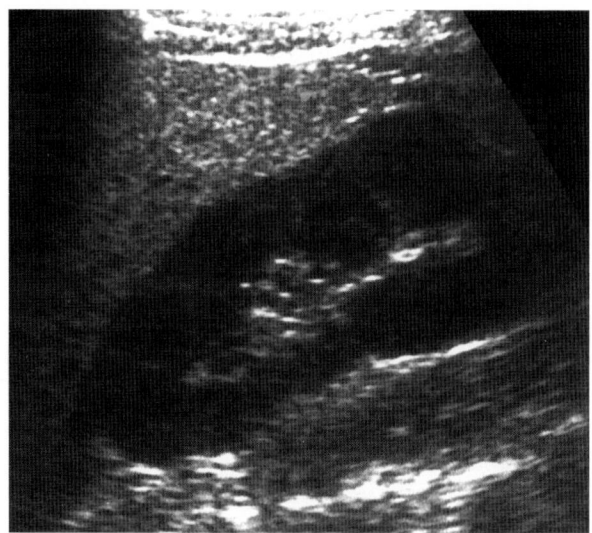

FIGURE 9-54. Renal lymphoma. Diffuse infiltration and parenchymal destruction are seen. The kidney is diffusely hypoechoic; however, reniform shape is maintained.

being more commonly affected. On **sonography,** a bladder wall mass is seen, usually covered by intact epithelium. If the mass is large, ulceration may occur (Fig. 9-56).

Leukemia

Leukemic involvement of the kidney may be diffuse or focal. In those with leukemia, renal infiltrates will be found in 65% at autopsy.[191] Although seen with great

frequency at autopsy, the sonographic changes may be hard to appreciate. On **sonography,** bilateral diffuse renal enlargement may occur; however, 15% of patients demonstrating enlargement will have no evidence of leukemic infiltrate.[192] The renal parenchyma may demonstrate a coarsened echopattern with distortion of the central sinus echo complex.[193] Alternatively, diffuse decreased echogenicity of the renal parenchyma may be seen. Focal masses may occur that may be single or multiple.[194] These patients are prone to renal, subcapsular, or perinephric hemorrhage.

Metastases

Kidney. Metastatic disease to the kidneys is common with metastases to the lung, liver, bone, and adrenal glands only surpassing the kidney in frequency.[195] Spread to the kidneys is via a hematogenous route. The most common primary tumors giving rise to renal metastases are (1) **lung carcinoma;** (2) **breast carcinoma;** and (3) **renal cell carcinoma** of the contralateral kidney.[104] Other tumors that may produce renal metastases include **colon, stomach, cervix, ovary, pancreas,** and **prostate.**[104] Most remain clinically silent, although some patients may develop hematuria or flank pain. Morphologically, the **pattern of renal metastases** may be (1) a solitary mass; (2) multiple masses; or (3) diffusely infiltrative masses enlarging the kidney with maintenance of reniform shape. Choyke et al.[196] evaluated 27 patients with renal metastases and found that metastases are usually multifocal; however, solitary large tumors may

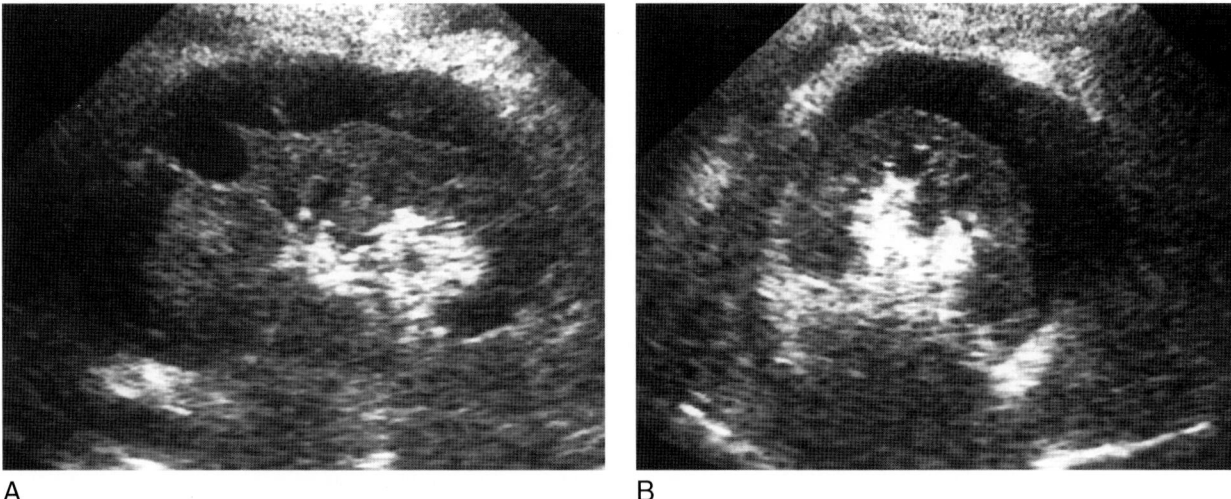

A   B

FIGURE 9-55. Perirenal lymphoma. A, Sagittal and **B**, transverse sonograms demonstrate a rind of hypoechoic tissue surrounding and indenting the renal margin.

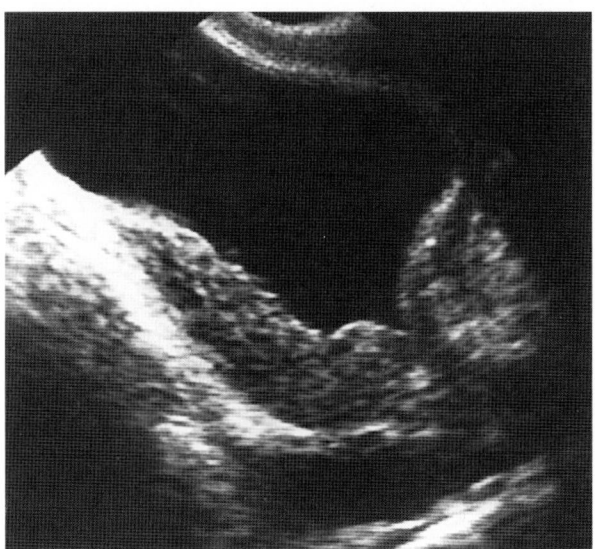

FIGURE 9-56. Bladder lymphoma. Sagittal transverse sonogram shows extensive bladder wall thickening with intact overlying mucosa.

occur that are otherwise indistinguishable from primary renal cell carcinoma. They also found that a new renal lesion in a patient with advanced cancer is more likely a metastatic tumor than a primary one. If a single renal lesion is discovered synchronously in a patient with a known primary tumor or a tumor in remission with no evidence of other metastases, renal biopsy is necessary to differentiate a primary renal cell carcinoma from a renal metastasis.

Contrast-enhanced CT is the best radiographic technique for detecting renal metastasis, although ultrasound is almost as sensitive.[196] On **sonography**, the appearance will depend on the pattern of involvement. A **solitary metastasis** will be seen as a solid mass indistinguishable from RCC (Fig. 9-57). This occurs often with colon carcinoma.[196] Central necrosis, hemorrhage, and calcification may be evident. **Multiple metastases** are usually small, poorly marginated hypoechoic masses. Involvement of the perinephric space is possible, particularly with malignant melanoma and lung cancer.[196] **Diffuse tumor infiltration** will be seen as renal enlargement with distorted architecture and loss of the normal corticomedullary differentiation (see Fig. 9-57). **Ureter.** Ureteric metastases are rare and evidence of diffuse metastases elsewhere will be seen in 90% of cases.[197] Metastatic disease to the ureter occurs either by hematogenous or lymphatic dissemination. Tumors that may secondarily involve the ureter include **melanoma, bladder, colon, breast, stomach, lung, prostate, kidney,** and **cervix**. Three types of ureteral involvement occur and these are (1) infiltration of the periureteral soft tissues; (2) transmural involvement of the ureteral wall; and (3) submucosal nodules. The first two types demonstrate stricture formation with or without an associated mass, whereas the third type demonstrates an intraluminal mass(es).[160] On **sonography**, the site of tumor involvement may be seen if a mass is present. Usually, the secondary sign of hydronephroureterosis is present.

Bladder. Metastases to the bladder may occur with **malignant melanoma, lung, gastric,** or **breast cancer**. This is a rare occurrence, however. **Sonographically**, a solid mass may be seen in the bladder wall (Fig. 9-58). Often, metastatic malignant melanoma will be recognized cystoscopically by its deep brown color.

Urachal Adenocarcinoma

The urachus measures 3 to 10 cm in length and represents the obliterated remnant of the allantois. It is lined by transitional epithelium and neoplasms of the

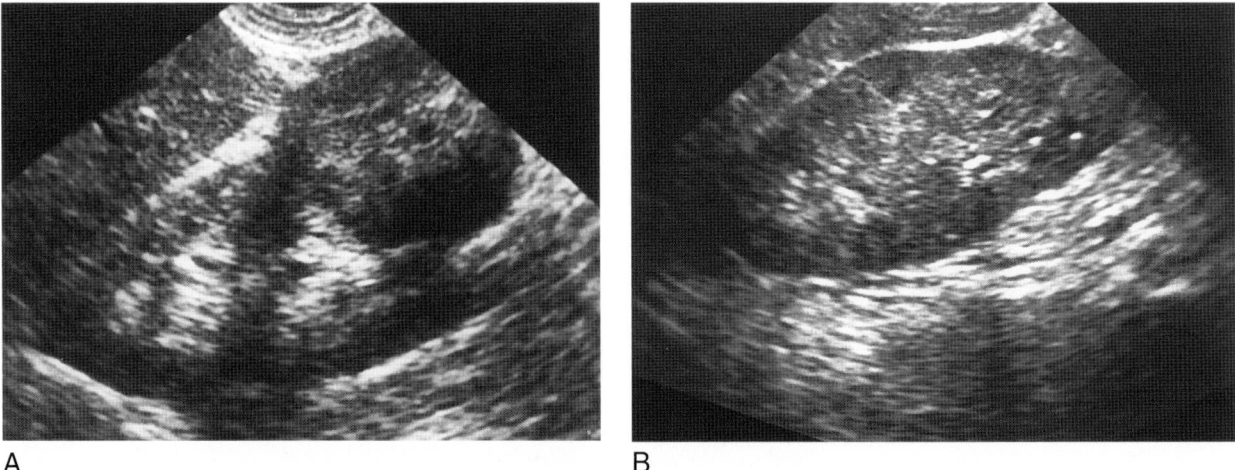

FIGURE 9-57. Renal metastases shown on sagittal sonograms in two patients. A, Solitary renal metastasis. This cannot be differentiated from renal cell carcinoma. **B,** Diffuse parenchymal tumor infiltration. Reniform shape is maintained.

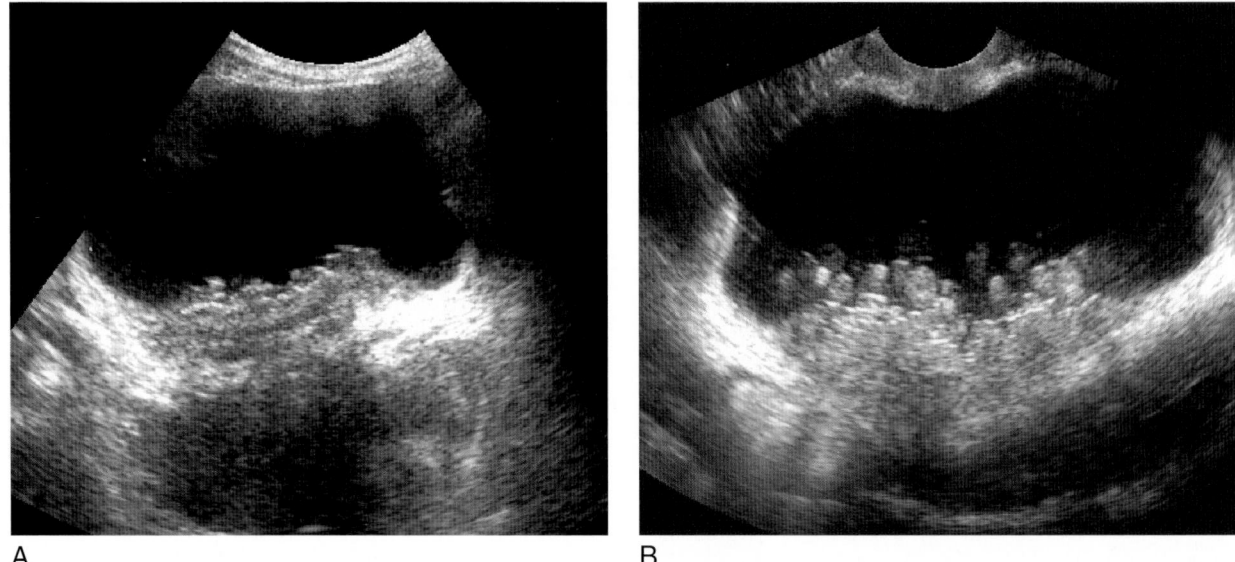

FIGURE 9-58. Bladder metastasis from gastric adenocarcinoma. A, Transverse suprapubic sonogram shows a papillary solid intraluminal mass with obvious bladder wall involvement. **B,** Confirmatory transvaginal scan shows the papillary nature of the tumor to better advantage.

urachus are rare. The urachal remnant is divided into supravesical, intramural, and intramucosal portions. Tumors usually arise in the upper part of the intramural portion or in the lower part of the extravesical portion of the bladder.[198] They represent 0.01% of all adult cancers, 0.17% to 0.34% of all bladder cancers, and 20% to 39% of all primary bladder adenocarcinomas.[199] Seventy-five percent of patients are men.[200] Most tumors arise at the bladder dome at the vesicourachal junction. The tumors have a poor prognosis and tend to invade the anterior abdominal wall. Most patients present with hematuria, although other common clinical presentations include frequency, dysuria, and mucosuria.[200] On **sonography**, a bladder dome mass is seen that is often calcified (50% to 70%). The mass may be solid, cystic, or complex in

nature. Tumor extension into the perivesical fat, space of Retzius, and the abdominal wall is common. Local recurrence following resection is common.

Rare Neoplasms

Kidney. Juxtaglomerular tumors are rare benign tumors that occur most frequently in women. They produce renin that causes hypertension. On **sonography**, they are usually small, solid, and hyperechoic.[201] Excision will alleviate the hypertension. **Leiomyomas** are benign tumors. They are usually discovered incidentally but may grow large enough to become clinically evident. On **sonography**, a solid, well-defined mass is seen. They may be peripheral, arising from the renal capsule. **Carcinoid tumor** is a rare renal tumor that tends to be solid, often showing peripheral or central calcification.[202] Other benign tumors have been described including **lipoma** and **hemangioma**.

Renal sarcomas represent approximately 1% of all malignant renal tumors. **Leiomyosarcoma** is the most common, accounting for 58% of all renal sarcomas. Patients have a poor prognosis. **Hemangiopericytoma** represents 20% of all renal sarcomas. On **sonography**, these tumors cannot be distinguished from renal cell carcinoma. **Liposarcoma** accounts for 20% of all renal sarcomas. Depending on the amount of mature fat present, these tumors can be quite hyperechoic and indistinguishable from an angiomyolipoma. Less common sarcomas include **rhabdomyosarcoma**, **fibrosarcoma**, and **osteogenic sarcoma**. **Wilms' tumor** may rarely occur in adults and cannot be differentiated radiologically from renal cell carcinoma.

Bladder. Mesenchymal bladder tumors are rare, accounting for 1% of all bladder tumors. **Leiomyoma** is the most common benign bladder tumor. Most leiomyomas arise from the submucosa near the bladder trigone.[203] These tumors may show intravesical (63%), intramural (7%), or extravesical (30%) growth.[203] On **sonography**, a well-defined round or oval solid mass will be seen. Cystic degeneration may occur. **Neurofibromas** of the bladder may be seen as an isolated finding or occur with diffuse systemic disease. Sonographically, these tumors are similar to leiomyomas. **Cavernous hemangiomas** are most commonly found in the dome and posterolateral bladder wall.[204] Cystoscopically, they are bluish-red in color. On **sonography**, two types have been described: (1) a round, well-defined, solid, hyperechoic, intraluminal mass that is highly vascular on color Doppler ultrasound; and (2) diffuse wall thickening with multiple hypoechoic spaces and calcification.[204] **Bladder pheochromocytomas** are rare and represent only 1% of all pheochromocytomas.[203] Patients may have symptoms including headache, sweating, and tachycardia related to bladder distention or voiding. These tumors arise in the submucosa and may be found anywhere in the bladder, although they are commonly found at the dome. **Sonographically**, a well-defined, solid, intramural bladder wall mass will be seen (Fig. 9-59). Malignant mesenchymal bladder tumors are rare. The most common ones include **leiomyosarcoma** and **rhabdomyosarcoma**. On **sonography**, a large, infiltrative mass is seen.

RENAL CYSTIC DISEASE

Cortical Cysts

Simple. **Simple renal cysts** are benign and fluid filled. Their exact pathogenesis is unknown, although they are believed to be acquired lesions. Their incidence increases with advancing age and they are found in at least 50%

APPROACH TO A SONOGRAPHICALLY DISCOVERED COMPLEX RENAL CYST

Internal Echoes

Follow-up with ultrasound if no other features of malignancy are present.
Perform computed tomography if associated features of malignancy are present (perceptible thickened wall, multiple or thick septations, or extensive septal calcification).

Septations

Follow-up with ultrasound if few and thin (≤1 mm).
Perform computed tomography if there is septal irregularity and nodularity, multiple complex septations, or solid elements at septal wall attachment.

Calcification

Follow-up with ultrasound if small amount of calcium or milk of calcium without associated soft tissue mass.
Perform computed tomography if thick, irregular, or amorphous calcification.
Perform computed tomography if calcification obscures adequate sonographic visualization.

Perceptible Defined Wall or Mural Nodularity

Presumed malignant, perform computed tomography.
Use a combination of ultrasound and computed tomography to analyze the internal features of a complex renal cyst to determine if more likely benign or malignant. Benign-type lesions can be followed with serial imaging, whereas malignant-type lesions will require surgical removal.

---

of people over the age of 50. Most are asymptomatic; however, if large, then flank pain and hematuria may occur. The **sonographic criteria** used to diagnose a simple cyst include

- anechoic
- acoustic enhancement
- sharply defined, imperceptible, smooth far wall
- round or ovoid shape

If all these sonographic criteria are met, further evaluation or follow-up of the cyst is not required (Fig. 9-60). If the renal cyst is large and symptomatic, cyst puncture and sclerosis may be performed. Several simple cysts may be found in both kidneys and, rarely, several simple cysts may involve only one kidney or a localized portion of one kidney (Fig. 9-61).

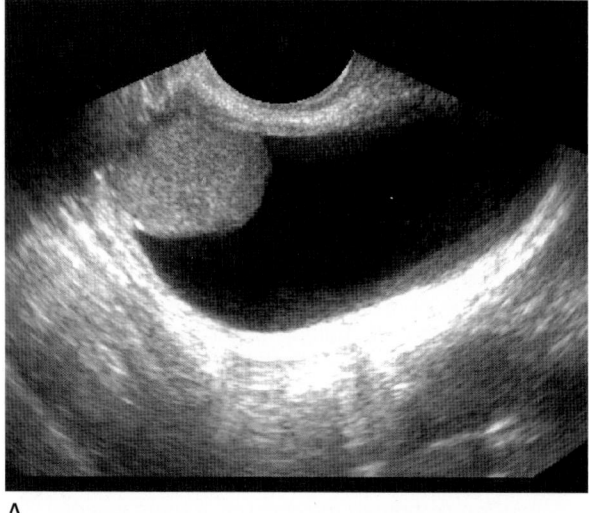

A

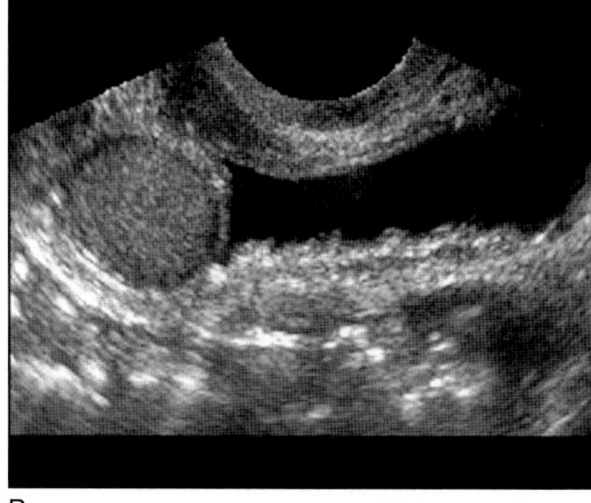

B

C

FIGURE 9-59. Bladder pheochromocytoma. A, Suprapubic image of the bladder shows a smooth surface to a solid bladder mass. **B,** Transvaginal scan with partial bladder emptying shows the mucosa is intact over the submucosal nodule. **C,** Color Doppler image confirms lesional vascularity. (From Damani N, Wilson S: Nongynecologic applications of transvaginal US. RadioGraphics 1999;19:S179-S200. Reproduced with permission.)

Complex. Complex renal cysts are those that do not meet the strict criteria of a simple renal cyst. These include cysts containing **internal echoes**, **septations**, **calcification**, **perceptible defined wall**, and **mural nodularity**. Depending on the degree of abnormality, most of these cysts require further imaging with CT. A combination of ultrasound and CT will help to determine whether or not a complex cystic lesion is more likely benign or malignant.

Internal echoes within a cyst are usually the result of hemorrhage or infection. Approximately 6% of cysts are complicated by hemorrhage.[205] Infection of a cyst may occur by hematogenous seeding, by vesicoureteric reflux, or iatrogenically following cyst puncture or surgical manipulation. **Sonographically,** infected cysts usually also demonstrate a thickened wall with a debris-fluid or gas-fluid level. Hemorrhagic cysts may be followed with serial ultrasound if other imaging features of malignancy are absent (Fig. 9-62). Infected cysts will require aspiration and drainage for diagnosis and treatment.

Septations may be seen within a renal cyst and they often occur following hemorrhage, infection, and percutaneous aspiration. Occasionally, two adjacent cysts sharing a wall may appear as a large septated cyst. If septa are thin (≤1 mm), smooth, and attach to the cyst wall without thickened elements, a benign cyst can be diagnosed (see Fig. 9-62).[206] If septal irregularity, thickness greater than 1 mm, or solid elements at the wall attachment are present, the lesion must be presumed malignant. Cyst aspiration is not indicated in these multiseptated cystic lesions.[206] Ultrasound is often better than CT in defining the internal characteristics of a cystic lesion.

Calcification of renal cysts may be fine and linear or amorphous and thick. If all other ultrasound and CT criteria for a cyst are met, the presence of a small amount of calcium or thin, fine areas of calcification in the wall or on a septum, without associated soft tissue mass or enhancement, likely represents a complicated cyst rather than malignancy (see Fig. 9-62).[207] Thick, irregular,

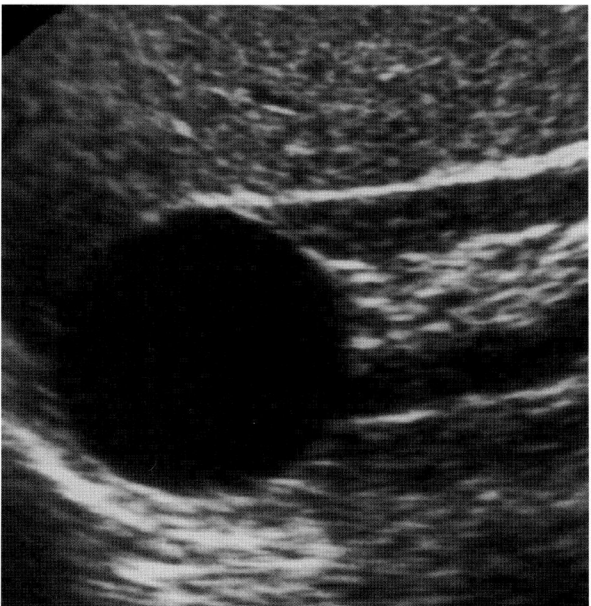

FIGURE 9-60. Renal cyst. A simple renal cyst shows a smooth wall, an echo-free center, and posterior acoustic enhancement.

amorphous calcification is more worrisome, however, and likely requires surgical removal to determine if the lesion is benign or malignant, especially if associated with enhancing solid components.[207] Calcium may also be present as milk of calcium with layering present (see Fig. 9-62). These cysts are always benign. Bright, echogenic foci with ringdown are seen frequently on septa and cyst walls (see Fig. 9-62). These foci are of no consequence and do not correspond with calcification on CT. **Perceptible, defined, thickened wall**, or **mural nodularity** essentially excludes a diagnosis of benign cyst (see Fig. 9-62). These lesions will all require surgical removal to exclude malignancy.

Parapelvic Cysts

Parapelvic cysts do not communicate with the collecting system and likely are lymphatic in origin or develop from embryologic rests.[208] Most are asymptomatic, although they may cause hematuria, hypertension, hydronephrosis, become infected or bleed.[209] On **sonography**, parapelvic cysts appear as well-defined anechoic renal sinus masses (Fig. 9-63). If they have hemorrhaged, internal echoes will be seen in the cysts (Fig. 9-63). It may be difficult to differentiate multiple parapelvic cysts from hydronephrosis (Fig. 9-63). When hydronephrosis is present, the anechoic fluid-filled calices and renal pelvis can be seen to communicate; whereas multiple parapelvic cysts often have haphazard orientation and are seen as noncommunicating renal sinus cystic masses. If differentiation between the two is not possible with sonography, either IVP or contrast-enhanced CT will easily resolve the dilemma (Fig. 9-64).

Medullary Cysts

Medullary Sponge Kidney. Medullary sponge kidney (MSK) is defined as dilated, ectatic collecting tubules. It may be focal or diffuse. The etiology is unknown. The incidence in the general population is not known, but it is found in up to 12% of patients with renal stones.[210] It usually occurs in the third to fourth decade of life.[190] There is an association with **hemihypertrophy, Ehlers-Danlos syndrome, congenital hypertrophic pyloric stenosis, hyperparathyroidism, Caroli's disease**, and **autosomal recessive polycystic disease**.[190] Uncomplicated MSK is usually not associated with symptoms; however, with stone formation, renal colic, hematuria, dysuria, and flank pain may occur.[211] On sonography, tubular ectasia may be difficult to recognize. When

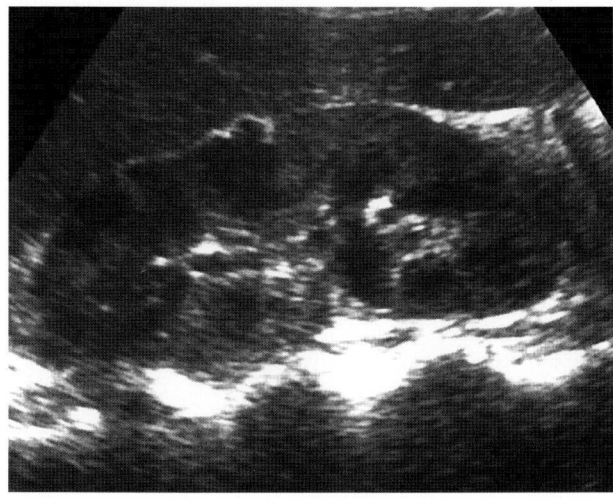

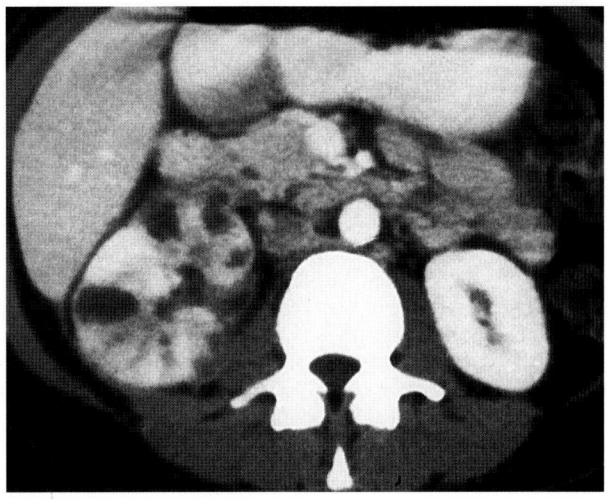

A B

FIGURE 9-61. Localized cystic disease. A, Sagittal sonogram shows multiple renal cysts in the right kidney. **B,** Confirmatory computed tomography shows multiple right renal cysts and a normal left kidney.

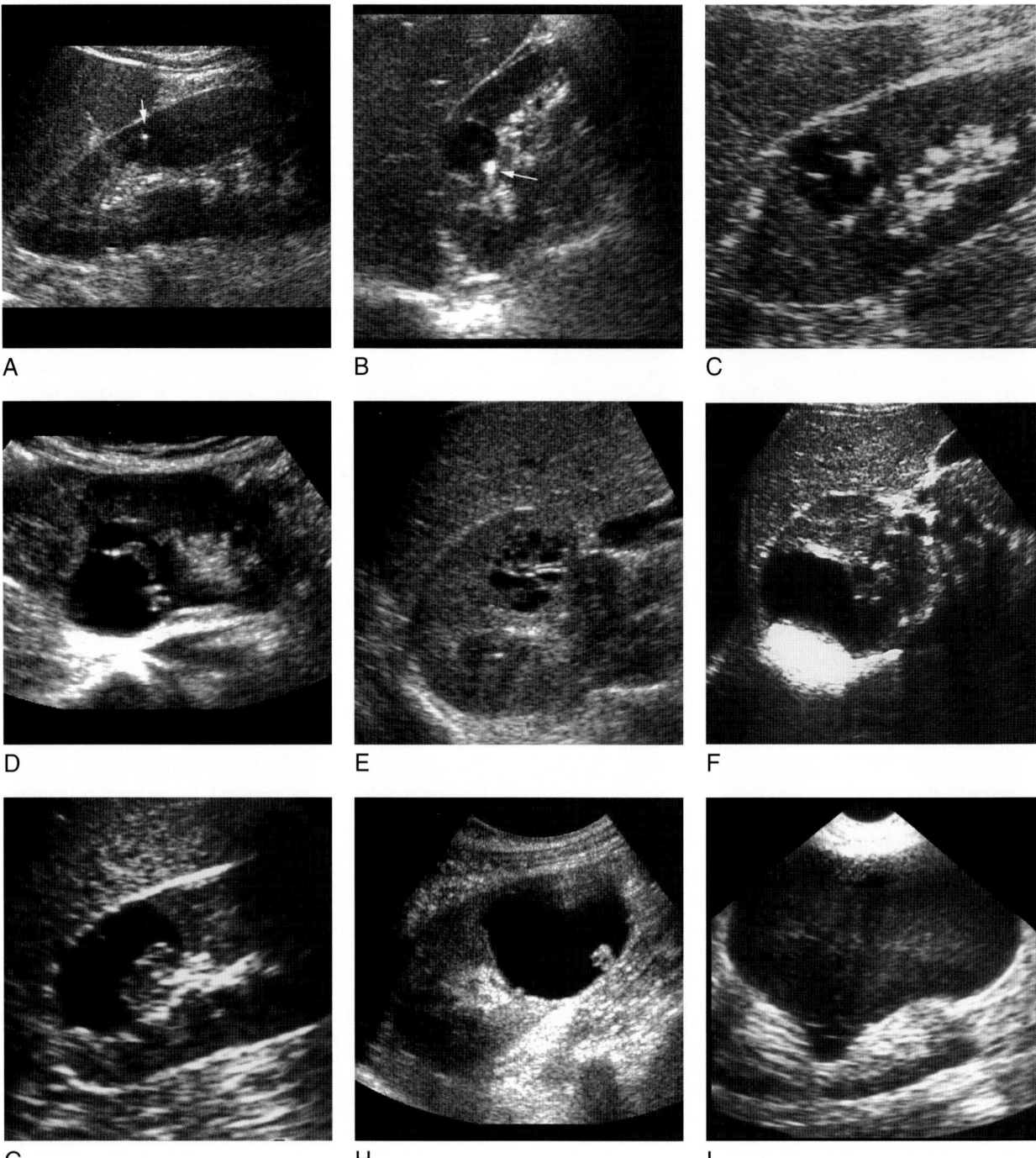

FIGURE 9-62. Complex renal cysts. **A,** Tiny renal cyst (*arrow*) in the anterior cortex is not resolved. A bright echogenic focus with ringdown artifact is the only visible abnormality. **B,** Discernible cyst shows a bright echogenic focus (*arrow*) with ringdown artifact. This echogenicity does not represent calcification. **C,** Complex benign cyst with a few thin septations. Ringdown artifact originates from the septations and the cyst wall. **D,** Complex cyst shows thick nodular septations. **E,** Cyst shows numerous internal thick and thin septations. **F,** Renal cyst with milk of calcium shown as dependent echogenic material that was mobile on real-time examination. **G** and **H,** Cyst with mural nodules. **I,** Large hemorrhagic cyst shows extensive internal debris within an otherwise simple-looking cyst.

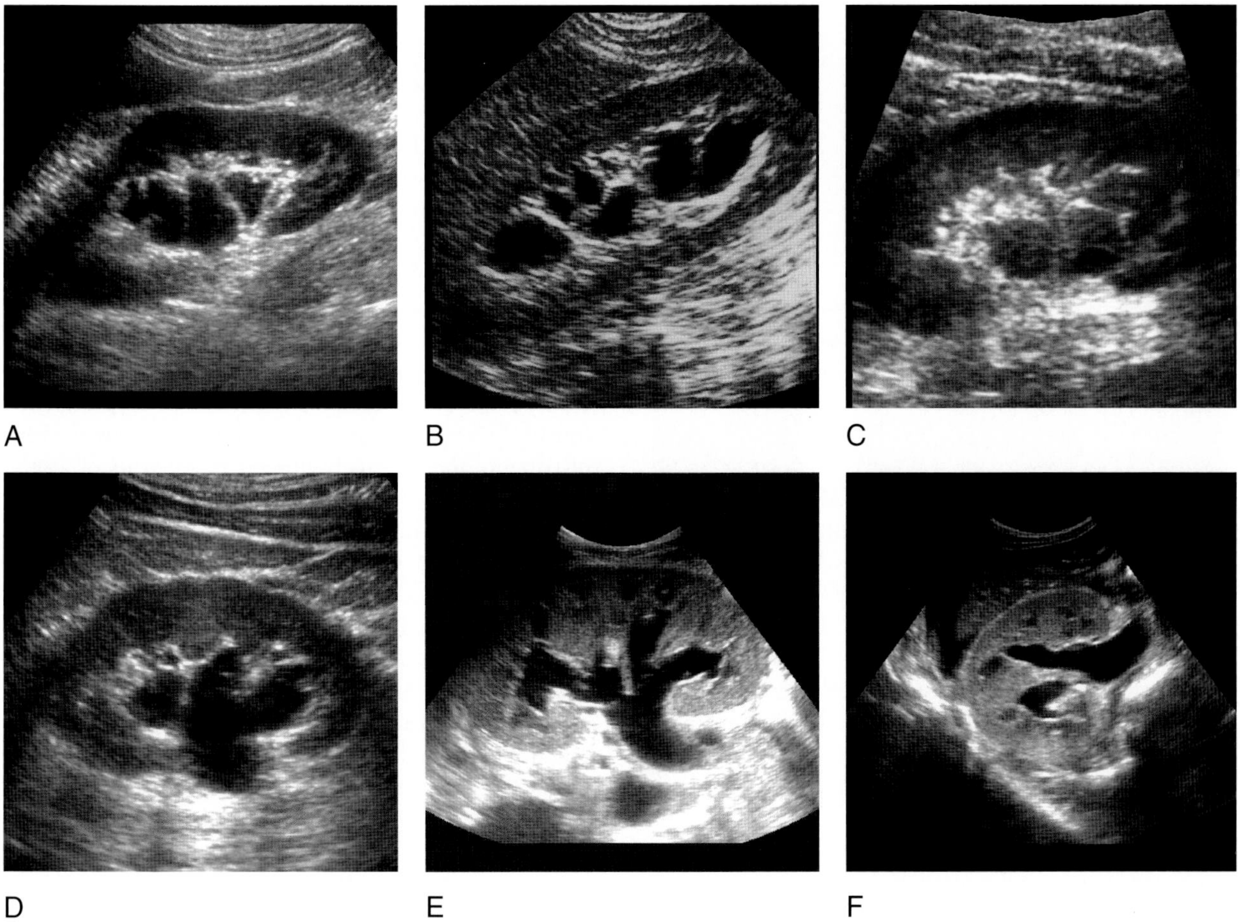

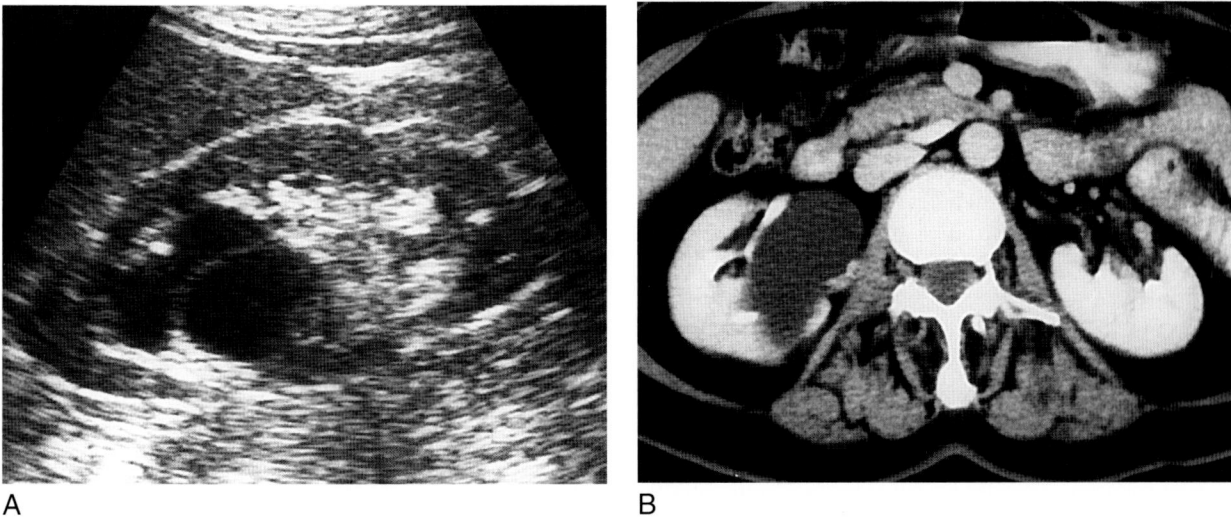

FIGURE 9-63. Central renal cysts—parapelvic cysts and hydronephrosis. A and **B** show multiple renal cystic masses with a haphazard arrangement indicative of parapelvic cysts. **C,** Same patient as in **B** at a different time showing low-level echoes within the parapelvic cysts related to hemorrhage. **D,** Parapelvic cysts simulating hydronephrosis. This, in fact, is rare on sonography. **E** and **F** are sagittal and transverse sonograms showing true hydronephrosis with communication of the central cystic components.

FIGURE 9-64. Parapelvic cysts. A, Sagittal sonogram shows hypoechoic masses in the renal sinus simulating a duplex collecting system with upper-moiety hydronephrosis. **B,** Confirmatory computed tomography shows a large central parapelvic cyst.

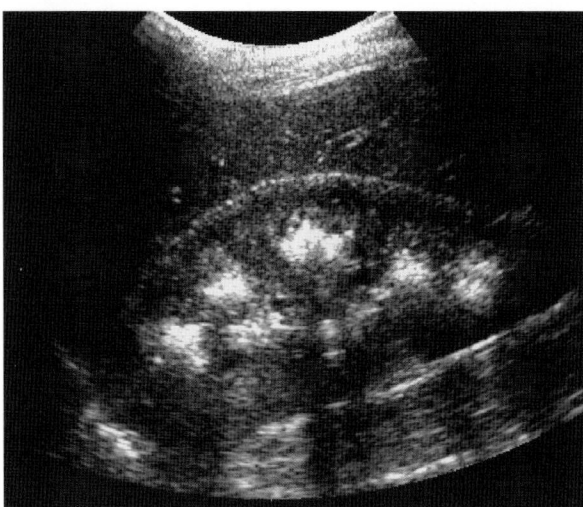

FIGURE 9-65. Medullary sponge kidney. Sagittal sonogram shows multiple echogenic foci representing calcifications localized to the medullary pyramids.

nephrocalcinosis is present, multiple echogenic shadowing foci are seen localized to the medullary pyramids (Fig. 9-65). If a focus of calcification has eroded into the collecting system, a stone will be seen that may or may not be obstructing.

Medullary Cystic Disease. This occurs as a result of progressive renal tubular atrophy. The kidneys are small or normal sized with tubulointerstitial fibrosis and cysts in the medulla or at the corticomedullary junction.[212] The pathogenesis is unknown. There is a childhood form inherited as an autosomal recessive disorder and an adult form inherited as an autosomal dominant disorder. On **sonography**, small echogenic kidneys with medullary cysts (0.1 to 1.0 cm) are seen.

Polycystic Kidney Disease

Autosomal Recessive Polycystic Kidney Disease (ARPKD). This disease is divided into four types, depending on the individual's age at onset of clinical manifestations and includes **perinatal**, **neonatal**, **infantile**, and **juvenile**. The disease is characterized pathologically by dilation of renal collecting tubules, hepatic cysts, and periportal fibrosis. Younger patients present predominantly with renal abnormality, whereas older patients have predominantly hepatic abnormality. ARPKD occurs in 1:6000 to 1:14,000 live births. Perinatal disease will demonstrate massive renal enlargement, hypoplastic lungs, and oligohydramnios. Death usually occurs as a result of renal failure and pulmonary hypoplasia. Older children will present with manifestations of portal hypertension. On sonography, massively enlarged, echogenic kidneys with lack of corticomedullary differentiation are seen. Occasionally, macroscopic cysts will be noted.

Autosomal Dominant Polycystic Kidney Disease (ADPKD). This is a disorder resulting in a large number of bilateral cortical and medullary renal cysts. The cysts may vary considerably in size and are often asymmetrical. ADPKD is the most common hereditary renal disorder with no gender predilection. It is found in 1:500 to 1:1000 individuals and accounts for 10% to 15% of patients on dialysis.[213] Up to 50% of patients will have no family history because the disease is characterized by variable expression and also occurs as a result of spontaneous mutation. Signs and symptoms of palpable mass(es), pain, hypertension, hematuria, and urinary tract infection usually do not develop until the fourth or fifth decade. Renal failure develops in 50% of patients and is usually present by 60 years of age.[213] Complications of ADPKD include infection, hemorrhage, stone formation, cyst rupture, and obstruction. Stone formation tends to occur in patients who have more cysts and a significantly larger predominant cyst size.[214] Associated anomalies occur including (1) **liver cysts** (30% to 60%); (2) **pancreatic cysts** (10%); (3) **splenic cysts** (5%); (4) **cysts in thyroid, ovary, endometrium, seminal vesicles, lung, brain, pituitary gland, breast,** and **epididymis**; (5) **cerebral berry aneurysms** (18% to 40%); (6) **abdominal aortic aneurysm**; (7) **cardiac lesions**; and (8) **colonic diverticula**. Patients with ADPKD who are not on dialysis do not have an increased incidence of renal cell carcinoma.[213]

On **sonography**, the kidneys are enlarged with multiple bilateral asymmetrical cysts of varying size (Fig. 9-66). Cysts complicated by hemorrhage or infection will demonstrate thick walls, internal echoes, and/or fluid-debris levels. Dystrophic calcification on cyst walls or stones may be seen as echogenic foci with distal sharp acoustic shadowing. Renal cysts in patients under the age of 30 are rare. Ravine et al.[215] modified the Bear[216] criteria and state that patients 30 years of age or younger with a family history of ADPKD require two renal cysts (unilateral or bilateral) to make the diagnosis of ADPKD disease. For patients 30 to 59 years of age, two cysts in both kidneys are required, and for those 60 years of age or older, four cysts in each kidney are needed. Ultrasound is the best imaging modality available for screening families of known affected individuals, as well as for routine follow-up of those patients with known disease.

Multicystic Dysplastic Kidney

Multicystic dysplastic kidney (MCDK) is a nonhereditary developmental anomaly also known as renal dysplasia, renal dysgenesis, and multicystic kidney. The kidney is small, malformed, and composed of multiple cysts with little, if any, normal renal parenchyma. It functions poorly if at all. The dysplastic change is usually unilateral and involves the entire kidney; however, it

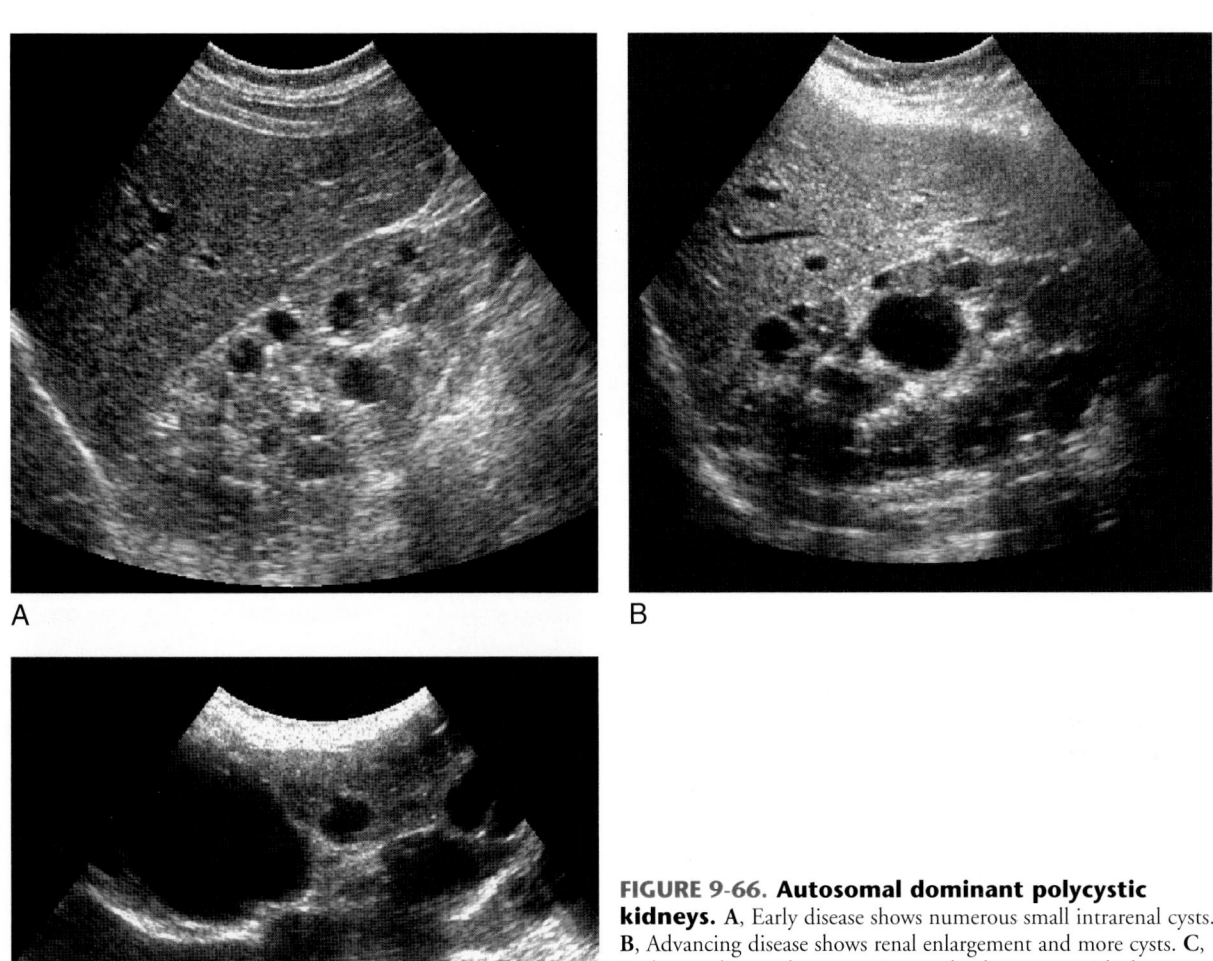

A

B

C

FIGURE 9-66. Autosomal dominant polycystic kidneys. **A**, Early disease shows numerous small intrarenal cysts. **B**, Advancing disease shows renal enlargement and more cysts. **C**, End stage disease shows massive renal enlargement with the parenchyma replaced completely by cysts.

rarely may be bilateral, segmental, or focal. If unilateral, the condition is asymptomatic; if bilateral, it is incompatible with life. Men and women are equally affected as are both sides. Up to 30% will have contralateral UPJ obstruction. The exact pathogenesis is obscure; however, 90% are associated with some form of urinary tract obstruction during embryogenesis. The severity of the malformation affects the spectrum of findings, which range from a large multicystic mass present at birth to a kidney with smaller cysts not discovered until adulthood.

On **sonography**, the findings include (1) multiple noncommunicating cysts; (2) absence of both normal parenchyma and normal renal sinus; and (3) focal echogenic areas representing primitive mesenchyma or

tiny cysts.[217] In adults, the cystic renal fossa mass is not large and cyst wall calcification is appreciated as echogenic foci with shadowing. Calcification may be so extensive that ultrasound visualization is impossible and CT is required to make the diagnosis. Segmental disease is usually seen in duplex kidneys and, if the cysts are very tiny, the mass may appear solid and echogenic.

Multilocular Cystic Nephroma

Multilocular cystic nephroma (MLCN) is an uncommon benign cystic neoplasm composed of multiple, noncommunicating cysts contained within a well-defined capsule. Occasionally, sarcomatous stroma is present, making this a more malignant lesion. MLCN

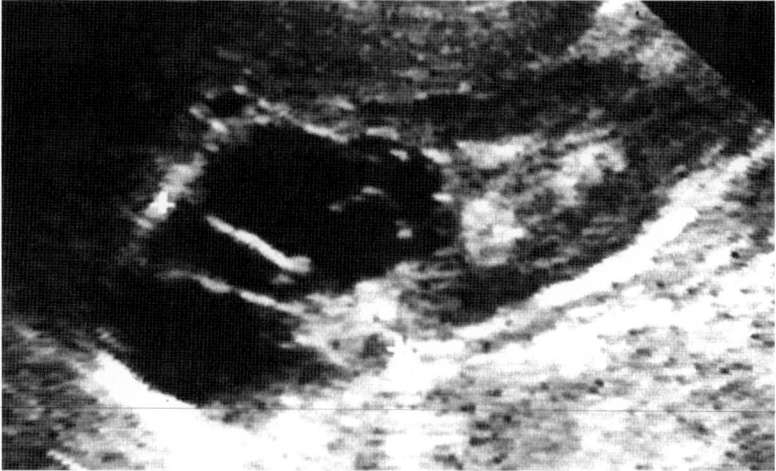

FIGURE 9-67. Multilocular cystic nephroma. Sagittal sonogram demonstrates a multiseptated, upper-pole renal mass with noncommunicating locules.

has no predilection for side and occasionally bilateral tumors are seen. These tumors are found in males less than 4 years of age and females between the ages of 4 and 20 or 40 and 60.[218] Most children present with an abdominal mass; whereas adults can be asymptomatic or present with abdominal pain, hematuria, hypertension, and urinary tract infection.

On **sonography**, the appearance of MLCN is quite variable depending on the number and size of the locules. If the locules are large, multiple, noncommunicating cysts will be seen within a well-defined mass (Fig. 9-67). If the locules are tiny, a more solid-appearing nonspecific echogenic mass will be present. Calcification of the capsule and septa is uncommon. With either appearance, it is impossible with imaging to differentiate it from cystic renal cell carcinoma.

Renal Cystic Disease Associated with Neoplasms

Acquired Cystic Kidney Disease (ACKD). This occurs in the native kidneys of patients with renal failure, who are undergoing either hemodialysis or peritoneal dialysis, with a frequency of 90% after 5 years of dialysis.[110,111,219] Renal cell carcinoma occurs in 4% to 10% of patients with ACKD.[219] The pathogenesis of ACKD is speculative. Epithelial hyperplasia caused by tubular obstruction that occurs as a result of toxic substances plays some role in the development of both cysts and tumors.[219] Pathologically multiple small cysts (0.5 to 3 cm) involving both renal cortex and medulla are found. Hemorrhage into cysts is common. Ultrasound, CT, and MRI are useful in the evaluation and follow-up of patients with ACKD and its complications.[110,111,220] Current data suggest that ACKD and tumor development persist even after successful renal transplantation. ACKD and tumors may develop in renal allografts during dialysis therapy.[221]

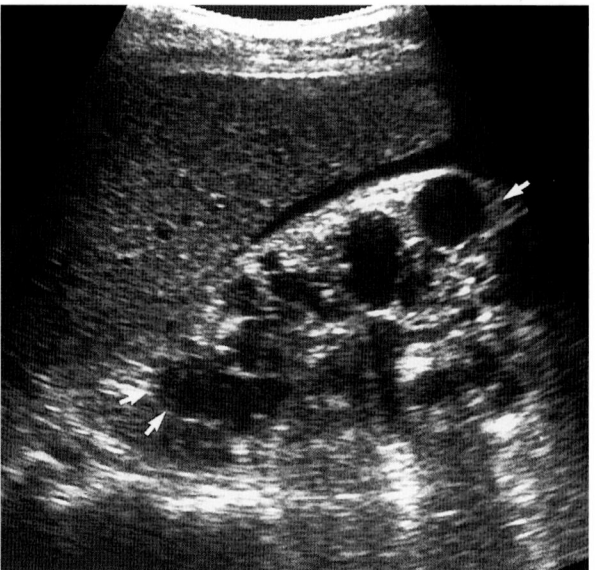

FIGURE 9-68. Acquired cystic kidney disease. Sagittal sonogram demonstrates an echogenic kidney (*arrows*) with parenchymal loss and multiple cysts. A small amount of intraperitoneal dialysate fluid is seen.

On **sonography**, three to five cysts in each kidney in a patient with chronic renal failure are diagnostic.[221] The cysts are usually small as are the kidneys, which usually are quite echogenic (Fig. 9-68). Internal echoes will be seen in cysts that have hemorrhaged. Tumors will be solid or cystic with mural nodules.

Von Hippel-Lindau Disease (VHL). This disease is transmitted as an autosomal dominant gene with variable expression and moderate penetrance. Its incidence is 1:35,000.[213] The predominant significant abnormalities include **retinal angiomatosis, CNS hemangioblastomas, pheochromocytomas,** and **renal cell carcinoma** (40%). Renal cell carcinoma in patients with VHL usually is multifocal (75% to 90%) and bilateral (75%). These patients are often offered

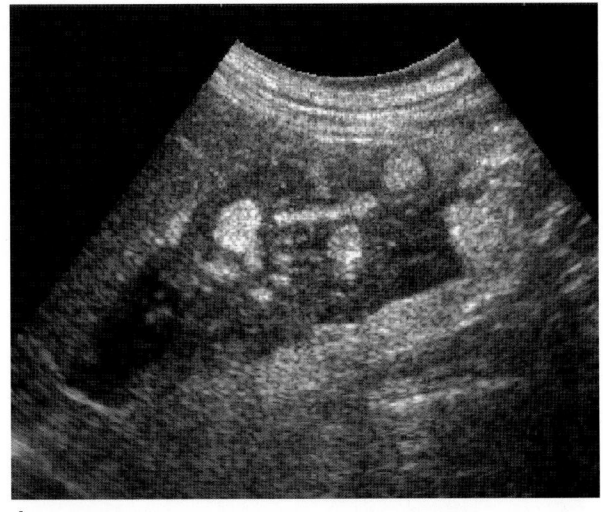

A

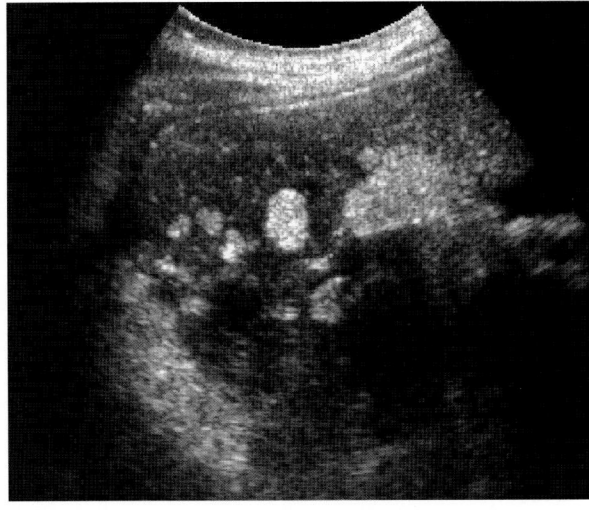

B

FIGURE 9-69. Tuberous sclerosis with multiple angiomyolipomas. A, Sagittal and **B**, transverse sonograms demonstrate multiple, well-defined echogenic tumors throughout the kidney. **C**, Confirmatory CT scan.

C

nephron-sparing surgery. In addition, **renal cysts**, which are the most common finding in this disease, are found in 76% of patients.[222] Cysts range in size from 0.5 to 3.0 cm and are mostly cortical in location. Sonography is good for screening these patients; however, CT is better for detection of the small multifocal bilateral tumors found in this disease.

Tuberous Sclerosis (TS). This is a genetically transmitted disease characterized by **mental retardation**, **seizures**, and **adenoma sebaceum**. Some cases are transmitted in an autosomal dominant fashion, although many cases result from spontaneous mutation. The incidence ranges from 1:9000 to 1:170,000.[223] Associated renal lesions include **cysts, angiomyolipomas (AML)**, and **renal cell carcinoma** (1% to 2%).[213] The renal cysts vary in size from microscopic to 3 cm. On **sonography**, if only cysts are present, it may be difficult to differentiate from ADPKD disease. If cysts and multiple AMLs are present and confirmed with CT,

tuberous sclerosis can be suggested (Fig. 9-69). Periodic CT screening is recommended to assess for AML growth and tumor development.

TRAUMA

Kidney

Traumatic injury to the kidney may be either blunt or penetrating. Most forms of blunt trauma to the kidney are relatively minor and heal without treatment. Penetrating injuries are usually the result of gunshot or stab wounds. Kidneys with cysts, tumors, and hydronephrosis are more prone to injury. **Renal injuries** are classified into four categories and include the following:

I—**Minor injury** (75% to 85%): contusions, subcapsular hematoma, small cortical infarct and lacerations that do not extend into the collecting system

II—**Major injury** (10%): renal lacerations that may extend into the collecting system and segmental renal infarct

III—**Catastrophic injury** (5%): vascular pedicle injury and shattered kidney

IV—**UPJ avulsion**[224]

Category I lesions are treated conservatively, whereas category III and IV lesions require urgent surgery. Category II lesions will be treated conservatively or surgically depending on severity.[224,225]

Computed tomography is regarded as the premier imaging modality for the evaluation of suspected renal trauma.[224] Because renal trauma is frequently accompanied by injuries to other organs, CT has the advantage of multiorgan imaging. Theoretically, sonography has the capability of evaluating traumatized kidneys; in reality, technical limitations usually hinder an adequate examination. Sonography does not provide information regarding renal function and is probably best used in the follow-up of patients with known renal parenchymal traumatic injury. **Renal hematomas** may be hypoechoic, hyperechoic, or heterogeneous. **Lacerations** will be seen as linear defects that may extend through the kidney if a fracture is present (Fig. 9-70). Associated **perirenal collections** consisting of blood and urine will be present if the kidney is fractured. **Subcapsular hematoma** may be seen as a perirenal fluid collection that flattens the underlying renal contour (Fig. 9-71). A **shattered kidney** will consist of multiple fragments of disorganized tissue with associated hemorrhage and urine collection in the renal bed. Color Doppler may be helpful in the assessment of **vascular pedicle injuries**.

Ureter

Traumatic injury of the ureter is most commonly iatrogenic related to gynecologic (70%) or urologic (30%) surgery.[226] Blunt and penetrating injuries are far less common. The treatment of these injuries is controversial. Many urologists suggest nephrostomy and ureteral stenting as an initial approach, if possible. Ureteral stents are left for 8 to 12 weeks to allow the ureter to heal.[227] Sonography is not useful in the assessment of these injuries, except to detect sizable fluid collections and/or hydronephrosis.

Bladder

Bladder injury may be the result of blunt, penetrating, or iatrogenic trauma. Bladder injury may result in extra- or intraperitoneal rupture, or a combination of the two. Sonography is usually not helpful in the assessment of these injuries except to identify large fluid collections or free intraperitoneal fluid.

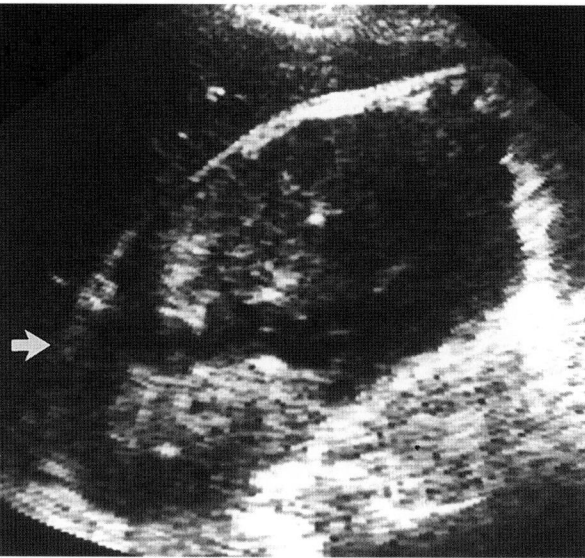

FIGURE 9-70. Fractured kidney. Sagittal sonogram demonstrates a linear hypoechoic tear through the renal sinus (*arrow*).

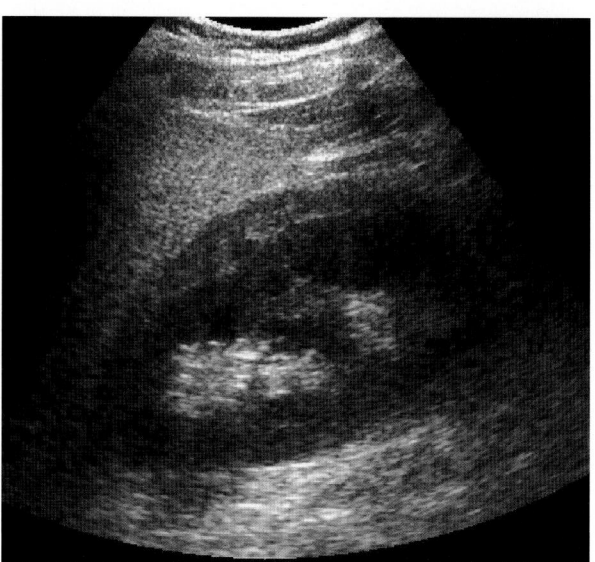

FIGURE 9-71. Acute subcapsular renal hematoma. Sagittal sonogram shows a large posttraumatic collection compressing the renal parenchyma. Acute hematomas may be echogenic or isoechoic relative to the parenchyma. Indentation of the renal cortex may be the only clue to their presence.

VASCULAR

Renal Vascular Doppler Sonography

The number and size of arteries supplying a kidney are quite variable. Duplex and color-imaging Doppler are able to demonstrate both normal and abnormal renal blood flow. Flow in the renal artery demonstrates a low resistance perfusion pattern on duplex Doppler indicative of continuous forward blood flow during diastole.

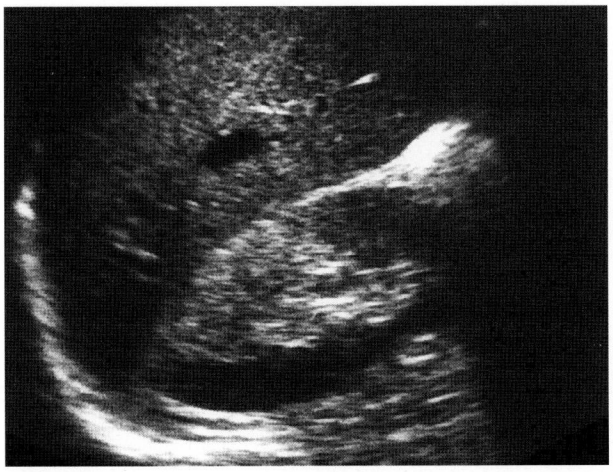
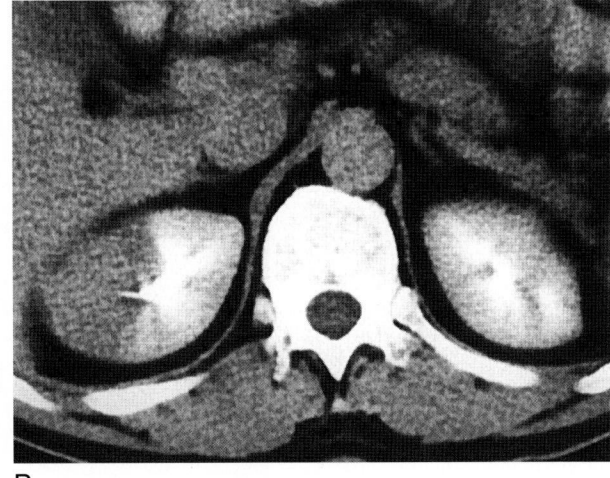

A   B

FIGURE 9-72. Renal infarct. A, Sagittal sonogram shows a wedge-shaped echogenic mass in the anterolateral renal cortex. **B,** Confirmatory computed tomography shows segmental infarction.

The measurement of resistance index (RI = peak systolic frequency – end diastolic frequency/peak systolic frequency) on duplex Doppler is used to assess arterial resistance. Keogan et al.[228] recommend averaging a number of RI measurements in a kidney before a single representative average is reported. The RI of native kidneys is normally 0.60 to 0.92.[229] Mostbeck et al.[230] reported that the RI, however, varies with heart rate and can range from 0.57 ± 0.06 (pulse 120/min) to 0.70 ± 0.06 (pulse 70/min). Variation in RI has been described in both native and transplant kidneys with the following: obstruction; medical renal disease; renal vein thrombosis; renal artery stenosis; and transplant rejection and dysfunction.

Color Doppler sonography is based on mean Doppler frequency shift, whereas power Doppler relies on the integrated Doppler power spectrum, which is related to the number of erythrocytes producing the Doppler shift. Power Doppler is subject to significant flash artifact; however, Bude et al.[231] demonstrated that in normal cooperative individuals, power Doppler is superior to conventional color Doppler in the demonstration of normal intrarenal vessels. Power Doppler also has the advantage of not being subject to aliasing and angle dependence; however, direction and velocity of motion are apparent only with color Doppler imaging.

Renal Arterial Occlusion and Infarction

Renal artery occlusion may occur with embolus or thrombosis. The degree of renal insult depends on the size and location of the occluded vessel. If the main renal artery is occluded, the entire kidney will be affected, whereas segmental and focal infarction may occur with peripherally located vascular occlusion. On gray-scale **sonography**, **acute** complete renal arterial occlusion may demonstrate a normal kidney. Duplex and color

Doppler sonography will not demonstrate flow to the kidney. Segmental or focal infarction may appear as a wedge-shaped mass indistinguishable from acute pyelonephritis (Fig. 9-72). With time, an echogenic mass[232] or scar may form. With **chronic** occlusion, an end-stage, small, scarred kidney will be seen.

Arteriovenous Fistula and Malformations

Abnormal arteriovenous communications may be acquired (75%) or congenital (25%). Acquired lesions are usually iatrogenic, although spontaneous abnormal arteriovenous communications may occur with eroding tumors. Most acquired lesions consist of a single, dominant feeding artery and a single, dominant draining vein. **Congenital malformations** consist of a tangle of small abnormal vessels. Gray-scale sonography may reveal no abnormality. The addition of duplex and color Doppler imaging has been helpful in defining these lesions.[233] Duplex Doppler demonstrates increased flow velocity, decreased resistivity (0.3 to 0.4), and turbulent diastolic flow in the arterial limb. Arterial pulsations in the draining vein are also observed. Spectral broadening is present. Color Doppler sonography may demonstrate a tangle of tortuous vessels with multiple colors indicative of the haphazard orientation and turbulent flow within the malformation (Fig. 9-73).

Renal Artery Stenosis

Hypertension may be primary (95% to 99%) or secondary (1% to 5%). The vast majority of patients with secondary hypertension suffer from renovascular disease. Renovascular disease is most commonly due to **atherosclerosis** (66%) with the majority of the remaining cases due to **fibromuscular dysplasia.**[234]

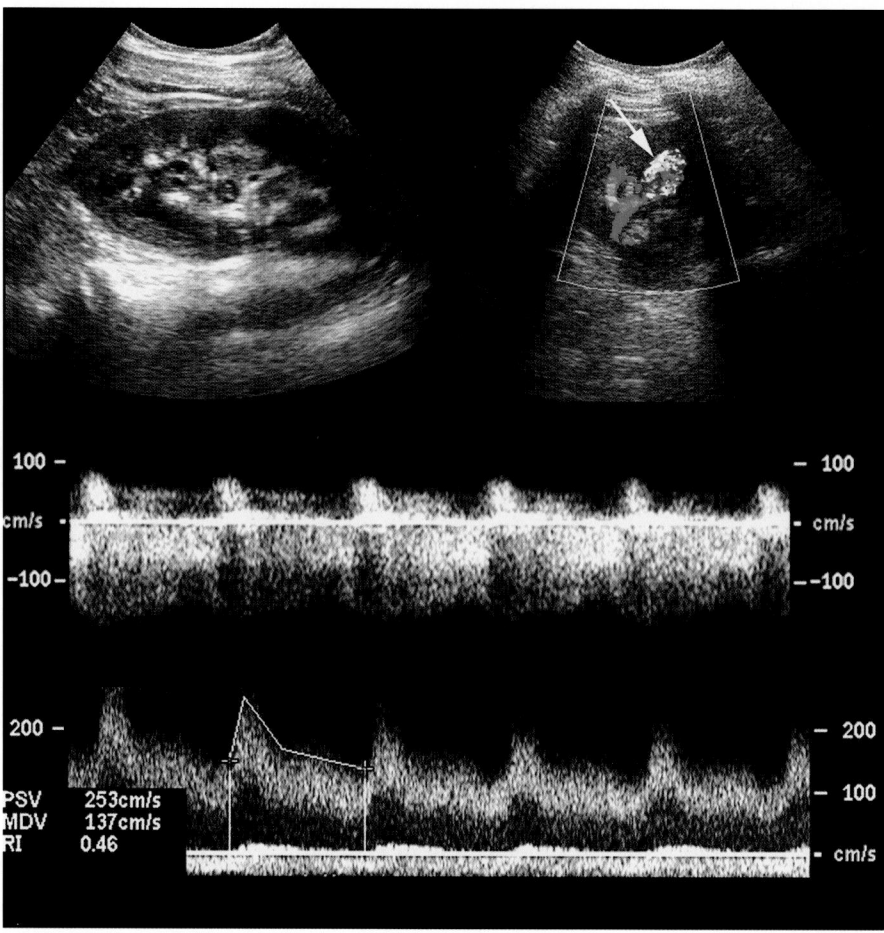

FIGURE 9-73. Renal arteriovenous malformation (AVM). Left image (*top line*) shows a normal sagittal image of the kidney. Right image (*top line*) shows a focus of color aliasing (*arrow*). The spectral waveform in the midline shows a high-velocity draining vein. The bottom spectral waveform shows an arterial signal from within the AVM showing a high-velocity low-impedance waveform consistent with arteriovenous shunting.

Many different imaging techniques have been used in an effort to detect patients with renovascular hypertension and include IV and intra-arterial digital subtraction angiography; captopril renal scintigraphy; duplex and color Doppler ultrasound; and magnetic resonance angiography.

There has been significant effort to use **duplex and color Doppler to diagnose renal artery stenosis** reliably. Despite this, use of this method remains controversial. The approach is twofold: (1) detection of abnormal Doppler signals at or just distal to the stenosis; or (2) detection of abnormal Doppler signals in the intrarenal vasculature. Evaluation of the main renal arteries in their entirety is usually impossible. It is estimated that the main renal arteries are not seen in up to 42% of patients.[235] Approximately 14% to 24% of patients will have accessory renal arteries that are usually not detected sonographically. Therefore, evaluation of the main renal arteries as a screening technique for renal artery stenosis fails. The second approach is to interrogate the intrarenal vasculature, which can be identified in virtually all patients. Normally, there is a steep upstroke in systole with a second small peak in early systole. A **tardus-parvus waveform** seen downstream from a stenosis refers to a slowed systolic acceleration with a low amplitude of the systolic peak (Fig. 9-74). To

evaluate the delayed upstroke, two measurements must be taken:

- **acceleration time**—time from start of systole to peak systole
- **acceleration index**—slope of the systolic upstroke

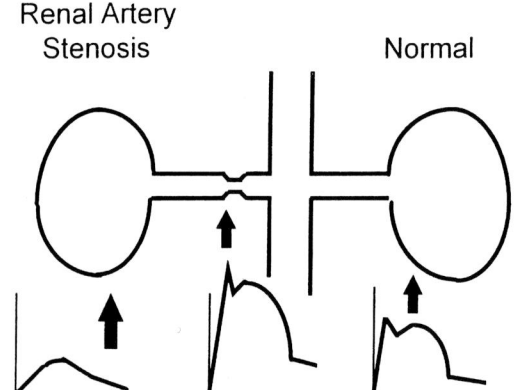

FIGURE 9-74. Schematic diagram of renal artery Doppler tracings. The tracing on the right side of the diagram is a normal renal artery. The tracing in the middle shows high-velocity flow measured at the stenosis. The tracing on the left side of the diagram shows the dampened tardus-parvus waveform downstream from the stenosis. (From Mitty HA, Shapiro RS, Parsons RB, et al: Renovascular hypertension. Radiol Clin North Am 1996;34(5):1017-1036.)

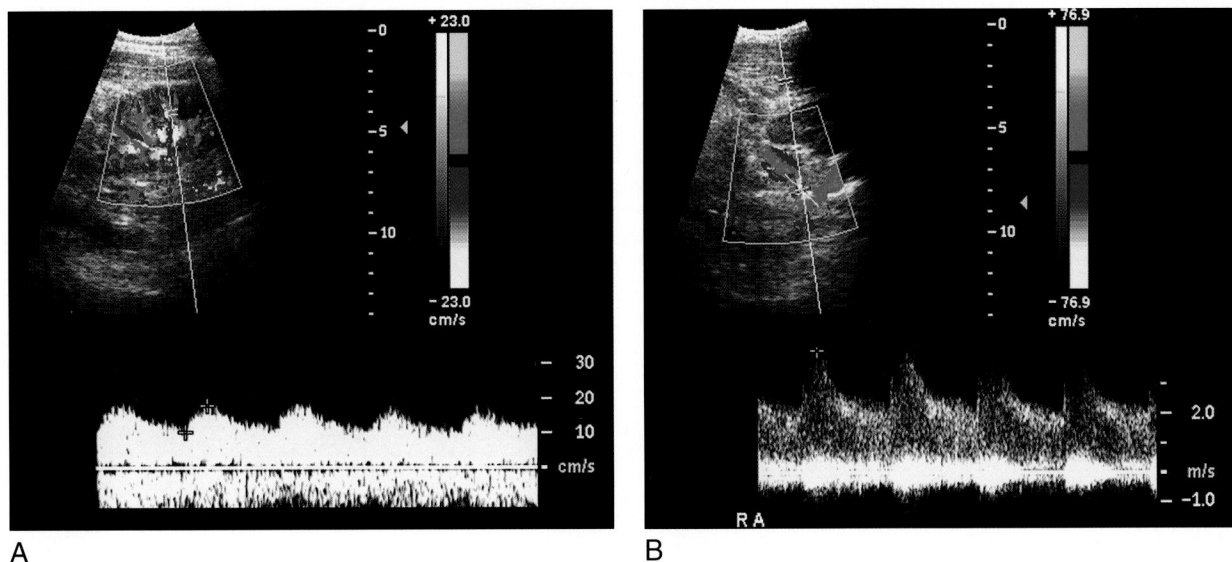

FIGURE 9-75. Renal artery stenosis. A, Intrarenal spectral waveform shows a tardus parvus signal with a prolonged acceleration time and a low resistance index. **B,** Waveform at the origin of the renal artery from the aorta shows a high peak velocity of 410 cm/second with an RI of 0.43.

An acceleration time greater than 0.07 second and a slope of systolic upstroke less than 3 m/s² are suggested as thresholds to assess for renal artery stenosis.[235] Simple recognition of the change in pattern may be adequate (Fig. 9-75).[236] Pharmacologic manipulation with captopril[237] may enhance the waveform abnormalities in patients with renal artery stenosis. Doppler sonography remains a controversial technique for the detection of native renal artery stenosis, however. The use of intravascular contrast agents increases the technical success rate for the evaluation of renal artery stenosis.[238] It may also play a role in the assessment and follow-up of patients undergoing renal artery angioplasty and stent placement.[239]

Renal Artery Aneurysm

Renal artery aneurysm is a saccular or fusiform dilation of the renal artery or one of its branches and it occurs with an incidence of 0.09% to 0.3%.[240] The etiology may be **congenital, inflammatory, traumatic, atherosclerotic, or related to fibromuscular disease**. If large (>2.5 cm), noncalcified, or associated with pregnancy, the possibility of rupture increases and treatment is recommended. On gray-scale **sonography,** a cystic mass may be seen. The addition of duplex and color Doppler imaging will readily demonstrate arterial flow within the cystic mass.

Renal Vein Thrombosis

Renal vein thrombosis (RVT) usually occurs because of underlying abnormality of the kidney, hydration, or coagulation status. Tumors of the kidney and left adrenal

gland may grow into the veins resulting in RVT. Extrinsic compression related to **tumors, retroperitoneal fibrosis, pancreatitis,** and **trauma** may cause RVT by attenuating the vessel and slowing flow. In adults, the most common etiology is **membranous glomerulonephritis**, and 50% of patients with this disease will have RVT. If thrombosis is acute, signs and symptoms of flank pain and hematuria will occur. With a more chronic onset and development of venous collaterals, symptoms are usually insignificant. The **sonographic features** of **acute RVT** are nonspecific and include an enlarged, edematous, hypoechoic kidney with loss of normal corticomedullary differentiation (Fig. 9-76).[241,242] Occasionally, thrombus will be seen within the renal vein, but acutely, it may be anechoic and invisible. The use of duplex and color Doppler ultrasound may help; however, lack of detectable flow in a patent renal vein is possible, especially if the flow is of low velocity. Absent or reversed end diastolic flow in the intraparenchymal native renal arteries may be a secondary sign of RVT. Platt et al.[243] evaluated 20 native kidneys in 12 patients with clinical findings suggestive of acute RVT. They found that normal arterial Doppler studies should not prevent further work-up if RVT is suspected, nor should absent or reversed diastolic signals be considered highly suggestive of RVT. If findings are equivocal, MRI should be performed. **Chronic RVT** usually results in a small, end-stage, echogenic kidney.

Ovarian Vein Thrombosis

Ovarian vein thrombosis is seen in postpartum women but it may also be seen as a result of pelvic inflammatory disease, Crohn's disease, or following gynecologic

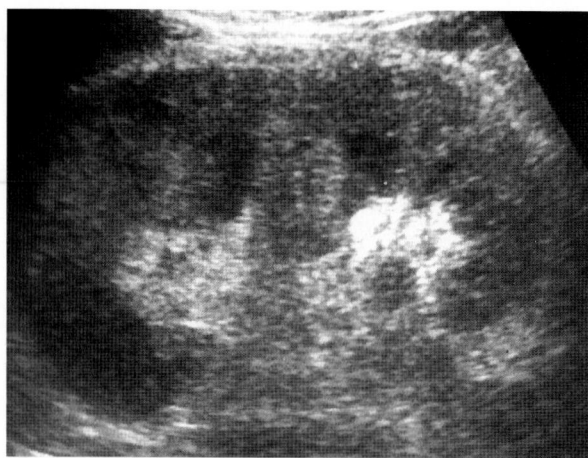
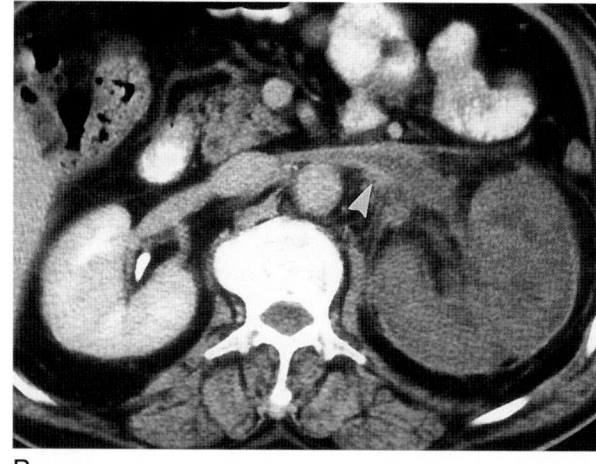

A   B

FIGURE 9-76. Renal vein thrombosis. A, Sagittal sonogram demonstrates a diffusely enlarged edematous left kidney with loss of corticomedullary differentiation. **B,** Confirmatory computed tomography shows a poorly functioning inhomogeneous kidney with thrombus in the left renal vein (*arrowhead*).

surgery. The right side is more commonly affected than the left. **Gray-scale, duplex, and color Doppler sonography** may reveal a long, tubular structure filled with thrombus extending from the region of the renal vein to deep within the pelvis. Patients are usually treated with anticoagulation and antibiotics.

MEDICAL DISEASES OF THE GENITOURINARY TRACT

Patients presenting with elevated creatinine levels are often sent to the ultrasound department for an initial screening test. The purpose is to rule out an underlying mechanical obstruction. If obstruction is not found, this often indicates a renal parenchymal abnormality. The kidney is able to react to insult in a limited number of ways. The kidney may look normal, swollen, shrunken, diffusely hypoechoic or echogenic. Sometimes various amounts of perirenal fluid will be observed. This fluid accumulation is thought to be a spontaneous subcapsular transudate as a result of sodium retention.[244] It is usually not possible to determine the cause, except to say that the patient has underlying medical renal disease. A percutaneous renal biopsy is often necessary to determine the etiology.

Acute Tubular Necrosis

Acute tubular necrosis (ATN) is the most common cause of acute reversible renal failure and is related to deposition of cellular debris within the renal collecting tubules. Both ischemic and toxic insults will cause tubular damage. Some of the initiating factors include **hypotension, dehydration, drugs, heavy metals,** and **solvent exposure.** The **sonographic appearance** of ATN depends on the underlying etiology. Hypotension-

causing ATN will often produce no sonographic abnormality, whereas drugs, metals, and solvents will cause enlarged, echogenic kidneys.

Prerenal disease and ATN account for 75% of all patients presenting with acute renal failure. Platt et al.[245] evaluated the usefulness of duplex Doppler in trying to differentiate these two common causes and found that most cases of acute renal failure will have elevated resistance index (RI >0.7). At the initial examination, duplex Doppler with elevated RI (>0.75) may be helpful in differentiating ATN from prerenal failure because most patients with prerenal failure will have RI less than 0.75. Patients with prerenal failure combined with severe liver disease (hepatorenal syndrome), who also exhibit elevated RI (>0.75), are the exception.

Acute Cortical Necrosis

Acute cortical necrosis (ACN) is a rare cause of acute renal failure caused by ischemic necrosis of the cortex with sparing of the medullary pyramids. The outermost aspect of cortex remains viable as a result of capsular blood supply. ACN occurs in association with **sepsis, burns, severe dehydration, snake bites,** and **pregnancy complicated by placental abruption or septic abortion.** The exact etiology is uncertain, although it is likely related to a transient episode of intrarenal vasospasm, intravascular thrombosis, or glomerular capillary endothelial damage. On **sonography,** the renal cortex is initially hypoechoic.[246] With time (mean = 2 months), calcification of the cortex becomes apparent.

Glomerulonephritis

Acute glomerulonephritis is a disease of the glomerulus with proliferative and necrotizing abnormality. Systemic diseases that also have acute glomerulonephritis as a feature

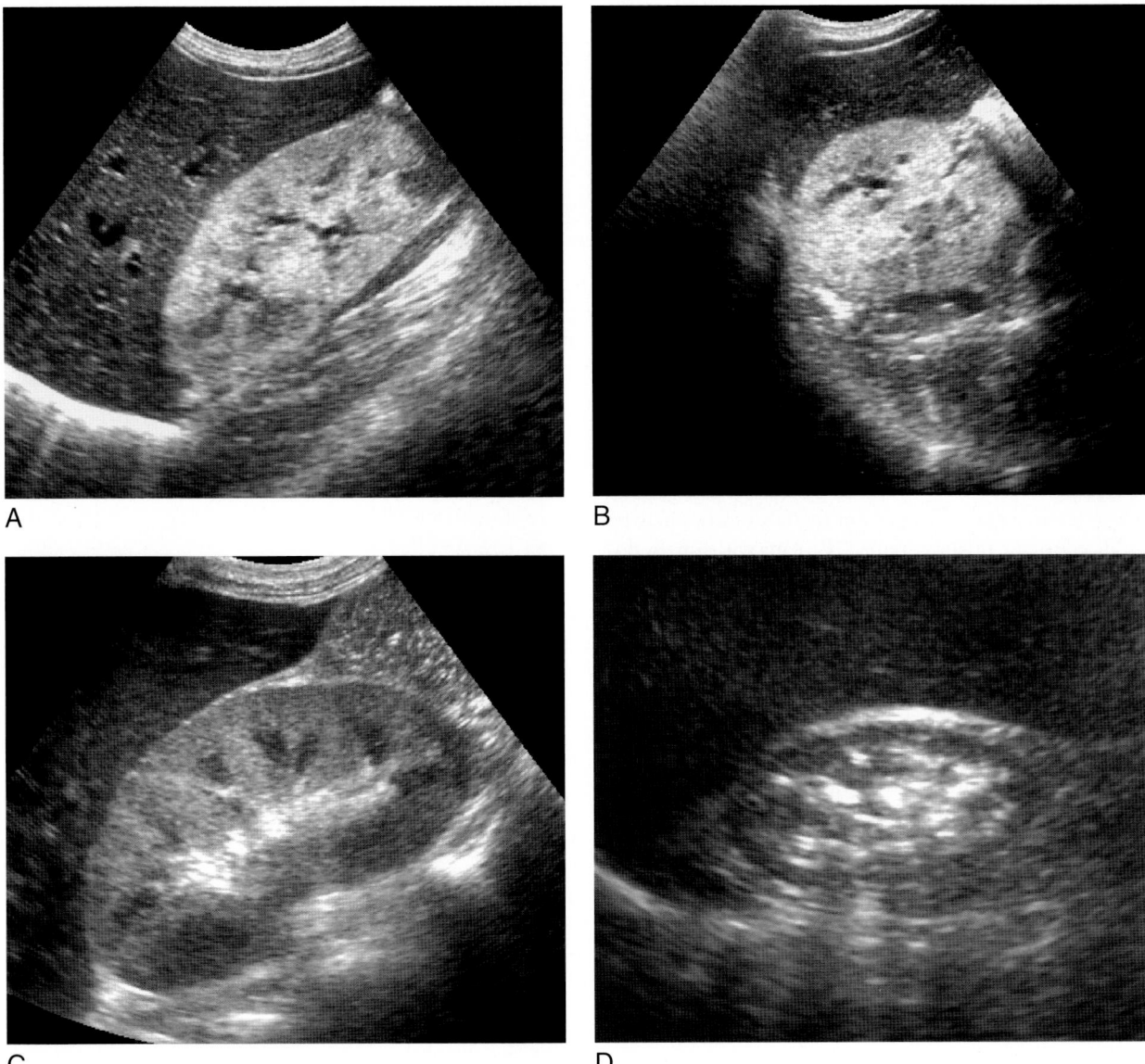

FIGURE 9-77. Medical renal disease in three patients. Acute. **A**, Sagittal and **B**, transverse sonograms show marked increase in cortical echogenicity with loss of corticomedullary differentiation. **C**, Very large kidney shows similar increased cortical echogenicity but to a lesser degree than in **A** and **B**. **D**, Small end-stage kidney shows parenchymal atrophy with fat filling the renal sinus.

include **polyarteritis nodosa, systemic lupus erythematosus, Wegener's granulomatosis, Goodpasture's syndrome, thrombocytopenic purpura,** and **hemolytic uremic syndrome**. Patients often present with hematuria, hypertension, and azotemia. On **sonography**, both kidneys are affected and the size may range from normal to markedly enlarged. The echopattern of the cortex is altered with medullary sparing and may be normal, hypoechoic, or hyperechoic (Fig. 9-77). With treatment, the kidneys may revert to normal size and echopattern. **Chronic glomerulonephritis** occurs with progression of acute disease and occurs over a period of weeks to months following an acute episode. Profound global symmetric parenchymal loss occurs. The calices and papillae are normal, and there is an increase in the

amount of peripelvic fat (see Fig. 9-77). Small, smooth, echogenic kidneys are seen with prominence of the central echo complex.

Acute Interstitial Nephritis

Acute interstitial nephritis (AIN) is an acute hypersensitivity reaction of the kidney most commonly related to drugs. Penicillin, methicillin, rifampin, sulfa-based drugs, nonsteroidal anti-inflammatory drugs (NSAIDs), cimetidine, furosemide, and thiazide drugs have been implicated. Usually, renal failure will resolve with cessation of drug therapy. On sonography, enlarged echogenic kidneys are noted.

Diabetes Mellitus

Diabetes mellitus is the most common cause of chronic renal failure. Diabetic nephropathy is believed to be related to glomerular hyperfiltration. Renal hypertrophy occurs. With time, diffuse intercapillary glomerulosclerosis develops,[247] causing progressive decrease in renal size. On **sonography**, the kidneys are enlarged and, with time, reduction in size and increase in cortical echogenicity with preservation of the corticomedullary junction are noted. With end-stage disease, the kidneys become smaller and more echogenic, and the medulla becomes as echogenic as the cortex.[247]

Amyloidosis

Amyloidosis may be primary or secondary and usually is a systemic disease. Ten percent to 20% of cases may be localized to one organ system.[248] Patients with amyloidosis often present with renal failure. Patients with primary disease are more often men, with a mean age of 60 years. Causes of secondary amyloidosis include **multiple myeloma** (10% to 15%), **rheumatoid arthritis** (20% to 25%), **tuberculosis** (50%), **familial Mediterranean fever** (26% to 40%), **renal cell carcinoma**, and **Hodgkin's disease**.[248] On **sonography**, acutely the kidneys may be symmetrically enlarged. With disease progression, the kidneys shrink in size and demonstrate cortical atrophy with increased cortical echogenicity. Focal renal masses, amorphous calcification, a central renal pelvic mass that may be a hemorrhage or amyloid deposit, and perirenal soft tissue masses may be seen. Similarly, involvement of the ureter and bladder may be localized or diffuse. Wall thickening or masses with or without calcification may be seen. The diagnosis is made with biopsy.

Endometriosis

Endometriosis occurs when endometrial tissue is found outside the uterus in women during the reproductive years. Patients typically present with pain, infertility, dysmenorrhea, dyspareunia, and menorrhagia. Approximately 1% of women with pelvic endometriosis will have urinary tract involvement, most frequently in the bladder. Most present with hematuria. **Bladder endometriosis** may be focal or diffuse. Less commonly, the ureter and rarely the kidney are affected. On **sonography**, patients with bladder endometriosis may present with a mural or intraluminal cyst, or a complex or solid lesion. Diagnosis is usually made cystoscopically with biopsy (Fig. 9-78).

Interstitial Cystitis

Interstitial cystitis is a chronic inflammation of the bladder wall of unknown etiology. It usually affects

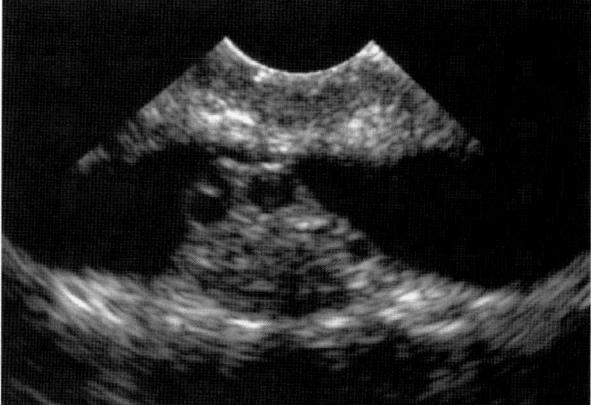

FIGURE 9-78. Bladder endometrioma. Transvaginal scan demonstrates cystic components in a mural mass that are typical for an endometrioma. (From Damani N, Wilson S: Nongynecologic applications of transvaginal US. RadioGraphics 1999;19:S179-S200.)

middle-aged women and has been associated with other systemic diseases including **systemic lupus**, **rheumatoid arthritis**, and **polyarteritis**.[68] Irritative voiding symptoms predominate and hematuria (30%) may occur.[249] On **sonography**, a small capacity, thick-walled bladder is seen (Fig. 9-79). Ureteric obstruction may be present. In some cases, it may be impossible to differentiate from diffuse transitional cell carcinoma of the bladder, and patients should have cystoscopy with biopsy for confirmation.

NEUROGENIC BLADDER

Voiding is a well-coordinated neurologic process controlled by areas within the cerebral cortex. These areas control the detrusor muscle of the bladder as well as both the internal and external urethral sphincters. For simplicity, lesions causing neurogenic bladder may be divided into those causing either **detrusor areflexia**—a lower motor neuron lesion—or **detrusor hyperreflexia**—lesions above the sacral reflux arc

On **sonography**, **detrusor areflexia** results in a smooth, large-capacity, thin-walled bladder. The bladder may extend high into the abdomen (Fig. 9-80). **Detrusor hyperreflexia** produces a thick-walled, vertical, trabeculated bladder often with associated upper-tract dilation (see Fig. 9-80). A large, postvoid residual will be seen.[250] If neurogenic bladder dysfunction is not properly diagnosed and treated, rapid deterioration of renal function may occur.

BLADDER DIVERTICULA

Bladder diverticula may be congenital or acquired. Congenital diverticula are known as **Hutch diverticula**

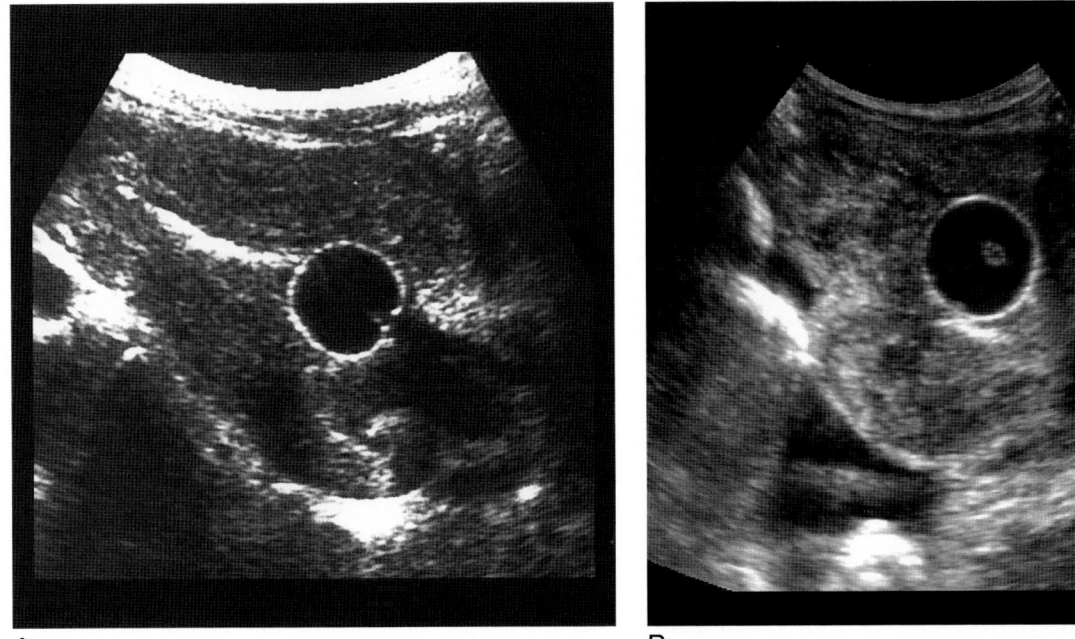

A   B

FIGURE 9-79. Diffuse bladder wall thickening in two patients who present with urinary retention. A,
Interstitial cystitis and **B,** diffuse transitional cell carcinoma both show gross mural thickening of the bladder wall surrounding a Foley
catheter. Cystoscopy and biopsy are required for differentiation.

and are located near the ureteral orifice. Most **acquired diverticula** result from bladder outlet obstruction. Bladder mucosa herniates through weak areas in the wall that are typically located posterolaterally near the ureteral orifices. The diverticular neck may be either narrow or wide. It is the narrow neck diverticula that lead to urinary stasis and give rise to complications including infection, stones, tumors, and ureteral obstruction. Tumors arising in a diverticulum have a poorer prognosis than tumors arising within the bladder. Diverticuli are composed only of mucosa and submucosa without the muscularis layer present. Tumors therefore grow and invade much more quickly into the surrounding perivesical fat.

On **sonography**, diverticuli appear as an outpouching sac from the bladder. The internal echogenicity of the diverticulum varies depending on its contents. The neck is often easily appreciated (Fig. 9-81). Urine may be seen flowing into and out of the diverticulum (see Fig. 9-81).

ULTRASOUND-GUIDED INTERVENTION

Intraoperative Ultrasound

Nephron-sparing surgery is being performed on patients with bilateral renal tumors, tumor in a solitary kidney, small renal tumors, indeterminate masses, and tumors in patients with underlying renal insufficiency. Real-time intraoperative ultrasound is useful because it can provide valuable information regarding the location and extent

of the lesion being resected. Intraoperative ultrasound can be used to localize small renal tumors and monitor ice ball formation during cryoablation (Fig. 9-82).[251] Intraoperative color Doppler sonography is useful for detecting renal artery complications (intimal flaps, thromboses, and anastomotic stenosis) during transaortic renal endarterectomy or bypass grafting.[252]

Biopsy

Biopsy of a native kidney, renal transplant, or renal mass can be performed safely with ultrasound guidance. If visualization with ultrasound is suboptimal, CT guidance may be used. Ultrasound guidance is preferable because it is quicker and allows real-time visualization of needle placement. Generally, an 18-gauge core biopsy is sufficient; however, for mass lesions a cytologic sample is also obtained. Potential complications include hemorrhage and pneumothorax. Needle tract seeding with 18-gauge needles or smaller is extremely rare and has been reported only in a single case.[253]

Abscess Drainage

The use of ultrasound and CT has greatly improved our ability to detect, characterize, and accurately localize intra-abdominal and retroperitoneal abscesses. The use of percutaneous drainage is well established as a mechanism to deal with these collections and is often curative, thereby obviating the need for surgery. Ultra-

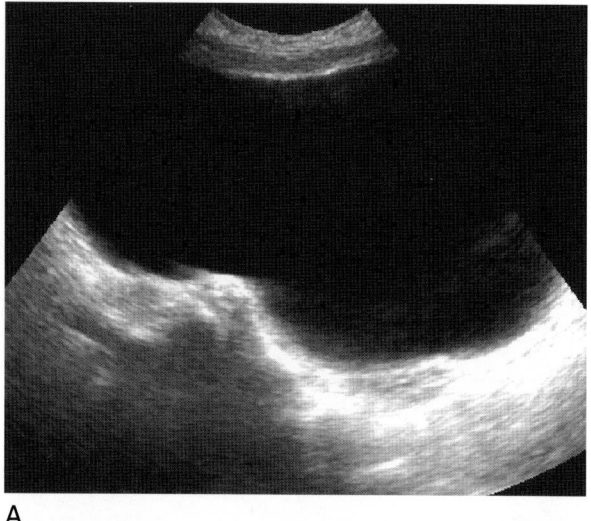

A

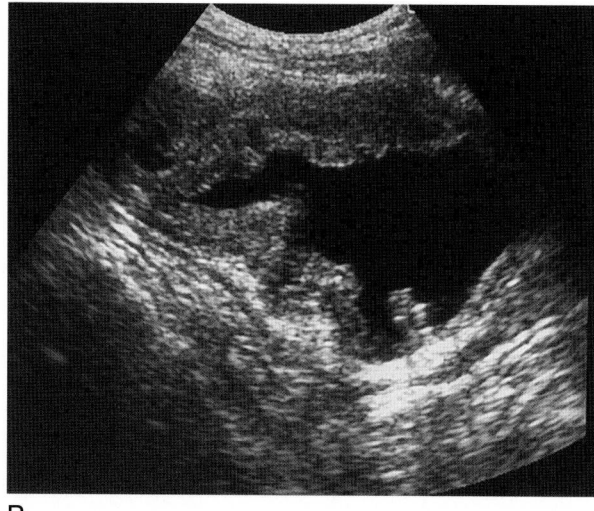

B

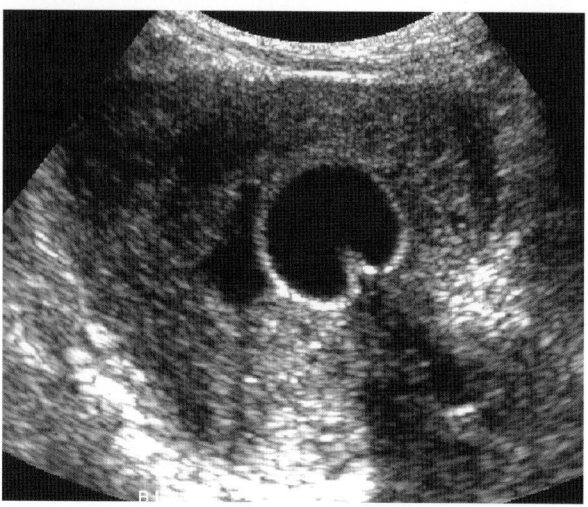

C

FIGURE 9-80. Neurogenic bladder. A, Detrusor areflexia (lower motor neuron lesion) shows a large volume, thin-walled bladder. **B** and **C,** two patients with detrusor hyperreflexia (upper motor neuron lesion) showing thick-walled trabeculated bladders.

sound guidance is a quick, effective way to guide needle placement using either ultrasound or fluoroscopy for final tube placement. It has the advantage of portability and can be performed at the bedside in critically ill intensive care unit patients.

Nephrostomy

Nephrostomy tube insertion is a relatively common procedure performed in patients for ureteric obstruction, urine leaks, access for percutaneous stone removal, and percutaneous endopyelotomy. The use of ultrasound to allow real-time guidance of the needle tip into a selected calix will save time as well as decrease radiation exposure to both the patient and the operator. If necessary, the procedure could be performed entirely with ultrasound guidance in critically ill, nonmobile, intensive care unit patients and in pregnant patients.

POSTSURGICAL EVALUATION

Kidney

When small tumors are wedged out during surgery, vascularized retroperitoneal fat is wedged into the defect. Postoperative appearance by both ultrasound and CT may simulate a focal renal mass. On sonography the mass may be hyperechoic or isoechoic (Fig. 9-83).[254,255] Being aware of this appearance will prevent unnecessary work-up.

Conduits

Urinary diversion is created for patients with nonfunctioning bladders or those patients who have had cystectomy. Recently, the trend has been to form continent urinary diversions. A portion of bowel is used

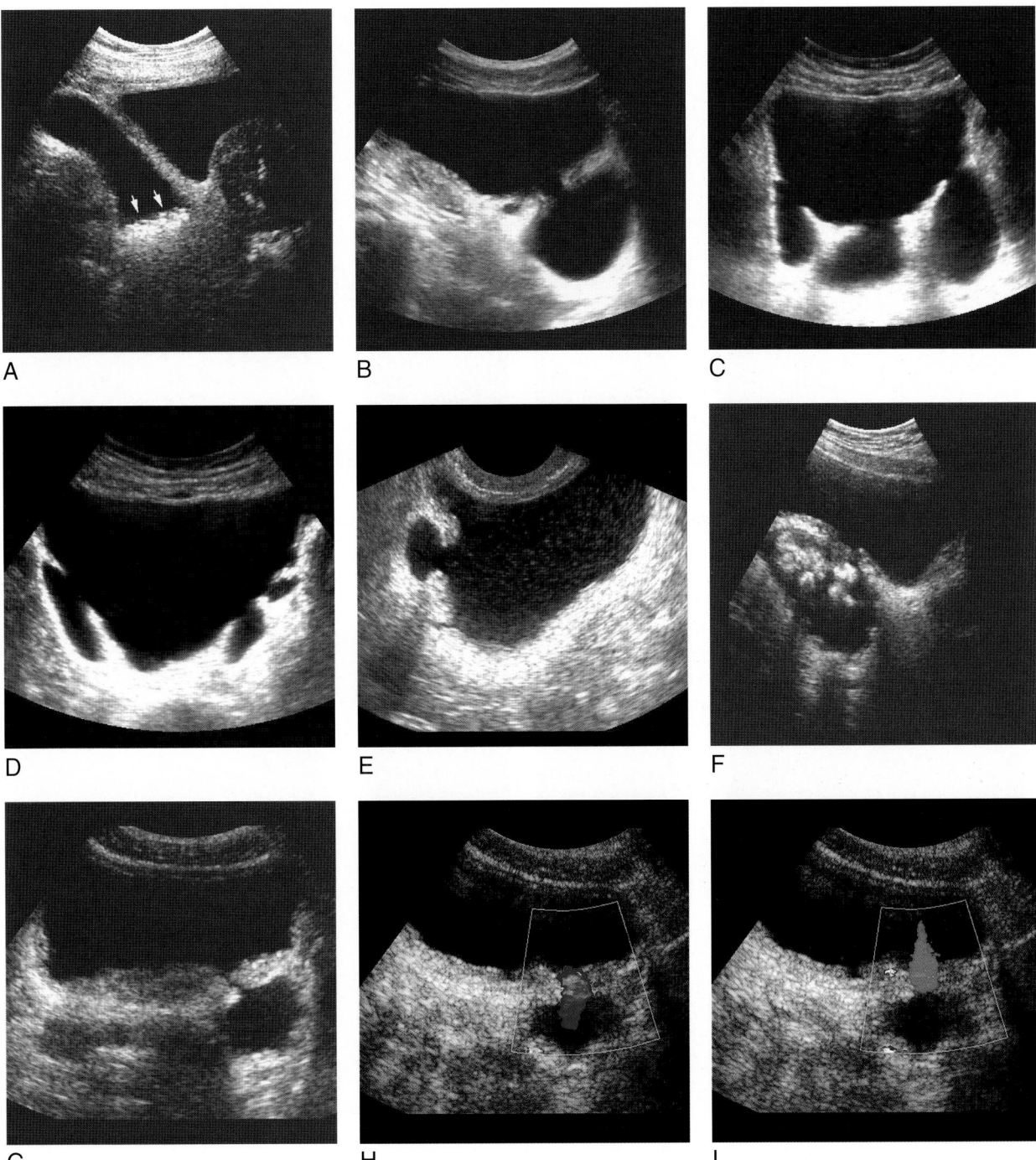

FIGURE 9-81. Bladder diverticula: spectrum of appearances. A, Large bladder diverticulum shows multiple stones (*arrows*). **B, Hutch diverticulum** arising in a posterolateral location. **C, Multiple** wide-necked diverticula. **D, Multiple** diverticula of variable size. **E,** Transvaginal sonogram shows an **unusual diverticulum** in a woman. There is debris in the bladder lumen. **F,** Large **transitional cell carcinoma** with extensive calcification fills the diverticulum. **G, H,** and **I** are in the same patient and show a narrow-necked diverticulum (**G**). **H** and **I** show urine flow into and out of the diverticulum.

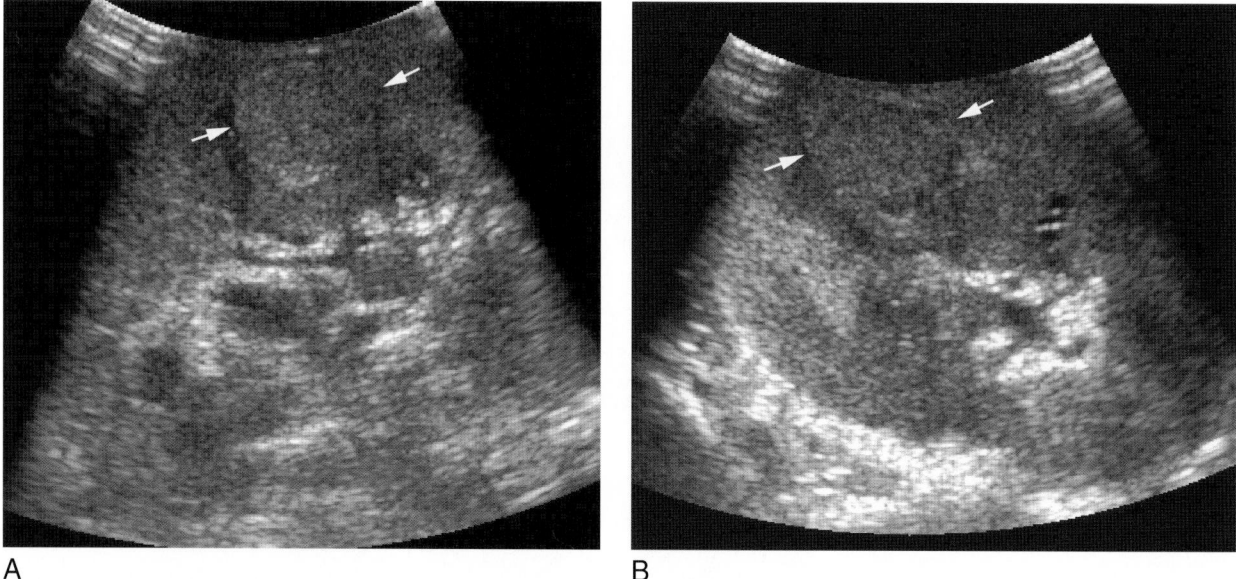

FIGURE 9-82. Intraoperative ultrasound to localize a renal tumor (*arrows*) for partial resection. **A**, Sagittal and **B**, transverse images are taken with the transducer on the kidney surface (*arrows*).

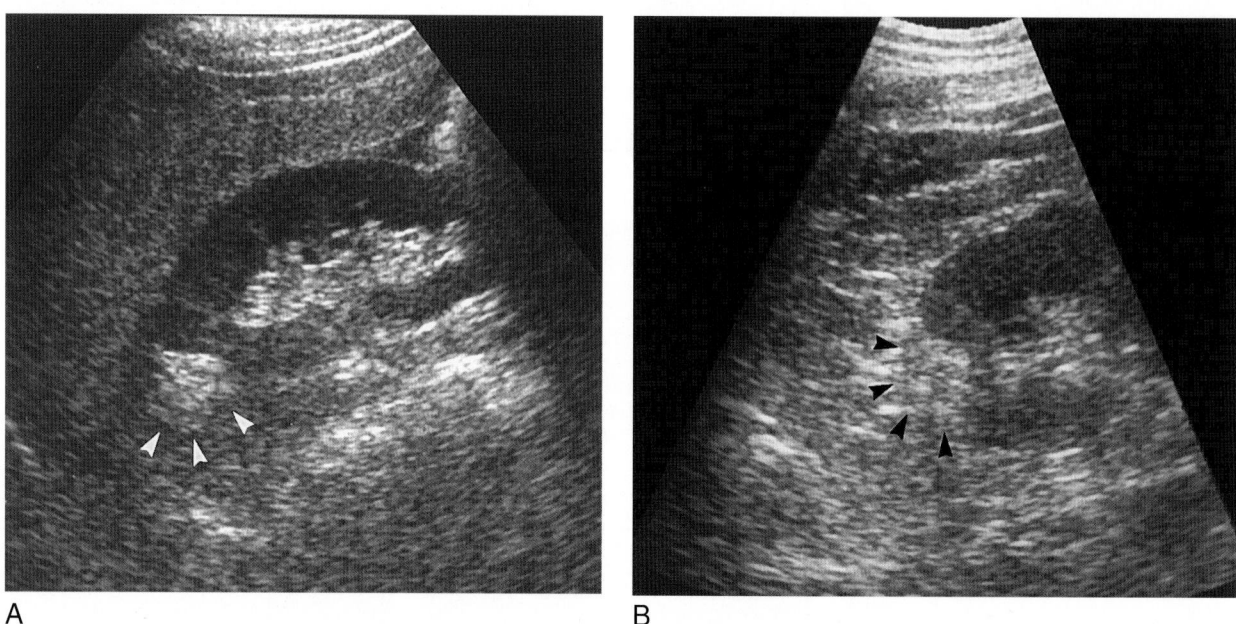

FIGURE 9-83. Postoperative renal ultrasound. **A**, Sagittal and **B**, transverse sonograms show a hyperechoic mass (*arrowheads*) at the site of previous tumor resection. This represents fat that was wedged into the defect at the time of surgery.

to create a pouch that can mimic normal bladder function. The pouch may attach to the abdominal wall (**cutaneous pouch**) or urethra (**orthotopic pouch**). Postoperative complications are similar for both and include urine extravasation, reflux, fistula formation, abscess, urinoma, hematoma, deep-vein thrombosis, ileus and small bowel obstruction.[256] The role of sonography is mostly in detecting complications rather than in evaluating the pouch itself. If the pouch is urine filled, sonographic assessment is possible (Fig. 9-84). Often, thickened or irregularly shaped bowel wall, pseudomasses, intraluminal mucus collections, and intussuscepted bowel segments can be seen.[256] Stone formation in a pouch may occur.

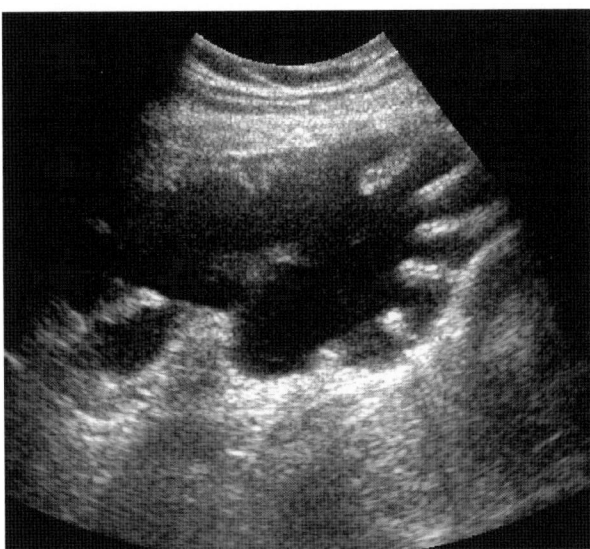

FIGURE 9-84. Ileal conduit. The bladder reservoir may show gut wall and variable filling.

Acknowledgment

The authors would like to thank Dr. Jenny Tomashpolskaya for her wonderful illustrations.

References

1. The kidney. In Cotran RS, Kumar V, Robbins SL (eds): Pathologic Basis of Disease. 5th ed. Philadelphia, WB Saunders, 1994, pp 927-989.

Embryology
2. The urogenital system. In Moore KL, Persaud TVN (eds): The Developing Human. 5th ed. Philadelphia, WB Saunders, 1993, pp 265-303.

Anatomy
3. Anatomy, structure, and embryology. In Netter FH: The CIBA Collection of Medical Illustrations. vol. 6. Kidneys, Ureters, and Urinary Bladder. CIBA Pharmaceutical, 1987, pp 2-35.
4. Emamian SA, Nielsen MB, Pedersen JF, et al: Kidney dimensions at sonography: Correlation with age, sex, and habitus in 665 adult volunteers. AJR 1993;160:83-86.
5. Platt JF, Rubin JM, Bowerman RA, et al: The inability to detect kidney disease on the basis of echogenicity. AJR 1988;151:317-319.
6. Carter AR, Horgan JG, Jennings TA, et al: The junctional parenchymal defect: A sonographic variant of renal anatomy. Radiology 1985;154:499-502.
7. Yeh HC, Halton KP, Shapiro RS, et al: Junctional parenchyma: Revised definition of hypertrophied column of Bertin. Radiology 1992;185:725-732.
8. Leekam RN, Matzinger MA, Brunelle M, et al: The sonography of renal columnar hypertrophy. J Clin Ultrasound 1983;11:491-494.
9. Middleton W, Lelan Melson G: Renal duplication artifact in US imaging. Radiology 1989;173:427-429.
10. Chesbrough RM, Burkhard TK, Martinez AJ, et al: Gerota versus Zuckerkandl: The renal fascia revisited. Radiology 1989;173:845-846.

11. Bechtold RE, Dyer RB, Zagoria RJ, et al: The perirenal space: Relationship of pathologic processes to normal retroperitoneal anatomy. RadioGraphics 1996;16:841-854.

Genitourinary Tract Sonography
12. Mortensson O, Duchek M: Translabial sonography in evaluating the lower female urogenital tract. AJR 1996;166:1327-1331.

Congenital Anomalies of the Genitourinary Tract
13. Congenital and hereditary disorders. In Netter FH: The CIBA Collection of Medical Illustrations, vol. 6. Kidneys, Ureters, and Urinary Bladder. CIBA Pharmaceutical 1987;223-249.
14. Congenital anomalies of the urinary tract. In Elkin M (ed): Radiology of the Urinary System. Boston, Little Brown, 1980, pp 62-147.
15. Friedland GW, Devries PA, Nino-Murcia M, et al: Congenital anomalies of the urinary tract. In Pollack HM (ed): Clinical Urography. An Atlas and Textbook of Urologic Imaging. Philadelphia, WB Saunders, 1990, pp 559-787.
16. Horgan JG, Rosenfield NS, Weiss RM, et al: Is renal ultrasound a reliable indicator of a nonobstructed duplication anomaly? Pediatric Radiology 1984; 14:388-391.
17. Shimoya K, Shimizu T, Hashimoto K, et al: Diagnosis of ureterocele with transvaginal sonography. Gynecol Obstet Invest 2002;54(1):58-60.
18. Madeb R, Shapiro I, Rothschild E, et al: Evaluation of ureterocele with Doppler sonography. J Clin Ultrasound 2000 Oct; 28(8):425-429.
19. Talner LB: Specific causes of obstruction. In Pollack HM (ed): Clinical Urography. An Atlas and Textbook of Urologic Imaging. Philadelphia: WB Saunders, 1990, pp 1629-1751.
20. Vargas B, Lebowitz RL: The coexistence of congenital megacalyces and primary megaureter. AJR 1986;147:313.
21. Tortora FL, Jr Lucey DT, Fried FA, et al: Absence of the bladder. J Urol 1983;129(6):1235-1237.
22. Spataro RF, Davis RS, McLachlan MSF, et al: Urachal abnormalities in the adult. Radiology 1983;149:659-663.
23. Schnyder PA, Candarjia G: Vesicourachal diverticulum. CT diagnosis in two adults. AJR 1981;137:1063-1065.

Infections of the Genitourinary Tract
24. Piccirillo M, Rigsby CM, Rosenfield AT: Sonography of renal inflammatory disease. Urol Radiol 1987;9:66-78.
25. Papanicolaou N, Pfister RC: Acute renal infections. Radiol Clin North Am 1996;34(5):965-995.
26. Talner LB, Davidson AJ, Lebowitz RL, et al: Acute pyelonephritis: Can we agree on terminology? Radiology 1994;192:297-305.
27. Farmer KD, Gellett LR: The sonographic appearance of acute focal pyelonephritis: 8 years' experience. Clin Radiol 2002;57(6):483-487.
28. Majd M, Nussbaum Blask AR, Markle BM, et al: Acute pyelonephritis: Comparison of diagnosis with 99mTc-DMSA, SPECT, spiral CT, MR imaging, and power Doppler US in an experimental pig model. Radiology 2001;218:101-108.
29. Thoumas D, Darmallaicq C, Pfister C, et al: Imaging characteristics of alkaline-encrusted cystitis and pyelitis. AJR 2002;178:389-392.
30. Lowe LH, Zagoria RJ, Baumgartner BR, et al: Role of imaging and intervention in complex infections of the urinary tract. AJR 1994;163:363-367.

31. Brun-Buisson C, Doyon F, Carlet J, et al: Incidence, risk factors and outcome of severe sepsis and septic shock in adults. JAMA 1995;274:968.

32. Yoder IC, Pfister RC, Lindfors KK, et al: Pyonephrosis imaging and intervention. AJR 1983;141:735-740.

33. Grayson DE, Abbott RM, Levy AD, et al: Emphysematous infections of the abdomen and pelvis: A pictorial review. Radiographics 2002;22:543-561.

34. Patel NP, Lavengood RW, Ernande SM, et al: Gas-forming infections in the genitourinary tract. Urology 1992;39:341-345.

35. Michaeli J, Mogle P, Perlberg S, et al: Emphysematous pyelonephritis. J Urol 1984;131:203-208.

36. Wan YL, Lee TY, Bullard MJ, et al: Acute gas-producing bacterial renal infection: Correlation between imaging findings and clinical outcome. Radiology 1996; 198:433-438.

37. Joseph RC, Amendola MA, Artze M, et al: Genitourinary tract gas: Imaging evaluation. RadioGraphics 1996;16:295-308.

38. Bhathena DB, Weiss JH, Holland NH, et al: Focal and segmental glomerular sclerosis in reflux nephropathy. Am J Med 1980;68:886.

39. Kay CJ, Rosenfield AT, Taylor KJW, et al: Ultrasonic characteristics of chronic atrophic pyelonephritis. AJR 1979;132:47-49.

40. Hartman DS, Davis CJ, Goldman SM, et al: Xanthogranulomatous pyelonephritis: Sonographic-pathologic correlation of the 16 cases. J Ultrasound Med 1984;3:481-488.

41. Anhalt MA, Cawood CD, Scott R: Xanthogranulomatous pyelonephritis: A comprehensive review with report of 4 additional cases. J Urol 1971;105:10-17.

42. Gammil S, Rabinowitz JG, Peace R, et al: New thoughts concerning xanthogranulomatous pyelonephritis. AJR 1975;125:154-163.

43. Tiu CM, Chou YH, Chiou HJ, et al: Sonographic features of xanthogranulomatous pyelonephritis. J Clin Ultrasound 2001;29(5):279-285.

44. Cousins C, Somers J, Broderick N, et al: Xanthogranulomatous pyelonephritis in childhood: Ultrasound and CT diagnosis. Pediatr Radiol 1994;24:210-212.

45. Davidson AJ: Chronic parenchymal disease. In Pollack HM (ed): Clinical Urography. An Atlas and Textbook of Urologic Imaging. Philadelphia: WB Saunders, 1990, pp 2277-2288.

46. Hoffman JC, Schnur MJ, Koenigsburg M: Demonstration of renal papillary necrosis by sonography. Radiology 1982;145:785-787.

47. Elkin M: Urogenital tuberculosis. In Pollack HM (ed): Clinical Urography. An Atlas and Textbook of Urologic Imaging. Philadelphia, WB Saunders, 1990, pp 1020-1052.

48. Das KM, Indudhara R, Vaidyanathan S: Sonographic features of genitourinary tuberculosis. AJR 1992; 158:327-329.

49. Pollack HM, Banner MP, Martinez LO, et al: Diagnostic considerations in urinary bladder wall calcification. AJR 1981;136:791.

50. Premkumar A, Lattimer J, Newhouse JH: CT and sonography of advanced urinary tract tuberculosis. AJR 1987;148:65-69.

51. Das KM, Vaidyanathan S, Rajwanshi A, et al: Renal tuberculosis: Diagnosis with sonographically guided aspiration cytology. AJR 1992;158:571-573.

52. Spring D: Fungal diseases of the urinary tract. In Pollack HM (ed): Clinical Urography. An Atlas and Textbook of Urologic Imaging. Philadelphia, WB Saunders, 1990, pp 987-998.

53. Shirkhoda A: CT findings in hepatosplenic and renal candidiasis. J Comput Assist Tomogr 1987;11:795.

54. Mindell HJ, Pollack HM: Fungal disease of the ureter. Radiology 1983;146:46.

55. Boldus RA, Brown RC, Culp DA: Fungus balls in the renal pelvis. Radiology 1972;102:555.

56. Stuck KJ, Silver TM, Jaffe HM, et al: Sonographic demonstration of renal fungus balls. Radiology 1981;142:473.

57. Palmer PES, Reeder MM: Parasitic disease of the urinary tract. In Pollack HM (ed): Clinical Urography. An Atlas and Textbook of Urologic Imaging. Philadelphia, WB Saunders, 1990, pp 999-1019.

58. Buchanan WM, Gelfand M: Calcification of the bladder in urinary schistosomiasis. Trans R Soc Trop Med Hyg 1970;64:593-596.

59. Diamond HM: Echinococcal disease of the kidney. J Urol 1976;115:742-744.

60. King DJ: Ultrasonography of echinococcal cysts. J Clin Ultrasound 1976;1:64-67.

61. Sabnis RB, Punekar SV, Desai RM, et al: Instillation of silver nitrate in the treatment of chyluria. Br J Urolog 1992;70:660-662.

62. Hamper UM, Goldblum LE, Hutchins GM, et al: Renal involvement in AIDS: Sonographic-pathologic correlation. AJR 1988;150:1321-1325.

63. Schaffer RM, Schwartz GE, Becker JA, et al: Renal ultrasound in acquired immune deficiency syndrome. Radiology 1984;153:511-513.

64. Pastor-Pons E, Martinez-Lon M, Alvarez-Bustos G, et al: Isolated renal mucormycosis in two patients with AIDS. AJR 1996;166:1282-1284.

65. Spouge AR, Wilson S, Gopinath N, et al: Extrapulmonary Pneumocystis carinii in a patient with AIDS. Sonographic findings. AJR 1990;155:76-78.

66. Towers MJ, Withers CE, Hamilton PA, et al: Visceral calcification in patients with AIDS may not always be due to Pneumocystis carinii. AJR 1991;156:745-747.

67. Falkoff GE, Rigsby CM, Rosenfield AT: Partial, combined cortical and medullary nephrocalcinosis: US and CT patterns in AIDS associated MAI infection. Radiology 1987;162:343-344.

68. Clayman RV, Weyman PJ, Bahnson RR: Inflammation of the bladder. In Pollack HM (ed): Clinical Urography. An Atlas and Textbook of Urologic Imaging. Philadelphia, WB Saunders, 1990, pp 902-924.

69. Stark GL, Feddersen R, Lowe BA, et al: Inflammatory pseudotumor (pseudosarcoma) of the bladder. J Urol 1989;141:610-612.

70. Kenney PJ, Breatnach ES, Stanley RJ: Chronic inflammation. In Pollack HM (ed): Clinical Urography. An Atlas and Textbook of Urologic Imaging. Philadelphia, WB Saunders, 1990, pp 822-843.

71. Lewin KJ, Fair WR, Steigbigel RT, et al: Clinical and laboratory studies into the pathogenesis of malacoplakia. J Clin Pathol 1976;29:354-363.

72. Curran FT: Malakoplakia of the bladder. Br J Urol 1987;59:559.

73. Kauzlauric D, Barmeir E: Sonography of emphysematous cystitis. J Ultrasound Med 1985;4:319-320.

74. Weiner DP, Koss LG, Sablay B, et al: The prevalence and significance of Brunn's nests, cystitis cystica and squamous metaplasia in normal bladders. J Urol 1979;122:317-321.

75. Lang EK, Fritzsche P: Fistulas of the genitourinary tract. In Pollack HM (ed): Clinical Urography. An Atlas and

Textbook of Urologic Imaging. Philadelphia, WB Saunders, 1990, pp 2579-2593.

76. Wilson S: The gastrointestinal tract. In Rumack CM, Wilson SR, Charboneau JW (eds): Diagnostic Ultrasound. St. Louis, Mosby-Year Book, 1991, pp 181-207.

77. Damani N, Wilson S: Nongynecologic applications of transvaginal US. RadioGraphics 1999;19:S179-S200.

78. Volkmer BG, Kuefer R, Nesslauer T, et al: Colour Doppler ultrasound in vesicovaginal fistulas. Ultrasound Med Biol 2000;26(5):771-775.

Genitourinary Tract Stones and Nephrocalcinosis

79. Sierakowski R, Finlayson B, Landes RR, et al: The frequency of urolithiasis in hospital discharge in the United States. Invest Urol 1978;15:438.

80. Spirnak JP, Resnick M, Banner MP: Calculus disease of the urinary tract, general considerations. In Pollack HM (ed): Clinical Urography. An Atlas and Textbook of Urologic Imaging. Philadelphia, WB Saunders, 1990, pp 1752-1758.

81. Middleton WD, Dodds WJ, Lawson TL, et al: Renal calculi: Sensitivity for detection with US. Radiology 1988;167:239-244.

82. Lee JY, Kim SH, Cho JY, et al: Color and power Doppler twinkling artifacts from urinary stones: Clinical observations and phantom studies. AJR 2001; 176:1441-1445.

83. Kimme-Smith C, Perrella RR, Kaveggia LP, et al: Detection of renal stones with real-time sonography: Effect of trans-ducers and scanning parameters. AJR 1991;157:975-980.

84. Sinclair D, Wilson S, Toi A, et al: The evaluation of suspected renal colic: Ultrasound scan versus excretory urography. Ann Emerg Med 1989;18:556-559.

85. Erwin BC, Carroll BA, Sommer FG: Renal colic: The role of ultrasound in initial evaluation. Radiology 1984;152:147-150.

86. Haddad MC, Sharif HS, Shahed MS, et al: Renal colic: Diagnosis and outcome. Radiology 1992;184:83-88.

87. Haddad MC, Sharif HS, Samihan AM, et al: Management of renal colic: Redefining the role of the urogram. Radiology 1992;184:35-36.

88. LeRoy A: Diagnosis and treatment of nephrolithiasis: Current perspectives. AJR 1994;163:1309-1313.

89. Cronan JJ, Tublin ME: Role of the resistance index in the evaluation of acute renal obstruction. AJR 1995; 164:377-378.

90. Patlas M, Farkas A, Fisher D, et al: Ultrasound versus CT for the detection of ureteric stones in patients with renal colic. Br J Radiol 2001;74(886):901-904

91. Laing FC, Benson CB, DiSalvo DN, et al: Distal ureteral calculi: Detection with vaginal US. Radiology 1994;192:545-548.

92. Hertzberg BS, Kliewer MA, Paulson EK, et al: Distal ureteral calculi: Detection with transperineal sonography. AJR 1994;163:1151-1153.

93. Burge HJ, Middleton WD, McClennan BL, et al: Ureteral jets in healthy subjects and in patients with unilateral ureteral calculi: Comparison with color Doppler US. Radiology 1991;180:437-442.

94. Price CI, Adler RS, Rubin JM: Ultrasound detection of differences in density: Explanation of ureteric jet phenomenon and implications for new ultrasound applications. Invest Radiol 1989;24:876-883.

95. Baker S, Middleton WD: Color Doppler sonography of ureteral jets in normal volunteers: Importance of relative specific gravity of urine in the ureter and bladder. AJR 1992;159:773-775.

96. Geavlete P, Georgescu D, Cauni V, et al: Value of duplex Doppler ultrasonography in renal colic. Eur Urol 2002;41(1):71-78.

97. Platt JF, Rubin JM, Ellis JH: Acute renal obstruction: Evaluation with intrarenal duplex Doppler and conventional US. Radiology 1993;186:685-688.

98. Tublin ME, Dodd GD, Verdile VP: Acute renal colic: Diagnosis with duplex Doppler US. Radiology 1994;193:697-701.

99. Katz DS, Lane MJ, Sommer FG: Unenhanced helical CT of ureteral stones: Incidence of associated urinary tract findings. AJR 1996;166:1319-1322.

100. Smith RC, Rosenfield AT, Choe KA, et al: Acute flank pain: Comparison of non-contrast-enhanced CT and intravenous urography. Radiology 1995;194:789-794.

101. Smith RC, Verga M, McCarthy S, et al: Diagnosis of acute flank pain: Value of unenhanced helical CT. AJR 1996;166:97-101.

102. Banner M: Nephrocalcinosis. In Pollack HM (ed): Clinical Urography. An Atlas and Textbook of Urologic Imaging. Philadelphia, WB Saunders, 1990, pp 1768-1775.

103. Patriquin H, Robitaille P: Renal calcium deposition in children: Sonographic demonstration of the Anderson-Carr progression. AJR 1986;146:1253-1256.

Tumors of the Genitourinary Tract

104. Bennington JL, Beckwith JB: Atlas of Tumor Pathology, 2nd series. Fascicle 12. Tumors of the kidney, renal pelvis and ureter. Washington, DC: Armed Forces Institute of Pathology, 1975, pp 25-162.

105. Bennington JL, Laubscher FA: Epidemiologic studies on carcinoma of the kidney. I. Association of renal adenocarcinoma with smoking. Cancer 1968;21:1069.

106. Cohen AJ, Li FP, Berg S, et al: Hereditary renal cell carcinoma associated with a chromosomal translocation. N Engl J Med 1979;301:592.

107. Choyke PL, Glenn GM, Walther MM, et al: Hereditary renal cancers. Radiology 2003;226:33-46.

108. Choyke PL, Glenn GM, Walther MM, et al: Von Hippel-Lindau disease: Genetic, clinical, and imaging features. Radiology 1995;194:629-642.

109. Choyke PL, Glenn GM, Walther MM, et al: The natural history of renal lesions in von Hippel-Lindau disease: A serial CT imaging study in 28 patients. AJR 1992;159:1229-1234.

110. Takase K, Takahashi S, Tazawa S, et al: Renal cell carcinoma associated with chronic renal failure: Evaluation with sonographic angiography. Radiology 1994;192:787-792.

111. Levine E, Grantham J, Slusher S, et al: CT of acquired cystic kidney disease and renal tumors in long-term dialysis patients. AJR 1984;142:125-131.

112. Kim JK, Kim TK, Ahn HJ, et al: Differentiation of subtypes of renal cell carcinoma on helical CT Scans. AJR 2002;178:1499-1506.

113. Skinner DG, Colvin RB, Vermillion CD, et al: Diagnosis and management of renal cell carcinoma. A clinical and pathologic study of 309 cases. Cancer 1971; 28:1165.

114. Sufrin G, Murphy GP: Renal adenocarcinoma. Urol Surv 1980;30:129.

115. Raval B, Lamki N: Computed tomography in detection of occult hypernephroma. J Comput Tomogr 1983; 7:199-207.

116. Curry N: Small renal masses (lesions smaller than 3 cm): Imaging evaluation and management. AJR 1995; 164:355-362.

117. Warshauer DM, McCarthy SM, Street L, et al: Detection of renal masses: Sensitivities and specificities of excretory urography/linear tomography, US and CT. Radiology 1988;169:363-365.

118. Jamis-Dow CA, Choyke PL, Jennings SB, et al: Small (≤3 cm) renal masses: Detection with CT versus US and pathologic correlation. Radiology 1996;198:785-788.

119. Szolar DH, Kammerhuber F, Altziebler S, et al: Multiphasic helical CT of the kidney: Increased conspicuity for detection and characterization of small (<3 cm) renal masses. Radiology 1997;202:211-217.

120. Urban B: The small renal mass. What is the role of multiphasic helical scanning? Radiology 1997;202:22-23.

121. Birnbaum BA, Jacobs JE, Ramchandani P: Multiphasic renal CT comparison of renal mass enhancement during the corticomedullary and nephrographic phases. Radiology 1996;200:753-758.

122. Zeman R, Zeiberg A, Hayes W, et al: Helical CT of renal masses: The value of delayed scans. AJR 1996; 167:771-776.

123. Campeau NG, Johnson CD, Felmlee JP, et al: MR imaging of the abdomen with a phased-array multicoil: Prospective clinical evaluation. Radiology 1995; 195:769-776.

124. Semelka RC, Hricak H, Stevens S, et al: Combined gadolinium-enhanced and fat-saturation MR imaging of renal masses. Radiology 1991;178:803-809.

125. Bosniak MA, Birnbaum BA, Krinsky GA, et al: Small renal parenchymal neoplasms: Further observations on growth. Radiology 1995;194:589-597.

126. Gervais DA, McGovern FJ, Arellano RS, et al: Renal cell carcinoma: Clinical experience and technical success with radio-frequency ablation of 42 tumors. Radiology 2003;226:417-424.

127. Charboneau JW, Hattery RR, Ernst EC, et al: Spectrum of sonographic findings in 125 renal masses other than benign simple cyst. AJR 1983;140:87-94.

128. Forman HP, Middleton WD, Melson GL, et al: Hyperechoic renal cell carcinomas: Increase in detection at US. Radiology 1993;188:431-434.

129. Yamashita Y, Takahashi M, Watanabe O, et al: Small renal cell carcinoma: Pathologic and radiologic correlation. Radiology 1992;184:493-498.

130. Yamashita Y, Ueno S, Makita O, et al: Hyperechoic renal tumors: Anaechoic rim and intratumoral cysts in US differentiation of renal cell carcinoma from angiomyolipoma. Radiology 1993;188:179-182.

131. Sniderman KW, Kreiger JN, Seligson GR, et al: The radiologic and clinical aspects of calcified hypernephroma. Radiology 1979;131:31-35.

132. Phillips TL, Chin FG, Palubinskas AJ: Calcifications in renal masses: An eleven year survey. Radiology 1963;80:786-794.

133. Kikkawa K, Lasser EC. "Ring-like" or "rim-like" calcification in renal cell carcinoma. AJR 1969; 107:737-742.

134. Daniels WW, Hartman GW, Witten DM, et al: Calcified renal masses: A review of ten years' experience at the Mayo Clinic. Radiology 1972;103:503-508.

135. Onitsuka H, Murakami J, Naito S, et al: Diffusely calcified renal cell carcinoma: CT features. J Comput Assist Tomogr 1992;16(4):654-656.

136. Weyman PJ, McClennan BL, Lee J, et al: CT of calcified renal masses. AJR 1982;138:1095-1099.

137. Press GA, McClennan BL, Melson GL, et al: Papillary renal cell carcinoma: CT and sonographic evaluation. AJR 1984;143:1005-1009.

138. Mancilla-Jimenez R, Stanley RJ, Blath RA: Papillary renal cell carcinoma. Cancer 1976;38:2469-2480.

139. Yamashita Y, Watanabe O, Miyazaki H, et al: Cystic renal cell carcinoma. Acta Radiologica 1994;35(1):19-24.

140. Hartman DS, Davis CJ, Johns T, et al: Cystic renal cell carcinoma. Urology 1986;28(2):145-153.

141. Zagoria RJ: Imaging of small renal masses: A medical success story. AJR 2000;175(4):945-955.

142. Silverman SG, Lee BY, Seltzer SE et al: Small (≤3 cm) renal masses: Correlation of spiral CT features and pathologic findings. AJR 1994;163:597-605.

143. Taylor KJ, Ramos I, Carter D, et al: Correlation of Doppler US tumor signals with neovascular morphologic features. Radiology 1988;166:57-62.

144. Taylor KJ, Ramos I, Morse SS, et al: Focal liver masses: Differential diagnosis with pulsed Doppler US. Radiology 1987;164:643-647.

145. Kier R, Taylor KJ, Feyock AL, et al: Renal masses: Characterization with Doppler US. Radiology 1990;176:703-707.

146. Ramos IM, Taylor KJ, Kier R, et al: Tumor vascular signals in renal masses: Detection with Doppler US. Radiology 1988;168:633-637.

147. Kuijpers D, Jaspers R: Renal masses: differential diagnosis with pulsed Doppler US. Radiology 1989;270:59-60.

148. McNichols DW, Segura JW, DeWeerd JH: Renal cell carcinoma: Long-term survival and late recurrence. J Urol 1981;126:17.

149. Zagoria RJ, Bechtold RE, Dyer RB: Staging of renal adenocarcinoma: Role of various imaging procedures. AJR 1995;164:363-370.

150. Habboub HK, Abu-Yousef MM, Williams RD, et al: Accuracy of color Doppler sonography in assessing venous thrombus extension in renal cell carcinoma. AJR 1997;168:267-271.

151. Fritzsche PJ, Millar C: Multimodality approach to staging renal cell carcinoma. Urol Radiol 1992;14:3-7.

152. Brierly RD, Thomas PJ, Harrison NW, et al: Evaluation of fine-needle aspiration cytology for renal masses. BJU Int 2000;85(1):14-18.

153. Campbell SC, Novick AC, Herts B, et al: Prospective evaluation of fine needle aspiration of small, solid renal masses: Accuracy and morbidity. Urology 1997; 50(1):25-29.

154. Lechevallier E, Andre M, Barriol D, et al: Fine-needle percutaneous biopsy of renal masses with helical CT guidance. Radiology 2000;216(2):506-510.

155. Buckley JA, Urban BA, Soyer P, et al: Transitional cell carcinoma of the renal pelvis: A retrospective look at CT staging with pathologic correlation. Radiology 1996;201:194-198.

156. Leder RA, Dunnick NR: Transitional cell carcinoma of the pelvicalices and ureter. AJR 1990;155:713-722.

157. Yousem DM, Gatewood OM, Goldman SM, et al: Synchronous and metachronous transitional cell carcinoma of the urinary tract: Prevalence, incidence and radiographic detection. Radiology 1988;167:613-618.

158. Dinsmore BJ, Pollack HM, Banner MP: Calcified transitional cell carcinoma of the renal pelvis. Radiology 1988;167:401-404.

159. Hartman DS, Pyatt RS, Daily E: Transitional cell carcinoma of the kidney with invasion into the renal vein. Urol Radiol 1983;5:83-87.

160. Winalski CS, Lipman JC, Tumeh SS: Ureteral neoplasms. RadioGraphics 1990;10:271-283.

161. Dershaw DD, Scher HI: Sonography in evaluation of carcinoma of the bladder. Urology 1987;29:454.

162. Dondalski M, White EM, Ghahremani G, et al: Carcinoma arising in urinary bladder diverticula: Imaging findings in six patients. AJR 1993;161:817-820.

163. Barentsz JO, Ruijs SHJ, Strijk SP: The role of MR imaging in carcinoma of the urinary bladder. AJR 1993;160:937-947.

164. Narumi Y, Sato T, Hori S, et al: Squamous cell carcinoma of the uroepithelium: CT evaluation. Radiology 1989;173:853-856.

165. Blacher EJ, Johnson DE, Abdul-Karim FW, et al: Squamous cell carcinoma of the renal pelvis. Urology 1985;25:124.

166. Mirone V, Prezioso D, Palombini S, et al: Mucinous adenocarcinoma of the renal pelvis. Eur Urol 1984;10:284.

167. Merino MJ, Livolsi VA: Oncocytomas of the kidney. Cancer 1982;50:1852.

168. Honda H, Bonsib S, Barloon T, et al: Unusual renal oncocytomas: Pathologic and CT correlations. Urol Radiol 1992;14:148-154.

169. Hartman GW, Hattery RR: Benign neoplasms of the renal parenchyma. In Pollack HM (ed): Clinical Urography. An Atlas and Textbook of Urologic Imaging. Philadelphia, WB Saunders, 1990, pp 1193-1215.

170. Davidson AJ, Hayes WS, Hartman DS, et al: Renal oncocytoma and carcinoma: Failure of differentiation with CT. Radiology 1993;186:693-696.

171. Goiney RC, Goldenberg L, Cooperberg P, et al: Renal oncocytoma: Sonographic analysis of 14 cases. AJR 1984;143:1001-1004.

172. Tikkakoski T, Paivansalo M, Alanen A, et al: Radiologic findings in renal oncocytoma. Acta Radiologica 1991;32(5):363-367.

173. Curry NS, Schabel SI, Garvin AJ, et al: Intratumoral fat in a renal oncocytoma mimicking angiomyolipoma. AJR 1190;154:307-308.

174. Schatz SM, Lieber MM: Update on oncocytoma. Curr Urol Rep 2003;(1):30-35.

175. Gentry LR, Gould HR, Alter AJ, et al: Hemorrhagic angiomyolipoma: Demonstration by CT. J Comput Assist Tomogr 1981;5(6):861-865.

176. Oesterling JE, Fishman EK, Goldman SM, et al: The management of renal angiomyolipoma. J Urol 1986;135:1121-1124.

177. Silverman SG, Pearson GD, Seltzer SE, et al: Small (≤3 cm) hyperechoic renal masses: Comparison of helical and conventional CT for diagnosing angiomyolipoma. AJR 1996;167:877-881.

178. Siegel CL, Middleton WD, Teefey SA, et al: Angiomyolipoma and renal cell carcinoma: US differentiation. Radiology 1996;198:789-793.

179. Arenson AM, Graham RT, Shaw P, et al: Angiomyolipoma of the kidney extending into the inferior vena cava: Sonographic and CT findings. AJR 1988;151:1159-1161.

180. Israel GM, Bosniak MA, Slywotzky CM, et al: CT differentiation of large exophytic renal angiomyolipomas and perirenal liposarcomas. AJR 2002;179:769-773.

181. Yamakado K, Tanaka N, Nakagawa T, et al: Renal angiomyolipoma: Relationships between tumor size, aneurysm formation, and rupture. Radiology 2002;225:78-82.

182. Lapeyre M, Correas JM, Ortonne N, et al: Color-flow Doppler sonography of pseudoaneurysms in patients with bleeding renal angiomyolipoma. AJR 2002;179:145-147.

183. Earthman WJ, Mazer MJ, Winfield AC: Angiomyolipomas in tuberous sclerosis: Selective embolotherapy with alcohol with long-term follow-up study. Radiology 1986; 160:437.

184. Richmond J, Sherman RS, Diamond HD, et al: Renal lesions associated with malignant lymphomas. Am J Med 1962;32:184.

185. Horii SC, Bosniak MA, Megibow AJ, et al: Correlation of computed tomography and ultrasound in the evaluation of renal lymphoma. Urol Radiol 1983;5:69-76.

186. Heiken JP, Gold RP, Schnur MJ, et al: Computed tomography of renal lymphoma with ultrasound correlation. J Comput Assist Tomogr 1983;7(2):245-250.

187. Gregory A, Behan M: Lymphoma of the kidneys: Unusual ultrasound appearances due to infiltration of the renal sinus. J Clin Ultrasound 1981;9:343-345.

188. Jafri SZ, Bree RL, Amendola MA, et al: CT of renal and perirenal non-Hodgkin lymphoma. AJR 1982; 138:1101-1105.

189. Deuskar V, Martin LFW, Leung W: Renal lymphoma: An unusual example. Can Assoc Radiol J 1987;38:133-135.

190. Binkovitz LA, Hattery RR, LeRoy AJ: Primary lymphoma of the bladder. Urol Radiol 1988;9:231-233.

191. Kirshbaum JD, Preuss FS: Leukemia: A clinical and pathological study of 123 fatal cases in 14,400 necropsies. Arch Int Med 1943;71:777.

192. Sternby NH: Studies in enlargement of leukemic kidneys. Acta Haemat 1955;14:354.

193. Kumari-Subaiya S, Lee WJ, Festa R, et al: Sonographic findings in leukemic renal disease. J Clin Ultrasound 1984;12:465-472.

194. Araki T: Leukemic involvement of the kidney in children: CT features. J Comput Assist Tomogr 1982;6:781.

195. Mitnick JS, Bosniak MA, Rothberg M, et al: Metastatic neoplasm to the kidney studied by computed tomography and sonography. J Comput Assist Tomogr 1985;9:43.

196. Choyke PC, White EM, Zeman RK, et al: Renal metastases: Clinicopathologic and radiologic correlation. Radiology 1987;162:359-363.

197. Ambos MA, Bosniak MA, Megibow AJ, et al: Ureteral involvement by metastatic disease. Urol Radiol 1979;1:105.

198. Mengiardi B, Wiesner W, Stoffel F, et al: Case 44: Adenocarcinoma of the urachus. Radiology 2002; 222:744-747.

199. Rao BK, Scanlan KA, Hinke ML: Abdominal case of the day. AJR 1986;146:1074-1079.

200. Brick SH, Friedman AC, Pollack HM, et al: Urachal carcinoma: CT findings. Radiology 1988;169:377-381.

201. Dunnick NR, Hartman DS, Ford KK, et al: The radiology of juxtaglomerular tumors. Radiology 1983;147:321-326.

202. McKeown DK, Nguyen GK, Rudrick B, et al: Carcinoid of the kidney: Radiologic findings. AJR 1988; 150:143-144.

203. Chen M, Lipson SA, Hricak H: MR imaging evaluation of benign mesenchymal tumors of the urinary bladder. AJR 1997;168:399-403.

204. Kogan MG, Koenigsberg M, Laor E, et al: US case of the day: Cavernous hemangioma of the bladder. RadioGraphics 1996;16:443-447.

Renal Cystic Disease

205. Jackman RJ, Stevens GM: Benign hemorrhagic renal cyst. Nephrotomography, renal arteriography and cyst puncture. Radiology 1974;110:7-13.

206. Bosniak M: The current radiological approach to renal cysts. Radiology 1986;158:1-10.

207. Israel GM, Bosniack MA: Calcification in cystic renal masses: Is it important in diagnosis? Radiology 2003;226:47-52.

208. Hidalgo H, Dunnick NR, Rosenberg ER, et al: Parapelvic cysts: Appearance on CT and sonography. AJR 1982;138:667-671.
209. Chan JC, Kodroff MB: Hypertension and hematuria secondary to parapelvic cyst. Pediatrics 1980;65:821-823.
210. Ginalski JM, Portmann L, Jaeger PH: Does medullary sponge kidney cause nephrolithiasis? AJR 1990; 155:299-302.
211. Goldman S, Hartman DS: Medullary sponge kidney. In Pollack HM (ed): Clinical Urography. An Atlas and Textbook of Urologic Imaging. Philadelphia, WB Saunders, 1990, pp 1167-1177.
212. Resnick JS, Hartman DS: Medullary cystic disease of the kidney. In Pollack HM (ed): Clinical Urography. An Atlas and Textbook of Urologic Imaging. Philadelphia, WB Saunders, 1990, pp 1178-1184.
213. Choyke PL: Inherited cystic diseases of the kidney. Radiol Clin North Am 1996;34(5):925-946.
214. Grampsas SA, Chandhoke PS, Fan J, et al: Anatomic and metabolic risk factors for nephrolithiasis in patients with autosomal dominant polycystic kidney disease. Am J Kidney Dis 2000;36(1):53-57.
215. Ravine D, Gibson RN, Walker RG: Evaluation of ultrasonographic diagnostic criteria. Lancet 1994;343:824.
216. Bear JC, McManamon P, Morgan J, et al: Age at clinical onset and at ultrasonographic detection of adult polycystic kidney disease: Data for genetic counseling. Am J Med Genet 1984;18:45-53.
217. Sanders RC, Hartman DS: The sonographic distinction between neonatal multicystic kidney and hydronephrosis. Radiology 1984;151:621-625.
218. Madewell JE, Goldman SM, Davis CJ, et al: Multilocular cystic nephroma: A radiographic-pathologic correlation of 58 patients. Radiology 1983;146:309-321.
219. Master U, Cruz C, Schmidt R, et al: Renal malignancy in peritoneal dialysis patients with acquired cystic kidney disease. Adv Perit Dial 1992;8:145-149.
220. Taylor AJ, Cohen EP, Erickson SJ, et al: Renal imaging in long-term dialysis patients: A comparison of CT and sonography. AJR 1989;153:765-767.
221. Levine E: Acquired cystic kidney disease. Radiol Clin North Am 1996;34(5):947-964.
222. Levine E, Collins DL, Horton WA, et al: CT screening of the abdomen in von Hippel-Lindau disease. AJR 1982;139:505-510.
223. Kuntz N: Population studies. In Gomez MR: Tuberous Sclerosis, 2nd ed. New York, Raven Press, 1988, p 214.

Trauma
224. Kawashima A, Sandler CM, Corl FM, et al: Imaging of renal trauma: A comprehensive review. Radiographics 2001;21:557-574.
225. Federle MP: Evaluation of renal trauma. In Pollack HM (ed): Clinical Urography. An Atlas and Textbook of Urologic Imaging. Philadelphia, WB Saunders, 1990, pp 1472-1494.
226. Lang EK: Ureteral injuries. In Pollack HM (ed): Clinical Urography. An Atlas and Textbook of Urologic Imaging. Philadelphia, WB Saunders, 1990, pp 1495-1504.
227. Titton RL, Gervais DA, Boland GW, et al: Renal trauma: Radiologic evaluation and percutaneous treatment of nonvascular injuries. AJR 2002;178:1507-1511.

Vascular
228. Keogan MT, Kliewer MA, Hertzberg BS, et al: Renal resistance indexes: Variability in Doppler US measurement in a healthy population. Radiology 1996;199:165-169.
229. Middleton WD, Kellman GM, Leland Melson GL, et al: Post biopsy renal transplant arteriovenous fistulas: Color Doppler US characteristics. Radiology 1989; 171:253-257.
230. Mostbeck GH, Gossinger HD, Mallek R, et al: Effect of heart rate on Doppler measurements of resistive index in renal arteries. Radiology 1990;175:511-513.
231. Bude RO, Rubin JM, Adler RS: Power versus conventional color Doppler sonography: Comparison in the depiction of normal intrarenal vasculature. Radiology 1994; 192:777-780.
232. Erwin BC, Carroll BA, Walter JF, et al: Renal infarction appearing as an echogenic mass. AJR 1982;138:759-761.
233. Takebayashi S, Aida N, Matsui K: Arteriovenous malformations of the kidneys: Diagnosis and follow-up with color Doppler sonography in six patients. AJR 1991;157:991-995.
234. Hillman BJ: Imaging advances in the diagnosis of renovascular hypertension. AJR 1989;15:4-14.
235. Mitty HA, Shapiro RS, Parsons RB, et al: Renovascular hypertension. Radiol Clin North Am 1996; 34(5):1017-1036.
236. Stavros AT, Parker SH, Yakes WF, et al: Segmental stenosis of the renal artery: Pattern recognition of tardus and parvus abnormalities with duplex sonography. Radiology 1992;184:487-492.
237. Rene PC, Oliva VL, Bui BT, et al: Renal artery stenosis: Evaluation of Doppler US after inhibition of angiotensin-converting enzyme with captopril. Radiology 1995;196:675-679.
238. Dowling RJ, House MK, King PM, et al: Contrast-enhanced Doppler ultrasound for renal artery stenosis. Australas Radiol 1999;43(2):206-209.
239. Sharafuddin MJA, Raboi CA, Abu-Yousef M, et al: Renal artery stenosis: Duplex US and angioplasty and stent placement. Radiology 2001;220:168-173.
240. Fleshner N, Johnston KW: Repair of an autotransplant renal artery aneurysm: Case report and literature review. J Urol 1992;148:389-391.
241. Rosenfield AT, Zeman RK, Cronan JJ, et al: Ultrasound in experimental and clinical renal vein thrombosis. Radiology 1980;137:735-741.
242. Braun B, Weilemann LS, Weigand W: Ultrasonographic demonstration of renal vein thrombosis. Radiology 1981;138:157-158.
243. Platt JF, Ellis JH, Rubin JM: Intrarenal arterial Doppler sonography in the detection of renal vein thrombosis of the native kidney. AJR 1994;162:1367-1370.

Medical Diseases of the Genitourinary Tract
244. Haddad MC, Medawar WA, Hawary MM, et al: Perirenal fluid in renal parenchymal medical disease ('floating kidney'): Clinical significance and sonographic grading. Clin Radiol 2001;56(12):979-983.
245. Platt JF, Ruben JM, Ellis JH: Acute renal failure: Possible role of duplex Doppler US in distinction between acute prerenal failure and acute tubular necrosis. Radiology 1991;179:419-423.
246. Sty JR, Starshak RJ, Hubbard AM: Acute renal cortical necrosis in hemolytic uremic syndrome. J Clin Ultrasound 1983;11:175-178.
247. Rodriguez-de-Velasquez A, Yoder IC, Velasquez P, et al: Imaging the effects of diabetes on the genitourinary system. RadioGraphics 1995;15:1051-1068.
248. Urban BA, Fishman EK, Goldman SM, et al: CT evaluation of amyloidosis: Spectrum of disease. RadioGraphics 1993;13:1295-1308.

249. Gomes CM, Sanchez-Ortiz RF, Harris C, et al: Significance of hematuria in patients with interstitial cystitis: Review of radiographic and endoscopic findings. Urology 2001;57(2):262-265.

Neurogenic Bladder

250. Amis ES, Blavas JG: Neurogenic bladder simplified. Radiol Clin North Am 1991;29(3):571-580.

Ultrasound-Guided Intervention

251. Lee DI, McGinnis DE, Feld R, et al: Retroperitoneal laparoscopic cryoablation of small renal tumors: Intermediate results. Urology 2003;61(1):83-88.
252. Lantz EJ, Charboneau JW, Hallett JW, et al: Intraoperative color Doppler sonography during renal artery revascularization. AJR 1994;162:859-863.

253. Bush WH, Burnett LL, Gibbons RP: Needle tract seeding of renal cell carcinoma. AJR 1977;129:725-727.

Postsurgical Evaluation

254. Papanicolaou N, Harbury OL, Pfister RC: Fat-filled postoperative renal cortical defects: Sonographic and CT appearance. AJR 1988;151:503-505.
255. Millward SF, Lanctin HP, Lewandowski BJ, et al: Fat-filled postoperative renal pseudotumor: Variable appearance in ultrasonography images. Can Assoc Radiol J 1992; 43:116-119.
256. Ng C, Amis ES: Radiology of continent urinary diversion. Radiol Clin North Am 1991;29(3):557-570.

10

THE PROSTATE

Ants Toi / Robert L. Bree

Chapter Outline

ROLE OF TRANSRECTAL PROSTATE ULTRASOUND

Transrectal ultrasound (TRUS) of the prostate was initially thought to be the pivotal imaging test for the prostate, providing clinically important information of benign and malignant conditions, including benign prostatic hyperplasia (BPH), prostatitis, obstructive infertility and prostate cancer evaluation including screening, diagnosis, biopsy, staging, and monitoring of response to therapy. Over time, the strengths and limitations of TRUS have become better defined. Most patients today are referred for TRUS related to cancer evaluation and biopsy. The contemporary literature regarding TRUS is totally dominated by its role in the assessment of prostate cancer.[1] Transrectal ultrasound was initially considered a primary screening test for prostate cancer. This role has now been replaced by prostate specific antigen (PSA) and digital rectal examination.[2-4]

Occasional patient referrals relate to infertility and prostatitis.

HISTORY OF PROSTATE ULTRASOUND

The prostate is located deep in the pelvis and is sonographically accessible from a transabdominal, transvesical approach. Correlative studies have shown that volumetric evaluation of the prostate with suprapubic ultrasound is accurate and that a gram of prostate tissue is equivalent to 1 mL of volume, hence volume could be converted to weight. The usefulness of the **transvesical** examination for detection of prostate cancer is limited because most prostate cancers occur posteriorly and their small size makes identification difficult. Most of the current interest in prostatic imaging relates to **transrectal** techniques. In 1974, Japanese[5] investigators were the first to publish their experience with a radial scanner situated on a chair. The

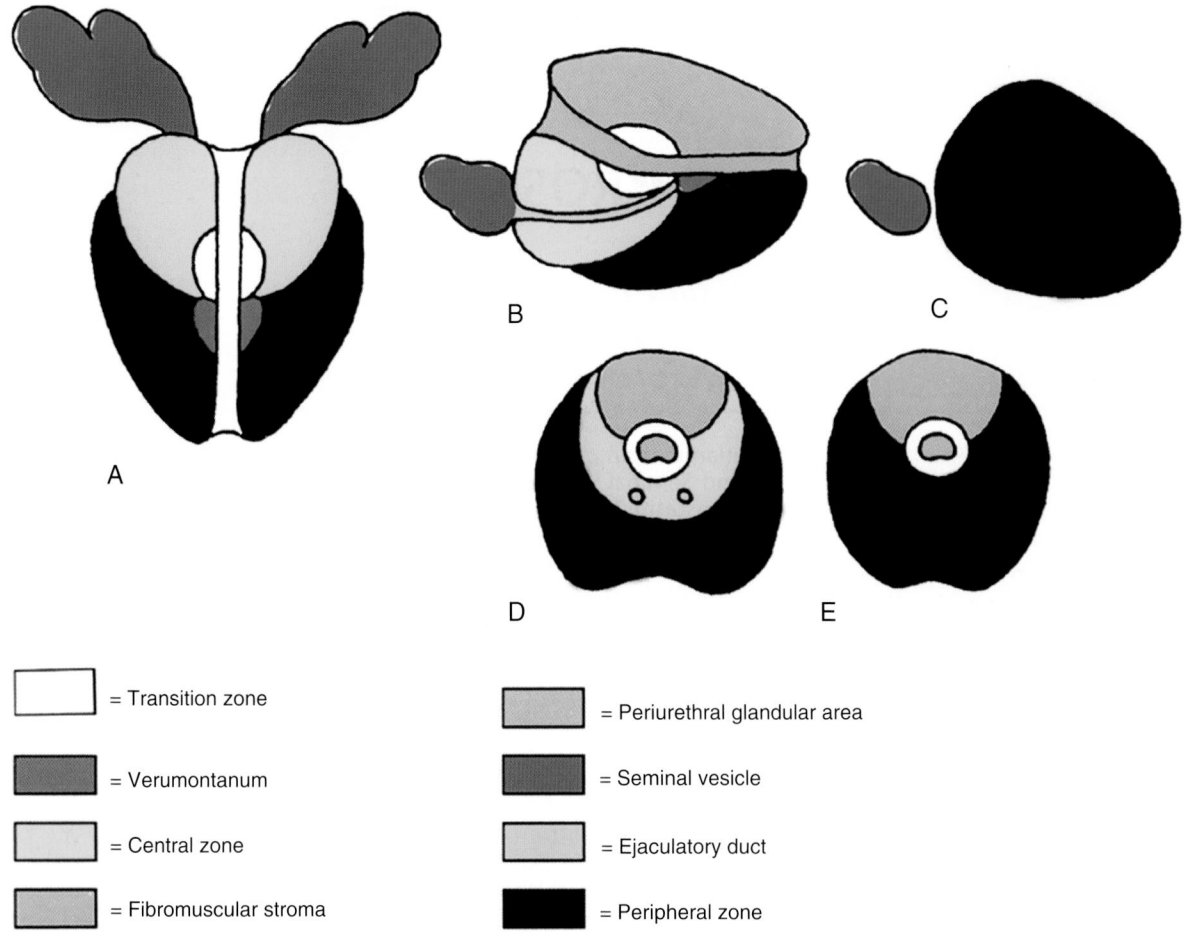

FIGURE 10-1. Diagram of prostate zonal anatomy. This is the anatomy in a young man as the transition zone (*white areas*) is small. The transition zone will undergo marked enlargement in older men with BPH. **A,** Coronal section midprostate level. **B,** Sagittal midline. **C,** Parasagittal section. **D,** Axial section through base. **E,** Axial section through apex.

☐ = Transition zone

■ = Verumontanum

▨ = Central zone

▨ = Fibromuscular stroma

▨ = Periurethral glandular area

■ = Seminal vesicle

▨ = Ejaculatory duct

■ = Peripheral zone

technique has evolved slowly since that time, with significant advances occurring with the development of gray-scale, real-time imaging, improved transducer crystal design, and, most recently, biplane probes that allow for prostatic assessment in both axial and longitudinal planes. Recently Doppler imaging techniques have been introduced.[6,7] Transrectal sonography, especially in the evaluation of cancer, should not be performed in isolation. It is important to have appropriate history, digital rectal examination results, and PSA results available before starting the examination.

GENERAL ANATOMY

Original textbook anatomic descriptions of the prostate referred to **lobar anatomy**, describing anterior, posterior, lateral, and median lobes. Although the concept of a median lobe bulging into the bladder may be useful in the evaluation of patients with benign prostatic hypertrophy, this lobar anatomy has not been useful in identification of carcinoma of the prostate.[1,8] Detailed

anatomic dissections of the prostate reveal **zonal anatomy**, whereby the prostate is divided into four glandular zones surrounding the prostatic urethra: the peripheral zone, transition zone, central zone, and the periurethral glandular area (Figs. 10-1, 10-2 and 10-3). In the normal young man's gland, however, sonography can rarely identify these zones unless a pathologic condition is present (see Fig. 10-2B and Fig. 10-4A). On sonography, it is more useful to separate the prostate into a peripheral or outer gland (peripheral zone + central zone) and inner gland (transition zone + anterior fibromuscular stroma + internal urethral sphincter) (Fig. 10-4A).[9-11]

The **peripheral zone**, the largest of the glandular zones, contains approximately 70% of the prostatic glandular tissue in a young man prior to onset of BPH and is the site for most prostate cancer. It surrounds the distal urethral segment and is separated from the transition zone and central zone by the **surgical capsule**, which is usually a hypoechoic line but may be echogenic, as corpora amylacea or calcifications frequently occur along this line. It is called the surgical capsule because, traditionally, urologists, at suprapubic resection or trans-

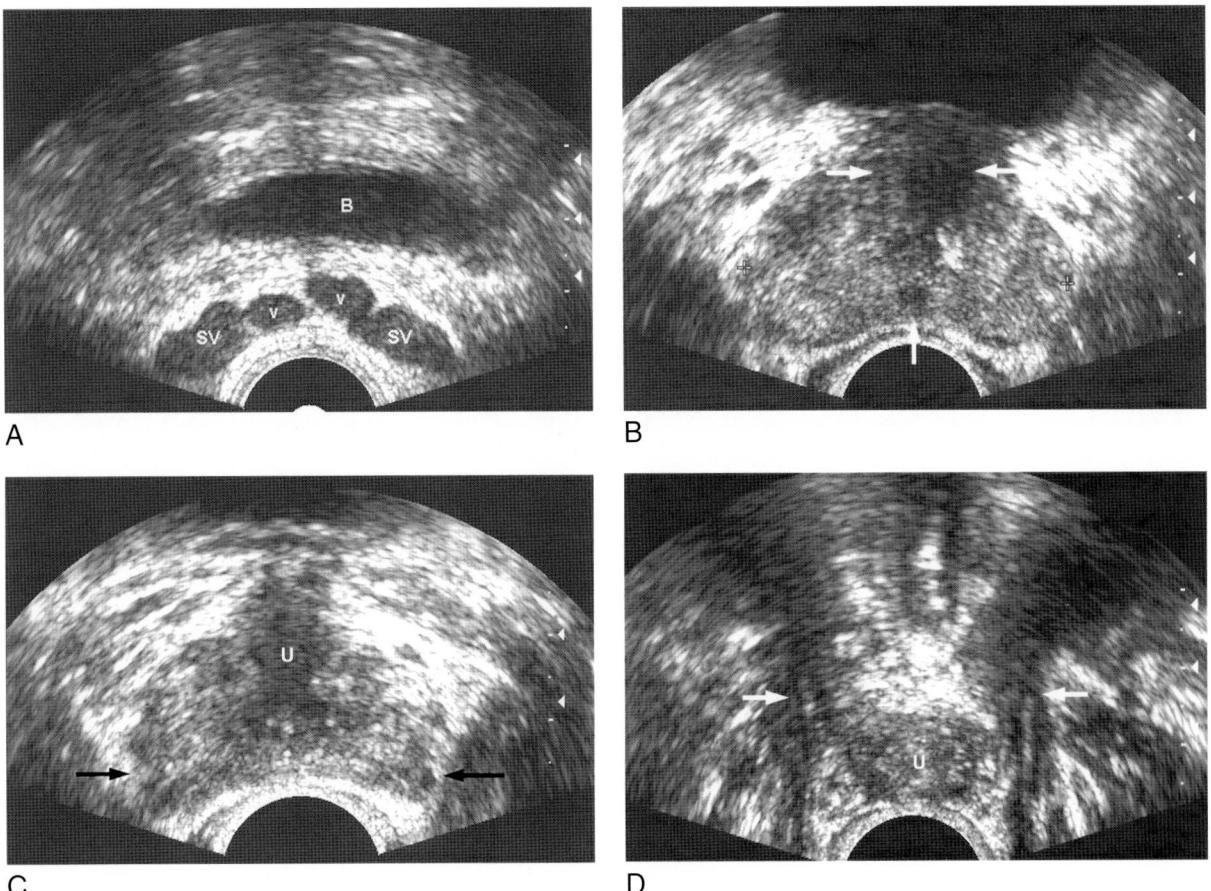

FIGURE 10-2. Axial sonograms of prostate. A, Transverse image above base showing the seminal vesicles (SV) and vas (V). **B,** Axial scan of prostate at midgland level. Note the normal hypoechoic muscular internal urethral sphincter (*horizontal arrows*) and the ejaculatory ducts (*vertical arrow*). **C,** Axial scan at lower third of prostate shows hypoechoic urethra (U). Most of the visible gland at this level is peripheral zone. Note the irregular outline at the posterolateral aspects (*arrows*), which is due to the entrance of the neurovascular bundles. **D,** Axial scan just below apex of prostate showing cross section of distal urethra (U). Pelvic sling muscles are visible (*arrows*).

urethral resection of the prostate (TURP), felt that they dissected to this line. The peripheral zone occupies the posterior, lateral, and apical regions of the prostate, extending somewhat anteriorly, much like an egg-cup holding the "egg" of the central gland (see Figs. 10-2A, 10-2B, 10-4A and 10-4B). The ducts of the peripheral zone enter the distal urethra.

The **transition zone** in the young man contains approximately 5% of the prostatic glandular tissue. It is seen as two small glandular areas located like saddle-bags adjacent to the proximal urethral sphincter, which is a muscular tube up to 2 cm in diameter. The transition zone is where benign prostatic hyperplasia originates. The ducts of the transition zone end in the proximal urethra at the level of the verumontanum, which bounds the transition zone caudally.

The **central zone** constitutes approximately 25% of the glandular tissue. It is located like a midline wedge at the prostatic base between the peripheral and transition zones. The ducts of the vas deferens and seminal vesicles enter the central zone, and the ejaculatory ducts pass through it as they go to the verumontanum (see Figs. 10-1, 10-2B, and 10-3A). The central zone is felt to be relatively resistant to disease processes because only 5% of prostate cancers start here. Central zone ducts terminate in the proximal urethra near the verumontanum. The periurethral glands form about 1% of the glandular volume. They are embedded in the longitudinal smooth muscle of the proximal urethra, also known as the internal prostatic sphincter (see Figs. 10-1, 10-2B, and 10-3A).[1,9,10]

Vascular Anatomy

Blood flow to the prostate is supplied by the prostaticovesical arteries arising from the internal iliac arteries on each side. These vessels then give rise to the prostatic artery and inferior vesical artery. The prostatic artery gives rise to the urethral and capsular arteries. The inferior vesical artery supplies the bladder base, seminal

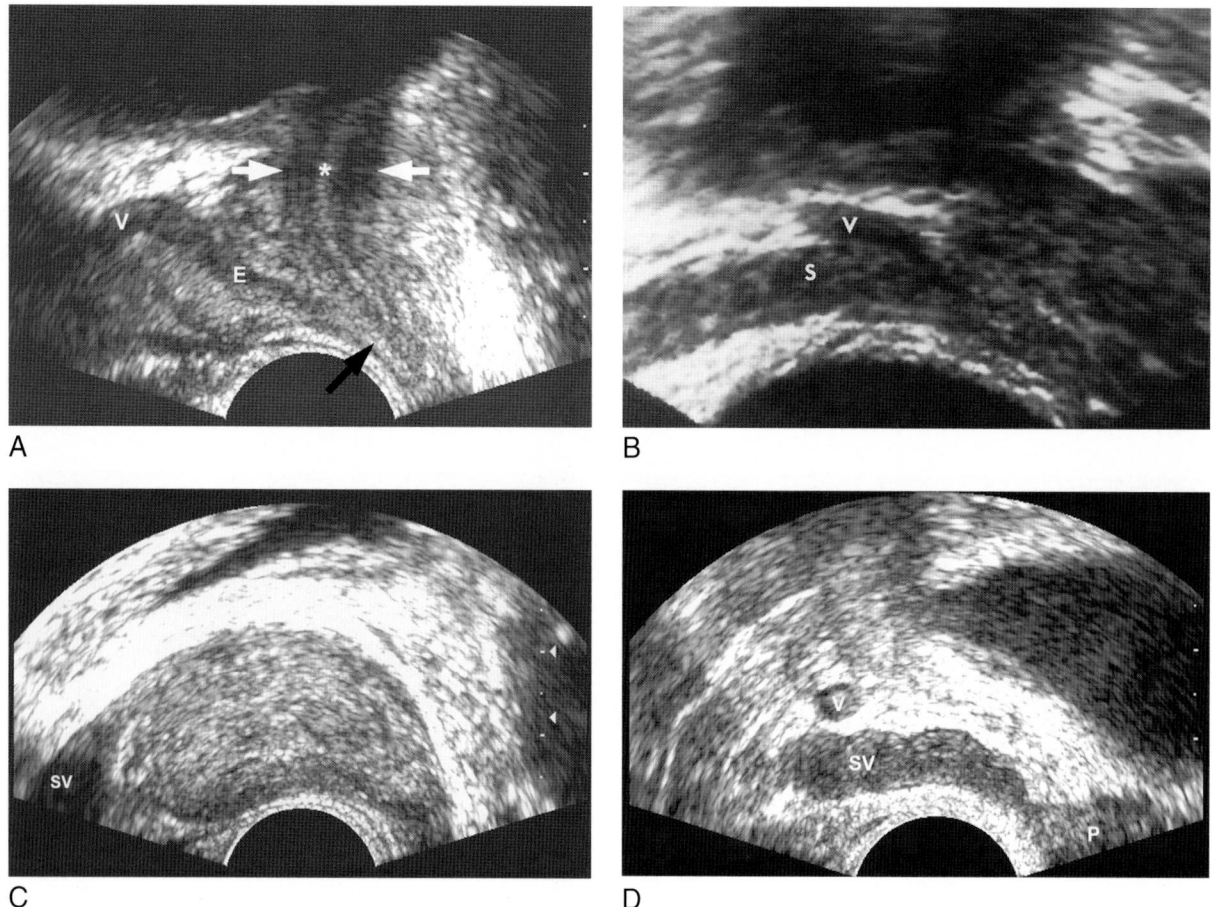

FIGURE 10-3. Sagittal views of prostate. A, Midsagittal view shows internal urethral sphincter (*arrows*), which contains the echogenic collapsed urethra (*). The ejaculatory ducts (E) course from the vas (V) to the verumontanum (*arrow*). **B,** Midsagittal view at base shows the vas (V) and adjacent seminal vesicles (SV) as they enter the prostate. **C,** Parasagittal view shows the lateral prostate, which is homogeneous and isoechoic and composed almost totally of peripheral zone tissue. Seminal vesicle (SV). **D,** Parasagittal view cephalad to the prostate shows the normal seminal vesicles (SV) and vas (V) in cross-section above the prostate (P).

vesicles, and ureter. The urethral artery supplies about one third of the prostate, whereas the capsular branches supply the remainder of the gland.[12]

With color Doppler, particularly using the power mode, the prostate is a moderately vascular structure. The capsular and urethral arteries are easily seen, and branches to the inner gland and peripheral zone may be prominent (Fig. 10-5). It is suggested that Doppler depiction of prostate vascular density varies with patient position, the dependent side being more vascular.[13]

Scan Orientation

Using a transrectal approach, various scanning orientations have been proposed. The most commonly used convention illustrated is similar to that for transabdominal sonography (see Figs. 10-1, 10-2, and 10-3). As if standing at the foot of a supine patient, looking up, the rectum is displayed at the bottom of the screen with the ultrasound beam emanating from within the rectum. On transverse imaging, the anterior abdominal wall is at the top of the screen with the right side of the patient on the left side of the image (see Fig. 10-2) In a sagittal plane, the anterior abdominal wall is again located at the top of the screen, and the head of the patient is on the left side of the image (see Fig. 10-3).

The most commonly used commercially available probes fire from the end and can be used for both transrectal and transvaginal imaging; longitudinal and axial scans are obtained by rotating the probe through 90-degrees. The sagittal and axial images are relatively more oblique than those obtained with side-firing probes. Therefore, axial images near the base of the gland are considered semicoronal in orientation. In addition, the prostate appears more elongated when imaged with an end-firing probe than when a true axial orientation is presented (see Fig. 10-2B). With end-firing probes, the top of the image is in an oblique direction toward the head, and the bottom of the image is in an oblique direction toward the feet. Because of these differences in probe design, the anatomy that is depicted may vary from machine to machine.

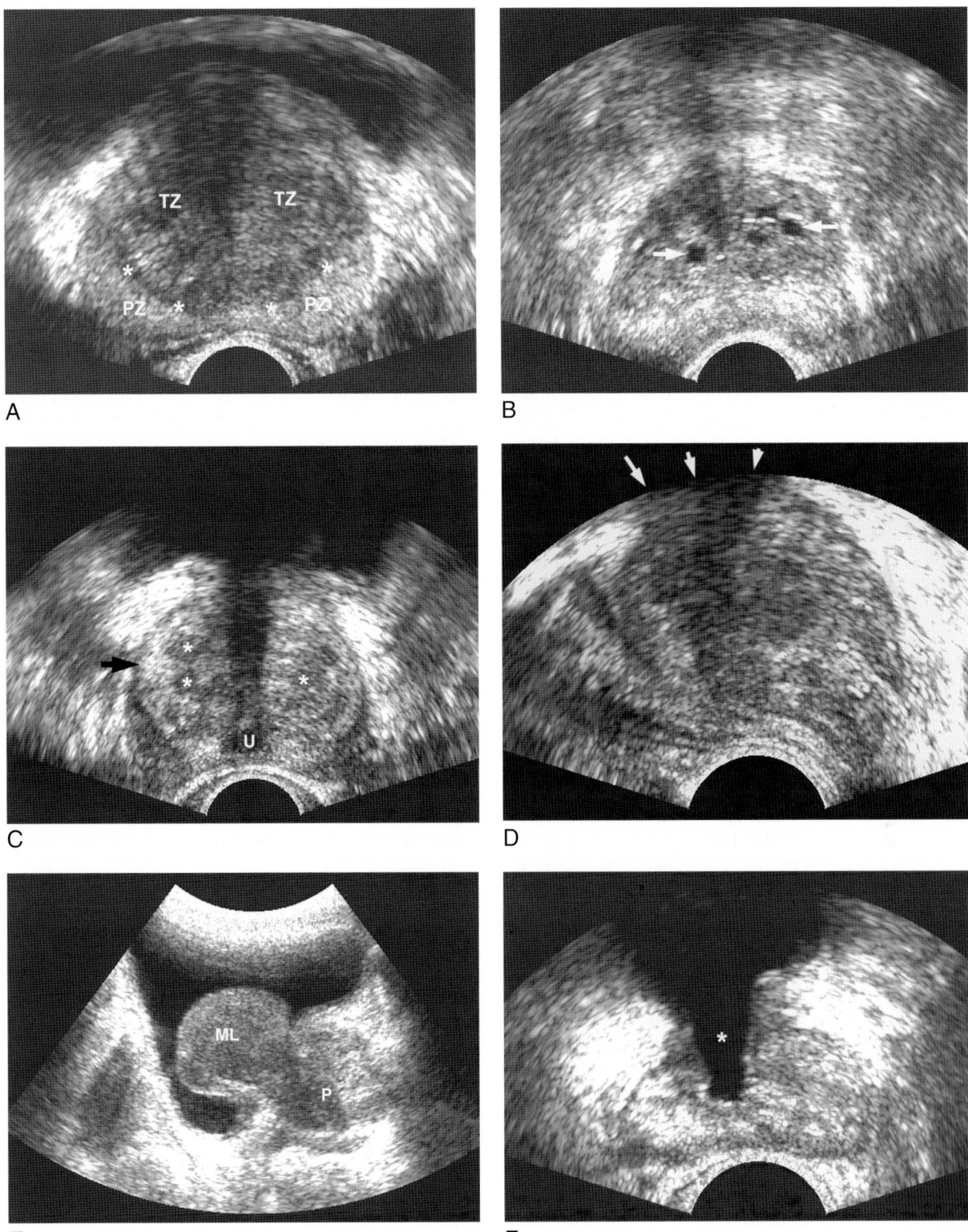

FIGURE 10-4. Benign prostatic hyperplasia (BPH). A, Axial view shows the markedly enlarged, slightly hypoechoic, **transition zone** (TZ), which compresses the more echogenic peripheral zone (PZ). Their interface is the surgical capsule (*). The region inside the surgical capsule (transition zone) is also called the "inner gland" and the region outside the surgical capsule the "outer gland," which is composed of peripheral zone plus central zone. **B, Benign degenerative cysts** in the transition zone (*arrows*) have no clinical significance. **C, Heterogeneous nature of hyperplasia in the transition zone**. Both hyperechoic (*black arrow*) and hypoechoic (*) areas are present. This makes cancer detection difficult. Urethra (U). **D, Prominent median lobe enlargement may be cut off and escape detection**. Sagittal view shows pitfall if the field-of-view is not deep enough (*arrows*). **E, Massive enlargement of the median lobe (ML) protruding into the bladder.** Transvesical midsagittal scan. Prostate (P). Evaluation for symptoms of prostatism is better done transvesically than transrectally with transrectal ultrasound (TRUS). **F, Typical transurethral resection of prostate (TURP) surgical defect.** Axial view (*).

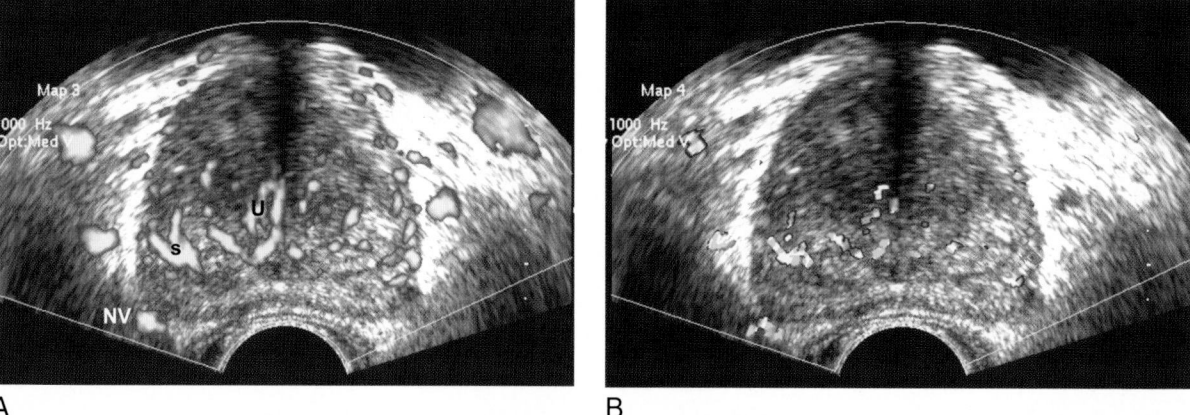

FIGURE 10-5. Normal Doppler anatomy in a patient with moderate BPH. A, Axial power Doppler shows the urethral vessels (U); some vessels along the surgical capsule (S); and the neurogenic bundle on one side (NV) with an average degree of vascularity. Note the large vessels, mostly veins, outside the prostate. Care must be taken when biopsy is performed outside the prostate to avoid injury to these vessels. **B,** Color flow Doppler scan for comparison. Vascular density is slightly harder to evaluate because the amount of color is more dependent on machine settings than it is with power Doppler.

Axial and Coronal Anatomy

The **seminal vesicles** are paired, relatively hypoechoic, multiseptated structures cephalad to the base of the prostate. (see Fig. 10-2A). They usually measure about 1 cm front to back, but occasionally can be thicker in normal men. In the axial plane, the anterior urethra and its surrounding smooth muscle and glandular area appear relatively hypoechoic and can be quite prominent measuring 2 cm in diameter. Because the **sphincter** is muscular, it frequently is very hypoechoic, especially in young men (see Figs. 10-2B and 10-3A). It can mimic the appearance of a TURP. Those uninitiated at transrectal and pelvic ultrasound can mistake the sphincter for tumor because both can be hypoechoic. The inner gland is separated from the peripheral zone by the surgical capsule (see Fig. 10-4A). The capsule becomes very obvious as BPH occurs and enlarges the transition zone. Often **corpora amylacea**, seen as echogenic foci, develop along the surgical capsule (Fig. 10-6C). Frequently, in young men, the separation between the zones on transverse imaging is only positional, and no distinct structures will be present to clarify the anatomy (see Fig. 10-2B). Typically, the peripheral zone is more uniform in texture and slightly more echogenic than the transition zone. The peripheral zone echogenicity is the standard for echogenicity in the prostate and is defined to be isoechoic. Echogenicity in other areas of the gland is compared to that of the peripheral zone.

Sagittal Anatomy

The most parasagittal images of the gland in the sagittal plane show **peripheral zone tissue** with uniform echogenicity. With BPH, the **transition zone** may extend laterally, compressing the peripheral zone posteriorly (see Figs. 10-4A and C). At the base of the gland, the **seminal vesicles** immediately adjoin the central and peripheral zone (see Fig. 10-3A). The entrance of the seminal vesicles and vas deferens into the **central zone** produces an invaginated extraprostatic space, which is one pathway for cancer to spread from the prostate into the seminal vesicle. The **ejaculatory ducts** can usually be seen coursing through the central zone from the seminal vesicles and joining the angle of the urethra at the verumontanum (see Fig. 10-3A). The **urethra** and surrounding glands and smooth muscle are most often hypoechoic, especially in young men (see Figs. 10-2A and 10-3A). On sagittal imaging, the anterior fibromuscular stroma may be visible anterior to the urethra but it generally just blends into the internal urethral sphincter and transition zone (see Fig. 10-3A).

Prostate "Capsule"

On transverse and sagittal imaging, the border of the prostate with the periprostatic fat appears sharply defined, except at the posterolateral margins where the neurovascular bundle enters the prostate and makes the margin look ragged (see Fig. 10-2C). Histologically, the prostate does not have a true membranous capsule but rather just condensed connective tissue through which the vessels and nerves course. Posteriorly, the periprostatic tissue is fibroadipose, and no true surrounding capsule exists.[14] In addition to the absence of a well-defined capsule, the presence of prominent vessels in the periprostatic soft tissues may make assessment of capsular integrity difficult in patients with prostate cancer (see Fig. 10-2C). At the apex of the gland, the rectourethralis muscle, the rectum, the urethra, and the prostate gland form a **fatty trapezoid area** that is an area of potential weakness for extraprostatic spread of cancer.[1,11]

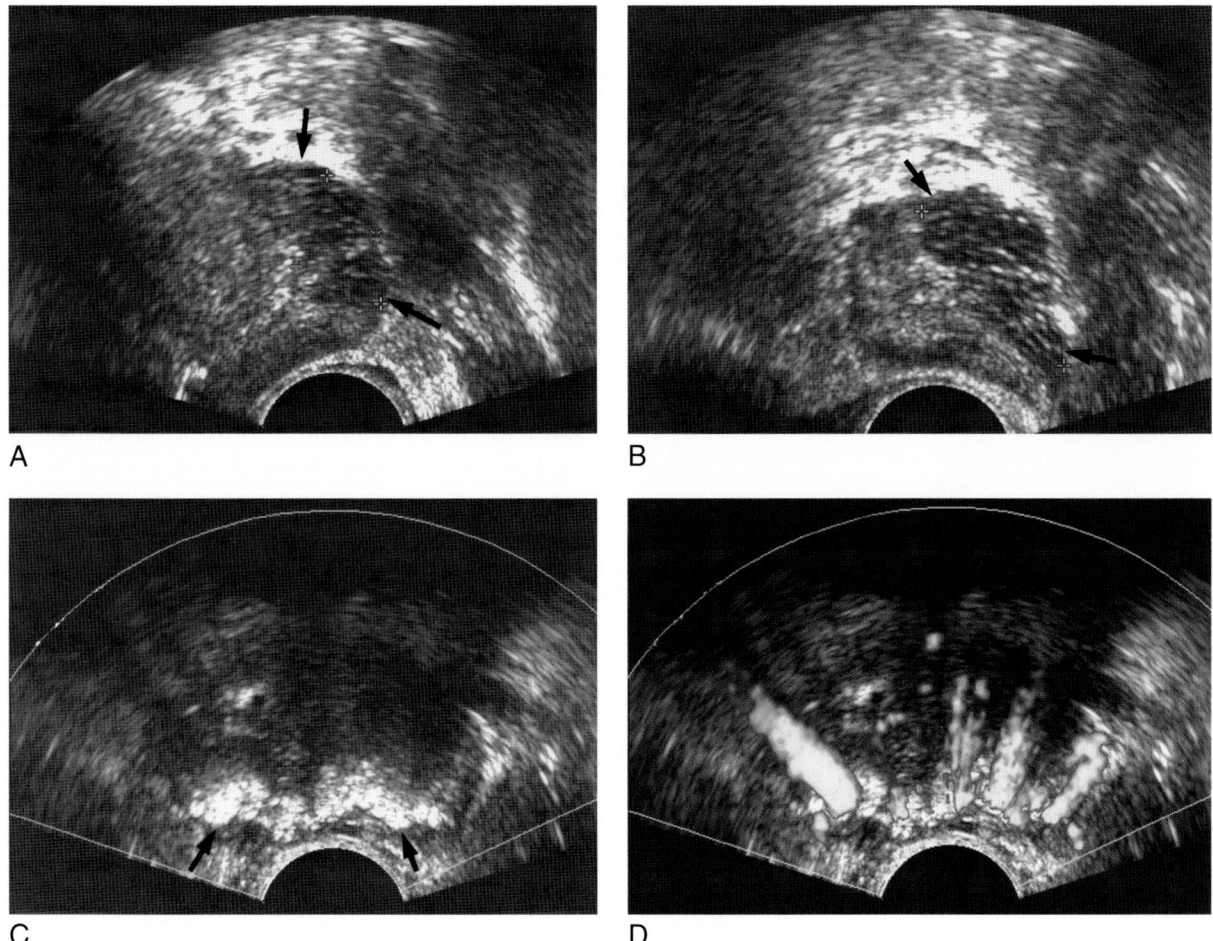

FIGURE 10-6. Normal anatomic variants. A, Axial view with **benign glandular ectasia,** seen as a peripheral hypoechoic area containing multiple radially oriented tubes. This should not be mistaken for cancer (*arrows*). **B,** Parasagittal view of **benign ectatic glands** (*arrows*). **C,** Axial view shows extensive echogenic material, both **calcifications and corpora amylacea** (*arrows*), along the surgical capsule and peripheral zone. This has no clinical significance, is usually not palpable, and hinders ultrasonic visibility. **D, Calcifications** cause extensive Doppler noise artifact in same patient.

EQUIPMENT AND TECHNIQUES

Most modern ultrasound machines have transrectal probes that have been developed to perform ultrasound of the prostate and rectum. Probes should be at least 5 MHz, and most are as high as 7 or 8 MHz. Probe design and biopsy attachments vary. It is best to use the thinnest probe that provides adequate imaging because there are a number of men with tight anal sphincters who cannot tolerate large probes.

Transducer Design

Following the initial development of linear array and rotating radial probe designs, manufacturers have now developed probes for biplane transrectal prostate scanning with either a single probe or multiple probes

on the same machine.[1] A convenient probe design is an **end-viewing transducer,** which allows for multiplanar imaging in semicoronal and axial projections (Fig. 10-7). Other probe designs include **360 degree radial** scanners paired with end-viewing probes for a sagittal image and paired side-viewing axial and sagittal probes. The advantages of end-viewing probe designs include patient convenience, ease of use, and biopsy capability at the time of the diagnostic examination.

Probes must be covered during the examination with condoms that have been developed to fit individual probes (see Fig. 10-7). Because they are often made of latex, nonlatex covers should be used in patients who have significant latex allergies. Between uses, the probes are washed and then soaked in an antiseptic solution following the manufacturer's recommendations.

Some probes use a **water path** between the crystal and the rectal mucosa. This decreases the near-field artifact

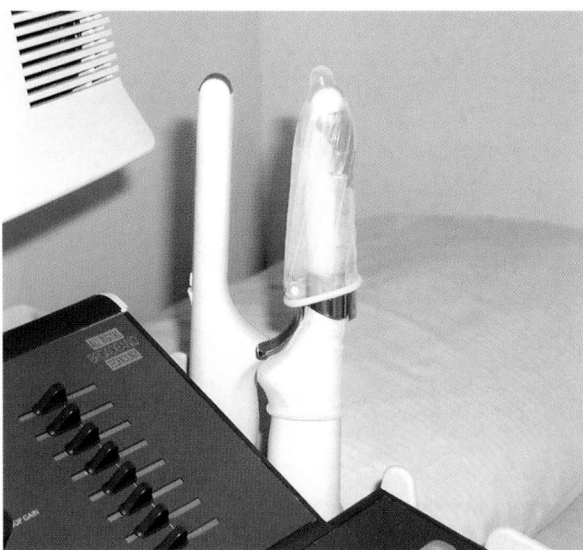

FIGURE 10-7. Typical ultrasound probes for transrectal and intracavitary work. The right probe is covered with inner condom, biopsy guide, and outer condom. Because most men present for biopsy, we start the examination with the biopsy guide in place.

and can be useful for examining the rectal wall itself or structures close to the rectal wall, but can create artifacts if air is allowed into the system.

Scanning Technique

In most instances, the patient lies in a **left lateral decubitus** position for the scan. Some examiners prefer a lithotomy position, particularly if the examination is done in conjunction with other urologic procedures. Rectal cleansing with laxatives or a self-administered enema is routinely used before scanning. It is routine to perform a digital rectal examination before probe insertion to ensure that there are no rectal abnormalities that could interfere with safe probe insertion and to correlate the imaging with palpable abnormalities. Using adequate lubrication, the probe is gently inserted into the rectum. End-firing probes allow imaging of the passage to facilitate easy insertion.

When examining the prostate gland, a systematic approach is necessary (see Figs. 10-2 and 10-3). If one begins in the transverse or semicoronal plane, the seminal vesicles are seen at the cephalad portion of the prostate gland above the prostatic base. These paired structures may be different in size and shape. They are generally hypoechoic and irregular and are usually symmetrical. Continuing in the transverse or semi-coronal plane, the base of the prostate is then examined with demonstration of the central zone, transition zone, and periurethral glandular area. The anterior fibro-muscular stroma is hyperechoic. In a semicoronal plane, the periurethral area may be very hypoechoic and simulate

a transurethral resection defect. The urethra and the ejaculatory ducts may be identified. At the level of the verumontanum, the ejaculatory ducts and urethra merge. Near the apex of the gland, most of the tissue is in the peripheral zone. It is often difficult in the normal young man's gland to separate the peripheral zone from the inner gland. With benign prostatic hyperplasia, the surgical capsule becomes more evident, separating the peripheral and central gland (see Figs. 10-4A and C).

By rotating the probe to the sagittal plane, the gland is systematically surveyed from right to midline to left (see Fig. 10-3). **Measurements** are taken as follows: **maximal transverse width** (right to left), **antero-posterior** (anterior midline to rectal surface), **length** (maximal head to foot). Glandular volumes can be estimated by volumetric techniques performed sonographically.[15] **Prostate volume** is calculated with the oblate spheroid formula: volume = $1.57(W \times AP \times L)$. Repeatability of the volume measurement is not perfect and most practitioners are only able to repeat within ±10%. Prostate volume can be converted to weight because the specific gravity of prostate tissue is about 1, thus 1 mL of prostate tissue is equivalent to 1 g. More precise and repeatable measurements can be obtained with the step-section technique, but this requires special side-firing probes and external stepping equipment.

Color or power Doppler is routinely used, particularly when cancer is suspected and biopsy is contemplated. Vascular density may be easier to appreciate with power Doppler than with color Doppler (see Fig. 10-5). Abnormal vascularity is not specific and can be seen with hypertrophy, inflammation, and cancer.

BENIGN CONDITIONS
Normal Variants

Benign ductal ectasia is seen in older men who develop atrophy and dilation of peripheral prostatic ducts. These are visible, either as single or grouped radially oriented 1 to 2 mm diameter tubular structures in the peripheral zone, starting at the capsule and radiating toward the urethra. When grouped, they can form a hypoechoic area that the unwary practitioner may mistake for prostate cancer. They have no clinical significance (see Figs. 10-6A and B).

Prostatic calcifications and corpora amylacea are a normal variant and are seen more commonly with advancing years. Both form bright echogenic foci or areas in the prostate. Corpora amylacea are simply proteinaceous debris in dilated prostatic ducts. They are most commonly seen in periurethral glands and along the surgical capsule but can occur anywhere in the prostate. When very dense, they can cause sound attenuation and prevent sonographic examination of the anterior parts of the prostate and also create tremendous

Doppler artifact (see Figs. 10-6C and D). Subclinical infections, inflammation, and atrophy may contribute to their formation. They have no clinical significance and even if very dense, they are usually not palpable. Peripheral zone calcifications should not be accepted as a cause for palpable firmness or nodules. Patients with palpable abnormality need further evaluation with biopsy.

Benign Prostatic Hyperplasia

Enlargement of the prostate gland is a common cause of symptoms in older men. The weight of the gland in a younger patient is approximately 20 g. From age 50, the doubling time of the weight of the prostate is approximately 10 years. Prostate glands weighing more than 40 g are generally considered enlarged in older men.[16]

The **sonographic appearance** of benign prostatic hyperplasia is varied and depends on the histopathologic changes. The typical sonographic feature of BPH is enlargement of the inner gland, which remains relatively hypoechoic relative to the peripheral zone. Inhomogeneity is common and with BPH, the transition zone can exhibit diffuse enlargement or distinct hypo-, iso- or hyperechoic nodules (see Fig. 10-4).[1] The specific echo pattern depends on the admixture of glandular and stromal elements because nodules may be fibroblastic, fibromuscular, muscular, hyperadenomatous, or fibroadenomatous.[1,17]

Other sonographic features of BPH include calcifications and well-circumscribed, rounded hyperechoic or hypoechoic nodules and degenerative or retention cysts in the transition zone (see Figs. 10-4B and C and Fig. 10-9A). Because of distortion of the gland in patients with BPH, these nodules may appear to be in the peripheral zone when they actually lie in the transition zone. Well-circumscribed transition zone hypoechoic nodules are virtually always benign.[18] BPH and hyperplastic nodules are generally felt to be confined to the transition zone. Occasionally, they can occur in the peripheral zone as an isoechoic nodule with a well-circumscribed halo very similar in appearance to those seen in the transition zone. When BPH nodules occur in the peripheral zone they are palpable as a firm nodule, and they should undergo biopsy to confirm their benign nature to avoid continuing concern.[19]

Prostate size correlates poorly with urinary obstruction and large prostates are often seen in asymptomatic patients, whereas other patients with severe voiding difficulties due to prostatic obstruction may have small glands. Also, remember that urinary dysfunction is multifactorial and can arise from abnormalities of the CNS, spine, bladder, prostate, and urethra. Patients with urinary dysfunction need evaluation of all these areas and not just the prostate. Investigation of the patient with symptoms of prostatism is best done transvesically.

Transvesical ultrasound can adequately assess prostate size and presence of median lobe enlargement. It also can aid in evaluating bladder volume and postvoid residual, bladder wall character, trabeculation, diverticula, tumors, and calculi. Transvesical ultrasound is useful in detecting hydronephrosis and masses in the kidneys and ureters (see Figs. 10-4D and E). Transrectal ultrasound plays little role in evaluation of BPH unless there is a clinical concern for prostate cancer. TRUS, however, should be employed if it is important to monitor gland size in patients undergoing drug therapy for prostatism because transrectal measurements are more accurate than those taken transvesically.

Patients who have TURP initially have a large surgical defect, but this rapidly decreases in size as the gland collapses into the defect. This can surprise unwary urologists who feel they have removed considerably more tissue than the visible defect suggests. Patients, however, are uniformly symptom free following these procedures, suggesting that the amount of prostatic tissue removed does not necessarily correlate with the success of the procedure (see Fig. 10-4F).

Inflammation of the Prostate and Seminal Vesicles (Prostatitis)

With the major emphasis of TRUS on diagnosis of carcinoma of the prostate, there have been few studies analyzing its usefulness in inflammatory diseases. There is a significant population incidence of acute and chronic prostatitis with varied symptoms. **Chronic prostatitis** may be associated with specific pathogens such as *Chlamydia* or *Mycoplasma* organisms. If no known etiologic factor can be found, the condition is then termed **prostatodynia**. The diagnosis is made clinically.[20] Patients with active prostatitis or abscess are in considerable pain and the rectum and prostate are very tender. Digital rectal examinations must be performed very gently.

Prostate sonography is normal in most patients with prostatitis. Sonographic findings that have been described with chronic prostatitis include focal masses of different degrees of echogenicity, ejaculatory duct calcifications, capsular thickening or irregularity, and periurethral glandular irregularity (Fig. 10-8). Dilation of periprostatic veins and distended seminal vesicles have been described with chronic prostatitis or prostatodynia. Sonographic-guided biopsy has been used to identify chronic prostatitis and to confirm the presence of bacteria.[21,22]

Chronic granulomatous prostatitis can mimic the sonographic features of prostatic carcinoma and show diffuse large and small hypoechoic zones or a solitary hypoechoic lesion. Patients undergoing **bacillus Calmette-Guérin** (BCG) instillation into the bladder to treat bladder cancer are at risk of development of granulomatous prostatitis (see Figs. 10-8C and D).[23]

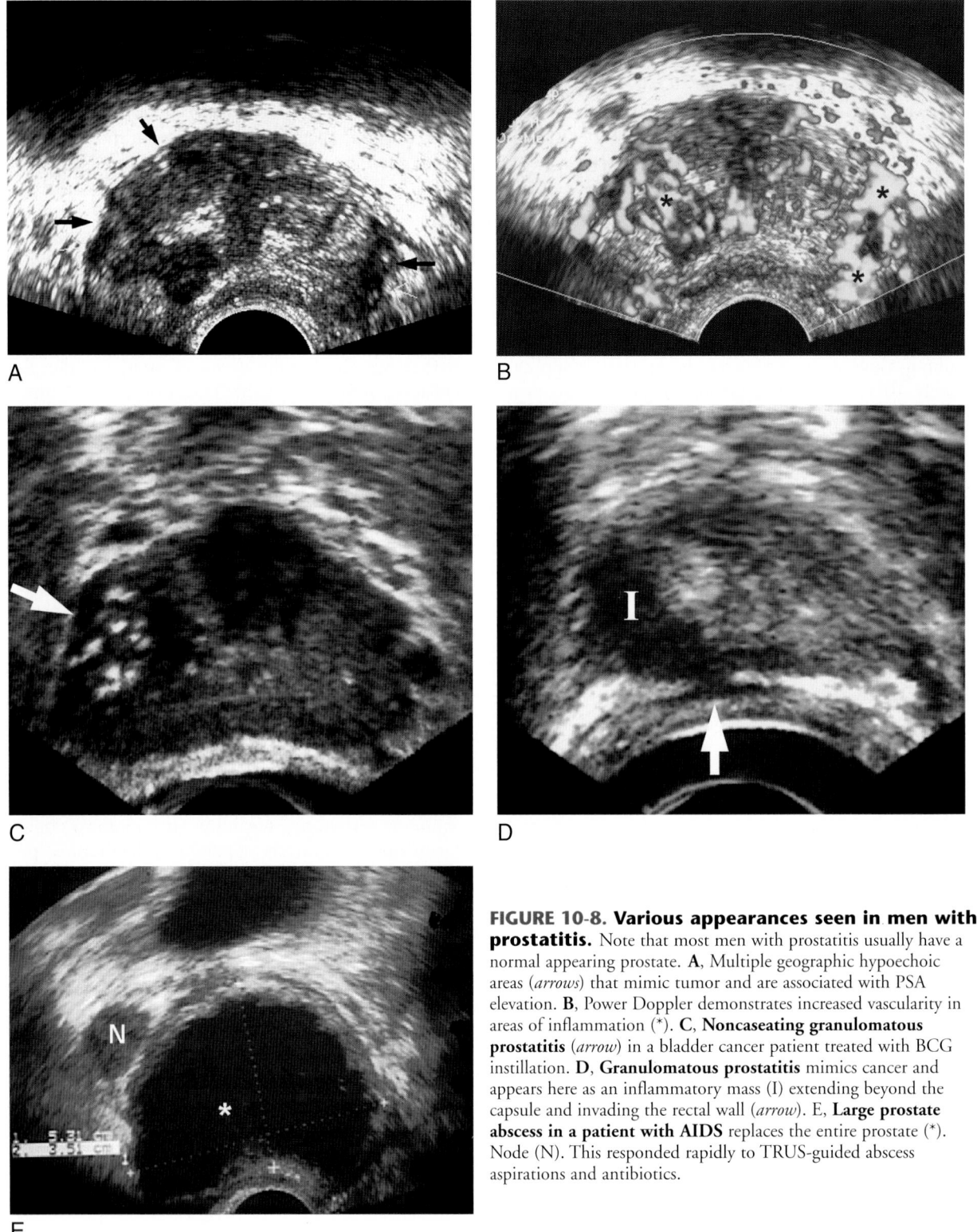

FIGURE 10-8. Various appearances seen in men with prostatitis. Note that most men with prostatitis usually have a normal appearing prostate. **A,** Multiple geographic hypoechoic areas (*arrows*) that mimic tumor and are associated with PSA elevation. **B,** Power Doppler demonstrates increased vascularity in areas of inflammation (*). **C, Noncaseating granulomatous prostatitis** (*arrow*) in a bladder cancer patient treated with BCG instillation. **D, Granulomatous prostatitis** mimics cancer and appears here as an inflammatory mass (I) extending beyond the capsule and invading the rectal wall (*arrow*). **E, Large prostate abscess in a patient with AIDS** replaces the entire prostate (*). Node (N). This responded rapidly to TRUS-guided abscess aspirations and antibiotics.

The roll of TRUS is limited in patients with **acute prostatitis**. Physical examination and placing the probe in the rectum are often difficult because of pain. Ultrasound may demonstrate significant abnormality, mimicking carcinoma. In general, the glands are hypoechoic and often show several geographic strikingly hypoechoic areas. As with other infections, color Doppler shows a very vascular focus in areas of prostatitis, mimicking carcinoma (see Fig. 10-8). Ultrasound can lead to an early diagnosis of a prostatic abscess. In a patient with acute prostatitis refractory to treatment, the development of an anechoic mass with or without internal echoes suggests the presence of an **abscess** (see Fig. 10-8E). Sonographic-guided aspiration and instillation of antibiotic into the abscess may be performed using a transrectal or transperineal approach.[24,25]

Prostatic and Seminal Vesicle Cysts

The most common cysts are degenerative or retention cysts in hyperplastic nodules in the transition zone. These have no clinical significance (Figs. 10-4B and 10-9A). Most patients with congenital cystic lesions in the prostate and seminal vesicle will be asymptomatic. Occasionally, these cysts can cause symptoms or become infected, particularly if they are large.

Congenital abnormalities are common in and around the prostate and seminal vesicles. The Müllerian tubercle gives rise to the prostatic utricle, a midline, small, blind-ending pouch that is situated near the summit of the colliculus seminalis, which is a mound on the posterior wall of the prostatic urethra. **Prostatic utricle cysts** are caused by dilation of the prostatic utricle (see Fig. 10-9B and C). Utricle cysts can be associated with unilateral renal agenesis and rarely contain spermatozoa. Utricle cysts are always in the midline and are usually small but can become quite large, measuring several centimeters in diameter (see Fig. 10-9B and C). **Müllerian duct cysts** may arise from remnants of the Müllerian duct. Müllerian duct cysts may extend laterally to the midline and can be large. They have no other associations and never contain spermatozoa. Like utricle cysts, they have a teardrop shape with the pointed end of the teardrop pointed toward the verumontanum, a thick visible wall, and occasional mural or contained calcifications (see Fig. 10-9E).[26,27] **Ejaculatory duct cysts** are usually small and probably represent cystic dilation of the ejaculatory duct, possibly as a result of obstruction. Alternatively, they may be diverticula of the duct. They tend to be fusiform in shape and are typically pointed at both ends. These cysts contain spermatozoa when aspirated. They can be associated with infertility and may be seen in patients with a low sperm count. They may cause perineal pain.[26,28]

Seminal vesicle cysts, when large and solitary, may be associated with ipsilateral renal agenesis. This is the result of a Wolffian duct anomaly because the Wolffian duct also gives rise to the ureter (Fig. 10-10C). Affected patients may benefit from aspiration when cysts are large and symptomatic.[27,28]

Infertility

Infertility is defined as failure to achieve pregnancy after one year of regular unprotected intercourse; it affects about 15% of couples. Male factors are solely responsible in about 20% of couples and contributory in another 30% to 40%. When male infertility is present, it is usually—but not always—detected by semen analysis. The American Urological Association has defined best practice policies for investigating male infertility.[29]

Transrectal sonography is indicated in azoospermic (lacking sperm in the ejaculate) patients with palpable vasa and low ejaculatory volume to evaluate for ejaculatory duct obstruction and anomalies (see Fig. 10-10). Only about 1% to 2% of infertile men have obstructive causes. Seminal vesicles over 1.5 cm in AP diameter, dilated ejaculatory ducts, and midline cysts can suggest obstruction. Absence of the vasa is a clinical diagnosis achieved by examining the scrotum. There is a strong association of bilateral absence of the vas with the presence of at least one cystic fibrosis (CFTR) gene.

Transrectal ultrasound findings in infertile men with low-volume azoospermia include normal appearances (25%), bilateral absence of vas deferens (34%), bilateral occlusion of the vas deferens, seminal vesicles, and ejaculatory ducts by calcification or fibrosis (16%), unilateral absence of the vas deferens (11%), obstructing cysts of the seminal vesicles, ejaculatory ducts, or prostate (9%), and ductal obstruction due to calculi (4%). Ultrasound is preferred to vasography, which can cause iatrogenic ductal injury. MRI is also being used. Surgically correctable causes of infertility are confined to lesions involving the distal two-thirds of the ejaculatory ducts and include cysts, fibrosis, and calcifications.[30]

Hematospermia

Hematospermia refers to blood in the seminal fluid. Acute blood is red, but old blood becomes dark brown. Hematospermia most commonly results from nonspecific inflammation in the prostate or seminal structures and resolves spontaneously over several weeks. It is rarely associated with any significant urologic pathology. Further evaluation is indicated if it persists, and investigation should be done to exclude tumors of the prostate and bladder and infection, including tuberculosis. Prostate biopsy commonly causes iatrogenic hematospermia that lasts several weeks to months and appears as dark seminal fluid discoloration.

TRUS should be the first imaging modality used to investigate men with hematospermia.[31,32] Possible causes

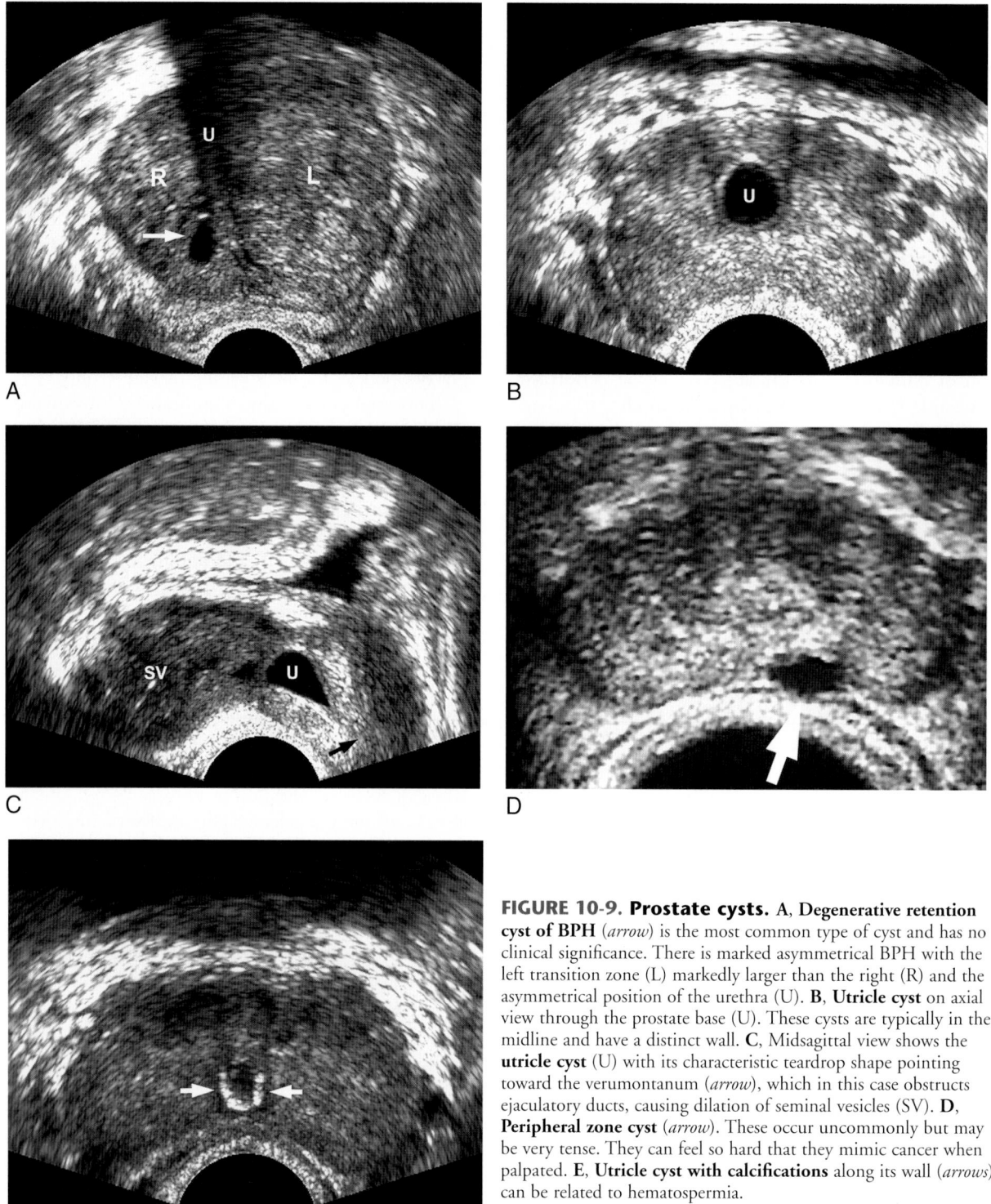

FIGURE 10-9. Prostate cysts. A, Degenerative retention **cyst of BPH** (*arrow*) is the most common type of cyst and has no clinical significance. There is marked asymmetrical BPH with the left transition zone (L) markedly larger than the right (R) and the asymmetrical position of the urethra (U). **B, Utricle cyst** on axial view through the prostate base (U). These cysts are typically in the midline and have a distinct wall. **C,** Midsagittal view shows the **utricle cyst** (U) with its characteristic teardrop shape pointing toward the verumontanum (*arrow*), which in this case obstructs ejaculatory ducts, causing dilation of seminal vesicles (SV). **D, Peripheral zone cyst** (*arrow*). These occur uncommonly but may be very tense. They can feel so hard that they mimic cancer when palpated. **E, Utricle cyst with calcifications** along its wall (*arrows*) can be related to hematospermia.

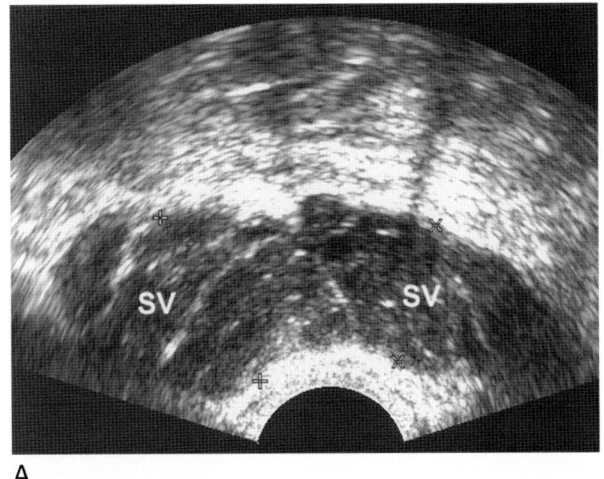

A

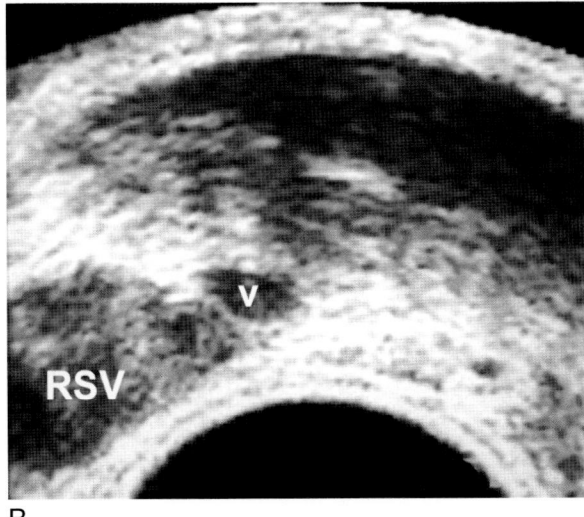

B

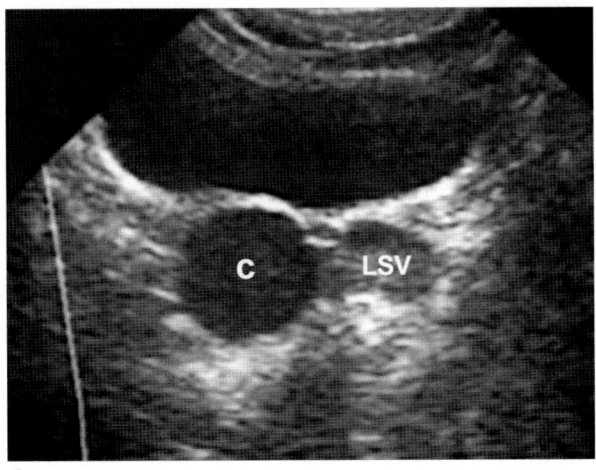

C

FIGURE 10-10. Infertility. A, Dilated seminal vesicles (SV) over 1.5 cm. This is presumptive evidence of mechanical obstruction to the ejaculatory ducts that may cause infertility. **B, Unilateral agenesis of the left seminal vesicle and vas.** Only the right side is intact (RSV, V). **C, Unilateral right seminal vesicle cyst** (C) at transvesical scan. This patient also had absence of the ipsilateral right kidney. Left seminal vesicle (LSV).

of hematospermia that can be seen with transrectal and Doppler ultrasound include prostatic and seminal vesicle cysts, seminal vesicle or ejaculatory calculi, and vascular malformations (see Fig. 10-9E).[33,34]

PROSTATE CANCER

Clinical Aspects

Epidemiology

The epidemiology of prostate cancer has changed dramatically since the advent of PSA screening programs. It has become the most commonly diagnosed cancer in men, leading lung and colorectal cancer by a factor of two to three times. It is a disease seen primarily in men over age 50. The death rate from prostate cancer has risen slightly, probably because of longer life span, and less likely because of increased virulence of the disease. After lung cancer, it is the second leading cause of cancer deaths in men. In the United States, it kills about 45,000 men each year. American men have an approximate 1 in 6 (17%) lifetime risk of developing prostate cancer and about a 1 in 30 chance of dying from it. The risk is higher in African-American men and in those with a family history of prostate cancer.[35-37]

Screening

The purpose of screening is to detect clinically significant prostate cancer in asymptomatic men at an early stage, when curative therapy can be offered.[35-38] Most screening programs recommend starting screening at age 50 years with an annual digital rectal examination and PSA (age 40 if there is a positive family history). PSA screening has allowed detection earlier in the stage of disease and the proportion of men presenting with metastatic disease has dropped markedly.

There is controversy regarding screening for prostate cancer. Microfocal clinically unimportant cancer is very common and up to 30% of men dying at age 50 years have microscopic cancer.[37] Concerns have been raised that screening programs and systematic biopsy protocols will detect many insignificant cancers. This fear has been proved false and most detected cancers are likely to cause morbidity and shorten life span. It is suggested that 16 of every 100 cases of prostate cancer detected through screening would be fatal if left untreated.[35,39,40]

Prostate cancer, on average, takes about 10 years to cause death. Men over age 50 years have many competing causes for mortality. As a result, most recommendations for screening start at age 50, but suggest that it be performed in reasonably healthy men with an expected life span of 10 years. This generally means screening to about age 75 years because life span after that age is likely to be less than a decade and treatment of prostate cancer would not provide health benefits or longevity.

The health and mortality benefits of prostate cancer screening in the general population have not been unequivocally established with large randomized trials. Case studies suggest improved outcomes. There are several North American and European studies underway to evaluate whether population screening provides the anticipated survival and health benefits. Until the results are available, most practitioners offer screening only after the risks and benefits of cancer detection and radical therapy have been discussed with the patient.

Staging and Histologic Grading of Prostate Cancer

The American Joint Committee on Cancer (AJCC) Tumor Node Metastasis (TNM)) staging classification is now almost universally used because of its international uniformity and ability to integrate clinical, imaging, and pathologic staging information (Table 10-1).[39,41] Previously the Jewett and Whitmore classification was in common use (Fig. 10-11).[42,43]

In addition to clinical staging, histologic grading is done using the Gleason scoring system, which analyzes the microscopic appearance of glandular differentiation and histologic aggressiveness; Grade 1 is well differentiated and Grade 5 is poorly differentiated. Most tumors are not uniform and show different Gleason patterns in different parts of the tumor. Gleason score is assigned by determining the primary dominant histologic pattern and the second most dominant pattern and then adding the two grades together to obtain a Gleason score between 2 and 10.[44] Scores 1 to 5 are considered well differentiated, 6 to 7 moderately differentiated, and 8 to 10 poorly differentiated. Most clinicians now use a combination of digital rectal examination, PSA, and Gleason score to define the tumor, estimate likelihood of extracapsular spread, and assign prognosis.[45,46]

Stage T1 (formerly A) tumors are not palpable clinically, either because they are soft or located in an anterior part of the gland that cannot be reached by palpation. This stage was initially used to describe cancers detected microscopically in chips obtained at transrectal prostatectomy. More recently, an additional T1c designation has been devised to stage tumors that are impalpable and not visible at TRUS but are found by needle biopsy done because of elevated PSA.[39,46] It has been suggested that at least 85% of T1c cancers are clinically significant and deserve treatment.[4,47,48]

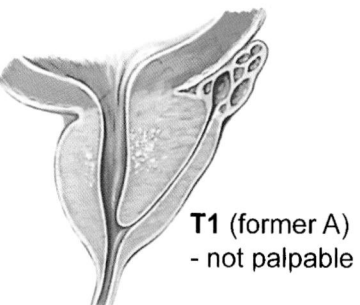

T1 (former A)
- not palpable

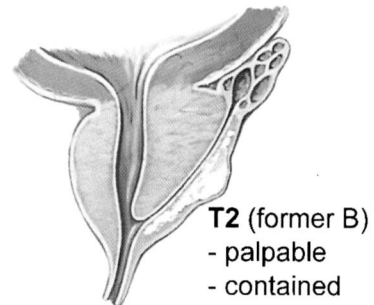

T2 (former B)
- palpable
- contained

FIGURE 10-11. Cancer staging.
Contemporary prostate cancer staging using the TNM classification.[39,41]

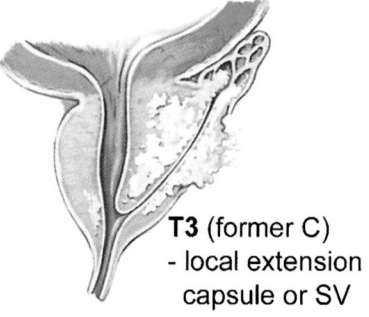

T3 (former C)
- local extension
  capsule or SV

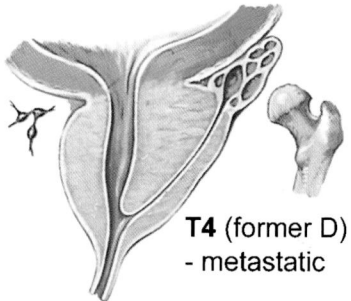

T4 (former D)
- metastatic

TABLE 10-1. AMERICAN JOINT COMMITTEE ON CANCER (AJCC) STAGING OF PROSTATE CANCER

Primary Tumor (T)

T1	**Clinically inapparent tumor not palpable on digital rectal examination nor visible by radiologic imaging. Tumor is confined to the prostate.**
T1a	Tumor incidental histologic finding in <5% of resected tissue
T1b	Tumor incidental histologic finding in >5% of resected tissue
T1c	Tumor identified by needle biopsy (often because of elevated PSA)
T2	**Clinically palpable tumor confined within the prostate**
T2a	Involves only one lobe
T2b	Involves both lobes
T3	**Tumor extends through the prostate capsule**
T3a	Extracapsular extension (unilateral or bilateral)
T3b	Seminal vesicle involvement
T4	**Tumor fixation or tumor invades adjacent structures**
T4a	Tumor involves bladder neck
T4b	Tumor involves external sphincter
T4c	Tumor involves rectum
T4d	Tumor involves levator muscles
T4e	Tumor extends to pelvic sidewall

Regional Lymph Nodes (N)

N0	No regional lymph node metastasis
N1	Metastasis in regional lymph nodes

Distant Metastasis (M)

M0	No distant metastasis
M1	Distant metastasis
M1a	Nonregional lymph node(s)
M1b	Bone(s)
M1c	Other site(s)

PSA, prostate specific antigen.

TNM classification modified from Nam RK, Jewett MAS, Krahn MD: Prostate cancer: 2. Natural history. CMAJ 1998;159(6):685-691 and Eng TY, Thomas CR, Herman TS: Primary radiation therapy for localized prostate cancer. Urol Oncol 2002;7:239-257.

Stage T2 (formerly B) tumors are palpable as a nodule by digital rectal examination and represent local cancer, typically in the peripheral zone.

Stage T3 (formerly C) tumors have local extension outside confines of the prostate into the seminal vesicles or periprostatic soft tissue.

Patients with clinical stages T1 to T3 have no evidence of metastatic disease at bone scan or other imaging techniques.

Stage T4 (formerly D) tumors represent cancer that has spread farther either in lymph nodes, distant organs, or bones.

With TNM staging, the local tumor T stage is modified with N (node status) and M (non-lymph node distant metastasis).

In the pre-PSA era, most cancers at time of initial presentation had already extended beyond the prostate (Stage T3 or T4) and only palliative care was possible. The advent of PSA screening has resulted in stage *migration*, meaning that most prostate cancer is being detected at an earlier stage (T1 and T2) when curative therapy is still an option.[36]

Therapy of Prostate Cancer

Once cancer is discovered, thought to be clinically significant, and judged to be treatable, there are several treatment options that include "watchful waiting," radical prostatectomy, and radiation therapy (external beam, brachytherapy). If the tumor has extended beyond the prostate, then palliative therapy can be provided, usually with hormone treatments.[37,49-51]

Prostate-Specific Antigen

Prostate-specific antigen (PSA) testing has been a tremendous advance in the diagnosis and management of prostate cancer.[4,52] PSA is a normally occurring enzyme secreted by the epithelial cells of prostate ducts. It functions to help liquefy the ejaculate. The normal level is accepted to be less than 4 ng/mL. The prostate is the main source of PSA and only trace, clinically unimportant amounts are found in other tissues in men and women. Some PSA leaks into the serum, where it can be measured.[53] In the serum it is partly unbound (free) and partly bound to proteins such as alpha-1-antitrypsin. The free-to-total PSA ratio (percent free PSA) has been found to be different in benign and malignant conditions. With cancer, the ratio tends to be low. Abnormal serum PSA levels result from excessive leak or excessive production. Cancer on average is felt to produce or be associated with 10 times as much PSA as a similar volume of benign tissue.

PSA is probably best considered to be a general non-specific test of prostate abnormality or irritation. Elevated levels occur with cancer and also benign conditions, including BPH, inflammation, prostate manipulation, biopsy, and cystoscopy. Digital rectal examination and TRUS without biopsy generally do not elevate PSA but it is prudent to draw the blood prior to disturbing the prostate. Not all prostate cancers can produce PSA and "normal" serum levels less than 4 ng/mL are found in about 20% to 30% of men with cancer. A normal PSA should not prevent proceeding to biopsy if the digital rectal examination or ultrasound findings are suspicious for cancer.

PSA levels can be artificially reduced with medications. Proscar (finasteride) reduces the level by a factor of about 2.[4] Unpredictably reduced levels are found with saw palmetto and other herbal medications. In past years, serum acid phosphatase was used to detect prostate cancer. Acid phosphatase becomes abnormal only when cancer has already metastasized. It is no longer used and has been totally replaced by PSA and imaging tests such as bone scan, CT, and MRI. Other serum tests are undergoing evaluation for their ability to detect and stage prostate cancer and may soon come into active clinical use.

Use of PSA to Direct Biopsy. As PSA increases, so does the likelihood of cancer being present. Normal PSA is accepted to be less than 4 ng/mL even though cancer is found in 4% to 9% of men at these levels if the digital rectal examination is negative and 10% to 21% if the digital rectal examination is positive. PSA greater than 10 ng/mL is sufficiently elevated to recommend biopsy even with negative digital rectal examination and TRUS.

A problem area has been in men with unexplained PSA of 4 to 10 ng/mL when digital rectal examination and TRUS are normal. The proportion of men that have cancer in this 4 to 10 ng/mL group is about 35%. In many men, the elevation is more likely due to BPH than to cancer, and many in this group will have negative biopsy. When cancer is found in this group, most (over 85%) are clinically significant.[48] There are several tactics that have been suggested to try to reduce the number of biopsies in the PSA 4 to 10 ng/mL group without missing cancer. All of these can decrease the number of biopsies, but will also result in cancer being missed.[37] More recently, some groups suggest biopsy starting at PSA greater than 4 ng/mL and even 2.5 ng/mL.[54] Others are continuing to try to decrease the number of

biopsies in the 4 to 10 ng/mL group without missing significant numbers of cancer with techniques as described below, including PSA density, age-specific PSA, PSA velocity, and free-to-total PSA ratio.[4] Men in whom biopsy is avoided will need continued clinical surveillance, generally with digital rectal examination and PSA.

PSA Density (Excess PSA, Predicted PSA). PSA production by benign tissue (normal and hyperplastic) is less than production by cancer. If there is an excess PSA level above that which is predicted from gland volume as measured by TRUS, then there is an increased chance of cancer. PSA density is determined by (PSA/volume). For example, with PSA 4.5 and gland volume 55 mL; PSA density = 4.5/55 = 0.08.

Restricting biopsy in the PSA 4 to 10 ng/mL group to those with PSA density greater than 0.12 will detect about 80% of those with cancer in this group and avoid many biopsies. In the above example, the PSA density is 0.08, which is less than 0.12. This suggests that the PSA level is consistent with the prediction from gland volume and not excessive and, hence, biopsy would be avoided with about 80% confidence that cancer is not present. Others have suggested PSA density ranging from 0.05 to 0.15. Remember that in all cases, a proportion of cancers will be missed and these men need continued surveillence.[55]

Age-Specific PSA. PSA normally increases with age.[4] It has been suggested that by using different threshold PSA levels at different ages, it may be possible to make PSA more sensitive in younger men, and less sensitive in older men.[56] Suggested ranges are: 40 to 49 years—0.0 to 2.5 ng/mL; 50 to 59 years—0.0 to 3.5; 60 to 69 years—0.0 to 4.5; 70 to 79 years—0.0 to 6.5. Although PSA does increase with age, the change is very slight. Most of the increase with age is due to the larger prostates due to BPH found in older men. Hence, age-specific PSA is really a surrogate for prostate volume and volume is better evaluated with TRUS. The suggested age specific ranges in the important 50- to 75-year age group close enough to 4.0 that 4.0 can continue to be used. We have not found the age specific to be useful.[7]

PSA Velocity. PSA levels in men with cancer usually rise more rapidly than with BPH. The rate of rise over time is termed *velocity*. If three PSA tests are done over 2 years and the rate of rise exceeds 0.75 ng/mL/year, then this rapid change (velocity) is claimed to distinguish subjects with CA from those with BPH with a specificity of 90%.[4,57] Many labs do not wait for two years and offer biopsy if there is an unexplained rise in the 4 to 10 ng/mL group of greater than 1 ng/mL between two tests less than a year apart.[7]

Free to Total PSA Ratio (Percent Free PSA). PSA in the blood is partly free and partly bound to proteins, especially α-1-antitrypsin. The usual PSA measurement is the total of the free PSA plus the bound PSA. Free to total is calculated as (free/total). Free/total ratio or percent PSA tends to be high with benign conditions and low with cancer, for reasons that have not been clearly explained.[4] In the 4 to 10 ng/mL PSA range, using a free/total ratio less than 20% will detect about 95% of cancer and reduce the number of biopsies by 30%. But this means that 5% of clinically significant cancer will be missed. An exact cutoff ratio has not yet been generally accepted. We feel that all men with elevated PSA should at least have TRUS to see if an impalpable nodule can be detected.

All of the above techniques can decrease the number of biopsies, but at the cost of missing clinically significant cancer. In practice, it is very unusual to see PSA greater than 2 ng/mL in a healthy man of any age. As a result, many physicians avoid these temporizing tactics and recommend biopsy in any man with unexplained PSA greater than 4 ng/mL and some even suggest biopsy for any man with PSA greater 2.5 ng/mL.[58] The above-mentioned techniques can be used to guide the urgency of *repeat* biopsy if the initial one is negative. Remember also that about 20% to 30% of men with clinically significant cancer have an entirely normal PSA. Biopsy is indicated even if PSA is normal when there is an obvious nodule at palpation or ultrasound.

Role of Transrectal Ultrasound with Prostate Cancer

Originally, it was thought that TRUS would be pivotal in men suspected to have cancer and help with screening, cancer detection, biopsy guidance, staging, therapy guidance, and monitoring response to treatment. Therapy guidance includes brachytherapy, insertion of fiducial markers to guide escalated dose external beam radiotherapy, cryotherapy, thermotherapy, and phototherapy. Experience has shown that TRUS today has two main roles with prostate cancer: (1) to guide biopsy, and (2) to guide therapy.

Screening is best done with digital rectal examination and PSA. Transrectal ultrasound by itself is not sufficiently sensitive to be used alone for cancer detection and diagnosis. Biopsy is needed. The number of labs using TRUS to calculate volume and PSA density to avoid biopsy is decreasing.

Transrectal ultrasound is not being generally used for staging to detect extracapsular disease. It is moderately accurate for staging and generally as accurate as CT and MRI.[59] Unfortunately, there is considerable interobserver variability with TRUS and, as a result, most clinical centers use multifactorial staging nomograms, such as proposed by Partin, which make use of digital rectal examination, PSA, and Gleason score.[60]

Monitoring therapy is better done with PSA, which is a better indicator of total tumor burden and neoplastic activity than is TRUS. However, TRUS is superb in guiding biopsy and in helping to guide therapy implements. These have become its main application in men suspected to have cancer.

Location of Prostate Cancer

About 70% of prostate cancers arise in the peripheral zone, 20% in the transition zone, and 10% in the central zone (see Figs. 10-1 and 10-11).[61] Surgical series have shown that prostate cancer is usually multifocal (83%), and 74% of lesions are in the peripheral zone, 15% are in both peripheral and transition zones, and only 2% are isolated in the transition zone.[62]

The homogeneous and isoechoic appearance of the peripheral and central zone tissue facilitates detection of textural changes associated with cancer (see Figs. 10-2B, C, 10-3C, 10-13A, C, E). Unfortunately, the transition zone has a very heterogeneous appearance at ultrasound and this makes detection of cancer in the transition zone very difficult (see Fig. 10-4A-C). The surgical capsule acts as a temporary anatomic barrier to spread into the inner gland, and many tumors spread laterally in the peripheral zone before entering the transition zone. Similarly, transition zone tumors may grow quite large before entering the peripheral zone (see Fig. 10-14D). In a large series of patients undergoing ultrasound and ultrasound-guided biopsy, only 13% of suspected lesions in the transition zone were malignant as opposed to 41% in the peripheral zone.[63]

Sonographic Appearances of Prostate Cancer

Overall, about 60% to 70% of prostate cancer is visible at TRUS. This sensitivity is similar to cancer detection by digital rectal examination, PSA, and MRI. CT cannot detect cancer until there is gross glandular distortion by extensive tumor growth.

It is important to remember that biopsy should be performed if the digital rectal examination or PSA is suspicious, even if TRUS is negative. Normal appearance at TRUS does not imply the absence of cancer and should not delay systematic biopsy because only about 60% to 70% of cancer is detectable by TRUS.

The sonographic appearance of prostate cancer has been debated extensively. Early investigators incorrectly thought that most prostate cancers were hyperechoic. With the development of higher-frequency transducers, it has been shown that 53% to 80% of peripheral zone cancers are **hypoechoic** to some extent (Figs. 10-12, 10-13 and 10-14).[1,64,65]

When attempting to correlate the echogenicity of neoplasms with the amount of stromal fibrosis, it was found that hypoechoic lesions had less stromal fibrosis than did their more echogenic counterparts (see Fig. 10-13). Also, hypoechoic lesions tended to have more aggressive behavior than isoechoic lesions.[1,65]

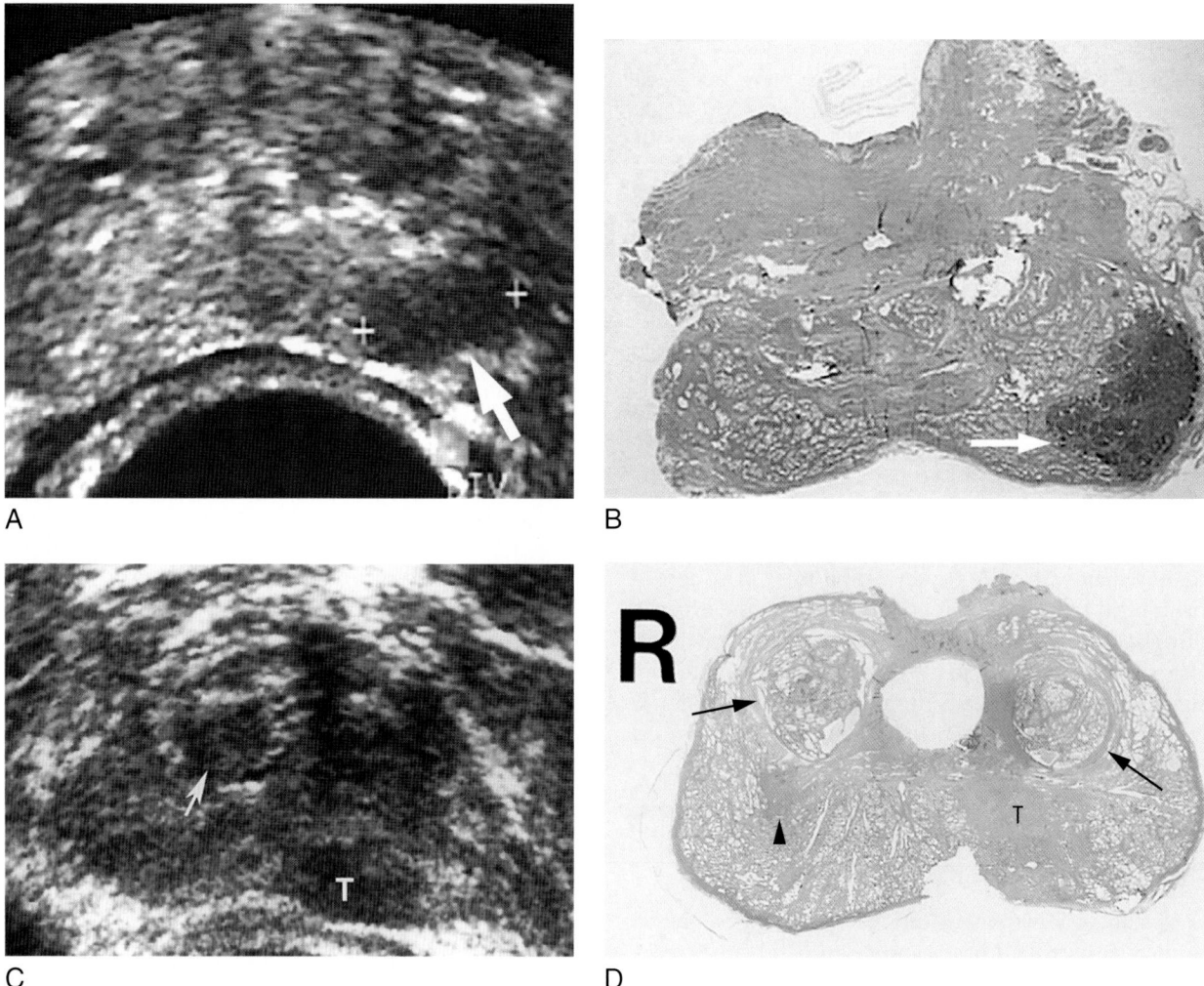

FIGURE 10-12. Prostate cancer, typical appearances. A, Typical appearance of a hypoechoic nodule in the peripheral zone along the capsule that cannot be attributed to benign causes (*arrow*). **B,** Pathology shows homogeneous solid cellular mass of tumor tissue (*arrow*), which reflects sound poorly compared to the adjacent prostate, which has multiple glandular interfaces. **C,** Typical hypoechoic peripheral zone cancer nodule (T). Note also the well-circumscribed hypoechoic BPH nodule in the right transition zone (*arrow*). **D,** Pathology shows the homogeneous tumor mass (T). There is a second small lesion on the right side (*arrowhead*). Note also the right and left BPH nodules seen on ultrasound (*arrow*).

Further research suggests that echogenicity varies with the presence of tumor glands with enlarged lumina as well as residual prostatic glands and stroma.[66]

Hyperechoic cancer, does occur but it is uncommon. With large cancers, the hyperechoic appearance may be caused by a desmoplastic response of the surrounding glandular tissue to the presence of the tumor or to infiltration of neoplasm into a background of benign prostatic hyperplasia with preexisting degenerative calcifications (see Fig. 10-11C).[67,68] Some histologic types of cancer, including the cribriform pattern and comedo-necrosis with focal calcifications, also correlate with echogenic cancer. Rare prostate cancers are associated with deposits of intraluminal crystalloid material, which also can produce increased echogenicity in a "starry sky" pattern where the focal calcifications appear

to twinkle as the probe is moved over the area (see Fig. 10-14C).[69] A few extensive large cancers have a hyperechoic appearance, probably as a result of the infiltration of the neoplasm into a background of benign prostatic hyperplasia. Biopsy of hyperechoic lesions with sonographic guidance is the only way in which it can be proved that the lesion seen represents a neoplasm.

A significant number of prostate cancers, about 30%, are difficult or impossible to detect with TRUS because they are **isoechoic** and do not contrast with the surrounding prostate gland (see Figs. 10-13C and 10-14A and E). When an isoechoic tumor is present, it can be detected only if secondary signs are appreciated, including glandular asymmetry, capsular bulging, and areas of attenuation.[70] This is often true of transition zone cancer (see Fig. 10-14D).

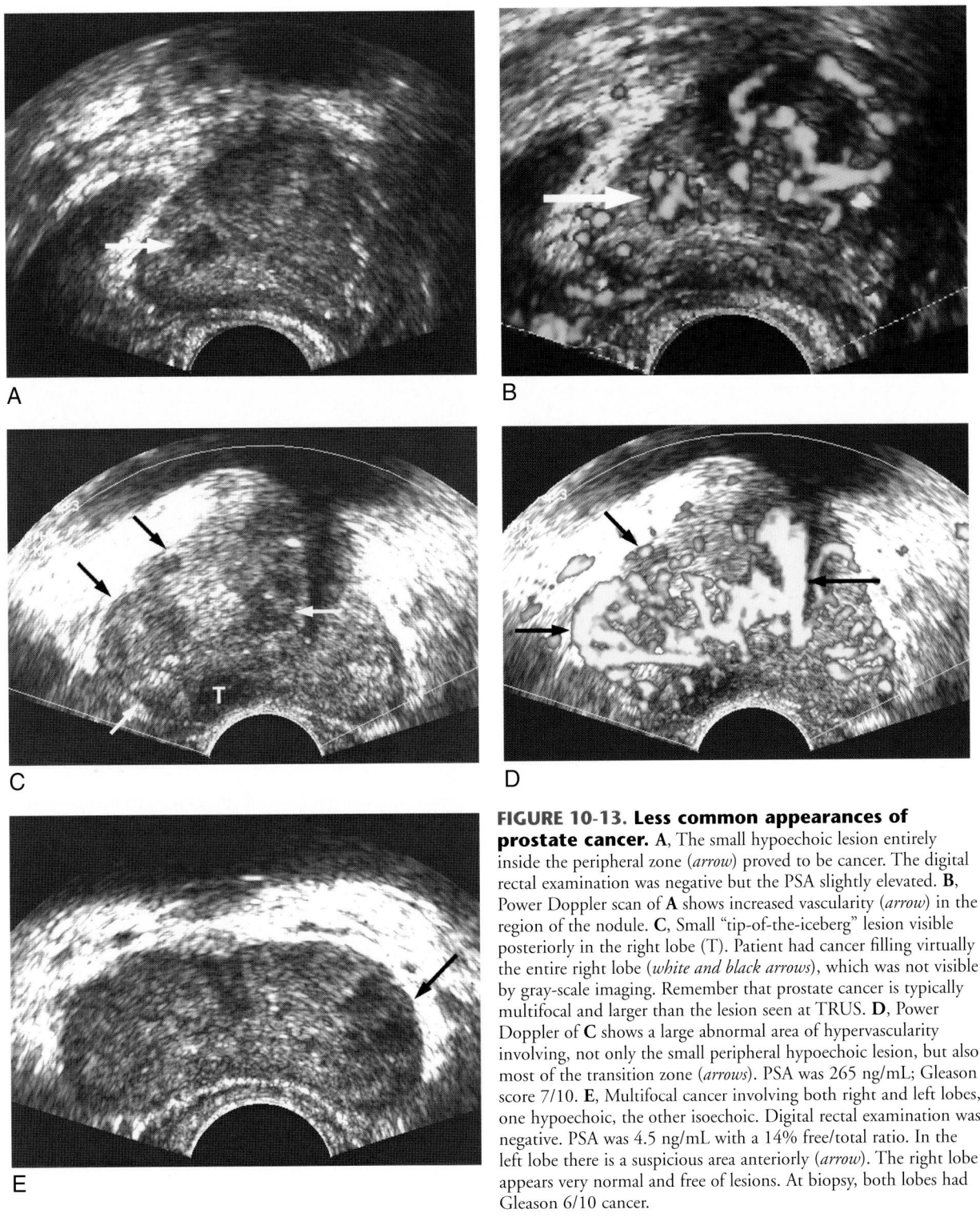

FIGURE 10-13. Less common appearances of prostate cancer. A, The small hypoechoic lesion entirely inside the peripheral zone (*arrow*) proved to be cancer. The digital rectal examination was negative but the PSA slightly elevated. **B,** Power Doppler scan of **A** shows increased vascularity (*arrow*) in the region of the nodule. **C,** Small "tip-of-the-iceberg" lesion visible posteriorly in the right lobe (T). Patient had cancer filling virtually the entire right lobe (*white and black arrows*), which was not visible by gray-scale imaging. Remember that prostate cancer is typically multifocal and larger than the lesion seen at TRUS. **D,** Power Doppler of **C** shows a large abnormal area of hypervascularity involving, not only the small peripheral hypoechoic lesion, but also most of the transition zone (*arrows*). PSA was 265 ng/mL; Gleason score 7/10. **E,** Multifocal cancer involving both right and left lobes, one hypoechoic, the other isoechoic. Digital rectal examination was negative. PSA was 4.5 ng/mL with a 14% free/total ratio. In the left lobe there is a suspicious area anteriorly (*arrow*). The right lobe appears very normal and free of lesions. At biopsy, both lobes had Gleason 6/10 cancer.

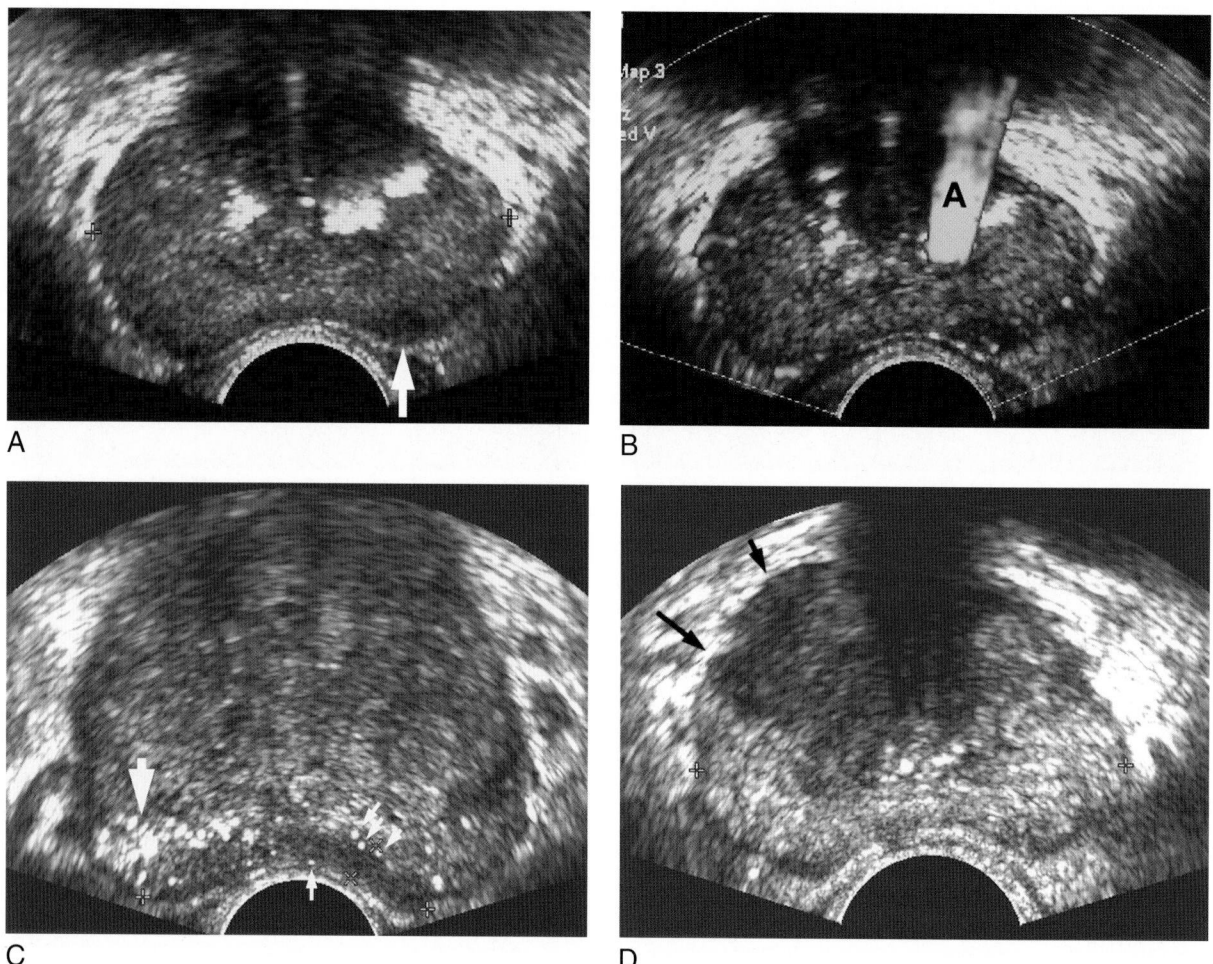

FIGURE 10-14. Other appearances of cancer. A, Almost isoechoic, nonvascular, nonpalpable cancer. PSA 6.08 ng/mL with 12% free/total ratio. Suspicious area at the left (*arrow*). Biopsy showed right-sided Gleason 7/10 cancer involving 25% of the tissue. On the left, where there is a visible lesion (*arrow*), the biopsy was only 15% cancer. **B,** Power Doppler of **A** shows almost no detectable signal, despite extensive bilateral cancer. The strong Doppler color signal is calcification artifact (A). **C, Extensive cancer with "starry sky" appearance** due to comedo-necrosis in the tumor. The malignant nodule extends across the peripheral zone from right to left (*between cursors*). On the right, the calcified clumps are normal corpora amylacea (*thick arrow*). On the left, the densities are small, more scattered, round, and very echogenic and will "twinkle" on probe movement (*arrows*), highly suggestive of comedo-necrosis in tumor. **D, Isolated transition zone cancer** visible as an amorphous hypoechoic bulge of the right anterior transition zone (*arrows*). Digital rectal examination was negative. PSA 12.0 ng/mL showed Gleason 6/10 cancer.

When the tumor replaces the entire peripheral zone, it will often be less echogenic than the inner gland, which is a reversal of the normal sonographic relationship. When the entire gland is replaced with tumor, on a background of hyperplasia, the gland may be diffusely inhomogeneous. Doppler imaging has been evaluated for detection of neovascularity associated with cancer, especially isoechoic cancer (see Fig. 10-13D). Neither color flow imaging nor power Doppler has shown a dramatic advantage over gray-scale imaging.[71] There is a slight increase in cancer detection but the improvement is small, allowing only 5% increased detection above gray-scale imaging. In addition, vascularity may be increased with nonmalignant conditions such as inflammation (see Fig. 10-8B). There is no increased

benefit for Doppler in the transition zone because BPH nodules can range from hypo- to hypervascular.

Doppler can be sensitive to patient position.[13] We prefer to use the power Doppler mode, which is more sensitive to flow detection, gives a more uniform display of vascular density, and provides more stable images with different equipment settings (see Fig. 10-5). There are pitfalls with Doppler. Not all cancers are vascular; the absence of vascularity should not prevent biopsy of an otherwise suspicious nodule (see Fig. 10-14A and B). The capsule of the prostate is very vascular, especially at the base and apex, and it can mimic neovascularity to the uninitiated. Prostate calcifications and corpora amylacea cause considerable Doppler artifact and may prevent diagnostic studies (see Figs. 10-6D and 10-14B). Investigations are underway using ultrasound contrast-enhanced imaging and specialized ultrasound imaging parameters, such as phase-inversion technology.[71] These allow slight increases in tumor detection, but false positive results are also seen.

Prostate Biopsy with Transrectal Ultrasound Guidance

Prostate biopsy and cancer diagnosis has been revolutionized by TRUS guidance and the biopsy gun. This approach has replaced the "blind" finger-guided transrectal and transperineal biopsy. Virtually all guided biopsies are now done transrectally (Fig. 10-15).[1,54]

Preparation. Prostate biopsy is usually performed in an ambulatory setting with little patient preparation.[1,54] Experience has shown that it is easier to schedule and prepare men for TRUS and biopsy at the same visit. This avoids the need for two visits. If TRUS shows a benign cause for the clinical findings, then the biopsy is simply cancelled.

Informed consent is obtained. Some advocate the use of cleansing enemas before performing the biopsy. A rapidly absorbed antibiotic is administered, such as ciprofloxacin in one dose just before and in several doses following the biopsy. Patients on anticoagulating agents (aspirin, nonsteroidal anti-inflammatory drugs, or warfarin [Coumadin]) should not undergo biopsy until these drugs have been discontinued for several days, depending on the agent. Aspirin is commonly taken by men in the prostate cancer age group. Even a "baby-aspirin" (81 mg) blocks platelet function irreversibly for 7 to 10 days. Some have suggested that aspirin-induced coagulation disturbance is not severe enough to prevent safe biopsy.[72] Nonetheless, bleeding complications can occur following prostate biopsy, and medical legal defense may be difficult if an elective procedure was performed with the knowledge of aspirin ingestion. Warfarin is discontinued and International Normalized Ratio (INR) is tested prior to biopsy with the help of the referring physician. Patients with **valvular heart disease** undergo endocarditis prophylaxis as recommended by the American Heart Association, using intravenous ampicillin (vancomycin for penicillin-allergic patients) and gentamicin.[73]

Technique. Transrectal ultrasound-guided prostate biopsy is performed with a transrectal approach.[1,54] Needle-guidance systems that clamp onto the side of the probe are available for end-firing and side-firing probes (see Figs. 10-7 and 10-15). Electronic guidelines direct the needle path (see Fig. 10-15D).

Local anesthesia is frequently used during the biopsy with 5 to 10 mL of 1% lidocaine (Xylocaine) without epinephrine. This is injected either into the neurovascular bundles at the base of the prostate or, more easily, into the gland itself at the biopsy sites.

With direct injections into the gland, anesthesia is instantaneous.

The automatic biopsy gun with 18-gauge needles has remarkable patient acceptance and safety.[72,74] Biopsy is best done by a single operator who controls both the probe and gun. With the gun cocked, the needle is "parked" in the guide, ensuring that the tip is safely inside the guide. The probe and contained needle are moved to the target by using the targeting line (see Fig. 10-15D). A simple, swift motion advances the gun and needle tip to the surface of the lesion. Once triggered, the needle advances approximately 2 to 3 cm with the push of a button. The inner needle advances, and the outer needle cuts the tissue core and traps it in the beveled chamber of the inner needle (see Fig. 10-15C). We avoid biopsy of the urethra and internal urethral sphincter, which can result in considerable urethral bleeding. **Cytology** rather than core tissue biopsy has been done in the past, but both false-positive and false-negative results can occur and Gleason scoring is not possible. Most physicians do not use cytology today.

Significant **complications** from prostate biopsy have been relatively low, regardless of the mode of guidance, needle size, or approach.[54,72] Minor side effects include blood in the urine, stool, and sperm and will be seen in most patients undergoing transrectal biopsy. This minor bleeding generally lasts only a few days but can continue for many weeks, and the ejaculate may remain discolored for many months. Major complications needing physician intervention are uncommon and occur in less than 1% to 2% of instances. These include sepsis, large hematomas, urinary retention, and significant rectal bleeding. With the use of prophylactic antibiotics, the incidence of septic complications requiring therapy should be less than 1%.[72] Tumor seeding is virtually unknown.

In our clinic about 1% of patients have a **vasovagal reaction** to the biopsy; others have found this in up to 5.8%.[72] It is characterized by pallor, sweating, nausea and vomiting, and there is bradycardia of 50 to 60 beats per minute associated with significant hypotension. This usually occurs within 30 to 60 minutes after biopsy. Many recover spontaneously, but some need intravenous atropine. We keep patients in the clinic for an hour after the biopsy to avoid problems with delayed vasovagal reactions. Biopsy should not be taken lightly. Some patients require hospitalization due to biopsy-related complications, and there are rare reports of patients dying because of biopsy-related complications.

Indications for Initial Biopsy. Biopsy is performed in patients in whom there is a clinical suspicion of cancer and in whom the results would alter clinical management (Table 10-2). The indications include:

- Abnormal digital rectal examination
- PSA >10 ng/mL (Some advocate reducing the PSA criterion to 4 or even 2.5 ng/mL.)

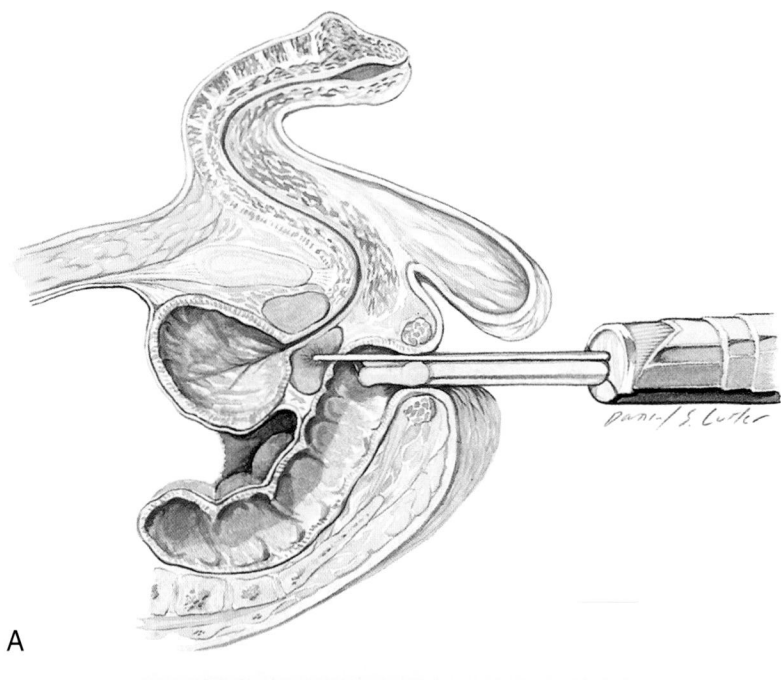

A

FIGURE 10-15. Prostate biopsy technique. A, Diagram showing TRUS guidance technique. **B,** Typical disposable biopsy "gun." **C,** Mechanism of needle function: (1) closed needle advanced to lesion; (2) on triggering, the inner chambered stylet enters the lesion; (3) the outer sheath advances and cuts off and encloses the sample.

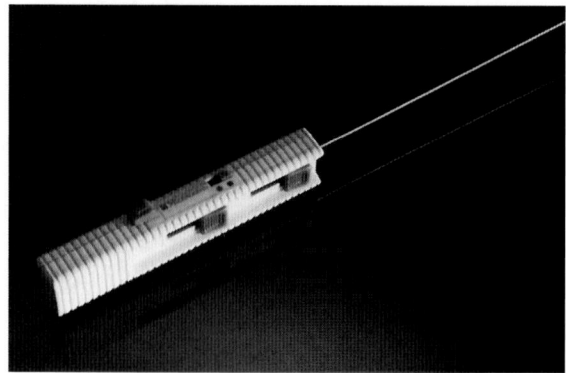

B

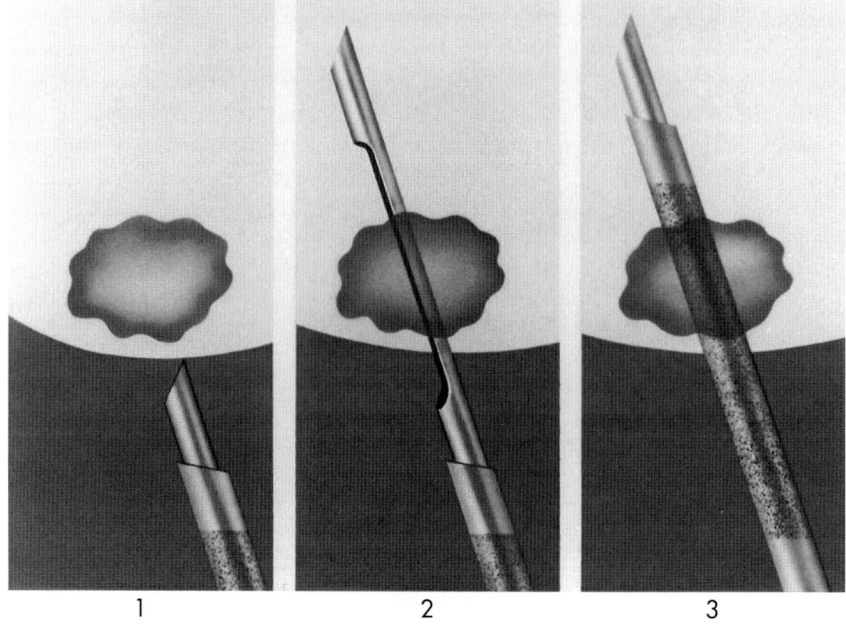

C   1   2   3

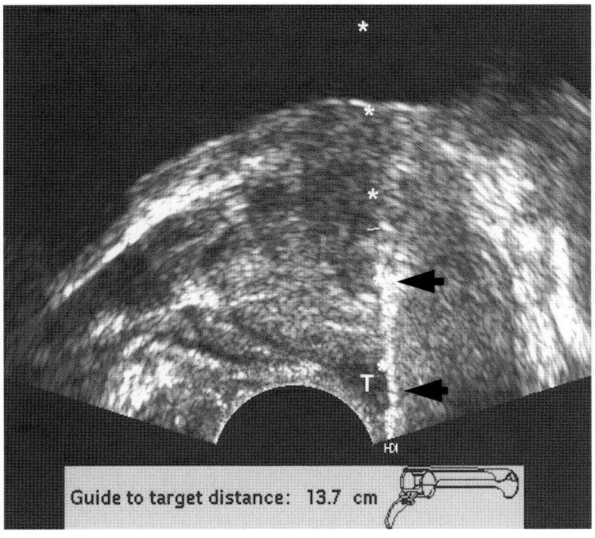
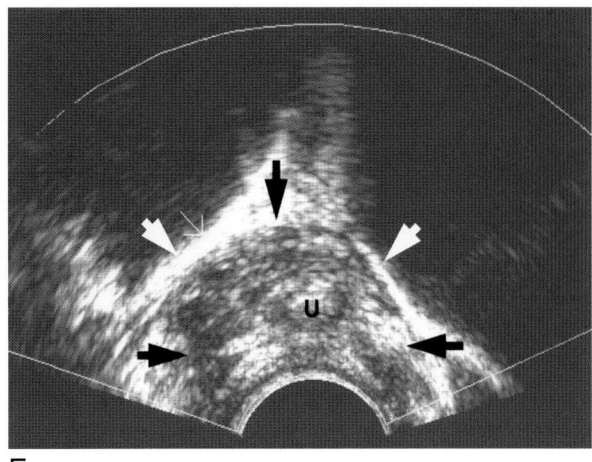

Guide to target distance: 13.7 cm

D

E

FIGURE 10-15, *cont'd.* **Prostate biopsy technique. D**, Biopsy needle as seen at TRUS (*arrows*). Targeting line dots are visible (*). T, nodule. **E**, Recurrent prostate cancer at anastomotic site following radical prostatectomy. The lesion (*black arrows*) is low in the pelvis behind the pubic arch bones (*white arrows*) and surrounds the urethra (U).

- Nodule visible at TRUS
- Excessive PSA velocity
- Positive chips at transurethral prostatectomy
- Men with metastatic adenocarcinoma in whom a primary is not evident

Any one of these indications is sufficient to perform biopsy. On the first occasion, the biopsy is performed using a systematic sextant (six cores) pattern with additional samples obtained from suspicious areas lying outside the sextant pattern (Fig. 10-16).[75,76]

Three samples are taken from each side of the peripheral zone at the level of the base, midgland, and apex, slightly favoring the lateral aspect of each lobe (six in total). Additional samples are taken from suspicious lesions or abnormally vascular areas that lie outside the sextant pattern (e.g., in the anterior part of the gland) (see Fig. 10-16). This approach following the above indications should result in an overall 30% to 60% positive biopsy rate and about 60% for lesions that appear suspicious on ultrasound.[1]

Indications for Repeat Biopsy. Biopsy is repeated, generally using a more extensive sampling pattern, in the following situations:

- Initial biopsy is negative, but there is continued strong clinical suspicion of cancer (palpable nodule, PSA >10 or continuing to rise).
- Initial biopsy shows suspicious histology that would not qualify for radical therapy (high grade prostate intraepithelial neoplasia [PIN], atypical cells, and microscopic cancer).

Because about 30% to 40% of cancers are not visible at TRUS, there is a chance that the initial samples missed

the cancer and it is reasonable to repeat the biopsy at intervals of 3 to 6 months up to two times if needed, especially if there is continuing unexplained rise in PSA, the PSA ratio is low, or initial results show changes that are precancerous or highly associated with cancer, such as prostate intraepithelial neoplasia or atypical cells (atypical small acinar proliferation).[77] In our hands, the first biopsy has yielded PIN in 7.3% and atypical cells in 4% and cancer in 46% of 2473 biopsies. Thus about

---

TABLE 10-2. INDICATIONS FOR PROSTATE BIOPSY TO INVESTIGATE CANCER

This group includes any patient whose histologic information would alter management and in whom the biopsy can be safely performed.

Initial Biopsy Indications

Abnormal digital rectal examination
Unexplained PSA elevation
Abnormal TRUS
Excessive PSA velocity
Positive chips at TURP
Metastatic adenocarcinoma where primary is not evident

Repeat Biopsy Indications

Initial biopsy is negative, strong continued clinical suspicion
PSA >10 ng/mL or continuing to rise
Suspicious digital rectal examination but initial biopsy negative
Initial suspicious histology (PIN, atypical cells, microscopic cancer)

PIN, Prostate intraepithelial neoplasia; PSA, prostate specific antigen; TRUS, transrectal ultrasonography; TURP, transurethral prostatectomy.

FIGURE 10-16. Biopsy sites viewed *en-face* from the posterior aspect of the prostate. Left sextant image shows the six standard sites (S). Additional samples are taken of any lesion that is evident outside the sextant pattern (+). Right image shows a typical extended pattern of biopsies—in this instance, a 13-core pattern. The sextant sites are sampled (S). In addition samples are taken from the lateral peripheral zones (L), deep in the anterior transition zone (T), and from the peripheral zone in the midline (M) at the base, cephalad to the verumontanum. (Right image from Babaian RJ, Toi A, Kamoi K, et al: A comparative analysis of sextant and an extended 11-core multisite directed biopsy strategy. J Urol 2000;163(1):152.)

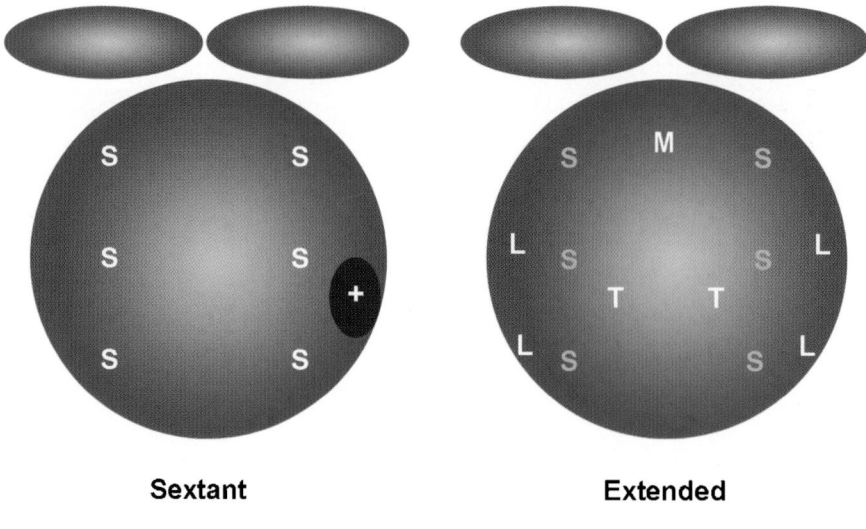

Sextant   **Extended**

11.3% of men would return for repeat biopsy because of suspicious cells.[78] Beyond three biopsy sessions, the yield becomes too small, and most laboratories will revert to about 1 year follow-up. Cancer detection rates on repeat biopsies one, two, three, and four are reported as 22% to 38%, 10%, 5%, and 4%, respectively.[54,79]

Repeat biopsies use a more extensive pattern of sampling (see Fig. 10-16).[80] The sites of cancer missed by the initial sextant pattern have been evaluated.[81] Several patterns for extended biopsy have been suggested.[54,82] We have found that a 13-core pattern modeled after Babaian[82] has been very effective with samples obtained as follows: for each lobe—lateral peripheral zone (two cores); medial peripheral zone (three cores = sextant sites); transition zone (one core), in addition, one from the midline just above the level of the verumontanum. Overall, 13 cores are obtained and cancer yield at repeat biopsy is about 42%. Most of the cancers will be found in the sextant sites or the lateral sites with only a small contribution from the transition zone and midline.[82] Color Doppler has slightly increased the sensitivity and specificity regardless of whether a gray-scale lesion is detected (see Fig. 10-13).

Biopsy After Radical Prostatectomy. Radical prostatectomy should reduce PSA to virtually undetectable levels. Recurrent disease is suspected if the PSA starts rising. Transrectal sonography is used to evaluate the anastomotic site and to look for local lymphadenopathy and pelvic masses (see Fig. 10-15E). If locally recurrent disease is found, then treatment with radiotherapy can be helpful. In these men, we perform biopsies of any nodelike masses and obtain two samples from either side of the anastomosis. Care must be taken not to mistake large pelvic vessels for masses. Doppler interrogation is important prior to biopsy.

Biopsy in Men with Absent Anus. Men who have had their anus closed because of abdominoperineal resection present a difficult group to manage when their PSA becomes elevated. We have tried transabdominal and transperineal ultrasound, but visibility is very restricted. Transperineal ultrasound-guided biopsy with local anesthesia is moderately successful in obtaining prostate tissue.[83] An alternative approach using MRI for lesion detection followed by CT trans-sciatic biopsy could be considered.

Role of Transrectal Ultrasound in Staging Prostate Cancer

Following the diagnosis of prostate cancer, definitive therapeutic decisions cannot be made unless the stage of prostate cancer is determined. Multiple avenues of therapy are available that need to be discussed with the patient, but all depend on knowing the extent of disease.[49] The current practice is to use a nomogram that includes clinical stage (digital rectal examination) + PSA + Gleason score to predict pathologic stage.[45,46] TRUS in good hands can make some contributions to cancer staging, but the considerable interobserver variability in detecting extracapsular extension had decreased its reliability. Only gross tumor extension is detectable; microscopic extension cannot be detected by any imaging technique, including CT and MRI.

In patients with less than 5% positive chips at transurethral prostatectomy (stage T1a) ultrasound-guided biopsy has been suggested instead of a repeat transurethral resection or blind needle biopsy to determine if they have a larger burden of disease. Therapy would be altered if a larger volume of cancer can be shown. For example, if a minimal amount of cancer were found

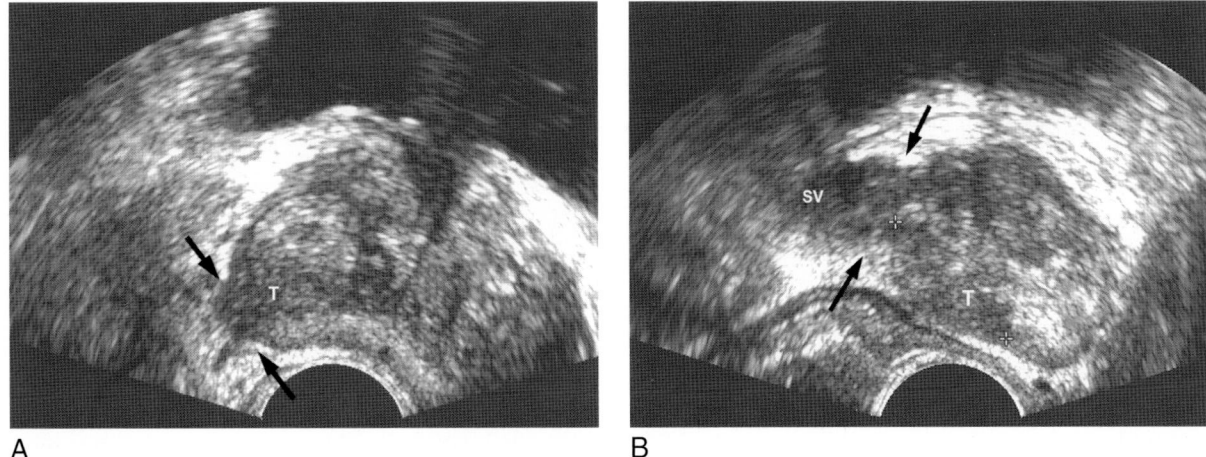

FIGURE 10-17. Staging of extensive prostate cancer. A, The cancer (T) has extended outside the prostate at the neurovascular bundle (*arrows*). Note how difficult it is to differentiate tumor extension from the normal irregularity caused by the neurovascular bundle, stage T3a. **B,** Parasagittal view shows cancer (T) extending (*arrows*) into the seminal vesicles (SV) above the prostate, stage T3c.

on a transurethral resection as the result of resection sampling of the edge of a large cancer, ultrasound could properly assess and determine the stage of cancer.[84] In these instances, a sextant biopsy is done and samples are taken from the transition zone adjacent to the TRUP cavity at its right, posterior, and left aspects. Cancer confined within the prostate, clinical stages T1 and T2 (localized and confined within the prostate), can be offered potentially curative radical prostatectomy or radiation therapy. If the disease has already metastasized, then local therapy is not helpful.

Controversy exists concerning the best therapy for locally invasive prostate cancer (stage T3). If microscopic invasion is found, surgery followed by radiation seems to be an acceptable approach. With macroscopic invasion there appears to be no advantage to surgery, and radiation therapy can be tried. In some instances TRUS can detect macroscopic local extension into the periprostatic fat or seminal vesicles (Fig. 10-17A, B).

The accuracy of TRUS and other imaging tests for staging has been evaluated. In general, TRUS and MRI are similar, though MRI with endorectal coils is slightly more accurate in determining seminal vesicle involvement. Overall, in determining extracapsular or seminal vesicle extension, TRUS has sensitivity 50% to 90%, specificity 46% to 91%, and overall accuracy 46% to 86%. For MRI, the figures are sensitivity 38% to 68%, specificity 72% to 95%, overall accuracy 51% to 91%. Large tumors can easily be seen to extend outside of the capsule as a result of the loss of symmetry and capsular irregularity but microscopic invasion cannot be seen. CT is a relatively poor staging technique for involvement of both local periprostatic structures and lymph nodes.[85,86] Seminal vesicle extension can be difficult to detect; affected seminal vesicles may appear normal. Invasion can be suspected if there is enlargement, cystic dilation,

asymmetry, anterior displacement, hyperechogenicity, and loss of the seminal vesicle beak.[87]

There is a role for staging biopsies in patients with known prostate cancer. Only a few reports have described the role of direct staging biopsies for prostate cancer and these have been directed toward the seminal vesicles. When seminal vesicle biopsy has been positive, 100% also have capsular penetration and 50% have positive nodes.[88,89] Occasionally, we have purposely performed staging pericapsular biopsies to attempt to prove extracapsular spread. When the pathologist sees tumor intermixed with fat, there is extracapsular invasion, probably of the macroscopic type.

Transrectal Ultrasound as a Guide to Prostate Cancer Therapy

Transrectal ultrasound is an effective tool to guide implements into the prostate for therapy. This includes standard treatments, such as radiotherapy (brachytherapy and escalated dose conformal radiotherapy),[41] and cryotherapy, as well as experimental treatments, such as thermotherapy,[90] gene therapy with viral injection,[91] and photodynamic therapy.[92]

For **escalated dose external beam conformal radiotherapy**, TRUS is used to guide placement of fiducial marker seeds (small gold wires about 5 × 0.5 mm) into the base, back, and apex of the prostate (Fig. 10-18). In conventional radiotherapy, the radiation fields are deliberately larger than the prostate to compensate for the significant changes in prostate position that are known to occur. This results in injury to collateral organs, which are included in the fields. With markers in the prostate, portal imagers (fluoroscopy units that can function at the high radiation levels used for therapy) can be used during radiotherapy to follow prostate

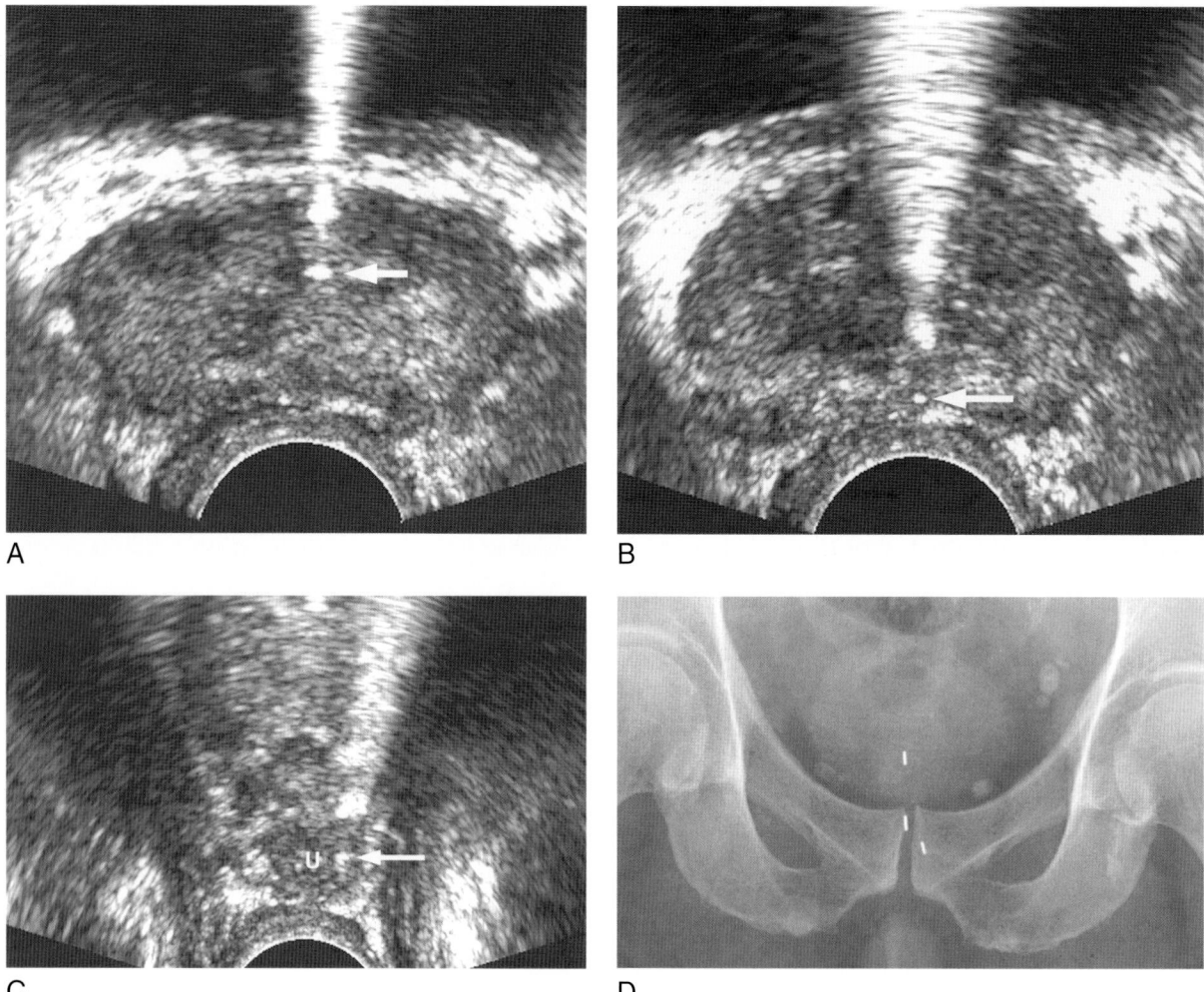

FIGURE 10-18. Fiducial marker seeds inserted with TRUS guidance and used to guide escalated dose external beam radiotherapy. A, Transverse image shows basal seed (*arrow*) with characteristic comet-tail reverberation artifact. **B,** Rectal surface seed (*arrow*). **C,** Apical seed (*arrow*) just beside the urethra (U). **D,** Pelvic radiograph shows the three marker seeds in place. TRUS, Transrectal ultrasound.

movement.[93] This allows the beam to be tightly conformed to the prostate and follow its movement. As a result, higher radiation doses can be focused directly on the prostate to improve outcomes and spare collateral organ injury.

Brachytherapy involves the direct placement of multiple radioactive seeds (usually ^{125}I) into the prostate via the transperineal approach.[94] This technique allows the highest possible intraprostatic radiation dose because all the seeds are within the prostate and adjacent organs are spared. Brachytherapy is suited to a select group of cancer patients with clinical stage T1 or T2, PSA <10, Gleason score <7, and prostate volume <50 mL. Transrectal ultrasound is used to estimate prostate size, plan seed locations, and then to guide seed placement transperineally using special guidance templates (Fig. 10-19).

Cryotherapy treats prostate cancer by freezing it with the use of thermal probes inserted transperineally with TRUS guidance. Transrectal ultrasound can determine the extent of the ablation process by following ice ball formation to the margins of the prostate and helps to decrease complications.[95]

Several **experimental** prostate cancer therapies are being tested. These require TRUS guidance to introduce the active elements into specific parts of the prostate. They include viral injection for gene therapy and photodynamic therapy, whereby malignant cells are labeled and destroyed by reagents that are activated by specific wavelengths of light, which is delivered into the prostate by optical fibers inserted with TRUS guidance.

Biopsy Following Nonsurgical Prostate Therapy

Many of the above therapies can alter the texture of the prostate, making it impossible to detect recurrent cancer with TRUS. We perform sextant biopsy of these patients when tissue is needed for patient management.

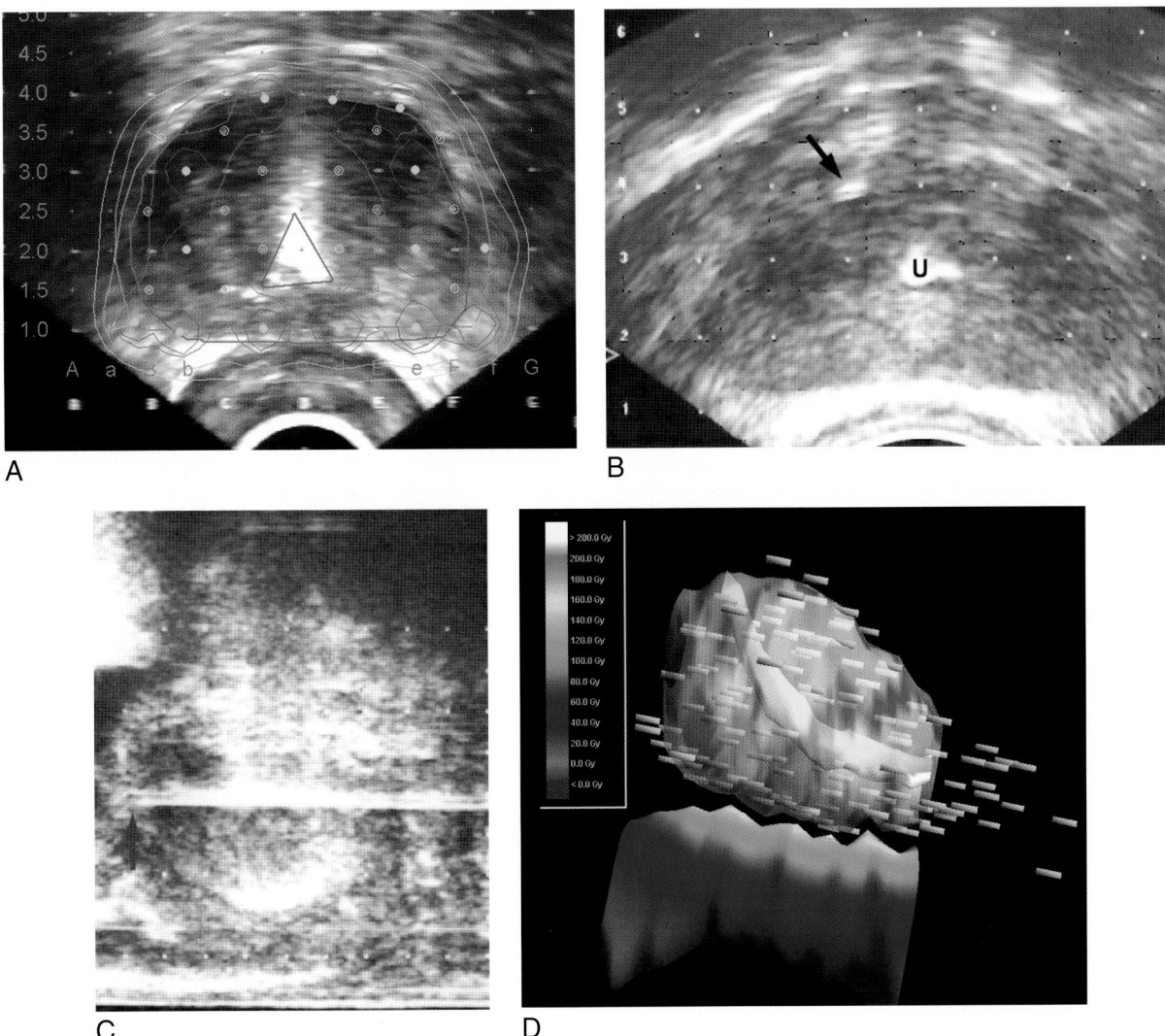

FIGURE 10-19. Transrectal ultrasound. TRUS is used to plan and guide brachytherapy (radioactive seed implantation) using a special stepping device and perineal needle template. **A**, One of multiple transverse prostate images used to plan seed sites (*dots*) and determine radiation isodose curves (*colored lines*). Urethral dose is avoided (*white central area inside the green triangle*). Note the grid markers at the bottom (A a B....) and left side (1, 1.5, 2.0....) and the grid dots superimposed on the field. **B**, TRUS-guided seed placement in the operating room. Transverse image shows the guiding grid dots and the tip of one inserting needle as a "hamburger-like" echo (*arrow*). U, urethra. **C**, Sagittal image shows brachytherapy needle inserted to base of prostate (*arrow*) to insert a row of seeds. **D**, Postprocedural CT reconstruction shows the position of the seeds (*green*). TRUS, transrectal ultrasound. (Images courtesy of Dr. Juanita Crook, Radiation Oncology, Princess Margaret Hospital, Toronto).

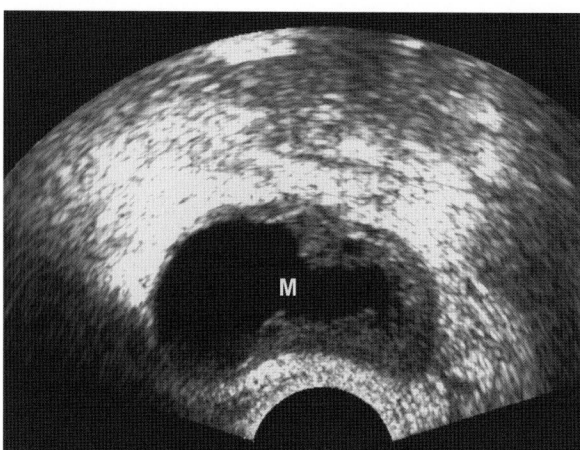

FIGURE 10-20. Woman with abnormal pelvic mass illustrates nonprostate uses of TRUS guidance and biopsy in men and women. This is a recurrent pelvic mass (M) following hysterectomy for uterine cancer. TRUS examination and biopsy provided the histologic proof that was needed prior to further therapy. The transrectal technique is useful for biopsy of any pelvic mass that can be reached by the probe. TRUS, transrectal ultrasound.

OTHER APPLICATIONS FOR TRANSRECTAL ULTRASOUND AND BIOPSY/ASPIRATION

In both men and women, the transrectal route is useful to evaluate and sample any pelvic mass that is within range of the probe and needle. Transrectal ultrasound also provides high resolution pelvic access in girls and women when transvaginal ultrasound is not possible (Fig. 10-20).

There are a few caveats. Because there are large vessels in the pelvis, it is important to use Doppler to interrogate any area where biopsy is contemplated. Remember that **pelvic kidneys** may mimic pathologic masses. Also, **anterior meningoceles** may mimic masses behind the rectum and should not be aspirated for fear of infection.

That aside, we have performed abscess drainages and done biopsies of numerous masses, including **ovarian masses**, **recurrent masses after diverse primary tumor surgery**, **periureteric masses**, **bladder masses,** and **pericolonic masses**. All these procedures have the same preparation and protocol as the basic prostate biopsy. The distal ureters and ureterovesical junctions are readily accessible to evaluation for distal ureteric obstructing lesions including **calculi**.

References

1. Scherr DS, Eastham J, Ohori M, et al: Prostate biopsy techniques and indications: When, where, and how? Semin Urol Oncol 2002;20(1):18-31.
2. Babaian RJ, Camps JL: The role of prostate-specific antigen as part of the diagnostic triad and as a guide when to perform a biopsy. Cancer 1991;68:2060-2063.
3. Meyer F, Yves F: Prostate cancer: 4. Screening. CMAJ 1998;159(8):968.
4. Polascik TJ, Oesterling JE, Partin AW: Prostate specific antigen: A decade of discovery—what we have learned and where are we going. J Urol 1999;162:293-306.
5. Watanabe H, Igari D, Tanahasi Y, et al: Development and application of new equipment for transrectal ultrasonography. J Clin Ultrasound 1974;2:91-98.
6. Aarnink RG, Beerlage HP, De la Rosette JJ, et al: Transrectal ultrasound of the prostate: Innovations and future applications. J Urol 1998;159:1568-1579.
7. Littrup PJ, Bailey SE: Prostate cancer: The role of transrectal ultrasound and its impact on cancer detection and management. Radiol Clin North Am 2000;38(1):87-113.
8. Lee F, Torp-Pedersen ST, Siders DB, et al: Transrectal ultrasound in the diagnosis and staging of prostatic carcinoma. Radiology 1989;170:609-615.
9. Kaye KW, Richter L: Ultrasonographic anatomy of normal prostate gland: Reconstruction by computer graphics. Urology 1990;35:12-17.
10. McNeal JE: The zonal anatomy of the prostate. Prostate 1981;2:35-49.
11. Ayala AG, Ro JY, Babaian R, et al: The prostatic capsule: Does it exist? Am J Surg Pathol 1989;13:21-27.
12. Leventis AK, Shariat SF, Utsunomia T, et al: Characteristics of normal prostate vascular anatomy as displayed by power Doppler. Prostate 2001;46:281-288.
13. Halpern EJ, Frauscher F, Forsberg F, et al: High-frequency Doppler US of the prostate: Effect of patient position. Radiology 2002;222(3):634-639.
14. Ayala AG, Ro JY, Babaian RJ, et al: The prostate capsule: Does it exist? Am J Surg Path 1989;13(1):21-27.
15. Hendrikx AJ, van Helvoort, van Dommelen CA, et al: Ultrasonic determination of prostatic volume: A cadaver study. Urology 1989;34(3):123-125.
16. Jacobsen H, Torp-Pedersen S, Juul N: Ultrasonic evaluation of age-related human prostatic growth and development of benign prostatic hyperplasia. Scand J Urol Nephrol 1988;107(suppl):26-31.
17. Shinohara K, Scardino PT, Carter S, et al: Pathologic basis of the sonographic appearance of the normal and malignant prostate. Urol Clin North Am 1989;16:675-691.
18. Burks DD, Drolshagen LF, Fleischer AC, et al: Transrectal ultrasound of benign and malignant prostatic lesions. AJR 1986;146:1187-1191.
19. Oyen RH, Van de Voorde QM, Van Poppel HP, et al: Benign hyperplastic nodules that originate in the peripheral zone of the prostate gland. Radiology 1993;189:707-711.
20. Thin RN: Diagnosis of chronic prostatitis: Overview and update. Int J STD AIDS 1997;8:475-481.
21. Doble A, Thomas BJ, Furr PM, et al: A search for infectious agents in chronic abacterial prostatitis using ultrasound guided biopsy. Br J Urol 1989;64:297-301.
22. Di Trapani D, Pavone C, Serretta V, et al: Chronic prostatitis and prostatodynia: Ultrasonographic alterations of the prostate, bladder neck, seminal vesicles and periprostatic venous plexus. Eur Urol 1988; 15:230-234.
23. Bude R, Bree RL, Adler RS, et al: Transrectal ultrasound appearance of granulomatous prostatitis. J Ultrasound Med 1990;9:677-680.
24. Cytron S, Weinberger M, Pitlik S, et al: Value of transrectal ultrasonography for diagnosis and treatment of prostatic abscess. Urology 1988;32(5):454-458.

25. Papanicolaou N, Pfister R, Stafford S, et al: Prostatic abscess: Imaging with transrectal ultrasound and magnetic resonance. AJR 1987;149:981-982.

26. Nghiem HT, Kellman GM, Sandberg SA, et al: Cystic lesions of the prostate. RadioGraphics 1990;10:635-650.

27. Shabsigh R, Lerner S, Fishman IJ, et al: The role of transrectal ultrasonography in the diagnosis and management of prostatic and seminal vesicle cysts. J Urol 1989;141:1206-1209.

28. Littrup PJ, Lee F, McLeary RD, et al: Transrectal ultrasound of the seminal vesicles and ejaculatory ducts: Clinical correlation. Radiology 1988;168:625-628.

29. Jarow JP, Sharlip ID, Belker AM, et al: Best practice policies for male infertility. J Urol 2002;167:2138-2144. See also AUA web site: ttps://shop.auanet.org/timssnet/products/guidelines/main_reports.cfm

30. Kuligowska E, Fenlon HM: Transrectal US in male infertility: Spectrum of findings and role in patient care. Radiology 1998;207:173-181.

31. Doble A, Thomas BJ, Furr PM, et al: A search for infectious agents in chronic abacterial prostatitis using ultrasound guided biopsy. Br J Urol 1989; 64:297-301.

32. Fuse H, Sumiya H, Ishii H, et al: Treatment of hemospermia caused by dilated seminal vesicles by direct drug injection guided by ultrasonography. J Urol 1988;140:991-992.

33. Worischeck JH, Parra RO: Chronic hematospermia: Assessment by transrectal ultrasound. Urology 1994;43(4):515-520.

34. Munkelwitz R, Krasnokutsky S, Lie J, et al: Current perspectives on hematospermia: A review. J Androl 1997;18(1):6-14

35. Levy IG, Iscoe NA, Klotz LH: Prostate cancer: 1. The descriptive epidemiology in Canada. CMAJ 1998;159(5):509.

36. Neal DE, Leung HY, Powell PH, et al: Unanswered questions in screening for prostate cancer. Euro J Cancer 2000;36:1316-1321.

37. Rietbergen JBW, Schroder FH: Screening for prostate cancer—More questions than answers. Acta Oncol 1998;37(6):515-532.

38. Thompson I, Carroll P, Coley C, et al: Prostate-specific antigen (PSA) best practice policy. Oncology 2000; 14(2):267-286. See also web site: https://shop.auanet.org/timssnet/products/guidelines/main_reports.cfm.

39. Nam RK, Jewett MAS, Krahn MD: Prostate cancer: 2. Natural history. CMAJ 1998;159(6):685-691.

40. Meyer F, Fradet Y: Prostate cancer: 4. Screening. CMAJ 1998;159(8):968-972.

41. Eng TY, Thomas CR, Herman TS: Primary radiation therapy for localized prostate cancer. Urol Oncol 2002;7:239-257.

42. Whitmore WF Jr: Natural history staging of prostate cancer. Urol Clin North Am 1984;11:205-220.

43. Garnick MB: Prostate Cancer: Screening, diagnosis and management. Ann Int Med 1993;118:804-818.

44. Gleason DF: Veterans Administration Cooperative Urological Research Group. Histologic Grading and Clinical Staging of Prostatic Carcinoma. Philadelphia, Lea & Febiger; 1977.

45. Partin AW, Yoo J, Carter HB, et al: The use of prostate specific antigen, clinical stage and Gleason score to predict pathological stage in men with localized prostate cancer. J Urol 1993;150:110-114.

46. Ross PL, Scardino PT, Kattan MW: A catalogue of prostate cancer nomograms. J Urol 2001;165:1562-1568.

47. Dugan JA, Bostwick DG, Myers RP, et al: The definition and preoperative prediction of clinically insignificant prostate cancer. JAMA 1996;275:288-294.

48. Etzioni R, Penson DF, Legler JM, et al: Overdiagnosis due to prostate-specific antigen screening: Lessons from U.S. prostate cancer incidence trends. J Nat Cancer Inst 2002;94(13):981-990.

49. Thompson IM: Counseling patients with newly diagnosed prostate cancer. Oncology 2000;14:119.

50. Goldenberg LS, Ramsey EW, Jewett MAS: Prostate cancer: 6. Surgical treatment of localized disease. CMAJ 1998;159(10):1265.

51. Warde P, Catton C, Gospodarowicz, M: Prostate cancer: 7. Radiation therapy for localized disease. CMAJ 1998;159(11):1381.

52. Thompson I, Carroll P, Coley C, et al: Prostate-specific antigen (PSA) best practice policy vol 14, No 2, from the American Urological Association. Oncology 2000; 14(2):267-286. See also web site: https://shop.auanet.org/timssnet/products/guidelines/main_reports.cfm.

53. Stenman UH, Leinonen J, Zhang WM, et al: Prostate-specific antigen. Semin Cancer Biol 1999;9:83-93.

54. Matlaga BR, Eskew A, McCullough DL: Prostate biopsy: Indications and technique. J Urol 2003;169:12-19.

55. Littrup P, Kane RA, Mellen CJ, et al: Cost effective prostate cancer detection. Reduction of low-yield biopsies. Cancer 1994;74:3146.

56. Oesterling JE, Jacobsen SJ, Chute CG, et al: Serum prostate-specific antigen in a community-based population of healthy men: Establishment of age-specific reference ranges. JAMA 1993;270(7):860-864.

57. Carter HB, Pearson JD, Metter EJ, et al: Longitudinal evaluation of prostate-specific antigen levels in men with and without prostate disease. JAMA 1992; 267(16):2215-2220.

58. Catalona WJ, Smith DS, Ornstein DK: Prostate cancer detection in men with serum PSA concentrations of 2.6-4.0 ng/ml and benign prostate examination. Enhancement of specificity with free PSA measurements. JAMA 1997;227(18):1452-1455.

59. Rifkin MD, Zerhouni EA, Gastsonis CA: Comparison of magnetic resonance imaging and ultrasound in staging early prostate cancer. N Engl J Med 1990;323(10): 621-626.

60. Partin AW, Kattan MW, Subong ENP, et al: Combination of prostate-specific-antigen, clinical stage, and Gleason score to predict pathological stage of localized prostate cancer: A multi-institutional update. JAMA 1997; 277(18):1445-1451.

61. McNeal JE, Redwine EA, Freiha FS, et al: Zonal distribution of prostatic adenocarcinoma. Am J Surg Pathol 1988;12:897-906.

62. Chen ME, Johnston DA, Tang K, et al: Detailed mapping of prostate carcinoma foci: Biopsy strategy implications. Cancer 2000;89(8):1800-1809.

63. Lee F, Torp-Pedersen S, Littrup PJ, et al: Hypoechoic lesions of the prostate: Clinical relevance of tumor size, digital rectal examination, and prostate-specific antigen. Radiology 1989;170:29-32.

64. Dahnert WF, Hamper UM, Eggleston JC, et al: Prostatic evaluation by transrectal ultrasound with histopathologic correlation: The echogenic appearance of early carcinoma. Radiology 1986;158:97-102.

65. Shinohara K, Wheeler TM, Scardino PT: The appearance of prostate cancer on transrectal ultrasonography: Correlation of imaging and pathological examinations. J Urol 1989;142:76-82.

66. Hasegawa Y, Sakamoto N: Relationship of ultrasonographic findings to histology in prostate cancer. Eur Urol 1994;26(1):10-17.

67. Rifkin MD, Dahnert W, Kurtz AB: State of the art: Endorectal sonography of the prostate gland. AJR 1990;154:691-700.
68. Dahnert WF, Hamper UM, Walsh PC, et al: The echogenic focus in prostatic sonograms, with xeroradiographic and histopathologic correlation. Radiology 1986;159:95-100.
69. Hamper UM, Sheth S, Walsh PC, et al: Bright echogenic foci in early prostatic carcinoma: Sonographic and pathologic correlation. Radiology 1990;176:339-343.
70. Dahnert WF: Ultrasonography of carcinoma of the prostate: A critical review. Appl Radiol 1988;17:39-44.
71. Frauscher F, Klauser A, Halpern EJ: Advances in ultrasound for the detection of prostate cancer. Ultrasound Quarterly 2002;18(2):135-142.
72. Rodriguez LV, Terris MK: Risks and complications of transrectal ultrasound guided needle biopsy: A prospective study and review of the literature. J Urol 1998; 160(6-I):2115-2120.
73. Dajani AS, Taubert KA, Wilson W, et al: Prevention of bacterial endocarditis. Recommendations by the American Heart Association. JAMA 1997;277(22):1794-801.
74. Clements R, Aideyan OU, Griffiths GJ, et al: Side effects and patient acceptability of transrectal biopsy of the prostate. Clin Radiol 1993;47:125-126.
75. Hodge KK, McNeal JE, Terris MK, et al: Random systematic versus directed ultrasound guided transrectal core biopsies of the prostate. J Urol 1989;142:71-75.
76. Dyke CH, Toi A, Sweet JM: Value of random ultrasound-guided transrectal prostate biopsy. Radiology 1990; 176:345-349.
77. Borboroglu PG, Sur RL, Roberts JL, et al: Repeat biopsy strategy in patients with atypical small acinar proliferation or high grade prostate intraepithelial neoplasia on initial prostate biopsy. J Urol 2001;166:866-870.
78. Princess Margaret Hospital Prostate Center biopsy results 2000-2002, unpublished data.
79. Djavan B, Ravery V, Zlotta A, et al: Prospective evaluation of prostate cancer detected on biopsies 1, 2, 3 and 4: When should we stop? J Urol 2001;166:1679-1683.
80. Djavan B, Remzi M, Schulman CC, et al: Repeat prostate biopsy: Who, how, when? Eur Urol 2002;42:93-103.
81. Chen ME, Troncoso P, Johnston DA, et al: Optimization of prostate biopsy strategy using computer based analysis. J Urol 1997;158(6):2168-2175.
82. Babaian RJ, Toi A, Kamoi K, et al: A comparative analysis of sextant and an extended 11-core multisite directed biopsy strategy. J Urol 2000;163(1):152.
83. Shinohara K, Gulati M, Koppie TM, Terris MK: Transperineal biopsy after abdominoperineal resection. J Urol 2003;169:141-144.
84. Parra RO, Gregory JG: Transrectal ultrasound in stage A1 prostate cancer. Urology 1989;34:344-346.
85. Platt J, Bree RL, Schwab RE: Accuracy of computed tomography in the staging of carcinoma of the prostate. AJR 1987;149:315-318.
86. Salo JO, Kivisaari L, Rannikko S, et al: Computerized tomography and transrectal ultrasound in the assessment of local extension of prostatic cancer before radical retropubic prostatectomy. J Urol 1987;137:435-438.
87. Terris MK, McNeal JE, Stamey TA: Invasion of the seminal vesicles by prostatic cancer: Detection with transrectal ultrasound. AJR 1990;155:811-815.
88. Stock RG, Stone NN, Ianuzzi C, et al: Seminal vesicle biopsy and laparoscopic pelvis lymph node dissection: Implications for patient selection in the radiotherapeutic management of prostate cancer. Int J Radiat Oncol Biol Phys 1995;33(4):815-821.
89. Vallancien G, Prapotnich D, Beillon B, et al: Seminal vesicle biopsies in the preoperative staging of prostatic cancer. Eur Urol 1991;19:196-200.
90. Lancaster C, Toi A, Trachtenberg J: Interstitial microwave thermotherapy for localized prostate cancer. Urology 1999;53:828-831.
91. Steiner MS, Gingrich JR, Chauhan RD: Prostate cancer gene therapy. Surg Oncol Clin N Am 2002;11(3): 607-620.
92. Chen Q, Huang Z, Luck D, et al: Preclinical studies in normal canine prostate of a novel palladium-bacteriopheophorbide (WST09) photosensitizer for photodynamic therapy of prostate cancers. Photochem Photobiol 2002;76(4):438-445.
93. Wu J, Haycocks T, Alasti H, et al: Positioning errors and prostate motion during conformal prostate radiotherapy using on-line isocentre set-up verification and implanted prostate markers. Radiother Oncol 2001;61:127-133.
94. Nag S, Beyer D, Friedland J, et al: American Brachytherapy Society (ABS) recommendations for transperineal permanent brachytherapy of prostate cancer. Int J Radiat Oncol Biol Phys 1999;44(4):789-799.
95. Saliken JC, Donnelly BJ, Rewcastle JC: The evolution and state of modern technology for prostate cryosurgery. Urology 2002;60(2 Suppl 1):26-33.

11

THE ADRENAL GLANDS

Wendy Thurston / Stephanie R. Wilson

Chapter Outline

The adrenal glands are the smallest paired organs found in the abdomen, weighing about 4 g each in a normal nonstressed adult.[1] Although they are small and tucked anteromedial to the upper pole of the kidneys, the adrenal glands play a significant role in the maintenance of homeostasis through hormone secretion.

Computed tomography (CT) has been regarded as the premier imaging modality to identify adrenal gland disease. However, sonography can be efficient and economical in the work-up of patients with suspected adrenal gland pathology. Because the adrenal glands may be involved with both local and systemic disease, a thorough understanding of the applications and limitations of all imaging techniques is necessary to direct the most appropriate imaging strategy.

EMBRYOLOGY

The adrenal gland is composed of two parts, a **cortex** and a **medulla**, which have different embryologic origins. The cortex develops from **mesoderm** tissue and the medulla from **neuroectodermal** tissue.

During the sixth week of fetal development there is rapid proliferation of mesenchymal cells, originating from the posterior abdominal wall peritoneal epithelium near the cranial end of the mesonephros (primitive kidney). These cells penetrate the retroperitoneal mesenchyme to become the **primitive adrenal cortex**.[2] Further mesenchymal cell proliferation occurs, and these cells envelop the primitive cortex more compactly to become the **permanent adrenal cortex**. By the end of the eighth gestational week the cortical mass separates from the posterior peritoneal surface and becomes surrounded by retroperitoneal connective tissue.

During the seventh week of development, cells originating from neuroectoderm migrate and invade the medial aspect of the developing primitive adrenal cortex. These cells differentiate into the chromaffin cells of the **adrenal medulla**.

At birth, the gland is composed predominantly of primitive fetal cortex and adrenal medulla. Immediately after birth, the primitive cortex begins to involute and disappears by 1 year of age. Simultaneously, the thin, compact, **permanent adrenal cortex** further differentiates into the three zones of the adult gland: **glomerulosa**, **fasciculata**, and **reticularis** (Fig. 11-1).[3]

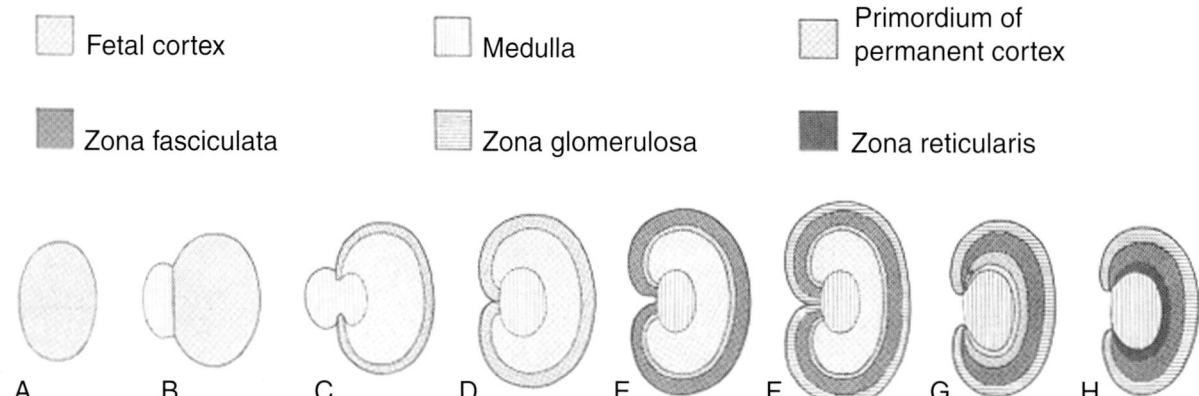

☐ Fetal cortex   ☐ Medulla   ☐ Primordium of permanent cortex

▨ Zona fasciculata   ▦ Zona glomerulosa   ▧ Zona reticularis

A   B   C   D   E   F   G   H

FIGURE 11-1. Adrenal gland embryology. A, Six weeks. **B**, Seven weeks. **C**, Eight weeks. **D** and **E**, Later stages of encapsulation of the medulla by the cortex. **F**, Newborn. **G**, One year showing fetal cortex has almost disappeared. **H**, Four years showing the adult pattern of the cortical zones. (Modified with permission from Moore KL (ed): The Developing Human: Clinically Oriented Embryology, 5th ed. Philadelphia, WB Saunders, 1993.)

NORMAL ANATOMY, MORPHOLOGY, AND PHYSIOLOGY

Anatomy

The adrenal glands are found at the level of the 11th or 12th thoracic rib, lateral to the first lumbar vertebrae (Fig. 11-2). Each measures from 2 to 3 cm in width, 4 to 6 cm in length, and 3 to 6 mm in thickness.[2] Each gland is composed of an **anteromedial ridge** and a **medial** and **lateral wing**. The glands are surrounded by fatty areolar tissue that has a thin, fibrous capsule and many fibrous extensions into the adrenal glands.[2] With their fascial support, the adrenals are relatively fixed, unlike the kidney, which is not anchored to the perinephric fascia. Thus, the adrenal glands have a more constant relationship with the abdominal great vessels than they do with the kidneys (Fig. 11-3). The adrenal gland and kidney will separate during deep inspiration or in the upright position. This may allow differentiation between renal and adrenal masses, particularly during sonographic examination.[4,6]

The **right adrenal gland** is located posterior to the inferior vena cava and cephalad to the upper pole of the right kidney (Fig. 11-4). Medially the crus of the diaphragm runs parallel to the medial wing of the gland, whereas the lateral wing is adjacent to the posteromedial aspect of the liver (see Fig. 11-3). The medial wing may extend caudally along the medial aspect of the upper pole of the kidney. The tip of the gland always terminates cephalad to the renal vessels.[7]

The **left adrenal gland** is positioned anteromedially to the kidney (Fig. 11-5). It may extend from above the superior pole of the kidney to the level of the renal hilum in 10% of persons.[8,9] The aorta and crus of the diaphragm are on the medial aspect of the adrenal. The cephalic two thirds of the gland are posterior to the

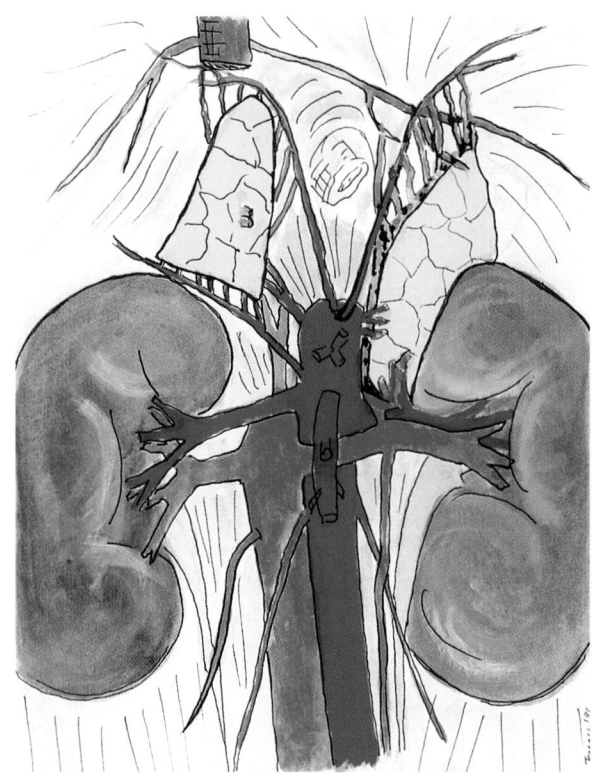

FIGURE 11-2. Anatomy and blood supply of the adrenal glands. (Courtesy of Jenny Tomash.)

stomach and, therefore, covered by peritoneum of the lesser sac. The caudal one third of the gland is related to the posterior aspect of the pancreatic body and splenic vasculature (see Fig. 11-3).[10]

On sonography, the adrenal gland is less echogenic than the surrounding perirenal fat, whereas the medulla is evident as a highly echogenic central linear structure. The echogenic linear medulla is most prominent in the fetus and newborn; however, it can be identified in thin adults.

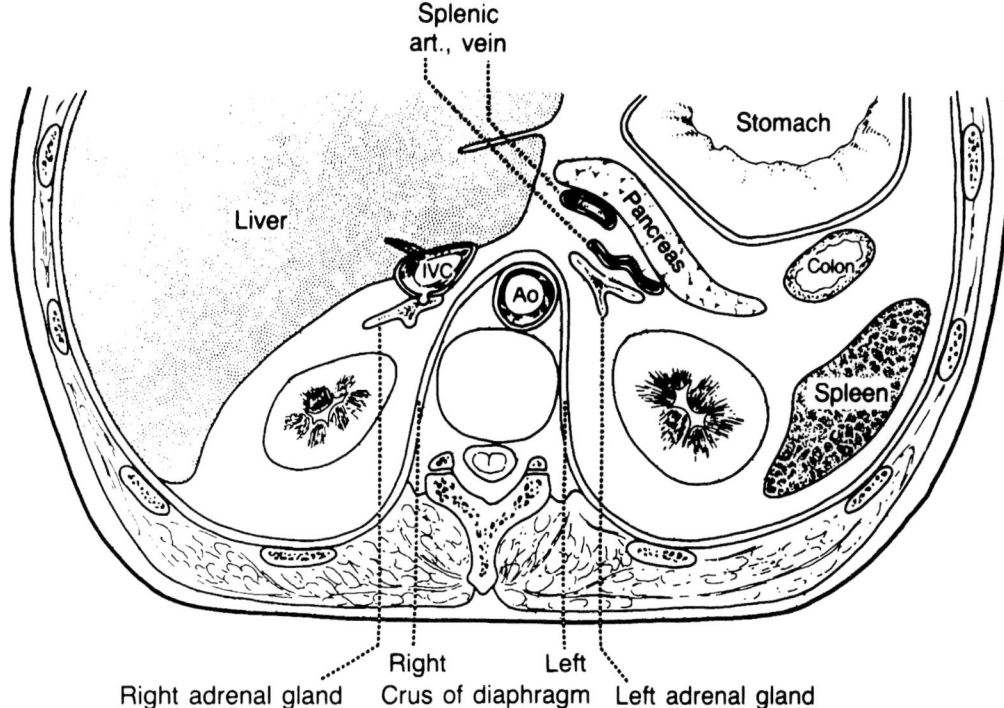

FIGURE 11-3. Cross-sectional anatomy of the adrenal glands. (From Mitty HA, Yeh HC: Radiology of the Adrenals with Sonography and CT. Philadelphia, WB Saunders, 1982.)

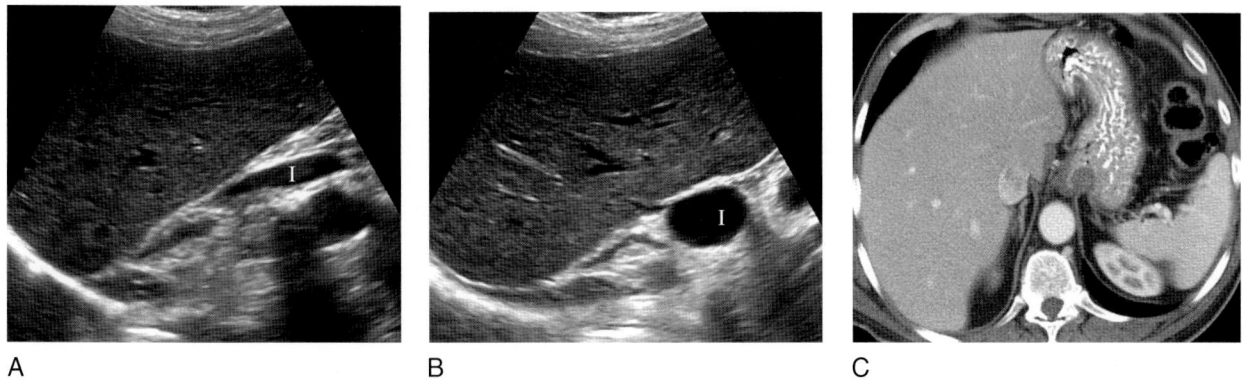

A   B   C

FIGURE 11-4. Normal adult right adrenal gland. A, Sagittal and **B,** transverse sonograms show the adrenal as a linear hypoechoic structure that lies deep to and slightly lateral to the inferior vena cava (*I*). The kidney lies caudal to the right adrenal gland and, therefore, is not seen in the same plane. **C,** CT scan confirms the retrocaval position of the right adrenal gland. Only the tip of the upper pole of the right kidney is seen. The left adrenal gland, by comparison, is located anterior to the left kidney.

Oppenheimer et al.[11] proposed that the medullary echogenicity in newborn infants is due to an increased amount of collagen around the central vessels and haphazard orientation of its cell population, resulting in multiple reflective interfaces.

Morphology

The **medial wing** of the adrenal gland is larger superiorly and smaller or absent inferiorly, whereas the **lateral wing** is larger inferiorly and smaller superiorly.[8] Complete visualization of the adrenal gland in a single sonographic plane is virtually impossible because of the complex shape of the organ.[12]

Physiology

The adrenal cortex secretes steroid hormones and the medulla secretes catecholamines. The **cortex** is subdivided into **three distinct zones**. The **zona glomeru-**

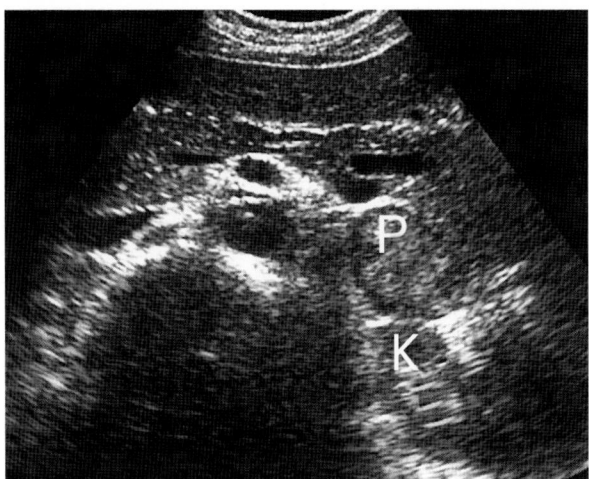

FIGURE 11-5. Left adrenal gland enlarged due to tumor. Visualization of this pheochromocytoma (*P*), via a ventral epigastric approach. Kidney (K).

losa, which is the outermost layer, produces and secretes the mineralocorticoid **aldosterone**. This hormone is part of a coordinated hormonal system (renin-angiotensin-aldosterone) involved in the homeostasis of fluid volume and blood pressure. The principal action of aldosterone is on the renal tubules, causing sodium retention. The **zona fasciculata** and **reticularis** act as a single unit and secrete **cortisol (glucocorticoid)** and **androgens**. The adrenal cortex in a nonstressed adult secretes about 20 mg per day of cortisol and with stressful stimuli may increase secretion up to 150 to 200 mg per day.[13] The physiologic significance of the adrenal androgens is not known. In excess, they may cause hirsutism or virilization in females and precocious pseudopuberty in males.[13]

The **adrenal medulla** is responsible for the synthesis and secretion of **catecholamines (epinephrine and norepinephrine)**. These hormones play an important role in an individual's response to actual or anticipated stress though they are not essential to life.[13]

ADRENAL SONOGRAPHY

Technical Aspects

Ability to visualize the adrenal glands sonographically is related to body habitus, operator experience, and type of equipment. With the introduction of high-resolution, real-time sector scanners, the adrenal glands have become easier to examine. Ideally the patient should fast for 6 to 8 hours prior to the examination in an attempt to reduce the amount of intervening bowel gas.

Marchal et al.[12] reported that the normal right and left adrenal glands were visualized by high-resolution real-time sonography in 92% and 71% of patients, respectively. Cortex and medulla were differentiated in 13% of patients. Alternatively, Günther et al.[14] studied

60 healthy subjects with high-resolution real-time sonography and identified adrenal glands in only one thin female. In newborn infants, real-time high-frequency scanning identified the right and left adrenal glands in 97% and 83% of patients, respectively.[11]

Scanning Techniques

Because of the complex shape of the adrenal gland, a comprehensive, systematic, multiplanar approach is necessary to fully evaluate it. The gland should be assessed in the transverse, coronal, and longitudinal plane, as well as in the supine, oblique, and lateral decubitus positions. **Right Adrenal Gland.** The right adrenal gland is best evaluated intercostally at the midaxillary or anterior axillary line.[8,12,14] The key to the identification of the right adrenal is to remember its suprarenal location and its relationship to the IVC (Fig. 11-6). The liver provides a good acoustic window. Alternatively, a subcostal oblique approach parallel to the rib cage at the midclavicular line can be used. Scanning from a direct anterior or posterior approach is typically poor because of overlying bowel gas or intervening muscle and fat interfaces (Fig. 11-7). **Left Adrenal Gland.** The left adrenal gland is best evaluated from the epigastrium or intercostally at the posterior axillary or midaxillary line through the spleen or kidney.[8,14] The key to the identification of the left adrenal is to remember it lies anterior to the upper pole of the left kidney (see Fig. 11-5). As with the right adrenal gland, a direct posterior approach is usually not helpful.

Pitfalls

When the scan plane is parallel to the anterior surface of the lateral wing, false enlargement may be observed.[5] This could lead to erroneous diagnosis of hyperplasia or a small mass. If this occurs, changing the angle of the insonating sound beam by altering the intercostal space should allow differentiation between real and false enlargement.

Structures that may **simulate adrenal masses** include a thickened diaphragmatic crus, an accessory spleen, the gastric fundus, a gastric diverticulum, the renal vein, retrocrural and retroperitoneal lymphadenopathy, upper pole renal cysts and tumors, pancreatic tumors, a hypertrophied caudate lobe of the liver, and interposition of a fluid-filled colon (see box).[8,14]

INFECTIOUS DISEASES

Tuberculosis, histoplasmosis, blastomycosis, meningococcus, echinococcus, cytomegalovirus, herpes, and pneumocystis are the most frequent infectious organisms that affect the adrenal gland.[15-17]

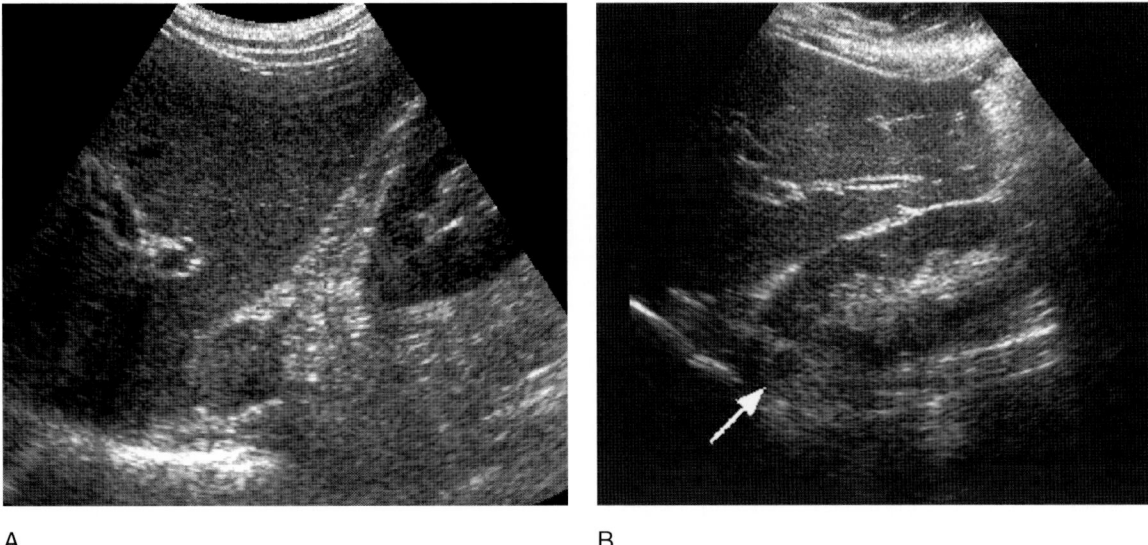

A   B

FIGURE 11-6. Importance of position in localization of pathology to the adrenal gland. A, Right adrenal mass. Sagittal sonogram shows a solid mass cephalad to the upper pole of the right kidney. **B,** Metastatic lymph node in a different patient. A sagittal sonogram shows a small solid nodule (*arrow*) posterior to the upper pole of the kidney. This location is not consistent with the adrenal.

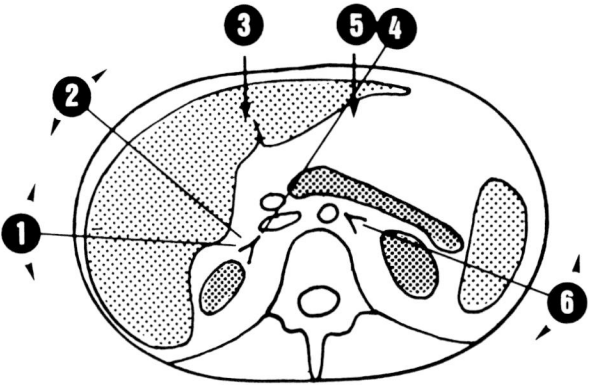

FIGURE 11-7. Scan planes for sonographic visualization of the adrenal glands. *1, 2* = Lateral approach (*right*): 1=midaxillary line; 2 = anterior axillary line. *3, 5* = Ventral approach (*right and left*): paramedian or midclavicular line. *4* = Ventral approach (right adrenal through the left liver lobe): longitudinal oblique scan. 6 = Lateral approach (*left*): posterior axillary line. (Modified from Günther RW, Kelbel C, Lenner V: Real-time ultrasound of normal adrenal glands and small tumors. J Clin Ultrasound 1984;12:211-217. Reprinted by permission of John Wiley & Sons, Inc.)

ADRENAL PSEUDOMASSES

Thickened diaphragmatic crus
Accessory spleen
Gastric fundus
Gastric diverticulum
Renal vein
Retrocrural and retroperitoneal adenopathy
Upper pole renal cysts and tumors
Pancreatic tumors
Hypertrophied caudate lobe of the liver
Fluid-filled colon interposed between stomach and
    kidney

Tuberculosis has a variable appearance, depending on the stage of infection. Acutely, there is bilateral diffuse enlargement, often inhomogeneous, due to caseous necrosis. Punctate calcification is a feature. Chronically, the glands become atrophic and calcified.[16,18] Tuberculosis and **histoplasmosis** are the two most common agents responsible for adrenal calcification in the adult population (Fig. 11-8).[18] Calcification in the absence of a soft tissue mass should suggest infection rather than neoplasm. When the adrenal glands are involved with

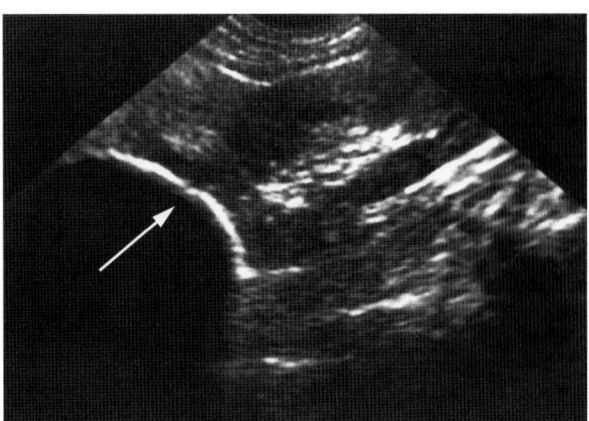

FIGURE 11-8. Adrenal gland calcification. Sagittal sonogram shows a large calcification of the adrenal gland with distal acoustic shadowing.

tuberculosis, chest radiographs and sputum cultures may be negative. Prior to development of antituberculous therapy, tuberculosis was the most common cause of Addison's disease (adrenal insufficiency). Autoimmune disorders predominate as the most common cause of adrenal insufficiency.

In association with **AIDS**, both infectious and neoplastic involvement of the adrenal gland are being found with increased frequency at autopsy. The most common offending organisms include fungi (histoplasmosis), mycobacteria, CMV, herpes, *Pneumocystis*, HIV, and toxoplasmosis.[16,17] Grizzle[17] described focal or diffuse damage of the glands by cytomegalovirus in 70% of patients who died with AIDS. Sonographically, these lesions are usually hypoechoic masses that may be heterogeneous and gas containing if abscess formation occurs.

Bacterial adrenal abscesses are found more commonly in the neonate and are relatively uncommon in adults.[19,20] In the neonate, hematogenous seeding of normal glands or those affected by hemorrhage can result in abscess formation.[20] As **organ transplantation** becomes more popular, patients receiving exogenous steroid for immunosuppression are also at increased risk for developing adrenal infection. Patients with **endogenous excess steroid production** also have an increased risk of developing adrenal infection.[17]

BENIGN ADRENAL NEOPLASMS

Adenoma

Adrenal adenomas can be regarded as either **hyperfunctioning** or **nonfunctioning**. Adrenal adenomas are found in about 3% of adult autopsies and most are nonfunctioning.[21] Ten percent of patients will have bilateral adrenal adenomas.[22] The incidence increases with advancing age.[22] Adenomas have been reported in patients with hypertension, diabetes, hyperthyroidism, renal cell carcinoma,[23] and hereditary adenomatosis of the colon and rectum.[24] Patients with hyperfunctioning adrenal adenomas will present with the manifestations of excess hormone secretion, whereas nonfunctioning adenomas are typically detected incidentally. Hyperfunctioning adrenal adenomas most commonly give rise to **Cushing's syndrome** or **Conn's disease**.

Cushing's Syndrome

Cushing's syndrome was described in 1932 by Harvey Cushing and is characterized by truncal obesity, hirsutism, amenorrhea, hypertension, weakness, and abdominal striae. This results from **excessive cortisol secretion**, which may occur with adrenal hyperplasia (70%), adenoma (20%), carcinoma (10%),[21] or from exogenous corticosteroid administration. **Cushing's**

disease is the result of hyperplastic adrenal glands excreting excessive cortisol due to elevated ACTH production from a pituitary adenoma. Biochemical profile with high plasma cortisol and urinary 17-hydroxycorticoid levels and low serum ACTH suggests an autonomous adrenal tumor (adenoma/carcinoma) as the source of excessive hormone.

Conn's Disease

Conn's disease results from **excessive secretion of aldosterone** and was first described in 1955.[25] Primary aldosteronism can result from adrenal adenoma (70%), adrenal hyperplasia (30%), and, rarely, adrenal carcinoma.[26] Clinically, hyperaldosteronism causes hypertension, muscular weakness, tetany, and ECG abnormalities. Patients with unexplained hypertension and hypokalemia should suggest excess secretion of aldosterone. Patients with hyperaldosteronism from an adenoma most typically are female,[27] whereas those with hyperaldosteronism from hyperplasia more commonly are male.[28] These tumors tend to be small, usually less than 2 cm in size. Biochemically, elevated urine and serum aldosterone levels, hypokalemia, hypernatremia, and elevated bicarbonate and low plasma pH levels are found. A suppressed renin level indicates primary hyperaldosteronism.

Pathologically, it may be difficult to differentiate nodules of hyperplasia from adrenal adenomas. Nodules greater then 1 cm are likely to be adenomas.[1] As well, it may be impossible histologically to differentiate adenoma from carcinoma with biologic behavior as the only defining feature. Histologically, nonhyperfunctioning adenomas are composed of lipid-filled cells indicative of their secretory inactivity.[1]

Patients with a small adrenal mass and evidence of excess hormone production usually require resection, which is often done laparoscopically. Size criteria are often used to direct further management with nonfunctioning adrenal masses. A nonfunctioning adrenal mass measuring 3 to 6 cm is usually considered potentially malignant.[29,30]

Imaging of Adrenal Adenoma. The majority of adrenal masses are discovered as an incidental finding on CT examination or as an isolated finding during the staging work-up in a patient with a known primary tumor. **The intracytoplasmic lipid** of adrenal adenomas has initiated the use of unenhanced CT attenuation values and opposed phase chemical shift MRI to allow their diagnosis.[31] Korobkin et al.[32] assessed the percentage of lipid-rich cortical cells histologically in 20 resected adrenal adenomas. They found an inverse linear relationship between the amount of lipid in adrenal adenomas and their unenhanced CT number. Many accumulated series have demonstrated that if an adrenal mass has unenhanced CT attenuation values of 10 HU or less, the overall sensitivity and specificity for the diagnosis of adrenal adenoma are 75% and 96%, respectively.[33] At 0 HU or less, the sensitivity and specificity are 47% and 100%, respectively.[33] It has also been shown that loss of signal in an adrenal mass on opposed phase chemical shift MRI is also related to the amount of intracytoplasmic lipid.[31,32,34] An optimal algorithm for characterizing an adrenal mass has not been firmly established; however, it appears that the use of unenhanced CT attenuation values or opposed phase chemical shift MRI allows characterization of an adrenal mass as benign without the need for other invasive procedures.[35]

On sonography, adrenal adenomas are solid, small, round, and well defined (Fig. 11-9). Sonography is often better than CT in determining organ of origin of a large mass, particularly in the right upper quadrant. Gore et al.[36] demonstrated that the right upper quadrant retroperitoneal fat reflection is displaced posteriorly by hepatic and subhepatic masses, whereas kidney and adrenal masses displace it anteriorly. This is best appreciated using a parasagittal plane (Fig. 11-10).

Myelolipoma

Adrenal myelolipomas are rare, benign, **nonfunctioning tumors** composed of varying proportions of fat and bone marrow elements.[37] The etiology and pathogenesis of these lesions are not known, although they are

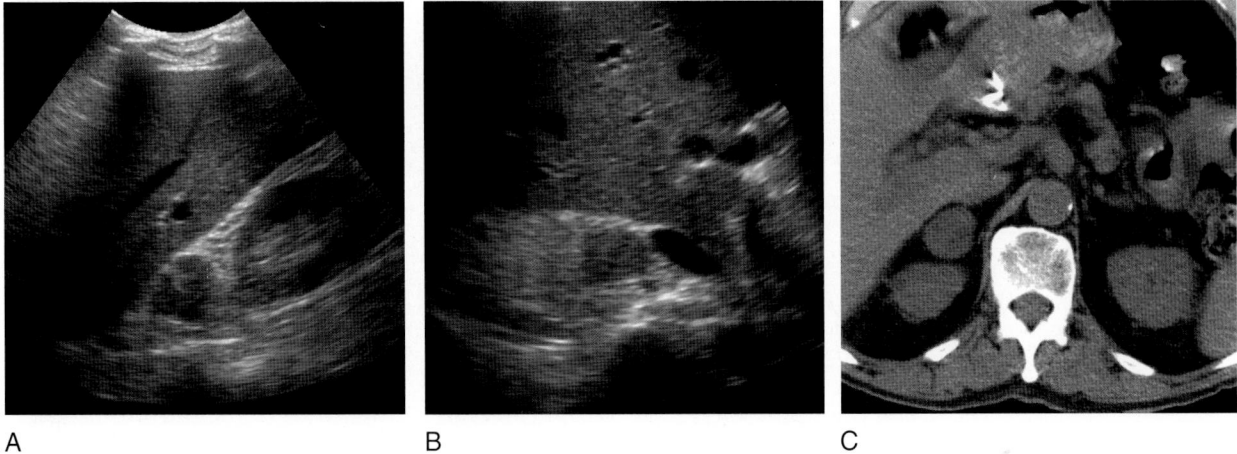

A   B   C

FIGURE 11-9. Adrenal adenoma. A, Sagittal and **B,** transverse sonograms show a small, solid right adrenal mass between the liver and the upper pole of the right kidney. **C,** Confirmatory CT scan demonstrates low attenuation of the right adrenal gland confirming adenoma.

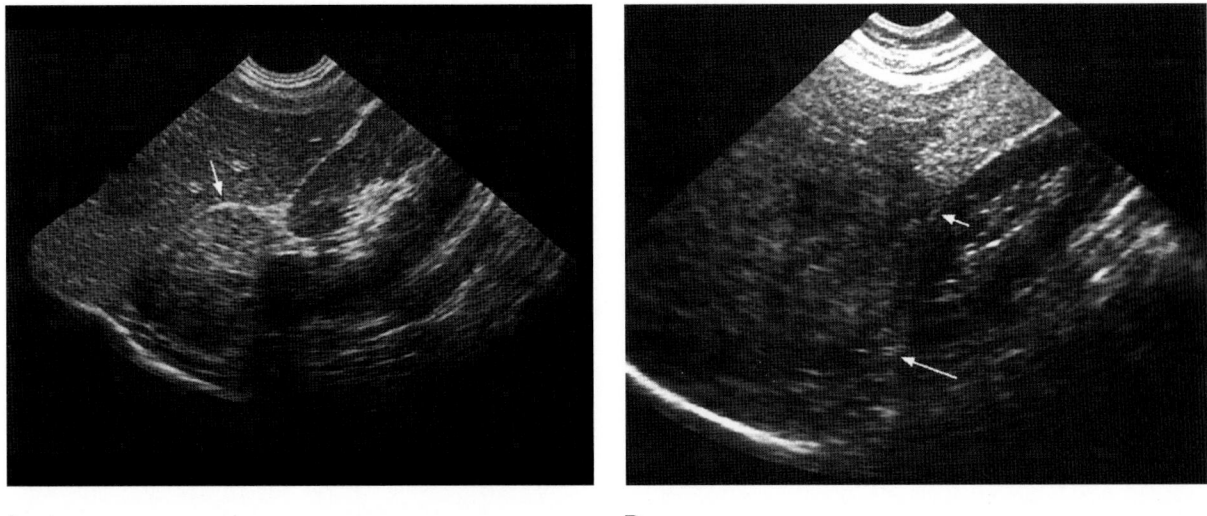

A   B

FIGURE 11-10. Retroperitoneal fat stripe displacement. Parasagittal sonograms demonstrating, **A,** anterior displacement of the retroperitoneal fat stripe (*arrow*) by a right adrenal cortical cancer, and **B,** posterior displacement of the retroperitoneal fat stripe (*arrows*) by a large hepatic adenoma.

thought to arise in the **zona fasciculata** of the adrenal cortex. Males and females are equally affected as are both glands. Tumors most commonly occur during the fifth or sixth decade of life. Myelolipomas are typically discovered incidentally in asymptomatic individuals with a frequency at autopsy of 0.08% to 0.2%.[38] Although tumors can range in size from microscopic to 30 cm, most are less than 5 cm in diameter.[39] If these tumors undergo hemorrhage, necrosis, or compress surrounding structures, symptoms may occur. Imaging features of myelolipoma depend on the varying proportion of fat, myeloid element, hemorrhage, and calcification/ossification present.

On sonography, these tumors are typically seen as an echogenic mass in the adrenal bed if a significant amount of fat is present (Fig. 11-11). When small, they may be hard to differentiate from the adjacent echogenic retroperitoneal fat. **Propagation speed artifact** occurs as a result of decreased sound velocity through fatty masses. Originally described by Richman et al.[40] with an adrenal myelolipoma, apparent diaphragmatic disruption was noted as a result of this velocity change (Fig. 11-12). The presence of this artifact is good evidence as to the fatty nature of a mass.[38,40] Musante et al.[38] found this artifact only when tumors were larger than 4 cm. The tumors may be homogeneous or heterogeneous and, if predom-

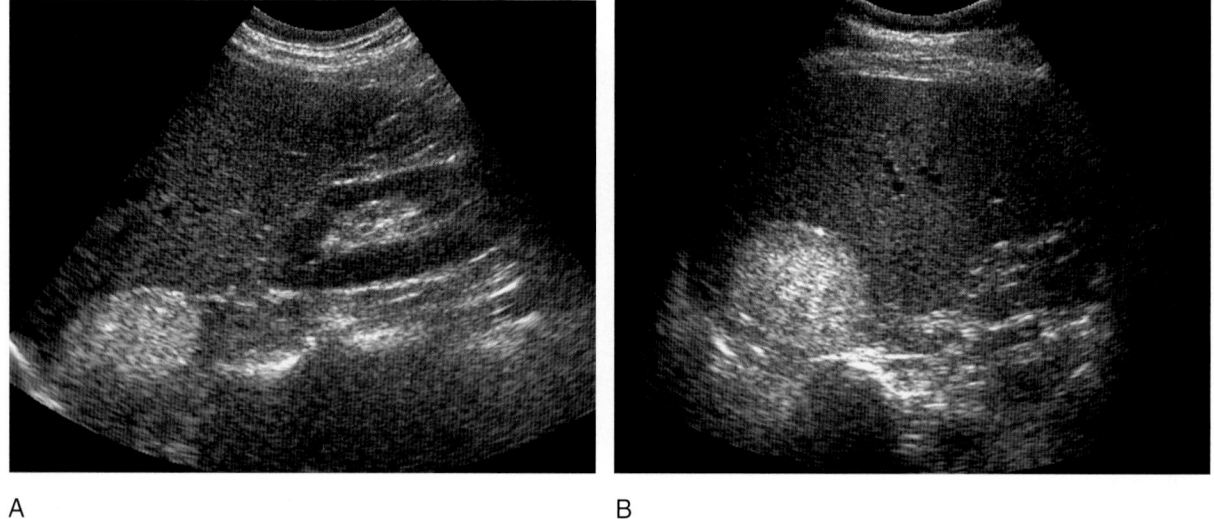

A   B

FIGURE 11-11. Myelolipoma. A, Sagittal and **B,** transverse sonograms show a homogeneous, highly echogenic, well-defined mass in the right adrenal gland.

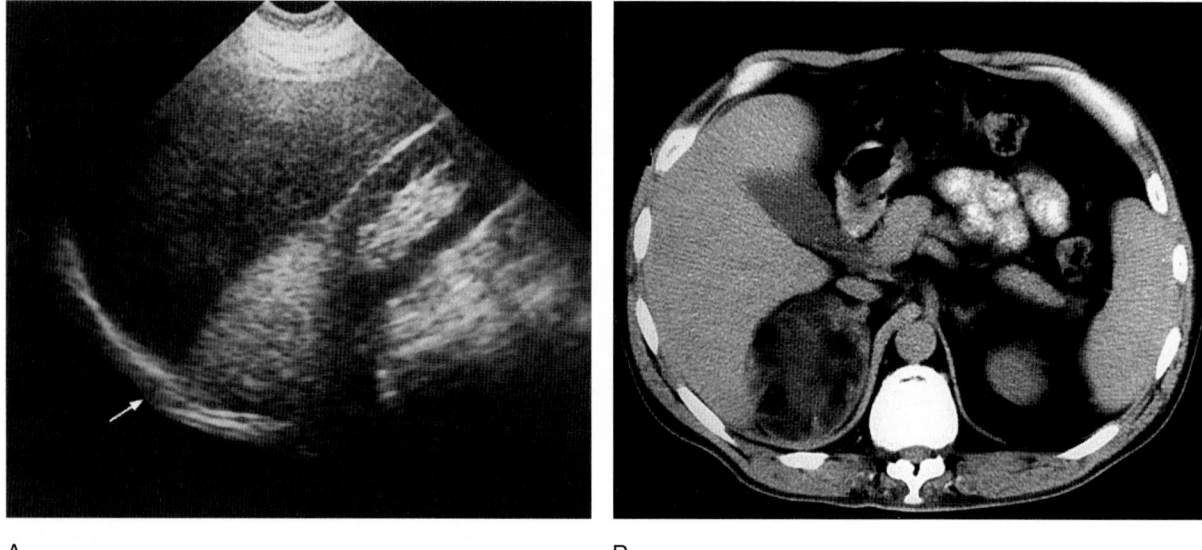

A   B

FIGURE 11-12. Myelolipoma. A, Sagittal sonogram shows a large echogenic adrenal mass with apparent diaphragmatic disruption as a result of **propagation speed artifact** (*arrow*). **B,** Confirmatory CT demonstrates the presence of fat within the right adrenal mass.

inantly of myeloid component, they will be isoechoic or hypoechoic. The heterogeneity may be due to internal hemorrhage, which is common. Focal areas of calcification may be seen.

CT is very sensitive for the diagnosis of adrenal myelolipomas and should be performed to confirm the presence of fat suspected sonographically (see Fig. 11-12). Musante et al.[38] found that unenhanced CT could explain confusing sonographic signs, including the demonstration of fat within sonographically isoechoic/hypoechoic myeloid predominant myelolipomas.

The differential diagnosis of a suprarenal fatty mass includes myelolipoma, renal angiomyolipoma, lipoma, retroperitoneal liposarcoma, lymphangioma, increased fat deposition, and teratoma.[41] If the adrenal origin of a fatty mass can be ascertained with imaging (US, CT, or MRI), the most likely diagnosis is adrenal myelolipoma. When large or atypical, fine-needle aspiration may be necessary to establish the diagnosis. The presence of mature fat cells and megakaryocytes is characteristic of adrenal myelolipoma.[41-43]

Pheochromocytoma

Pheochromocytoma was first described by Frankel in 1886. Pheochromocytomas are usually **hyperfunctioning tumors** that secrete **norepinephrine** and **epinephrine** into the blood. It is the excess secretion of these catecholamines that gives rise to the clinical manifestations of hypertension, pounding or severe headache, palpitations often with tachycardia, and excessive inappropriate perspiration.[44] These symptoms are often episodic.

These tumors typically arise from the **neuroectodermal tissue** of the **adrenal medulla**. They are usually solitary but 10% are bilateral. Ectopic extra-adrenal pheochromocytomas occur in 10% of patients and have been described in the organ of Zuckerkandl, the sympathetic nerve chains, the aortic and carotid chemoreceptors, the bladder, the prostate, and the chest. Multiple or extra-adrenal pheochromocytomas are more common in children.[45] Ten to thirteen percent of intra-adrenal pheochromocytomas and 40% of extra-adrenal pheochromocytomas are malignant.[15] Metastatic disease is the only reliable indicator of malignancy. Pheochromocytomas are associated with many **neuroectodermal disorders**, including tuberous sclerosis, neurofibromatosis, Hippel-Lindau disease, and multiple endocrine neoplasia (MEN) IIa (50%) and IIb (90%).[15] Autopsy incidence of pheochromocytomas is about 0.1%, and the frequency in hypertensive patients is 0.4% to 2%.[46] This rare tumor occurs most commonly in adults between the fourth and sixth decades of life and is a curable cause of hypertension.

Biochemical screening is essential to confirm the diagnosis of pheochromocytoma. This is accomplished by measuring the level of **urinary catecholamines** and its metabolites **vanillylmandelic acid** (**VMA**) and **total metanephrines**.

Pathologically, pheochromocytomas are well encapsulated, weigh 90 to 100 g, and measure 5 to 6 cm in diameter.[46] The right gland is affected twice as frequently as the left gland. These tumors have a red-to-brown color on cut surface and microscopically demonstrate large pleomorphic cells with abundant cytoplasm and irregular nuclei. Calcification may be seen. Neurosecretory granules are seen ultrastructurally.[44]

Sonography has proved accurate in detecting adrenal pheochromocytomas, particularly because most are large and well marginated. Bowerman et al.[46] found in a series of eight surgically confirmed cases of pheochromocytoma that most were either heterogeneous or homogeneously solid. Those that were heterogeneous had areas of necrosis or hemorrhage (Fig. 11-13). Two tumors were predominantly cystic, which corresponded to old blood and necrotic debris, and one of these demonstrated a fluid-fluid level.

Extra-adrenal pheochromocytoma thought to lie in the retroperitoneum may be more difficult to localize with sonography because of body habitus and overlying bowel gas. In these patients, CT or MRI may be extremely useful for localization. For patients with suspected recurrent or metastatic disease, iodine-131-MIBG scintigraphy can play a significant role in screening.[47]

Multiple Endocrine Neoplasia

Multiple endocrine neoplasia (MEN) is a **familial** disease that is categorized into **three types**:

- MEN I affects pancreatic islets, the adrenal cortex, and pituitary and parathyroid gland;
- MEN IIa (Sipple's syndrome) includes medullary thyroid carcinoma, parathyroid hyperplasia, and pheochromocytoma; and
- MEN IIb (III) includes all features of IIa with marfanoid facies, mucosal neuromas, and gastrointestinal ganglioneuromatosis.

MEN II is inherited as an autosomal dominant trait and believed to be caused by a genetic defect in the neural crest.[48] Pheochromocytomas in MEN syndromes most typically are:

- in the adrenal gland;
- usually bilateral (65%);[49]
- multicentric within the gland;
- more often malignant; and
- frequently asymptomatic.

Patients diagnosed with MEN II should be screened biochemically and with imaging on a routine basis as they will eventually develop bilateral adrenal pheochromocytomas.

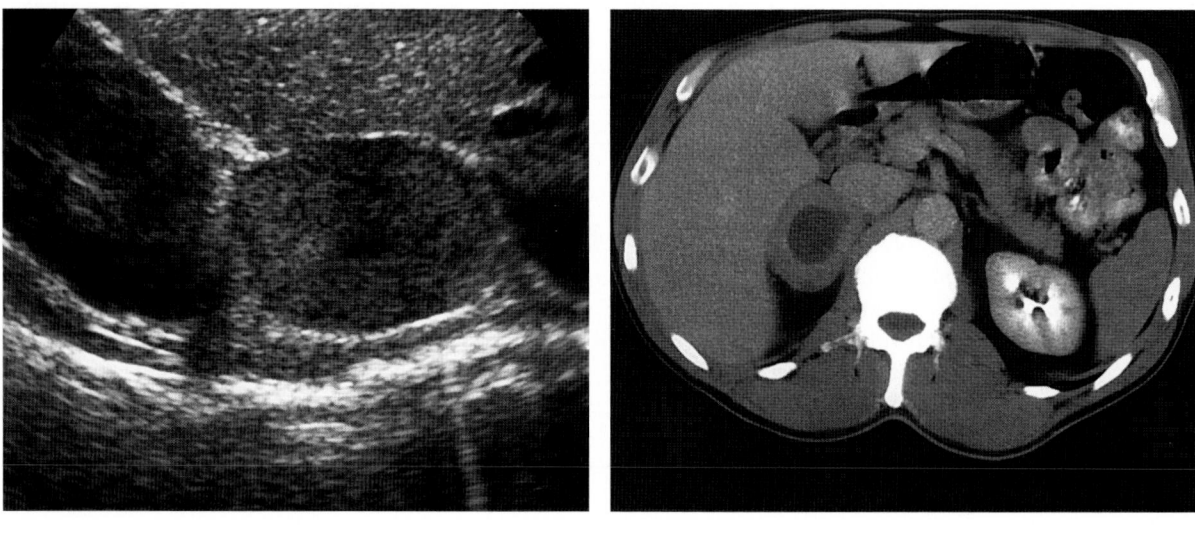

A   B

FIGURE 11-13. Pheochromocytoma. A, Transverse sonogram shows a solid right adrenal mass situated between the kidney and inferior vena cava. A central hypoechoic area corresponds to an area of necrosis. **B,** CT scan shows the large, partially necrotic tumor intimate to the posterior aspect of the inferior vena cava.

Rare Benign Adrenal Neoplasms

Ganglioneuromas are benign tumors occurring most frequently in adults.[50] They are composed of **ganglion** and **Schwann cells** and arise most frequently in the sympathetic chain, with 30% arising in the adrenal gland.[50] They are slow growing and usually clinically silent unless pressure phenomenon occurs. Rarely, they increase urinary catecholamine levels with symptoms of diarrhea, hypertension, and sweating.[50] Sonographically, they are solid and homogeneous and, because of their soft consistency, are pliable and change shape rather than displace organs.[51] The diagnosis can only be made histologically.

Hemangiomas of the adrenal gland are rare, benign, **nonfunctioning** tumors. Most are small and discovered incidentally at autopsy. They may grow large and range from 2 to 15 cm in diameter.[52] Histologically, these hemangiomas resemble hemangiomas elsewhere in the body and consist of **multiple dilated, endothelial-lined, blood-filled channels.**[53] Sonographically, they have a nonspecific structural pattern with cystic, solid, and complex appearances. Calcification in the form of phleboliths may be seen (Fig. 11-14).[54] MRI has been useful in the differentiation of liver hemangiomas and perhaps may play a role here if the diagnosis is suspected. With time and growth, these lesions often hemorrhage; therefore, surgical treatment is warranted.

Other rare adrenal gland tumors, such as **teratomas, lipomas, fibromas, leiomyomas, osteomas,** and **neurofibromas,** have been reported. Radiologic findings are nonspecific. Most typically, the diagnosis is made histologically.

MALIGNANT ADRENAL NEOPLASMS

Adrenal Cortical Cancer

Primary adrenal cortical cancer is a rare malignancy and accounts for only 0.2% of all deaths from cancer.[55] It may arise from any of the layers in the adrenal cortex. Tumors may be **hyperfunctioning** (54%) or **nonfunctioning** (46%).[55] Hyperfunctioning tumors are detected earlier because of their clinical manifestations of excess hormone production, which include:

- Cushing's syndrome (most common)
- Adrenogenital syndrome (virilization or feminization)
- Precocious puberty
- Conn's syndrome (rare)

Hyperfunctioning tumors occur more commonly in females, whereas nonfunctioning tumors are more common in males. Overall, adrenal cortical cancer occurs more commonly in females. These tumors occur most commonly in the fourth decade with equal frequency bilaterally. Tumors range in size from small to very large at the time of presentation. On cut surface they are predominantly yellow with larger lesions exhibiting areas of hemorrhage and necrosis. Adrenal cortical cancer is a highly malignant tumor and has a tendency to invade the adrenal vein, inferior vena cava, and lymphatics[56] and to recur following surgery.

The **sonographic appearance** is variable, depending on the size of the mass. Hyperfunctioning tumors tend to be smaller when discovered and usually demonstrate a homogeneous echo pattern similar to renal cortex. The

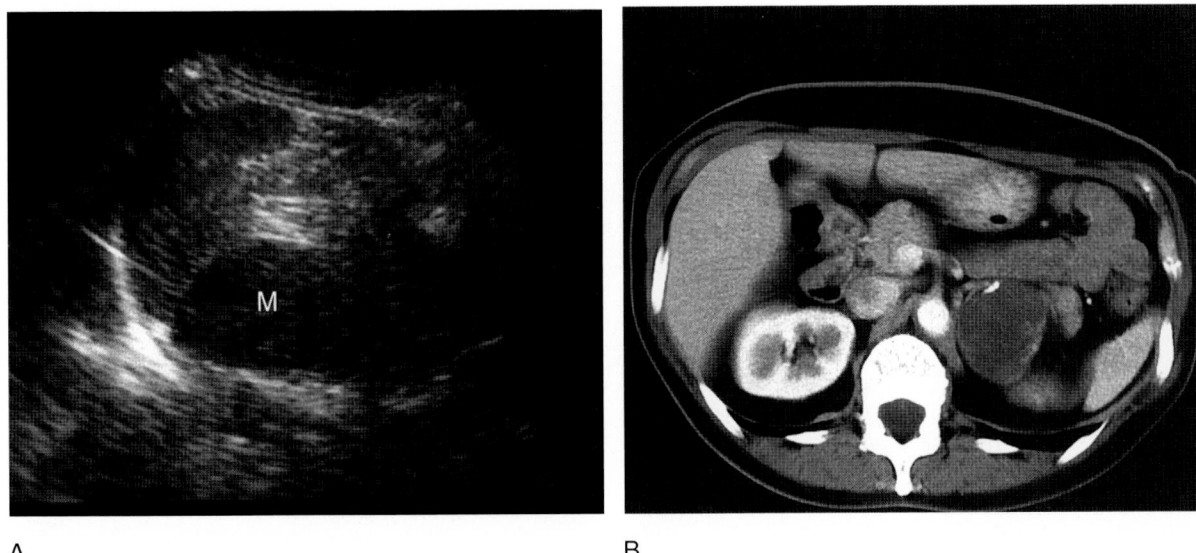

FIGURE 11-14. Adrenal gland hemangioma. A, Sagittal sonogram demonstrates a nonspecific solid mass, *M*, in the left adrenal gland. **B,** CT shows a nonspecific enhancing heterogeneous left adrenal mass with focal calcification.

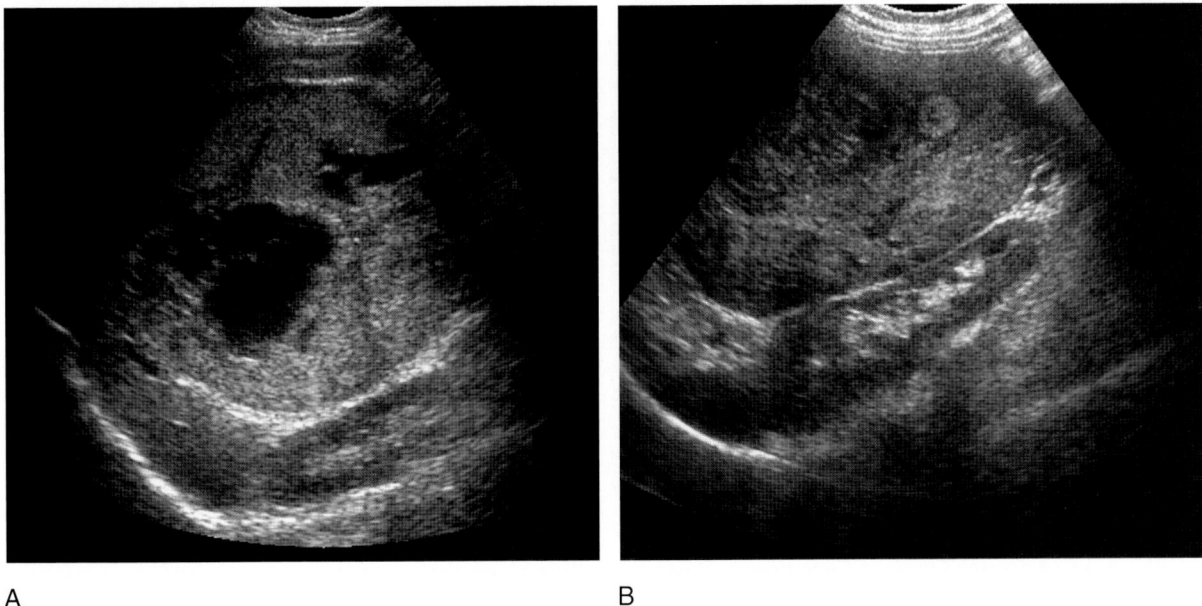

FIGURE 11-15. Large adrenal tumors. A, Adrenal pheochromocytoma. Sagittal sonogram of the left flank shows a large complex mass with cystic components lying anterior to the left kidney. **B,** Adrenal cortical carcinoma. Sagittal sonogram of the left flank shows an inhomogeneous solid mass anterior to the left kidney.

larger, nonfunctioning lesions are more heterogeneous, with central areas of necrosis and hemorrhage. Nineteen percent will demonstrate calcification. All lesions tend to be well defined with a lobulated border. Occasionally, a surrounding echogenic, capsule-like, thin rim is seen (27%).[55] Fishman et al.[57] have suggested that this may represent a well-vascularized portion of the adrenal cortical cancer and may be specific for this diagnosis.

Unfortunately, the sonographic appearance of adrenal masses does not allow differentiation between adenoma, carcinoma, pheochromocytoma, and metastases (Fig. 11-15). Smaller lesions are more likely benign, and larger masses with hemorrhage, necrosis, and calcification are more likely malignant (Fig. 11-16). If a large, necrotic, calcified adrenal mass is noted as an isolated finding, in the absence of a known primary tumor, adrenal cortical cancer should be suspected. Sonography is an excellent screening method that allows rapid, noninvasive confirmation and localization of a lesion in patients suspected of having an adrenal tumor on clinical grounds. Duplex and color Doppler may be helpful to interrogate the veins for venous tumor extension.

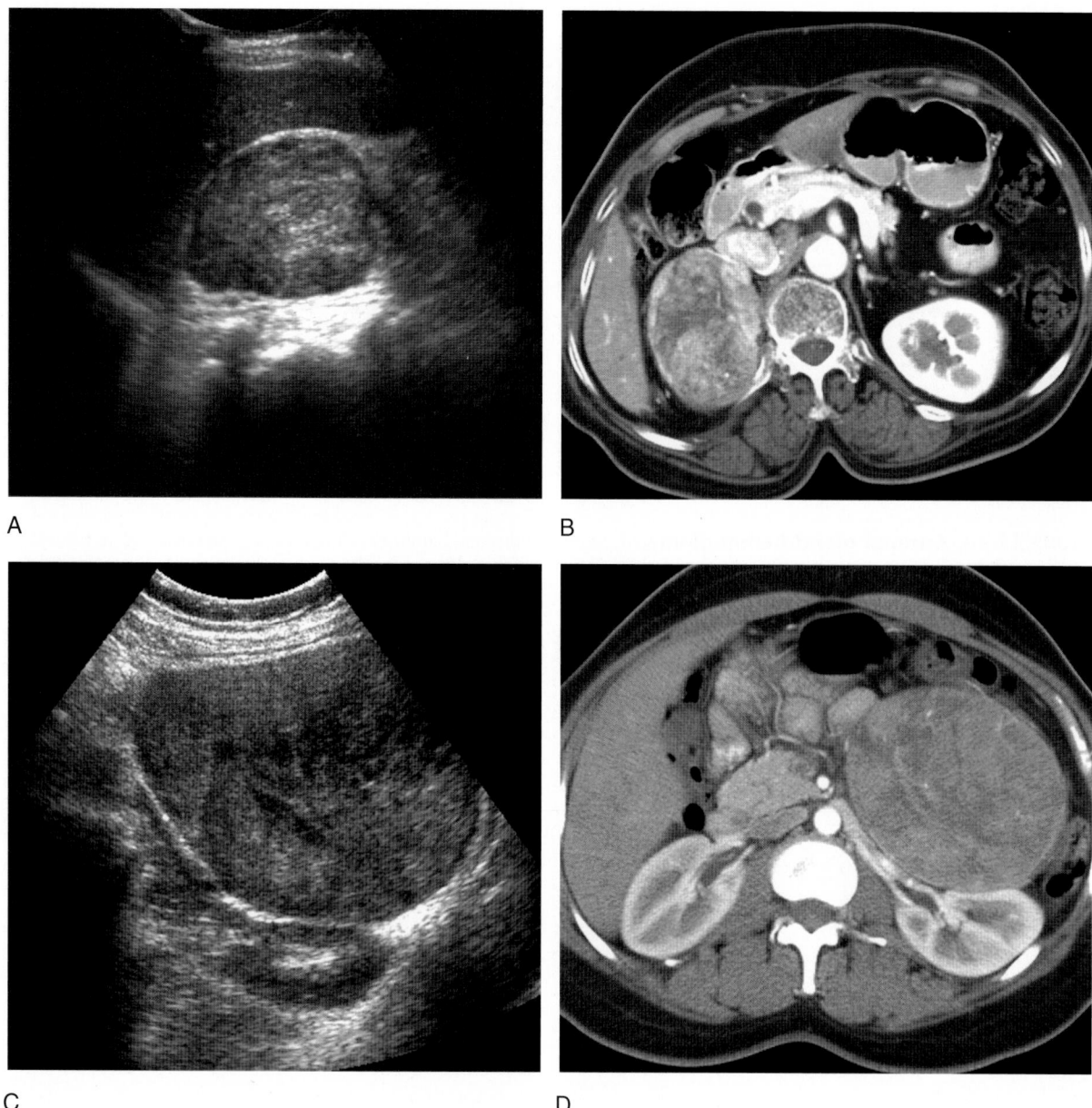

FIGURE 11-16. Adrenal Cortical Carcinoma. Value of localizing a large flank mass to the adrenal gland. **A,** Transverse sonogram and **B,** corresponding CT scan show a large, solid heterogeneous mass, which is above the right kidney and impinging on the posterior aspect of the inferior vena cava. Right adrenal masses commonly lie cephalad to the right kidney. **C,** Transverse sonogram and **D,** corresponding CT scan show a large solid mass anterior to the left kidney. Left renal masses are commonly seen lying anterior to the left kidney.

Ultrasound can be used to assess for metastatic spread, as well as for guided fine-needle aspiration. Fine-needle aspiration can be difficult when trying to differentiate adenoma from well-differentiated carcinoma.

Lymphoma

Primary lymphoma of the adrenal gland is rare but may occur. It may arise from heterotrophic lymphoid elements that are occasionally found in normal adrenal glands.[58] More commonly, however, adrenal gland involvement is due to **contiguous spread** from bulky retroperitoneal disease. **Non-Hodgkin disease** is the most common cell type with 4% of patients exhibiting discrete adrenal masses, often bilateral (46%).[59,60] At autopsy, adrenal involvement will be seen in 24%.[59] Following therapy, isolated adrenal gland recurrence may be seen. Necrosis and calcification within adrenal gland lymphoma are rare without prior treatment.[59]

On sonography, intranodal and extranodal lymphoma most typically appears as a discrete or conglomerate hypoechoic mass (Fig. 11-17). This is likely related to

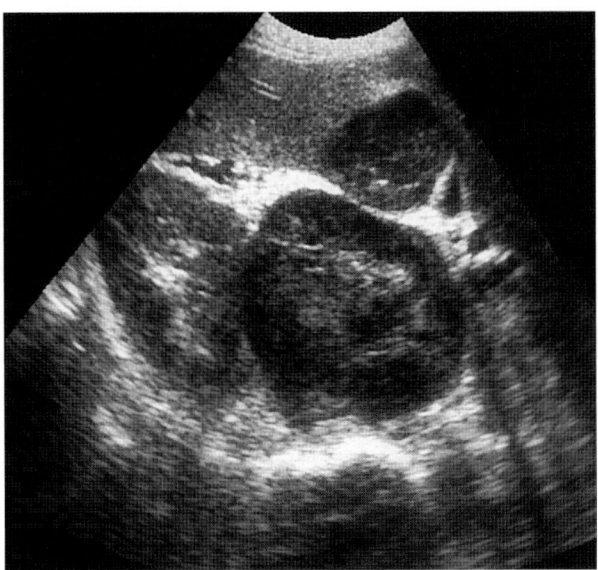
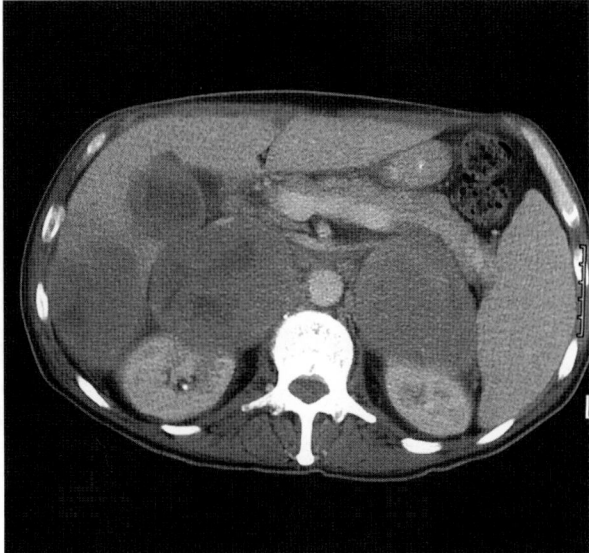

A　　　　　　　　　　　　　　　　　B

FIGURE 11-17. Adrenal lymphoma. A, Transverse sonogram shows a large, solid right adrenal mass as well as a large, solid hepatic mass in this AIDS patient. **B,** CT shows bilateral solid adrenal masses, hepatic masses, and splenomegaly.

the internal monotonous cell population within the tumor. Masses may be so hypoechoic as to simulate cysts; however, lack of appropriate through-transmission will indicate their solid nature.

Kaposi's Sarcoma

The adrenal glands of patients with **AIDS** demonstrate an increased incidence of both **opportunistic infection** (CMV, histoplasmosis, *Candida*, *Cryptococcus*, herpes, *Pneumocystis*, *Mycobacterium avium intracellulare*, HIV, and toxoplasmosis)[16,17,61,62] and **neoplasm** (Kaposi's sarcoma and lymphoma). If 90% or more of adrenal tissue is damaged by infection or tumor, frank adrenal insufficiency occurs.[63] This is often a late manifestation in AIDS patients.[61,62]

Sonographically, Kaposi's sarcoma of the adrenal gland is not well documented in the literature. A non-specific solid mass with or without necrosis may be seen in the adrenal bed. Biopsy is necessary for confirmation (Fig. 11-18).

Metastases

The adrenal gland is the **fourth** most frequent site of metastatic disease after lung, liver, and bone. The most common **primary tumors** giving rise to adrenal metastases include lung, breast, melanoma, kidney, thyroid, and colon cancer. Most are clinically silent. The discovery of an adrenal mass in a patient with a known primary malignancy is equally likely to be an adenoma or metastasis.

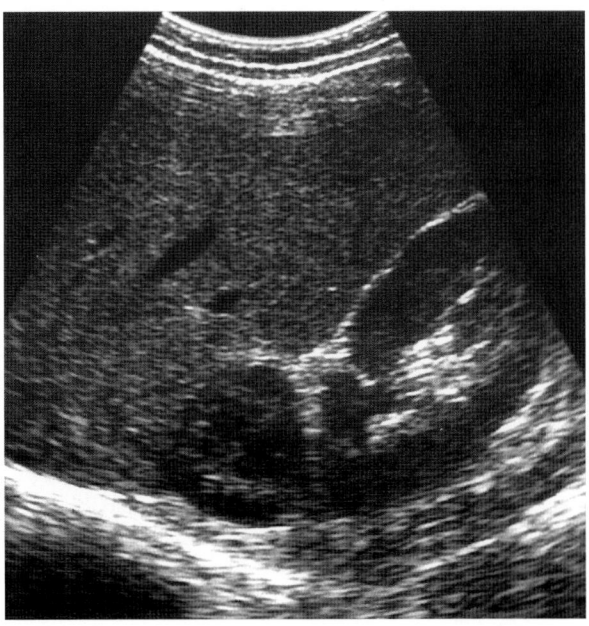

FIGURE 11-18. Kaposi's sarcoma. Sagittal sonogram shows a heterogeneous, predominantly solid right adrenal mass.

Adrenal metastases may be unilateral or bilateral and are variable in size, ranging from microscopic deposits to enormous masses. Central necrosis and hemorrhage may occur. Calcification in metastases is rare.[35]

The use of unenhanced CT attenuation values and opposed phase chemical shift MRI has shown its ability to differentiate adrenal adenomas from metastatic lesions.[31-35,64] Unenhanced CT attenuation values of 20 or greater and lack of signal loss on opposed phase

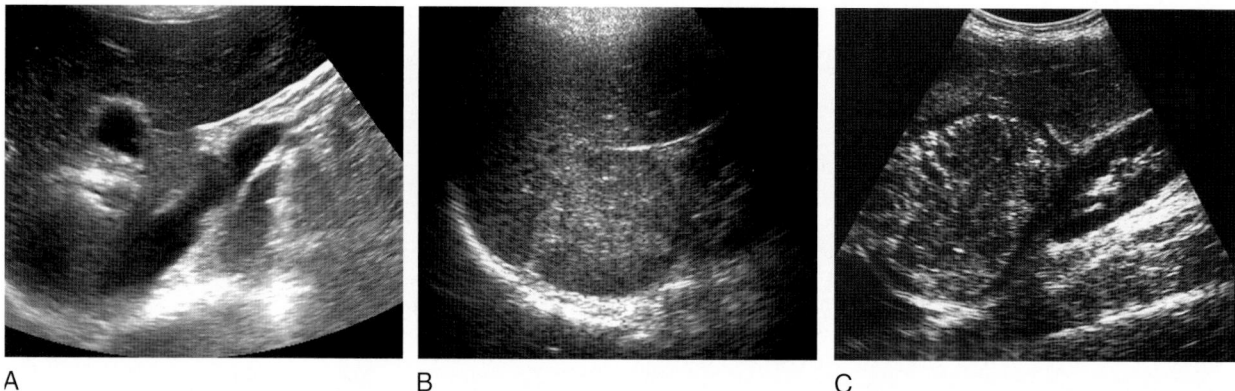

A   B   C

FIGURE 11-19. Right adrenal metastases in different patients. A, Sagittal sonogram shows a thickened adrenal that retains the shape of an adrenal limb. **B**, Sagittal sonogram shows a moderate-sized solid mass superior to the kidney. **C**, Sagittal sonogram shows a large inhomogeneous mass with a hypoechoic rim between the liver and the upper pole of the kidney.

chemical shift imaging indicate a non–lipid-rich mass, favoring a metastasis. Percutaneous biopsy is necessary to confirm or exclude metastases.

Sonographically, the masses are solid and may demonstrate inhomogeneity due to necrosis or hemorrhage (Fig. 11-19). Percutaneous needle biopsy may be performed with either ultrasound or CT guidance.

ADRENAL CYSTS

Adrenal cysts are rare benign lesions and are discovered most frequently as an incidental finding at autopsy with a frequency of 0.06%.[65] They are found with equal frequency on both sides and are typically unilateral. They may be bilateral in up to 15%.[66] They may occur at any age but most commonly are found in the third through fifth decades. There is a 3:1 female preponderance.[67]

Most adrenal cysts are asymptomatic but with growth may cause symptoms related to displacement or compression of adjacent structures. These include abdominal pain or discomfort, nausea, vomiting, and back pain.

Adrenal cysts are classified into **four types** based on origin.[53,68-70]

1. **Endothelial** (45%): angiomatous, lymphangiectatic, and hamartomatous;
2. **Pseudocysts** (39%): secondary to hemorrhage into a normal adrenal gland or tumor;
3. **Epithelial** (9%); and
4. **Parasitic** (7%): most commonly echinococcal infection.

Sonographically, these cysts have the same characteristics as cysts elsewhere in the body (Fig. 11-20). They are usually round or oval with a thin, smooth wall. Good through-transmission is present, but often internal

debris is noted. Fifteen percent will display peripheral curvilinear wall calcification, usually in the pseudocysts and parasitic adrenal cysts.

Percutaneous cyst aspiration showing **adrenal steroids** or **cholesterol** may be helpful to determine an adrenal origin if imaging techniques fail to do so.[67]

Adrenal cysts are benign and can be followed with serial imaging. If they are large and symptomatic, percutaneous aspiration, with or without sclerosis, or surgery may be necessary.

ADRENAL HEMORRHAGE
Spontaneous Hemorrhage

Spontaneous adrenal hemorrhage in the adult population is uncommon.[71] It is usually associated with **severe stress**, including septicemia, burns, trauma, and hypotension. It may also occur in patients with **hematologic abnormalities**, including thrombocytopenia and disseminated intravascular coagulation (DIC). Patients on **anticoagulation therapy** are also susceptible to adrenal hemorrhage, which usually occurs within the first 3 weeks following initiation of therapy.[53] It has also been recently recognized that ligation and division of the right adrenal vein during **orthotopic liver transplantation** may cause venous congestion and hemorrhagic infarction or hematoma formation in the right adrenal gland.[72] The resulting congested gland may rupture, causing excessive hemorrhage requiring reoperation.

Posttraumatic Hemorrhage

Posttraumatic adrenal hemorrhage may be present in up to 25% of severely injured patients.[73] Most patients will have ipsilateral thoracic, abdominal, or retroperitoneal injury.[74] The right adrenal gland is affected more often

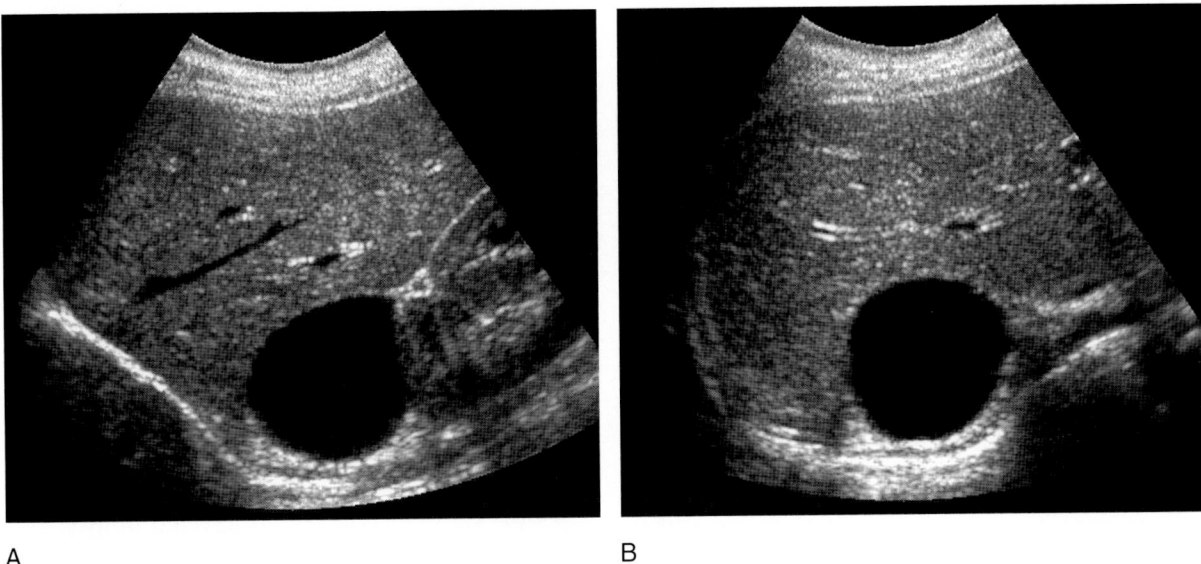

A   B

FIGURE 11-20. Adrenal cyst. A, Sagittal and B, transverse sonograms show a large, well-defined anechoic cyst with through transmission.

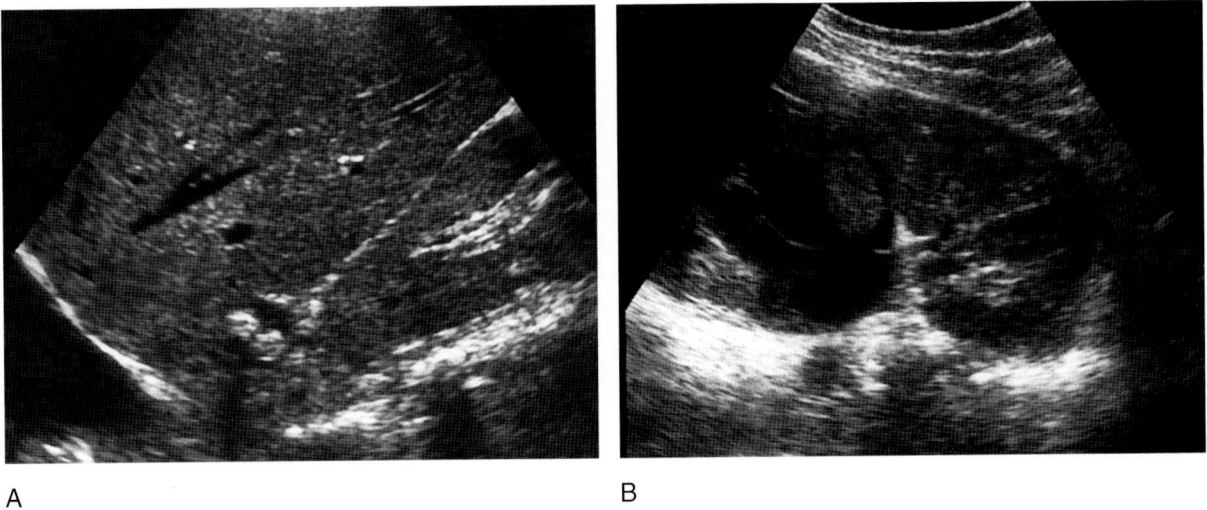

A   B

FIGURE 11-21. Spontaneous adrenal hemorrhage in two patients. A, **Chronic hemorrhage.** Sagittal sonogram shows two echogenic foci representing clotted blood in an enlarged right adrenal gland. B, **Acute hemorrhage.** Sagittal sonogram shows a large complex mass displacing the left kidney inferior and anterior.

than is the left. **Three mechanisms** have been proposed to explain traumatic adrenal hemorrhage:

- Direct compression of the gland with rupture of sinusoids and venules;
- Inferior vena cava (IVC) compression elevating right adrenal venous pressure as its vein drains directly into the IVC; and
- Deceleration forces causing shearing of small vessels perforating the adrenal capsule.[73,74]

Most typically, the **sonographic appearance** of acute adrenal hemorrhage is a bright, echogenic mass in the adrenal bed, which becomes smaller and anechoic with time. Occasionally, an adrenal hemorrhage will initially

appear as an anechoic mass becoming more echogenic with time (Fig. 11-21). This likely is because the initial hemorrhage consists of unclotted blood. With resolution of an adrenal hematoma, focal areas of calcification may develop. Most traumatic adrenal hematomas (83%) have a round or oval appearance and occur predominantly in the **medulla**.[74] The central hemorrhage may stretch or disrupt the cortex, resulting in periadrenal hemorrhage.

Unilateral adrenal hemorrhage has little clinical significance; however, patients with bilateral hemorrhage are at increased risk for development of acute adrenal insufficiency. It is crucial to exclude hemorrhage into a preexisting underlying neoplasm and, therefore, serial follow-up studies are necessary to document resolution of the adrenal hemorrhage. Most hematomas will resolve with time, requiring no intervention.

DISORDERS OF METABOLISM

Hemochromatosis

Hemochromatosis may be **primary (idiopathic)** or **secondary** following repeated blood transfusions. Patients with **idiopathic hemochromatosis** have a defect in their intestinal mucosa, which allows increased iron absorption and subsequent excess deposition in liver, pancreas, heart, spleen, kidneys, lymph nodes, endocrine glands, and skin. Clinically they present with cirrhosis, diabetes mellitus, and hyperpigmentation.[75] Patients with **secondary hemochromatosis** have increased iron deposition in the reticuloendothelial cells of the spleen, liver, and bone marrow. Organ dysfunction does not usually occur.[75]

Excessive iron deposition in the adrenal glands often leads to mild adrenocortical insufficiency, but Addison's disease is rare.[76] The adrenal glands are usually small and may show increased attenuation on CT scan.

Wolman's Disease

Wolman's disease is a rare **autosomal-recessive lipid storage disease** caused by a deficiency of liposomal acid lipase. Most patients die within 6 months of birth. The disease is characterized by marked hepatosplenomegaly and massive adrenal gland enlargement. The adrenal glands demonstrate diffuse punctate calcification.

ULTRASOUND-GUIDED ADRENAL INTERVENTION

Biopsy

Welch et al.[77] reviewed their experience of adrenal biopsy over a 10-year time period, which included 277 percutaneous biopsies in 270 patients. Sensitivity was 81%, specificity 99%, and accuracy 90%. Positive predictive value was 99%, and negative predictive value was 80%. Complication rate was 2.8%. Potential complications of percutaneous adrenal biopsy depend on the approach and include hematoma (0.05% to 2.5%),[78] pneumothorax (most common),[78] pancreatitis (6%),[79] sepsis, and needle tract seeding. Needle biopsy of a pheochromocytoma may precipitate a hypertensive crisis and should be avoided.[80]

Most commonly, biopsies of the adrenal glands are performed with CT guidance. However, if the lesion is visible and readily accessible, ultrasound may be used to guide the procedure. Often a transhepatic approach is chosen on the right to avoid the pleural space (Fig. 11-22). On the left a posterior, lateral, or anterior

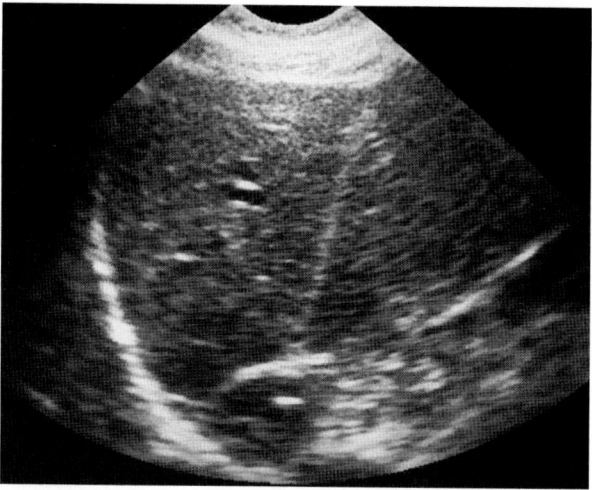

FIGURE 11-22. Percutaneous adrenal biopsy. Sagittal sonogram shows transhepatic placement of a needle (echogenic line) into a small right adrenal metastasis in a patient with lung cancer.

approach is chosen, depending on the lesion size and available safe access. A posterior approach is preferable to an anterior approach on the left in an attempt to avoid development of acute pancreatitis.

Drainage

Percutaneous drainage of an adrenal abscess or drainage and sclerosis of an adrenal cyst is possible provided safe access for catheter placement exists. Choice of catheter size depends on the viscosity of the material to be drained. Because of the deep location of the adrenal gland, these procedures are most frequently performed with CT guidance.

INTRAOPERATIVE ULTRASOUND

Intraoperative ultrasound with a 7.5-MHz transducer may be helpful when partial adrenalectomy is being performed. The exposed adrenal gland is scanned to allow precise localization of the pathology, which therefore allows the surgeon to obtain clear resection margins.

References

1. The endocrine system. In Cotran RS, Kumar V, Robbins SL (eds): Pathologic Basis of Disease, 5th ed. Philadelphia, WB Saunders, 1994, pp 1149-1165.

Embryology

2. The suprarenal glands (adrenal glands). In Netter FH: The CIBA Collection of Medical Illustrations. Vol 4: Endocrine System and Selected Metabolic Diseases. Summit, NJ, CIBA Pharmaceutical, 1981, pp 77-108.

3. The urogenital system. In Moore KL (ed): The Developing Human: Clinically Oriented Embryology, 5th ed. Philadelphia, WB Saunders, 1993, pp 265-303.

Normal Anatomy, Morphology, and Physiology

4. Mitty HA, Yeh HC: Radiology of the Adrenals with Sonography and CT. Philadelphia, WB Saunders, 1982.
5. Yeh HC: Sonography of the adrenal glands: Normal glands and small masses. AJR 1980;135:1167-1177.
6. Yeh HC, Mitty HA, Rose JR, et al: Ultrasonography of adrenal masses-usual features. Radiology 1978;27:467.
7. Brownlie K, Kreel L: Computer assisted tomography of normal suprarenal glands. J Comput Assist Tomogr 1978;2:1-20.
8. Yeh H: Ultrasonography of the adrenals. Semin Roentgenol 1988;23:250-258.
9. Yeh H: Adrenal and retroperitoneal sonography. In Leopold GR (ed): Ultrasound in Breast and Endocrine Disorders. New York, Churchill Livingstone, 1984.
10. Mitty HA: Adrenal embryology, anatomy, and imaging techniques. In Pollack HM (ed): Clinical Urography: An Atlas and Textbook of Urologic Imaging. Philadelphia, WB Saunders, 1990, pp 2291-2305.
11. Oppenheimer DA, Carroll BA, Yousem S: Sonography of the normal neonatal adrenal gland. Radiology 1983;146:157-160.
12. Marchal G, Gelin J, Verbeken E, et al: High resolution real-time sonography of the adrenal glands, a routine examination. J Ultrasound Med 1986;5:65-68.
13. Lurie SN, Neelon FA: Physiology of the adrenal gland. In Pollack HM (ed): Clinical Urography: An Atlas and Textbook of Urologic Imaging. Philadelphia, WB Saunders, 1990, pp 2306-2312.
14. Günther RW, Kelbel C, Lenner V: Real-time ultrasound of normal adrenal glands and small tumors. J Clin Ultrasound 1984;12:211-217.

Infectious Diseases

15. Shumam WP, Moss AA: The adrenal glands. In Moss AA, Gamsu G, Genant H (eds): Computed Tomography of the Body with Magnetic Resonance Imaging. Philadelphia, WB Saunders, 1992,1021-1057.
16. Rezneck RH, Armstrong P: The adrenal gland. Clin Endocrinol 1994;40:561-576.
17. Grizzle WE: Pathology of the adrenal gland. Semin Roentgenol 1988;23:323-331.
18. Dunnick NR: The adrenal gland. In Taveras JM, Ferrucci T (eds): Radiology. Philadelphia, JB Lippincott, 1990, p 4.
19. O'Brien WM, Coyke PL, Copeland PL, et al: Computed tomography of adrenal abscesses. J Comput Assist Tomograph 1987;11:550-551.
20. Atkinson GO, Kodroff MB, Gay BB, et al: Adrenal abscess in the neonate. Radiology 1985;155:101-104.

Benign Adrenal Neoplasms

21. Dunnick NR: Adrenal imaging: Current status. AJR 1990; 154:927-936.
22. Commons RR, Callaway CP: Adenomas of the adrenal cortex. Arch Intern Med 1948;81:37-41.
23. Ambos MA, Bosniak MA, Lefleur RS, et al: Adrenal adenoma associated with renal cell cancer. AJR 1981;136:81-84.
24. Painter TA, Jagelman DG: Adrenal adenomas in association with hereditary adenomatosis of the colon and rectum. Cancer 1985;55:2001-2004.
25. Conn JW: Primary aldosteronism. J Lab Clin Med 1955; 45:661.

26. Slee PH, Schaberg A, Van Brummelen P: Carcinoma of the adrenal cortex causing primary aldosteronism. Cancer 1983;51:2341-2345.
27. Conn JW, Knopf RF, Nesbit RM: Clinical characteristics of primary aldosteronism from an analysis of 145 cases. Am J Surg 1964;107:159-172.
28. Grant CS, Carpenter P, Van Heerden JA, et al: Primary aldosteronism. Arch Surg 1984;119:585-589.
29. Hubbard MM, Husami TW, Abumrad NN: Non-functioning adrenal tumors: Dilemmas in management. Am J Surg 1989;5:516-522.
30. Bitter DA, Ross DS: Incidentally discovered adrenal masses. Am J Surg 1989;58:159-161.
31. McNicholas MMJ, Lee MJ, Mayo-Smith WW, et al: An imaging algorithm for the differential diagnosis of adrenal adenomas and metastases. AJR 1995;165:1453-1459.
32. Korobkin M, Giordano TJ, Brodeur FJ, et al: Adrenal adenomas: Relationship between histologic lipid and CT and MR findings. Radiology 1996;200:743-747.
33. Korobkin M, Brodeur FJ, Yutzy GG, et al: Differentiation of adrenal adenomas from nonadenomas using CT attenuation values. AJR 1996;166:531-536.
34. Outwater EK, Siegelman ES, Huang AB, et al: Adrenal masses: Correlation between CT attenuation value and chemical shift ratio at MR imaging with in-phase and opposed phase sequences. Radiology 1996;200:749-752.
35. Dunnick NR, Korobkin M, Frances I: Adrenal radiology: Distinguishing benign from malignant adrenal masses. AJR 1996;167:861-867.
36. Gore RM, Callen PW, Filly RA: Displaced retroperitoneal fat: Sonographic guide to right upper quadrant mass localization. Radiology 1982;142:701-705.
37. Rao P, Kenney PJ, Wagner BJ, et al: Imaging and pathologic features of myelolipoma. RadioGraphics 1997;17:1375-1385.
38. Musante F, Derchi LE, Zappasodi F, et al: Myelolipoma of the adrenal gland: Sonographic and CT features. AJR 1988;151:961-964.
39. Nobel MJ, Montague DK, Levin HS: Myelolipoma: an unusual surgical lesion of the adrenal gland. Cancer 1982;49:952-958.
40. Richman TS, Taylor KJW, Kremkau FW: Propagation speed artifact in a fatty tumor (myelolipoma): Significance for tissue differential diagnosis. J Ultrasound Med 1983;2:45-47.
41. Vick CW, Zeman RK, Mannes E, et al: Adrenal myelolipoma: CT and ultrasound findings. Urol Radiol 1984;6:7-13.
42. De Blois GG, DeMay RM: Adrenal myelolipoma diagnosis by computed-tomography-guided fine-needle aspiration. Cancer 1985;55:848-850.
43. Galli L, Gaboardi F: Adrenal myelolipoma: Report of diagnosis by fine needle aspiration. J Urol 1986;136:655-657.
44. Korobkin M: Pheochromocytoma. In Pollack HM (ed): Clinical Urography: An Atlas and Textbook of Urologic Imaging. Philadelphia, WB Saunders, 1990, pp 2347-2361.
45. Manger W, Gifford R, Jr: Pheochromocytoma: Diagnosis and management. NY State J Med 1980;80:216.
46. Bowerman RA, Silver TM, Jaffe MH, et al: Sonography of adrenal pheochromocytomas. AJR 1981;137:1227-1231.
47. Quint LE, Glazer GM, Francis IR, et al: Pheochromocytoma and paraganglioma: Comparison of MR imaging with CT and I-131 MIBG scintigraphy. Radiology 1987;165:89-93.
48. Cho KJ, Freier DT, McCormick TL, et al: Adrenal

medullary disease in multiple endocrine neoplasia type II. AJR 1980;134:23-29.

49. Brunt LM, Wells SA, Jr: The multiple endocrine neoplasia syndromes. Invest Radiol 1985;20:916-927.

50. Silverman ML, Lee AK: Anatomy and pathology of the adrenal glands. Urol Clin North Am 1989;16(3):417-432.

51. Bosniak M: Neoplasms of the adrenal medulla. In Pollack HM (ed): Clinical Urography: An Atlas and Textbook of Urologic Imaging. Philadelphia, WB Saunders, 1990, pp 2344-2346.

52. Vergas AD: Adrenal hemangioma. Urology 1980;16:389-390.

53. Rumanick WM, Bosniak MA: Miscellaneous conditions of the adrenals and adrenal pseudotumors. In Pollack HM (ed): Clinical Urography: An Atlas and Textbook of Urologic Imaging. Philadelphia, WB Saunders, 1990, pp 2399-2412.

54. Derchi L, Rapaccini GL, Banderali A, et al: Ultrasound and CT findings in two cases of hemangioma of the adrenal gland. J Comput Assist Tomogr 1989;13(4):659-661.

Malignant Adrenal Neoplasms

55. Hamper UM, Fishman EK, Harman DS, et al: Primary adrenocortical carcinoma: Sonographic evaluation with clinical and pathologic correlation in 26 patients. AJR 1987;148:915-919.

56. Ritchey ML, Kinard R, Novicki DE: Adrenal tumors: Involvement of the inferior vena cava. J Urol 1987;138:1134-1136.

57. Fishman EK, Deutch BM, Hartman DS, et al: Primary adrenal cortical carcinoma: CT evaluation with clinical correlation. AJR 1987;148:531-535.

58. Glazer HS, Lee JKT, Balfe DM, et al: Non-Hodgkin lymphoma: Computed tomographic demonstration of unusual extranodal involvement. Radiology 1983;149:211-217.

59. Vicks BS, Perusek M, Johnson J, et al: Primary adrenal lymphoma: CT and sonographic appearances. J Clin Ultrasound 1987;15:135-139.

60. Feldberg MAM, Hendriks MJ, Klinkhamer AC: Massive bilateral non-Hodgkin's lymphoma of the adrenals. Urol Radiol 1986;85-88.

61. Freda PU, Wardlaw SL, Brudney K, et al: Clinical case seminar: Primary adrenal insufficiency in patients with the acquired immunodeficiency syndrome: A report of five cases. J Clin Endocrinol Metab 1994;79(6):1540-1545.

62. Donovan DS, Dluhy RG: AIDS and its effect on the adrenal gland. Endocrinologist 1991;1(4):227-232.

63. Findling JW, Buggy BP, Gilson IH, et al: Longitudinal evaluation of adrenocortical function in patients infected with the human immunodeficiency virus. J Clin Endocrinol Metab 1994;79(4):1091-1096.

64. Schwartz LH, Panicek DM, Koutcher JA, et al: Adrenal masses in patients with malignancy: Prospective comparison of echo-planar, fast spin-echo and chemical shift MR imaging. Radiology 1995;197:421-425.

Adrenal Cysts

65. Wahl HR: Adrenal cysts. Am J Pathol 1951;27:758.

66. Scheible W, Coel M, Siemers PT, et al: Percutaneous aspiration of adrenal cysts. AJR 1977;128:1013-1016.

67. Tung TA, Pfister RC, Papanicolaou N, et al: Adrenal cysts: Imaging and percutaneous aspiration. Radiology 1989;173:107-110.

68. Kearney GP, Mahoney EM: Adrenal cysts. Urol Clin North Am 1977;4:273-283.

69. Abeshouse GA, Goldstein RB, Abeshouse BS: Adrenal cysts: Review of the literature and report of three cases. J Urol 1959;81:711.

70. Barron SH, Emanual B: Adrenal cysts: Case report and review of pediatric literature. J Pediatr 1961;59:592.

Adrenal Hemorrhage

71. Kawashima A, Sandler CM, Ernst RD, et al: Imaging of nontraumatic hemorrhage of the adrenal gland. Radiographics 2000;174:319-321.

72. Bowen A, Keslar P, Newman B, et al: Adrenal hemorrhage after liver transplantation. Radiology 1990;176:85-88.

73. Murphy BJ, Casillas J, Yrizarry JM: Traumatic adrenal hemorrhage: Radiologic findings. Radiology 1988;169:701-703.

74. Burks DW, Mirvis SE, Shanmuganathan K: Acute adrenal injury after blunt abdominal trauma: CT findings. AJR 1992;158:503-507.

Disorders of Metabolism

75. Baron RL, Freeny PC, Moss AA: The liver. In Moss AA, Gamsu G, Genant HK (eds): CT of the Body with Magnetic Resonance Imaging. Philadelphia, WB Saunders, 1992, pp 735-821.

76. Doppman JL: Adrenal cortical hypofunction. In Pollack HM (ed): Clinical Urography: An Atlas and Textbook of Urologic Imaging. Philadelphia, WB Saunders, 1990, pp 2338-2343.

Ultrasound-Guided Adrenal Intervention

77. Welch TJ, Sheedy PF II, Stephens DH, et al: Percutaneous adrenal biopsy: Review of a 10-year experience. Radiology 1994;193:341-344.

78. Zornoza J: Fine-needle biopsy of lymph nodes, adrenal glands and periureteral tissues. In Pollack HM (ed): Clinical Urography: An Atlas and Textbook of Urologic Imaging. Philadelphia, WB Saunders, 1990, pp 2854-2860.

79. Kane NM, Korobkin M, Francis IR, et al: Percutaneous biopsy of left adrenal masses: Prevalence of pancreatitis after anterior approach. AJR 1991;157:777-780.

80. Casola G, Nicolet V, Van Sonnenberg E, et al: Unsuspected pheochromocytoma: Risk of blood-pressure alterations during percutaneous adrenal biopsy. Radiology 1986;159:733-735.

12

THE RETROPERITONEUM AND GREAT VESSELS

Dónal B. Downey

Chapter Outline

RETROPERITONEUM

The retroperitoneum is a large, posterior abdominal area that is challenging to evaluate clinically. Retroperitoneal disease symptoms are usually nonspecific; physical examination is difficult; the tissues there react less severely and less acutely to insults than most other anatomic regions; and so many retroperitoneal masses, fluid collections, and inflammatory and vascular disorders are large at the time of diagnosis.

Ultrasound has many useful roles in retroperitoneal assessments. It screens for disease rapidly, safely, and inexpensively; it detects incidental primary retroperitoneal pathology and retroperitoneal complications of both adjacent organ pathology and diffuse diseases such as lymphoma; it locates pathology accurately to a specific organ or anatomic space; it characterizes lesions based on their B mode, Doppler, and contrast agent enhancement characteristics; it accurately guides diagnostic and therapeutic interventions; and it measures retroperitoneal organs and pathologic process such as abdominal aortic aneurysms (AAAs) accurately and precisely.

Several anatomic and physiologic factors combine to make the retroperitoneum harder to scan well than almost any other anatomic region. Ultrasound beam disrupters including bowel gas, thick muscles, fat, ribs, the lower lungs, and the uterus combine with physiologic respiratory, bowel, and cardiac motion to degrade image quality. The area is large and deep and cannot be seen in its entirety from any one perspective. Ultrasound frequently has difficulty directly demonstrating the thin fascia, which divides the area into compartments. Correctly locating a large mass or fluid collection to a given compartment is even harder when the fascia is severely attenuated, displaced, or destroyed by that pathologic process.

To minimize these difficulties operators must consistently and continuously optimize patient factors and machine settings and use excellent scanning technique.

Scanning Technique

Ideally, patients should be scanned after an overnight fast. Pancreatic and left upper quadrant retroperitoneal visibility may be improved by having patients drink water or oral ultrasound contrast material,[1] but neither is usually needed.

If there is a choice of machines, the one that gives the best visibility of deep structures should be used. The examiner should use the highest frequency transducer that gives adequate penetration. For adults, gray-scale scanning frequencies of 5 MHz and lower are usually necessary. Recently available technical advances such as tissue harmonic imaging[2-6] and compound imaging[7] will frequently improve visibility in obese patients.

The general scanning principles of knowing what is clinically suspected and doing a "general" abdominal and pelvic survey usually with a lower-frequency curved-array transducer is particularly important in the retro-peritoneum. Then it is usually best to evaluate the site of any known or suspected disease because retroperitoneal pathologic processes typically spread in a predictable manner. For example, a renal colic patient should have the ipsilateral perirenal space evaluated for the presence of a urinoma before the rest of the retroperitoneum is viewed.

One scanning technique that helps to ensure that the entire retroperitoneum is scanned involves dividing the area into subsegments based on easily identifiable sono-graphic landmarks. These include the **aorta** (Fig. 12-1), the **diaphragmatic crura** (Figs. 12-1 and 12-2), the **kidneys,** the **iliac vessels,** the **superior mesenteric artery** (SMA) (see Fig. 12-1), the **inferior vena cava** (IVC), the **psoas muscles** (Fig. 12-3), and the **common femoral vessels** at the **inguinal ligaments.** The land-mark organ or blood vessel is first evaluated in at least two different planes, preferably perpendicular to each other. Next, the fibrous and fatty tissue in the neighboring anatomic spaces and adjacent structures are scanned. If one gets lost, orientation may be regained by returning to the sonographic landmark. One must adopt a very flexible approach to patient movement, transducer position, and respiration, because visibility is extremely variable.

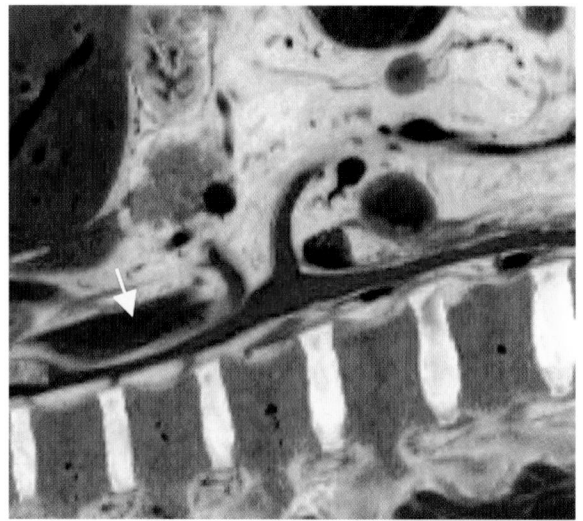

A

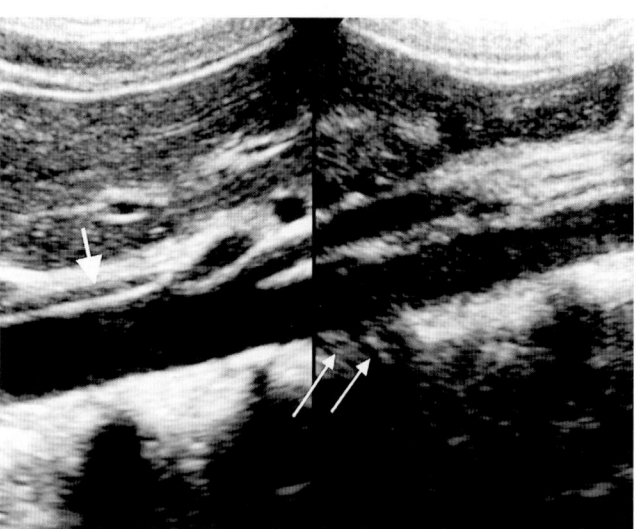

B

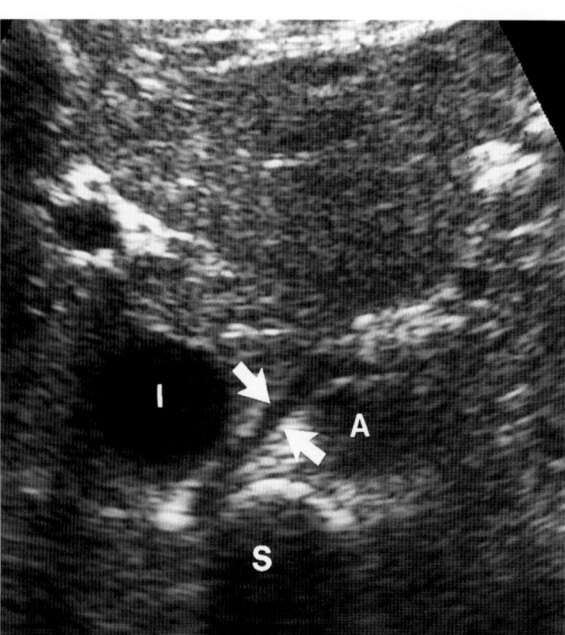

C

FIGURE 12-1. Normal midline anatomy. A, Midline longitudinal section through the "visible human" shows the abdominal aorta and the celiac and superior mesentery artery (SMA) branches filled with blue contrast agent. Note right diaphragmatic crus *(arrow).* **B,** Longitudinal midline scan also shows the diaphragmatic crus *(arrow),* the celiac artery, and the SMA origins. Two right renal arteries are noted *(small arrows).* **C,** Transverse upper abdominal scan shows the diaphragmatic crus *(arrows)* between the aorta (A) and the inferior vena cava (I). S, spine. (All "visible human" images courtesy of Dr. Victor Spitzer, Visible Human Project, University of Colorado School of Medicine, and the National Library of Medicine.)

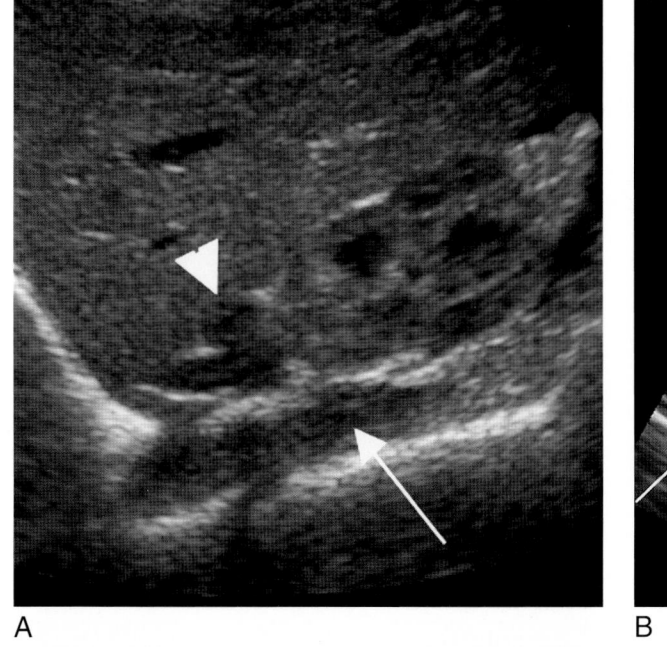

A

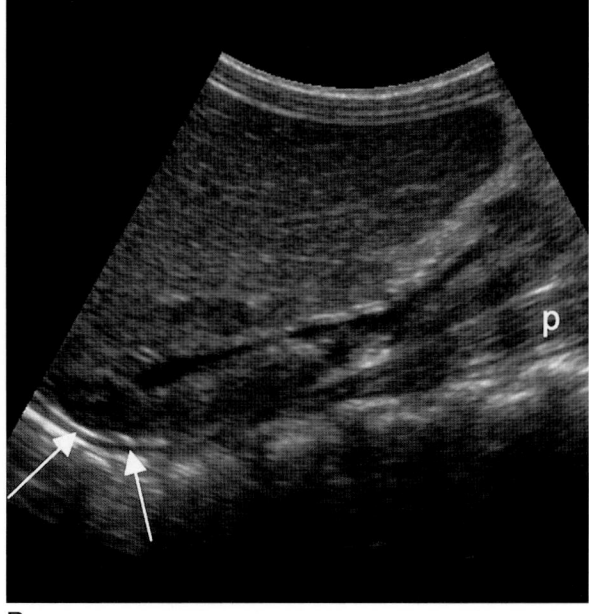

B

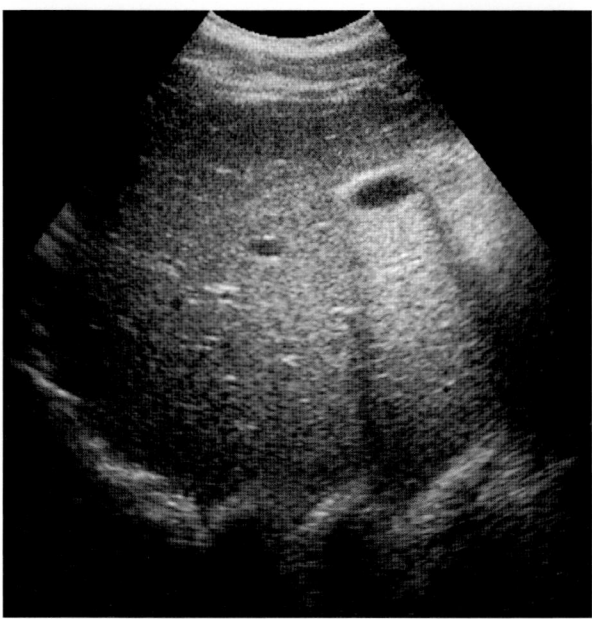

C

FIGURE 12-2. Sonographic appearance of the diaphragm. A, The right diaphragmatic crus *(arrow)* is bulky in this child. Adrenal *(arrowhead)* is noted over the right kidney. **B,** Longitudinal right flank scan in an adult with renal failure shows the lateral portion of the diaphragm as a thin curvilinear line *(arrows).* p, psoas muscle. **C,** Longitudinal oblique view of the right side of the liver shows the diaphragmatic slips posteriorly.

A firm, slow, graded compression technique similar to that used for the diagnosis of appendicitis[8] often allows improved retroperitoneal visibility because it moves bowel loops out of the way without patient discomfort. It is important that the operator ensure that a portion of the heel of the hand touches the patient's skin to ensure that unnecessary painful pressure is not put on ribs or other sensitive structures by the transducer. The area between the rectus abdominis muscles and immediately lateral to them usually provides an adequate acoustic window when the patient is supine (see Fig. 12-1B). A coronal perspective through the flank, with the patient in a supine or decubitus position, is often useful in the middle and lower retroperitoneum (see Fig. 12-3).[9] The immediate perirenal areas are scanned with the patient in the identical position as for renal ultrasound: supine, oblique, decubitus, and rarely prone.

Because intraoperative[10-12] and laparoscopic ultrasound[11-13] are being increasingly employed in retroperitoneal diagnoses and treatment,[14-16] ultrasound professionals are being called on to participate in these procedures in a variety of different ways. The transducers are typically high-frequency (5 to 15 MHz) linear or curved arrays and usually have an excellent near-field focusing ability and produce excellent image detail (Fig. 12-4). They typically have a more limited field of view than standard abdominal transducers, and this can make interpretation challenging because it may not be

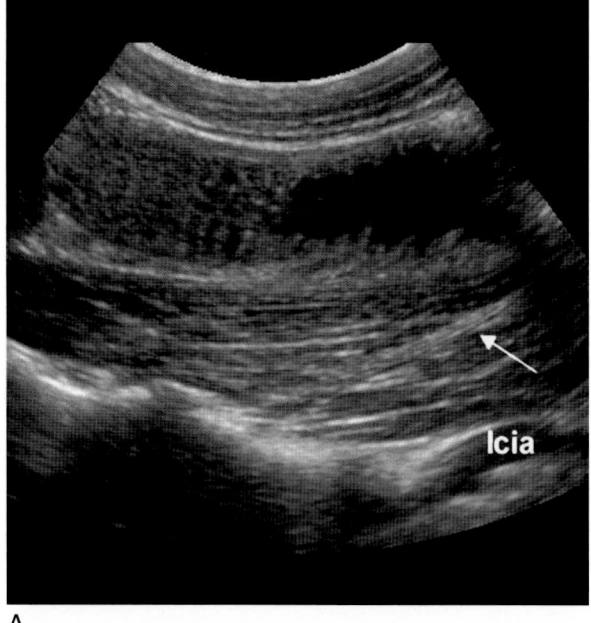

A

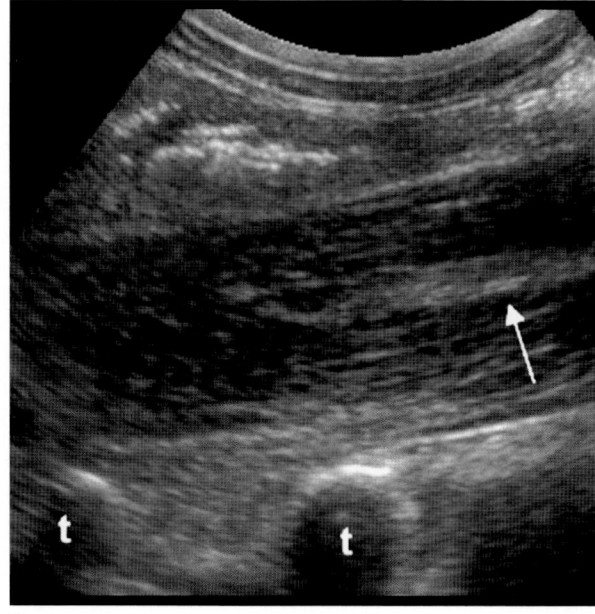

B

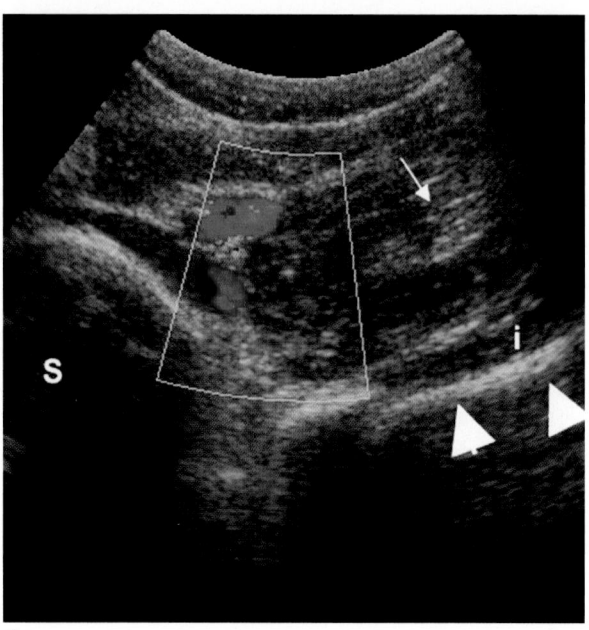

C

FIGURE 12-3. Normal psoas muscle. A, Left flank coronal sonogram of the psoas muscle. The psoas tendon *(arrow)* is echogenic and becomes prominent in the distal third of the muscle. lcia, left common iliac artery. **B,** The mid psoas muscle with its tendon *(arrow)* is shown with its relationship with the vertebral transverse processes (t). **C,** The distal psoas muscle in transverse plane is shown with its echogenic central tendon *(arrow)* and the left common iliac artery overlying the left common iliac vein. S, spine. *Arrowheads,* iliac bone; i, iliacus muscle.

clear where a detected lesion is in the retroperitoneum (Fig. 12-5). Some steps that have been found helpful in setting up a **successful laparoscopic or intraoperative program** include the following:

- Full commitment is necessary between the laparoscopist/surgeon and the sonographer to develop a process that works locally.
- Attainment of laparoscopic principles by the sonographer and ultrasound principles by the laparoscopist is essential.
- The process should be meticulously planned.

- Participants should develop a common nomenclature, especially relating to location in space.
- A clear understanding should be had of who is responsible for what.
- Practice in a laparoscopy training facility benefits all.
- All available films should be reviewed before the clinical procedure to understand where each laparoscopic port will be positioned.
- Participation of an experienced colleague for the first few cases is helpful, and debriefing should occur after every case.

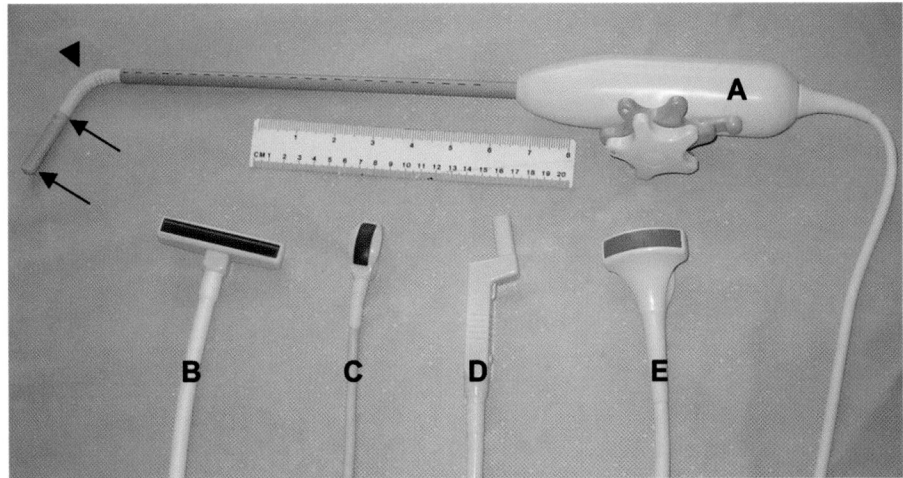

FIGURE 12-4. Operative and laparoscopic transducers. A, Laparoscopic transducer. This is designed to insert through a laparoscopic port in the abdominal wall to enter either the retroperitoneum or the abdominal cavity. The two knobs on the handle can rotate the linear ray transducer at the tip through an east/west and north/south group of planes. *Arrows* indicate the length of the linear ray transducer. *Arrowhead* indicates the swivel point of the tip. **B,** Linear ray transducer. This is suitable for intraoperative use and provides excellent near-field visibility. Its retroperitoneal usefulness is limited by its size. **C,** Curved ray transducer is designed for placing longitudinally between the operator's index and middle fingers. This is an extremely flexible intraoperative probe with a small footprint and good deep visibility. Its near-field resolution is not as good as that of the linear ray transducer. **D,** This end-firing small transducer was designed for use through bur holes. It can be used in the retroperitoneum when a very focused area is under evaluation. **E,** This curved ray transducer is oriented in an east/west orientation compared with a north/south orientation of probe C. Being a curved ray, it has similar advantages and disadvantages to probe C, although it is slightly bigger.

Anatomy of the Retroperitoneum

The retroperitoneum[17-35] (Figs. 12-6 and 12-7) is a posterior abdominal anatomic segment that lies between the transversalis fascia and the parietal peritoneum. It is limited cranially by the diaphragm and caudad by the pelvic brim. In normal patients, it contains relatively small amounts of fibrous and fatty tissue whose volume varies with the degree of obesity. It contains a large amount of "potential space" that can fill with solid and cystic material in different disease processes.

The thinner anterior perirenal fascia[17,28] (Gerota's fascia or Toldt's fascia) and the thicker posterior perirenal fascia[17,28] (Zuckerkandl's fascia) are dense, collagenous, elastic connective tissue sheaths that lie approximately parallel to each other in the coronal plane parallel to the anterior surface of the psoas muscle (Figs. 12-6 to 12-8).[28] They fuse laterally to form the lateral conal fascia.[17] Medially, the anterior perirenal fascia fuses with anterior perirenal fascia on the opposite side (see Fig. 12-6B). The posterior perirenal fascia merges with the fascia overlying the quadratus lumborum and the psoas[28] and forms the medial border of the posterior pararenal space (see Fig. 12-6B). These perirenal fascia divide the retroperitoneum coronally into three compartments[20] (see Fig. 12-7): the posterior pararenal space, the perirenal space, and the anterior pararenal space.

The **posterior pararenal space** (see Figs. 12-7 and 12-9A) lies between the fascia covering the quadratus lumborum and the psoas muscle[17] and the posterior perirenal fascia. It contains no solid organs and relative little fat.[17,28] The posterior pararenal space communicates with the properitoneal space anteriorly and laterally. Caudad, it communicates with the pelvic extraperitoneal space. It also usually communicates with the anterior pararenal space near the pelvic brim.[18,20]

The **perirenal space** (see Figs. 12-6A and B, 12-7, and 12-9B) lies between the two layers of perirenal fascia and contains the kidney, adrenal gland, proximal ureter, and an inverted cone-shaped mass of fat that allows the renal outline to be seen on plain radiographs. The lateral conal fascia bounds it laterally. There is ongoing debate about whether its upper border, lower border, and inferomedial borders are intact. Cadaveric and cross-sectional imaging studies have shown that at least in some people there is a connection between the left perirenal space and the left subdiaphragmatic retroperitoneal space and the right perirenal space and the "bare area" of the liver. Several studies have shown that contrast medium injected into the perinephric space of some cadavers will track to the other perinephric space through a conduit anterior to the aorta and IVC but posterior to the anterior pararenal space.[35] There is also debate as to whether large collections can track inferiorly out of the perirenal space into the pelvic extraperitoneal space. The consensus seems to be that although this does not occur often clinically, cadaveric studies indicate that contrast medium injected into the perirenal space usually tracks readily into the pelvic extraperitoneal space.[35]

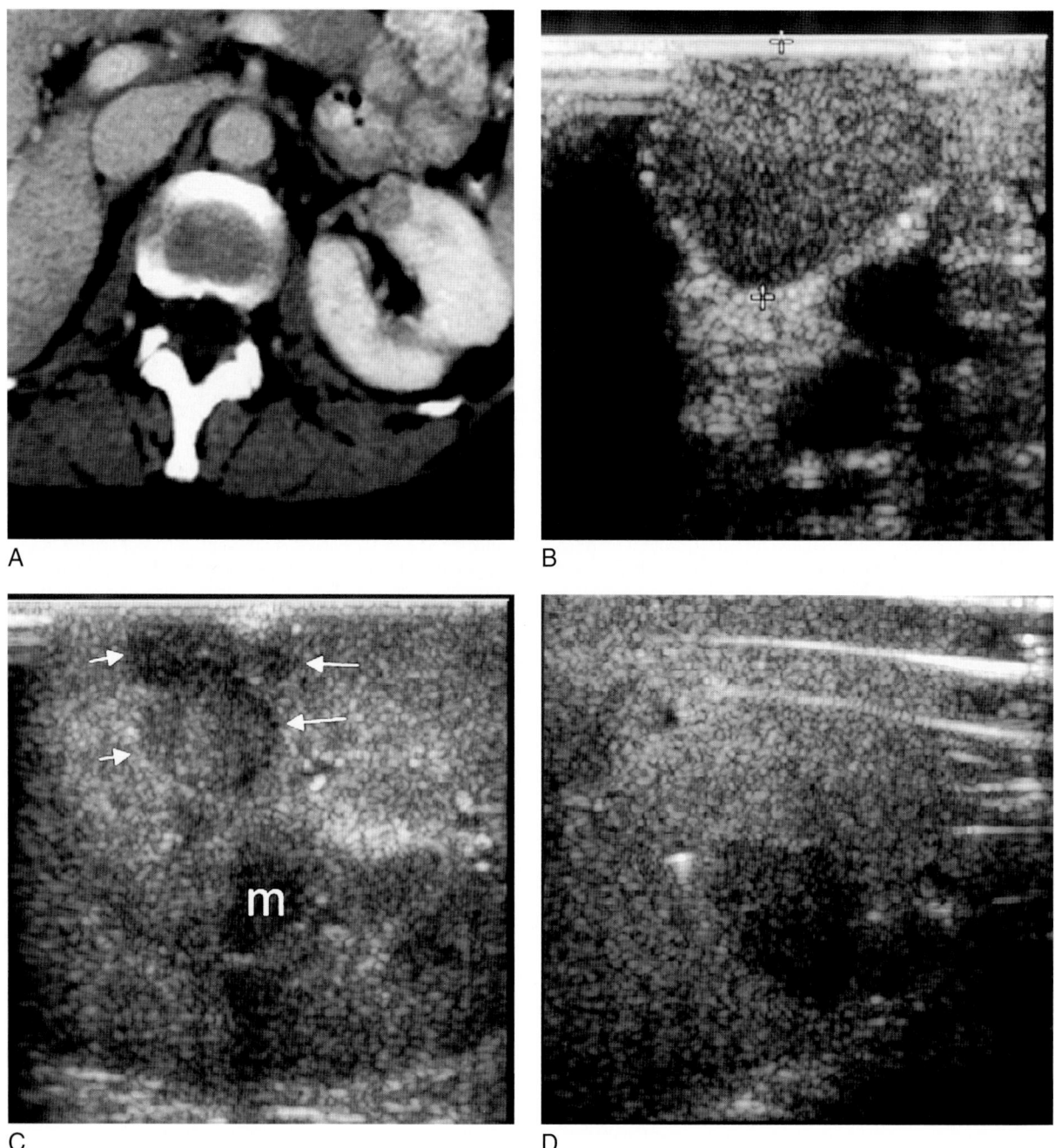

A

B

C

D

FIGURE 12-5. Laparoscopic ultrasound discovering tiny renal lesions. A, CT scan of a 52-year-old woman who previously had a right nephrectomy to treat six renal cell carcinomas (RCCs). She had two previous RCCs on the left side resected also. CT shows a further RCC forming anteriorly. **B,** Laparoscopic ultrasound shows the same lesion with the hilar vessels deep to it. **C,** Laparoscopic ultrasound finds a further bilobed (<1 cm) small nodule (*arrows*) in the lower pole. m, medullary pyramid. **D,** The same lesion has been located for the surgeon by positioning two needles (echogenic centers on either side of the lesion) to facilitate its removal.

The **anterior pararenal space** (see Figs. 12-6B and 12-9C to E) lies between the posterior parietal peritoneum and the anterior perirenal fascia. It is bounded laterally by the lateral conal fascia, and it contains the ascending and descending colon; the second, third, and fourth parts of the duodenum; the pancreas and arguably portions of the proximal superior mesenteric artery and vein; and the hepatic and splenic vessels.[1,3] It communicates with the anterior pararenal space on the opposite side through a plane that tracks both anterior and posterior to the pancreas (see Fig. 12-6B). Inferiorly it connects with the pelvic extraperitoneal space and the posterior pararenal space. There is considerable debate about its superior border. Meyers[17] claims that it is open, whereas others have claimed it is closed, allowing no access to either the bare area of the liver on the right and the left retroperitoneal subdiaphragmatic area.[28]

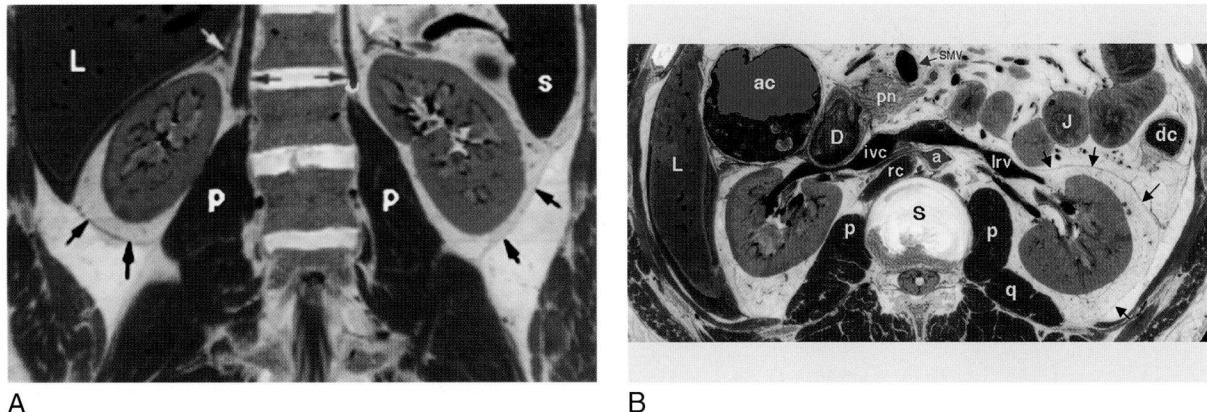

FIGURE 12-6. Normal retroperitoneal anatomy. A, Coronal slice through the "visible human" at the level of the kidneys. **B,** Transaxial slice through the "visible human" at the level of the renal vein. *Arrows,* Gerota's fascia and posterior perirenal fascia; *blue arrows,* crura of diaphragm; *yellow arrows,* adrenal glands; L, liver; s, spleen; p, psoas; ivc, inferior vena cava; a, aorta; lrv, left renal vein; smv, superior mesenteric vein; dc, descending colon; ac, ascending colon; J, jejunum; q, quadratus lumborum; pn, pancreas; rc, right crus of diaphragm; S, spine; D, duodenum.

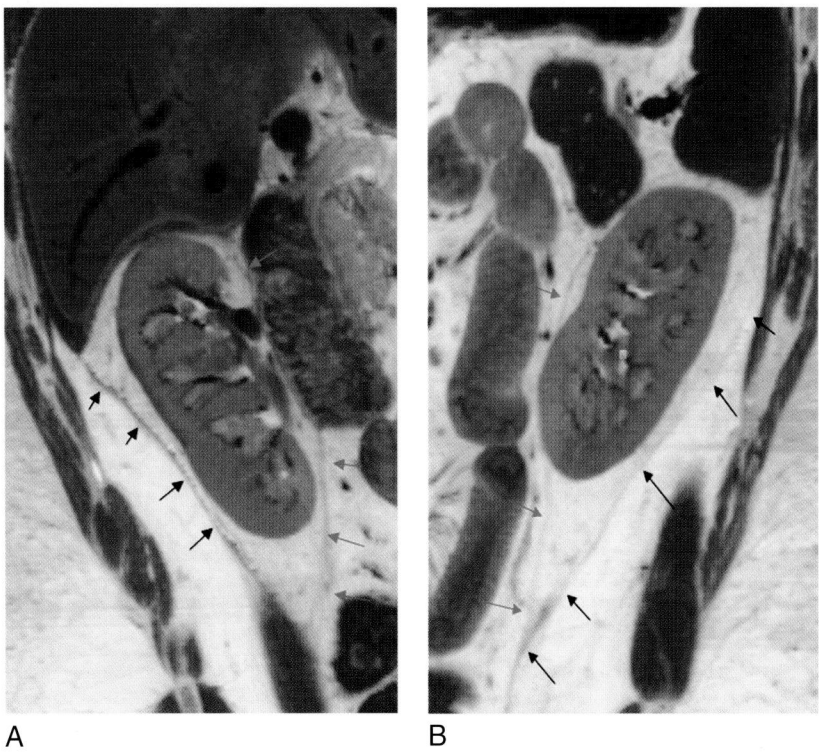

FIGURE 12-7. Retroperitoneal perirenal fascia. "Visible human" sagittal oblique cuts through (**A**) right retroperitoneum and (**B**) left retroperitoneum. The posterior perirenal, or Zuckerkandl's, fascia *(black arrows)* and the anterior perirenal, or Gerota's, fascia are incompletely demonstrated *(red arrows)*.

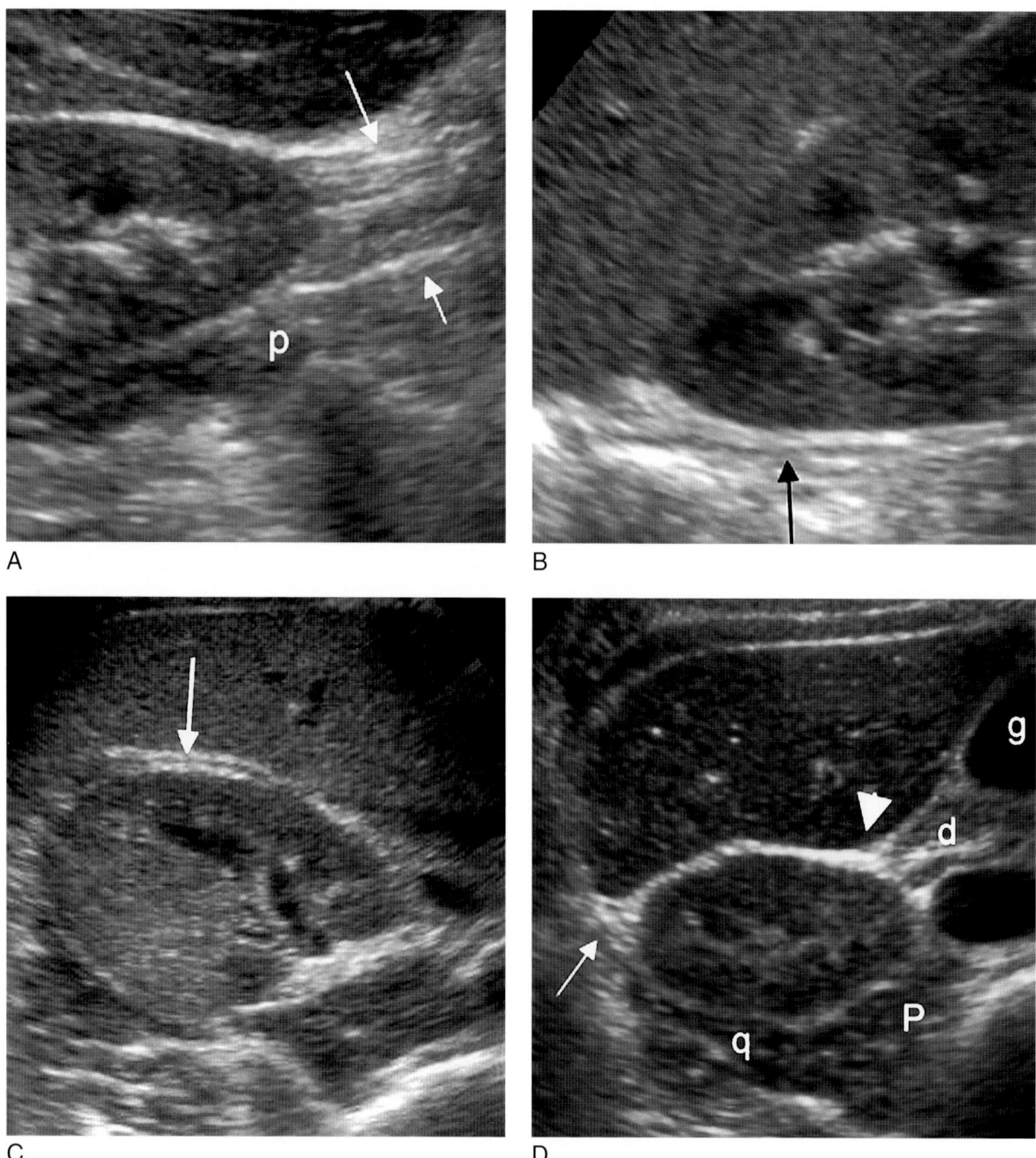

FIGURE 12-8. Ultrasound of the perirenal fascia. A, Longitudinal right flank sonogram shows the inverted cone of relatively hypoechoic fat *(arrows)* in the perinephric space caudad to the right kidney. p, psoas muscle. Longitudinal (**B**) and transverse (**C**) right flank scans of a patient with acute lobar nephronia demonstrate the posterior perirenal Zuckerkandl's fascia and the anterior perirenal Gerota's fascia *(arrows)*. **D,** Transverse upper abdominal scan shows the lateral conal fascia *(arrow)*. q, quadratus lumborum muscle; P, psoas muscle; d, duodenum; g, gallbladder; *arrowhead,* Morrison's pouch.

The correct compartmental anatomic location for the great vessels is also controversial. It has been proposed that the **aorta and IVC** lie in a fascial plane between medial extensions of the anterior and posterior layers of the posterior perirenal or Zuckerkandl's fascia.[36] From a practical standpoint it is probably better not to include the great vessels in either of the three main compart-ments but to understand that they are closely associated with all three on both sides.

The **retrofascial space**[37] contains the **psoas** and **quadratus lumborum** muscles (see Figs. 12-6 and 12-7), which are frequently included in descriptions of the retroperitoneum.[37] They lie posterior to the retroperito-neum and are covered by their own fascia. The quadratus

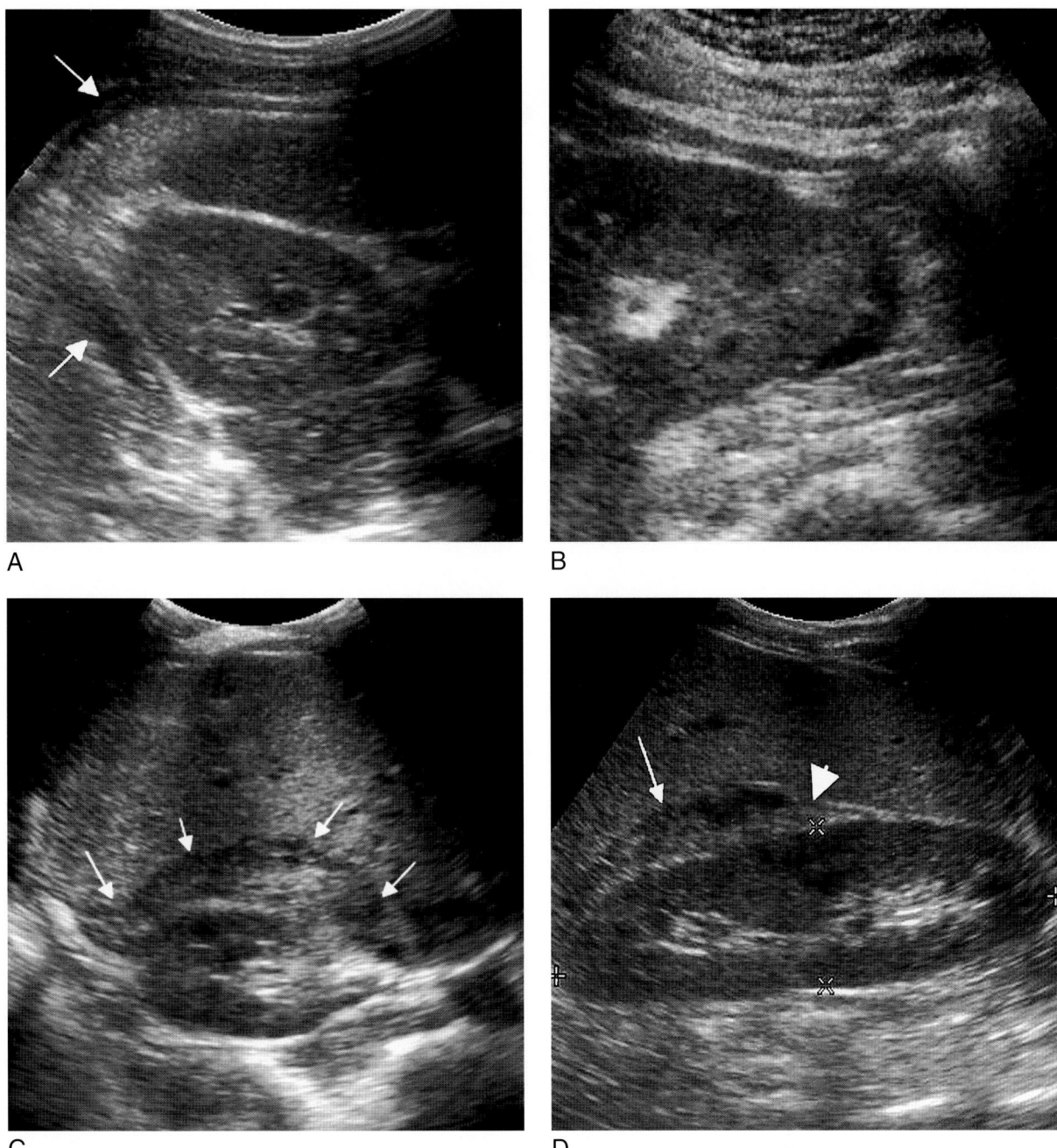

FIGURE 12-9. Retroperitoneal collections. A, Transverse right-sided sonogram shows fluid in the posterior pararenal space tracking anteriorly *(arrows).* **B,** Tiny amount of perinephric fluid is evident at the caudal aspect of the right kidney. Transverse (**C**) and longitudinal (**D**) right flank scans show a complex collection *(small arrows)* predominantly in the anterior pararenal space. *Arrowhead* shows anterior perirenal fascia or Gerota's fascia. Because it is minimally elevated from the kidney this suggests there is also some perirenal complex fluid present.

lumborum (see Figs. 12-6B and12-8D) is roughly quadrilateral, being wider cranially than caudad.[38,39] It arises from the medial part of the 12th rib and attaches to the vertebral transverse process before fusing into the iliac crest and the iliolumbar ligament. The **psoas muscle** (see Figs. 12-3 and 12-6A) is frequently made up of two conjoined muscles, the dominant psoas major and the smaller psoas minor, which is present in 60% of people. They take origin from the lumbar vertebrae and

transverse process and insert into the lesser trochanter of the femur.[39] Near the inguinal ligament they receive fibers from the iliacus muscle.[39]

The **diaphragmatic crura** (see Figs. 12-1A and D, 12-2, and 12-6) are the linear muscular portions of the diaphragm that border the aortic hiatus and attach to the lateral aspect of the lumbar vertebrae (see Figs. 12-1, 12-2, and 12-6A).[39] The right crus is bigger, longer, and more lobular. It attaches to the anterior bodies and

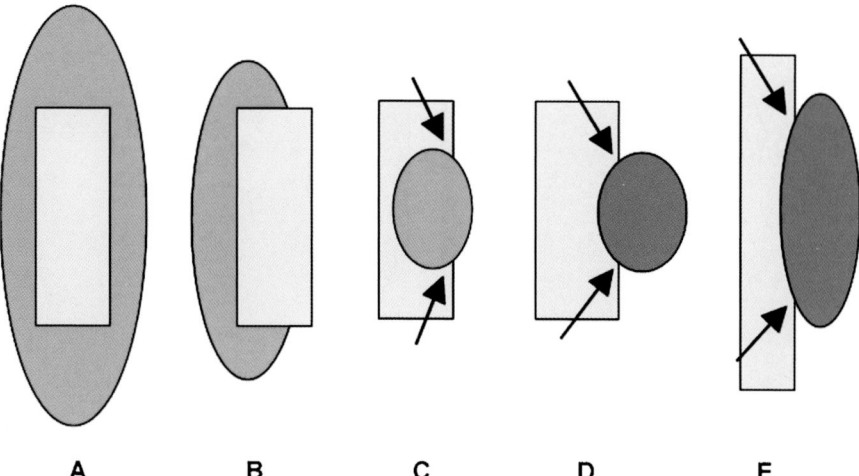

FIGURE 12-10. Schematic showing possible relationships of retroperitoneal masses (ovals) to retroperitoneal organs (rectangles). A, Mass completely surrounds and envelops the organ. The organ is typically not seen sonographically, resulting in the "phantom" sign. **B,** The organ is embedded in the mass. This results in the "embedded organ" sign. **C,** The mass is arising from the organ. The acute angle *(arrows)* the organ makes with the mass is called the "claw" sign or "beak" sign and when present it indicates that the lesion is arising from within the organ. **D,** The mass is making an obtuse angle with the organ *(arrows).* This is a negative "beak" or "claw" sign, indicating the mass is arising outside the organ. **E,** The mass is being compressed tightly against the organ. Both structures are compressed, but the "beak" or "claw" sign is negative *(arrows).*

intervertebral discs from L1 to L3. The **left crus** attaches to L1 and L2 and that intervertebral disc.[17,39] The **right crus** lies posterior to the inferior vena cava, right renal artery, right adrenal, and liver (see Figs. 12-1 and 12-6).[39]

Sonographic Appearance of the Retroperitoneum

The kidneys, inferior vena cava, pancreas, duodenum, aorta, and hepatic and splenic vessels are readily identified on ultrasound (see Figs. 12-1 to 12-3 and 12-9) and, occasionally, the perirenal fascial planes may be visible (see Figs. 12-7 to 12-9).

The diaphragmatic crura (see Figs. 12-1 and 12-2A) are useful anatomic landmarks, but they may be mistaken for pathologic processes, especially if they are thickened (see Fig. 12-2A).[40-42] On transverse scanning, the right crus is identified in about 90% of cases (see Fig. 12-1C), the left in about 50%. They are usually hypoechoic and surrounded by echogenic (fibrous fatty) tissue (see Figs. 12-1 and 12-2A).[40-42] On longitudinal scanning, the right crus is seen in about 50% of cases (see Figs. 12-1B and 12-2A). The quadratus lumborum (see Figs. 12-6B and 12-8D) is usually hypoechoic relative to the adjacent fat and can mimic fluid collections, especially in obese patients.[38] Scanning the opposite side is often helpful, because the muscles are usually symmetrical. The psoas muscles are usually easy to see by scanning coronally through the flanks and angling the upper portion of the transducer posteriorly to follow the plane of the muscle (see Fig. 12-3).[9,43] The caudal part of the psoas is usually easy to see in a transverse plane (see Fig. 12-3C), whereas its upper portions are often obscured by gas.[43] The muscles are hypoechoic with vertically oriented echogenic lines in them; caudad, they have an echogenic central tendon (see Fig. 12-3).

The overlying parietal peritoneum is almost never seen on ultrasound unless it is involved by a pathologic process (Fig. 12-9).

The mesentery extends anteriorly from the retroperitoneum and contains the splanchnic blood vessels and the attached small bowel.[17] It is difficult to see on ultrasound but is identified when there is lymphadenopathy present within it. The leaves of the mesentery are irregularly seen as echogenic lines.[44]

Retroperitoneal Pathology

The most common manifestation of retroperitoneal pathology is the presence of a mass (see Figs. 12-10 to 12-18).[45] Other sonographic signs of disease include the displacement of normal structures to an abnormal location (see Figs. 12-10E, 12-12B, 12-15, and 12-16), direct invasion of adjacent organs (see Fig. 12-17), asymmetry of normal structures, silhouetting of normal structures by disease (see Fig. 12-12A), and loss of retroperitoneal detail.

On finding a retroperitoneal mass the examiner should[46]:

- Assess it in two dimensions and ensure it is real.
- Trace its entire circumference and measure it.
- Assess for the presence of air or calcium.
- Assess whether it is fixed or free.

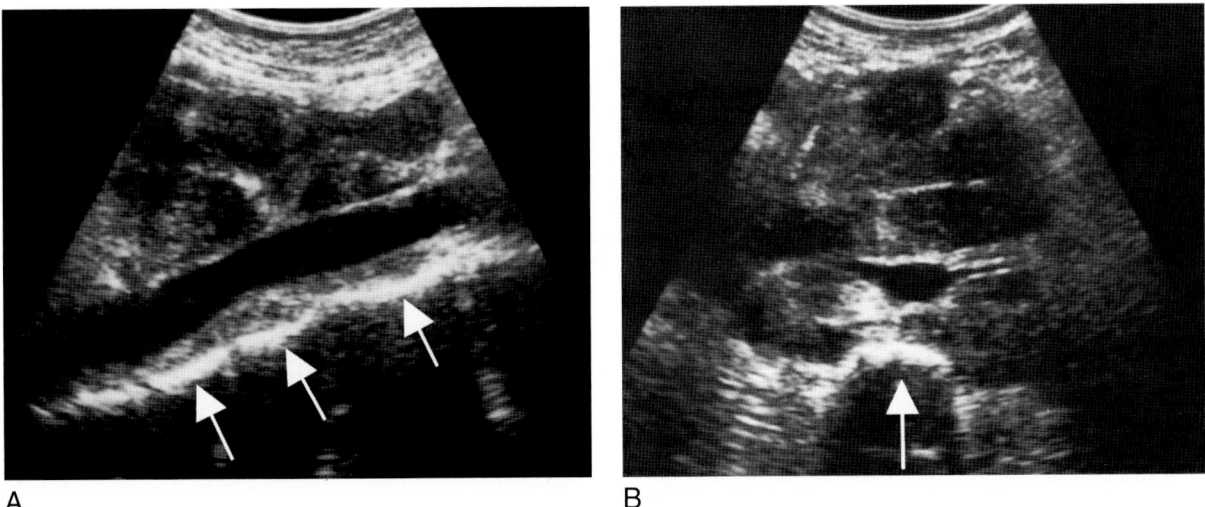

FIGURE 12-11. Para-aortic lymph nodes. Multiple hypoechoic masses surround the aorta and aortic branches. Aorta is displaced likely anteriorly from the spine *(arrows)* from the retroaortic nodes. Sagittal (**A**) and transverse (**B**) scans. (Courtesy of Stephanie R. Wilson, MD, University of Toronto.)

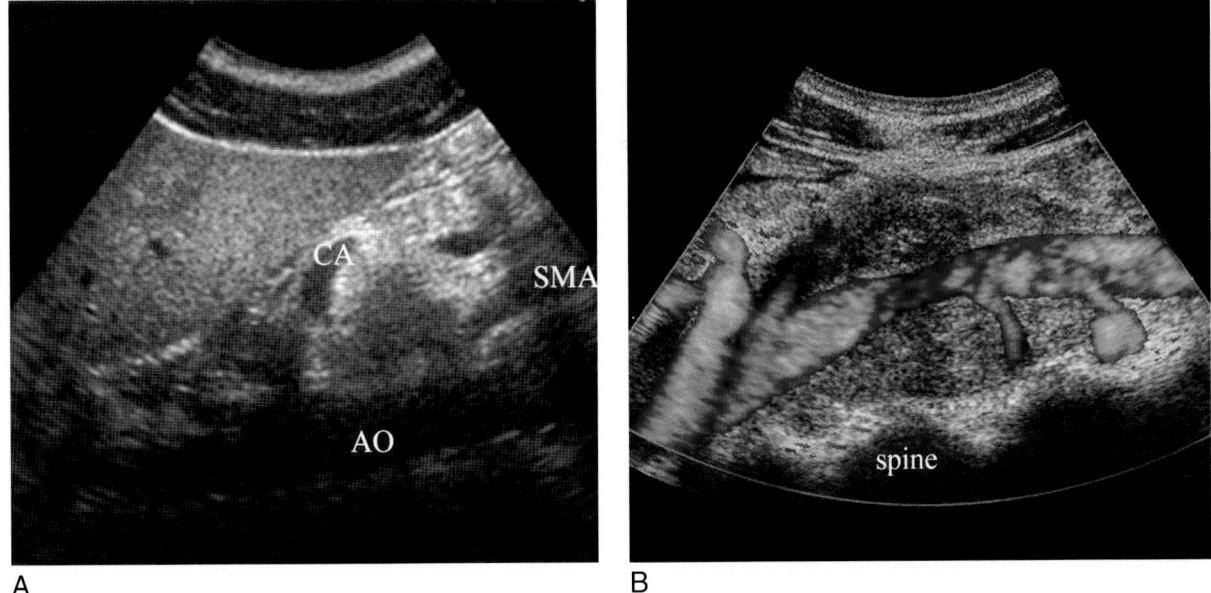

FIGURE 12-12. Malignant involvement of the retroperitoneum in two patients. A, Sagittal image of the aorta (AO). The origins of the celiac axis (CA) and the superior mesenteric artery (SMA) are engulfed in poorly defined soft tissue density, which also silhouettes the anterior border of the aorta. **B,** Sagittal image of the inferior vena cava. It is elevated from the spine *(spine),* which is posterior. A soft tissue mass surrounding and narrowing the cava is retroperitoneal lymphadenopathy. (**A,** Courtesy of Stephanie R. Wilson, MD, University of Toronto; **B,** courtesy of J. W. Charboneau, MD, Mayo Clinic.)

- Determine its internal echogenicity and blood flow.
- Discover whether it is cystic, solid, or vascular.
- Determine the relationship of a mass to other organs, blood vessels, and structures.
- Seek its origin.
- Check for the "beak sign," "embedded organ" sign and "phantom organ" sign (see Fig. 12-10).

Solid Masses

These are usually classified into lymphadenopathy, primary malignancies, secondary malignancies, infections, and other lesions that masquerade as solid masses on sonography. It is frequently not possible to clearly assign masses to a particular class based on the ultrasound appearance alone.

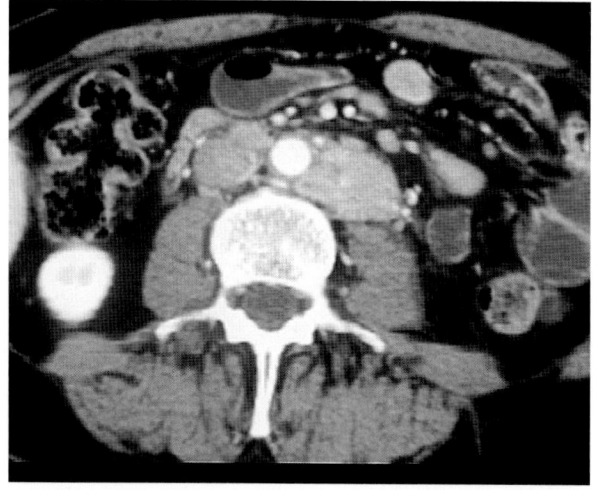

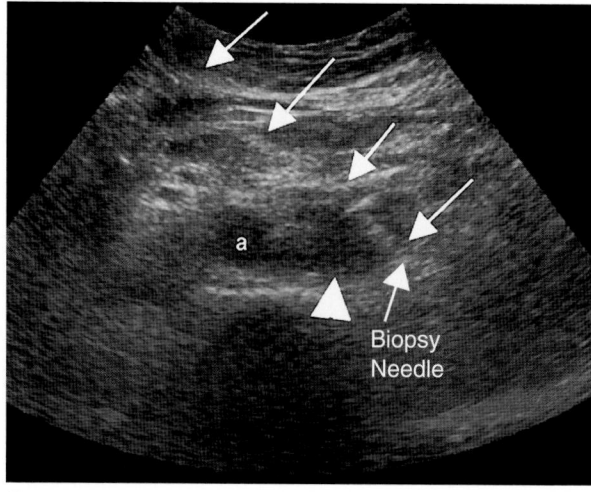

A   B

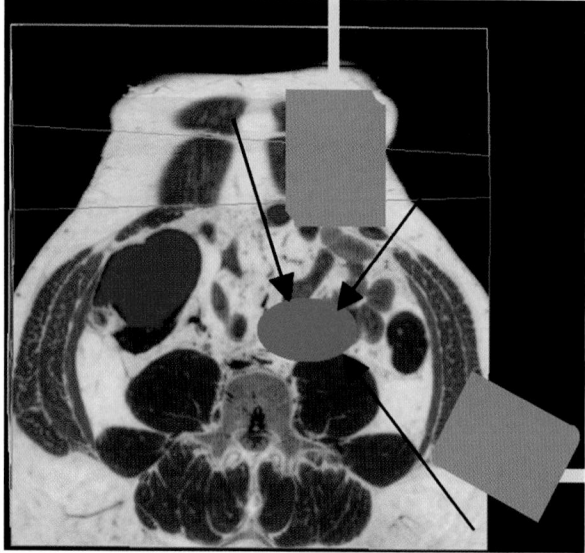

C

FIGURE 12-13. Retroperitoneal nodes. CT scan (**A**) and transverse lower abdominal midline sonogram (**B**) show a large hypoechoic mass *(arrowhead)* lying immediately to the left of the aorta (a) on the left psoas muscle. *Arrows* demonstrate the path of a core needle biopsy, which showed lymphoma. **C,** A transverse section through the "visible human" has a theoretical lesion *(pink oval)* positioned over the left psoas. *Arrows* show possible directions of needle insertion with transducer positions also outlined.

Lymphadenopathy. The aim of ultrasound is to detect enlarged retroperitoneal lymph nodes, characterize them, and measure them accurately (see Figs. 12-11, 12-13, and 12-14).[47] Although ultrasound is superior to CT in some thin patients for detecting retroperitoneal adenopathy, CT is usually the imaging procedure of choice because it provides a standard and repeatable view of the retroperitoneum that is not degraded by bowel gas. Measurement of the size of the retroperitoneal node is more easily repeatable on CT, and enlarged intraperitoneal nodes, which are present in 50% of non-Hodgkin's lymphoma patients at presentation,[47,48] are easier to appreciate on CT.

In the abdomen, the most useful criterion for assessing nodal disease is node size.

Disease will be missed if size is the only criterion applied to abdominal nodes; approximately 10% of lymphoma patients are found to have disease in normal-sized nodes. At sonography, **malignant nodes** are usually round or oval and have a longitudinal/transverse ratio of less than 2. Eccentric cortical widening and a narrow or absent echogenic hilus also suggest malignancy.[49] Malignancy is suggested on color Doppler imaging when avascular intranodal regions are shown and intranodal vessels are displaced or distorted.[50]

CRITERIA FOR ASSESSING NODAL DISEASE

Anatomic Location	Size	Classification
Abdomen	<1.0 cm	= normal
	>1.0 cm, single	= suspicious
	>1.5 cm, single	= abnormal
	>1.0 cm, multiple	= abnormal
Retrocrural	>0.6 cm	= abnormal
Pelvic	>1.5 cm	= abnormal

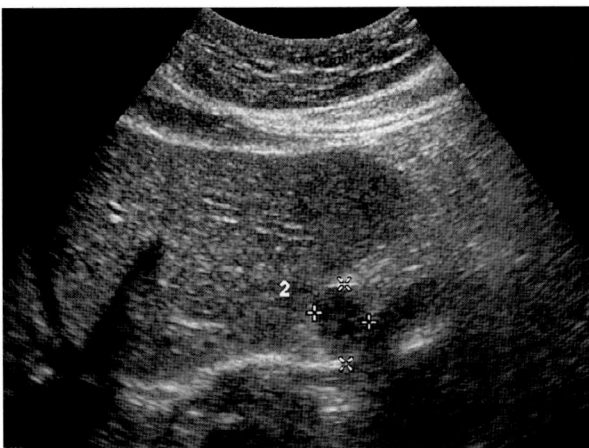

FIGURE 12-14. Metastatic stomach adenocarcinoma. Transverse left upper abdominal sonogram shows a small left retroperitoneal mass *(cursors and the number 2)* on the surface of left diaphragm behind the left lobe of the liver that proved to be metastatic stomach adenocarcinoma on biopsy. The hypoechoic lesion in the overlying left lobe is also a metastasis.

Whereas needle biopsy of nodal disease will rarely give the pathologist all the information required to make a full histologic diagnosis in patients with lymphoma, ultrasound-guided biopsy is useful for distinguishing lymphoma from other diseases, for assessing the response

to treatment of known disease, and for diagnosing some infections.[51,52] A variety of different approaches can be used (see Fig. 12-13C). In general, it is best to choose the shortest, least obstructed path to the lesion to facilitate good sonographic visibility and to use a standard technique.[53] It is usually prudent to assess patients with retroperitoneal adenopathy for more superficial nodes that may afford an easier route to biopsy.

Retroperitoneal adenopathy is most commonly seen in **lymphoma** (see Figs. 12-11 and 12-13A and B); para-aortic adenopathy is present in 25% of patients newly diagnosed with Hodgkin's disease and in 50% of patients with non-Hodgkin's lymphoma.[48,54] Ultrasound is between 80% and 90% accurate in detecting retroperitoneal nodal lymphoma, and it can also detect extranodal disease.[47] Its sonographic appearance is variable. Most commonly, discrete hypoechoic masses or anechoic masses are seen both anterior and posterior to the great vessels (see Fig. 12-11). These nodes have poor sound transmission and, unlike cysts, they do not have increased through-transmission.[47] Sometimes the nodes fuse to form a **hypoechoic mantle** of tissue that surrounds the aorta and that may elevate it from the spine (see Fig. 12-11). Extranodal lymphoma is also typically hypoechoic and may spread directly from the nodes to the solid organs or may arise de novo in the retroperitoneal space and retrofascial muscles. This is

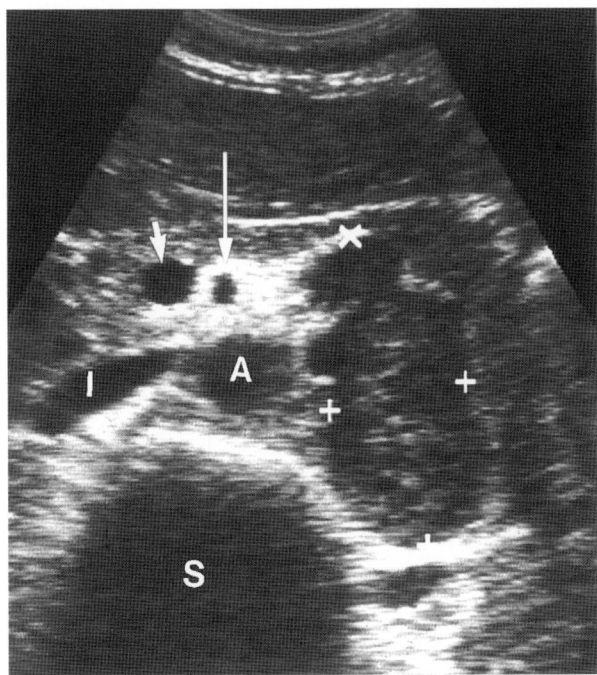

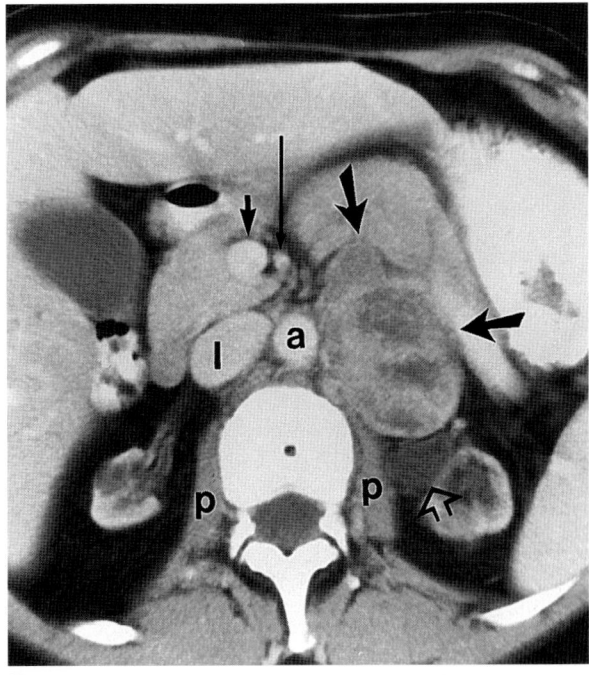

A   B

FIGURE 12-15. Metastatic sarcomatoid renal cell carcinoma originating in a left lower quadrant transplant kidney with spread cephalad in the retroperitoneum. Transverse ultrasound (**A**) and contrast medium–enhanced CT scan (**B**) showing a large left retroperitoneal, anterior pararenal space, lobulated mass *(large arrows or +)* displacing the stomach, pancreas, and bowel anteriorly. It displaces the aorta (A) slightly to the right. The native kidneys are small, and the left one is hydronephrotic *(open arrow). Long thin arrow* (on **A**) and *short arrow* (on **B**), superior mesenteric artery; I, inferior vena cava; a, aorta; p, psoas.

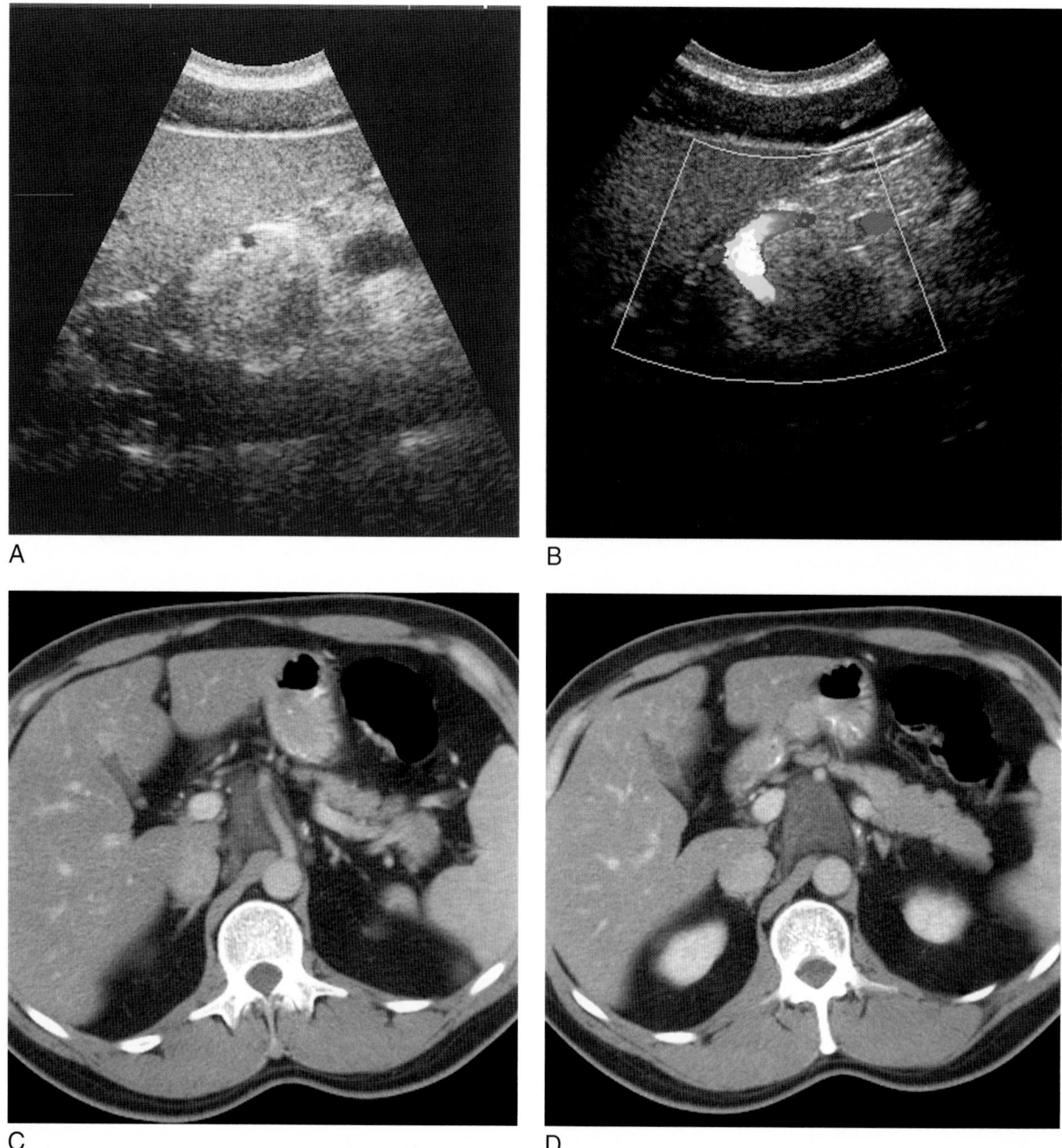

FIGURE 12-16. Neuroma arising from the sympathetic nerve chain at the celiac axis. Sagittal gray-scale image (**A**) and color Doppler image (**B**) of the aorta at the level of the celiac axis. A well-defined and solid mass is seen intimate to the celiac axis, which is shown in color. **C** and **D,** Confirmatory CT scans showing the solid and well-defined mass adjacent to the celiac axis, which remains patent and uninvolved. (Courtesy of Stephanie Wilson, MD, University of Toronto.)

particularly true of the **AIDS-related lymphoma** and of lymphoma that occurs in other immunosuppressed patients. The sonographic morphology has not been found to correlate with any particular histologic pattern.[55] If the mass silhouettes the aortic border as opposed to coming close to it (see Fig. 12-11A), it is reasonable to assume that the nodes are truly retroperitoneal, and radiation ports may be adjusted accordingly.[47]

Retroperitoneal metastases occur either by lymphatic or hematogenous spread or by direct extension from other solid organs or the adjacent peritoneal cavity. They may stay confined within lymph nodes or spread beyond their confines. Metastatic deposits from testicular tumors and pelvic tumors are most common, although lung, melanoma, and gastrointestinal metastases also occur. Direct invasion of the retroperitoneum is also commonly associated with pancreatic cancer (see Fig. 12-12A).

Sonographic appearances of **nonlymphomatous malignant nodal disease** are variable, although such

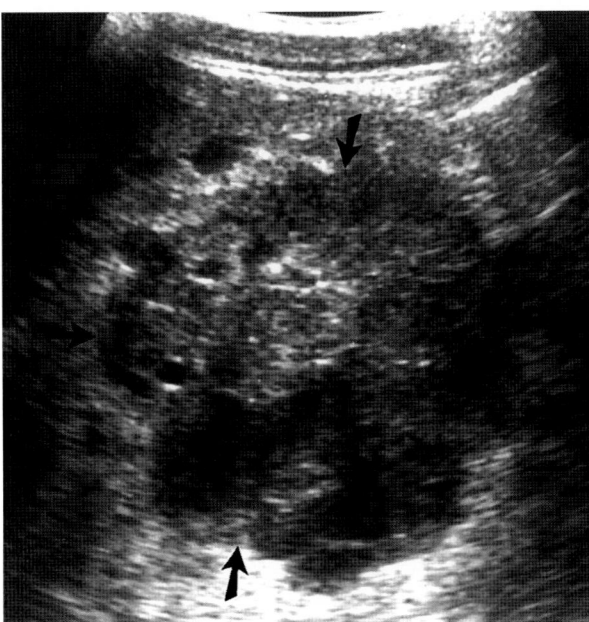

FIGURE 12-17. Retroperitoneal leiomyosarcoma. Longitudinal sonogram of the left retroperitoneum shows an extensive complex tumor *(arrows)* that is more solid anteriorly and cystic posteriorly.

nodes are less likely to be as intensely hypoechoic as those with lymphoma, and they are often more echogenic and heterogeneous. Ultrasound is less accurate in assessing metastatic nodal disease than in assessing lymphoma; a 31% sensitivity and an 87% specificity were reported in patients with testicular tumors.[56]

Infection can also cause lymphadenopathy, as can AIDS and AIDS-related lymphoma. Sonographic appearances are, again, nonspecific.

One of the more important, although rare, tumors that occurs in the retroperitoneum is the **germ cell tumor.**[57,58] Most of them are secondary lesions. When a retroperitoneal primary germ cell tumor is thought to have been found, it is essential to check the scrotum carefully.[57,58] The lesions can be benign or malignant; they are generally heterogeneous. **Teratomas** may be suspected in the pediatric population if a fat-fluid level or a large area of calcification is seen.[59]

Primary Retroperitoneal Tumors. Primary retroperitoneal tumors are rare neoplasms that arise and develop in the retroperitoneal space but are not attached to the adjacent retroperitoneal organs.[60] Most are of mesenchymal origin (see Figs. 12-15 and 12-17), and between 70% and 90% of those that occur in adults are malignant. Three times as many men as women are affected, and the 5-year survival varies between 22% and 50%.[61,62] **Liposarcoma, leiomyosarcoma** (see Fig. 12-17), and **malignant fibrous histiocytoma** are the most common.[18,61,62] Fixation of the tumor and invasion of adjacent structures are the worst prognostic features. Complete surgical excision offers the best hope of cure, although this is often technically very difficult.[60-62]

Ultrasound rarely produces a specific diagnosis, because there is considerable overlap in the sonographic appearances of retroperitoneal tumors, with most lesions being large and heterogeneous and many containing cysts (see Figs. 12-17 and 12-18).[46] Increased echogenicity within the retroperitoneal masses may be related to fat, calcification,[59] increased vascularity,[63] or hemorrhage.[64,65] Tumors of muscle origin are more likely to be hypoechoic (see Fig. 12-17), whereas isoechoic masses may represent lipomas in which the fat is indistinguishable from adjacent retroperitoneal fat.

Whereas CT will often give a better overview of a retroperitoneal lesion (see Fig. 12-15A), ultrasound may give a better appreciation of whether the lesion is fixed or has invaded adjacent structures, both important features

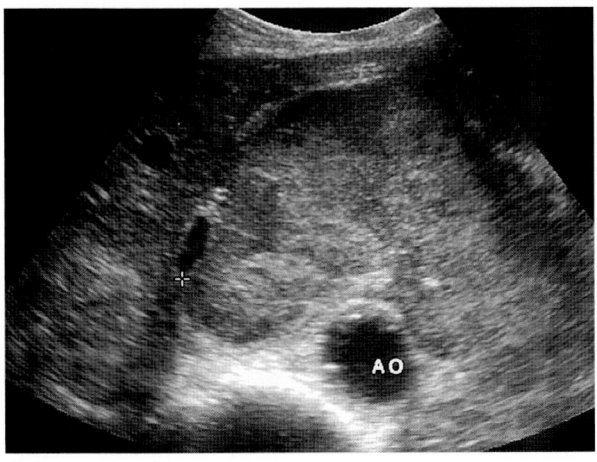

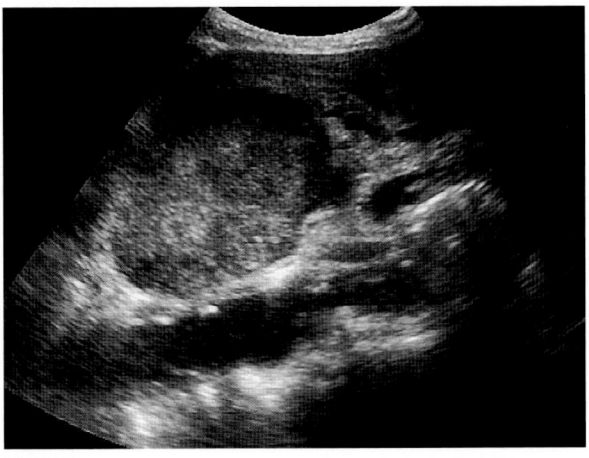

A   B

FIGURE 12-18. Mixed cell type sarcoma. Transverse upper abdominal scan (**A**) and sagittal longitudinal scan (**B**) show a large retroperitoneal mass in the midline and left upper quadrant that proved to be a malignant sarcoma of mixed cell type. Note also the metastatic deposit in the liver posteriorly on the transverse scan. AO, aorta.

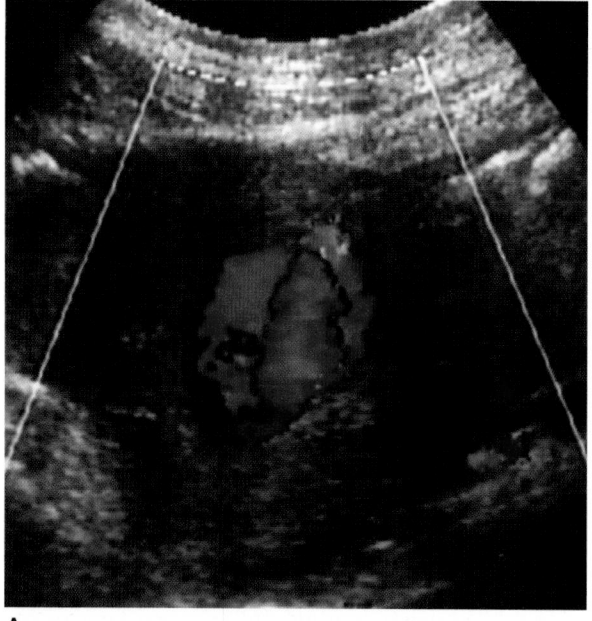

A

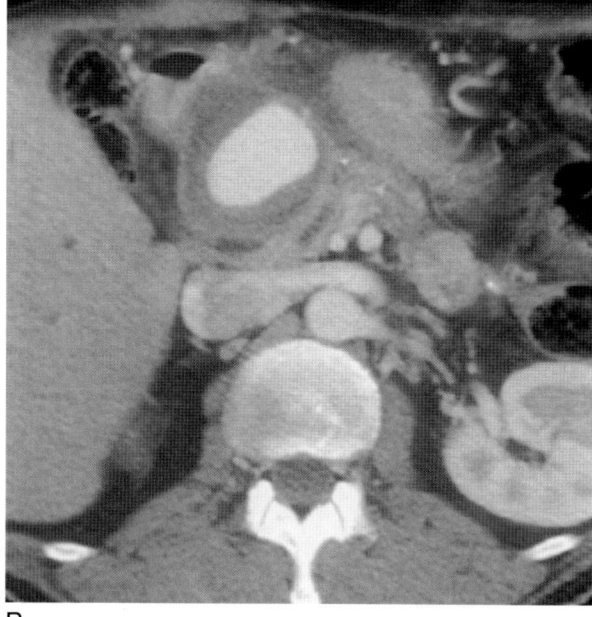

B

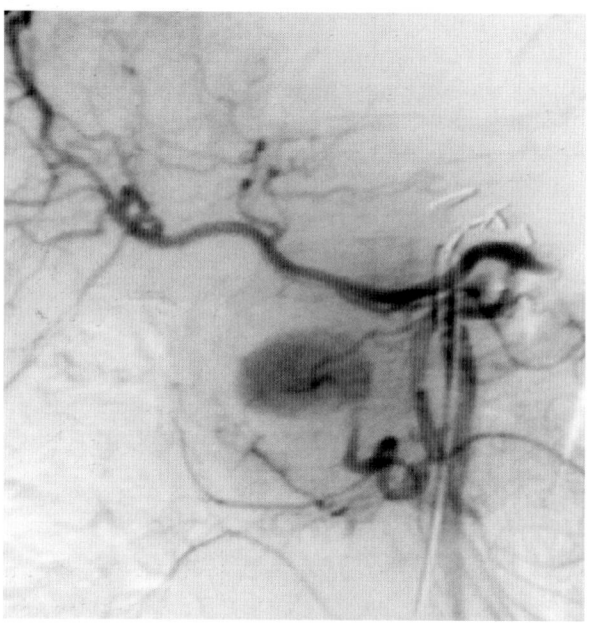

C

FIGURE 12-19. Pancreatic pseudoaneurysm. Transverse right upper quadrant color Doppler image (**A**) and contrast medium–enhanced CT scan (**B**) show a large, thick-walled pseudoaneurysm lying slightly ventral and to the right of the head of the pancreas. **C,** Angiogram shows it filled from an inferior branch of the gastroduodenal artery. This pseudoaneurysm was successfully treated by embolization.

for prognosis and surgical planning.[61,62] Ultrasound also allows rapid and accurate biopsy of retroperitoneal masses (see Fig. 12-13C). It is prudent to evaluate with Doppler imaging all retroperitoneal masses before biopsy to avoid sampling or draining an **aneurysm** (Fig. 12-19).[66]

Retroperitoneal Fibrosis. Retroperitoneal fibrosis (Ormond's disease) (Figs. 12-20 and 12-21) is idiopathic in 68% of cases. In 8% it is associated with malignancy **(infiltrating secondary neoplasia of the stomach, lung, breast, colon, prostate, and kidney)** and in 12% it is associated with **methysergide** use. Less frequent associations include **Crohn's disease, Riedel's struma,** **sclerosing cholangitis, radiation therapy, aneurysm surgery** or **leakage, retroperitoneal infection,** and **urine leakage.**[67-70]

When the process occurs around the aorta it is called an inflammatory aneurysm and its exact cause is unknown.[71,72] Pathologic changes seen in both conditions include clumps of fibrous tissue with associated inflammatory infiltrate on the anterior aspect of the aorta, IVC, and psoas muscles.[69,70] It is an important diagnosis to make because, if unrecognized, it can lead to renal failure or can be mistaken for more serious pathology. It usually responds well to medical therapy.

PRIMARY RETROPERITONEAL TUMORS

Mesenchymal Origin	Neurogenic Origin	Embryonic Rest
Lipoma/liposarcoma	Neurilemmoma	Teratoma
Leiomyoma/	Neurofibroma	Seminoma
Leiomyosarcoma	Malignant schwannoma	Yolk sac tumor
Hemangiopericytoma/	Neuroblastoma/	Wilms' tumor
Angiosarcoma	Ganglioneuroblastoma	
Fibroma/fibrosarcoma	Ganglioneuroma	
Rhabdomyoma/	Paraganglioma/	
Rhabdomyosarcoma	Pheochromocytoma	
Malignant fibrous histiocytoma		
Mesothelioma		
Chondrosarcoma		
Osteosarcoma		
Hemangioma		

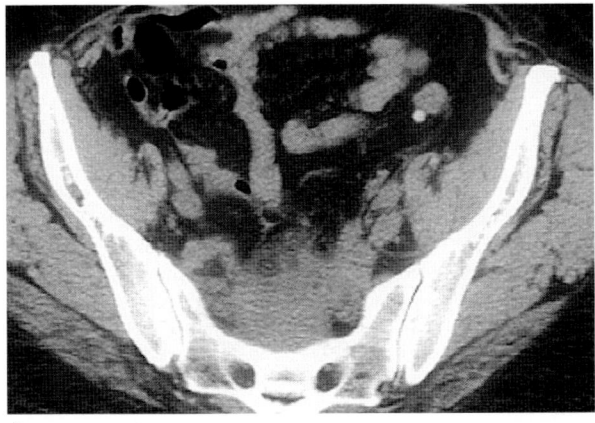
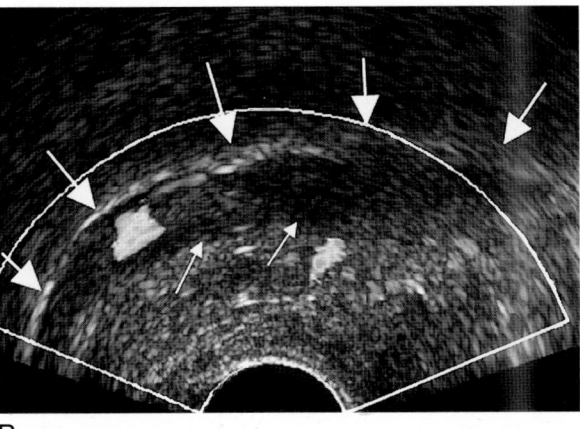

A   B

FIGURE 12-20. Retroperitoneal fibrosis. A, CT scan shows a poorly defined area of increased radiodensity immediately ventral to the sacrum in a patient with bilateral hydronephrosis. **B,** Transrectal scan with the same orientation shows the sacrum *(large arrows)*. Immediately ventral to it is a hypoechoic area *(small arrows)*, and the tissue between the probe and the small arrows was hypervascular. Ultrasound-guided biopsy showed retroperitoneal fibrosis.

Sonographically, the appearances are nonspecific. The fibrous clumps are mostly hypoechoic, smoothly marginated, and homogeneous masses that often appear as plaque around the distal aorta (see Fig. 12-21). In cases in which the clumps of fibrosis are not obvious, the characteristic medial deviation of the ureters may suggest the diagnosis. Whereas CT is the diagnostic modality of choice,[70] ultrasound can be used to follow the response of the ureters and the masses to corticosteroids and other interventions.

Other Retroperitoneal Masses and Pseudomasses. Benign masses such as **horseshoe kidneys** (Fig. 12-22), ptotic kidneys, bowel duplication cysts, and a **low-lying pancreas** should be considered as possible explanations for a retroperitoneal mass. Perhaps the most frequent problem with sonography occurs when a loop of **aperistaltic bowel** mimics a true mass. The distinction can usually be made by changing the patient's position during the examination and watching the area while the patient drinks. **Acute retroperitoneal hemorrhage,** a potentially lethal condition,[73] may be quite echogenic and may appear to be a focal mass (Figs. 12-23 and 12-24).[65] **Varices** can also mimic solid lesions[74] as can **extramedullary hematopoiesis, splenules,** and **splenosis.**

Fluid Collections

These are commonly found in the retroperitoneum. They include **hematomas** (see Figs. 12-23 and 12-24),[75] **lymphoceles,**[76-78] **abscesses,**[79-81] **urinomas** (see Fig. 12-9B),[21,23] **cystic tumors,**[59] **germ cell tumors,**[58] **primary retroperitoneal cysts,**[82] **exophytic renal cysts, lymphangiomas,**[83-85] **cystic hamartomas,**[86] **venous varices,**[74,87] and **dilated renal collecting systems** (see Fig. 12-21C). Many of these pathologic processes appear

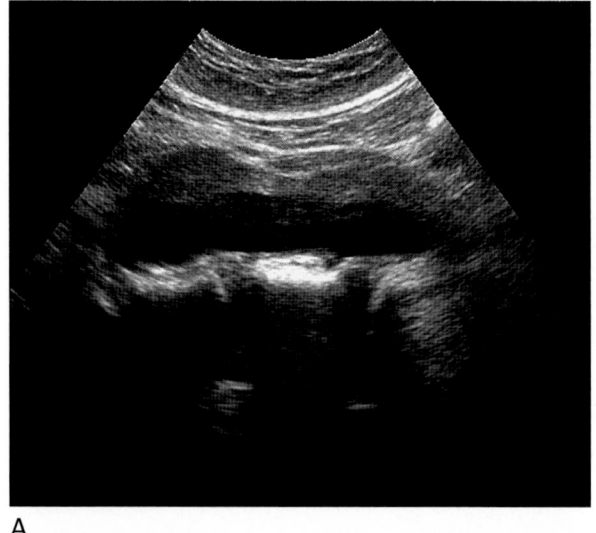

A

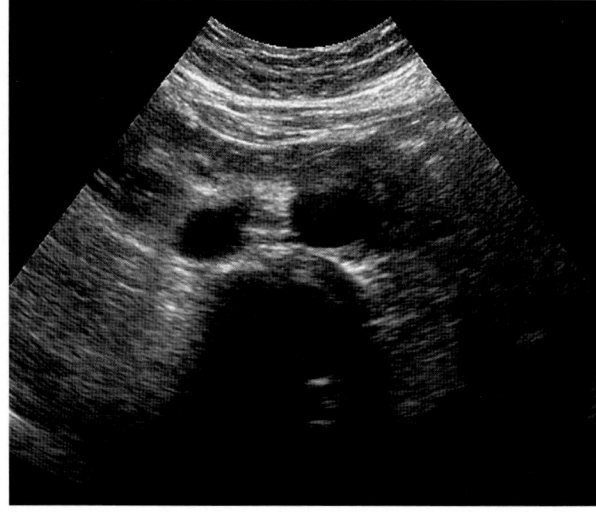

B

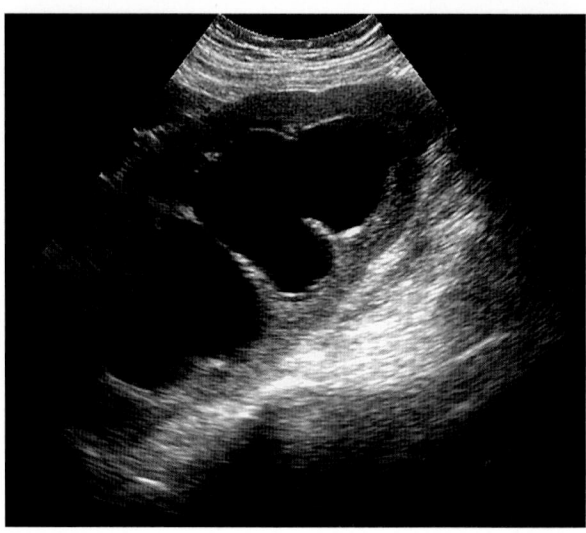

C

FIGURE 12-21. Retroperitoneal fibrosis with hydronephrosis of the kidney. Sagittal (**A**) and transverse (**B**) images of the aorta show a soft tissue mass anterior and to the left of the aorta. The soft tissue mass is smooth and otherwise resembles lymphadenopathy. **C,** Right kidney shows grade III hydronephrosis related to ureteric entrapment. (Courtesy of Stephanie Wilson, MD, University of Toronto.)

similar at sonography, and localization of the fluid to a given compartment is helpful in diagnosing both their nature and their origin.

Primary Cysts and Lymphangiomas. Primary retroperitoneal cysts are frequently large and usually have the sonographic appearance of simple cysts.[82] Lymphangiomas[83-85] are congenital malformations of the lymphatic system and are seen as elongated unilocular or multilocular cysts with thick septations; 44% contain some debris. The diagnosis is important, because incompletely removed lesions can give rise to severe chylous ascites or local recurrence.

Lymphoceles. Lymphoceles[13,34,76,78,88,89] are common after surgical procedures. They have been reported in between 10% and 27% of patients after staging lymphadenectomy[76] and are frequently found adjacent to transplanted kidneys.[76] Most are small, develop within 10 to 21 days after surgery, and resolve spontan-

eously. Treatment of larger lesions includes surgery, percutaneous drainage, and the injection of sclerosing agents.[77]

Most lymphoceles are anechoic and resemble simple cysts.[78,90] Between 20% and 50% present as complex masses with septations that are usually not of clinical significance. Most lymphoceles occur lateral to the bladder and within 3 cm of the abdominal wall, but they can occur anywhere in the abdomen and pelvis.[76] Their differentiation from abscess, hematoma, or urinoma is often difficult, especially if debris is present. Localized tenderness and increasing size should make one suspicious of infection.[91]

Urinomas. In many medical centers, urinomas most often arise after iatrogenic intervention, although they also occur after high-grade ureteric obstruction and trauma.[92] Persisting urinomas may induce fibrosis or become infected. They usually resolve after drainage of

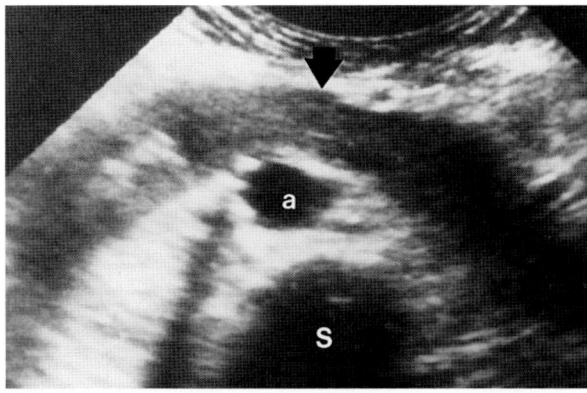

FIGURE 12-22. Horseshoe kidney. Transverse scan shows the isthmus *(arrow)* of a horseshoe kidney lying over the distal aorta (a). S, spine.

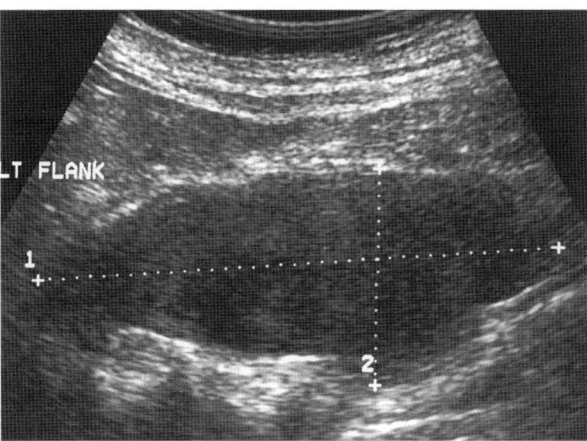

FIGURE 12-23. Postangiogram hematoma. Linear isoechoic mass on left psoas. Longitudinal scan was taken 3 hours after an angiographic procedure. The extensive retroperitoneal hematoma *(cursors)* is of medium echogenicity.

the collecting system with or without ureteric stenting.[92] Classically, they present as hypoechoic retroperitoneal collections often conforming to the shape of the compartment in which they are located (see Fig. 12-9B).

Varices. Varices may appear cystic or echogenic on B-mode examination. Doppler imaging usually confirms the diagnosis, but it is important to adjust the Doppler parameters appropriately to show the slow flow.

Pancreatic Pseudocysts. Pseudocysts are well-demarcated pockets of fluid that develop around the pancreas after pancreatitis. The anterior pararenal space is most frequently involved (see Fig. 12-9C),[93] although the other retroperitoneal spaces may be involved, especially if pancreatic fluid dissolves the fascia.[22,25,32] Diagnostic aspiration is often very helpful in differentiating them from other clear fluid collections and may help in the treatment.

Retroperitoneal Hemorrhage. Retroperitoneal hemorrhage occurs through a defect in the patient's coagulation process,[75] spontaneous vascular rupture,[94] traumatic vascular rupture, or medical intervention,[73,95,96] or it occurs secondary to tumor bleeding or vessel invasion. It has also been reported after lithotripsy.[97] Common sites of bleeding include the psoas muscle and the perinephric space (see Figs. 12-23 and 12-24). Psoas hematoma may be very difficult to diagnose, especially in early stages.

Acute retroperitoneal hemorrhage may be catastrophic,[73] but often it is confined by the fascial layers, which may tamponade the process and obviate the need for surgery. In the acute situation, it is essential that the patient's condition be stable before any imaging is undertaken. CT is preferable to ultrasound, because it is both more sensitive and more specific in identifying the presence and extent of disease.[98]

The sonographic appearances of retroperitoneal hemorrhage are variable (see Figs. 12-23 and 12-24). Solid or cystic masses are the most common sonographic findings. Cystic lesions vary from being entirely sonolucent, like a urinoma (see Fig. 12-9B), to being markedly echogenic and indistinguishable from adjacent fat in the acute or chronic state (see Fig. 12-24A and C). Cellular debris may layer dependently in a hematoma, making its differentiation from an abscess difficult. The character of blood clots changes over time. Some researchers suggest that the age of the clot can be crudely estimated based on its echogenicity,[65,99] because dense fibrin clots, which occur later in disease processes, are more echogenic than are loose fibrin clots,[99] which are more common at the start of the coagulation process.[65]

Retroperitoneal Infections

These infections may be primary or may be caused by spread from an adjacent organ, such as the kidney, bowel, or spine. A preexisting fluid collection such as a pancreatic pseudocyst may also be secondarily infected. Paraspinal infections may arise with disc or vertebral body infection. Diverticulitis and Crohn's disease are the major antecedent bowel conditions that spread inflammatory processes into the retroperitoneum. Predisposing factors include diabetes mellitus, ureteral obstruction, AIDS, trauma or surgery, and alcohol and drug abuse.

Percutaneous drainage is an important diagnostic test and is also the treatment of choice in most cases of retroperitoneal infection. In many cases it may be the only treatment required.

The appearances on ultrasound are rarely specific, so distinguishing abscesses from other collections or masses is challenging. Air within an abscess may be difficult to discern on sonography, and, where suspected, a plain film or a CT scan of the abdomen should be performed. Also, distinguishing **aperistaltic bowel loops, dilated ureters, thrombosed aneurysms,** and **vessels** from abscesses is often challenging, because these conditions may produce pseudocollections.

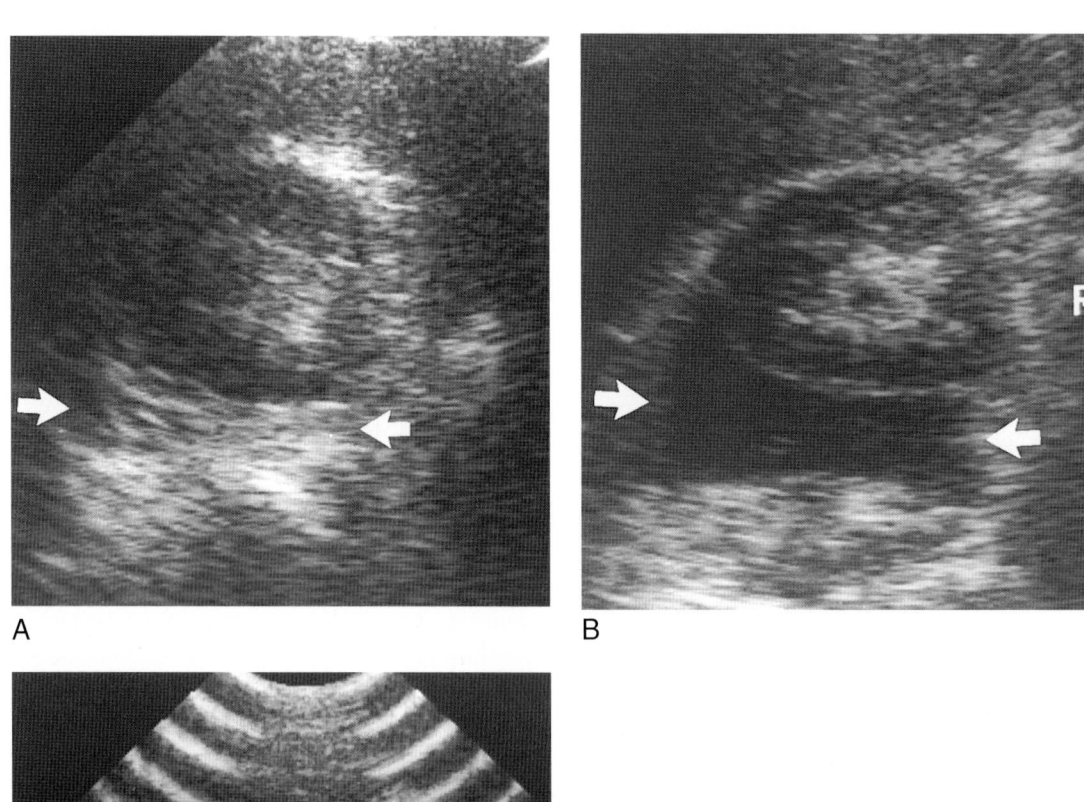

A

B

C

FIGURE 12-24. Retroperitoneal hemorrhage over time. Sequential transverse sonograms of the right kidney in a patient who suffered a small renal laceration and a combined perirenal and posterior pararenal hematoma *(arrows)* after a motor vehicle accident. **A,** Two days post accident. **B,** Twelve days post accident. **C,** Twenty-two days post accident. Initially, the combined perirenal and posterior pararenal hematoma is very hard to detect, because it is echogenic and similar to the adjacent echogenicity of the perirenal fat. As the hematoma liquefies (**B**) it is easily detectable, and after 3 weeks (**C**), with increasing fibrosis, it becomes more echogenic and decreases in size.

Xanthogranulomatous Pyelonephritis. Xanthogranulomatous pyelonephritis is an unusual chronic renal infection that results in enlargement of the kidney, destruction of the normal parenchyma, and severe infiltration of the kidney by lipid-laden macrophages.[100,101] Stones are present in over 80% of cases, and obstruction is common. It usually involves a whole kidney, and there is an intense surrounding fibrotic reaction. The perirenal and pararenal spaces are usually involved; the kidney often contains a staghorn calculus. The enlarged kidney is usually clearly seen on ultrasound, as are adjacent abscesses, when present. The calculi are often not as obvious as one might expect, because the perirenal fibrosis attenuates the ultrasound beam. Ill-defined hypoechoic areas may be seen in the collecting systems.[100]

GREAT VESSELS

Aorta

The abdominal aorta supplies arterial blood to the digestive organs, the kidneys, the adrenals, the gonads, the abdominal and paraspinal musculature, and the pelvis and lower limbs.[39]

Anatomy

The aorta enters the abdomen through the aortic hiatus of the diaphragm, immediately anterior to the 12th dorsal vertebra (see Figs. 12-1, 12-6 and 12-11A).[39] It descends anterior to and slightly to the left of the

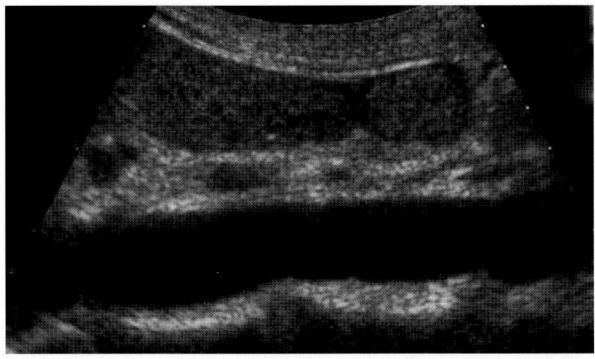

A

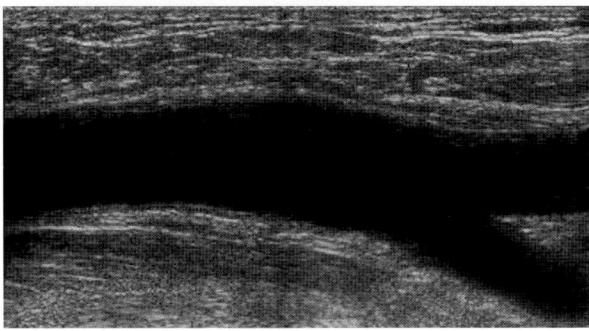

B

FIGURE 12-25. Normal aorta. A and **B,** Sagittal images of the aorta in the upper abdomen and at the iliac bifurcation, respectively. The wall is smooth and the lumen appears echo free. (Courtesy of J. W. Charboneau, MD, Mayo Clinic.)

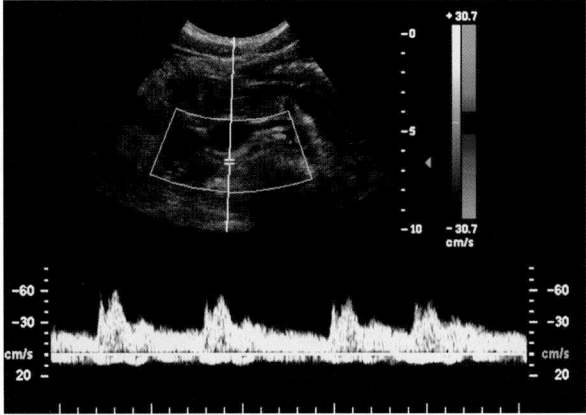

FIGURE 12-26. Renal artery Doppler. Normal color and B-mode Doppler tracing from a right renal artery demonstrate the usual "early systolic spike" that is seen in normal patients.

vertebral bodies. Superiorly, it lies posterior and slightly to the left of the gastroesophageal junction. The median arcuate ligament of the diaphragm abuts its anterior surface, and it is flanked on either side by the diaphragmatic crura. To its right lies the azygous vein and thoracic duct; on its left lies the hemiazygous vein. Below the level of the crura, it lies immediately to the left of the IVC and posterior to the celiac artery, SMA, inferior mesenteric artery, left renal vein, gonadal vessels, and root of the mesentery. At the L4 level, it bifurcates into the paired common iliac arteries,[39] which are about 5 cm long and generally run slightly anterior to the corresponding veins (Fig. 12-25). The common iliac arteries bifurcate into the external and the internal iliac arteries. The external iliac artery lies just on the medial aspect of the psoas.

The main aortic branches[39] that are frequently seen on ultrasound are the celiac artery (see Fig. 12-1), the paired renal arteries (Fig. 12-26; see also Fig. 12-6), the SMA (Fig. 12-27; see also Fig. 12-1), and the common iliac arteries. The celiac artery is the first major abdominal aortic branch, and typically it bifurcates into the hepatic and splenic arteries within 3 cm of its origin. It has a T-shaped or a Y-shaped configuration in the transverse plane. The left gastric artery is given off superiorly and is sometimes seen. The internal iliac arteries have

numerous branches immediately after the common iliac artery bifurcation, but they are rarely seen on routine sonograms. The external iliac artery gives off the inferior epigastric artery and the deep circumflex iliac artery before continuing below the inguinal ligament as the common femoral artery.[39]

Other aortic branches not usually identified include the paired inferior diaphragmatic (inferior phrenic) branches, the paired middle suprarenal arteries, the paired gonadal arteries, the inferior mesenteric artery, and the paired first to fourth lumbar arteries. At the aortic termination, the middle sacral artery is given off posteroinferiorly.[39] Identification of an aberrant branch may aid the diagnosis of some entities.

Aortic Sonography

The **indications for an aortic sonogram** include a pulsatile abdominal mass, hemodynamic compromise in the lower limb arterial system, abdominal pain, and an abdominal bruit. Its examination is an integral part of the "routine" abdominal scan, and it is prudent to at least survey the aorta during limited abdominal scans performed for other indications. Two recent prospective trials indicated that monitoring small (<5.5 cm in diameter) abdominal aortic aneurysms with ultrasound is as effective as early surgery in preventing mortality and carries a lower morbidity and cost.[102-105] There is increasing evidence that it is worthwhile and cost effective to screen selected populations for aortic aneurysms with "screening" ultrasound examinations.[106-112]

Good acoustic windows for scanning the abdominal aorta include:

- The midline in the upper abdomen
- The left flank, with the patient supine (or right lateral decubitus)

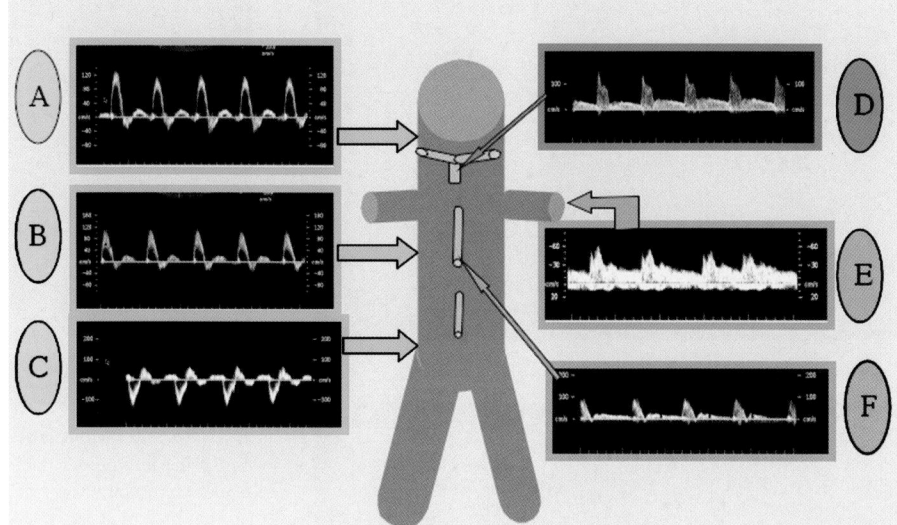

FIGURE 12-27. Normal Doppler tracings. A to **C,** Tracings from the proximal, mid, and distal aorta in a healthy 16-year-old volunteer. The peak velocity decreases and the tracing widens as the wave progresses distally. **E,** Typical low-resistance renal artery pattern with the characteristic "early systolic spike" typical of normal people. Celiac artery (**D**) and superior mesenteric artery (**F**) tracings are typically of a low resistance type postprandially and a higher resistance type during fasting.

- Along the lateral aspect of the lower rectus abdominis muscle for evaluating the iliac vessels

Objectives of aortic sonography include:

- Visualization of the entire aorta and its main branches
- Detection of atheromatous stenoses, aneurysms, dissections, or other pathologic processes
- Measurements, including any dilated segments
- Evaluation of adjacent organs and structures

The entire aorta should be seen in transverse and longitudinal planes and its maximum anteroposterior and transverse diameter measured accurately.[113] It is shown as a hypoechoic tubular structure with echogenic walls (see Fig. 12-1A). It is seen just to the left of the midline, although it is variable in position when it becomes ectatic. It is frequently difficult to visualize well at the level of the renal arteries because of overlying bowel gas.

Normal Aortic Measurements. The abdominal aorta tapers from its cranial to its caudal extent in 95% of people and usually measures less than 2.3 cm in diameter for men and 1.9 cm for women.[114,115] It increases in diameter by approximately 24% between ages 25 and 71, and both the overall diameter and the rate of increase in diameter are greater in men than in women.[116,117] The upper limit of normal for aortic diameter varies with age, because the diameter normally increases by up to 25% in the seventh and eighth decades. In one study, the maximum normal diameter was 2.4 cm for a 60-year-old and 3.7 cm for a 75-year-old.[115] The maximum diameter of the common iliac artery is 1.4 to 1.5 cm for men and 1.2 cm for women.[114,116]

Aortic Doppler Analysis. The abdominal aorta is a compliant elastic tube[116,117] that plays a major role in maintaining the forward flow of blood during diastole.

INDICATIONS FOR AN AORTIC SONOGRAM

Pulsatile abdominal mass
Hemodynamic compromise in the lower limb arterial system
Abdominal pain
Abdominal bruit

In systole, it acts as a reservoir of fluid in response to the very pulsatile inflow it receives from the left ventricle. It decreases in size during diastole by discharging blood into the rest of the circulation in a much less pulsatile manner.[118] The normal flow pattern in the aorta is classified as "plug flow," a situation in which most of the blood in that section of the aorta is moving at the same velocity (see Fig. 12-27).[118] The blood flow pattern in the aorta and iliac arteries is classified as being of a "high-resistance" type (see Fig. 12-27). There is a sharp increase in its antegrade velocity during systole, followed by a rapid decrease in velocity and culminating in a brief period of reversed flow. During the remainder of diastole there may be some low velocity, antegrade flow. Spectral Doppler analysis shows the peak antegrade velocity decreases and the amount of retrograde flow increases as one progresses from the proximal aorta to the iliac system (see Fig. 12-25). The blood flow patterns in the main aortic branches to the kidney, the liver, and the postprandial bowel are of a "low-resistance" type with a lower resistive index and a lower pulsatility index (see Figs. 12-26 and 12-27E). This blood flow pattern is characterized by continuous forward flow throughout the cardiac cycle and a more variable velocity pattern across the blood vessel, which results in the thickness of the spectral line being broadened.

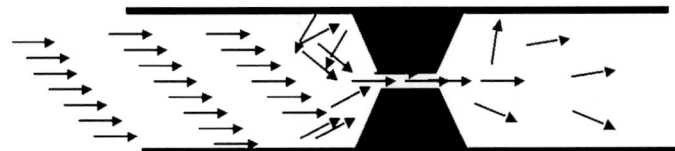
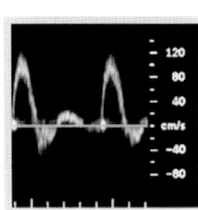
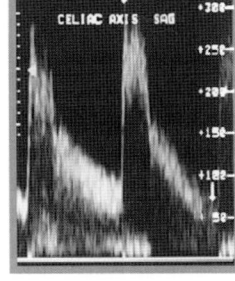
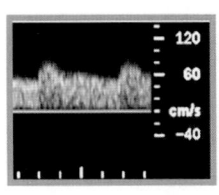

Pre Stenosis Stenosis Post Stenosis

FIGURE 12-28. Doppler tracings about stenoses. A, Prestenosis. Forward flow of blood is impeded by the narrowing, resulting in a high resistance or aortic type tracing. **B,** At the stenosis. Flow is typically of a high velocity and turbulent with disruption of the normal laminar flow pattern. **C,** Post stenosis there is typically relatively little blood relative to the size of the vessel, so flow has a "parvus tardus" pattern.

Objectives of aortic Doppler sonography include:

- Validation of the entire aorta and its main branches, determining their patency with color Doppler imaging
- Detection of atheromatous stenoses, aneurysms, dissections, or other pathologic processes by showing altered intraluminal flow on color Doppler imaging
- Characterization of these abnormalities with spectral Doppler tracings
- Definition of flow in the examined vessels as a "high resistance" or "low resistance" type, which might suggest an upstream or downstream pathologic process

Color Doppler analysis can rapidly confirm that the aorta and its main branches are patent. If color Doppler aliasing occurs, a Doppler spectral tracing helps to determine whether a true stenosis is present (Fig. 12-28). Angle-corrected spectral Doppler analysis at stenosis typically shows increased pulsatility (increased pulsatility index and resistive index) proximal to the stenosis, increased peak systolic and peak diastolic velocity immediately at the stenosis, turbulence immediately post stenosis, and dampening of the waveform farther distal

to the stenoses (see Fig. 12-28).[119,120] Stenoses should be mapped and waveform and peak systolic velocity documented.[113]

Aortic Pathology

The abdominal aorta and its main branches are affected by atheroma,[121] aneurysm formation,[113] connective tissue disorders,[122,123] rupture,[94,105] thrombosis, infections,[124] and displacement by and invasion from diseases in adjacent structures.

Atheromatous Disease. Atheroma, or arteriosclerosis, is a vascular wall disorder characterized by the presence of lipid deposits in the intima (Fig. 12-29). The atheromatous plaque is a soft, porridge-like material that may discharge into the vessel lumen, causing a distal embolus or a local thrombus or both. Plaques cause mural irregularity and frequently narrow the vessel

---

EVIDENCE OF STENOSIS ON SPECTRAL DOPPLER ANALYSIS

Increased pulsatility proximal to the stenosis
Increased pulsatility index and resistive index
Increased peak systolic velocity at the stenosis
Increased peak diastolic velocity at the stenosis
Turbulence immediately post stenosis
Dampening of the waveform farther distal to the stenosis

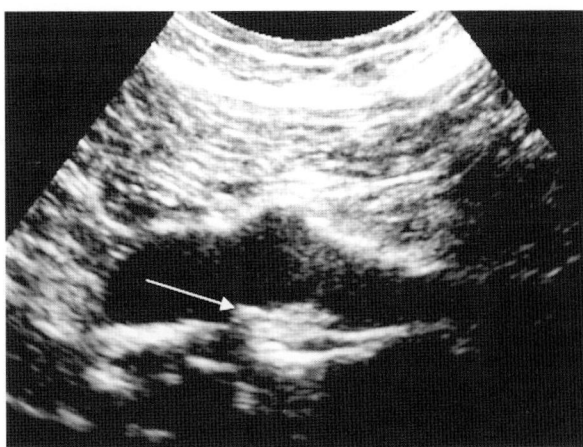

FIGURE 12-29. Aortic aneurysm with eccentric plaque. A focal area of plaque *(arrow)* has developed some thrombus around it and now protrudes into the lumen. This is seen to "flutter" in the lumen during real-time scanning and is a potential source of emboli.

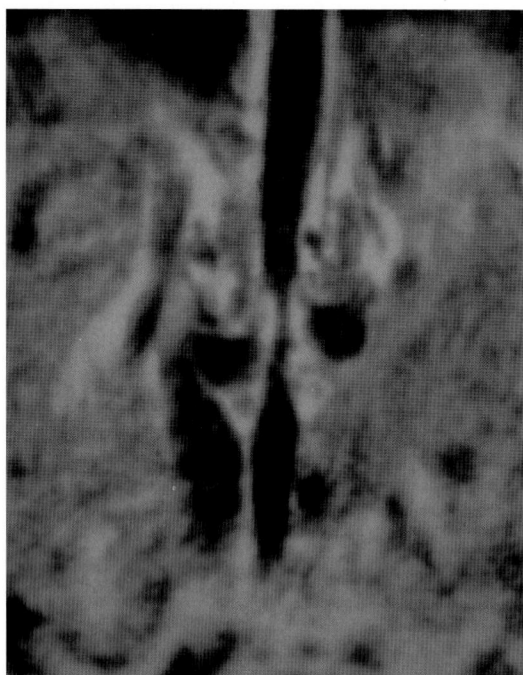

FIGURE 12-30. Takayasu's disease. Coronal MRI shows midabdominal narrowing of the aorta, the second most common manifestation of this disease.

lumen, with resulting distal ischemia.[121] Stenotic or occlusive disease most often occurs in the infrarenal portion of the aorta. Atheroma may also be associated with mural weakening and aneurysm formation.[121]

The incidence of atheromatous disease increases with age and affects more men than women.[121] It involves both the aorta, the iliac arteries, and the other aortic branch arteries and is most common on the posterior wall in the aortoiliac area.[121] It is associated with cigarette smoking, diabetes mellitus, hypertension, and increased levels of the low-density lipoprotein fraction of serum cholesterol.[120]

If significant lower limb pain is present, it is prudent to assess the entire lower limb arterial tree to rule out emboli and to look for further stenoses.[113] Similarly, in lower limb analysis the presence of a dampened waveform in the common femoral artery should provoke a search for a stenotic lesion more proximal in the arterial tree (Fig. 12-30).

Ectasia occurs when the aorta increases not only in transverse diameter but also in vertical length, causing the distal abdominal aorta to kink, usually anteriorly and to the left.

An **aneurysm** is any swelling in a blood vessel, either focal or diffuse (Fig. 12-31).[125] Histologically, they are classified into true aneurysms (see Figs. 12-31B, 12-32 and 12-33), which are lined by all three layers of the aorta, and false aneurysms (pseudoaneurysms), which are not (see Figs. 12-31C, 12-34, and 12-35). **True**

aneurysms form when the tensile strength of the wall decreases (see Fig. 12-31B). A minority of true aneurysms are due to clearly identified underlying diseases that predispose affected patients to aneurysm formation, such as Marfan's syndrome, Ehlers–Danlos syndrome (Fig. 12-36), annuloaortic ectasia, familial aortic dissection, and intimomedial mucoid degeneration. Most true aneurysms, however, are idiopathic.[54,122,123]

In **false, or pseudo, aneurysms,** blood escapes through a hole in the innermost vessel lining (the intima) but is contained by the deeper layers of the aorta or by the adjacent tissue (see Figs. 12-31C, 12-34, and 12-35). Most pseudoaneurysms are round or oval protuberances from the artery; blood circulates into them in systole and out of them in diastole (see Fig. 12-34). They can be caused by infection (mycotic[124]) or can result from trauma, surgery, or interventional radiology procedures (see Figs. 12-34 and 12-35).[126-130]

Abdominal Aortic Aneurysms. Idiopathic abdominal aortic aneurysms (AAAs) are true aneurysms (see Fig. 12-31B), 95% of which are infrarenal. Of patients with AAAs, 30% to 60% are asymptomatic and the rest present with abdominal, back, or leg pain.[113] They may also present after leakage or rupture. While AAAs are strongly associated with atherosclerosis, their **origin is likely to be multifactorial**[131-136] because most people with atheroma do not develop aneurysms.[113,136] Furthermore, AAA patients frequently have arteriomegaly, with vessels 40% to 50% bigger than those with atheromatous aortic occlusive disease (see Fig. 12-24).[131,132] There is an increased risk of the disease in close relatives[136,137] (an estimated 11% to 18% increased risk in a first-degree relative), and it also appears that proper innervation of the aorta may also help to stop aneurysm formation, because the aorta is bigger in patients with spinal injury.[135]

The **true incidence** of AAAs is unknown, but studies suggest a 5% to 10% prevalence in men older than 60.[107,113,138-141] The incidence is highest in elderly men, with between 70% and 90% of AAAs occurring in men older than 65.[113] Various cases have been made for screening entire groups of elderly people or subgroups at high risk,[94,106,107,111,136,139,140,142-148] but as yet there is no consensus.

Several studies have found that ultrasound measurements of AAA (Fig. 12-37) are both accurate and repeatable.[112,149-151]

The recognized **complications** of idiopathic AAAs include rupture, thrombosis, dissection, distal embolism, infection, and obstruction and invasion of adjacent structures.[131] The most common complications of AAAs are branch artery occlusions or stenoses,[113] which have more to do with the atheroma than with the aneurysm. They can occur anywhere but are most commonly seen in the inferior mesenteric artery and the renal arteries. A **dissecting aneurysm**[113,152] is a special type of pseudoaneurysm in which blood leaves the lumen through an

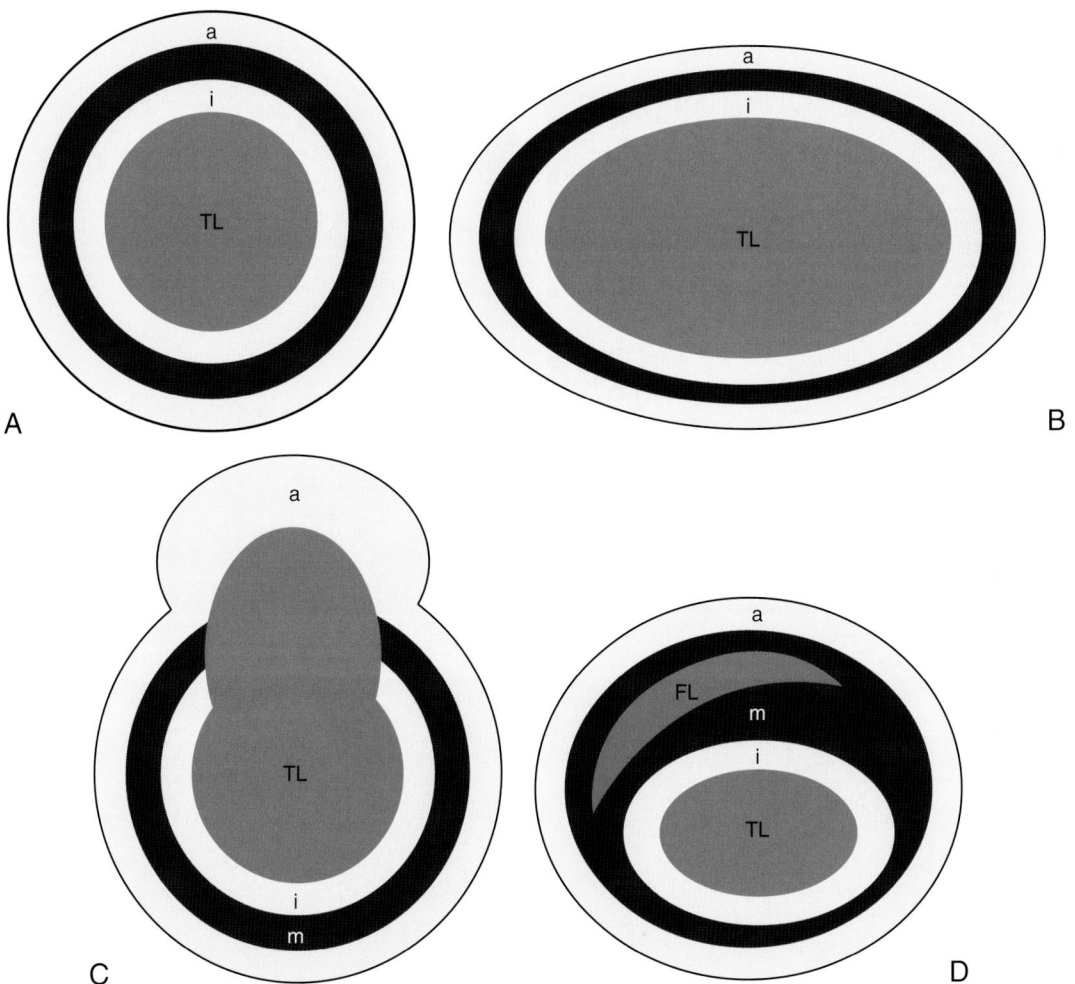

FIGURE 12-31. Schematics of the layers of the normal aorta. A, Normal. There are three layers: the inner intima *(beige [i]),* the middle media *(brown [m]),* and the outer adventitia *(light blue [a]).* TL, true lumen. **B,** True aneurysm: the vessel enlarges, as do all three mural layers. **C,** False aneurysm: the vessel enlarges but part of the protruding portion of the true lumen is covered only by adventitia (a). It has herniated through the intima (i) and the media (m). **D,** Dissecting aneurysm: while the outer diameter of the aorta has increased, the diameter of the true lumen is unchanged. However, a new lumen, or "false lumen" (FL), has opened within the media and is not lined by intima.

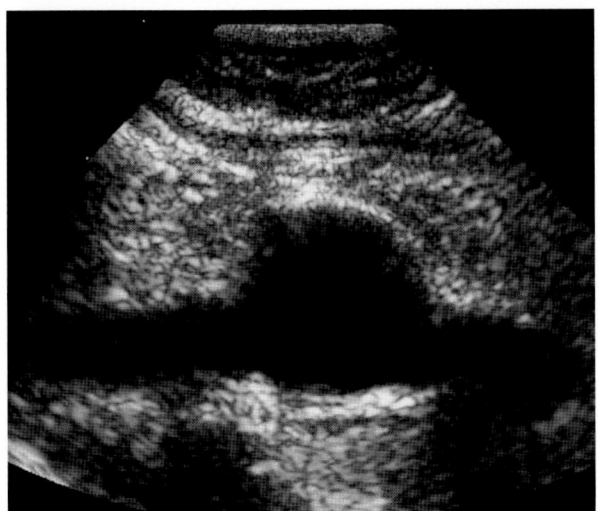

FIGURE 12-32. Saccular abdominal aortic aneurysm. Sagittal sonogram shows a focal saccular aneurysm. Above and below this diameter increase, the aorta is quite normal in caliber. (Courtesy of J. W. Charboneau, MD, Mayo Clinic.)

intimal defect, courses a variable distance in the wall, and reenters the aorta farther distal in the arterial system (Fig. 12-31D).

Aortic Rupture. The most catastrophic of aortic aneurysm complications is aortic rupture, which has a mortality rate of at least 50%. Most aneurysms that rupture have not been recognized before rupture.[132,133] Natural history indicates a cumulative incidence of rupture of 25% over 8 years for aneurysms greater than 5 cm in anteroposterior diameter (Figs. 12-33C and 12-33D).[132] There is a 5% cumulative incidence of rupture over the same time period for abdominal aortic aneurysms with an anteroposterior diameter between 3.5 and 4.9 cm (Figs. 12-32, 12-33A and B) and a 0% incidence for aneurysms less than 3.5 cm in antero-posterior diameter.[132,133,153-155] The average rate at which an aneurysm enlarges varies between 0.2 to 0.4 or 0.5 cm per year, depending on the study.[131-133,155-157] However, there is considerable interpersonal variation, so the optimal time interval for screening these patients

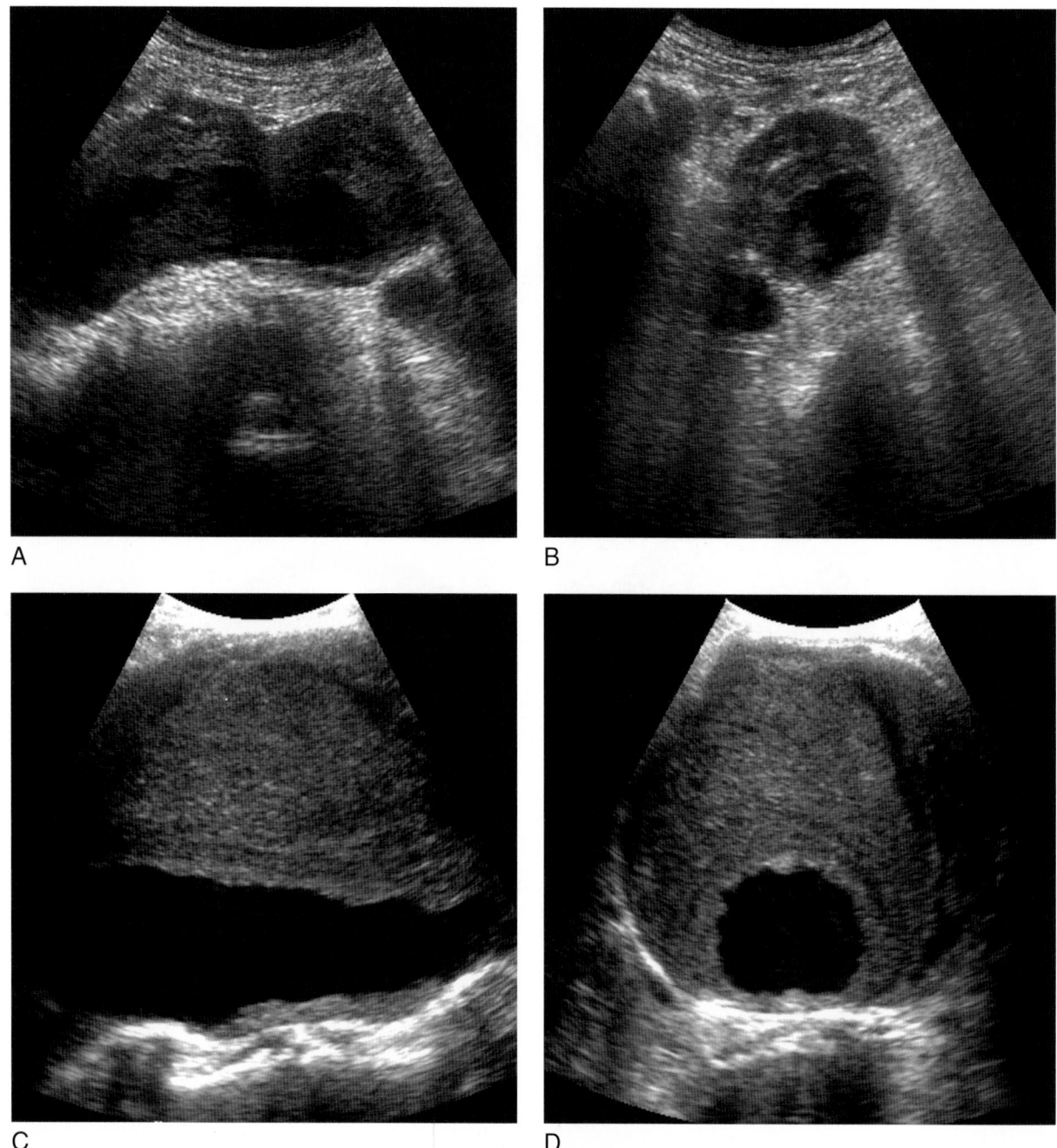

FIGURE 12-33. Abdominal aortic aneurysms in two patients. A and **C,** Sagittal images. **B** and **D,** Corresponding transverse images. The aneurysm on the top line is dumbbell shaped, arising below the renal arteries. There is a moderate amount of anterior thrombus. The aneurysm on the bottom line is very large, measuring 8 cm in maximal diameter. There is again extensive anterior thrombus. This aneurysm has a significant risk of life-threatening rupture. (Courtesy of Stephanie Wilson, MD, University of Toronto.)

is unclear. One suggested protocol is to scan larger aneurysms at 6-month intervals and smaller ones at 12-month intervals.

Aortic rupture is a surgical emergency; and if any imaging is done, CT is the test of choice.[113] It is better at detecting acute hemorrhages, is not hampered by bowel gas, and provides a greater overall perspective. Some aortic ruptures may be contained in the retro-

peritoneum and are referred to as chronic ruptures.[158] If patients with this condition do come to ultrasound, retroperitoneal complex fluid collections are the most common findings.[113,159]

The aneurysm may compress, displace, or invade the ureter, the bowel, the IVC, and the kidney and renal arteries.[131,159,160] The left kidney is more frequently affected than the right.[131] Iliac aneurysms

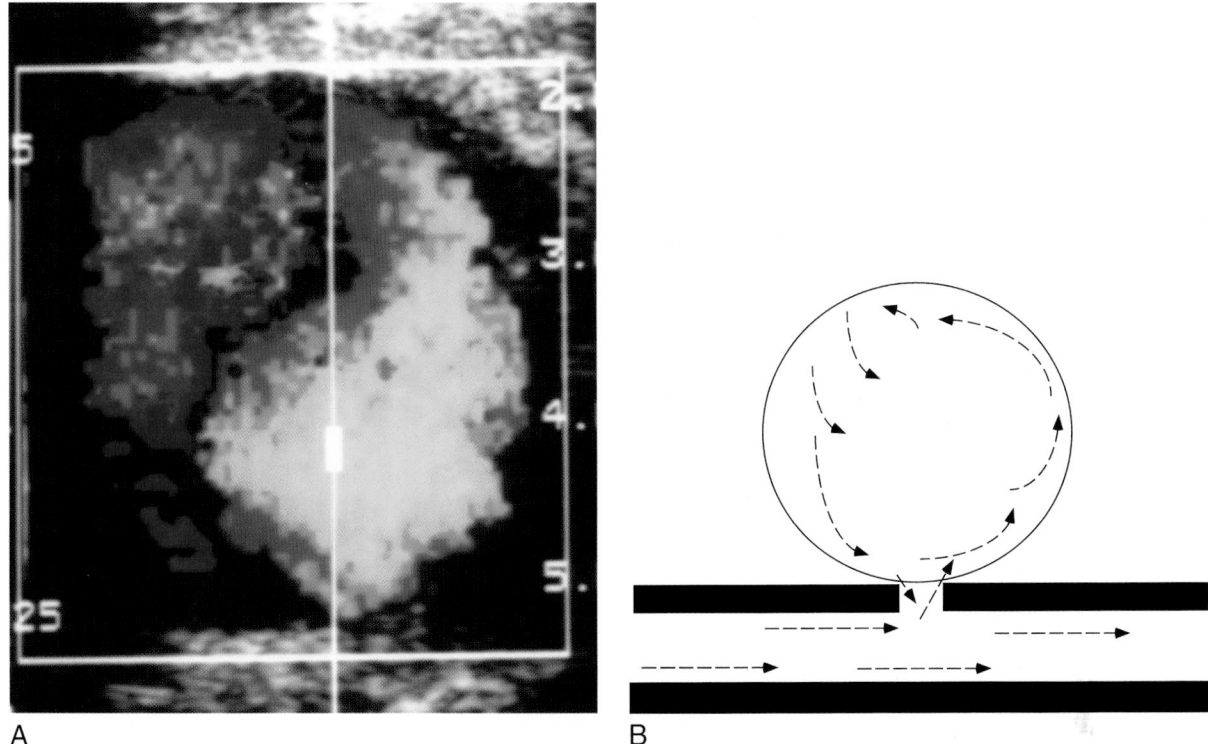

A   B

FIGURE 12-34. Postangiographic pseudoaneurysm. Longitudinal sonograms of the right groin. **A,** Color Doppler shows the typical ying/yang appearance and the relatively low-velocity flow within the lesion. **B,** Diagram demonstrates how blood circulates in these pseudoaneurysms. The entry jet is invariably pulsatile. The blood swirling in the pseudoaneurysm may have variable waveforms and is often monophasic and nonpulsatile. This may be incorrectly interpreted as a venous waveform.

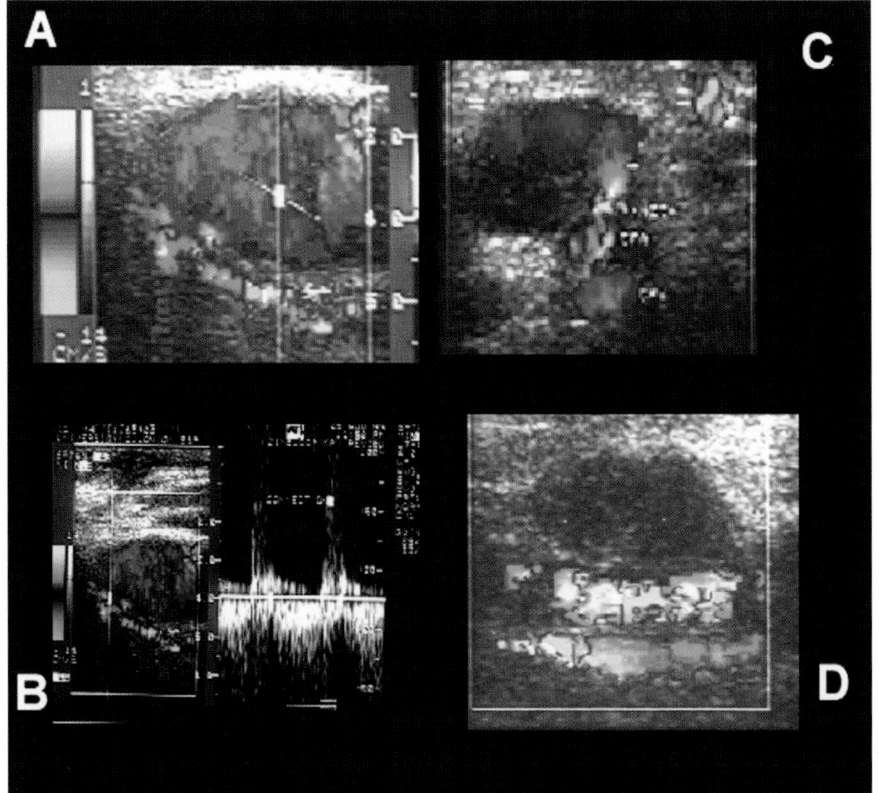

FIGURE 12-35. Thrombin injection of groin pseudoaneurysm. A, Video capture shows a classic pseudoaneurysm just below the inguinal ligament lying ventral to the groin vessels. **B,** Spectral tracing confirms the "in and out" directional flow in the neck of the aneurysm. **C,** Video capture obtained during the injection of 600 IU of activated bovine thrombin. **D,** Video capture taken seconds later shows the entire pseudoaneurysm thrombosed with patent vessels deep to it. (Courtesy of David J. Peck, MD, University of Western Ontario.)

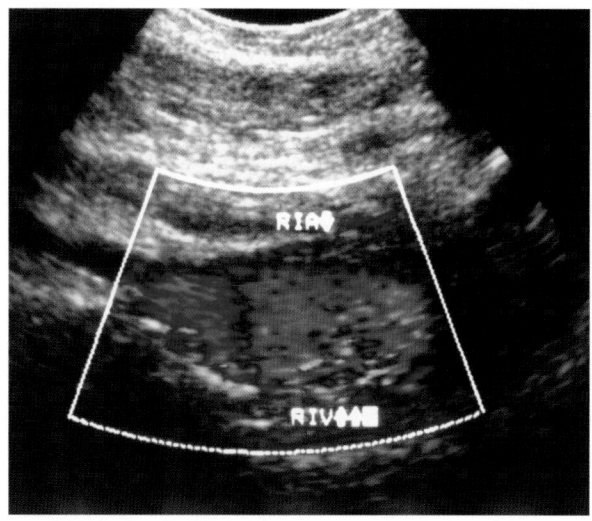

A

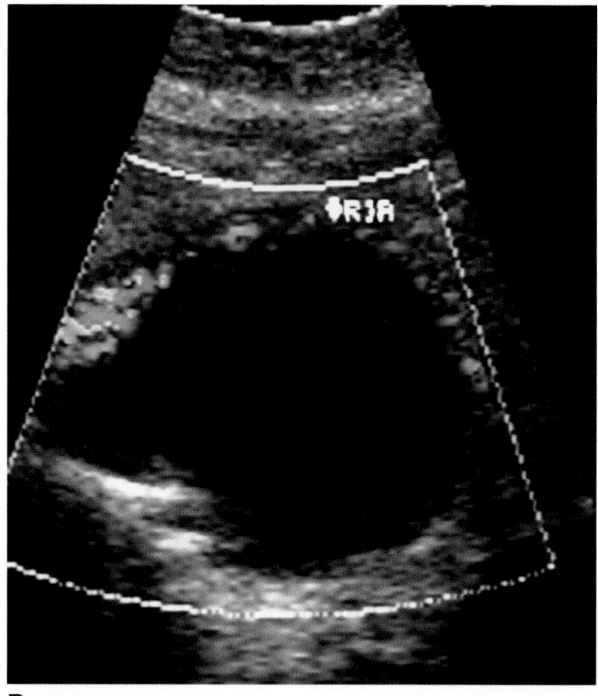

B

FIGURE 12-36. Ehlers-Danlos syndrome. A, Color Doppler diagram showing focal fusiform pseudoaneurysm of the right common iliac artery (RIA). RIV, right iliac vein. **B,** Appearance post spontaneous thrombosis of that pseudoaneurysm.

may rupture into the ureter, the rectosigmoid colon, and the iliac vein.[159]

Mural Thrombus. Mural thrombus in AAAs is prevalent in most large lesions and is frequently circumferential but eccentric (see Figs. 12-33 and 12-37). This thrombus is often poorly attached and friable and is an important source of distal emboli (see Fig. 12-29).[113] The thrombus within an aneurysm is usually not organized and therefore adds no tensile strength to the vessels. The volume of thrombus has no bearing on the risk of rupture.[160]

Inflammatory Aortic Aneurysms. Inflammatory aortic aneurysms are a variant of atherosclerotic AAAs in which the wall of the aneurysm is thickened and surrounded by fibrosis and adhesions of a type similar to those seen in retroperitoneal fibrosis (see Fig. 12-21A and B).[71,106,161] Their surgical repair is associated with a higher mortality and morbidity than is standard aneurysm surgery, so diagnosis before surgery is desirable.[71,106,161] Of AAAs, 4% to 23% are estimated to be inflammatory in origin.[71,161] They are very difficult to diagnose, because they often present as pain and may mimic a retroperitoneal hemorrhage.[161] Whereas less than 25% of idiopathic AAAs present as pain, pain was present in 84% of patients with inflammatory aneurysms.

Sonographic Appearances of Abdominal Aortic Aneurysms. In experienced hands, the diagnosis of aortic aneurysms on sonography is close to 100%.[112,142] The diagnosis is made by finding any focal dilatation of the aorta or a generalized dilatation bigger than 3 cm.[113] *Arteriomegaly* is a term given to generalized enlargement of the arteries (Fig. 12-39). Aneurysms elongate as they

grow; and because the lower end of the aorta rarely moves significantly caudad, most AAAs deflect to the left side or kink anteriorly, or both, as they enlarge (see Fig. 12-37C). The anterior and posterior borders of the aneurysm are usually better seen than its lateral borders, which may be indistinct (see Fig. 12-37B).[151] The adventitia is usually continuous with adjacent fibrofatty tissue and is echogenic (see Fig. 12-37A and B). Mural thrombus, which frequently makes up most of the wall, is usually of low to medium echogenicity (see Figs. 12-33, 12-37A and B), and it may or may not have a lamellated appearance. The intimal lining may be smooth or irregular, and calcification may also be present (see Fig. 12-29).

Sonographic measurement of these AAAs may be challenging, and it is important to get an accurate outer-layer-to-outer-layer measurement in a plane perpendicular to the long axis of the vessels (see Fig. 12-37C).[113] The mean difference between the aortic diameter as measured at surgery and as measured by ultrasound was 2.9 mm in one study.[164]

Analysis of an AAA would include its maximum true length, width, and transverse dimensions; documentation of its shape; and documentation of its location, including suprarenal extension or involvement of the common iliac vessels. By convention, measurements should be given in the order length by width by height. This analysis is of great practical importance, because different surgical approaches are used with the different types of aneurysms. The etiology, complication rate, and postprocedure morbidity are also quite distinct. The nature and type of the wall thickening should be

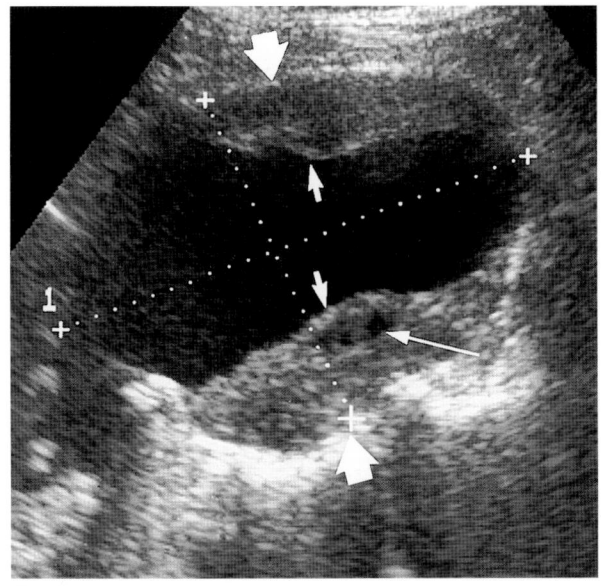

A

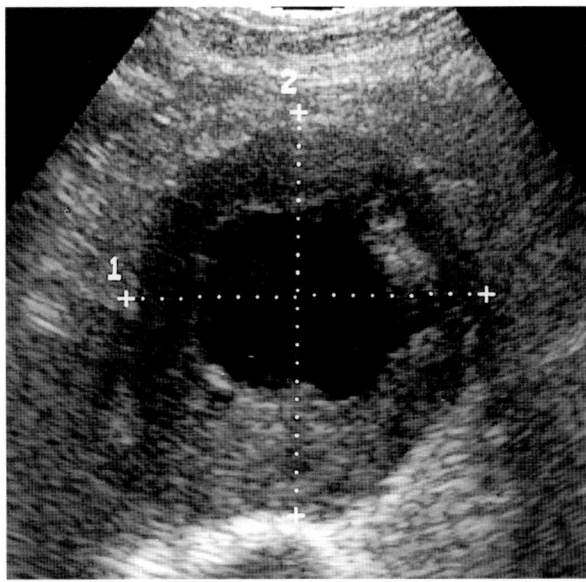

B

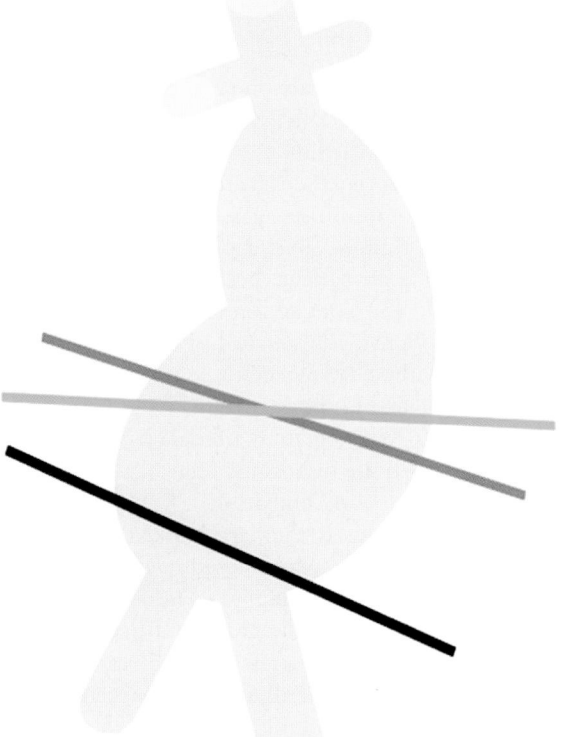

C

FIGURE 12-37. Infrarenal aortic aneurysm. Longitudinal (**A**) and transverse (**B**) images show extensive atheromatous plaque and thrombus with an area of ulceration *(narrow arrow)* in the intima with some cystic change in the wall. Combined plaque and mural thrombus *(larger arrows)*. Cursors are on the margins of the aneurysm, which measures 11 × 7.3 cm. **C,** Aneurysm measurement technique. Line diagram shows a typical infrarenal abdominal aortic aneurysm. Three scan planes are shown. Green line is incorrect, because it is not perpendicular to the main axis of the vessel. Red line is correct. Black line is in the correct plane but not in the widest part of the aneurysm.

assessed: is it calcified plaque, flowing blood, soft plaque, or well-established plaque? The patent channel should be found and the flow pattern characterized. An effort should be made to detect any dissection and to evaluate hypoechoic channels for flow with Doppler imaging. Both kidneys should always be examined, their size measured, and pelvocaliectasis excluded.[113] Doppler evaluation of the renal artery is not part of a "routine" aortic scan, but it should be considered if there is a shrunken kidney or if the patient has hypertension.[113]

The following **descriptive terms** and **sonographic criteria** are commonly used for idiopathic abdominal aortic aneurysms:

- *Bulbous:* sharp junction between normal and abnormal (see Fig. 12-32)
- *Fusiform:* gradual transition between normal and abnormal (see Fig. 12-36)
- *Saccular:* sharp, sudden transition between normal and abnormal (see Fig. 12-32)

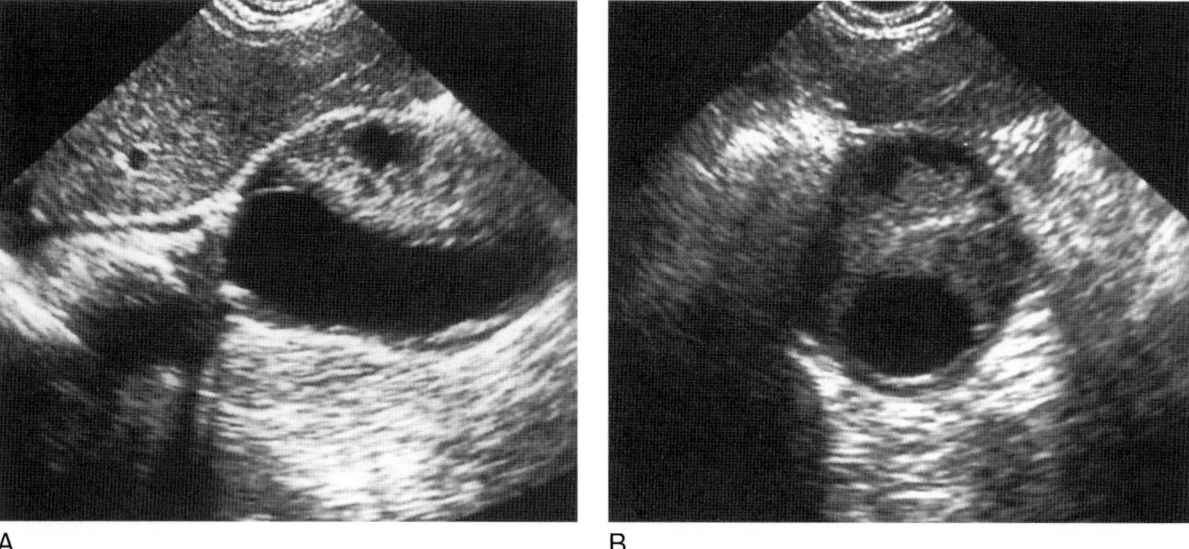

FIGURE 12-38. Atheromatous dissection and pseudodissection. Sagittal (**A**) and transverse (**B**) sonograms on a different patient show hypoechoic zones near the outer margin of laminated thrombus. Clot in this area is recent, as compared with more echogenic laminated thrombus closer to liver. (Courtesy of Stephanie R. Wilson, MD, University of Toronto.)

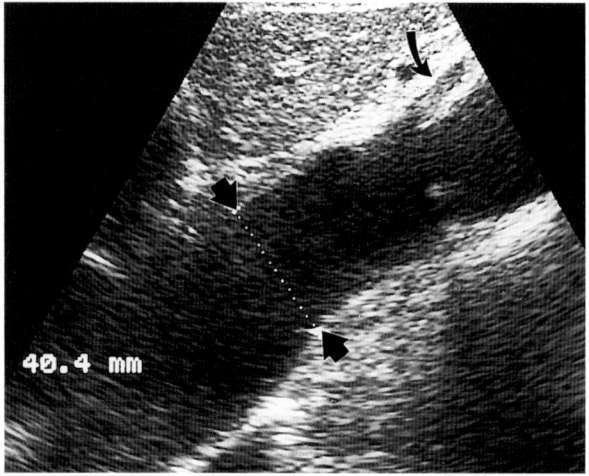

FIGURE 12-39. Arteriomegaly with associated atheroma and distal aneurysm formation. Longitudinal midline scan shows a diffusely widened upper abdominal aorta *(wide arrows)*. *Curved arrow,* superior mesenteric artery.

- *Dumbbell:* Figure-of-eight appearance to the aneurysm (see Fig. 12-33A and B)

Sonographic evaluation of a patient with a known or suspect aneurysm should allow for the following:

- Diagnosis of the aneurysm
- Identification of any complications
- Provision of information that will allow the surgeon to decide whether to intervene surgically
- Monitoring the effects of any therapy given for the AAA

The **decision to operate** on an aneurysm is based on the absolute size, especially when the diameter is over 6 cm, documented enlargement over time, associated pain or tenderness, associated distal emboli, renal obstruction or vascular compromise, gastrointestinal bleeding, and suspected rupture. This decision must be carefully considered in each patient, because these patients are often at risk for concomitant disease. One study reported a 73% five-year survival of patients with small aneurysms, with most mortality coming from diseases not directly related to the aneurysm.[165]

Aortic Grafts. At sonography, arterial grafts (Figs. 12-40 to 12-42) are quite echogenic and have a textured appearance (Figs. 12-42 and 12-43).[113] They are usually named after the vessels they are hooked up with (see Fig. 12-40) and can be anastomosed in either an end-to-side or an end-to-end manner. The native aorta is usually wrapped around the graft, and fluid frequently accumulates between the graft and the vessel wall (see Fig. 12-43). The vessel wall is often thickened at the anastomotic site as a result of puckering at the site of the sutures. Endoprosthetic grafts are gaining popularity for less invasive treatment of aortic aneurysms (see Fig. 12-44).

Some surgeons are using intraoperative ultrasound to assess the vessels during surgery, because ultrasound has been shown to be ideally suited to monitoring vascular reconstructions.[166]

When scanning post procedurally it is essential to:

- Assess the upper and lower anastomoses.
- Check these sites for stenoses, aneurysms, and pseudoaneurysm formations with Doppler imaging.

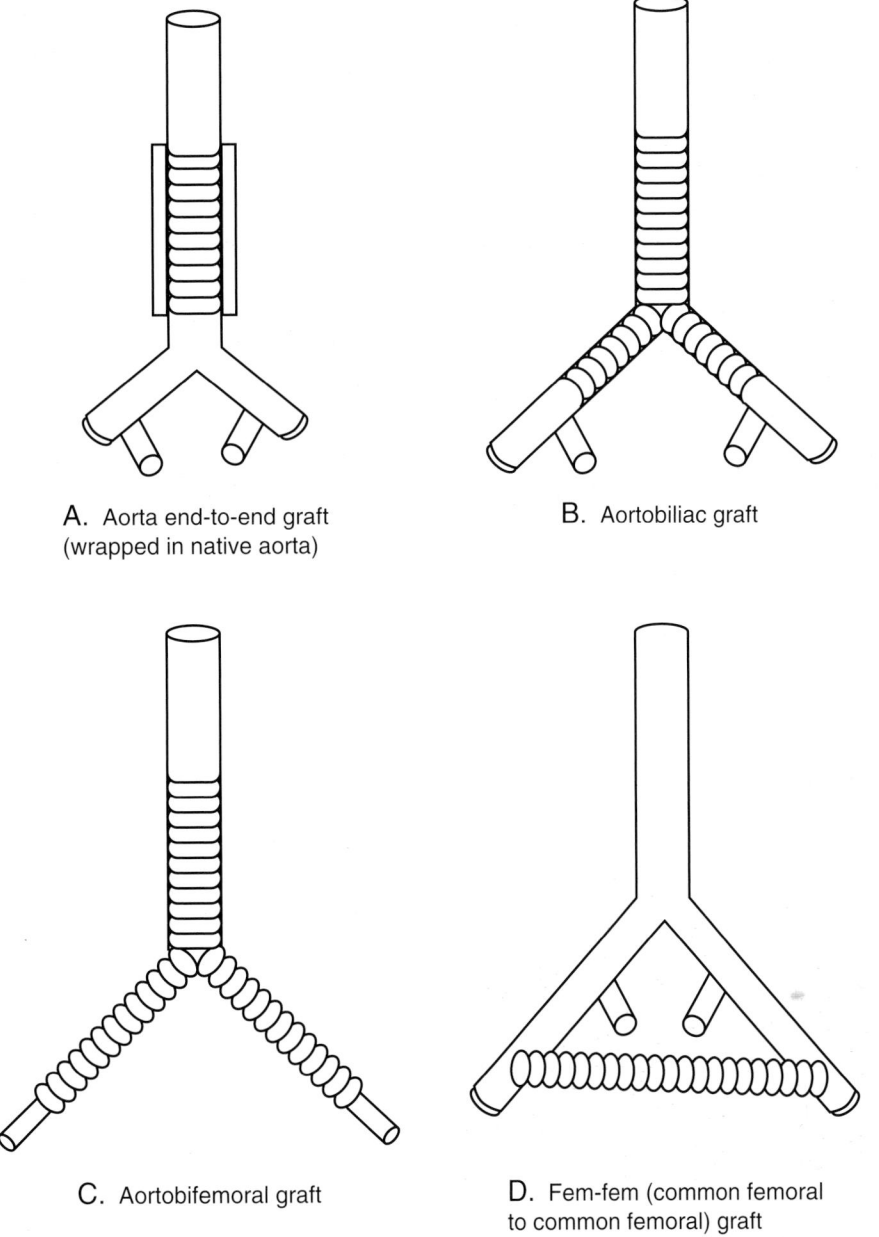

A. Aorta end-to-end graft
(wrapped in native aorta)

B. Aortobiliac graft

C. Aortobifemoral graft

D. Fem-fem (common femoral
to common femoral) graft

FIGURE 12-40. Diagram of common types of prosthetic aortic grafts.

- Identify and measure fluid collections around the graft and elsewhere in the abdomen.
- Check blood flow distally.

The most common finding sonographically is fluid collections around the grafts (see Fig. 12-43).[113] These may be hematomas, lymphoceles, seromas, or abscesses. Distinguishing among the different causes is difficult. If the collection is large, echogenic, increasing in size, or far away from the graft, then infection must be considered,[113] and fine-needle aspiration is indicated.[167] Lymphocele around the graft may be very hypoechoic and may simulate a dissection.[168] Color and spectral Doppler analyses are very useful in these instances. They are also useful for assessment of endoprosthetic grafts to assess for leaks (Fig. 12-44).

Iliac/Suprarenal Aneurysms. Of patients with distal aortic aneurysms, 5% will have an associated iliac artery aneurysm.[134,159] Most occur in the common iliac segment, with the next most common area being the external iliac just beyond the bifurcation. Patients with iliac artery aneurysms have a much higher incidence of aneurysms elsewhere in the body.[134,137] Such aneurysms are of great concern if they exist independently, because they are very difficult to diagnose.[113]

Trauma, syphilis, and mycotic disease should all be

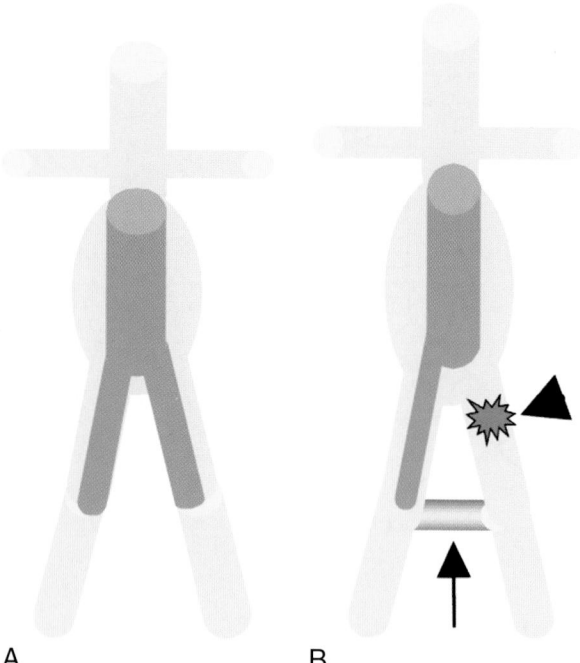

FIGURE 12-41. Intravascular grafts. A, The commonly performed graft in which a component inserts itself up into the abdominal aortic aneurysm and widens and stabilizes the lumen and the lower limbs are lodged in both common iliac arteries. **B,** Similar situation, but the left common iliac vessel is blocked. In this situation, a single iliac limb is inserted and a fem-fem graft *(arrow)* is performed to ensure the other limb remains viable.

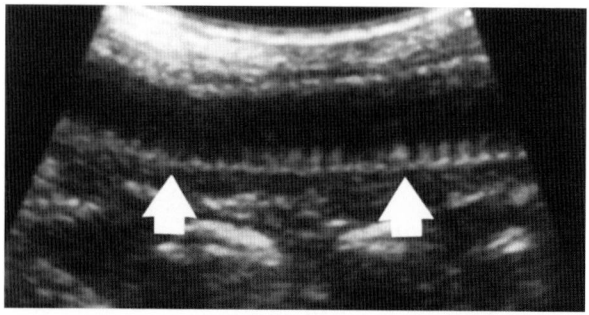

FIGURE 12-42. Vascular graft. Longitudinal scan along the patient's flank region shows subcutaneous vascular axillofemoral graft *(arrows).*

considered potential causes if aneurysms are discovered suprarenally.

Dissection. For an aortic dissection to occur, a defect must exist in the intima and an internal weakness must exist in the wall (see Fig. 12-31D).[113] Most are idiopathic, but some are related to Marfan's disease, pregnancy, bicuspid aortic valve, trauma, focal stenoses, or hypertension.[169] Aortic dissection typically begins in the thorax and extends into the abdomen, with less than 5% occurring primarily in the abdomen. It may

extend into the iliac vessels and the other aortic branch vessels. It may also occlude aortic branch vessels. Dissection may also occur within the thickened wall of an atheromatous AAA.

A special type of dissection is the iatrogenic, post-angiographic type in which the dissection is more localized and the amount of blood flow in the false lumen is usually much less.

Aortic dissection is easily recognized on sonography, with the classic appearance being a thin membrane "fluttering" in the lumen at different phases of the cardiac cycle (Fig. 12-45). Color Doppler imaging shows blood flow in both channels, although flow rates frequently differ between the channels (Fig. 12-46).

Every effort should be made to distinguish a true dissection from a pseudodissection (see Fig. 12-38), which is caused by liquefaction of aneurysm thrombus.[152] The distinguishing features include no fluttering of the intravascular membrane, no flow in one lumen, and a thick membrane in pseudolesions.

Infection. This rare condition is difficult to diagnose and often results in mycotic aneurysms. Septic emboli, which are frequently associated with valvular heart disease or other cardiac anomalies and group D streptococci,[51] often cause the disease. Infection may also result from the hematogenous spread of organisms, especially staphylococci and *Salmonella.*[132] Staphylococci or streptococci may invade a preceding idiopathic aneurysm and produce a focal abscess. Infection may also be secondary to previous surgery or other intervention[170] or may result from the spread of an infection in adjacent structures. Sonography alone will rarely indicate a diagnosis, but by combining the findings with clinical information one can suggest the diagnosis in many cases. The disease itself can result in thrombosis, arterial rupture, distal ischemia, and invasion into adjacent structures.[171]

Pseudoaneurysms/Arteriovenous Fistula. Although these may occur post infection and post trauma, most pseudoaneurysms result from problems at the site of angiographic puncture (see Fig. 12-34) or at the site of a surgical anastomosis. They have a spectacular sonographic appearance on color Doppler examination (see Fig. 12-34), where a pulsatile jet is seen as blood enters the aneurysm during systole, with turbulent blood flow in diastole. Recently, the trend of treating these pseudoaneurysms with ultrasound-guided compression[172,173] has been replaced by treating them with ultrasound-guided thrombin injection (see Fig. 12-35).[127-130] The neck of the pseudoaneurysm is identified on sonography. A needle is introduced, and a minimal amount of bovine-activated thrombin is injected into the pseudoaneurysm well away from its neck. The pseudoaneurysm is monitored with color Doppler imaging, and thrombosis is confirmed. The procedure is well tolerated and

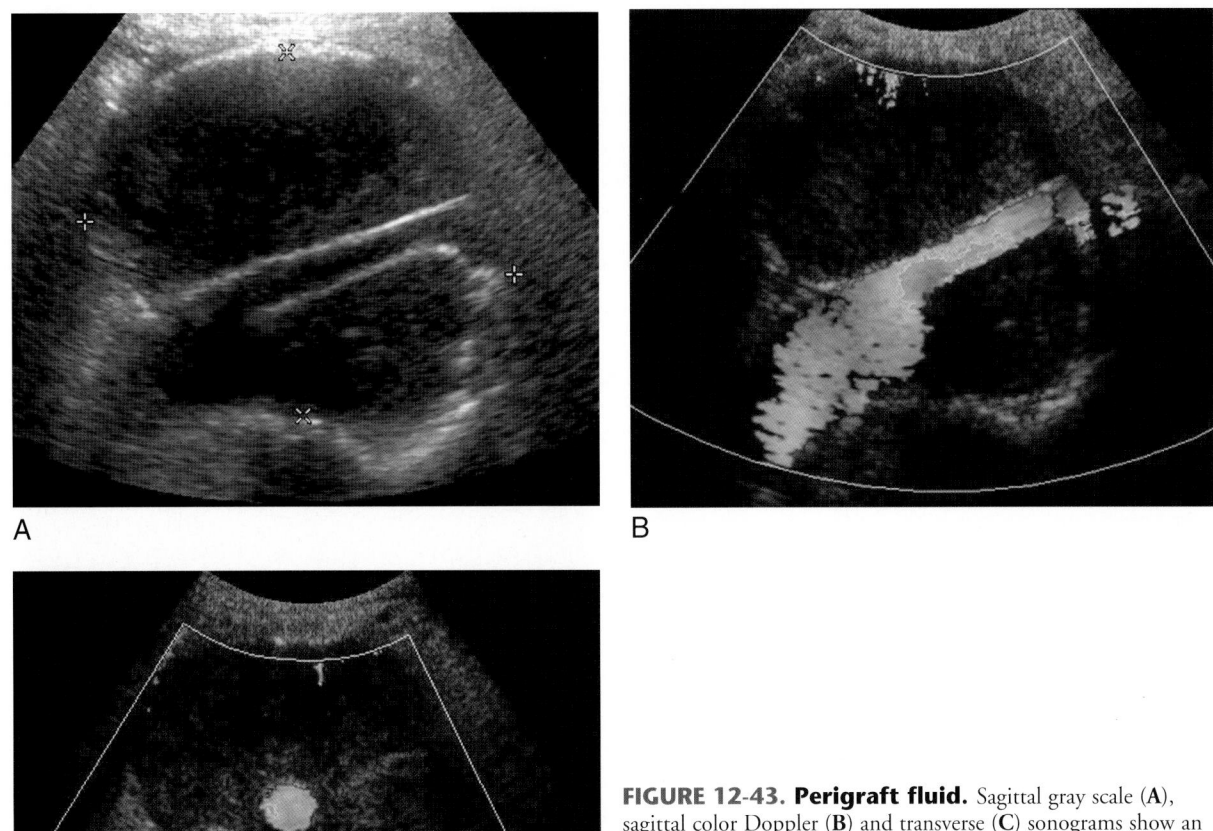

FIGURE 12-43. Perigraft fluid. Sagittal gray scale (**A**), sagittal color Doppler (**B**) and transverse (**C**) sonograms show an aortobifemoral graft surrounded by hypoechoic fluid collection.

works effectively in the majority of patients, although there is a minimal risk of allergic reaction to the thrombin.

Occasionally, post angiography, post surgery, or, spontaneously, an arteriovenous fistula may form. It is also possible for one to arise in association with a tumor. These are not typically suitable for treatment with thrombin injection or direct compression.

Aortic Branches

Celiac/Mesenteric Arteries. Classically, the celiac artery has a high-resistive pattern at its origin, with a small amount of reversed early diastolic flow (see Fig. 12-27). As one goes more distally, it loses the reversed early diastolic flow component, and the hepatic and splenic arteries usually have a low-resistive type of pattern. The celiac artery has continuous forward flow throughout the

cardiac cycle of the low-resistance type. The hepatic artery arises solely from the celiac axis 72% of the time. The SMA gives off the common hepatic artery in 4% of cases, the right hepatic artery in 11% of cases, and the left hepatic artery in 10% of cases. The splenic artery is frequently tortuous, producing spectral broadening without any increase in peak systolic velocity.[119]

The SMA begins about 1 cm caudad to the celiac axis, has a short component that proceeds anteriorly, and then has a long portion that extends inferiorly (see Fig. 12-1B). The flow pattern and the Doppler spectral trace pattern in the SMA vary depending on whether the patient is fasting. In the fasting state, the pattern is of high resistance with a small amount of reversed flow in early diastole. After eating, in a normal person the peak systolic and diastolic velocities increase dramatically. The reversed diastolic flow disappears, a low-resistive pattern develops, and the systolic spectral peaks become

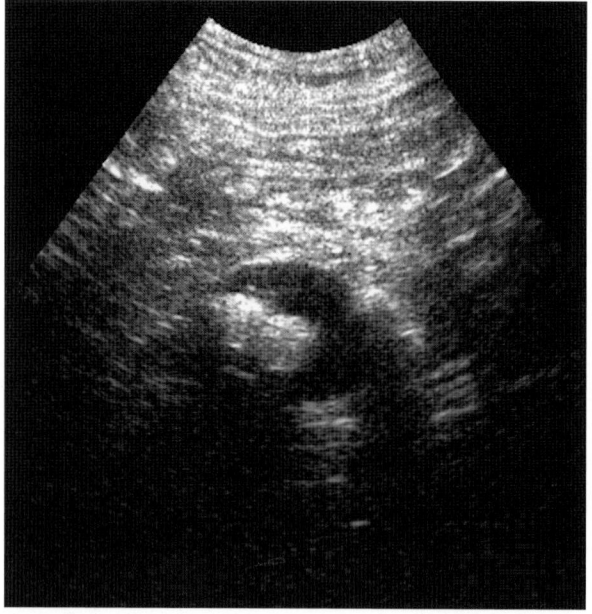

A

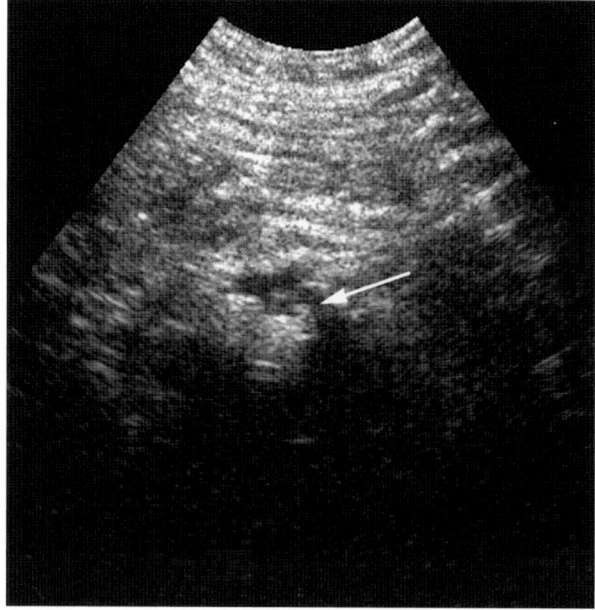

B

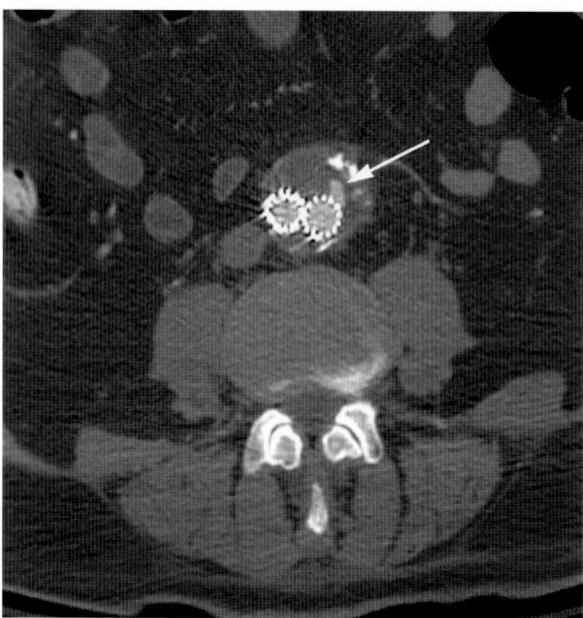

C

FIGURE 12-44. Leak of endoprosthesis at distal end of stent, shown on contrast medium–enhanced sonography (taken with Definity enhancement and pulse inversion imaging). A, Transverse image of the aortic bifurcation shows the two adjacent lumens of the graft limbs with a wraparound that is hypoechoic. The lumen of the graft is filled with contrast agent and appears bright white. **B,** Transverse image taken just caudad to the first image and corresponding with the CT scan shown in **C.** Both **B** and **C** show contrast medium extravasation *(arrows)* outside the lumen of the prosthetic graft. (Courtesy of Marcus Dill-Macky, University of Toronto.)

FIGURE 12-45. Dissection of abdominal aorta. Sagittal (**A**) and transverse (**B**) sonograms show the intimal flap anteriorly separating the true lumen from the false lumen. (Courtesy of Stephanie R. Wilson, MD, University of Toronto.)

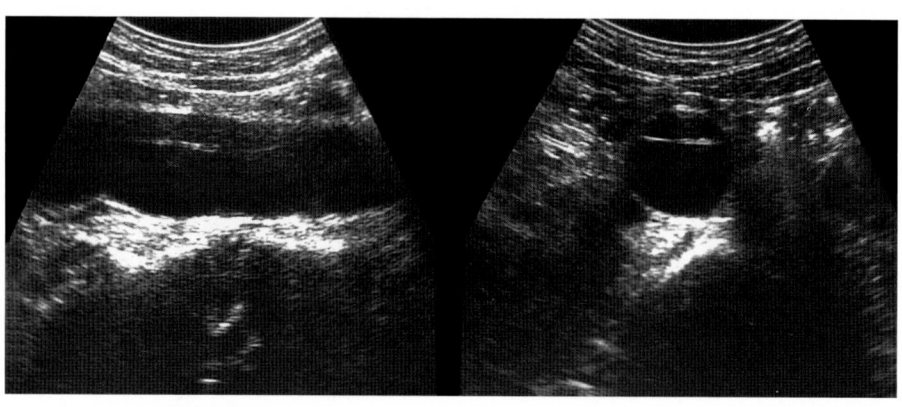

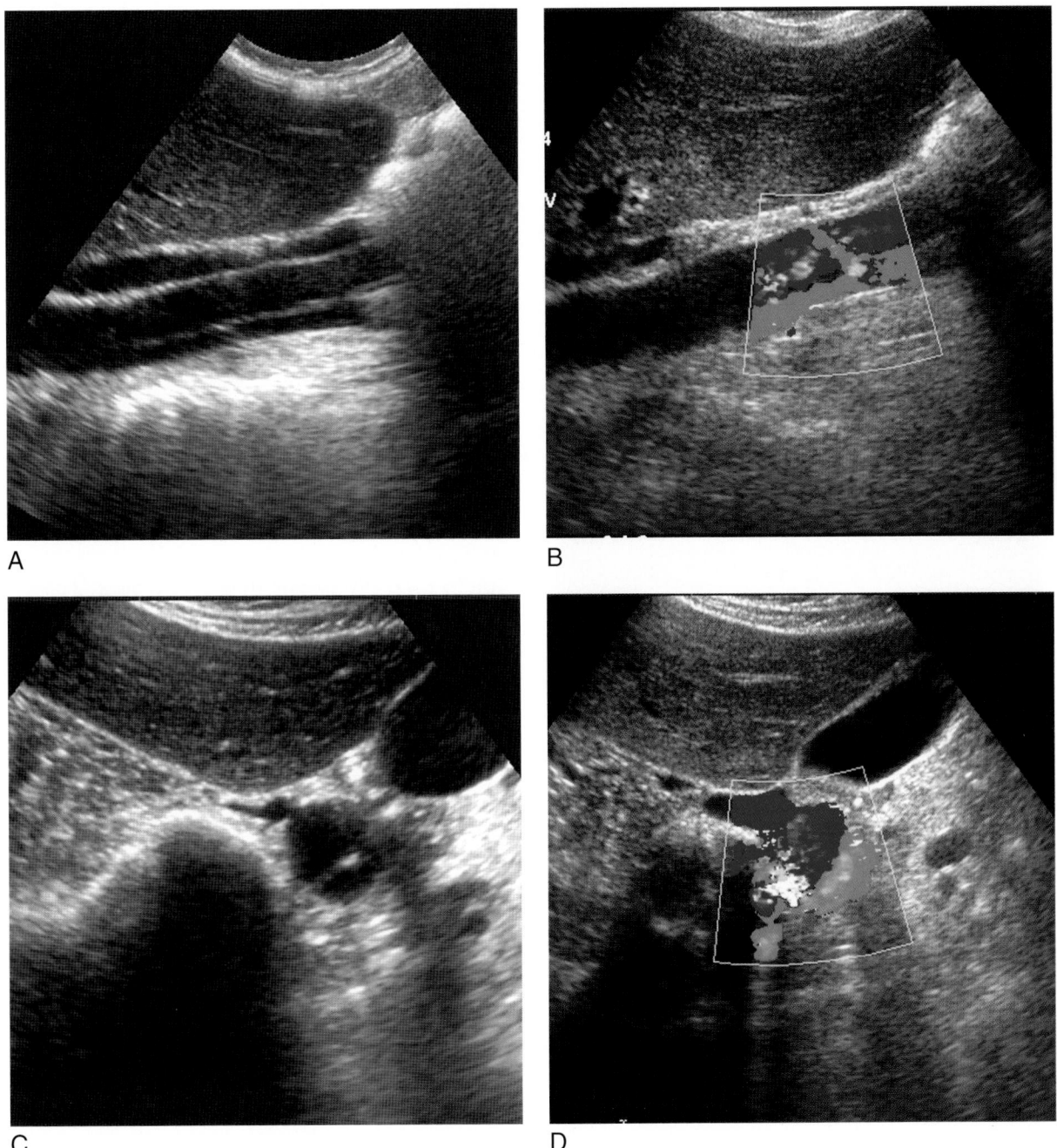

FIGURE 12-46. Aortic dissection. A and **C,** Sagittal and transverse gray-scale images of the aorta. There is a membrane within the lumen of the vessel throughout its length. **B** and **D,** Corresponding color Doppler images show flow on both sides of the membrane. (Courtesy of Stephanie Wilson, MD, University of Toronto.)

broadened. This pattern is most prominent 45 minutes postprandially and is dependent on the type and amount of food ingested.[174]

Intestinal ischemia is a clinical disease with a variety of different symptoms, so it is difficult to diagnose. It is caused by a deficiency of blood delivery to the bowel and usually requires significant narrowing or obstruction of both the celiac axis and the SMA. Although sonography helps with the diagnosis in many cases, the exact sensitivity and specificity of ultrasound are unknown.[174]

Some authors have devised complex protocols to assess the pattern postprandially in greater detail by scanning at standard intervals after standardized meals.[174]

Splanchnic aneurysms may be congenital, atherosclerotic, post-traumatic, mycotic, or inflammatory. About 10% of patents with chronic pancreatitis develop these pseudoaneurysms (see Fig. 12-19), which occur in the hepatic artery, splenic artery, SMA, gastroduodenum, or inferior mesenteric artery. They may be saccular or fusiform and usually have no reverse flow within

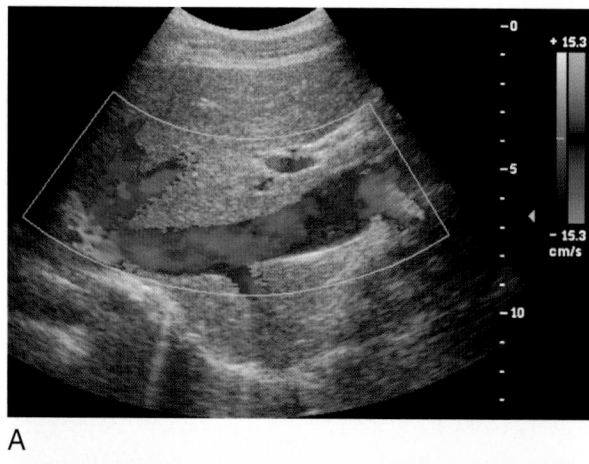

A

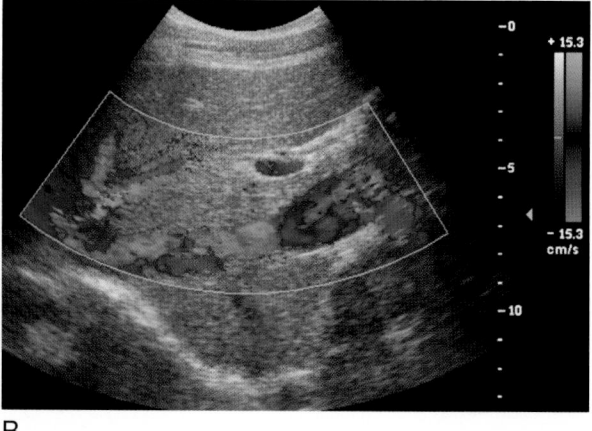

B

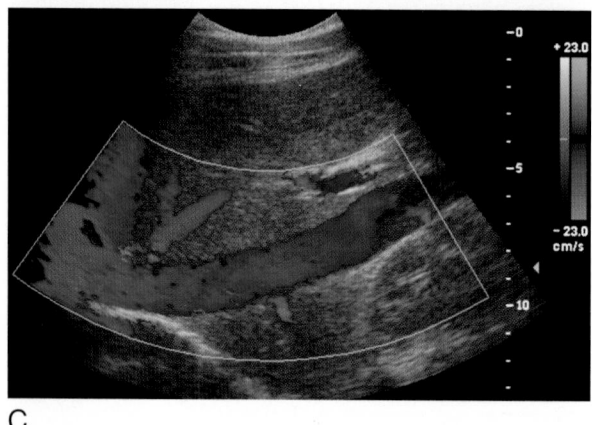

C

FIGURE 12-47. IVC phasic flow. A to **C,** Images show the phasicity of venous blood flow at different phases of the cardiac cycle.

them. They may have layers of thrombus on the walls. They present a significant risk to the interventional radiologist, because they may be mistaken for simple abscesses.[66] It is probably prudent to evaluate with Doppler imaging all collections before drainage.

Renal Arteries. The renal arteries arise within 1.5 cm of the origin of the SMA[113] and can be sonographically identified in 86% of cases (see Figs. 12-6, 12-26, and 12-27).[175] Twenty-two percent of patients have two renal arteries (see Fig. 12-1B), and 2% have three or more.[176] Doppler tracings should be obtained from within the renal artery and also from within the kidney. The Doppler tracings are typically of a low-resistance type, with the peak systolic and diastolic readings decreasing as one goes farther into the kidney.[119]

Renal Artery Stenosis. Renal artery stenosis produces a rare (2%) but treatable cause of hypertension and may be due to atherosclerotic disease or fibromuscular hyperplasia, a rare disease typically affecting young women.[177] Whereas both are treatable with angioplasty, the latter has a much better prognosis.

Renal Aneurysms and Arteriovenous Fistula. Most of these are acquired problems and may be post-traumatic or post large-bore needle biopsy. The aneurysms are usually pseudoaneurysms and sonographically. They resemble those that arise from the external iliac artery or the common femoral artery. One fourth of arteriovenous fistulas are congenital, and less than 5% result from malignancy. On sonography, they usually produce a mosaic of color in the kidney.

Inferior Vena Cava

Anatomy

The inferior vena cava (see Fig. 12-47) is a large vein that returns blood from the lower limbs, pelvis, and abdomen to the right atrium. It is formed by the paired common iliac veins on the anterior surface of the L5 vertebral body and lies anteriorly and slightly to the right of the spine.[39] It traverses the diaphragm and enters the right atrium at the level of the eighth thoracic vertebra. Its main branches are the hepatic veins, the renal veins, and the common iliac veins.[39] The walls of the IVC are much thinner than those of the aorta, and the pressure of blood it deals with is also much lower.

Sonography

The intrahepatic portion of the IVC is routinely viewed by using the liver as an acoustic window (Fig. 12-48; see also Fig. 12-47). The remainder of the vessel is

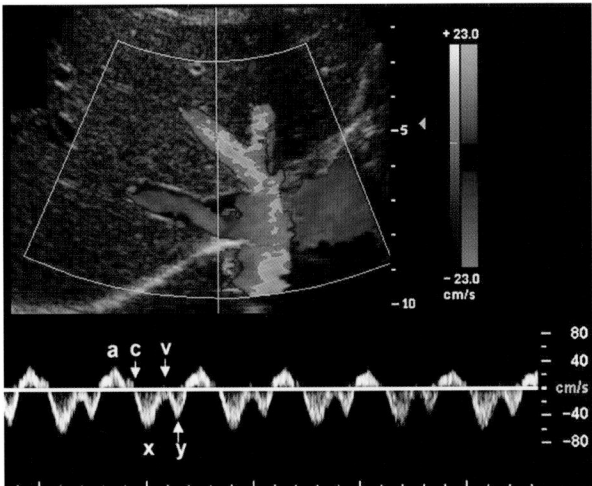

FIGURE 12-48. Hepatic vein phasic Doppler flow.
This Doppler tracing shows the classic waveform seen in the hepatic veins and the inferior vena cava. Within the venous Doppler waveform, "a" represents atrial contraction or systole, "x descent" corresponds with atrial relaxation, "c" is a small positive deflection caused by the start of right ventricular contraction, "v" corresponds with rapid atrial filling post ventricular systole, and "y" is rapid emptying of the atria into the ventricles after atrioventricular valves open.

inconsistently seen because it is intermittently flat and oval and may be obscured by overlying bowel gas and pannus. Common iliac veins and external iliac veins are seen inconsistently with their corresponding arteries on the lateral aspect of the pelvic brim. The IVC lumen is usually anechoic, although with slow-flowing blood it becomes more echogenic and may show swirling. This is seen with right-sided heart failure, fluid overload, and caudad to an IVC obstruction. The appearance varies with respiration. With deep inspiration, venous return decreases and the IVC dilates. With deep expiration, venous return improves and the IVC diameter decreases. When performing a Valsalva maneuver, venous return is blocked and flow temporarily reversed in the IVC, causing it to bulge. The IVC transmits both cardiac and respiratory pulsations; the transmissions are more noticeable sonographically the closer one comes to the heart (see Figs. 12-47 and 12-48). The classic tracing has a sawtooth pattern similar to what is described in detail below for the hepatic veins. Most distally and in the common iliac veins there is a more phasic pattern similar to the pattern in the proximal limbs.

Pathology

Congenital Abnormalities. Most abnormalities occur at or below the level of the renal veins.[178] The IVC, azygos, and hemiazygos vessels form in the embryo from the paired cardinal veins. The most frequent congenital anomalies are duplication (0.2% to 3%) and transposition (0.2% to 0.5%) (Fig. 12-49).[119] Both of these form a normal vein at the level of the renal hilum. Interruption of the IVC by azygos or hemiazygos continuation is caused by the failure of the hepatic veins to form, which occurs in about 0.6% of cases.[119] In these

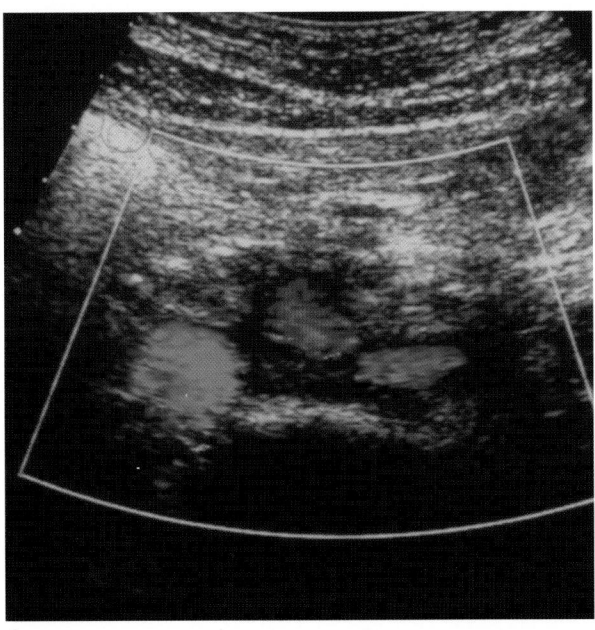

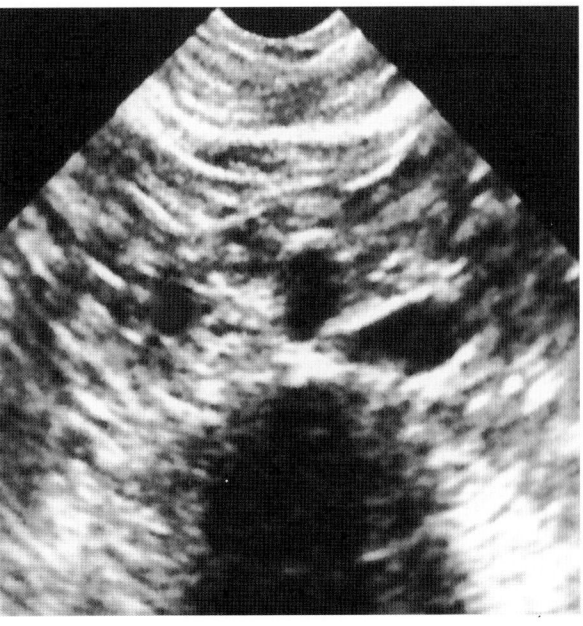

A   B

FIGURE 12-49. A, Transverse lower abdominal scan shows a left-sided inferior vena cava (IVC) adjacent to the aorta in addition to a normal right-sided IVC. **B,** Transverse scan just above umbilicus shows normal round aorta on the right and more flattened IVC on the left. (Courtesy of Stephanie R. Wilson, MD, University of Toronto.)

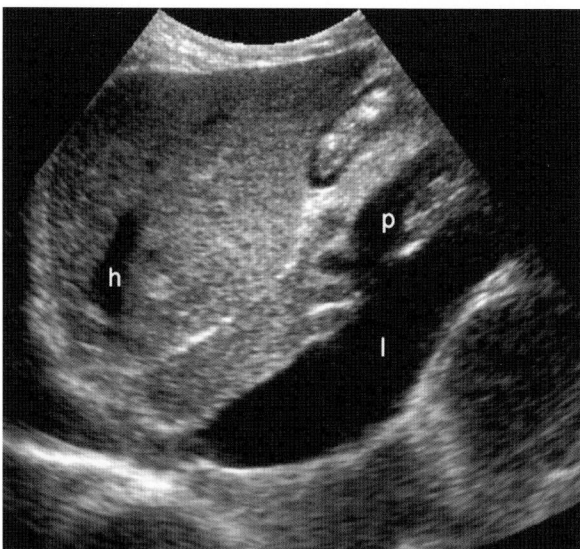

FIGURE 12-50. Portacaval shunt. The portal vein (p) has been surgically anastomosed to the inferior vena cava (I), which is widened cranial to this. One of the hepatic veins (h) is also shown.

instances the hepatic veins drain directly into the right atrium. These IVC anomalies are often associated with other cardiac malformations.

Acquired Abnormalities. Portosystemic shunts are sometimes fashioned to decrease portal venous pressure (Fig. 12-50) in patients with portal hypertension.

Thrombosis. The most commonly encountered intraluminal anomaly of the IVC is thrombus, which usually spreads from another vein in the pelvis, lower limb, liver, or kidney. IVC thrombosis is sonographically diagnosed as an intraluminal filling defect that usually expands the diameter of the vessel (Fig. 12-51). The echogenicity of a thrombus depends on its age; chronic thrombi may calcify. If a thrombus is hypoechoic or isoechoic with the liver, color Doppler imaging is very helpful in making the diagnosis, because color frequently surrounds the thrombus.

Spectral Doppler analysis produces no signal from uncomplicated thrombus. An arterial-type tracing may be seen within tumor thrombi. In obese patients, B-mode artifact may produce a pseudolesion on the images. In these patients, color Doppler analysis is very helpful in confirming vessel patency.

The presence of IVC tumor thrombus is usually diagnosed readily. The kidney is the most likely site of origin.

A variety of vena caval filters are now being inserted in the IVC to prevent distal venous thrombi from going on to pulmonary embolism (Fig. 12-52). Ultrasound can sometimes see these as echogenic structures within the IVC and can also monitor complications that may occur at their site of insertion.[179]

Mural Lesions/IVC Rupture. Mural-based lesions include adherent thrombus and tumor. Primary tumors are rare, but, of them, the leiomyosarcoma is the most common. Leiomyosarcoma of the wall of the IVC is the most common type and location of mural tumor in the venous system (60%).[60,180-183] It occurs most commonly in older women, and surgery is the treatment of choice. The location and extent of the disease determine the resectability of the lesion, so every effort should be made to document it accurately.[184] Metastatic lesions include direct spread from lymphoma, hepatocellular carcinoma, breast, and renal cell carcinoma. Mural IVC lesions can exert mass effect and affect structures like the ureter (retrocaval ureter), or the lesions can spread into IVC branches, such as the renal veins and the hepatic veins.

IVC rupture usually follows severe abdominal trauma or surgical or interventional therapy. It frequently results in large retroperitoneal hemorrhages, and it is associated with damage to other structures from the same preceding cause.

Cardiac Failure/Fluid Overload. Cardiac failure and fluid overload increase the diameter of the IVC and hepatic veins and exaggerate the normal Doppler flow pattern.

Inferior Vena Cava Branches and Tributaries

Renal Veins. The right renal vein is very short, whereas the left renal vein has a much longer course as it travels between the aorta and the SMA to reach the IVC (see Fig. 12-6B). Both are usually best scanned on the transverse plane.[176,185] The renal veins (especially the left) frequently collect blood from varices in patients with portal hypertension.

Circumaortic veins are rare. The left renal vein retroaortic variant, which occurs in about 2% of patients, is of great importance when contemplating surgery.[185]

Renal veins may be displaced and compromised by retroperitoneal hemorrhage, aortic aneurysms, tumors, and aberrant vessels. Malignant extension into the renal veins can occur in renal cell carcinoma, renal lymphoma, transitional cell carcinoma, Wilms' tumor, and adrenal carcinoma.[186]

Renal vein thrombosis is associated with acute glomerulonephritis, lupus, amyloidosis, hypercoagulable states, sepsis, trauma, and dehydration.[186] Of those who have undergone renal transplants, 1% develop this problem. On sonography, one may see dilation of the vein proximal to the occlusion. The kidney enlarges, and there is decreased echogenicity secondary to edema in the kidney.[187] In the neonate, chronic cases may go on to calcify.[188,189] Doppler study shows no renal vein flow and a high-resistive arterial pattern.

Hepatic Veins. There are usually three hepatic veins, which lie between the hepatic segments and drain

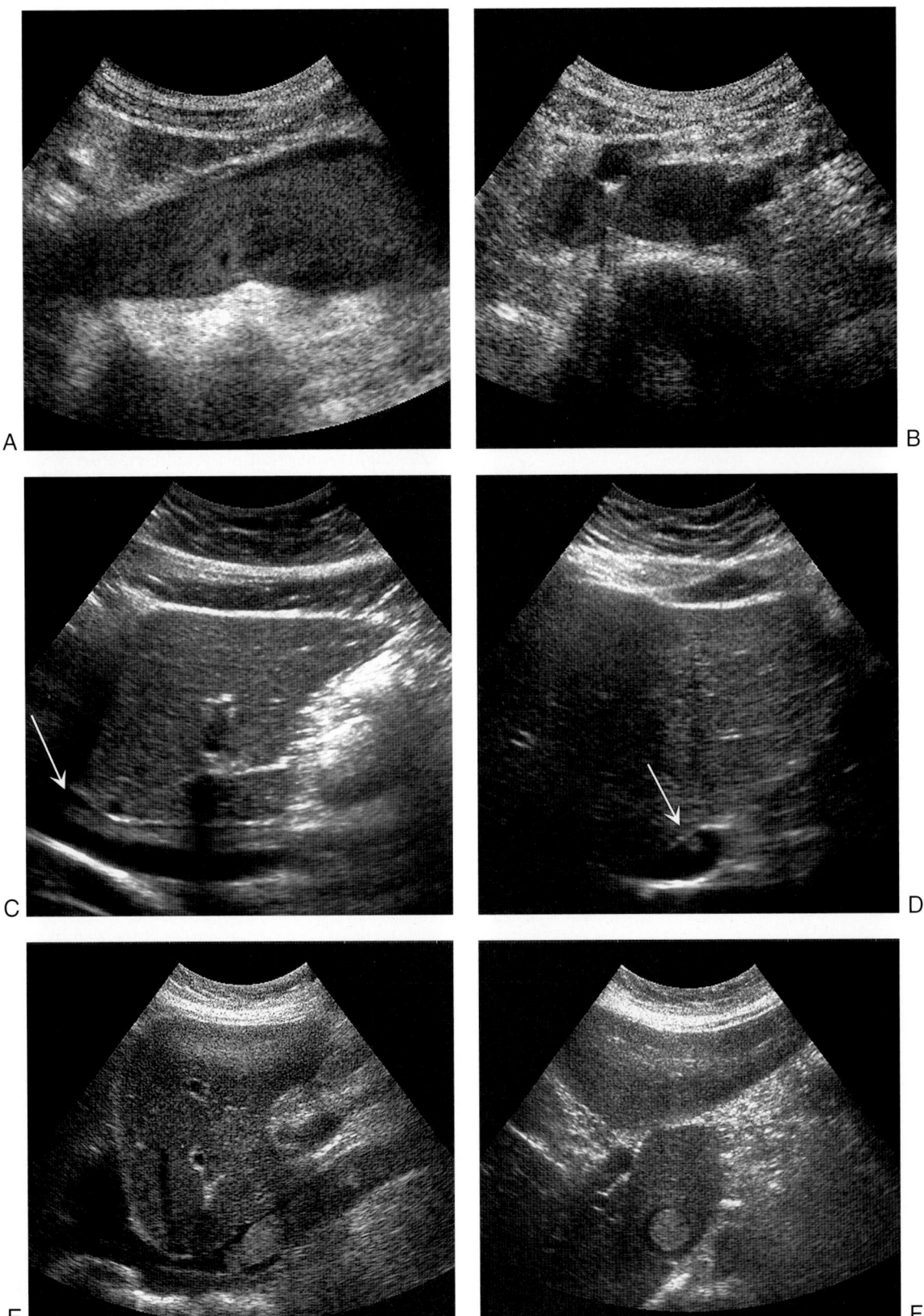

FIGURE 12-51. Inferior vena cava thrombus in three patients. Left images are sagittal and right images are corresponding transverse images. **A** and **B,** Long, thin nonocclusive thrombus. **C** and **D,** Larger nonocclusive thrombus *(arrows).* **E** and **F,** Large expansive occlusive thrombus. The transverse image in **F** is taken at the confluence of the right and left iliac veins, which are both large and echogenic compared with the normal right and left iliac arteries. (Courtesy of Stephanie Wilson, MD, University of Toronto.)

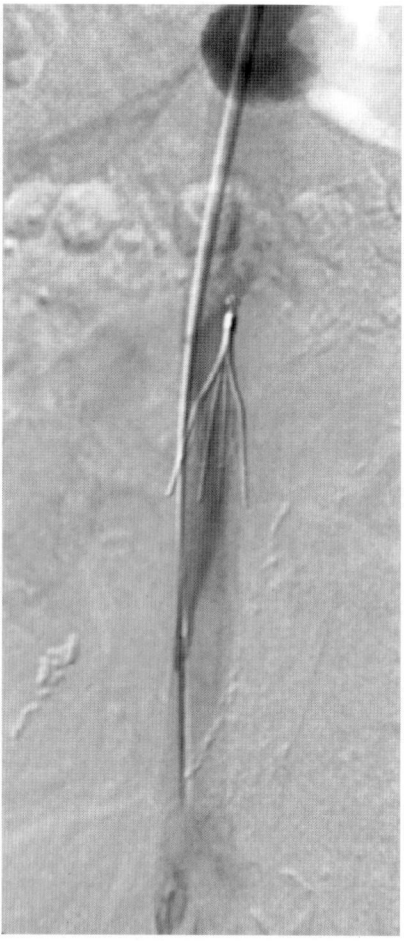

FIGURE 12-52. Inferior vena cava filter. Digital subtraction venogram shows an inferior vena cava filter in position.

posteriorly into the IVC close to the diaphragm (see Fig. 12-48). In most people the middle and left hepatic veins fuse just before joining the IVC,[190] and other congenital variants are possible but infrequently recognized sonographically.[190] Hepatic vein Doppler spectral tracings are usually triphasic and pulsatile, reflecting transmitted cardiac pulsations (see Fig. 12-48). This pattern is abolished in about 20% of cases of cirrhosis and portal hypertension, and it is exaggerated in right-sided heart failure.[137]

Iliac/ovarian Veins. The common and external iliac veins run with the adjacent arteries (see Fig. 12-3C). They are predominantly medial and anterior at the inguinal ligament, and they become posterior and lateral to the accompanying arteries close to the IVC. They have a respiratory phasicity and can be compressed by adjacent structures and pathology, including lymphoceles, hematoma, transplant kidneys, abscess, and aneurysm. They collapse with a Valsalva maneuver because of their intra-abdominal position but increase in diameter after augmentation by a squeezing of the leg or by elevation.[191] It occurs most often on the right side, and sonographic detection should include evaluation of the expected entry of the vein directly into the IVC.

Ovarian vein thrombosis (Fig. 12-53) usually occurs postpartum and is associated with endometritis and surgery. Sonography frequently shows massive enlargement of all or part of the ovarian vein, often with an echogenic thrombus within.[191] It usually occurs on the right side. Sonographic detection should include evaluation of the expected entry of the vein directly into the IVC.

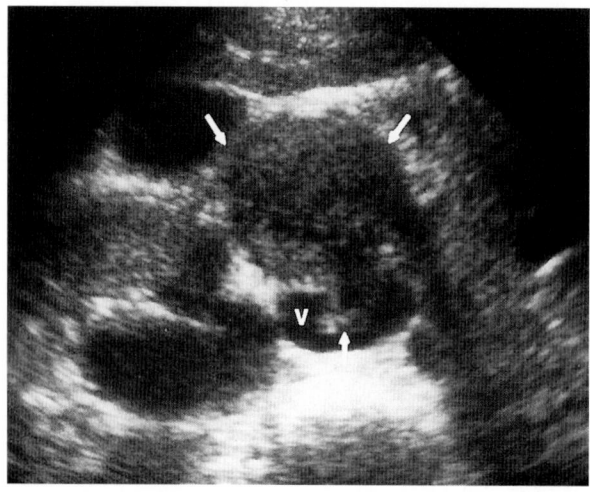

A

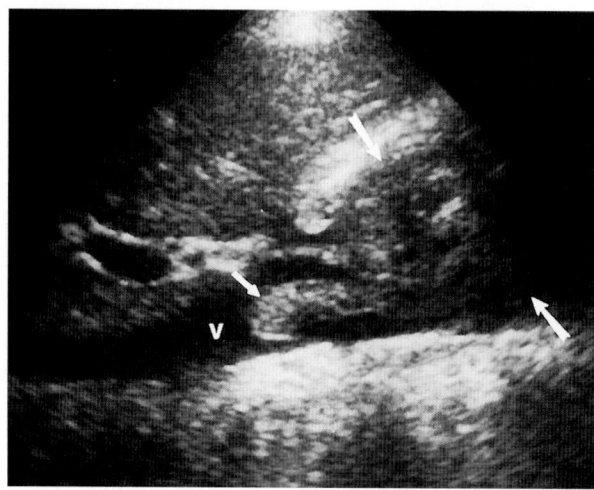

B

FIGURE 12-53. Ovarian vein thrombosis. A tubular hypoechoic, inhomogeneous mass was seen arising out of the pelvis in a patient after cesarean delivery. Transverse (**A**) and longitudinal (**B**) sonograms show the superior extent of this large thrombus *(arrows)* that extends into the inferior vena cava (v) from its anterior aspect.

References

1. Lev-Toaff AS, Langer JE, Rubin DL, et al: Safety and efficacy of a new oral contrast agent for sonography: A phase II trial. AJR Am J Roentgenol 1999;173:431-436.
2. Blaivas M, DeBehnke S, Sierzenski PR, et al: Tissue harmonic imaging improves organ visualization in trauma ultrasound when compared with standard ultrasound mode. Acad Emerg Med 2002;9:48-53.
3. Choudhry S, Gorman B, Charboneau JW, et al: Comparison of tissue harmonic imaging with conventional US in abdominal disease. Radiographics 2000; 20:1127-1135.
4. Desser TS, Jeffrey RB Jr, Lane MJ, et al: Tissue harmonic imaging: Utility in abdominal and pelvic sonography. J Clin Ultrasound 1999;27:135-142.
5. Ortega D, Burns PN, Hope Simpson D, et al: Tissue harmonic imaging: Is it a benefit for bile duct sonography? AJR Am J Roentgenol 2001;176:653-659.
6. Yucel C, Ozdemir H, Asik E, et al: Benefits of tissue harmonic imaging in the evaluation of abdominal and pelvic lesions. Abdom Imaging 2003;28:103-109.
7. Entrekin RR, Porter BA, Sillesen HH, et al: Real-time spatial compound imaging: Application to breast, vascular, and musculoskeletal ultrasound. Semin Ultrasound CT MRI 2001;22:50-64.
8. Puylaert JB: Acute appendicitis: US evaluation using graded compression. Radiology 1986;158:355-360.
9. Creagh-Barry M, Adam EJ, Joseph AE: The value of oblique scans in the ultrasonic examination of the abdominal aorta. Clin Radiol 1986;37:239-241.
10. Luck AJ, Maddern GJ: Intraoperative abdominal ultrasonography. Br J Surg 1999;86:5-16.
11. Bezzi M, Silecchia G, De Leo A, et al: Laparoscopic and intraoperative ultrasound. Eur J Radiol 1998;27(Suppl 2):S207-S214.
12. Kolecki R, Schirmer B: Intraoperative and laparoscopic ultrasound. Surg Clin North Am 1998;78:251-271.
13. Matin SF, Gill IS: Laparoscopic ultrasonography. J Endourol 2001;15:87-92.
14. Dibenedetto LM, Lei Q, Gilroy AM, et al: Variations in the inferior pelvic pathway of the lateral femoral cutaneous nerve: Implications for laparoscopic hernia repair. Clin Anat 1996;9:232-236.
15. Hsu TH, Su LM, Ong A: Anterior extraperitoneal approach to laparoscopic retroperitoneal lymph node dissection: A novel technique. J Urol 2003;169:258-260.
16. Ogan K, Lotan Y, Koeneman K, et al: Laparoscopic versus open retroperitoneal lymph node dissection: A cost analysis. J Urol 2002;168:1945-1949; discussion 1949.
17. Meyers M: The extraperitoneal spaces: Normal and pathologic anatomy. In Meyers M (ed): Dynamic Radiology of the Abdomen: Normal and Pathologic Anatomy, 5th ed. New York, Springer-Verlag, 2000, pp 219-342.
18. Davidson AJ: The retroperitoneum. In Davidson AJ (ed): Radiology of the Kidney. Philadelphia, WB Saunders, 1994, pp 671-714.
19. Davidson AJ, Hartman DS: Imaging strategies for tumors of the kidney, adrenal gland, and retroperitoneum. CA Cancer J Clin 1987;37:151-164.
20. Dunnick NR, Sandler CM, Newhouse JH, et al: Anatomy and Embryology: Textbook of Uroradiology, 3rd ed. Philadelphia, Lippincott Williams & Wilkins, 2001, pp 1-14.
21. Aizenstein RI, Owens C, Sabnis S, et al: The perinephric space and renal fascia: Review of normal anatomy, pathology, and pathways of disease spread. Crit Rev Diagn Imaging 1997;38:325-367.
22. Auh YH, Rubenstein WA, Schneider M, et al: Extraperitoneal paravesical spaces: CT delineation with US correlation. Radiology 1986;159:319-328.
23. Bechtold RE, Dyer RB, Zagoria RJ, et al: The perirenal space: Relationship of pathologic processes to normal retroperitoneal anatomy. Radiographics 1996;16:841-854.
24. Chesbrough RM, Burkhard TK, Martinez AJ, et al: Gerota versus Zuckerkandl: The renal fascia revisited. Radiology 1989;173:845-846.
25. Dodds WJ, Darweesh RM, Lawson TL, et al: The retroperitoneal spaces revisited. AJR Am J Roentgenol 1986;147:1155-1161.
26. Hureau J, Pradel J, Agossou-Voyeme AK, et al: The posterior interparieto-peritoneal or retroperitoneal spaces: II. Pathological x-ray computed tomographic image. J Radiol (French) 1991;72:205-227.
27. Korobkin M, Silverman PM, Quint LE, et al: CT of the extraperitoneal space: Normal anatomy and fluid collections. AJR Am J Roentgenol 1992;159:933-942.
28. Lim JH, Kim B, Auh YH: Anatomical communications of the perirenal space. Br J Radiol 1998;71:450-456.
29. Mindell HJ, Mastromatteo JF, Dickey KW, et al: Anatomic communications between the three retroperitoneal spaces: Determination by CT-guided injections of contrast material in cadavers. AJR Am J Roentgenol 1995;164:1173-1178.
30. Raptopoulos V, Lei OF, Touliopoulos P, et al: Why perirenal disease does not extend into the pelvis: The importance of closure of the cone of the renal fasciae. AJR Am J Roentgenol 1995;164:1179-1184.
31. Raptopoulos V, Touliopoulos P, Lei QF, et al: Medial border of the perirenal space: CT and anatomic correlation. Radiology 1997;205:777-784.
32. Rubenstein WA, Whalen JP: Extraperitoneal spaces. AJR Am J Roentgenol 1986;147:1162-1164.
33. Snady H: Vascular anatomy: How to identify the major retroperitoneal vessels. Gastrointest Endosc Clin North Am 1995;5:497-506.
34. Szolar DH, Uggowitzer MM, Kammerhuber FH, et al: [Benign non–organ-related diseases of the retroperitoneal space]. Rofo Fortschr Geb Rontgenstr Neuen Bildgeb Verfahr 1997;167:107-121.
35. Thornton FJ, Kandiah SS, Monkhouse WS, et al: Helical CT evaluation of the perirenal space and its boundaries: A cadaveric study. Radiology 2001;218:659-663.
36. Gore RM, Balfe DM, Aizenstein RI, et al: The great escape: Interfascial decompression planes of the retroperitoneum. AJR Am J Roentgenol 2000;175:363-370.
37. Simons GW, Sty JR, Starshak RJ: Retroperitoneal and retrofascial abscesses: A review. J Bone Joint Surg Am 1983;65:1041-1058.
38. Callen PW, Filly RA, Marks WM: The quadratus lumborum muscle: A possible source of confusion in sonographic evaluation of the retroperitoneum. J Clin Ultrasound 1979;7:349-352.
39. Gray H: Gray's Anatomy, 31st ed. London, Longmans, 1954, pp 589-590.
40. Callen PW, Filly RA, Sarti DA, et al: Ultrasonography of the diaphragmatic crura. Radiology 1979;130:721-724.
41. Yeh HC, Halton KP, Gray CE: Anatomic variations and abnormalities in the diaphragm seen with US. Radiographics 1990;10:1019-1030.
42. Crespi G, Zappasodi F, Cicio G, et al: Ultrasonography features of the diaphragmatic crura: Normal anatomy and its variants. Radiol Med (Torino) 2000;99:426-431.

43. King AD, Hine AL, McDonald C, et al: The ultrasound appearance of the normal psoas muscle. Clin Radiol 1993;48:316-318.

44. Derchi LE, Solbiati L, Rizzatto G, et al: Normal anatomy and pathologic changes of the small bowel mesentery: US appearance. Radiology 1987;164:649-652.

45. Filly RA, Marglin S, Castellino RA: The ultrasonographic spectrum of abdominal and pelvic Hodgkin's disease and non-Hodgkin's lymphoma. Cancer 1976;38:2143-2148.

46. Nishino M, Hayakawa K, Minami M, et al: Primary retroperitoneal neoplasms: CT and MR imaging findings with anatomic and pathologic diagnostic clues. Radiographics 2003;23:45-57.

47. Jing BS: Diagnostic imaging of abdominal and pelvic lymph nodes in lymphoma. Radiol Clin North Am 1990;28:801-831.

48. Castellino RA: The non-Hodgkin lymphomas: Practical concepts for the diagnostic radiologist. Radiology 1991;178:315-321.

49. Vassallo P, Wernecke K, Roos N, et al: Differentiation of benign from malignant superficial lymphadenopathy: The role of high-resolution US. Radiology 1992;183:215-220.

50. Tschammler A, Wirkner H, Ott G, et al: Vascular patterns in reactive and malignant lymphadenopathy. Eur Radiol 1996;6:473-480.

51. Nobrega J, Dos Santos G: Aspirative cytology with fine-needle in the abdomen, retroperitoneum and pelvic cavity: A seven year experience of the Portuguese Institute of Oncology, Center of Porto. Eur J Surg Oncol 1994; 20:37-42.

52. Al-Mofleh IA: Ultrasound-guided fine needle aspiration of retroperitoneal, abdominal and pelvic lymph nodes: Diagnostic reliability. Acta Cytol 1992;36:413-415.

53. Downey DB, Wilson SR: Ultrasonographically guided biopsy of small intra-abdominal masses. Can Assoc Radiol J 1993;44:350-353.

54. Castellino RA, Billingham M, Dorfman RF: Lymphographic accuracy in Hodgkin's disease and malignant lymphoma with a note on the "reactive" lymph node as a cause of most false-positive lymphograms. Invest Radiol 1990;25:412-422.

55. Hillman BJ, Haber K: Echographic characteristics of malignant lymph nodes. J Clin Ultrasound 1980;8:213-215.

56. Bussar-Maatz R, Weissbach L: Retroperitoneal lymph node staging of testicular tumours. TNM Study Group. Br J Urol 1993;72:234-240.

57. Bohle A, Studer UE, Sonntag RW, et al: Primary or secondary extragonadal germ cell tumors? J Urol 1986;135:939-943.

58. Choyke PL, Hayes WS, Sesterhenn IA: Primary extragonadal germ cell tumors of the retroperitoneum: Differentiation of primary and secondary tumors. Radiographics 1993;13:1365-1375; quiz 1377-1378.

59. Davidson AJ, Hartman DS, Goldman SM: Mature teratoma of the retroperitoneum: Radiologic, pathologic, and clinical correlation. Radiology 1989;172:421-425.

60. Hartman DS, Hayes WS, Choyke PL, et al: From the archives of the AFIP. Leiomyosarcoma of the retroperitoneum and inferior vena cava: Radiologic-pathologic correlation. Radiographics 1992; 12:1203-1220.

61. Dalton RR, Donohue JH, Mucha P Jr, et al: Management of retroperitoneal sarcomas. Surgery 1989;106:725-732; discussion 732-733.

62. Solla JA, Reed K: Primary retroperitoneal sarcomas. Am J Surg 1986;152:496-498.

63. Koci TM, Worthen NJ, Phillips JJ, et al: Perirenal hemangioendothelioma in a newborn: Sonograph and MR findings. J Comput Assist Tomogr 1989;13:145-147.

64. Goldman SM, Davidson AJ, Neal J: Retroperitoneal and pelvic hemangiopericytomas: Clinical, radiologic, and pathologic correlation. Radiology 1988;168:13-17.

65. Sigel B, Feleppa EJ, Swami V, et al: Ultrasonic tissue characterization of blood clots. Surg Clin North Am 1990;70:13-29.

66. Lee MJ, Saini S, Geller SC, et al: Pancreatitis with pseudoaneurysm formation: A pitfall for the interventional radiologist. AJR 1991;156:97-98.

67. Baker LR, Mallinson WJ, Gregory MC, et al: Idiopathic retroperitoneal fibrosis: A retrospective analysis of 60 cases. Br J Urol 1987;60:497-503.

68. Degesys GE, Dunnick NR, Silverman PM, et al: Retroperitoneal fibrosis: Use of CT in distinguishing among possible causes. AJR Am J Roentgenol 1986;146:57-60.

69. Sanders RC, Duffy T, McLoughlin MG, et al: Sonography in the diagnosis of retroperitoneal fibrosis. J Urol 1977;118:944-946.

70. Fagan CJ, Larrieu AJ, Amparo EG: Retroperitoneal fibrosis: Ultrasound and CT features. AJR Am J Roentgenol 1979;133:239-243.

71. Fitzgerald EJ, Blackett RL: "Inflammatory" abdominal aortic aneurysms. Clin Radiol 1988;39:247-451.

72. Cullenward MJ, Scanlan KA, Pozniak MA, et al: Inflammatory aortic aneurysm (periaortic fibrosis): Radiologic imaging. Radiology 1986;159:75-82.

73. Lodge JP, Hall R: Retroperitoneal haemorrhage: A dangerous complication of common femoral arterial puncture. Eur J Vasc Surg 1993;7:355-357.

74. Kedar RP, Cosgrove DO: Case report: Retroperitoneal varices mimicking a mass: Diagnosis on color Doppler. Br J Radiol 1994;67:661-662.

75. Graif M, Martinovitz U, Strauss S, et al: Sonographic localization of hematomas in hemophilic patients with positive iliopsoas sign. AJR Am J Roentgenol 1987; 148:121-123.

76. Spring DB, Schroeder D, Babu S, et al: Ultrasonic evaluation of lymphocele formation after staging lymphadenectomy for prostatic carcinoma. Radiology 1981;141:479-483.

77. Akhan O, Cekirge S, Ozmen M, et al: Percutaneous transcatheter ethanol sclerotherapy of postoperative pelvic lymphoceles. Cardiovasc Intervent Radiol 1992; 15:224-227.

78. Oyen O, Siwach V, Line PD, et al: Improvement of post-transplant lymphocele treatment in the laparoscopic era. Transpl Int 2002;15:406-410.

79. Lee YT, Lee CM, Su SC, et al: Psoas abscess: A 10-year review. J Microbiol Immunol Infect 1999;32:40-46.

80. De Jesus Lopes Filho G, Matone J, Arasaki CH, et al: Psoas abscess: Diagnostic and therapeutic considerations in six patients. Int Surg 2000;85:339-343.

81. Dib M, Bedu A, Garel C, et al: Iliopsoas abscess in neonates: Treatment by ultrasound-guided percutaneous drainage. Pediatr Radiol 2000;30:677-680.

82. Derchi Le, Rizzatto G, Banderali A, et al: Sonographic appearance of primary retroperitoneal cysts. J Ultrasound Med 1989;8:381-384.

83. Davidson AJ, Hartman DS: Lymphangioma of the retroperitoneum: CT and sonographic characteristic. Radiology 1990;175:507-510.

84. Iyer R, Eftekhari F, Varma D, et al: Cystic retroperitoneal lymphangioma: CT, ultrasound and MR findings. Pediatr Radiol 1993;23:305-306.

85. Breidahl WH, Mendelson RM: Retroperitoneal lymphangioma. Australas Radiol 1995;39:187-191.
86. De Lange EE, Black WC, Mills SE: Radiologic features of retroperitoneal cystic hamartoma. Gastrointest Radiol 1988;13:266-270.
87. Sussman SK, Jacobs JE, Glickstein MF, et al: Cross-sectional imaging of idiopathic solitary renal vein varix: Report of two cases. Urol Radiol 1991;13:98-102.
88. Kim JK, Jeong YY, Kim YH, et al: Postoperative pelvic lymphocele: Treatment with simple percutaneous catheter drainage. Radiology 1999;212:390-394.
89. Duepree HJ, Fornara P, Lewejohann JC, et al: Laparoscopic treatment of lymphoceles in patients after renal transplantation. Clin Transplant 2001; 15:375-379.
90. Secin FP, Rovegno AR, Marrugat RE, et al: Value of gray scale ultrasonography in the early diagnosis of urologic complications of renal transplantation. Arch Esp Urol (Spanish) 2002;55:395-404.
91. Rifkin MD, Needleman L, Kurtz AB, et al: Sonography of nongynecologic cystic masses of the pelvis. AJR Am J Roentgenol 1984;142:1169-1174.
92. Dunnick NR: Genitourinary trauma. In McClennan BL (ed): A Categorical Course in Genitourinary Radiology. Oak Brook, Radiological Society of North America, 1994, pp 95-102.
93. Jeffrey RB Jr, Laing FC, Wing VW: Extrapancreatic spread of acute pancreatitis: New observations with real-time US. Radiology 1986;159:707-711.
94. Graham M, Chan A: Ultrasound screening for clinically occult abdominal aortic aneurysm. Can Med Assoc J 1988;138:627-629.
95. Castoldi MC, Del Moro RM, D'urbano ML, et al: Sonography after renal biopsy: Assessment of its role in 230 consecutive cases. Abdom Imaging 1994;19:72-77.
96. Lumsden AB, Miller JM, Kosinski AS, et al: A prospective evaluation of surgically treated groin complications following percutaneous cardiac procedures. Am Surg 1994;60:132-137.
97. Papanicolaou N, Stafford SA, Pfister RC, et al: Significant renal hemorrhage following extracorporeal shock wave lithotripsy: Imaging and clinical features. Radiology 1987;163:661-664.
98. Belville JS, Morgentaler A, Loughlin KR, et al: Spontaneous perinephric and subcapsular renal hemorrhage: Evaluation with CT, US, and angiography. Radiology 1989;172:733-738.
99. Tomaru T, Uchida Y, Masuo M, et al: Experimental canine arterial thrombus formation and thrombolysis: A fiberoptic study. Am Heart J 1987;114:63-69.
100. Kenney PJ: Chronic renal infections. In McClennan BL (ed): Syllabus: A categorical course in genitourinary radiology. Oak Brook, Radiological Society of North America, 1994, pp 51-54.
101. Hayes WS, Hartman DS, Sesterbenn IA: From the archives of the AFIP. Xanthogranulomatous pyelonephritis. Radiographics 1991;11:485-498.
102. Health service costs and quality of life for early elective surgery or ultrasonographic surveillance for small abdominal aortic aneurysms. UK Small Aneurysm Trial Participants. Lancet 1998;352:1656-1660.
103. Mortality results for randomised controlled trial of early elective surgery or ultrasonographic surveillance for small abdominal aortic aneurysms. The UK Small Aneurysm Trial Participants. Lancet 1998;352:1649-1655.
104. United Kingdom Small Aneurysm Trial Participants. Long-term outcomes of immediate repair compared with surveillance of small abdominal aortic aneurysms. N Engl J Med 2002;346:1445-1452.
105. Lederle FA, Wilson SE, Johnson GR, et al: Immediate repair compared with surveillance of small abdominal aortic aneurysms. N Engl J Med 2002; 46(19): 1437-1444.
106. Collin J, Araujo L, Walton J, et al: Oxford screening programme for abdominal aortic aneurysm in men aged 65 to 74 years. Lancet 1988;2:613-615.
107. Lucarotti M, Shaw E, Poskitt K, et al: The Gloucestershire aneurysm screening programme: The first 2 years' experience. Eur J Vasc Surg 1993;7:397-401.
108. Lindholt JS, Vammen S, Juul S, et al: The validity of ultrasonographic scanning as screening method for abdominal aortic aneurysm. Eur J Vasc Endovasc Surg 1999;17:472-475.
109. Connelly JB, Hill GB, Millar WJ: The detection and management of abdominal aortic aneurysm: A cost-effectiveness analysis. Clin Invest Med 2002;25:127-133.
110. Lee TY, Korn P, Heller JA, et al: The cost-effectiveness of a "quick-screen" program for abdominal aortic aneurysms. Surgery 2002; 132R:399-407.
111. Vardulaki KA, Walker NM, Couto E, et al: Late results concerning feasibility and compliance from a randomized trial of ultrasonographic screening for abdominal aortic aneurysm. Br J Surg 2002;89:861-864.
112. Wilmink AB, Forshaw M, Quick CR, et al: Accuracy of serial screening for abdominal aortic aneurysms by ultrasound. J Med Screen 2002;9:125-127.
113. Zwiebel WJ: Aortic and iliac aneurysm. Semin Ultrasound CT MR 1992;13:53-68.
114. Pedersen OM, Aslaksen A, Vik-Mo H: Ultrasound measurement of the luminal diameter of the abdominal aorta and iliac arteries in patients without vascular disease. J Vasc Surg 1993;17:596-601.
115. Grimshaw GM, Thompson JM: The abnormal aorta: A statistical definition and strategy for monitoring change. Eur J Vasc Endovasc Surg 1995;10:95-100.
116. Lanne T, Sonesson B, Bergqvist D, et al: Diameter and compliance in the male human abdominal aorta: Influence of age and aortic aneurysm. Eur J Vasc Surg 1992;6:178-184.
117. Sonesson B, Hansen F, Stale H, et al: Compliance and diameter in the human abdominal aorta—the influence of age and sex. Eur J Vasc Surg 1993;7:690-697.
118. Burns PN: Hemodynamics. In Taylor KJW, Burns PN, Wells PNT (eds): Clinical Applications of Doppler Ultrasound, 2nd ed. New York, Raven Press, 1995, pp 35-53.
119. Zwiebel WJ, Fruechte D: Basics of abdominal and pelvic duplex: instrumentation, anatomy, and vascular Doppler signatures. Semin Ultrasound CT MR 1992;13:3-21.
120. Polak JF: Pathophysiology. In Polak JF (ed): Peripheral Vascular Sonography: A Practical Guide. Baltimore, Williams & Wilkins, 1992, pp 59-72.
121. Allison DJ: Arteriography. In Grainger RG, Allison DJ (eds): An Anglo-American Textbook of Imaging. Edinburgh, Churchill Livingstone, 1986, pp 2014-2015.
122. Recchia D, Sharkey AM, Bosner MS, et al: Sensitive detection of abnormal aortic architecture in Marfan syndrome with high-frequency ultrasonic tissue characterization. Circulation 1995;91:1036-1043.
123. Abdool-Carrim AT, Robbs JV, Kadwa AM, et al: Aneurysms due to intimomedial mucoid degeneration. Eur J Vasc Endovasc Surg 1996;11:324-329.
124. Lobe TE, Richardson CJ, Boulden TF, et al: Mycotic thromboaneurysmal disease of the abdominal aorta in

preterm infants: Its natural history and its management. J Pediatr Surg 1992;27:1054-1059; discussion 1059-1060.

125. Halloran BG, Baxter BT: Pathogenesis of aneurysms. Semin Vasc Surg 1995;8:85-92.

126. Erturk H, Erden A, Yurdakul M, et al: Pseudoaneurysm of the abdominal aorta diagnosed by color duplex Doppler sonography. J Clin Ultrasound 1999;27:202-205.

127. Taylor BS, Rhee RY, Muluk S, et al: Thrombin injection versus compression of femoral artery pseudoaneurysms. J Vasc Surg 1999;30:1052-1059.

128. Mohler ER III, Mitchell ME, Carpenter JP, et al: Therapeutic thrombin injection of pseudoaneurysms: A multicenter experience. Vasc Med 2001;6:241-244.

129. Olsen DM, Rodriguez JA, Vranic M, et al: A prospective study of ultrasound scan-guided thrombin injection of femoral pseudoaneurysm: A trend toward minimal medication. J Vasc Surg 2002;36:779-782.

130. Maleux G, Hendrick S, Vaninbrouk J, et al: Percutaneous injection of human thrombin to treat iatrogenic femoral pseudoaneurysms: Short- and mid-term ultrasound follow-up. Eur Radiol 2003;13:209-212.

131. Ballard DJ, Hallett, JW: Natural history of aneurysms. In Strandness DE Jr, Vanbreda A (eds): Vascular Diseases: Surgical and Interventional Therapy. New York, Churchill Livingstone, 1994, pp 565-569.

132. Nevitt MP, Ballard DJ, Hallett JW Jr: Prognosis of abdominal aortic aneurysms: A population-based study. N Engl J Med 1989;321:1009-1014.

133. Kaufman JA, Bettmann MA: Prognosis of abdominal aortic aneurysms: A population-based study. Invest Radiol 1991;26:612-614.

134. Dent TL, Lindenauer SM, Ernst CB, et al: Multiple arteriosclerotic arterial aneurysms. Arch Surg 1972;105:338-344.

135. Gordon IL, Kohl CA, Arefi M, et al: Spinal cord injury increases the risk of abdominal aortic aneurysm. Am Surg 1996;62:249-252.

136. Johansen K, Koepsell T: Familial tendency for abdominal aortic aneurysms. JAMA 1986;256:1934-1936.

137. Cohen JR, Hallett JW: Pathophysiology of arterial aneurysm development. In Strandness DE Jr, Vanbreda A (eds): Vascular Diseases: Surgical and Interventional Therapy. New York, Churchill Livingstone, 1994, pp 559-564.

138. Dowson HM, Montgomery BS: Prevalence of abdominal aortic aneurysms in urology patients referred for ultrasound. Ann R Coll Surg Engl 2000;82:146.

139. Krohn CD, Kullmann G, Kvernebo K, et al: Ultrasonographic screening for abdominal aortic aneurysm. Eur J Surg 1992;158:527-530.

140. Lederle FA, Walker JM, Reinke DB: Selective screening for abdominal aortic aneurysms with physical examination and ultrasound. Arch Intern Med 1988;148:1753-1756.

141. Joyce JW: Preoperative evaluation of aneurysms. In Strandness DE Jr, Vanbreda A (eds): Vascular Diseases: Surgical and Interventional Therapy. New York, Churchill Livingstone, 1994, pp 579-588.

142. Quill DS, Colgan MP, Sumner DS: Ultrasonic screening for the detection of abdominal aortic aneurysms. Surg Clin North Am 1989;69:713-720.

143. Russell JG: Is screening for abdominal aortic aneurysm worthwhile? Clin Radiol 1990;41:182-184.

144. Axelrod DA, Diwan A, Stanley JC, et al: Cost of routine screening for carotid and lower extremity occlusive disease in patients with abdominal aortic aneurysms. J Vasc Surg 2002;35:754-758.

145. Lindholt JS: Screening for abdominal aortic aneurysm. Ugeskr Laeger 2002;164:157-159.

146. Law M: Screening for abdominal aortic aneurysms. Br Med Bull 1998;54:903-913.

147. Vazquez C, Sakalihasan N, D'harcour JB, et al: Routine ultrasound screening for abdominal aortic aneurysm among 65- and 75-year-old men in a city of 200,000 inhabitants. Ann Vasc Surg 1998;12:544-549.

148. Beebe HG, Kritpracha B: Screening and preoperative imaging of candidates for conventional repair of abdominal aortic aneurysm. Semin Vasc Surg 1999;12:300-305.

149. Van Essen JA, Gussenhoven EJ, Van Der Lugt A, et al: Accurate assessment of abdominal aortic aneurysm with intravascular ultrasound scanning: Validation with computed tomographic angiography. J Vasc Surg 1999;29:631-638.

150. Wilmink AB, Hubbard CS, Quick CR: Quality of the measurement of the infrarenal aortic diameter by ultrasound. J Med Screen 1997;4:49-53.

151. Schmidt MH, Mitchell JR, Downey DB: Sonographic surveillance of abdominal aortic aneurysms: What is the smallest change in measured diameter that reliably reflects aneurysm growth? Can Assoc Radiol J 1999;50:241-246.

152. King PS, Cooperberg PL, Madigan SM: The anechoic crescent in abdominal aortic aneurysms: Not a sign of dissection. AJR Am J Roentgenol 1986;146:345-348.

153. Guirguis EM, Barber GG: The natural history of abdominal aortic aneurysms. Am J Surg 1991; 162:481-483.

154. Glimaker H, Holmberg L, Elvin A, et al: Natural history of patients with abdominal aortic aneurysm. Eur J Vasc Surg 1991;5:125-130.

155. Bernstein EF, Chan EL: Abdominal aortic aneurysm in high-risk patients: Outcome of selective management based on size and expansion rate. Ann Surg 1984; 200:255-263.

156. Cronenwett JL, Murphy TF, Zelenock GB, et al: Actuarial analysis of variables associated with rupture of small abdominal aortic aneurysms. Surgery 1985;98:472-483.

157. Sterpetti AV, Schultz RD, Feldhaus RJ, et al: Abdominal aortic aneurysm in elderly patients: Selective management based on clinical status and aneurysmal expansion rate. Am J Surg 1985;150:772-776.

158. Moran KT, Persson AV, Jewell ER: Chronic rupture of abdominal aortic aneurysms. Am Surg 1989;55:485-487.

159. Richardson JW, Greenfield LJ: Natural history and management of iliac aneurysms. J Vasc Surg 1988; 8:165-171.

160. Scott RA, Wilson NM, Ashton HA, et al: Is surgery necessary for abdominal aortic aneurysm less than 6 cm in diameter? Lancet 1993;342:1395-1396.

161. Pennell RC, Hollier LH, Lie JT, et al: Inflammatory abdominal aortic aneurysms: A thirty-year review. J Vasc Surg 1985;2:859-869.

162. Fiorani P, Bondanini S, Faraglia V, et al: Clinical and therapeutical evaluation of inflammatory aneurysms of the abdominal aorta. Int Angiol 1986;5:49-53.

163. Berletti R, D'andrea P, Cavagna E, et al: Inflammatory and fibrotic changes in the periaortic regions: Integrated US, CT and MR imaging in three cases. Radiol Med (Torino) 2002;103:427-432.

164. Maloney JD, Pairolero PC, Smith SF Jr, et al: Ultrasound evaluation of abdominal aortic aneurysms. Circulation 1977;56(3 Suppl):I180-I185.

165. Zollner N, Zoller WG, Spengel F, et al: The spontaneous course of small abdominal aortic aneurysms: Aneurysmal growth rates and life expectancy. Klin Wochenschr 1991;69:633-639.

166. Okuhn SP, Stoney RJ: Intraoperative use of ultrasound in arterial surgery. Surg Clin North Am 1990;70:61-70.

167. Guinet C, Buy JN, Ghossain MA, et al: Aortic anastomotic pseudoaneurysms: US, CT, MR, and angiography. J Comput Assist Tomogr 1992;16:182-188.

168. Puyau FA, Adinolfi MF, Kerstein MD: Lymphocele around aortic femoral grafts simulating a false aneurysm. Cardiovasc Intervent Radiol 1985;8:195-198.

169. Hillman BJ: Disorders of the renal artery circulation and renal vascular hypertension. In Pollack HM (ed): Clinical Urology. Philadelphia, WB Saunders, 1990, pp 2127-2185.

170. Wilson SE, Van Wagenen P, Passaro E Jr: Arterial infection. Curr Probl Surg 1978;15:1-89.

171. Calligaro KD, Bergen WS, Savarese RP, et al: Primary aortoduodenal fistula due to septic aortitis. J Cardiovasc Surg (Torino) 1992;33:192-198.

172. Fellmeth BD, Roberts AC, Bookstein JJ, et al: Postangiographic femoral artery injuries: Nonsurgical repair with US-guided compression. Radiology 1991;178:671-675.

173. Feld R, Patton GM, Carabasi RA, et al: Treatment of iatrogenic femoral artery injuries with ultrasound-guided compression. J Vasc Surg 1992;16:832-840.

174. Flinn WR, Rizzo RJ, Park JS, et al: Duplex scanning for assessment of mesenteric ischemia. Surg Clin North Am 1990;70:99-107.

175. Avasthi PS, Voyles WF, Greene ER. Noninvasive diagnosis of renal artery stenosis by echo-Doppler velocimetry. Kidney Int 1984;25:824-829.

176. Urban BA, Ratner LE, Fishman EK: Three-dimensional volume-rendered CT angiography of the renal arteries and veins: Normal anatomy, variants, and clinical applications. Radiographics 2001;21:373-386; questionnaire 549-555.

177. Stavros AT, Parker SH, Yakes WF, et al: Segmental stenosis of the renal artery: Pattern recognition of tardus and parvus abnormalities with duplex sonography. Radiology 1992;184:487-492.

178. Mathews R, Smith PA, Fishman EK, et al: Anomalies of the inferior vena cava and renal veins: Embryologic and surgical considerations. Urology 1999;53:873-880.

179. Mewissen MW, Erickson SJ, Foley WD, et al: Thrombosis at venous insertion sites after inferior vena caval filter placement. Radiology 1989;173:155-157.

180. Khalfallah N, Zermani R, Ben Miled K, et al: Leiomyosarcomas of the inferior vena cava: Two cases. Tunis Med 1992;70:493-498.

181. Parrilla M, Montilla Y, Alvarez C, et al: Leiomyosarcoma of the vena cava inferior: The correlation: ultrasound and fine-needle puncture biopsy. G E N (Spanish) 1992;46:336-340.

182. Singh-Panghaal S, Karcnik TJ, Wachsberg RH, et al: Inferior vena caval leiomyosarcoma: Diagnosis and biopsy with color Doppler sonography. J Clin Ultrasound 1997;25:275-278.

183. Hemant D, Krantikumar R, Amita J, et al: Primary leiomyosarcoma of inferior vena cava, a rare entity: Imaging features. Australas Radiol 2001;45:448-451.

184. Ridwelski K, Rudolph S, Meyer F, et al: Primary sarcoma of the inferior vena cava: Review of diagnosis, treatment, and outcomes in a case series. Int Surg 2001;86:184-190.

185. Beckmann CF, Abrams HL: Renal venography: Anatomy, technique, applications, analysis of 132 venograms, and a review of the literature. Cardiovasc Intervent Radiol 1980;3:45-70.

186. Mellins HZ: Clinical urology. In Pollack HM (ed): Clinical Urology. Philadelphia, WB Saunders, 1990, pp 2119-2126.

187. Hibbert J, Howlett DC, Greenwood KL, et al: The ultrasound appearances of neonatal renal vein thrombosis. Br J Radiol 1997;70:1191-1194.

188. Brill PW, Mitty HA, Strauss L: Renal vein thrombosis: A cause of intrarenal calcification in the newborn. Pediatr Radiol 1977;6:172-175.

189. Jayogapal S, Cohen HL, Brill PW, et al: Calcified neonatal renal vein thrombosis demonstration by CT and US. Pediatr Radiol 1990;20:160-162.

190. Patriquin HB, Lafortune MA: Doppler sonography of the child's abdomen. In Taylor KJW, Burns PN, Wells PNT (eds): Clinical Application of Doppler Ultrasound. New York, Raven Press, 1995.

191. Adkins J, Wilson S: Unusual course of the gonadal vein: A case report of postpartum ovarian vein thrombosis mimicking acute appendicitis clinically and sonographically. J Ultrasound Med 1996;15:409-412.

13

THE ABDOMINAL WALL

Khanh T. Nguyen / Eric E. Sauerbrei / Robert L. Nolan /
Bernard J. Lewandowski

Chapter Outline

A common indication for scanning the abdominal wall is the presence of a palpable mass. Is the mass in the wall or inside the abdominal cavity? Is it cystic or solid? Sonography can readily give the answer to these questions. Occasionally, an abnormality is found in the abdominal wall during routine scanning of the intra-abdominal organs.

SCANNING TECHNIQUES

Because the skin is "out of focus" with even the highest-frequency transducers, scanning the skin requires various stand-off techniques to obtain the best resolution and to avoid the "bang effect" of direct transducer placement on the skin. Flotation pads that are liquid-filled microcell sponges (Reston Flotation Pad, 3M Company, Minneapolis, MN.), synthetic polymer blocks (Kitecko, 3M Company, St. Paul, MN.), and silicone elastomer blocks (Echomould, AHS/Belgium, Steenweg op Zellick 30, B-1080, Brussels, Belgium) are commercially available. These substances are dense enough to stand unsupported and have a uniform consistency to minimize artifacts.

Scanning the abdominal wall requires no special patient preparation. The examination can be performed over surgical wounds by applying an adhesive plastic membrane (Op-site, Smith and Nephew, Welwyn Garden City, Hertfordshire, UK) over the wound after removing the dressing.[1] The adhesive is sterile and prevents both contamination of the wound by the transducer and contamination of the transducer by an infected wound or draining sinus. Gentle pressure with the transducer is applied, but excessive pressure should be avoided over wounds and other tender areas. The highest frequency possible that allows penetration to the area of interest should be used; this usually is accomplished with a high-frequency linear array probe.

ANATOMY

The abdominal wall is divided into anterior, antero-lateral, and posterior parts and is best appreciated on a transverse computed tomography (CT) scan (Fig. 13-1) or in schematic form (Fig. 13-2). The anterior abdominal wall is a laminated structure. From the outermost layer working in, the wall includes the skin, the superficial fascia, the subcutaneous fat, the muscle layers, the transversalis fascia, and a layer of extraperitoneal fat. The anterior muscle layer is composed of the paired midline rectus muscles and the anterolaterally situated external oblique, the internal oblique, and transversus abdominis muscles. The rectus abdominis muscles insert

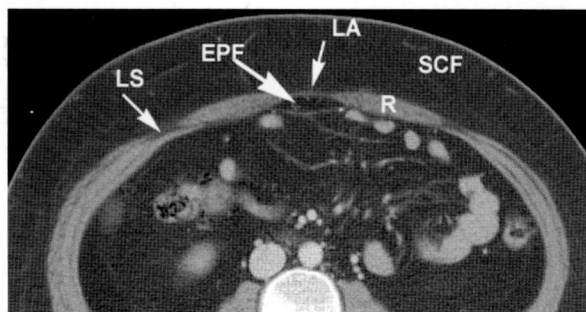

FIGURE 13-1. CT of abdomen showing the normal anatomy of anterior abdominal wall. Extraperitoneal fat, epf; LA, linea alba; LS, linea semilunaris; R, rectus muscle; scf, subcutaneous fat.

superiorly into the fifth, sixth, and seventh ribs and extend inferiorly to the pubic crest. They are enclosed anteriorly and posteriorly by the rectus sheath, which is formed by the aponeuroses of the internal oblique, external oblique, and transversus muscles. The posterior caudal aspect of the sheath ends at the arcuate line, which is situated usually midway between the umbilicus and the symphysis pubis. Distal to the arcuate line, the aponeuroses of all three muscles pass in front of the rectus muscle, which is then separated posteriorly from the peritoneum only by the transversalis fascia.[2] At the medial border of the rectus, the aponeuroses fuse to form the linea alba, which separates the rectus muscles in the midline.

The normal epidermis is a highly reflective layer measuring 1 to 4 mm in thickness.[3] The subcutaneous fat layer is of variable thickness. A significant amount of work has been done to determine the usefulness of this sonographic measurement to predict total body density

and to compare the ability of ultrasound assessment with traditional caliper techniques in measuring subcutaneous fat. Real-time sonography has proven as effective as caliper techniques in cadaver experiments,[4] as well as in young male and obese subjects, whereas A-mode scanning is less effective but probably more convenient than CT scanning.[5-8] One report, however, concluded that total abdominal circumference provides a better estimate of body fat in obese women than does ultrasound measurement of subcutaneous fat because ultrasound does not measure the deep fat. Nonetheless, these measurements are important in sports medicine and in obesity clinics.

Over the years there have been conflicting reports concerning the echogenicity of fat. Some fatty tissues (e.g., breast lipomas) are relatively anechoic, and subcutaneous fat is relatively hypoechoic; however, fat in the liver is echogenic.[9] The spectrum of echogenicity displayed by fat and fatty tissues can be explained by the water content within the fat. In an in vitro experiment, margarine (containing 85% vegetable oil and 15% water) scanned in a water bath was echogenic and attenuated sound, whereas when the margarine melted, floating echogenic globules were seen. When the margarine was heated until the water vaporized and then rescanned after cooling, the substance was anechoic.[9] The authors concluded that not only is pure fat anechoic, but that a mixture of fat and water is echogenic. Because water and fat are immiscible, there are multiple fat/water and water/fat interfaces, each with a significant acoustic impedance mismatch that causes the marked echogenicity.[10]

The musculofascial layer is usually more echogenic than the subcutaneous fat layer (Fig. 13-3A). With high-

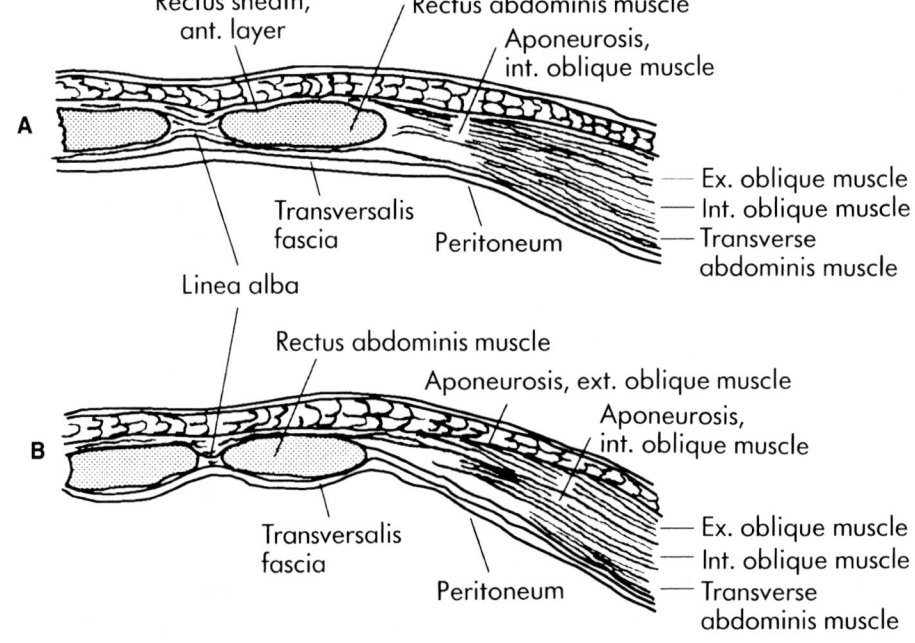

FIGURE 13-2. Schema of anterior abdominal wall. **A,** Above arcuate line and **B,** below arcuate line.

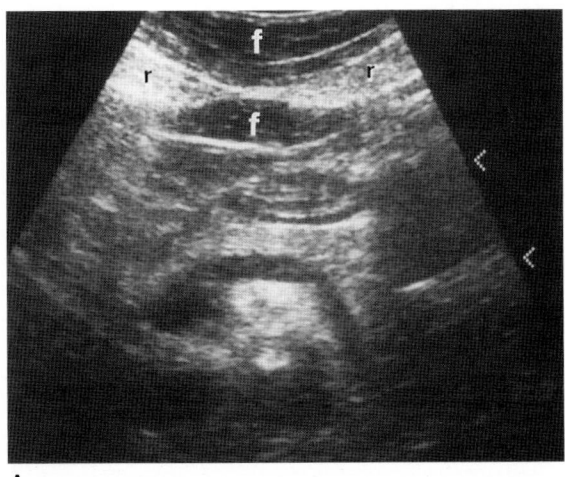
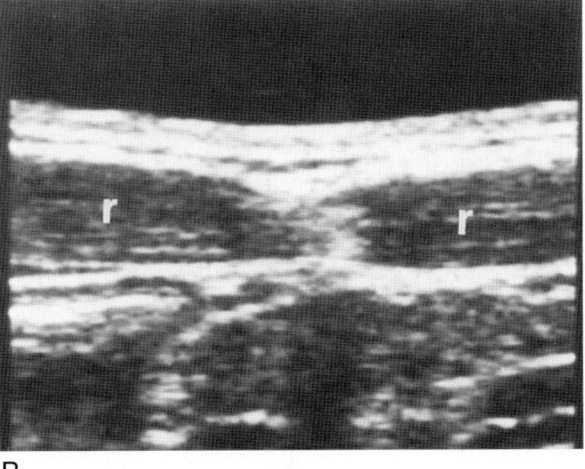

A   B

FIGURE 13-3. Anterior abdominal wall. A, Transverse scan. The muscles appear echogenic. The fat (f) appears hypoechoic. Note the prominent extraperitoneal fat collection that appears lens-shaped. **B,** Sagittal scan. The individual muscle bundles (r) appear hypoechoic in this thin patient.

resolution probes, individual muscle bundles can be identified that show fairly uniform texture and orientation (see Fig. 13-3B). Because the muscles of the back are thicker, they are more difficult to visualize in detail than the muscles of the anterolateral walls.

The extraperitoneal fat collection posterior to the muscles appears thick in many people, particularly those who are obese, at the level of the linea alba and linea semilunaris (see Fig. 13-3A). This acts as the source of the split image artifact, which will be discussed later in this chapter. It should not be mistaken for a tumor.

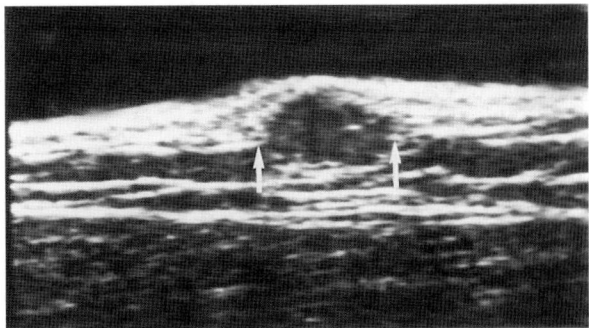

FIGURE 13-4. Subcutaneous metastatic melanoma. The nodule appears hypoechoic. Note disruption of the skin layer (*arrows*).

PATHOLOGY

Cutaneous Lesions

Sonographic evaluation of the skin has been used to detect clinically occult foci of recurrent or metastatic melanoma and has been used to guide fine-needle aspiration biopsies of these lesions.[11,12] Pigmented nevi and malignant melanomas are clearly demarcated from normal skin (Fig. 13-4). Most melanomas are hypoechoic and demonstrate enhancement through transmission. Although malignant melanoma is rarely found on the anterior abdominal wall, almost 75% of patients with melanoma develop cutaneous or subcutaneous metastases.[12] More importantly, the nodules may be found in unexpected locations.

Hernias

Ventral Hernia

Ventral hernias may be acquired or congenital. Acquired hernias are more frequently seen in patients who are obese or elderly or in those with previous trauma or

surgery. The typical locations are at points of weakness where no muscle is present, along the linea alba in the midline or the linea semilunaris on each side (spigelian hernia), and in the inferior lumbar space.[13-15] The fascial defect and the herniated contents (omental fat or bowel) are usually identified by careful scanning with a 7.5 MHz linear array transducer. Seen in cross section, herniated bowel loops appear as target lesions with strong reflective central echoes representing air in the lumen. When obstructed, they appear as tubular, fluid-filled structures containing valvulae conniventes (small bowel) or fecal material (colon). Congenital ventral hernias consist of gastroschisis and omphalocele. Gastroschisis (Fig. 13-5) occurs in about 1 per 174,000 births and usually as an isolated anomaly. The abdominal wall defect is usually on the right side of the umbilical cord insertion, with herniation of small bowel not covered by a membrane. In contrast, omphalocele (Fig. 13-6) occurs directly at the site of the umbilical cord insertion. It is three times more common than gastroschisis and is associated with other organ mal-

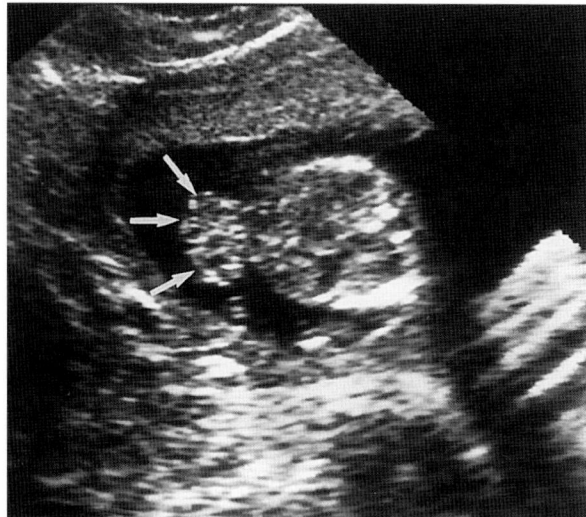

FIGURE 13-5. Gastroschisis seen *in utero* at 17 weeks' menstrual age. Note the mass of herniated bowel (*arrows*) in this transverse view of the fetus.

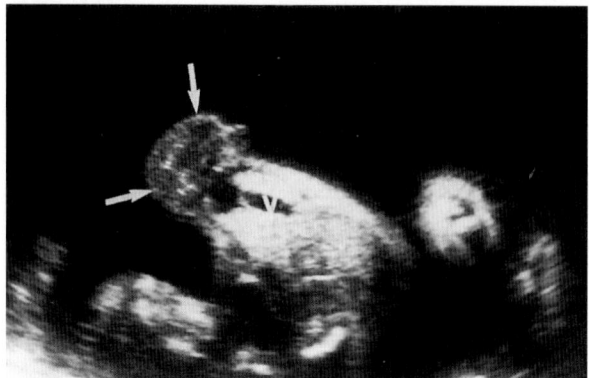

FIGURE 13-6. Omphalocele seen *in utero* at 18 weeks' menstrual age. Note the umbilical vein (v) running into the omphalocele (*arrows*), which is covered by a membrane.

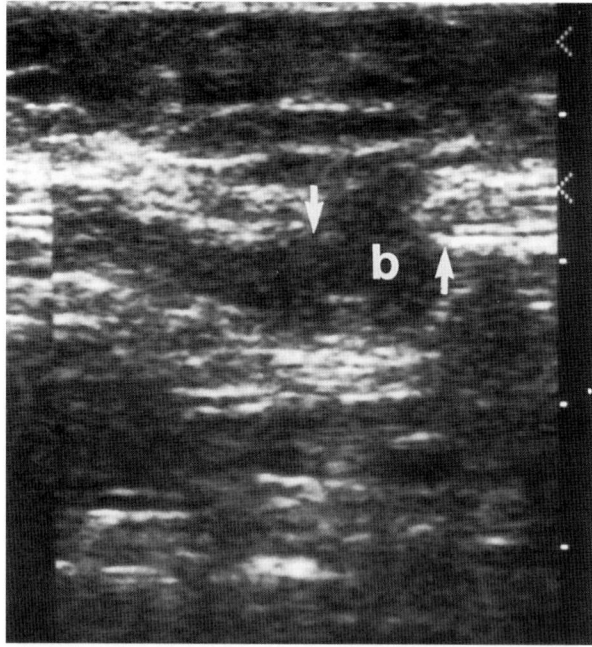

A

B

FIGURE 13-7. Spigelian hernia. A, Ultrasound appearance. Bowel (b) is seen herniating through the fascial defect (*arrows*). **B,** CT appearance. Note the hernia orifice (*arrow*).

formations. The hernia sac usually contains liver and/or bowel. Both conditions may be detected by sonography in the fetus *in utero* as early as 18 weeks' menstrual age.[16]

Spigelian Hernia

Spigelian hernia, the only spontaneous hernia of the lateral abdominal wall, was first described in the year 1721.[17,18] It consists of a defect in the aponeurosis of the transversus abdominis muscle lateral to the rectus sheath. The most common location of spigelian hernias is at or near the junction of linea semilunaris and the arcuate line. Before the use of high-resolution sonography, the diagnosis of spigelian hernia was missed in 50% of cases preoperatively because the classic findings are often missing.[19,20] The sonographic diagnosis of a spigelian hernia depends on the demonstration of a defect at any point in the linea semilunaris that represents the hernial orifice (Fig. 13-7).[21] If associated with protrusion of deep tissues, the hernia is usually bounded anteriorly by the external oblique aponeurosis. The external aponeurosis is so thick at this level that only 15 of 876 patients have been reported to have a subcutaneous hernial sac. More than 280 articles and 5 medical theses have been published on spigelian hernias, yet a review of the literature by Spangen revealed that only 876 patients had undergone surgery.[22] It should be noted that all patients with a spigelian hernia have tenderness over the orifice on palpation.

Lumbar Hernia

Lumbar hernias are uncommon and are most often acquired rather than congenital.[23,24] Spontaneous hernias occur in two areas of weakness in the flank: the inferior (Petit's hernia) and superior (Grynfeltt's hernia) lumbar triangles. Acquired lumbar hernias are usually posttraumatic or iatrogenic.[25,26]

Lumbar hernias are usually asymptomatic. Because the neck of the hernia is wide, strangulation is uncommon, occurring in about 10% of cases. It is postulated that they are more common in females because of the wider pelvis.[27] The diagnosis depends on cross-sectional imaging, usually CT.[28-30] There has been, however, at least one case report in which the diagnosis was made sonographically.[31] In this case, sonography showed fluid-filled loops of small bowel extending from the peritoneal cavity into a midflank mass.

Incisional Hernia

Incisional hernias are delayed complications of abdominal surgery, and they occur in 0.5% to 14% of patients[32-34]; the current rate is about 4%. Because almost two million abdominal operations are performed in the United States every year, the problem is not a trivial one.[35,36] Enlargement of these hernias will usually manifest within the first year; however, 5% to 10% will remain silent.[37] Clinically unsuspected incisional hernias are often detected by CT scan.[38] Sonography may occasionally identify a herniated bowel loop at the incision site.

Inguinal Hernia

The inguinal canal extends from the deep inguinal ring to the superficial inguinal ring. The deep inguinal ring is a defect in the transversalis fascia anterior to the femoral vessels and above the inguinal ligament. The superficial inguinal ring is an opening in the aponeurosis of the external oblique muscle. Hesselbach's triangle is formed by the lateral border of the rectus sheath medially, the inferior epigastric artery laterally, and the inguinal ligament inferiorly. Direct inguinal hernias protrude through a weakened inguinal canal floor medial to the inferior epigastric artery, whereas an indirect hernia exits via the deep inguinal ring (i.e., lateral to the inferior epigastric artery) and courses through the inguinal canal. Both direct and indirect inguinal hernias can extend into the scrotum (Fig. 13-8).

Because both the superficial inguinal ring and the inferior epigastric artery are not easily seen sonographically, ultrasound has not been helpful in distinguishing direct from indirect inguinal hernias. However, sonography can distinguish hernias from other inguinal canal masses, such as undescended testicles or varicoceles.[39] Inguinal sonography can be useful in delineating the superior aspect of a scrotal mass[40] and defining the presence of intestine and/or omentum in a hernial sac.

Sonography can detect complications of inguinal herniorrhaphy. The most common acute complication is hematoma extending from the inguinal canal into the scrotum. Less common complications include epididymitis and ischemic orchitis. Delayed scrotal swelling (several months after surgery) is usually secondary to a

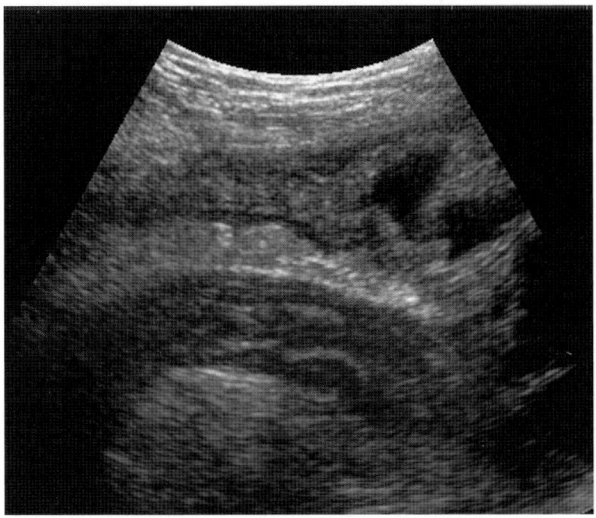
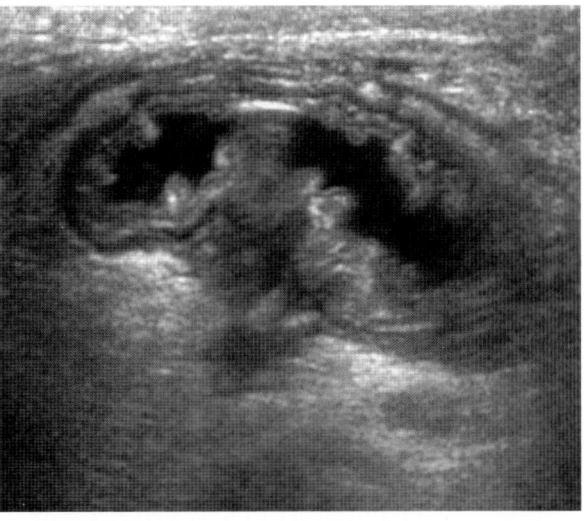

A   B

FIGURE 13-8. Inguinal hernia containing loop of bowel. A, Sonogram over the inguinal canal shows an elongated structure within the inguinal canal. **B**, High frequency transducer shows the structure is a loop of bowel with a fluid-filled lumen and a laminated wall. (Courtesy Anthony Hanbidge, University of Toronto.)

small hydrocele.[41] One theory is that inguinal herniorrhaphy aggravates an existing hydrocele by disturbing the lymphatic drainage.[42]

Femoral Hernia

Sonography is recommended in patients with groin pain and no palpable mass,[43] questionable palpable masses, and elderly obese patients with unexplained abdominal pain.[44] Up to 70% of nonobstructed femoral hernias are misdiagnosed by nonsurgical practitioners,[45] and 25% of femoral hernias are misdiagnosed surgically because they can be incarcerated and yet be impalpable.[46] The boundaries of the femoral canal are the femoral vein laterally, the superior pubic ramus posteriorly, and the ileopubic tract anteromedially. The sonographic detection of a femoral hernia depends on the demonstration of a mass medial to the femoral vein (Fig. 13-9A, B). The mass must then be differentiated from other masses found in the femoral triangle, which include hematomas, pseudoaneurysms, arteriovenous (AV) fistulae, lipomas, lymph nodes, hydroceles, saphenous varices, and inguinal hernias.

Rectus Sheath Hematoma

Rectus sheath hematomas are either posttraumatic or spontaneous. The traumatic causes include direct trauma, surgery, or sudden vigorous abdominal contractions that may occur with seizures, and paroxysms of coughing,[47] sneezing, defecation, urination, and intercourse.[48,49] Recently a single case of rectus sheath hematoma as a complication of tetanus has been reported.[50] Anticoagulant therapy is the most common cause of spontaneous rectus sheath hematoma. Other less common associations include collagen diseases, steroid therapy, pregnancy,[51] and bleeding disorders.[52] Bleeding is usually secondary to either the rupture of the epigastric artery or veins or a primary tear of the muscle fibers.[53] The bleeding is usually intramuscular but may be extramuscular and confined by the rectus sheath. The tamponade effect of the sheath usually limits the size of the hematoma; however, there is a case report of a massive hematoma where the bleeding site was identified sonographically.[54] Clinical findings include abdominal pain, palpable mass, ecchymosis, and the Fothergill sign,[55,56,57] which involves palpating the suspected abdominal mass while the patient tenses the abdominal muscles. An abdominal wall mass will remain fixed whereas an intra-abdominal mass will become less apparent. The sonographic appearance depends on the location of bleed with respect to the arcuate line, its age, and the transducer frequency. Above the arcuate line, the linea alba prevents the spread of hematoma across the midline; thus the hematomas are ovoid transversely and biconcave in the long axis.[58,59] Below the arcuate line, blood can spread to the pelvis or cross the midline, forming a large mass that indents on the dome of the urinary bladder (Fig. 13-10).

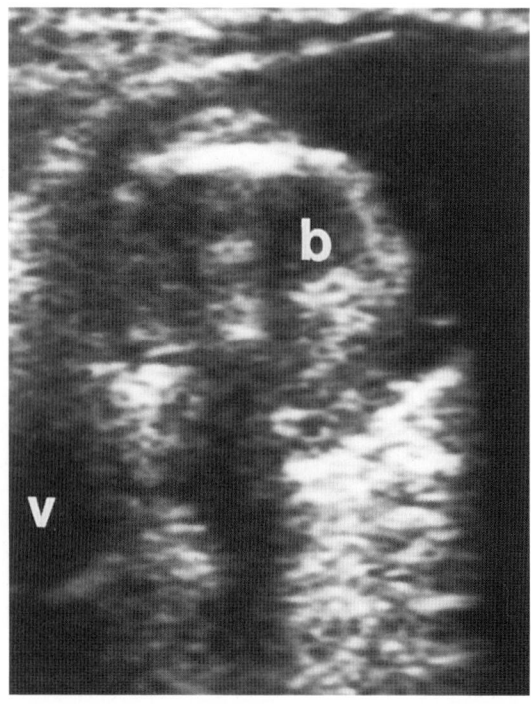

A

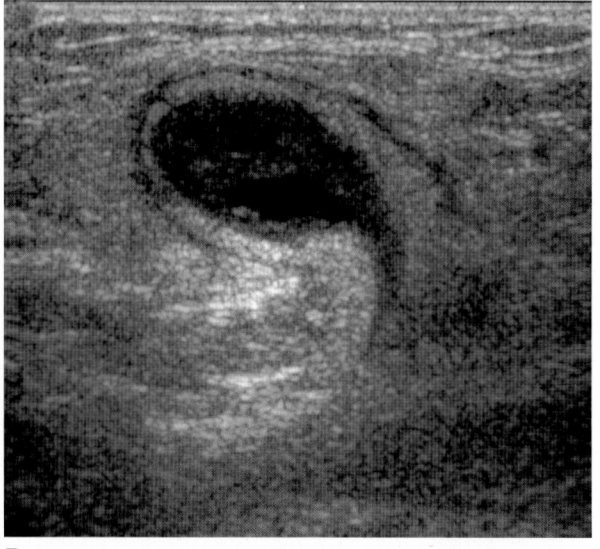

B

FIGURE 13-9. Strangulated femoral hernia. A, Transverse scan. Note the target appearance typical of a dilated bowel loop (b) medial to the vessels (v). **B,** Sonogram over the femoral canal shows a well-defined cystic structure protruding through the canal from the peritoneal cavity in a patient with ascites. (Courtesy J. W. Charboneau, M.D., Mayo Clinic.)

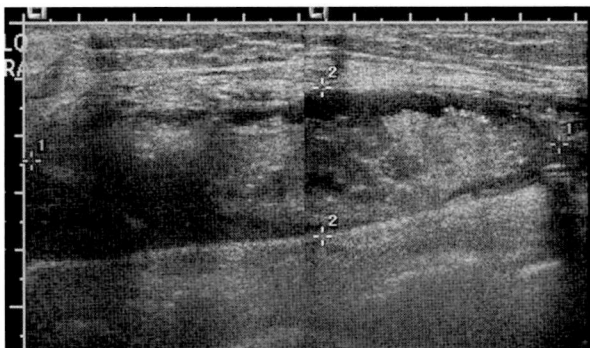

FIGURE 13-10. Rectus sheath hematoma. Split screen image.

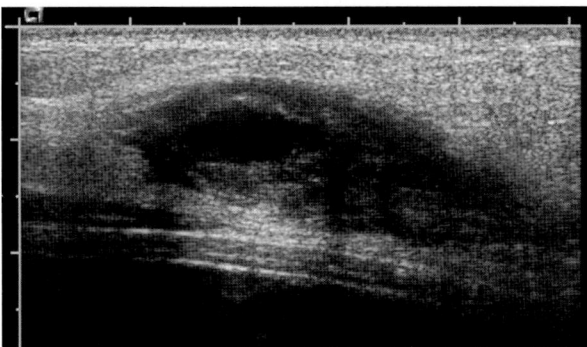

FIGURE 13-11. Subcutaneous hematoma in the abdominal wall. There is a focal hypoechoic elongated mass in the abdominal wall with a liquefied center. Appearance is classic for a maturing hematoma.

Fluid Collections

Fluid collections are usually seromas, liquefying hematomas, or abscesses related to previous surgery or trauma. Occasionally, a urachal cyst may be seen extending from the umbilicus to the dome of the urinary bladder.[39] A urachal cyst may be complicated by hemorrhage or infection (urachal abscess).[59] Uncommonly, tumors may arise in the urachus in children or young adults.[60]

Sterile fluid collections are usually echo free. When complicated by hemorrhage or infection, they appear more complex, with septations and/or layering, low-level echoes representing blood cells or debris (Fig. 13-11). Fluid collections may be aspirated percutaneously under sonographic guidance, with the specimen sent for Gram stain and culture and sensitivity.

Vascular Lesions

Subcutaneous Arterial Bypass Grafts. High-resolution sonography is ideal in imaging subcutaneous axillofemoral and femorofemoral arterial bypass grafts.[61-64] Postoperatively, the grafts demonstrate transient, small, perigraft fluid collections at the level of the surgical tunnels, which disappear as the graft is incorporated into the subcutaneous tissues. Persistent perigraft fluid collections or localized collections are abnormal and are usually seromas or abscesses.[65] Any abnormal perigraft fluid collection should be followed until it resolves or a definitive diagnosis is made. Although loss of pulsatility within the graft may indicate thrombosis,[66] duplex Doppler and color flow Doppler imaging make the diagnosis easier. Other reported complications include graft aneurysms due to failure of the graft and pseudoaneurysms.

Pseudoaneurysms and Arteriovenous Fistulas

Most femoral artery pseudoaneurysms involve the common femoral artery and are secondary to vascular reconstruction.[67,68] Pseudoaneurysm is also a well-known but uncommon complication of femoral artery catheterization, with an incidence of 0.1%.[69] Arteriovenous (AV) fistulas are considerably rarer. A pseudoaneurysm is a pulsatile hematoma secondary to bleeding into the soft tissue, with fibrous encapsulation and a persistent communication between the vessel and the fluid space. The vessel wall does not heal, and the blood flows back and forth between the two spaces during the cardiac cycle.[70-72] Most hematomas and pseudoaneurysms are within 2 cm of the arterial injury. The real-time criteria of pseudoaneurysm include echogenic swirls within a cystic cavity, expansile pulsatility, hypoechoic mass, and a visible tract.[73] When present, echogenic swirls are diagnostic of a pseudoaneurysm. Unfortunately, they are not often seen. Similarly, expansile pulsatility is difficult to evaluate and has not always been helpful.[74] A fistulous tract is the least observed sonographic finding. Thus, the ultrasound findings alone may not be sufficient to distinguish a hematoma from a pseudoaneurysm.[75] Duplex Doppler and color flow Doppler imaging have increased our ability to distinguish these entities.[76] The Doppler characteristics of a pseudoaneurysm include arterial flow within a mass, separate from the artery, and to-and-fro flow between the artery and the mass. One author states that demonstration of to-and-fro flow at the neck of the pseudoaneurysm is not a necessary condition for the diagnosis of a pseudoaneurysm and reports sensitivities of 94% and specificities of 97%, with an accuracy of 96% using the first criterion alone.[77] With duplex Doppler imaging, the sample volume should interrogate the cavity and not an adjacent small vessel, whereas with color flow Doppler imaging, a perivascular color flow artifact should not be interpreted as representing abnormal flow within a pseudoaneurysm.[78] A false-positive diagnosis using color Doppler has been reported in a case of necrotizing lymphadenitis where the mass was mistaken for a false aneurysm on the basis of a jet within the hilum of the inflamed inguinal lymph node.[79]

Varices

A recanalized umbilical vein seen in portal hypertension, saphenous varices, and varicoceles found in the femoral triangle and inguinal area are easily identified because they are characteristically compressible and have typical venous Doppler characteristics.

Lymph Nodes

Ultrasound can be used to detect lymphadenopathy when there is no palpable mass, or when it can be used to categorize a palpable groin mass as lymphadenopathy. Although it was originally thought that normal lymph nodes are not detected sonographically because they are indistinguishable from subcutaneous fat,[80] high-resolution sonography can detect pathologically proven normal superficial lymph nodes. Most nodes are ovoid in shape and are variable in size. Very few are homogeneous. They vary in echogenicity, depending on the degree of central lipomatosis.[81] Thus, the center of the node is echogenic, and the periphery is hypoechoic. With extensive lipomatosis, the node may become indistinguishable from the surrounding subcutaneous tissue. Ultrasound is more effective in demonstrating lymphadenopathy than is clinical palpation,[82-84] and it is useful for staging lymphoma and for monitoring therapy.[85] There is no criterion to distinguish malignant from inflammatory lymphadenopathy, and the metastatic inference must be confirmed by biopsy. Although not all enlarged nodes are malignant and not all malignant nodes are enlarged, there are some sonographic clues available to help distinguish malignant from inflamed nodes. Lymphomatous nodes are extremely hypoechoic and may even be anechoic, especially in non-Hodgkin's lymphoma.[80] A recent study of patients with palpable lymph nodes suggests that a 1 to 3 mm central artery can be seen within enlarged lymphomatous nodes, whereas in lymph nodes with carcinomatous involvement, the central artery is not seen sonographically because it is infiltrated and destroyed on microscopy.[86] As discussed in the section on pseudoaneurysms, this central artery has been identified in one case of lymphadenitis.

Undescended Testicles

Cryptorchidism is the most common congenital anomaly of the male reproductive system, with an incidence of between 0.23% and 0.8% in the adult population.[87] It is bilateral in 10% to 25% of all cases.[88,89] Testicular descent can stop at any point between the hilum of the ipsilateral kidney to the external inguinal ring.[90,91] Of all undescended testicles,

80% are palpable and 20% are not palpable. Of those that are not palpable, 80% are in the inguinal canal and the remaining 20% are intra-abdominal[92,93]; the testicle is absent in 4% of cases when it is not palpable. Sonography is useful in the detection of undescended testicles. The undescended testis often appears smaller than the normal testis. It usually appears ovoid, and its long axis is usually parallel to the inguinal canal. Visualization of the echogenic hilum of the lymph node should distinguish the structure from a testicle. Unfortunately, although sonography can often detect testicles that are in the inguinal canal, it is less successful in detecting intra-abdominal testicles.[94-96]

Neoplasms

The abdominal wall is an uncommon site for neoplastic disease (Fig. 13-12). The most common primary neoplasms are desmoid tumors, which arise from fascia or aponeurosis of muscles (Fig. 13-13). The most common location is in the anterior abdominal wall. Desmoid tumors are usually seen in patients with previous abdominal surgery and often occur at the site of the previous laparotomy scar. They also occur in patients with familial polyposis and are often associated with pregnancy. Of patients with desmoid tumors, 70% are between 20 to 40 years of age. There is a 3:1 female preponderance.[97-102] CT and ultrasound are ideal methods to demonstrate both the site and extent of the mass.[99] Lipoma (Fig. 13-14A, B, C), neuroma, and neurofibroma are occasionally seen.

The most frequent malignant subcutaneous nodules are metastatic melanoma. Secondary malignancies from lymphoma or carcinoma of the lung, breast, ovary, and colon are less frequent.[39,59] The metastasis may occur as an isolated finding (Fig. 13-15), but more often it is seen in patients with widespread metastatic disease elsewhere. The abdominal wall may also be locally invaded by malignancies arising from the pleura, peritoneum, diaphragm (mesothelioma, rhabdomyosarcoma, or fibrosarcoma), or intra-abdominal organs such as the colon.

ARTIFACTS

The anatomic arrangement of the lower abdominal wall has been implicated in an important artifact observed deep in the pelvis. It has been called a *ghost artifact* (named after the "ghosting" seen in television images) or, more appropriately, the split-image artifact.[103-105]

The split-image artifact arises because of the presence of extraperitoneal fat deep to the linea alba and rectus abdominis muscles. In transverse scan planes at the

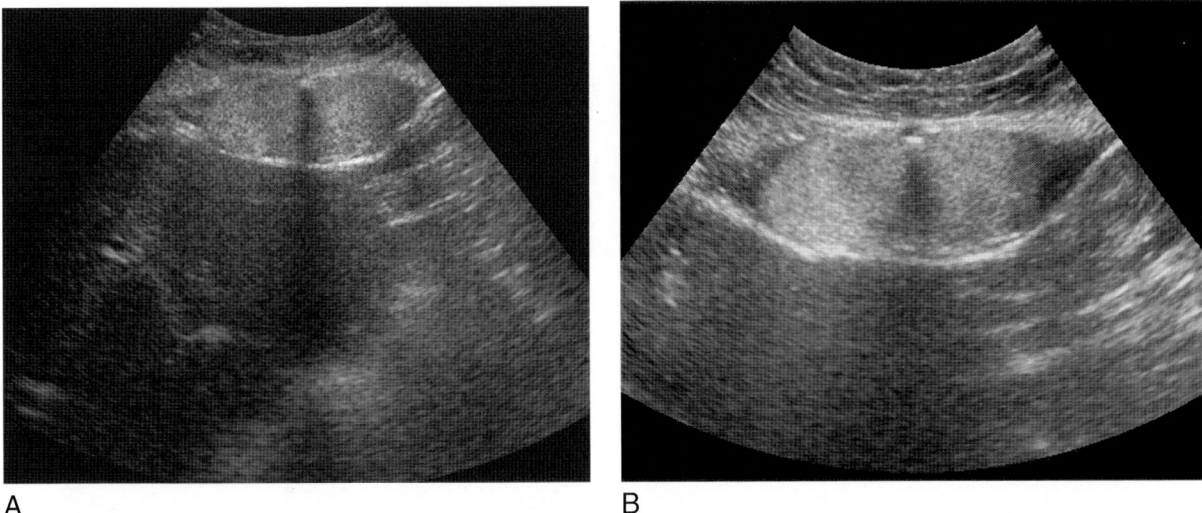

A   B

FIGURE 13-12. Localization of a mass to the abdominal wall. A, Transverse image shows an echogenic mass superficial to the left lobe of the liver, suggesting a superficial location. **B,** Magnified view in the same location shows, in addition, posterior displacement of the peritoneal line that appears as a bright and echogenic line. This confirms that the echogenic mass is within the abdominal wall.

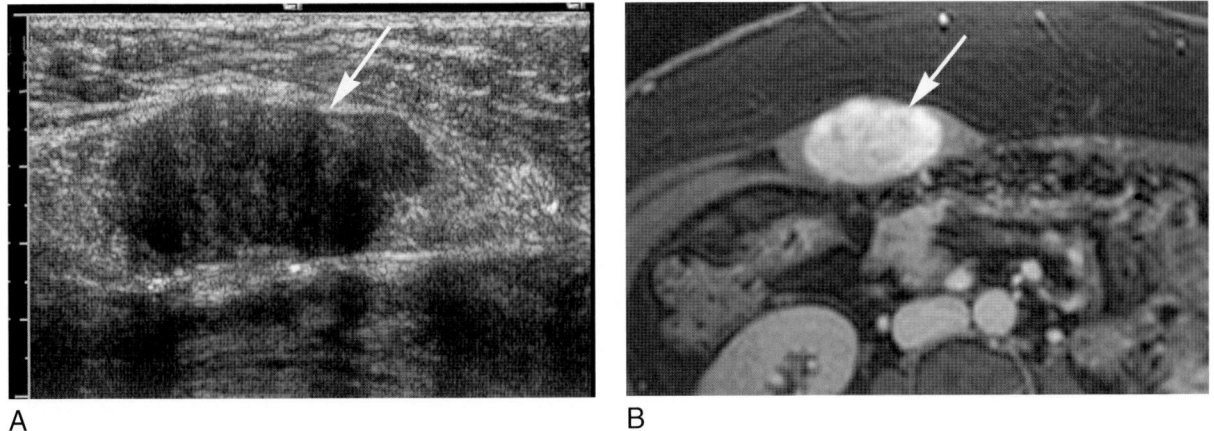

A   B

FIGURE 13-13. Desmoid tumor of anterior abdominal wall. A, Transverse sonogram shows a lobulated soft tissue solid mass just superficial to the peritoneal line. **B,** Confirmatory CT scan. (Courtesy J.W. Charboneau, M.D., Mayo Clinic.)

midline, sound rays are refracted at the muscle/fat interfaces in such a way that smaller structures in the abdomen or pelvis may be completely duplicated. For example, a small gestational sac may appear as two sacs, one small embryo may appear as two embryos, one aorta may appear as two aortas, and so on. The effect is usually seen only when the collection of fat beneath the linea

alba is large (and thus, the muscle/fat interfaces lie in an oblique orientation) and the structure of interest is deep below the abdominal wall.

Scanning in sagittal and oblique scan planes will fail to demonstrate the duplicated images seen in the transverse scans and thereby resolve the ambiguity (Fig. 13-16).

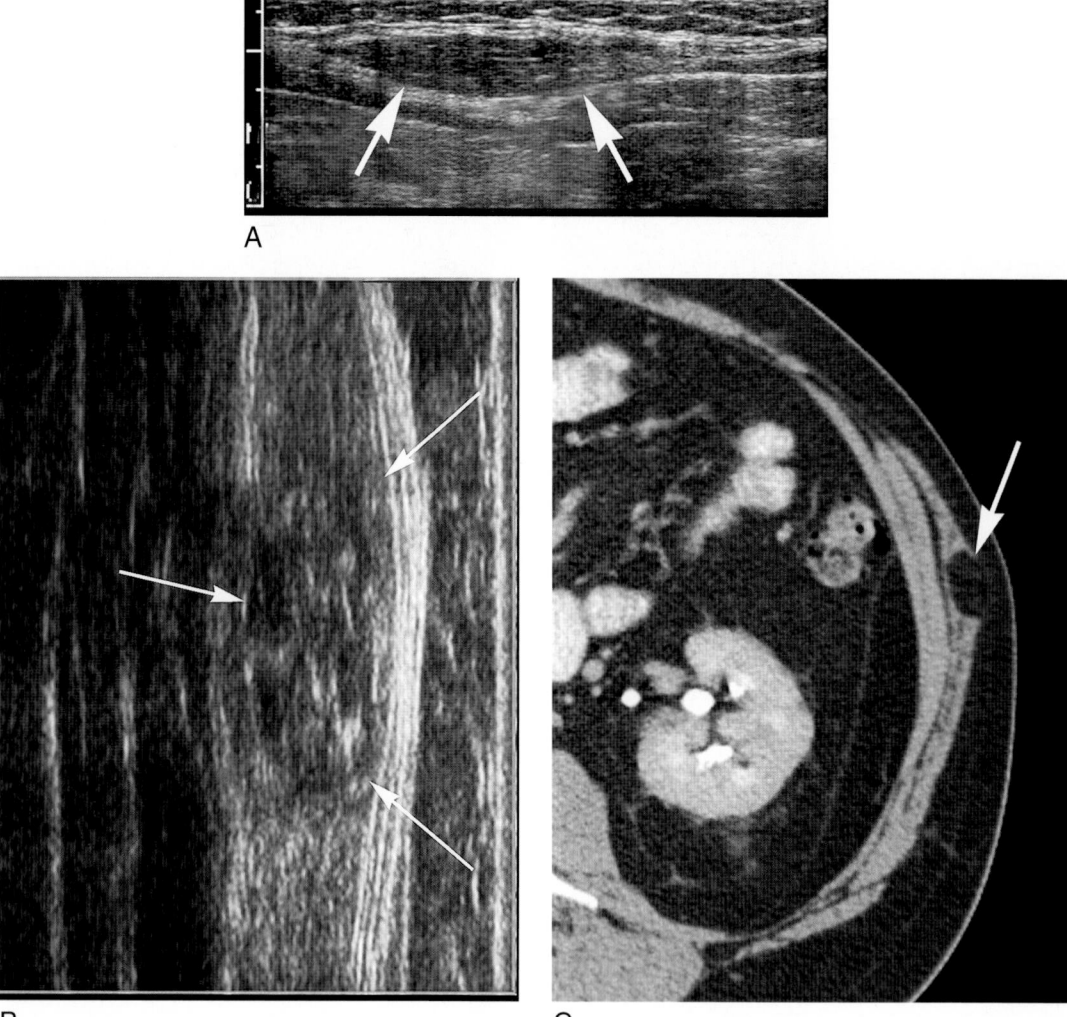

FIGURE 13-14. Lipomas in the muscular layer of the abdominal wall. A, Lesion is well encapsulated and hypoechoic lipomas (*arrows*). **B,** Sonogram shows a focal mixed echogenic subtle mass (*arrows*) in the muscular layer deep to the subcutaneous fat. Orientation is changed to match the CT scan. **C,** Confirmatory CT scan (*arrow*). (Courtesy of J. W. Charboneau, M.D., Mayo Clinic.)

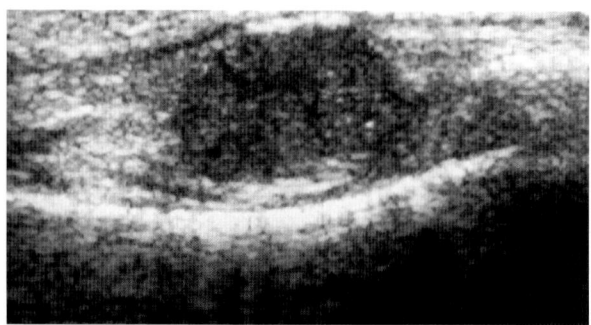

FIGURE 13-15. Metastasis in anterior abdominal wall. A hypoechoic nodule, a metastatic tumor from renal cell carcinoma, is seen superficial to the peritoneum, which shows as a strong white line. (Courtesy of Stephanie R. Wilson, M.D., University of Toronto.)

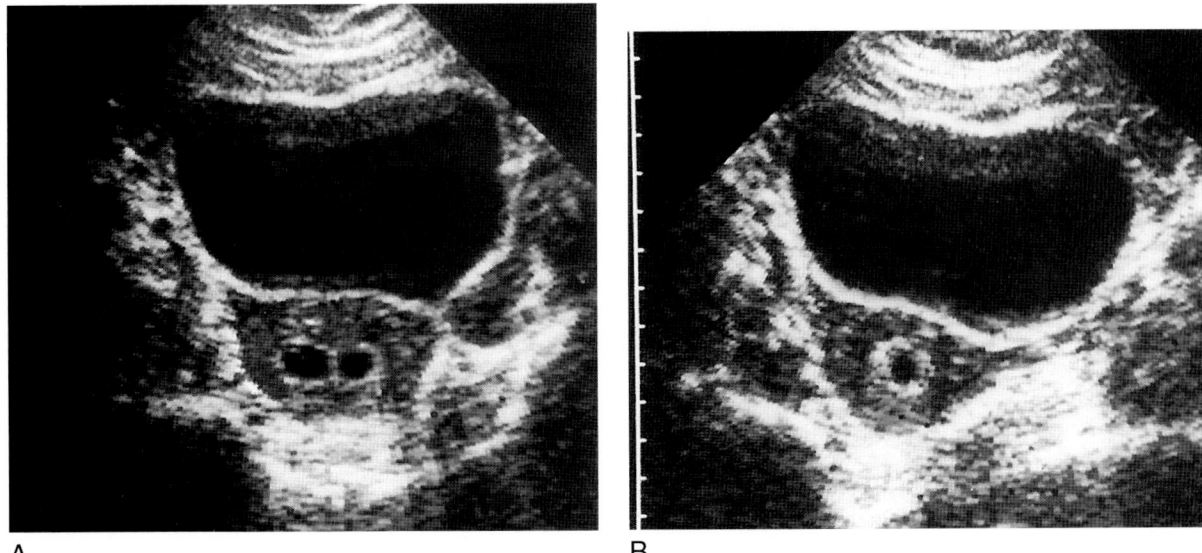

A   B

FIGURE 13-16. Split-image artifact. A, Two gestational sacs were seen in this transverse scan of the pelvis. **B,** In fact, only one gestational sac was present. When the transducer is angled or the parasagittal plane is scanned, the artifact will disappear. In the upper abdomen, a double aorta or double superior mesenteric artery may be seen because of this artifact.

References

Scanning Techniques

1. Fataar S, Goodman H, Tuft R, et al: Postoperative abdominal sonography using a trans-sonic sealing membrane. AJR 1983;141:565-566.

Anatomy

2. Warwick R, Williams PL, eds: Gray's Anatomy. Edinburgh, Longman Group Ltd, 1978, pp 519-527.
3. Shafir R, Itzchak Y, Heymen Z, et al: Preoperative ultrasonic measurements of the thickness of cutaneous malignant melanoma. J Ultrasound Med 1984;3:205-208.
4. Jones PR, Davies PS, Norgan NG: Ultrasonic measurements of subcutaneous adipose tissue in man. Am J Phys Anthropol 1986;73:359-363.
5. Weits T, van der Beek EJ, Wedel M: Comparison of skinfold caliper measurements of subcutaneous fat tissue. Int J Obesity 1986;10:161-168.
6. Kuczmarski RJ, Fanelli MT. Ultrasonic assessment of body composition in obese adults: overcoming the limitations of the skinfold caliper. Am J Clin Nutr 1987;45:717-724.
7. Chumlea WC, Roche AF: Ultrasonic and skinfold caliper measures of subcutaneous adipose tissue thickness in elderly men and women. Am J Phys Anthropol 1986;71:351-357.
8. Black D, Vora J, Hayward M, et al: Measurement of subcutaneous fat thickness with high frequency pulsed ultrasound: comparison with a caliper and a radiographic technique. Clin Phys Physiol Measure 1988;9:57-64.
9. Behan M, Kazam E: The echogenic characteristics of fatty tissues and tumors. Radiology 1978;129:143-151.
10. Errabolu RL, Sehgal CM, Bahn RC, et al: Measurement of ultrasonic nonlinear parameter in excised fat tissues. Ultrasound Med Biol 1988;14:137-146.

Pathology

11. Fornage BD: Fine-needle aspiration biopsy with a vacuum test tube. Radiology 1988;169:553.

12. Fornage BD, Lorigan JG: Sonographic detection and fine-needle aspiration biopsy of nonpalpable recurrent or metastatic melanoma in subcutaneous tissues. J Ultrasound Med 1989;8:421-424.
13. Thomas JL, Cunningham JJ. Ultrasonic evaluation of ventral hernias disguised as intra-abdominal neoplasms. Arch Surg 1978;113:589-590.
14. Rubio PA, Del Castillo H, Alvaraz A: Ventral hernia in a massively obese patient: Diagnosis by computed tomography. South Med J 1981;10:1307-1308.
15. Spangen L: Ultrasound as a diagnostic aid in ventral abdominal hernia. J Clin Ultrasound 1975;3:211-213.
16. Sauerbrei EE, Nguyen TK, Nolan RL: The fetus. In Sauerbrei EE (ed): A Practical Guide to Ultrasound in Obstetrics and Gynecology. New York, Raven Press, 1987, pp 111-159.
17. La Chausse BI: De hernia ventrali 1746. In Haller: Disputations Chirurgicales. Bosquet (Lausanne) 1755;3:181-211.
18. LeDran HF: Observation de Chirurgie. Paris, C. Osmont; 1771, p 143.
19. Weiss Y, Lernau O, Nissan S: Spigelian hernia. Ann Surg 1974;180:836-839.
20. Deitch EA, Engel JM: Spigelian hernia: An ultrasound diagnosis. Arch Surg 1980;115:193.
21. Spangen L: Spigelian hernia. Acta Chir Scand (Suppl) 1976;462.
22. Spangen L: Spigelian hernia. World J Surg 1989;13:573-580.
23. Swartz WT: Lumbar hernia. In: Nyhus LM, Condon RE (eds): Hernia, 2nd ed. Philadelphia, JB Lippincott, 1978, pp 409-426.
24. Ponka JL: Lumbar hernia. In: Ponka JL: Hernias of the Abdominal Wall. Philadelphia, WB Saunders, 1980, pp 465-477.
25. Quick CR: Traumatic lumbar hernia. Br J Surg 1982;69:160-162.
26. Castelein RM, Sauter AJ: Lumbar hernia in an iliac bone graft. Acta Orthop Scand 1985;56:2273-2274.

27. Light HG: Hernia of the inferior lumbar space: A cause of back pain. Arch Surg 1983;118:1077-1080.
28. Lawdahl R, Moss CN, Van Dyke JA: Inferior lumbar (Petit's) hernia. AJR 1986;147:744-745.
29. Baker ME, Weinerth JL, Andriani RT, et al: Lumbar hernia: Diagnosis by CT. AJR 1987;148:565-567.
30. Chenoweth J, Vas W: Computed tomography demonstration of inferior lumbar (Petit's) hernia. Clin Imag 1989;13:164-166.
31. Siffring PA, Forrest TS, Frick MP: Hernia of the inferior lumbar space: Diagnosis with US. Radiology 1989;170:190.
32. Fischer JD, Turner FW: Abdominal incisional hernias—a 10 year review. Can J Surg 1974;17:202-204.
33. Bucknall TE, Cox PJ, Ellis H: Burst abdomen and incisional hernia: A prospective study of 1129 major laparotomies. Br Med J 1982;284:931-933.
34. Baker RJ: Incisional hernia. In: Nyhus LM, Condon RE (eds): Hernia. 2nd ed. Philadelphia, JB Lippincott, 1978:329-341.
35. Larson GM, Vandertoll DJ: Approaches to repair of ventral hernia and full thickness losses of the abdominal wall. Surg Clin North Am 1984;64:335-349.
36. Ghahremani GG, Meyers MA: Iatrogenic abdominal hernias. In Meyers MA, Ghahremani GG: Iatrogenic Gastrointestinal Complications. New York, Springer-Verlag, 1981, pp 269-278.
37. Ellis H, Gajraj H, George CD: Incisional hernias: When do they occur? Br J Surg 1983;70:290-291.
38. Ghahremani GG, Jimenez MA, Rosenfeld M, et al: CT diagnosis of occult incisional hernias. AJR 1987;148:139-142.
39. Engel JM, Deitch EE: Sonography of the anterior abdominal wall. AJR 1981;137:73-77.
40. Subramanyam BR, Balthazar EJ, Raghavendra BN, et al: Sonographic diagnosis of scrotal hernia. AJR 1982;139:535-538.
41. Archer A, Choyke PL, O'Brien W, et al: Scrotal enlargement following inguinal herniorrhaphy: Ultrasound evaluation. Urol Radiol 1988;9:249-252.
42. Wantz GE: Complications of inguinal hernia repair. Surg Clin North Am 1984;64:287-298.
43. Ekberg O, Abrahamsson P, Kesek P: Inguinal hernia in urological patients: The value of herniography. J Urol 1988;139:1253-1255.
44. Deitch EA, Soncrant M: The value of ultrasound in the diagnosis of nonpalpable femoral hernias. Arch Surg 1981;116:185-187.
45. Waddington RT: Femoral hernia: A recent appraisal. Br J Surg 1971;59:920-922.
46. Ponka PL, Brush BE: Problem of femoral hernia. Arch Surg 1971;102:411-413.
47. Lee TM, Greenberger PA, Nahrwold DL, et al: Rectus sheath hematoma complicating an exacerbation of asthma. J Allergy Clin Immunol 1986;78:290-292.
48. Lee PWR, Bark M, Macfie J, et al: The ultrasound diagnosis of rectus sheath haematoma. Br J Surg 1977;64:633-634.
49. Manier JW: Rectus sheath haematoma. Six case reports and a literature review. Am J Gastroenterol 1972;54:433-435.
50. Suhr GM, Green AE: Rectus abdominis sheath hematoma as a complication of tetanus: diagnosis by computed tomography scanning. Clin Imag 1989;13:82-86.
51. Torpin R, Coleman J, Handkins JR: Hematoma of the rectus abdominis muscle in pregnancy, labor, or puerperium: Report of three cases. J Med Assoc Ga 1969;58:158-159.
52. DeLaurentis DA, Rosemond GP: Hematoma of the rectus abdominis muscle complicated by anticoagulant therapy. Am J Surg 1966;112:359.
53. Henzel JH, Pories WJ, Smith JL, et al: Pathogenesis and management of abdominal wall haematomas. Arch Surg 1966;93:929-935.
54. Savage PE, Joseph AEA, Adam EJ: Massive abdominal wall hematoma: Real-time ultrasound localization of bleeding. J Ultrasound Med 1985;4:157-158.
55. Gocke JE, MacCarty RL, Faulk WT: Rectus sheath hematoma: Diagnosis by computed tomography scanning. Mayo Clin Proc 1981;56:757-761.
56. Fisch AE, Brodey PA. Computed tomography of the anterior abdominal wall: Normal anatomy and pathology. J Comput Assist Tomogr 1981;5:728-733.
57. Tromans A, Campbell N, Sykes P: Rectus sheath haematoma. Diagnosis by ultrasound. Br J Surg 1981;68:518-519.
58. Kaftori JK, Rosenberger A, Pollack S, et al: Rectus sheath hematoma: Ultrasonographic diagnosis. AJR 1977;128:283-285.
59. Diakoumakis EE, Weinberg B, Seife B: Unusual case studies of anterior wall mass as diagnosed by ultrasonography. J Clin Ultrasound 1984;12:351-354.
60. Kwok-Liu JP, Zikman JM, Cockshott WP: Carcinoma of the urachus: The role of computed tomography. Radiology 1980;137:731-734.
61. Gooding GAW, Herzog KA, Hedgecock NW, et al: B-mode ultrasonography of prosthetic vascular grafts. Radiology 1978;127:763-766.
62. Gooding GA, Effeney DJ, Goldstone J: The aortofemoral graft: Detection and identification of healing complications by ultrasonography. Surgery 1981;89:94-101.
63. Clifford PC, Skidmore R, Bird DR, et al: Pulsed Doppler and real-time "duplex" imaging of Dacron arterial grafts. Ultrason Imaging 1980;2:381-390.
64. Wolson AH, Kaupp HA, McDonald K: Ultrasound of arterial graft surgery complications. AJR 1979;133:869-875.
65. Gooding GAW, Effeney DJ: Sonography of axillofemoral and femorofemoral subcutaneous arterial bypass grafts. AJR 1985;144:1005-1008.
66. Gooding GAW, Effeney DJ: Static and real-time scanning B-mode sonography of arterial occlusions. AJR 1982;139:949-952.
67. Lang EK: A survey of the complications of percutaneous retrograde arteriography: Seldinger technique. Radiology 1973;81:257-263.
68. Szilagyi DE, Smith RE, Elliot JP, et al: Anastomotic aneurysms after vascular reconstruction problems of incidence, etiology and treatment. Surgery 1975;78:800-816.
69. Brener BJ, Couch NP: Peripheral arterial complications of left heart catheterization and their management. Am J Surg 1973;125:521-525.
70. Rapoport S, Sniderman KW, Morse SS, et al: Pseudo-aneurysm: complication of faulty technique in femoral arterial puncture. Radiology 1985;154:529-530.
71. Quera LA, Flinn WR, Yao JST, et al: Management of peripheral arterial aneurysms. Surg Clin North Am 1979;59:693-706.
72. Perl S, Wener L, Lyon WS: Pseudoaneurysms after angiography. Med Ann Dist Columbia 1973;42:173-175.
73. Abu-Yousef MM, Wiese JA, Shamma AR: Case report. The "to-and-fro" sign: Duplex Doppler evidence of femoral artery pseudoaneurysm. AJR 1988;150:632-634.

74. Mitchell DG, Needleman L, Bezzi M, et al: Femoral artery pseudoaneurysm: Diagnosis with conventional duplex and color Doppler US. Radiology 1987;164:687-690.

75. Sandler MA, Alpern MB, Madrazo BL, et al: Inflammatory lesions of the groin: Ultrasonic evaluation. Radiology 1984;151:747-750.

76. Sacks D, Robinson MD, Perlmutter GS: Femoral arterial injury following catheterization duplex evaluation. J Ultrasound Med 1989;8:241-246.

77. Coughlin BF, Paushter DM: Peripheral pseudoaneurysms: Evaluation with duplex US. Radiology 1988; 168:339-342.

78. Middleton WD, Erickson S, Melson GL: Perivascular color artifact: Pathologic significance and appearance on color Doppler US images. Radiology 1989;171:647-652.

79. Morton MJ, Charboneau JW, Banks PM: Inguinal lymphadenopathy simulating a false aneurysm on color-flow Doppler sonography. AJR 1988;151:115-116.

80. Hillman BJ, Haber K: Echographic characteristics of malignant lymph nodes. J Clin Ultrasound 1980;8:213-215.

81. Marchal G, Oyen R, Verschakelen J, et al: Sonographic appearance of normal lymph nodes. J Ultrasound Med 1985;4:417-419.

82. Bruneton JN, Roux P, Caramella E, et al: Ear, nose, and throat cancer: Ultrasound diagnosis of metastasis to cervical lymph nodes. Radiology 1984;142:771-773.

83. Bruneton JN, Normand F: Cervical lymph nodes. In Bruneton JN (ed): Ultrasonography of the Neck. Berlin, Springer-Verlag, 1987, pp 81-92.

84. Bruneton JN, Caramella E, Hery M, et al: Axillary lymph node metastases in breast cancer: Preoperative detection with US. Radiology 1986;158:325-326.

85. Bruneton JN, Normand F, Balu-Maestro C, et al: Lymphomatous superficial lymph nodes: US detection. Radiology 1987;165:233-235.

86. Majer MC, Hess CF, Kolbel G, et al: Small arteries in peripheral lymph nodes: A specific sign of lymphomatous involvement. Radiology 1988;168:241-243.

87. Martin DC: The undescended testis—evolving concepts in management. J Cont Ed Urol 1977;1:17-31.

88. Glickman MG, Weiss RM, Itzchak Y: Testicular venography for undescended testicles. AJR 1977;129:67-70.

89. Pinch L, Aceto T, Meyer-Bahlburg HF: Cryptorchidism: A paediatric review. Urol Clin North Am 1974;1:573-592.

90. Diamond AB, Meng CH, Kodroff M, et al: Testicular venography in the nonpalpable testis. AJR 1977;129:71-75.

91. Levitt SB, Kogan SJ, Schneider KM, et al: Endocrine tests in phenotypic children with bilateral impalpable testes can reliably predict "congenital" anorchism. Urology 1978;11:11-14.

92. Kogan SJ, Gill B, Bennett B, et al: Human monorchism: A clinicopathological study of unilateral absent testes in 65 boys. J Urol 1986;135:758-761.

93. Madrazo BL, Klugo RC, Parks JA, et al: Ultrasonographic demonstration of undescended testes. Radiology 1979;133:181-183.

94. Wolverson MK, Jagannadharao B, Sundaram M, et al: CT in localization of impalpable cryptorchid testes. AJR 1980;134:725-729.

95. Wolverson MK, Houttuin E, Heiberg E, et al: Comparison of computed tomography with high-resolution real-time ultrasound in the localization of the impalpable undescended testis. Radiology 1983;146:133-136.

96. Weiss RM, Carter AR, Rosenfield AT: High-resolution real-time ultrasonography in the location of the undescended testis. J Urol 1986;135:936-938.

97. Pasciak RM, Kozlowski JM: Mesenteric desmoid tumor presenting as an abdominal mass following salvage cystectomy for invasive bladder cancer. J Urol 1987;138:145-146.

98. McAdam WA, Goligher JC: The occurrence of desmoids in patients with familial polyposis coli. Br J Surg 1970;57:618-631.

99. Baron RL, Lee JK: Mesenteric desmoid tumors: Sonographic and computed tomographic appearance. Radiology 1981;140:777-779.

100. Brasfield RD, Das Gupta TK: Desmoid tumors of the anterior abdominal wall. Surgery 1969;65:241-246.

101. Mantello MT, Haller JO, Marquis JR. Sonography of abdominal desmoid tumors in adolescents. J Ultrasound Med 1989;8:467-470.

102. Magid D, Fishman EK, Bronwyn J, et al: Desmoid tumors in Gardner's syndrome: Use of computed tomography. AJR 1984;142:1141-1145.

Artifacts

103. Buttery B, Davison G: The ghost artifact. J Ultrasound Med 1984;3:49-52.

104. Muller N, Cooperberg PL, Rowley VA, et al: Ultrasonic refraction by the rectus abdominis muscles: The double image artifact. J Ultrasound Med 1984;3:515-519.

105. Sauerbrei EE: The split image artifact in pelvic sonography: The anatomy and physics. J Ultrasound Med 1985;4:29-34.

14

THE PERITONEUM

Anthony E. Hanbidge / Stephanie R. Wilson

Chapter Outline

𝒰ltrasound of the abdomen and pelvis has become an extension of the physical examination when evaluating patients with abdominal symptoms and signs. It is accurate, safe, readily available, and relatively inexpensive. Evaluations have traditionally focused on assessing the solid viscera, the gallbladder, and bile ducts. Frequently, images of only these organs will be recorded and the peritoneal cavity is often neglected or subjected to only a cursory evaluation. There is a general belief that ultrasound is not particularly helpful at imaging the peritoneum because of technical limitations, such as poor visibility and interference from bowel gas. There is also unfamiliarity with the common sonographic features encountered with peritoneal disease. This is reflected in the literature where there are extensive publications on ultrasound of the liver, gallbladder, bile ducts, pancreas, spleen, kidneys, bladder, and reproductive organs. By comparison, little has been written on sonographic evaluation of the peritoneum and peritoneal cavity. As a result, little time is spent on teaching optimal sonographic technique to evaluate these areas.

If there is clinical concern regarding peritoneal pathology, computed tomography (CT)[1] or, more recently, magnetic resonance imaging (MRI)[2-4] is generally used to investigate the possibility. It is our belief that ultrasound can also be sensitive and specific in this regard.[5] To be successful, however, **two criteria** must be met: (1) the operator performing the examination must be aware of the potential involvement of the peritoneum and peritoneal cavity with a disease process; and (2) a thorough sonographic assessment of these areas must be carried out.

APPEARANCE OF NORMAL PERITONEUM, OMENTUM, AND MESENTERY

The **peritoneum** is a serous membrane lined with epithelial cells. It is divided into the parietal and visceral peritoneum. The **parietal peritoneum** lines the anterior and posterior walls of the abdominal cavity and is visible with ultrasound as a thin, smooth, echogenic line in the deepest layer of the anterior abdominal wall. Bowel loops can usually be seen deep to the parietal peritoneum, moving independent of it with respiration. The **visceral peritoneum**, on the other hand, covers the intra-abdominal organs and is not visible with ultrasound in its normal state. The potential space between these two layers is known as the **peritoneal cavity**, which usually contains a small volume of fluid that acts as a lubricant.[6]

The **small bowel mesentery** is a specialized, fan-shaped, peritoneal fold extending from the second lumbar vertebra to the right iliac fossa. It connects the jejunum and ileum to the posterior abdominal wall. It is composed of a double layer of peritoneum, blood vessels, nerves, lacteals, lymph nodes, and a variable amount of fat. Normal bowel mesentery is best assessed with ultrasound in the presence of ascites; it appears as freely floating, smooth leaves separated by fluid, directed toward the center of the abdomen, away from small bowel loops (Fig. 14-1). In the absence of ascites, the mesentery is more difficult to appreciate but has been described as a series of elongated, aperistaltic structures separated from each other by specular echoes, best appreciated in the left lower quadrant.[7] It is frequently difficult to localize a disease process to the mesentery and the relationship to other anatomic landmarks may be helpful. For example, lymphoma may be correctly localized to the mesentery if a mass is seen that encases the mesenteric vessels.

The **omenta** are also specialized peritoneal folds. They are composed of a double layer of peritoneum, blood vessels, lymphatics, and a variable amount of fat. The **lesser omentum** connects the lesser curvature of the stomach and proximal duodenum with the liver. The **greater omentum** descends from the greater curvature of the stomach, anterior to the abdominal contents, often as low as the pelvis, and then reflects back on itself to form a four-layered structure that ascends and separates to enclose the transverse colon. A potential space exists between the two layers of the greater omentum, which is continuous with the lesser sac.

In the normal state the omenta may be extremely difficult or impossible to distinguish with ultrasound. In the presence of ascites, the free inferior edge of the normal greater omentum may be visible floating in the fluid with variable thickness, depending on the fat content. In disease, the greater omentum may become infiltrated, thickened, and nodular. Its superficial location allows for careful sonographic evaluation with high frequency transducers, and disease processes may often be correctly identified and localized to the greater omentum even in the absence of ascites.

TECHNIQUE

Sonographic assessment of the peritoneum requires a motivation to evaluate, as far as possible, the parietal and visceral peritoneum, the mesentery, the omentum, and the peritoneal cavity. The **initial survey** of the peritoneum and peritoneal cavity is performed with a standard frequency, 3.5 MHz or 5 MHz, transducer (Fig. 14-2A). The **field of view (FOV)** is set to include the full depth of the peritoneal cavity, but no more. This adds perspective to the image. The **focal zone** is continually adjusted to evaluate in detail different depths within the FOV. The **power and gain** settings are also adjusted using a high gain setting to characterize free fluid as anechoic or particulate and a low gain setting to optimally visualize hypoechoic nodules or masses. Once the initial survey is complete, **higher frequency transducers** are used to more carefully evaluate and characterize abnormalities in the near field (see Fig. 14-2B). When scanning transabdominally, graded compression is used to displace bowel gas. Determination of the site of origin of a peritoneal process may be aided by several techniques. Palpation of an abnormal mass, either with the transducer or with the free hand, will determine both the compliance and the mobility of a mass. Masses arising from the parietal peritoneum are often fixed, whereas masses arising from the visceral peritoneum may be mobile. This distinction may also be demonstrated by changing the patient's position or with changes in respiration. For example, in the right upper quadrant, a lesion in the near field is likely to be located on the

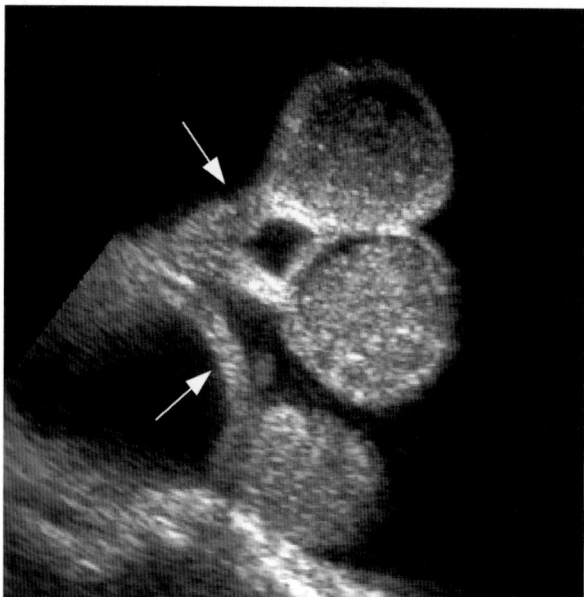

FIGURE 14-1. Normal mesentery with gross ascites. A sagittal oblique ultrasound image of the midabdomen shows the normal small bowel mesenteric leaves (*arrows*) outlined by fluid.

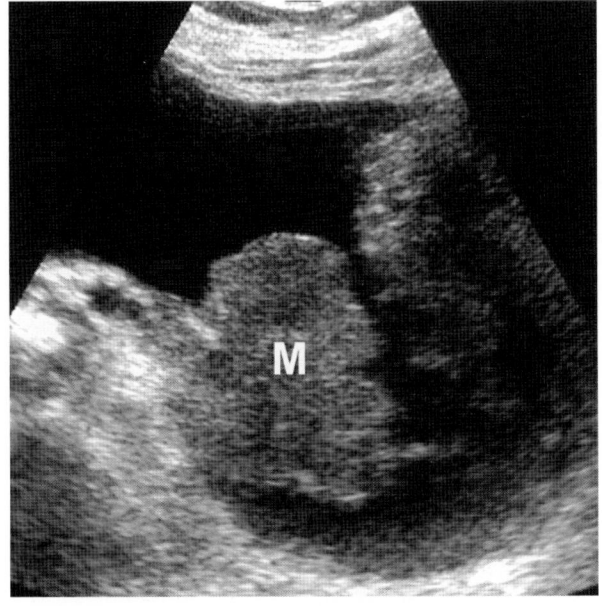

A

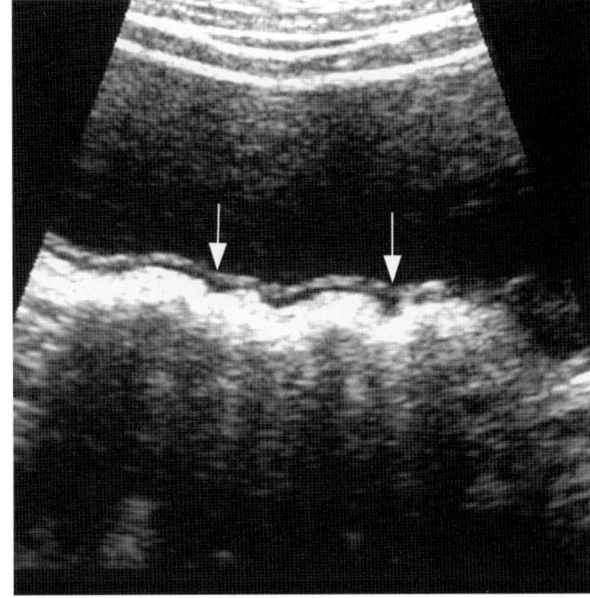

B

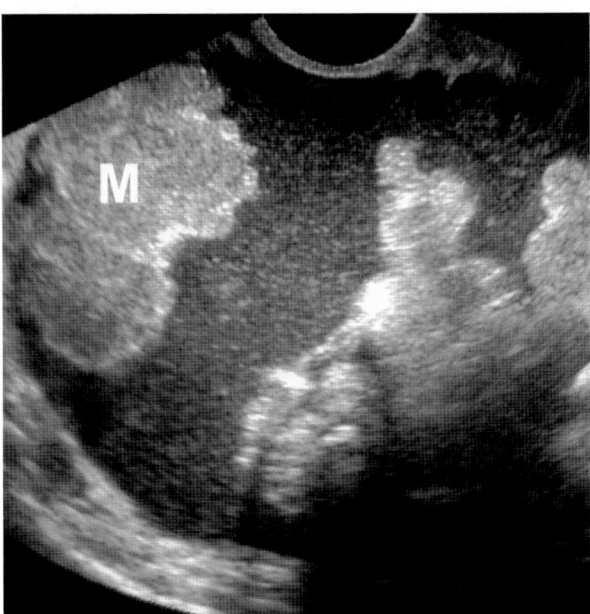

C

FIGURE 14-2. Optimization of technique. Stage 3 papillary serous adenocarcinoma of the ovary. **A,** Suprapubic, sagittal image of the right adnexa using a 5-2 MHz curvilinear transducer, taken at the time of the initial survey, shows ascites and a solid, lobulated, hypoechoic mass (M). The field of view includes the full depth of the peritoneal cavity but no more. **B,** Transabdominal, sagittal image of the left flank using a higher frequency, 7-4 MHz, curvilinear transducer shows ascites and hypoechoic seeding on the serosal surface of the descending colon (*arrows*). A low gain setting is used to optimize visualization of the seeding, seen as a thin continuous line on the serosal surface of the gut, which contains shadowing air. **C,** Transverse transvaginal image of the right adnexa using an 8-4 MHz transvaginal probe shows the right adnexal mass (M) and particulate ascites. A high gain setting is used to better characterize the particulate ascites.

parietal peritoneum if the liver moves independent of it with respiration.

Performing a **transvaginal ultrasound** examination on all female patients suspected of having, or who are at risk for, peritoneal disease is critical (see Fig. 14-2C), because the pelvic pouch of Douglas is a common site of involvement, particularly in carcinomatosis and acute conditions. This technique allows exquisite assessment of both the parietal and visceral pelvic peritoneum.[8,9] In addition to assessing the uterus and ovaries, the probe should be directed to the pouch of Douglas, by elevating the examining hand, and to both pelvic side-walls. The transvaginal scan may also facilitate improved visualization of pelvic bowel loops and the urinary bladder.

ASCITES

One of the earliest uses of sonography in the abdomen and pelvis involved the **detection of ascites.**[10] Normally, 50 to 75 mL of free fluid are present in the peritoneal cavity, acting as a lubricant. Ascites occurs with excess accumulation of peritoneal fluid. Ascites can be classified as transudate or exudate depending on the protein content. In North America today, cirrhosis, peritoneal

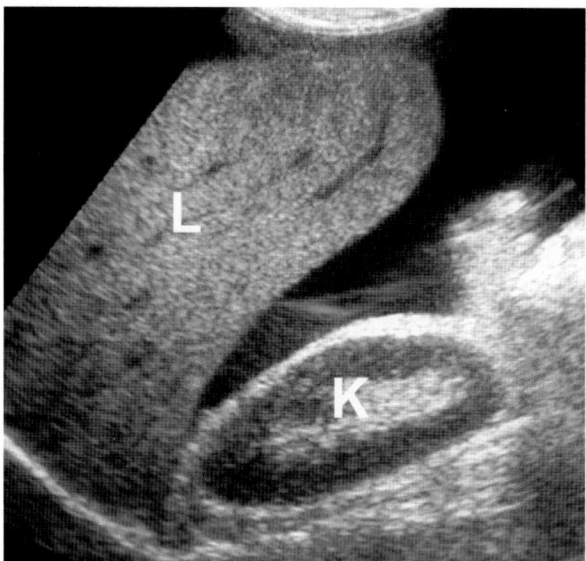

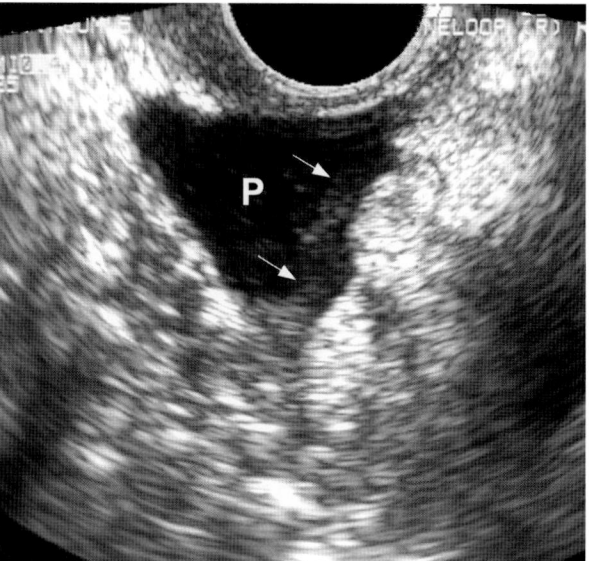

FIGURE 14-3. Cirrhosis of the liver with portal hypertension. A sagittal image of the right upper quadrant readily demonstrates a large amount of ascites surrounding an enlarged, bulbous, fatty liver (L). Right kidney (K).

FIGURE 14-4. Grade 2/3 ovarian mucinous cystadenocarcinoma. Transverse, transvaginal image of the right adnexa shows a small amount of particulate free fluid (P) and serosal seeding (*arrows*) on loops of bowel in the pelvis. This was visible only on the transvaginal scan.

carcinomatosis, congestive heart failure, and tuberculosis account for 90% of all cases. Accumulations of blood, urine, chyle, bile, or pancreatic juice are more unusual causes.

Ascites can be detected with physical examination when the volume reaches 500 mL. Transabdominal ultrasound can readily detect large volumes of ascites (Fig. 14-3). Transvaginal ultrasound is more sensitive in this regard, and volumes of free fluid as small as 0.8 mL can be demonstrated with the transvaginal probe (Fig. 14-4).[11] With the patient lying supine, free fluid tends to accumulate in the paracolic gutters and pelvis,[12] particularly the superior end of the right paracolic gutter and Morison's pouch. These areas should, therefore, be carefully assessed when ascites is suspected. Ultrasound is also accurate at quantifying[13] and localizing ascites and may be used to guide both diagnostic and therapeutic paracentesis.

In addition to its excellent capability to quantify ascites, ultrasound can also characterize ascites as anechoic or particulate. This may be helpful at determining the cause because **particulate ascites** suggests the presence of blood, pus, or neoplastic cells in the fluid. The observation of particulate ascites should prompt a more detailed assessment of the peritoneum with ultrasound,[14,15] further imaging with CT/MRI, and/or therapeutic paracentesis.

Hemoperitoneum has many causes, including trauma, ruptured aneurysm, ruptured ectopic pregnancy, ruptured liver mass (e.g., adenoma or hepatoma), and postsurgical bleeding. Spontaneous hemorrhage may occur in patients on anticoagulants. The appearance

of acute blood is varied, including anechoic or particulate free fluid (Fig. 14-5). A fluid debris level may develop if the patient has maintained a stable position for a period of time. **Massive hemorrhage** often results in a large echogenic mass that may become more heterogeneous as lysis occurs over time (Figs. 14-6 and 14-7).

Focused Assessment with Sonography for Trauma (FAST) has become an accepted screening modality for intra-abdominal injuries in the traumatized patient.[16-20] The primary focus of this limited study is to detect free intraperitoneal fluid with ultrasound in the trauma room. If fluid is detected in this setting, it strongly suggests significant intra-abdominal injury requiring urgent laparotomy. FAST has replaced peritoneal lavage in many centers.

Chylous ascites is an unusual condition wherein lymph accumulates within the peritoneal cavity. The causes are varied, including trauma, surgery, lymphangioma, lymphoma, intestinal lymphangiectasia, or cystic hygroma. Sonography may show particulate ascites or a fluid-fluid level because of layering of the lymphatic fluid.[21,22]

It is sometimes difficult to decide if fluid visualized in the peritoneal cavity is **free** or **loculated**. Altering the patient's position may be helpful to establish if the fluid moves under the force of gravity. For example, free fluid in the right paracolic gutter with the patient lying supine may move from this location if the patient lies in a left lateral decubitus position. The morphology of the fluid collection may also be helpful. Free fluid tends to conform to the surrounding organs and will frequently

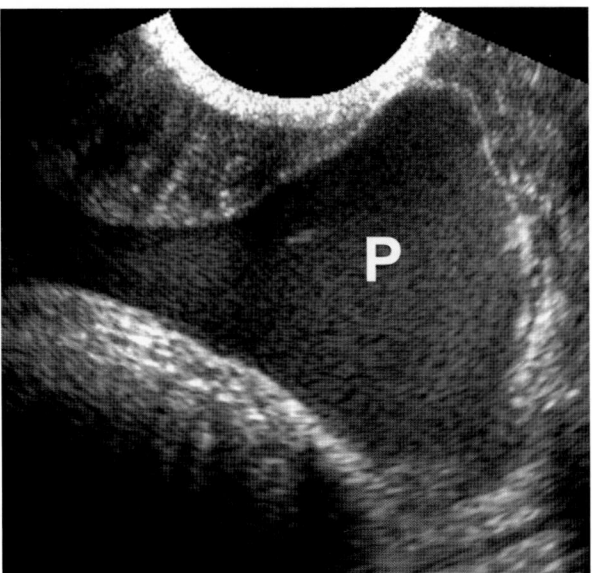

FIGURE 14-5. Hemoperitoneum in ruptured ectopic pregnancy. Transverse, oblique transvaginal ultrasound image of the left adnexa shows particulate free fluid (P).

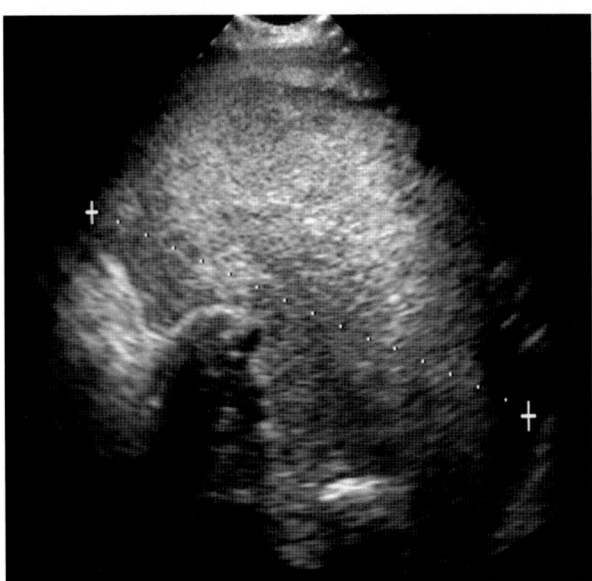

FIGURE 14-6. Acute blood clot. Acute blood clot, secondary to rupture of a pseudoaneurysm at the hepatic artery anastomosis post liver transplantation. Sagittal ultrasound image of the left lower quadrant shows a solid, heterogeneous mass (*calipers*).

exhibit acute angles when in contact with surrounding structures such as bowel loops. Loculated fluid, on the other hand, tends to have rounded margins and show mass effect, frequently displacing surrounding structures from their usual location. Loculated fluid collections can occur anywhere in the abdomen and pelvis. Characterization of fluid and the demonstration of complexity of localized or generalized peritoneal fluid collections are

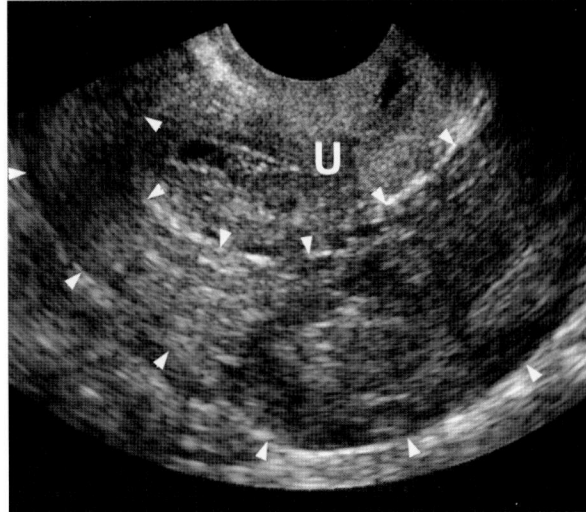

FIGURE 14-7. Pelvic hematoma two days following surgery in a female patient on anticoagulants. Midline, sagittal, transvaginal ultrasound image shows the uterus (U), with fluid in the endometrial canal, surrounded by a large, hypoechoic, heterogeneous hematoma (*arrowheads*).

strengths of ultrasound, and ultrasound is superior to CT scan in this regard (Fig. 14-8A, B).

PERITONEAL INCLUSION CYSTS (BENIGN ENCYSTED FLUID)

The fluid produced by active ovaries in premenopausal patients is usually absorbed by the peritoneum. This balance can be upset by disease processes involving the pelvis, such as previous surgery, trauma, pelvic inflammatory disease, inflammatory bowel disease, or endometriosis. In these situations, the fluid produced by the ovaries may not be absorbed but may become trapped by adhesions. Over time, an **inclusion cyst** forms that frequently encases the ovary and may cause pelvic pain and pressure. Inclusion cysts vary in size and complexity and may be relatively simple or contain internal echoes and septations.[23-25] They often cause confusion when imaging is performed and may be misinterpreted as representing ovarian cysts, parovarian cysts, hydrosalpinges, or even ovarian cancer. The key to the correct diagnosis is to suspect this condition based on the patient's profile and then to demonstrate a **normal ovary,** either within or on the margin of the inclusion cyst, most often with the transvaginal scan (Fig. 14-9A, B).[26]

MESENTERIC CYSTS

Mesenteric cysts are rare intra-abdominal masses that are often discovered incidentally at the time of imaging.

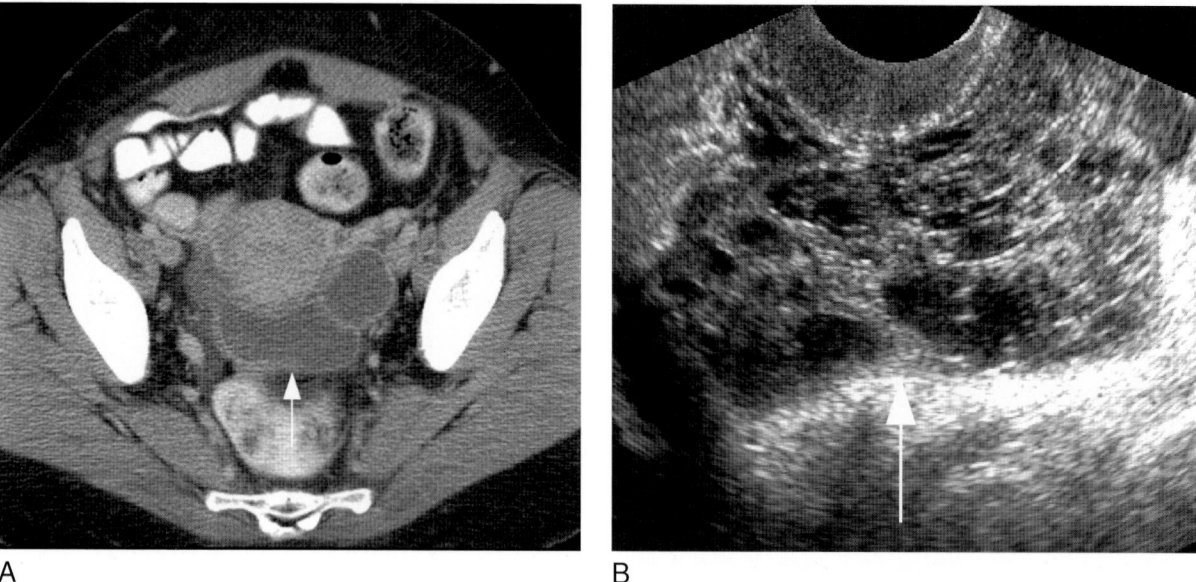

A   B

FIGURE 14-8. Fibrinous peritonitis. A, Axial, oral, and intravenously enhanced CT image through the midpelvis of a female patient shows loculated fluid in the pouch of Douglas and left adnexa with an enhancing rim (*arrow*). **B,** Transverse, transvaginal ultrasound image taken the same day as **A** shows the high degree of complexity of this fluid (*arrow*) to much better advantage.

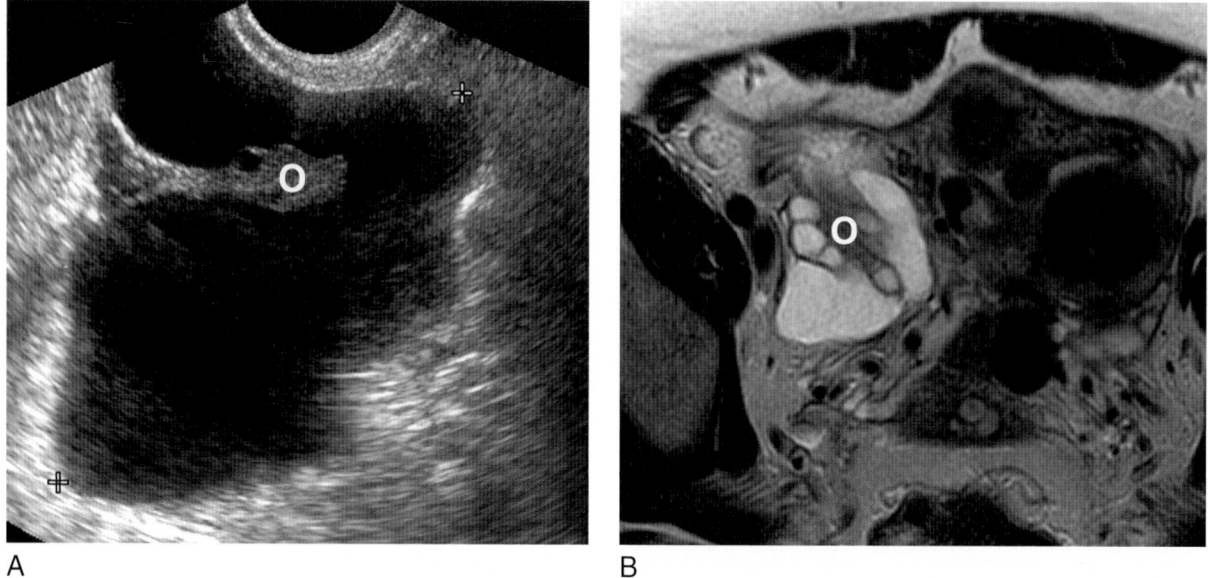

A   B

FIGURE 14-9. Peritoneal inclusion cyst. A, Transverse, transvaginal ultrasound image of the right adnexa and **B,** axial, T2 weighted MRI image through the midpelvis show the normal, right ovary (O) surrounded by encysted fluid, conforming to the contours of the peritoneal cavity.

They may, however, present clinically with abdominal distention because of their size or acutely with pain because of a complication such as hemorrhage, rupture, or torsion. These cysts are most often of lymphatic (**lymphangioma**) or mesothelial origin, but cysts of enteric (**enteric duplication cyst**) and urogenital origin may also be encountered. **Dermoid cysts** and **pseudocysts** (infectious, inflammatory, or traumatic) are also seen.[27] Mesenteric cysts vary in size from less than 1 cm to greater than 25 cm, filling the entire peritoneal cavity.

They may be entirely simple to highly complex with extensive internal septations as is sometimes seen with lymphangiomas (Fig. 14-10A to D).[28,29] Smaller mesenteric cysts are frequently mobile, changing location with palpation or with changes in the patient's position. Asymptomatic cysts are frequently managed conservatively, particularly if they are simple or if they have a typical appearance of a lymphangioma. Surgery is usually reserved to alleviate pressure symptoms or to address acute complications.

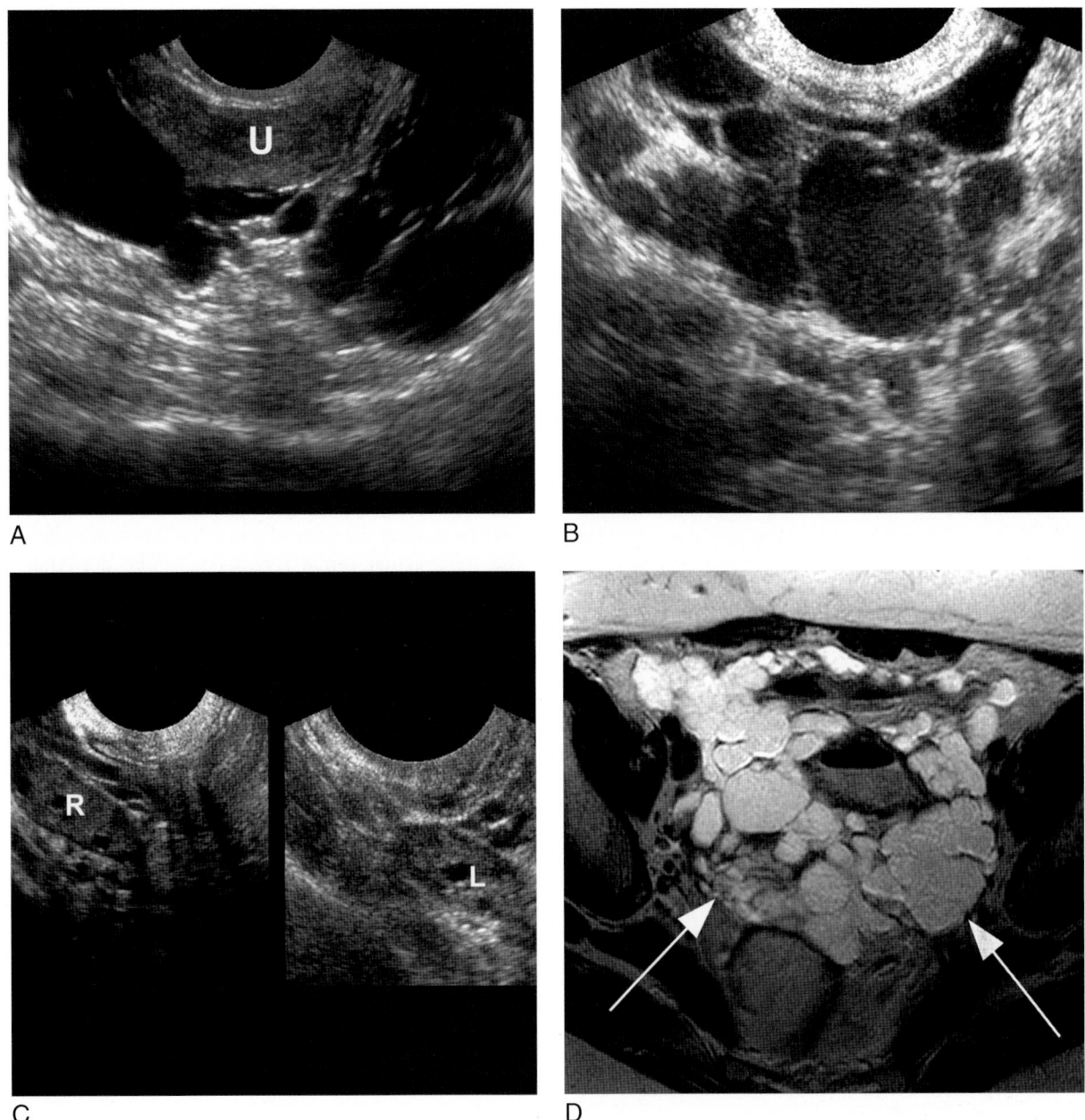

FIGURE 14-10. Pelvic lymphangioma in an asymptomatic woman. A, Transverse transvaginal ultrasound image shows the normal uterus (U) in cross section, surrounded by innumerable cystic spaces with thin septations separating the fluid-filled components. There is no identified nodularity. Real-time examination suggested that these cysts were soft and compliant. **B,** Transvaginal image taken lateral to the uterus shows that the cystic changes are extensive. Their distribution and extent do not suggest an ovarian origin. **C,** Two transvaginal images shown side by side show a normal right (R) and a normal left (L) ovary. This excludes the ovaries as a source of the pathology. **D,** T2-weighted MR image confirms the extensive intraperitoneal cystic masses that show as high signal intensity areas on the scan (*arrows*). The septations between the fluid components are thin.

PERITONEAL TUMORS

Tumors involving the peritoneum are commonly encountered with ultrasound and are generally malignant. **Metastatic tumors** are much more common than **primary peritoneal tumors**. In females, the ovary is the primary site of disease in the vast majority of patients. Other sites of primary disease with a propensity to spread to the peritoneum include the stomach, colon, breast, pancreas, kidney, bladder, uterus, and skin (melanoma).

PERITONEAL CARCINOMATOSIS

Peritoneal carcinomatosis is the term used to describe diffuse involvement of the peritoneum with metastatic disease. Carcinomatous seeding involving the parietal (Fig. 14-11) or visceral peritoneum (Fig. 14-12) may produce discrete hypoechoic nodules, irregular masses, or hypoechoic rindlike thickening of the peritoneum.[15] Ascites is common and may be the only finding. The

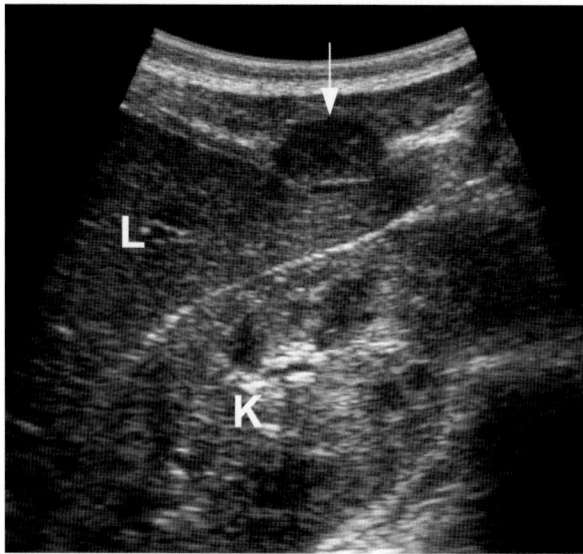

FIGURE 14-11. Parietal peritoneal metastasis from squamous cell carcinoma of the lung. Sagittal image of the right upper quadrant shows a hypoechoic nodule (*arrow*) anterior to the liver (L). With respiration the liver moved freely and independent of the nodule, which stayed stationary, correctly suggesting its location on the parietal peritoneum. (Kidney [K]).

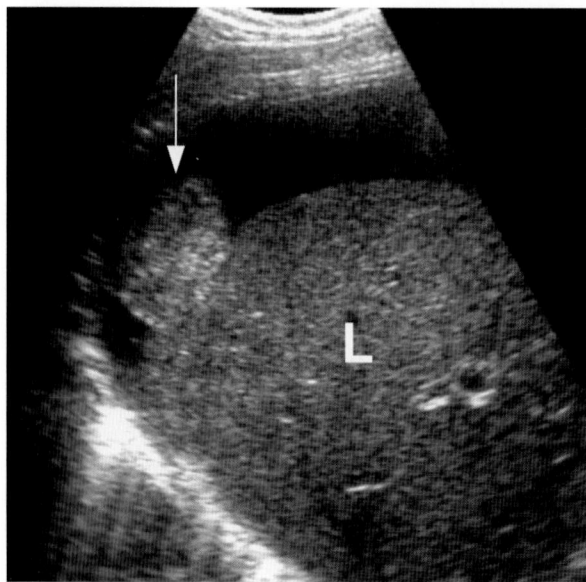

FIGURE 14-12. Visceral peritoneal metastasis from adenocarcinoma of the colon. Sagittal, oblique image of the right upper quadrant shows an echogenic nodule (*arrow*) on the surface of the liver (L), surrounded by ascites. With respiration the nodule moved in concert with the liver, correctly suggesting its location on the visceral peritoneum.

pouch of Douglas, greater omentum, Morison's pouch, and the right subphrenic space are commonly involved sites[30] and, therefore, any sonographic evaluation of the peritoneum for metastatic disease should include careful and detailed assessment of these areas (Figs. 14-13A to E).[26] The parietal peritoneal line is often preserved on sonography with small seeds but is often lost as the lesion increases in size. Growth of a lesion is usually inward, toward the peritoneal cavity, but growth outward with invasion of the abdominal wall can occur (Fig. 14-14). If **psammomatous calcification** occurs within a peritoneal nodule, it appears echogenic with ultrasound, and if the calcification is dense, it may demonstrate posterior acoustic shadowing (Fig. 14-15).

Peritoneal carcinomatosis can be detected with ultrasound in the absence of ascites (Figs. 14-16 and 14-17A, B), but its presence greatly enhances the detection of peritoneal lesions, where nodules as small as 2 to 3 mm may be seen on the parietal and visceral peritoneum with the transvaginal probe (Fig. 14-18). The detection of omental involvement is also enhanced by ascites. Infiltration of the omentum leads to an **"omental cake"**[31] which may float freely in the ascitic fluid (Fig. 14-19).[26] Alternatively, the omentum may be adherent to the parietal peritoneum in the near field (Fig. 14-20) or be deeper in the peritoneal cavity, adherent to the visceral peritoneum and surrounding small bowel loops (Fig. 14-21). **Thickening of the mesentery, mesenteric nodules,** and **lymphadenopathy** are other possible features of carcinomatosis.

After the full extent of peritoneal involvement has been documented with ultrasound, a careful search should be made for the primary lesion within the abdomen and pelvis if it has not already been identified. This search should not be limited to the solid organs, gallbladder, and bile ducts but should also include assessment of the stomach and bowel.

PRIMARY TUMORS OF THE PERITONEUM

Primary tumors of the peritoneum are extremely rare and **primary peritoneal serous papillary carcinoma (PPSPC), malignant mesothelioma,** and **lymphoma** are the most common. PPSPC is a multicentric peritoneal tumor that is morphologically identical to ovarian serous papillary carcinoma (OSPC) of equivalent grade but that can spare or minimally invade the ovaries.[32] Women with PPSPC are more likely to present with ascites than women with OSPC and have a worse three-year survival rate.[33] With imaging the typical features of peritoneal carcinomatosis may be demonstrated but no obvious primary site will be seen. (Fig. 14-22A-D).[26,34-36] The ovaries are generally normal in size but may be enlarged by surface involvement.

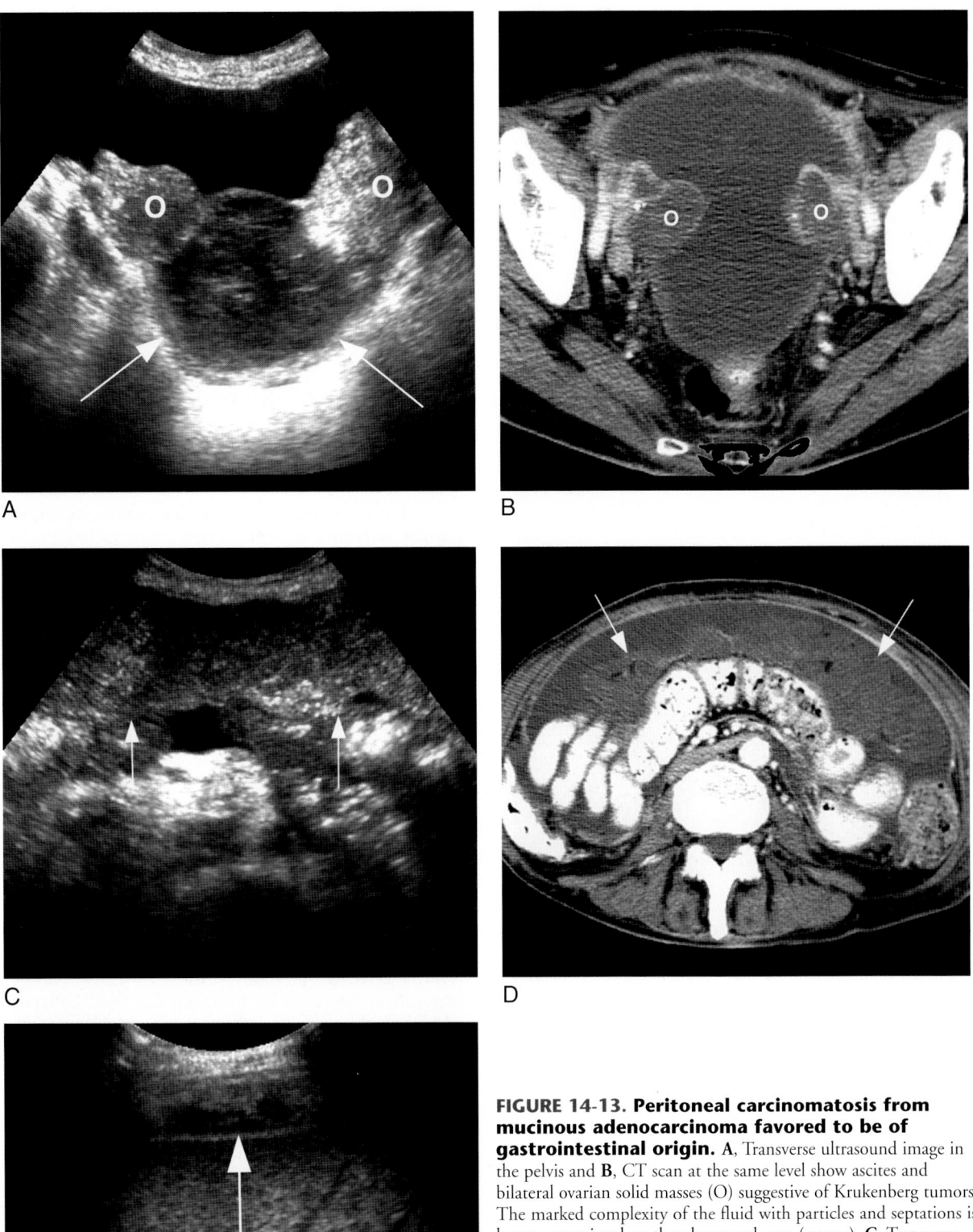

A

B

C

D

E

FIGURE 14-13. Peritoneal carcinomatosis from mucinous adenocarcinoma favored to be of gastrointestinal origin. A, Transverse ultrasound image in the pelvis and **B,** CT scan at the same level show ascites and bilateral ovarian solid masses (O) suggestive of Krukenberg tumors. The marked complexity of the fluid with particles and septations is better appreciated on the ultrasound scan (*arrows*). **C,** Transverse midabdominal ultrasound image and **D,** corresponding CT scan both show a thick omental cake (*arrows*) displacing bowel loops posteriorly in the peritoneal cavity. There is also a small volume of free fluid. **E,** Sagittal ultrasound image in the right upper quadrant shows a rim of complex, mixed echogenic material overlying and indenting the convexity of the liver (*arrow*). There is echogenic nodularity on the parietal peritoneum of the diaphragm. This did not move with the liver with respiration, confirming its origin from the parietal peritoneum.

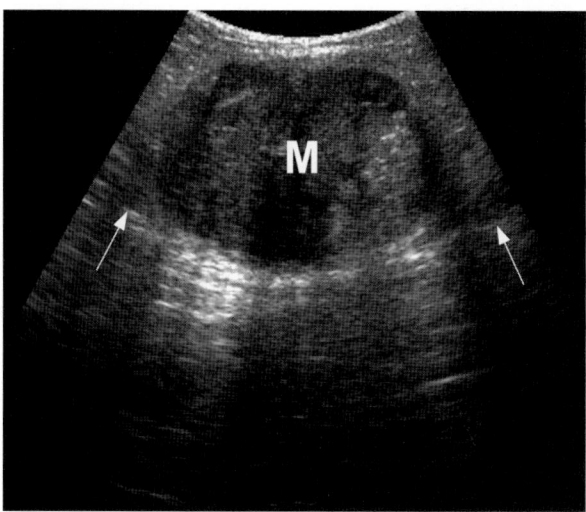

FIGURE 14-14. Abdominal wall seed in a patient with known peritoneal carcinomatosis. Transverse ultrasound image of the midabdomen shows a hypoechoic solid mass (M) in the anterior abdominal wall, superficial to the parietal peritoneum (*arrows*).

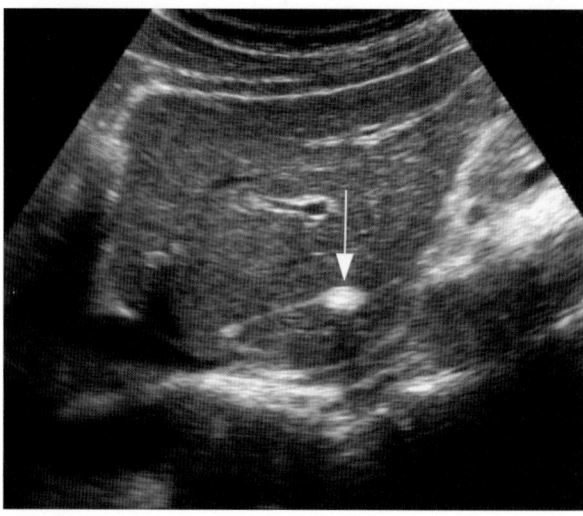

FIGURE 14-15. Stage 3, well-differentiated papillary serous ovarian cancer. Sagittal ultrasound image through the liver shows a calcified implant (*arrow*) in the ligamentum venosum, with posterior acoustic shadowing.

Primary peritoneal mesothelioma accounts for 33% of all cases of mesothelioma[37] and is most common in middle-aged men. The tumor proves invariably fatal and like mesothelioma of the pleura, there is an association with asbestos exposure. Up to 65% of chest radiographs show evidence of asbestos exposure at the time of diagnosis. In this condition, the parietal and visceral peritoneum are diffusely thickened or are extensively involved by tumor plaques or nodules. These plaques and nodules may aggregate to form discrete masses. The viscera may be encased or invaded by tumor. Ascites is a common finding and is seen in up to 90% of cases.[38] As with peritoneal carcinomatosis, the nodules and

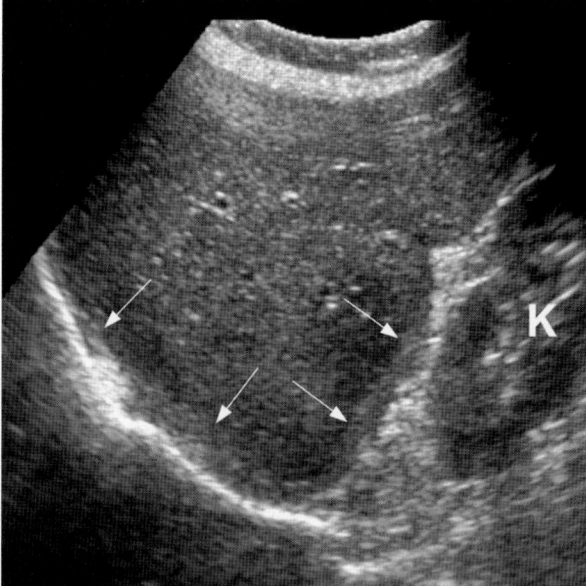

FIGURE 14-16. Stage 3 papillary serous ovarian cancer without ascites. Sagittal ultrasound image in the right upper quadrant shows a subtle, thin, echogenic "rind" of seeding (*arrows*) on the surface of the liver, extending into Morison's pouch. (Kidney [K]).

plaques are often hypoechoic (Fig. 14-23A to C). Pleural effusions and pleural plaques may also be appreciated with ultrasound. The solid organs should be evaluated for direct invasion or metastases. Ultrasound-guided biopsy can be performed to confirm the diagnosis.[39] Generally, core biopsies from a number of locations are required because of difficulty sometimes encountered in establishing the diagnosis.

Primary lymphoma of the peritoneum is extremely rare and is the non-Hodgkin's variety.[40] There is an increased incidence in AIDS patients.[41] Again features include diffuse peritoneal seeding, often with more focal masses. Lymphomatous masses may be extremely hypoechoic and can be mistaken for fluid collections with cursory assessment (Fig. 14-24A, B).

Pseudomyxoma Peritonei

Pseudomyxoma peritonei (PP) is a rare, often fatal intra-abdominal disease characterized by dissecting gelatinous ascites and multifocal peritoneal implants of columnar epithelium that secrete copious globules of extracellular mucin.[42] Controversy surrounds the origin of PP. Some studies suggest synchronous ovarian and appendiceal tumors in 90% of patients,[43] whereas most now believe that the condition nearly always originates from a perforated appendiceal epithelial tumor.[44] The disease process tends to remain localized to the peritoneal cavity, and extraperitoneal spread is rare. The disease encompasses benign, borderline, and malignant mucinous neoplasms resulting in a variable and poorly

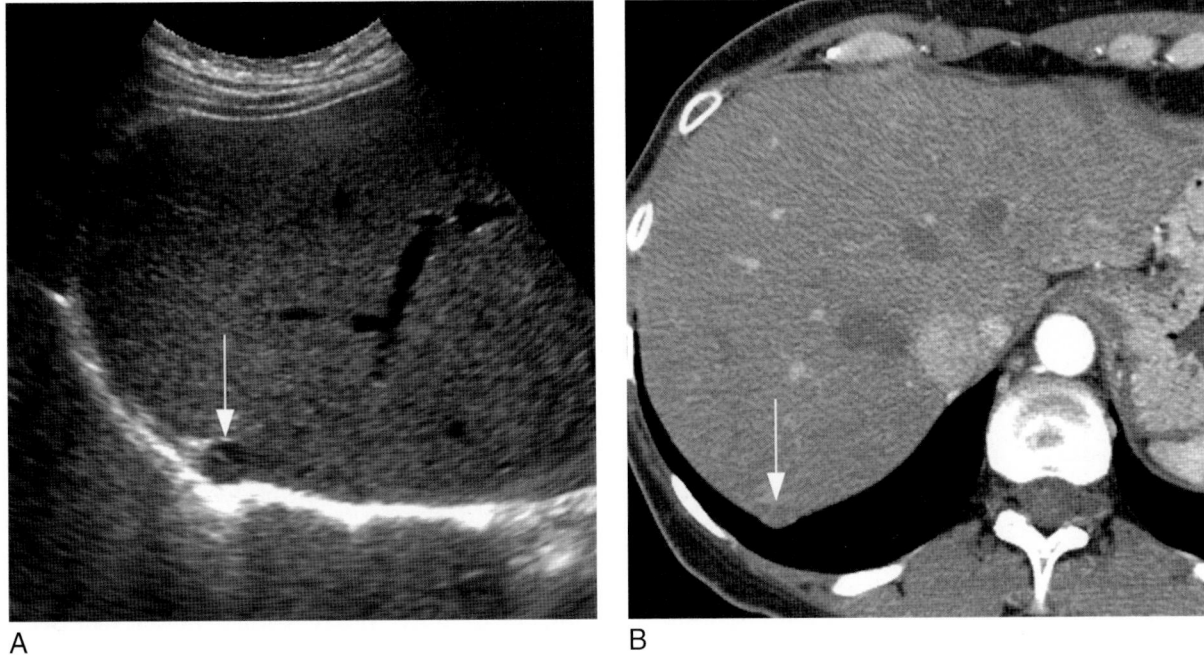

FIGURE 14-17. Peritoneal implant without ascites. A, Transverse ultrasound image and **B,** axial CT image of the right upper quadrant show a small peritoneal implant (*arrow*) overlying segment 7 of the liver. Note that the implant is better appreciated on the ultrasound image.

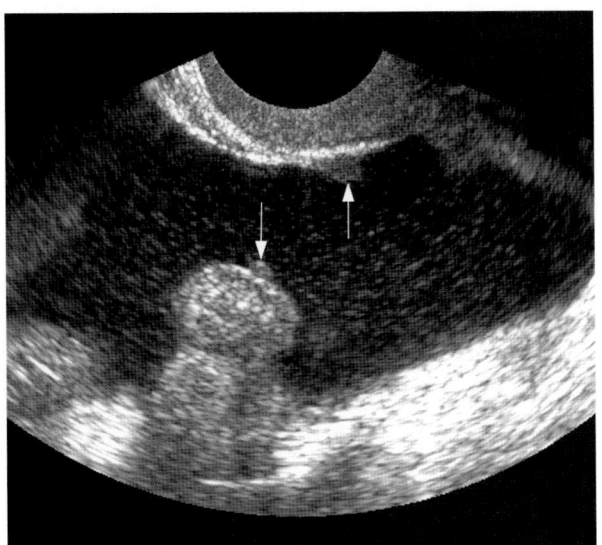

FIGURE 14-18. Peritoneal carcinomatosis from ovarian cancer. Sagittal, oblique, transvaginal ultrasound image shows small (<5 mm), parietal (near-field), and visceral (far-field) peritoneal implants (*arrows*), surrounded by particulate ascites.

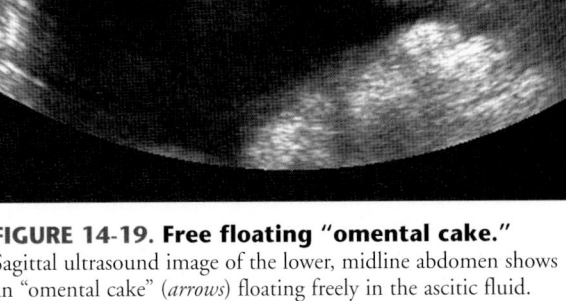

FIGURE 14-19. Free floating "omental cake." Sagittal ultrasound image of the lower, midline abdomen shows an "omental cake" (*arrows*) floating freely in the ascitic fluid. Note the free edge of the abnormal greater omentum inferiorly.

predictable prognosis. An overall 5-year survival of 40% to 50% is suggested from the literature, depending on cell type.[45]

Patients present with abdominal pain and distention. Ultimately the bowel becomes encased with mucinous material and bowel obstruction may occur. Repeated surgical intervention to remove the accumulated mucinous material remains the treatment of choice.[46] Perioperative intraperitoneal chemotherapy may add additional benefit.[47] Because patients present with abdominal symptoms, the diagnosis is frequently made preoperatively by ultrasound or CT.[48] Sonography frequently shows complex ascites reflecting the gelatinous nature of the fluid. The echogenic foci within the

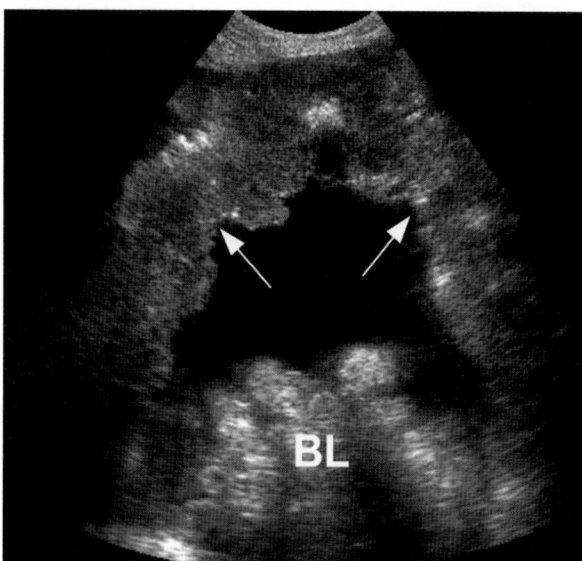

FIGURE 14-20. "Omental cake" adherent to the parietal peritoneum. Transverse ultrasound image of the midabdomen shows an "omental cake" (*arrows*) in the near-field, adherent to the parietal peritoneum. Small bowel loops (BL) are visible in the far-field outlined by ascites.

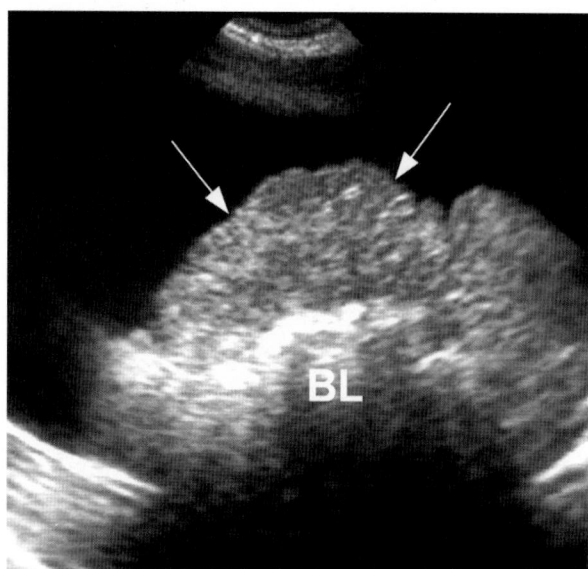

FIGURE 14-21. "Omental cake" adherent to the visceral peritoneum. Transverse ultrasound image of the midabdomen shows a thick omental cake (*arrows*) adherent to the visceral peritoneum and encasing gas-filled, small bowel loops (BL).

fluid are nonmobile and the bowel loops, instead of floating freely, are displaced centrally and posteriorly by the surrounding mass, giving a characteristic **"starburst"** appearance (Fig. 14-25A to I).[26] **Scalloping** of the liver is another typical feature of PP.[49] Ultrasound may be helpful to guide paracentesis in these patients, because less viscous areas may be identified, with a greater likelihood of successful aspiration.

INFLAMMATORY DISEASE OF THE PERITONEUM

Peritonitis is defined as diffuse inflammation of the parietal and visceral peritoneum and can occur as a result of infectious and noninfectious causes. **Infectious causes** include bacteria (including tuberculosis [TB]), viruses, fungi, and parasites. **Noninfectious causes** are less common and include chemical peritonitis (secondary to gastric or pancreatic juice or bile), granulomatous peritonitis (secondary to foreign bodies such as talc), and sclerosing peritonitis associated with continuous ambulatory peritoneal dialysis (CAPD).

Most cases of infective peritonitis are bacterial, secondary to complications of disease processes involving intra-abdominal organs. Common causes include **bowel necrosis secondary to ischemia, perforated appendicitis, perforated diverticulitis, perforated duodenal ulcer, inflammatory bowel disease**, or **postoperative leaks**. Culture of the exudate generally reveals a **mixed flora** in this setting, with gram-negative bacilli and anaerobes predominating.

Primary or **spontaneous bacterial peritonitis (SBP)** is much less common. It occurs predominantly in association with cirrhosis and nephrotic syndrome. The clinical findings are often subtle, and correct diagnosis requires a high index of suspicion. It should be considered in any cirrhotic patient with ascites, fever, and an unexplained clinical deterioration. Culture of the ascitic fluid will characteristically reveal a single organism, usually *Escherichia coli*.

The sonographic appearance of infective peritonitis varies but may include particulate ascites (Fig. 14-26A), loculated ascites or ascitic fluid containing septations (Fig. 14-27A to C), debris, or gas.[50] Diffuse thickening of the parietal and visceral peritoneum (see Fig. 14-26B), mesentery, and omentum may also be observed, and heterogeneous exudate may be seen interposed between bowel loops.

Peritonitis secondary to viruses, fungi, or parasites is rare and usually occurs in immunocompromised patients or those on CAPD. **Echinococcal disease** may involve the peritoneum.[51] A hepatic or splenic cyst may rupture, resulting in diffuse seeding of the peritoneal cavity. Ultrasound may reveal one or more of the typical appearances of hydatid cysts, including daughter cysts, the sonographic "water lily sign," or multiple, closely folded echogenic membranes within the cyst cavity.

Abscess

Abscesses may occur at the site of a localized perforation or as a result of delayed treatment of peritonitis, in which case they often develop in dependent areas of the abdomen and pelvis. The subphrenic or subhepatic

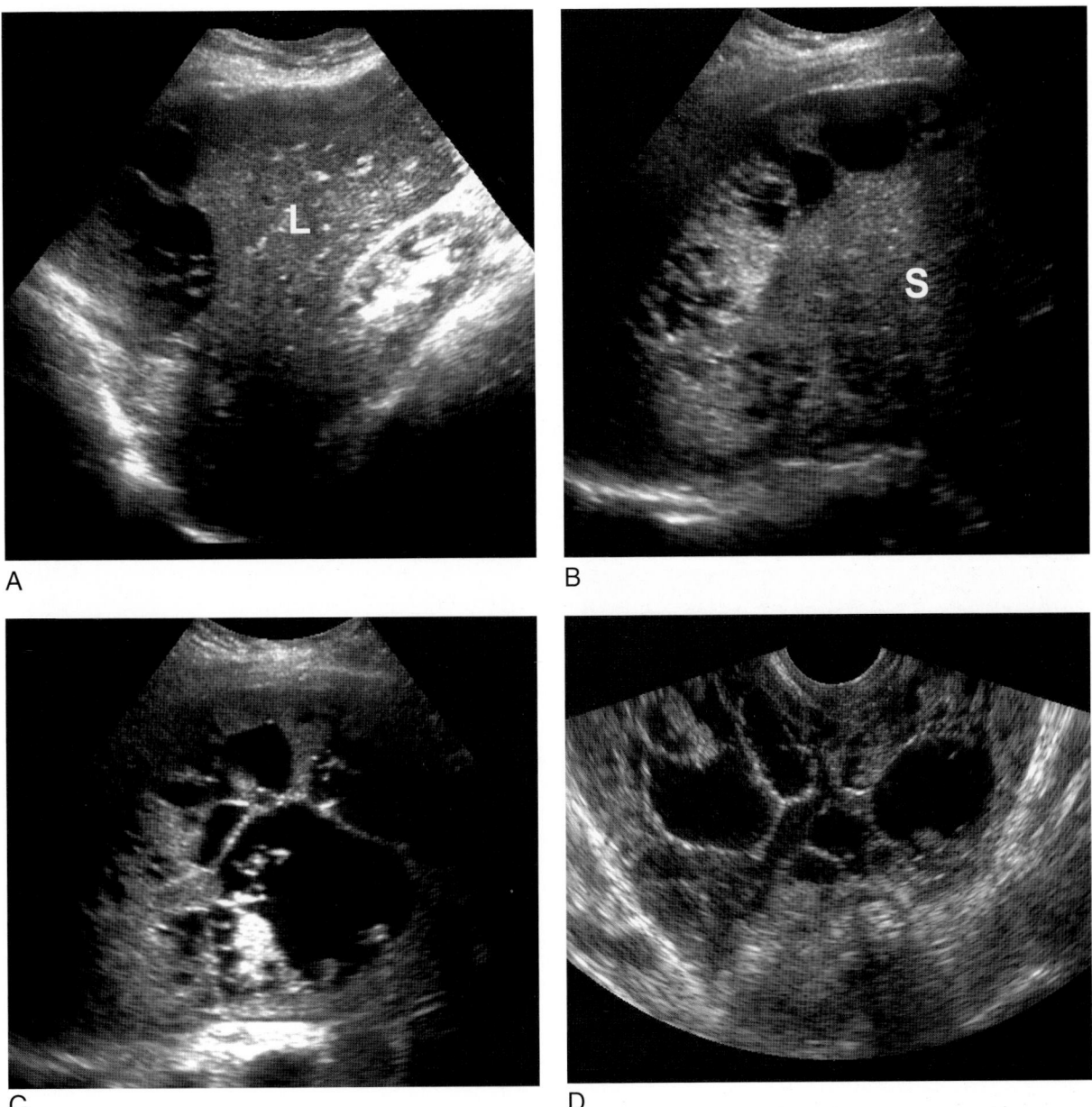

FIGURE 14-22. Primary peritoneal serous papillary carcinoma. A, Sagittal ultrasound image shows a highly complex peritoneal mass between the right hemidiaphragm and the liver (L). The liver border is scalloped. **B,** Sagittal ultrasound image in the left upper quadrant shows a similar complex peritoneal mass over the convexity of the spleen (S). **C,** Midabdominal image shows a complex peritoneal cystic and solid mass of enormous size. **D,** Transvaginal image taken in the pouch of Douglas shows no normal tissue. The entire pouch is filled with a complex cystic and solid tumor.

spaces and the pouch of Douglas are common locations. Ultrasound is often limited in detecting intra-abdominal abscesses, particularly in postoperative patients. These patients are less mobile because of their recent surgery and frequently have open wounds and dressings, limiting access for the ultrasound probe. In addition, visibility is often limited by extensive bowel gas, a result of paralytic ileus. In this setting, it may prove extremely difficult to distinguish between a dilated, aperistaltic, fluid- or gas-filled bowel loop and an extraluminal abscess collection.

Recognized features of intra-abdominal abscesses include round or oval fluid collections with well-defined and irregular walls. They commonly contain internal debris and septations (Figs. 14-28 and 14-29) and occasionally small pockets of gas that appear as echogenic

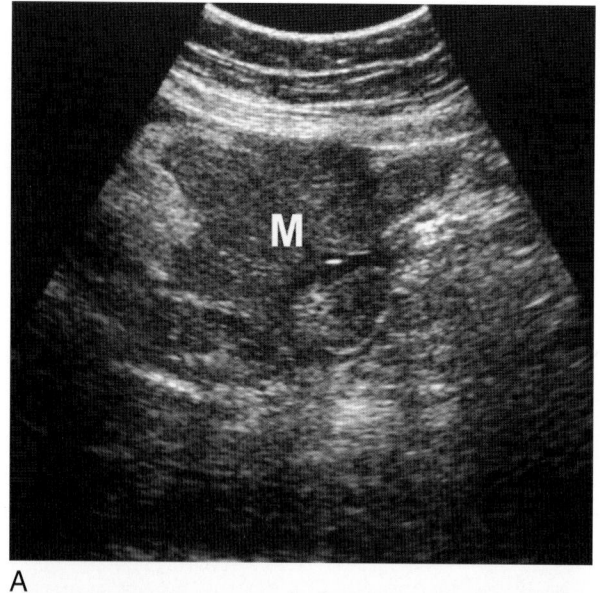

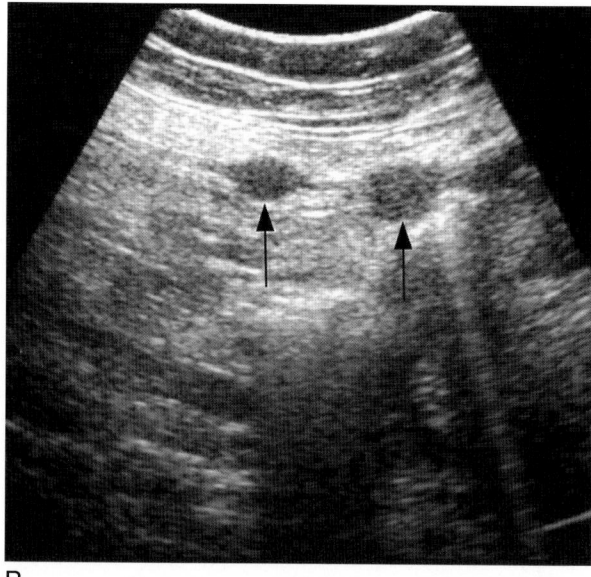

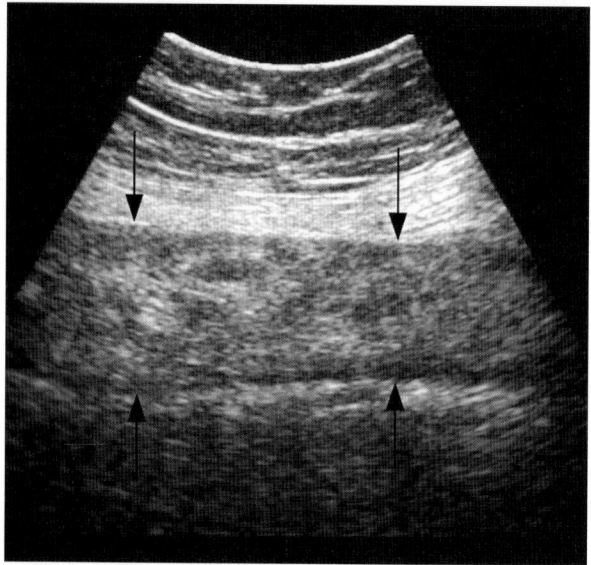

FIGURE 14-23. Peritoneal mesothelioma. A, Sagittal ultrasound image of the left upper quadrant shows a lobulated, heterogeneous mass (M) involving the greater omentum. **B,** Sagittal image in the lower abdomen shows two small, hypoechoic implants in the near-field (*arrows*). **C,** Sagittal image of the right lower quadrant shows an omental cake (*arrows*). Note absence of ascites.

foci with ultrasound, often with posterior reverberation artifact. The presence of gas within a collection is virtually diagnostic of infection.[52] Ultrasound- or CT-guided percutaneous drainage is generally the treatment of choice, and follow-up sonographic examinations are helpful at assessing response to therapeutic intervention.

Tuberculous Peritonitis

Tuberculosis (TB) is still prevalent in developing countries and there has been a recent resurgence in the developed world, particularly among AIDS patients and among the immigrant population.[53] Others at risk include alcoholics and those with cirrhosis. Of all non-AIDS patients with TB, extrapulmonary disease occurs

in only 10% to 15%. This incidence of extrapulmonary disease rises to over 50% in those with AIDS.[54] The peritoneum is a common site of extrapulmonary involvement, and the chest radiograph in these patients will show evidence of pulmonary TB in only 14% of cases. Therefore, a high index of suspicion, particularly in high risk groups, and knowledge of the sonographic features commonly encountered, allow for earlier diagnosis of this potentially curable disease, thus reducing morbidity and mortality.

There are no pathognomonic **sonographic features** for TB peritonitis but, in the right clinical setting, a diffuse peritoneal process may strongly suggest the diagnosis. Ascites is frequently present and may be free or loculated. It may be anechoic or—more frequently—

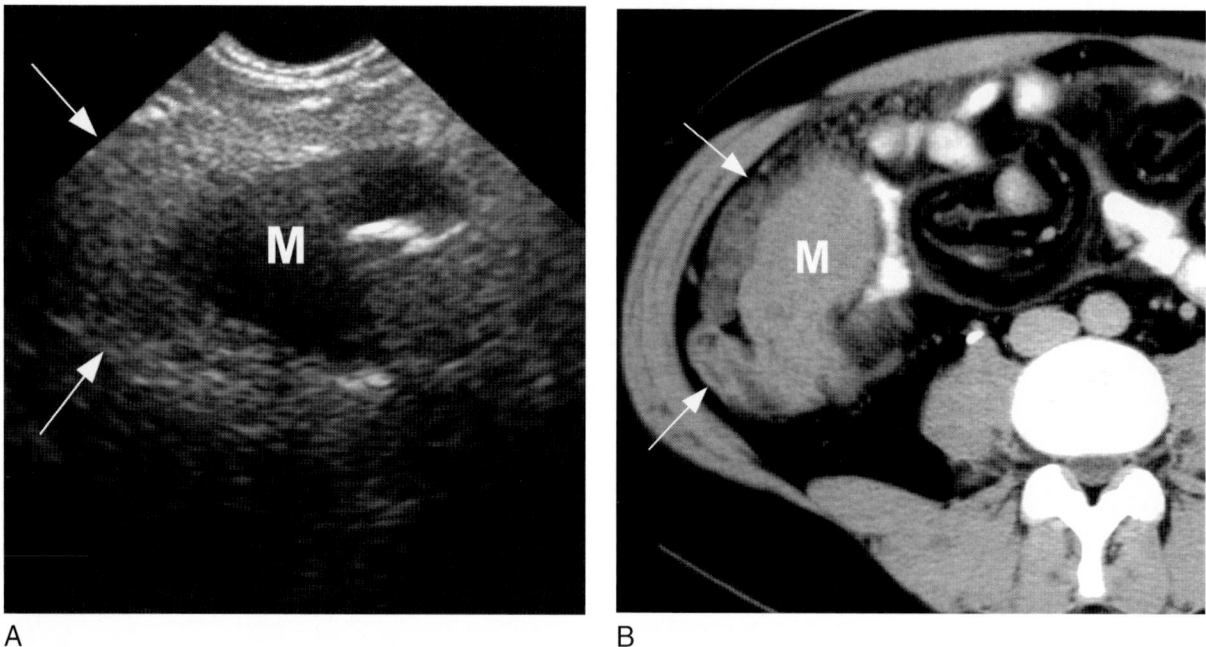

FIGURE 14-24. Non-Hodgkin's lymphoma of the peritoneum. A, Transverse ultrasound image and **B,** axial CT image of the right lower quadrant show a mass (M) displacing bowel loops medially. Infiltrated fat (*arrows*) is seen lateral to mass as echogenic mass-effect on the sonogram.

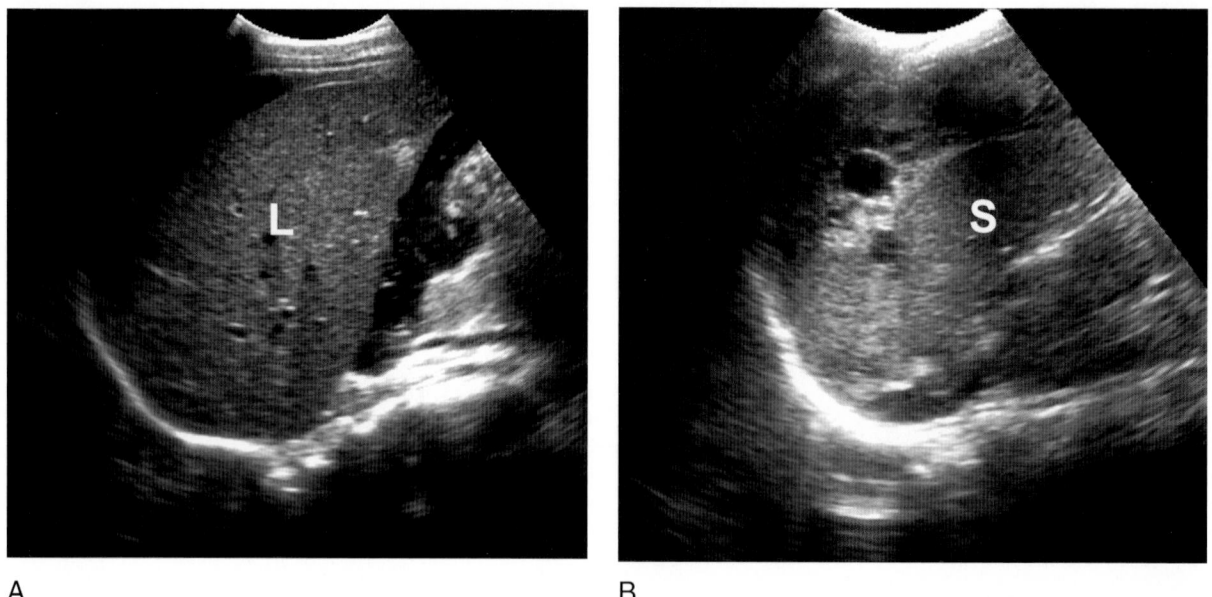

FIGURE 14-25. Pseudomyxoma peritonei. A, Sagittal ultrasound image of the right upper quadrant shows complex fluid surrounding the liver (L). There is very mild and subtle scalloping of the deep border of the liver. **B,** Sagittal ultrasound image of the left upper quadrant shows the spleen (S) surrounded by highly complex and echogenic fluid. The echogenic components of the fluid do not move with gravity. There is an indentation on the convexity of the spleen where the peritoneal process appears to invaginate the splenic parenchyma.

Continued

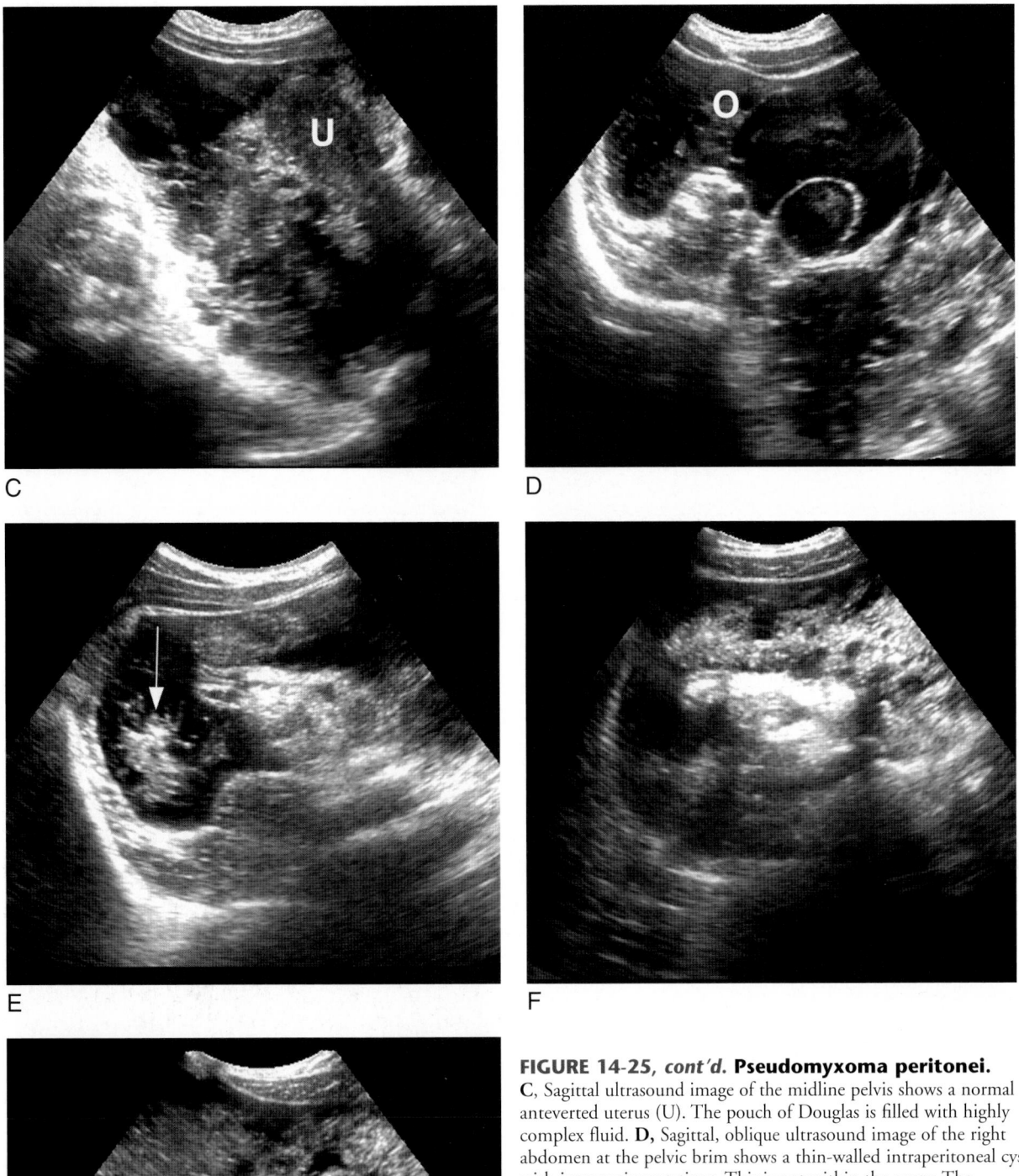

FIGURE 14-25, *cont'd.* **Pseudomyxoma peritonei.**
C, Sagittal ultrasound image of the midline pelvis shows a normal anteverted uterus (U). The pouch of Douglas is filled with highly complex fluid. **D,** Sagittal, oblique ultrasound image of the right abdomen at the pelvic brim shows a thin-walled intraperitoneal cyst with intracystic septations. This is not within the ovary. The normal right ovary (O) with small follicles is seen adjacent to the intraperitoneal cyst. The normal left ovary was seen elsewhere.
E, Transverse image in the right paracolic gutter shows a starburst appearance within the fluid *(arrow)*. This is associated, in our experience, with the presence of mucin in the peritoneal cavity.
F, Shows a highly echogenic plaquelike structure anteriorly representing a very thick and abnormal omentum, an "omental cake." There are hypoechoic nodules within the cake that are highly suggestive of tumor deposits. **G,** Also taken in the peritoneal cavity, this image shows that the loops of bowel are compressed deep into the abdomen by the overlying abnormal and thick fluid and the omental cake.

Continued

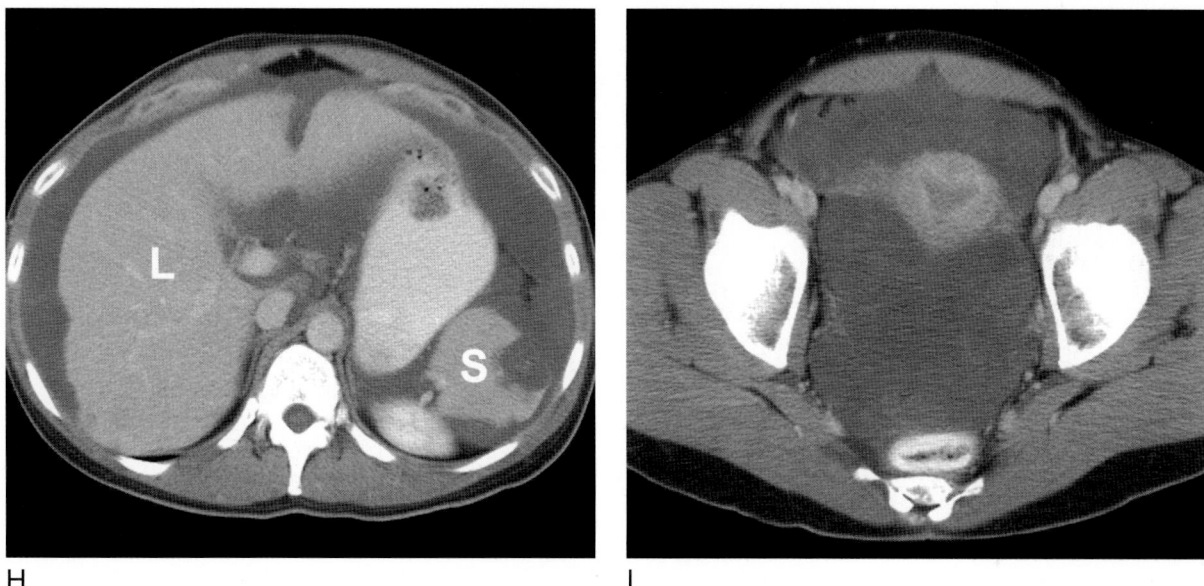

FIGURE 14-25, cont'd. Pseudomyxoma peritonei. H and I are CT images taken in the upper abdomen and the pelvis, respectively (liver [L], spleen [S]). They confirm the extensive peritoneal process, the organ scalloping, and the pouch of Douglas full of complex fluid.

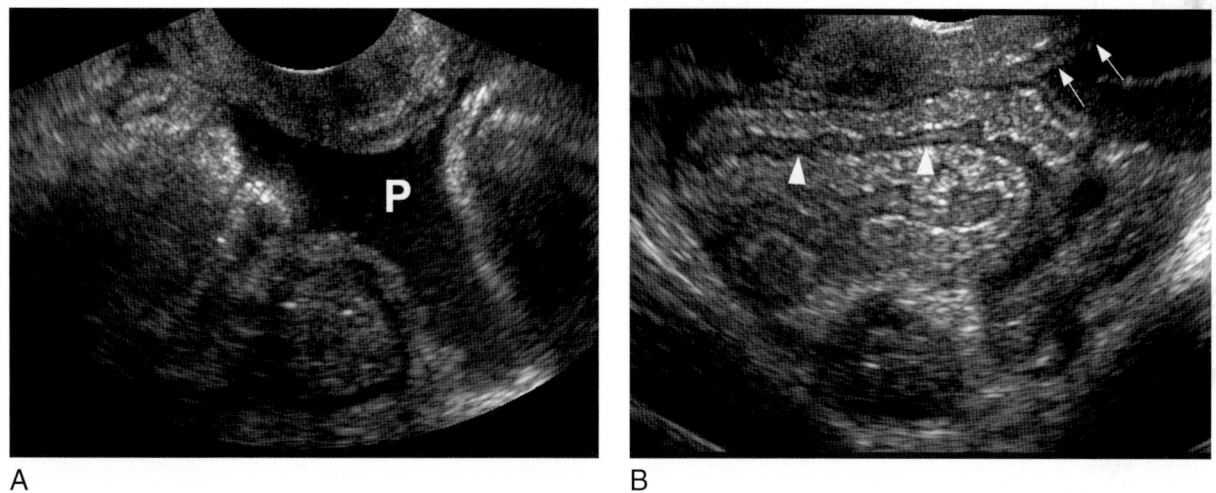

FIGURE 14-26. Suppurative peritonitis. A, Transverse, transvaginal ultrasound image of the pouch of Douglas shows particulate free fluid (P). B, Transverse transvaginal ultrasound image more anteriorly in the pelvis shows diffuse thickening of both the parietal (*arrows*) and visceral (*arrowheads*) peritoneum. An S-shaped, small bowel loop is seen meandering through the thickened visceral peritoneum.

particulate and contain fine mobile strands composed of fibrin (Fig. 14-30A, B). These strands may produce a latticelike pattern. Irregular and nodular hypoechoic thickening of the peritoneum, mesentery, and omentum is another feature.[55] Associated lymphadenopathy in the mesentery and retroperitoneum is a very common feature and is more common than in peritoneal carcinomatosis.[56,57] The nodes may be discrete or conglomerate due to periadenitis. Caseation may give rise to a hypoechoic center within the node, although a similar appearance can be seen with metastatic lymph nodes undergoing necrosis. Echogenic nodes due to fat deposi-

tion may suggest the diagnosis of TB. Sonographic assessment of the solid viscera may show involvement, particularly hypoechoic masses in the spleen. Ultrasound is very helpful at guiding diagnostic paracentesis in this condition and may also guide fine-needle aspiration of enlarged nodes. It can also readily document response to treatment.

Sclerosing Peritonitis

Sclerosing peritonitis is a major complication of CAPD and is characterized by the formation of a connective

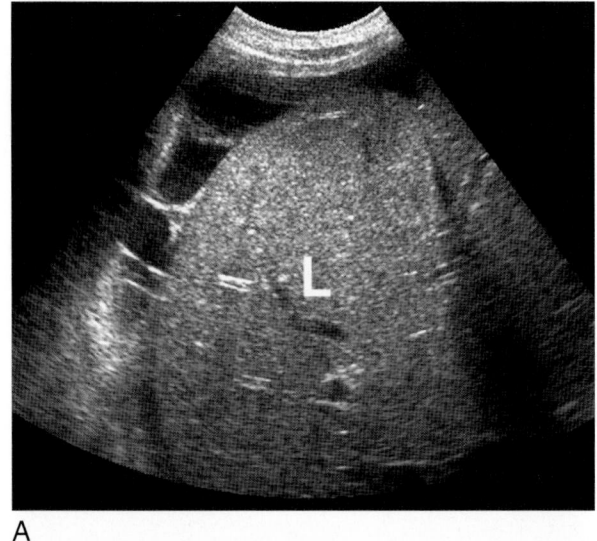

A

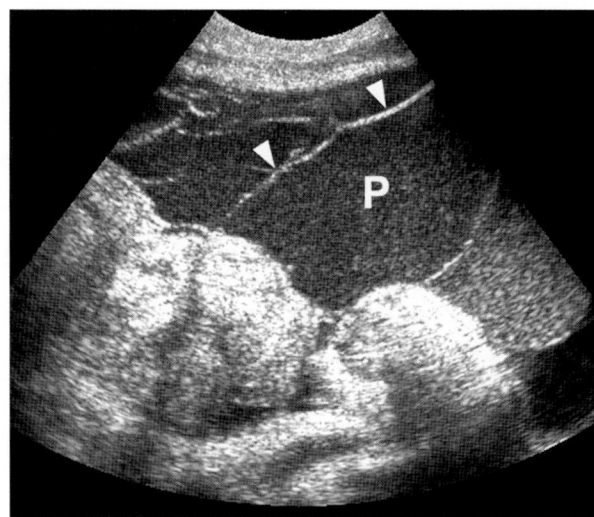

B

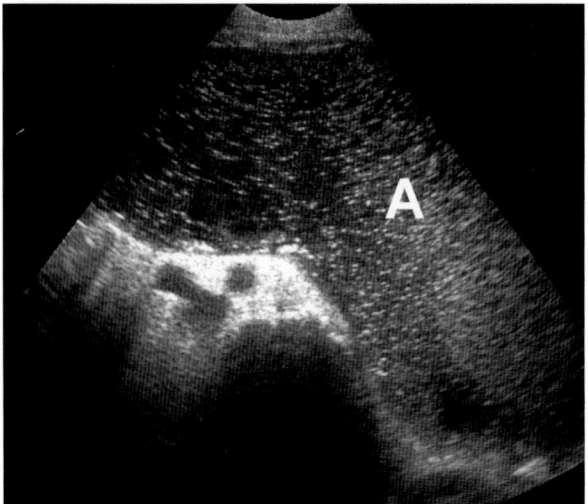

C

FIGURE 14-27. Spontaneous bacterial peritonitis.
A, Transverse, oblique ultrasound image of the right upper quadrant shows ascites with septations surrounding the right lobe of the liver (L). **B,** Sagittal and **C,** transverse images of the mid/lower abdomen show particulate fluid (P) with extensive septations (*arrowheads*). Bowel loops are displaced posteriorly.

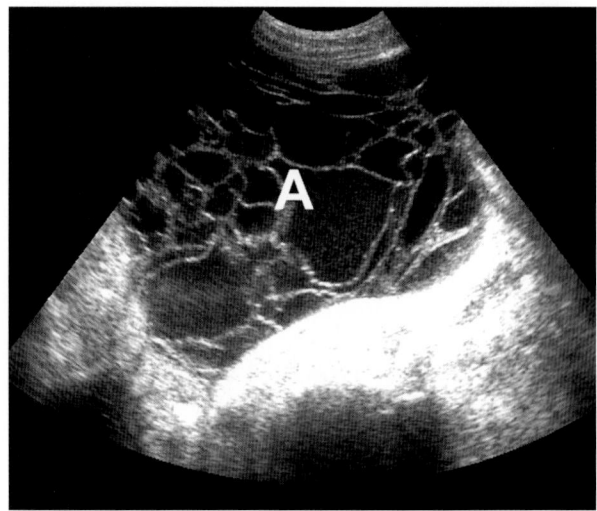

FIGURE 14-28. Abscess. Transverse ultrasound image of the midabdomen shows a large abscess collection (A).

FIGURE 14-29. Abscess. Sagittal ultrasound image of the right lower quadrant shows a large abscess collection with internal septations (A).

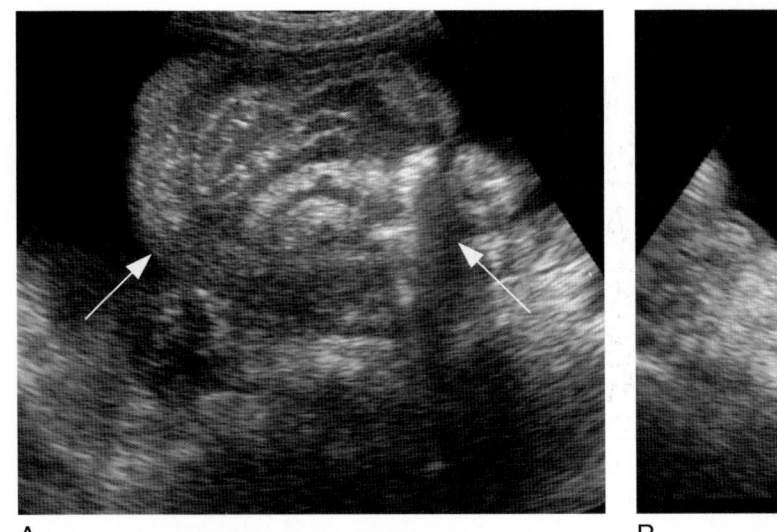

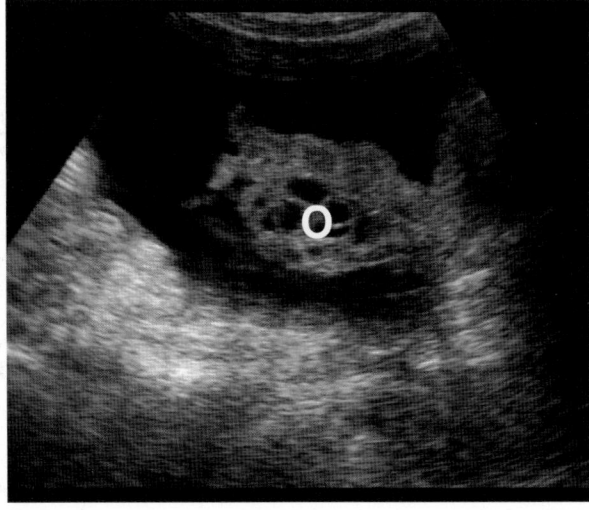

A   B

FIGURE 14-30. Tuberculous peritonitis. A, Transverse, midline ultrasound image shows "matted" bowel loops (*arrows*) surrounded by ascites. Note thickening of the visceral peritoneum. **B,** Sagittal ultrasound image of the left adnexa shows the ovary (O) embedded in thickened visceral peritoneum and surrounded by ascites.

tissue membrane covering the peritoneum and eventually encasing and strangulating bowel loops.[58,59] Patients initially complain of abdominal pain and loss of ultrafiltration. Ultimately, bowel obstruction occurs. Surgery is often difficult in these patients and the prognosis is poor. Early diagnosis of the disease may be important in reducing mortality.

Ultrasound is very helpful in diagnosing this condition.[60] Increased peristalsis in multiple bowel loops is one of the earliest findings. Ascites, both free and loculated, is common. With time, the fluid becomes more complex with stranding (Fig. 14-31). Bowel loops become matted together and are tethered to the posterior abdominal wall by a characteristic **enveloping membrane**. This membrane can be seen with ultrasound as a uniformly echogenic layer measuring 1 to 4 mm in thickness.

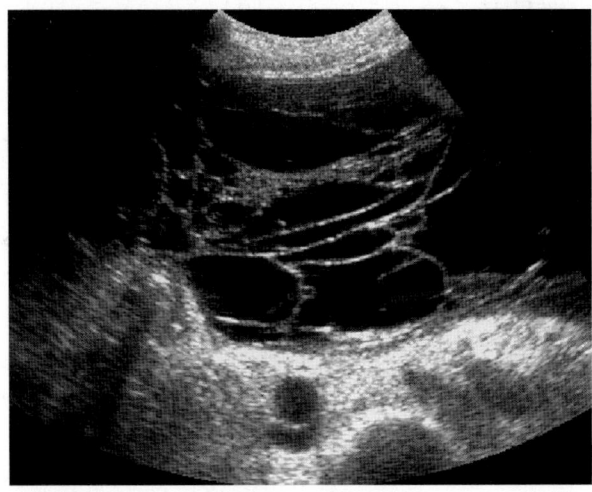

FIGURE 14-31. Sclerosing peritonitis. Transverse ultrasound image of the midabdomen shows extensive, complex, septated ascites.

LOCALIZED INFLAMMATORY PROCESS OF THE PERITONEAL CAVITY

The CT appearance and significance of inflamed peritoneal fat is well known to imagers. If ultrasound is to be successful at investigating patients with abdominal symptoms, the sonographic appearance of inflamed fat must be as familiar.

Inflamed perienteric fat appears as an **echogenic "mass effect"** with ultrasound frequently displacing bowel loops out of the scanning plane. Compression sonography may greatly enhance the detection of focally inflamed fat, and gentle palpation with the transducer over this area will frequently show that it is the site of the patient's maximal tenderness. Frequently, there will be an associated, underlying abnormality, such as an abnormal bowel segment, that can be identified with ultrasound (Fig. 14-32).[61] **Appendicitis** and **diverticulitis** are the most common acute processes giving rise to focally inflamed fat. Other possibilities include **inflammatory bowel disease, pancreatitis,** and **complicated acute cholecystitis.** Progression to phlegmon typically shows development of a hypoechoic region within the echogenic fat without fluid content (Fig. 14-33). If untreated this may progress to abscess formation. Color Doppler imaging frequently shows increased blood flow in the area of inflammation.[62]

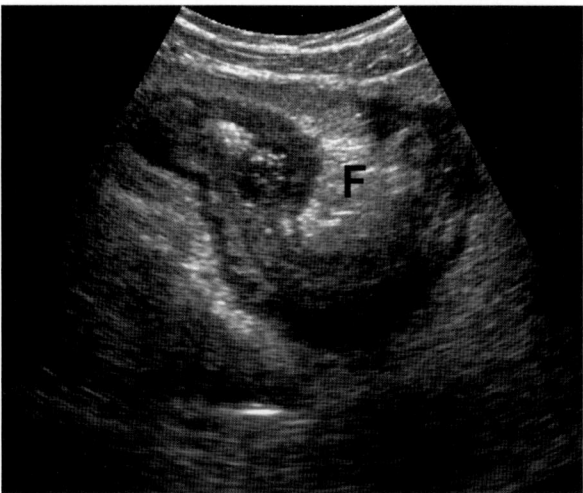

FIGURE 14-32. Inflamed fat. Transverse ultrasound image of the right lower quadrant shows echogenic, inflamed fat (F) associated with a long segment of thickened terminal ileum in a patient with Crohn's disease.

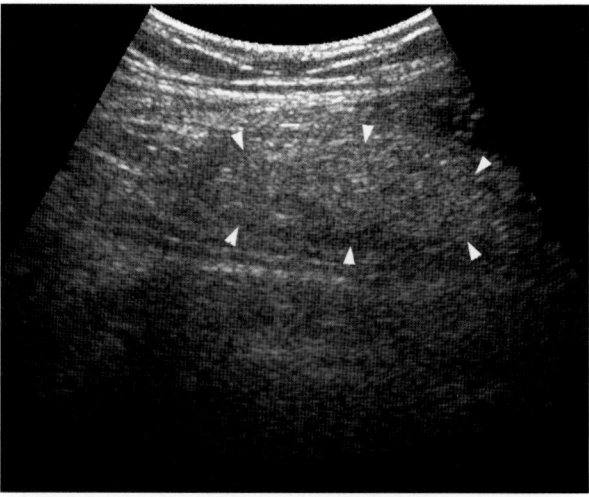

FIGURE 14-34. Right-sided segmental omental infarction. Sagittal image of the right midabdomen shows an ovoid echogenic mass (*arrowheads*). This was the site of the patient's maximal tenderness.

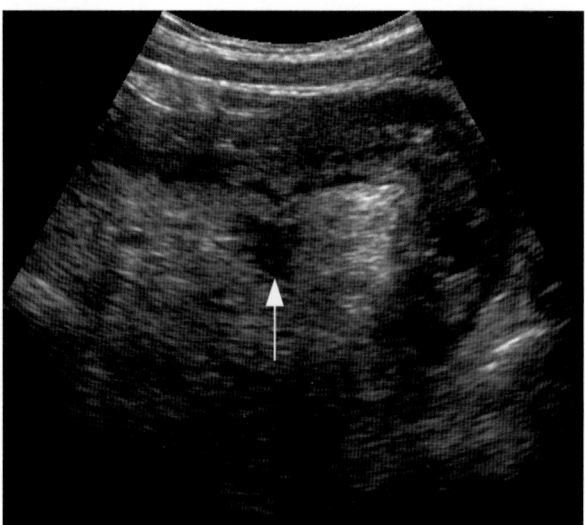

FIGURE 14-33. Inflamed fat with phlegmon. Sagittal, oblique ultrasound image of the right lower quadrant shows the thickened terminal ileum with echogenic, inflamed fat and hypoechoic, perienteric phlegmon formation (*arrow*).

RIGHT-SIDED SEGMENTAL OMENTAL INFARCTION

Right-sided segmental omental infarction is a rare clinical entity that usually presents with right-sided abdominal pain and is often mistaken for appendicitis. It is important to make the correct diagnosis because the condition is self limiting and resolves spontaneously with supportive measures. It occurs in all age groups and is thought to result from an embryologic variant in the blood supply to the right inferior portion of the

omentum leaving it prone to infarction. Precipitating factors include straining and eating a large meal.

Ultrasound reveals an echogenic, ovoid, or **cake-like mass** in the right midabdomen at the site of the patient's tenderness (Fig. 14-34).[63,64] Careful assessment will reveal no underlying bowel abnormality. The typical location of this abnormality is anterolateral to the hepatic flexure of the colon, and it corresponds with a circumscribed fatty mass on CT with areas of stranding. The mass often adheres to the parietal peritoneum with bowel moving deep to it on respiration.

ENDOMETRIOSIS

Endometriosis is a common condition affecting predominantly premenopausal women and occurs when functional endometrium is located outside of the uterus. Patients may be asymptomatic but frequently present with pelvic pain, dyspareunia, and/or infertility. The ovaries and suspensory ligaments of the uterus are the most commonly affected sites, but endometriotic implants can involve the bowel, urinary bladder, peritoneum, chest, or soft tissues.[65]

Sonographic evaluation will often be normal in patients with endometriosis. If endometriomas are present, transvaginal ultrasound is very sensitive at detecting and characterizing the masses, often showing the typical **chocolate cysts** with uniform low-level internal echoes. There may be associated complex free fluid with stranding. Occasionally tiny echogenic foci may be identified along the pelvic peritoneal surfaces. These foci are not specific for this condition but may also be seen with papillary serous ovarian neoplasms. Clinical correlation is essential and occasionally laparo-

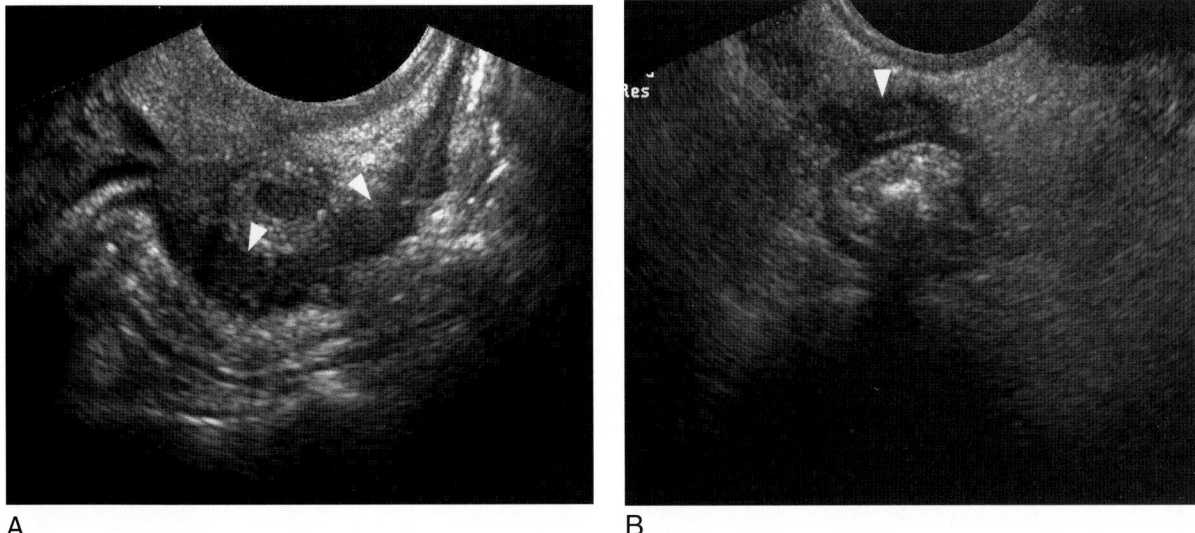

FIGURE 14-35. Endometriotic plaque. A, Sagittal and **B,** transverse transvaginal ultrasound images show hypoechoic endometriotic plaque (*arrowheads*) along one serosal surface of the sigmoid colon.

scopic evaluation may be necessary, with biopsy of the peritoneum to rule out tumor.

Another possible sonographic finding in endometriosis is the presence of **hypoechoic plaques** on the serosal surface of pelvic bowel loops or urinary bladder. These plaques may tether the wall of the affected organ and show flow with color Doppler imaging. They are best demonstrated with the transvaginal probe (Fig. 14-35A, B).

LEIOMYOMATOSIS PERITONEALIS DISSEMINATA

Leiomyomatosis peritonealis disseminata (LPD) is a relatively rare clinical entity, which is characterized by the presence of **multiple nodules**, mainly due to smooth muscle proliferation over the surface of the peritoneal cavity.[66] It often mimics a malignant process, but the diagnosis of LPD is easily made with biopsy.

LPD is usually an incidental finding at the time of imaging or during procedures such as laparoscopy, cesarean section, laparotomy, and postpartum tubal ligation. It occurs mainly in women, primarily during the reproductive period. Exposure to estrogen seems to play an etiologic role. Many patients have uterine leiomyomas as well. Conservative care is generally indicated. When LPD occurs during pregnancy or with the use of birth control pills, it may regress spontaneously after delivery or with discontinuation of the pills. Whether malignant transformation of LPD occurs remains uncertain. In a few isolated cases malignant leiomyosarcomas have been described shortly after the diagnosis of LPD was made. A clear association, however, has not been established. **Sonographic evaluation** may show multiple, small hypoechoic nodules throughout the peritoneal cavity (Fig. 14-36).

PNEUMOPERITONEUM

CT is regarded as the standard for detecting, localizing, and quantifying free air.[67] Plain radiographs are also sensitive at detecting free air with as little as 1 mL being potentially visible on an erect chest radiograph. **Ultrasound**, however, is often the initial imaging modality requested for the investigation of abdominal pain, so the identification of free air is an extremely important finding.

Sonographic technique is critical when assessing for free air. The patient should be scanned in the supine and steep left posterior oblique positions, paying particular attention to the epigastrium and right upper quadrants, respectively.[68,69] Free air in the epigastrium, with the patient lying supine, will frequently shift to the right upper quadrant with the patient lying in a left posterior oblique position (Fig. 14-37A-C). Free air is most often seen just deep to the parietal peritoneum, is best appreciated with a linear array transducer, and appears as **enhancement of the parietal peritoneal line**—often with posterior reverberation artifact.[70] Another sonographic sign of pneumoperitoneum in patients with ascites is the presence of **gas bubbles** within the ascitic fluid. They may appear as tiny floating echogenic foci and have a high association with gut perforation and infection of the peritoneal fluid. When free air is detected, ultrasound will frequently reveal the underlying cause, so the remainder of the abdomen and pelvis should be carefully assessed for evidence of inflammation or tumor.[68]

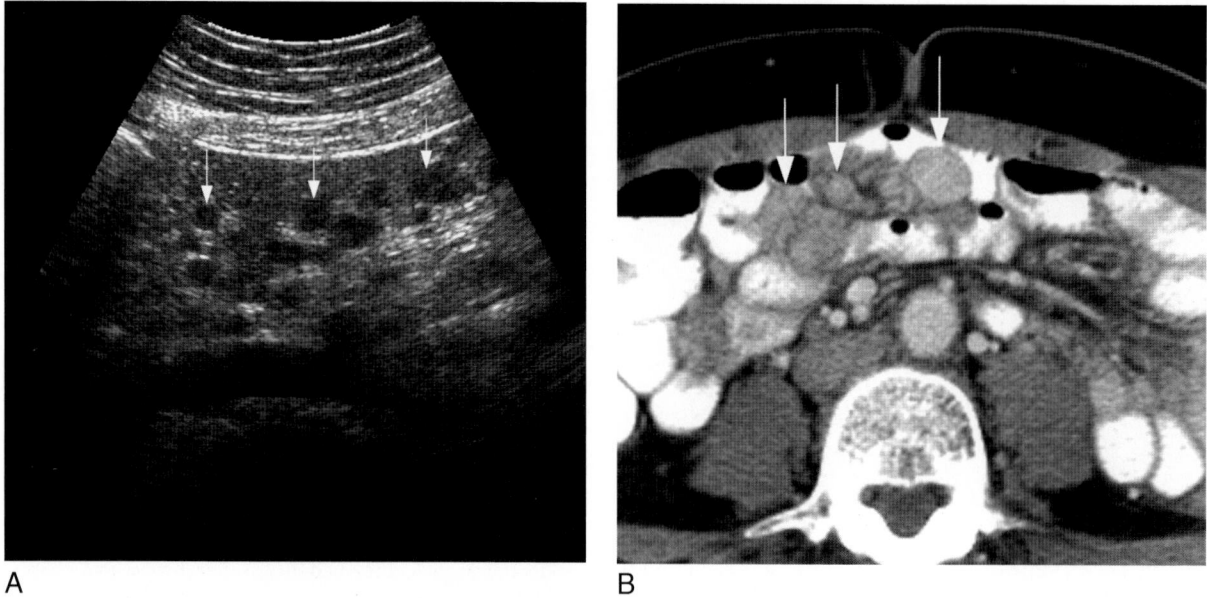

FIGURE 14-36. Leiomyomatosis peritonealis disseminata. A, Sagittal ultrasound and **B,** axial CT image showing multiple, small, hypoechoic, enhancing peritoneal nodules (*arrows*).

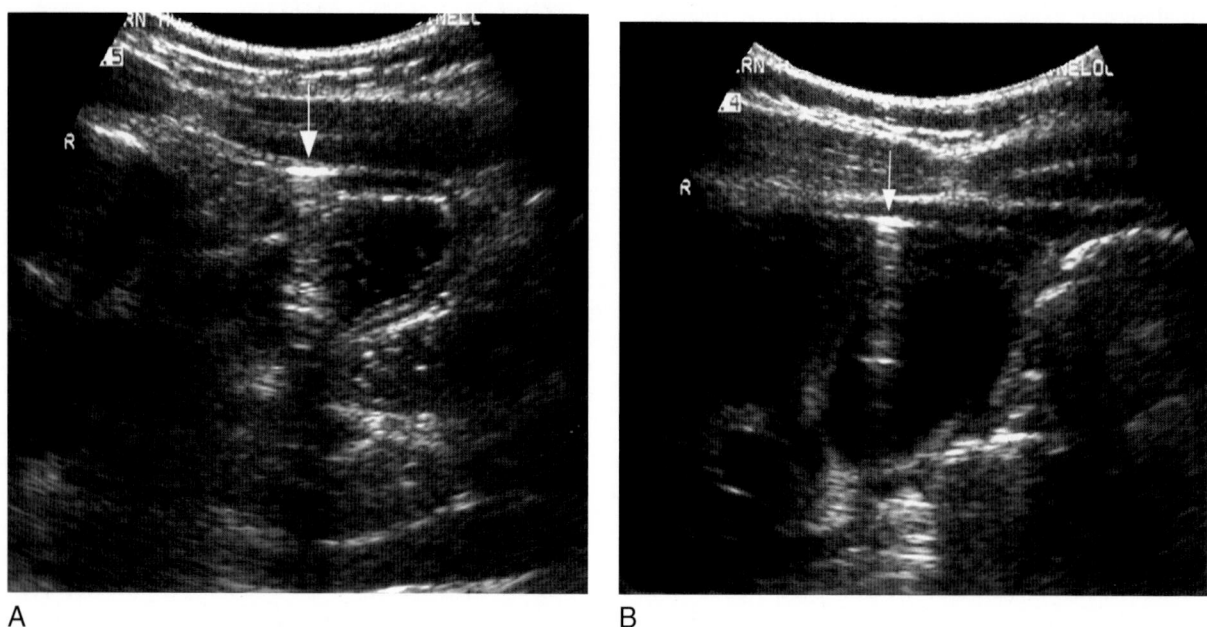

FIGURE 14-37. Pneumoperitoneum. A, Sagittal, upper midline image with the patient supine shows a small area of enhancement of the parietal peritoneal stripe (*arrow*) with ringdown artifact from free air. **B,** Sagittal image of the right upper quadrant, with the patient in left decubitus oblique position, shows that the small area of enhancement of the peritoneal stripe (*arrow*) by free air has moved to lie anterior to the liver.

Continued

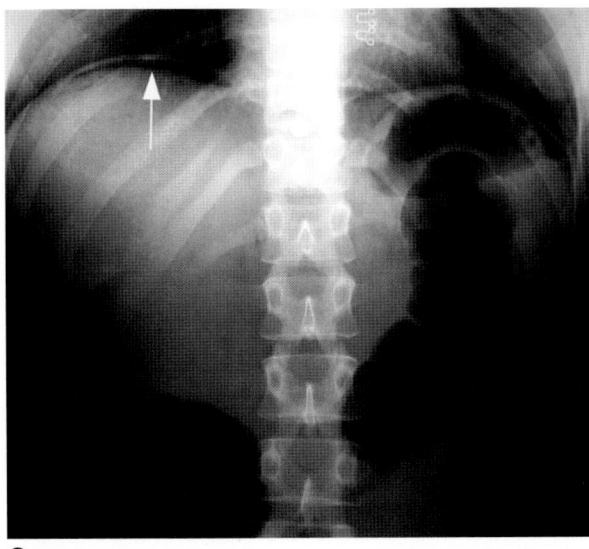

C

FIGURE 14-37, *cont'd.* **Pneumoperitoneum.** C, Upright, frontal radiograph of the abdomen confirms free air under the right hemidiaphragm (*arrow*).

CONCLUSION

Assessment of the peritoneum is easily performed with ultrasound in the majority of patients and should not add significantly to scanning time when the peritoneum is normal. There are **limitations** in markedly obese and postoperative patients but, in general, most peritoneal diseases can be readily detected and characterized with ultrasound. Many of the patterns of peritoneal disease are nonspecific, however, and **sonographic findings** must be interpreted in light of the patient's clinical symptoms, physical findings, and laboratory investigations. Where fluid or tissue is required to reach a specific diagnosis, ultrasound is a very efficient and cost-effective modality for **guidance**.[71] It is also a safe, readily available, and relatively inexpensive modality for **monitoring** disease progression and response to treatment. In patients with ovarian cancer, ultrasound is invariably performed as part of the patient's initial clinical work-up. Because peritoneal dissemination is the major determinant of both prognosis and treatment choices, **we recommend including** the peritoneal cavity in the sonographic assessment of this patient population.

References

1. Raptopoulos V, Gourtsoyiannis N: Peritoneal carcinomatosis. Eur Radiol 2001;11(11):2195-2206.
2. Low RN: Gadolinium-enhanced MR imaging of liver capsule and peritoneum. Magn Reson Imaging Clin N Am 2001;9(4):803-819.
3. Tempany CM, Zou KH, Silverman SG, et al: Staging of advanced ovarian cancer: Comparison of imaging modalities—Report from the Radiological Diagnostic Oncology Group. Radiology 2000;215(3):761-767.
4. Coakley FV, Hricak H: Imaging of peritoneal and mesenteric disease: Key concepts for the clinical radiologist. Clin Radiol 1999;54(9):563-574.
5. Hanbidge AE, Lynch D, Wilson SR: Ultrasound of the peritoneum. Radiographics, 2003;23(3):663–684.
6. Healy JC, Reznek RH: The peritoneum, mesenteries and omenta: Normal anatomy and pathological processes. Eur Radiol 1998;8(6):886-900.
7. Derchi LE, Solbiati L, Rizzatto G, et al: Normal anatomy and pathological changes of the small bowel mesentery: US appearance. Radiology 1987;164(3):649-652.
8. Damani N, Wilson SR: Nongynecologic applications of transvaginal US. Radiographics 1999;19 Spec No:S179-200; quiz S265-266.
9. Serafini G, Gandolfo N, Gandolfo N, et al: Transvaginal ultrasonography of nongynecologic pelvic lesions. Abdom Imaging 2001;26(5):540-549.
10. Goldberg BB, Goodman GA, Clearfield HR: Evaluation of ascites by ultrasound. Radiology 1970;96(1):15-22.
11. Nichols JE, Steinkampf MP: Detection of free peritoneal fluid by transvaginal sonography. J Clin Ultrasound 1993;21(3):171-174.
12. Meyers MA. The spread and localization of acute intraperitoneal effusions. Radiology 1970;95(3):547-554.
13. Inadomi J, Cello JP, Koch J: Ultrasonographic determination of ascitic volume. Hepatology 1996; 24(3):549-551.
14. Edell SL, Gefter WB: Ultrasonic differentiation of types of ascitic fluid. AJR 1979;133(1):111-114.
15. Goerg C, Schwerk WB: Peritoneal carcinomatosis with ascites. AJR 1991;156(6):1185-1187.
16. Kimura A, Otsuka T: Emergency center ultrasonography in the evaluation of hemoperitoneum: A prospective study. J Trauma 1991;31(1):20-23.
17. Rozycki GS, Ochsner MG, Schmidt JA, et al: A prospective study of surgeon-performed ultrasound as the primary adjuvant modality for injured patient assessment. J Trauma 1995;39(3):492-500.
18. Wherrett LJ, Boulanger BR, McLellan BA, et al: Hypotension after blunt abdominal trauma: The role of emergent abdominal sonography in surgical triage. J Trauma 1996;41(5):815-820.
19. Chiu WC, Cushing BM, Rodriquez A, et al: Abdominal injuries without hemoperitoneum: A potential limitation of focused abdominal sonography for trauma (FAST). J Trauma 1997;42(4):617-625.
20. Sirlin CB, Casola G, Brown MA, et al: Patterns of fluid accumulation on screening ultrasonography for blunt abdominal trauma: Comparison with site of injury. J Ultrasound Med 2001;20(4):351-357.
21. Franklin JT, Azose AA: Sonographic appearance of chylous ascites. J Clin Ultrasound 1984;12(4):239-240.
22. Hibbeln JF, Wehmueller MD, Wilbur AC: Chylous ascites: CT and ultrasound appearance. Abdom Imaging 1995;20(2):138-140.
23. Sohaey R, Gardner TL, Woodward PJ, et al: Sonographic diagnosis of peritoneal inclusion cysts. J Ultrasound Med 1995;14(12):913-917.
24. Hoffer FA, Kozakewich H, Colodny A, Goldstein DP: Peritoneal inclusion cysts: Ovarian fluid in peritoneal adhesions. Radiology 1988;169(1):189-191.
25. Kim JS, Lee HJ, Woo SK, et al: Peritoneal inclusion cysts and their relationship to the ovaries: Evaluation with sonography. Radiology 1997;204(2):481-484.
26. Wilson SR: Gastrointestinal Disease Test and Syllabus

(Sixth Series). Reston, VA: American College of Radiology, in press.

27. de Perrot M, Brundler M, Totsch M, et al: Mesenteric cysts. Toward less confusion? Diag Surg 2000;17(4):323-328.

28. Egozi EI, Ricketts RR: Mesenteric and omental cysts in children. Am Surg 1997;63(3):287-290.

29. Konen O, Rathaus V, Dlugy E, et al: Childhood abdominal cystic lymphangioma. Pediatr Radiol 2002;32(2):88-94.

30. Meyers MA, Oliphant M, Berne AS, et al: The peritoneal ligaments and mesenteries: Pathways of intraabdominal spread of disease. Radiology 1987;163(3):593-604.

31. Rioux M, Michaud C: Sonographic detection of peritoneal carcinomatosis: A prospective study of 37 cases. Abdom Imaging 1995;20(1):47-57.

32. Koutselini HA, Lazaris AC, Thomopoulou G, et al: Papillary serous carcinoma of peritoneum: Case study and review of the literature on the differential diagnosis of malignant peritoneal tumors. Adv Clin Path 2001;5(3):99-104.

33. Halperin R, Zehavi S, Langer R, et al: Primary peritoneal serous papillary carcinoma: A new epidemiologic trend? A matched-case comparison with ovarian serous papillary cancer. Int J Gynecol Cancer 2001;11(5):403-408.

34. Furukawa T, Ueda J, Takahashi S, et al: Peritoneal serous papillary carcinoma: Radiological appearance. Abdom Imaging 1999;24(1):78-81.

35. Chopra S, Laurie LR, Chintapalli KN, et al: Primary papillary serous carcinoma of the peritoneum: CT-pathologic correlation. J Comput Assist Tomogr 2000;24(3):395-399.

36. Zissin R, Hertz M, Shapiro-Feinberg M, et al: Primary serous papillary carcinoma of the peritoneum: CT findings. Clin Radiol 2001;56(9):740-745.

37. Moertel CG: Peritoneal mesothelioma. Gastroenterology 1972;63(2):346-350.

38. Guest PJ, Reznek RH, Selleslag D, et al: Peritoneal mesothelioma: The role of computed tomography in diagnosis and follow-up. Clin Radiol 1992;45(2):79-84.

39. Reuter K, Raptopoulos V, Reale F, et al: Diagnosis of peritoneal mesothelioma: Computed tomography, sonography, and fine-needle aspiration biopsy. AJR 1983;140(6):1189-194.

40. Runyon BA, Hoefs JC: Peritoneal lymphomatosis with ascites. A characterization. Arch Intern Med 1986;146(5):887-888.

41. Lynch MA, Cho KC, Jeffrey RB Jr, et al: CT of peritoneal lymphomatosis. AJR 1988;151(4):713-715.

42. O'Connell JT, Tomlinson JS, Roberts AA, et al: Pseudomyxoma peritonei is a disease of MUC2-expressing goblet cells. Am J Pathol 2002;161(2):551-564.

43. Hart WR: Ovarian epithelial tumors of borderline malignancy (carcinomas of low malignant potential). Hum Pathol 1977;8(5):541-549.

44. Yan H, Pestieau SR, Shmookler BM, et al: Histopathologic analysis in 46 patients with pseudomyxoma peritonei syndrome: Failure versus success with a second-look operation. Mod Pathol 2001;14(3):164-171.

45. Fox H. Pseudomyxoma peritonei. Br J Obstet Gynaecol 1996;103(3):197-198.

46. Mann WJ Jr, Wagner J, Chumas J, et al: The management of pseudomyxoma peritonei. Cancer 1990;66(7):1636-1640.

47. Sugarbaker PH: Cytoreductive surgery and perioperative intraperitoneal chemotherapy as a curative approach to pseudomyxoma peritonei syndrome. Tumori 2001;87(4):S3-5.

48. Walensky RP, Venbrux AC, Prescott CA, et al: Pseudomyxoma peritonei. AJR 1996;167(2):471-474.

49. Seshul MB, Coulam CM: Pseudomyxoma peritonei: Computed tomography and sonography. AJR 1981;36(4):803-806.

50. Yeh HC, Wolf BS: Ultrasonography of ascites. Radiology 1977;124(3):783-790.

51. Prousalidis J, Tzardinoglou K, Sgouradis L, et al: Uncommon sites of hydatid disease. World J Surg 1998;22(1):17-22.

52. Gazelle GS, Mueller PR: Abdominal abscess. Imaging and intervention. Radiol Clin North Am 1994;32(5):913-932.

53. Sneider DE Jr, Roper WL: The new tuberculosis. N Engl J Med 1992;5;326(10):703-705.

54. Marshall JB: Tuberculosis of the gastrointestinal tract and peritoneum. Am J Gastroenterol 1993;88(7):989-999.

55. Akhan O, Pringot J: Imaging of abdominal tuberculosis. Eur Radiol 2002;12(2):312-323.

56. Kedar RP, Shah PP, Shivde RS, et al: Sonographic findings in gastrointestinal and peritoneal tuberculosis. Clin Radiol 1994; 49(1):24-29.

57. Lee DH, Lim JH, Ko YT, et al: Sonographic findings in tuberculous peritonitis of the wet-ascitic type. Clin Radiol 1991;44(5):306-310.

58. Hollman AS, McMillan MA, Briggs JD, et al: Ultrasound changes in sclerosing peritonitis following continuous ambulatory peritoneal dialysis. Clin Radiol 1991;43(3):176-179.

59. Cohen O, Abrahamson J, Ben-Ari J, et al: Sclerosing encapsulating peritonitis. J Clin Gastroenterol 1996;22(1):54-57.

60. Krestin GP, Kacl G, Hauser M, et al: Imaging diagnosis of sclerosing peritonitis and relation of radiologic signs to the extent of the disease. Abdom Imaging 1995; 20(5):414-520.

61. Sarrazin J, Wilson SR: Manifestations of Crohn disease at US. Radiographics 1996;16(3):499-521.

62. McDonnell CH 3rd, Jeffrey RB Jr, Vierra MA: Inflamed pericholecystic fat: Color Doppler flow imaging and clinical features. Radiology 1994;193(2):547-550.

63. Puylaert JB: Right-sided segmental infarction of the omentum: Clinical, US and CT findings. Radiology 1992;185(1):169-172.

64. McClure MJ, Khalili K, Sarrazin J, et al: Radiological features of epiploic appendagitis and segmental omental infarction. Clin Radiol 2001;56(10):819-827.

65. Woodward PJ, Sohaey R, Mezzetti TP Jr: Endometriosis: Radiologic-pathologic correlation. Radiographics 2001;21(1):193-216; questionnaire 288-294.

66. Bekkers RL, Willemsen WN, Schijf CP, et al: Leiomyomatosis peritonealis disseminata: Does malignant transformation occur? A literature review. Gynecol Oncol 1999;75(1):158-163.

67. Baker SR. Imaging of pneumoperitoneum. Abdom Imaging 1996;21(5):413-414.

68. Lee DH, Lim JH, Ko YT, et al: Sonographic detection of pneumoperitoneum in patients with acute abdomen. AJR 1990;154(1):107-109.

69. Braccini G, Lamacchia M, Boraschi P, et al: Ultrasound versus plain film in the detection of pneumoperitoneum. Abdom Imaging 1996;21(5):404-412.

70. Muradali D, Wilson S, Burns PN, et al: A specific sign of pneumoperitoneum on sonography: Enhancement of the peritoneal stripe. AJR 1999;173(5):1257-1262.

71. Gottlieb RH, Tan R, Widjaja J, et al: Extravisceral masses in the peritoneal cavity: Sonographically guided biopsies in 52 patients. AJR 1998;171(3):697-701.

15

GYNECOLOGIC ULTRASOUND

Shia Salem / Stephanie R. Wilson

Chapter Outline

Sonography plays an integral role in the evaluation of gynecologic disease. It can determine the organ or site of abnormality and provide a diagnosis or short differential diagnosis in the vast majority of patients. Both the transabdominal and transvaginal approaches are now well-established techniques for assessing the female pelvic organs. Transvaginal sonography is now considered an essential part of almost all pelvic ultrasound examinations. Color and spectral Doppler sonography have evolved to play a role in assessing normal and pathologic blood flow. Doppler can also distinguish vascular structures from nonvascular structures, such as dilated fallopian tubes or fluid-filled bowel loops. The more recent addition of sonohysterography has provided more detailed evaluation of the endometrium, allowing differentiation among intracavitary, endometrial, and submucosal lesions. Sonography also plays an important role in guiding interventional procedures. Magnetic resonance imaging (MRI), because of its excellent tissue characterization, can occasionally be helpful when sonography is inconclusive and in the staging of pelvic malignancies. Computed tomography (CT) has a limited role but is used for cancer staging.

NORMAL PELVIC ANATOMY

The **uterus** is a hollow, thick-walled muscular organ. Its internal structure consists of a muscular layer, or **myometrium**, which forms most of the substance of the uterus, and a mucous layer, the **endometrium**, which is firmly adherent to the myometrium. The uterus is located between the two layers of the broad ligament laterally, the bladder anteriorly, and the rectosigmoid colon posteriorly. It is divided into two major portions, the **body** and the **cervix**, by a slight narrowing at the level of the internal os. The **fundus** is the superior area of the body above the entrance of the fallopian tubes. The area of the body where the tubes enter the uterus is called the **cornua**. The anterior surface of the uterine fundus and body is covered by peritoneum. The peritoneal space anterior to the uterus is the **vesico-uterine pouch** or **anterior cul-de-sac**. This space is usually empty, but may contain bowel loops. Posteriorly, the peritoneal reflection extends to the posterior fornix of the vagina, forming the **rectouterine recess (posterior cul-de-sac)**. Laterally, the peritoneal reflection forms the **broad ligaments**, which extend from the lateral aspect of the uterus to the lateral pelvic sidewalls. The **round ligaments** arise from the uterine cornua anterior to the fallopian tubes in the broad ligaments, extend anterolaterally, and course, through the inguinal canals, to insert into the fascia of the labia majora.

The **cervix** is located posterior to the angle of the bladder and is anchored to the bladder angle by the parametrium. The cervix opens into the upper vagina through the external os. The **vagina** is a fibromuscular canal that lies in the midline and runs from the cervix to the vestibule of the external genitalia. The cervix projects into the proximal vagina, creating a space between the vaginal walls and the surface of the cervix called the **vaginal fornix**. Although the space is continuous, it is divided into anterior, posterior, and two lateral fornices.[1]

The two **fallopian tubes** run laterally from the uterus in the upper free margin of the broad ligament. Each tube varies from 7 to 12 cm in length and is divided into intramural, isthmic, ampullary, and infundibular portions.[2] The **intramural** portion, which is approx-imately 1 cm long, is contained within the muscular wall of the uterus and is the narrowest part of the tube. The **isthmus**, constituting the medial third, is slightly wider, round, cordlike, and continuous with the **ampulla**, which is tortuous and forms approximately one half the length of the tube.[1] The ampulla terminates in the most distal portion, the **infundibulum**, or fimbriated end, which is funnel shaped and opens into the peritoneal cavity (Fig. 15-1).

The **ovaries** are elliptical in shape, with the long axis usually oriented vertically. The surface of the ovary is not covered by peritoneum but by a single layer of cuboidal or columnar cells called the **germinal epithelium** that becomes continuous with the peritoneum at the hilum of the ovary. The internal structure of the ovary is divided into an outer cortex and inner medulla. The **cortex** consists of an interstitial framework, or stroma, which is composed of reticular fibers and spindle-shaped cells and which contains the ovarian follicles and corpus lutea. Beneath the germinal epithelium, the connective tissue of the cortex is condensed to form a fibrous capsule, the **tunica albuginea**. The **medulla**, which is smaller in volume than the cortex, is composed of fibrous tissue and blood vessels, especially veins. In the nulliparous female, the ovary is located in a depression on the lateral pelvic wall called the **ovarian fossa**, which is bound anteriorly by the obliterated umbilical artery, posteriorly by the ureter and the internal iliac artery, and superiorly by the external iliac vein.[1] The fimbriae of the fallopian tube lie superior and lateral to the ovary. The anterior surface of the ovary is attached to the posterior surface of the broad ligament by a short mesovarium. The lower pole of the ovary is attached to the uterus by the **ovarian ligament**, whereas the upper pole is attached to the lateral wall of the pelvis by the lateral extension of the broad ligament known as the **suspensory (infundibulopelvic) ligament** of the ovary. The suspensory ligament contains the ovarian vessels and nerves. These ligaments are not rigid and, therefore,

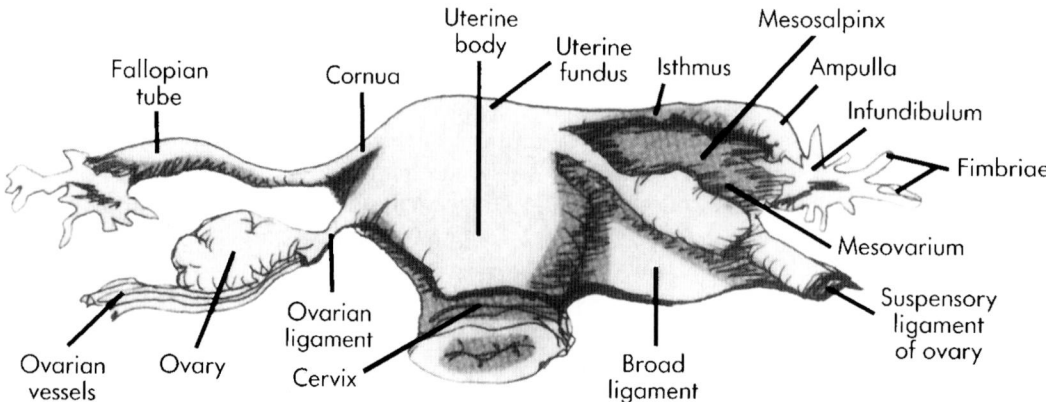

FIGURE 15-1. Normal gynecologic organs. Diagram of uterus, ovaries, tubes, and related structures. On left side, broad ligament has been removed. (Courtesy of Jocelyne Salem.)

the ovary can be quite mobile, especially in women who have had pregnancies.

The **arterial blood supply** to the uterus comes primarily from the **uterine artery**, a major branch of the anterior trunk of the internal iliac artery. The uterine artery ascends along the lateral margin of the uterus in the broad ligament and, at the level of the uterine cornua, runs laterally to anastomose with the ovarian artery. The uterine arteries anastomose extensively across the midline through the anterior and posterior arcuate arteries, which run within the broad ligament and then enter the myometrium.[1,2] The uterine plexus of veins accompanies the arteries.

The **ovarian arteries** arise from the aorta laterally, slightly inferior to the renal arteries. They cross the external iliac vessels at the pelvic brim and run medially within the suspensory ligament of the ovary. After giving off branches to the ovary, they continue medially in the broad ligament to anastomose with the branches of the uterine artery. The **ovarian veins** leave the ovarian hilum and form a plexus of veins in the broad ligament that communicate with the uterine plexus of veins. The right ovarian vein drains into the inferior vena cava inferior to the right renal vein, whereas the left ovarian vein drains directly into the left renal vein.[1]

The **lymphatic drainage** of the pelvic organs is variable but tends to follow recognizable patterns. The lymph vessels of the ovary accompany the ovarian artery to the lateral aortic and periaortic lymph nodes. The lymphatics of the fundus and upper uterine body and fallopian tube accompany those of the ovary. The lymphatics of the lower uterine body course laterally to the external iliac lymph nodes, whereas those of the cervix course in three directions—laterally, to the external iliac lymph nodes; posterolaterally, to the internal iliac lymph nodes; and posteriorly, to the lateral sacral lymph nodes. The lymphatics of the upper vagina course laterally with the branches of the uterine artery to the external and internal iliac lymph nodes, whereas those of the middle vagina follow the vaginal artery branches to the internal iliac lymph nodes. The lymphatic vessels of the lower vagina near the orifice join those of the vulva and drain to the superficial inguinal lymph nodes.[1]

SONOGRAPHIC TECHNIQUE

The **transabdominal sonogram** is performed with a distended urinary bladder, which provides an acoustic window to view the pelvic organs and serves as a reference standard for evaluating cystic structures. The distended bladder displaces the bowel out of the pelvis and displaces the pelvic organs 5 to 10 cm from the anterior abdominal wall. The highest frequency transducer possible should be used. In practice, most sonograms are performed using a 5.0-MHz or a 3.5-MHz transducer. The urinary bladder is considered ideally filled when it covers the entire fundus of the uterus. Overdistention may distort the anatomy by compression and may also push the pelvic organs beyond the focal zone of the transducer, limiting detail.

Imaging of the uterus and adnexa is performed in both sagittal and transverse planes. The long axis of the uterus is identified in the sagittal plane, and a somewhat oblique angulation is often necessary to visualize the entire uterus and cervix. The adnexa may be imaged by scanning obliquely from the contralateral side, although in many instances visualization can be achieved by scanning directly over the adnexa, especially when an overdistended bladder pushes the adnexa beyond the focal zone of the transducer. Gentle pressure on the transducer may be necessary to bring the area of interest within the focal zone.

For **transvaginal sonography**, the bladder must be empty to bring the pelvic organs into the focal zone of the transvaginal transducer. An empty bladder also provides patient comfort during the examination. The examination must be explained to the patient and verbal consent obtained before beginning the examination. If the examiner is a male, it is essential to have a female staff member in the room during the entire examination to act as a chaperone. Contraindications include virginal patients and patients who do not willingly consent to the examination. In patients with a narrow introitus or vagina, who experience discomfort at attempted insertion of the transducer, the examination should be discontinued.

The transducer is prepared with ultrasound coupling gel and then covered with a protective sheath, usually a condom. Air bubbles should be eliminated to avoid artifacts. An external lubricant is then applied to the outside of the protective covering. If the examination is part of an **infertility study**, saline or water should be used as a lubricant because coupling gel may adversely affect sperm motility. The transducer is inserted into the vagina with the patient supine, knees gently flexed and hips elevated slightly on a pillow. The elevated hips allow free movement of the transducer by the operator. A slightly reversed Trendelenburg position may be helpful in lowering the pelvic organs to enhance visualization. It is important to avoid placing the patient in the Trendelenburg position, as small amounts of pelvic fluid may be missed.

With gentle rotation and angulation of the transducer, both sagittal and coronal images can be obtained. Slight anterior angulation of the transducer will bring the fundus of an anteverted uterus into view. To visualize the cervix, the transducer must be pulled slightly outward, away from the external os. Extreme angulation may be needed to visualize the entire adnexa and cul-de-sac. The tip of the transducer can be used to evaluate for areas of focal tenderness. Abdominal palpation may be helpful in bringing adnexal structures closer to the transducer. Movement of an adnexal mass with transducer pressure may aid in determining the organ of origin in uncertain cases. Following the examination, the transducer is removed from the vagina with the sheath intact. The sheath is discarded and the transducer is cleaned of gel. The transducer is then immersed in a disinfectant according to the manufacturer's preferred method.

Image orientation may be confusing initially as the sagittal images are displayed 90 degrees counterclockwise from their actual orientation, whereas the coronal scans are similarly rotated in their craniocaudad direction but correctly displayed as to right-left orientation (Fig. 15-2).

Sonohysterography involves the instillation of sterile saline into the endometrial cavity under ultrasound guidance. The procedure is explained to the patient and verbal consent is obtained. A sterile speculum is inserted into the vagina and the cervix is cleansed with an antiseptic solution. A special catheter, or a 5-F pediatric feeding tube, is inserted into the uterine cavity to the level of the uterine fundus. The catheter should be prefilled with saline prior to insertion to minimize air artifact. A hysterosalpingography catheter with a balloon may be necessary in women with a patulous or incom-

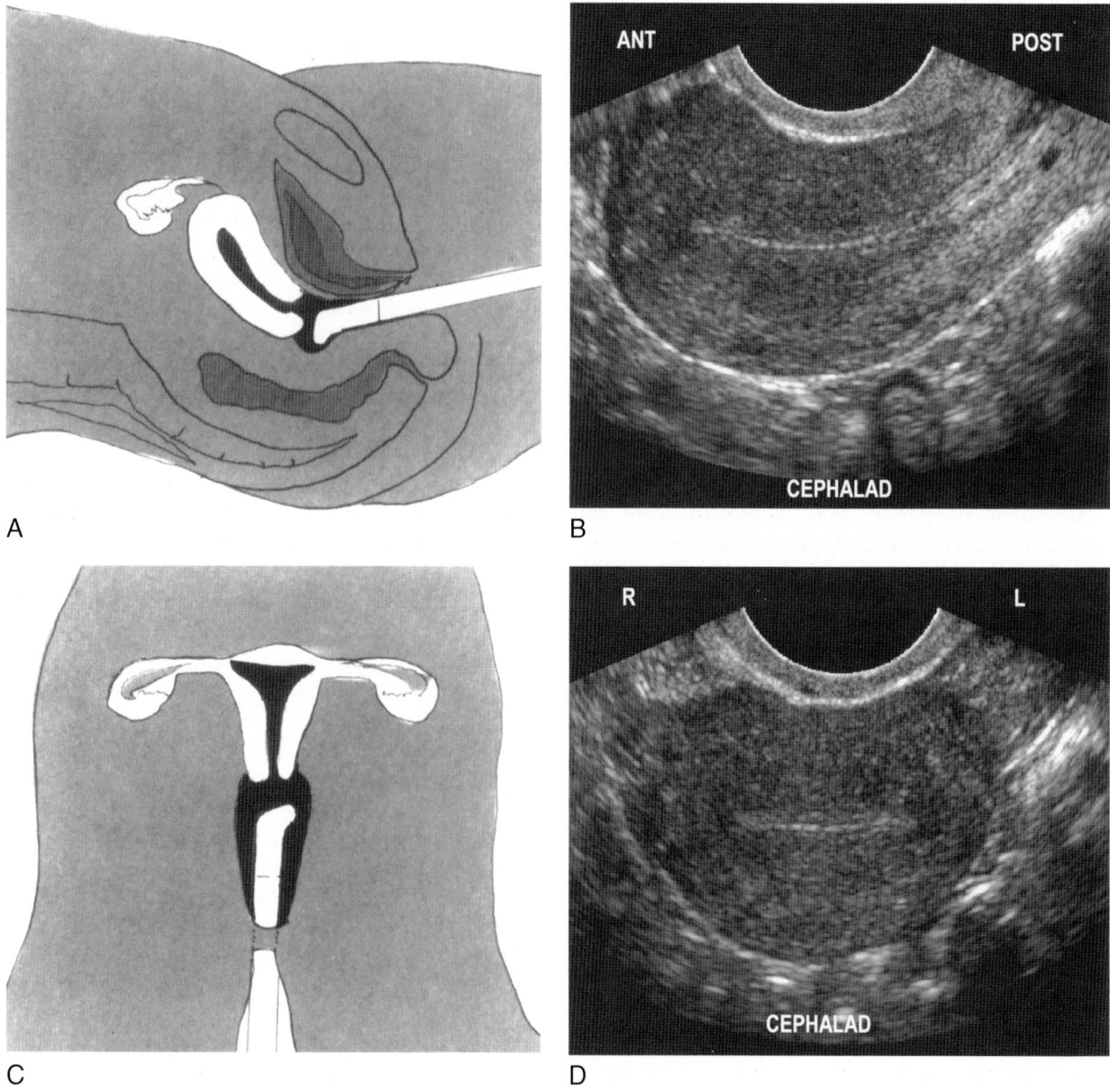

FIGURE 15-2. Transvaginal sonography orientation. **A**, Illustration of transvaginal scanning in sagittal plane. **B**, Corresponding sagittal sonogram of uterus. **C**, Illustration of transvaginal scanning in coronal plane. **D**, Corresponding coronal sonogram of uterus. R indicates right; L, left. (A and C, courtesy of Jocelyne Salem.)

petent cervix to prevent retrograde leakage of saline into the vagina. The balloon should be placed as close to the internal os as possible and inflated with saline, not air.

The speculum is then removed and the transvaginal transducer is inserted into the vagina. The catheter position in the endometrial cavity is identified and repositioned if necessary. Sterile saline is then injected slowly through the catheter under continuous sonographic control. The uterus is scanned systematically in sagittal and coronal planes to delineate the entire endometrial cavity and appropriate images are recorded.

In premenopausal women with regular cycles, the procedure is usually performed between days 6 to 10 of the menstrual cycle to avoid the possibility of disrupting an early pregnancy. For women with irregular cycles, the procedure is performed soon after the cessation of bleeding. In postmenopausal women on sequential hormone replacement therapy, sonohysterography is performed shortly after the monthly bleeding period. In postmenopausal women, who are not on sequential hormone replacement, the procedure can be performed at any time. The procedure is not performed in women with acute pelvic inflammatory disease. In most cases, there is no special patient preparation. Prophylactic antibiotics are given to women with chronic pelvic inflammatory disease and to women with a history of mitral valve prolapse or other cardiac disorders.[3]

Transabdominal versus Transvaginal Scanning

Transabdominal and transvaginal sonography are complementary techniques; both are used extensively in evaluation of the female pelvis. The **transabdominal approach** visualizes the entire pelvis and gives a global overview. Its main **limitations** include the examination of patients who are unable to fill their bladders, the examination of obese patients, the evaluation of a retroverted uterus in which the fundus may be located beyond the focal zone of the transducer, and less optimal characterization of adnexal masses. Because of the proximity of the transducer to the uterus and adnexa, **transvaginal sonography** allows the use of higher-frequency transducers, producing much better resolution. However, because of the higher frequencies, the **field-of-view is limited**, and that is the major disadvantage of this technique. Large masses may fill or extend out of the field-of-view, making orientation difficult, and superiorly or laterally placed ovaries or masses may not be visualized. Transvaginal sonography better distinguishes adnexal masses from bowel loops and provides greater detail of the internal characteristics of a pelvic mass because of its improved resolution. Thus, the two techniques complement each other. Several studies comparing the two techniques in a variety of pelvic disorders have shown that transvaginal

---

ADVANTAGES OF TRANSVAGINAL SONOGRAPHY

Use of higher-frequency transducers with better resolution
Examination of patients who are unable to fill their bladders
Examination of obese patients
Evaluation of a retroverted uterus
Better distinction between adnexal masses and bowel loops
Better characterization of the internal characteristics of a pelvic mass
Better detail of a pelvic lesion
Better detail of the endometrium

---

sonography provides better anatomic detail and image quality.[4-8] This is not surprising because of the higher-frequency transducers used.

Many women will require both transabdominal and transvaginal studies; however, if the initial study is completely normal or a well-defined abnormality is detected, no further study is usually necessary. The second study is added if the pelvic organs are not well visualized. In our laboratory, we begin with a transabdominal scan to look for large masses or any obvious abnormalities, but do not ask the patient to fill her bladder. If the bladder is full, we will do a complete scan. If the bladder is empty, we will proceed directly with the transvaginal scan.

Transvaginal sonography should always be performed in women with suspected endometrial disorders in patients who have a high risk of disease, such as a strong family history of ovarian cancer, and to assess the internal characteristics of a pelvic mass. For follow-up examinations, only the more efficient diagnostic technique is needed.

UTERUS

Normal Sonographic Anatomy

The uterus lies in the true pelvis between the urinary bladder anteriorly and the rectosigmoid colon posteriorly (Fig. 15-3). Uterine position is variable and changes with varying degrees of bladder and rectal distention. The cervix is fixed in the midline, but the body is quite mobile and may lie obliquely on either side of the midline. **Flexion** refers to the axis of the uterine body relative to the cervix, whereas **version** refers to the axis of the cervix relative to the vagina. The uterus is usually anteverted and anteflexed, but it may appear straight or slightly retroflexed on transabdominal sonograms due to posterior displacement by the distended bladder. The uterus may also be retroflexed when the

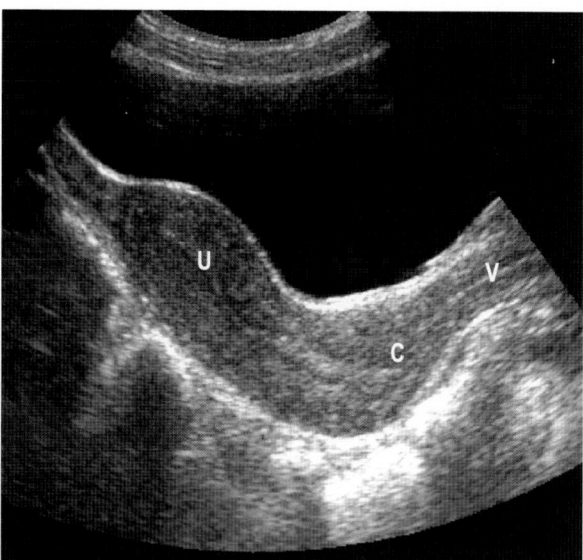

FIGURE 15-3. Normal uterus (U), cervix (C), and vagina (V). Sagittal scan. Central linear echo representing apposed surfaces of vaginal mucosa (V).

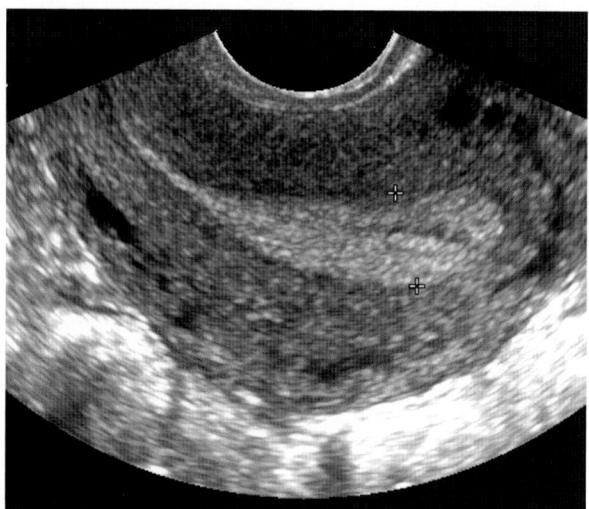

FIGURE 15-4. Retroverted uterus. Sagittal transvaginal scan. Secretory endometrium outlined by cursors.

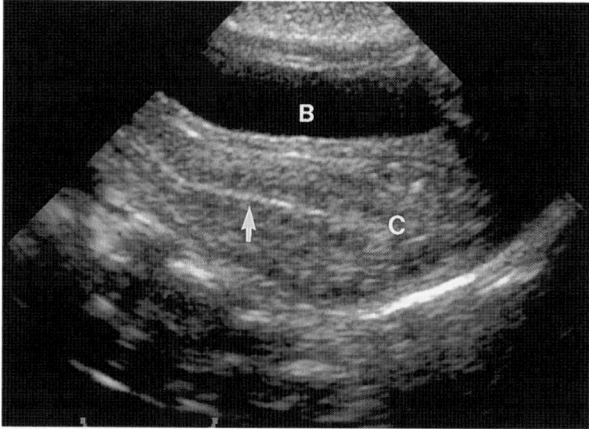

FIGURE 15-5. Normal neonatal uterus. Sagittal scan. Inverse pear shape with cervix (C) having greater AP diameter and length than body. The endometrium (*arrow*) is thin and normal B, Bladder.

body is tilted posteriorly (relative to the cervix) or retroverted when the entire uterus is tilted backward (relative to the vagina) (Fig. 15-4). The fundus of a retroverted or retroflexed uterus is frequently difficult to assess by transabdominal sonography. Because this portion of the uterus is situated at a distance from the transducer, it may appear hypoechoic and simulate a fibroid. Transvaginal sonography has proved to be excellent for assessing the retroverted or retroflexed uterus because the transducer is close to the posteriorly located fundus.[8]

The **size** and **shape** of the normal uterus vary throughout life and are related to age, hormonal status, and parity. The infantile or **prepubertal uterus** ranges from 2.0 to 3.3 cm (mean = 2.8 cm) in length, with the cervix accounting for two thirds of the total length, and 0.5 to 1.0 cm (mean = 0.8 cm) in anteroposterior (AP) diameter.[9] The prepubertal uterus has a tubular or inverse pear-shaped appearance, with the AP diameter of the cervix being greater than that of the fundus.[10] In the immediate neonatal period, because of residual maternal hormone stimulation, the **neonatal uterus** is slightly larger varying in length from 2.3 to 4.6 cm (mean = 3.4 cm) and AP diameter from 0.8 to 2.1 cm (mean = 1.2 cm).[11] Also because of residual maternal hormone stimulation, an echogenic endometrium is seen in nearly all neonatal uteri (Fig. 15-5). A small amount of endometrial fluid may be present in up to 25% of neonatal uteri.[12] There is little growth of the prepubertal uterus from infancy until approximately 8 years of age, when the uterus gradually increases in size until puberty.[13] At this time, there is a more dramatic increase in size with more pronounced growth in the body until it reaches the eventual adult, pear-shaped appearance, with the diameter and length of the body being approximately double that of the cervix.[10] The normal postpubertal, or **adult, uterus** varies considerably in size. The maximal dimensions of the nulliparous uterus are approximately 8 cm in length by 5 cm in width by 4 cm in AP diameter. Parity increases the normal size by more than 1 cm in each dimension.[14-16] Merz et al. also found a significant difference in uterine length between primiparas and multiparas, with an increase of approximately 1 cm in primiparas and approximately 2 cm in multiparas.[15] After menopause, the uterus atrophies, with the most rapid decrease in size occurring in the first 10 years following cessation of menstruation.[14] In patients over the age of 65 years, the uterus ranges from 3.5 to 6.5 cm in length and 1.2 to 1.8 cm in AP diameter.[16]

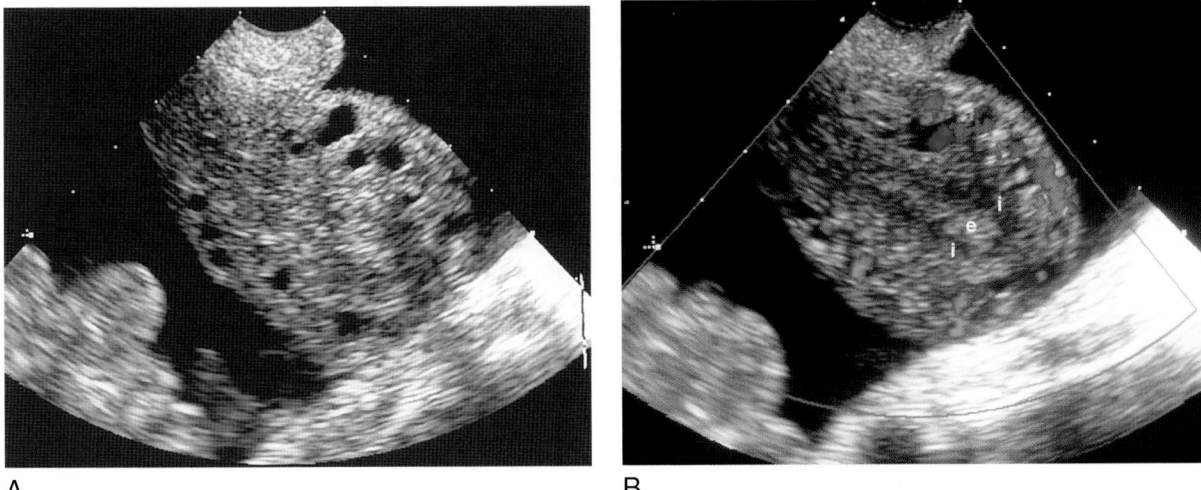

A   B

FIGURE 15-6. Uterine veins. A, Transvaginal sagittal scan of uterus surrounded by ascites shows multiple peripheral anechoic areas. **B,** Confirmation by color Doppler. Endometrium (e), hypoechoic inner layer of myometrium (i). The outer layer of myometrium is separated from the intermediate layer by the arcuate veins.

The normal **myometrium** consists of three layers that can be distinguished by sonography. The **intermediate layer** is the thickest and has a uniformly homogeneous texture of low to moderate echogenicity. The **inner layer** of myometrium is thin, compact, and relatively hypovascular.[17,18] This inner layer, which is hypoechoic and surrounds the relatively echogenic endometrium, has also been referred to as the **subendometrial halo**. The thin **outer layer** is slightly less echogenic than the intermediate layer and is separated from it by the arcuate vessels.

The **arcuate arteries** lie between the outer and intermediate layers of the myometrium and branch into the radial arteries which run in the intermediate layer to the level of the inner layer. The radial arteries then branch into the spiral arteries, which enter the endometrium and supply the functional layer. The uterine veins are larger than the accompanying arcuate arteries and are frequently identified as small focal anechoic areas by both transabdominal and transvaginal sonography.[19] This can be confirmed by Doppler examination (Fig. 15-6). **Calcification** may be seen in the arcuate arteries in postmenopausal women because of Monkeberg's sclerosis.[20,21] On sonography, such calcification appears as peripheral linear echogenic areas with shadowing; they should be distinguished from calcified leiomyomas (Fig. 15-7). This is a normal aging process that may be accelerated in diabetic patients.

Small, highly echogenic foci in the inner layer of myometrium may be seen in normal women. These foci, measuring only a few millimeters, may be single or multiple and are usually nonshadowing. They are thought to represent dystrophic calcification related to previous instrumentation, such as dilation and curettage

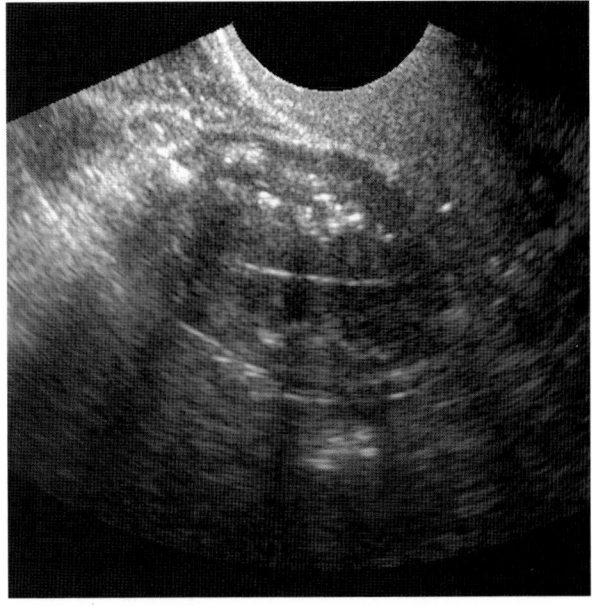

FIGURE 15-7. Arcuate artery calcification. Transvaginal sagittal scan shows multiple small peripheral linear hyperechoic foci.

or endocervical biopsy.[22] They are of no clinical significance.

Uterine perfusion can be assessed by duplex Doppler or color Doppler sonography of the uterine arteries. In normal women, the Doppler waveform usually shows a high-velocity, high-resistance pattern.

The normal **endometrial cavity** is seen as a thin echogenic line as a result of specular reflection from the interface between the opposing surfaces of the endometrium.[23] The sonographic appearance of the endometrium varies during the menstrual cycle (Fig. 15-8A-D) and has been correlated with histology.[17,24,25] The endometrium is composed of a **superficial functional layer** and a **deep basal layer**. The functional layer thickens throughout the menstrual cycle and is shed with menses. The basal layer remains intact during the cycle and contains the spiral arteries, which become tortuous and elongate to supply the functional layer as it thickens. The **proliferative phase** of the cycle before ovulation is under the influence of estrogen, whereas progesterone is mainly responsible for maintenance of the endometrium in the **secretory phase** following ovulation.

The **menstrual phase** endometrium consists of a thin echogenic line. During the **proliferative phase**, the endometrium thickens, reaching 4 to 8 mm. The endometrium is best measured on a midline sagittal scan of the uterus and should include both anterior and posterior portions of the endometrium. It is important not to include the thin hypoechoic inner layer of myometrium in this measurement. A relatively hypoechoic region that represents the functional layer can be seen around the central echogenic line. In the early proliferative phase, this hypoechoic area is thin, but it increases and becomes more clearly defined in the later proliferative phase (**periovulatory**), probably as a result of edema. The hypoechoic appearance of the proliferative endometrium has been related to the relatively homogeneous histologic structure because of the orderly arrangement of the glandular elements. Following ovulation, the functional layer of the endometrium changes from hypoechoic to hyperechoic as the endometrium progresses to the **secretory phase**.[24,25] The endometrium in this phase measures 7 to 14 mm in thickness. The hyperechoic texture in the secretory endometrium is related to increased mucus and glycogen within the glands, as well as to the increased number of interfaces caused by the tortuosity of the spiral arteries. Acoustic enhancement may be seen posterior to the secretory endometrium, but it is not specific because it has also been seen with the proliferative endometrium, although not as frequently.[25]

Following menopause, the endometrium becomes **atrophic** as it is no longer under hormonal control.

THE PREMENOPAUSAL ENDOMETRIUM

Menstrual phase	Thin broken echogenic line
Proliferative phase	Hypoechoic thickening 4 to 8 mm
Periovulatory phase	Triple layer 6 to 10 mm
Secretory phase	Hyperechoic thickening 7 to 14 mm

Sonographically, the endometrium is seen as a thin echogenic line measuring no more than 8 mm (see Fig. 15-8F).

Congenital Abnormalities

Congenital uterine abnormalities are associated with an increased incidence of spontaneous abortion and other obstetric complications.[26] The fused caudal ends of the two Müllerian (paramesonephric) ducts form the uterus, cervix, and upper vagina, whereas the unfused cranial ends form the paired fallopian tubes. Fusion occurs in a cephalad direction, and the median septum formed by the medial walls of the Müllerian ducts resorbs, leaving a single uterine cavity.[2]

Uterine malformations (Figs. 15-9, 15-10 and 15-11) may be due to the following:

- Arrested development of the Müllerian ducts;
- Failure of fusion of the Müllerian ducts; or
- Failure of resorption of the median septum

Arrested development of the Müllerian ducts may be either unilateral or bilateral. Arrested bilateral development is extremely rare and results in congenital absence of the uterus or **uterine aplasia**. Arrested unilateral development results in a **uterus unicornis unicollis** (one uterine horn and one cervix). Hypoplasia of one Müllerian duct may result in a rudimentary uterine horn. The rudimentary horn may be noncavitary or cavitary, either communicating or noncommunicating with the other horn.[27] Most rudimentary horns are noncommunicating and are connected to the opposite cornua by fibrous bands. If the endometrium in a rudimentary horn is nonfunctional, no clinical symptoms occur, but if a functional endometrium is present, retention of menstrual blood in the rudimentary horn may occur.

Failure of fusion of the Müllerian ducts may be complete, resulting in a **uterus didelphys** (two vaginas, two cervices, and two uteri), or partial, which may result in either a **uterus bicornis bicollis** (one vagina, two cervices, and two uterine horns) or a **uterus bicornis unicollis** (one vagina, one cervix, and two uterine horns). **Uterus arcuatus** is the mildest fusion anomaly, resulting in a partial indentation of the uterine fundus with a relatively normal endometrial cavity and is considered either a very mild form of the bicornuate uterus or a normal variant.

Failure of resorption of the median septum results in a **septate** or **subseptate uterus**, depending on whether the failure is complete or partial, respectively. This results in complete or partial duplication of the uterine cavities without duplication of the uterine horns and is the most common uterine abnormality. The septate or subseptate uterus can be distinguished from the bicornuate uterus by looking at the external contour of the uterus.

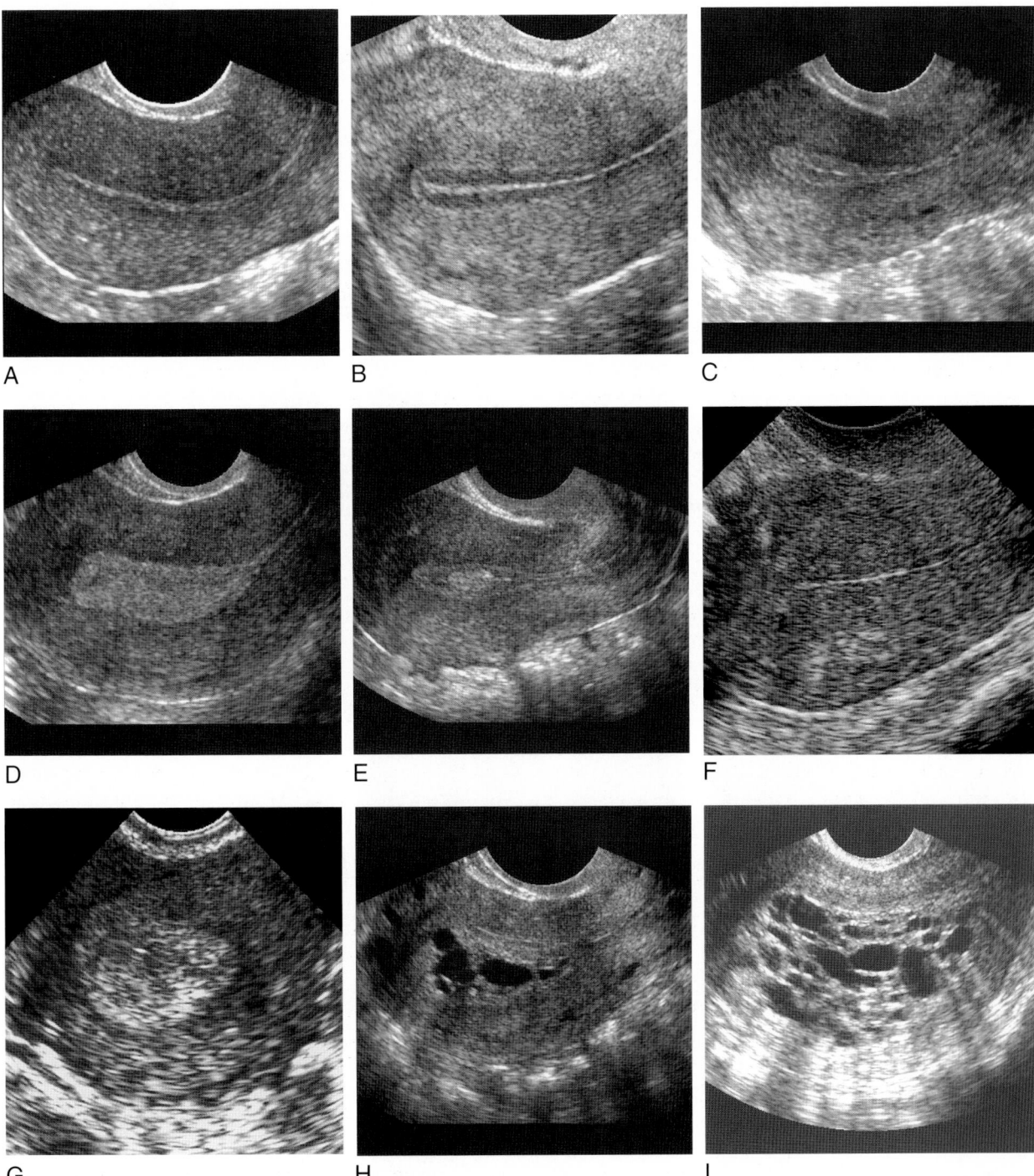

FIGURE 15-8. Endometrium—spectrum of appearances. Transvaginal scans. **A,** Normal, thin early proliferative endometrium. **B,** Normal late proliferative endometrium with triple-layer appearance. Central echogenic line due to opposed endometrial surfaces surrounded by thicker hypoechoic functional layer, bounded by outer echogenic basal layer. **C,** Normal, early secretory phase endometrium. The functional layer surrounding the echogenic line has become hyperechoic. **D,** Normal, thick hyperechoic late secretory endometrium. **E,** Oval, well-defined polyp which is more hyperechoic than surrounding periovulatory endometrium. **F,** Normal, thin postmenopausal endometrium. **G,** Thickened endometrium due to multiple small polyps proved on sonohysterogram. **H,** Thick, cystic endometrium due to **hyperplasia** in patient on tamoxifen. **I,** Thick, cystic endometrium due to **large polyp** in patient on tamoxifen.

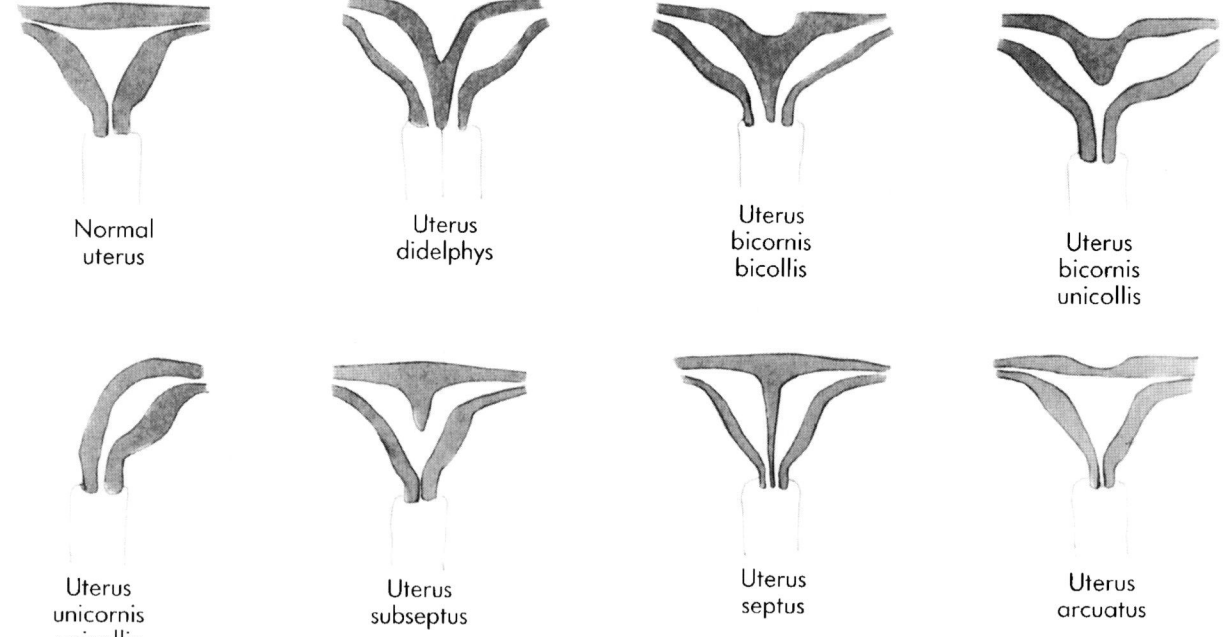

Normal uterus

Uterus didelphys

Uterus bicornis bicollis

Uterus bicornis unicollis

Uterus unicornis unicollis

Uterus subseptus

Uterus septus

Uterus arcuatus

FIGURE 15-9. Congenital uterine abnormalities. Diagram of common types. (Courtesy of Jocelyne Salem.)

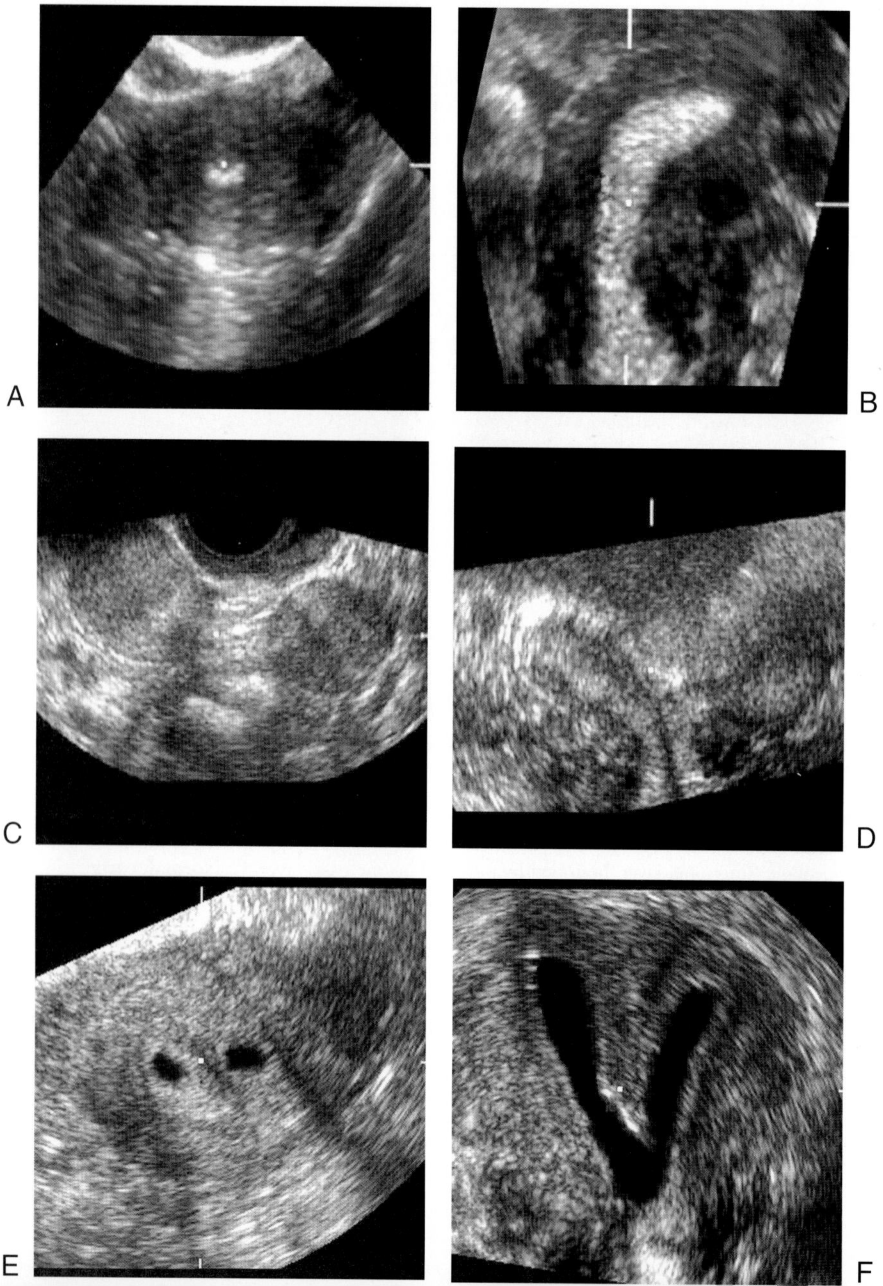

A

B

C

D

FIGURE 15-10. Congenital uterine abnormalities. A, B, **Unicornuate uterus** (3-Dimensional reconstruction). **A,** Transverse scan. **B,** 3-D Coronal reconstruction. **C, D,** **Didelphys uterus.** **C,** Transverse scan. **D,** 3-D Coronal reconstruction. **E, F,** **Subseptate uterus**. **E,** Transverse sonohysterogram. **F,** 3-D Coronal reconstruction.

E

F

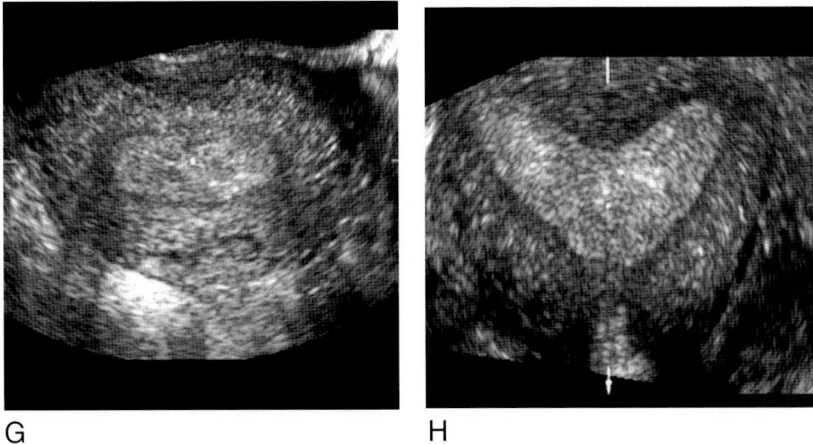

FIGURE 15-10, *cont'd.* **Congenital uterine abnormalities. G, H, Arcuate uterus. G,** Transverse scan. **H,** 3-D Coronal reconstruction. (Courtesy of Anna Lev-Toaff, M.D.)

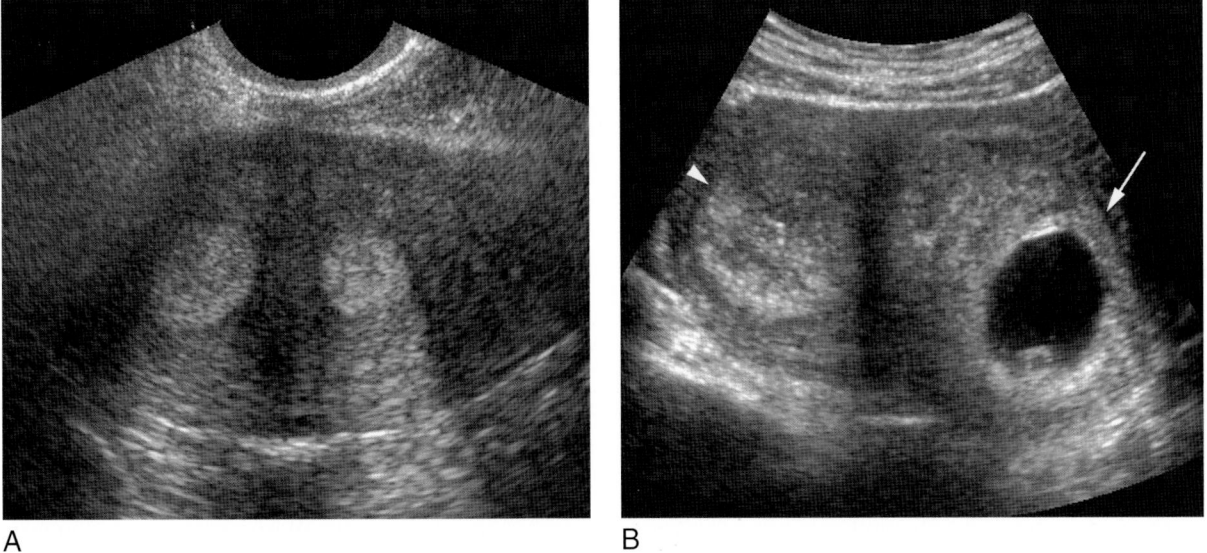

FIGURE 15-11. Bicornuate uterus. A, Transvaginal transverse scan through fundus of a bicornuate uterus shows two endometria separated by uterine musculature. **B,** Transabdominal transverse scan through fundus of a bicornuate uterus shows gestational sac (*arrow*) in left horn and decidual reaction (*arrowhead*) in right horn.

There is a high association between **uterine malformations** and **congenital renal abnormalities,** especially renal agenesis and ectopia.[28] The most common uterine anomaly associated with renal agenesis is the uterus bicornis bicollis with a partial vaginal septum in which one side has no outlet for menstrual blood, resulting in a unilateral hematometrocolpos.[29] In all patients with uterine malformations, the kidneys should be evaluated sonographically. In females with an absent or ectopic kidney, the uterus should be scanned for malformations. The abnormalities are always on the same side.

Most uterine anomalies can be detected by sonography.[30] Two endometrial echo complexes may be seen in the bicornuate or septate uterus. Sonography can also outline the external contour of the uterus. In the **didelphys** and **bicornuate uterus,** the endometrial cavities are widely separated, and there is a deep indentation on the fundal contour. The **septate uterus,** in contrast, has a relatively normal outline, and the two endometrial cavities are closer together and are separated by a thin, fibrous septum. The septum has a poor blood supply and contains little, if any, myometrium.[31] Sonography, combined with hysterosalpingography, has a high level of accuracy in distinguishing between the septate and the bicornuate uterus.[32] It is important to differentiate these two conditions because the septate uterus can be treated by outpatient hysteroscopic incision of the fibrous septum. Because the bicornuate uterus consists of two separate uterine horns, each containing a full complement of myometrium and endometrium, correction requires abdominal surgery.

The **unicornuate uterus** is difficult to differentiate from the normal uterus by sonography. It may be suspected when the uterus appears small and laterally positioned. Hydrometra in the opposite rudimentary horn may be seen and mistaken for a uterine or adnexal mass. The bicornuate uterus may also be confused with a uterine or adnexal mass if the central endometrial echo complex is not seen in one horn. In many instances, the bicornuate uterus is first diagnosed incidentally in early pregnancy when a gestational sac is present in one horn and there is decidual reaction in the other (see Fig. 15-11B).

Three-dimensional ultrasound with multiplanar imaging has been shown to be quite valuable in detecting and classifying uterine anomalies (see Fig. 15-10).[33] The coronal view through the entire uterus, which cannot be obtained on routine two-dimensional ultrasound due to the limited mobility of the transducer in the vagina, is essential for diagnosis. MRI is also highly accurate in demonstrating uterine anomalies.[34] However, because of the relatively high cost of MRI, it is usually reserved for the more complicated anomalies.

Uterine abnormalities have also been seen in patients who have had *in utero* **exposure to diethylstilbestrol**. Diethylstilbestrol given during the first trimester crosses the placenta and exerts a direct effect on the Müllerian system of the fetus. Sonography may demonstrate a diffuse decrease in the size of the uterus and an irregular T-shaped uterine cavity.[35,36]

Abnormalities of the Myometrium

Leiomyoma

Leiomyomas (fibroids) are the most common neoplasms of the uterus. They occur in approximately 20% to 30% of females over the age of 30 years[37] and are more common in black women. They are usually multiple and are the most common cause of enlargement of the nonpregnant uterus. Although frequently asymptomatic, women with leiomyomas can experience pain and uterine bleeding. Leiomyomas may be classified as **intramural**, confined to the myometrium; **submucosal**, projecting into the uterine cavity and displacing or distorting the endometrium; or **subserosal**, projecting from the peritoneal surface of the uterus.

LEIOMYOMA CLASSIFICATION

Intramural
    Confined to the myometrium
Submucosal
    Projecting into the uterine cavity
Subserosal
    Projecting from the peritoneal surface

Intramural fibroids are the most common. Submucosal fibroids, although less common, produce symptoms most frequently. Subserosal fibroids may be pedunculated and present as an adnexal mass. They may also project between the leaves of the broad ligament, where they are referred to as intraligamentous. Cervical fibroids account for approximately 8% of all fibroids.

Fibroids are **estrogen dependent** and may increase in size during anovulatory cycles as a result of unopposed estrogen stimulation[38] and during pregnancy, although about one half of all fibroids show little significant change during pregnancy.[39] Fibroids identified in the first trimester are associated with an elevated risk of pregnancy loss, and this risk is higher in patients with multiple fibroids than in those with a single fibroid.[40] Large fibroids do not interfere with pregnancy or normal vaginal delivery except when they are located in the lower uterine segment or the cervix. Leiomyomas rarely develop in postmenopausal women, and most stabilize or decrease in size following menopause. They may increase in size in postmenopausal patients who are undergoing hormone replacement therapy. Tamoxifen has also been reported to cause growth in leiomyomas.[41] A rapid increase in fibroid size, especially in a postmenopausal patient, should raise the possibility of sarcomatous change.[2]

Pathologically, leiomyomas are composed of spindle-shaped, smooth muscle cells arranged in whorl-like patterns separated by variable amounts of fibrous connective tissue. The surrounding myometrium may become compressed to form a pseudocapsule. As they enlarge, leiomyomas may outgrow their blood supply, resulting in ischemia and cystic degeneration.

Sonographically, leiomyomas have variable appearances (Fig. 15-12A-H). The uterus may be enlarged, with a globular outline and heterogeneous echotexture resulting from small, diffuse leiomyomas. Localized leiomyomas are most commonly hypoechoic or heterogeneous in echotexture. They frequently distort the external contour of the uterus. Minimal contour irregularity at the interface between the uterus and bladder may be a subtle diagnostic sign.[42] Many leiomyomas demonstrate areas of **acoustic attenuation** or **shadowing** without a discrete mass, making it impossible to estimate size. The attenuation is thought to be due to dense fibrosis within the substance of the tumor. Kliewer et al. have suggested that posterior shadowing arising from within the substance of a leiomyoma (but not from echogenic foci) originates from transitional zones between apposed tissues.[43] Histologically, the transitional zone includes the margins of the leiomyoma with adjacent normal myometrium, the borders between fibrous tissue and smooth muscle, and the edges of whorls and bundles of smooth muscle.[43] This type of shadowing is a very useful diagnostic feature in distinguishing a pedunculated or exophytic leiomyoma from other types of adnexal masses.[44]

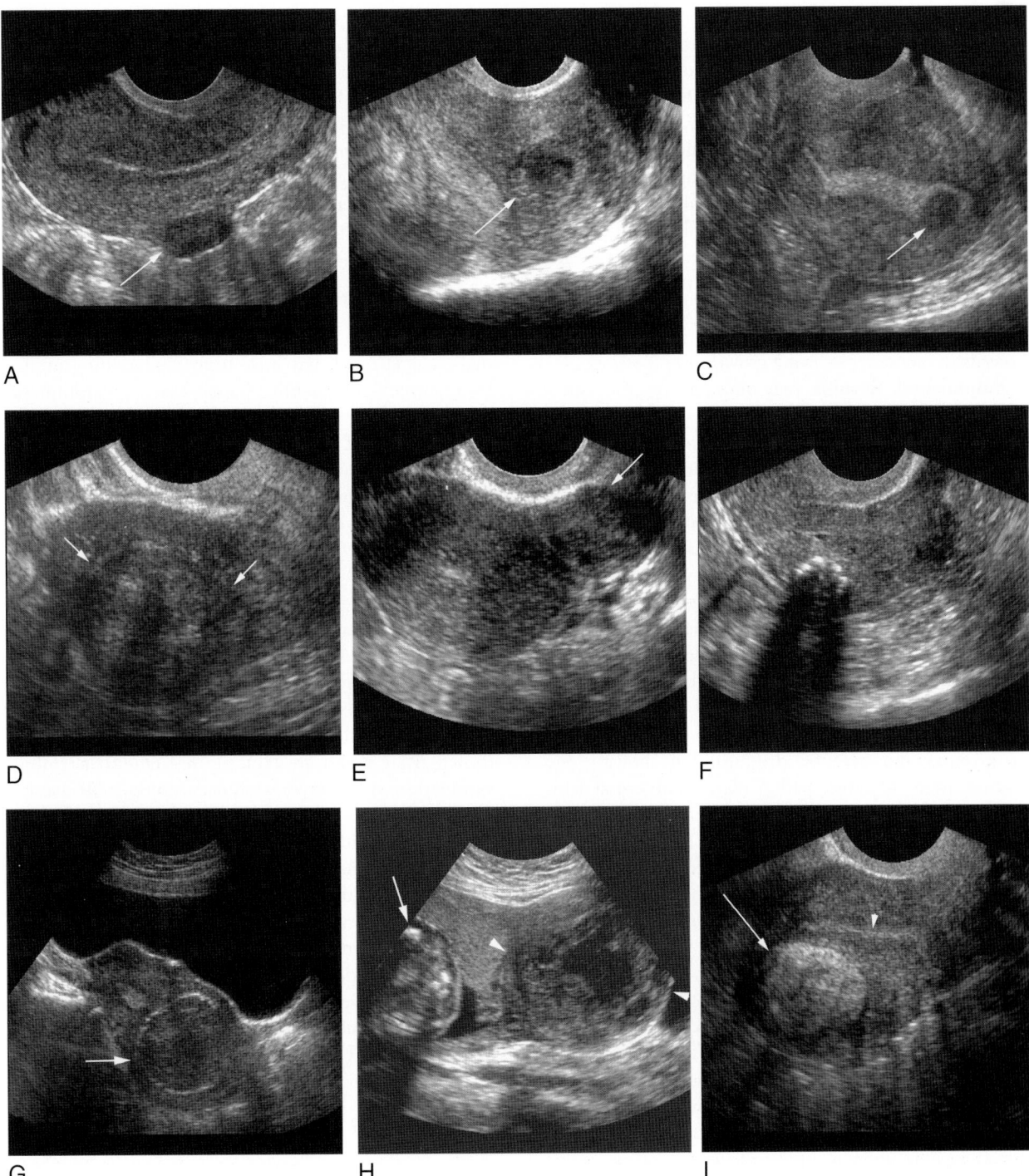

FIGURE 15-12. Uterine fibroids—spectrum of appearances. A-F and I, Transvaginal scans. **G, H,** Transabdominal scans. **A,** Localized hypoechoic **subserosal fibroid** (*arrow*). **B,** Localized hypoechoic **intramural fibroid** (*arrow*). **C,** Hypoechoic **submucosal fibroid** (*arrow*). **D,** Marked attenuation of sound beam by fibroid (*arrows*). **E, Pedunculated subserosal fibroid** (*arrow*) presenting as solid left adnexal mass. **F, Fibroid with calcification** causing posterior shadowing. **G, Calcified fibroid** with curvilinear peripheral calcification (*arrow*) mimicking a fetal head. **H,** Fibroid with **cystic degeneration** (*arrowheads*) in pregnancy. Patient presented with pain and tenderness over degenerating fibroid. Fetus (*arrow*). **I, Lipoleiomyoma.** Highly echogenic mass within myometrium (*arrow*) with posterior attenuation. Endometrium (*arrowhead*).

Calcification may occur in older females, frequently appearing as focal areas of increased echogenicity with shadowing or as a curvilinear echogenic rim, which may simulate the outline of a fetal head.[45] **Degeneration** and **necrosis** produce areas of decreased echogenicity or cystic spaces within the fibroid. This tends to occur more commonly during pregnancy, affecting approximately 7% to 8% of pregnant patients with fibroids, who may present with pain over this area.[39] Giant leiomyomas with multiple cystic spaces due to edema have been described.[46] Doppler should be used to assess the vascularity of fibroids. It has been suggested that vascularity is useful as a predictor of growth, with 46% of vascular fibroids in one series showing growth over 1 year.[47]

Submucosal fibroids may impinge on the endometrium, distorting the cavity with varying degrees of intracavitary extension. Transvaginal sonography allows better differentiation between a submucosal and an intramural lesion and its relationship to the endometrial cavity.[48] Sonohysterography is very helpful to determine the exact location and relationship of the fibroid to the endometrium, amount of intracavitary extension, and its potential resectability.[49] In some cases, sonohysterography may also be necessary to distinguish a submucosal leiomyoma from an endometrial lesion. Submucosal fibroids are usually broad-based hypoechoic solid masses with an overlying layer of echogenic endometrium. Transvaginal sonography can detect very small leiomyomas and may be diagnostic in showing the uterine origin of large, pedunculated, subserosal leiomyomas that simulate adnexal masses. However, **subserosal** or **pedunculated fibroids** may be missed if the transvaginal approach alone is used, because of the limited field-of-view.[50] Leiomyomas in the fundus of a retroverted uterus are much better delineated by transvaginal sonography.

Lipomatous Uterine Tumors

Lipomatous uterine tumors (lipoleiomyoma) are uncommon, benign neoplasms consisting of variable portions of mature lipocytes, smooth muscle, or fibrous tissue. Histologically, these tumors comprise a spectrum including pure lipomas, lipoleiomyomas, and fibrolipo-

myomas. **Sonographically**, the finding of a highly echogenic, attenuating mass within the myometrium is virtually diagnostic of this condition (see Fig. 15-12I).[51] Color Doppler shows complete absence of flow within the mass.[52] It is important to identify the lesion within the uterus so as not to confuse it with the more common, similar-appearing, fat-containing ovarian dermoid.[53] Because lipomatous uterine tumors are usually asymptomatic, they do not require surgery.

Leiomyosarcoma

Leiomyosarcoma is rare, accounting for 1.3% of uterine malignancies, and may arise from a preexisting uterine leiomyoma.[37] Frequently, patients are asymptomatic, although uterine bleeding may occur. This condition is rarely diagnosed preoperatively. **Sonographically**, the appearance is similar to that of a rapidly growing or degenerating leiomyoma, except when there is evidence of local invasion or distant metastases (Fig. 15-13).

Adenomyosis

Adenomyosis is a condition characterized pathologically by the presence of endometrial glands and stroma within the myometrium, which are associated with adjacent myometrial hypertrophy. It is usually more extensive in the posterior wall.[37] The endometrial glands arise from the basal layer and are typically resistant to hormonal stimulation. Adenomyosis can occur in both **diffuse** and **nodular** forms. The more common diffuse form is composed of widely scattered adenomyosis foci within the myometrium, whereas the nodular form is composed of circumscribed nodules called adenomyomas. The clinical presentation is usually nonspecific, consisting of uterine enlargement, pelvic pain, dysmenorrhea, and menorrhagia. Adenomyosis is more commonly seen in women who have had children.

Sonographically, the diagnosis has been considered to be difficult. Using transabdominal sonography, this diagnosis may be suggested if there is **diffuse uterine enlargement** with a normal contour, normal endo-

---

SONOGRAPHIC FEATURES OF LEIOMYOMAS

Variable appearance
Hypoechoic or heterogeneous mass
Distortion of external uterine contour
Attenuation or shadowing without discrete mass
Calcification
Degeneration or necrosis

SONOGRAPHIC FEATURES OF ADENOMYOSIS

Diffuse uterine enlargement
Diffusely heterogeneous myometrium
Asymmetrical thickening of myometrium
Inhomogeneous hypoechoic areas
Myometrial cysts
Poor definition of endometrial myometrial border
Focal tenderness elicited by vaginal transducer
Subendometrial echogenic linear striations
Subendometrial echogenic nodules

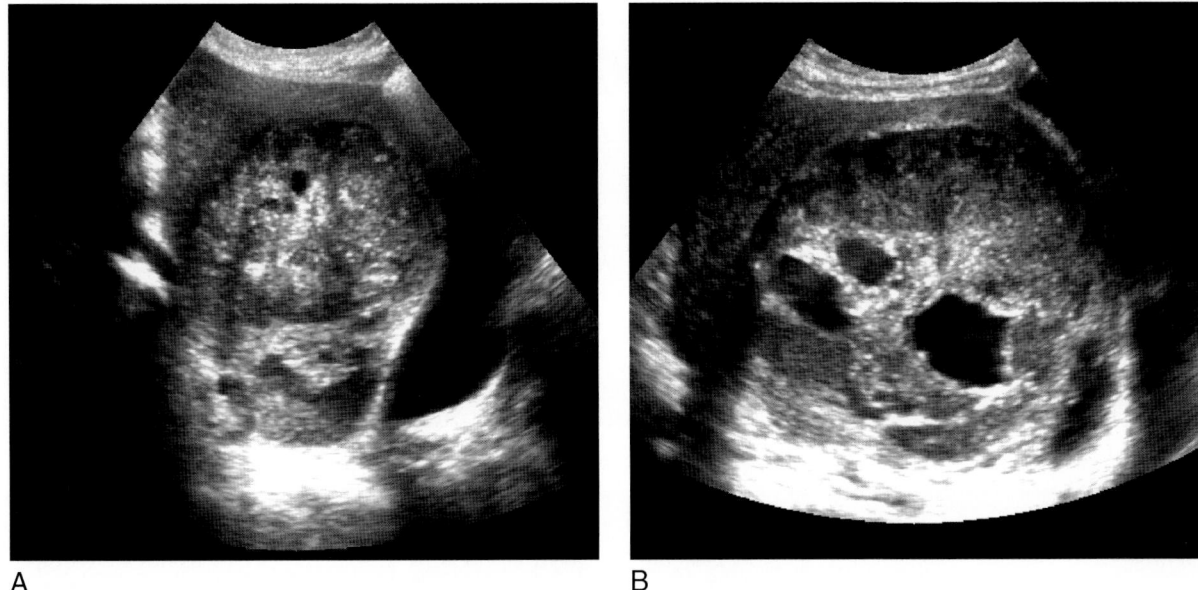

FIGURE 15-13. Leiomyosarcoma. A, Sagittal and **B**, transverse transabdominal scans show a large heterogeneous uterine mass with cystic areas. There is a rim of remaining normal myometrium.

metrial texture, and normal myometrial texture.[54] Thickening of the posterior myometrium, with the involved area being slightly more anechoic than normal myometrium, has also been described.[55] Transvaginal sonography is more accurate in diagnosing this condition, which is now being detected with increasing frequency (Fig. 15-14).[56-59] The uterus may be enlarged, having a globular configuration with a diffusely heterogeneous-appearing myometrium. The myometrium may be asymmetrically thickened. The endometrial-myometrial border may be poorly defined. Focal uterine tenderness may be elicited by the transvaginal transducer. Inhomogeneous hypoechoic areas within the myometrium, having indistinct margins, have also been described.

Small myometrial cysts, frequently subendometrial, may also be present within the myometrium and have been shown histologically to represent dilated glands in ectopic endometrial tissue.[57] Adenomyosis is the most common cause of myometrial cysts, although cysts within the myometrium may also be congenital in origin or may be seen in leiomyomas undergoing cystic degeneration. Subendometrial echogenic linear striations and subendometrial echogenic nodules have recently been described and reported to improve the specificity and positive predictive value in diagnosing adenomyosis.[60]

Localized adenomyomas may be seen by transvaginal sonography as inhomogeneous, circumscribed areas in the myometrium, having indistinct margins and containing anechoic lacunae.[61,62] However, they are usually difficult to distinguish from leiomyomas, and these two conditions frequently occur together. The presence of fibroids has been shown to limit the ability

to diagnose the severity of adenomyosis.[59] The variable sonographic appearance is related to the distribution of the heterotopic endometrial tissue, the degree of associated muscle hypertrophy, and the presence and size of the cysts within the heterotopic endometrial tissue.[60]

MRI is highly accurate in demonstrating adenomyosis, which appears as ill-defined areas of decreased signal intensity within the myometrium or diffuse or focal thickening of the junctional zone on T2-weighted images.[63-65] Reinhold et al. found MRI and sonography to be of comparable accuracy in the diagnosis of adenomyosis.[65]

Arteriovenous Malformations

Uterine arteriovenous malformations (AVMs) (Fig. 15-15) consist of a vascular plexus of arteries and veins without an intervening capillary network. They are rare lesions, usually involving the myometrium and, at times, the endometrium. Although they may be congenital, most cases are acquired due to pelvic trauma, surgery, and gestational trophoblastic neoplasia. Patients, typically young women in the childbearing years, present with metrorrhagia with hemoglobin-dropping blood loss. Diagnosis is critical, as dilation and curettage may lead to catastrophic hemorrhage.

On **sonography**, uterine AVMs may be nonspecific, with minimal findings. They may be seen as multiple serpiginous, anechoic structures within the pelvis and may be confused with multiloculated ovarian cysts, fluid-filled bowel loops, and hydrosalpinx.[66] Color Doppler is diagnostic, showing abundant blood flow within the anechoic structures.[67,68] There is a florid color mosaic, which is more extensive than the gray-scale

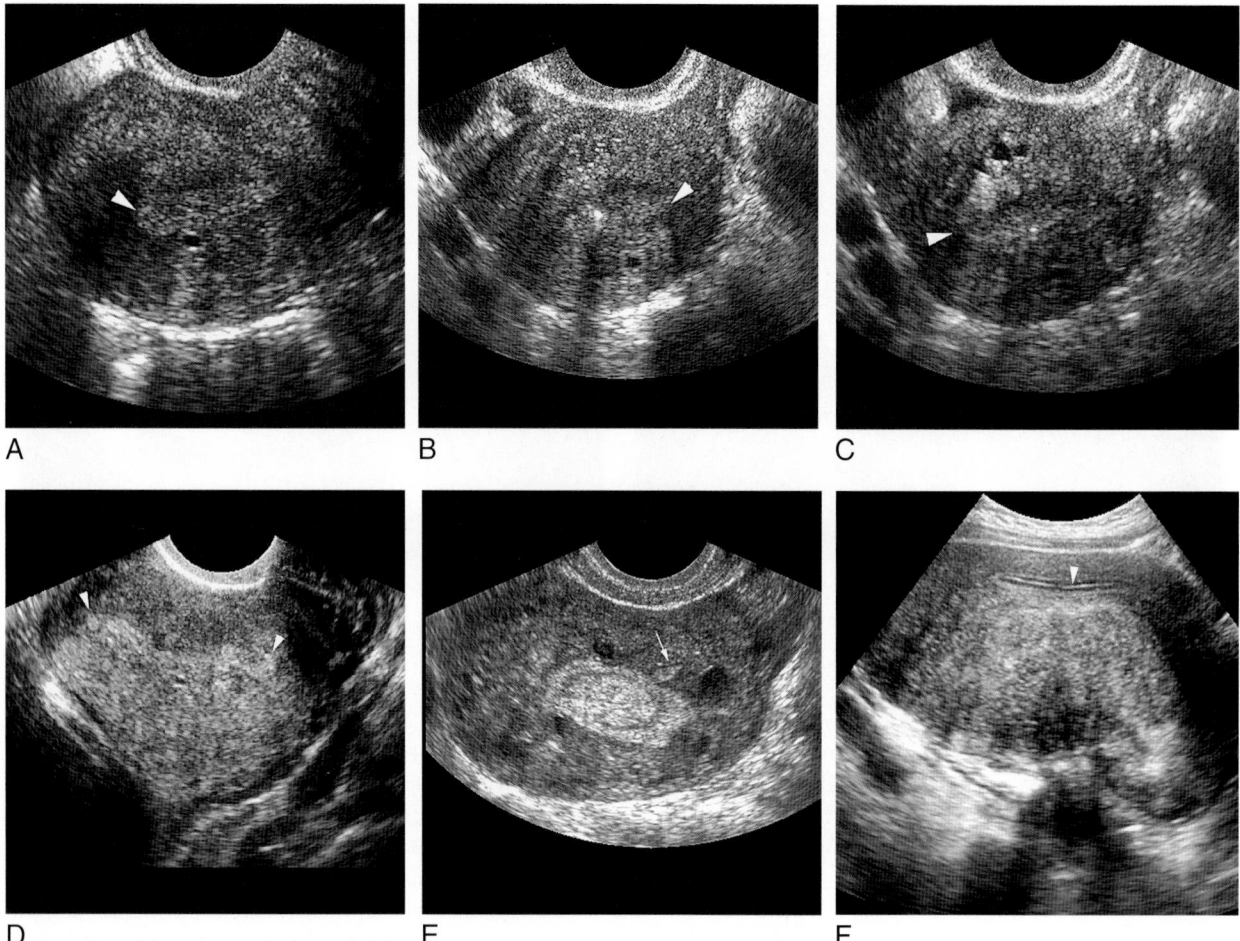

FIGURE 15-14. Adenomyosis on transvaginal scans—spectrum of appearances. A, Subendometrial cyst (*arrow*). **B, Cysts** with heterogeneity in both anterior and posterior myometrium. **C, Cysts** with heterogeneity in anterior myometrium. **D, Myometrial heterogeneity** with ill-defined endometrial borders (*arrowheads*). **E,** Multiple **subendometrial cysts** and **echogenic nodule** (*arrow*). **F,** Large area of **myometrial heterogeneity** producing a focal mass effect and displacing endometrium (*arrowhead*). This may mimic a fibroid.

abnormality. **Spectral Doppler** shows high-velocity, low-resistance arterial flow with high-velocity venous flow often being indistinguishable from the arterial signal.[68] Treatment and confirmation include angiography with embolic therapy.

Abnormalities of the Endometrium

Because of its improved resolution, transvaginal sonography is better able to image and depict subtle abnormalities within the endometrium and to clearly define the endometrial-myometrial border.[69] Knowledge of the normal sonographic appearance of the endometrium allows for earlier recognition of endometrial pathologic conditions manifested by endometrial thickening with well defined or poorly defined, irregular margins (see box). Many endometrial pathologies, such as **hyperplasia, polyps, and carcinoma,** can cause abnormal bleeding, especially in the postmenopausal patient. All of these conditions can have similar sonographic appearances. A hyperechoic line partially or completely surrounding the endometrium has been described as a sign of a focal intracavitary process and is felt to be due to the interface between the intraluminal mass and the surrounding endometrium or the endometrium itself.[70]

Sonohysterography has been shown to be of great value in further evaluating the abnormally thickened endometrium.[71-75] It can distinguish between focal and diffuse endometrial abnormalities and determine further management. If the abnormality is diffuse, a blind non-directed biopsy can be done, but if the process is focal, hysteroscopy with directed biopsy or excision should be done.[75,76] Sonohysterography may also be able to distinguish benign from malignant endometrial processes.[77,78] Patients with endometrial cancer may have poorly distensible endometrial cavities, despite successful cervical os cannulation.[78]

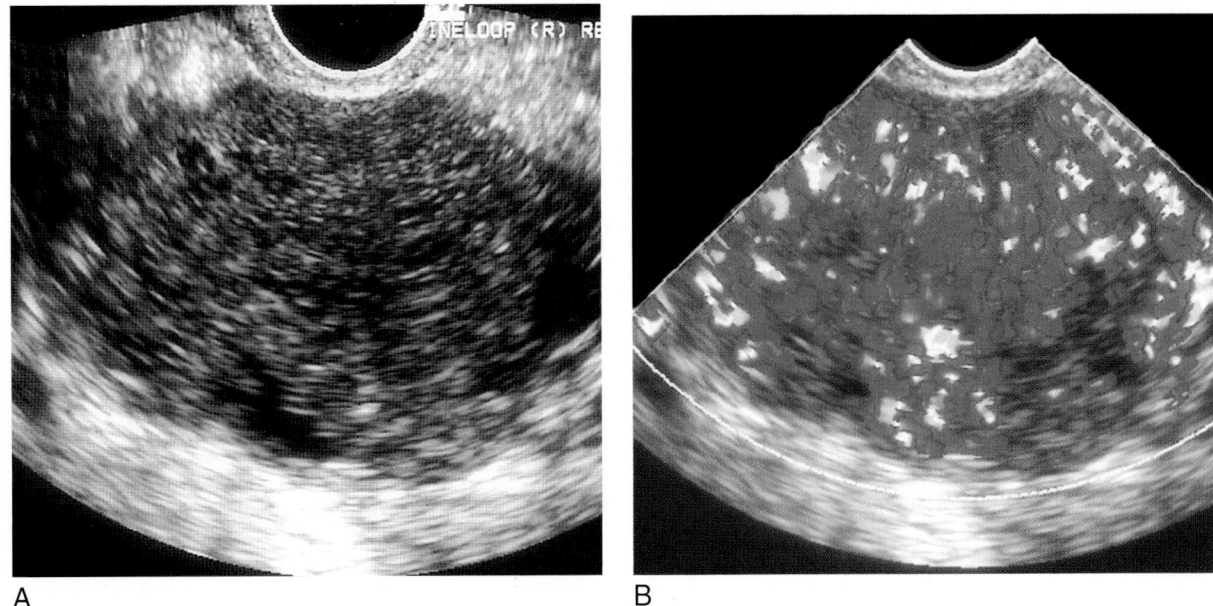

FIGURE 15-15. Uterine arteriovenous malformation. A, Transverse transvaginal sonogram shows a textural inhomogeneity in the uterine fundus. **B,** Color Doppler image shows a floridly colored mosaic pattern with apparent flow reversals and areas of color aliasing. (From Huang M, Muradali D, Thurston WA, et al: Uterine arteriovenous malformations (AVMs): Ultrasound and Doppler features with MRI correlation. Radiology 1998;206;115-123.)

CAUSES OF ENDOMETRIAL THICKENING

Early intrauterine pregnancy
Incomplete abortion
Ectopic pregnancy
Retained products of conception
Trophoblastic disease
Endometritis
Adhesions
Hyperplasia
Polyps
Carcinoma

Postmenopausal Endometrium

Postmenopausal bleeding is considered to be any vaginal bleeding that occurs in a postmenopausal woman other than the expected cyclic bleeding with sequential hormone replacement therapy. Because the prevalence of endometrial cancer is low, the negative predictive value of a thin endometrium is high and, therefore, a thin endometrium can be reliably used to exclude cancer. Several studies have shown that in patients with postmenopausal bleeding who have had endometrial sampling, an **endometrial measurement of either 4 mm or less**[79-82] **or 5 mm or less**[83-85] **can be considered normal.** The bleeding in these patients is usually due to an **atrophic endometrium.** In a large study of 1168 women with postmenopausal bleeding, in whom 114

endometrial cancers were found, no women with endometrial cancer had an endometrium measuring less than 5 mm.[81]

A meta-analysis of 35 published studies that included 5892 women showed that an endometrial thickness greater than 5 mm detected 96% of endometrial cancer and 92% of any endometrial disease.[86] A recent multi-specialty consensus conference sponsored by the Society of Radiologists in Ultrasound to discuss the role of sonography in women with postmenopausal bleeding using the above meta-analysis concluded that an endometrial thickness of greater than 5 mm is abnormal.[87] However, Doubilet, in a commentary on these conclusions, recommends using 4 mm rather than 5 mm because that will have a higher sensitivity and miss fewer cancers.[88] Because the prevalence of endometrial cancer is low, the presence of a **thin endometrium can be used reliably to exclude cancer.**

Transvaginal assessment of endometrial thickness has been shown to be highly reproducible with excellent intraobserver and good interobserver agreement.[89] If the endometrium cannot be visualized in its entirety, the examination should be considered nondiagnostic and lead to further investigation.[87]

The consensus conference also addressed the issue of when sonohysterography or hysteroscopy should be used in the evaluation of postmenopausal bleeding. There was agreement that either is appropriate if a focal abnormality is suspected on transvaginal sonography and that sonohysterography is more sensitive than transvaginal sonography alone in detecting focal abnormalities in women with postmenopausal bleeding. Some authors have recommended that all women with postmenopausal bleeding should undergo sonohysterography, even if the transvaginal sonogram is normal.[90,91] Neele et al. found 30% of 111 healthy asymptomatic postmenopausal women with a normal transvaginal sonogram had endometrial abnormalities detected on sonohysterography.[92] The important question is whether finding and treating these benign conditions improves the patient's quality of life, morbidity, and survival. Further investigation into this issue is warranted.[87]

Further studies have assessed the endometrium in **asymptomatic postmenopausal patients**, and it is felt that an **endometrium of less than 9 mm can be considered normal**.[93-95] Most of these reports have included a mixed group of patients, some of whom were undergoing hormone replacement therapy and some of whom were not. Many postmenopausal patients are now on hormone replacement therapy, as estrogen replacement decreases the risk of osteoporosis and relieves menopausal symptoms. However, unopposed estrogen replacement is associated with an increased risk of endometrial hyperplasia and carcinoma. Therefore, estrogen therapy is frequently combined with progesterone, in continuous combined or in sequential regimens. Patients on sequential hormone therapy have a changing endometrial appearance on sonography similar to the premenopausal endometrium. If noncyclic bleeding occurs, endometrial hyperplasia, polyps, and malignancy must be considered. In these patients, it is important that sonography be done 4 to 5 days after completion of the cyclic bleeding when the endometrium is at its thinnest.[96]

A small amount of **fluid within the endometrial canal**, detected by transvaginal sonography, may be a normal finding in asymptomatic patients (Fig. 15-16).[97] Larger amounts of fluid may be associated with benign conditions, most often related to cervical stenosis, or with malignancy.[98,99] The fluid should be excluded when measuring the endometrium. Because the fluid allows better detail of the endometrium, it is extremely important to assess the endometrium carefully for irregularities and polypoid masses.[100]

Hydrometrocolpos and Hematometrocolpos

Obstruction of the genital tract results in the accumulation of secretions, blood, or both in the uterus and/or vagina, with the location depending on the amount of obstruction. Before menstruation, the accumulation of secretions in the vagina and uterus is referred to as hydrometrocolpos. Following menstruation, hematometrocolpos results from the presence of retained menstrual blood. The obstruction may be congenital and is most commonly due to an **imperforate hymen**. Other congenital causes include a **vaginal septum**,

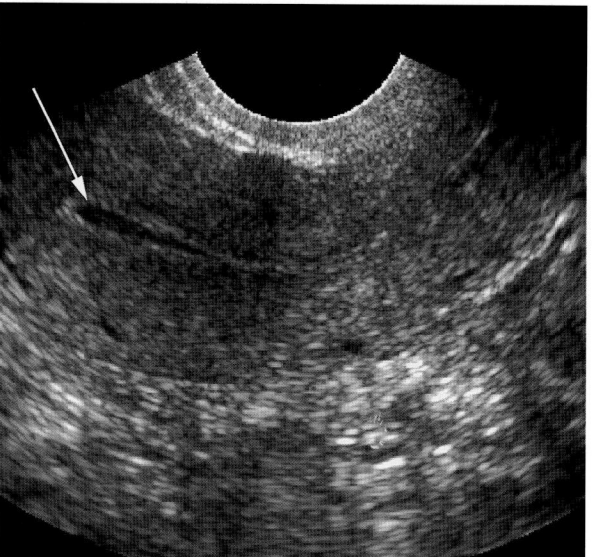

FIGURE 15-16. Transvaginal scan. Small amount of fluid (*arrow*) in postmenopausal endometrial canal.

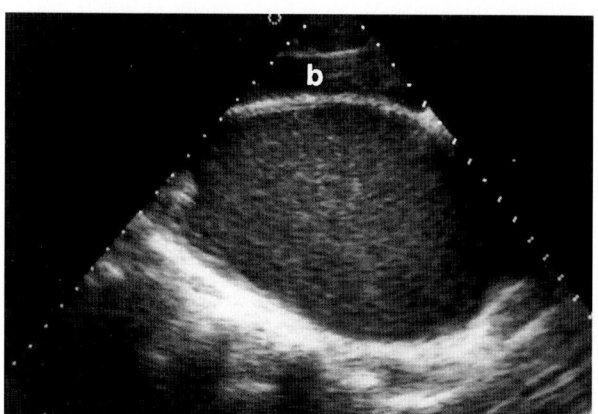

FIGURE 15-17. Hematocolpos in young patient with imperforate hymen. Sagittal scan shows distended vagina filled with echogenic material and compressing the bladder (b) anteriorly.

vaginal atresia, or a **rudimentary uterine horn**.[101] Hydrometra and hematometra may also be acquired as a result of cervical stenosis from **endometrial or cervical tumors** or from **postirradiation fibrosis**.[98,102]

Sonographically, if the obstruction is at the vaginal level, there is marked distention of the vagina and endometrial cavity with fluid. If seen before puberty, the accumulation of secretions is anechoic. Following menstruation, the presence of old blood results in echogenic material in the fluid (Fig. 15-17). There may also be layering of the echogenic material, resulting in a fluid-fluid level.

Acquired hydrometra or hematometra usually shows a distended, fluid-filled endometrial cavity which may contain echogenic material (Fig. 15-18). Superimposed

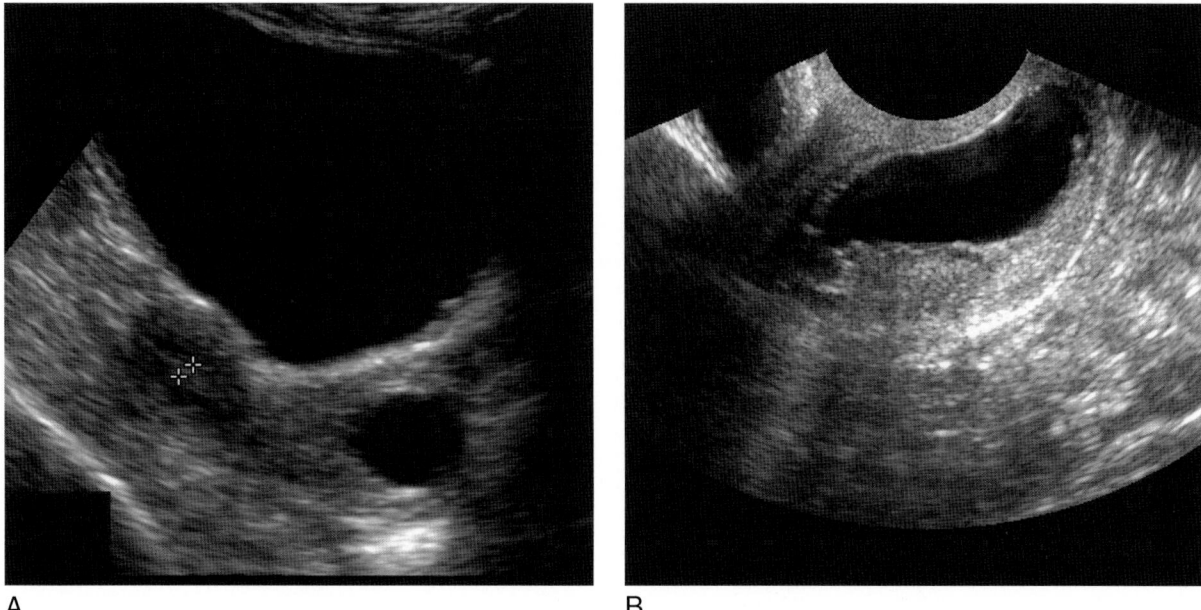

FIGURE 15-18. Hematometra in patient with cervical stenosis secondary to cervical carcinoma. A, Transabdominal sagittal scan shows small postmenopausal uterus with fluid-filled cervical canal. Endometrium outlined by cursors. **B,** Transvaginal scan shows distended cervical canal filled with fluid and echogenic material, as a result of blood and debris.

infection (pyometra) is difficult to distinguish from hydrometra on sonography, and this diagnosis is usually made clinically in the presence of hydrometra.[102]

Endometrial Hyperplasia

Hyperplasia of the endometrium is defined as a proliferation of glands of irregular size and shape, with an increase in the gland/stroma ratio when compared with the normal proliferative endometrium.[37] The process is diffuse but may not involve the entire endometrium. Histologically, endometrial hyperplasia can be divided into hyperplasia without cellular atypia and hyperplasia with cellular atypia (atypical hyperplasia). Long-term follow-up studies have shown that about 25% of atypical hyperplasia will progress to carcinoma, as opposed to less than 2% of hyperplasia without cellular atypia.[37] Each of these types may be further subdivided into simple (cystic) or complex (adenomatous) hyperplasia, depending on the amount of glandular complexity and crowding. In simple (cystic) hyperplasia, the glands are cystically dilated and surrounded by abundant cellular stroma, whereas in complex (adenomatous) hyperplasia, the glands are crowded together with little intervening stroma.

Endometrial hyperplasia is a common cause of abnormal uterine bleeding. Hyperplasia develops from unopposed estrogen stimulation; in postmenopausal and perimenopausal women, it is usually due to **unopposed estrogen hormone replacement therapy**. Hyperplasia is less commonly seen during the reproductive years, but it may occur in women with **persistent anovulatory cycles, polycystic ovarian disease**, and in **obese women** with increased production of endogenous estrogens. Hyperplasia may also be seen in women with estrogen-producing tumors, such as **granulosa cell tumors** and **thecomas of the ovary**.

Sonographically, the endometrium is usually diffusely thick and echogenic, with well-defined margins (Fig. 15-19). Focal or asymmetrical thickening can also occur. Small cysts may be seen within the endometrium in **cystic hyperplasia**; however, a similar appearance may be seen in **cystic atrophy**, and cystic changes can also be seen in **endometrial polyps**. These cystic areas have been shown to represent the dilated cystic glands seen at histology.[103,104] Although cystic changes within a thickened endometrium are more frequently seen in benign conditions, they can also be seen in **endometrial carcinoma**.[105] Because hyperplasia has a nonspecific sonographic appearance, biopsy is necessary for diagnosis.

Endometrial Atrophy

The majority of women with postmenopausal uterine bleeding have endometrial atrophy.[80-85,106] On transvaginal sonography, an atrophic endometrium is usually thin, measuring less than 5 mm, and in these patients, no further investigation or therapy is necessary. Histologically, the endometrial glands may be dilated, but the cells are cuboidal or flat and the stroma is fibrotic. A thin endometrium with cystic changes on transvaginal

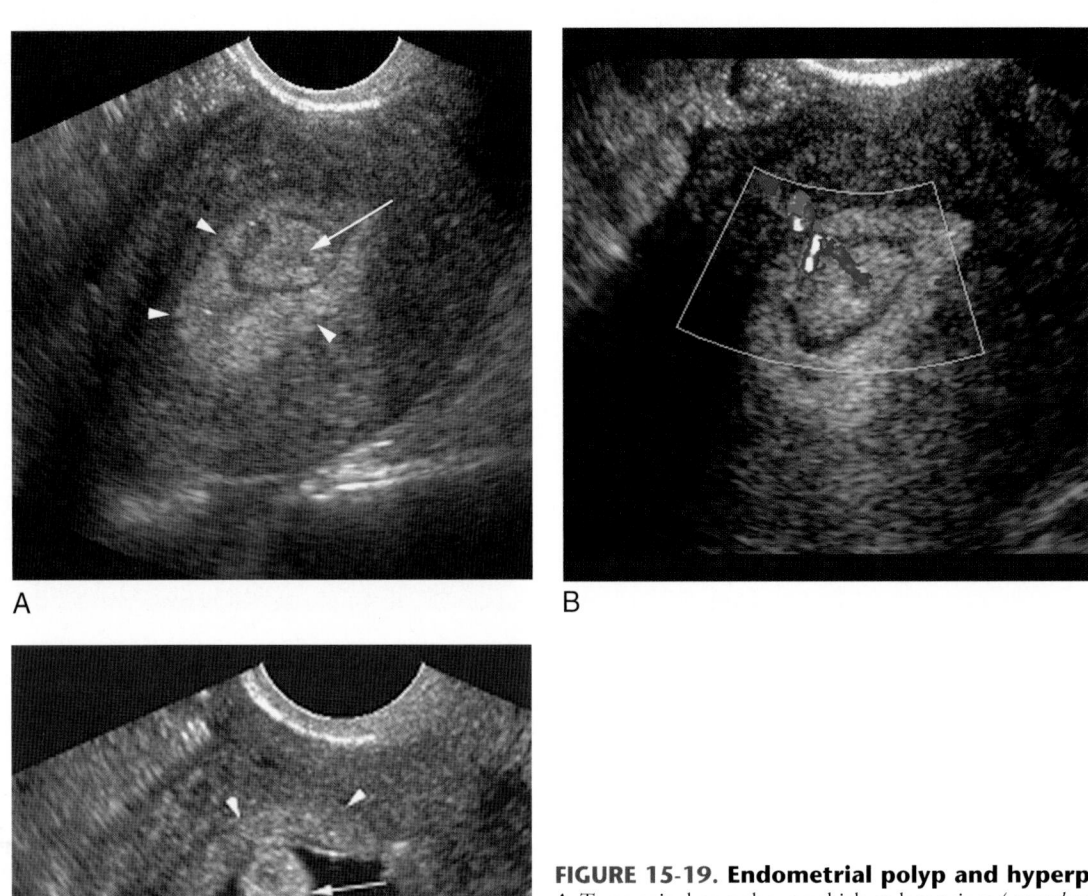

FIGURE 15-19. Endometrial polyp and hyperplasia.
A, Transvaginal scan shows a thick endometrium (*arrowheads*) with central round polyp (*arrow*). **B**, Color Doppler shows feeding vessel. **C**, Sonohysterogram confirms polyp (*arrow*) and thick endometrium (*arrowheads*) due to hyperplasia.

sonography is consistent with a diagnosis of cystic atrophy, but when the endometrium is thick, the appearance is indistinguishable from that of cystic hyperplasia.[105]

Endometrial Polyps

Endometrial polyps are common lesions that are more frequently seen in perimenopausal and postmenopausal women. They may cause uterine bleeding, although most are asymptomatic. In the menstruating woman, endometrial polyps may be associated with intermenstrual bleeding or menometrorrhagia and may be a cause of infertility. Histologically, polyps are localized overgrowths of endometrial tissue covered by epithelium, and they contain a variable number of glands, stroma, and blood vessels.[37] They may be pedunculated, or broad

based, or have a thin stalk. Approximately 20% of endometrial polyps are multiple. Malignant degeneration is uncommon. Occasionally, a polyp will have a long stalk, allowing it to protrude into the cervix or even into the vagina.

On **sonography**, polyps may appear as nonspecific echogenic endometrial thickening, which may be diffuse or focal (see Fig. 15-8G). However, they may also appear as a focal, round, echogenic mass within the endometrial cavity (see Figs. 15-8E and 15-19).[107] This appearance is much more easily identified when there is fluid within the endometrial cavity outlining the mass. Because fluid is instilled into the endometrial cavity during **sonohysterography**, this technique is ideal for demonstrating polyps (Figs. 15-20A-F). Sonohysterography is also a valuable technique when transvaginal sonography is unable to differentiate an **endometrial polyp** from a

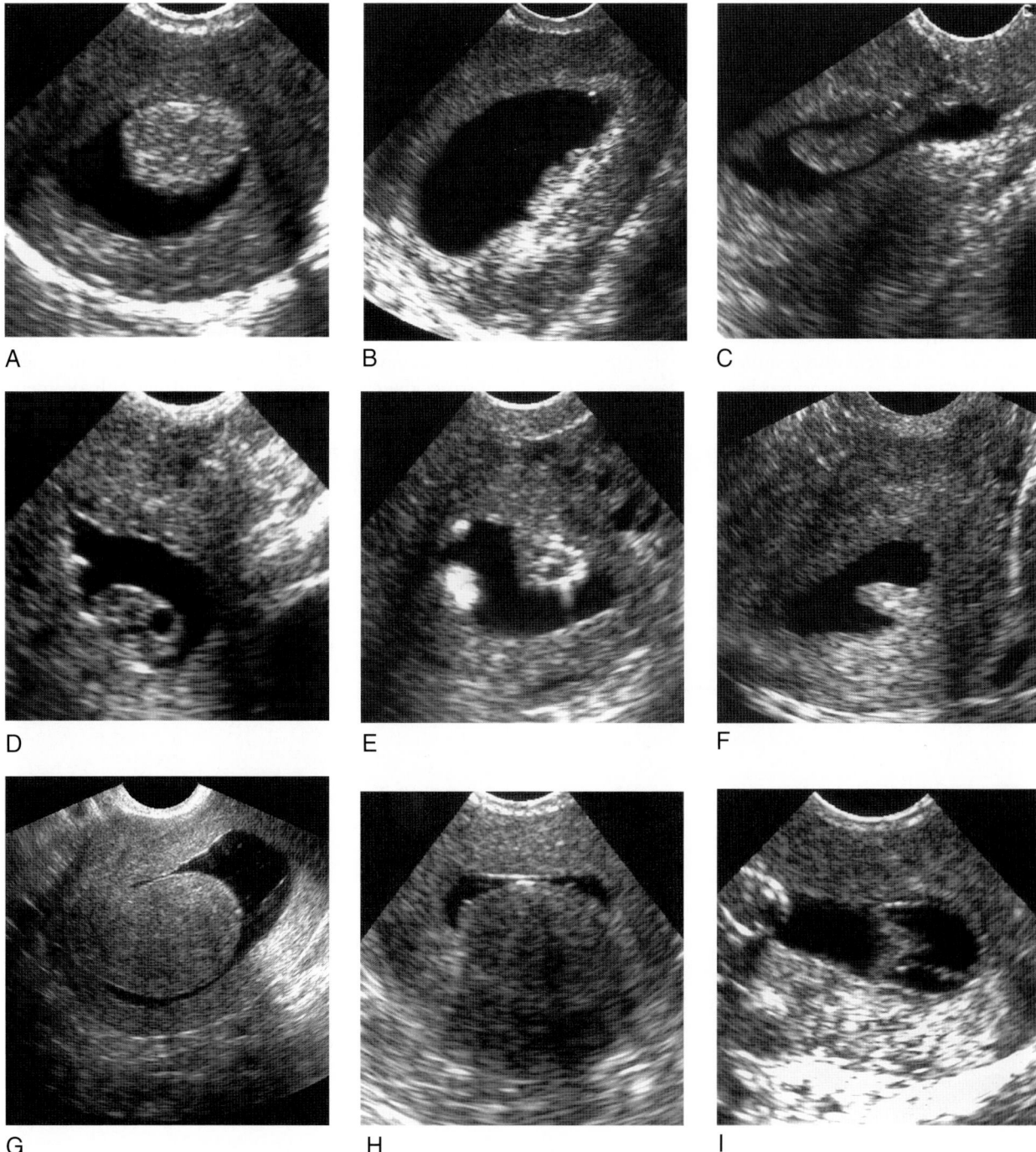

FIGURE 15-20. Sonohysterograms. A, Well-defined, round echogenic polyp. **B**, Carpet of small polyps. **C**, Polyp on a stalk. **D**, Polyp with cystic areas. **E**, Small polyp. **F**, Small polyp. **G**, Hypoechoic submucosal fibroid. **H**, Hypoechoic attenuating submucosal fibroid. **I**, Endometrial adhesions. Note bridging bands of tissue within fluid-filled endometrial canal.

submucosal leiomyoma (see Figs. 15-20G and H). The polyp can be seen arising from the endometrium, whereas a normal layer of endometrium is seen overlying the submucosal fibroid. Cystic areas may be seen within a polyp (see Fig. 15-8I), representing the histologically dilated glands.[103,104] A feeding artery in the pedicle may be seen with color Doppler (see Fig. 15-19B).

Endometrial polyps may not be diagnosed on dilation and curettage, as a polyp on a pliable stalk may be missed by the curette. If abnormal bleeding persists after a nondiagnostic dilation and curettage in a postmenopausal woman with an endometrial thickness greater than 8 mm, then hysteroscopy with direct visualization of the endometrial cavity is recommended.[108]

Endometrial Carcinoma

Endometrial carcinoma is the most common gynecologic malignancy in North America, and its incidence has been rising. It occurs in approximately 3% of women, yet it accounts for less than 1.5% of cancer deaths because more than 75% of the carcinomas are confined to the uterus at the time of clinical presentation. Most—75% to 80%—endometrial carcinomas occur in postmenopausal women. The most common clinical presentation is uterine bleeding, although only **10% of women with postmenopausal bleeding will have endometrial carcinoma**. There is a strong association with replacement estrogen therapy. In the premenopausal woman, anovulatory cycles and obesity are also considered risk factors, as in endometrial hyperplasia. Approximately 25% of patients with atypical endometrial hyperplasia will progress to well-differentiated endometrial carcinoma.[37]

Sonographically, a thickened endometrium must be considered cancer until proven otherwise. The thickened endometrium may be well defined, uniformly echogenic, and indistinguishable from hyperplasia and polyps. Cancer is more likely when the endometrium has a heterogeneous echotexture with irregular or poorly defined margins (Fig. 15-21). Cystic changes within the endometrium are more commonly seen in endometrial atrophy, hyperplasia, and polyps but can also be seen with carcinoma.[105] Endometrial carcinoma may also obstruct the endometrial canal, resulting in hydrometra

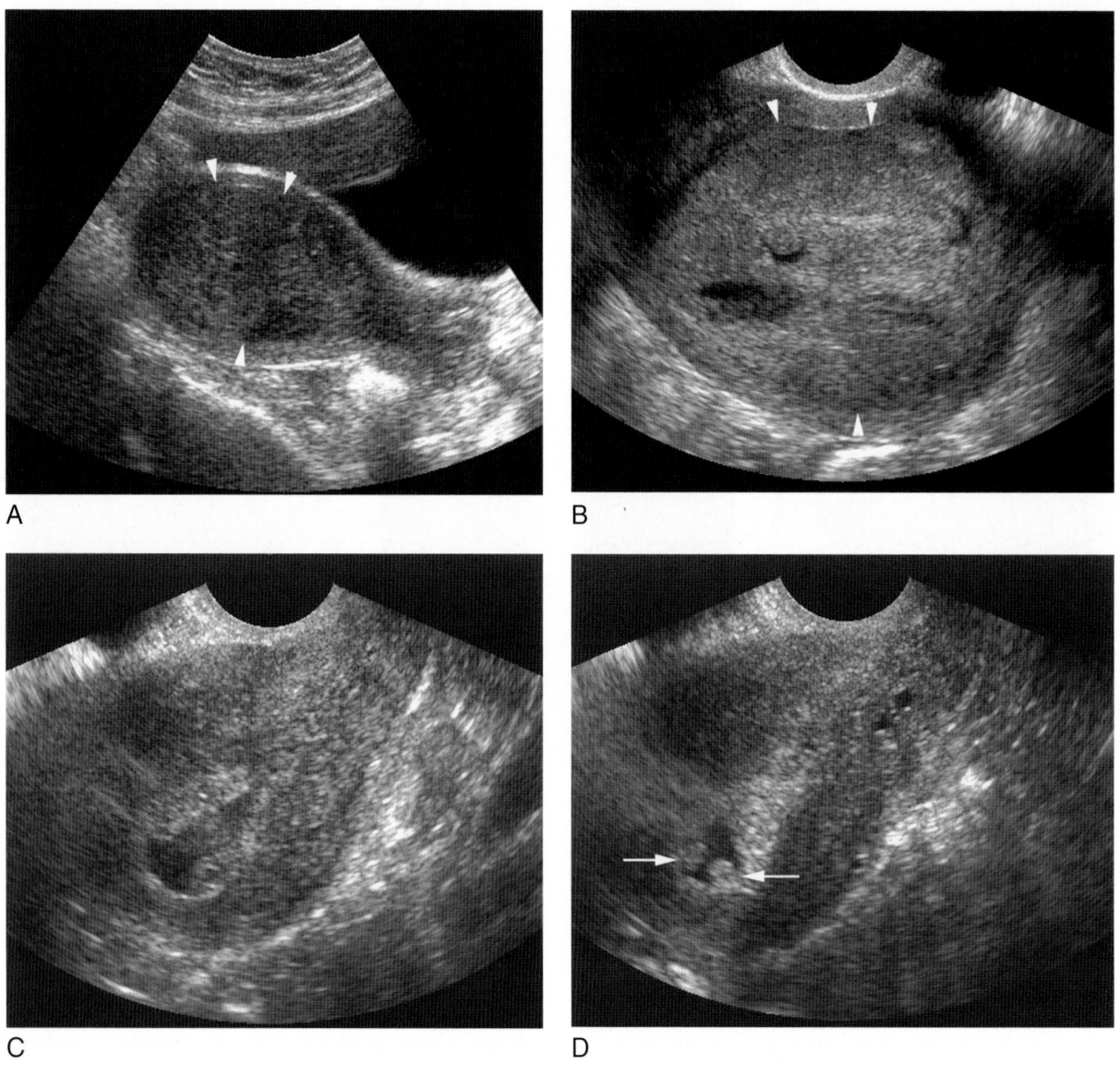

FIGURE 15-21. Endometrial carcinoma, varying appearances in two patients. A, Transabdominal scan.
B, Transvaginal scans show a large heterogeneous endometrial mass (*arrowheads*) compressing the surrounding myometrium. **C** and **D** are transvaginal images showing a localized irregular endometrial thickening with echogenic polypoid projections (*arrows*) into the fluid-filled endometrial canal.

or hematometra. Although certain sonographic appearances tend to favor a benign or malignant etiology, there are overlapping features, and endometrial biopsy is usually required for a definite diagnosis.

The role of color and spectral **Doppler** in the diagnosis of endometrial carcinoma is still **controversial**. Initial studies using transvaginal color and spectral Doppler suggested that endometrial carcinoma could be differentiated from a normal or benign postmenopausal endometrium by the presence of low-resistance flow in the uterine arteries in women with endometrial cancer, as compared with high-resistance flow in women with normal or benign endometria.[109,110] Subsequent reports, however, have shown no significant difference in uterine blood flow between benign and malignant endometrial processes.[111-113] Low-resistance flow in the uterine artery has also been reported in association with uterine fibroids.[110] Other reports have assessed subendometrial and endometrial blood flow as well, and some investigators have found a significant difference between benign and malignant endometrial lesions, with malignancies demonstrating low-resistance flow in the subendometrial and endometrial arteries.[95,114] Others, in evaluating these arteries, have found no statistically significant difference.[112,113,115] Blood flow is difficult to detect in the normal endometrium. Sladkevicius et al. thought endometrial thickness to be a better method for discriminating between normal and pathologic or benign and malignant endometrium than Doppler of the uterine, subendometrial, or intraendometrial arteries.[113] Further studies with large numbers of patients are necessary to determine whether Doppler will play a role in differentiating benign from malignant endometrial processes.

Sonography may be used in the preoperative evaluation of a patient with endometrial carcinoma by determining myometrial invasion.[116-118] Intactness of the subendometrial halo (the inner layer of myometrium) usually indicates superficial invasion, whereas obliteration of the halo is indicative of deep invasion.[116] MRI may also be helpful in assessing myometrial invasion. Transvaginal sonography and unenhanced T2-weighted MRI have been reported to have similar accuracy,[119] but contrast-enhanced MRI has been shown to be superior to both in demonstrating myometrial invasion.[120-122] MRI can also assess cervical extension. Sonography may be helpful in staging carcinoma and in distinguishing between tumors limited to the uterus (stages I and II) and those with extrauterine extension (stages III and IV).[117] Both MRI and CT are useful in staging by demonstrating lymphadenopathy and distant disease (stages III or IV).

Tamoxifen, a nonsteroidal antiestrogen compound, is widely used for adjuvant therapy in pre- and postmenopausal women with breast cancer. Tamoxifen acts by competing with estrogen for estrogen receptors. In premenopausal women, it has an antiestrogen effect, but in postmenopausal women it may have estrogenic effects. An **increased risk of endometrial carcinoma** has been reported in patients on tamoxifen therapy,[123] as well as an **increased risk of endometrial hyperplasia and polyps.**[124,125] On sonography, tamoxifen-related endometrial changes are nonspecific and similar to those described in hyperplasia, polyps, and carcinoma.[125-127] Cystic changes within the thickened endometrium are frequently seen (Figs. 15-8H and I). Polyps are frequently seen and have a higher incidence in women on tamoxifen therapy than in untreated women, and these polyps can be quite large.[128,129] It has been reported that there is a correlation between increased endometrial thickness and duration of tamoxifen therapy longer than 5 years.[129] In some patients on tamoxifen therapy, the cystic changes actually have been shown to be subendometrial in location and represent abnormal adenomyosis-like changes in the inner layer of myometrium.[130] Because it may be difficult to distinguish the endometrial-myometrial border in many of these patients, sonohysterography is valuable in determining whether an abnormality is endometrial or subendometrial.[131,132]

Endometritis

Endometritis may occur postpartum, following dilation and curettage, or in association with pelvic inflammatory disease. **Sonographically**, the endometrium may appear thick, irregular, or both, and the cavity may or may not contain fluid (Fig. 15-22). Gas with distal acoustic shadowing may be seen within the endometrial canal. Gas can be seen in up to 21% of clinically normal women, however, following uncomplicated vaginal delivery in the first 3 weeks post partum.[133] Clinical correlation is necessary when endometrial gas is seen in the postpartum patient.

Endometrial Adhesions

Endometrial adhesions (synechiae, Asherman's syndrome) are posttraumatic or postsurgical in nature and may be a cause of infertility or recurrent pregnancy loss. The sonographic diagnosis is difficult unless fluid is distending the endometrial cavity. The endometrium usually appears normal on transabdominal and transvaginal sonograms, although adhesions may be seen transvaginally as irregularities or a hypoechoic bridgelike band within the endometrium.[134] This is best seen during the secretory phase when the endometrium is more hyperechoic. **Sonohysterography** is an excellent technique for demonstrating adhesions and should be performed in all cases of suspected adhesions.[135] Adhesions appear as bridging bands of tissue that distort the cavity (see Fig. 15-20I) or as thin, undulating membranes best seen on real-time sonography.[3] Thick,

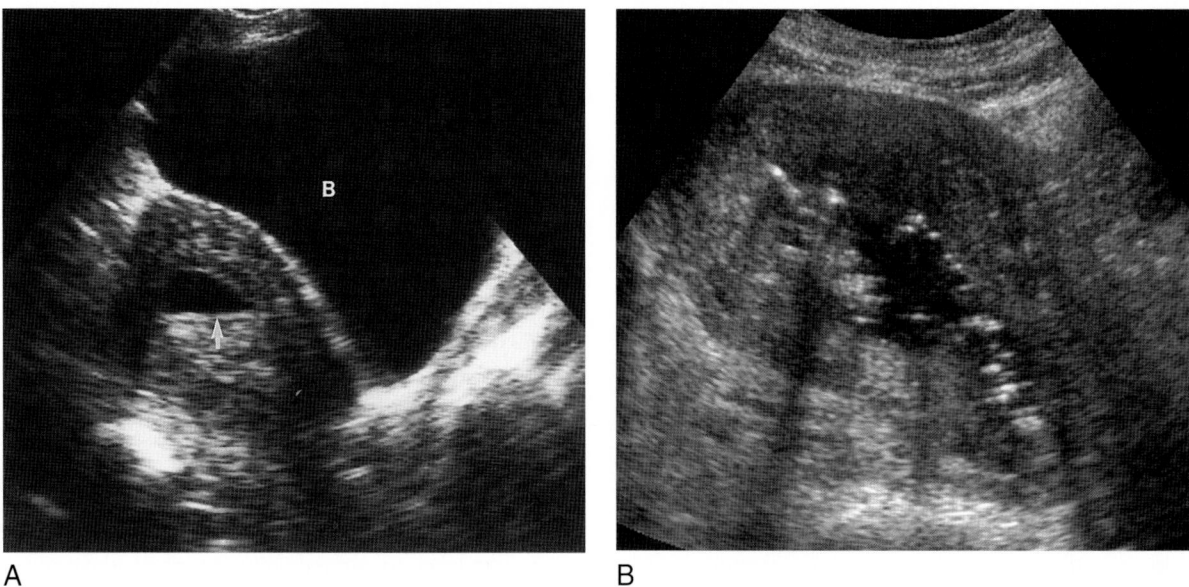

FIGURE 15-22. Endometritis. Varying appearances in two patients on transabdominal sagittal scans is shown. **A, Fluid-fluid level** (*arrow*) within endometrial canal in patient with pelvic inflammatory disease. This resolved following antibiotic therapy. Bladder (B). **B, Multiple linear hyperechogenic foci with shadowing due to gas** are seen within a distended endometrial canal in a febrile postpartum patient.

broad-based adhesions may prevent distention of the uterine cavity.[71] The adhesions can be divided under hysteroscopy.

Intrauterine Contraceptive Devices

Intrauterine contraceptive devices (IUCDs) are readily demonstrated on both transabdominal and transvaginal sonography (Fig. 15-23). They appear as highly echo-genic linear structures in the endometrial cavity in the body of the uterus. Several types of IUCDs demonstrate a characteristic appearance on sonography, reflecting their gross appearance. One must be able to distinguish the IUCD from the normal, high-amplitude central endometrial cavity echo. Acoustic shadowing from the IUCD is usually demonstrated, and two parallel echoes (entrance-exit reflections), representing the anterior and posterior surfaces of the IUCD, may also be observed (see Fig. 15-23A).[136] Sonography can demonstrate malposition, perforation, and incomplete removal. Eccentric position of an IUCD suggests myometrial penetration. If the IUCD is not seen on sonography, a radiograph should be taken to assess whether it is lying free in the peritoneal cavity or is not present, having been previously expelled. The IUCD may be hidden by coexisting intrauterine abnormalities, such as blood clots or an incomplete abortion. When an IUCD is present in the uterus in association with an intrauterine pregnancy, it can be seen reliably early in the first trimester, but it is rarely identified thereafter. In the first trimester, the device can usually be removed safely under ultrasound guidance.

Abnormalities of the Cervix

The cervix may be difficult to assess adequately by transabdominal sonography because it lies low in the pelvis, posterior to the bladder. Better visualization is obtained by transvaginal sonography, which can reliably diagnose normal and benign cervical conditions.[137]

Nabothian (inclusion) cysts of the cervix are commonly seen during routine sonography (Fig. 15-24). They may vary in size from a few millimeters to 4 cm. They may be single or multiple and are usually diagnosed incidentally, although they may be associated with healing chronic cervicitis. Occasionally, nabothian cysts may have internal echoes that may be caused by hemorrhage or infection. Multiple cysts may be a cause of benign enlargement of the cervix.[138]

Cervical polyps are a frequent cause of vaginal bleeding and may be seen on sonography. The diagnosis is usually made clinically, however. Approximately 8% of **leiomyomas** arise in the cervix. They may be pedunculated and prolapse into the vagina. In patients who have had a hysterectomy, the cervical stump may occasionally simulate a mass. Transvaginal sonography is usually diagnostic; it can demonstrate a normal cervix. **Cervical stenosis** may be secondary to previous radiation therapy, previous cone biopsy, postmenopausal cervical atrophy, or cervical carcinoma.

Cervical carcinoma is usually diagnosed clinically and patients are rarely referred for sonographic evaluation. Sonography may demonstrate a solid retrovesical mass, which may be indistinguishable from a cervical fibroid (Fig. 15-25). **Adenoma malignum,**

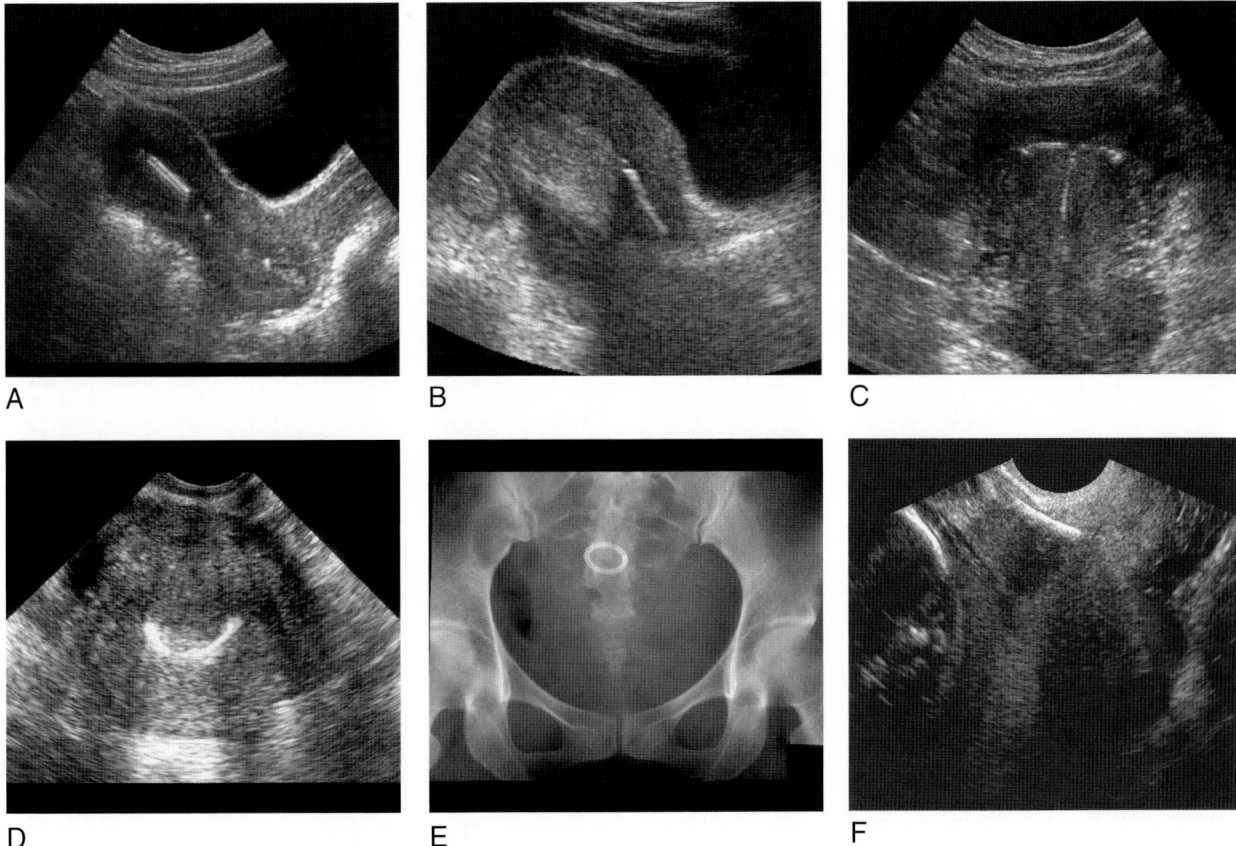

FIGURE 15-23. Intrauterine contraceptive devices. A, Highly echogenic linear structure in normal location within endometrial canal in body of uterus. **B,** IUCD abnormally positioned in lower uterine segment. **C,** Typical appearance of copper T type of IUCD. **D,** Unusual Chinese ring IUCD, **E,** Radiograph of **D. F,** IUCD in a 30-week gravid uterus. **A, B, C,** Transabdominal scans. **D** and **E,** Transvaginal scan.

which is also termed "minimal deviation adeno-carcinoma," is a rare cervical neoplasm arising from the endocervical glands and is often associated with Peutz-Jeghers syndrome.[139] Multiple cystic areas are seen within a solid cervical mass (Fig. 15-26).[139,140] This condition should be easily differentiated from deep nabothian cysts because nabothian cysts do not have an associated mass. Sonography may be used for staging cervical carcinoma, but CT and MRI are preferable.

VAGINA

The vagina runs anteriorly and caudally from the cervix between the bladder and rectum. It is best seen on midline sagittal sonograms with a slight caudal angulation of the transducer. It appears as a collapsed hypoechoic tubular structure with a central, high-amplitude, linear echo representing the apposed surfaces of the vaginal mucosa (see Fig. 15-2). The most common congenital abnormality of the female genital tract is an **imperforate hymen** resulting in **hemato-colpos**. Occasionally, sonography is used to characterize a vaginal mass. **Gartner's duct cysts** are remnants of the

caudal end of the mesonephric duct that form single or multiple cysts along the lateral or anterolateral wall of the vagina. These are the most common cystic lesions of the vagina and are usually found incidentally during sonographic examination. They are usually small and asymptomatic and may be associated with renal and ureteral abnormalities.[141] Solid masses of the vagina are rare. Two cases of **neurofibroma** of the vagina that appear as solid masses have been described.[142] As in carcinoma of the cervix, sonography is not used for diagnosis of carcinoma of the vagina, but it may play a role in staging.

In patients who have had a hysterectomy, a **vaginal cuff** should not be mistaken for a mass. The upper limit of normal for the anteroposterior diameter of the vaginal cuff is 2.1 cm.[143] A cuff that is larger than 2.1 cm or that contains a definite mass suggests malignancy. Nodular areas may be due to postirradiation fibrosis.[143]

RECTOUTERINE RECESS

The rectouterine recess (**posterior cul-de-sac**) is the most posterior and inferior reflection of the peritoneal

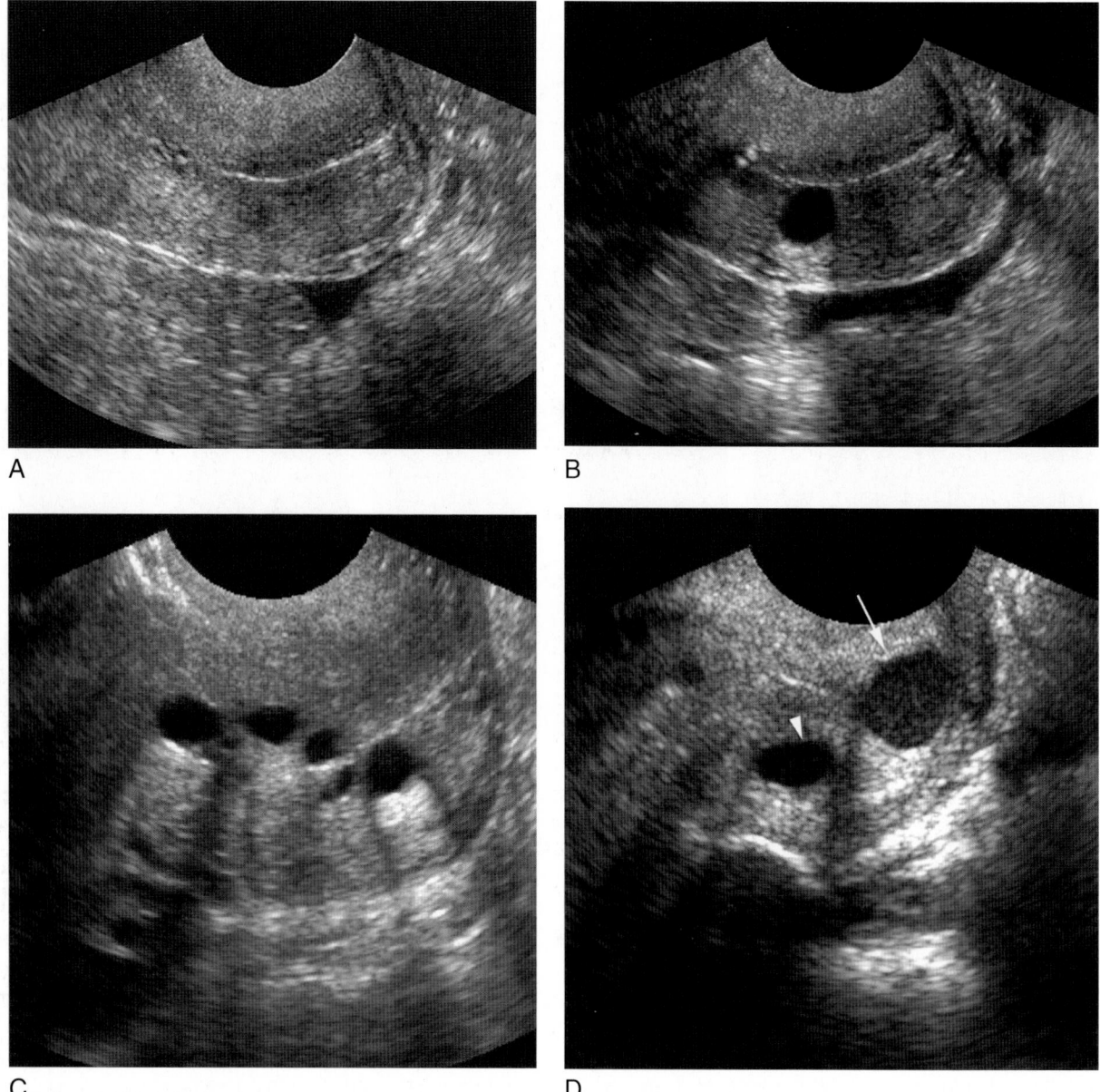

FIGURE 15-24. Nabothian cysts on transvaginal scans. A, Normal cervix. **B**, Single nabothian cyst in cervix. **C**, Multiple nabothian cysts. **D**, Hemorrhagic nabothian cyst (*arrow*) and simple nabothian cyst (*arrowhead*).

cavity. It is located between the rectum and vagina and is also known as the *pouch of Douglas*. The posterior fornix of the vagina is closely related to the posterior cul-de-sac and is separated by the thickness of the vaginal wall and the peritoneal membrane. The posterior cul-de-sac is a potential space, and because of its location, it is frequently the initial site for intraperitoneal fluid collection. As little as 5 mL of fluid have been detected by transvaginal sonography.[144]

Fluid in the cul-de-sac is a normal finding in asymptomatic women and can be seen during all phases of the menstrual cycle. Possible sources have been postulated, including blood or fluid caused by follicular

rupture, blood caused by retrograde menstruation, and increased capillary permeability of the ovarian surface caused by the influence of estrogen.[145,146]

Pathologic fluid collections in the pouch of Douglas may be seen in association with generalized **ascites**, **blood** resulting from a ruptured ectopic pregnancy or hemorrhagic cyst, or **pus** resulting from infection. **Sonography** may aid in differentiating the type of fluid because blood, pus, mucin, and malignant exudates usually contain echoes within the fluid, whereas serous fluid (either physiologic or pathologic) is usually anechoic. Clotted blood may be very echogenic.[147] Transvaginal sonography can demonstrate echoes

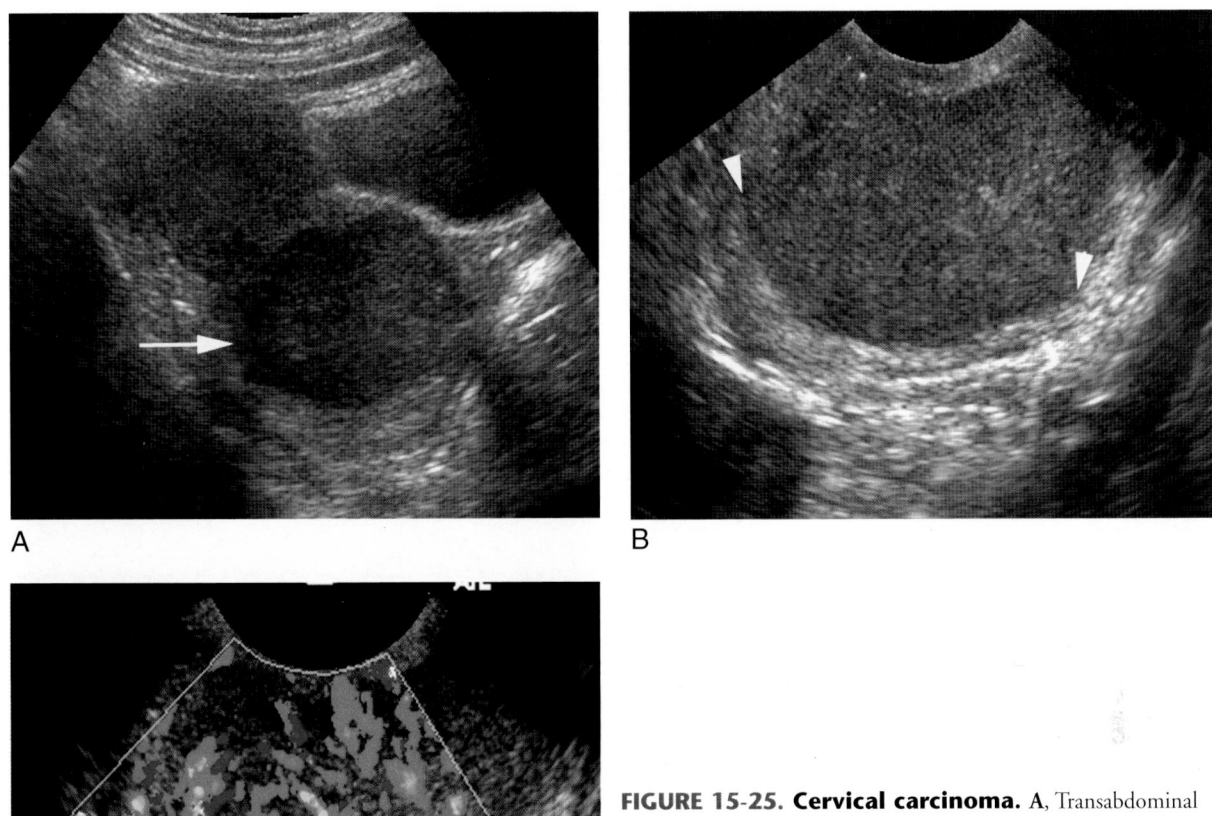

A

B

C

FIGURE 15-25. Cervical carcinoma. A, Transabdominal sagittal and **B,** transvaginal scans show a large cervical mass (*arrow*). The margin of the mass with the rim of normal tissue is marked (*arrowheads*) in **B. C,** Color Doppler shows hypervascularity of the mass.

within the fluid more frequently because of its improved resolution (Fig. 15-27). Pelvic abscesses and hematomas can also occur in the cul-de-sac.

OVARY

Normal Sonographic Anatomy

Uterine location influences the position of the ovaries. The normal ovaries are usually identified laterally or posterolaterally to the anteflexed midline uterus. When the uterus lies to one side of the midline (a normal variant), the ipsilateral ovary often lies superior to the uterine fundus. In a retroverted uterus, the ovaries tend to be located laterally and superiorly, near the uterine fundus. When the uterus is enlarged, the ovaries tend to be displaced more superiorly and laterally. Following hysterectomy, the ovaries tend to be located more medially and directly superior to the vaginal cuff.

Because of the laxity of the ligamentous attachments, the ovary can be quite variable in position and may be located high in the pelvis or in the cul-de-sac. Because of their **variable position**, superiorly or extremely laterally placed ovaries may not be visualized by the transvaginal approach because they are out of the field-of-view. The ovaries are ellipsoid in shape, with their craniocaudad axes paralleling the internal iliac vessels, which lie posteriorly and serve as a helpful reference (Fig. 15-28). In patients with uterine leiomyomas, some investigators have been able to visualize the ovaries more frequently by transvaginal sonography than by the transabdominal method.[7,8]

On **sonography**, the **normal ovary** has a relatively homogeneous echotexture with a central, more echogenic medulla. Well-defined, small anechoic or cystic follicles may be seen peripherally in the cortex. The appearance of the ovary changes with age and with the phase of the menstrual cycle. During the early **proli-**

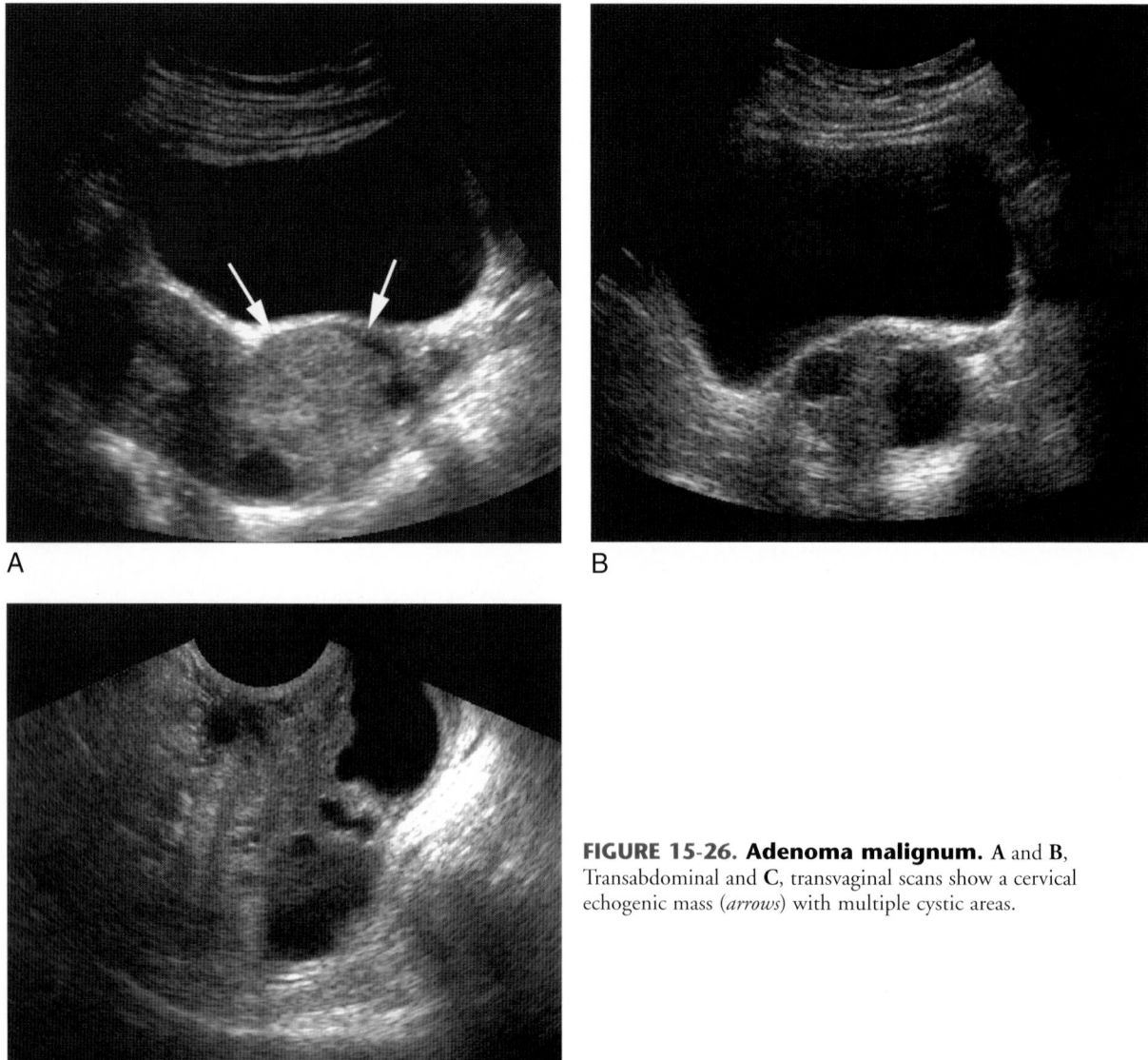

FIGURE 15-26. Adenoma malignum. A and **B**, Transabdominal and **C**, transvaginal scans show a cervical echogenic mass (*arrows*) with multiple cystic areas.

ferative phase, many follicles that are stimulated by both follicle-stimulating hormone (FSH) and luteinizing hormone (LH) develop and increase in size until about day 8 or 9 of the menstrual cycle. At that time one follicle becomes dominant, destined for ovulation, and increases in size, reaching up to 2.0 to 2.5 cm at the time of ovulation. The other follicles become atretic. A **follicular cyst** develops if the fluid in one of these nondominant follicles is not resorbed. Following ovulation, the **corpus luteum** develops and may be identified sonographically as a small hypoechoic or isoechoic structure peripherally within the ovary. The corpus luteum involutes before menstruation.

Because of the variability in shape, **ovarian volume** has been considered the best method for determining ovarian size. The volume measurement is based on the formula for a prolate ellipse (0.523 × length × width × height). Studies have shown that ovarian volumes are larger than previously thought. In the first 2 years of life, the mean ovarian volume is slightly greater than 1 cc in the first year and 0.7 cc in the second year.[148] The upper limit of normal has been reported as 3.6 cc in the first 3 months, 2.7 cc from 4 to 12 months, and 1.7 cc in the second year.[148] Ovarian volume remains relatively stable up to 5 years of age and then gradually increases up to menarche when the mean volume is 4.2 ± 2.3 cc, with an upper limit of 8.0 cc.[10] Small follicles or cysts are frequently seen in neonatal and premenarchal ovaries. One study showed follicle activity in 87% of prepubertal girls.[13] These follicles usually measure less than 9 mm but may be as large as 17 mm.[149]

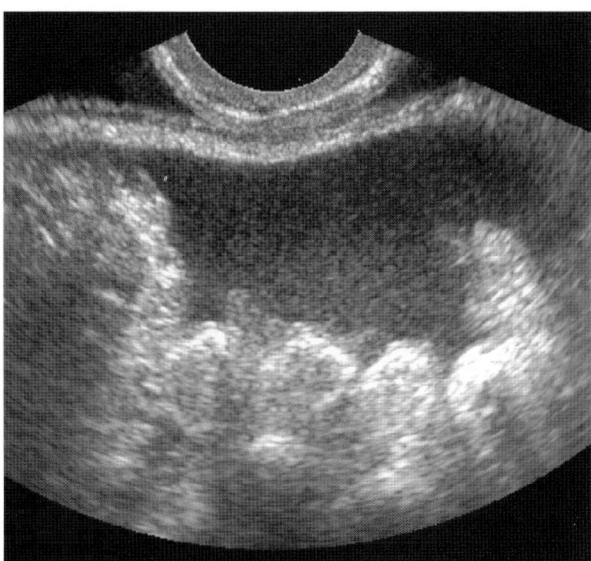

FIGURE 15-27. Echogenic fluid in cul-de-sac due to blood on transvaginal scan.

In the adult menstruating female, a normal ovary may have a volume as large as 22 cc. Cohen et al. assessed 866 normal ovaries by transabdominal sonography and reported a mean ovarian volume of 9.8 ± 5.8 cc, with an upper limit of 21.9 cc.[150] Another study of 406 patients with normal ovaries used transvaginal sonography and reported a mean ovarian volume of 6.8 cc, with an upper limit of 18.0 cc.[151] There is no significant parity-related change in ovarian volume in premenopausal women.[15]

Echogenic ovarian foci are commonly seen in an otherwise normal-appearing ovary (Fig. 15-29). These are tiny (1 to 3 mm) nonshadowing foci, usually multiple and peripherally located, although they can be diffuse. They were thought to represent inclusion cysts and associated psammomatous calcifications.[152] Muradali et al., in a study with histopathologic correlation in seven normal ovaries with echogenic foci, showed that these foci are caused by a specular reflection from the walls of tiny unresolved cysts below the spatial resolution of ultrasound rather than calcification.[153] As these echogenic foci do not indicate significant underlying disease, no further investigations or follow-up is necessary.

Focal calcification may occasionally be seen in an otherwise normal-appearing ovary and is thought to represent stromal reaction to previous hemorrhage or infection.[154] However, the calcification may be the initial or early manifestation of a neoplasm, so follow-up sonography is recommended.

Postmenopausal Ovary

Following menopause, the ovary atrophies and the follicles disappear over the subsequent few years, with the ovary decreasing in size with increasing age.[15,155-157] Due to its smaller size and lack of follicles, the postmenopausal ovary may be difficult to visualize sonographically (Fig. 15-30). A stationary loop of bowel may be mistaken for a normal ovary; therefore, scanning must be done slowly to look for peristalsis. **Sonographic visualization** of normal postmenopausal ovaries varies greatly in the literature, from a low of 20% to a high of 99%, using either the transabdominal or transvaginal approach.[151,155-160] The variation is likely due to differences in technique and length of time since menopause. The ovary decreases in size with increasing age and, therefore, the ability to see the ovaries decreases with lengthening time since menopause.[161] Also, the absence of the uterus may play a role because the ovaries

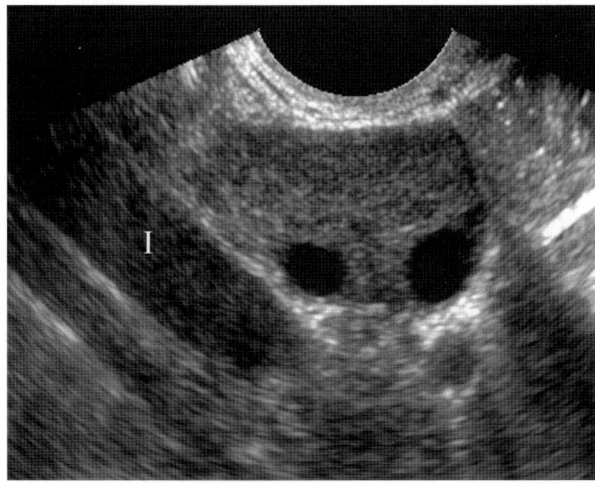

A

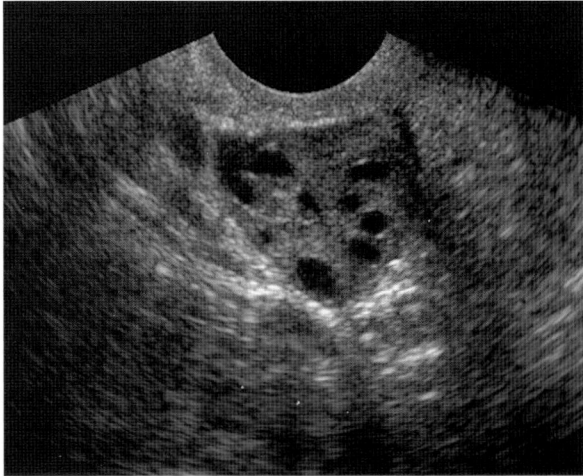

B

FIGURE 15-28. Normal ovary. **A** and **B**, Transvaginal scans show normal ovaries with a few follicles in two patients. Internal iliac vein (I) is seen posterior to ovary.

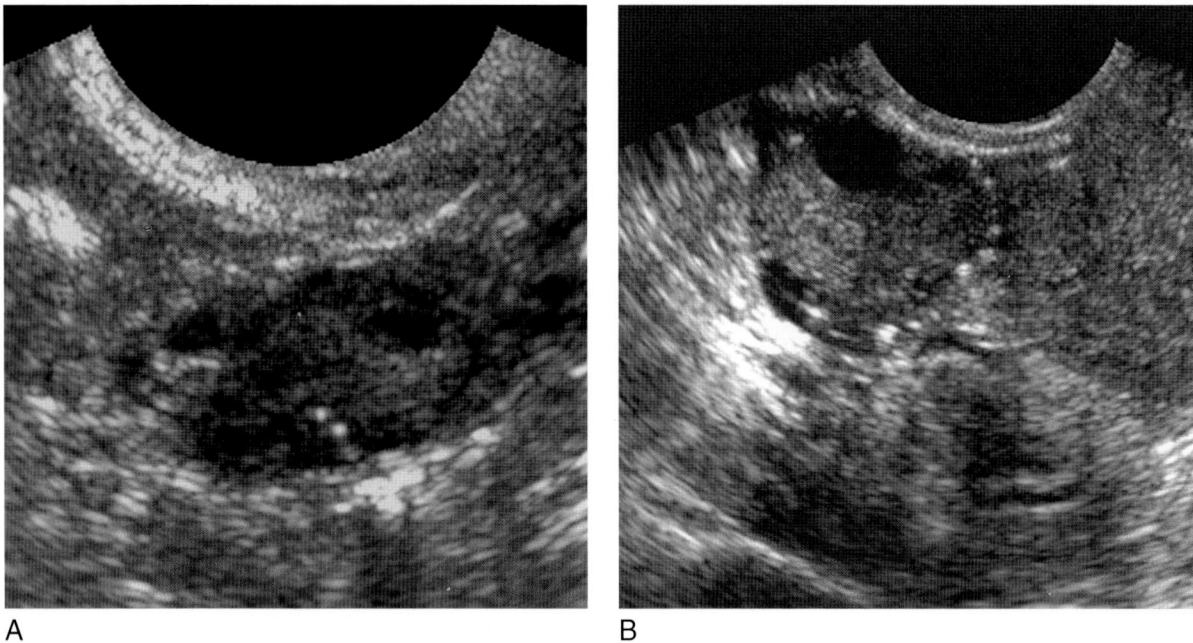

A   B

FIGURE 15-29. Ovarian echogenic foci. Transvaginal scans in two patients show **A,** Two tiny echogenic foci in normal appearing ovary and **B,** multiple peripheral tiny echogenic foci.

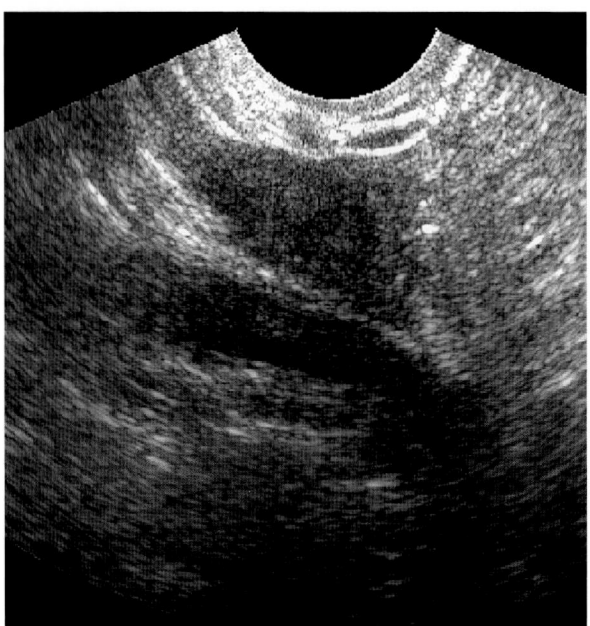

FIGURE 15-30. Normal postmenopausal ovary. Transvaginal scan shows a normal postmenopausal ovary (o). Note small size and lack of follicles.

are less likely to be seen following hysterectomy due to the loss of normal anatomical landmarks. Wolf et al., in a study of 290 postmenopausal ovaries known to be present, using both transabdominal and transvaginal sonography, visualized only 41% of ovaries transvaginally and 58% transabdominally. Using both techniques resulted in their visualizing more ovaries than when they used either technique alone (68%).[161] Highly placed

ovaries may be out of the field-of-view of transvaginal transducers, and transabdominal sonography may not image very small or deeply placed ovaries. Nonvisualization of an ovary does not exclude the possibility of an ovarian lesion.

Mean ovarian volume ranges are reported from 1.2 cc to 5.8 cc.[150,151,155-159] The mean values in these studies may be somewhat high because nonvisualized ovaries were not included. One study assessing 563 patients with normal postmenopausal ovaries by transvaginal sonography reported a mean ovarian volume of 2.0 cc with an upper limit of normal of 8.0 cc.[151] An **ovarian volume of more than 8.0 cc is definitely considered abnormal.** Some authors have suggested that an ovarian volume more than twice that of the opposite side should also be considered abnormal, regardless of the actual size.[156,158]

Postmenopausal Cysts

Small anechoic cysts (less than 3 cm in diameter) may be seen in up to 15% of postmenopausal ovaries and are not related to age, length of time since menopause, or hormone use.[161] These cysts are more frequently seen by transvaginal sonography due to its improved resolution, but in some women, especially those who have had a hysterectomy or those with highly placed ovaries, the cysts may be seen only by transabdominal sonography. These cysts can disappear or change in size over time (Fig. 15-31).[162]

Several studies have shown a very low incidence of malignancy in unilocular postmenopausal cysts that

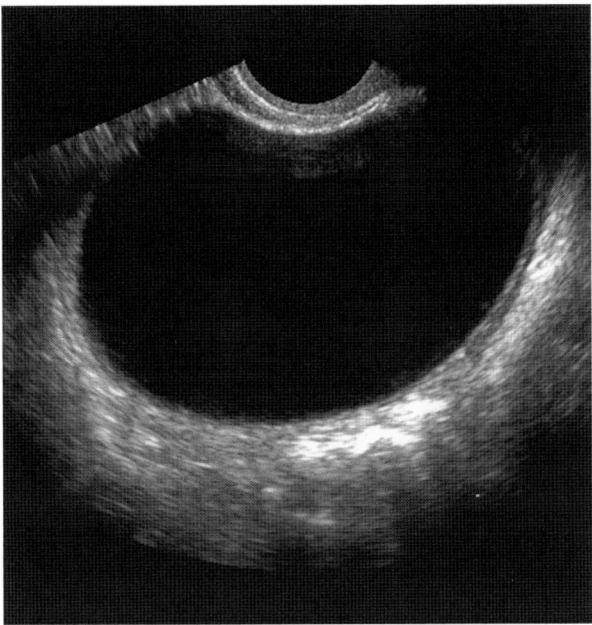

FIGURE 15-31. Postmenopausal large ovarian cyst. Transvaginal scan shows a 7 cm ovarian cyst that contains no internal echoes or septations and had not changed in size over 4 years.

measure less than 5 cm in diameter and are without septation or solid components.[163-168] It is recommended that these patients be followed by serial sonographic examinations without surgical intervention unless there is an increase in size or change in the characteristics of the lesion.[166-168] Surgery is generally recommended for postmenopausal cysts greater than 5 cm and for those containing internal septations and/or solid nodules.

Nonneoplastic Lesions

Functional Cysts

Functional cysts of the ovary include follicular, corpus luteum, and theca-lutein cysts. A **follicular cyst** occurs when a mature follicle fails to ovulate or to involute. Follicular cysts range from 1.0 cm to 20.0 cm in size. However, because normal follicles can vary from a few millimeters to 2.0 cm and can reach up to 2.5 cm at maturity, a follicular cyst cannot be diagnosed with certainty until it is greater than 2.5 cm.[169] They are usually unilateral, asymptomatic, and frequently detected incidentally on sonographic examination. Follicular cysts usually regress spontaneously.

The **corpus luteal cyst** results from failure of absorption or from excess bleeding into the corpus luteum. They are less common than follicular cysts but tend to be larger and more symptomatic. Pain is the major symptom. These cysts are usually unilateral and more prone to hemorrhage and rupture. If the ovum is fertilized, the corpus luteum continues as the corpus luteum of pregnancy, which may become enlarged and

cystic. Maximum size is reached at 8 to 10 weeks, and by 16 weeks the cyst has usually resolved.

Sonographically, these functional cysts are typically unilocular, anechoic structures with well-defined thin walls and posterior acoustic enhancement. Corpus luteal cysts may have a thicker wall with a crenulated appearance. They may also have a peripheral rim of color around the wall on color Doppler.

Hemorrhagic Cysts

Internal hemorrhage may occur in both types of functional cysts, although it is much more frequently seen in corpus luteal cysts. Women with hemorrhagic cysts frequently present with acute onset of pelvic pain. Hemorrhagic cysts show a spectrum of findings as a result of the variable sonographic appearance of blood (Fig. 15-32). The **sonographic appearance** depends on the amount of hemorrhage and the time of the hemorrhage relative to the time of the sonographic examination.[170-172] The internal characteristics are much better appreciated on transvaginal sonography because of its improved resolution. An **acute hemorrhagic cyst** is usually hyperechoic and may mimic a solid mass. However, it usually has a smooth posterior wall and shows posterior acoustic enhancement, indicating the cystic nature of the lesion. Diffuse low-level internal echoes may be seen, but this appearance is more commonly seen in endometriomas. As the clot hemolyzes, the internal pattern becomes more complex, with a reticular-type pattern containing internal echoes and interdigitating septations. Color Doppler sonography will show no flow within the clot. As the clot retracts, a curvilinear demarcation line or fluid-fluid level between the clot and the fluid component may be seen. The echogenic clot may also settle to the dependent portion of the cyst. The presence of echogenic free intraperitoneal fluid in the cul-de-sac can help confirm the diagnosis of a leaking or ruptured hemorrhagic cyst. Rupture of a hemorrhagic cyst may mimic a ruptured ectopic pregnancy, both clinically and sonographically.

Functional cysts are the **most common cause of ovarian enlargement in young women.**[169] Because most functional cysts typically resolve within one to two menstrual cycles, follow-up is usually not required for small, simple cysts or typically appearing hemorrhagic cysts. However, follow-up of larger cysts can be performed at a different time of the menstrual cycle, usually in 6 weeks, to show a changing appearance or resolution.

Theca-luteal cysts are the largest of the functional cysts and are associated with high levels of human chorionic gonadotropin (HCG). These cysts typically occur in patients with gestational trophoblastic disease but can also be seen in the ovarian hyperstimulation syndrome as a complication of drug therapy for

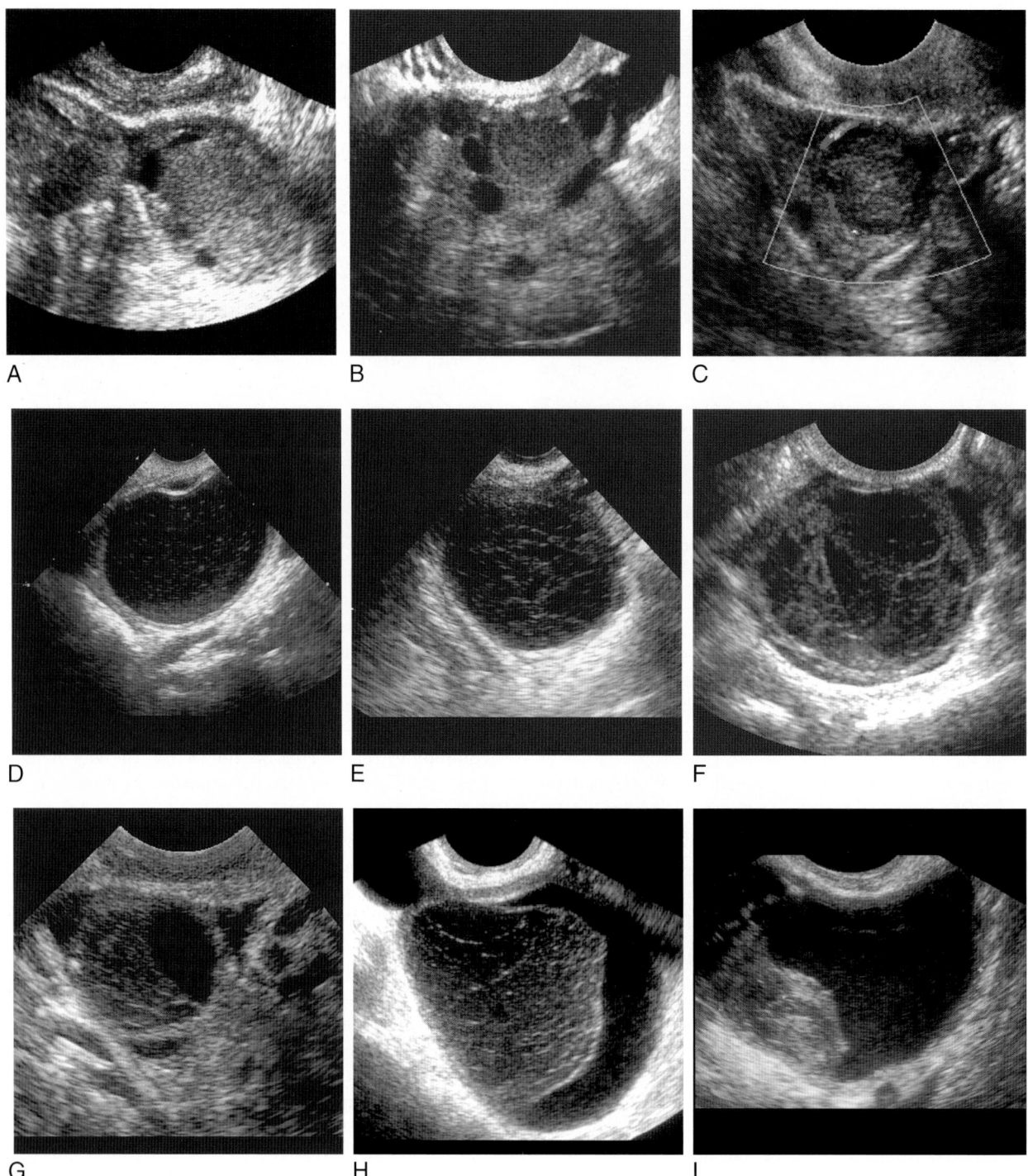

FIGURE 15-32. Hemorrhagic cysts on transvaginal scans—spectrum of appearances. A, Acute hyperechoic hemorrhagic cyst. **B,** Acute hemorrhagic cyst mimicking a solid lesion. **C,** Color Doppler shows peripheral ring of vascularity, but no vascularity within the cyst. **D,** Large cyst containing multiple internal low-level echoes. **E,** Reticular pattern of internal echoes and septations within cyst. **F,** Reticular pattern. **G, H,** and **I** show variations in clot retraction. The clot in **I** suggests a solid mass. Lack of color Doppler signal supports its benign nature.

infertility. Sonographically, theca-luteal cysts are usually bilateral, multilocular, and very large. They may undergo hemorrhage, rupture, and torsion.

Surface epithelial inclusion cysts are nonfunctional cysts commonly seen in postmenopausal women, although they may be seen at any age and are usually located peripherally in the cortex. They arise from cortical invaginations of the ovarian surface epithelium.[37] They are usually tiny unilocular, thin-walled cysts, but can measure up to several centimeters in

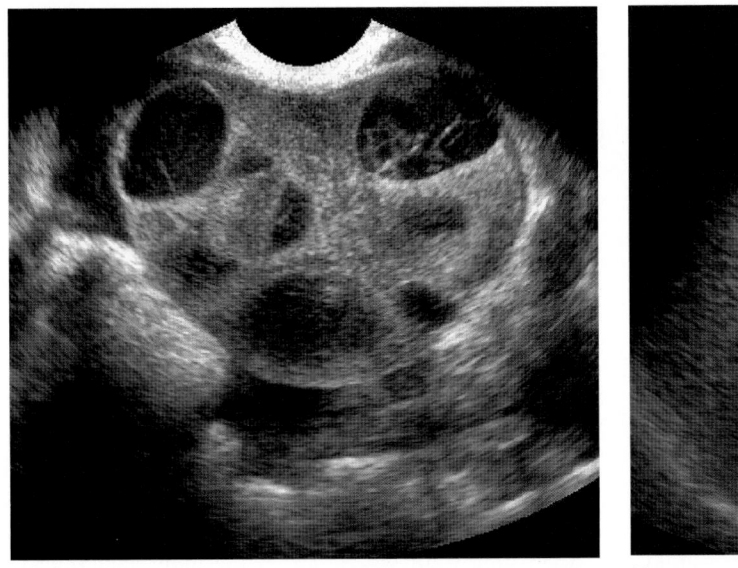 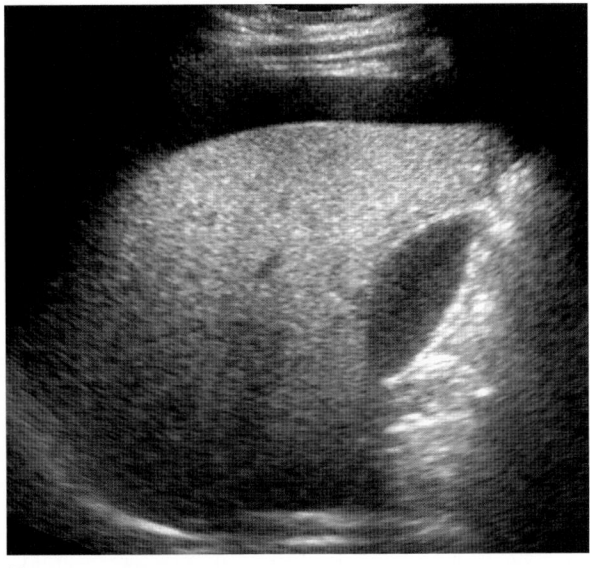

A   B

FIGURE 15-33. Ovarian hyperstimulation. A is a transvaginal image showing a markedly enlarged and round ovary with multiple complicated cysts. **B** is a sagittal image in the right upper quadrant showing large volume of free intraperitoneal fluid.

diameter. Occasionally, these cysts may be hemorrhagic, particularly if torsion has occurred.

Ovarian Hyperstimulation Syndrome

Ovarian hyperstimulation syndrome (OHS) (Fig. 15-33) is a frequent iatrogenic complication of ovulation induction. Clinically, three degrees of OHS are described: mild, moderate, and severe. The mild form is associated with lower abdominal discomfort, but no significant weight gain. The ovaries are enlarged, but less than 5 cm in average diameter. With severe hyperstimulation, there is weight gain and the patient complains of severe abdominal pain and distention. The ovaries are markedly enlarged (greater than 10 cm in diameter) and contain numerous large, thin-walled cysts, which may replace most of the ovary. There are associated ascites and pleural effusions, which lead to depletion of intravascular fluids and electrolytes, resulting in hemoconcentration with hypotension, oliguria, and electrolyte imbalance. Severe OHS is usually treated conservatively to attempt to correct the depleted intravascular volume and electrolyte imbalance and usually resolves within 2 to 3 weeks.

Ovarian Remnant Syndrome

Infrequently, a cystic mass may be encountered in a patient who has undergone bilateral oophorectomy in which a small amount of residual ovarian tissue has been unintentionally left behind. The surgery has usually been technically difficult because of adhesions from endometriosis, pelvic inflammatory disease, or tumor.[173] The residual ovarian tissue can become functional and produce pelvic pain or extrinsic compression of the distal ureter, or both. Sonographically, the cysts vary from small to relatively large completely cystic or complex masses.[174,175] A thin rim of ovarian tissue is usually present in the wall of the cyst.[175]

Parovarian Cysts

Parovarian (paratubal) cysts account for about 10% of all adnexal masses. They are found in the broad ligament and are usually of mesothelial or paramesonephric origin, or rarely, of mesonephric origin.[176] They may occur at any age but are most common in the third and fourth decades of life. They vary in size, and on sonography have the typical appearance of cysts. Parovarian cysts show no cyclic changes. They are frequently located superior to the uterine fundus[176] and may contain internal echoes as a result of hemorrhage.[177] The cyst may undergo torsion and rupture similar to other cystic masses. Benign neoplasms such as cystadenomas and cystadenofibromas of parovarian origin are uncommon. On sonography, they may appear as simple cysts or contain small nodular areas and occasionally have septations.[178] Malignancy has been reported in 2% to 3% of parovarian cystic masses studied by histopathology[179,180] but is even less frequent in masses less than 5 cm.[181] A specific diagnosis of a parovarian cyst is possible only by demonstrating a normal ipsilateral ovary close to, but separate from, the cyst.[182]

Peritoneal Inclusion Cysts

Peritoneal inclusion cysts occur predominantly in premenopausal women with a history of previous abdominal surgery, but they may also be seen in patients with a history of trauma, pelvic inflammatory disease, or endometriosis. The ovaries are the main producers of peritoneal fluid in women.[146] In patients with peritoneal adhesions, fluid may accumulate within the adhesions and entrap the ovaries, resulting in a large adnexal mass.[183,184] Peritoneal inclusion cysts are lined with mesothelial cells; this condition has also been referred to as ***benign cystic mesothelioma*** or ***benign encysted fluid***. Clinically, most patients present with pain and/or a pelvic mass.

On **sonography**, peritoneal inclusion cysts are multi-loculated cystic adnexal masses (Fig. 15-34). The diagnostic finding is the presence of an intact ovary amid septations and fluid.[184-186] This indicates the extra-ovarian origin of the mass. The ovary may be located centrally or displaced peripherally, and although it may appear distorted, it is easily identified. The septations represent the mesothelial and fibrous strands seen pathologically. The fluid is usually anechoic but may contain echoes in some compartments as a result of hemorrhage or proteinaceous fluid. Peritoneal inclusion cysts must be differentiated from parovarian cysts and hydrosalpinx. While these conditions are all extra-ovarian, parovarian cysts are separate from the ovary, whereas the ovary lies inside or in the wall of a peritoneal inclusion cyst.[184,185] **Parovarian cysts** are usually round

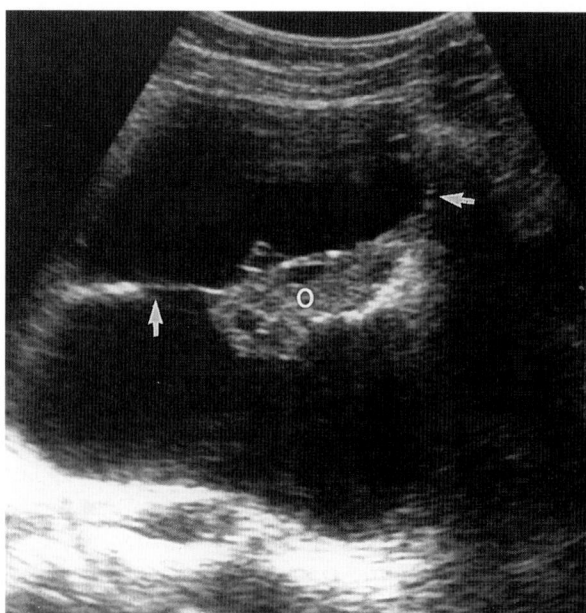

FIGURE 15-34. Peritoneal inclusion cyst. Trans-abdominal scan shows multiple fluid-filled cystic areas with linear septations (*arrows*) representing adhesions attached to normal ovary (O).

or ovoid and not associated with a history of pelvic surgery, trauma, or inflammation. **Hydrosalpinx** appears as a tubular or ovoid cystic structure with often visible folds, and the ovary is shown to be outside of the cystic structure. Accurate diagnosis of peritoneal inclusion cysts is important because the risk of recurrence after surgical resection is 30% to 50%.[187] Conservative therapy, such as ovarian suppression with oral contraceptives or fluid aspiration, is recommended. Peritoneal inclusion cysts have no malignant potential.

Endometriosis

Endometriosis is defined as the presence of functioning endometrial tissue outside the uterus. Endometriosis most commonly occurs in the ovary, fallopian tube, broad ligament, and posterior cul-de-sac, but it can also occur almost anywhere else in the body, including the bladder and bowel. Two forms have been described: **diffuse** and **localized** (**endometrioma**). The diffuse form, which is more common, consists of minute endometrial implants involving the pelvic viscera and their ligamentous attachments. The ectopic endometrium is hormonally responsive and undergoes bleeding during the menses, resulting in a local inflammatory reaction with adhesions. This diffuse form is rarely diagnosed by sonography because the implants are too small to be imaged.[188] Endometriosis commonly affects women during the reproductive years, and clinical symptoms include dysmenorrhea, dyspareunia, and infertility.

The localized form consists of a discrete mass referred to as an **endometrioma**, or **chocolate cyst**. Although endometriosis is frequently associated with infertility, an endometrioma may occasionally be seen in a pregnant patient. Endometriomas are usually asymptomatic and are frequently multiple. The characteristic sonographic appearance is that of a well-defined unilocular or multi-locular, predominantly cystic mass containing diffuse homogeneous, low-level, internal echoes (Fig. 15-35). This is much better appreciated on transvaginal sonography.[189] These low-level internal echoes may be seen diffusely throughout the mass or in the dependent portion. Occasionally, a fluid-fluid level can be seen. Small linear hyperechoic foci may be present in the wall of the cyst and are thought to be due to cholesterol deposits accumulating in the cyst wall.[190] An adnexal mass with diffuse low-level internal echoes and absence of neoplastic features is highly likely to be an endometrioma, especially if multilocularity or hyperechoic wall foci are present, whereas an endometrioma is highly unlikely when no component of the mass contains low-level echoes.[190]

The appearance of an endometrioma may be similar to a hemorrhagic ovarian cyst because both are cystic masses that contain blood of variable age.[191] However, a

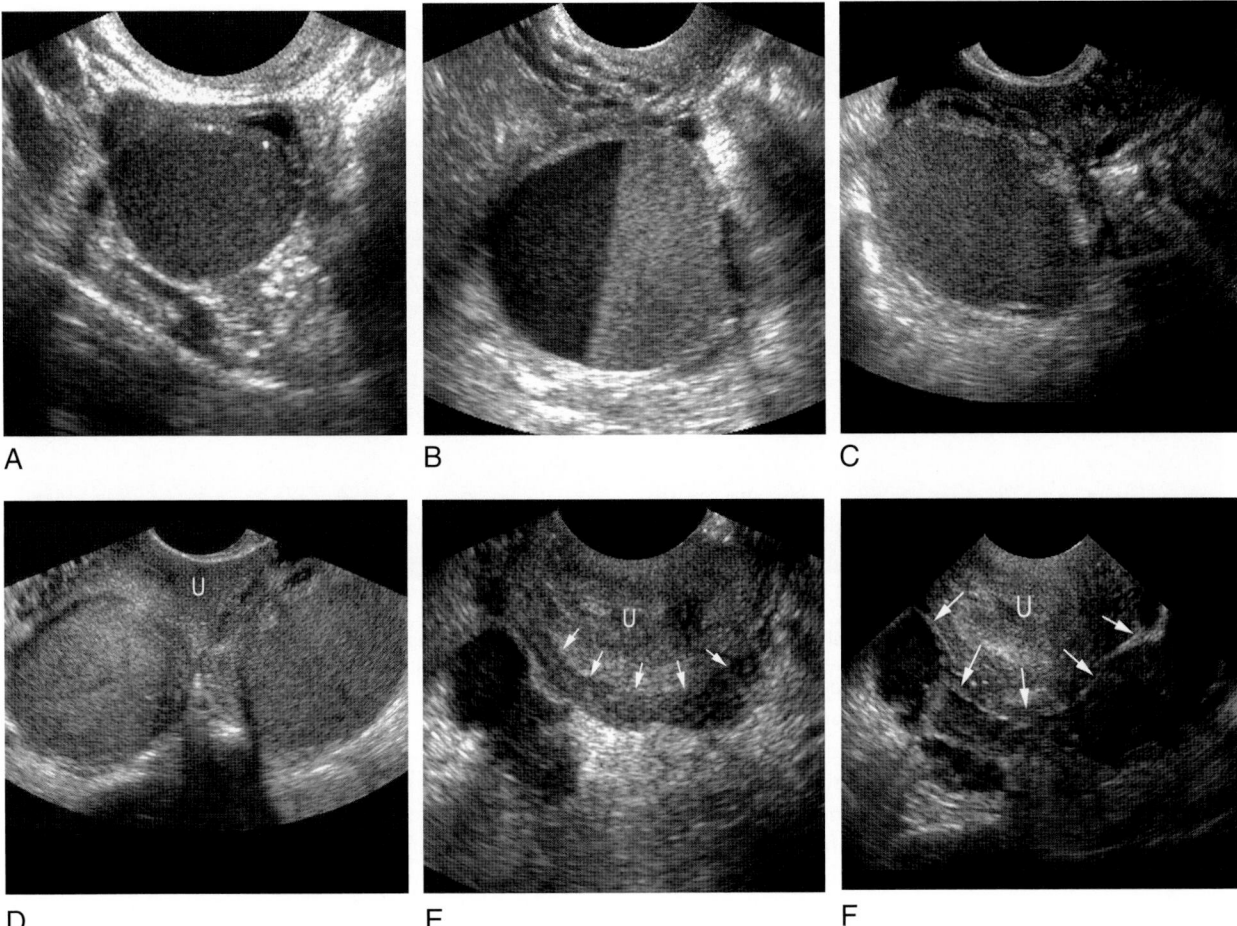

FIGURE 15-35. Endometriosis—spectrum of appearances. Transvaginal scans. Images **A** to **D** show uniform low-level echoes within a cystic ovarian mass. **A** shows typical peripheral echogenic foci. **B** shows a fluid-fluid level. **C** shows avascular marginal echogenic nodules, and **D** shows bilateral disease. **E** shows endometriotic plaque on the posterior surface of the uterus (*arrows*) and in **F**, filling the pouch of Douglas (*arrows*). U, Uterus.

hemorrhagic cyst more frequently demonstrates a reticular internal pattern and is more frequently associated with free fluid in the cul-de-sac. A hemorrhagic cyst will resolve or show a significant decrease in size over the next few menstrual cycles, whereas endometriomas tend to show little change in size and internal echo pattern. Endometriomas or hemorrhagic cysts showing less typical features may be confused with an ovarian neoplasm or tubo-ovarian abscess. Clinically, most women with an acute hemorrhagic cyst present with acute pelvic pain, whereas women with an endometrioma are asymptomatic or have more chronic discomfort associated with their menses.

Polycystic Ovarian Disease

Polycystic ovarian disease (PCOD) is a complex endocrinologic disorder resulting in chronic anovulation. An imbalance of LH and FSH results in abnormal estrogen and androgen production.[169] The serum LH level is elevated and the FSH level is depressed; an elevated LH/FSH ratio is a characteristic finding. Pathologically, the ovaries contain an increased number of follicles in various stages of maturation and atresia, and there is an increased local concentration of androgens, producing stromal abnormality. PCOD is a common cause of infertility and a higher-than-usual rate of early pregnancy loss.[192,193] There is a wide spectrum of clinical manifestations of PCOD, ranging from mild signs of hyperandrogenism in thin, normally menstruating women to the classic Stein-Leventhal syndrome (oligo- or amenorrhea, hirsutism, and obesity).

The typical sonographic findings are those of bilaterally enlarged ovaries containing multiple small follicles and increased stromal echogenicity (Fig. 15-36). The ovaries have a more rounded shape, with the follicles usually located peripherally, although they can also occur randomly throughout the ovarian parenchyma. Transvaginal sonography, because of its superior resolution, is more sensitive in detecting the small follicles. The follicles measure from 0.5 to 0.8 cm in size with more than five in each ovary.[194] However, these

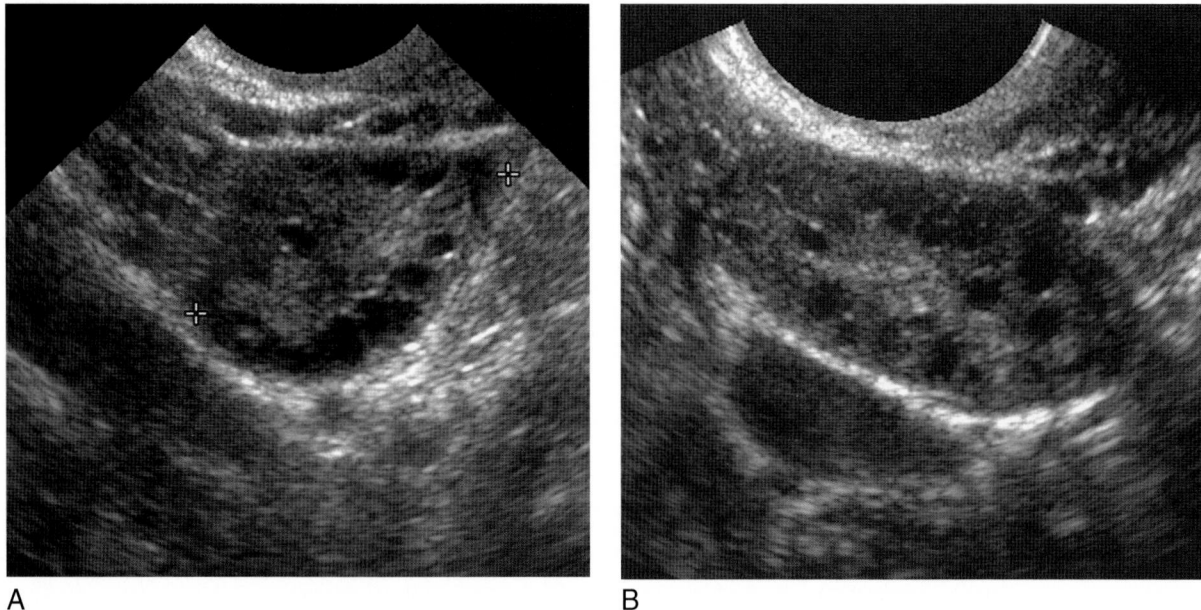

FIGURE 15-36. Polycystic ovarian disease, typical appearances on transvaginal scans. A, Enlarged round ovary (outlined by cursors) with mildly increased stromal echogenicity and multiple peripheral follicles; "string of pearls" sign. **B,** Enlarged ovary with multiple peripheral and central follicles.

typical findings are seen in fewer than 50% of patients with this condition. Ovarian volume is normal in approximately 30%.[194,195] A combination of mean follicular size and ovarian volume has been found to be more sensitive and specific than either feature alone.[196] Using transvaginal sonography, increased stromal echogenicity is believed to be the most sensitive and specific sign of PCOD.[196,197] In a small number of patients with PCOD, the sonographic findings may be unilateral.[193,198] The diagnosis of PCOD is usually made biochemically, but sonography is useful. Because ovulation does not occur, the follicles will persist on serial studies. Long-term follow-up is recommended in these patients because the unopposed high estrogen levels appear to be associated with an increased risk of endometrial and breast carcinoma.[169]

Ovarian Torsion

Torsion of the ovary is an acute abdominal condition requiring prompt surgical intervention. It is caused by partial or complete rotation of the ovarian pedicle on its axis. This results in compromise of the lymphatic and venous drainage, causing congestion and edema of the ovarian parenchyma and leading to eventual loss of arterial perfusion and resultant infarction. Torsion may occur in normal ovaries or in association with a preexisting ovarian cyst or mass. The mass is almost always benign.[199] Torsion of a normal ovary usually occurs in children and younger females with especially mobile adnexa, allowing torsion at the mesosalpinx.[200] Torsion usually occurs in childhood and during the

reproductive years. There is an increased risk during pregnancy. Clinically, there is severe pelvic pain, nausea, and vomiting. A palpable mass may be present. Torsion occurs more frequently on the right side, and the pain may clinically mimic acute appendicitis. This has been thought to be due to the decreased space on the left side which is occupied by the sigmoid colon.[201]

The **sonographic findings** are variable, depending on the duration and degree of vascular compromise and whether an adnexal mass is present (Figs. 15-37 and 15-38). The ovary is enlarged. Multiple cortical follicles in an enlarged ovary are considered a specific sign, although they are not always present.[200] The multi-follicular enlargement is the result of transudation of fluid into the follicles from the circulatory impairment. Free fluid in the cul-de-sac is commonly seen.[202] Color and spectral Doppler examination may show absent flow in the affected ovary. However, Doppler findings may vary depending on the degree and chronicity of the torsion and whether or not there is an associated adnexal mass.[203] The presence of Doppler arterial waveforms and color flow has been reported in surgically proven cases of torsion.[204,205] The possible explanations proposed are that venous thrombosis leads to symptoms before arterial occlusion occurs and that persistent adnexal arterial flow is related to the dual ovarian arterial blood supply (from the ovarian artery and ovarian branches of the uterine artery).[205] A twisted vascular pedicle (consisting of the broad ligament, fallopian tube, and adnexal and ovarian branches of the uterine artery and vein) may be demonstrated as a round hyperechoic structure with multiple concentric hypoechoic stripes (**target**

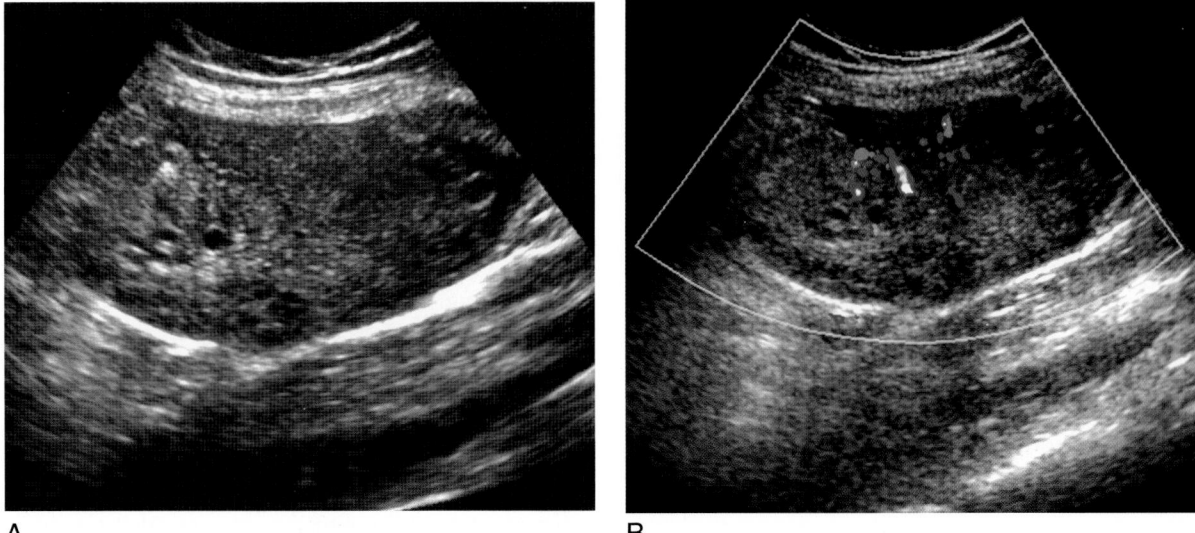

FIGURE 15-37. Ovarian torsion. A and **B** are transabdominal images on a pregnant patient with acute lower abdominal pain. They show a markedly enlarged ovary with some peripheral follicles. On color Doppler evaluation, sparse flow in this ovary was much less than on the normal side. Detection of blood flow does not eliminate the possibility of ovarian torsion.

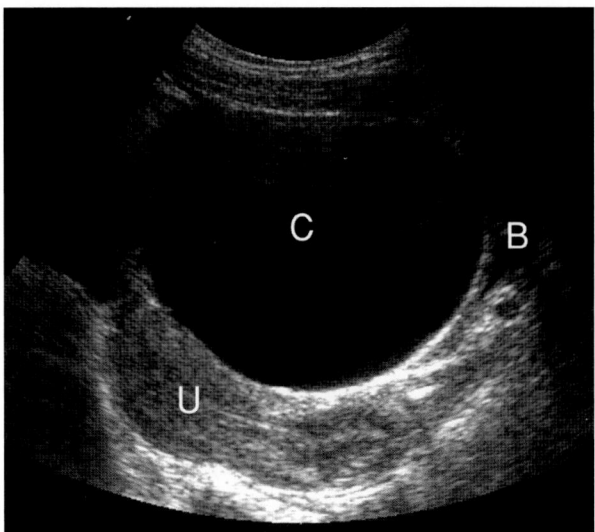

FIGURE 15-38. Ovarian torsion. A transabdominal sagittal image of a young woman with acute pain shows a large simple cyst (C) which lies anterior to the uterus (U) and cephalad to the bladder (B). This unusual position should raise the suspicion of torsion. No blood flow could be detected in the ovary on color Doppler.

appearance) or as an **ellipsoid** or **tubular structure** with internal heterogeneous echoes.[206] When flow within the vascular pedicle is seen on color Doppler, the presence of circular or coiled twisted vessels (**whirlpool sign**) is helpful in diagnosing torsion.[206] The presence of arterial or venous flow or both does not exclude the diagnosis of torsion. Decreased flow may be present. Comparison with the morphologic appearance and flow patterns of the contralateral ovary may aid in the diagnosis.[202]

Massive Edema of the Ovary

This is a rare condition resulting from partial or intermittent torsion of the ovary, causing venous and lymphatic obstruction but not arterial occlusion. This results in ovarian enlargement due to marked stromal edema. The few cases described on sonography show a large, predominantly multicystic adnexal mass.[207-209]

Neoplasms

Ovarian Cancer

Ovarian cancer is the fourth leading cause of cancer death among women in the United States. The American Cancer Society estimates 25,400 new cases of ovarian cancer in the United States in 2003, and about 14,300 deaths. Between 1989 and 1999, the incidence has decreased at a rate of 0.7% a year. Ovarian cancer comprises 25% of all gynecologic malignancies, with its peak incidence occurring in the sixth decade of life. Although only the third most common gynecologic malignancy, it has the highest mortality rate as a result of late diagnosis. As there are few clinical symptoms, approximately 60% to 70% of women have advanced disease (stages III or IV) at the time of diagnosis. The overall 5-year survival rate is 20% to 30%, but with early detection in stage I, the rate rises to 80% to 90%. Therefore, efforts have been directed at developing methods of early diagnosis of this condition.

Increasing age, nulliparity, a history of breast, endometrial, or colon cancer, or a family history of ovarian cancer have been associated with a higher risk of developing ovarian cancer. **Family history** is considered to be the most important risk factor. The lifetime risk of a woman developing ovarian cancer is 1 in 70 (1.4%). However, if a woman has a first-degree relative (mother, daughter, sister) or second-degree relative (aunt or grandmother) who has had ovarian cancer, the risk is 5%. With two or more relatives, the lifetime risk increases to 7%.[210] About 3% to 5% of women with a family history of ovarian cancer will have a hereditary ovarian cancer syndrome. The three main hereditary syndromes associated with ovarian cancer are the **breast-ovarian cancer syndrome**, the most common, in which there is a high frequency of both cancers; the **hereditary nonpolyposis colorectal cancer syndrome** (Lynch II) in which ovarian cancer occurs in association with nonpolyposis colorectal cancer or endometrial cancer, or both; and **site-specific ovarian cancer syndrome** without an excess of breast or colorectal cancer, the least common.[211] Heredity ovarian cancer syndromes are thought to have an autosomal-dominant inheritance, and the lifetime risk of ovarian cancer in these patients is approximately 40% to 50%. They have an earlier age of onset (10 to 15 years) than do other ovarian cancers.[211]

A number of **clinical screening trials** of asymptomatic, predominantly postmenopausal women have been reported.[212-215] These trials have focused on biologic tumor markers such as CA 125 and on sonography, initially transabdominal and more recently transvaginal. CA 125 is a high-molecular-weight glycoprotein recognized by the OC 125 monoclonal antibody. It has proved extremely useful in following the clinical course of patients undergoing chemotherapy and in detecting recurrent subclinical disease.[216,217] Although serum CA 125 is elevated in approximately 80% of women with epithelial ovarian cancer, it detects less than 50% of stage I disease and is insensitive to mucinous and germ-cell tumors.[217] Other malignancies, as well as several benign conditions, may be associated with elevated serum CA 125.[217,218] Therefore, the use of serum CA 125 as a screening test has been disappointing. Studies combining CA 125 with sonography have been more encouraging.[213] More recent screening trials have included color and pulsed Doppler sonography in addition to transvaginal sonography in asymptomatic women,[219] in women with a family history of ovarian or other cancer,[220,221] and in women with previous breast cancer.[222] At present, the use of sonography for ovarian cancer screening must still be considered to be in the research stage and cannot be recommended for routine clinical use. An NIH consensus conference on ovarian cancer, held in 1994, concluded that there is no evidence that the current screening modalities of CA 125 and transvaginal sonography can be effectively used for widespread screening to reduce mortality from ovarian cancer or that their use will result in decreased rather than increased morbidity and mortality. Routine screening has resulted in unnecessary surgery with its attendant potential risks.[223]

Histologically, epithelial neoplasms comprise 65% to 75% of ovarian tumors and 90% of ovarian malignancies.[37] The remaining neoplasms consist of germ cell tumors (15% to 20%), sex cord-stromal tumors (5% to 10%), and metastatic tumors (5% to 10%) (Table 15-1).

TABLE 15-1. HISTOLOGIC OUTLINE OF OVARIAN NEOPLASMS

Type		Incidence (%)	Example
I	Surface epithelial-stromal tumors	65-75	Serous cystadenoma (carcinoma)
			Mucinous cystadenoma (carcinoma)
			Endometrioid carcinoma
			Clear cell carcinoma
			Transitional cell tumor
II	Germ cell tumors	15-20	Teratoma
			Dermoid
			Immature
			Dysgerminoma
			Yolk sac tumor
III	Sex cord-stromal tumors	5-10	Granulosa cell tumor
			Sertoli-Leydig cell tumor
			Thecoma and fibroma
IV	Metastatic tumors	5-10	Genital primary
			Uterus
			Extragenital primary
			Stomach
			Colon
			Breast
			Lymphoma

Sonographically, ovarian cancer usually presents as an adnexal mass. Sonography reflects the gross morphologic condition of the tumor but not the histology. Therefore, it has been difficult to distinguish benign from malignant ovarian tumors by sonography. Well-defined anechoic lesions are more likely to be benign, whereas lesions with irregular walls, thick, irregular septations, mural nodules, and solid echogenic elements favor malignancy.[224,225]

Scoring systems based on the morphologic characteristics have been proposed.[226-230] These systems assign a numeric value for individual sonographic findings; the higher the score, the higher the likelihood of malignancy. Ferrazzi et al. in a prospective multicenter study of 330 adnexal masses, used four previously published morphologic scoring systems and a new multicenter score[231] that had a higher accuracy than the other systems, mainly due to two criteria that allowed correction for typical dermoids and endohemorrhagic corpora lutea. However, they concluded that a completely reliable differentiation of benign from malignant masses cannot be obtained by morphologic criteria alone.

Doppler Findings in Ovarian Cancer

Color and pulsed Doppler sonography have been advocated for distinguishing benign from malignant ovarian masses. Support is based on the premise that malignant masses, because of internal neovascularization, will have high diastolic flow that can be detected on spectral Doppler waveforms. Malignant tumor growth is dependent on angiogenesis with the development of abnormal tumor vessels.[232] These abnormal vessels lack smooth muscle within their walls which, along with arteriovenous shunting, leads to decreased vascular resistance and thus higher diastolic flow velocity. Two angle-independent indexes, the pulsatility index (PI) and the resistive index (RI), have been predominantly used to analyze the Doppler waveform pattern. The PI is the peak systolic velocity minus the end-diastolic velocity divided by the mean velocity; the RI is the peak systolic velocity minus the end-diastolic velocity divided by the peak systolic velocity.

Initial studies using transvaginal color and pulsed Doppler reported both high sensitivity and high specificity in distinguishing benign from malignant ovarian masses, with malignant masses having a PI of less than 1.0 or an RI of less than 0.4.[233-236] Numerous subsequent articles have been unable to reproduce such high sensitivity and specificity, however, and have shown considerable overlap between benign and malignant lesions.[237-247] In categorizing lesions, most authors have used the lowest PI or RI obtained, assuming the worst-case value because this may correspond to the only histologic evidence of malignancy.[236,237]

In menstruating women, the ovarian arterial waveform varies according to the phase of the menstrual cycle. During the menstrual and proliferative phase, there is a high-resistance flow pattern. With development of the corpus luteum at midcycle, a low-resistance waveform pattern is seen because of newly formed vessels along the wall of the corpus luteum. These vessels also lack smooth muscle and demonstrate low-resistance, high-diastolic flow similar to tumor neovascularity. In menstruating women, it is recommended that Doppler studies be done between days 3 and 10 of the menstrual cycle to avoid confusion with normal luteal flow.

Although most reports have found a tendency for both PI and RI to be lower in malignant lesions, there has been too much overlap to differentiate reliably between benign and malignant lesions in the individual patient. Some authors have found no specific cut-off value for either PI or RI that had both high sensitivity and high specificity.[238-240] Absence of flow within a lesion usually indicates a benign lesion, but several reports have shown absent flow within malignant lesions as well.[234,235,238-241]

Other parameters, such as vessel location and the presence of a diastolic notch, have been suggested to improve the specificity of Doppler assessment of ovarian masses.[248] Malignant lesions tend to have more central flow, whereas benign lesions tend to have more peripheral flow. Stein et al. however, found considerable overlap, with 21% of malignant lesions having only peripheral flow and 31% of benign lesions having central flow.[240] Guerriero et al. found a higher accuracy in predicting malignancy when color Doppler demonstrated arterial flow within the solid portions of the mass.[249] The presence of a diastolic notch indicates normal smooth muscle within the arterial wall that is absent in malignant lesions. This finding is frequently absent in benign lesions as well, so its absence has no diagnostic significance.

Some reports have compared the morphologic features on sonography with the Doppler findings and found that Doppler did not add any more diagnostic information than did morphologic assessment alone.[241-243,250] Valentin concluded that, in experienced hands, morphologic assessment is the best method for discriminating between benign and malignant masses—with the main advantage of adding Doppler being to increase the confidence with which a correct diagnosis is made.[250] Others have found that Doppler, when added to sonographic morphologic assessment, improves specificity and positive predictive value.[245-247,251] Brown et al. proposed a multiparameter scoring system using three gray-scale and one Doppler feature developed by means of a stepwise logistic regression analysis.[252] A nonhyperechoic solid component was the most statistically significant predictor of malignancy. Additional features that were statistically discriminatory in decreasing order of importance were location of flow on color Doppler (central), amount of free intraperitoneal fluid, and presence and thickness of septations. Schelling et al. also found that a solid component in an adnexal mass with central vascularity achieved high accuracy, sensitivity, and specificity in predicting malignancy. [253] A meta-analysis of 46 published studies concluded that ultrasound techniques that combine morphologic assessment with color Doppler flow imaging is significantly better in characterizing ovarian masses than morphologic assessment, color Doppler flow imaging, or Doppler indexes alone.[254]

The results of the many studies using Doppler are quite variable and confusing. It is difficult to compare studies due to many factors, such as the lack of standardization of equipment, equipment settings, examination techniques, and differences in patient populations. Doppler is probably not needed if the mass has a characteristic benign morphology, as morphologic assessment is highly accurate in this group of lesions.[240,244] Doppler is likely valuable in assessing the mass that is morphologically indeterminant or suggestive of malignancy. However, the Doppler findings should not be used in isolation but should be combined with morphologic assessment, clinical findings, patient age, and phase of menstrual cycle to best evaluate an adnexal mass.[255]

Surface Epithelial-Stromal Tumors

Surface epithelial-stromal tumors (Fig. 15-39) are generally considered to arise from the surface epithelium that covers the ovary and the underlying ovarian stroma. These tumors can be divided into five broad categories based on epithelial differentiation: **serous, mucinous, endometrioid, clear cell, and transitional cell (Brenner)**.[37] This group of tumors accounts for 65% to 75% of all ovarian neoplasms and 80% to 90% of all ovarian malignancies. There is an intermediate group of approximately 10% to 15% of each serous and mucinous tumors that are histologically categorized as **borderline** or of **low malignant potential**. These tumors have cytologic features of malignancy but do not invade the stroma and, although malignant, have a much better prognosis. The mode of spread of the malignant tumors is primarily intraperitoneal, although direct extension to contiguous structures and lymphatic spread are not uncommon. Lymphatic spread is predominantly to the paraortic nodes. Hematogenous spread usually occurs late in the course of the disease.

Serous Cystadenoma and Cystadenocarcinoma. Serous tumors are the most common, comprising 30% of all ovarian neoplasms. Approximately 50% to 70% of serous tumors are benign. Serous cystadenomas account for 20% to 25% of all benign ovarian neoplasms, and serous cystadenocarcinomas account for 40% to 50% of all malignant ovarian neoplasms.[37] The peak incidence of serous cystadenomas is in the fourth and fifth decades, whereas serous cystadenocarcinomas most frequently occur in perimenopausal and postmenopausal women. Approximately 20% of benign serous tumors and 50% of malignant serous tumors are bilateral. Their sizes vary greatly, but in general, they are smaller than mucinous tumors.

Sonographically, serous cystadenomas are usually large, thin-walled, unilocular cystic masses that may contain thin septations (see Fig. 15-39A, B, and C). Papillary projections are occasionally seen. Serous cystadenocarcinomas may be quite large and usually present as multilocular cystic masses containing multiple papillary projections arising from the cyst walls and septae (see Fig. 15-39G, H, and I). The septae and walls may be thick. Echogenic solid material may be seen within the loculations. Papillary projections may form on the surface of the cyst and surrounding organs, resulting in fixation of the mass. Ascites is frequently seen.

Mucinous Cystadenoma and Cystadenocarcinoma. Mucinous tumors are the second most common ovarian epithelial tumor, accounting for 20% to 25% of ovarian neoplasms. Mucinous cystadenomas constitute 20% to 25% of all benign ovarian neoplasms, and mucinous cystadenocarcinomas make up 5% to 10% of all primary malignant ovarian neoplasms.[37] Mucinous cystadenomas occur most often in the third to fifth decades, but may be seen in very young women, whereas mucinous cystadenocarcinomas most frequently occur in the fourth to seventh decades. Mucinous tumors are less frequently bilateral than are their serous counterparts, with only 5% of the benign and 15% to 20% of the malignant lesions occurring on both sides. Approximately 80% to 85% of mucinous tumors are benign.

On sonographic examination, mucinous cystadenomas can be huge cystic masses, measuring up to 15 to 30 cm and filling the entire pelvis and abdomen (see Figs. 15-39D and 15-40). Multiple thin septae are present and low-level echoes caused by the mucoid material may be seen in the dependent portions of the mass (see Fig. 15-39E). Papillary projections are less frequently seen than in the serous counterpart. Mucinous cystadenocarcinomas (see Fig. 15-39F) are usually large, multiloculated cystic masses containing papillary projections and echogenic material; they generally have a sonographic appearance similar to that of serous cystadenocarcinomas.

Penetration of the tumor capsule or rupture may lead to intraperitoneal spread of mucin-secreting cells that fill the peritoneal cavity with a gelatinous material. This condition, known as **pseudomyxoma peritonei**, may be similar sonographically to ascites or may contain multiple septations in the fluid that fills much of the pelvis and abdomen. Low-level echogenic material may be seen within the fluid. This condition may occur in

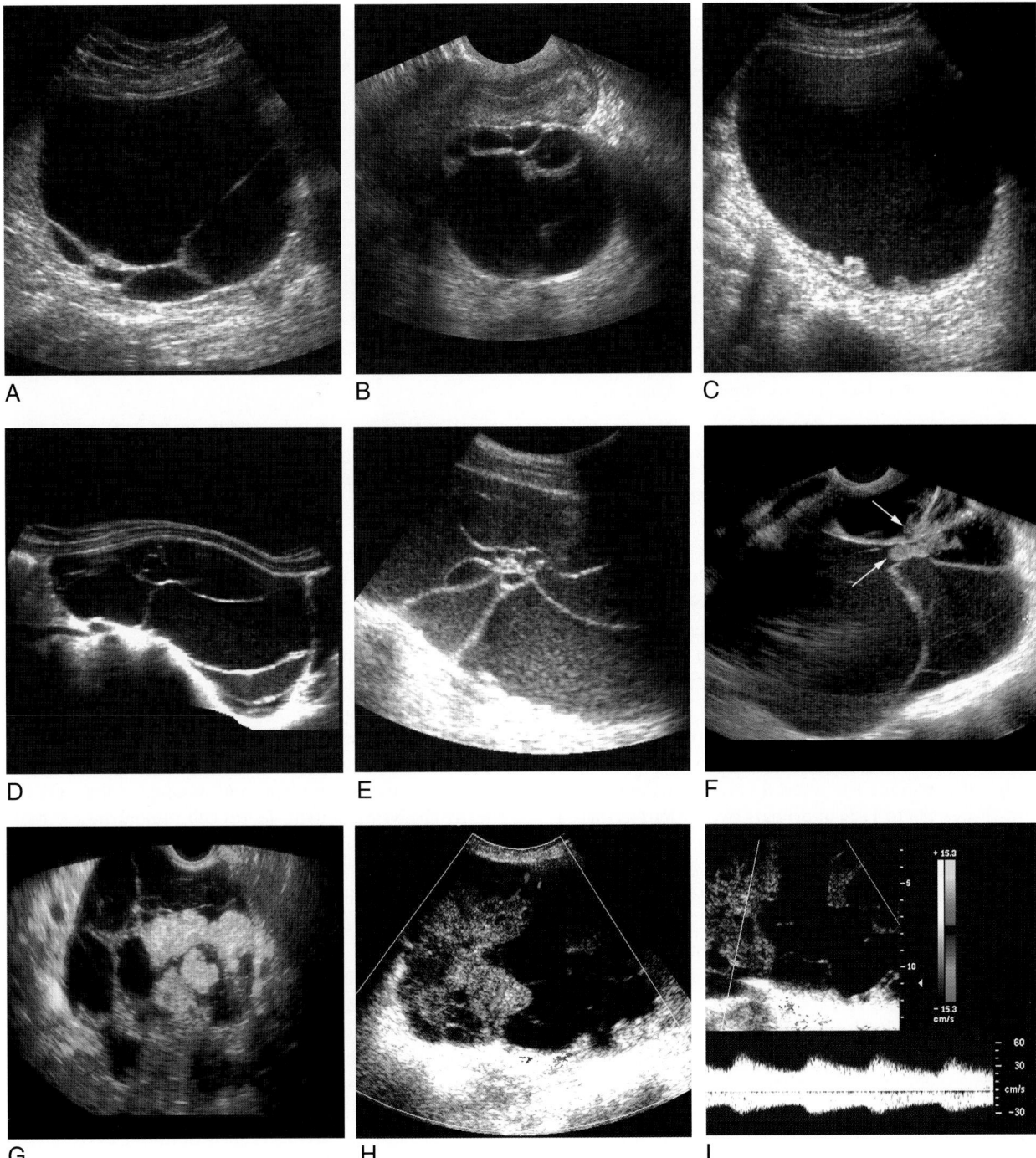

FIGURE 15-39. Epithelial ovarian neoplasms—spectrum of appearances. A, B, and C show **serous cystadenomas**. In **A**, septations within a cystic mass are fairly thin. In **B**, septations are thicker, and in **C**, there are low-level echogenic particles and small mural nodules. **D** and **E** are **mucinous cystadenomas**, and **F** is a **mucinous cystadenocarcinoma**. Large size and septations are characteristic; septal nodularity is marked in **F** (*arrows*). **G**, **H**, and **I** are images in a single patient with a **serous cystadenocarcinoma**. Extensive nodularity shows vascularity confirming the morphologic suspicion of a malignant mass. There is high diastolic flow resulting in a low resistive index.

mucinous cystadenomas and in mucinous cystadeno-carcinomas. A ruptured mucocele of the appendix and mucinous tumors of the appendix and colon can also lead to pseudomyxoma peritonei.

Endometrioid Tumor. Nearly all endometrioid tumors are malignant. They are the second most common

epithelial malignancy, comprising 20% to 25% of ovarian malignancies.[37] Approximately 25% to 30% are bilateral, and they occur most frequently in the fifth and sixth decades. Their histologic characteristics are identical to those of endometrial adenocarcinoma, and approximately 30% of patients with this condition have

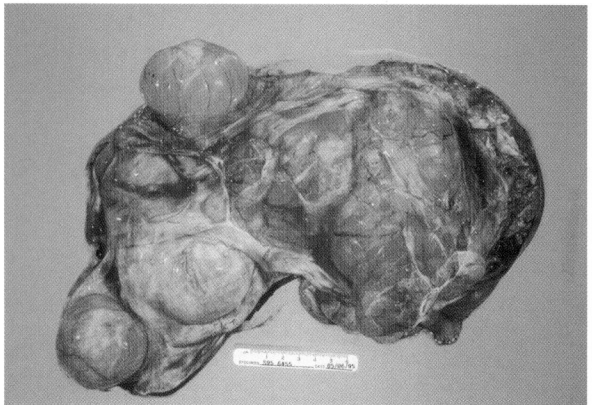

FIGURE 15-40. Mucinous cystadenoma. Gross pathologic specimen shows multiple cystic loculations.

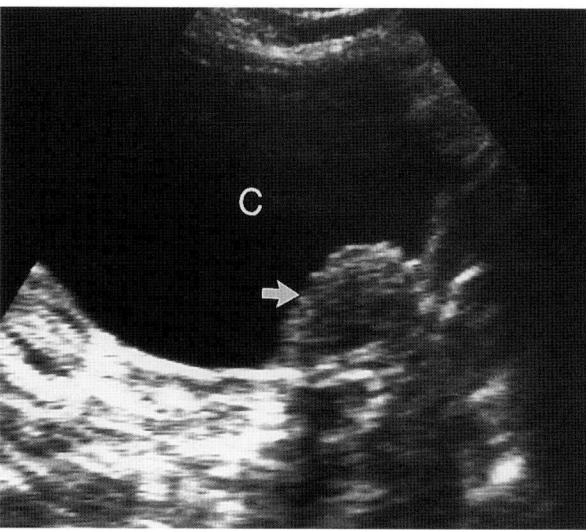

FIGURE 15-41. Brenner's tumor in wall of a mucinous cystadenoma. Transabdominal scan shows a large, well-defined cystic mass (C) with a solid hypoechoic mural nodule (*arrow*). Pathology showed a Brenner's tumor within wall of a large mucinous cystadenoma.

associated endometrial adenocarcinoma, which is thought to represent an independent primary tumor. The endometrioid tumor has a better prognosis than do other epithelial malignancies, which is probably related to diagnosis at an earlier stage. **Sonographically**, it usually presents as a cystic mass containing papillary projections, although in some cases there is a predominantly solid mass that may contain areas of hemorrhage or necrosis.[256,257]

Clear Cell Tumor. This tumor is considered to be of Müllerian duct origin and to be a variant of endometrioid carcinoma. It is nearly always malignant and constitutes 5% to 10% of primary ovarian carcinomas. It occurs most frequently in the fifth to seventh decades and is bilateral in about 20% of patients. Associated pelvic endometriosis is present in 50% to 70% of clear cell carcinomas, and approximately 25% arise from the lining of endometriotic cysts.[37] **Sonographically**, it usually presents as a nonspecific, complex, predominantly cystic mass.[256,257]

Transitional Cell Tumor. This tumor, also known as **Brenner's tumor,** is derived from the surface epithelium that undergoes metaplasia to form typical uroepithelial-like components.[37] It is uncommon, accounting for 1% to 2% of all ovarian neoplasms, and is nearly always benign; 6% to 7% are bilateral. Most patients are asymptomatic, and the tumor is discovered incidentally on sonographic examination or at surgery. Thirty percent are associated with cystic neoplasms, usually serous or mucinous cystadenomas or cystic teratomas, frequently in the ipsilateral ovary (Fig. 15-41).[258] **Sonographically**, Brenner tumors are hypoechoic solid masses. Calcification may occur in the outer wall. Cystic areas are unusual and when present are usually due to a coexistent cystadenoma.[257] Pathologically, they are solid tumors composed of dense fibrous stroma. They appear similar to ovarian fibromas and thecomas and to uterine leiomyomas, both sonographically and pathologically.

Germ Cell Tumors

Germ cell tumors are derived from the primitive germ cells of the embryonic gonad. They account for 15% to 20% of ovarian neoplasms, with approximately 95% being benign cystic teratomas. The others, including dysgerminomas and endodermal sinus (yolk sac) tumors, occur mainly in children and young adults and are nearly always malignant. Germ cell tumors are the most common ovarian malignancies in children and young adults. When a large, predominantly solid ovarian mass is present in a girl or young woman, the diagnosis of a malignant germ cell tumor should be strongly considered.[259]

Cystic Teratoma. Cystic teratomas make up approximately 15% to 25% of ovarian neoplasms; 10% to 15% are bilateral. They are composed of well-differentiated derivatives of the **three germ layers**—ectoderm, mesoderm, and endoderm. Because **ectodermal elements** generally predominate, cystic teratomas are virtually always benign and are also called **dermoid cysts**. Cystic teratomas and serous cystadenomas are the two most common ovarian neoplasms. In contrast to surface epithelial-stromal tumors, cystic teratomas are more commonly seen in the active reproductive years, but they can occur at any age and are not infrequently seen in postmenopausal women. These tumors may present as a clinically palpable mass. They are usually asymptomatic and often discovered incidentally during sonography. In 10% of cases, the tumor is diagnosed during pregnancy.[37] Complications include torsion and rupture. Torsion is the most common complication, whereas rupture is uncommon, occurring in approximately 1% of cases and causing a secondary chemical peritonitis.

Malignant transformation is also uncommon, occurring in approximately 2% of cases, usually in older women.[37]

Sonographically, cystic teratomas have a variable appearance ranging from completely anechoic to completely hyperechoic. However, certain features are considered specific (Figs. 15-42 and 15-43). These include a predominantly cystic mass with an echogenic mural nodule, the **"dermoid plug."**[260] The dermoid

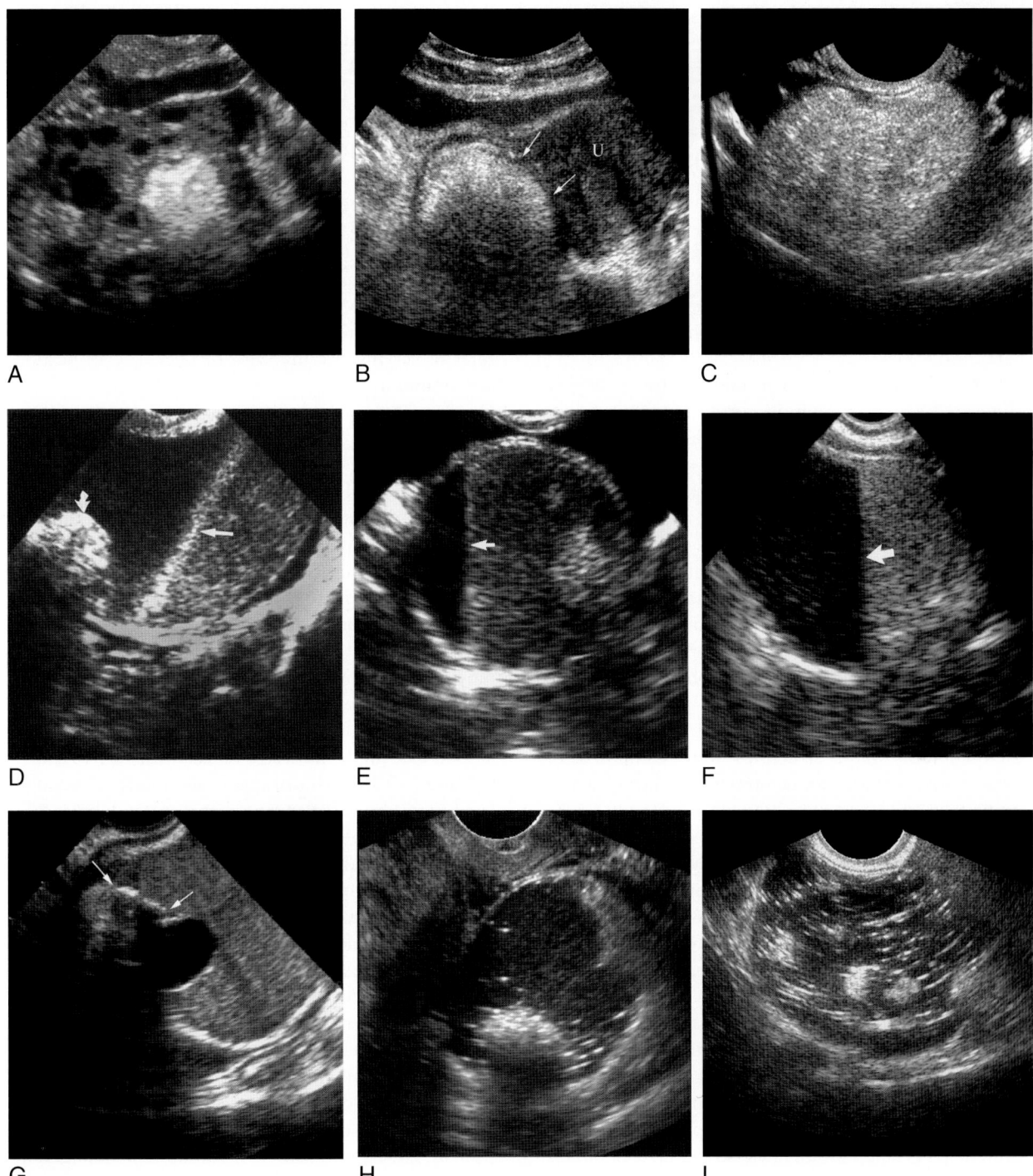

FIGURE 15-42. Dermoid cysts—spectrum of appearances. A shows a **small, highly echogenic mass** in an otherwise normal ovary. **B** is a transverse transabdominal scan showing the uterus (U). In the right adnexal region there is a **highly echogenic and attenuating mass** (*arrows*). This is a *tip-of-the-iceberg sign.* **C** shows a highly echogenic intraovarian mass with no normal ovarian tissue. **D**, Mass of varying echogenicity with hair-fluid level (*straight arrow*) and highly echogenic fat-containing dermoid plug (*curved arrow*) with shadowing. **E**, Predominantly echogenic mass with fat-fluid level (*arrow*). **F**, Mass with fat-fluid level (*arrow*). **G**, Mass containing uniform echoes, small cystic area, and calcification (*arrows*) with shadowing. **H**, Combination of ***dermoid mesh*** and dermoid plug appearances. **I**, ***Dermoid mesh***, multiple linear hyperechogenic interfaces floating within cystic mass.

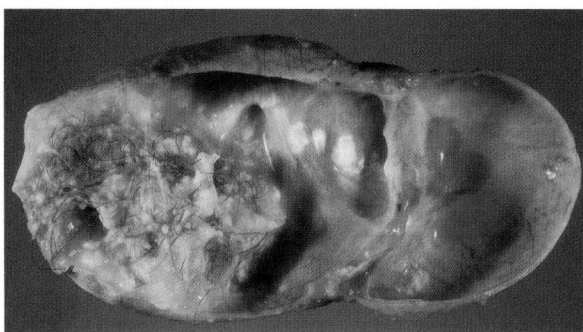

FIGURE 15-43. Cystic teratoma. Pathologic specimen shows large ovarian mass containing fluid, fat, hair, and teeth.

plug usually contains hair, teeth, or fat and frequently casts an acoustic shadow. Correlation with CT images has shown that in many cases the cystic component is pure sebum (which is liquid at body temperature) rather than fluid.[261]

A mixture of matted hair and sebum is highly echogenic because of multiple tissue interfaces, and it produces ill-defined acoustic shadowing that obscures the posterior wall of the lesion. This has been termed the **"tip-of-the-iceberg"** sign.[262] Highly echogenic foci with well-defined acoustic shadowing may arise from other elements, including teeth and bone. Multiple linear hyperechogenic interfaces may be seen floating within the cyst and have been shown to be hair fibers.[263] This is also considered a specific sign and has been referred to as the **"dermoid mesh."**[264] A **fat-fluid** or **hair-fluid level** may also be seen. Multiple mobile spherical echogenic structures floating in a large cystic pelvic mass has been recently described as a characteristic feature.[265] Microscopically these structures were composed of desquamative keratin containing fibrin, hemosiderin, and hair.

Patel et al. in a study of 252 adnexal masses, 74 of which were cystic teratomas, found that 55 of the cystic teratomas showed two or more sonographic dermoid features. None of the other adnexal masses showed more than one feature giving a positive predictive value of 100% for an adnexal mass showing two or more sonographic dermoid features.[266]

Pitfalls in the diagnosis of cystic teratomas have been described.[267] Acute hemorrhage into an ovarian cyst or an endometrioma may be so echogenic that it resembles a dermoid plug. However, posterior sound enhancement is usually seen with acute hemorrhage, whereas the dermoid plug tends to attenuate sound. Other pitfalls include pedunculated fibroids, especially lipoleiomyomas, and perforated appendicitis with an appendicolith.[267] An echogenic dermoid may appear similar to bowel gas and may be overlooked. If a definite pelvic mass is clinically palpable and the sonogram appears normal, the patient should be reexamined, with the intention of looking carefully for a dermoid.

Struma ovarii is a teratoma that is composed entirely or predominantly of thyroid tissue. It occurs in 2% to 3% of teratomas. Color Doppler sonography detected central blood flow in solid tissue in four reported cases of struma ovarii compared with absent central blood flow in benign cystic teratomas.[268] This is likely due to the highly vascularized thyroid tissue compared to the avascular fat and hair found in benign cystic teratomas. Although associated hormonal effects are rare, sonography may be valuable in identifying a pelvic lesion in a hyperthyroid patient when there is no evidence of a thyroid lesion in the neck.[269]

Immature teratoma is uncommon representing less than 1% of all teratomas and contains immature tissue from all three germ-cell layers. It is a rapidly growing malignant tumor that most commonly occurs in the first two decades of life. Sonographically, the tumor usually presents as a solid mass, but cystic structures of varying size may also be seen.[259] Calcifications are commonly seen.

Dysgerminoma. Dysgerminomas are malignant germ cell tumors that constitute approximately 1% to 2% of primary ovarian neoplasms and 3% to 5% of ovarian malignancies.[37] They are composed of undifferentiated germ cells and are morphologically identical to the male testicular seminoma. They are highly radiosensitive and have a five-year survival rate of 75% to 90%. This tumor occurs predominantly in women under 30 and is bilateral in approximately 15% of cases. The dysgerminoma and the serous cystadenoma are the two most common ovarian neoplasms seen in pregnancy.[37] **Sonographically**, they are solid masses that are predominantly echogenic but may contain small anechoic areas caused by hemorrhage or necrosis (Fig. 15-44).[259] CT and MR have shown these solid masses to be lobulated with fibrovascular septa between the lobules.[270] A report using color Doppler in three dysgerminomas showed prominent arterial flow within the fibrovascular septa of a multilobulated, solid, echogenic mass.[271]

Yolk Sac Tumor. This rare, rapidly growing tumor, also called **endodermal sinus tumor**, with a poor prognosis is the second most common malignant ovarian germ cell neoplasm after dysgerminoma. It is thought to arise from the undifferentiated and multipotential embryonal carcinoma by selective differentiation toward yolk sac and vitelline structures.[37] It usually occurs in females under 20 years of age and is almost always unilateral. Increased levels of serum α-fetoprotein (AFP) may be seen in association with this tumor. The sonographic appearance is similar to that of the dysgerminoma.[256,259]

Sex Cord-Stromal Tumors

Sex cord-stromal tumors arise from the sex cords of the embryonic gonad and/or from the ovarian stroma. The main tumors in this group include the granulosa cell

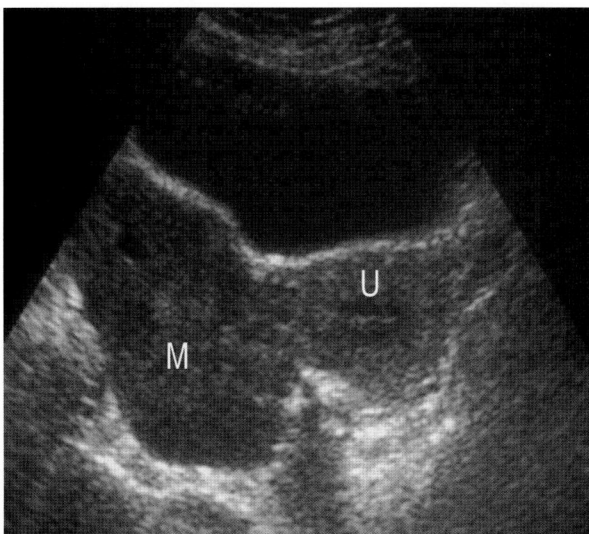

FIGURE 15-44. Dysgerminoma. Transverse transabdominal scan in a young woman shows a large, solid pelvic mass (M) adjacent to the uterus (U). The most common explanation for a solid adnexa mass is a pedunculated uterine fibroid.

tumor, Sertoli-Leydig cell tumor (androblastoma), thecoma, and fibroma. This group accounts for 5% to 10% of all ovarian neoplasms and 2% of all ovarian malignancies.

Granulosa Cell Tumor. This tumor makes up approximately 1% to 2% of ovarian neoplasms and has a low malignancy potential. Ninety-five percent are of the adult type and occur predominantly in postmenopausal women; nearly all are unilateral. They are the most common estrogenically active ovarian tumor,[37] and clinical signs of estrogen production can occur. Approximately 10% to 15% of patients with this tumor eventually develop endometrial carcinoma. The juvenile type comprises 5% of granulosa cell tumors and occur mainly in patients younger than 30 years and in children. In premenarchal girls, these tumors usually produce sexual precocity as a consequence of estrogen secretion. **Sonographically**, adult granulosa cell tumors have a variable appearance, ranging from small solid masses to tumors with variable degrees of hemorrhage or fibrotic changes to multilocular cystic lesions.[272] The solid masses may have an echogenicity similar to that of uterine fibroids, while the cystic masses may have an appearance similar to that of cystadenomas.[256] Metastases, although uncommon, appear as peritoneal-based masses similar to epithelial neoplasms or as cystic liver masses.[273]

Sertoli-Leydig Cell Tumor. This rare tumor, also called **androblastoma**, constitutes less than 0.5% of ovarian neoplasms. It generally occurs in women under 30 years of age; almost all are unilateral. Malignancy occurs in 10% to 20% of these tumors. The malignant tumors tend to recur relatively soon after initial diagnosis, with

relatively few recurrences occurring after five years.[274] Clinically, signs and symptoms of virilization occur in about 30% of patients, although about half will have no endocrine manifestations.[37] Occasionally, these tumors may be associated with estrogen production. **Sonographically**, they usually appear as solid hypoechoic masses or may have an appearance similar to that of granulosa cell tumors.[274]

Thecoma and Fibroma. Both these tumors arise from the ovarian stroma and may be difficult to distinguish from each other pathologically. Tumors with an abundance of thecal cells are classified as thecomas, whereas those with fewer thecal cells and abundant fibrous tissue are classified as thecofibromas and fibromas. **Thecomas** comprise approximately 1% of all ovarian neoplasms, and 70% occur in postmenopausal females. They are unilateral, almost always benign, and frequently show clinical signs of estrogen production. **Fibromas** comprise approximately 4% of ovarian neoplasms, are benign, usually unilateral, and occur most commonly in menopausal and postmenopausal women. Unlike thecomas, they are rarely associated with estrogen production and therefore are frequently asymptomatic, despite reaching a large size. Ascites has been reported to be present in up to 50% of patients with fibromas larger than 5 cm in diameter.[275] **Meigs' syndrome** (associated ascites and pleural effusion) occurs in 1% to 3% of patients with ovarian fibromas but is not specific, having been reported in association with other ovarian neoplasms as well. Fibromas also occur in approximately 17% of patients with the basal cell nevus (Gorlin) syndrome. In this condition, the fibromas are commonly bilateral, calcified, and occur in younger women with a mean age of 30 years.[274]

Sonographically, these tumors have a characteristic appearance (Fig. 15-45). A hypoechoic mass with marked posterior attenuation of the sound beam is seen as a result of the homogeneous fibrous tissue in these tumors.[275] The main differential diagnosis is that of a Brenner tumor or pedunculated uterine fibroid. Not all fibromas and thecomas show this characteristic appearance, and a variety of sonographic appearances have been noted, probably as a result of the tendency for edema and cystic degeneration to occur within these tumors.[276]

Metastatic Tumors

Approximately 5% to 10% of ovarian neoplasms are metastatic in origin. The most common primary sites of ovarian metastases are tumors of the breast and gastrointestinal tract. The term *Krukenberg tumor* should be reserved for those tumors containing the typical mucin-secreting "signet ring" cells, usually of gastric or colonic origin. Endometrial carcinoma frequently metastasizes to the ovary, but it may be difficult to

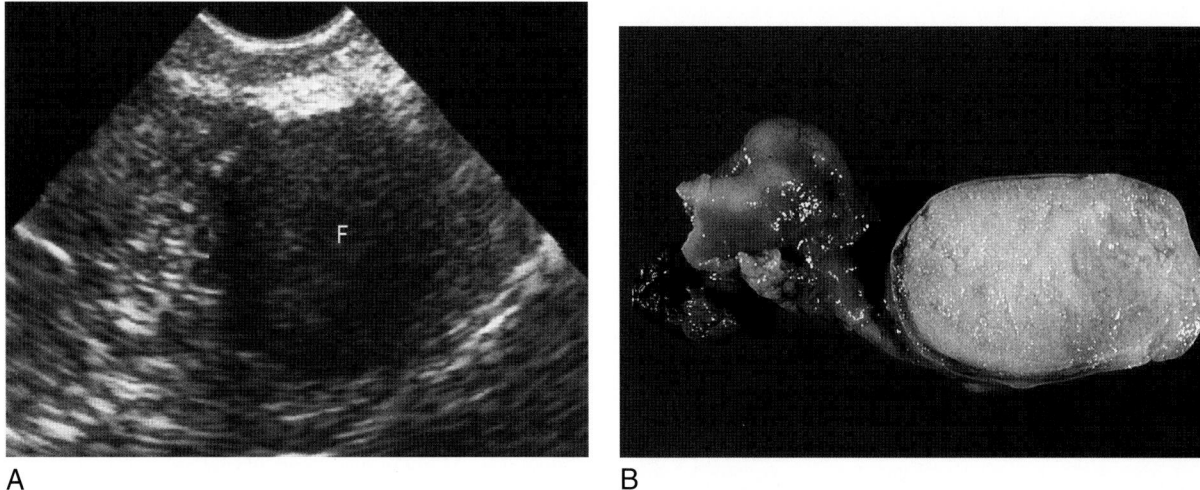

FIGURE 15-45. Ovarian fibroma. A, Transvaginal scan shows hypoechoic solid mass (F) with some posterior attenuation. **B**, Pathologic specimen shows homogeneous solid nature of fibroma.

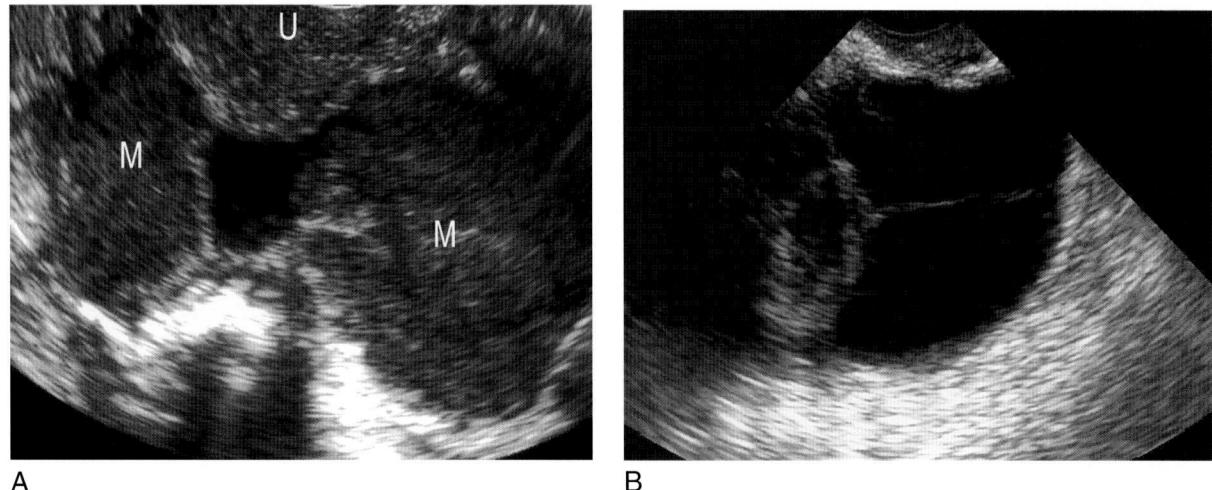

FIGURE 15-46. Ovarian metastases from carcinoma of the colon in two patients. A is from a young woman and shows bilateral solid ovarian masses (M) or Krukenberg tumors. Uterus (U). **B** is a postmenopausal woman showing a complex predominantly cystic mass with septations and nodules mimicking a primary ovarian cystadenocarcinoma.

distinguish from primary endometrioid carcinoma, as discussed earlier. **Sonographically**, ovarian metastases are usually bilateral solid masses, but they may become necrotic and have a complex, predominantly cystic appearance that simulates primary cystadenocarcinoma (Fig. 15-46).[277,278] Ascites may be seen in either primary or metastatic tumors. **Lymphoma** may involve the ovary, usually in a diffuse, disseminated form that is frequently bilateral. The sonographic appearance is that of a solid hypoechoic mass similar to lymphoma elsewhere in the body.

FALLOPIAN TUBE

The normal fallopian tube is difficult to identify by transabdominal or transvaginal sonography unless it is surrounded by fluid. The normal fallopian tube is an undulating echogenic structure of approximately 8 to 10 mm in width, running posterolaterally from the uterus to lie within the cul-de-sac near the ovary. The lumen is not seen unless it is fluid filled.[279] Developmental abnormalities of the tube are rare. Abnormalities of the tube include pregnancy, infection, and neoplasm.

Pelvic Inflammatory Disease

Pelvic inflammatory disease (PID) is a common condition that is increasing in frequency. It is usually due to sexually transmitted diseases, most commonly associated with gonorrhea and chlamydia. The infection commonly spreads by ascent from the cervix and endometrium. Less common causes include direct extension from appendiceal, diverticular, or postsurgical abscesses that have ruptured into the pelvis, as well as puerperal and postabortion complications. Hematogenous spread is rare but can occur from tuberculosis. PID is usually bilateral, except when it is caused by direct extension of an adjacent inflammatory process, when it is most commonly unilateral. The presence of an intrauterine contraceptive device increases the risk of PID. Long-term sequelae include chronic pelvic pain, infertility, and an increased risk of ectopic pregnancy.

Sexually transmitted PID spreads along the mucosa of the pelvic organs, initially infecting the cervix and uterine endometrium (endometritis), the fallopian tubes (acute salpingitis), and finally, the region of both ovaries and the peritoneum. A pyosalpinx develops as a result of occlusion of the tube. The patients usually present clinically with pain, fever, pelvic tenderness, and vaginal discharge. A pelvic mass may be palpated.

Sonographic Findings of PID

The sonographic findings may be normal early in the course of the disease.[280] As the disease progresses or becomes chronic, a spectrum of findings may occur (Figs. 15-47 and 15-48). Endometrial thickening or fluid may indicate **endometritis**. Pus may be demonstrated in the cul-de-sac; it contains echogenic particles,

---

SONOGRAPHIC FINDINGS OF PID

ENDOMETRITIS

Endometrial thickening or fluid

PUS IN CUL-DE-SAC

Particulate fluid

PERIOVARIAN INFLAMMATION

Enlarged ovaries with multiple cysts and indistinct margins

PYOSALPINX OR HYDROSALPINX

Fluid-filled fallopian tube with or without internal echoes

TUBO-OVARIAN COMPLEX

Fusion of the inflamed dilated tube and ovary

TUBO-OVARIAN ABSCESS

Complex multiloculated mass with variable septations, irregular margins, and scattered internal echoes

---

which distinguish it from serous fluid in this region. Enlarged ovaries with multiple cysts and indistinct margins may be seen as a result of periovarian inflammation.[280] On transabdominal sonography, dilated tubes appear as complex, predominantly cystic masses that are often indistinguishable from other adnexal masses. However, transvaginal sonography recognizes the fluid-filled tube by its tubular shape, somewhat folded configuration, and well-defined echogenic walls.[281] The dilated tube can be distinguished from a fluid-filled bowel loop by the lack of peristalsis. Low-level internal echoes may be seen within the fluid-filled tube as a result of pus (**pyosalpinx**), and a fluid-pus level may occasionally be seen. Anechoic fluid within the tube indicates hydrosalpinx. A thickened tubal wall (5 mm or more) is indicative of acute disease.[282,283] In assessing 14 acute and 60 chronic cases of PID, Timor-Tritsch et al. described three appearances of tubal wall structure: (1) "cogwheel" sign, defined as an anechoic cogwheel-shaped structure visible in the cross-section of the tube with thick walls, which was seen mainly in acute disease; (2) "beads on a string" sign, defined as hyperechoic mural nodules measuring 2 to 3 mm and seen on the cross-section of the fluid-filled distended tube. This is due to degenerated and flattened endosalpingeal fold remnants and was seen only in chronic disease; and (3) incomplete septa, defined as hyperechoic septa that originate as a triangular protrusion from one of the walls, but do not reach the opposite wall. This feature was seen frequently in both acute and chronic disease and was not discriminatory.[283]

As the infection worsens, periovarian adhesions may form, with fusion of the inflamed dilated tube and ovary, which is called the **tubo-ovarian complex**. The ovary cannot be separated from the tube by pushing with the vaginal transducer.[283] Further progression results in a **tubo-ovarian abscess** that appears sonographically as a complex multiloculated mass with variable septations, irregular margins, and scattered internal echoes. There is usually posterior acoustic enhancement, and a fluid-debris level or gas may occasionally be seen within the mass. The sonographic appearance may be indistinguishable from other benign and malignant adnexal masses, and clinical correlation is necessary for suggesting the correct diagnosis. Because the ovaries are relatively resistant to infection, areas of recognizable ovarian tissue may be seen within the inflammatory mass by transvaginal sonography.[144]

Both transabdominal and transvaginal sonography are useful in assessing patients with PID. The transabdominal approach is helpful in assessing the extent of the disease, whereas the transvaginal approach is sensitive to detecting dilated tubes, periovarian inflammatory change, and the internal characteristics of tubo-ovarian abscesses.[280,284] Sonography is also useful in following the response to antibiotic therapy. Tubo-ovarian

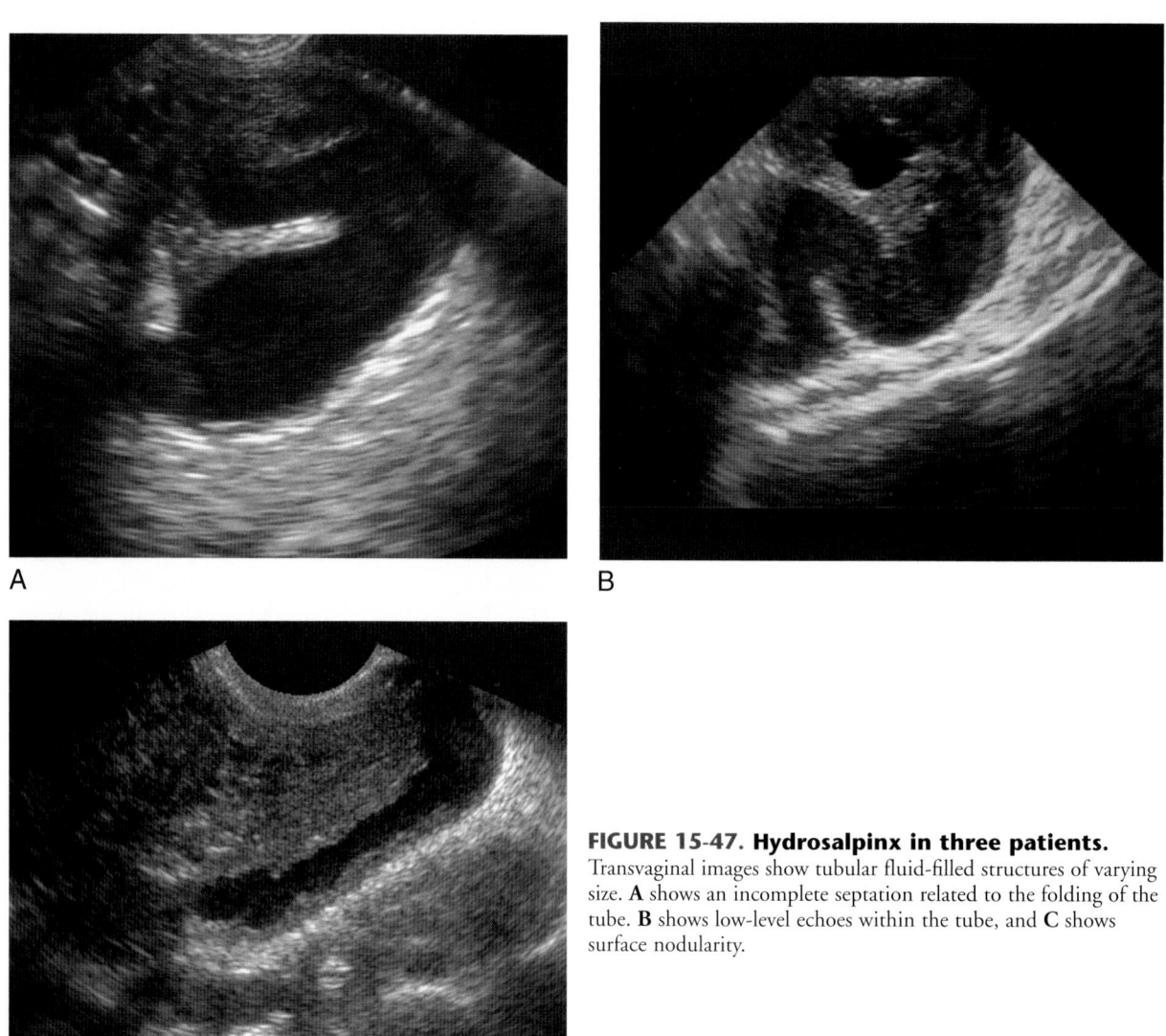

FIGURE 15-47. Hydrosalpinx in three patients.
Transvaginal images show tubular fluid-filled structures of varying size. **A** shows an incomplete septation related to the folding of the tube. **B** shows low-level echoes within the tube, and **C** shows surface nodularity.

abscesses may be treated by sonographically guided transvaginal aspiration and drainage.[285,286] Catheter drainage is used if the aspirate is frankly purulent, whereas complete aspiration without catheter drainage may be done if the aspirate is not purulent.[286]

In **chronic PID**, extensive fibrosis and adhesions may obscure the margins of the pelvic organs, which blend into a large, ill-defined mass. Isolated torsion of the fallopian tube is uncommon, but it occurs in association with chronic hydrosalpinx.[287] The patient presents with abrupt onset of severe pelvic pain. Hydrosalpinx and tubal torsion have also been reported as a late complication in patients undergoing tubal ligation.[288]

Carcinoma

Carcinoma of the fallopian tube is the least common (less than 1%) of all gynecologic malignancies, with adenocarcinoma being the most common histologic type. It occurs most frequently in postmenopausal women in their sixth decade who present clinically with pain, vaginal bleeding, and a pelvic mass. A minority of patients will have a profuse watery discharge, known as *hydrops tubae profluens*. The tumor usually involves the distal end, but it may involve the entire length of the tube. **Sonographically,** carcinoma of the fallopian tube has been described as a sausage-shaped, solid, or cystic

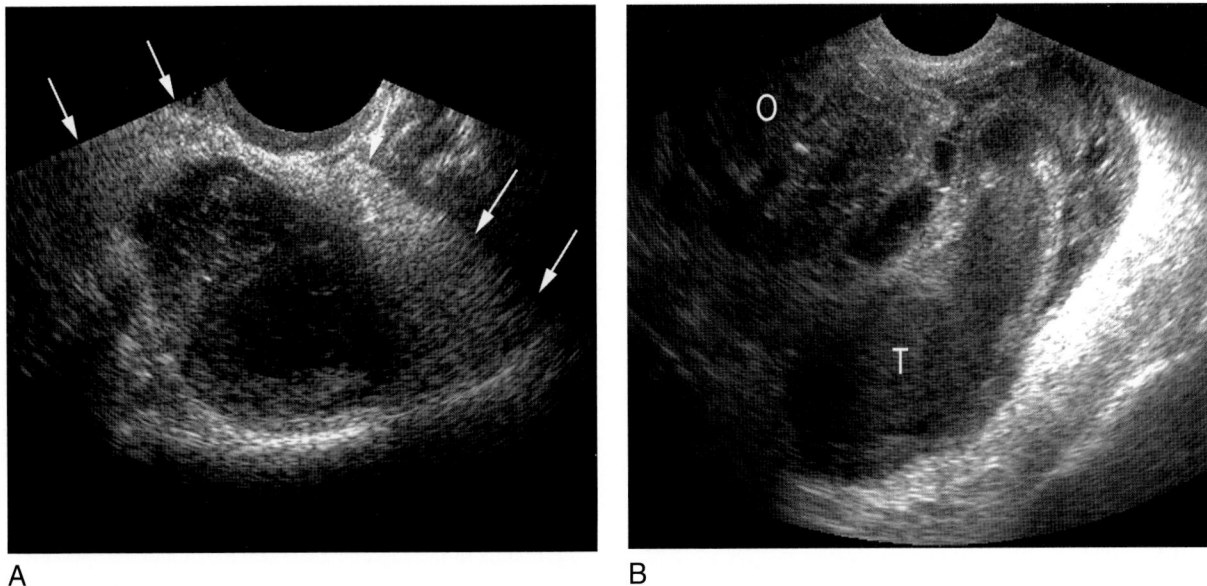

FIGURE 15-48. Pelvic inflammatory disease in two patients. A, Transvaginal image shows a very large ovary surrounded by a rim of highly echogenic and inflamed fat (*arrows*). There are complex fluid collections within the ovary. There is no normal architecture. **B,** The tube (T) is distended and elongated and filled with debris representing pus. The ovary (O) is similarly filled with pus with indistinct borders showing a tubo-ovarian complex.

TABLE 15-2. OVARIAN MASSES

Sonographic Characteristics	Suggestive of Benign Disease	Suggestive of Malignant Disease
Size	Small: <5cm	Large: >10 cm
External contour	Thin wall	Thick wall
	Well-defined borders	Ill-defined or irregular borders
Internal consistency	Purely cystic	Solid or complex
	Thin septations	Thick or irregular septations
		Echogenic solid nodules
		Papillary projections
Doppler	High-resistance or no flow	Low-resistance flow
	Avascular nodules	Vascular nodules
Associated findings		Ascites
		Peritoneal implants

mass with papillary projections.[289-292] The clinical and sonographic findings are similar to those of ovarian carcinoma, so a delay in diagnosis and treatment is unusual.[292]

SONOGRAPHIC EVALUATION OF A PELVIC MASS IN ADULT WOMEN

Sonography is commonly used to evaluate a pelvic mass (Table 15-2). Clinical features such as patient age, symptoms, menstrual status, and family history should also be considered when evaluating the mass. Comparison with previous examinations, if available, should be done to determine if the mass was previously present and if there has been any change in size or internal characteristics.

When a mass is found on sonography, it should be characterized by the following:

- Location (uterine or extrauterine)
- Size
- External contour (well-defined, ill-defined, or irregular borders)
- Internal consistency (cystic, complex predominantly cystic, complex predominantly solid, or solid)

Generally, uterine masses are mainly solid as opposed to ovarian masses, which are mainly cystic. If the mass can be shown to arise from the uterus it is usually a benign leiomyoma. Leiomyomas are common causes of solid adnexal masses, in which case showing their origin from the uterus is diagnostic. Occasionally, it may be impossible to determine the exact origin of the mass by sonography, and MRI may be helpful.

The vast majority of ovarian masses are functional in nature. Ovarian masses that are purely cystic and have well-defined borders are nearly always benign. The size of the mass is important. In premenopausal women, simple cysts or typical hemorrhagic cysts less than 3 cm can be considered functional and no follow-up is required. Simple cysts greater than 3 cm are also likely functional but resolution should be confirmed with a follow-up examination. In postmenopausal women, cysts less than 5 cm are usually benign. Larger masses, especially those greater than 10 cm, have a higher incidence of malignancy. Solid ovarian masses are usually malignant, except for teratomas, fibromas, and transitional cell (Brenner) tumors, which frequently have a specific sonographic appearance. Complex masses may be either benign or malignant and should be further assessed for wall contour, septations, and mural nodules. Irregular borders, thick irregular septations, papillary projections, and echogenic solid nodules favor malignancy. Color and spectral Doppler may demonstrate vascularity within the septae or nodules. High-resistance flow strongly suggests benign disease, whereas low-resistance flow suggests malignancy, although it can also be seen with benign disease. Although ascites may be associated with benign masses, it is much more frequently seen with malignant disease. Malignant ascites frequently contains echogenic particulate matter.

If a pelvic mass is suspected of being malignant, the abdomen should also be evaluated for evidence of ascites and peritoneal implants, obstructive uropathy, lymphadenopathy, and hepatic and splenic metastases. Hepatic and splenic metastases are uncommon in ovarian carcinoma, but when they occur, they are usually peripheral on the surface of the liver or spleen as a result of peritoneal implantation. Hematogenous metastases within the liver or splenic parenchyma may occur late in the course of the disease.

NONGYNECOLOGIC PELVIC MASSES

Pelvic masses and pseudomasses may not be of gynecologic origin. To make this diagnosis, it is important to visualize the uterus and ovaries separately from the mass (Fig. 15-49). This is frequently not possible because of displacement of the normal pelvic structures by the mass. Nongynecologic pelvic masses most commonly originate from the gastrointestinal or urinary tract or may develop after surgery.

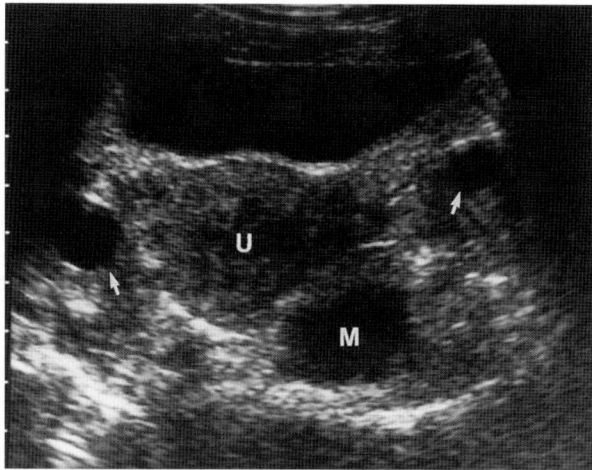

FIGURE 15-49. Extramedullary hematopoiesis. Transverse scan in 44-year-old asymptomatic woman with thalassemia shows anechoic mass (M) to left and separate from uterus (U) and both ovaries, which contain cysts (*arrows*). Diagnosis made by percutaneous biopsy under computed tomography guidance.

Postoperative Pelvic Masses

Postoperative masses may be **abscesses, hematomas, lymphoceles, urinomas,** or **seromas.** Sonographically, **abscesses** are ovoid-shaped, anechoic masses with thick, irregular walls and posterior acoustic enhancement. Variable internal echogenicity may be seen, and high-intensity echoes with shadowing caused by gas may be demonstrated. **Hematomas** show a spectrum of sonographic findings, varying with time.[293] During the initial acute phase, hematomas are anechoic. Following organization and clot formation, they become highly echogenic. With lysis of the clot, hematomas become more complex, until finally, with complete lysis, they are again anechoic. It is frequently not possible to distinguish an abscess from a hematoma sonographically, and clinical correlation is usually necessary.

Pelvic lymphoceles occur following surgical disruption of lymphatic channels, usually after pelvic lymph node dissection or renal transplantation. Sonographically, lymphoceles are cystic, having an appearance similar to that of **urinomas,** which are localized collections of urine, or **seromas,** which are collections of serum. Sonography-guided aspiration may be necessary to differentiate these conditions.

Gastrointestinal Tract Masses

The most frequent pelvic pseudomasses are fecal material in the rectum simulating a complex mass in the cul-de-sac and a fluid-filled rectosigmoid colon presenting as a cystic adnexal mass. Transvaginal sonography can usually distinguish the pseudomass from a true mass, but when it cannot, a repeat examination or

MRI may be necessary. **Bowel neoplasms**, especially those involving the rectosigmoid, cecum, and ileum, may simulate an adnexal mass. These tumors frequently show the characteristic target sign of a gastrointestinal mass, consisting of a central echogenic focus caused by air within the lumen, surrounded by a thickened hypoechoic wall.[294] **Abscesses** related to inflammatory disease of the gastrointestinal tract may also present as an adnexal mass. On the right side, this is most frequently caused by appendicitis or Crohn's disease, whereas abscesses on the left side are usually caused by diverticular disease and are seen in an older age group.

Urinary Tract Masses

Patients with a **pelvic kidney** may present with a clinically palpable mass. This is readily recognized sonographically by the typical reniform appearance and the absence of a kidney in the normal location. Occasionally, a markedly distended bladder may be mistaken for an ovarian cyst. When a cystic pelvic mass is identified, it is imperative that the bladder be seen separately from the mass. **Bladder diverticula** may also simulate a cystic adnexal mass. The diagnosis can be confirmed by demonstrating communication with the bladder and a changing appearance after voiding. **Dilated distal ureters** may simulate adnexal cysts on transverse scans; however, sagittal scans show their tubular appearance and continuity with the bladder.

POSTPARTUM PELVIC PATHOLOGIC CONDITIONS

The uterus is enlarged during the postpartum period and gradually returns to a nongravid size within 6 to 8 weeks. Pathologic states in the postpartum period are usually the result of infection and hemorrhage. Specific pathologic conditions occurring in the postpartum period include endometritis, retained products of conception, and ovarian vein thrombophlebitis. **Endometritis** is more frequent following cesarean section than vaginal delivery. It usually occurs in patients who have had prolonged labor or premature rupture of membranes or who have retained products of conception. The most common source of organisms is the normal vaginal flora. Clinically, there is pelvic pain or unexplained fever.

Retained Products of Conception

Retained placental tissue following delivery may cause secondary postpartum hemorrhage or may serve as a nidus for infection. **Sonographically**, an echogenic mass in the endometrial cavity (Fig. 15-50A) strongly supports this diagnosis.[295,296] Calcifications may be seen within the mass.[297] A heterogeneous mass may be seen, but it can also be caused by blood clots or infected or necrotic material without the presence of placental tissue.[296] Vascularity within the mass is additional evidence that the mass represents vascularized placental tissue rather than blood clot.[297] Occasionally, definitive placental tissue may be identified (see Figs. 15-50B and C).

Ovarian Vein Thrombophlebitis

Puerperal ovarian vein thrombosis or thrombophlebitis is an uncommon but potentially life-threatening condition (Fig. 15-51). Patients present with fever, lower abdominal pain, and a palpable mass, usually 48 to 96 hours postpartum. The underlying cause is venous stasis and spread of bacterial infection from endometritis. The right ovarian vein is involved in 90% of cases. Retrograde venous flow occurs in the left ovarian vein during the puerperium, which protects this side from bacterial spread from the uterus.[37] This condition may be diagnosed by sonography, CT, or MRI.[298,299] **Sonography** may demonstrate an inflammatory mass lateral to the uterus and anterior to the psoas muscle. The ovarian vein may be seen as a tubular, anechoic structure directed cephalad from the mass and containing echogenic thrombus. The thrombus commonly affects the most cephalic portion of the right ovarian vein and can usually be demonstrated sonographically at the junction of the right ovarian vein with the inferior vena cava, sometimes extending into the inferior vena cava.[300] Thrombus in the inferior vena cava may also be seen. Doppler may demonstrate absence of flow in these veins.[301] Most patients respond to anticoagulant and antibiotic therapy, and follow-up sonography may show resolution of the thrombus and normal flow on duplex Doppler imaging.

Cesarean Section Complications

A lower uterine transverse incision site is commonly used for cesarean section. On sonographic examination, the **incision site** can be identified as an oval, symmetrical region of hypoechogenicity relative to the myometrium, located between the posterior wall of the bladder and the lower uterine segment.[302] **Sutures** within the incision site may be recognized as small, punctate high-amplitude echoes (Fig. 15-52).

Hematomas may develop from hemorrhage at the incision site (bladder flap hematomas) or within the prevesical space (subfascial hematomas). **Bladder flap hematomas** can be diagnosed sonographically when a complex or anechoic mass greater than 2 cm in diameter is located adjacent to the scar and between the lower uterine segment and the posterior bladder wall

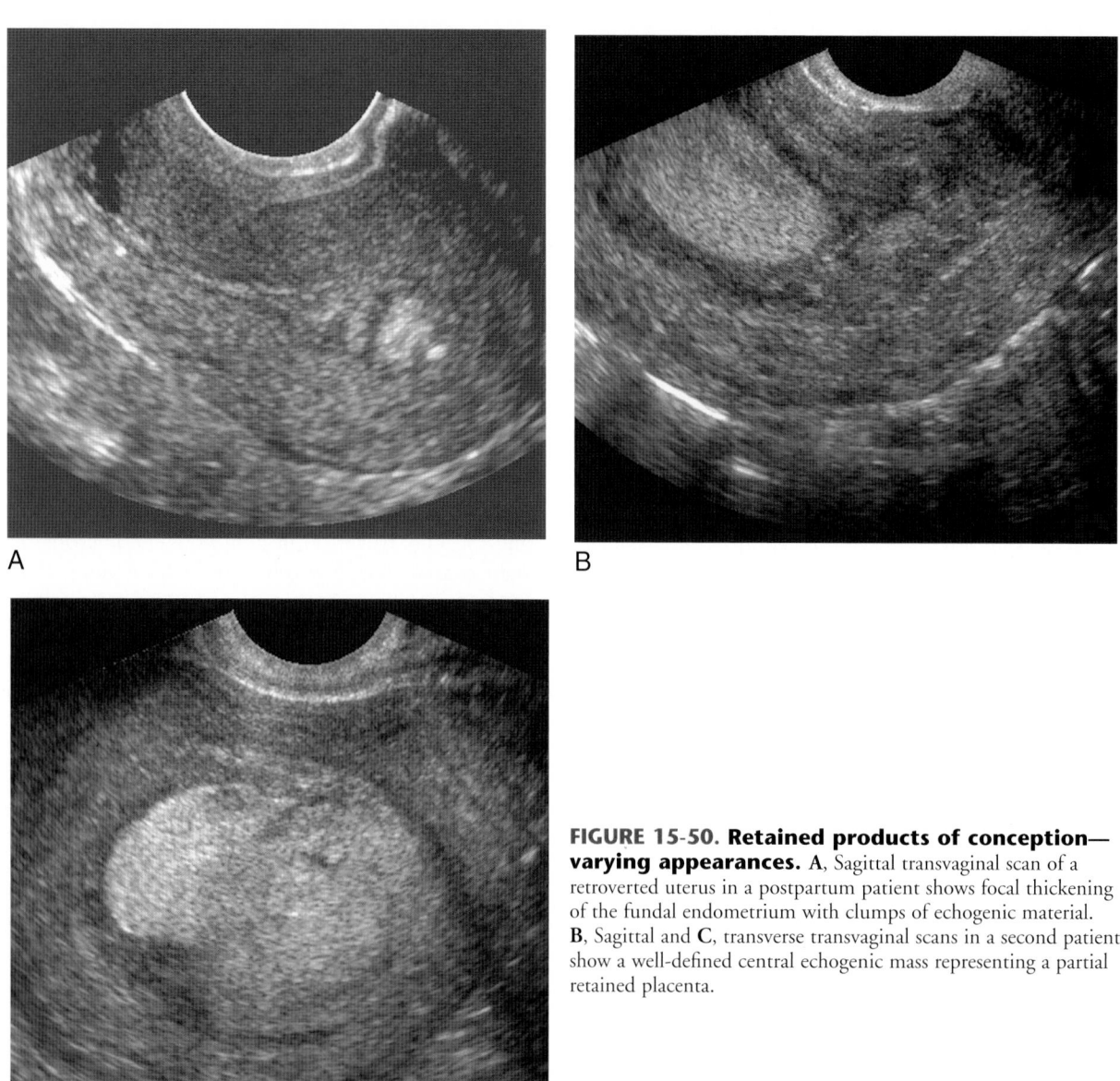

A

B

C

FIGURE 15-50. Retained products of conception—varying appearances. A, Sagittal transvaginal scan of a retroverted uterus in a postpartum patient shows focal thickening of the fundal endometrium with clumps of echogenic material. **B,** Sagittal and **C,** transverse transvaginal scans in a second patient show a well-defined central echogenic mass representing a partial retained placenta.

(Fig. 15-53). The echogenicity varies depending on the amount of organization within the hematoma.[293] The presence of air within the mass is highly suggestive of an infected hematoma.[303] **Subfascial hematomas** are extraperitoneal in location, contained within the prevesical space, and caused by disruption of the inferior epigastric vessels or their branches during cesarean section[304] or traumatic vaginal delivery.[305] Sonographically, a complex or cystic mass is seen anterior to the

bladder. High frequency, short-focus transducers are frequently necessary to recognize the superficial mass. It is important to identify the rectus muscle in order to distinguish the **superficial wound hematoma**, which is located anterior to the rectus muscle, from the subfascial hematoma located posterior to it.[304] Bladder flap and subfascial hematomas may be seen together in the same patient; however, they have different sources of bleeding and should be treated as separate conditions.

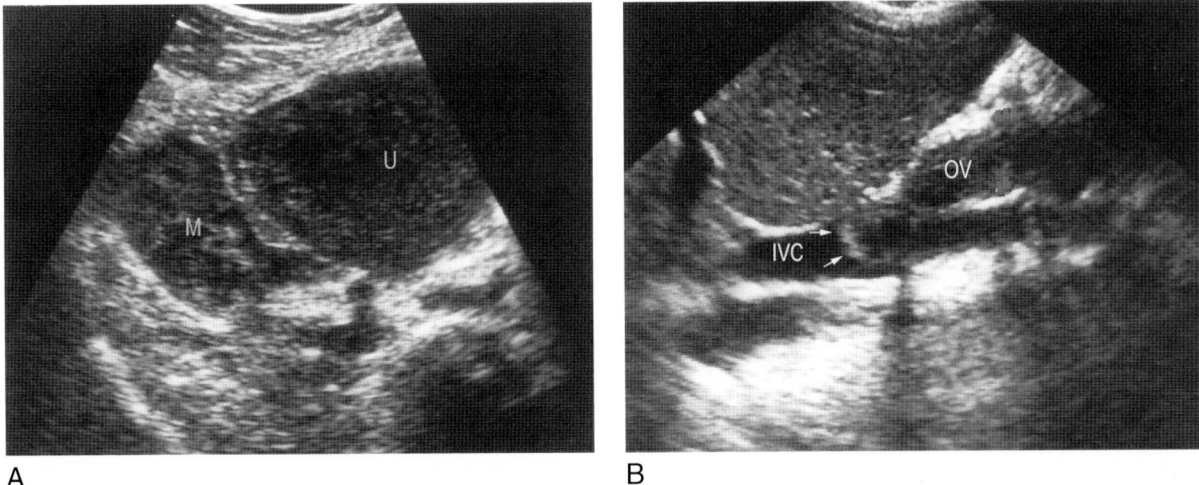

FIGURE 15-51. Ovarian vein thrombophlebitis. A, Transverse scan in patient with fever and right lower abdominal pain 4 days following cesarean section shows mass (M) to right of postpartum uterus (U). **B,** Sagittal scan of abdomen shows echogenic thrombus in distended right ovarian vein (OV). Thrombus (*arrows*) is seen extending into inferior vena cava (IVC).

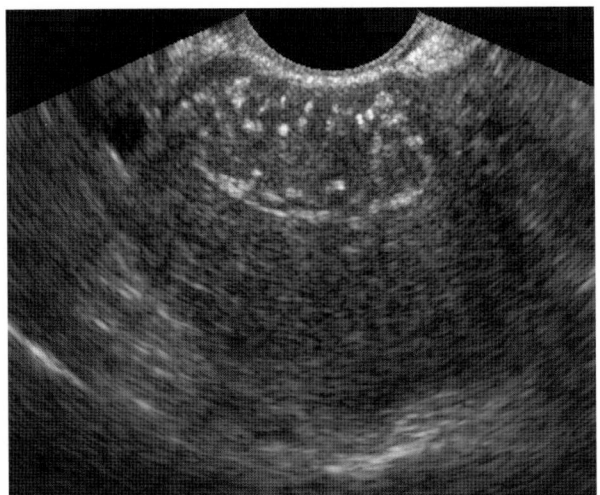

FIGURE 15-52. Cesarean section sutures. Transverse transvaginal image shows multiple bright echogenic foci in the surgical site.

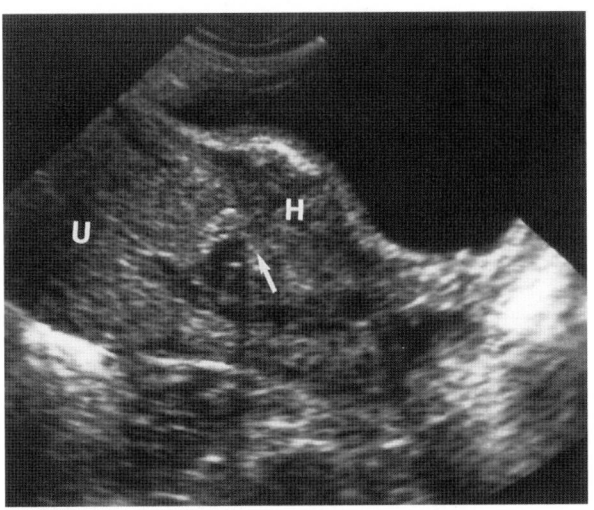

FIGURE 15-53. Bladder-flap hematoma. Sagittal scan in patient with fever and lower abdominal pain 8 days following cesarean section shows hematoma (H) between bladder and cesarean section scar (*arrow*). U, Uterus.

References

Normal Pelvic Anatomy

1. Williams PL, Warwick R: Gray's Anatomy. 37th ed. Edinburgh, Churchill Livingstone, 1989.
2. Jones HW III, Wentz AC, Burnett LS: Novak's Textbook of Gynecology, 11th ed. Baltimore, Williams & Wilkins, 1988.

Technique

3. Cullinan JA, Fleischer AC, Kepple DM, et al: Sonohysterography: A technique for endometrial evaluation. RadioGraphics 1995;15:501-514.
4. Mendelson EB, Bohm-Velez M, Joseph N, et al: Gynecologic imaging: Comparison of transabdominal and transvaginal sonography. Radiology 1988;166:321-324.
5. Lande IM, Hill MC, Cosco FE, et al: Adnexal and cul-de-sac abnormalities: Transvaginal sonography. Radiology 1988;166:325-332.
6. Leibman AJ, Kruse B, McSweeney MB: Transvaginal sonography: Comparison with transabdominal sonography in the diagnosis of pelvic masses. AJR 1988;151:89-92.
7. Tessler FN, Schiller VL, Perrella RR, et al: Transabdominal versus endovaginal pelvic sonography: prospective study. Radiology 1989;170:553-556.
8. Coleman BG, Arger PH, Grumbach K, et al: Transvaginal and transabdominal sonography: Prospective comparison. Radiology 1988;168:639-643.

Uterus

9. Sample WF, Lippe BM, Gyepes MT: Gray-scale ultrasonography of the normal female pelvis. Radiology 1977;125:477-483.

10. Orsini LF, Salardi S, Pilu G, et al: Pelvic organs in premenarcheal girls: Real-time ultrasonography. Radiology 1984;153:113-116.

11. Nussbaum AR, Sanders RC, Jones MD: Neonatal uterine morphology as seen on real-time US. Radiology 1986;160:641-643.

12. Siegel MJ: Pediatric gynecologic sonography. Radiology 1991;179:593-600.

13. Holm K, Mosfeldt E, Laursen V, et al: Pubertal maturation of the internal genitalia: An ultrasound evaluation of 166 healthy girls. Ultrasound Obstet Gynecol 1995;6:175-181.

14. Platt JF, Bree RL, Davidson D: Ultrasound of the normal nongravid uterus: Correlation with gross and histopathology. J Clin Ultrasound 1990;18:15-19.

15. Merz E, Miric-Tesanic D, Bahlmann F, et al: Sonographic size of uterus and ovaries in pre- and postmenopausal women. Ultrasound Obstet Gynecol 1996;7:38-42.

16. Miller EI, Thomas RH, Lines P: The atrophic postmenopausal uterus. J Clin Ultrasound 1977;5:261-263.

17. Fleischer AC, Kalemeris GC, Machin JE, et al: Sonographic depiction of normal and abnormal endometrium with histopathologic correlation. J Ultrasound Med 1986;5:445-452.

18. Farrer-Brown G, Beilby JOW, Tarbit MH: The blood supply of the uterus. 2. venous pattern. Br J Obstet Gynecol Comm 1970;77:682-689.

19. DuBose TJ, Hill LW, Hennigan HW Jr, et al: Sonography of arcuate uterine blood vessels. J Ultrasound Med 1985;4:229-233.

20. Occhipinti K, Kutcher R, Rosenblatt R: Sonographic appearance and significance of arcuate artery calcification. J Ultrasound Med 1991;10:97-100.

21. Atri M, de Stempel J, Senterman MK, et al: Diffuse peripheral uterine calcification (manifestation of Monckeberg's arteriosclerosis) detected by ultrasonography. J Clin Ultrasound 1992;20:211-216.

22. Burks DD, Stainken BF, Burkhard TK, et al: Uterine inner myometrial echogenic foci: Relationship to prior dilatation and curettage and endocervical biopsy. J Ultrasound Med 1991;10:487-492.

23. Callen PW, DeMartini WJ, Filly RA: The central uterine cavity echo: A useful anatomic sign in the ultrasonographic evaluation of the female pelvis. Radiology 1979;131:187-190.

24. Fleischer AC, Kalemeris GC, Entman SS: Sonographic depiction of the endometrium during normal cycles. Ultrasound Med Biol 1986;12:271-277.

25. Forrest TS, Elyaderani MK, Muilenburg MI, et al: Cyclic endometrial changes: US assessment with histologic correlation. Radiology 1988;167:233-237.

26. Pennes DR, Bowerman RA, Silver TM: Congenital uterine anomalies and associated pregnancies: Findings and pitfalls of sonographic diagnosis. J Ultrasound Med 1985;4:531-538.

27. Brody JM, Koelliker SL, Frishman GN: Unicornuate uterus: Imaging appearance, associated anomalies and clinical implications. AJR 1998;171:1341-1347.

28. Fried AM, Oliff M, Wilson EA, et al: Uterine anomalies associated with renal agenesis: Role of gray scale ultrasonography. AJR 1978;131:973-975.

29. Wiersma AF, Peterson LF, Justema EJ: Uterine anomalies associated with unilateral renal agenesis. Obstet Gynecol 1976;47:654-657.

30. Nicolini U, Bellotti M, Bonazzi B, et al: Can ultrasound be used to screen uterine malformations? Fertil Steril 1987;47:89-93.

31. Yoder IC: Diagnosis of uterine anomalies: Relative accuracy of MR imaging, endovaginal sonography, and hysterosalpingography. Radiology 1992;185:343.

32. Reuter KL, Daly DC, Cohen SM: Septate versus bicornuate uteri: Errors in imaging diagnosis. Radiology 1989;172:749-752.

33. Jurkovic D, Geipel A, Gruboeck K, et al: Three-dimensional ultrasound for the assessment of uterine anatomy and detection of congenital anomalies: A comparison with hysterosalpingography and two-dimensional sonography. Ultrasound Obstet Gynecol 1995;5:233-237.

34. Pellerito JS, McCarthy SM, Doyle MB, et al: Diagnosis of uterine anomalies: Relative accuracy of MR imaging, endovaginal sonography and hysterosalpingography. Radiology 1992;183:795-800.

35. Viscomi GN, Gonzalez R, Taylor KJW: Ultrasound detection of uterine abnormalities after diethylstilbestrol (DES) exposure. Radiology 1980;136:733-735.

36. Lev-Toaff AS, Toaff ME, Friedman AC: Endovaginal sonographic appearance of a DES uterus. J Ultrasound Med 1990;9:661-664.

37. Kurman RJ: Blaustein's Pathology of the Female Genital Tract, 4th ed. New York, Springer-Verlag, 1994.

38. Smith JP, Weiser EB, Karnei RF Jr, et al: Ultrasonography of rapidly growing uterine leiomyomata associated with anovulatory cycles. Radiology 1980;134:713-716.

39. Lev-Toaff AS, Coleman BG, Arger PH, et al: Leiomyomas in pregnancy: Sonographic study. Radiology 1987;164:375-380.

40. Benson CB, Chow JS, Chang-Lee W, et al: Outcome of pregnancies in women with uterine leiomyomas identified by sonography in the first trimester. J Clin Ultrasound 2001;29:261-264.

41. Dilts PV Jr, Hopkins MP, Chang AE, et al: Rapid growth of leiomyoma in patient receiving tamoxifen. Am J Obstet Gynecol 1992;166:167-168.

42. Gross BH, Silver TM, Jaffe MH: Sonographic features of uterine leiomyomas: Analysis of 41 proven cases. J Ultrasound Med 1983;2:401-406.

43. Kliewer MA, Hertzberg BS, George PY, et al: Acoustic shadowing from uterine leiomyomas: Sonographic-pathologic correlation. Radiology 1995;196:99-102.

44. Caoili EM, Hertzberg BS, Kliewer MA, et al: Refractory shadowing from pelvic masses on sonography: A useful diagnostic sign for uterine leiomyomas. AJR 2000;174:97-101.

45. Baltarowich OH, Kurtz AB, Pennell RG, et al: Pitfalls in the sonographic diagnosis of uterine fibroids. AJR 1988;151:725-728.

46. Moore L, Wilson S, Rosen B: Giant hydropic uterine leiomyoma in pregnancy: Unusual sonographic and Doppler appearance. J Ultrasound Med 1994;13:416-418.

47. Tsuda H, Kawabata M, Nakamoto O, et al: Clinical predictors in the natural history of uterine leiomyoma: preliminary study. J Ultrasound Med 1998;17:17-20.

48. Fedele L, Bianchi S, Dorta M, et al: Transvaginal ultrasonography versus hysteroscopy in the diagnosis of uterine submucous myomas. Obstet Gynecol 1991;77:745-748.

49. Becker E Jr, Lev-Toaff AS, Kaufman EP, et al: The added value of transvaginal sonohysterography over transvaginal sonography alone in women with known or suspected leiomyoma. J Ultrasound Med 2002;21:237-247.

50. Karasick S, Lev-Toaff AS, Toaff ME: Imaging of uterine leiomyomas. AJR 1992;158:799-805.

51. Dodd GD III, Budzik RF Jr: Lipomatous uterine tumors: Diagnosis by ultrasound, CT and MR. J Comput Assist Tomogr 1990;14:629-632.

52. Serafini G, Martinoli C, Quadri P, et al: Lipomatous tumors of the uterus: Ultrasonographic findings in 11 cases. J Ultrasound Med 1996;16:195-199.

53. Hertzberg BS, Kliewer MA, George P, et al: Lipomatous uterine masses: Potential to mimic ovarian dermoids on endovaginal sonography. J Ultrasound Med 1995;14:689-692.

54. Siedler D, Laing FC, Jeffrey RB Jr, et al: Uterine adenomyosis: A difficult sonographic diagnosis. J Ultrasound Med 1987;6:345-349.

55. Bohlman ME, Ensor RE, Sanders RC: Sonographic findings in adenomyosis of the uterus. AJR 1987;148:765-766.

56. Fedele L, Bianchi S, Dorta M, et al: Transvaginal ultrasonography in the diagnosis of diffuse adenomyosis. Fertil Steril 1992;58:94-97.

57. Reinhold C, Atri M, Mehio A, et al: Diffuse uterine adenomyosis: Morphologic criteria and diagnostic accuracy of endovaginal sonography. Radiology 1995;197:609-614.

58. Bromley B, Shipp TD, Benacerraf B: Adenomyosis: Sonographic findings and diagnostic accuracy. J Ultrasound Med 2000;19:529-534.

59. Hulka CA, Hall DA, McCarthy K, et al: Sonographic findings in patients with adenomyosis: Can sonography assist in predicting extent of disease? AJR 2002;179:379-383.

60. Atri M, Reinhold C, Mehie AR, et al: Adenomyosis: US features with histologic correlation in an in vitro study. Radiology 2000;215:783-790.

61. Fedele L, Bianchi S, Dorta M, et al: Transvaginal ultrasonography in the differential diagnosis of adenomyoma versus leiomyoma. Am J Obstet Gynecol 1992;167:603-606.

62. Botsis D, Kassanos D, Antoniou G, et al: Adenomyoma and leiomyoma: Differential diagnosis with transvaginal sonography. J Clin Ultrasound 1998;26:21-25.

63. Togashi K, Ozasa H, Konishi I, et al: Enlarged uterus: Differentiation between adenomyosis and leiomyoma with MR imaging. Radiology 1989;171:531-534.

64. Ascher SM, Arnold LL, Patt RH, et al: Adenomyosis: Prospective comparison of MR imaging and transvaginal sonography. Radiology 1994;190:803-806.

65. Reinhold C, McCarthy S, Bret PM, et al: Diffuse adenomyosis: Comparison of endovaginal US and MR imaging with histopathologic correlation. Radiology 1996;199:151-158.

66. Torres WE, Stones PJ Jr, Thames FM: Ultrasound appearance of pelvic arteriovenous malformation. J Clin Ultrasound 1979;7:383-385.

67. Musa AA, Hata T, Hata K, et al: Pelvic arteriovenous malformation diagnosed by color flow Doppler imaging. AJR 1989;152:1311-1312.

68. Huang M, Muradali D, Thurston WA, et al: Uterine arteriovenous malformations (AVMs): Ultrasound and Doppler features with MRI correlation. Radiology 1998;206:115-123.

69. Mendelson EB, Bohm-Velez M, Joseph N, et al: Endometrial abnormalities: Evaluation with transvaginal sonography. AJR 1988;150:139-142.

70. Baldwin MT, Dudiak KM, Gorman B, et al: Focal intracavitary masses recognized with the hyperechoic line sign at endovaginal US and characterized with hysterosonography. Radiographics 1999;19:927-935.

71. Parsons AK, Lense JJ: Sonohysterography for endometrial abnormalities: Preliminary results. J Clin Ultrasound 1993;21:87-95.

72. Gaucherand P, Piacenza JM, Salle B, et al: Sonohysterography of the uterine cavity: Preliminary investigations. J Clin Ultrasound 1995;23:339-348.

73. Dubinsky TJ, Parvey HR, Gormaz G, et al: Transvaginal hysterosonography in the evaluation of small endoluminal masses. J Ultrasound Med 1995;14:1-6.

74. Lev-Toaff AS, Toaff ME, Liu JB, et al: Value of sonohysterography in the diagnosis and management of abnormal uterine bleeding. Radiology 1996;201:179-184.

75. Jorizzo JR, Riccio GJ, Chen MYM, et al: Sonohysterography: The next step in the evaluation of the abnormal endometrium. Radiographics 1999;19:S117-S130.

76. Davis PC, O'Neill MJ, Yoder IC, et al: Sonohysterographic findings of endometrial and subendometrial conditions. Radiographics 2002;22:803-816.

77. Dubinsky TJ, Stroehlein K, Abu-Ghazzeh Y, et al: Prediction of benign and malignant endometrial disease: Hysterosonographic-pathologic correlation. Radiology 1999;210:393-397.

78. Laifer-Narin SL, Ragavendra N, Lu DSK, et al: Transvaginal saline hysterosonography: Characteristics distinguishing malignant and various benign conditions. AJR 1999;172:1513-1520.

79. Varner RE, Sparks JM, Cameron CD, et al: Transvaginal sonography of the endometrium in postmenopausal women. Obstet Gynecol 1991;78:195-199.

80. Osmers R, Völkson M, Schauer A: Vaginosonography for early detection of endometrial carcinoma? Lancet 1990;335:1569-1571.

81. Karlsson B, Granberg S, Wikland M, et al: Transvaginal ultrasonography of the endometrium in women with postmenopausal bleeding: A Nordic multicenter study. Am J Obstet Gynecol 1995;172:1488-1494.

82. Ferrazzi E, Torri V, Trio D, et al: Sonographic endometrial thickness: A useful test to predict atrophy in patients with postmenopausal bleeding. An Italian multicenter study. Ultrasound Obstet Gynecol 1996;7:315-321.

83. Granberg S, Wickland M, Karlsson B, et al: Endometrial thickness as measured by endovaginal ultrasonography for identifying endometrial abnormality. Am J Obstet Gynecol 1991;164:47-52.

84. Nasri MN, Shepherd JH, Setchell ME, et al: The role of vaginal scan in measurement of endometrial thickness in postmenopausal women. Br J Obstet Gynaecol 1991;98:470-475.

85. Goldstein SR, Nachtigall M, Snyder JR, et al: Endometrial assessment by vaginal ultrasonography before endometrial sampling in patients with postmenopausal bleeding. Am J Obstet Gynecol 1990;163:119-123.

86. Smith-Bindman R, Kerlikowske K, Feldstein VA, et al: Endovaginal ultrasound to exclude endometrial cancer and other endometrial abnormalities. JAMA 1998;280:1510-1517.

87. Goldstein RB, Bree RL, Benson CB, et al: Evaluation of the woman with postmenopausal bleeding. Society of Radiologists in Ultrasound-sponsored consensus conference statement. J Ultrasound Med 2001;20:1025-1036.

88. Doubilet PM: Society of Radiologists in Ultrasound consensus conference statement on postmenopausal bleeding. Commentary. J Ultrasound Med 2001;20:1037-1042.

89. Deslisle MF, Villeneuve M, Boulvain M: Measurement of endometrial thickness with transvaginal ultrasonography: Is it reproducible? J Ultrasound Med 1998;17:481-484.

90. Bree RL, Bowerman RA, Bohm-Velez M, et al: US evaluation of the uterus in patients with postmenopausal bleeding: A positive effect on diagnostic decision making. Radiology 2000;216:260-264.

91. Laifer-Narin S, Ragavendra N, Parmenter EK, et al: False-normal appearance of the endometrium on conventional transvaginal sonography: Comparison with saline hysterosonography. AJR 2002;178:129-133.

92. Neele SJM, Marchien Van Baal W, Van Der Mooren MJ, et al: Ultrasound assessment of the endometrium in healthy asymptomatic early post-menopausal women: Saline infusion sonohysterography versus transvaginal ultrasound. Ultrasound Obstet Gynecol 2000;16:254-259.

93. Shipley CF III, Simmons CL, Nelson GH: Comparison of transvaginal sonography with endometrial biopsy in asymptomatic postmenopausal women. J Ultrasound Med 1994;13:99-104.

94. Lin MC, Gosink BB, Wolf SI, et al: Endometrial thickness after menopause: Effect of hormone replacement. Radiology 1991;180:427-432.

95. Aleem F, Predanic M, Calame R, et al: Transvaginal color and pulsed Doppler sonography of the endometrium: A possible role in reducing the number of dilatation and curettage procedures. J Ultrasound Med 1995;14:139-145.

96. Levine D, Gosink BB, Johnson LA: Change in endometrial thickness in postmenopausal women undergoing hormone replacement therapy. Radiology 1995;197:603-608.

97. Lewit N, Thaler I, Rottem S: The uterus: A new look with transvaginal sonography. J Clin Ultrasound 1990;18:331-336.

98. Breckenridge JW, Kurtz AB, Ritchie WGM, et al: Post-menopausal uterine fluid collection: Indicator of carcinoma. AJR 1982;139:529-534.

99. McCarthy KA, Hall DA, Kopans DB, et al: Postmenopausal endometrial fluid collections: Always an indicator of malignancy? J Ultrasound Med 1986;5:647-649.

100. Goldstein SR: Postmenopausal endometrial fluid collections revisited: Look at the doughnut rather than the hole. Obstet Gynecol 1994;83:738-740.

101. Wilson DA, Stacy TM, Smith EI: Ultrasound diagnosis of hydrocolpos and hydrometrocolpos. Radiology 1978;128:451-454.

102. Scott WW Jr, Rosenshein NB, Siegelman SS, et al: The obstructed uterus. Radiology 1981;141:767-770.

103. Sheth S, Hamper UM, Kurman RJ: Thickened endometrium in the postmenopausal woman: Sonographic-pathologic correlation. Radiology 1993;187:135-139.

104. Hulka CA, Hall DA, McCarthy K, et al: Endometrial polyps, hyperplasia and carcinoma in postmenopausal women: Differentiation with endovaginal sonography. Radiology 1994;191:755-758.

105. Atri M, Nazarnia S, Aldis AE, et al: Transvaginal US appearance of endometrial abnormalities. RadioGraphics 1994;14:483-492.

106. Choo YC, Mak KC, Hsu C, et al: Postmenopausal uterine bleeding of nonorganic cause. Obstet Gynecol 1985;66:225-228.

107. Kupfer MC, Schiller VL, Hansen GC, et al: Transvaginal sonographic evaluation of endometrial polyps. J Ultrasound Med 1994;13:535-539.

108. Karlsson B, Granberg S, Hellberg P, et al: Comparative study of transvaginal sonography and hysteroscopy for the detection of pathologic endometrial lesions in women with postmenopausal bleeding. J Ultrasound Med 1994;13:757-762.

109. Bourne TH, Campbell S, Steer CV, et al: Detection of endometrial cancer by transvaginal ultrasonography with color flow imaging and blood flow analysis: A preliminary report. Gynecol Oncol 1991;40:253-259.

110. Weiner Z, Beck D, Rottem S, et al: Uterine artery flow velocity waveforms and color flow imaging in women with perimenopausal and postmenopausal bleeding: Correlation to endometrial histopathology. Acta Obstet Gynecol Scand 1993;72:162-166.

111. Chan FY, Chau MT, Pun TC, et al: Limitations of transvaginal sonography and color Doppler imaging in the differentiation of endometrial carcinoma from benign lesions. J Ultrasound Med 1994;13:623-628.

112. Carter JR, Lau M, Saltzman AK, et al: Gray scale and color flow Doppler characterization of uterine tumors. J Ultrasound Med 1994;13:835-840.

113. Sladkevicius P, Valentin L, Marsal K: Endometrial thickness and Doppler velocimetry of the uterine arteries as discriminators of endometrial status in women with postmenopausal bleeding: A comparative study. Am J Obstet Gynecol 1994;171:722-728.

114. Kurjak A, Shalan H, Sosic A, et al: Endometrial carcinoma in postmenopausal women: Evaluation by transvaginal color Doppler ultrasonography. Am J Obstet Gynecol 1993;169:1597-1603.

115. Sheth S, Hamper UM, McCollum ME, et al: Endometrial blood flow analysis in postmenopausal women: Can it help differentiate benign from malignant causes of endometrial thickening? Radiology 1995;195:661-665.

116. Fleischer AC, Dudley BS, Entman SS, et al: Myometrial invasion by endometrial carcinoma: Sonographic assessment. Radiology 1987;162:307-310.

117. Cacciatore B, Lehtovirta P, Wahlström T, et al: Preoperative sonographic evaluation of endometrial cancer. Am J Obstet Gynecol 1989;160:133-137.

118. Gordon AN, Fleischer AC, Reed GW: Depth of myometrial invasion in endometrial cancer: Preoperative assessment by transvaginal ultrasonography. Gynecol Oncol 1990;39:321-327.

119. DelMaschio A, Vanzulli A, Sironi S, et al: Estimating the depth of myometrial involvement by endometrial carcinoma: Efficacy of transvaginal sonography vs MR imaging. AJR 1993;160:533-538.

120. Yamashita Y, Mizutani H, Torashima M, et al: Assessment of myometrial invasion by endometrial carcinoma: Transvaginal sonography vs. contrast-enhanced MR imaging. AJR 1993;161:595-599.

121. Kinkel K, Kaji Y, Yu KK, et al: Radiologic staging in patients with endometrial cancer: A meta-analysis. Radiology 1999;212:711-718.

122. Frei KA, Kinkel K, Bonél HM, et al: Prediction of deep myometrial invasion in patients with endometrial cancer: Clinical utility of contrast-enhanced MR imaging—a meta-analysis and bayesian analysis. Radiology 2000;216:444-449.

123. Malfetano JH: Tamoxifen-associated endometrial carcinoma in postmenopausal breast cancer patients. Gynecol Oncol 1990;39:82-84.

124. Kedar RP, Bourne TH, Powles TJ, et al: Effects of tamoxifen on uterus and ovaries of postmenopausal women in a randomised breast cancer prevention trial. Lancet 1994;343:1318-1321.

125. Lahti E, Blanco G, Kauppila A, et al: Endometrial changes in postmenopausal breast cancer patients receiving tamoxifen. Obstet Gynecol 1993;81:660-664.

126. Cohen I, Rosen DJD, Tepper R, et al: Ultrasonographic evaluation of the endometrium and correlation with

endometrial sampling in postmenopausal patients treated with tamoxifen. J Ultrasound Med 1993;5:275-280.

127. Hulka CA, Hall DA: Endometrial abnormalities associated with tamoxifen therapy for breast cancer: Sonographic and pathologic correlation. AJR 1993;160:809-812.

128. Ascher SM, Imaoka I, Lage JM: Tamoxifen-induced uterine abnormalities: The role of imaging. Radiology 2000;214:29-38.

129. Hann LE, Giess CS, Bach AM, et al: Endometrial thickness in tamoxifen-treated patients: Correlation with clinical and pathologic findings. AJR 1997;168:657-661.

130. Goldstein SR: Unusual ultrasonographic appearance of the uterus in patients receiving tamoxifen. Am J Obstet Gynecol 1994;170:447-451.

131. Hann LE, Gretz EM, Bach AM, et al: Sonohysterography for evaluation of the endometrium in women treated with tamoxifen. AJR 2001;177:337-342.

132. Fong K, Kung R, Lytwyn A, et al: Endometrial evaluation with transvaginal US and hysterosonography in asymptomatic postmenopausal women with breast cancer receiving tamoxifen. Radiology 2001;220:765-773.

133. Wachsberg RH, Kurtz AB: Gas within the endometrial cavity at postpartum US: A normal finding after spontaneous vaginal delivery. Radiology 1992;183: 431-433.

34. Fedele L, Bianchi S, Dorta M, et al: Intrauterine adhesions: Detection with transvaginal US. Radiology 1996;199:757-759.

135. Salle B, Gaucherand P, de Saint Hilaire P, et al: Transvaginal sonohysterographic evaluation of intrauterine adhesions. J Clin Ultrasound 1999;27:131-134.

136. Callen PW, Filly RA, Munyer TP: Intrauterine contraceptive devices: Evaluation by sonography. AJR 1980;135:797-800.

137. Bajo J, Moreno-Calvo FJ, Uguet-de-Resayre C, et al: Contribution of transvaginal sonography to the evaluation of benign cervical conditions. J Clin Ultrasound 1999;27:61-64.

138. Fogel SR, Slasky BS: Sonography of nabothian cysts. AJR 1982;138:927-930.

139. Choi GC, Kim SH, Kim JS, et al: Adenoma malignum of uterine cervix in Peutz-Jeghers syndrome: CT and US features. J Comput Assist Tomogr 1993;17:819-821.

140. Yamashita Y, Takahashi M, Katabuchi H, et al: Adenoma malignum: MR appearances mimicking nabothian cysts. AJR 1994;162:649-650.

Vagina

141. Sherer DM, Abulafia O: Transvaginal ultrasonographic depiction of a Gartner duct cyst. J Ultrasound Med 2001;20:1253-1255.

142. McCarthy S, Taylor KJW: Sonography of vaginal masses. AJR 1983;140:1005-1008.

143. Schoenfeld A, Levavi H, Hirsch M, et al: Transvaginal sonography in postmenopausal women. J Clin Ultrasound 1990;18:350-358.

Rectouterine Recess

144. Mendelson EB, Bohm-Velez M, Neiman HL, et al: Transvaginal sonography in gynecologic imaging. Semin Ultrasound CT MR 1988;9:102-121.

145. Davis JA, Gosink BB: Fluid in the female pelvis: Cyclic patterns. J Ultrasound Med 1986;5:75-79.

146. Koninckx PR, Renaer M, Brosens IA: Origin of peritoneal fluid in women: An ovarian exudation product. Br J Obstet Gynaecol 1980;87:177-183.

147. Jeffrey RB, Laing FC: Echogenic clot: A useful sign of pelvic hemoperitoneum. Radiology 1982;145:139-141.

Ovary

148. Cohen HL, Shapiro MA, Mandel FS, et al: Normal ovaries in neonates and infants: A sonographic study of 77 patients 1 day to 24 months old. AJR 1993;160:583-586.

149. Cohen HL, Eisenberg P, Mandel F, et al: Ovarian cysts are common in premenarchal girls: A sonographic study of 101 children 2-12 years old. AJR 1992;159:89-91.

150. Cohen HL, Tice HM, Mandel FS: Ovarian volumes measured by US: Bigger than we think. Radiology 1990;177:189-192.

151. Van Nagel JR Jr, Higgins RV, Donaldson ES, et al: Transvaginal sonography as a screening method for ovarian cancer. Cancer 1990;65:573-577.

152. Kupfer MC, Ralls PW, Fu YS: Transvaginal sonographic evaluation of multiple peripherally distributed echogenic foci of the ovary: Prevalence and histologic correlation. AJR 1998;171:483-486.

153. Muradali D, Colgin T, Hayeems E, et al: Echogenic ovarian foci without shadowing: Are they caused by psammomatous calcifications? Radiology 2002;224:429-435.

154. Brandt KR, Thurmond AS, McCarthy JL: Focal calcifications in otherwise ultrasonographically normal ovaries. Radiology 1996;198:415-417.

155. Goswamy RK, Campbell S, Royston JP, et al: Ovarian size in postmenopausal women. Br J Obstet Gynaecol 1988;95:795-801.

156. Granberg S, Wikland M: A comparison between ultrasound and gynecologic examination for detection of enlarged ovaries in a group of women at risk for ovarian carcinoma. J Ultrasound Med 1988;7:59-64.

157. Andolf E, Jörgensen C, Svalenius E, et al: Ultrasound measurement of the ovarian volume. Acta Obstet Gynecol Scand 1987;66:387-389.

158. Hall DA, McCarthy KA, Kopans DB: Sonographic visualization of the normal postmenopausal ovary. J Ultrasound Med 1986;5:9-11.

159. Fleischer AC, McKee MS, Gordon AN, et al: Transvaginal sonography of postmenopausal ovaries with pathologic correlation. J Ultrasound Med 1990;9:637-644.

160. DiSantis DJ, Scatarige JC, Kemp G, et al: A prospective evaluation of transvaginal sonography for detection of ovarian disease. AJR 1993;161:91-94.

161. Wolf SI, Gosink BB, Feldesman MR, et al: Prevalence of simple adnexal cysts in postmenopausal women. Radiology 1991;180:65-71.

162. Levine D, Gosink BB, Wolf SI, et al: Simple adnexal cysts: The natural history in postmenopausal women. Radiology 1992;184:653-659.

163. Hall DA, McCarthy KA: The significance of the postmenopausal simple adnexal cyst. J Ultrasound Med 1986;5:503-505.

164. Rulin MC, Preston AL: Adnexal masses in postmenopausal women. Obstet Gynecol 1987;70:578-581.

165. Andolf E, Jörgensen C: Simple adnexal cysts diagnosed by ultrasound in postmenopausal women. J Clin Ultrasound 1988;16:301-303.

166. Goldstein SR, Subramanyam B, Snyder JR, et al: The postmenopausal cystic adnexal mass: The potential role of ultrasound in conservative management. Obstet Gynecol 1989;73:8-10.

167. Conway C, Zalud I, Dilena M, et al: Simple cyst in the postmenopausal patient: Detection and management. J Ultrasound Med 1998;17:369-372.

168. Bailey CL, Ueland FR, Land GL, et al: The malignant potential of small cystic ovarian tumors in women over 50 years of age. Gynecol Oncol 1998;69:3-7.

169. Hall DA: Sonographic appearance of the normal ovary, of polycystic ovary disease, and of functional ovarian cysts. Semin Ultrasound 1983;4:149-165.

170. Baltarowich OH, Kurtz AB, Pasto ME, et al: The spectrum of sonographic findings in hemorrhagic ovarian cysts. AJR 1987;148:901-905.

171. Yoffe N, Bronshtein M, Brandes J, et al: Hemorrhagic ovarian cyst detection by transvaginal sonography: The great imitator. Gynecol Endocrinol 1991;5:123-129.

172. Jain KA: Sonographic spectrum of hemorrhagic ovarian cysts. J Ultrasound Med 2002;21:879-886.

173. Price FV, Edwards R, Buchsbaum HJ: Ovarian remnant syndrome: Difficulties in diagnosis and management. Obstet Gynecol Surv 1990;45:151-156.

174. Phillips HE, McGahan JP: Ovarian remnant syndrome. Radiology 1982;142:487-488.

175. Fleischer AC, Tait D, Mayo J, et al: Sonographic features of ovarian remnants. J Ultrasound Med 1998;17:551-555.

176. Athey PA, Cooper NB: Sonographic features of parovarian cysts. AJR 1985;144:83-86.

177. Alpern MB, Sandler MA, Madrazo BL: Sonographic features of parovarian cysts and their complications. AJR 1984;143:157-160.

178. Korbin CD, Brown DL, Welch, WR: Paraovarian cystadenomas and cystadenofibromas: Sonographic characteristics in 14 cases. Radiology 1998;208:459-462.

179. Honore LH, O'Hare KE: Serous papillary neoplasms arising in paramesonephric parovarian cysts. Acta Obstet Gynecol Scand 1980;59:525-528.

180. Genadry R, Parmley T, Woodruff JD: The origin and clinical behavior of the parovarian tumor. Am J Obstet Gynecol 1977;129:873-880.

181. Stein AL, Koonings PP, Schlaerth JB, et al: Relative frequency of malignant parovarian tumors: Should parovarian tumors be aspirated? Obstet Gynecol 1990;75:1029-1031.

182. Kim JS, Woo SK, Suh SJ, et al: Sonographic diagnosis of parovarian cysts: Value of detecting a separate ipsilateral ovary. AJR 1995;164:1441-1444.

183. Hoffer FA, Kozakewich H, Colodny A, et al: Peritoneal inclusion cysts: Ovarian fluid in peritoneal adhesions. Radiology 1988;169:189-191.

184. Sohaey R, Gardner TL, Woodward PJ, et al: Sonographic diagnosis of peritoneal inclusion cysts. J Ultrasound Med 1995;14:913-917.

185. Kim JS, Lee HJ, Woo SK, et al: Peritoneal inclusion cysts and their relationship to the ovaries: Evaluation with sonography. Radiology 1997;204:481-484.

186. Jain KA: Imaging of peritoneal inclusion cysts. AJR 2000;174:1559-1563.

187. Ross MJ, Welch WR, Scully RE: Multilocular peritoneal inclusion cysts (so-called cystic mesotheliomas). Cancer 1989;64:1336-1346.

188. Friedman H, Vogelzang RL, Mendelson EB, et al: Endometriosis detection by US with laparoscopic correlation. Radiology 1985;157:217-220.

189. Kupfer MC, Schwimmer SR, Lebovic J: Transvaginal sonographic appearance of endometriomata: Spectrum of findings. J Ultrasound Med 1992;11:129-133.

190. Patel MD, Feldstein VA, Chen DC, et al: Endometriomas: Diagnostic performance of US. Radiology 1999;210:739-745.

191. Athey PA, Diment DD: The spectrum of sonographic findings in endometriomas. J Ultrasound Med 1989;8:487-491.

192. Balen AH, Tan S, Jacobs HS: Hypersecretion of luteinising hormone: A significant cause of infertility and miscarriage. Br J Obstet Gynaecol 1993;100:1082-1089.

193. Eden JA, Warren P: A review of 1019 consecutive cases of polycystic ovary syndrome demonstrated by ultrasound. Australas Radiol 1999;43:41-46.

194. Yeh HC, Futterweit W, Thornton JC: Polycystic ovarian disease: US features in 104 patients. Radiology 1987;163:111-116.

195. Hann LE, Hall DA, McArdle CR, et al: Polycystic ovarian disease: Sonographic spectrum. Radiology 1984;150:531-534.

196. Pache TD, Wladimiroff JW, Hop WCJ, et al: How to discriminate between normal and polycystic ovaries: Transvaginal US study. Radiology 1992;183:421-423.

197. Ardaens Y, Robert Y, Lemaitre L, et al: Polycystic ovarian disease: Contribution of vaginal endosonography and reassessment of ultrasonic diagnosis. Fertil Steril 1991;55:1062-1068.

198. Battaglia C, Regnani G, Petraglia F, et al: Polycystic ovary syndrome: It is always bilateral? Ultrasound Obstet Gynecol 1999;14:183-187.

199. Sommerville M, Grimes DA, Koonings PP, et al: Ovarian neoplasms and the risk of adnexal torsion. Am J Obstet Gynecol 1991;164:577-578.

200. Graif M, Itzchak Y: Sonographic evaluation of ovarian torsion in childhood and adolescence. AJR 1988;150:647-649.

201. Warner MA, Fleischer AC, Edell SI, et al: Uterine adnexal torsion: Sonographic findings. Radiology 1985;154:773-775.

202. Albayram F, Hamper UM: Ovarian and adnexal torsion: Spectrum of sonographic findings with pathologic correlation. J Ultrasound Med 2001;20:1083-1089.

203. Fleischer AC, Stein SM, Cullinan JA, et al: Color Doppler sonography of adnexal torsion. J Ultrasound Med 1995;14:523-528.

204. Stark JE, Siegel MJ: Ovarian torsion in prepubertal and pubertal girls: Sonographic findings. AJR 1994;163:1479-1482.

205. Rosado WM, Trambert MA, Gosink BB, et al: Adnexal torsion: Diagnosis by using Doppler sonography. AJR 1992;159:1251-1253.

206. Lee EJ, Kwon HC, Joo HJ, et al: Diagnosis of ovarian torsion with color Doppler sonography:depiction of twisted vascular pedicle. J Ultrasound Med 1998;17:83-89.

207. Kapadia R, Sternhill V, Schwartz E: Massive edema of the ovary. J Clin Ultrasound 1982;10:469-471.

208. Lee AR, Kim KH, Lee BH, et al: Massive edema of the ovary: Imaging findings. AJR 1993;161:343-344.

209. Hill LM, Pelekanos M, Kanbour A: Massive edema of an ovary previously fixed to the pelvic side wall. J Ultrasound Med 1993;12:629-632.

210. Kerlikowske K, Brown JS, Grady DG: Should women with familial ovarian cancer undergo prophylactic oophorectomy? Obstet Gynecol 1992;80:700-707.

211. Lynch HT, Watson P, Lynch JF, et al: Hereditary ovarian cancer: Heterogeneity in age at onset. Cancer 1993;71:573-581.

212. Einhorn N, Sjövall K, Knapp RC, et al: Prospective evaluation of serum CA125 levels for early detection of ovarian cancer. Obstet Gynecol 1992;80:14-18.

213. Jacobs I, Davies AP, Bridges J, et al: Prevalence screening for ovarian cancer in postmenopausal women by CA 125 measurement and ultrasonography. BMJ 1993;306:1030-1034.

214. Campbell S, Bhan V, Royston P, et al: Transabdominal ultrasound screening for early ovarian cancer. BMJ 1989;299:1363-1367.

215. DePriest PD, Gallion HH, Pavlik EJ, et al: Transvaginal sonography as a screening method for the detection of early ovarian cancer. Gynecol Oncol 1997;65:408-414.

216. Bast RC Jr, Klug TL, St. John E, et al: A radioimmunoassay using a monoclonal antibody to monitor the course of epithelial ovarian cancer. N Engl J Med 1983;309:883-887.

217. Jacobs I, Bast RC Jr: The CA 125 tumor-associated antigen: A review of the literature. Hum Reprod 1989;4:1-12.

218. Taylor KJW, Schwartz PE: Screening for early ovarian cancer. Radiology 1994;192:1-10.

219. Kurjak A, Shalan H, Kupesic S, et al: An attempt to screen asymptomatic women for ovarian and endometrial cancer with transvaginal color and pulsed Doppler sonography. J Ultrasound Med 1994;13:295-301.

220. Bourne TH, Campbell S, Reynolds KM, et al: Screening for early familial ovarian cancer with transvaginal ultrasonography and color blood flow imaging. BMJ 1993;306:1025-1029.

221. Karlan BY, Raffel LJ, Crvenkovic G, et al: A multidisciplinary approach to the early detection of ovarian carcinoma: Rationale, protocol design, and early results. Am J Obstet Gynecol 1993;169:494-501.

222. Weiner Z, Beck D, Shteiner M, et al: Screening for ovarian cancer in women with breast cancer with transvaginal sonography and color flow imaging. J Ultrasound Med 1993;12:387-393.

223. NIH Consensus Development Panel on Ovarian Cancer: Ovarian cancer: Screening, treatment, and follow-up. JAMA 1995;273:491-497.

224. Moyle JW, Rochester D, Sider L, et al: Sonography of ovarian tumors: Predictability of tumor type. AJR 1983;141:985-991.

225. Granberg S, Wikland M, Jansson I: Macroscopic characterization of ovarian tumors and the relation to the histologic diagnosis: Criteria to be used for ultrasound evaluation. Gynecol Oncol 1989;35:139-144.

226. Finkler NJ, Benacerraf B, Lavin PT, et al: Comparison of serum CA 125, clinical impression, and ultrasound in the preoperative evaluation of ovarian masses. Obstet Gynecol 1988;72:659-664.

227. Granberg S, Norstrom A, Wikland M: Tumors in the lower pelvis as imaged by vaginal sonography. Gynecol Oncol 1990;37:224-229.

228. Sassone AM, Timor-Tritsch IE, Artner A, et al: Transvaginal sonographic characterization of ovarian disease: Evaluation of a new scoring system to predict ovarian malignancy. Obstet Gynecol 1991;78:70-76.

229. DePriest PD, Shenson D, Fried A, et al: A morphology index based on sonographic findings in ovarian cancer. Gynecol Oncol 1993;51:7-11.

230. Lerner JP, Timor-Tritsch IE, Federman A, et al: Transvaginal ultrasonographic characterization of ovarian masses with an improved weighted scoring system. Am J Obstet Gynecol 1994;170:81-85.

231. Ferrazzi E, Zanetta G, Dordoni D, et al: Transvaginal ultrasonographic characterization of ovarian masses: Comparison of five scoring systems in a multicenter study. Ultrasound Obstet Gynecol 1997;10:192-197.

232. Folkman J, Watson K, Ingber D, et al: Induction of angiogenesis during the transition from hyperplasia to neoplasia. Nature 1989;339:58-61.

233. Bourne T, Campbell S, Steer C, et al: Transvaginal color flow imaging: A possible new screening technique for ovarian cancer. Br Med J 1989;299:1367-1370.

234. Kurjak A, Zalud I, Alfirevic Z: Evaluation of adnexal masses with transvaginal color ultrasound. J Ultrasound Med 1991;10:295-297.

235. Weiner Z, Thaler I, Beck D, et al: Differentiating malignant from benign ovarian tumors with transvaginal color flow imaging. Obstet Gynecol 1992;79:159-162.

236. Fleischer AC, Rodgers WH, Rao BK, et al: Assessment of ovarian tumor vascularity with transvaginal color Doppler sonography. J Ultrasound Med 1991;10:563-568.

237. Hamper UM, Sheth S, Abbas FM, et al: Transvaginal color Doppler sonography of adnexal masses: Differences in blood flow impedance in benign and malignant lesions. AJR 1993;160:1225-1228.

238. Tekay A, Jouppila P: Validity of pulsatility and resistance indices in classification of adnexal tumors with transvaginal color Doppler ultrasound. Ultrasound Obstet Gynecol 1992;2:338-344.

239. Brown DL, Frates MC, Laing FC, et al: Ovarian masses: Can benign and malignant lesions be differentiated with color and pulsed Doppler US? Radiology 1994;190:333-336.

240. Stein SM, Laifer-Narin S, Johnson MB, et al: Differentiation of benign and malignant adnexal masses: Relative value of gray-scale, color Doppler, and spectral Doppler sonography. AJR 1995;164:381-386.

241. Jain KA: Prospective evaluation of adnexal masses with endovaginal gray-scale and duplex and color Doppler US: Correlation with pathologic findings. Radiology 1994;191:63-67.

242. Levine D, Feldstein VA, Babcook CJ, et al: Sonography of ovarian masses: Poor sensitivity of resistive index for identifying malignant lesions. AJR 1994;162:1355-1359.

243. Bromley B, Goodman H, Benacerraf BR: Comparison between sonographic morphology and Doppler waveform for the diagnosis of ovarian malignancy. Obstet Gynecol 1994;83:434-437.

244. Salem S, White LM, Lai J: Doppler sonography of adnexal masses: The predictive value of the pulsatility index in benign and malignant disease. AJR 1994;163:1147-1150.

245. Carter J, Saltzman A, Hartenbach E, et al: Flow characteristics in benign and malignant gynecologic tumors using transvaginal color flow Doppler. Obstet Gynecol 1994;83:125-130.

246. Buy JN, Ghossain MA, Hugol D, et al: Characterization of adnexal masses: Combination of color Doppler and conventional sonography compared with spectral Doppler analysis alone and conventional sonography alone. AJR 1996;166:385-393.

247. Reles A, Wein U, Lichtenegger W: Transvaginal color Doppler sonography and conventional sonography in the preoperative assessment of adnexal masses. J Clin Ultrasound 1997;25:217-225.

248. Fleisher AC, Rodgers WH, Kepple DM, et al: Color Doppler sonography of ovarian masses: A multiparameter analysis. J Ultrasound Med 1993;12:41-48.

249. Guerriero S, Alcazar JL, Coccia ME, et al: Complex pelvic mass as a target of evaluation of vessel distribution by color Doppler sonography for the diagnosis of adnexal malignancies: Results of a multicenter European study. J Ultrasound Med 2002;21:1105-1111.

250. Valentin L: Prospective cross-validation of Doppler ultrasound examination and gray-scale ultrasound imaging for discrimination of benign and malignant pelvic masses. Ultrasound Obstet Gynecol 1999;14:273-283.

251. Fleischer AC, Cullinan JA, Kepple DM, et al: Conventional and color Doppler transvaginal sonography of pelvic masses: A comparison of relative histologic specificities. J Ultrasound Med 1993;12:705-712.

252. Brown DL, Doubilet PM, Miller FH, et al: Benign and malignant ovarian masses: Selection of the most discriminating gray-scale and Doppler sonographic features. Radiology 1998;208:103-110.

253. Schelling M, Braun M, Kuhn W, et al: Combined transvaginal B-mode and color Doppler sonography for differential diagnosis of ovarian tumors: Results of a multivariate logistic regression analysis. Gynecol Oncol 2000;77:78-86.

254. Kinkel K, Hricak H, Lu Y, et al: US characterization of ovarian masses: A meta-analysis. Radiology 2000;217:803-811.

255. Laing FC: US analysis of adnexal masses: The art of making the correct diagnosis. Radiology 1994;191:21-22.

256. Williams AG, Mettler FA, Wicks JD: Cystic and solid ovarian neoplasms. Semin Ultrasound 1983;4:166-183.

257. Wagner BJ, Buck JL, Seidman JD, et al: Ovarian epithelial neoplasms: Radiologic-pathologic correlation. Radiographics 1994;14:1351-1374.

258. Athey PA, Siegel MF: Sonographic features of Brenner tumor of the ovary. J Ultrasound Med 1987;6:367-372.

259. Brammer HM III, Buck JL, Hayes WS, et al: Malignant germ cell tumors of the ovary: Radiologic-pathologic correlation. Radiographics 1990;10:715-724.

260. Quinn SF, Erickson S, Black, WC: Cystic ovarian teratomas: The sonographic appearance of the dermoid plug. Radiology 1985;155:477-478.

261. Sheth S, Fishman EK, Buck JL, et al: The variable sonographic appearances of ovarian teratomas: Correlation with CT. AJR 1988;151:331-334.

262. Guttman PH Jr: In search of the elusive benign cystic ovarian teratoma: Application of the ultrasound "tip of the iceberg" sign. J Clin Ultrasound 1977;5:403-406.

263. Bronshtein M, Yoffe N, Brandes JM, et al: Hair as a sonographic marker of ovarian teratomas: Improved identification using transvaginal sonography and simulation model. J Clin Ultrasound 1991;19:351-355.

264. Malde HM, Kedar RP, Chadha D, et al: Dermoid mesh: A sonographic sign of ovarian teratoma. Letter AJR 1992;159:1349-1350.

265. Kawamoto S, Katsuhiko S, Matsumoto H, et al: Multiple mobile spherules in mature cystic teratoma of the ovary. AJR 2001;176:1455-1457.

266. Patel M, Feldstein VA, Lipson SD, et al: Cystic teratoma of the ovary: Diagnostic value of sonography. AJR 1998;171:1061-1065.

267. Hertzberg BS, Kliewer MA: Sonography of benign cystic teratoma of the ovary: Pitfalls in diagnosis. AJR 1996;167:1127-1133.

268. Zalel Y, Caspi B, Tepper R: Doppler flow characteristics of dermoid cysts: Unique appearance of struma ovarii. J Ultrasound Med 1997;16:355-358.

269. O'Malley BP, Richmond H: Struma ovarii. J Ultrasound Med 1982;1:177-178.

270. Tanaka YO, Kurosaki Y, Nishida M, et al: Ovarian dysgerminoma: MR and CT appearance. J Comput Assist Tomogr 1994;18:443-448.

271. Kim SH, Kang SB: Ovarian dysgerminoma: Color Doppler ultrasonographic findings and comparison with CT and MR imaging findings. J Ultrasound Med 1995;14:843-848.

272. Ko SF, Wan YL, Ng SH: Adult ovarian granulosa cell tumors: Spectrum of sonographic and CT findings with pathological correlation. AJR 1999;172:1227-1233.

273. Neste MG, Francis IR, Bude RO: Hepatic metastases from granulosa cell tumor of the ovary: CT and sonographic findings. AJR 1996;166:1122-1124.

274. Outwater EK, Wagner BG, Mannion C, et al: Sex cord-stromal and steroid cell tumors of the ovary. Radiographics 1998;18:1523-1546.

275. Stephenson WM, Laing FC: Sonography of ovarian fibromas. AJR 1985;144:1239-1240.

276. Athey PA, Malone RS: Sonography of ovarian fibromas/thecomas. J Ultrasound Med 1987;6:431-436.

277. Athey PA, Butters HE: Sonographic and CT appearance of Krukenberg tumors. J Clin Ultrasound 1984;12:205-210.

278. Shimizu H, Yamasaki M, Ohama K, et al: Characteristic ultrasonographic appearance of the Krukenberg tumor. J Clin Ultrasound 1990;18:697-703.

Fallopian Tube

279. Timor-Tritsch IE, Rottem S: Transvaginal ultrasonographic study of the fallopian tube. Obstet Gynecol 1987;70:424-428.

280. Patten RM, Vincent LM, Wolner-Hanssen P, et al: Pelvic inflammatory disease: Endovaginal sonography with laparoscopic correlation. J Ultrasound Med 1990;9:681-689.

281. Tessler FN, Perrella RR, Fleischer AC, et al: Endovaginal sonographic diagnosis of dilated fallopian tubes. AJR 1989;153:523-525.

282. Taipale P, Tarjanne H, Ylöstalo P: Transvaginal sonography in suspected pelvic inflammatory disease. Ultrasound Obstet Gynecol 1995;6:430-434.

283. Timor-Tritsch IE, Lerner JP, Monteagudo A, et al: Transvaginal sonographic markers of tubal inflammatory disease. Ultrasound Obstet Gynecol 1998;12:56-66.

284. Bulas DI, Ahlstrom PA, Sivit CJ, et al: Pelvic inflammatory disease in the adolescent: Comparison of transabdominal and transvaginal sonographic evaluation. Radiology 1992;183:435-439.

285. VanSonnenberg E, D'Agostino HB, Casola G, et al: US-guided transvaginal drainage of pelvic abscesses and fluid collections. Radiology 1991;181:53-56.

286. Feld R, Eschelman DJ, Sagerman JE, et al: Treatment of pelvic abscesses and other fluid collections: Efficacy of transvaginal sonographically guided aspiration and drainage. AJR 1994;163:1141-1145.

287. Sherer DM, Liberto L, Abramowicz JS, et al: Endovaginal sonographic features associated with isolated torsion of the fallopian tube. J Ultrasound Med 1991;10:107-109.

288. Russin LD: Hydrosalpinx and tubal torsion: A late complication of tubal ligation. Radiology 1986;159:115-116.

289. Subramanyam BR, Raghavendra BN, Whalen CA, et al: Ultrasonic features of fallopian tube carcinoma. J Ultrasound Med 1984;3:391-393.

290. Ajjimakorn S, Bhamarapravati Y: Transvaginal ultrasound and the diagnosis of fallopian tubal carcinoma. J Clin Ultrasound 1991;19:116-119.

291. Kurjak A, Kupesic S, Ilijas M, et al: Preoperative diagnosis of primary fallopian tube carcinoma. Gynecol Oncol 1998;68:29-34.

292. Slanetz PJ, Whitman GJ, Halpern EF, et al: Imaging of fallopian tube tumors. AJR 1997;169:1321-1324.

Nongynecologic Pelvic Masses

293. Wicks JD, Silver TM, Bree RL: Gray scale features of hematomas: An ultrasonic spectrum. AJR 1978;131:977-980.

294. Salem S, O'Malley BP, Hiltz CW: Ultrasonographic appearance of gastrointestinal masses. J Can Assoc Radiol 1980;31:163-167.

Postpartum Pelvic Pathology
295. Lee CY, Madrazo B, Drukker BH: Ultrasonic evaluation of the postpartum uterus in the management of postpartum bleeding. Obstet Gynecol 1981;58:227-232.
296. Hertzberg BS, Bowie JD: Ultrasound of the postpartum uterus: Prediction of retained placental tissue. J Ultrasound Med 1991;10:451-456.
297. Zuckerman J, Levine D, McNicholas MMJ, et al: Imaging of pelvic postpartum complications. AJR 1997;168:663-668.
298. Wilson PC, Lerner RM: Diagnosis of ovarian vein thrombophlebitis by ultrasonography. J Ultrasound Med 1983;2:187-190.
299. Savader SJ, Otero RR, Savader BL: Puerperal ovarian vein thrombosis: Evaluation with CT, US, and MR imaging. Radiology 1988;167:637-639.
300. Grant TH, Schoettle BW, Buchsbaum MS: Postpartum ovarian vein thrombosis: Diagnosis by clot protrusion into the inferior vena cava at sonography. AJR 1993;160:551-552.
301. Baran GW, Frisch KM: Duplex Doppler evaluation of puerperal ovarian vein thrombosis. AJR 1987;149:321-322.
302. Baker ME, Kay H, Mahony BS, et al: Sonography of the low transverse incision, cesarean section: A prospective study. J Ultrasound Med 1988;7:389-393.
303. Baker ME, Bowie JD, Killam AP: Sonography of post-cesarean-section bladder-flap hematoma. AJR 1985;144:757-759.
304. Wiener MD, Bowie JD, Baker ME, et al: Sonography of subfascial hematoma after cesarean delivery. AJR 1987;148:907-910.
305. Al-Naib S: Sonographic appearance of postpartum retropubic hematoma. J Clin Ultrasound 1990;18:520-521.

16

GESTATIONAL TROPHOBLASTIC NEOPLASIA

Margaret A. Fraser-Hill / Stephanie R. Wilson

Chapter Outline

*G*estational **trophoblastic neoplasia** (GTN) is a spectrum of disorders characterized by abnormal proliferation of pregnancy-related trophoblasts with progressive malignant potential.[1] GTN includes molar pregnancy, invasive mole, choriocarcinoma, and placental-site trophoblastic tumor (PSTT). Collectively, the last three conditions are referred to as **persistent trophoblastic neoplasia**, or PTN.

In a normal pregnancy, one of the primary functions of placental trophoblast is to gain access to the maternal circulation. Normal trophoblast infiltrates maternal tissues, invades vessels, and can even be transported to the lungs.[2] This capacity for invasion is shared by all trophoblastic tumors and is responsible for many of the distinctive pathologic, clinical, and imaging features of this fascinating group of lesions. GTN has been known since ancient times. Hippocrates described molar pregnancy as "dropsy of the uterus" and attributed it to unhealthy water. The term hydatidiform mole has been recognized for more than 3 centuries and refers to cystic degeneration of chorionic villi in molar pregnancy. Prior to the middle of this century, malignant GTN was uniformly fatal. Remarkably, it is now the **most curable gynecologic malignancy** as the result of several important advances, including the availability of a sensitive and reliable tumor marker (human chorionic gonadotropin, or hCG); the exquisite sensitivity of most lesions to antifolic chemotherapy; and the use of

aggressive multimodality regimens combining chemotherapy, radiation therapy, and surgery in selected patients unresponsive to conventional protocols.[1,3] In general, once the diagnosis of GTN has been established, therapeutic decisions rest mainly on clinical criteria. Diagnostic imaging has an important role to play in diagnosis and management.

MOLAR PREGNANCY

Molar pregnancy is the most common and benign form of GTN, with an incidence of 1 in 1000 pregnancies in North America.[1,3-5] Advancing maternal age, prior history of molar pregnancy, and Asian ancestry are established risk factors.[4,5] Molar pregnancy has the distinctive histologic characteristics of cystic or grapelike (hydatidiform) degeneration of chorionic villi, absent or inadequate vascularization of chorionic villi, and abnormal proliferation of placental trophoblast.[1,3,5-12] Hydatidiform mole is classified as either complete molar pregnancy or partial molar pregnancy on the basis of cytogenetic, morphologic, and clinical features.

Complete Molar Pregnancy

Complete molar pregnancy is characterized by a diploid karyotype of 46,XX in approximately 70% to

589

85% of cases. In complete molar pregnancy, chromosomal DNA is exclusively paternal in origin. This occurs when an ovum with absent or inactive maternal chromosomes is fertilized by a normal haploid sperm. Endoreduplication of paternal chromosomes produces a **diploid karyotype** of 46,XX (46,YY is lethal). Occasionally, fertilization of an empty ovum by two haploid sperm results in the 46,XY pattern.[10-12] At pathology, there is **no fetal development** in complete molar pregnancy. The placenta is entirely replaced by abnormal, hydropic chorionic villi with excessive trophoblastic proliferation.[1-3,8,9] Although the degree of trophoblastic proliferation ranges from mild to severe, up to 50% of cases are severe.[8,9] Excessive trophoblastic proliferation results in **classic symptoms and signs** that frequently suggest the diagnosis. These include excessive uterine size for dates, markedly elevated serum hCG (greater than 100,000 mIU/mL), hyperemesis gravidarum, toxemia, hyperthyroidism, and respiratory failure. Theca lutein cysts of the ovaries occur in approximately 15% to 30% of cases and reflect excessive hCG levels. Vaginal bleeding, present in over 90% of cases, is the most frequent symptom at presentation.[7-9] Passage of vesicles (hydropic villi) occurs in up to 80% of cases and is considered specific for the condition.[7] Today, the frequent use of ultrasound for any patient with spotting in pregnancy allows for early diagnosis and few patients show the classic features of hyperemesis and toxemia.[13,14]

Partial Molar Pregnancy

In contrast, **partial molar pregnancy** has a **triploid karyotype** of 69,XXX, 69,XXY, or 69,XYY. Most partial moles have one set of maternal chromosomes and two sets of paternal chromosomes resulting from fertilization of a normal ovum by two haploid sperm. This condition, in which the extra set of chromosomes is paternally derived, is known as diandric triploidy. Triploidy of maternal origin is not associated with GTN.[10-12] At pathology, partial molar pregnancy has well-developed but generally **anomalous (triploid) fetal tissues**. Hydropic degeneration of placental villi is focal, interspersed with normal placental villi. Trophoblastic proliferation is mild.[1-3,7] The clinical diagnosis of partial molar pregnancy is rarely made prospectively. Symptoms and signs are less frequent and less severe because trophoblastic proliferation is mild. Missed or incomplete abortion is the most common clinical diagnosis.[8,9]

Diagnosis and Management

The diagnosis of molar pregnancy should be considered in patients presenting with first trimester vaginal bleeding, rapid uterine enlargement, excessive uterine size for dates, hyperemesis gravidarum, and preeclampsia before 24 weeks. Serum hCG levels in molar pregnancy are abnormally elevated, commonly over 100,000 mIU/mL, in contrast to normal pregnancy levels of less than 60,000 mIU/mL.[7]

Sonographic Features. The **classic sonographic features of complete molar pregnancy** are well known and include an enlarged uterus containing echogenic tissue that expands the endometrial canal (Fig. 16-1A). Hydropic villi within molar tissue appear as innumerable, diffusely and uniformly distributed cystic spaces ranging in size from a few millimeters to 2 to 3 cm.[15-18] In the second trimester, transabdominal sonographic diagnosis is highly accurate. Transvaginal scans may not add significant diagnostic information or improve outcome.[19] However, early molar gestations may possess atypical features that make transabdominal diagnosis more difficult. In first trimester molar gestations, molar tissue appears as a predominantly solid and echogenic mass because very tiny hydropic villi are not adequately resolved by transabdominal sonography. This appearance is nonspecific, simulated by incomplete abortion or blood clot.[20] Transvaginal ultrasound (US) is more sensitive than transabdominal sonography and may depict hydropic villi earlier and to better advantage than transabdominal US (see Fig. 16-1B).[21,22] Transvaginal sonography of early molar pregnancy may also depict a solid, echogenic mass within a gestational sac.[23] In complete moles, a fetus is absent except in the rare event of a coexistent twin pregnancy (Fig. 16-2). In such cases, sonography is accurate in establishing the diagnosis. Differentiation from partial molar pregnancy rests on identifying a separate, normal placenta (see Fig. 16-2).[24] The ovaries may be greatly enlarged in complete molar pregnancy by multiple, bilateral theca lutein cysts. These may be clear or hemorrhagic and can be a source of pelvic pain.[7,22] The sonographic appearance is similar to that seen in ovarian hyperstimulation from ovulation induction therapy. Theca lutein cysts represent an in vivo bioassay for endogenous hCG and are most marked when trophoblastic proliferation is severe.

The **sonographic features of partial molar pregnancy** are less frequently described and they overlap with other conditions. Partial molar pregnancy is commonly mistaken for missed or incomplete abortion.[20] In partial molar pregnancy, the placenta is excessive in size and contains numerous cystic spaces distributed in a nonuniform manner. A gestational sac is present and is frequently deformed in shape.[15,16] A growth-retarded fetus is present and may show anomalies of triploidy, including syndactyly and hydrocephalus (Fig. 16-3).[1,7,15] Placental hydropic degeneration (unrelated to trophoblastic neoplasia) can also possess similar sonographic features.[15,17] Hydropic degeneration is a common occurrence in first trimester abortion of any cause. The associated cystic spaces may be difficult or impossible

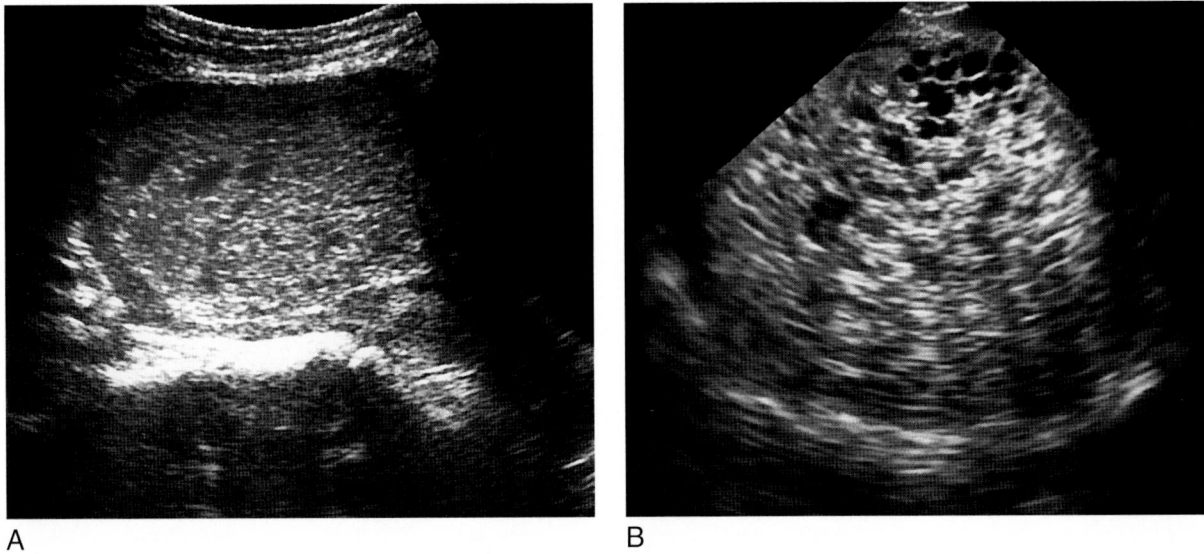

FIGURE 16-1. Complete molar pregnancy, classic appearance. A, Transabdominal scan shows a vesicular echogenic mass filling the endometrial canal. **B,** Transvaginal high-resolution sonogram shows innumerable uniformly distributed cystic spaces that correspond to hydropic chorionic villi at pathology.

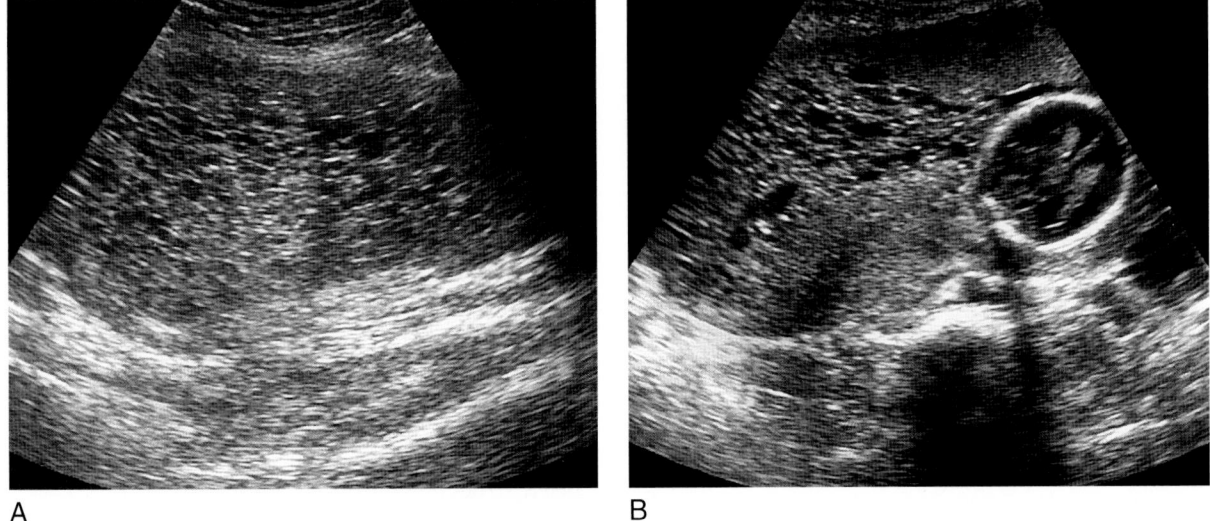

FIGURE 16-2. Complete mole with a coexistent fetus in an 18-weeks' gestation. A, Sagittal scan of right side of uterus shows a large echogenic mass with innumerable tiny cystic spaces, the classic morphology for a complete mole. **B,** Transverse image shows the mole on the left side of the image. There is a normal fetus, head shown here, and a normal anterior placenta. This condition has a poor prognosis.

to differentiate from an early mole. Therefore, careful evaluation of the products of conception should be recommended to avoid the possibility of missing a diagnosis of mole in cases with equivocal ultrasound features.

Therapy and Prognosis. Therapy of molar pregnancy is uterine evacuation, and the majority are adequately treated in this fashion. Approximately 80% of complete moles and 95% of partial moles will subsequently follow a benign course.[7-9,25] However, accurate diagnosis and classification of molar pregnancy are important because of the risk of PTN. For this reason, all patients with

molar pregnancy are monitored with weekly serum hCG determinations and are counseled to avoid pregnancy for at least 1 year.

PERSISTENT TROPHOBLASTIC NEOPLASIA

Persistent trophoblastic neoplasia is a life-threatening complication of pregnancy that encompasses invasive mole, choriocarcinoma, and the extremely rare PSTT. PTN occurs most commonly in the setting of molar

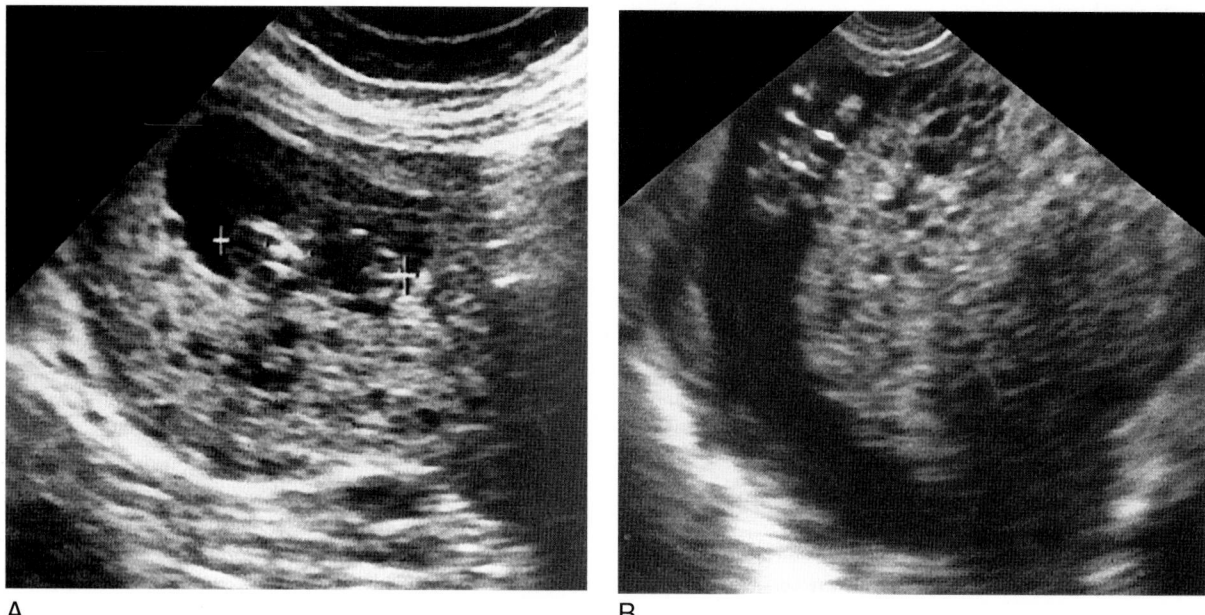

FIGURE 16-3. Partial mole at 16 weeks. A, Suprapubic scan shows a gravid uterus. There is a small, dead, growth-retarded fetus of approximately 12-week size. The placental tissue is large and has multiple vesicular spaces consistent with hydropic villi. There is no normal placenta. **B,** Transvaginal scan shows the small fetus relative to the large, abnormal posterior placenta.

pregnancy; up to 20% of complete moles develop persistent disease requiring additional therapy.[4,7-9,26-28] Complete moles with severe degrees of trophoblastic proliferation are at the highest risk. Persistent disease develops in 50% or more of these cases.[4,7,8,26,27] The risk is similarly high for complete molar pregnancy with a coexisting fetus, probably because of delayed diagnosis.[24] The risk of persistent disease after partial molar pregnancy is much lower, occurring in approximately 5% of cases.[9,11,16,26,28] Uncommonly, PTN develops in the setting of a normal term delivery, spontaneous abortion, or, very rarely, ectopic pregnancy.[4,6,7,11]

Invasive Mole

Invasive mole (chorioadenoma destruens) is the most common form of PTN, accounting for 80% to 95% of cases.[26] It is defined histologically by the presence of formed chorionic villi and proliferating trophoblast deep in the myometrium.[1,2,7] It is considered biologically benign and is usually confined to the uterus; however, uterine penetration or perforation can occur, with the potential for death from severe hemorrhage.[1,2,7,28] Lesions can invade beyond the uterus to parametrial tissues, adjacent organs, and blood vessels.[1,2,7] Invasive molar villi may embolize to distant sites including lung and brain.

Choriocarcinoma

Choriocarcinoma is a very rare malignancy with an incidence of 1 in 30,000 pregnancies.[1,7] As with other forms of PTN, the most important risk factor for choriocarcinoma is molar pregnancy. Molar gestations precede 50% to 80% of cases, and 1 in 40 molar pregnancies gives rise to choriocarcinoma. Choriocarcinoma is a purely cellular lesion defined histologically by the absence of formed villi and the invasion of the myometrium by abnormal, proliferating trophoblast.[1,6] Vascular invasion, hemorrhage, and necrosis are prominent features.[6] Distant metastases are common and most frequently affect the lungs, followed by the liver and brain, gastrointestinal tract, and kidney. Respiratory compromise may be the initial presentation.[7,29] Venous invasion and retrograde metastases to the vagina and pelvic structures are also common.[5,29]

Placental-Site Trophoblastic Tumor

Placental-site trophoblastic tumor is the rarest and most fatal form of GTN.[2,3,30] Like choriocarcinoma and invasive mole, PSTT can follow any type of gestation but most commonly follows term delivery.[6] PSTT may be confined to the uterus, may be locally invasive in the pelvis, or distantly metastatic to the lungs, lymph nodes, peritoneum, liver, pancreas, or brain. Vaginal bleeding is the most common symptom at presentation.[6] Surgical therapy is recommended because these lesions tend to be resistant to chemotherapy, and the risk of metastases is high. Unlike choriocarcinoma, PSTT does not prominently feature necrosis, vascular invasion, and hemorrhage.[2,3,6] Histologically, PSTT is distinct from other forms of trophoblastic neoplasia. It arises from nonvillus, "intermediate" trophoblast that infiltrates the decidua, spiral arteries, and myometrium at the placental bed.[2,6] PSTT presents a diagnostic challenge because it is frequently difficult to distinguish from the normal intermediate trophoblastic infiltration at the placental site. Unlike other forms of PTN, serum hCG is not a reliable marker for PSTT. Histochemical staining of intermediate trophoblast for hCG is weak or absent, whereas staining for human placental lactogen (hPL) is strongly positive. Unfortunately, serum hPL is not a reliable predictor of tumor behavior.[5,30]

Diagnosis and Management

Because PTN arises most commonly in the setting of molar pregnancy, the diagnosis is usually based on abnormal regression of hCG after uterine evacuation. A histologic diagnosis is not considered mandatory. Curettage risks uterine perforation and does not significantly alter management or outcome.[28] Patients are treated on the basis of clinical staging that includes computed tomography of the brain, chest, abdomen, and pelvis.[28,29] While the diagnosis of PTN is straight-forward in most cases, there are instances when PTN may go unrecognized. This most commonly occurs when inadequate pathologic examination fails to detect hydatidiform mole in a first trimester abortion. PTN developing in such cases or after nonmolar gestations will be mistaken for incomplete abortion or retained products of conception. Recognition of PSTT is further complicated by negative or low hCG levels. In addition, patients with PTN may present with a confusing variety of nongynecologic problems, including respiratory compromise and cerebral, gastrointestinal, or urologic hemorrhage.[26,29] In difficult cases, imaging may be the first to suggest the diagnosis. In all cases, sonography has an important role to play in staging disease and in monitoring response to therapy.

Human Chorionic Gonadotropin. With the exception of PSTT, hCG is a sensitive and specific marker for detecting and monitoring PTN. Elaborated by placental trophoblast, hCG is composed of α- and β-subunits that must combine to form the biologically active parent hormone. While the α-subunit of hCG is similar to that of pituitary glycoprotein hormones, luteinizing hormone (LH), follicle stimulating hormone (FSH), and thyroid stimulating hormone (TSH), the β-subunit is unique and confers the specific biologic activity on hCG.[31-33]

Quantitative measurements of hCG employ **radio-immunoassay** (RIA), an exquisitely sensitive technique that quantifies the amount of hormone present in small samples of serum or other body fluids. Care must be exercised when choosing an assay to diagnose PTN and monitor response to therapy. Assays that measure total hCG or β-hCG are recommended for these patients.[32,34]

Normal mean disappearance time of hCG in benign moles ranges from 7 to 14 weeks, with a median of 11 weeks. The maximum disappearance time can be as long as 60 weeks. Clinical criteria for abnormal hCG regression have not been uniformly defined. Some clinicians institute therapy when hCG levels plateau or increase for 2 to 4 weeks or have not returned to normal by 8 weeks. Others treat when hCG has not regressed completely by 6 months. These empirical criteria account for the variation in the reported frequency of PTN following molar pregnancy. **Standardized regression curves** constructed from large numbers of patients provide a more objective means of diagnosing persistent disease and monitoring response to therapy (Fig. 16-4A, B).[34] By 6 weeks, hCG levels deviate beyond the 95th percentile of the standard curve in 50% of cases of PTN. By 14 weeks, over 90% of cases are detected in this fashion. Standardized curves avoid the misdiagnosis of PTN in benign moles with minor, transitory plateaus or increases in hCG that remain in the normal range. When hCG continues to be positive after 6 months, expectant management is recommended as long as levels continue to fall. In general, PTN should be diagnosed and treated when hCG levels plateau or increase for 3 consecutive weeks with at least one measurement outside the normal regression corridor. Once hCG levels have normalized, the risk of PTN is low (less than 1% of cases); however, it is recommended that all patients with molar pregnancy be followed for at least 1 year.[34]

Sonography and Duplex Color Doppler. Sonography is currently the best imaging modality for assessing uterine and pelvic disease in PTN.[35] It is well tolerated, accessible, inexpensive, and reproducible—ideal for serial examinations. **Sonographic features of PTN** are less familiar than those of primary molar pregnancy. Whereas transvaginal sonography is frequently unnecessary for the diagnosis of primary molar pregnancy,[23] it is an essential diagnostic tool in PTN. The small, myometrial lesions typical of this condition may not be apparent through transabdominal scanning.[15,36-39]

Invasive mole, choriocarcinoma, and PSTT may appear similar sonographically.[15,17,40-43] Morphologic features reflect tissue invasion, necrosis, and hemorrhage. The most frequently described sonographic abnormality in PTN is a **focal, echogenic myometrial nodule** (Fig. 16-5).[15,16,18,29,37-43] The lesion usually lies close to the endometrial canal, but it may be found deep in the myometrium. Lesions may appear solid and uniformly echogenic, hypoechoic, or complex and multicystic, similar to molar tissue. Anechoic regions resulting from tissue necrosis and hemorrhage appear as thick-walled, irregular cavities within solid tumors (Fig. 16-6).[37,41,42] In other cases, echo-free areas within lesions represent vascular spaces (Fig. 16-7A, B).[40] Patients with PTN may also present with **bulky uterine enlargement** when tumor replaces the entire myometrium (Fig. 16-8). In these cases, the myometrium assumes a heterogeneous, lobulated appearance (Fig. 16-9). There may be exten-

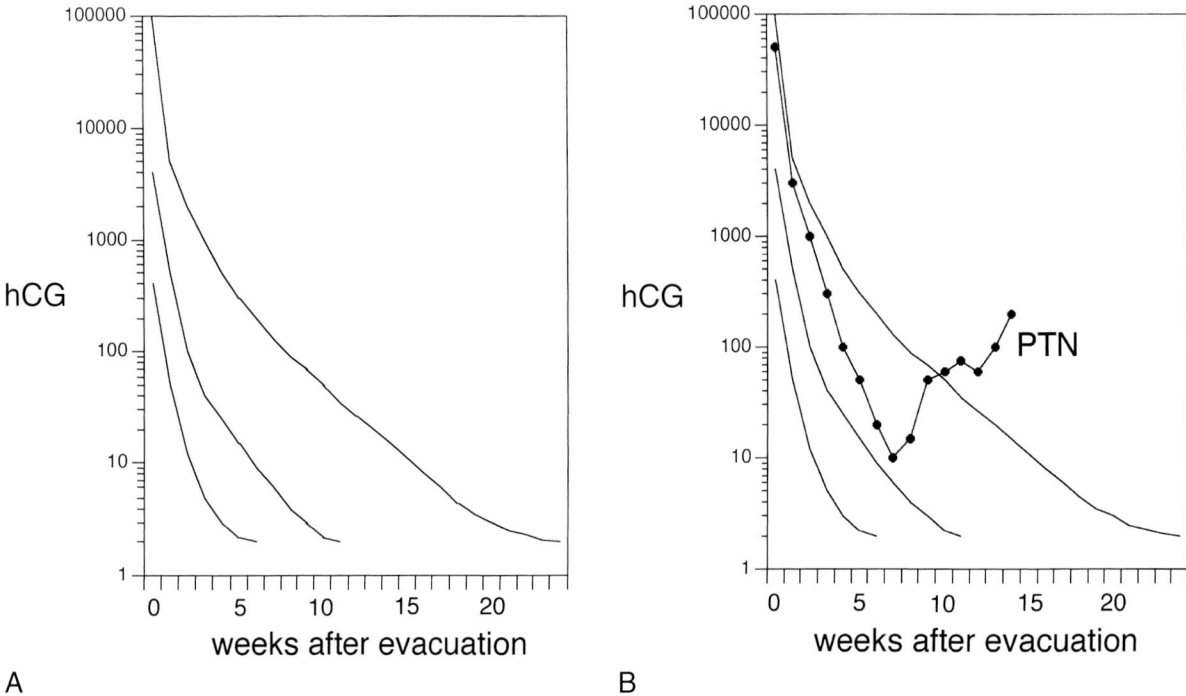

FIGURE 16-4. Human chorionic gonadotropin (hCG) regression curve. A, Normal regression curve for serum hCG following molar pregnancy. Lines (*from top to bottom*) represent the 95th, 50th, and 5th percentiles of spontaneous hCG regression in patients with benign moles. Median disappearance time is 11 weeks. **B,** In 90% of cases, PTN shows abnormal hCG regression by 14 weeks. The dotted line represents abnormal serum hCG regression in a patient with postmolar PTN. Standardized regression curves are a more objective means of identifying persistent disease than are empirical clinical criteria. PTN, persistent trophoblastic neoplasia. (From Yedema KA, Verheijen RH, Kenemans PK, et al: Identification of patients with persistent trophoblastic disease by means of a normal human chorionic gonadotropin regression curve. Am J Obstet Gynecol 1993;168[3]:787-792.)

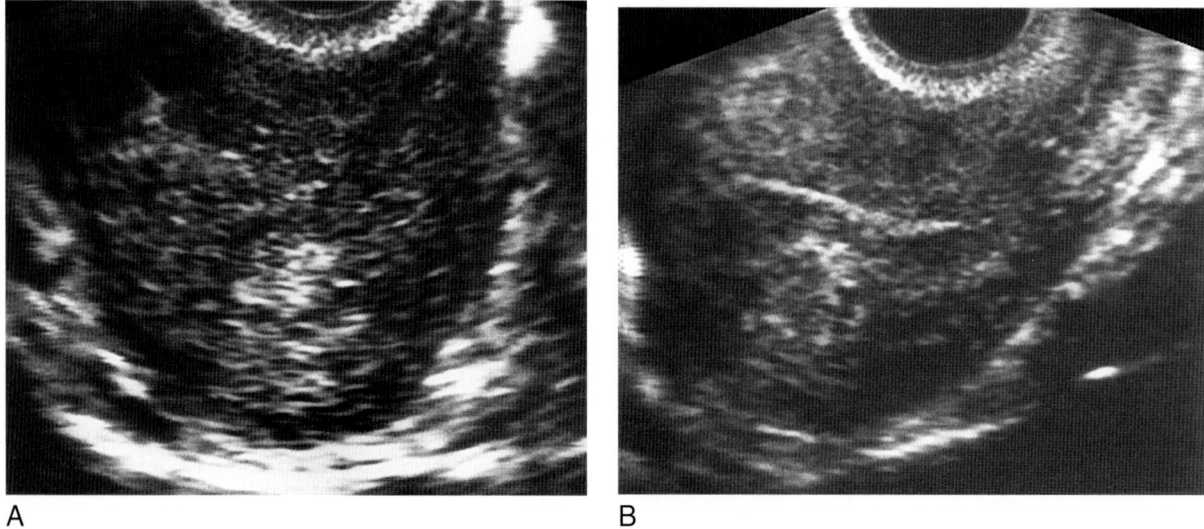

FIGURE 16-5. Focal echogenic myometrial nodule of persistent trophoblastic neoplasia (PTN). A, Transverse transvaginal sonogram shows central focal uterine echogenicity that could be mistaken for a thick endometrium. **B,** Sagittal image shows that the echogenic area lies within the myometrium posterior to a normal endometrial canal. (From Fraser-Hill MA, Burns PN, Wilson SR: Transvaginal ultrasound and duplex color Doppler of persistent trophoblastic neoplasia. Radiology 1993;189[P]:374-375.)

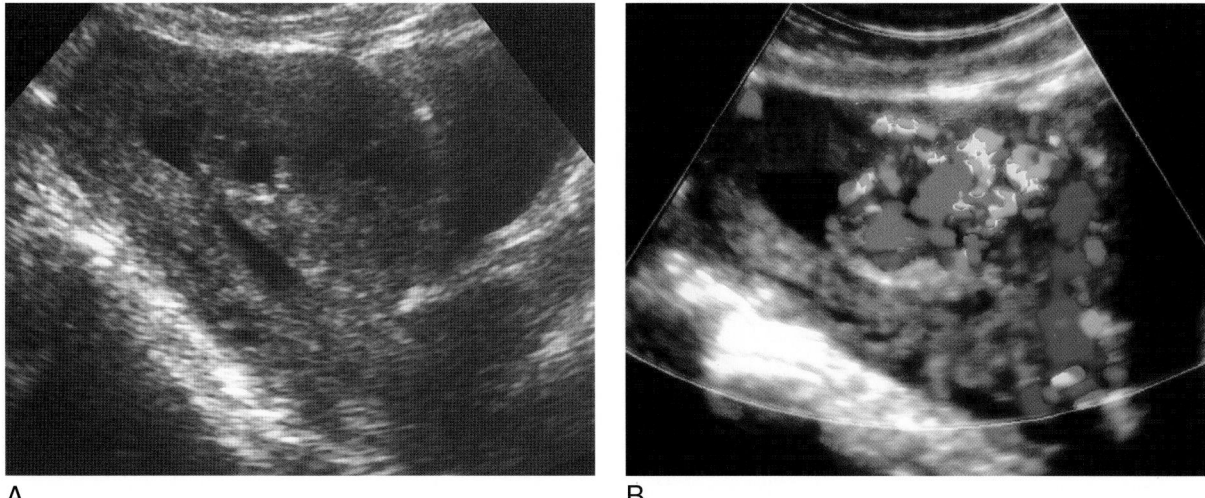

FIGURE 16-6. Cystic spaces representing vessels and hemorrhage in persistent trophoblastic neoplasia (PTN). A, Sagittal sonogram shows a bulky uterus with a complex anterior myometrial mass and blood in the endometrial cavity. **B**, Color Doppler shows a florid color mosaic pattern in the anterior myometrial tumor and blood in the endometrial cavity. (From Fraser-Hill MA, Burns PN, Wilson SR: Transvaginal ultrasound and duplex color Doppler of persistent trophoblastic neoplasia. Radiology 1993;189[P]:374-375.)

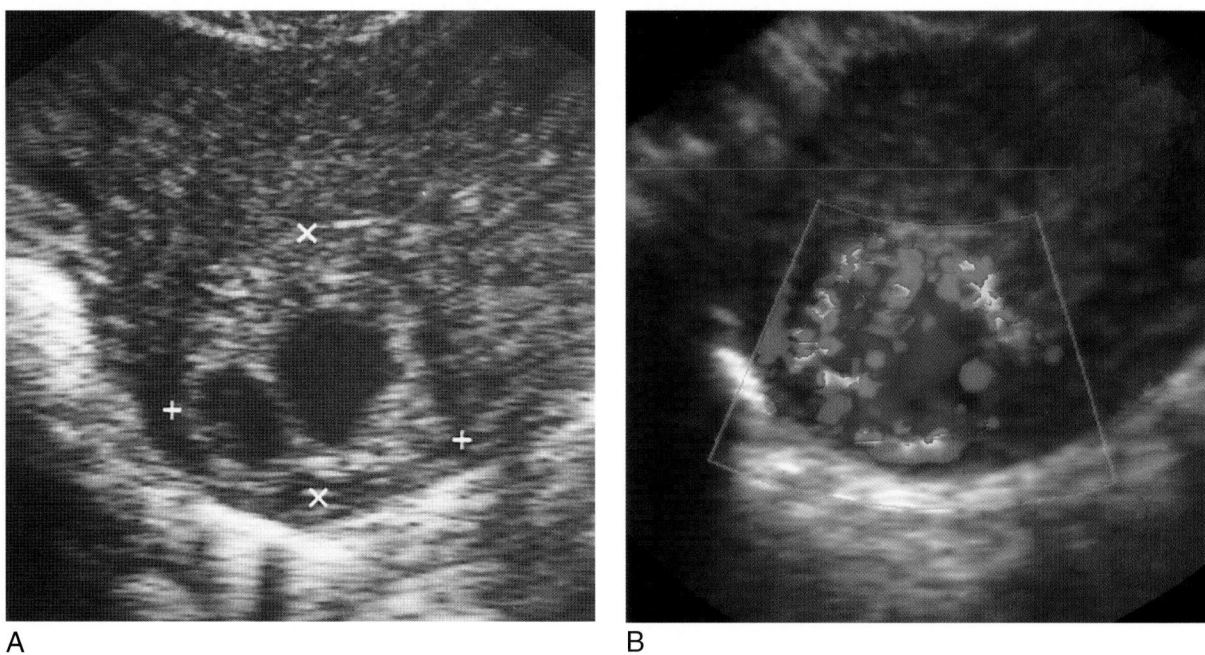

FIGURE 16-7. Cystic myometrial mass with vascular spaces in persistent trophoblastic neoplasia (PTN). A, Sagittal transvaginal sonogram shows a focal echogenic nodule with well-defined cystic spaces. **B**, Color Doppler shows a florid color mosaic pattern with aliasing. The cystic spaces fill in with color, confirming their vascular nature. (From Fraser-Hill MA, Burns PN, Wilson SR: Transvaginal ultrasound and duplex color Doppler of persistent trophoblastic neoplasia. Radiology 1993;189[P]:374-375.)

sion beyond the uterus to the parametrium, pelvic side wall, and adjacent organs. In extreme cases, PTN appears as a **large, undifferentiated pelvic mass** (Fig. 16-10). In the correct setting (e.g., recent molar pregnancy, rising serum hCG, and a previously documented normal sonogram), sonography can be diagnostic; however, sonography is not completely specific. Common, benign conditions, including adenomyosis and fibroids, may appear similar to PTN.[18,44,45] Accurate diagnosis depends on correlation with clinical findings and serum hCG levels.

After effective therapy, sonographic abnormalities usually resolve and uterine morphology returns to normal. Lesions become progressively more hypoechoic

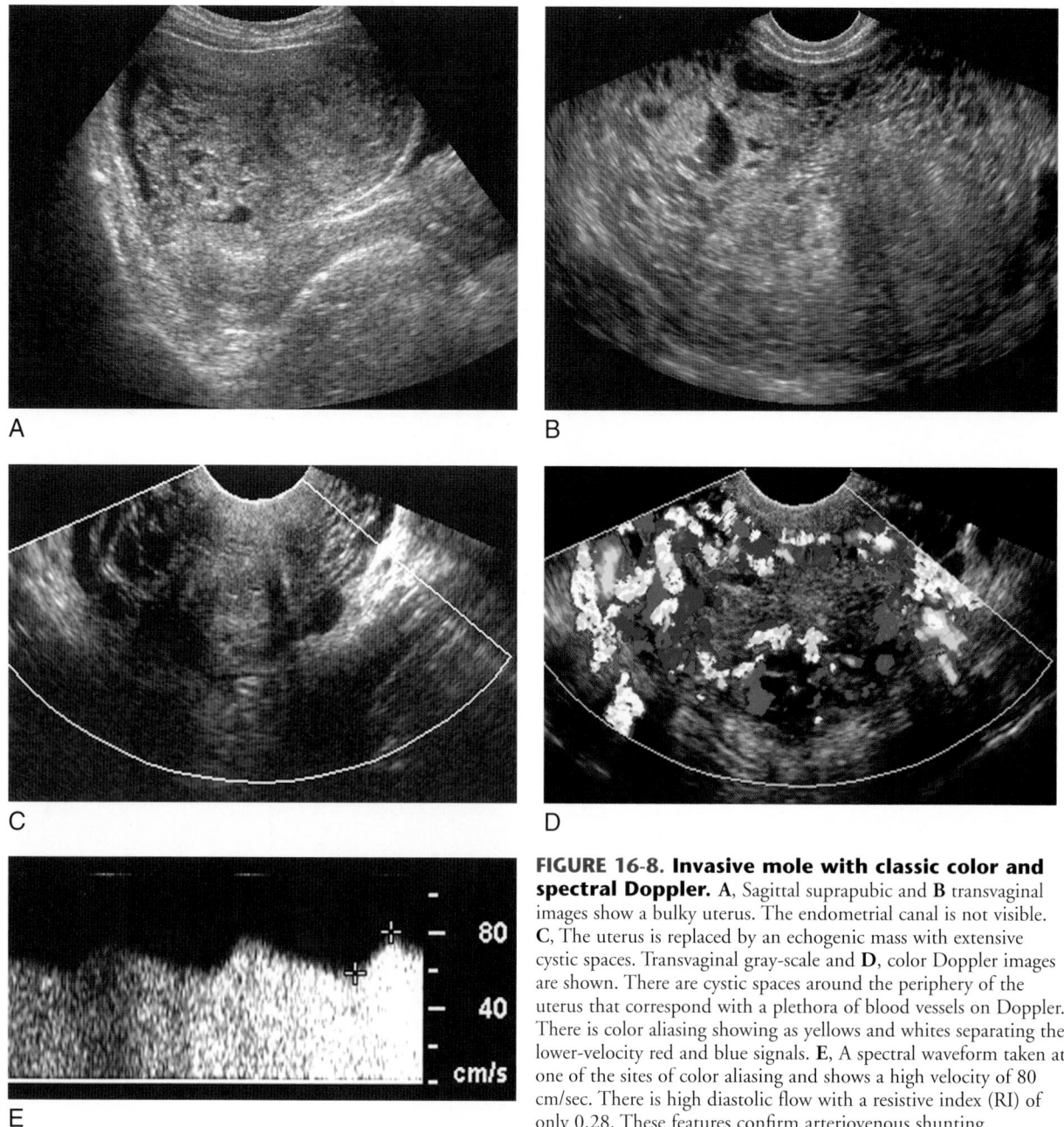

FIGURE 16-8. Invasive mole with classic color and spectral Doppler. A, Sagittal suprapubic and **B** transvaginal images show a bulky uterus. The endometrial canal is not visible. **C,** The uterus is replaced by an echogenic mass with extensive cystic spaces. Transvaginal gray-scale and **D,** color Doppler images are shown. There are cystic spaces around the periphery of the uterus that correspond with a plethora of blood vessels on Doppler. There is color aliasing showing as yellows and whites separating the lower-velocity red and blue signals. **E,** A spectral waveform taken at one of the sites of color aliasing and shows a high velocity of 80 cm/sec. There is high diastolic flow with a resistive index (RI) of only 0.28. These features confirm arteriovenous shunting.

and smaller in size (see Fig. 16-9C). Eventually, no residual abnormality is apparent in many cases.[37,39] However, up to 50% of patients will have persistent abnormalities after therapy that may be difficult to distinguish from active lesions sonographically.[40]

Normal Uterine Blood Flow. In the normal uterus, myometrial vascularity is always visible on color Doppler. Color flow is generally limited to discrete, regularly arranged vessels in the peripheral one half to one third of the myometrium. Smaller vessels radiate at intervals toward the endometrium. Duplex Doppler sonography shows signals of low velocity and high impedance. Myometrial color flow can appear increased in normal subjects with prominent parametrial vascular complexes and in conditions such as fibroids and adenomyosis. In pregnancy, myometrial color vascularity may be focally increased in the region of placental implantation. Endometrial color flow, usually absent in the nongravid uterus, is nonspecific and is seen in normal pregnancy, incomplete abortion, retained products of conception, endometrial polyps, cancer, and PTN.

Duplex and color Doppler features of PTN reflect the marked hypervascularity of invasive trophoblast.[36,45-50] The extreme vascularity of trophoblastic

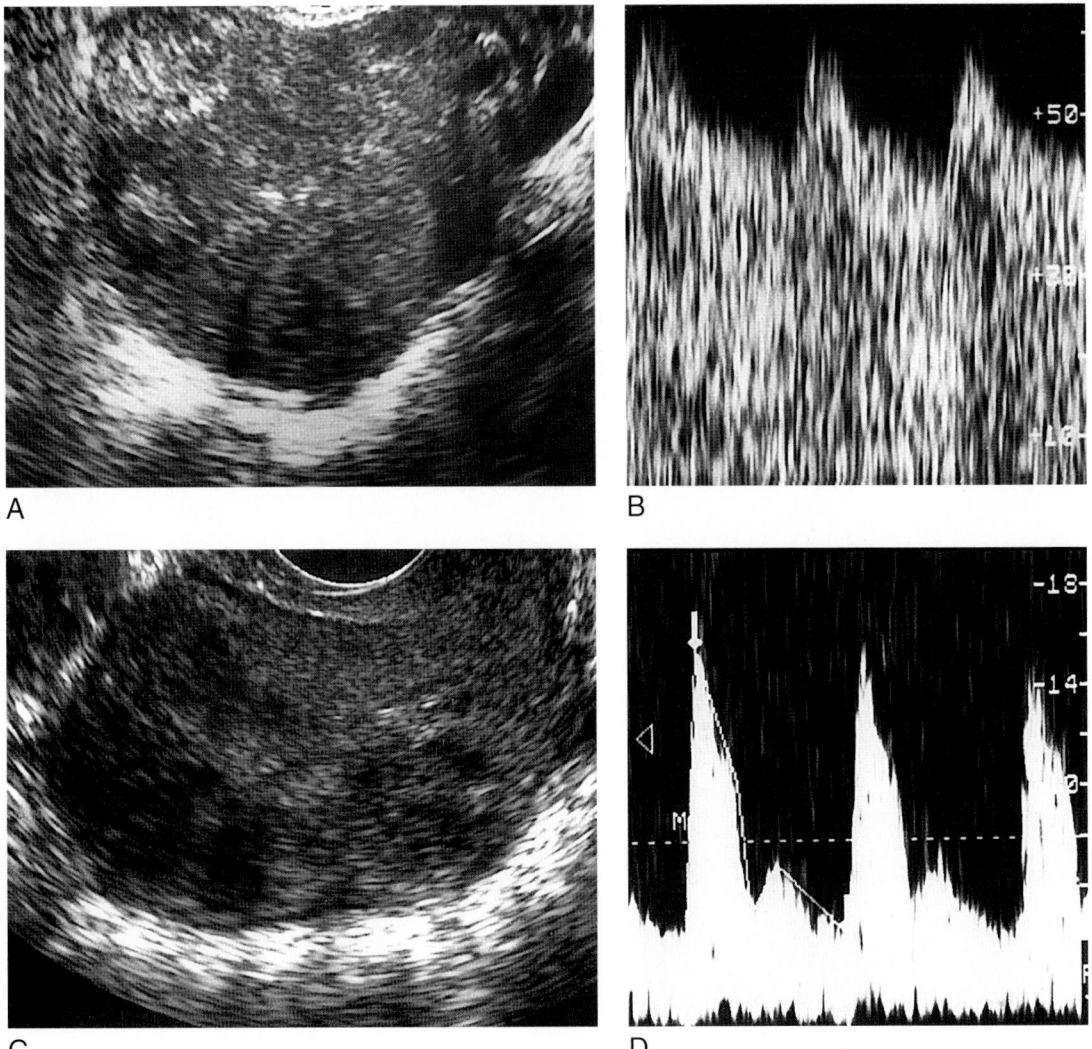

FIGURE 16-9. Bulky, lobulated uterus mimicking fibroids in persistent trophoblastic neoplasia (PTN); Doppler improves specificity. A, Transvaginal sonogram shows a bulky nonhomogeneous uterus with several areas suggesting fibroids. Color Doppler showed florid diffuse color with aliasing. **B,** Spectral waveforms show high-velocity, low-resistance flow PSV 70 cm/sec, PI 0.35, RI 0.29. **C** and **D,** Postchemotherapy, β-hCG was negative. PTN was gone. **C,** Transvaginal sonogram has improved, but uterus maintains a somewhat bulky and lobulated contour. Focal nodules are not as evident. Color Doppler showed minimal blood flow. **D,** Spectral waveform shows normal low-velocity, high-impedance flows. PSV 15 cm/sec, PI 1.43, RI 0.74, pulsatility index; PI, PSV, peak systolic velocity; RI, resistant index. (From Fraser-Hill MA, Burns PN, Wilson SR: Transvaginal ultrasound and duplex color Doppler of persistent trophoblastic neoplasia. Radiology 1993;189[P]:374-375.)

neoplasia has long been known from angiography.[50] Uterine spiral arteries feed directly into prominent vascular spaces that then communicate with draining veins.[3,50] These **functional arteriovenous shunts** produce abnormal uterine hypervascularity and high-velocity, low-impedance blood flow on duplex interrogation.[45,46,48] **Color Doppler features** typical of PTN include extensive color aliasing, admixture of color signals, loss of discreteness of vessels, and chaotic vascular arrangement. Regions of abnormal color Doppler frequently appear larger than corresponding sonographic abnormalities (see Fig. 16-8).[36]

Duplex Doppler features of PTN relate to the arteriovenous shunting. "Trophoblastic" blood flow has characteristic high peak systolic velocity (PSV) and low resistance index (RI).[36,45,50] PSV is usually greater than 50 cm/sec and is often over 100 cm/sec. RI is usually less than 0.50 and is often well below 0.40 (see Fig. 16-8).[6,45,50] In contrast, normal myometrial blood flow usually has a PSV of less than 50 cm/sec and an RI in the range of 0.70. Endometrial blood flow normally has a low-resistance pattern but is distinguished from trophoblastic flow by low peak velocity in the range of 10 to 15 cm/sec.[36] The sensitivity and specificity of Doppler in PTN are yet to be determined by a large prospective series.

Duplex and color Doppler are noninvasive and reliable alternatives to conventional angiography for

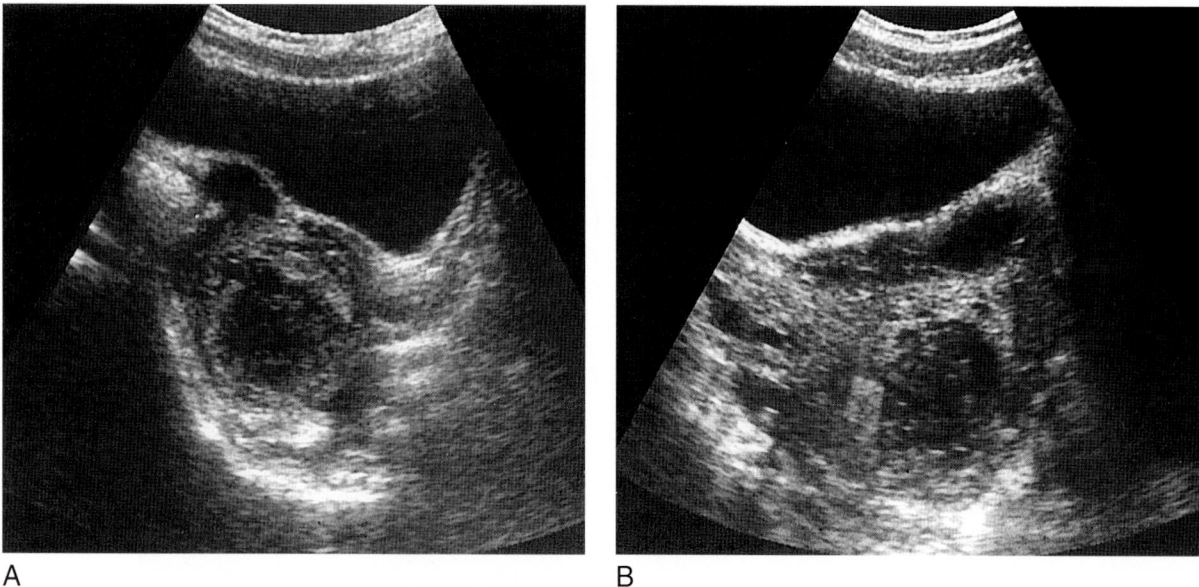

A   B

FIGURE 16-10. Choriocarcinoma. Choriocarcinoma after a normal term pregnancy, producing a large, ill-defined pelvic mass in persistent trophoblastic neoplasia (PTN). **A,** Sagittal and **B,** transverse sonograms show a large, poorly defined, complex pelvic mass with both cystic and solid components. The uterus could not be identified. Doppler showed trophoblastic signals everywhere within this mass. PTN was not suspected clinically or on sonography until Doppler was performed. (From Fraser-Hill MA, Burns PN, Wilson SR: Transvaginal ultrasound and duplex color Doppler of persistent trophoblastic neoplasia. Radiology 1993;189[P]:374-375.)

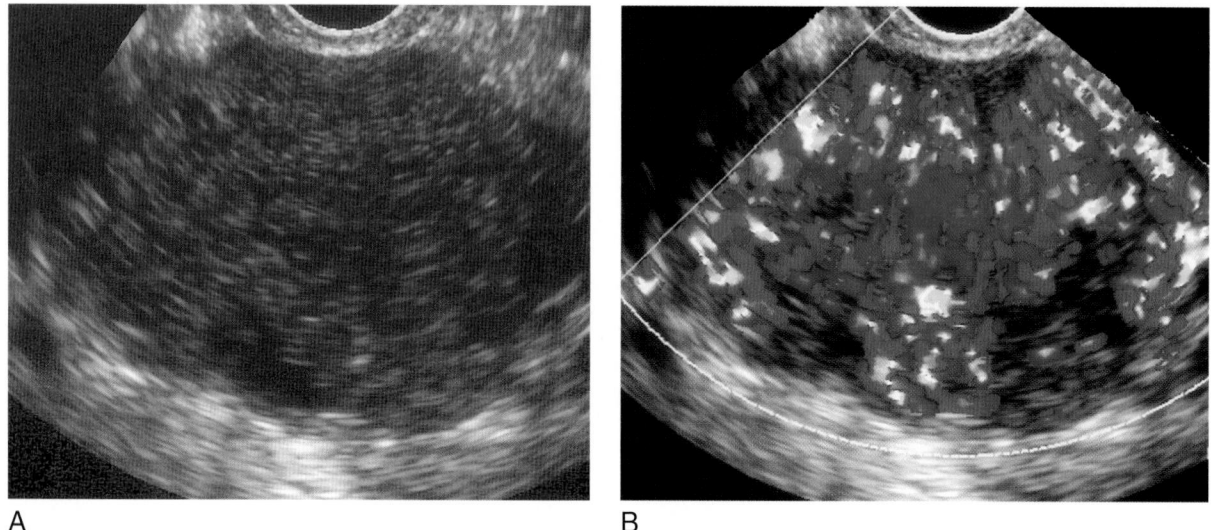

A   B

FIGURE 16-11. Arteriovenous malformation. Arteriovenous malformation (AVM) of the uterus in a young woman with severe menorrhagia following spontaneous abortion with dilation and curettage. Beta hCG was negative. AVM was treated successfully with embolotherapy. **A,** Transvaginal transverse sonogram shows a vague, subtle abnormality of the entire myometrium. **B,** Color Doppler image shows a florid mosaic pattern with color aliasing and prominent parametrial vessels. The sonographic and Doppler features are indistinguishable from PTN. Only β-hCG is discriminatory. (From Huang M, Muradali D, Thurston W, et al: Uterine arteriovenous malformations [AVM]: Ultrasound features with MRI correlation. Radiology 1998;206[1]:115-123.)

detecting and staging pelvic PTN.[48,51] In our experience, the contribution of Doppler is greater in patients with PTN than in patients with primary molar gestation. Abnormal vascularity may be difficult or impossible to detect in primary molar pregnancy but it is a major feature of PTN. Qualitative assessments of vascularity on color Doppler are not diagnostic of PTN. However, the extreme degree of myometrial vascularity in PTN is matched by few other conditions. We have not seen similar color Doppler hypervascularity except in extremely rare uterine arteriovenous malformations (Fig. 16-11), a potential pitfall.[52]

45. Taylor KJW, Schwartz PE, Kohorn EI: Gestational trophoblastic neoplasia: Diagnosis with US. Radiology 1987;165:445-448.

46. Desai RK, Desberg AL: Diagnosis of gestational trophoblastic disease: Value of endovaginal color flow Doppler sonography. AJR 1991;157:787-788.

47. Shimamoto K, Sakuma S, Ishigaki T, et al. Intratumoral blood flow: Evaluation with color flow echography. Radiology 1987;165:683-685.

48. Dobkin GR, Berkowitz RS, Goldstein DP, et al: Duplex ultrasonography for persistent gestational trophoblastic tumor. J Reprod Med 1991;36(1):14-16.

49. Chan FY, Chau MT, Pun TC, et al: A comparison of color Doppler sonography and the pelvic arteriogram in assessment of patients with gestational trophoblastic disease. Br J Obstet Gynaecol 1995;102(9):720-725.

50. Hendrickse JPV, Cockshott WP, Evans KTL et al: Pelvic angiography in the diagnosis of malignant trophoblastic disease. N Engl J Med 1964;271:859-865.

51. Yalcin OT, Ozalp SS, Tanir HM: Assessment of gestational trophoblastic disease by Doppler ultrasonography. Eur J Obstet Gynecol Reprod Biol 2002;103(1):83-87.

52. Huang M, Muradali D, Thurston W, et al: Uterine arteriovenous malformations (AVM): Ultrasound features with MRI correlation. Radiology 1998;206(1):115-123.

53. Kurjak A, Zalud I, Schulman H: Ectopic pregnancy: Transvaginal color Doppler of trophoblastic flow in questionable adnexa. J Ultrasound Med 1991;10:685-689.

54. Taylor KJ, Ramos IM, Feyock AL, et al: Ectopic pregnancy: Duplex Doppler evaluation. Radiology 1989;173:93-97.

55. Pellerito JS, Taylor KJ, Quedens-Case C, et al: Ectopic pregnancy: Evaluation with color flow imaging. Radiology 1992;183:407-411.

56. Feldman S, Goldstein DP, Berkowitz RS: Low-risk metastatic gestational trophoblastic tumors. Semin Oncol 1995;22(2):166-171.

57. Lurain JR: High-risk metastatic gestational trophoblastic tumors. Current management. J Reprod Med 1994;39(3):217-222.

17

THE THORAX

William E. Brant

Chapter Outline

$\mathcal{S}$onography is used to evaluate and diagnose a wide range of perplexing clinical problems in the thorax.[1] Although the ribs, spine, and air-filled lung act as barriers to ultrasound visualization, the presence of fluid in the pleural space and tumor, consolidation, or atelectasis in the lung provides ample sonographic windows for evaluation of most disease processes. When film radiography is unable to clarify a chest abnormality, sonography may further characterize the abnormality and limit the differential diagnosis. Sonography can be used to differentiate pleural from parenchymal lesions, to visualize diseased parenchyma hidden by pleural effusion, and to detect pleural septations and other pleural abnormalities not even suspected by other imaging modalities.[2] Ultrasound clearly demonstrates the diaphragm and differentiates subpulmonic effusion from subphrenic abscess. Because ultrasound equipment is portable, it can be readily used at the bedside of critically ill patients to evaluate thoracic disease and to provide safe and accurate guidance for interventional

procedures in the intensive care unit.[3] The patient can be examined in any position, minimizing the need for moving patients who are on life support devices. Cooperative patients can be maneuvered into a variety of positions to optimize sonographic visualization of the mediastinum and deep thoracic structures. Ultrasound is effectively used to guide a variety of interventional procedures in the thorax.[4] Most needle placements can be performed under direct and constant visualization, maximizing accuracy and patient safety. Ultrasound guidance improves the safety of thoracentesis and is effective in obtaining biopsies of virtually any lesion that can be visualized.

PLEURAL SPACE

The pleural space is superficial and is readily examined by ultrasound using either a direct intercostal or an abdominal approach. A high-frequency (5- to 7.5-MHz) linear transducer applied directly to the chest (direct intercostal approach) provides a broad, near field-of-view that allows excellent visualization of the pleural space. The lower reaches of the pleural space may be effectively examined by use of sector or convex-array (3.5-MHz) transducers directed superiorly from the abdomen (abdominal approach). The liver and spleen provide sonographic windows from the abdomen to the thorax. Sector transducers may be unsatisfactory for examination of the pleural space when applied directly to the chest (Fig. 17-1). The sector scanner has a narrow view in the near field, and near-field artifacts frequently obscure the pleural space.

Normal Pleural Space

Direct Intercostal Approach. The normal pleural space is readily identified when the ribs are used as sonographic landmarks (Fig. 17-2). With a linear-array transducer oriented perpendicular to the intercostal spaces, the ribs are displayed as rounded echogenic interfaces with prominent acoustic shadowing. Intercostal muscle is visualized between the rib shadows. The location and depth of the ribs are noted, and the thickness of the subcutaneous tissues and the overlying muscles of the chest wall are determined. The **pleural space** is located within 1 cm of depth from the rib interface. The

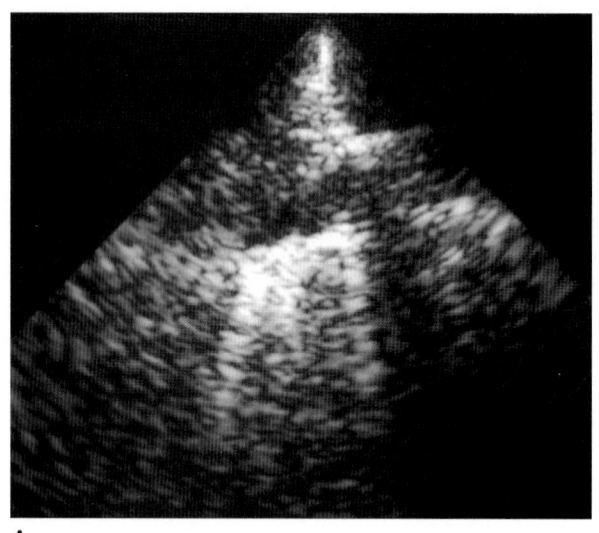
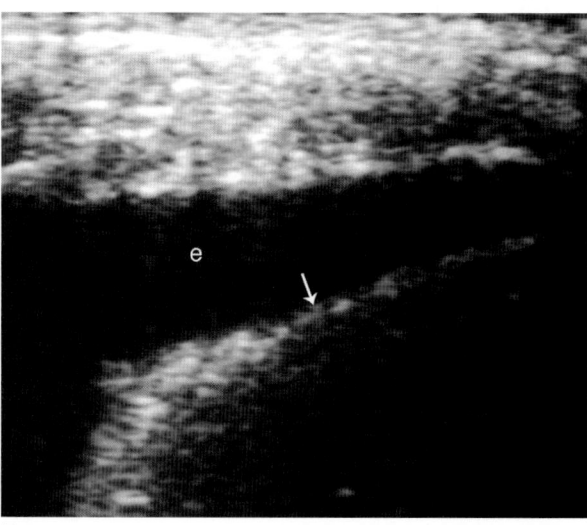

A   B

FIGURE 17-1. Linear array versus sector transducer. A, A 3.5-MHz sector transducer applied directly to the chest in the intercostal space produces a confusing appearance of reverberation artifacts with little anatomic detail. The pleural space is obscured by artifacts in the narrow near field-of-view. **B,** A 5.0-MHz linear array transducer applied in the same intercostal space shows a small pleural effusion (e). The air-filled lung produces a bright surface reflection (*arrow*) that moves with respiration.

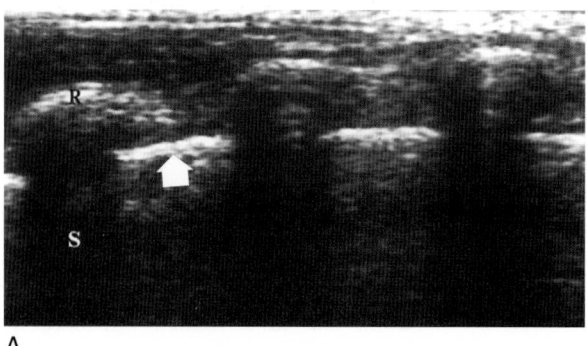
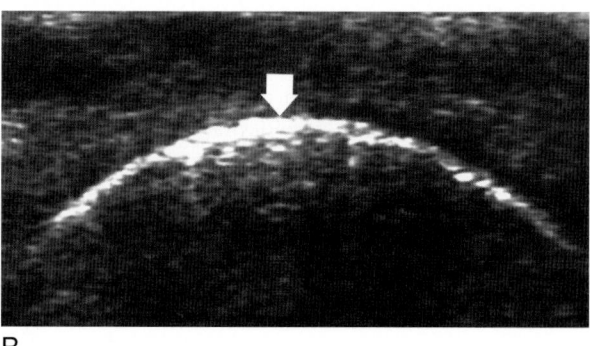

A   B

FIGURE 17-2. Normal pleural space (direct intercostal approach). A, The ribs (R) serve as sonographic landmarks to the pleural space. On this longitudinal image with the transducer applied directly to the chest wall, the ribs (R) appear as curving bright interfaces that cast dense acoustic shadows (S). The lung surface (*arrow*) is seen as a bright echogenic line that moves with respiration, **"the gliding sign."** The air-filled lung covered by visceral pleura reflects nearly all of the energy of the ultrasound beam. Echoes seen deep to the lung surface are artifactual reverberations that lack anatomic information. The spaces between the ribs are occupied by intercostal muscle that allows sound transmission. The parietal pleura is located approximately 1 cm deep to the echogenic rib interface. **B,** An image with the transducer placed within the intercostal space produces an unobstructed view of the lung surface (*arrow*) and pleural space.

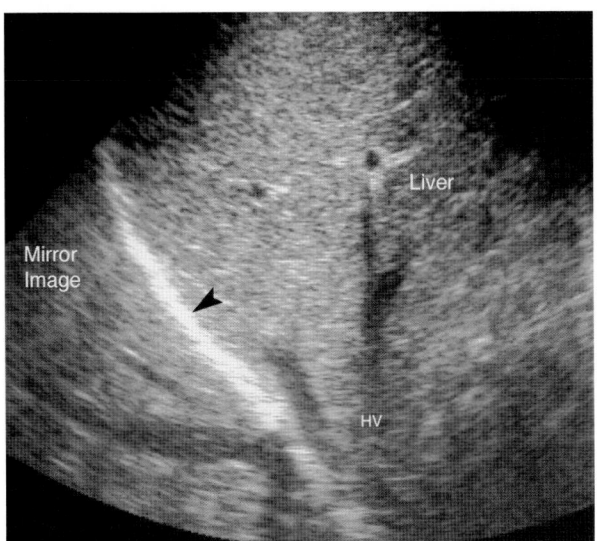
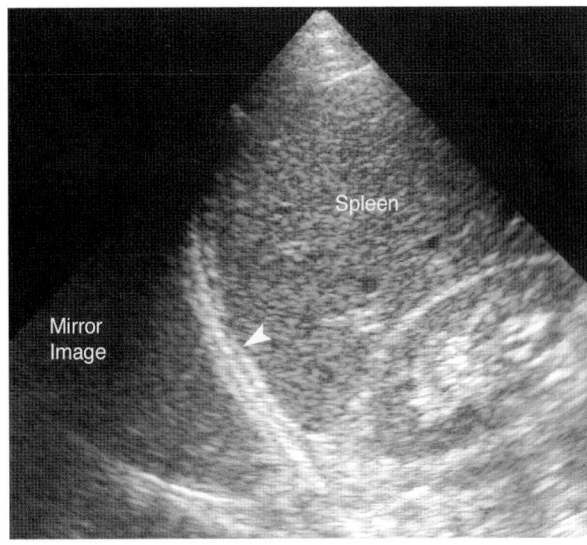

A B

FIGURE 17-3. Normal pleural space (abdominal approach). A, Longitudinal image through the liver shows the diaphragm (*arrowhead*) as a curving bright echogenic line, which can be observed to move with respiration. Because the lung above the diaphragm is air filled and the pleural space is normal, a **mirror-image refection of the liver** is displayed above the diaphragm. The mirror image even reproduces the hepatic veins (HV). **B,** Longitudinal image through the spleen shows a 5-line appearance of the **diaphragm** (*arrowhead*). The muscle of the diaphragm is seen as a thin hypoechoic line sandwiched between two echogenic lines representing the membranous coverings of the diaphragm. Because the left lower lobe of the lung is air filled and the left pleural space is normal, a detailed mirror image is produced above the diaphragm, which reproduces the hypoechoic line of muscle of the diaphragm and its echogenic coverings and the spleen. The presence of mirror-image artifact on scans of the thorax obtained from an abdominal approach is evidence of normal pleural space and normal air-filled base of the lung.

air-filled lung, covered by **visceral pleura**, is a potent reflector of the ultrasound beam, blocking sound penetration deeper into the chest and producing a bright, linear interface that moves with respiration. The normal back-and-forth movement of the lung surface with respiration is called the **"gliding sign."** The bright, linear interface of the lung surface is the sonographic marker of the visceral pleura. A thin, dark line of **pleural fluid** is normally present, separating the parietal pleura from the visceral pleura. The **parietal pleura** appears as a less distinct, weakly echogenic line, often obscured by reverberation artifact. Its location is inferred by its relationship to the ribs and the visceral pleura.

Abdominal Approach. When imaged from the abdomen, the diaphragm appears as a bright, curving, thick echogenic line that moves with respiration (Fig. 17-3). The normal diaphragm is approximately 5 mm thick and is covered by parietal pleura on its thoracic side and by peritoneum on its abdominal side. Often, the muscle of the diaphragm is shown as a thin, hypoechoic line just above the much brighter echo of its inferior surface. When the lung above the diaphragm is air filled, the curved surface of the diaphragm-lung interface acts as a **specular** (mirrorlike) **reflector.** An **artifactual, mirror-image reflection** of the liver or spleen is displayed above the diaphragm. The presence of this mirror image, although easily recognized as an artifact, should also be viewed as definitive evidence of

the presence of air-filled lung and absence of pleural fluid above the diaphragm.

Pleural Fluid

Before embarking on a search for pleural fluid by ultrasound, the patient's most recent chest radiograph or chest CT scan should be reviewed. The location of pleural lesions should be noted for correlation with the ultrasound examination. Areas of suspected loculated pleural fluid or pleural thickening can then be carefully examined.

Direct Intercostal Approach. Even minute amounts of pleural fluid can be detected by using a high-resolution linear-array transducer applied directly to the chest (Fig. 17-4). Sector transducers may be used when pleural effusions are large to image deep into the thorax, but the near-field pleural space is best shown by high frequency linear array transducers. Most pleural fluid is relatively anechoic and is easily recognized as an area of echo-lucency separating the parietal and visceral pleura.[5] The parietal pleura is identified by its position approximately 1 cm deep to the ribs. The visceral pleura is identified by observing motion of the lung as the patient breathes. The **quantity** of pleural fluid can be estimated by measuring the maximum perpendicular distance between the lung surface and the chest wall.[6] The scan is performed with the patient in the supine position and

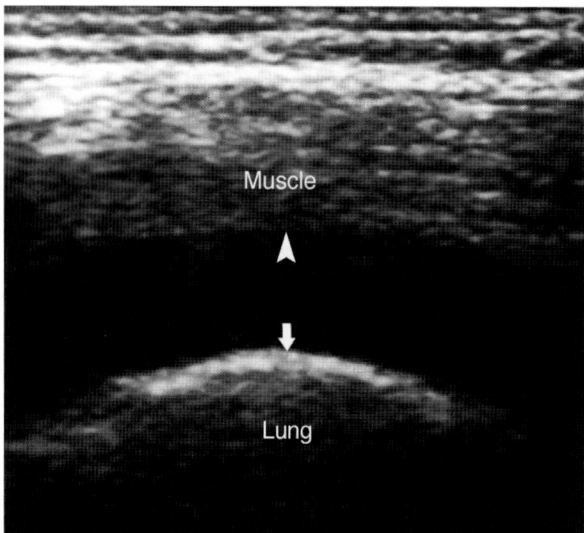

FIGURE 17-4. Pleural effusion (direct intercostal approach). Image obtained in an intercostal space using a linear array transducer shows a pleural effusion as an anechoic space between the parietal pleura (*arrowhead*) covering intercostal muscle and the visceral pleura (*arrow*) covering the lung surface. The lung is observed to move with respiration.

SONOGRAPHIC SIGNS OF PLEURAL FLUID VIA INTERCOSTAL VIEW

Hypoechoic fluid separating the visceral and parietal pleura
Floating echogenic particles
Moving septations within the pleural space
Moving lung suspended within fluid

holding maximum inspiration. Measurement is made just above the level of the diaphragm. A 20 mm width has a mean volume of 380 mL ±130 mL. A 40 mm measurement corresponded to a mean volume of 1000 mL ±330 mL.

Abdominal Approach. Pleural effusions are commonly detected during routine sonographic examinations of the abdomen (Fig. 17-5). Because the air-filled lung will block transmission of sound, the ribs and inside of the bony thorax are not normally visualized above the diaphragm when scanning from the abdomen. The presence of pleural fluid allows transmission of sound and visualization of these structures. Artifactual duplication of the diaphragm must not be mistaken for visualization of the inside of the bony thorax. The inside of the bony thorax forms a relatively straight line with rib shadows, whereas the artifactual reflection of the diaphragm is curved and rib shadows are absent.

Pleural Fluid Versus Pleural Thickening. Complex pleural fluid may be difficult to differentiate from solid

SONOGRAPHIC SIGNS OF PLEURAL FLUID VIA ABDOMINAL VIEW

Hypoechoic fluid above the diaphragm
Inside of the thorax seen through the fluid collection
Absence of the mirror-image reflection of the liver or spleen above the diaphragm
Inversion of the diaphragm with large effusions

SIGNS OF PLEURAL FLUID

Pleural lesion that changes shape with respiration
Echodensities that float and move with respiration (within the pleural lesion)
Presence of septations within the pleural lesion (that move with respiration)
"Fluid-color" sign—color Doppler signal within pleural fluid (during respiration with heart motion)

tissue in the pleural space when the fluid is echogenic (see Fig. 17-7). Alternatively, pleural thickening or pleural masses may be hypoechoic and difficult to distinguish from pleural fluid. Sonographic features indicating that a pleural lesion is fluid that can be aspirated include hypoechoic fluid above diaphragm, inside of the thorax seen through fluid, pleural lesion that changes shape with respiration, echodensities that float and move with respiration, presence of septations within the pleural lesions, and "fluid-color" sign.[7] In some cases, sonographic differentiation may not be possible, and thoracentesis must be attempted for clarification.

Transudate Versus Exudate. Transudative pleural effusions are essentially ultrafiltrates of plasma and are caused by an imbalance in the homeostatic forces that control the movement of fluid across pleural membranes. They result from an increase in capillary hydrostatic pressure or a decrease in colloid osmotic pressure. Pleural membranes are usually normal. **Exudative pleural effusions** are rich in protein and other constituents of whole blood, indicating disease of the pleural membranes and disruption of the integrity of the pleural blood vessels. Most exudates are caused by inflammatory and neoplastic processes. The common causes of transudative and exudative pleural effusions are listed in Table 17-1.

The sonographic appearance of pleural fluid is helpful in differentiating transudates from exudates (Fig. 17-6).[8] Pleural fluid that is anechoic (see Fig. 17-4) is usually a **transudate**, although occasionally anechoic fluid may prove to be an exudate. Fluid that is echogenic, contains

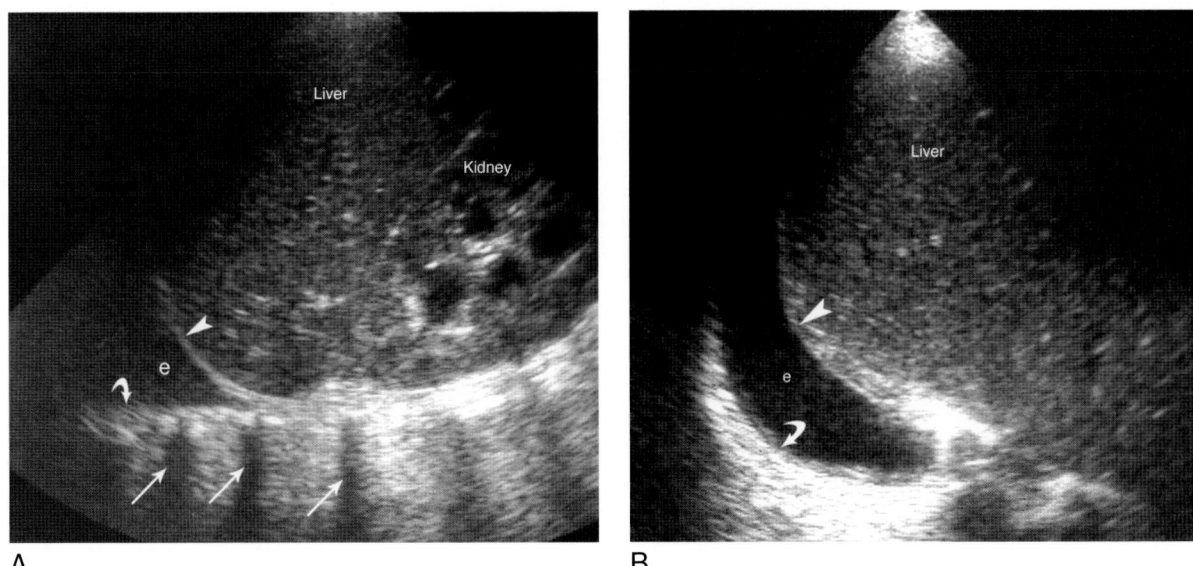

FIGURE 17-5. Pleural effusion (abdominal approach). **A,** A right pleural effusion (e) is seen as a triangular-shaped hypoechoic space above the diaphragm (*arrowhead*) on this longitudinal image. The presence of the effusion allows the ultrasound beam to traverse the lower chest and produce an image of the inside of the thorax (*curved arrow*). The chest wall is identified by the presence of rib shadows (*long arrows*). **B,** A transverse image shows a hypoechoic pleural effusion (e) between the diaphragm (*arrowhead*) and the chest wall (*curved arrow*).

TABLE 17-1. CAUSES OF TRANSUDATIVE AND EXUDATIVE PLEURAL EFFUSIONS

Transudates	Exudates
Increased Hydrostatic Pressure	**Infections**
Congestive heart failure	Parapneumonic effusion
Superior vena cava obstruction	Empyema
Constrictive pericarditis	Tuberculosis
Decreased Oncotic Pressure	Fungi (*Nocardia*, actinomycosis)
Cirrhosis with ascites	**Neoplasms**
Peritoneal dialysis	Pleural metastases (lung, breast, stomach, ovary)
Acute glomerulonephritis	Pleural mesothelioma
Nephrotic syndrome	Bronchogenic carcinoma
Urinary tract obstruction	Lymphoma
Hypoalbuminemia	**Vascular**
Overhydration	Pulmonary emboli
Hypothyroidism	**Collagen Vascular Disease**
Miscellaneous	Systemic lupus erythematosus
Misplaced venous catheter	Rheumatoid arthritis
	Abdominal Disease
	Subphrenic abscess
	Pancreatitis
	Trauma
	Hemothorax
	Miscellaneous
	Drug-induced effusion

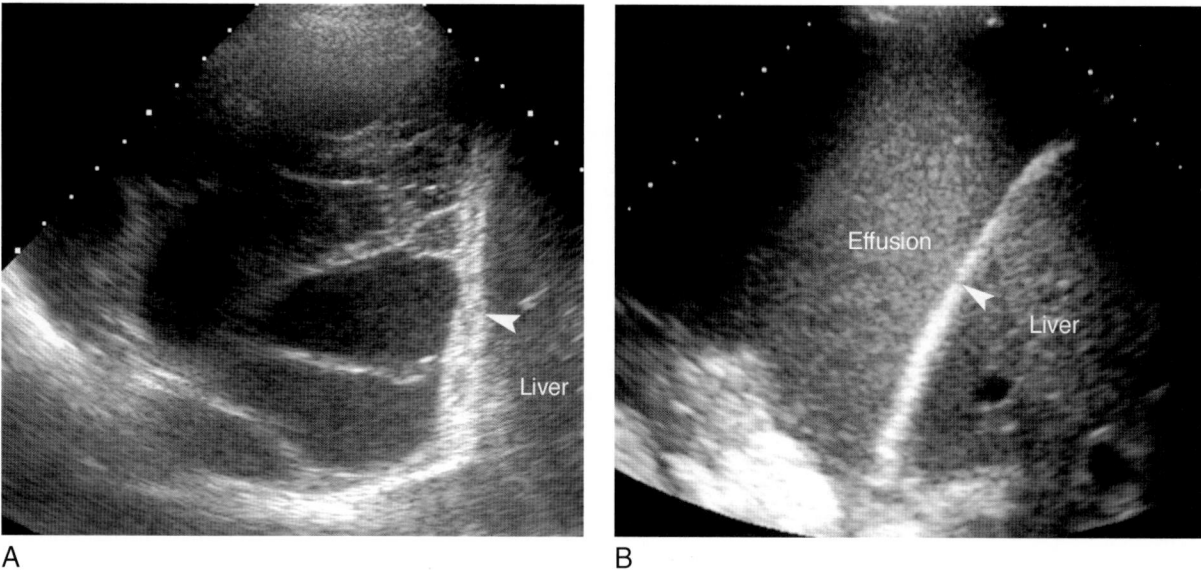

FIGURE 17-6. Exudative pleural effusions caused by inflammatory processes. A, Prominent septations associated with a parapneumonic pleural effusion are evidence of exudative effusion. The diaphragm (*arrowhead*) is flattened by the mass effect of the large pleural effusion. **B,** An empyema produces echogenic particulate matter in this large pleural effusion. This diaphragm (*arrowhead*) is also somewhat flattened.

TABLE 17-2. TRANSUDATIVE VERSUS EXUDATIVE PLEURAL EFFUSIONS

Transudate	Exudate
Clinical signs	
Pleural fluid protein/serum protein ratio <0.5	Pleural fluid protein/serum protein ratio >0.5
Pleural fluid LDH/serum LDH ratio <0.6	Pleural fluid LDH/serum LDH ratio >0.6
Pleural fluid LDH <2/3 upper limit of normal serum LDH	Pleural fluid LDH >two-thirds upper limit of normal serum LDH
Sonographic signs	
Anechoic fluid	Anechoic fluid
	Echogenic fluid
	Floating echodensities
	Septations
	Fibrin strands
	Pleural nodules
	Thickened pleura (>3 mm)

LDH, lactate dehydrogenase.

floating particulate matter, septations,[9] or fibrin strands, or is associated with pleural nodules or pleural thickening greater than 3 mm, is an **exudate**.[10] Definitive diagnosis is made by thoracentesis and analysis of the fluid obtained (Table 17-2).[11]

Parapneumonic Effusion and Empyema. A **parapneumonic effusion** is an exudative pleural effusion associated with pneumonia or lung abscess. The visceral pleura is inflamed, and inflammatory cells and fluid leak into the pleural space. Thoracentesis yields fluid with high protein concentration and an elevated white blood cell count but no bacteria. About 40% of bacterial pneumonias have an associated parapneumonic effusion.

Gross pus with bacteria or other infectious organisms in the pleural space define an **empyema**. Most empyemas occur by extension of infection from pneumonia. Trauma, surgery, thoracentesis, esophageal rupture, and subdiaphragmatic abscesses are other causes.

Parapneumonic effusions and empyemas commonly progress to a **fibropurulent stage** characterized by fibrin deposition on the pleura with loculation of fluid and formation of limiting membranes. These **fibrin membranes** are easily demonstrated by ultrasound. The final organization stage produces an inelastic membrane around the lung called a **pleural peel**. Pleurocutaneous or bronchopleural fistulas may further complicate the process. Many of these complicated effusions require catheter drainage for resolution even if bacteria do not actually contaminate the pleural space.

Pleural Thickening

Diffuse Pleural Thickening. Diffuse thickening of the pleura usually indicates pleural fibrosis (**fibrothorax, pleural peel**) or **pleural malignancy**. Diffuse pleural fibrosis most commonly involves the visceral pleura, entrapping the lung and causing restriction of ventilation. It may result from any **exudative pleural effusion, asbestos-related effusion, hemothorax,** or **empyema. Metastatic disease** to the pleura may cause diffuse lobulated pleural thickening or multiple discrete pleural masses. Calcification associated with diffuse pleural thickening favors tuberculosis or empyema as the cause. Ultrasound demonstrates solid, smooth, or lobulated pleural tissue that displaces air-filled lung away from the chest wall (Fig. 17-7). Pleural thickening is more apparent when a pleural effusion is present.

Pleural Plaques. Focal pleural thickening usually indicates fibrosis, which commonly occurs as a result of inflammation. Common causes of pleural plaques include pneumonia, asbestos exposure, pulmonary infarction, trauma, chemical pleurodesis, and drug-related pleural disease. Plaques resulting from asbestos exposure are usually confined to the parietal pleura. Ultrasound demonstrates pleural plaques as **smooth, elliptical, hypoechoic pleural thickenings. Visceral pleural plaques** are differentiated from **parietal pleural plaques** by observing the gliding sign during respiration. Calcified pleural plaques are irregular, echogenic, and produce acoustic shadowing and comet-tail artifacts. Calcified pleural plaques are commonly associated with asbestos exposure.[8]

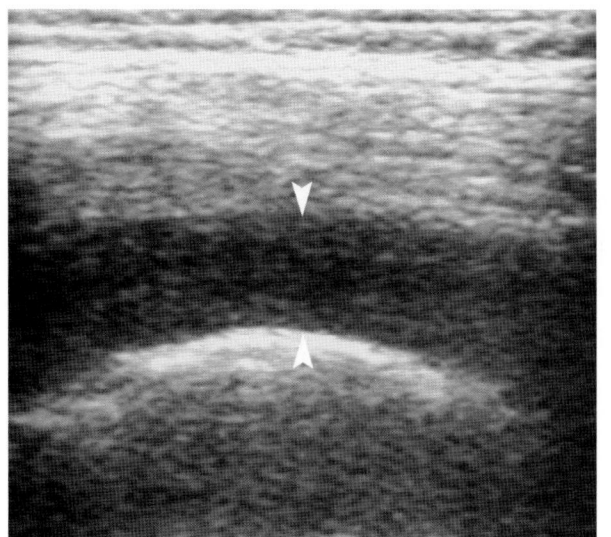

A

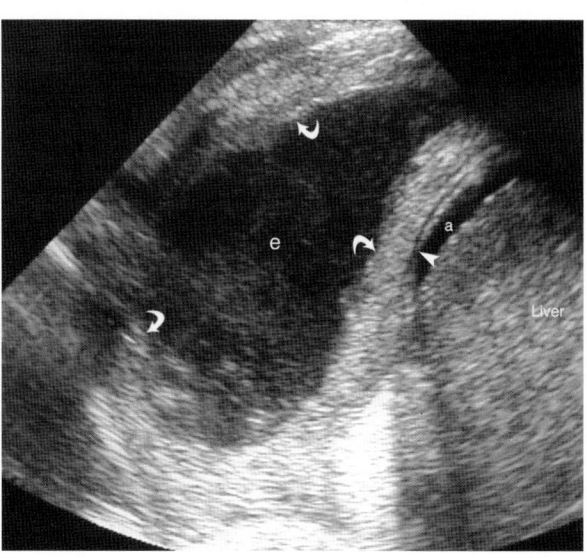

B

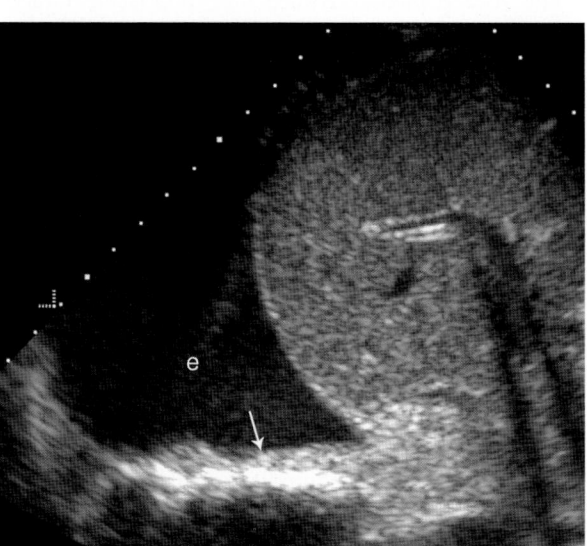

C

FIGURE 17-7. Pleural thickening. A, Pleural thickening (*between arrowheads*) in a patient with fibrothorax closely resembles a pleural effusion. The echoes in the thickened pleura did not move with respiration. **B,** A rind of pleural thickening (*curved arrows*) encases an echogenic pleural effusion (e) in a patient with empyema. A small volume of ascites (a) is seen between the liver and the diaphragm (*arrowhead*). **C,** Pleural thickening (*arrow*) lines the chest wall in a patient with lymphoma and a pleural effusion (e).

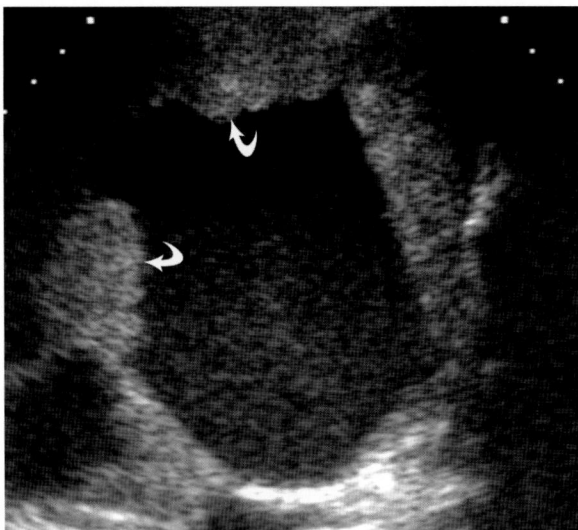

FIGURE 17-8. Pleural metastases. Metastases from malignant melanoma cause nodular masses (*curved arrows*), pleural thickening, and effusion.

Pleural Masses

Pleural Metastases. In patients older than 50 years, metastatic disease is second only to congestive heart failure as a cause of pleural effusion. Pleural effusion associated with malignant disease may result from[12]: (1) malignant cell implantation on the pleura, commonly associated with lung, breast, and gastrointestinal cancer; (2) obstruction of pleural or pulmonary lymphatics, commonly caused by lymphoma and breast cancer; (3) obstruction of pulmonary veins, usually caused by lung cancer; (4) malignant cells shed freely into the pleural space (lung and breast cancer), and (5) obstruction of the thoracic duct (usually caused by lymphoma), resulting in chylous effusion. Sonographic findings that favor malignant disease as a cause of pleural effusion are solid nodules in the pleural space (Fig. 17-8), circumferential pleural thickening, nodular pleural thickening, pleural thickening >1 cm, and pleural thickening involving the mediastinal parietal pleura.[12,14,15]

Localized Fibrous Tumors. Localized fibrous tumors are rare and usually are found in asymptomatic patients.[13,14] Most (80%) arise on the visceral pleura. They appear as solitary, spherical, or ovoid, noncalcified masses 2 to 30 cm in size.[16]

Pleural Mesothelioma. Malignant mesothelioma is a rare and usually fatal pleural tumor.[17] Most cases (80%) are associated with asbestos exposure. Imaging findings (Fig. 17-9) are (1) diffuse pleural thickening, often nodular and irregular (86%); (2) calcifications in thickened pleura (20%); (3) pleural effusion (74%); and (4) focal pleural mass (25%). Rib destruction occurs with advanced disease. Ultrasound-guided biopsy can be used in most cases to confirm the diagnosis.[18]

SONOGRAPHIC SIGNS OF MALIGNANT DISEASE

Solid nodules in the pleural space
Circumferential pleural thickening
Nodular pleural thickening
Pleural thickening >1 cm
Pleural thickening involving the mediastinal parietal pleura

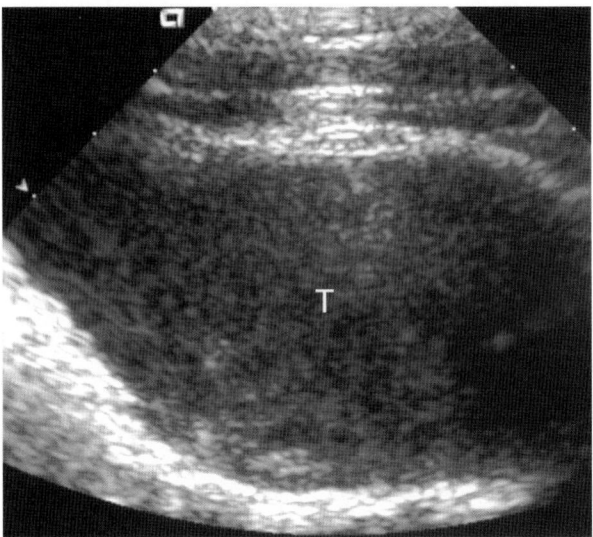

FIGURE 17-9. Localized fibrous tumor of the pleura and mesothelioma. A malignant mesothelioma shows a hypoechoic pleural mass (T). Benign fibrous tumors may show a similar appearance.

Pneumothorax

Pneumothorax is a diagnosis that can be made by sonography with careful attention to detail (Fig. 17-10).[8,19] The visceral pleura-air-filled lung interface produces a bright echogenic line of ultrasound reflection that characteristically moves with respiratory motion. In contrast, **free air** within the pleural space produces a similar bright echogenic line of sound reflection that **does not move with respiratory motion**. Disappearance of a lung or pleural lesion previously visualized during an ultrasound-guided interventional procedure also suggests the development of a pneumothorax. When both air and fluid are present in the pleural space, an air-fluid level can be identified (Fig. 17-11).[20]

Invasive Procedures in the Pleural Space

Sonography has become the imaging method of choice for guidance of many interventional procedures in the pleural space.

Diagnostic Thoracentesis. Sonographic guidance of diagnostic thoracentesis should be performed whenever

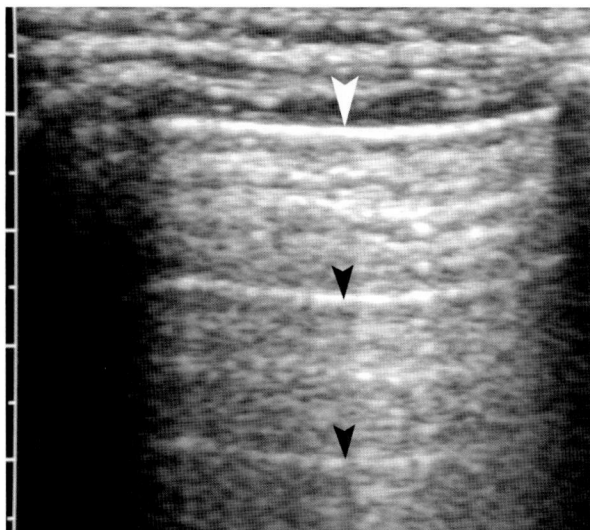

FIGURE 17-10. Pneumothorax. Air in the pleural space produces a bright linear interface (*white arrowhead*). Near complete sound reflection at the soft tissue–air interface of the pneumothorax results in a series of reverberation artifacts (*black arrowheads*) that reproduce the white line of the initial reflection. These reverberation artifacts diminish in intensity as they are repeated at deeper levels within the image. Reflection from air-filled lung produces a similar appearance. The lung surface moves back and forth with respiration (the gliding sign), whereas the reflection from a pneumothorax does not move with respiration.

clinically guided thoracentesis is unsuccessful or is judged to be difficult. Ultrasound guidance adds accuracy and safety to the procedure.[21] The incidence of pneumothorax is 18% for clinically guided thoracentesis and 3% for sonographically guided thoracentesis. The

physician first examines the chest radiograph or CT to determine size and location of the pleural fluid. The patient is then examined sonographically to identify the largest and most accessible pocket of pleural fluid. The location and depth of the fluid and its relationship to the lung are determined. Vital structures such as the heart and aorta are identified and avoided. A safe site for thoracentesis is chosen, based on careful diagnostic ultrasound examination. Actual puncture of the pleural space can then be performed blindly as long as the patient does not change position. For bedside thoracentesis in patients who are difficult to move, needle guides attached to the transducer are useful to direct accurate needle placement. Puncture of the pleural space under continuous ultrasound observation is not possible in all cases because the pleural space is so close to the transducer and the needle is difficult to track from the skin surface. The optimal patient position for diagnostic thoracentesis is the erect sitting position with the patient's arms resting comfortably on a bedside table. However, if the patient is unable to sit, the procedure may be performed with the patient in the lateral decubitus or supine position.

The puncture site is chosen in the intercostal space so that the needle crosses the top of the rib and avoids the neurovascular bundle coursing along the undersurface of the rib. The puncture site and surrounding area are cleansed with povidone-iodine solution. A local anesthetic, 1% to 2% lidocaine solution, is infiltrated subcutaneously at the puncture site. A 22-gauge needle attached to a 12 mL syringe is adequate for most diagnostic aspirations. A flexible 5F "centesis" catheter with end and side holes is useful for larger volume thora-

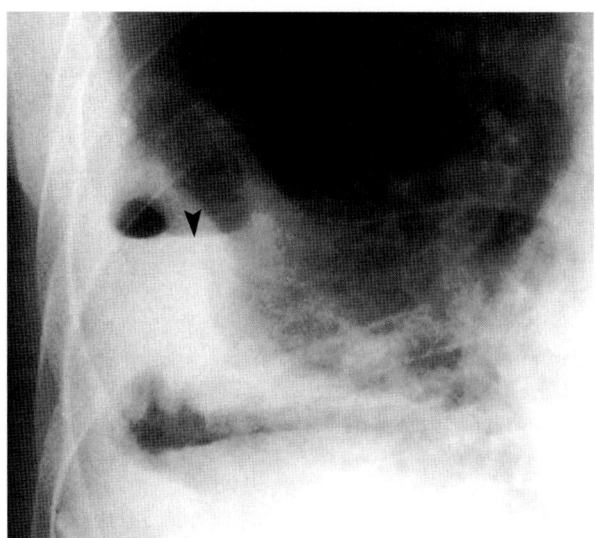

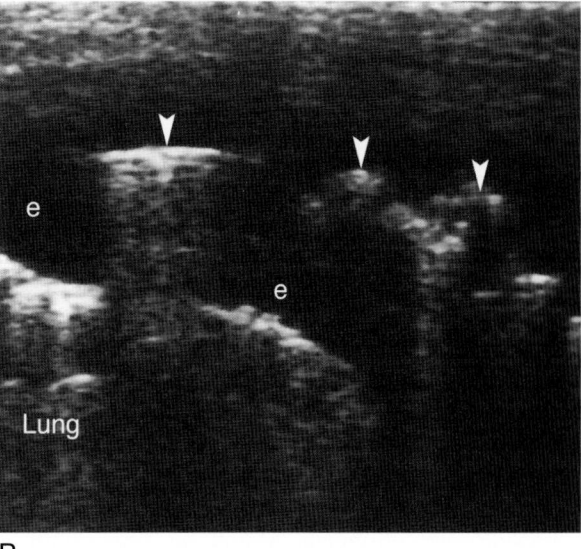

A   B

FIGURE 17-11. Hydropneumothorax. Correlate the appearance of a hydropneumothorax with multiple air-fluid levels (*arrowhead*) on a chest radiograph (**A**) with its appearance on an ultrasound image (**B**) obtained in an intercostal space. Locules of air (*arrowheads*) produce bright linear interfaces, with reverberation artifacts, with the anechoic fluid of pleural effusion (e). The air-filled lung is displaced away from the chest wall by the fluid and air in the pleural space.

centesis. If cytologic examination is planned, at least 100 mL volume of fluid should be obtained. The needle is directed perpendicular to the chest wall to puncture the pleural space. Mild suction is applied while the needle is advanced into the fluid. A characteristic "pop" can usually be felt as the needle punctures the parietal pleura. Care is taken to keep the needle tip well short of the measured depth of the lung surface. The aspirated pleural fluid is inspected for color, clarity, and smell, and is sent to the laboratory for Gram stain, bacterial culture, cell count, cytology, chemistries, and any special studies warranted by the patient's clinical condition.

Occasionally the pleural fluid may be too viscous to aspirate through a 22-gauge needle. When the sonographic diagnosis of pleural effusion is secure but fluid cannot be aspirated, the physician must first reexamine the patient to determine the accurate location of the needle within the fluid, then try larger needles (18-gauge).

Therapeutic Thoracentesis. Large pleural effusions may cause chest pain, dyspnea, or hypoxemia because of impaired gas exchange. These symptoms can be relieved by drainage of most or all of the pleural fluid. Ultrasound can be used to optimize positioning of the drainage catheter and to assess the completeness of fluid removal. To minimize patient discomfort and the risk of infecting the pleural space, complete drainage accomplished as one procedure is preferred to leaving an indwelling catheter. When large pleural effusions are present, the volume of fluid removed at any one setting should generally not exceed one liter. Removal of larger amounts may result in complications of acute mediastinal shift, including acute pulmonary edema, shock, and vasovagal syncope. Therapeutic drainage is accomplished as an extension of diagnostic thoracentesis with placement of a **flexible catheter** into the pleural space to minimize the possibility of trauma to the lung. Specially designed 15-cm-long, 5F thoracentesis catheters with side holes are especially useful for this procedure. The needle-catheter assembly with syringe attached is advanced into the pleural space. Suction is applied to ensure easy withdrawal of fluid. While fixating the needle, the catheter is advanced over the needle into the pleural fluid. The needle is then withdrawn, leaving only the flexible catheter within the pleural space. The catheter is connected to a three-way stopcock to which is connected a syringe for aspiration and a bag for fluid collection. This arrangement provides a closed system for repeated aspiration that limits the possibility of contamination of the pleural space. One liter vacuum bottles may be attached to the system to provide low continuous suction for large volume thoracentesis. Sonography is used to assess the volume and location of remaining fluid. The patient's position can be altered to access any remaining fluid. Separate loculations of fluid may be removed by additional

puncture. A small volume of fluid should be left in place to provide a cushion between the visceral and parietal pleura. Patients with neoplastic and infectious etiologies for pleural effusion generally have inflamed pleura that will cause chest pain with respiratory motion if all the pleural fluid is withdrawn and the inflamed surfaces rub together. When adequate drainage is attained, the catheter is removed. Immediate and four-hour follow-up chest radiographs are usually obtained after thoracentesis procedures to detect pneumothorax.

Catheter Drainage of Pleural Effusions. Numerous studies have documented the advantages of image-directed catheter placement over surgically placed catheters for drainage of empyema and complicated parapneumonic effusion. Catheter placement with ultrasound guidance is easier, causes fewer complications and less patient discomfort, and has high success rates. Image-guided percutaneous catheter placement is successful in treating empyema in 72% to 92% of cases, whereas success rates reported with surgically placed chest tubes are 35% to 80%.

Ultrasound is used to identify the largest fluid pocket for catheter placement. Direct puncture of the pleural cavity using the **trocar method** is quicker and easier than using guidewire and catheter exchange techniques. A relatively **stiff catheter** is needed for retention within the pleural space because the continued motion of respiration will place traction on the catheter, resulting in buckling and ineffective drainage.[22] Several catheter systems designed for empyema drainage are commercially available in 10 to 14 Fr sizes.

To introduce the catheter, the puncture site is infiltrated with local anesthetic and a nick is made in the skin with a scalpel. The catheter-cannula-trocar assembly is advanced directly into the pleural space. The trocar is removed and fluid aspiration attempted. If no fluid is aspirated, the catheter position is adjusted with ultrasound guidance until fluid is easily aspirated. The cannula is directed downward and held firmly in place while the catheter is advanced into the most dependent portion of the pleural space. The cannula is removed and the catheter is attached to a three-way stopcock and drainage bag. Aspiration is performed until ultrasound examination confirms that nearly all fluid has been removed. The pleural cavity is then irrigated several times with sterile saline solution to remove particulate matter. The catheter is sutured to the skin and connected to a standard underwater seal pleural drainage system. The catheter is placed to continuous negative suction (-20 cm water pressure), and the volume of fluid drainage is monitored. When less than 10 mL of fluid drains from the pleural space in 24 hours, the catheter can be removed.

Loculations in the pleural space may prevent complete catheter drainage of pleural fluid. Transcatheter instillation of urokinase or streptokinase has been reported to be useful in lysing fibrin membranes to facilitate drainage.[9,23] Bronchopleural fistula should be suspected when both air and fluid persist in the pleural space. Iodinated contrast agents can be injected into the pleural space to perform contrast sinography and demonstrate this complication.

Sclerosis of the Pleural Space. Malignant pleural effusions are a common cause of progressively disabling dyspnea, cough, and chest pain. Treatment is aimed at relieving symptoms, because most malignant pleural effusions are not curable. Simple thoracentesis and chest tube drainage may provide temporary relief, but nearly all malignant effusions recur within 1 month. Chemical pleurodesis is used to induce adhesion of the visceral and parietal pleural surfaces to prevent accumulation of fluid and air in the pleural space. A variety of agents have been used with varying success (60% to 80%).

Sonographic guidance is used to ensure accurate catheter placement for thoracentesis and instillation of the chemical agents, to assess adequacy of drainage and reaccumulation of fluid, and to identify loculated fluid collections. Therapeutic thoracentesis with a small catheter is performed to remove all pleural fluid. The sclerotherapy agent is injected into the pleural space, and the patient is asked to roll over three or four times to coat the pleural space. The chest catheter is clamped for 24 hours. The patient is instructed to change body position frequently to spread the agent over all pleural surfaces. Ultrasound is used to check for reaccumulation of fluid at 24 hours. If no fluid is present, the catheter is removed. If fluid has reaccumulated, sclerotherapy may be repeated. Current choices of sclerotherapy agents include suspension of sterile talc (2 to 10 g in 50 mL sterile saline),[24] doxycycline in repeated 500 mg doses, and minocycline (300 mg doses).[25]

Pleural Biopsy. Pleural masses and focal areas of pleural thickening are frequently hidden from fluoroscopic view by accompanying pleural fluid.[26] Ultrasound is effective in demonstrating these lesions and in guiding needle placement for biopsy. Pleural masses and thickened pleura can usually be biopsied using standard biopsy needles for histologic or cytologic examination.[27] Normal-thickness pleura in areas of loculated pleural effusion can be biopsied using a reverse-bevel pleural biopsy needle.[28]

Complications of Pleural Invasive Procedures. Complications of invasive procedures in the pleural space include pneumothorax, hemothorax from laceration of an intercostal artery or vein, vasovagal reaction, infection of the pleural space, and improper placement of needle or catheter into lung, liver, spleen, or kidney. Removal of large amounts of fluid (more than one liter) may cause re-expansion pulmonary edema.

Pneumothorax is the most frequent complication associated with invasive procedures of the thorax. Pneumothorax rates approach 9% for invasive procedures in the pleural space. Most pneumothoraces are small, self-limiting, and produce minimal symptoms. Some result in progressive loss of lung volume, causing respiratory distress or even respiratory failure in patients with underlying lung disease. The physician performing invasive procedures in the thorax must be familiar with catheter placement for the treatment of pneumothorax.

LUNG PARENCHYMA

Normal Sonographic Appearance

Air-filled lung, covered by visceral pleura, causes a highly reflective interface that blocks transmission of the ultrasound beam into the chest (see Figs. 17-2 and 17-3). The ultrasound image will display a pattern of bright echoes caused by **acoustic reverberation artifact**. These echoes are usually intense but formless, and they diminish in intensity with distance from the transducer. Whenever the ultrasound beam is directly perpendicular to the visceral-pleura-lung interface, however, the bright linear surface of the air-filled lung will be repeatedly duplicated on the image as a series of bright lines at fixed intervals. The strength of this pattern of reverberation artifacts also diminishes with increasing distance from the transducer. The normal lung surface is identified by its motion, gliding back and forth with inspiration and expiration, the **gliding sign.** Irregularities of the surface of the lung may cause transient **comet-tail artifacts** that emanate from the lung surface.[29] Although these artifacts may be prominent and confusing on the ultrasound image, they are to be expected and should be recognized as indicators of air-filled lung.

Consolidation

With consolidation, the air spaces of the lung are filled with fluid and inflammatory cells. The highly reflective aerated lung is converted into a firm, dense, solid mass with good sound transmission (Fig. 17-12).[30] Consolidated lung is hypoechoic as compared with highly reflective aerated lung, and, because of its high fluid content, is usually hypoechoic when compared with the liver and spleen. The consolidated lung is generally wedge shaped.[31] Air within bronchi surrounded by consolidated lung produces strongly reflective linear branching echoes that can be recognized as **sonographic air bronchograms.**[32] Aerated alveoli, surrounded by consolidated lung, produce highly reflective globular echoes that can be recognized as **sonographic air alveolograms**. The high-amplitude echoes produced by trapped air may cause acoustic shadows and reverberation artifacts. Fluid-filled bronchi produce multiple, branching, anechoic tubular structures within the consolidated lung that can be recognized as **sonographic fluid bronchograms.**[33] Pulmonary vessels can also be

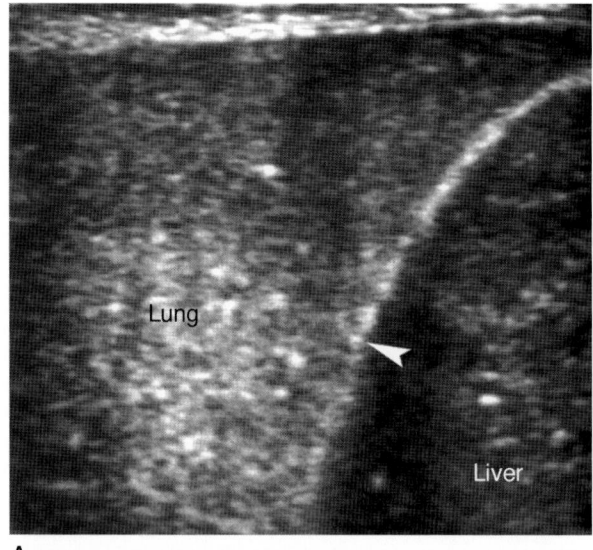

A

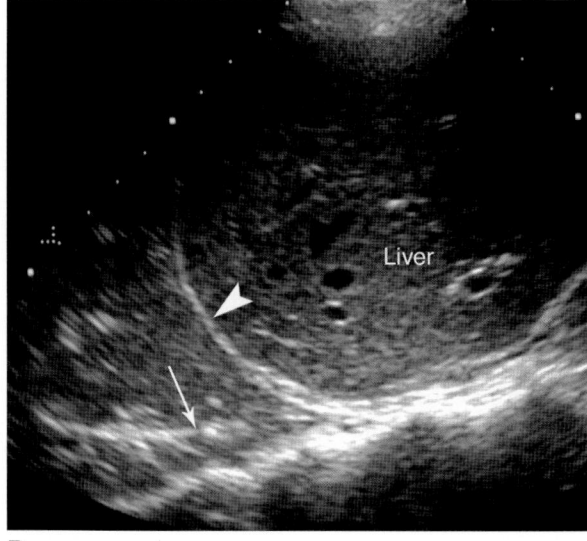

B

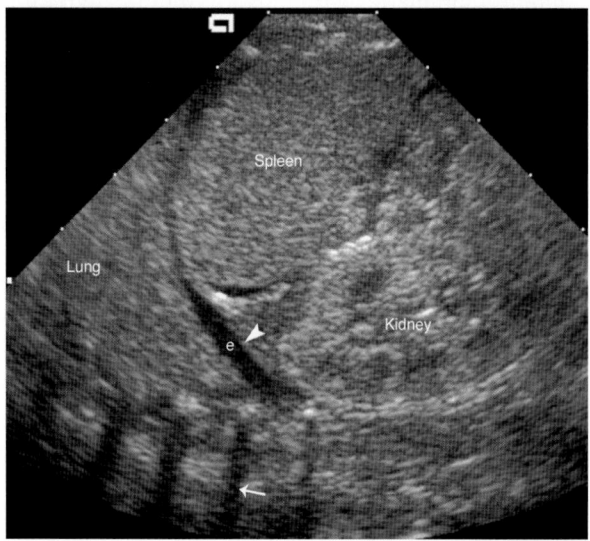

C

FIGURE 17-12. Consolidation. A, The right lower lobe of the lung is converted to a solid mass (consolidated) by filling of the air spaces with purulent material in this patient with pneumonia. The diaphragm (*arrowhead*) separates the consolidated lung and the liver. **B,** An image of the lower chest, taken from an abdominal approach through the liver, reveals an unsuspected right lower lobe pneumonia in a patient presenting with right upper quadrant abdominal pain. The diaphragm (*arrowhead*) separates the liver from the nearly isoechoic consolidated lung. Sonographic air bronchograms (*long arrow*) are seen as bright linear branching echoes. **C,** Consolidation of the left lung in a premature newborn infant with hyaline membrane disease allows sound to penetrate the lung and produce an image of the chest wall with rib shadows (*arrow*). A tiny pleural effusion (e) is seen as an anechoic band above the diaphragm (*arrowhead*).

recognized as branching tubular structures. Vessels can be differentiated from bronchi by observing their pulsatility, by tracing their origin to the pulmonary artery, and by the use of Doppler or color-flow imaging. Identification of sonographic air bronchograms, air alveolograms, fluid bronchograms, and pulmonary vasculature helps to differentiate consolidated lung from parenchymal masses and pleural lesions. Ultrasound also is useful to differentiate pneumonia alone from pneumonia with pleural effusion or empyema.

Atelectasis

Atelectasis refers to the absence of air in all or part of the lung with associated collapse of alveoli, resulting in loss of lung volume and crowding of lung blood vessels.

SONOGRAPHIC SIGNS OF CONSOLIDATION

Solidification of lung tissue, allowing sound transmission
Homogeneous, hypoechoic, wedge-shaped lung
Poor definition centrally where consolidation merges with air-filled lung
Sharp definition peripherally, defined by pleural surfaces
Sonographic air bronchograms
Sonographic fluid bronchograms
Sonographic air alveolograms
Visualization of intraparenchymal pulmonary arteries and veins
Appropriate motion with respiration

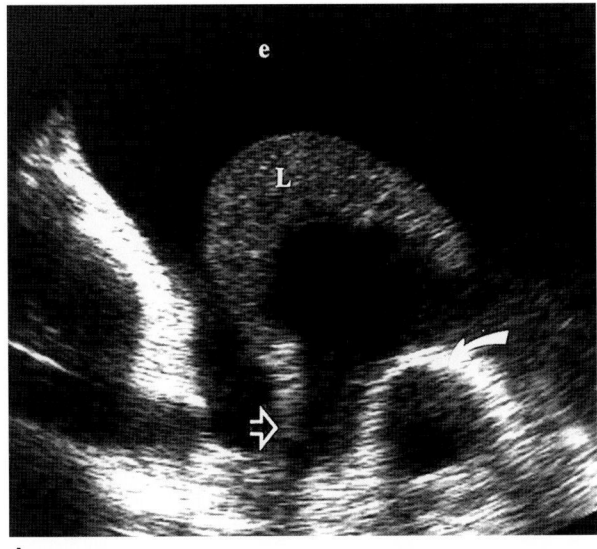

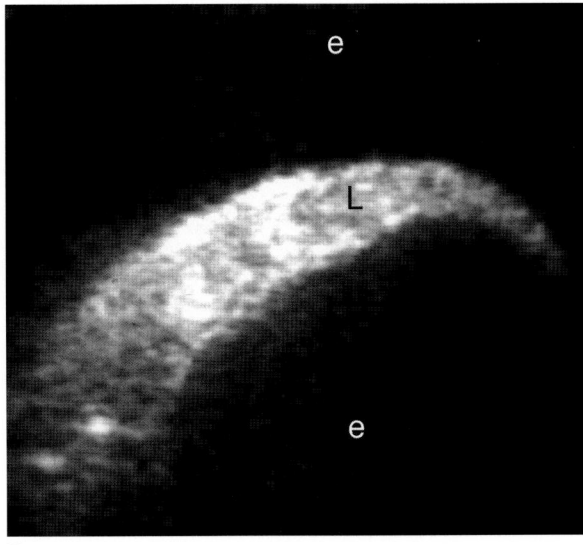

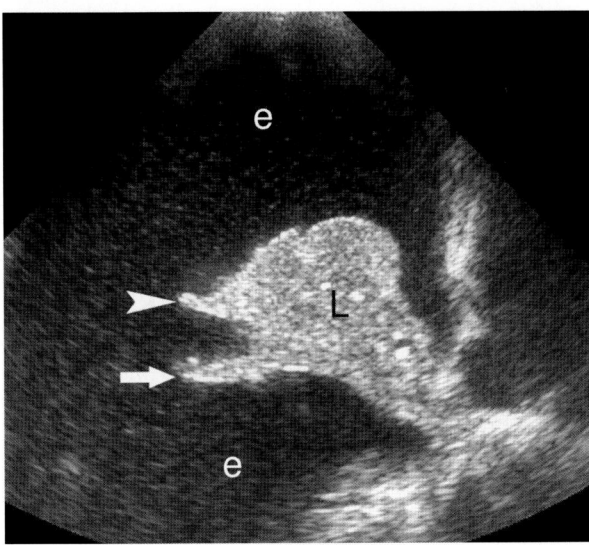

FIGURE 17-13. Atelectasis. A, Compressed collapsed lung (L) is suspended in a large anechoic pleural effusion (e). The lung sways gently back and forth with respiratory motion. The inferior pulmonary ligament (*open arrow*) and the descending thoracic aorta (*curved arrow*) are well visualized. **B**, The characteristic sickle shape of collapsed lung (L) is evident in a large pleural effusion (e). The surface of the collapsed lung is sharply defined by its covering of visceral pleura. **C**, A posterior intercostal image of the right thorax in a patient with a huge pleural effusion (e) shows total collapse of the right lung (L). The edge of the right lower lobe (*arrowhead*) and the right middle lobe (*arrow*) are evident. The presence of particulate matter within the effusion indicates that the effusion is an exudate.

Atelectasis is caused by obstruction of supplying bronchi or pressure on the lung due to a mass in the pleural space. Reflexive atelectasis always accompanies pleural effusion. Fluid in the pleural space breaks the normal adhesive forces that hold the lung open and adherent to the parietal pleura lining the thorax. Elastic tissue in the lung reflexively collapses the lung. Atelectatic lung appears as a wedge-shaped density moving through the pleural fluid in time with the patient's respirations[30] (Fig. 17-13). The echogenicity of collapsed lung is usually higher than that of consolidated lung because of lower fluid content. Crowding of fluid-filled bronchi and blood vessels may be seen within the collapsed portion of the lung. Sonographic air bronchograms are usually not present when bronchial obstruction is the cause of the atelectasis.

SONOGRAPHIC FINDINGS IN ATELECTASIS

Wedge-shaped echogenic lung
Sharp borders defined by visceral pleura
Decreased volume of affected lung
Crowding of bronchi and pulmonary blood vessels
Sonographic fluid bronchograms
Absence of sonographic air bronchograms with bronchial obstruction
Appropriate motion of affected lung with respiration

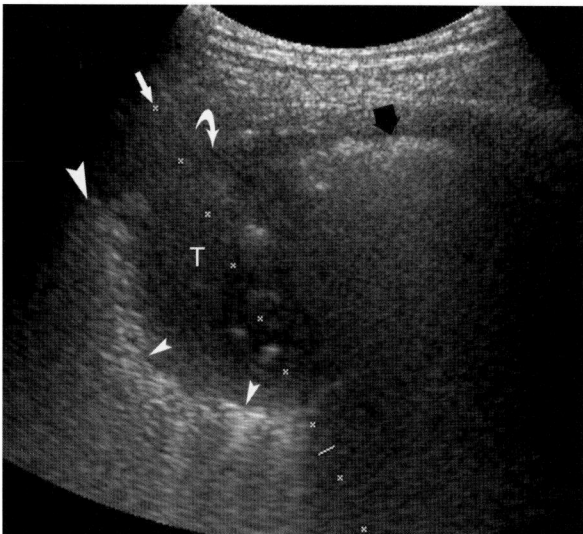
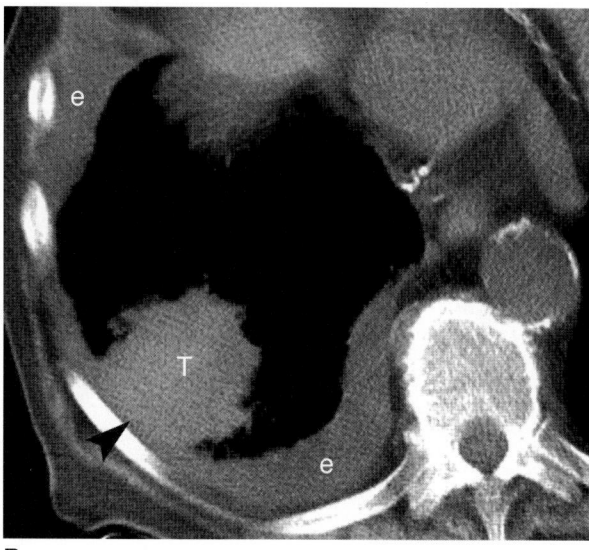

A   B

FIGURE 17-14. Peripheral lung mass. A, A peripheral lung carcinoma (T) appears as a hypoechoic mass surrounded by echogenic air-filled lung (*white arrowheads*). A rib shadow (*black arrow*) partially obscures the tumor. The tumor that abuts the pleural surface (*curved white arrow*) is hypoechoic and lacks the bright surface reflection that is characteristic of aerated lung. This mass was biopsied using ultrasound guidance. The markers (*straight white arrow*) of the needle guidance system are displayed on the image. Ultrasound guidance allows precise direction of the needle into the tumor while avoiding aerated lung and greatly diminishing the risk of pneumothorax. **B**, Confirming CT scan. CT scan demonstrates the tumor (T) partially surrounded by aerated lung. A small pleural effusion (e) is evident.

Lung Tumors

Lung tumors that abut the pleural surface appear as hypoechoic mass densities partially surrounded by highly reflective aerated lung (Fig. 17-14). The deep margins of the tumor are often well defined, as compared with the poorly defined deep margin seen with consolidation. The tumor stands out in strong relief compared to the surrounding air-filled lung. The linear surface-reflection echo produced by visceral pleura–air-filled lung interface is absent where the tumor abuts the visceral pleura. Echo enhancement is often present deep to the lesion because the tumor is a better sound transmitter than is aerated lung. Lesions smaller than 5 cm are usually hypoechoic compared to aerated lung, whereas lesions larger than 5 cm may be isoechoic compared to aerated lung. The increased echogenicity of larger lesions may be caused by internal hemorrhage or necrosis.[34] Cavitary lesions have irregular hyperechoic walls with central echolucent areas. Foci of calcification within lung masses are easily demonstrated by sonography as bright echogenic foci with acoustic shadowing. Ultrasound may help define tumor extension to pleura and adjacent structures by observing obliteration of the pleural surface echo and lack of gliding movement of the tumor with respiration.[35]

Centrally located lung tumors near the pulmonary hilum may be visualized by sonography when they are associated with peripheral lung consolidation (Fig. 17-15).[36] When the lung tumor causes obstruction to the airways, the tumor is visualized as a mass at the tip

---

SONOGRAPHIC SIGNS OF PULMONARY TUMORS

Hypoechoic mass within echogenic aerated lung
Absence of linear lung surface reflection echo
Relatively well-defined deep margin
Absence of tapered edges
Absence of sonographic air bronchograms
Mass within hypoechoic consolidated lung
Fixation of peripheral tumor during breathing
   (suggesting tumor invasion of the chest wall)

---

of the resulting triangular area of consolidation. Tumors surrounded by consolidated lung appear as a mass within hypoechoic fluid-filled lung.

Lung Abscess

A lung abscess is a localized suppurative process characterized by **necrosis** of lung tissue. **Primary lung abscesses** are caused by aspiration, necrotizing pneumonia, septic emboli, or a complication of chronic lung disease. These abscesses are amenable to cure by percutaneously placed drainage catheters. **Secondary lung abscesses** caused by lung carcinoma, pulmonary sequestration, lung cyst, or bronchoesophageal fistula generally require surgical intervention. Lung abscesses have thick, irregular walls with echogenic debris and air within the internal fluid (Fig. 17-16).[37]

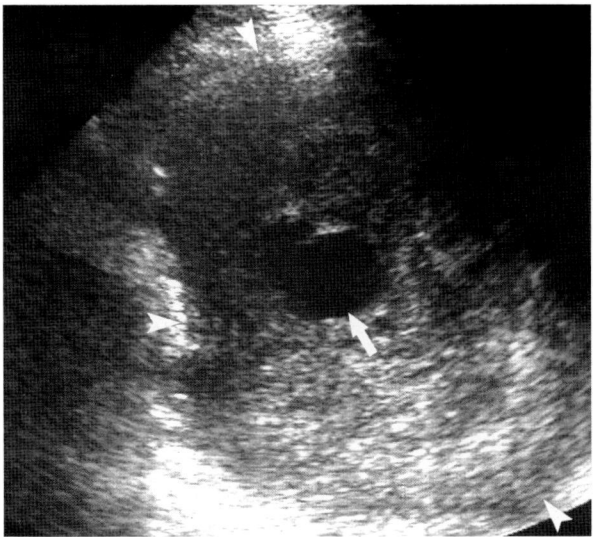

FIGURE 17-15. Lung tumors with cavitation. A large squamous cell carcinoma of the lung appears as a hypoechoic mass (*arrowheads*) surrounded by echogenic lung. Central necrosis (*arrow*) is a frequent finding with squamous cell carcinoma.

SONOGRAPHIC FINDINGS OF LUNG ABSCESSES

Irregular, thick, echogenic walls
Hypoechoic central cavity
Air echoes within central cavity
Air-fluid level within central cavity

Differentiating lung abscess from empyema is frequently a radiographic challenge. Empyemas are confined within the pleural space and tend to have smooth walls of uniform thickness. Lung parenchyma is compressed and displaced. Lung abscesses destroy lung parenchyma, are associated with surrounding areas of lung consolidation, and have irregular walls of varying thickness. With real-time sonography, a **lung abscess** will demonstrate expansion of its entire circumference with inspiration. With **empyema** only the internal wall, the visceral pleura, will show motion with inspiration.

Pulmonary Sequestration

Pulmonary sequestrations are uncommon congenital anomalies that consist of nonfunctioning lung tissue that does not communicate with the tracheobronchial tree. Most of these masses occur at the lung bases where they can be evaluated with ultrasound (Fig. 17-17). Diagnosis is made by demonstration of **systemic arterial blood supply** to the sequestered lung tissue.[38] Sonography can demonstrate the supplying systemic artery in most cases.[39] **Intralobar sequestrations** are contained within

SONOGRAPHIC FINDINGS OF PULMONARY SEQUESTRATION

Homogeneous solid mass in lower hemithorax
Fluid-filled cysts occasionally present
No bronchi are identified
Feeding artery identified arising from aorta (key finding)
Draining vein to systemic veins with extralobar sequestration
Draining vein to pulmonary veins with intralobar sequestration
Air within the sequestration will obscure ultrasound visualization

visceral pleura and have venous drainage via the pulmonary veins. **Extralobar sequestrations** are covered by their own pleura and have venous drainage via systemic veins.

Invasive Procedures in Lung Parenchyma

Lung Mass Biopsy. Sonography offers a number of advantages over CT or fluoroscopic guidance for percutaneous transthoracic biopsy of lung lesions (see Fig. 17-14).[40,41] Ultrasound-guided biopsy is quick, convenient, and safe. Biopsies can generally be performed more rapidly because real-time imaging allows for dynamic visualization of lung lesions that move with respiration. Blood vessels in the chest wall and lung can be visualized with real-time color Doppler flow ultrasound. Because sonography can visualize aerated lung adjacent to pleural-based lung nodules better than fluoroscopy and continuous visualization of the needle tip is easier than with CT, the aerated lung can be avoided more accurately. The incidence of pneumothorax for biopsy of pleural-based nodules is 2% with ultrasound guidance, as compared with 10% to 15% with CT or fluoroscopic guidance. Ultrasound, CT, and fluoroscopic guidance each have a reported 90% to 97% sensitivity for the diagnosis of lung cancer. Sonography is particularly useful in guiding biopsy of peripheral lung tumors obscured by pleural effusion. The obvious limitation of using ultrasound is that the target lesion must be visualized by ultrasound. A portion of the lesion must extend to the pleural surface to allow ultrasound detection. Lesions that are entirely surrounded by air-filled lung are not amenable to ultrasound-guided biopsy.

Preliminary inspection of the chest radiograph is essential in planning the approach to ultrasound-guided biopsy. Most lung lesions may be visualized and biopsied through the intercostal space. Lesions at the lung apex may be approached from either above or below the

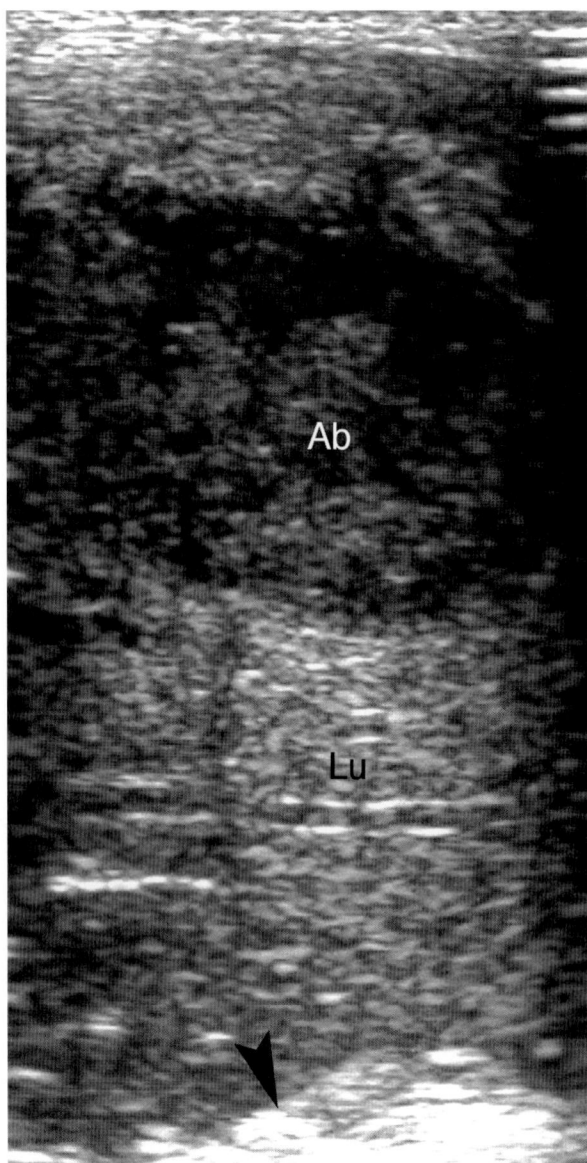

A

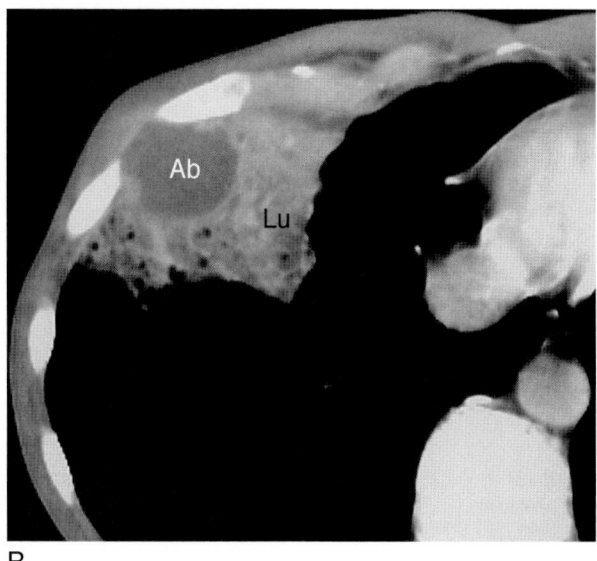

B

FIGURE 17-16. Lung abscess. A, Intercostal ultrasound image shows a lung abscess (Ab) as an hypoechoic cystic mass with echogenic internal debris that was observed to shift in location with changes in patient position. Adjacent lung (Lu) shows dense consolidation. Aerated lung produces a bright reflection (*arrowhead*). **B,** Corresponding CT scan shows the abscess (Ab) and the consolidated lung (Lu).

clavicle. Lesions on the diaphragm may be visualized and biopsied using an upward angle through the liver. Once the lesion is visualized, a safe course for the needle is determined. Needle entry into the lesion is performed either freehand or by using a needle guidance attachment to the transducer. The patient is asked to suspend respiration while the needle is being advanced into the lesion. The patient may then resume shallow respiration while the needle is allowed to swing freely. The patient is again asked to stop breathing while the biopsy is taken. Fine-needle aspiration (FNA) specimens are given to a cytopathologist for immediate examination for adequacy. Biopsies are repeated until diagnostic tissue is obtained. Cutting needle biopsies, up to 14-gauge for histology, provide an additional safe option.[42,43] The presence of a cytopathologist in the biopsy suite is essential to maximize diagnostic yield from FNA while

minimizing the number of needle passes. Core biopsy samples for histology can be obtained from large lesions.
Catheter Drainage of Lung Abscess. Most lung abscesses are successfully treated with antibiotics and bronchoscopic internal drainage. Treatment failures are considered candidates for lobectomy. External drainage by catheter was successfully used prior to availability of antibiotics and has been reaffirmed as a successful treatment method with a low complication rate. Ultrasound guidance may be used to accurately direct placement of a large-bore surgical tube or to place a smaller "radiology" catheter. The technique for catheter placement is the same as that used for empyema drainage.
Complications of Invasive Procedures in the Lung Parenchyma. Pneumothorax and minor bleeding are the most frequent complications of lung biopsy. The significance of pneumothorax is greatest in patients with

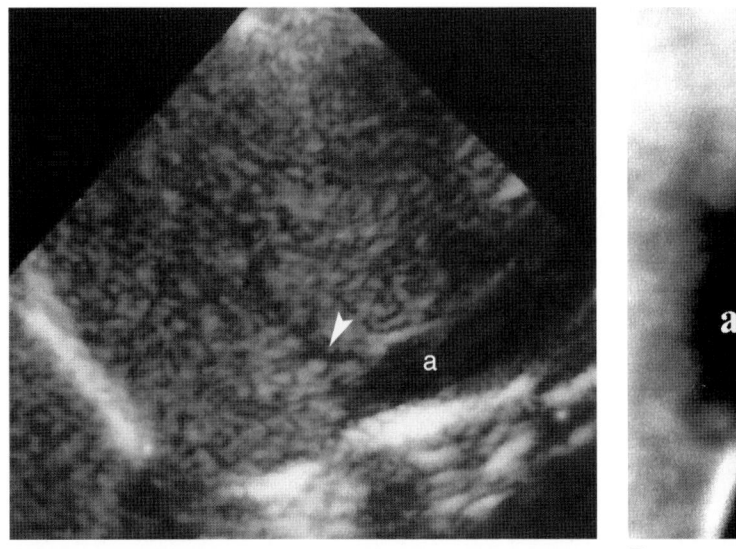
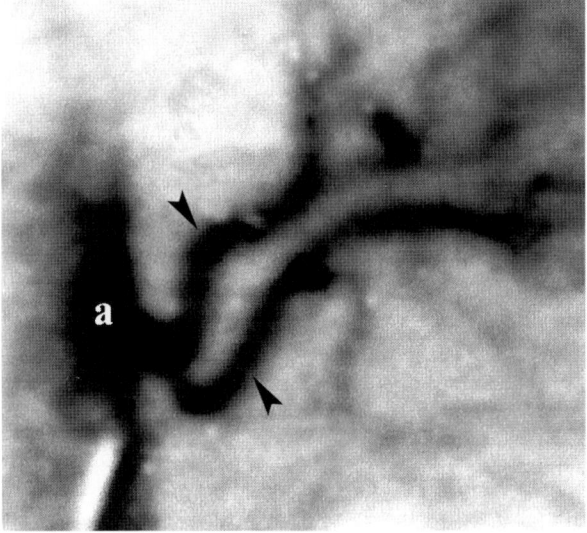

A

B

FIGURE 17-17. Pulmonary sequestration. A, Ultrasound reveals a homogeneous solid mass representing a pulmonary sequestration. A systemic artery (*arrowhead*) arising from the aorta (a) supplies the pulmonary mass. **B,** Arteriography shows two systemic arteries (*arrowheads*) arising from the aorta (a) to supply the mass.

severely compromised pulmonary function. The risk of bleeding is increased in patients with coagulopathy. Rare complications include major bleeding, air embolism, and neoplastic seeding of the needle tract.

MEDIASTINUM

Because the mediastinum is surrounded by shadowing bone and reflective lung, it offers a challenge to sonographic evaluation. However, with careful attention to technique and patient positioning, most areas of the mediastinum can be effectively examined. Ultrasound is best for examination of the superior and anterior mediastinum and is less useful for the posterior mediastinum and paravertebral region.[44] When abnormalities are detected, sonographic guidance can be used for biopsy. The ability to visualize the needle continually as it courses to the lesion is a significant advantage because this area is so rich with major vascular structures. Detailed knowledge of the three-dimensional anatomy of the mediastinum is critical because the planes of sonographic examination are usually oblique and not readily related to the standard orthogonal planes of computed tomography and magnetic resonance imaging.

Normal Sonographic Appearance

The upper mediastinum is accessible to sonographic investigation by use of a **suprasternal approach** (Fig. 17-18).[45] Patients are examined in a supine position with a pillow placed beneath the shoulders and the neck extended. The transducer is placed at the base

of the neck and angled caudally behind the manubrium. Oblique sagittal and coronal plane images can be obtained. The innominate veins and common carotid, brachiocephalic, and subclavian arteries are examined. Each vessel is identified by its location and Doppler characteristics. Tortuous vessels, which cause abnormal widening of the mediastinum on chest radiographs, are easily recognized. Mediastinal masses are precisely localized and characterized as solid, cystic, vascular, or calcified. The relationship of masses to cardiac and vascular structures can be accurately defined.

Parasternal scanning of the mediastinum is aided by placing the patient in the appropriate lateral decubitus position.[46] Gravity enlarges the sonographic window by swinging the mediastinum downward. The ascending aorta, anterior mediastinum, and subcarinal region are best imaged from a **right parasternal approach** with the patient lying with the right side down. The pulmonary trunk and left side of the anterior mediastinum are best imaged with a **left parasternal approach** (Fig. 17-19) with the patient in a left lateral decubitus position.

Large posterior masses may be imaged from a **posterior paravertebral approach**. Lesions near the diaphragm are evaluated from the abdomen through the liver or spleen. Large masses displace lung and may be imaged directly through the intercostal spaces.

The **thymus** (see Fig. 17-19) is a prominent normal anterior mediastinal structure in children up to 8 years of age.[47,48] The thymus has two well-defined, triangle-shaped lobes with homogeneous echogenicity slightly less than the thyroid gland.[49] The normal gland is closely applied to mediastinal vessels and may completely encircle the left innominate vein. In infants less than 2

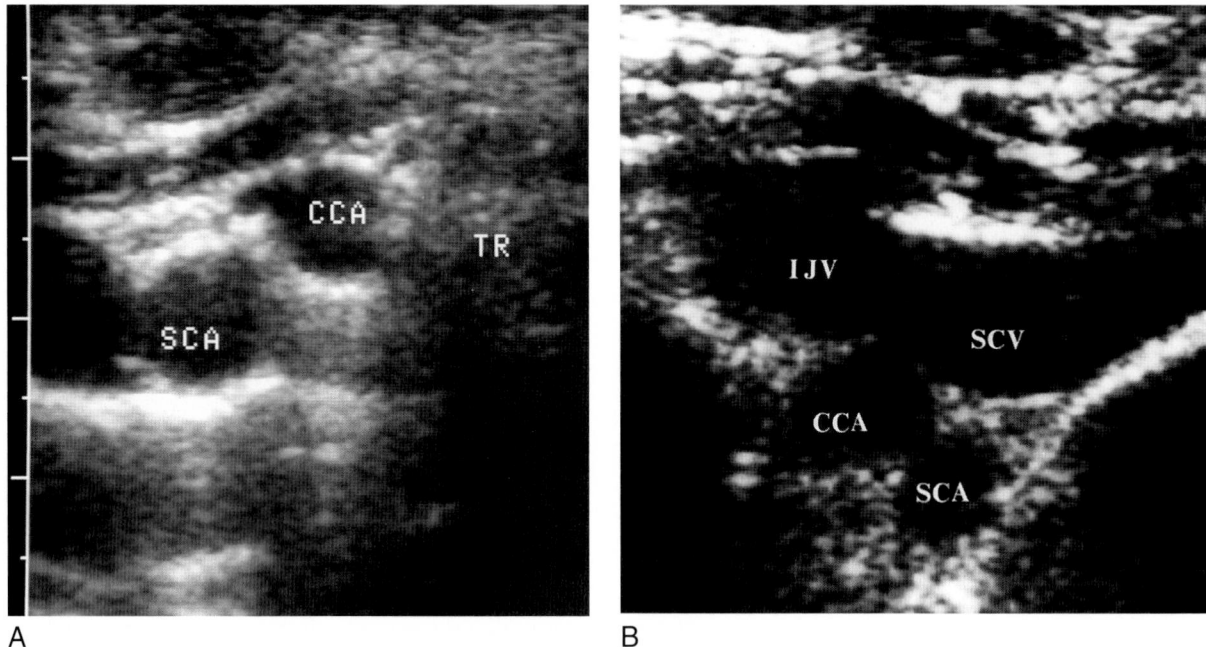

FIGURE 17-18. The upper mediastinum, suprasternal approach. A, A suprasternal view of the right superior mediastinum shows the right subclavian artery (SCA) and right common carotid artery (CCA) just lateral to the trachea (TR). This image is taken just above the bifurcation of the brachiocephalic artery. **B,** A suprasternal view of the left superior mediastinum shows the left internal jugular vein (IJV) at its junction with the left subclavian vein (SCV). The left common carotid artery (CCA) and left subclavian artery (SCA) are also visualized. Identification of blood vessels is made by anatomic position and is confirmed by Doppler characteristics.

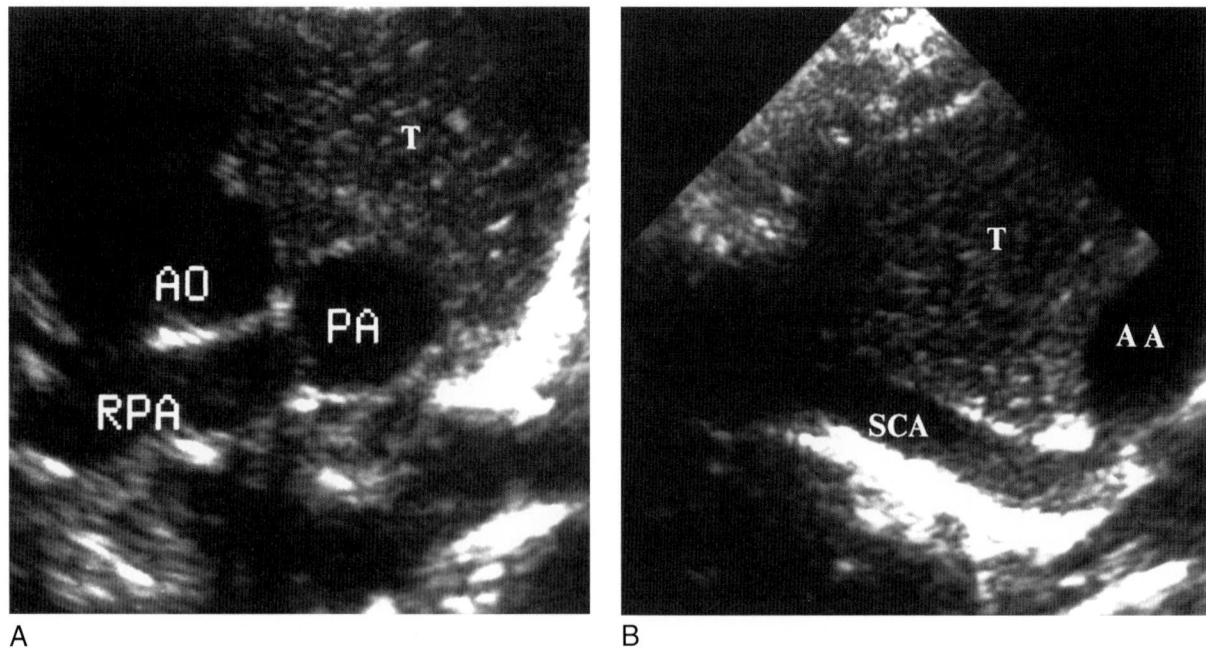

FIGURE 17-19. The anterior mediastinum, left parasternal approach. A, Transverse scan obtained in an intercostal space from a left parasternal approach reveals a prominent thymus (T) in a 2-year-old patient. The ascending aorta (AO), main pulmonary artery (PA), and right pulmonary artery (RPA) are also seen. **B,** Longitudinal scan in the same position as in **A** shows the aortic arch (AA) and the origin of the left subclavian artery (SCA). The thymus (T) serves as an excellent sonographic window.

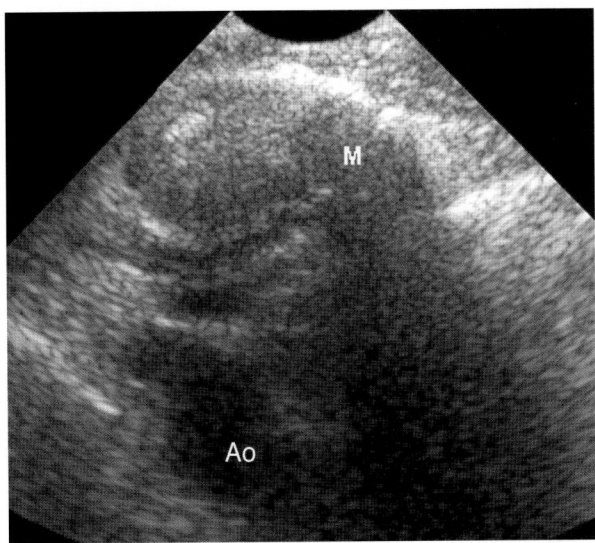 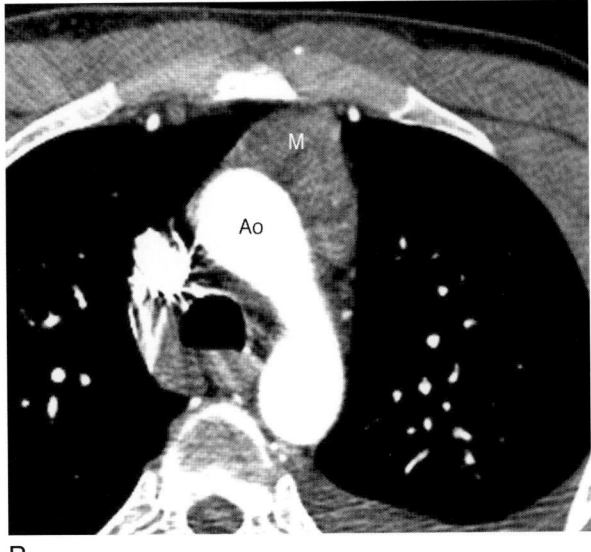

FIGURE 17-20. Mediastinal lymphoma. A, Lymphoma in the anterior mediastinum coalesces involved lymph nodes into a relatively homogeneous mass (M) anterior to the ascending aorta (Ao). **B,** Corresponding CT scan shows the mass (M) and the aorta (Ao). Core biopsy using ultrasound guidance confirmed the diagnosis of lymphoma.

years old, the normal thymus extends from the thoracic inlet to the base of the heart. From age 2 to 8 years, the thymus remains a prominent sonographic landmark when scanning the mediastinum, even though it is less obvious on chest radiographs. Progressive fatty replacement makes the thymus blend with mediastinal fat and become sonographically invisible in older children and adults. Sonographic visualization of the thymus in an adult suggests neoplastic disease.

Lymphadenopathy

Because normal mediastinal lymph nodes are generally not seen sonographically, every visualized lymph node (see Fig. 17-15B) should be considered to be abnormally enlarged due to an inflammatory or neoplastic process. Most **inflammatory nodes** are hypoechoic.[50] **Neoplastic nodes** tend to be hypoechoic when small (<2 cm) and complex and septated when large. **Calcified nodes** are echogenic and cast acoustic shadows. **Lymphoma** characteristically causes coalescence of individual nodes into a large, homogeneous, solid mass (Fig. 17-20). With response to therapy, the lymphomatous mass shrinks and becomes more echogenic.

Solid Masses

Accurate sonographic diagnosis of solid mediastinal masses is usually not possible.[50,51] The major role of sonography is to differentiate solid from cystic from vascular masses and to guide biopsy procedures.[52] However, extension of thyroid tissue into the mediasti-

CAUSES OF SOLID MEDIASTINAL MASSES

Thymic masses
  Normal thymus
  Hyperplastic thymus
  Thymoma
  Thymolipoma
  Thymic lymphoma
Lymph Nodes
  Lymphoma
  Metastases
  Granulomatous disease
  Lymph node hyperplasia
Thyroid Masses
  Goiter
  Thyroid adenoma
  Thyroid carcinoma
  Thyroiditis
Germ Cell Tumors
  Teratoma
  Embryonal cell carcinoma
  Choriocarcinoma
  Seminoma
Parathyroid Masses
  Ectopic parathyroid adenoma
Neurogenic Masses
  Schwannoma
  Neurofibroma
  Paraganglioma
Primary Tumors
  Esophageal carcinoma
  Tracheal/bronchial tumor
  Mesenchymal tumor

num is usually easily demonstrated sonographically by noting continuity with the thyroid gland in the neck.

Vascular Lesions

Ultrasound is an excellent, noninvasive method of diagnosing masses of vascular origin in the mediastinum.[53] Many abnormalities seen on chest radiographs and suspected of being of vascular origin can be definitively evaluated by ultrasound using real-time imaging supplemented by color-flow and spectral Doppler.

Cystic Masses

Cystic lesions account for about 21% of all primary mediastinal masses. Ultrasound is used to characterize wall thickness, septations, vascularity, appearance of internal fluid, location, and relationship to adjacent structures. Differential diagnosis includes thymic masses, germ cell tumors, thyroid masses, and bronchogenic and pericardial cysts.

CAUSES OF VASCULAR MASSES IN THE MEDIASTINUM

Arterial Causes
  Tortuous brachiocephalic artery
  Aneurysm of the aorta
  Aneurysm of the sinus of Valsalva
  Right-sided aortic arch
  Double aortic arch
Venous Causes
  Dilated superior vena cava
  Esophageal varices
  Enlarged azygous vein
  Enlarged hemiazygos vein
  Congenital anomalies

CAUSES OF CYSTIC MEDIASTINAL MASSES

Thymic Mass
  Thymoma (cystic degeneration)
  Thymic cyst
  Thymic lymphoma (cystic degeneration)
Germ Cell Tumors
  Dermoid cyst
Thyroid Mass (cystic degeneration)
  Adenomatous degeneration
  Carcinoma
  Adenomatous hyperplasia
Bronchogenic Cyst
Pericardial Cyst

Invasive Procedures in the Mediastinum

Ultrasound is a fully accepted image-guidance method for percutaneous aspiration or needle biopsy of mediastinal lesions in the anterior and superior mediastinum.[54] The simplicity, accuracy, and safety of sonographic guidance are significant advantages for accessible lesions.[55] Large lesions that abut the chest wall are most amenable to ultrasound-directed biopsy. Ultrasound-guided FNA biopsy is reported to be 77% sensitive for malignancy. Sensitivity is improved to 84% with ultrasound-guided core biopsies for histologic rather than cytologic diagnosis.

The patient is positioned to optimize ultrasonographic visualization of the lesion and to achieve continuous visualization of the needle path. Adjacent vital structures are visualized and avoided. Pneumothorax, hemoptysis, and hemorrhage are the most common complications reported with mediastinal biopsy procedures.

References

1. Brant WE: Chest Ultrasound. In Brant WE: The Core Curriculum—Ultrasound. Philadelphia, Lippincott Williams & Wilkins, 2001, pp 433-456.
2. Yuan A, Yang PC, Chang YC, et al: Value of chest sonography in the diagnosis and management of acute chest disease. J Clin Ultrasound 2001;29:78-86.
3. Yu C, Yang P, Chang D, Luh K: Diagnostic and therapeutic use of chest sonography: Value in critically ill patients. AJR 1992;159:695-701.
4. Klein JS, Schultz S, Heffner JE: Interventional radiology of the chest: image-guided percutaneous drainage of pleural effusions, lung abscesses, and pneumothorax. AJR 1995;164:581-588.
5. McLoud T, Flower C: Imaging the pleura: Sonography, CT, and MR imaging. AJR 1991;156:1145-1153.
6. Eibenberger K, Dock W, Ammann M, et al: Quantification of pleural effusions: Sonography versus radiography. Radiology 1994;191:681-684.
7. Wu R, Yang P, Kuo S, Luh K: Fluid color sign: A useful indicator for discrimination between pleural thickening and pleural effusion. J Ultrasound Med 1995;14:767-769.
8. Wernecke K: Sonographic features of pleural disease. AJR 1997;168:1061-1066.
9. Chen KY, Liaw YS, Wang HC, et al: Sonographic septation: A useful prognostic indicator of acute thoracic empyema. J Ultrasound Med 2000;19:837-843.
10. Yang PC, Luh KT, Chang DB, et al: Value of sonography in determining the nature of pleural effusion: Analysis of 320 cases. AJR 1992;159:29-33.
11. Kuhlman J, Singha N: Complex disease of the pleural space: Radiographic and CT evaluation. Radiographics 1997;17:63-79.
12. Matthay R, Coppage L, Shaw C, Filderman A: Malignancies metastatic to the pleura. Invest Radiol 1990;25:601-619.
13. Ferretti G, Chiles C, Choplin R, Coulomb M: Localized benign fibrous tumors of the pleura. AJR 1997;169:683-686.
14. Dynes M, White E, Fry W, Ghahremani G: Imaging manifestations of pleural tumors. Radiographics 1992;12:1191-1201.

15. Goerg C, Schwerk WB, Goerg K, et al: Pleural effusions: An "acoustic window" for sonography of pleural metastases. J Clin Ultrasound 1991;19:93-97.

16. Tublin M, Tessler F, Rifkin M: US case of the day. Radiographics 1998;18:523-525.

17. Miller B, Rosado-de-Christenson M, Mason A, et al: Malignant pleural mesothelioma: Radiologic-pathologic correlation. Radiographics 1996;16:613-644.

18. Heilo A, Stenwig A, Solheim O: Malignant pleural mesothelioma: US-guided histologic core-needle biopsy. Radiology 1999;211:657-659.

19. Wernecke K, Galanski M, Peters P, Hansen H: Pneumothorax: Evaluation by ultrasound—preliminary results. J Thorac Imag 1987;2:76-78.

20. Targhetta R, Bourgeois J, Chavagneux R, et al: Ultrasonographic approach to diagnosing hydropneumothorax. Chest 1992;101:931-934.

21. Weingardt J, Guico R, Nemcek A Jr, et al: Ultrasound findings following failed, clinically directed thoracentesis. J Clin Ultrasound 1994;22:419-426.

22. Silverman S, Mueller P, Saini S, Hahn P: Thoracic empyema: Management with image-guided catheter drainage. Radiology 1988;169:5-9.

23. Park C, Chung W, Lim M, Cho C: Transcatheter instillation of urokinase into loculated pleural effusion: Analysis of treatment effect. AJR 1996;167:649-652.

24. Marom E, Erasmus J, Herndon II J, et al: Usefulness of imaging-guided catheter drainage and talc sclerotherapy in patients with metastatic gynecologic malignancies and symptomatic pleural effusions. AJR 2002;179:105-108.

25. Patz E, McAdams H, Goodman P, et al: Ambulatory sclerotherapy for malignant pleural effusions. Radiology 1996;199:133-135.

26. Hsu W, Chiang C, Hsu J, Chen C: Value of ultrasonically guided needle biopsy of pleural masses: An under-utilized technique. J Clin Ultrasound 1997;25:119-125.

27. Adams RF, Gleeson FV: Percutaneous image-guided cutting-needle biopsy of the pleura in the presence of a suspected malignant effusion. Radiology 2001;219:510-514.

28. Mueller P, Saini S, Simeone J, et al: Image-guided pleural biopsies: Indications, technique, and results in 23 patients. Radiology 1988;169:1-4.

29. Lim J, Lee K, Kim T, Chung M: Ring-down artifacts posterior to the right hemidiaphragm on abdominal sonography: Sign of pulmonary parenchymal abnormalities. J Ultrasound Med 1999;18:404-410.

30. Kim O, Kim W, Kim M, et al: US in the diagnosis of pediatric chest disease. Radiographics 2000;20:653-671.

31. Targhetta R, Chavagneux R, Bourgeois J, et al: Sonographic approach to diagnosing pulmonary consolidation. J Ultrasound Med 1992;11:667-672.

32. Weinberg B, Diakoumakis E, Kass E, et al: The air bronchogram: Sonographic demonstration. AJR 1986;147:593-595.

33. Dorne H: Differentiation of pulmonary parenchymal consolidation from pleural disease using the sonographic fluid bronchogram. Radiology 1986;158:41-42.

34. Ablin D, Azouz E, Jain K: Large intrathoracic tumors in children: Imaging Findings. AJR 1995;165:925-934.

35. Suzuki N, Saitoh T, Kitamura S: Tumor invasion of the chest wall in lung cancer: Diagnosis with US. Radiology 1993;187:39-42.

36. Yang P, Luh K, Wu H, et al: Lung tumors associated with obstructive pneumonitis: US studies. Radiology 1990;174:717-720.

37. Yang P, Luh K, Lee Y, et al: Lung abscesses: US examination and US-guided transthoracic aspiration. Radiology 1991;180:171-175.

38. Ko SF, Ng SH, Lee TY, et al: Noninvasive imaging of bronchopulmonary sequestration. AJR 2000;175:1005-1012.

39. Hernanz-Schulman M, Stein S, Neblett W, et al: Pulmonary sequestration: Diagnosis with color Doppler sonography and a new theory of associated hydrothorax. Radiology 1991;180:817-821.

40. Sheth S, Hamper U, Stanley D, et al: US guidance for thoracic biopsy: A valuable alternative to CT. Radiology 1999;210:721-736.

41. Ikezoe J, Morimoto S, Arisawa J, et al: Percutaneous biopsy of thoracic lesions: Value of sonography for needle guidance. AJR 1990;154:1181-1185.

42. Morvay Z, Szabo E, Tiszlavicz L, et al: Thoracic core needle biopsy using ultrasound guidance. Ultrasound Quarterly 2001;17:113-121.

43. Liao W, Chen M, Chang Y, Wu H: US-guided transthoracic cutting biopsy for peripheral thoracic lesions less than 3 cm in diameter. Radiology 2000;217:685-691.

44. Wernecke K, Vassallo P, Pötter R, et al: Mediastinal tumors: Sensitivity of detection with sonography compared with CT and radiography. Radiology 1990;175:137-143.

45. Wernecke K, Peters P, Galanski M: Mediastinal tumors: Evaluation with suprasternal sonography. Radiology 1986;159:405-409.

46. Wernecke K, Pötter R, Peters PE, et al: Parasternal mediastinal sonography: Sensitivity in the detection of anterior mediastinal and subcarinal tumors. AJR 1988;150:1021-1026.

47. Adam EJ, Ignotus PI: Sonography of the thymus in healthy children: Frequency of visualization, size, and appearance. AJR 1993;161:153-155.

48. Han B, Babcock D, Oestreich A: Normal thymus in infancy: Sonographic characteristics. Radiology 1989;170:471-474.

49. Tashjian J, Teel G, Engeler C, et al: The radiographic spectrum of thymic lesions. The Radiologist 1996;3:167-177.

50. Dietrich C, Chichakli M, Bargon J, et al: Mediastinal lymph nodes demonstrated by mediastinal sonography: Activity marker in patients with cystic fibrosis. J Clin Ultrasound 1999;27:9-14.

51. Wu T, Wang H, Chang Y, Lee Y: Mature mediastinal teratoma—sonographic imaging patterns and pathologic correlation. J Ultrasound Med 2002;21:759-765.

52. Wernecke K, Diederich S: Sonographic features of mediastinal tumors. AJR 1994;163:1357-1364.

53. O'Laughlin M, Huhta J, Murphy DJ: Ultrasound examination of extracardiac chest masses in children—Doppler diagnosis of a vascular etiology. J Ultrasound Med 1987;6:151-157.

54. Gupta S, Gulati M, Rajwanshi A, et al: Sonographically guided fine-needle aspiration biopsy of superior mediastinal lesions by the suprasternal route. AJR 1998;171:1303-1306.

55. Rubens DJ, Strang JG, Fultz PJ, Gottlieb RH: Sonographic guidance of mediastinal biopsy: An effective alternative to CT guidance. AJR 1997;169:1605-1610.

18

ULTRASOUND-GUIDED BIOPSY AND DRAINAGE OF THE ABDOMEN AND PELVIS

Thomas D. Atwell / J. William Charboneau / Carl C. Reading / John P. McGahan

Chapter Outline

*U*ltrasound-guided percutaneous biopsy and abscess drainage have become invaluable diagnostic and therapeutic procedures for the management of patients. Growing experience with ultrasound and technical advances have significantly broadened the applications of ultrasound as a guidance procedure for interventional techniques. An approach to this topic requires knowledge of the current fundamental methods and applications of these procedures and of specific anatomic locations.

ULTRASOUND-GUIDED BIOPSY

Ultrasound-guided needle biopsy is an important diagnostic technique in radiology practices throughout the world. It has become an accurate, safe, and widely accepted technique for confirmation of suspected

malignant masses and characterization of many benign lesions in various intra-abdominal locations.[1-6] It also decreases patient costs by obviating the need for an operation, decreasing the duration of hospital stay, and decreasing the number of examinations necessary during a diagnostic evaluation.[7,8]

Traditionally, ultrasound-guided needle biopsy has been used for the biopsy of large, superficial, and cystic masses. Currently, however, because of improvements in instrumentation and biopsy techniques, small, deeply located, and solid masses can also undergo accurate biopsy.

Indications and Contraindications

Most needle biopsies are performed to confirm suspected malignancy before nonsurgical treatment, such as chemotherapy or radiation therapy, is begun. For example, a liver biopsy could be performed to confirm hepatic metastases in a patient with a known primary malignancy. Less often, needle biopsy is performed to determine the nature of an indeterminate lesion, such as a solitary indeterminate solid hepatic mass in a patient with no history of malignancy. Occasionally, needle biopsy is performed on a mass suspected to be benign but in which benignity must be established.[9] Relative contraindications to needle biopsy include **uncorrectable coagulopathy**, **lack of a safe biopsy route**, and an **uncooperative patient**.

To assess for **coagulopathy**, the primary information comes from the patient's medical history.[10] If the bleeding history is unremarkable, most superficial procedures can be performed without additional laboratory testing. However, if the history suggests a bleeding disorder, prothrombin time, partial thromboplastin time, and platelet count should be obtained.[11] The role of bleeding time measurement is of uncertain value in determining bleeding risk. For most cases, there is no good evidence to support the value of a bleeding time to predict bleeding.[12,13] One exception may be the uremic patient in whom bleeding tendency may be associated with the duration and severity of the uremic syndrome.[14] A selective, individually tailored, preprocedural testing, versus pretesting every patient, has been estimated to result in an annual savings of 20 to 30 million dollars in health care costs.[15]

Mild coagulopathies may occur secondary to the use of aspirin and some antibiotics. If present, the procedure may be delayed and the drug discontinued until coagulation measurements become normal.[16] Most coagulopathies can be sufficiently improved by the administration of the appropriate blood products to allow biopsy to be performed. Desmopressin (DDAVP) can be given to a uremic patient or a patient with a history of recent aspirin therapy in order to improve functioning platelet activity.[17] Postbiopsy embolization of the needle tract has been reported to control hemorrhage in patients whose coagulopathy is uncorrectable and in whom the need for biopsy outweighs any risks.[18,19]

The second relative contraindication is the **lack of a safe biopsy route**. Although biopsies performed through the inferior vena cava using small caliber needles have been reported,[20] a biopsy path extending through large vessels such as the extrahepatic portal or splenic vein increases the risk of hemorrhage. A biopsy path free of overlying stomach or bowel is also a preferable route. Nevertheless, puncture of an overlying loop of bowel is not an absolute contraindication if a small-caliber (21 gauge) needle is used.[21] Biopsy done through ascites has also proved to be safe.[22,23]

The third relative contraindication to needle biopsy is an **uncooperative patient** in whom uncontrolled motion during needle placement increases the risk of unanticipated tissue injury and hemorrhage. This is a common problem in pediatric patients and, to overcome it, occasionally it is necessary to administer sedatives.

Imaging Method

Both ultrasound and computed tomography (CT) can be used as guidance methods for percutaneous needle insertion. The choice of method depends on multiple factors, including lesion size and location, relative visibility of the lesion by the two imaging methods, and equipment availability. Biopsy of many masses can be done with ease under either ultrasound or CT guidance. In these cases, the choice of modality is determined by the personal preference and experience of the radiologist performing the biopsy.

Ultrasound

Ultrasound has several strengths as a biopsy guidance system. It is readily available, relatively inexpensive, and portable. Ultrasound uses no ionizing radiation and can provide guidance in multiple transverse, longitudinal, or oblique planes. The greatest advantage, however, is that it allows the real-time visualization of the needle tip as it passes through tissue into the target. This allows precise needle placement and avoidance of important intervening structures. Angled approaches are also easily performed with ultrasound guidance. In addition, color flow Doppler imaging can help prevent complications of needle placement by identifying the vascular nature of a mass and by allowing the clinician to avoid vascular structures lying within the needle path.[24,25]

Ultrasound guidance can be used for the biopsy of many organs and regions of the body. The technique is optimal for lesions located superficially or at moderate depth in a thin- to average-sized person. Biopsy of deep masses and masses in obese patients can be problematic with ultrasound because of the difficulty in lesion visualization resulting from sound attenuation in the soft tissues. Similarly, lesions located within or behind bone or gas-filled bowel cannot be visualized because of nearly complete reflection of sound from the bone or air interface.

Theoretically, any mass that is well visualized on a sonogram is amenable to ultrasound-guided needle biopsy. In our practice, most liver and kidney biopsies are performed with ultrasound guidance, as are most neck biopsies for thyroid, parathyroid, and cervical nodes. Sometimes, the pancreas and other sites in the abdomen and pelvis undergo biopsy with ultrasound guidance if lesion visualization is adequate.[5,21] Compared to CT, ultrasound-guided procedures require less time to perform and can be more cost effective.[26-28] Ultrasound-guided biopsy has been shown to be more accurate than CT, with a lower false-negative biopsy rate.[28,29]

Computed Tomography

CT is well established as an accurate guidance method for percutaneous biopsy of most regions in the body. It provides excellent spatial resolution of all structures between the skin and the lesion, and it provides an accurate image of the needle tip. In addition, lesions located deep in the abdomen, retroperitoneum, or within bone are all better seen with CT than with ultrasound. In our practice, many pelvic, adrenal, pancreatic, retroperitoneal, and musculoskeletal biopsies are performed with CT guidance because these structures are often best seen with this imaging method.[5,30]

Historically, CT has been limited by its lack of continuous visualization of the needle during insertion and biopsy. In the last several years, however, the introduction of CT fluoroscopy has allowed real-time visualization of needle positioning. This has reduced the time required for interventional CT procedures, at the cost of increased radiation dosage.[31]

Needle Selection

A variety of needles with a broad spectrum of calibers, lengths, and tip designs is commercially available for use in percutaneous biopsy.[30,32-37] Conceptually, needles can be grouped into small-caliber (20 to 25 gauge) and large-caliber (14 to 19 gauge) sizes. **Small-caliber needles** are used primarily to obtain specimens for cytologic analysis. However, small pieces of tissue may be obtained for histologic examination as well. With these needles, masses behind loops of bowel can be punctured with minimal likelihood of infection. Small-caliber needles are often used to simply confirm tumor recurrence or metastasis in a patient known to have a previous primary malignancy. Even if the sample is small, the pathologist is usually able to make an accurate diagnosis by comparing the biopsy specimen with the previously obtained tissue.

Large-caliber needles can be used to obtain greater amounts of material for more thorough histologic as well as cytologic analysis.[34,37] Their use may be necessary to obtain an adequate histologic specimen to confidently diagnose and subtype some types of malignancies (such as lymphoma), many benign lesions, and most chronic diffuse parenchymal disease processes (such as hepatic cirrhosis, renal glomerulonephritis, or renal allograft rejection).[38,39] The large-caliber tissue sample can also be used to generate an additional "touch preparation" specimen for more rapid cytologic analysis. This is performed by simply gently passing the soft-tissue core across a glass slide, leaving a cellular sample for subsequent analysis.

The preference and level of expertise of the pathologist involved in the interpretation of biopsy specimens are considerations in the selection of needle size and type. Cytopathologists deal with small specimens and are trained to diagnose on the basis of only a few cells. Unfortunately, some institutions do not offer cytopathologic interpretation. Histopathologists, in contrast, often prefer a large biopsy specimen for interpretation. For example, a large biopsy specimen from a metastatic lesion often allows a more reliable prediction of the likely primary site of the malignancy than does either a tiny sample or a cytologic aspirate. Determination of the probable site of primary malignancy is important in that it allows the oncologist to optimally tailor subsequent treatment.

Biopsy Procedure

Before percutaneous abdominal biopsy is performed, the procedure, risks, alternatives, and benefits should be explained in terms the patient can understand, and informed consent should be obtained. Most patients undergoing abdominal biopsy have a known or suspected malignancy and are concerned about the possible pathologic results. Physicians must be empathetic of patient apprehension regarding pain and possible complications of abdominal biopsy. After the procedure is discussed with the patient, any questions the patient might have should be answered fully.

Biopsies are frequently performed on an outpatient basis. Discomfort from the procedure is rarely severe and usually is controlled by local anesthesia at the biopsy site after the skin is cleaned and draped. Premedication is usually not necessary. Sedatives and analgesics, such as midazolam hydrochloride (Versed) or fentanyl citrate (Sublimaze) can be administered parenterally during the procedure, if necessary.[40,41] Such sedation should be administered only after legal consent is obtained. An intravenous access may be established before the biopsy is begun in the event that parenteral administration of sedatives, analgesics, or other medications or fluids is required during or after the biopsy procedure. If the patient's history suggests a bleeding disorder, coagulation studies should be reviewed before biopsy. In patients with increased risk of bleeding, a larger or second intravenous access site should be considered.

For **sterility**, the transducer can be covered with a sterile plastic sheath, but this may degrade image quality and make the transducer more difficult to handle. We prefer to clean the transducer with povidone-iodine (Betadine) and place it directly on the skin.[6] Sterile gel is used as an acoustic coupling agent. After the biopsy procedure, the transducer is soaked for 10 minutes in a bactericidal dialdehyde solution. Caturelli et al. reviewed their 3-year experience using a freehand technique and a similar degree of antisepsis and found no increase in postbiopsy infection.[42]

Most ultrasound-guided biopsies are performed under continuous real-time visualization. Several needle-

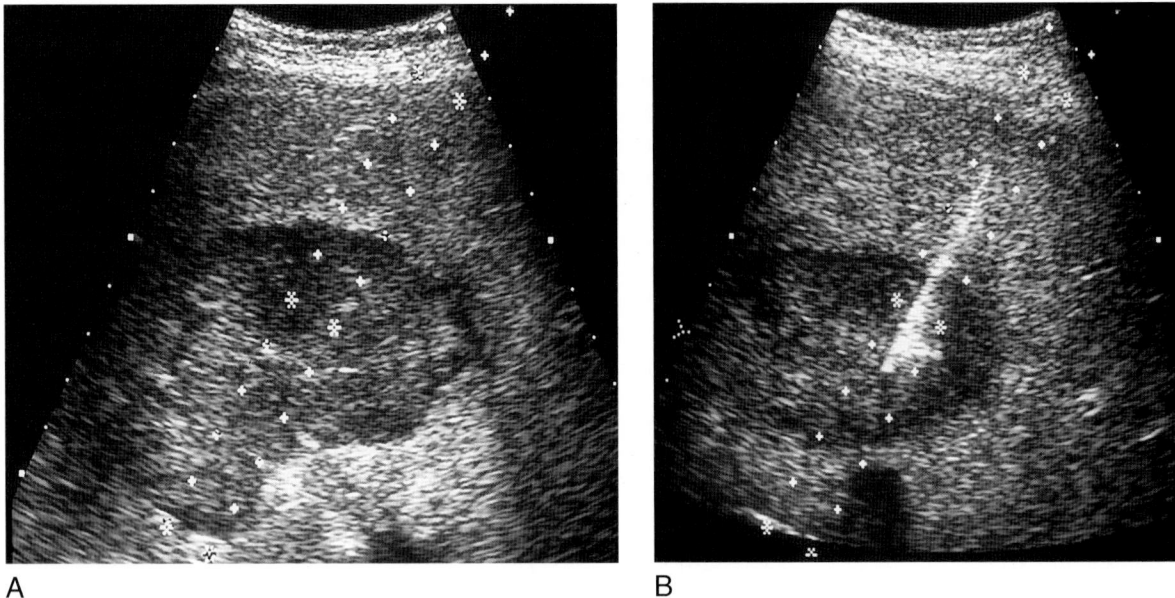

FIGURE 18-1. Ultrasound-guided biopsy with a needle guide. A, Ultrasound of the liver shows a mass in the right lobe of the liver. **B,** The needle is seen within the preselected angle boundaries with the tip within the mass.

guidance systems designed to facilitate proper needle advancement are commercially available. These guides direct the needle to various depths from the transducer surface, depending on the preselected angle of the guide relative to the transducer (Fig. 18-1).[43-45] Many radiologists prefer a "freehand" approach in which the needle is freely inserted through the skin directly into the view of the transducer without the use of a guide.[4,6] This approach provides great flexibility to the radiologist and allows subtle adjustments to be made during the course of the biopsy, thereby compensating for improper trajectory or patient movement.

When the tip is visualized within the lesion of interest, the biopsy specimen is obtained. If an automated, spring-loaded biopsy device (biopsy gun) that fires both the central stylet and cutting sheath in a rapid forward motion is used, careful attention should be paid to the expected excursion length of the biopsy device. Often the needle tip can be placed at the near edge of the target lesion to avoid the needle passing through the deep margin of the mass into an adjacent critical structure (Fig. 18-2). Some biopsy guns fire only the cutting sheath and not the central stylet. When this type of gun is used, the stylet can be advanced first to the desired depth within the mass. When the gun is fired, the cutting sheath advances over the stylet, but there is no additional forward motion of the stylet.

Most biopsies are performed by making one or more passes into a mass with a single needle. Occasionally, two needles are used in a coaxial manner, whereby a large needle is placed into the mass, the stylet is removed, and a longer, smaller-caliber needle is placed through the lumen of the first needle, which serves as a guide.

Multiple samples can then be obtained with the smaller needle without the need to reposition the larger needle. This technique allows a large amount of tissue to be obtained with only one puncture of the organ capsule, which may decrease the risk of hemorrhage. In addition, precise needle placement is performed only once, which saves time in the biopsy of lesions in deep or difficult locations.[46] In our practice, this coaxial technique is used frequently with CT-guided biopsies in deep locations and less often with ultrasound-guided biopsies.

After the biopsy is performed, the patient is observed in the radiology department for 1 to 2 hours, with vital signs checked frequently. In many medical centers, initial cytologic results are available within this time. If the results of the initial cytologic analysis are not conclusive, then a repeat biopsy is usually performed immediately. When core biopsy samples are obtained with needles such as biopsy guns, immediate interpretation of the core biopsy sample can be performed by traditional frozen-section diagnosis. Additional tissue samples are necessary if permanent fixation is needed. Alternatively, touch preparation cytology offers rapid diagnosis from one core biopsy sample and preserves the core material for subsequent permanent fixation for histologic diagnosis.[47,48]

Needle Visualization

One of ultrasound's greatest strengths as a biopsy-guidance method is its ability to continuously monitor needle-tip advancement under real-time visualization. However, this is frequently the most technically difficult aspect of ultrasound-guided biopsy for many radio-

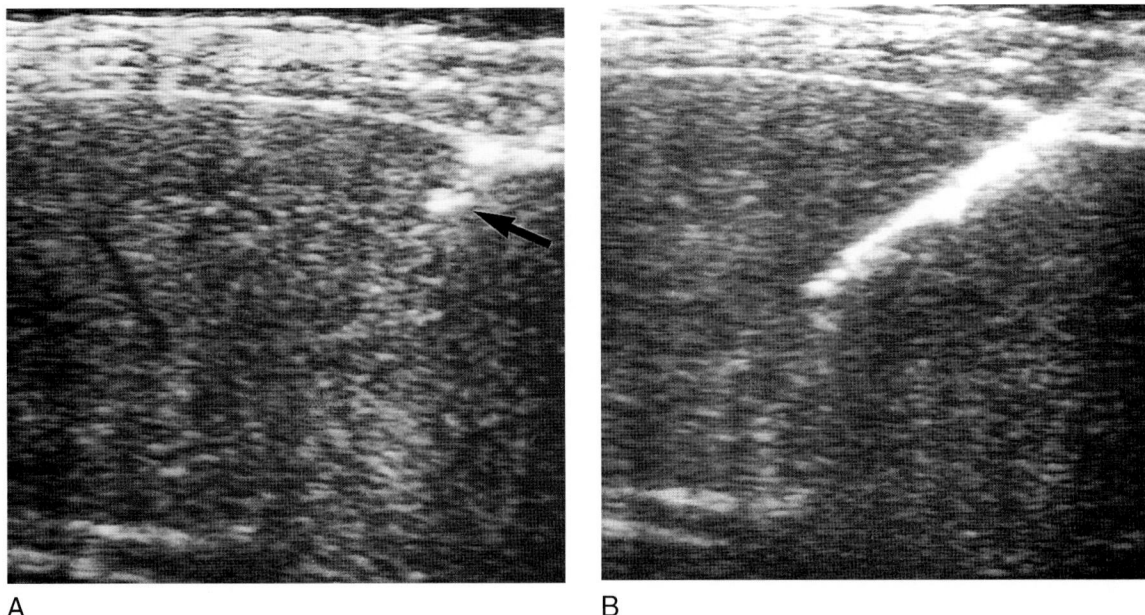

A   B

FIGURE 18-2. Ultrasound-guided liver parenchymal biopsy using an automated spring-loaded biopsy device. A, Longitudinal sonogram of the liver shows the needle tip (*arrow*) 1 cm into the liver parenchyma. **B**, Real-time image shows forward excursion of the needle tip during biopsy.

logists. Beginners may wish to practice on a homemade ultrasound biopsy phantom to develop the coordination necessary for ultrasound-guided procedures.[49-51]

The most common reason for nonvisualization of the needle tip is **improper alignment** of the needle tip and transducer.[5] To visualize the entire needle, the needle and the central ultrasound beam of the transducer must be in the same plane. This allows the entire shaft of the needle to be visualized. Such parallel placement can be challenging using the freehand technique. Often the radiologist must frequently look at the alignment of the needle with the transducer. When a mechanical needle guide is used, the needle is usually maintained within this central plane.

When the needle is not visualized, it is usually because the needle is misaligned—either initially aligned off-center relative to the central beam of the transducer or angled away from the central beam of the transducer (Fig. 18-3). Occasionally, the needle is deviated from the expected path by intervening structures. A **"bobbing" or in-and-out jiggling movement** of the biopsy needle during insertion improves needle visualization. This bobbing motion causes deflection of the soft tissues adjacent to the needle and makes the trajectory of the needle much more discernible within the otherwise stationary field. Alternatively, if one is using a coaxial system, the inner, smaller needle can be "pumped" or moved in and out within the larger introducer. Although this maneuver may require a second pair of hands, it minimizes trauma of the adjacent tissues.

Needle visualization can also be improved by **increasing the reflectivity** of the biopsy needle. Large-caliber needles are more readily visualized than small-caliber needles. Keeping the bevel of the needle up may also increase the conspicuity of the needle tip. Various modifications in needle-tip design have been tried to enhance needle visualization, including scoring the needle tip and using a screw stylet.[52-54] Extra-reflective needles specifically designed for ultrasound guidance are commercially available. Most needles, however, are sufficiently visible sonographically as long as the needle and transducer are aligned.

The echogenicity of the parenchyma of the organ undergoing biopsy also affects the visibility of the biopsy needle. If the parenchyma is relatively hypoechoic, such as liver, kidney, or spleen, an echogenic needle usually can be identified. Conversely, if the organ is relatively hyperechoic, it is usually difficult to visualize the echogenic needle tip in this background. This factor is responsible for poor needle visualization in biopsies of retroperitoneal structures or in obese patients.

Linear or curved-array transducers are frequently used for guiding procedures because of their good near-field resolution, which allows visualization of the needle after relatively little tissue penetration. The **focal zone** of the ultrasound beam should also be placed in the **near field** for better needle visualization. Sector transducers are often used if there is a small acoustic window or if there is a deep lesion situated at steep angles. Some authors have found color flow Doppler imaging helpful to visualize needle motion.[55,56] In our experience, however, color flow Doppler imaging has not been helpful in needle-tip localization.

Clear visualization of the biopsy needle is an

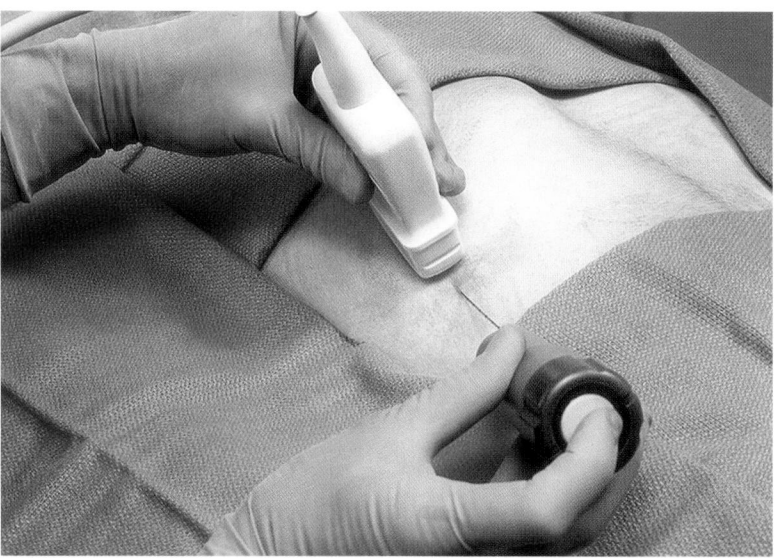

A

FIGURE 18-3. Freehand alignment of biopsy needle with the ultrasound transducer. A, Correct alignment for optimal sonographic visualization. Biopsy needle is aligned precisely within the central plane of the transducer. **B,** Incorrect alignment. Biopsy needle is aligned off-center relative to the transducer. **C,** Incorrect alignment. Biopsy needle is aligned correctly with the center of the transducer but is angled away from the central plane.

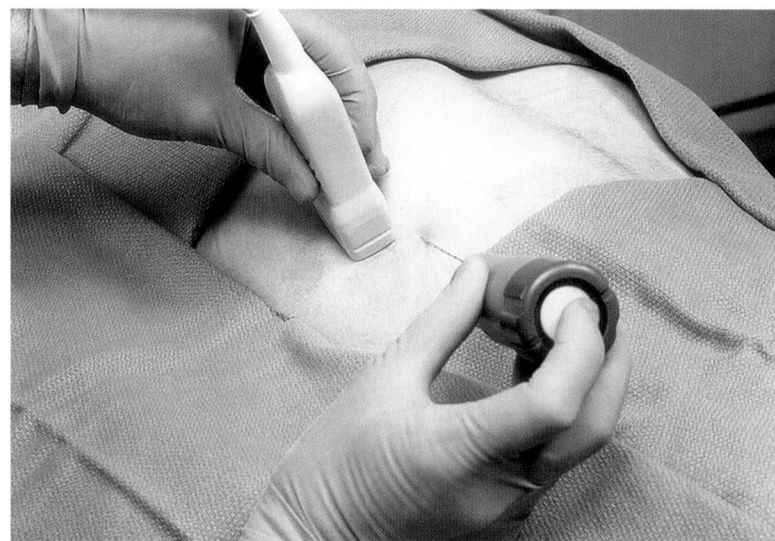

B

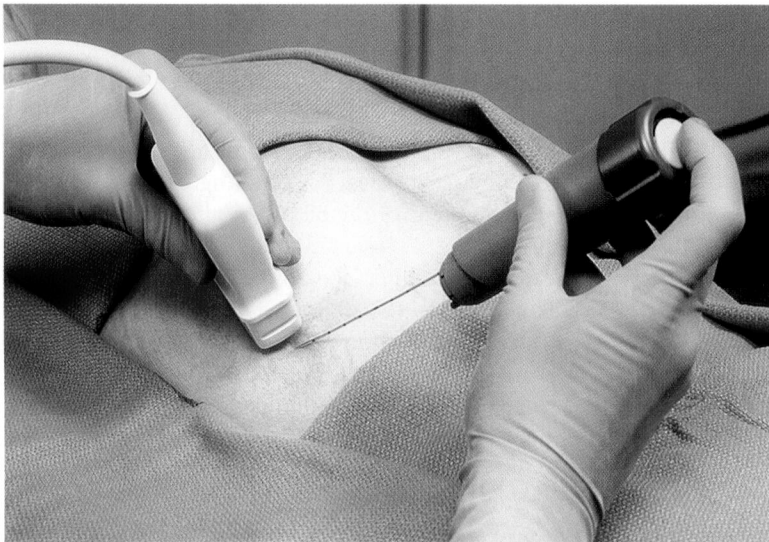

C

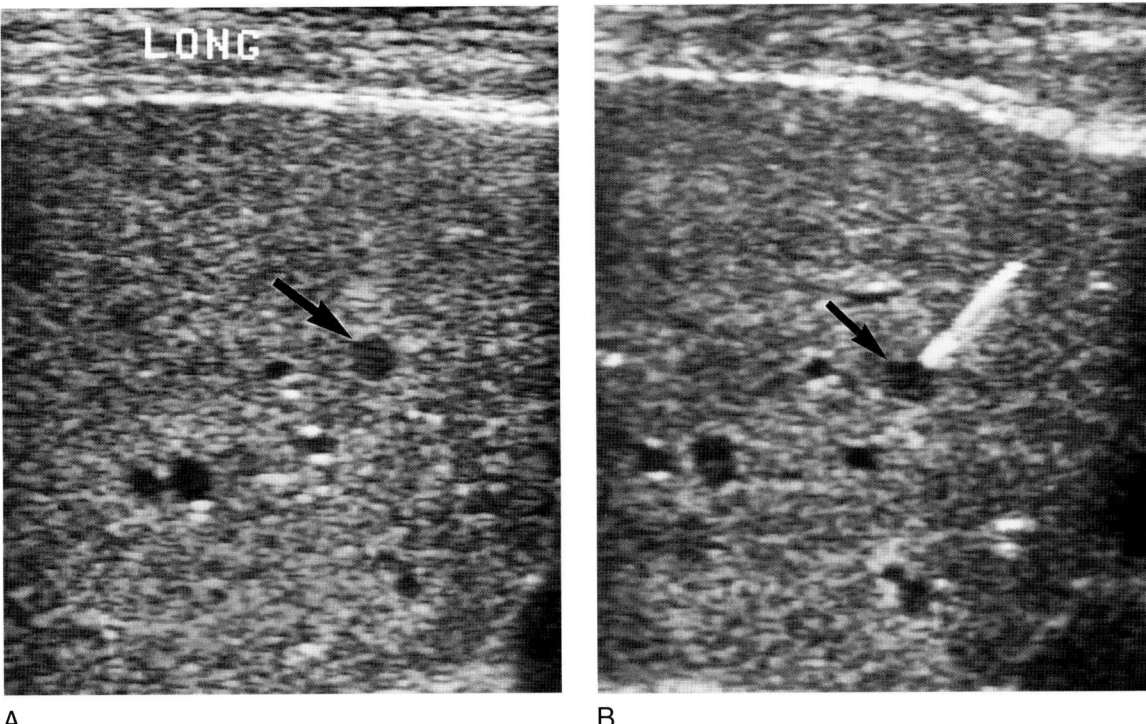

A   B

FIGURE 18-4. Ultrasound-guided biopsy of a small, metastatic lesion in the liver from transitional cell carcinoma of bladder. A, Longitudinal image of the right lobe of liver shows 0.5-cm mass in midportion (*arrow*). **B**, Ultrasound-guided biopsy with an 18-gauge biopsy needle (*arrow*).[5]

important element in the success of ultrasound-guided needle biopsies. The various techniques that have been described can be used to enhance needle visualization. However, considerable real-time scanning experience remains the key factor to the successful performance of ultrasound-guided biopsies.

SPECIFIC ANATOMIC APPLICATIONS

Liver

The liver is the abdominal organ for which percutaneous biopsy is most frequently used. Common indications for biopsy include nonsurgical confirmation of metastatic disease, characterization of focal liver mass(es) with inconclusive imaging, and diagnosis of progression of diffuse parenchymal abnormality. In our practice, liver biopsy is usually performed under ultrasound guidance because of the real-time needle visualization.[5,8] The advantage of real-time needle guidance becomes especially obvious when there is significant movement of the organ from respiratory variation. Biopsy of large or superficial lesions is easiest. With experience, deep lesions and lesions as small as 0.5 cm can undergo biopsy with high accuracies (Fig. 18-4).[5,6,57] In a retrospective study of 2091 ultrasound-guided hepatic biopsies, Buscarini et al. reported an overall accuracy of 95.1% for core hepatic biopsies.[58]

Lesions in the left lobe and in the inferior portion of the right lobe can usually undergo biopsy through a subcostal approach. Lesions located superiorly in the dome of the liver present a technical challenge for CT-guided biopsy, but biopsy can be done safely with ultrasound guidance by angling the needle from inferior to superior, usually using an intercostal approach (Fig. 18-5). Although the intercostal approach may enter the pleural space, aerated lung is rarely violated because it is well visualized sonographically and can be avoided (Fig. 18-6). We usually place the patient in the left posterior oblique rather than the supine position when an intercostal approach is used to improve visibility of the liver through the intercostal spaces. If one is working along the right side of the patient, such a position also prevents the patient from watching needle manipulation.

As feasible, **orienting the transducer along the longitudinal axis of the patient** is preferable. This allows both constant visualization of both the lesion and the needle with patient respiration. Benign hepatic lesions such as atypical cavernous hemangiomas, focal fatty infiltration, and focal areas of normal liver within a fatty infiltrated liver can occasionally mimic the appearance of malignancy on imaging studies. Biopsy of these processes can be done with ultrasound guidance to exclude malignancy and to confirm their benign nature (Fig. 18-7).[9] Although cavernous hemangiomas are vascular lesions, there have been multiple series in which

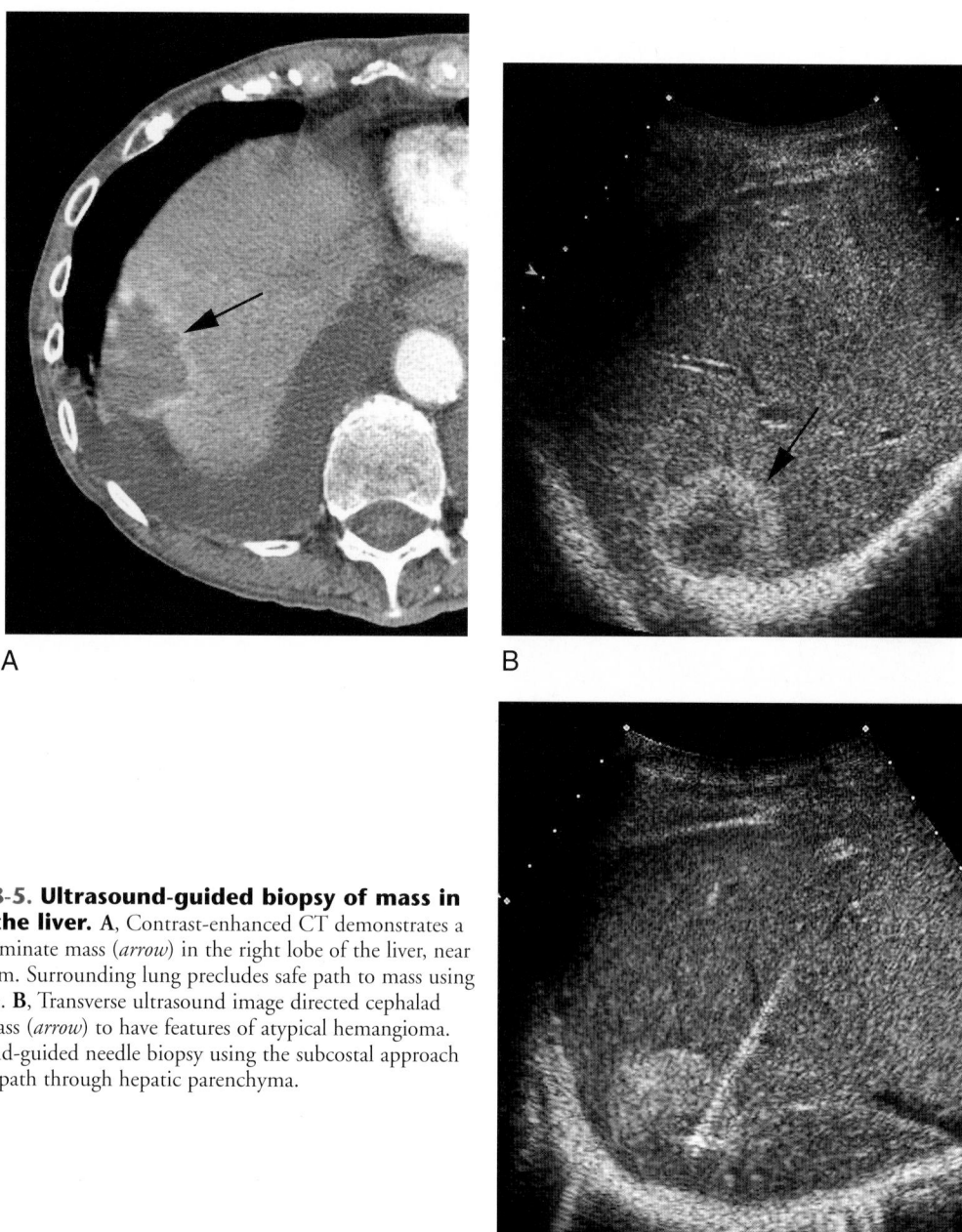

FIGURE 18-5. Ultrasound-guided biopsy of mass in dome of the liver. A, Contrast-enhanced CT demonstrates a 3 cm indeterminate mass (*arrow*) in the right lobe of the liver, near the diaphragm. Surrounding lung precludes safe path to mass using CT-guidance. **B,** Transverse ultrasound image directed cephalad shows the mass (*arrow*) to have features of atypical hemangioma. **C,** Ultrasound-guided needle biopsy using the subcostal approach shows a safe path through hepatic parenchyma.

these masses have undergone successful percutaneous biopsy without significant complications.[8,58-62] There is a case report, however, of a death due to hemorrhage after percutaneous biopsy of a large, subcapsular, hepatic hemangioma with a 21 gauge needle under CT guidance.[63] In this particular case, the needle was inserted directly into the mass through the liver capsule without any interposed normal hepatic parenchyma. If **normal liver can be interposed between the mass and liver capsule**, this may provide a potential tamponade effect if bleeding occurs.

Percutaneous ultrasound-guided **biopsy of portal vein thrombus** has proved to be a safe and accurate diagnostic procedure for the staging of hepatocellular carcinoma.[64,65] Accurate staging of hepatocellular carcinoma is necessary to determine appropriate treatment. In particular, neoplastic invasion of the main portal vein is a contraindication for hepatic resection or transplantation. Establishing the benign or malignant nature of portal vein thrombosis is, therefore, critical to patient management.

Complication rates are low. Liver biopsies are relatively safe. The overall significant complication rate of liver biopsy is 0.2% to 0.3%.[66-68] Of the complications, hemorrhage is the most common, occurring in 0.03% to 0.1% of patients.[30,58,66,67] Such significant

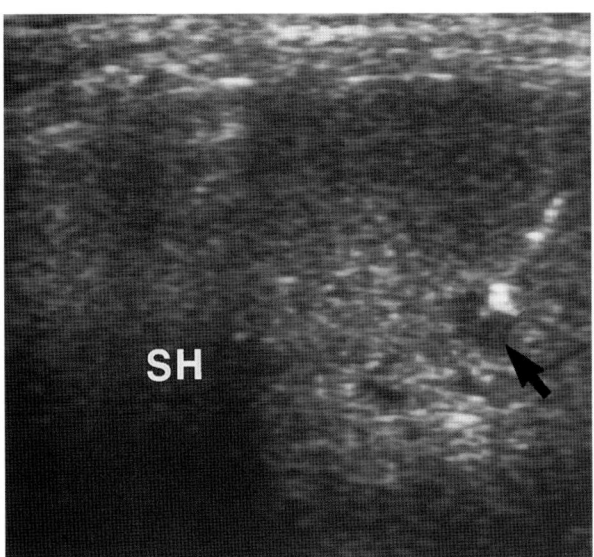

FIGURE 18-6. Avoidance of lung. Oblique ultrasound of right lobe of liver shows biopsy needle with 1 cm metastatic lesion (*arrow*). The aerated lung causes posterior acoustic shadowing (SH).

bleeding complications are more likely to occur in the biopsy of patients with malignancy and in those with chronic active hepatitis or cirrhosis.[66,69] Most complications occur soon after the biopsy procedure; 61% within 2 hours and 82% within 10 hours of the procedure, with rare fatal hemorrhage occurring within 6 hours.[66] The mortality rate of percutaneous liver biopsy is approximately 3 in 10,000 patients.[68]

Pancreas

Most pancreatic biopsies are performed in patients with ductal adenocarcinoma when it is considered to be unresectable because of tumor encasement of adjacent major vascular structures, such as the celiac axis or superior mesenteric artery. Occasionally, a pancreatic biopsy is performed to distinguish benign disease, such as chronic pancreatitis, from malignancy. At our institution, most pancreatic biopsies are done with CT guidance because the depth of the pancreas plus the presence of overlying bowel gas and hyperechoic abdominal fat can render ultrasound visualization of the needle difficult. Nevertheless, biopsy of pancreatic masses in normal-sized and slender patients can be done accurately under ultrasound guidance (Fig. 18-8). A particular advantage of ultrasound over CT is the capacity to biopsy pancreatic masses in an off-axis plane, which is very useful if overlying vessels are present on CT. A review of 211 CT-guided and 58 ultrasound-guided biopsies of pancreatic lesions demonstrated a CT-guided accuracy of 86% and an ultrasound-guided accuracy of 95%.[21]

In some reported series, the biopsy success rate for the diagnosis of pancreatic carcinoma has been lower than the success rate for the diagnosis of malignant lesions in other organs of the abdomen.[21,70,71] However, an increased success rate can be expected when ultrasound guidance is used if the needle is placed into the **central hypoechoic portion of the pancreatic mass**, which should represent tumor, rather than the adjacent echogenic regions, which are more likely to be nonmalignant pancreatic parenchyma or desmoplastic inflammatory change. In addition, carcinoma of the pancreas is often well-differentiated adenocarcinoma that is difficult to distinguish from normal pancreatic cells on cytologic sample alone.[72,73] Therefore, core specimens obtained with larger-bore needles are useful for histologic analysis.

The differentiation between benign serous and potentially malignant mucinous pancreatic tumors has important implications in patient management. Although the imaging findings can often be highly suggestive of tumor type, frequently a tissue diagnosis is required. Unfortunately, cystic pancreatic malignancies are difficult to diagnose accurately by percutaneous biopsy. In one study, a definitive diagnosis was achieved in only 11 of 18 (61%) patients.[74] In biopsying a cystic pancreatic lesion, **it is critical to obtain epithelial cells**, either in the wall of the lesion or within the cyst fluid.[74] Analysis of **percutaneous fluid aspirates** from cystic lesions has also been proposed as an aid to distinguish cystic neoplasms from pseudocysts.[74-76] A high amylase level is consistent with a pseudocyst. The presence of tumor markers within the cyst fluid may also be helpful in suggesting a cystic neoplasm.

The safety of percutaneous biopsy of the pancreas has been well established. Although complications are rare, with cited rates from 1.1% to 6.7%, six deaths have been reported.[21,77] Five of these deaths were attributed to pancreatitis and one to sepsis. No pancreatic cancer was found in either the biopsy specimen or postmortem examination of these patients, suggesting an increased risk for developing pancreatitis after biopsy of normal pancreas.[78]

The **gastrointestinal tract may be traversed** when biopsying the pancreas. With ultrasound, the stomach or bowel is either displaced or compressed. Brandt et al. demonstrated the safety of traversing bowel in performing percutaneous biopsies.[21] Sixty-six of the biopsies were performed by traversing the gastrointestinal tract, including the small bowel in 18 cases and the colon in 7 cases. Most of these biopsies were performed using a 21-gauge needle and there were no complications related to the biopsy route in these patients. Other investigators have also demonstrated the safety of biopsying through bowel.[78]

The **potential risk of tumor seeding** along the needle track has caused some authorities to recommend that the procedure not be performed in patients who

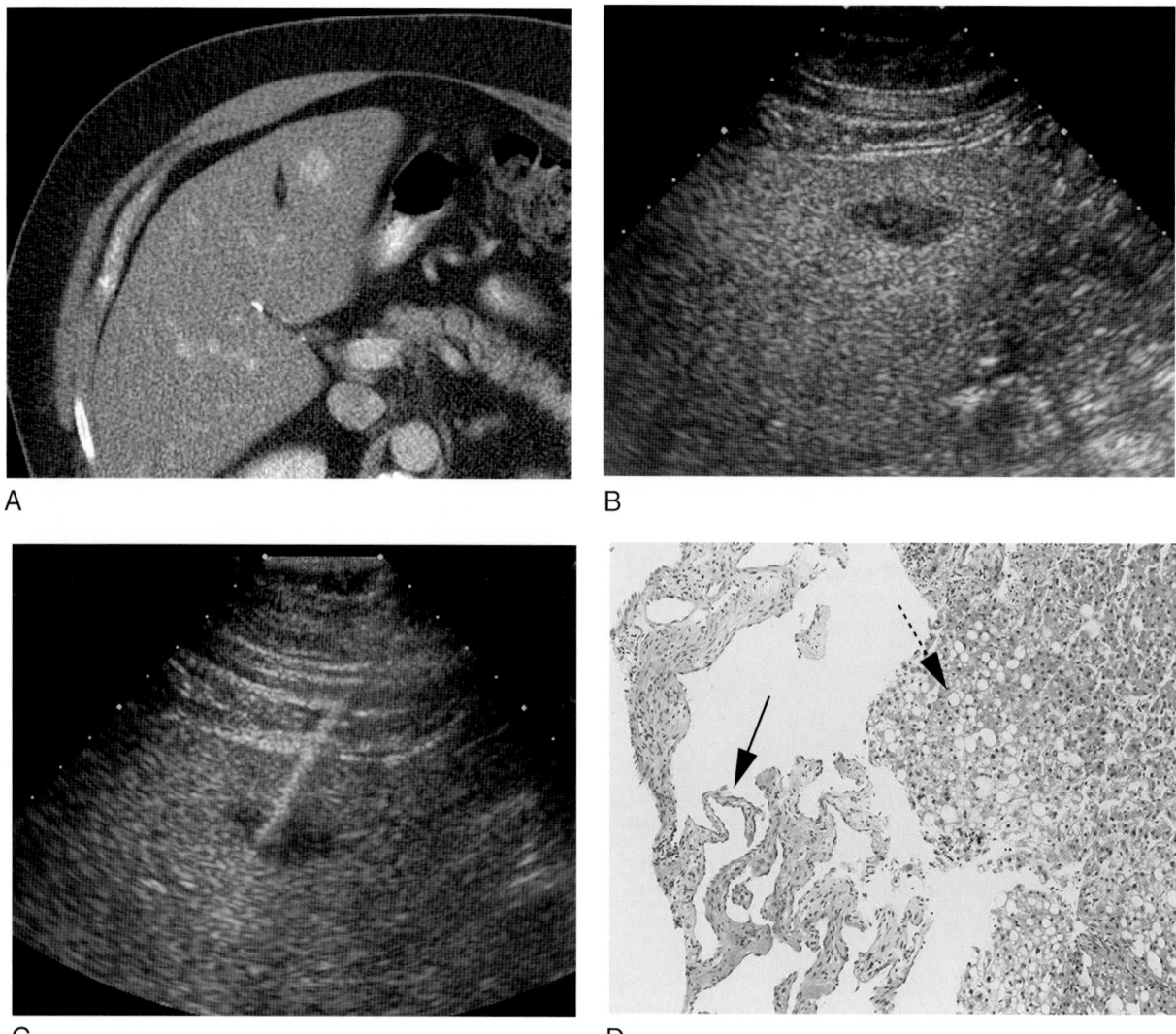

FIGURE 18-7. Biopsy of cavernous hemangioma. A, Contrast-enhanced CT shows a 1.5-cm vascular mass in the left lobe of the liver. **B,** Transverse ultrasound demonstrates a hypoechoic ellipsoid mass in a fatty infiltrated liver. **C,** Ultrasound-guided biopsy using an 18-gauge needle. **D,** Histologic specimen shows endothelial lined vascular spaces (*arrow*), diagnostic of cavernous hemangioma, as well as small round fat globules (*dashed arrow*) within hematoxylin and eosin-stained hepatocytes.

are considered potential surgical candidates.[79] Of 23 reported instances of needle-track seeding in a large review, 10 have occurred after biopsy of pancreatic malignancies.[77]

Kidney

Solid Masses

There is a limited role of percutaneous biopsy in the diagnosis of a solid renal mass. In general, about 85% of solid renal masses represent renal cell carcinoma. Therefore, when a solitary solid mass is discovered, it is usually removed without prior biopsy. While biopsy may be considered for the diagnosis of a solid renal mass, such tissue sampling is associated with a marginal

sensitivity of 82% and specificity of 33% to 60% with a nondiagnostic rate of 20%.[80] Thus, there is debate regarding the routine preoperative biopsy of a solid renal mass.

There are two scenarios in which percutaneous biopsy may be warranted. If the patient is **not a surgical candidate** or if there is a **strong suspicion of metastatic disease**, biopsy of the mass may provide tissue confirmation of presumed malignancy. This rare patient with multiple solid renal masses often undergoes biopsy to distinguish the potential causes of multiple masses: metastases, lymphoma, or multiple renal cell carcinomas (Fig. 18-9). Although these lesions can be similar in appearance, their treatments differ widely. Biopsy may effect a change in clinical management in approximately 40% of patients.[81]

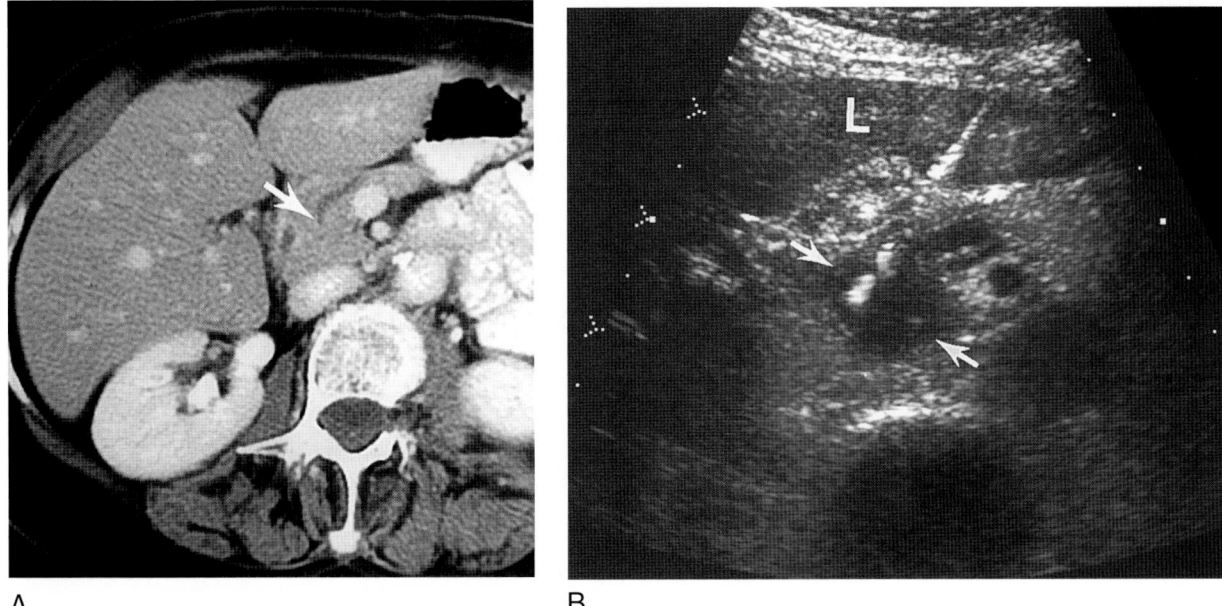

FIGURE 18-8. Ultrasound-guided pancreatic biopsy. A, Contrast-enhanced CT scan shows a mildly dilated pancreatic duct with abrupt termination in the head of the pancreas (*arrow*). No definite mass is identified on CT scan. **B,** Ultrasound for guided biopsy shows a 19-gauge needle passing through the left lobe of the liver (L), with needle tip within a 2-cm hypoechoic mass in the head of the pancreas (*arrows*). The biopsy was positive for adenocarcinoma.

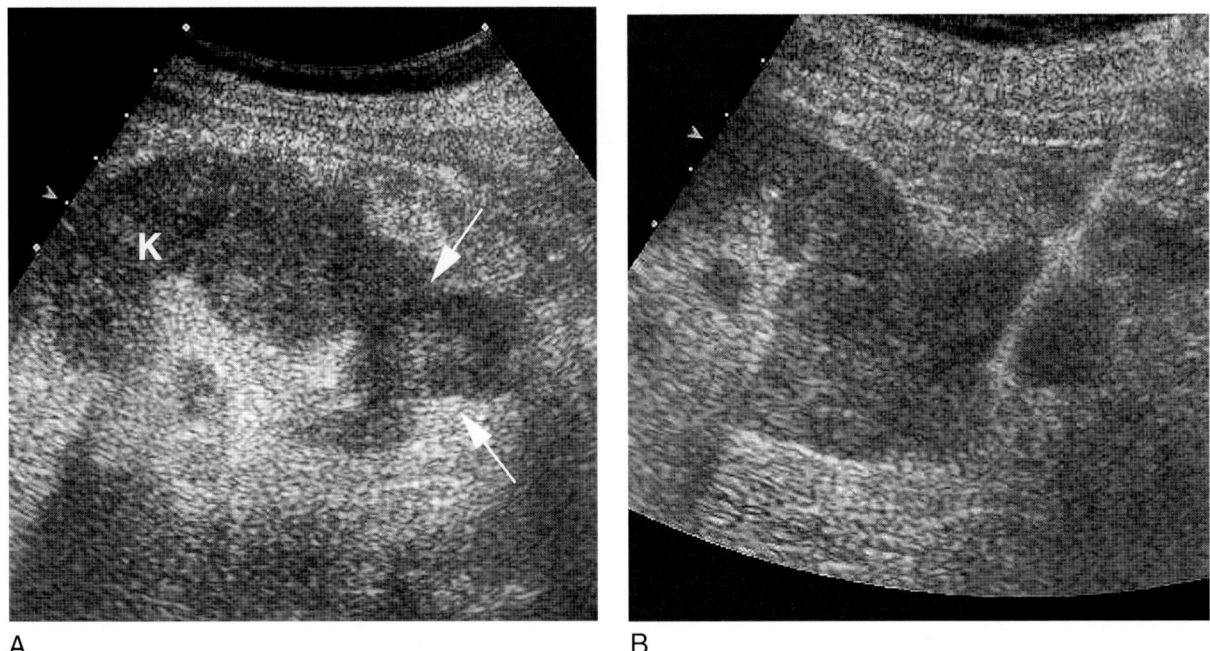

FIGURE 18-9. Ultrasound-guided biopsy of renal mass. A, Longitudinal image shows a 2-cm solid mass extending from the lower pole of the left kidney (K). **B,** Mass was biopsied using an 18-gauge biopsy device, confirming renal cell carcinoma.

Historically, an **atypical cystic renal mass** with internal debris, solid components, or a thick irregular wall could be aspirated and a biopsy of the solid elements could be done under ultrasound guidance in an attempt to distinguish a complicated benign cyst from renal cell carcinoma. However, with improved imaging tech-

niques, we are now able to better characterize cystic renal lesions as nonsurgical or surgical lesions, obviating the need for biopsy.

Sonographic guidance can also be used in the biopsy of kidneys with **diffuse parenchymal disease**. Insertion of the needle into the cortex of the lower-pole renal

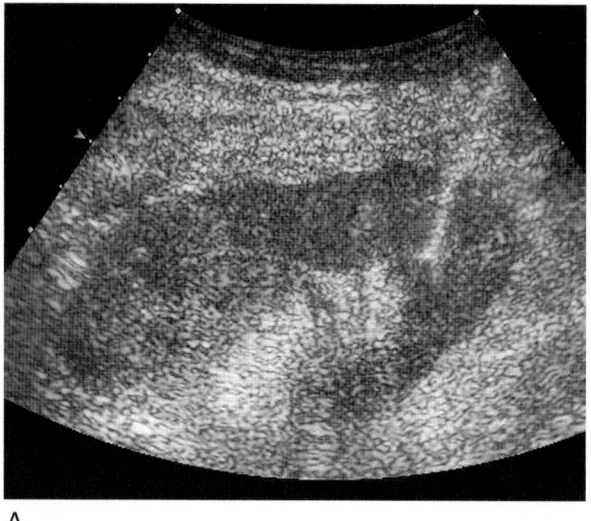

A

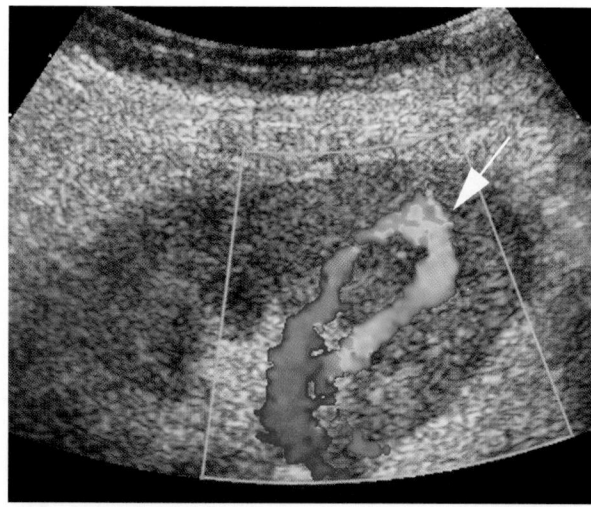

B

RENAL TX

1.1

3.0

m/s

C

FIGURE 18-10. Arteriovenous (A-V) fistula following renal transplant biopsy. A, Longitudinal ultrasound image of renal transplant demonstrates an 18 gauge needle in the lower pole. **B,** Color Doppler ultrasound 3 weeks later demonstrates focal communication between a renal artery and vein indicating A-V fistula. **C,** Spectral Doppler image demonstrates the high velocity and low resistance waveform of A-V fistula. Most A-V fistulas either spontaneously thrombose or are of no clinical significance.

parenchyma under continuous real-time guidance results in few complications and produces a tissue sample of excellent quality for microscopic analysis.[82-84] Ultrasound-guided biopsy of renal transplants with an **18 gauge automated cutting needle** provides a biopsy specimen that is equivalent in diagnostic quality to the biopsy specimen obtained by the traditional 14 gauge cutting needle.[85] In addition, there were substantially fewer complications with the 18 gauge biopsy gun than with the 14 gauge needle in this series.

In a large review of 1090 ultrasound-guided parenchymal renal biopsies performed with 18 gauge biopsy devices, Hergesell et al. found a 98.8% success rate in obtaining diagnostic tissue.[84] Only four (0.36%) patients had a serious bleeding complication necessitating transfusion or interventional radiology management, although 2% of patients did have a clinically occult hematoma larger than 2 cm on subsequent ultrasound. Small, insignificant **arteriovenous fistulas** detected by ultrasound occurred in 9% of patients (Fig. 18-10).

Adrenal Gland

The most common indication for adrenal biopsy is to **confirm metastatic disease** in a patient with an adrenal mass and a known primary malignancy elsewhere.[86] In the last several years, the CT and MRI characteristics of adrenal masses have approached diagnostic value in establishing benignity in an adrenal mass. Occasionally, however, histologic diagnosis is required. Guidance by CT is often preferable for the biopsy of small adrenal masses.

The **right adrenal gland** is more accessible to ultrasound-guided biopsy than the left adrenal gland because of the sonographic window of the right lobe of the liver (Fig. 18-11). Brightly echogenic fat containing adrenal masses and homogeneous, thin-walled, fluid-filled adrenal masses may not need to undergo biopsy because these should represent benign adrenal myelo-lipomas and cysts, respectively. CT can be performed to confirm this prior to considering biopsy.

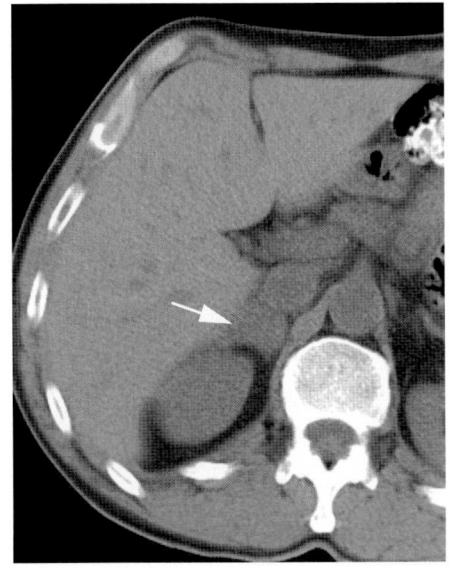

A

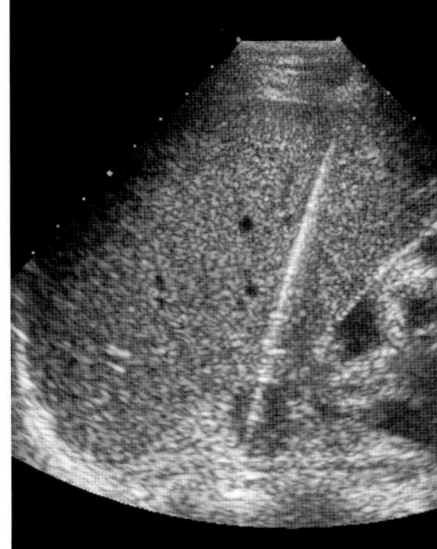

B

FIGURE 18-11. Ultrasound-guided biopsy of adrenal mass. A, CT scan without contrast demonstrates a 2 cm mass (*arrow*) in the right adrenal gland. **B**, Longitudinal ultrasound image shows the value of the liver as a biopsy path to the right adrenal gland.

Large Adrenal Masses. Although benign adenomas can be larger than 3 cm, the likelihood of silent adrenal carcinoma increases significantly if an incidentally discovered mass is larger than 5 cm.[87] However, needle biopsy may not be accurate in these patients because the histologic diagnosis of carcinoma requires the demonstration of adrenal capsular breakthrough and invasion of vascular structures by tumor. Therefore, surgical exploration rather than biopsy is often warranted for asymptomatic adrenal masses larger than 5 cm.[88]

Pheochromocytoma. Radiologists performing adrenal biopsies should be familiar with the management of a hypertensive crisis from the inadvertent biopsy of a pheochromocytoma.[89,90] If the clinical history suggests pheochromocytoma, further laboratory tests should establish the diagnosis rather than biopsy. If biopsy is necessary, pretreatment with a-adrenergic blockers should be considered.

Spleen

The main clinical reason for performing percutaneous biopsy of the spleen is to **differentiate recurrent lymphoma, metastasis, and infection** in a patient who has a new splenic mass but no disease elsewhere in the abdomen. Particularly in the immune-compromised patient with lymphoma or leukemia, differentiation between malignancy and fungal infection can be critical in patient management. Biopsy of a splenic mass will yield a specific diagnosis in up to 89% to 91% of patients.[91,92]

The spleen is the abdominal organ that undergoes biopsy least often. First, it is rare for the spleen to be the only organ in the abdomen involved with a pathologic process, such as metastasis (Fig. 18-12). In most cases, when the splenic lesion is visualized, there is also concomitant disease in other abdominal organs, such as the liver or lymph nodes, in which a biopsy can be done.

Second, the spleen is a highly vascular organ and the risk of hemorrhage from needle biopsy would seem to be high. The reported rate of significant hemorrhage from spleen biopsy is variable, ranging from 0% to 8%.[91-96] In a series of 20 splenic biopsies performed using 18- to 22-gauge needles, there were no complications and no pain reported by patients.[91] This contrasts with an 8% incidence of significant hemorrhage in a series of splenic biopsies published recently.[92] A single complication of a self-resolving pneumothorax has been reported in a review of 50 fine-needle aspiration biopsies using 20- to 22-gauge needles, but no bleeding complications.[95]

Lung

Percutaneous biopsy of lung lesions has been performed for decades. This is often the mainstay of differentiating benign from malignant disease in the chest. Typically, such biopsies are performed with fluoroscopic or CT guidance. However, ultrasound has proved to be effective in the biopsy of masses that abut the chest wall, thus preventing imaging interference of aerated lung parenchyma (Fig. 18-13).[97] Such lesions include pulmonary, pleural, and mediastinal masses. Advantages of ultrasound in this arena include real-time guidance during patient respiration, ability to biopsy in the off-axial plane, ability to biopsy lesions in patients who would otherwise have difficulty cooperating with the procedure, and absence of ionizing radiation.[98] Ultrasound-guided biopsy of mediastinal masses can be performed if the mass is visible. Mediastinal vessels in the path of the needle may be avoided with the use of color Doppler ultrasound prior to needle advancement.

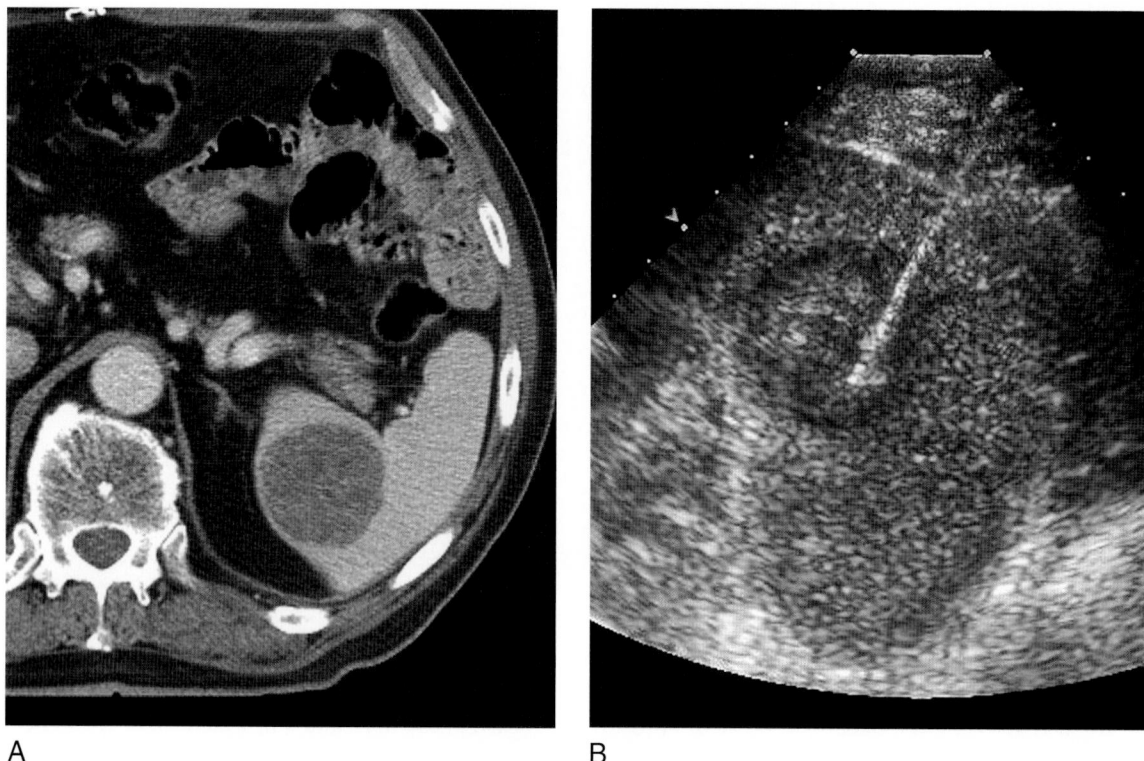

FIGURE 18-12. **Ultrasound-guided biopsy of melanoma metastasis to the spleen.** A, Contrast-enhanced CT shows a 4 cm mass in the spleen. B, Transverse ultrasound demonstrates the 18 gauge biopsy needle within the mass.

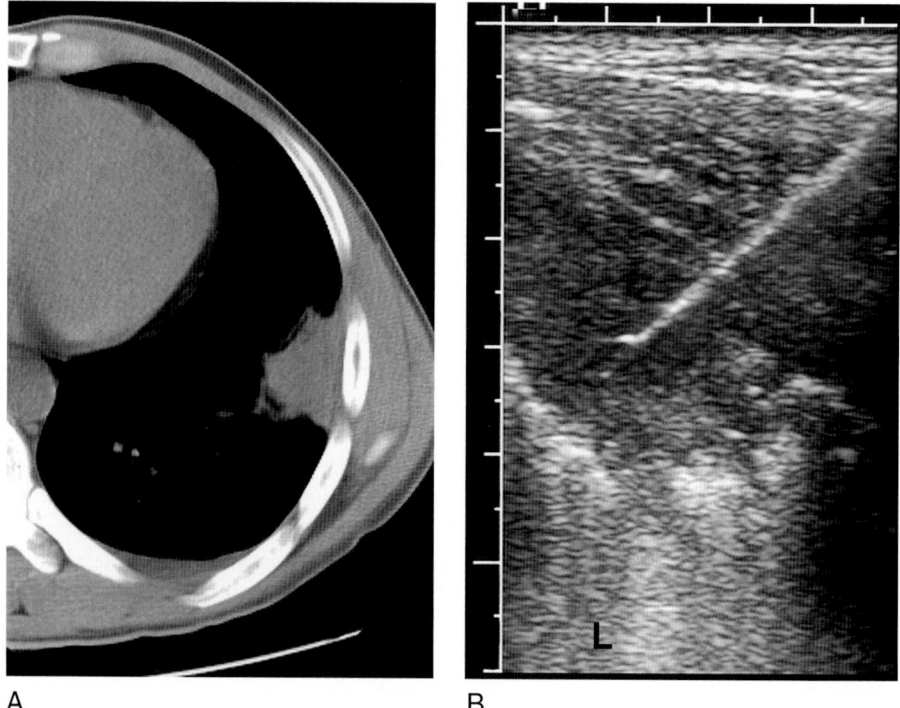

FIGURE 18-13. **Ultrasound-guided biopsy of peripheral lung mass.** A, Noncontrast CT demonstrates an indeterminate peripheral left lung mass. B, Oblique ultrasound image shows a 20 gauge biopsy needle isolated within the hypoechoic mass, which is surrounded by aerated lung (L). Biopsy confirmed histoplasmosis.

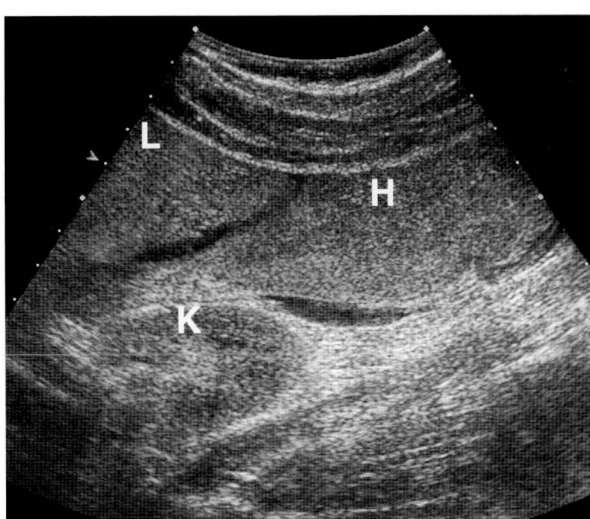

FIGURE 18-14. Isoechoic hematoma following biopsy of pancreas transplant. A large intraperitoneal hematoma (H) developed following biopsy. This fresh hematoma is isoechoic with the adjacent liver (L) and right kidney (K). Newly evolving clot (less than 30 minutes) can be echogenic and, therefore, overlooked.

COMPLICATIONS

Radiologically guided percutaneous needle biopsy has widely expanded, in part because of its well-documented safety, with rare and usually minor complications. Several large reviews obtained by multi-institutional questionnaires have reported mortality rates of 0.008% to 0.038% and major complication rates of 0.05% to 0.19%.[77,99-101]

Although rare, **hemorrhage** is the most common major complication of solid-organ biopsy and accounts for most deaths in these series. If hemorrhage is suspected after biopsy and the patient is hemodynamically stable, a CT should be obtained. CT is more accurate than ultrasound to evaluate for acute hemorrhage. On ultrasound, fresh blood has an echogenicity similar to that of surrounding organs and can be overlooked (Fig. 18-14).

Other major complications secondary to biopsy include **pneumothorax**, **pancreatitis**, **bile leakage**, **peritonitis**, **infection** (Fig. 18-15), and **needle-track seeding**. Needle-track seeding is a rare complication with an estimated frequency of 0.003%.[77] Seeding has occurred from biopsy of a wide variety of malignancies, including pancreas, prostate, liver, kidney, lung, neck, pleura, breast, eye, and retroperitoneum.[102-113] Because seeding is such a rare complication, it should not affect the decision to perform percutaneous biopsy.

Minor complications more commonly encountered include **vasovagal reactions** and **pain**, with **transient hematuria** and **tiny self-resolving pneumothoraces** in the appropriate context. The differences in the complication rates associated with the use of larger-caliber cutting needles and small-caliber needles may be overestimated. An early comparative study found complication rates of 0.8% with small-caliber (22 gauge) and 1.4% with large-caliber cutting needles (18 gauge and 19 gauge); this difference was not statistically significant.[112] Welch et al. found equal rates of complications from the use of 18 gauge and 21 gauge biopsy needles (0.3%).[30]

ULTRASOUND-GUIDED DRAINAGE

Like needle biopsy, percutaneous aspiration and drainage procedures have gained wide acceptance in clinical practice because of their safety, simplicity, and effectiveness. Modalities such as ultrasound and CT allow for

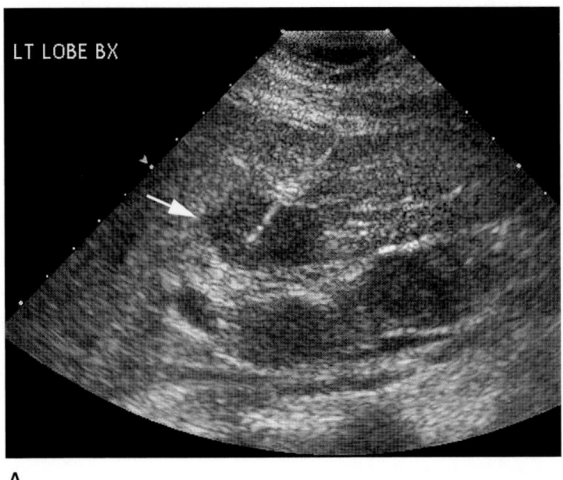

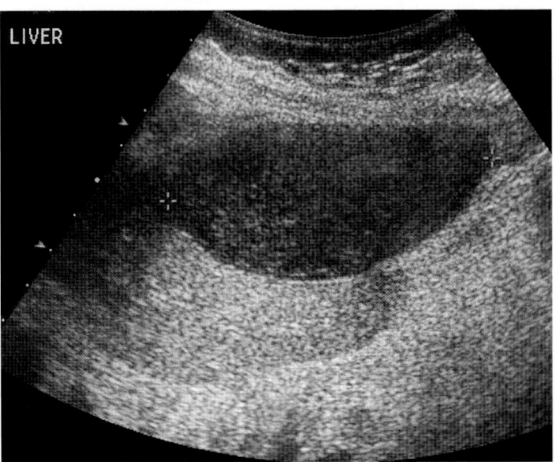

A

B

FIGURE 18-15. Abscess following liver mass biopsy. A, Transverse ultrasound image shows an 18 gauge biopsy needle in a 3 cm metastasis (*arrow*). **B,** Longitudinal image obtained 2 weeks later demonstrates a 6 cm debris-containing fluid collection, anterior to the left lobe of the liver, at the biopsy site. Subsequent aspiration and drain placement confirmed abscess.

precise needle placement for superficial and deep abdominal fluid collections or abscesses.[114]

Although needle puncture and aspiration were first described in 1930, the development of improved guidance methods and refinement of catheters was responsible for a more general acceptance of percutaneous procedures in the early 1980s.[115-117] This acceptance has continued to progress. In one large U.S. center, nonvascular interventional caseloads have increased nearly 11% per year.[118]

Indications and Contraindications

The indications for image-guided percutaneous abscess drainage continue to expand. Initial criteria specified that the fluid collection be unilocular with no communications, and surgical backup was considered essential.[117,119] Currently, percutaneous abscess drainage is performed safely for solitary, multilocular, and multifocal fluid collections with or without communication to the gastrointestinal tract.[119,120] Such collections include complex solid organ abscesses, enteric-related abdominal abscesses (e.g., due to appendicitis and diverticulitis), tubo-ovarian abscesses, and percutaneous cholecystostomy for an inflamed gallbladder.

Most percutaneous abscess drainage is performed to facilitate a cure and thus obviate the risks and morbidity of general anesthesia and operation. Other times it is a temporizing procedure that either postpones the definitive operation until the patient is stable, such as periappendiceal abscess drainage, or permits a single-stage surgery versus a multistage surgery, such as peridiverticular abscess drainage. This is particularly desirable in elderly, high-risk patients who present with sepsis. Poorly defined fluid in the peritoneum with an underlying surgically correctable abnormality, such as perforated colon with generalized peritonitis, should not be drained percutaneously and is best treated surgically.

Contraindications to image-guided percutaneous catheter drainage are all relative and are similar to those of percutaneous biopsy discussed earlier in this chapter. **Lack of a safe route** for percutaneous drainage precludes the procedure; this is uncommon, however. Unlike percutaneous biopsy, wherein bowel may be traversed without complications, fluid aspiration and percutaneous abscess drainage through bowel should be avoided. Initial advancement of the drain through normally contaminated bowel may seed a sterile fluid collection, resulting in iatrogenic infection. In addition, drain placement through bowel may not only cause significant perforation, but may also result in enteric fistula. **Bleeding diathesis** should be maximally corrected prior to drain placement, and appropriate sedation (local and systemic) should be given to an **uncooperative patient**.

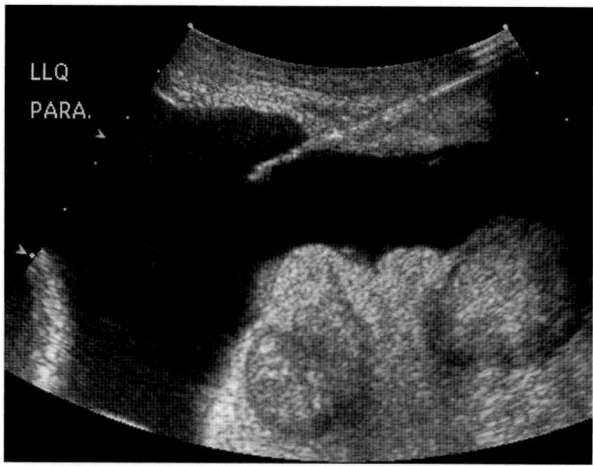

FIGURE 18-16. Ultrasound-guided paracentesis.
Longitudinal image shows a 5-French angiocatheter with side holes within the left lower peritoneal cavity during the course of a paracentesis.

Imaging Method

Selection of an imaging modality, whether ultrasound, CT, or fluoroscopy, for guidance of aspiration and drainage is influenced by several factors, including the location of the fluid collection as well as the strengths and weaknesses of each imaging modality as discussed earlier in this chapter. For instance, a **simple paracentesis** is best performed under ultrasound guidance (Fig. 18-16). More complicated drainage procedures in the retroperitoneum or pelvis are best performed with CT guidance. More **superficial abdominal fluid collections** may be performed easily with ultrasound guidance; however, obtaining a CT scan before the procedure provides an anatomic map for planning a safe access route.

In certain anatomic areas such as the gallbladder, biliary tract, and kidneys, combined **ultrasound-fluoroscopic guidance** of catheter placement may be preferred. The combined use of ultrasound for initial needle placement and fluoroscopy for catheter placement, via the guidewire exchange technique, optimizes the strengths of both guidance systems. Fluoroscopy may then be used to opacify the area drained and to confirm final catheter placement and the adequacy of drainage.[121,122]

No single method of guidance for percutaneous guidance is appropriate for all abdominal fluid collections or abscesses. Part of the intrigue in implementing abdominal interventional procedures is that each case is different. The approach to any fluid collection or potential abscess must be tailored to the patient, procedure, and specific circumstances.

Catheter Selection

Various catheters and introducing systems are available for percutaneous abscess drainage.[123] The catheter and introducing system chosen depend most on personal preference. As with most interventional procedures, it is important for the radiologist to be familiar and comfortable with the system. In general, thicker fluid is best drained with larger-caliber catheters. A 10 to 14 French catheter provides adequate drainage for virtually all abscesses. Smaller (6 to 8 French) catheters are adequate for less viscous collections. Catheters with retention devices, such as locking Cope loop catheters, are frequently used to prevent catheter dislodgment.

Patient Preparation

The procedure and risks should be explained to the patient and informed consent should be obtained. The patient's hemostatic status should be assessed through clinical history, and recent coagulation studies should be available. We routinely require platelets and prothrombin time in drainage procedures. Intravenous access is obtained in all patients for the administration of medications and for emergency access in case the patient develops complications from the procedure, such as hemorrhage or sepsis/hypotension. Patients often receive broad-spectrum antibiotics intravenously to decrease the possibility of sepsis. Satisfactory analgesia is necessary throughout the procedure to provide optimal patient comfort and cooperation. Local anesthesia is usually sufficient for needle aspiration; however, intravenous administration of sedatives and analgesics such as midazolam hydrochloride (Versed) or fentanyl citrate (Sublimaze) is beneficial for percutaneous catheter insertion. Dilation of the drain tract can be very painful to the patient.

Diagnostic Aspiration

Because fluid collections often have a nonspecific appearance, diagnostic aspiration is the first step. A fine needle is guided into the fluid collection by the selected imaging modality. This needle insertion defines a precise and safe route to the fluid collection. A small amount of fluid is aspirated and sent for appropriate microbiologic evaluation. The resulting culture and sensitivity data are used to modify the antibiotic therapy. If the fluid does not appear infected (i.e., clear, colorless, and odorless), the radiologist may elect to completely aspirate the cavity and not perform the drainage procedure. This is important, because a catheter placed in a sterile fluid collection will eventually serve as a nidus of infection with subsequent infection of the fluid collection. If pus is aspirated, care should be taken to aspirate only a small amount of fluid because any decrease in the cavity size may make subsequent catheter placement more difficult.

Catheter Placement

Catheter insertion can be performed using the trocar or Seldinger technique, and the decision to use one or the other usually depends on the preference of the operator. In the **trocar technique**, the catheter fits over a stiffening cannula, and a sharp inner stylet is placed within the cannula for insertion. The catheter assembly is advanced into the fluid collection. The catheter is then pushed from the cannula, and the distal loop is formed and tightened to secure the catheter within the fluid collection. This method works best for large and superficial fluid collections.

With the **Seldinger technique** (guidewire exchange technique), a guidewire is advanced through the aspiration needle and coiled within the fluid collection. The needle is then removed, and the guidewire is used as an anchor for passage of a dilator to widen the catheter track. The catheter-cannula assembly is placed over the guidewire into the fluid collection. The guidewire and inner cannula are removed while the catheter is simultaneously advanced. The distal locking loop of the catheter is reformed to prevent catheter dislodgment. If the catheter is difficult to see with ultrasound, the use of color flow Doppler imaging may improve conspicuity. During aspiration or irrigation, Doppler shifts improve catheter visualization (Fig. 18-17).

Final positioning of the catheter is important in maximizing effectiveness of drainage. For this purpose, ultrasound and CT are very complementary and should be used in conjunction with one another. CT provides an anatomic roadmap for ideal catheter placement. Because this ideal position seldom lies in the true axial plane, ultrasound can be used to direct the needle, guidewire, and catheter into the ideal position. Final placement can be then verified with CT.

Drainage

After the drainage catheter is placed, the cavity is **completely aspirated** and gently irrigated. Care should be taken not to distend the cavity during the irrigation because this may increase the risk of bacteremia. Repeat images are obtained to determine the size of the residual cavity, the position of the drainage tube, and whether the entire abscess communicates with the drainage tube. If the abscess cavity has not completely resolved, the drainage catheter may need to be repositioned or a second drain may need to be placed. Such manipulations are often performed under fluoroscopy the day after initial drain placement. Correct catheter position and adequate catheter size are the most important factors for successful drainage.[124]

Follow-Up Care

All drains must be **irrigated regularly**. Injection and aspiration of 10 mL isotonic saline three or four times a day is usually sufficient. If drainage is especially tenacious or the abscess is large, more frequent irrigations

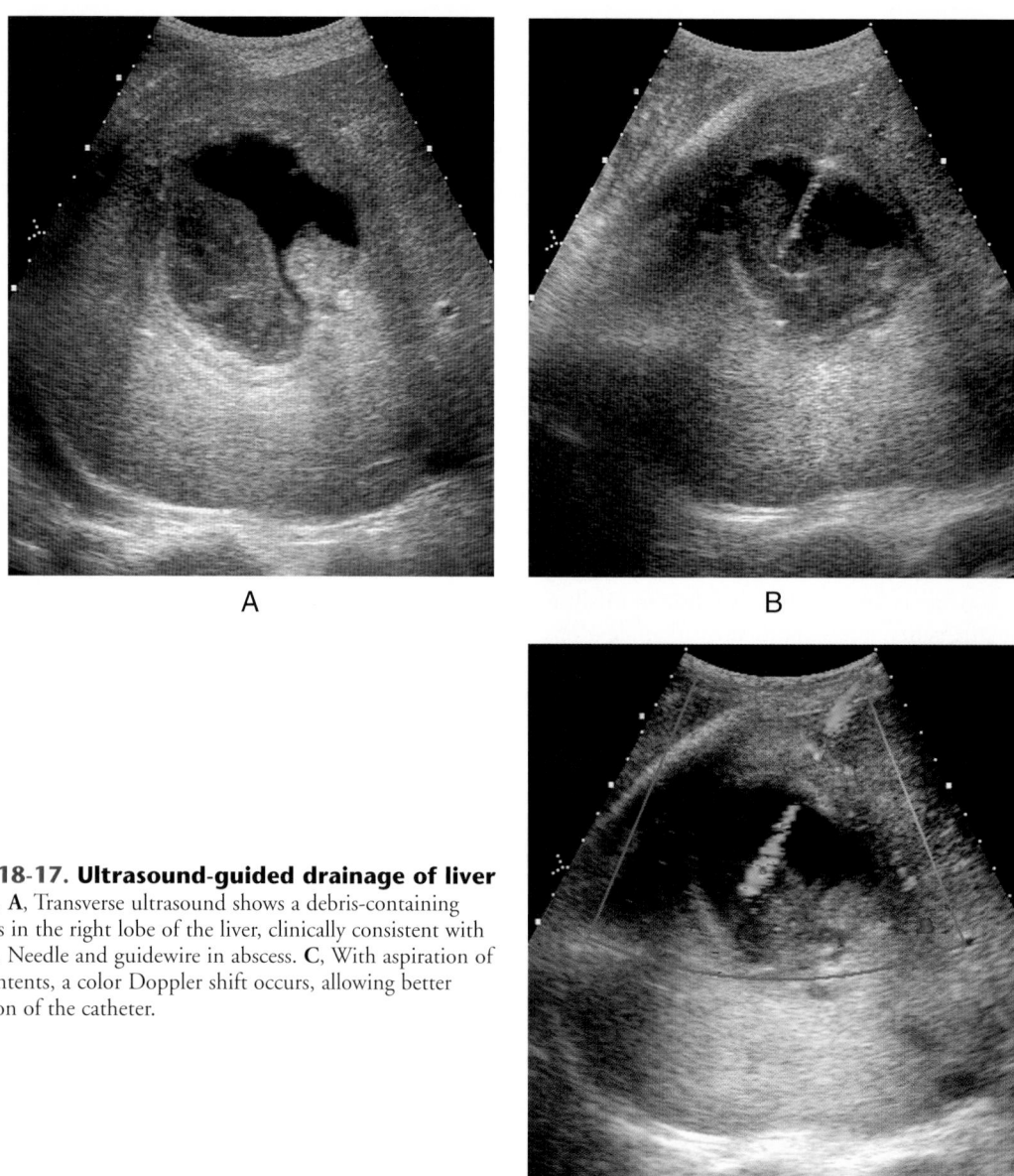

FIGURE 18-17. Ultrasound-guided drainage of liver abscess. A, Transverse ultrasound shows a debris-containing cystic mass in the right lobe of the liver, clinically consistent with abscess. **B**, Needle and guidewire in abscess. **C**, With aspiration of abscess contents, a color Doppler shift occurs, allowing better visualization of the catheter.

with greater volumes of saline may be necessary. The fluid collection can be drained either dependently or by low intermittent suction. The character and volume of the output should be recorded each nursing shift and checked daily on rounds by the radiology service.[125] If the drainage changes significantly in volume or character or if fever recurs, the patient should be reexamined to check for fistulas, catheter blockage, reaccumulation of the abscess, or a previously undiagnosed collection.

Twenty-four to 48 hours after tube placement, a sinogram should be performed to look at the abscess cavity size, completeness of drainage, and catheter position, and to look for fistulas. Simple abscess cavities may drain for 5 to 10 days. Abscesses secondary to fistulas from bowel, biliary, or urinary tracts may drain for 6 weeks or

longer. As long as drainage persists, sinograms are performed every 3 to 4 days and the drains are left in place. Outpatient care is possible for selected patients.

Catheter Removal

There are three criteria for catheter removal:

- Negligible drainage in 24 hours
- Afebrile patient
- Minimal residual cavity

Drains in small, superficial abscess cavities can be pulled all at once, whereas drains in large, deeper cavities may be removed gradually over a few days, which promotes healing by secondary intention.

Abdominal and Pelvic Abscesses

Most abdominal and pelvic abscesses are secondary to operation or related to underlying bowel abnormality. Percutaneous abscess drainage for postoperative abdominal abscesses has become the accepted primary treatment of choice, with cure being the procedural goal.[119] Percutaneous drainage has also played a principal role in the treatment of diverticular, appendiceal, and Crohn's-related abscesses.[126-132] Drainage of abscesses in these acutely ill patients can help alleviate sepsis and permit the necessary curative surgical treatment on an elective basis.

Drainage of abdominal abscesses is often best performed with CT guidance, which allows for the best visualization and avoidance of adjacent bowel loops. CT also provides an overview of the entire abdomen, which is essential to be certain that all collections are drained. Ultrasound can also provide excellent guidance for percutaneous abscess drainage; however, careful review of CT scans assists in planning an optimal approach free of intervening bowel. As opposed to CT, ultrasound is especially valuable in the treatment of critically ill patients who cannot be transported to the radiology department.[133]

Pelvic abscesses are of variable origin and have been notoriously difficult to access because of their deep location, overlying bowel, blood vessels, bony pelvis, and bladder. Traditional approaches include an anterior transperineal approach or a posterior transgluteal approach. The transgluteal approach is relatively painful, and care must be taken to avoid the sciatic nerve. Small, deep, pelvic abscesses may be difficult to access safely via traditional approaches.

Experience with **ultrasound-guided transrectal and transvaginal drainage** is growing, and these techniques appear to be effective and well-tolerated procedures in appropriate patients (Fig. 18-18).[134-140] Needle guides are available for endovaginal probes that help guide the needle into the fluid collection. The use of the Seldinger technique and the combination of ultrasound and fluoroscopic guidance has been found by some authors to improve the technical ease of transvaginal and transrectal ultrasound drainage.[137,139,141] The trocar technique may also be successfully used for endovaginal drain placement.

For **nonpurulent collections**, immediate catheter drainage is not necessarily indicated. Most of these patients respond to a one-step aspiration, lavage, and antibiotic therapy based on results of cultures of the aspirates.[139,140] With regard to tubo-ovarian abscesses, ultrasound-guided transvaginal drainage has also been shown to be a successful alternative to operation in patients who fail standard initial antibiotic treatment.[137,142]

Enteric abscesses often have **communication with the gastrointestinal tract**. For these abscesses to be drained successfully, one must first recognize that such a communication exists, and the communication must be allowed to close before removal of the catheter.[119] Fistulas will not close if there is distal obstruction, tumor, or persistent infection. Unfortunately, even with the most aggressive techniques, success in treating abscesses with enteric communication is lower than for noncommunicating abscesses.[143,144]

Successful percutaneous treatment of **Crohn's-related abscesses** can be particularly challenging. Obviating surgery in the short term can be achieved in only 50% to 56% of Crohn's patients with abscesses, with a much lower success rate in patients with pre-existing bowel fistulas.[145,146] Nevertheless, the placement of a percutaneous drainage catheter may allow the surgeon to perform a single-stage operation, as opposed to a two-stage surgery where the abscess is evacuated surgically, with bowel resection performed at a later date. Enterocutaneous fistulas can occur along the catheter tract in these patients.[145,146]

SPECIFIC ANATOMIC APPLICATIONS
Liver

Percutaneous catheter drainage is considered the initial treatment of choice for pyogenic liver abscesses (see Fig. 18-17). Pyogenic liver abscesses are most often due to seeding from intestinal sources, such as appendicitis or diverticulitis; as a direct extension from cholecystitis or cholangitis (Fig. 18-19); or secondary to surgery or trauma. Like abscesses elsewhere in the body, the sonographic appearance of hepatic abscesses is usually one of a complex fluid collection, although they can also appear as a solid hypoechoic mass. Both ultrasound and CT provide excellent guidance for percutaneous drainage of hepatic abscesses. The cure rate ranges from 67% to 94%.[143,147-149]

Complications of percutaneous hepatic abscess catheter drainage include sepsis, hemorrhage, and catheter transgression of the pleura. Because of these complications, some authors have suggested treating pyogenic liver abscesses with antibiotics and percutaneous needle aspiration alone, without catheter drainage, although multiple aspiration procedures may be required.[150] Such an approach is particularly reasonable in smaller (less than 6 cm) abscesses.[151] Multiple, small (< 1 cm) microabscesses are typically treated with antibiotics alone after diagnostic aspiration.[152] Ultimate cure often depends on identification and appropriate treatment of the infectious source.

Amebic liver abscesses are caused by *Entamoeba histolytica*. Most amebic liver abscesses are effectively treated with metronidazole alone with 85% to 95% success.[151,153] However, percutaneous abscess drainage of amebic abscesses is indicated if the diagnosis is

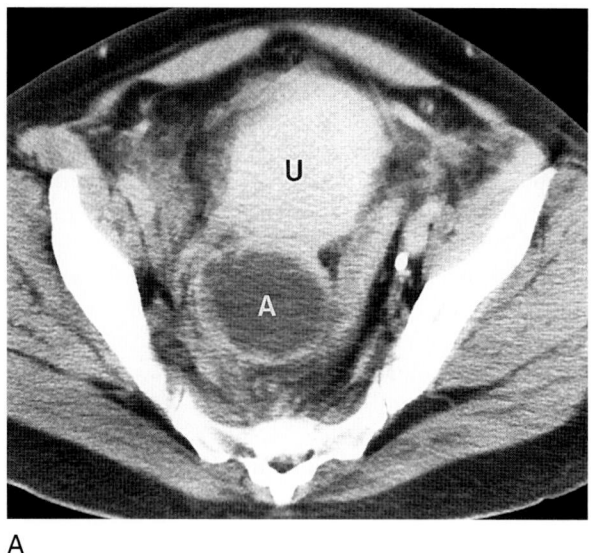

A

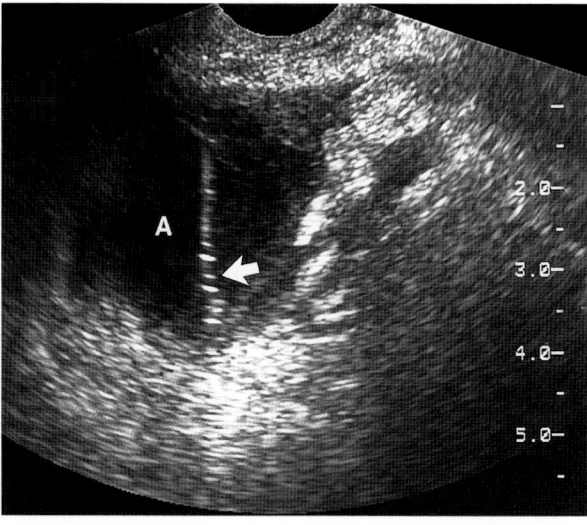

B

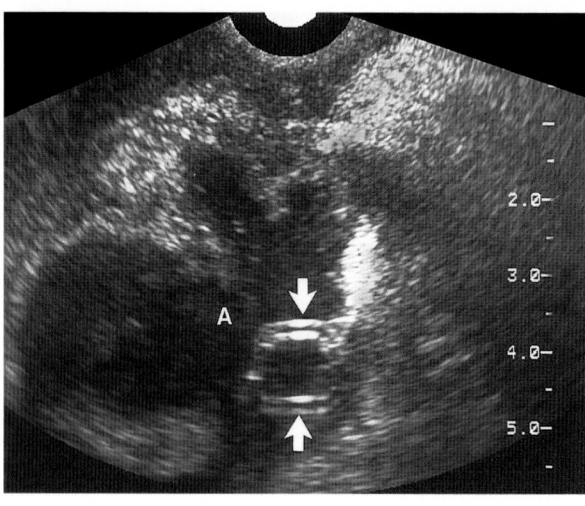

C

FIGURE 18-18. Ultrasound-guided transvaginal drainage of pelvic abscess. A, Contrast-enhanced CT scan shows an abscess (A) deep in the pelvis, posterior to the uterus (U). **B,** Transvaginal ultrasonogram shows needle tip (*arrow*) in abscess cavity (A). **C,** With the catheter exchange technique, a locking loop catheter (*arrows*) was placed into the abscess cavity for drainage.

uncertain, the cavity is larger than 10 cm, the patient is not responding to medical treatment, or there are signs of abscess cavity rupture.[149,150] Catheter drainage in these situations is safe and generally provides a rapid cure; the catheter can often be removed within a few days.[119,153,154]

Previously, **liver hydatid abscesses** caused by *Echinococcus granulosus* were considered a contraindication to percutaneous abscess drainage because of the concern of **anaphylactic reaction to cyst contents**. More recently, these abscesses have been successfully treated with percutaneous aspiration combined with appropriate antihelmintic therapy.[155] The procedure is typically divided into three steps with partial aspiration of the cyst contents, followed by the instillation of a scolicidal agent such as silver nitrate or hypertonic saline, and then subsequent complete aspiration of the cyst. In three studies, there were no treatment failures.[156-158] In these studies, successfully treated anaphylactic reactions

occurred in 2% to 4% of patients. While the most important treatment modality for liver hydatid disease remains surgery, percutaneous aspiration may have a role in select cases, including those in a deep, critical liver location or type I to II cysts, with consideration given to type III cysts.[159,160]

Biliary Tract

Gallbladder

Percutaneous cholecystostomy has evolved into a favorable alternative to surgery in critically ill patients with acute calculous and acalculous cholecystitis. There are conflicting reports concerning the management of patients with acute cholecystitis, especially with regard to optimal time for intervention. Some surgeons prefer emergency cholecystectomy, but others advocate delaying cholecystectomy until the patient is in a less

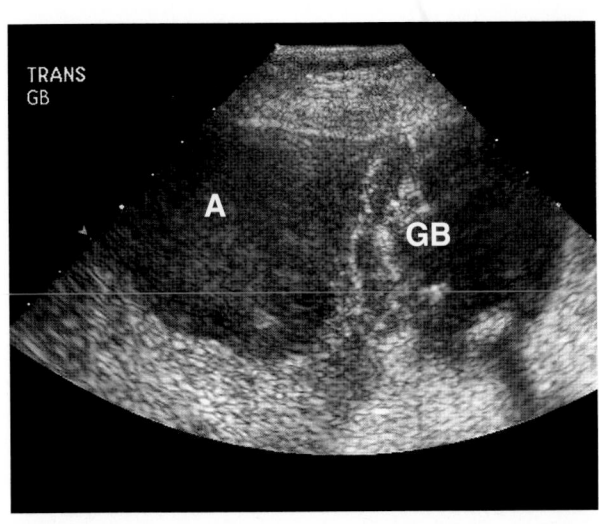

A

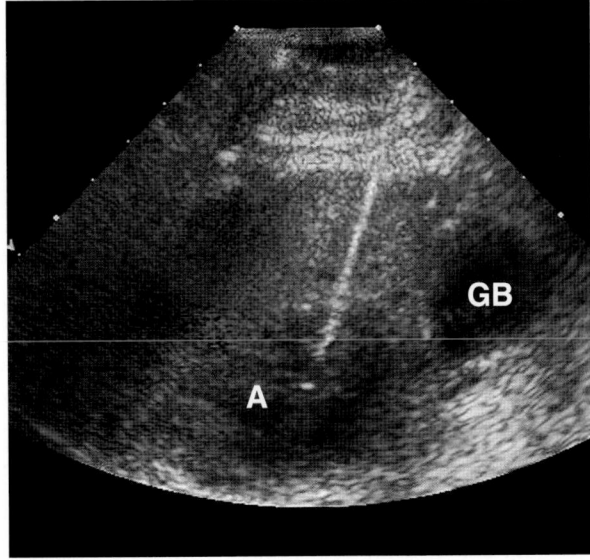

B

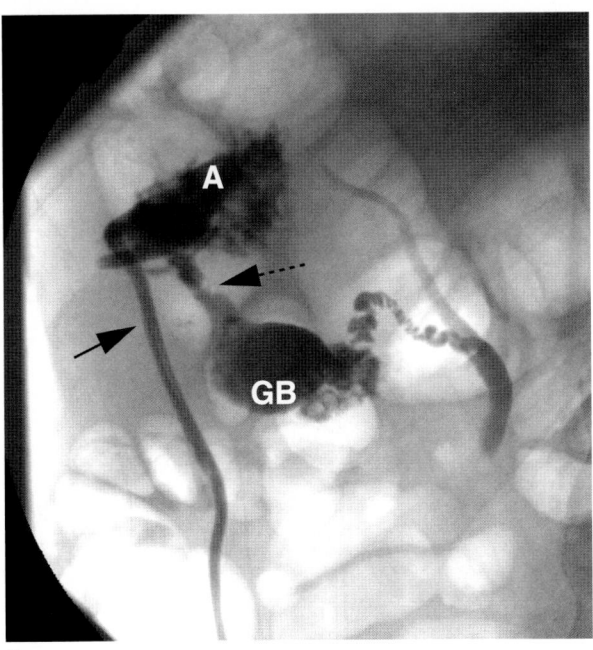

C

FIGURE 18-19. Ultrasound-guided drainage of pyogenic liver abscess secondary to cholecystitis. **A,** Longitudinal ultrasound shows cholelithiasis, complex thickening of the gallbladder (GB) wall, and adjacent debris-containing fluid collection (A) in the liver. **B,** Drainage catheter within the abscess. **C,** Subsequent sinogram through drainage catheter (*arrow*) shows communication (*dashed arrow*) between the gallbladder (GB) and abscess (A).

toxic condition. Emergency cholecystectomy has been shown to have a mortality rate as high as 19% in the elderly.[161] This high mortality is most certainly a reflection of not only the cholecystitis but also the poor overall medical condition of these patients. Emergency surgical cholecystostomy has been championed as a lifesaving, although temporizing, procedure in the elderly, debilitated, or critically ill patient; yet it, too, may be associated with high mortality because of the underlying medical problems in this group of patients.[162]

A major advantage of ultrasound-guided cholecystostomy is that the procedure may be performed at the patient's bedside. Thus, critically ill patients need not be

moved to surgery or the radiology department. Similar to other drainage catheter placement, the cholecystostomy is easily placed with ultrasound guidance via a transhepatic route, using either the trocar method or guidewire exchange technique (Fig. 18-20).

Cholecystostomy placement can be successfully performed in up to 100% of cases with rapid clinical improvement seen in 56% to 95% of patients.[163-165] A review of 182 percutaneous ultrasound-guided cholecystostomies indicates that complications are few; there were 18 technical problems or complications (8%) and one reported death.[166] Many of the technical problems were due to dislodgment of early catheters designed

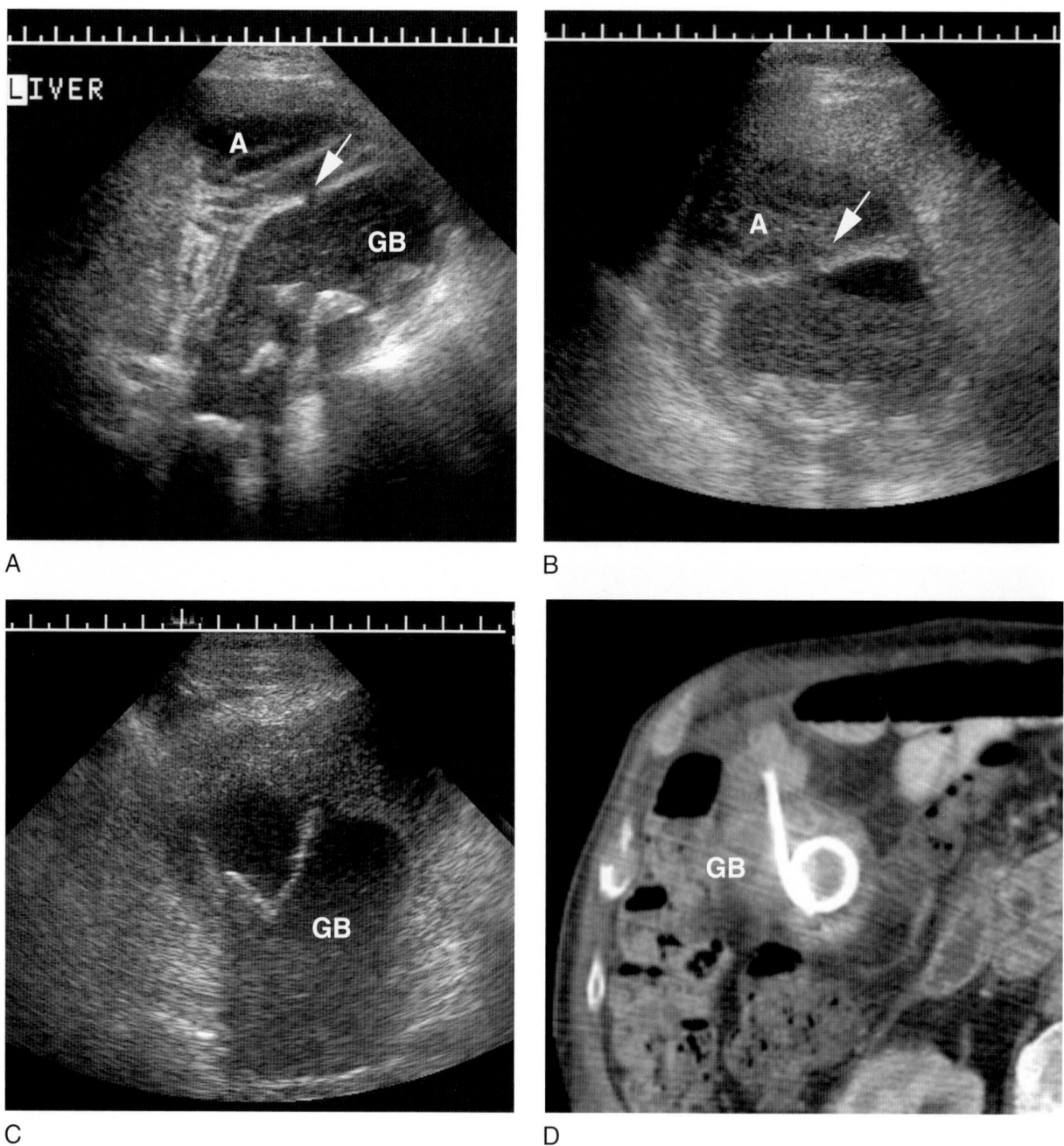

FIGURE 18-20. Cholecystostomy using ultrasound guidance. A, Longitudinal and **B**, Transverse ultrasound images show stones within the gallbladder (GB) and adjacent debris-containing fluid collection representing abscess (A). Perforation of gallbladder wall is identified (*arrow*). **C**, Drainage catheter was placed using ultrasound guidance. **D**, Subsequent CT confirms catheter placement within gallbladder lumen.

without a securing device. Most catheters now include some type of **securing device such as a locking loop**. Due to the severe comorbidities of these patients, the periprocedural mortality rate can be very high. Mortality rates of 36% to 59% have been reported in hospitalized patients following tube placement.[163,166]

Gallbladder aspiration alone may also be considered in treating the noncritically ill patient with acute cholecystitis who is a high surgical risk (Fig. 18-21).

Given that positive bile cultures are present in less than 50% of patients with acute cholecystitis, continuous drainage may not be as critical in the management of this condition.[167] In fact, Chopra et al. achieved a 77% clinical response in high-risk surgical patients using aspiration alone, compared with 90% response in those treated with percutaneous cholecystostomy.[167] Of important note is the absence of complications with aspiration in this study, compared to a 14% complica-

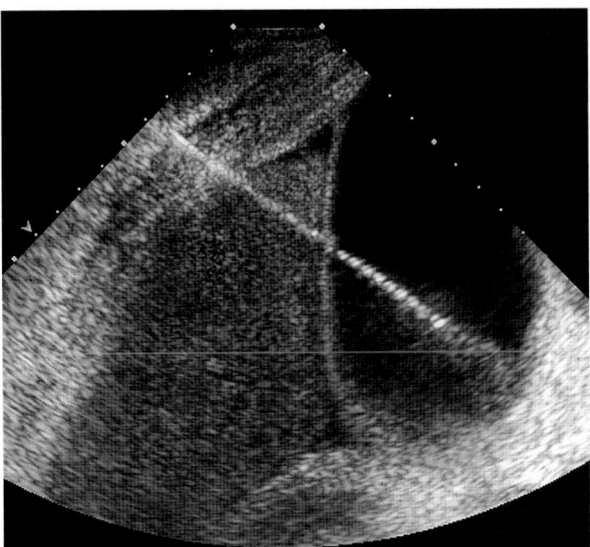

FIGURE 18-21. Ultrasound-guided gallbladder aspiration. Using freehand technique, a needle is advanced transhepatically into the lumen of a sludge-filled gallbladder.

tion rate in those treated with tube drainage. Those patients who failed aspiration were subsequently treated with a cholecystostomy tube. Care must be taken to avoid direct puncture of the gallbladder wall in those with biliary obstruction because significant bile leak may occur.[168]

Bile Ducts

Percutaneous transhepatic cholangiography and drainage is traditionally performed using "blind" cholangiography with fluoroscopy for initial needle placement. However, the combined use of **ultrasound for the initial needle puncture and fluoroscopy for final catheter placement** via the guidewire exchange technique optimizes the advantages of both guidance systems for performance of percutaneous transhepatic cholangiography, biliary drainage, and other invasive procedures.[121] Selected ducts may be punctured under ultrasound guidance for percutaneous transhepatic cholangiography or as the site of definitive catheter placement. In patients with segmental biliary obstruction, a "blind" technique allows initial opacification of the biliary system only by chance. However, ultrasound may allow direct puncture of the appropriate biliary duct. Some authors have advocated the use of ultrasound alone for percutaneous transhepatic biliary drainage.[169] These authors used complete ultrasound guidance for percutaneous transhepatic cholangiography and drainage in patients with hilar cholangiocarcinoma. Ultrasound guidance was successful for percutaneous puncture and drainage in these patients. There was only one major complication in this group in which one patient with ascites and severe cholangitis developed bacterial peritonitis.

Pancreas

The role of percutaneous management of **pancreatitis-related fluid collections** is controversial. Percutaneous aspiration of a significant pancreatic fluid collection is reasonable and effective to exclude infection.[170] Although CT is superior to ultrasound in evaluation of acute pancreatitis, ultrasound provides easy guidance for percutaneous interventional procedures, such as fluid aspiration, in these patients.[171] Nevertheless, CT is often necessary to access deep-seated pancreatitis-related fluid collections.

Percutaneous drainage of **pancreatic abscesses** is effective and can result in cure in up to 86% to 92% of patients (Fig. 18-22).[172,173] Key in the management of these often complex collections is optimized placement of the drain within the infected cavity and frequent monitoring of drain function and cavity size. Frequent drain manipulations are often necessary, with drains varying in size from 8 to 30 French.[172] Drainage catheters may be in place for several weeks to several months.

Although historically considered a surgically managed condition, **infected pancreatic necrosis** may be treated with percutaneous drainage to provide short-term control of sepsis in almost 75% of patients and cure in almost 50% of patients.[174] Such a procedure typically involves very large-bore catheters with frequent, vigorous irrigation, essentially resulting in a "percutaneous necrosectomy."[174]

Pancreatic pseudocysts arise in about 6% of patients following an episode of acute pancreatitis.[173] About half of these pseudocysts will resolve spontaneously.[175] Simple aspiration of these pseudocysts is associated with a high rate of recurrence; therefore, percutaneous catheter drainage is preferred in select cases.[176,177]

Indications for treatment of pseudocysts are well established in the literature and outlined by Neff:[176]

1. Recurrent pain on attempts at feeding following the acute phase of pancreatitis
2. Pseudocyst enlargement
3. Pseudocyst infection
4. Intracystic hemorrhage
5. Secondary biliary or bowel obstruction
6. Pseudocyst cannot be differentiated from neoplastic cyst

Only one third of pseudocysts larger than 6 cm will resolve spontaneously; therefore, many of these large persistent collections require percutaneous drainage.[178] Success of percutaneous pseudocyst drainage ranges from 70% to 100%.[176] Van Sonnenberg et al. published their experience with percutaneous drainage of pseudocysts with excellent results.[179] The cure rate by catheter drainage alone was 90.1%; this includes 48 of 51 infected pseudocysts (94%) and 43 of 50 noninfected pseudocysts (86%). In most of these patients, CT, rather

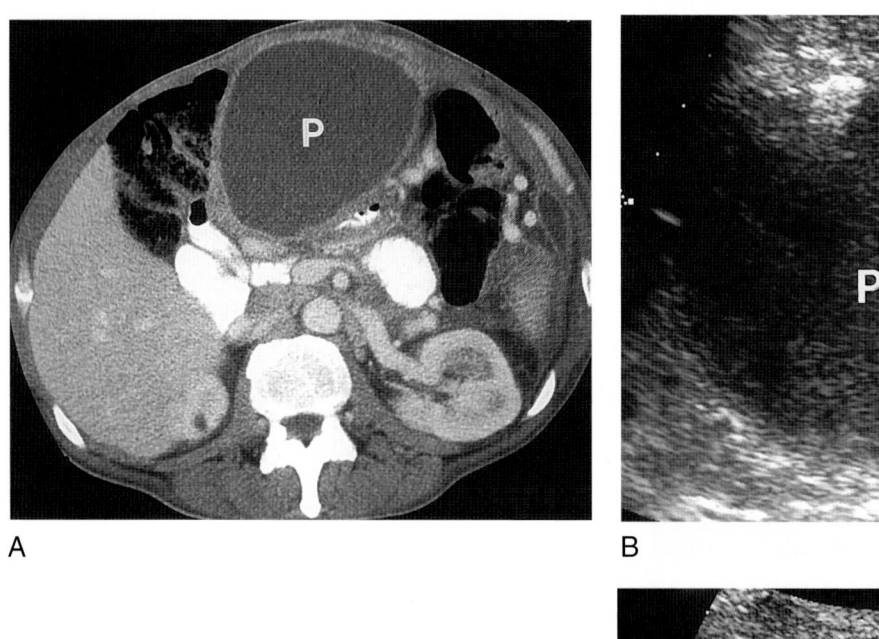

A

B

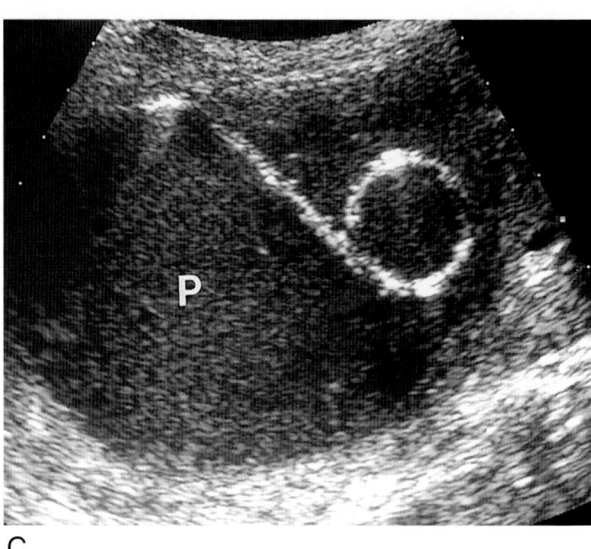

C

FIGURE 18-22. Ultrasound-guided pancreatic pseudocyst drainage. A, Contrast-enhanced CT scan shows a large fluid collection pseudocyst (P) anterior and superior to the pancreas. **B,** Ultrasound shows aspiration needle (*arrow*) in the pseudocyst, which contains echogenic debris. **C,** With the catheter exchange technique, a locking loop catheter was placed into pancreatic pseudocyst for drainage.

than ultrasound, was the primary method of guidance, although ultrasound may be used for guidance of drainage (see Fig. 18-22). Overall success of percutaneous drainage may be related to the integrity of the pancreatic duct.[180]

Spleen

Splenic abscesses are very uncommon and have historically been managed surgically. However, with increasing experience in percutaneous abscess management, imaging-guided drain placement into select splenic abscesses has been successfully performed in up to 100% of patients.[181,182] With smaller (<3.5 cm) infected splenic fluid collections, a trial of simple aspiration may be reasonable, with drain placement considered if reaccumulation of fluid occurs. More complex, multi-loculated abscesses or deep-seated collections should be managed surgically. The risk of bleeding during splenic

drainage is not trivial, occurring in one of seven drainages in one series.[92]

Kidney

Abscess

Renal abscesses may be successfully treated with percutaneous drainage combined with systemic antibiotics (Fig. 18-23). The size of the abscess should be considered when determining the type of treatment. In a review of 52 patients with renal abscesses, Siegel et al. determined that percutaneous drainage of renal abscesses measuring 3 to 5 cm resulted in a 92% cure rate.[183] For abscesses larger than 5 cm, a cure rate of 73% was achieved using percutaneous drainage, although two drainage procedures were required in one third of these patients. Abscesses smaller than 3 cm can be treated with antibiotics alone.

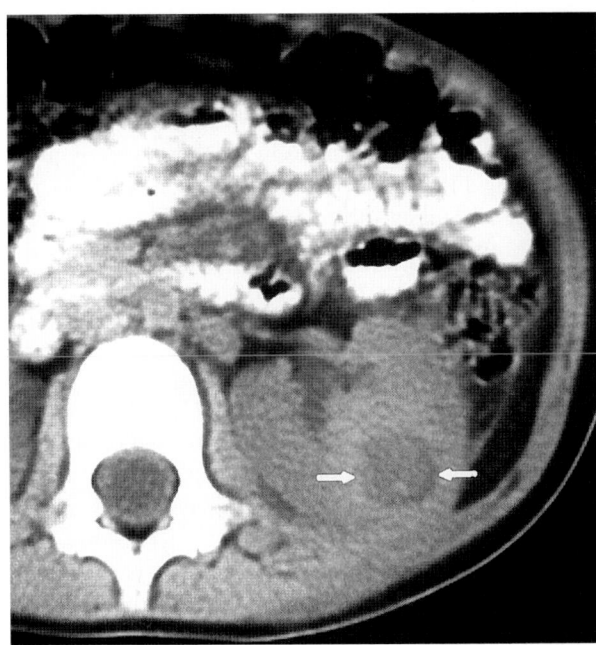

A

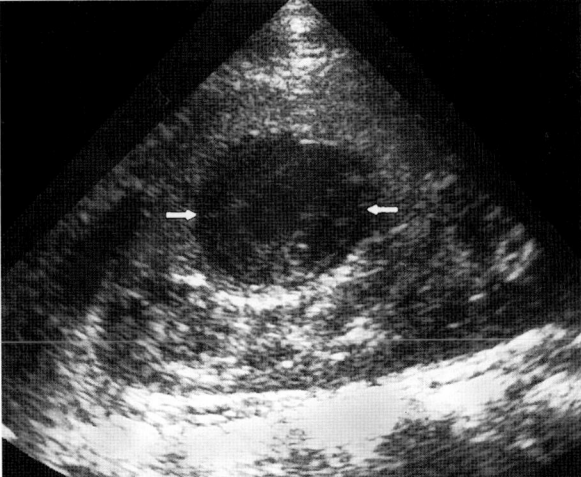

B

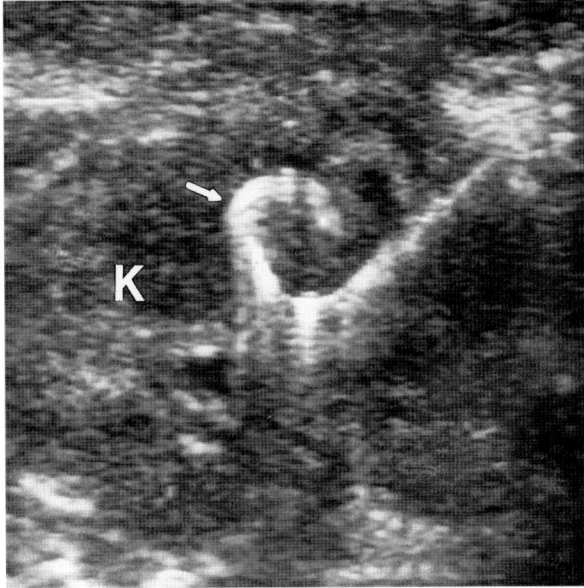

C

FIGURE 18-23. Renal abscess drainage. A, CT scan with orally administered contrast material shows a small 2.5 cm, low-attenuating mass (*arrows*) in the mid-left kidney. **B,** Longitudinal ultrasound of the left kidney shows a 2.5 cm cystic mass with internal debris (*arrows*). **C,** Transverse image of the kidney (K). Using the Seldinger technique, a locking loop catheter (*arrow*) was placed into the renal abscess.

Percutaneous Nephrostomy

Ultrasound has gained wide acceptance as the imaging modality for initial needle placement for percutaneous nephrostomy (Fig. 18-24). After the dilated collecting system is accessed, a catheter is placed via the Seldinger technique using fluoroscopic control.[184,185] Color flow Doppler imaging is useful in supplementing ultrasound guidance in renal biopsies, nephrostomies, and renal cyst punctures.[185] Puncture of intrarenal vessels can be avoided by using color flow Doppler imaging in performance of these interventional procedures.

Perinephric Abscesses or Fluid Collections

Fluid collections that occur in the retroperitoneal space include **abscesses, urinomas, lymphoceles,** and **hematomas.** CT is usually performed to identify the fluid collection and its extent. Either ultrasound or CT may be used for aspiration or drainage of these fluid collections. If drainage is needed, the Seldinger technique may be used with ultrasound for initial needle placement and fluoroscopy for catheter placement.

PERCUTANEOUS CYST MANAGEMENT—WHEN TO CONSIDER ABLATION

Renal Cyst

Simple aspiration of large symptomatic or obstructing renal cysts is ineffective in the long-term management of renal cysts due to rapid reaccumulation of cyst fluid within the cavity.[186] For this reason, there has been interest in aspiration combined with sclerosis in order to provide more permanent ablation of the cyst.

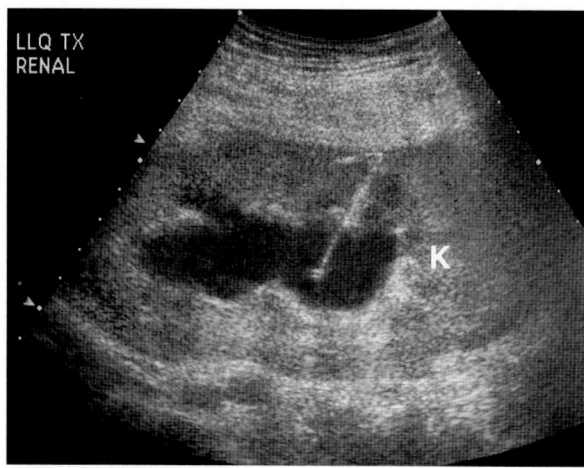

FIGURE 18-24. Ultrasound-guided nephrostomy tube placement in renal transplant. Longitudinal image shows moderate pyelocaliectasis of the renal transplant (K). Needle is visible within the dilated renal pelvis.

Permanent Ablation of a Cyst. The procedure involves placing a 7 to 8 French drain into the cyst with aspiration of the cyst fluid. This fluid is sent for cytology and other chemical markers to confirm a serous nature of the fluid.[187] If there is no evidence of malignancy, the cyst is then injected with contrast material under fluoroscopy to **exclude a communication with the urinary collecting system**; sclerosis should not be performed if such a communication exists. The cyst is then injected with 95% alcohol at one half of the cyst volume, not to exceed 100 mL.[188] Twenty mL of 2% lidocaine may be injected with the alcohol to minimize the burning pain that often accompanies alcohol injection. The patient is turned in various positions over a 20-minute period to facilitate exposure of the cyst wall to the sclerosing agent. The alcohol is aspirated and the drain is removed or placed to continuous suction. Repeat injections are often performed over the next 2 to 3 days to maximize sclerosis.

Fontana et al. successfully treated 68 of 70 renal cysts using 95% ethanol as a sclerosing agent with no recurrence at mean follow-up of 48 months.[186] Their technique included two repeat alcohol injections performed over 24 hours following the initial sclerosis session. Two cysts could not be treated due to communication with the collecting system and hemorrhage into the cyst following percutaneous puncture. While alcohol is a commonly used sclerosing agent, other agents include tetracycline, doxycycline, talc, and iodine.

Liver Cyst

In a fashion similar to that for renal cysts, hepatic cysts can be effectively sclerosed to provide long-term relief of symptoms. A **communication to the biliary tract must**

be excluded by injecting the cyst with contrast under fluoroscopy. Using alcohol and/or tetracycline or doxycycline, van Sonnenberg et al. were able to successfully treat 21 of 24 (88%) symptomatic hepatic cysts.[189] Frequently, multiple sclerosing sessions were required, including 11 sessions over 44 days in one patient. Such treatment resulted in a reduction in the cyst to 5% to 15% of its original size.

Ovarian Cyst

Historically, surgical extirpation of symptomatic ovarian cysts has been the standard of care. Percutaneous management has been discouraged due to the concern of seeding of malignant cells in the inadvertent aspiration of a low-grade neoplasm and the poor sensitivity in characterizing aspirated cyst fluid.[190,191] However, given the well-recognized sonographic criteria of benign ovarian cysts, the confidence level in percutaneous aspiration of such symptomatic simple cysts has improved.

Ultrasound-guided aspiration of symptomatic, benign ovarian cysts is highly effective in alleviating patient symptoms.[192] A thorough ultrasound examination should be performed initially to fully characterize the symptomatic cyst. If the cyst can be confidently characterized as benign with no worrisome features, aspiration can be performed. Some authors recommend that preprocedural serum tumor markers be obtained to help exclude malignancy.[193] Using either a transabdominal or endovaginal approach, a 20 or 22 gauge needle can be used to completely aspirate the cyst, with 100% relief reported in one series.[192] Fluid should be sent for appropriate studies, including cytology. An 11% to 26% recurrence rate can be expected.[194,195]

References

1. Bernardino M: Percutaneous biopsy. AJR 1984;142:41-45.
2. Grant E, Richardson J, Smirniotopoulos J, et al: Fine-needle biopsy directed by real-time sonography: Technique and accuracy. AJR 1983;141:29-32.
3. Gazelle G, Haaga J: Guided percutaneous biopsy of intraabdominal lesions. AJR 1989;153:929-935.
4. Matalon T, Silver B: US guidance of interventional procedures. Radiology 1990;174:43-47.
5. Charboneau J, Reading C, Welch T: CT and sonographically guided needle biopsy: Current techniques and new innovations. AJR 1990;154:1-10.
6. Reading CC, Charboneau JW, James EM, et al: Sonographically guided percutaneous biopsy of small (3 cm or less) masses. AJR Am J Roentgenol 1988;151:189-192.
7. Mitty H, Efremidis S, Yeh H: Impact of fine-needle biopsy on management of patients with carcinoma of the pancreas. AJR 1981;137:1119-1121.
8. Bret PM, Sente JM, Bretagnolle M, et al: Ultrasonically guided fine-needle biopsy in focal intrahepatic lesions: Six years' experience. Can Assoc Radiol J 1986;37:5-8.
9. Spamer C, Brambs H, Koch H, et al: Benign circumscribed lesions of the liver diagnosed with

ultrasonically guided fine-needle biopsy. J Clin Ultrasound 1986;14:83-88.

10. Rapaport S: Preoperative hemostatic evaluation: Which tests, if any? Blood 1983;61:229-231.

11. Silverman S, Mueller P, Pfister R: Hemostatic evaluation before abdominal interventions: An overview and proposal. AJR 1990;154:233-238.

12. Channing Rodgers R, Levin J: A critical appraisal of the bleeding time. Sem Thromb Hemostasis 1990;16:1-20.

13. Peterson P, Hayes T, Arkin C, et al: The preoperative bleeding time test lacks clinical benefit: College of American Pathologists' and American Society of Clinical Pathologists' position article. Arch Surg 1998;133:134-139.

14. Mattix H, Singh A: Is the bleeding time predictive of bleeding prior to a percutaneous renal biopsy? Curr Opin Neph Hyp 1999;8:715-718.

15. Murphy T, Dorfman G, Becker J: Use of preprocedural tests by interventional radiologists. Radiology 1993;186:213-220.

16. Rapaport S: Assessing hemostatic function before abdominal interventions. AJR 1990;154:239-240.

17. Peter FW, Benkovic C, Muehlberger T, et al: Effects of desmopressin on thrombogenesis in aspirin-induced platelet dysfunction. Br J Haematol 2002;117:658-663.

18. Zins M, Vilgrain V, Gayno S, et al: US-guided percutaneous liver biopsy with plugging of the needle track: A prospective study in 72 high-risk patients. Radiology 1992;184:841-843.

19. Crummy A, McDermott J, Wojtowycz M: A technique for embolization of biopsy tracts. AJR 1989;153:67-68.

20. Gupta S, Ahrar K, Morello F, et al: Masses in or around the pancreatic head: CT-guided coaxial fine-needle aspiration biopsy with a posterior transcaval approach. Radiology 2002;222:63-69.

21. Brandt K, Charboneau J, Stephens D, et al: CT- and US-guided biopsy of the pancreas. Radiology 1993;187:99-104.

22. Murphy F, Barefield K, Steinberg H, et al: CT- or sonography-guided biopsy of the liver in the presence of ascites: Frequency of complications. AJR 1988;151:485-486.

23. Little AF, Ferris JV, Dodd GD, 3rd, et al: Image-guided percutaneous hepatic biopsy: Effect of ascites on the complication rate. Radiology 1996;199:79-83.

24. Longo J, Bilbao J, Barettino M, et al: Percutaneous vascular and nonvascular puncture under US guidance: Role of color Doppler imaging. Radiographics 1994;14:959-972.

25. McGahan J, Anderson M: Pulsed Doppler sonography as an aid in ultrasound-guided aspiration biopsy. Gastrointest Radiol 1987;12:279-284.

26. Sheafor D, Paulson E, Kleiwer M, et al: Comparison of sonographic and CT guidance techniques: Does CT fluoroscopy decrease procedure time? AJR 2000;174:939-942.

27. Kleiwer M, Sheafor D, Paulson E: Percutaneous liver biopsy: A cost-benefit analysis comparing sonographic and CT guidance. AJR 1999;173:1199-1202.

28. Sheafor DH, Paulson EK, Simmons CM, et al: Abdominal percutaneous interventional procedures: Comparison of CT and US guidance. Radiology 1998;207:705-710.

29. Dameron R, Paulson E, Fisher A, et al: Indeterminate findings on imaging-guided biopsy. AJR 1999;173:461-464.

30. Welch T, Sheedy PI, Johnson C, et al: CT-guided biopsy: Prospective analysis of 1,000 procedures. Radiology 1989;171:493-496.

31. Kirchner J, Kickuth R, Laufer U, et al: CT fluoroscopically-assisted puncture of thoracic and abdominal masses: A randomized trial. Clin Radiol 2002;57:188-192.

32. Isler R, Ferruci JJ, Wittenberg J, et al: Tissue core biopsy of abdominal tumors with a 22 gauge cutting needle. AJR 1981;136:725-728.

33. Wittenberg J, Mueller P, Ferruci JJ, et al: Percutaneous core biopsy of abdominal tumors using 22 gauge needles: Further observations. AJR 1982;139:75-80.

34. Andrioloe J, Haaga J, Adams R, et al: Needle characteristics assessed in the laboratory. Radiology 1983;148:659-662.

35. Lieberman R, Hafez G, Crummy A: Histology from aspiration biopsy: Turner needle experience. AJR 1982;138:561-564.

36. Pagani JJ: Biopsy of focal hepatic lesions. Comparison of 18 and 22 gauge needles. Radiology 1983;147:673-675.

37. Haaga JR, LiPuma JP, Bryan PJ, et al: Clinical comparison of small- and large-caliber cutting needles for biopsy. Radiology 1983;146:665-667.

38. Ubhi CS, Irving HC, Guillou PJ, et al: A new technique for renal allograft biopsy. Br J Radiol 1987;60:599-600.

39. Erwin BC, Brynes RK, Chan WC, et al: Percutaneous needle biopsy in the diagnosis and classification of lymphoma. Cancer 1986;57:1074-1078.

40. Miller DL, Wall RT: Fentanyl and diazepam for analgesia and sedation during radiologic special procedures. Radiology 1987;162:195-198.

41. Hurlbert B, Landers D: Sedation and analgesia for interventional radiologic procedures in adults. Semin Interven Radiol 1987;4:151-160.

42. Caturelli E, Giacobbe A, Facciorusso D, et al: Free-hand technique with ordinary antisepsis in abdominal US-guided fine-needle punctures: Three-year experience. Radiology 1996;199:721-723.

43. Rizzatto G, Solbiati L, Croce F, et al: Aspiration biopsy of superficial lesions: Ultrasonic guidance with a linear-array probe. AJR Am J Roentgenol 1987;148:623-625.

44. Buonocore E, Skipper GJ: Steerable real-time sonographically guided needle biopsy. AJR Am J Roentgenol 1981;136:387-392.

45. Reid MH: Real-time sonographic needle biopsy guide. AJR Am J Roentgenol 1983;140:162-163.

46. Moulton JS, Moore PT: Coaxial percutaneous biopsy technique with automated biopsy devices: Value in improving accuracy and negative predictive value. Radiology 1993;186:515-522.

47. Hahn PF, Eisenberg PJ, Pitman MB, et al: Cytopathologic touch preparations (imprints) from core needle biopsies: Accuracy compared with that of fine-needle aspirates. AJR Am J Roentgenol 1995;165:1277-1279.

48. Miller DA, Carrasco CH, Katz RL, et al: Fine needle aspiration biopsy: The role of immediate cytologic assessment. AJR Am J Roentgenol 1986;147:155-158.

49. McNamara MP, Jr, McNamara ME: Preparation of a homemade ultrasound biopsy phantom. J Clin Ultrasound 1989;17:456-458.

50. Fornage BD: A simple phantom for training in ultrasound-guided needle biopsy using the freehand technique. J Ultrasound Med 1989;8:701-703.

51. Georgian-Smith D, Shiels WE, 2nd: From the RSNA refresher courses. Freehand interventional sonography in the breast: Basic principles and clinical applications. Radiographics 1996;16:149-161.

52. Heckemann R, Seidel KJ: The sonographic appearance and contrast enhancement of puncture needles. J Clin Ultrasound 1983;11:265-268.

53. McGahan JP: Laboratory assessment of ultrasonic needle and catheter visualization. J Ultrasound Med 1986;5:373-377.

54. Reading CC, Charboneau JW, Felmlee JP, et al: US-guided percutaneous biopsy: Use of a screw biopsy stylet to aid needle detection. Radiology 1987;163:280-281.

55. Hamper UM, Savader BL, Sheth S: Improved needle-tip visualization by color Doppler sonography. AJR Am J Roentgenol 1991;156:401-402.

56. Cockburn JF, Cosgrove DO: Device to enhance visibility of needle or catheter tip at color Doppler US. Radiology 1995;195:570-572.

57. Downey DB, Wilson SR: Ultrasonographically guided biopsy of small intra-abdominal masses. Can Assoc Radiol J 1993;44:350-353.

58. Buscarini L, Fornari F, Bolondi L, et al: Ultrasound-guided fine-needle biopsy of focal liver lesions: Techniques, diagnostic accuracy and complications. A retrospective study on 2091 biopsies. J Hepatol 1990;11:344-348.

59. Cronan JJ, Esparza AR, Dorfman GS, et al: Cavernous hemangioma of the liver: Role of percutaneous biopsy. Radiology 1988;166:135-138.

60. Caturelli E, Rapaccini GL, Sabelli C, et al: Ultrasound-guided fine-needle aspiration biopsy in the diagnosis of hepatic hemangioma. Liver 1986;6:326-330.

61. Tung GA, Cronan JJ: Percutaneous needle biopsy of hepatic cavernous hemangioma. J Clin Gastroenterol 1993;16:117-122.

62. Heilo A, Stenwig AE: Liver hemangioma: US-guided 18-gauge core-needle biopsy. Radiology 1997;204:719-722.

63. Terriff BA, Gibney RG, Scudamore CH: Fatality from fine-needle aspiration biopsy of a hepatic hemangioma. AJR Am J Roentgenol 1990;154:203-204.

64. Dodd GD, 3rd, Carr BI: Percutaneous biopsy of portal vein thrombus: A new staging technique for hepatocellular carcinoma. AJR Am J Roentgenol 1993;161:229-233.

65. Vilana R, Bru C, Bruix J, et al: Fine-needle aspiration biopsy of portal vein thrombus: Value in detecting malignant thrombosis. AJR Am J Roentgenol 1993;160:1285-1287.

66. Piccinino F, Sagnelli E, Pasquale G, et al: Complications following percutaneous liver biopsy. A multicentre retrospective study on 68,276 biopsies. J Hepatol 1986;2:165-173.

67. Van Thiel DH, Gavaler JS, Wright H, et al: Liver biopsy. Its safety and complications as seen at a liver transplant center. Transplantation 1993;55:1087-1090.

68. Garcia-Tsao G, Boyer JL: Outpatient liver biopsy: How safe is it? Ann Intern Med 1993;118:150-153.

69. McGill DB, Rakela J, Zinsmeister AR, et al: A 21-year experience with major hemorrhage after percutaneous liver biopsy. Gastroenterology 1990;99:1396-1400.

70. Lees WR, Hall-Craggs MA, Manhire A: Five years' experience of fine-needle aspiration biopsy: 454 consecutive cases. Clin Radiol 1985;36:517-520.

71. Hall-Craggs MA, Lees WR: Fine-needle aspiration biopsy: Pancreatic and biliary tumors. AJR Am J Roentgenol 1986;147:399-403.

72. Jennings PE, Donald JJ, Coral A, et al: Ultrasound-guided core biopsy. Lancet 1989;1:1369-1371.

73. Mitchell ML, Carney CN: Cytologic criteria for the diagnosis of pancreatic carcinoma. Am J Clin Pathol 1985;83:171-176.

74. Carlson SK, Johnson CD, Brandt KR, et al: Pancreatic cystic neoplasms: The role and sensitivity of needle aspiration and biopsy. Abdom Imaging 1998;23:387-393.

75. Lewandrowski K, Lee J, Southern J, et al: Cyst fluid analysis in the differential diagnosis of pancreatic cysts: A new approach to the preoperative assessment of pancreatic cystic lesions. AJR Am J Roentgenol 1995;164:815-819.

76. Yong WH, Southern JF, Pins MR, et al: Cyst fluid NB/70K concentration and leukocyte esterase: Two new markers for differentiating pancreatic serous tumors from pseudocysts. Pancreas 1995;10:342-346.

77. Smith EH: Complications of percutaneous abdominal fine-needle biopsy. Review. Radiology 1991;178:253-258.

78. Mueller PR, Miketic LM, Simeone JF, et al: Severe acute pancreatitis after percutaneous biopsy of the pancreas. AJR Am J Roentgenol 1988;151:493-494.

79. Warshaw AL, Fernandez-del Castillo C: Pancreatic carcinoma. N Engl J Med 1992;326:455-465.

80. Dechet CB, Zincke H, Sebo TJ, et al: Prospective analysis of computerized tomography and needle biopsy with permanent sectioning to determine the nature of solid renal masses in adults. J Urol 2003;169:71-74.

81. Wood BJ, Khan MA, McGovern F, et al: Imaging guided biopsy of renal masses: Indications, accuracy and impact on clinical management. J Urol 1999;161:1470-1474.

82. Yoshimoto M, Fujisawa S, Sudo M: Percutaneous renal biopsy well-visualized by orthogonal ultrasound application using linear scanning. Clin Nephrol 1988;30:106-110.

83. Rapaccini GL, Pompili M, Caturelli E, et al: Real-time ultrasound guided renal biopsy in diffuse renal disease: 114 consecutive cases. Surg Endosc 1989;3:42-45.

84. Hergesell O, Felten H, Andrassy K, et al: Safety of ultrasound-guided percutaneous renal biopsy-retrospective analysis of 1090 consecutive cases. Nephrol Dial Transplant 1998;13:975-977.

85. Bogan ML, Kopecky KK, Kraft JL, et al: Needle biopsy of renal allografts: Comparison of two techniques. Radiology 1990;174:273-275.

86. Welch TJ, Sheedy PF, 2nd, Stephens DH, et al: Percutaneous adrenal biopsy: Review of a 10-year experience. Radiology 1994;193:341-344.

87. Dunnick NR, Heaston D, Halvorsen R, et al: CT appearance of adrenal cortical carcinoma. J Comput Assist Tomogr 1982;6:978-982.

88. Bernardino ME: Management of the asymptomatic patient with a unilateral adrenal mass. Radiology 1988;166:121-123.

89. Casola G, Nicolet V, Van Sonnenberg E, et al: Unsuspected pheochromocytoma: Risk of blood-pressure alterations during percutaneous adrenal biopsy. Radiology 1986;159:733-735.

90. McCorkell SJ, Niles NL: Fine-needle aspiration of catecholamine-producing adrenal masses: A possibly fatal mistake. AJR Am J Roentgenol 1985;145:113-114.

91. Keogan MT, Freed KS, Paulson EK, et al: Imaging-guided percutaneous biopsy of focal splenic lesions: Update on safety and effectiveness. AJR Am J Roentgenol 1999;172:933-937.

92. Lucey BC, Boland GW, Maher MM, et al: Percutaneous nonvascular splenic intervention: A 10-year review. AJR Am J Roentgenol 2002;179:1591-1596.

93. Jansson SE, Bondestam S, Heinonen E, et al: Value of liver and spleen aspiration biopsy in malignant diseases when these organs show no signs of involvement in sonography. Acta Med Scand 1983;213:279-281.

94. Solbiati L, Bossi MC, Bellotti E, et al: Focal lesions in the spleen: Sonographic patterns and guided biopsy. AJR Am J Roentgenol 1983;140:59-65.

95. Caraway NP, Fanning CV: Use of fine-needle aspiration biopsy in the evaluation of splenic lesions in a cancer center. Diagn Cytopathol 1997;16:312-316.

96. Soderstrom N: How to use cytodiagnostic spleen puncture. Acta Med Scand 1976;199:1-5.

97. Sheth S, Hamper UM, Stanley DB, et al: US guidance for thoracic biopsy: A valuable alternative to CT. Radiology 1999;210:721-726.

98. Douglas BR, Charboneau JW, Reading CC: Ultrasound-guided intervention: Expanding horizons. Radiol Clin North Am 2001;39:415-428.

99. Livraghi T, Damascelli B, Lombardi C, et al: Risk in fine-needle abdominal biopsy. J Clin Ultrasound 1983;11:77-81.

100. Fornari F, Civardi G, Cavanna L, et al: Complications of ultrasonically guided fine-needle abdominal biopsy. Results of a multicenter Italian study and review of the literature. The Cooperative Italian Study Group. Scand J Gastroenterol 1989;24:949-955.

101. Nolsoe C, Nielsen L, Torp-Pedersen S, et al: Major complications and deaths due to interventional ultrasonography: A review of 8000 cases. J Clin Ultrasound 1990;18:179-184.

102. Bergenfeldt M, Genell S, Lindholm K, et al: Needle-tract seeding after percutaneous fine-needle biopsy of pancreatic carcinoma. Case report. Acta Chir Scand 1988;154:77-79.

103. Caturelli E, Rapaccini GL, Anti M, Fabiano A: Malignant seeding after fine-needle aspiration biopsy of the pancreas. Diagn Imaging Clin Med 1985;54:88-91.

104. Haddad FS, Somsin AA: Seeding and perineal implantation of prostatic cancer in the track of the biopsy needle: Three case reports and a review of the literature. J Surg Oncol 1987;35:184-191.

105. Greenstein A, Merimsky E, Baratz M, et al: Late appearance of perineal implantation of prostatic carcinoma after perineal needle biopsy. Urology 1989;33:59-60.

106. Onodera H, Oikawa M, Abe M, et al: Cutaneous seeding of hepatocellular carcinoma after fine-needle aspiration biopsy. J Ultrasound Med 1987;6:273-275.

107. Kiser GC, Totonchy M, Barry JM: Needle tract seeding after percutaneous renal adenocarcinoma aspiration. J Urol 1986;136:1292-1293.

108. Muller NL, Bergin CJ, Miller RR, et al: Seeding of malignant cells into the needle track after lung and pleural biopsy. Can Assoc Radiol J 1986;37:192-194.

109. Fajardo LL: Breast tumor seeding along localization guide wire tracks. Radiology 1988;169:580-581.

110. Glasgow BJ, Brown HH, Zargoza AM, et al: Quantitation of tumor seeding from fine needle aspiration of ocular melanomas. Am J Ophthalmol 1988;105:538-546.

111. Hidai H, Sakuramoto T, Miura T, et al: Needle tract seeding following puncture of retroperitoneal liposarcoma. Eur Urol 1983;9:368-369.

112. Raftopoulos Y, Furey WW, Kacey DJ, et al: Tumor implantation after computed tomography-guided biopsy of lung cancer. J Thorac Cardiovasc Surg 2000;119:1288-1289.

113. Shinohara S, Yamamoto E, Tanabe M, et al: Implantation metastasis of head and neck cancer after fine needle aspiration biopsy. Auris Nasus Larynx 2001;28:377-380.

114. McGahan JP, Hanson F: Ultrasonographic aspiration and biopsy techniques. In Dublin A (ed): Outpatient Invasive Radiologic Procedures: Diagnostic and Therapeutic. Philadelphia, WB Saunders, 1989, pp 79-113.

115. Blady J: Aspiration biopsy of tumors in obscure or difficult locations under roentgenoscopic guidance. AJR 1939;42:515-524.

116. Gronvall S, Gammelgaard J, Haubek A, et al: Drainage of abdominal abscesses guided by sonography. AJR Am J Roentgenol 1982;138:527-529.

117. Haaga JR, Alfidi RJ, Havrilla TR, et al: CT detection and aspiration of abdominal abscesses. AJR Am J Roentgenol 1977;128:465-474.

118. Hahn PF, Gervais DA, O'Neill MJ, et al: Nonvascular interventional procedures: Analysis of a 10-year database containing more than 21,000 cases. Radiology 2001;220:730-736.

119. Van Sonnenberg E, D'Agostino HB, Casola G, et al: Percutaneous abscess drainage: Current concepts. Radiology 1991;181:617-626.

120. Gazelle GS, Mueller PR: Abdominal abscess. Imaging and intervention. Radiol Clin North Am 1994;32:913-932.

121. McGahan JP, Raduns K: Biliary drainage using combined ultrasound fluoroscopic guidance. J Intervent Radiol 1990;5:33-37.

122. McGahan JP: Aspiration and biopsy—advantages of sonographic guidance. In McGahan JP (ed): Controversies in Ultrasound: Clinics in Diagnostic Ultrasound. Vol. 20. New York, Churchill Livingstone, 1987, pp 249-270.

123. McGahan JP, Brant W: Principles, instrumentation, and guidance systems. In McGahan JP (ed): Interventional Ultrasound. Baltimore, Williams & Wilkins, 1990, pp 1-20.

124. Deveney CW, Lurie K, Deveney KE: Improved treatment of intra-abdominal abscess. A result of improved localization, drainage, and patient care, not technique. Arch Surg 1988;123:1126-1130.

125. Goldberg MA, Mueller PR, Saini S, et al: Importance of daily rounds by the radiologist after interventional procedures of the abdomen and chest. Radiology 1991;180:767-770.

126. Casola G, Van Sonnenberg E, Neff CC, et al: Abscesses in Crohn disease: Percutaneous drainage. Radiology 1987;163:19-22.

127. Safrit HD, Mauro MA, Jaques PF: Percutaneous abscess drainage in Crohn's disease. AJR Am J Roentgenol 1987;148:859-862.

128. Mueller PR, Saini S, Wittenburg J, et al: Sigmoid diverticular abscesses: Percutaneous drainage as an adjunct to surgical resection in 24 cases. Radiology 1987;164:321-325.

129. Stabile BE, Puccio E, Van Sonnenberg E, et al: Preoperative percutaneous drainage of diverticular abscesses. Am J Surg 1990;159:99-104.

130. Neff CC, Van Sonnenberg E, Casola G, et al: Diverticular abscesses: Percutaneous drainage. Radiology 1987;163:15-18.

131. Van Sonnenberg E, Wittich GR, Casola G, et al: Periappendiceal abscesses: Percutaneous drainage. Radiology 1987;163:23-26.

132. Jeffrey RB, Jr, Tolentino CS, Federle MP, et al: Percutaneous drainage of periappendiceal abscesses: Review of 20 patients. AJR Am J Roentgenol 1987;149:59-62.

133. McGahan JP, Anderson MW, Walter JP: Portable real-time sonographic and needle guidance systems for aspiration and drainage. AJR Am J Roentgenol 1986;147:1241-1246.

134. Nosher JL, Needell GS, Amorosa JK, et al: Transrectal pelvic abscess drainage with sonographic guidance. AJR Am J Roentgenol 1986;146:1047-1048.

135. Nosher JL, Winchman HK, Needell GS: Transvaginal pelvic abscess drainage with US guidance. Radiology 1987;165:872-873.

136. Abbitt PL, Goldwag S, Urbanski S: Endovaginal

sonography for guidance in draining pelvic fluid collections. AJR Am J Roentgenol 1990;154:849-850.

137. Van Sonnenberg E, D'Agostino HB, Casola G, et al: US-guided transvaginal drainage of pelvic abscesses and fluid collections. Radiology 1991;181:53-56.

138. Alexander AA, Eschelman DJ, Nazarian LN, et al: Transrectal sonographically guided drainage of deep pelvic abscesses. AJR Am J Roentgenol 1994;162:1227-1232.

139. Feld R, Eschelman DJ, Sagerman JE, et al: Treatment of pelvic abscesses and other fluid collections: Efficacy of transvaginal sonographically guided aspiration and drainage. AJR Am J Roentgenol 1994;163:1141-1145.

140. Kuligowska E, Keller E, Ferrucci JT: Treatment of pelvic abscesses: Value of one-step sonographically guided transrectal needle aspiration and lavage. AJR Am J Roentgenol 1995;164:201-206.

141. Kastan DJ, Nelsen KM, Shetty PC, et al: Combined transrectal sonographic and fluoroscopic guidance for deep pelvic abscess drainage. J Ultrasound Med 1996;15:235-239.

142. Nelson AL, Sinow RM, Renslo R, et al: Endovaginal ultrasonographically guided transvaginal drainage for treatment of pelvic abscesses. Am J Obstet Gynecol 1995;172:1926-1935.

143. Lambiase RE, Deyoe L, Cronan JJ, et al: Percutaneous drainage of 335 consecutive abscesses: Results of primary drainage with 1-year follow-up. Radiology 1992;184:167-179.

144. Schuster MR, Crummy AB, Wojtowycz MM, et al: Abdominal abscesses associated with enteric fistulas: Percutaneous management. J Vasc Interv Radiol 1992;3:359-363.

145. Gervais DA, Hahn PF, O'Neill MJ, et al: Percutaneous abscess drainage in Crohn disease: Technical success and short- and long-term outcomes during 14 years. Radiology 2002;222:645-651.

146. Sahai A, Belair M, Gianfelice D, et al: Percutaneous drainage of intra-abdominal abscesses in Crohn's disease: Short and long-term outcome. Am J Gastroenterol 1997;92:275-278.

147. Johnson RD, Mueller PR, Ferrucci JT, Jr, et al: Percutaneous drainage of pyogenic liver abscesses. AJR Am J Roentgenol 1985;144:463-467.

148. Van Sonnenberg E, Mueller PR, Ferrucci JT, Jr: Percutaneous drainage of 250 abdominal abscesses and fluid collections. Part I: Results, failures, and complications. Radiology 1984;151:337-341.

149. Wong WM, Wong BC, Hui CK, et al: Pyogenic liver abscess: Retrospective analysis of 80 cases over a 10-year period. J Gastroenterol Hepatol 2002;17:1001-1007.

150. Giorgio A, Tarantino L, Mariniello N, et al: Pyogenic liver abscesses: 13 years of experience in percutaneous needle aspiration with US guidance. Radiology 1995;195:122-124.

151. Krige JE, Beckingham IJ: ABC of diseases of liver, pancreas, and biliary system. BMJ 2001;322:537-540.

152. Shankar S, Van Sonnenberg E, Silverman SG, et al: Interventional radiology procedures in the liver. Biopsy, drainage, and ablation. Clin Liver Dis 2002;6:91-118.

153. Van Sonnenberg E, Mueller PR, Schiffman HR, et al: Intrahepatic amebic abscesses: Indications for and results of percutaneous catheter drainage. Radiology 1985;156:631-635.

154. Van Allan RJ, Katz MD, Johnson MB, et al: Uncomplicated amebic liver abscess: Prospective evaluation of percutaneous therapeutic aspiration. Radiology 1992;183:827-830.

155. Khuroo MS, Zargar SA, Mahajan R: Echinococcus granulosus cysts in the liver: Management with percutaneous drainage. Radiology 1991;180:141-145.

156. Khuroo MS, Wani NA, Javid G, et al: Percutaneous drainage compared with surgery for hepatic hydatid cysts. N Engl J Med 1997;337:881-887.

157. Aygun E, Sahin M, Odev K, et al: The management of liver hydatid cysts by percutaneous drainage. Can J Surg 2001;44:203-209.

158. Odev K, Paksoy Y, Arslan A, et al: Sonographically guided percutaneous treatment of hepatic hydatid cysts: Long-term results. J Clin Ultrasound 2000;28:469-478.

159. Sahin M, Aksoy F: Percutaneous drainage for liver hydatid cysts (letter to ed.). Can J Surg 2002;45:70.

160. Sayek I, Onat D: Diagnosis and treatment of uncomplicated hydatid cyst of the liver. World J Surg 2001;25:21-27.

161. Houghton PW, Jenkinson LR, Donaldson LA: Cholecystectomy in the elderly: A prospective study. Br J Surg 1985;72:220-222.

162. Jurkovich GJ, Dyess DL, Ferrara JJ: Cholecystostomy. Expected outcome in primary and secondary biliary disorders. Am Surg 1988;54:40-44.

163. Davis CA, Landercasper J, Gundersen LH, et al: Effective use of percutaneous cholecystostomy in high-risk surgical patients: Techniques, tube management, and results. Arch Surg 1999;134:727-732.

164. Granlund A, Karlson BM, Elvin A, et al: Ultrasound-guided percutaneous cholecystostomy in high-risk surgical patients. Langenbecks Arch Surg 2001;386:212-217.

165. Sugiyama M, Tokuhara M, Atomi Y: Is percutaneous cholecystostomy the optimal treatment for acute cholecystitis in the very elderly? World J Surg 1998;22:459-463.

166. McGahan JP, Lindfors KK: Percutaneous cholecystostomy: An alternative to surgical cholecystostomy for acute cholecystitis? Radiology 1989;173:481-485.

167. Chopra S, Dodd GD, 3rd, Mumbower AL, et al: Treatment of acute cholecystitis in non-critically ill patients at high surgical risk: Comparison of clinical outcomes after gallbladder aspiration and after percutaneous cholecystostomy. AJR Am J Roentgenol 2001;176:1025-1031.

168. Phillips G, Bank S, Kumari-Subaiya S, et al: Percutaneous ultrasound-guided puncture of the gallbladder (PUPG). Radiology 1982;145:769-772.

169. Lameris JS, Hesselink EJ, Van Leeuwen PA, et al: Ultrasound-guided percutaneous transhepatic cholangiography and drainage in patients with hilar cholangiocarcinoma. Semin Liver Dis 1990;10:121-125.

170. Rau B, Pralle U, Mayer JM, et al: Role of ultrasonographically guided fine-needle aspiration cytology in the diagnosis of infected pancreatic necrosis. Br J Surg 1998;85:179-984.

171. Kumar P, Mukhopadhyay S, Sandhu M, et al: Ultrasonography, computed tomography and percutaneous intervention in acute pancreatitis: A serial study. Australas Radiol 1995;39:145-152.

172. Van Sonnenberg E, Wittich GR, Chon KS, et al: Percutaneous radiologic drainage of pancreatic abscesses. AJR Am J Roentgenol 1997;168:979-984.

173. Beger HG, Rau B, Mayer J, et al: Natural course of acute pancreatitis. World J Surg 1997;21:130-135.

174. Freeny PC, Hauptmann E, Althaus SJ, et al: Percutaneous CT-guided catheter drainage of infected acute necrotizing pancreatitis: Techniques and results. AJR Am J Roentgenol 1998;170:969-975.

175. Pitchumoni CS, Agarwal N: Pancreatic pseudocysts. When and how should drainage be performed? Gastroenterol Clin North Am 1999;28:615-639.

176. Neff R: Pancreatic pseudocysts and fluid collections: Percutaneous approaches. Surg Clin North Am 2001;81:399-403.

177. Grosso M, Gandini G, Cassinis MC, et al: Percutaneous treatment (including pseudocystogastrostomy) of 74 pancreatic pseudocysts. Radiology 1989;173:493-497.

178. Yeo CJ, Bastidas JA, Lynch-Nyhan A, et al: The natural history of pancreatic pseudocysts documented by computed tomography. Surg Gynecol Obstet 1990;170:411-417.

179. Van Sonnenberg E, Wittich GR, Casola G, et al: Percutaneous drainage of infected and noninfected pancreatic pseudocysts: Experience in 101 cases. Radiology 1989;170:757-761.

180. Nealon WH, Walser E: Main pancreatic ductal anatomy can direct choice of modality for treating pancreatic pseudocysts (surgery versus percutaneous drainage). Ann Surg 2002;235:751-758.

181. Chou YH, Tiu CM, Chiou HJ, et al: Ultrasound-guided interventional procedures in splenic abscesses. Eur J Radiol 1998;28:167-170.

182. Thanos L, Dailiana T, Papaioannou G, et al: Percutaneous CT-guided drainage of splenic abscess. AJR Am J Roentgenol 2002;179:629-632.

183. Siegel JF, Smith A, Moldwin R: Minimally invasive treatment of renal abscess. J Urol 1996;155:52-55.

184. Pedersen H, Juul N: Ultrasound-guided percutaneous nephrostomy in the treatment of advanced gynecologic malignancy. Acta Obstet Gynecol Scand 1988;67:199-201.

185. Saitoh M: Color Doppler flow imaging in interventional ultrasound of the kidney. Scand J Urol Nephrol Suppl 1991;137:59-64.

186. Fontana D, Porpiglia F, Morra I, et al: Treatment of simple renal cysts by percutaneous drainage with three repeated alcohol injections. Urology 1999;53:904-907.

187. Bozkurt FB, Boyvat F, Tekin I, et al: Percutaneous sclerotherapy of a giant benign renal cyst with alcohol. Eur J Radiol 2001;40:64-67.

188. Lohela P: Ultrasound-guided drainages and sclerotherapy. Eur Radiol 2002;12:288-295.

189. Van Sonnenberg E, Wroblicka JT, D'Agostino HB, et al: Symptomatic hepatic cysts: Percutaneous drainage and sclerosis. Radiology 1994;190:387-392.

190. Higgins RV, Matkins JF, Marroum MC: Comparison of fine-needle aspiration cytologic findings of ovarian cysts with ovarian histologic findings. Am J Obstet Gynecol 1999;180:550-553.

191. Martinez-Onsurbe P, Ruiz Villaespesa A, Sanz Anquela JM, et al: Aspiration cytology of 147 adnexal cysts with histologic correlation. Acta Cytol 2001;45:941-947.

192. Troiano RN, Taylor KJ: Sonographically guided therapeutic aspiration of benign-appearing ovarian cysts and endometriomas. AJR Am J Roentgenol 1998;171:1601-1605.

193. Mathevet P, Dargent D: Role of ultrasound guided puncture in the management of ovarian cysts. J Gynecol Obstet Biol Reprod (Paris) 2001;30:Suppl 1:S53-58.

194. Balat O, Sarac K, Sonmez S: Ultrasound guided aspiration of benign ovarian cysts: An alternative to surgery? Eur J Radiol 1996;22:136-137.

195. Lee CL, Lai YM, Chang SY, et al: The management of ovarian cysts by sono-guided transvaginal cyst aspiration. J Clin Ultrasound 1993;21:511-514.

19

ORGAN TRANSPLANTATION

Derek Muradali / Stephanie Wilson

Chapter Outline

Organ transplantation is the preferred treatment for patients with end-stage liver, renal, and pancreatic disease. Patients with fulminant liver failure have no other treatment option apart from orthotopic liver transplantation. Although patients with renal and/or pancreatic failure may be treated with either dialysis or medical therapy, their long-term survival and quality of life are far superior with organ transplantation. Recent improvements in graft survival have been attributed to a combination of better donor-recipient matching,[1] more effective immunosuppressive therapy, improvements in surgical technique,[2] and early recognition of transplant-related complications. These improvements have resulted in a 1-year patient survival rate of over 80% for each of these organ transplants.[3,4,5]

Because the clinical presentation of post-transplant complications varies widely and is often nonspecific, imaging studies are essential for monitoring the status of the allograft. Should there be a delay in diagnosis, the function of the allograft may be permanently compromised, and in severe cases with complete loss of function, retransplantation may be warranted. However, the chronic shortage of suitable donor organs may delay or preclude immediate retransplantation, with devastating clinical consequences. Therefore, preservation of the allograft function and early detection of complications, with institution of appropriate treatment, is essential in the clinical management of these patients.

Ultrasound has revolutionized the practice of organ transplantation because gray-scale sonography permits optimal assessment of the textural and morphologic changes of the parenchyma and color and spectral Doppler permit evaluation of both parenchymal perfusion, as well as the status of the major transplanted artery and vein. However, during routine transplant sonography, multiple ultrasound artifacts are encountered that may be related to either the intrinsic property of the structure being insonated, or to the scanning technique of the sonographer. Differentiation of these pseudolesions from true pathology is dependent on an understanding of the physical basis of the artifact. As well, awareness of the spectrum of ultrasound appearances of common transplant-related complications is requisite knowledge. This chapter will focus on the ultrasound appearances of the normal organ transplant, acute and chronic transplant-related complications, and potential errors of misinterpretation that can lead to misdiagnoses.

LIVER TRANSPLANTATION

In the United States, more than 5000 liver transplants were performed in 2001, with a 1-year patient survival rate of 87% and a 1-year graft survival rate of 80.3%. **Patients are selected for transplantation** when their life expectancy without transplantation is less than their life expectancy following the procedure. **Hepatitis C** is the most common disease requiring transplantation followed by **alcoholic liver disease** and **cryptogenic cirrhosis**. Other end-stage liver disorders treated by transplantation include chronic cholestatic diseases, such as **primary biliary cirrhosis** and **primary sclerosing cholangitis**; metabolic diseases, including **hemachromatosis** and **Wilson's disease**; other hepatitides, such as **autoimmune hepatitis, chronic hepatitis B**, and **acute liver failure**. Patients with end-stage **hepatitis B cirrhosis** were initially regarded as poor transplant candidates due to the high recurrence rate of infection in the implant associated with rapid progression to cirrhosis. The use of hyperimmunoglobulins and nucleoside analogs has changed these expectations to a more favorable outcome.[6]

Most centers consider transplantation only in patients with **early stage hepatocellular carcinoma** (HCC) or, rarely, **neuroendocrine metastases**. The generally accepted guidelines for transplanting patients with hepatocellular carcinoma are the Milan criteria of no lesion greater than 5 cm in diameter or no more than 3 lesions of greater than 3 cm in diameter.[6,7]

Contraindications for liver transplantation include compensated cirrhosis without complications, extrahepatic malignancy, cholangiocarcinoma, active untreated sepsis, advanced cardiopulmonary disease, active alcoholism or substance abuse, or an anatomic abnormality precluding the surgical procedure. Although portal vein thrombosis is not an absolute contraindication to liver transplanta-

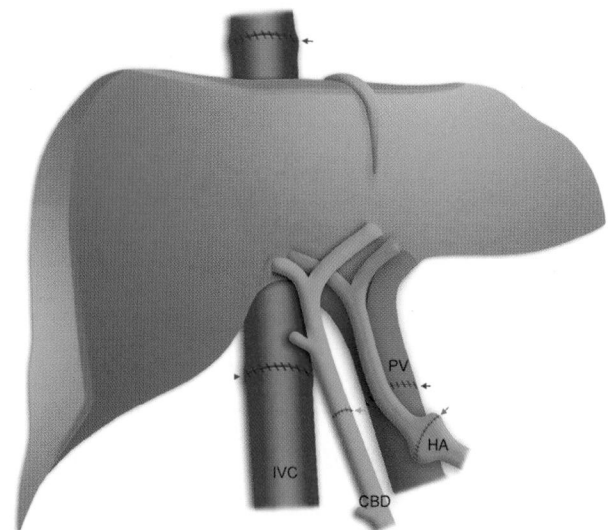

FIGURE 19-1. Normal liver transplant: surgical approach. The transplanted liver shows four vascular anastomoses and a biliary anastomosis. The inferior vena cava (IVC–*blue*) is transplanted with a suprahepatic and infrahepatic anastomosis. An end-to-end anastomosis is often used for the common bile duct (CBD–*green*) and portal vein (PV–*purple*), while the hepatic artery (HA–*red*) is reconstructed with a fish-mouth anastomosis.

tion, its presence makes the surgery more complex, and post-transplantation patients show higher morbidity and mortality rates.[6,8]

Surgical Technique

Traditionally, most adult liver transplants involve explantation of the recipient liver, and replacement with a cadaveric allograft. The surgery requires **four** vascular anastomoses (suprahepatic and infrahepatic vena cava, hepatic artery, and portal vein) as well as a biliary anastomosis (Fig. 19-1).

The **hepatic artery** is reconstructed with a fish-mouth anastomosis between the donor celiac artery **and** either the bifurcation of the right and left hepatic arteries or the branch point of the gastroduodenal and proper hepatic artery of the recipient. In cases where the native hepatic artery is either small in diameter or shows minimal flow, a donor iliac artery interposition graft may be anastomosed directly to the supraceliac or infrarenal aorta.[9]

The **portal vein** anastomosis is usually end-to-end between the donor and recipient portal veins. In cases of extensive recipient portal vein thrombosis, a venous jump graft from the donor portal vein or the iliac vein may be utilized or, as a last resort, an anastomosis between both the portal vein and hepatic artery of the donor and the arterial vessels of the recipient may be performed.[9,10]

Most commonly, during hepatectomy, the inferior vena cava (**IVC**) of the recipient is transected above and below the intrahepatic portion. The donor IVC is then anastomosed with two end-to-end suprahepatic and infrahepatic anastomoses. In an attempt to preserve the recipient retrohepatic IVC, some newer techniques advocate creation of an anastomosis between the donor and recipient IVCs in an end-to-side or side-to-side configuration or an end-to-end anastomosis between the donor IVC and a common stump of the three hepatic veins.[9]

The donor and recipient **common bile duct** are usually anastomosed in an end-to-end fashion, after a cholecystectomy. A T-tube may be left in place for cholangiography or other biliary procedures. A choledochojejunostomy is performed in those cases where the recipient common hepatic duct is diseased (e.g., sclerosing cholangitis), too short, or too narrow in diameter.[9]

The growing discrepancy between the number of patients awaiting transplantation and the lack of available cadaveric donor organs has led to a progressive increase in the number of **living related donor transplantations**. In this technique, the recipient liver is replaced with the right lobe of a living donor. In the pediatric population, the lateral segment of the left lobe, or the entire left lobe has been used successfully; the relative small size of the left lobe is not sufficient, however, to sustain adequate liver function in an adult. Another advantage of using a right lobe as the donor portion for transplantation, as opposed to the left, is the relative ease of positioning the right lobe in the right subphrenic space, which permits for a technically less challenging hepatic venous anastomosis and a decrease in the incidence of torsion, compared to left lobe grafts.[11]

For living related transplants, the **donor operation** consists of a cholecystectomy followed by a right hepatectomy, removing segments V, VI, VII, and VIII as well as the right hepatic vein. Occasionally an extended right hepatectomy may be done to include a portion of segment IV and the middle hepatic vein. However, most surgeons prefer not to remove the middle hepatic vein, but to leave it intact in the donor due to the intimate relationship of the middle and left hepatic veins near their drainage into the IVC.[11]

Regardless of the type of liver transplantation, routine **imaging evaluation of each anastomosis** must be assessed with gray-scale ultrasound, color Doppler, and spectral Doppler interrogation. In order to interpret the gray-scale appearance and Doppler features of these anastomotic regions, the sonographer should be aware of the surgical techniques utilized in liver transplantation.

Normal Liver Transplant Ultrasound

The **normal** liver transplant has a homogeneous or slightly heterogeneous echotexture on gray-scale ultrasound, appearing identical to a normal non-transplanted liver. In the early postoperative period, there is usually a small amount of free intraperitoneal fluid or small perihepatic seromas/hematomas, which tend to resolve within 7 to 10 days.

The **biliary tree** should have a normal appearance, with an anechoic lumen and thin imperceptible walls. If a T-tube is in situ, the adjacent duct wall may appear mildly prominent secondary to irritation and edema. Ideally, the biliary anastomosis (end-to-end or biliary-enteric) should be visualized and inspected for changes in caliber or wall thickness.

Pneumobilia is commonly observed in patients in whom a choledochojejunostomy has been performed, and appears as bright echogenic foci with or without posterior acoustic shadowing, within the bile duct lumen. The disappearance of previously documented pneumobilia should alert the sonographer to possible interval development of a biliary stricture at the biliary-enteric anastomosis. In addition, the sonographer should be aware that intraductal air may be confused with tiny biliary stones or adjacent hepatic arterial calcifications because these structures can all appear identical on gray-scale imaging (Fig. 19-2).

Vascular patency of the transplanted vessels (hepatic artery, portal vein, hepatic veins, IVC) is assessed by direct inspection for narrowing of the diameter, and the presence of thrombus within the vessel lumen, as well as documentation of normal spectral waveforms with appropriate directional flow. Particular attention should be paid to the anastomotic regions because these areas have a higher propensity to develop a hemodynamically significant stenosis compared to the remaining vessel. Because intrahepatic segmental stenoses or occlusions can develop, the hepatic artery and main portal vein, as well as their major right and left branches, should be interrogated with color and spectral Doppler.

The **normal hepatic artery** shows a rapid systolic upstroke with an acceleration time (time from end diastole to the first systolic peak) of less than 100 msec and continuous flow throughout diastole with a restive index between 0.5 and 0.7 (Fig. 19-3A). The **portal veins** show continuous hepatopedal flow with mild velocity variations due to respiration (see Fig. 19-3B). The Doppler appearance of the **hepatic veins** shows a phasic waveform reflecting physiologic changes in blood flow during the cardiac cycle (see Fig. 19-3C).

Abnormal Liver Transplant: Biliary Complications

Biliary tract complications are a significant cause of morbidity and mortality in 15% to 30% of orthotopic liver transplantations and may be seen in up to 25% of all transplants.[12-14] Complications related to biliary-enteric anastomoses usually present within the first month of surgery, and include anastomotic breakdown, bleeding, and an increased risk of ascending cholangitis from bacterial overgrowth. Choledochocholedochostomy-related complications most frequently present after the

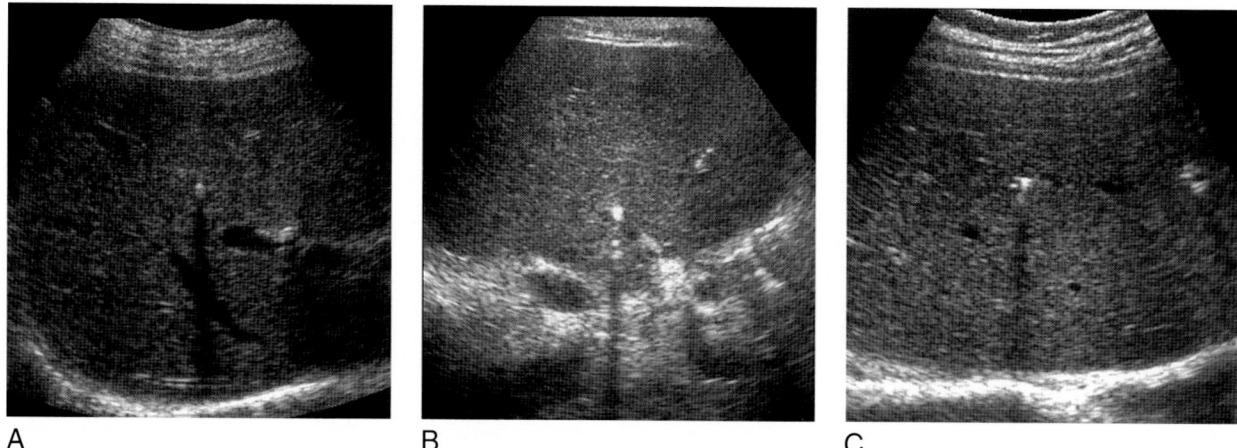

FIGURE 19-2. Echogenic foci in liver transplant. Transverse sonograms show similar bright echogenic foci with posterior acoustic shadowing secondary to **A**, intrahepatic calcification, **B**, hepatic arterial calcifications, and **C**, pneumobilia.

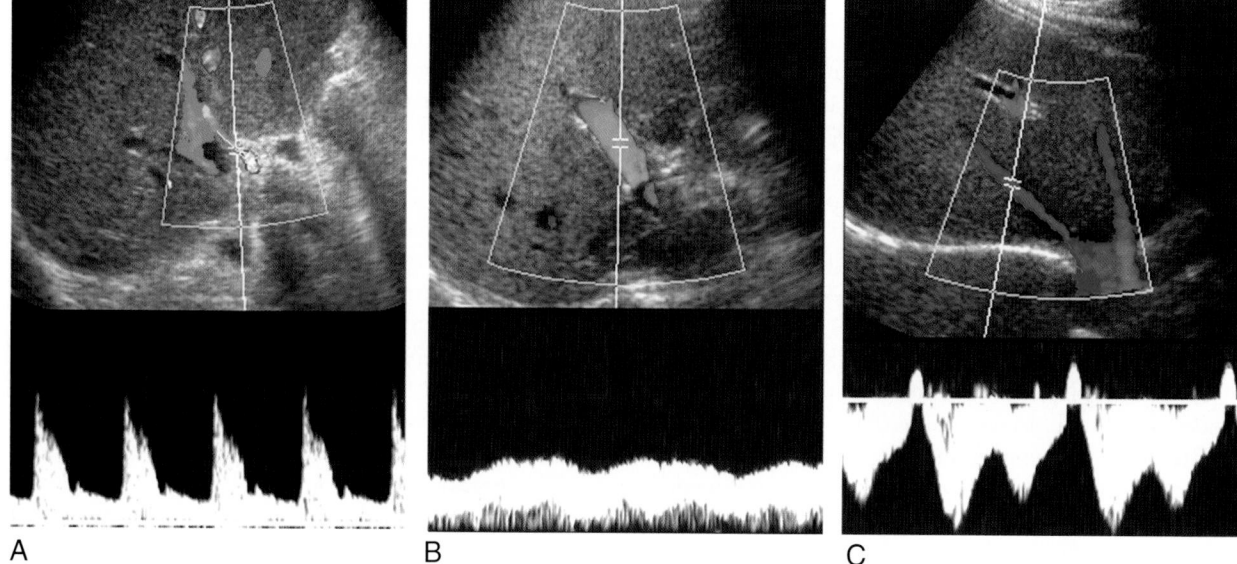

FIGURE 19-3. Normal liver transplant: color and spectral Doppler. Color and spectral Doppler images of normal **A**, hepatic artery, **B**, main portal vein, and **C**, right hepatic vein. (Reprinted with permission from Crossin J, Muradali D, Wilson SR: US of liver transplants: normal and abnormal. Radiographics 2003;23(5):1093-1114.)

first post-transplantation month, and are often managed by endoscopic retrograde cholangiopancreatography (ERCP).[13] Regardless of the type of anastomoses utilized, biliary tract complications can be broadly classified as those related to leaks, strictures, intraluminal sludge or stones, dysfunction of the sphincter of Oddi, and recurrent disease.

Biliary Stricture

Early diagnosis of biliary tree complications may be difficult as transplant recipients do not typically experience colic because the transplanted liver has a poor supply of nerves.[15] Therefore, patients with biliary strictures may be asymptomatic, present with painless

obstructive jaundice, or manifest with abnormalities in liver function tests.[13] These strictures can be categorized based on location and pathophysiology as **anastomotic (extrahepatic)** and **intrahepatic** strictures.

Anastomotic strictures are the most common cause of biliary obstruction after transplantation[16,17] and arise from postsurgical scarring, resulting in retraction of the duct wall and narrowing of the luminal diameter.[18] On ultrasound, a focal narrowing can sometimes be observed at the anastomoses, associated with dilation of the intrahepatic bile ducts, with a normal- or near normal-sized distal common bile duct (Fig. 19-4).

Intrahepatic strictures occur proximal to the anastomosis and may be either unifocal or multifocal. The arterial supply of the distal common bile duct

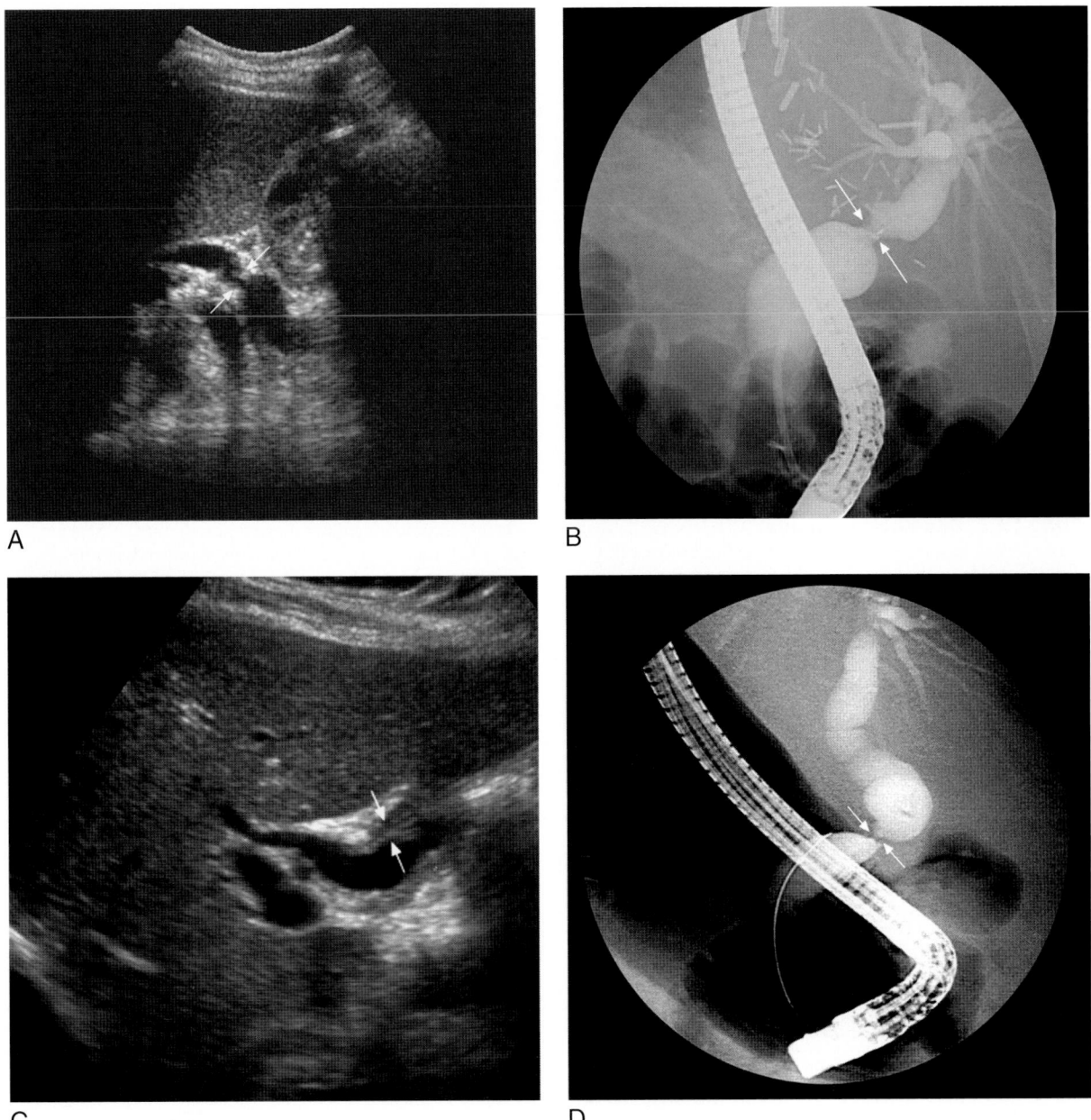

FIGURE 19-4. Bile duct: anastomotic stricture. A, Gray-scale sonogram of common bile duct shows anastomotic stricture (*arrows*), which is confirmed on endoscopic retrograde cholangiopancreatography (**B**) (ERCP—*arrows*). **C,** Second patient with grossly thickened common bile duct (CBD) walls (*arrows*), secondary to ascending cholangitis, which was a consequence of an anastomotic stricture, and **D,** as shown on the correlative ERCP (*arrows*). In both ERCPs the CBD distal to the stricture appears dilated due to the pressure of contrast injection during the procedure. (**A** and **B,** Reprinted with permission from Crossin J, Muradali D, Wilson SR: US of liver transplants: normal and abnormal. Radiographics 2003;23(5):1093-1114.)

(recipient duct) is rich because of prominent collateral flow, whereas the reconstructed hepatic artery is the only blood supply to the proximal common bile duct and intrahepatic bile ducts (donor ducts).[13,19] Therefore, most intrahepatic duct strictures result from ischemia caused by hepatic artery occlusion (thrombosis or significant stenosis). In rare instances, biliary duct ischemia may be caused by prolonged cold preservation time of the donor organ.[18,20]

Ultrasound findings include focal areas of narrowing in the intrahepatic or proximal common bile duct and segmental dilation of the intrahepatic bile ducts without evidence of an obstructing mass. The presence of echogenic intraluminal material within a dilated biliary tree is an ominous sign, sometimes caused by severe biliary ischemia, resulting in sloughing of the entire biliary epithelium. In this scenario, the intraluminal echogenic material represents a combination of biliary sludge or

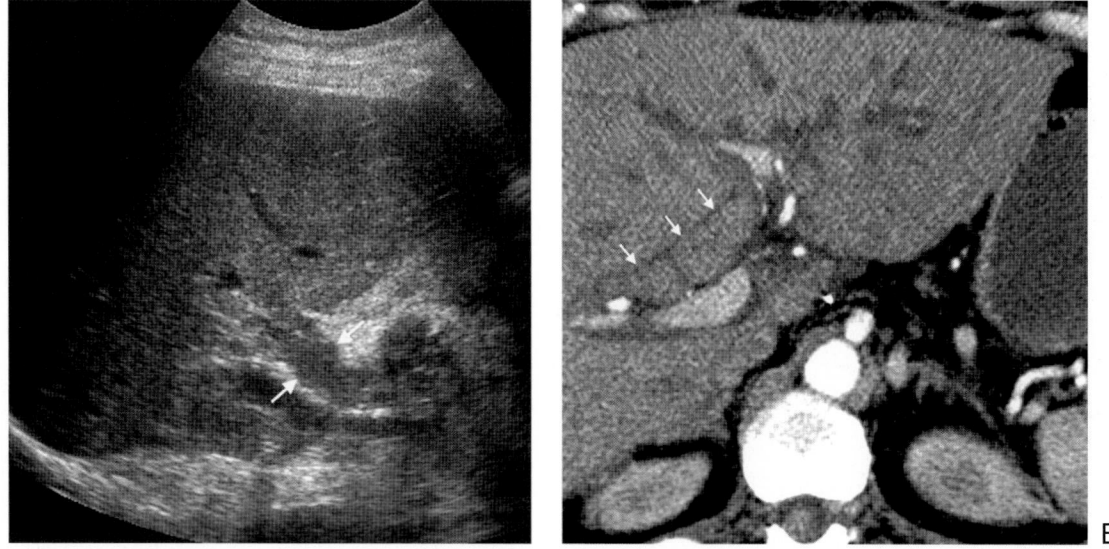

FIGURE 19-5. Bile duct: ischemia. A, Transverse sonogram of ischemic common bile duct showing intraluminal echogenic material (*arrow*) secondary to blood and sloughed mucosa. **B,** Corresponding CT scan shows intraluminal debris extending into the central intrahepatic bile ducts (*arrows*).

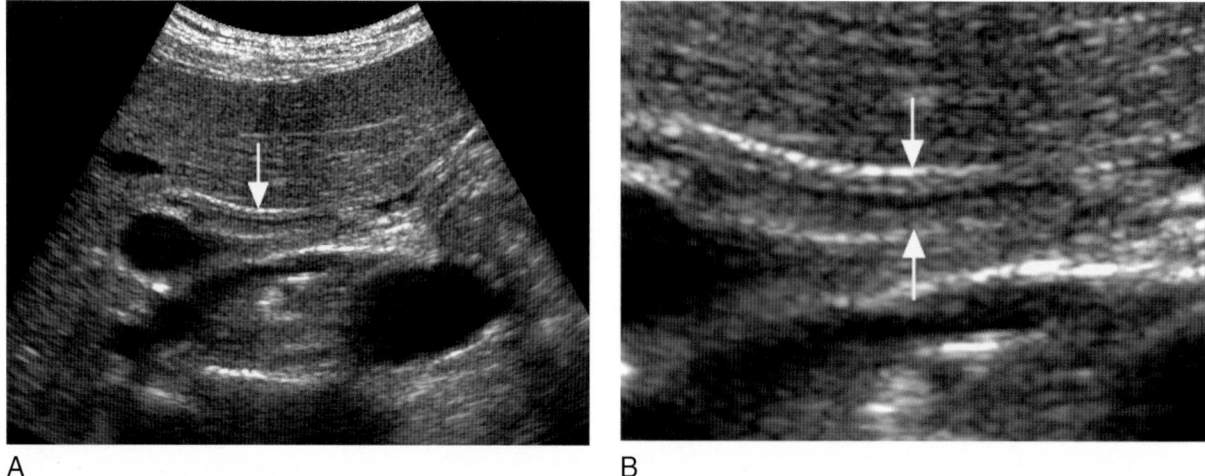

FIGURE 19-6. Bile duct: recurrent sclerosing cholangitis. A and **B,** Transverse sonograms at different magnifications show diffuse thickening and beading of the common hepatic duct (*arrows*). (Reprinted with permission from Crossin J, Muradali D, Wilson SR: US of liver transplants: normal and abnormal. Radiographics 2003;23(5):1093-1114.)

stones, sloughed biliary epithelium, and intraluminal hemorrhage (Fig. 19-5). Other causes of nonanastomotic strictures resulting in intrahepatic duct dilation include chronic rejection, ascending cholangitis, and recurrent sclerosing cholangitis.[18]

Recurrent Sclerosing Cholangitis

This condition occurs in up to 20% of recipients undergoing orthotopic transplantation for sclerosing cholangitis, with a mean interval time of 350 days.[6,10,21] **Ultrasound** findings include diffuse mural thickening of the intrahepatic and/or common bile duct and diverticulum-like outpouchings of the common bile duct (Fig. 19-6).[18,22] Recurrent disease should be

suspected in patients transplanted for end-stage primary sclerosing cholangitis presenting with biliary dilation and mural thickening in the presence of a normal hepatic arterial waveform.

Occasionally, patients with **ascending cholangitis** may present with an identical ultrasound appearance. Infectious etiologies include both enteric flora as well as opportunistic infections, such as cytomegalovirus and *Cryptosporidium*.[18]

Biliary Sludge and Stones

Biliary sludge can be detected within the hepatobiliary tree in up to 10% to 29% of liver transplant patients, as early as 6 days, or as late as 8.5 years postsurgery. The

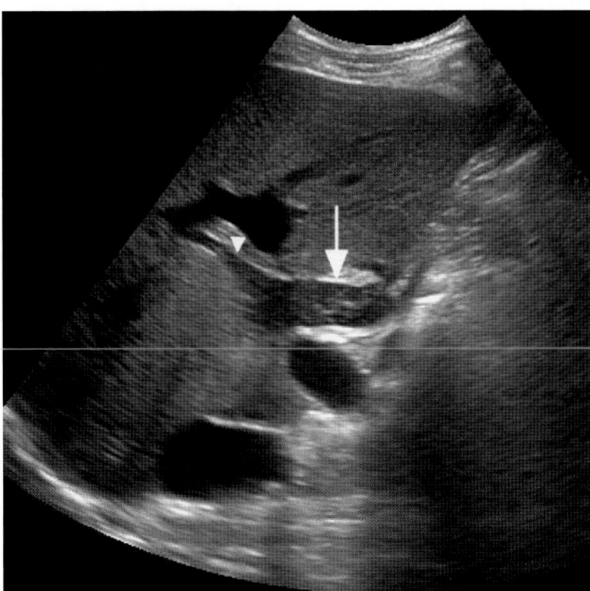

FIGURE 19-7. Bile duct: sludge. Oblique sonogram showing intraluminal sludge, secondary to ascending cholangitis, in the common bile duct (*arrow*), with extension into the right hepatic duct (*arrowhead*).

pathogenesis of biliary sludge in these patients is uncertain, although it has been related to ischemia, infection, rejection, mechanical obstruction, and biliary leaks.[15] Once sludge is present within either the donor or recipient biliary tree, it has the potential to produce biliary obstruction and life-threatening ascending cholangitis (Fig. 19-7). The detection of biliary sludge is an ominous sign that should prompt meticulous evaluation of the common bile duct to exclude the possibility of an obstructing lesion or leak; the hepatic artery to ensure an optimal arterial supply, and a detailed clinical assessment to determine if there is infection.

Intraductal stones are rare, but may result from cyclosporine-induced changes in bile composition inciting crystal formation in the common bile duct, with subsequent stone development. Other causes include retained donor stones, and stones secondary to biliary stasis from mechanical obstruction (e.g., stricture, dysfunctional T tubes, mucocele formation in a cystic duct remnant, and kinking in a redundant common bile duct) (Fig. 19-8).[23-25]

Dysfunction of the Sphincter of Oddi

In a minority of patients, hepatic dysfunction is observed in the presence of diffuse dilation of the donor and recipient bile ducts in the absence of biliary stenosis. The cause of this is uncertain, but may be related to devascularization or denervation of the ampulla of Vater resulting in dysfunction of the sphincter of Oddi. Patients are usually treated with ERCP-guided sphincterotomy, which has been shown to normalize liver function tests and decompress the biliary tree.[13,16]

Arterial Complications

At the time of explantation, extrahepatic arterial vessels that supply the liver, such as the parabiliary arteries, are disrupted.[26] **This results in the transplanted hepatic artery becoming the only arterial blood supply to intrahepatic biliary epithelium.** Any compromise of the hepatic arterial perfusion can result in biliary ischemia and, potentially, to biliary necrosis. While biliary necrosis is incompatible with graft survival and is an absolute indication for retransplantation, uncomplicated biliary ischemia (i.e., no necrosis) may be reversible if hepatic arterial flow can be reinstituted.[27] **The detection of hepatic arterial dysfunction prior to the development of biliary necrosis is paramount in the management of liver transplant patients.**

Hepatic Artery Thrombosis

This is the most significant vascular complication of liver transplantation occurring in up to 12% of adult patients.[4] The pathophysiology is often difficult to decipher. Risk factors include those patients requiring complex vascular reconstruction (due to multiple arterial supply to the liver or small donor and recipient vessels), rejection, severe stenosis, increased cold ischemic time of the donor liver, and ABO blood type incompatibility.[4,10,27]

After transplantation, the donor bile duct is entirely dependent on the transplanted hepatic artery, particularly the right, for its arterial blood supply. Therefore, patients with **hepatic artery thrombosis can present clinically with delayed biliary leak, fulminant hepatic failure, or intermittent episodes of sepsis** thought to be secondary to liver abscess formation within infarcted tissue.[4]

Ultrasound has been shown to detect up to 92% of cases of hepatic artery thrombosis.[28] Gray-scale sonography may show the hepatic artery at the porta hepatis with absence of flow on color or spectral Doppler. Occasionally, a **tardus parvus arterial waveform** (RI < 0.5, AT > 100 ms) may be obtained within the hepatic parenchyma (Fig. 19-9). This waveform is produced by collateral arterial vessels, which may develop as early as two weeks postsurgery. Sources of collateralization include the superior mesenteric artery, splenic artery, right inferior phrenic artery, and through adhesions to the diaphragm, omentum, and bowel.[4,29] The presence of collateral vessels has significant implications for patient survival, because these vessels may preserve tissue viability in the presence of complete hepatic artery thrombosis.

A **false positive** diagnosis of hepatic artery thrombosis may occur with severe hepatic edema, systemic hypotension, and high-grade hepatic artery stenosis.[10] In situations with poor visibility of the porta hepatis due to abdominal girth or overlying bowel gas, lack of

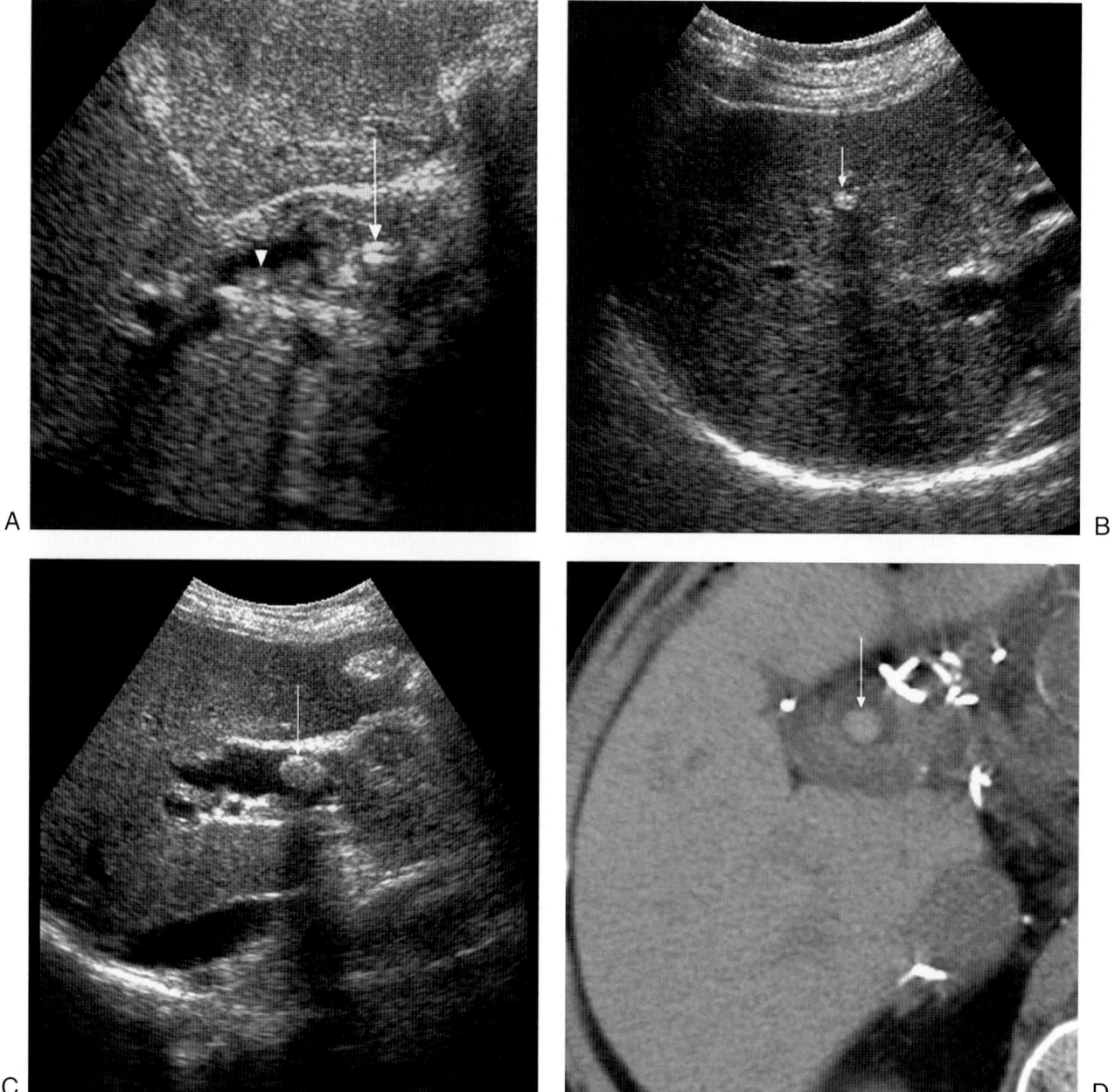

FIGURE 19-8. Bile duct: stones. Transverse sonograms from three patients show **A**, Multiple stones (*arrowhead*) in the right hepatic duct, which is obstructed by a coiled biliary stent (*arrow*), and **B**, nonobstructing intrahepatic stone. **C**, Sonogram and **D**, correlative CT scan show a large obstructing stone (*arrows*) in common hepatic duct. (**C** and **D** reprinted with permission from Crossin J, Muradali D, Wilson SR: US of liver transplants: normal and abnormal. Radiographics 2003;23(5):1093-1114.)

detectable flow within the hepatic artery should be viewed with caution and confirmed on CT angiography.

Hepatic Artery Stenosis

This complication has been reported in up to 11% of transplant recipients and occurs most commonly at the surgical anastomosis.[4] Risk factors for development include faulty surgical technique, clamp injury, rejection, and intimal trauma caused by perfusion

catheters.[27] Clinically, patients may present with biliary ischemia or abnormal liver function tests.

Doppler ultrasound may provide either *direct* or *indirect* evidence of hepatic artery stenosis. **Direct evidence of hepatic artery stenosis** involves identifying and localizing a hemodynamically significant narrowing within the vessel. The porta hepatis should be initially screened with color Doppler in order to detect a focal region of color aliasing within the hepatic artery, which would indicate the presence of high velocity turbulent

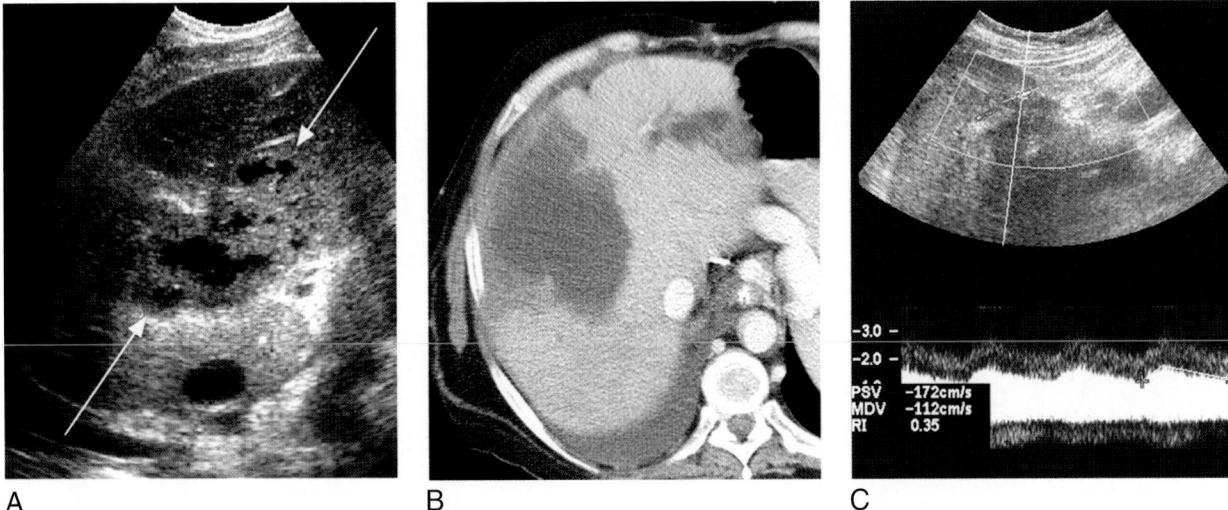

FIGURE 19-9. Hepatic artery: thrombosis. A, Transverse sonogram shows a right lobe infarct appearing as a solid-cystic region (*arrows*), resulting from hepatic arterial thrombosis. **B**, Corresponding CT scan shows the infarct as a low attenuating wedge-shaped region. **C**, On spectral Doppler, no flow could be detected in the main hepatic artery. A tardus parvus waveform detected within the liver indicates an upstream hepatic arterial problem: in this case, hepatic artery thrombosis with collateral arterial vessels supplying the hepatic tissue.

flow produced by the stenotic segment. If the stenosis is hemodynamically significant, spectral tracing will reveal peak systolic velocities of greater than 2 to 3 m/sec, with associated turbulent flow distally. **Indirect evidence of hepatic artery stenosis** includes a tardus parvus waveform anywhere within the hepatic artery (RI < 0.5, AT > 100 msec). This waveform suggests the presence of a more proximally located stenotic region (Fig. 19-10).[27] Indirect evidence of stenosis is far more common in clinical practice than is the actual documentation of the stenosis itself.

Mild degrees of hepatic artery narrowing may be present without Doppler abnormalities. Therefore, if clinical suspicion is high, a normal Doppler study should not preclude further investigation with angiography, although, in such cases, the stenosis, if detected, may be of a mild degree.

Hepatic Artery Pseudoaneurysms

These are an uncommon complication of transplantation occurring most frequently at the vascular anastomosis. Intrahepatic pseudoaneurysms are rare, usually peripherally located, and associated with percutaneous needle biopsies, infection, or biliary procedures. These aneurysms are often asymptomatic, but have the potential to cause life-threatening arterial hemorrhage, or in mycotic pseudoaneurysms, produce fistulas between the aneurysm and the biliary tree or portal veins.[10]

Gray-scale ultrasound shows a cystic (anechoic) periportal structure, with intense swirling flow on color Doppler and a **disorganized spectral waveform** (Fig. 19-11). Management options include surgery, transcatheter embolization, or stent insertion.

Celiac Artery Stenosis

Celiac artery stenosis may be due to **atheromatous disease** or impingement of the celiac axis by the **median arcuate ligament** of the diaphragm, and if severe, can potentially result in decreased arterial flow to the allograft. Patients are often asymptotic prior to transplantation, presumably due to the presence of rich collateral networks, usually through the pancreaticoduodenal arcade. Post-transplantation, patients may become symptomatic, presenting with evidence of biliary ischemia and abnormalities in serum liver function tests, due to the greater flow demand imposed on the celiac artery by the newly transplanted liver.

Doppler ultrasound may be normal, or may reveal a low resistance tardus parvus waveform in the transplanted hepatic artery and/or a high velocity jet across the celiac stenosis. Patients are treated with either division of the median arcuate ligament or, in the case of atheromatous disease, an aortohepatic interposition bypass graft (Fig. 19-12).[30,31]

Portal Vein Complications

Portal vein stenosis or **thrombosis** is uncommon, with a reported incidence of 1% to 13%.[4,32,33] Risk factors include faulty surgical technique, misalignment or excessive vessel length, hypercoagulable states, or previous portal vein surgery.[4] Clinical presentations include hepatic failure and/or signs of portal hypertension (gastrointestinal hemorrhage from varices or massive ascites).

Gray-scale ultrasound of portal vein stenosis may show narrowing of the vessel lumen, usually at the anasto-

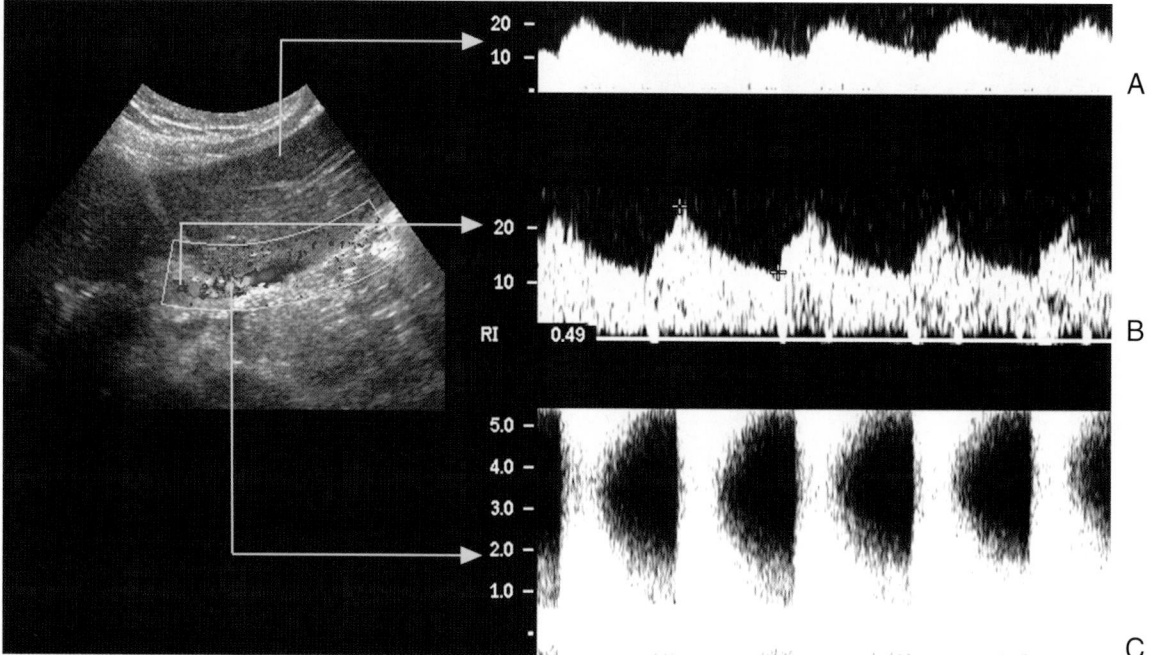

FIGURE 19-10. Hepatic artery: stenosis. A, Intrahepatic spectral waveform and **B,** hepatic artery waveform at porta hepatis show a prolonged acceleration time and low resistance, a tardus parvus waveform, suggesting an upstream problem. **C,** Spectral waveform at the anastomosis shows high velocity flow greater than 400 cm/sec. The corresponding color Doppler shows aliasing as turquoise and yellow between the red and blue at the stenosis, with turbulence beyond.

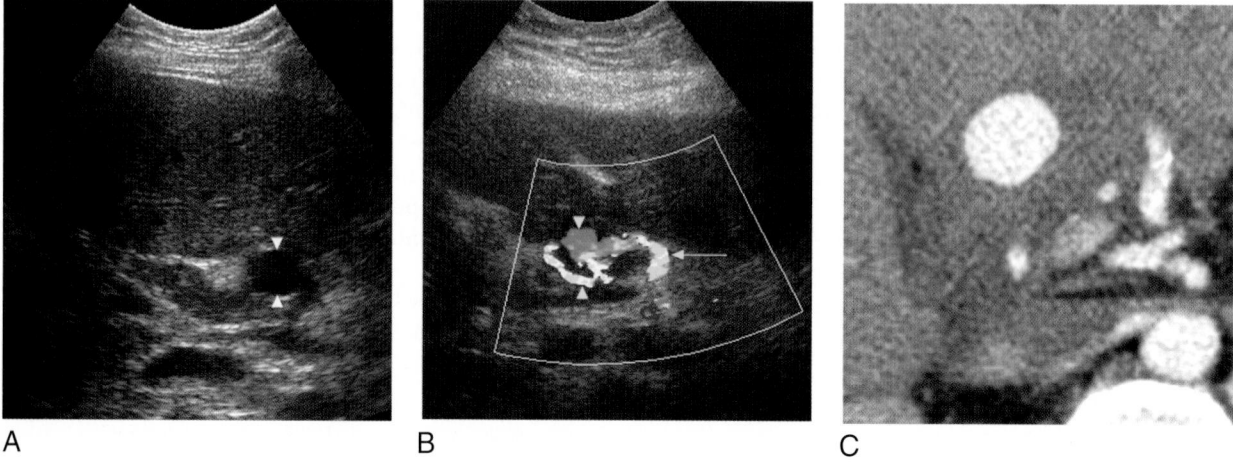

FIGURE 19-11. Hepatic artery: pseudoaneurysm. A, Gray-scale sonogram shows a small cystic mass close to the porta hepatis (*arrowheads*). **B,** Color Doppler confirms vascularity within the pseudoaneurysm (*arrowheads*) arising from the hepatic artery (*arrow*). **C,** Corresponding enhanced CT scan confirms the pseudoaneurysm arising at the hepatic artery anastomosis. (Reprinted with permission from Crossin J, Muradali D, Wilson SR: US of liver transplants: normal and abnormal. Radiographics 2003;23(5): 1093-1114.)

mosis. Doppler interrogation shows a focal region of color aliasing, reflecting turbulent, high velocity flow, with a three- to fourfold velocity increase at the site of stenosis relative to the prestenotic segment, on spectral interrogation (Figs. 19-13 and 19-14).[34]

Portal vein thrombosis presents as echogenic solid material within the portal vein lumen (Figs. 19-15 and 19-16). In the acute state, the thrombus may be anechoic, making detection difficult on gray-scale ultrasound. In this scenario, the thrombus is only evident by the lack of portal venous flow on color and spectral Doppler, emphasizing the necessity for careful gray-scale and Doppler assessment of the entire portal venous system. As with portal vein thrombosis in the native liver, the thrombus may decrease in size, and eventually recanalize showing multiple venous flow channels within the thrombus. Treatment of portal vein thrombosis or stenosis includes thrombectomy, segmental portal vein resection, percutaneous thrombolysis, stent placement, or balloon angioplasty.

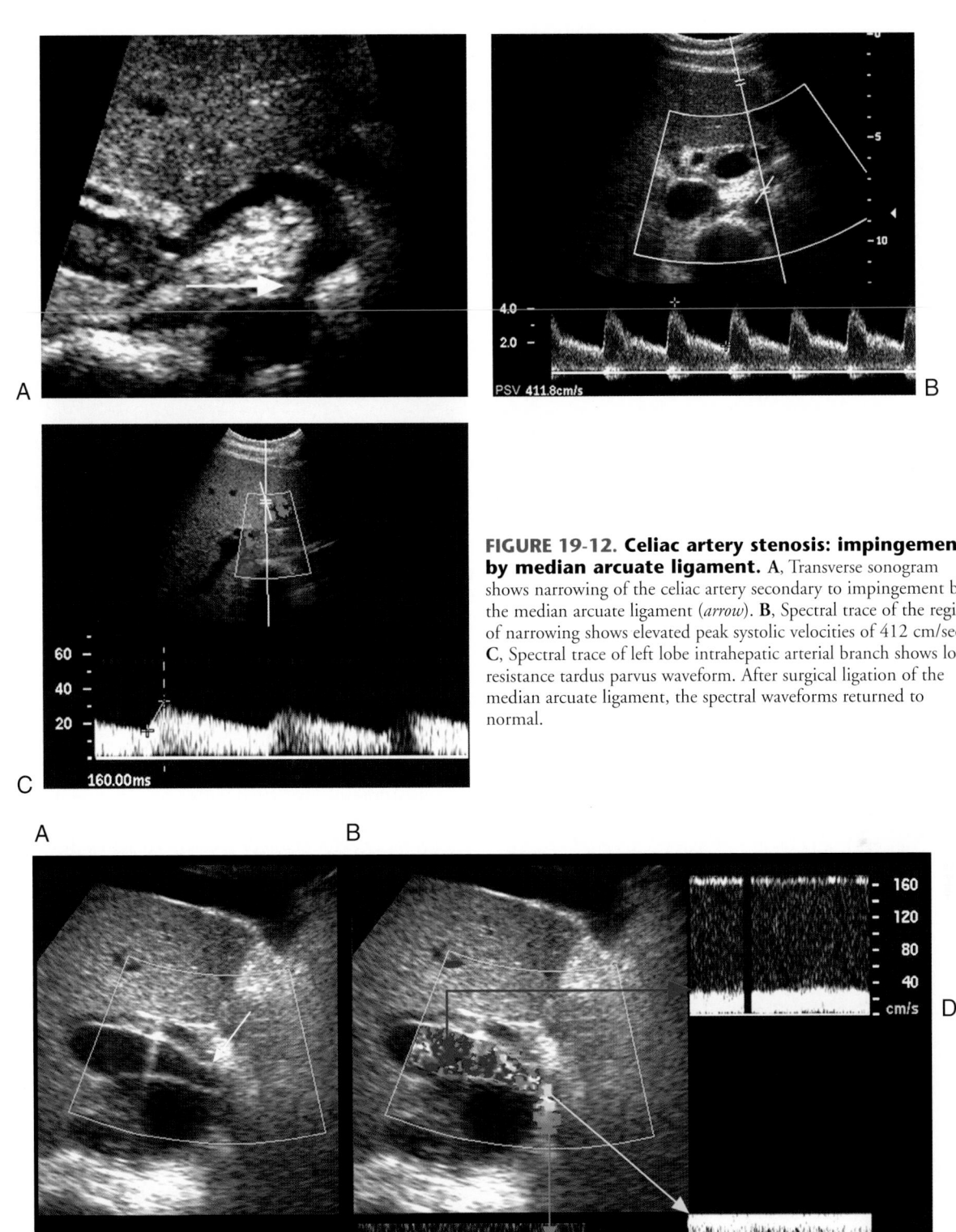

FIGURE 19-12. Celiac artery stenosis: impingement by median arcuate ligament. **A**, Transverse sonogram shows narrowing of the celiac artery secondary to impingement by the median arcuate ligament (*arrow*). **B**, Spectral trace of the region of narrowing shows elevated peak systolic velocities of 412 cm/sec. **C**, Spectral trace of left lobe intrahepatic arterial branch shows low resistance tardus parvus waveform. After surgical ligation of the median arcuate ligament, the spectral waveforms returned to normal.

FIGURE 19-13. Portal vein stenosis: anastomotic stricture. **A**, Gray-scale sonogram of main portal vein shows narrowing at the anastomosis (*arrow*). **B**, Color Doppler shows aliasing at the region of narrowing due to high velocity turbulent flow. **C**, Spectral Doppler shows velocities (*yellow arrow*) greater than 300 cm/sec at the anastomotic stricture, **D**, while velocities (*blue arrow*) distal to and, **E**, (*red arrow*) proximal to the stricture are significantly less, measuring 40 cm/sec and 50 cm/sec, respectively. This sixfold velocity gradient across the anastomosis indicates that the stenosis is hemodynamically significant.

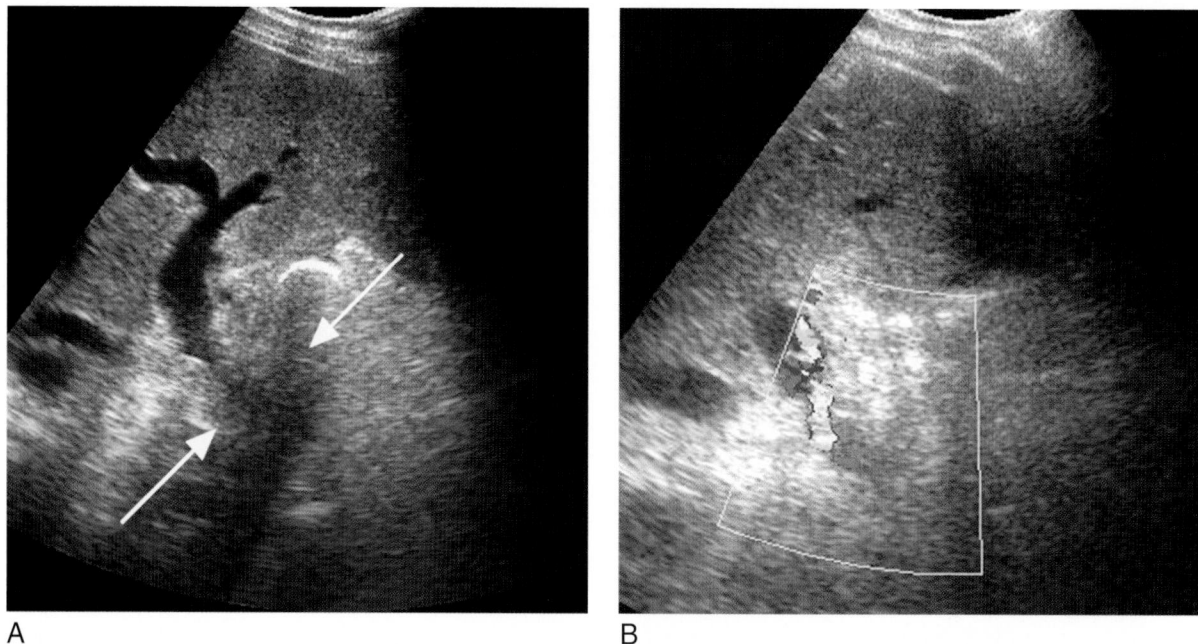

A   B

FIGURE 19-14. Portal vein stenosis secondary to extrinsic compression. A, Gray-scale sonogram of the distal portal vein shows a tapered narrowing of the vessel lumen related to an ill-defined mass (*arrows*), secondary to post-transplant lymphoproliferative disease. **B,** Color Doppler of the main portal vein shows aliasing at the region of encasement.

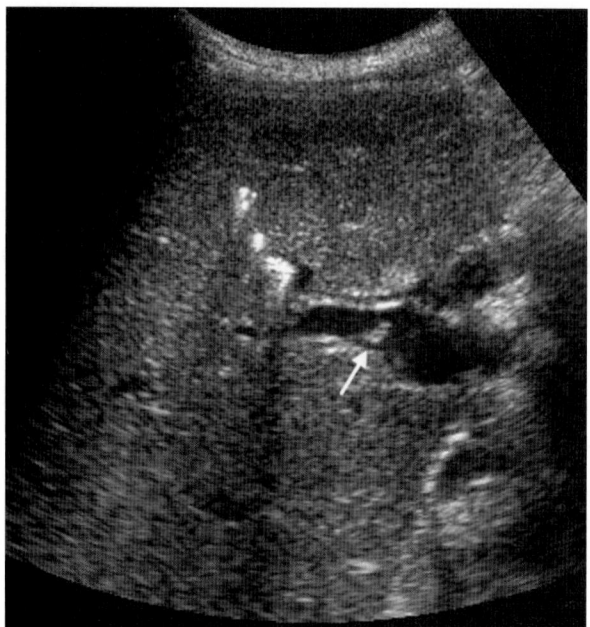

FIGURE 19-15. Portal vein: bland thrombus.
Sagittal sonogram shows a small nonocclusive mass (*arrow*) in the main portal vein. The intraluminal thrombus subsequently resolved 1 month later. Bright echogenic foci represent pneumobilia.

Inferior Vena Cava Complications

Stenosis of the IVC is a rare complication of liver transplantation and may occur at either the suprahepatic or infrahepatic anastomosis. It has been reported to occur more frequently in pediatric recipients and in patients undergoing retransplantation.[35] Causes of IVC stenosis include anastomotic discrepancy, IVC kinking, fibrosis, or neointimal hyperplasia. On gray-scale ultrasound, the IVC may show obvious narrowing at the site of anastomosis, associated with a focal region of aliasing on color Doppler. On spectral interrogation, a three- to fourfold velocity gradient is observed across the stenosis, compared to the prestenotic segment. The hepatic veins may show reversal of flow or lose their normal phasicity, with a monophasic waveform (Figs. 19-17 and 19-18).[10]

Inferior vena cava thrombosis has been reported in less than 3% of recipients and is caused by technical difficulties at surgery, hypercoagulable states, or by compression from adjacent fluid collections.[26,35] Gray-scale ultrasound shows echogenic thrombus within the IVC that may continue into the hepatic veins. In cases of recurrent hepatocellular carcinoma, tumor thrombus may extend from the hepatic veins into the IVC (Fig. 19-19).

Extrahepatic Fluid Collections

Perihepatic fluid collections and ascites are frequently observed post-transplantation. In the early postoperative period, a small amount of free fluid or a right pleural effusion may be observed, but these usually resolve in a few weeks. Fluid collections and hematomas are **common in the areas of vascular anastomosis** (hepatic hilum and adjacent to the IVC), biliary anastomosis, in the lesser sac, and in the peri- and subhepatic spaces.[9] Because the peritoneal reflections surrounding the liver are ligated at transplantation, fluid collections can occur

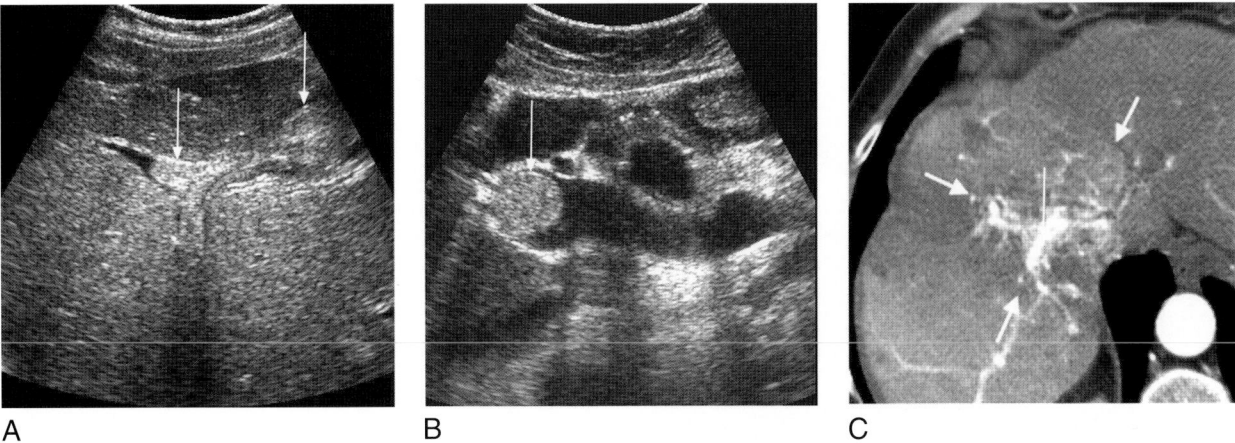

FIGURE 19-16. Portal vein: malignant thrombus. A, Transverse sonogram of malignant thrombus (*arrows*) in right portal vein with **B,** extension into main portal vein (*arrow*). **C,** Triphasic CT scan of the liver shows the recurrent hepatocellular carcinoma (*arrows*) that accounts for the portal vein thrombus. (Reprinted with permission from Crossin J, Muradali D, Wilson SR: US of liver transplants: normal and abnormal. Radiographics 2003;23(5):1093-1114.)

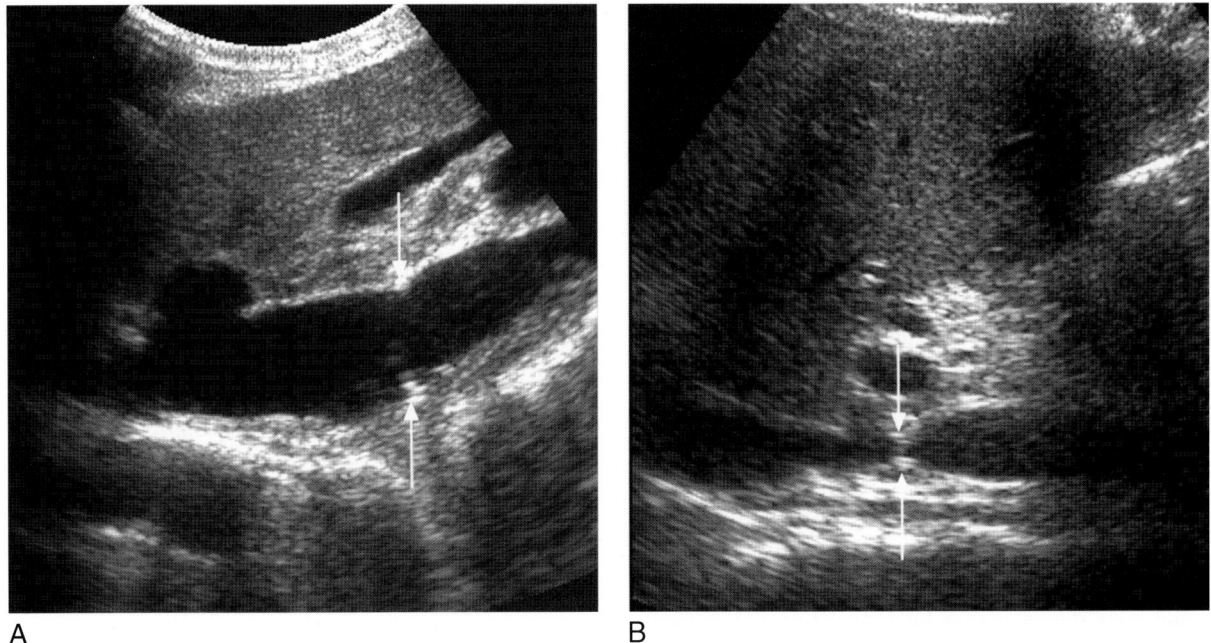

FIGURE 19-17. Inferior vena cava (IVC) infrahepatic anastomosis: normal and abnormal in two patients. Sagittal sonograms of IVC show **A,** a normal caliber at the anastomosis (*arrows*) and **B,** narrowing at the anastomosis (*arrows*).

around the **bare area of the liver**, a location not encountered in the preoperative liver (Fig. 19-20).[6]

Ultrasound is highly sensitive in detecting these fluid collections, although it lacks specificity because bile, blood, pus, and lymphatic fluid may all have a similar sonographic appearance. The presence of internal echoes in a fluid collection, although nonspecific, is suggestive of either blood or infection. Particulate ascites may also be observed in peritoneal carcinomatosis, although this would seem less likely in the transplant recipient population.[6]

Adrenal Hemorrhage

Right-sided adrenal hemorrhage may be observed in the immediate postoperative period and occurs from either venous engorgement caused by ligation of the right adrenal vein during the removal of a portion of the IVC, or from a coagulopathy caused by the patient's preexisting liver disease.[26] On ultrasound adrenal bleeds may present as a hypoechoic nodular structure, or as a fluid collection in the right suprarenal region (Fig. 19-21).

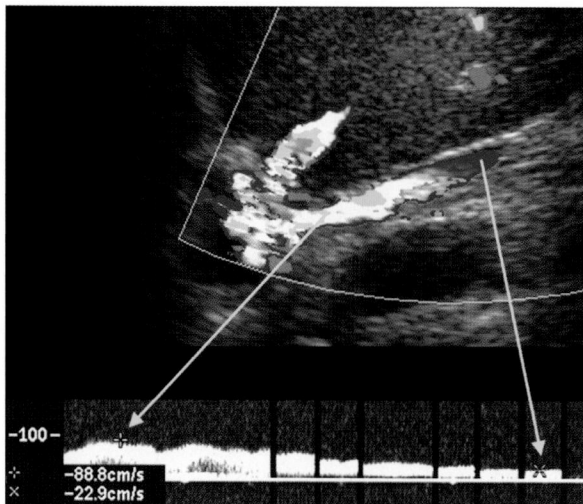

**FIGURE 19-18. Inferior vena cava (IVC)
suprahepatic anastomotic stricture.** Sagittal color
Doppler sonogram of a stenosed segment of the IVC shows
aliasing produced by high velocity turbulent flow in both the
IVC and the hepatic vein. Spectral tracing shows a greater than
threefold velocity increase at the stenotic region (*left arrow*).

Intrahepatic Fluid Collections

Sterile postoperative fluid collections are often located
along the falciform ligament and ligamentum venosum,
usually appearing as fluid-filled anechoic structures
surrounding the echogenic ligaments (Fig. 19-22).
Bilomas may present as a hypoechoic, round structure
or a complex cyst. **Intraparenchymal hematomas** may
occur as a result of the transplant surgery, percutaneous
biopsy, or may be a sequela of trauma experienced by the
donor, such as those donors involved in a motor vehicle
accident.

Abscess versus Infarct

**In the early stages, it may be difficult to differentiate
a liver abscess from an infarct.** Initially, both abscesses
and infarcts may appear as a subtle, hypoechoic region,
associated with a localized coarsening of the parenchymal echotexture. **Infarcts** may subsequently organize
into avascular round or wedge-shaped lesions, which can
eventually develop central hypoechoic areas reflecting
liquefaction and necrosis. When considering the
diagnosis of a focal liver infarct, there should also be
accompanying Doppler evidence of hepatic arterial
compromise.

   As with infarcts, the ultrasound appearance of a liver
abscess also varies with its maturation. The classic
appearance of a mature transplant liver abscess is that of
a complex, cystic structure with thick, irregular walls and
particulate internal fluid—with or without associated
septations.

Both infarcts and abscesses may contain bubbles of
air, occurring as bright echogenic foci with or without
posterior acoustic shadowing (Fig. 19-23). Occasionally,
bubbles of air within the lumen of an intraparenchymal
abscess can be confused with benign pneumobilia or
may be mistaken for air outside of the liver within the
gastrointestinal tract. A high index of suspicion is critical
in patients at risk for either abscess or infarct to avoid
these misinterpretations.

Intrahepatic Solid Masses

The differential diagnosis of a solitary mass in the
transplanted liver is similar to that in the native liver. For
example, benign lesions, such as hemangiomas and cysts,
are relatively common in the transplanted liver with the
same range of appearances as described in the native
liver. There are, however, several pathologies unique to
the transplanted liver that may also present with a solid
or complex mass on gray-scale ultrasound, including
infarcts (Fig. 19-24), abscesses, hematomas, recurrent/
metastatic hepatocellular carcinoma ,and post-transplant
lymphoproliferative disease (PTLD).

   Recurrent hepatocellular carcinoma is a serious complication that can potentially develop post-transplantation
in patients with a preoperative history of end-stage
cirrhosis with known or occult hepatomas. The most
common site of recurrent hepatocellular carcinoma is
the lung, presumably caused by embolization with
tumor cells through the hepatic veins before or during
transplantation. The second most common location of
recurrent hepatomas is within **the allograft**, followed by
regional or distant lymph nodes. Early detection of
recurrent hepatomas within the transplanted liver is
essential to facilitate early resection, ablation, or chemotherapy (Fig. 19-25).[26,36] One should note that transplant recipients might develop any type of primary or
secondary neoplasm within the liver, as in the general
population.

RENAL TRANSPLANTATION

Transplantation is the treatment of choice for many
patients with chronic renal failure severe enough to
warrant dialysis. The only **contraindications** for transplantation are unsuitability for general anesthesia or
surgery, preexisting infection or malignancy, and a risk of
recurrent renal disease (e.g., active vasculitis or oxalosis).
Prior to transplantation, a suitable donor must be
obtained with appropriate human lymphocytic antigen
(HLA) matching with the recipient.[37]

   As the number of patients with chronic renal failure
continues to rise, the major limitation for expanding
transplant programs is the continuing shortage of
suitable donor kidneys. This organ shortage has resulted

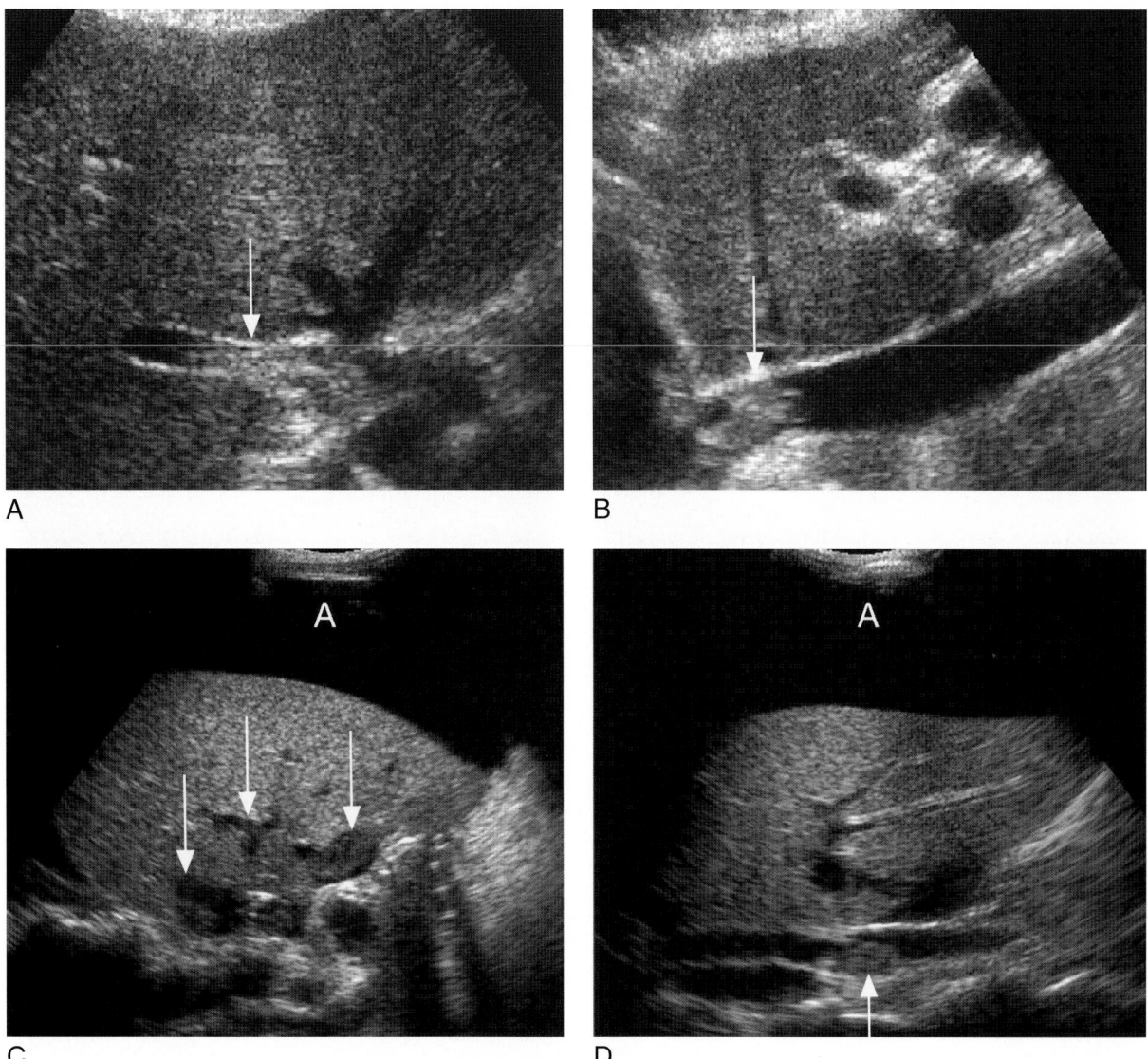

FIGURE 19-19. Inferior vena cava (IVC) thrombosis in two patients. A, Transverse and **B,** sagittal sonograms show malignant IVC and hepatic vein thrombus (*arrows*) in a patient with recurrent hepatocellular carcinoma following transplantation. **C,** Transverse sonogram of the hepatic veins and **D,** sagittal sonogram of IVC show bland thrombus (*arrows*) in each (A—ascites). (**A** and **B,** Reprinted with permission from Crossin J, Muradali D, Wilson SR: US of liver transplants: normal and abnormal. Radiographics 2003;23(5):1093-1114.)

in an increasing number of renal transplantations from **living-related donors**. These donors may include family members or close friends with a long-standing close personal relationship with the recipient. The average life expectancy for a cadaveric allograft is 7 to 10 years, and a live-donor allograft is 15 to 20 years.[37]

Regardless of whether a cadaveric or live donor allograft is used, the cost-benefit of a functioning successful transplant far outweighs that of a patient with persistent chronic renal failure, and so, multiple health care resources are targeted to ensure that high rates of success are achieved. Ultrasound is unequivocally the most valuable noninvasive imaging modality used in monitoring the renal transplant.

Normal Renal Transplant Ultrasound

Surgical Technique

Detailed sonography of the renal transplant requires a thorough knowledge of the basic surgical procedure utilized in most institutions as well as the postsurgical anatomic relationships. The right or left lower quadrant is selected for the incision, based on the patient's prior surgical history and the preference of the surgeon. At the time of harvesting, the hilar fat and adventitia surrounding the ureter are preserved in an attempt to maximize the blood supply to these areas. Most commonly, the **vascular supply** is created from an **end-to-side** anastomosis of donor artery and vein to the

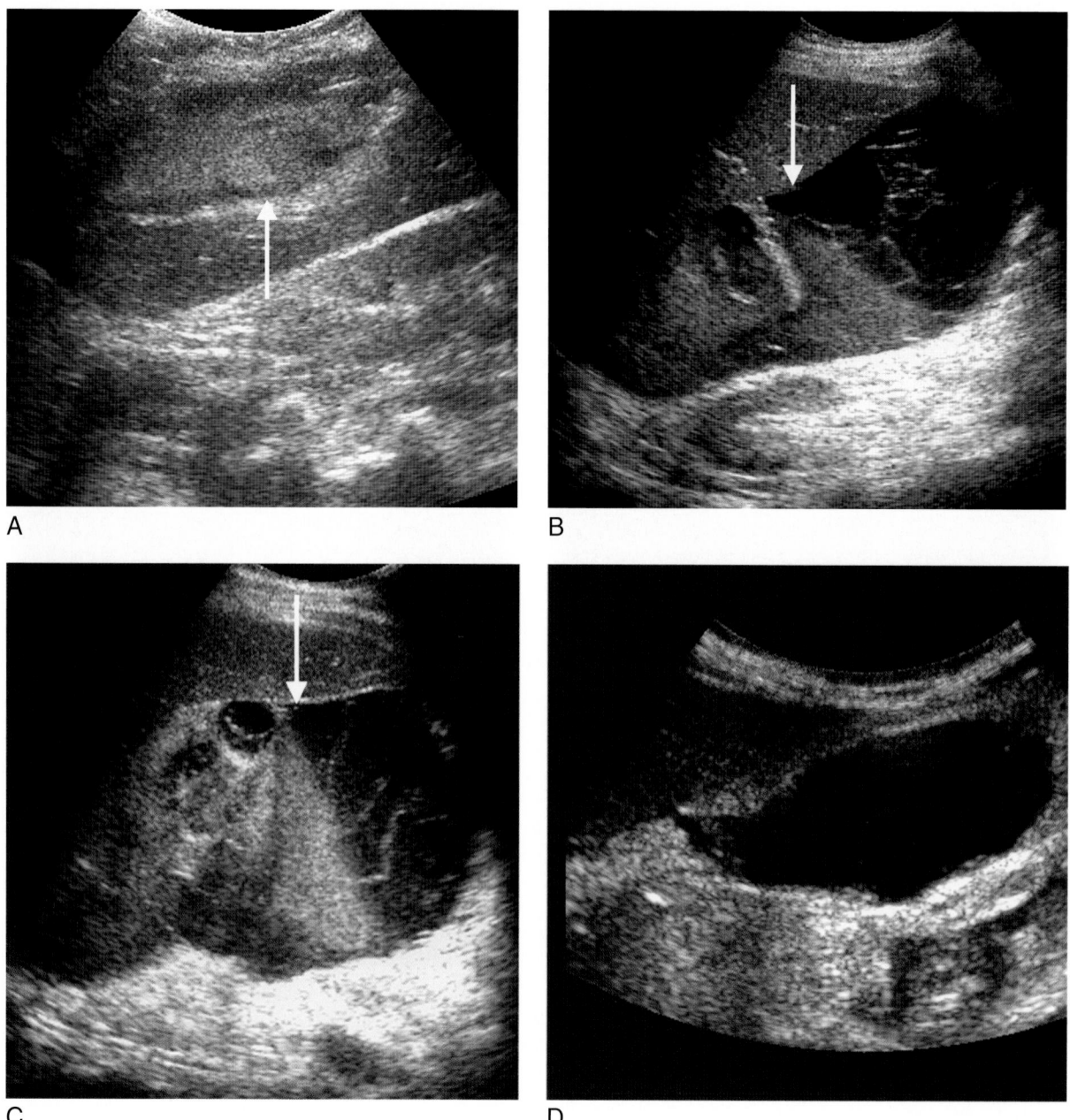

FIGURE 19-20. Extrahepatic fluid collection. Hematoma at surgical margin of a right lobe living related transplant. Transverse sonogram shows **A,** acute hematoma that appears echogenic, heterogeneous, and solid. **B** and **C,** hematoma liquefies after 3 weeks with internal strands and a fluid-debris level and **D,** after 2 months, there is further liquefaction of the hematoma to appear as a smaller anechoic collection. *Arrows* mark boundary of hematomas with liver.

external iliac artery and vein, respectively. Occasionally the common iliac vessels may be used instead. Multiple donor arteries may be anastomosed as a Carrel patch, or anastomosed separately to the external iliac vessels. The **ureter** is anastomosed to the superolateral wall of the urinary bladder via a neocystostomy in order to prevent reflux to the transplant. For patients undergoing repeat surgery on the collecting system, or in those cases with complex surgeries, the recipient's ureter may be used as a conduit to the bladder (Fig. 19-26).[38]

Due to the chronic shortage of donor organs, paired cadaveric kidneys from young (<5 years old) donors may be transplanted *en bloc* in an attempt to provide a functional renal mass that would be analogous to the renal mass of a single cadaveric kidney transplanted from an adult. At harvesting, both kidneys are removed *en bloc* with preservation of the ureters, main renal arteries and veins, as well as segments of the suprarenal and infrarenal abdominal aorta and IVC. The donor aorta and IVC are oversewn just cephalad to the origin of the

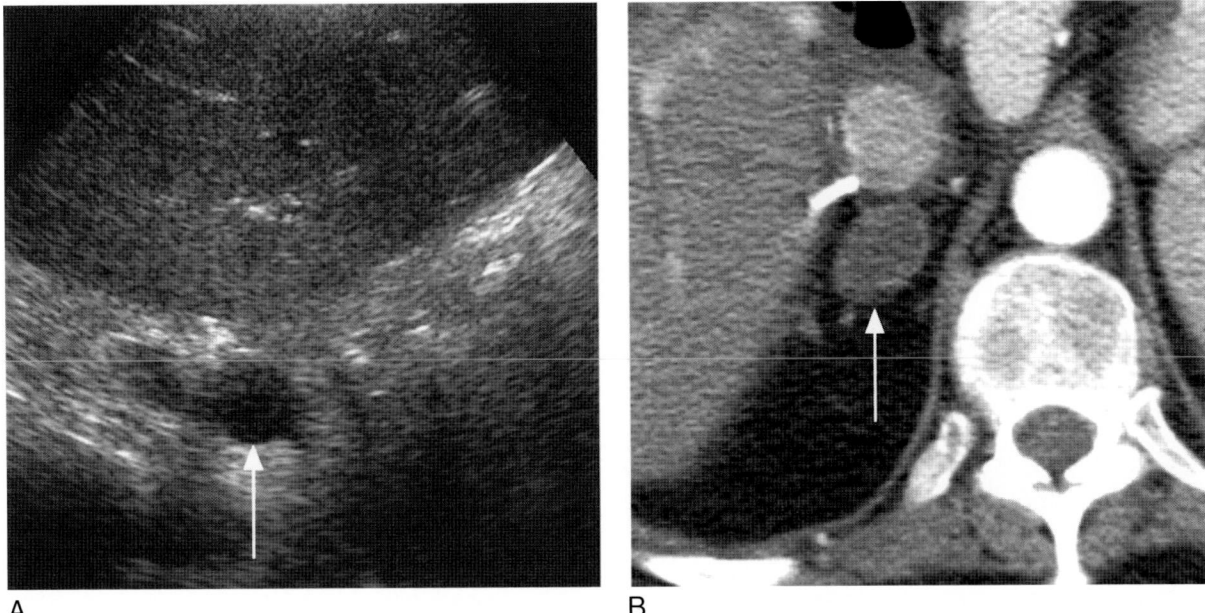

FIGURE 19-21. Right adrenal hemorrhage. A, Sagittal sonogram and **B,** CT scan show a small right adrenal mass (*arrows*). (Reprinted with permission from Crossin J, Muradali D, Wilson SR: US of liver transplants: normal and abnormal. Radiographics 2003;23(5):1093-1114.)

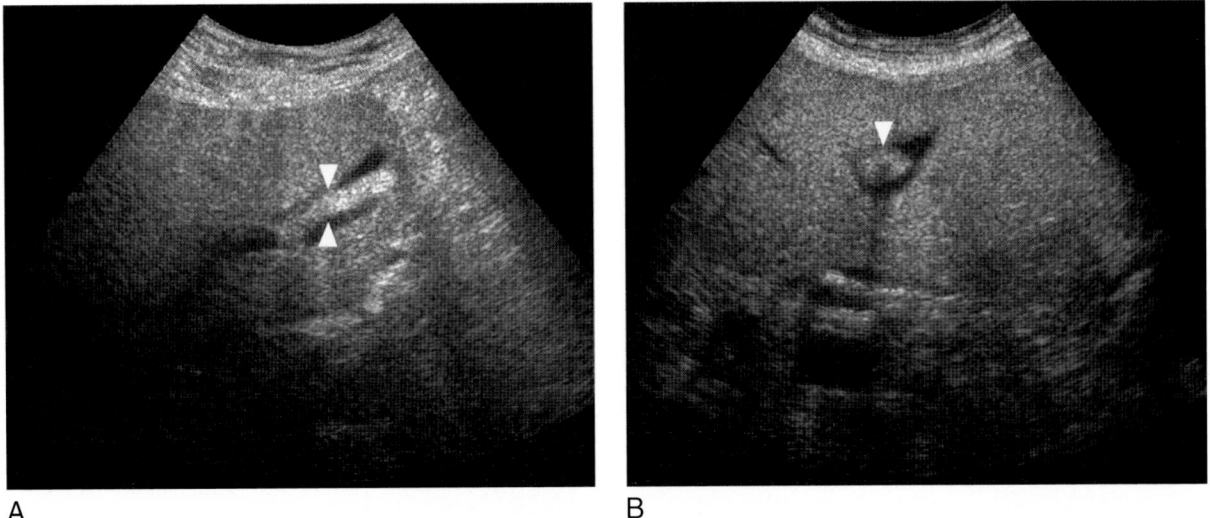

FIGURE 19-22. Intrahepatic fluid collection. A, Transverse and **B,** sagittal sonograms show anechoic fluid surrounding echogenic falciform ligament (*arrowheads*).

renal arteries and veins, and the caudal ends anastomosed end-to-side to the recipient's external iliac artery and vein. The donor ureters are implanted into the urinary bladder through individual or common ureteroneocystostomies.[39] This surgery is more commonly performed in the pediatric population than in adults.

Gray-Scale Assessment of the Renal Transplant

Sonography of the renal transplant is usually easily performed due to the superficial location of the kidney in either the right or left lower quadrant. Because the allograft is held in place by its pedicle, a variety of orientations may be encountered. Most commonly, the kidney is aligned with its long axis parallel to the surgical incision, with the hilum oriented inferiorly and posteriorly. Occasionally, in obese patients, the long axis may lie in an anterior to posterior plane.[40]

Longitudinal and transverse (width × depth) **measurements of the transplant** should be obtained with the kidney imaged through the hilum in the sagittal and transverse planes, respectively. While there are no normative data for comparison, these measurements

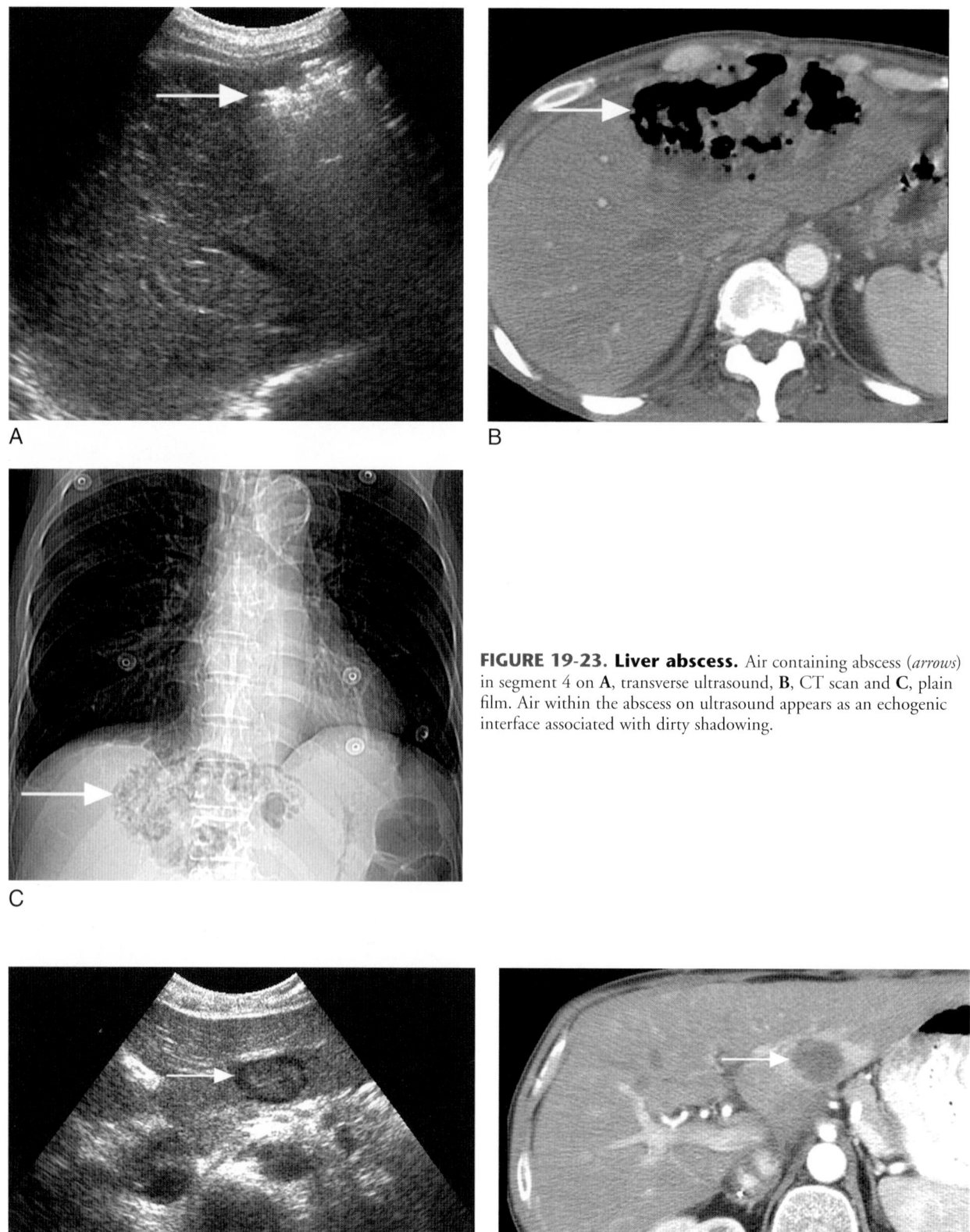

FIGURE 19-23. Liver abscess. Air containing abscess (*arrows*) in segment 4 on **A**, transverse ultrasound, **B**, CT scan and **C**, plain film. Air within the abscess on ultrasound appears as an echogenic interface associated with dirty shadowing.

FIGURE 19-24. Atypical infarct. A, Transverse sonogram shows an atypical infarct (*arrow*) appearing as a round mass associated with a surrounding hypoechoic halo. **B**, Correlative CT scan shows that the infarct (*arrow*) is avascular, with a surrounding parenchymal blush. (Reprinted with permission from Crossin J, Muradali D, Wilson SR: US of liver transplants: normal and abnormal. Radiographics 2003;23(5):1093-1114.)

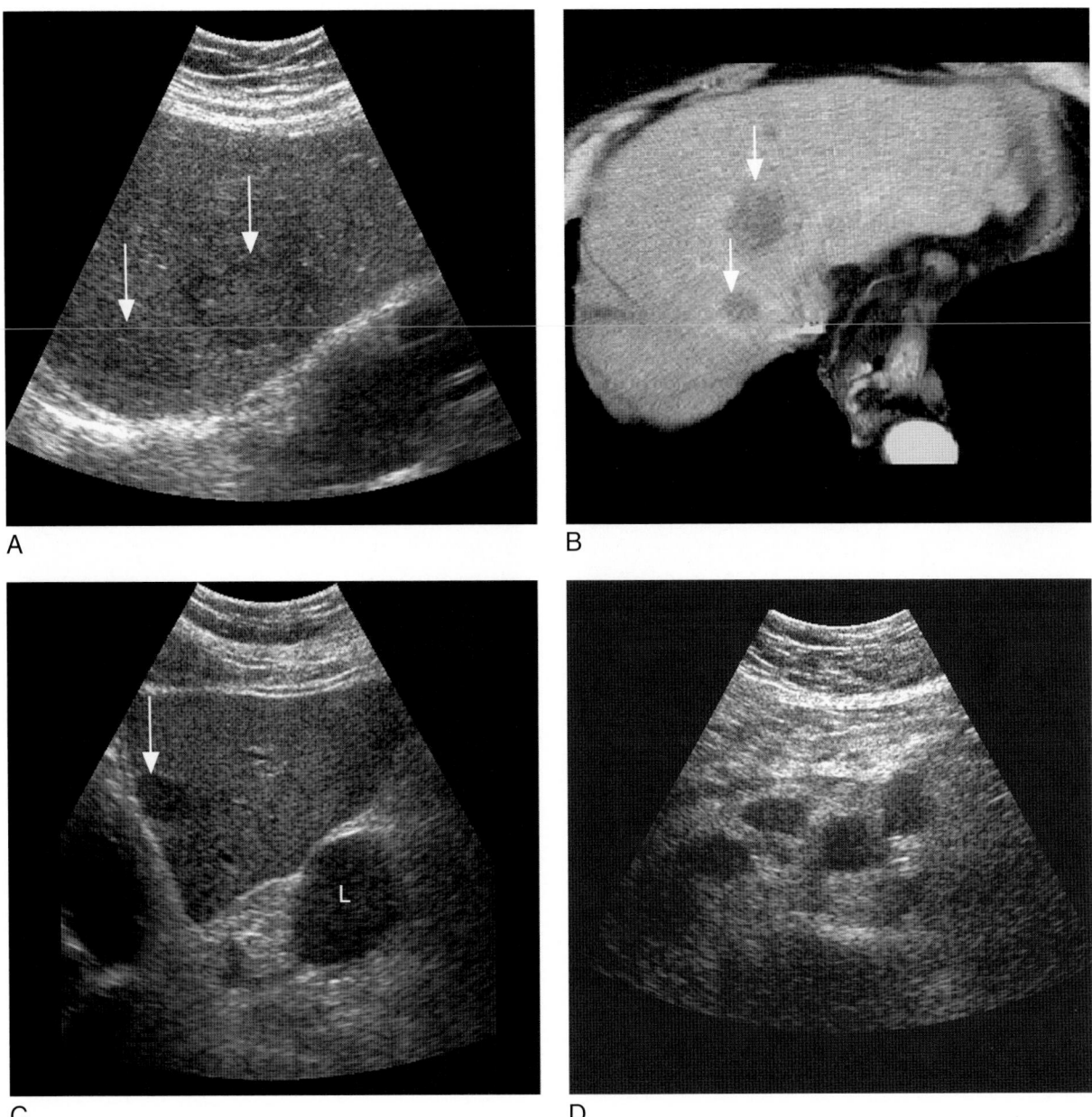

FIGURE 19-25. Recurrent hepatocellular carcinoma. **A**, Transverse sonogram shows two malignant-appearing masses (*arrows*) secondary to recurrent hepatocellular carcinoma (HCC). **B**, Correlative arterial phase CT scan shows peripheral enhancement of the masses (*arrows*). **C**, Sagittal sonogram shows a third HCC in the medial segment of the left lobe (*arrow*) and a large metastatic lymph node (L). **D**, Transverse midline sonogram shows multiple enlarged metastatic lymph nodes. (Reprinted with permission from Crossin J, Muradali D, Wilson SR: US of liver transplants: normal and abnormal. Radiographics 2003;23(5):1093-1114.)

serve as a useful baseline for future reference to assess for interval changes in volume of the allograft. The normal kidney may hypertrophy by up to 15% within the first 2 weeks after surgery, and eventually, may increase in volume by 40%, with the final size attained at approximately 6 months.[41-43]

The transplanted kidney appears morphologically similar to the native kidney, with many of the subtle differences attributed to the improved resolution due to the close proximity of the allograft to the skin surface

(Fig. 19-27). The normal renal cortex is well defined, hypoechoic, and easily differentiated from the highly reflective central echogenic renal sinus fat. Apart from this improved corticomedullary differentiation, the renal pyramids of the allograft are more easily visualized than in the native kidney, appearing as wedge-shaped structures that are hypoechoic to the surrounding parenchyma.[37]

The sonographer should always be aware that the transplanted kidney might show **intrinsic pathology in the donor kidney**. In our clinical practice, we have

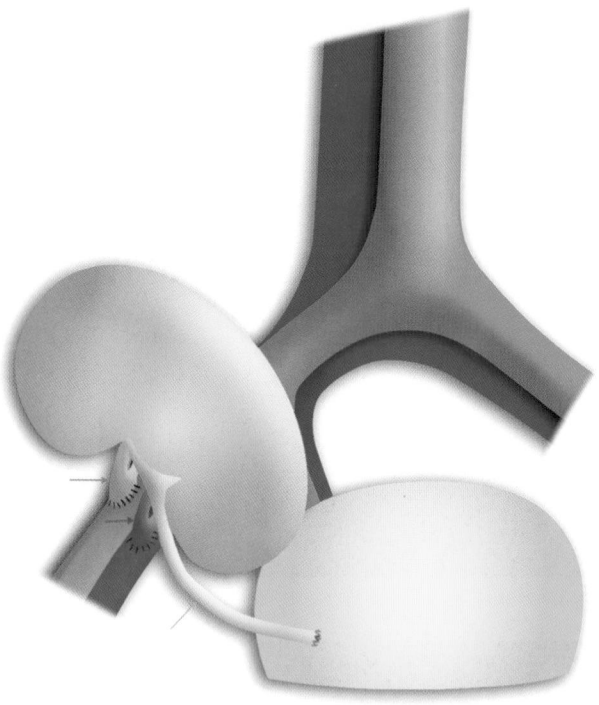

FIGURE 19-26. Surgery: single cadaveric transplant. The main renal artery (*red*) and main renal vein (*purple*) are anastomosed to the external iliac artery and vein, respectively. The ureter (*brown*) is anastomosed to the superolateral bladder wall.

observed a host of donor pathologies in the transplanted kidney, ranging from angiomyolipomas to medullary sponge kidney (Fig. 19-28).

Doppler Assessment of the Renal Transplant

Color Doppler gives a global assessment of the intra-parenchymal perfusion and is useful in localizing the

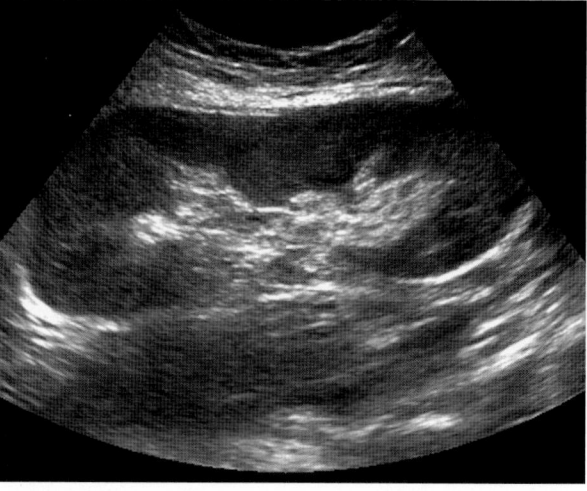

FIGURE 19-27. Normal gray-scale ultrasound of renal transplant.

main renal artery and vein. The renal parenchyma should be screened initially with color Doppler to determine if there are focal regions of hypoperfusion, as well as to locate the interlobar arteries for spectral inter-rogation.[37] **Spectral traces** of the **interlobar arteries** should be obtained from the upper-, mid- and lower-pole regions with low filter settings, maximal gain, and the smallest scale demonstrating the peak systolic velocity. The normal waveform is low impedance with a brisk upstroke and continuous diastolic flow. A resistive index (RI) of 0.6 to 0.8 is normal, 0.8 to 0.9 equivocal, and greater than 0.9 is abnormal, suggesting increased intraparenchymal resistance. Provided that flow in the recipient common iliac vein is normal, the velocity of the transplanted main renal artery should be less than 200 cm/sec (Fig. 19-29).

The intra- and extraparenchymal **renal veins** show either monophasic continuous flow, or phasicity with

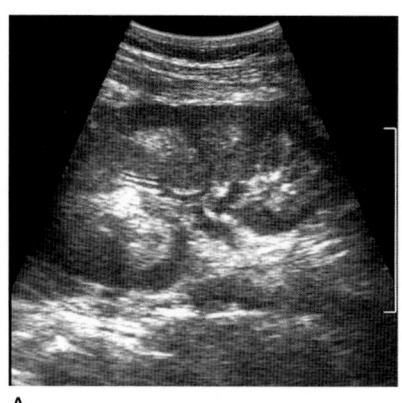
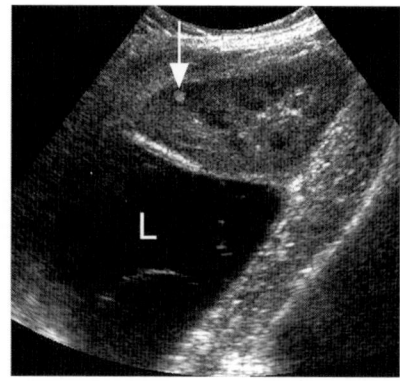
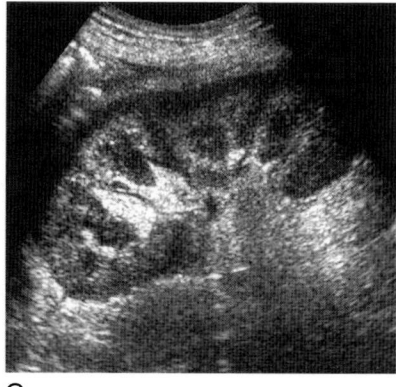

A   B   C

FIGURE 19-28. Donor pathology in three patients. Sagittal sonograms of transplant kidneys show **A**, nephrocalcinosis with calcifications in the renal medulla, **B**, a tiny angiomyolipoma (*arrow*, L–lymphocele) and **C**, Anderson-Carr morphology with echogenic borders around the medullary pyramids.

Parenchymal Pathology

Acute Tubular Necrosis and Acute Rejection

Acute tubular necrosis (ATN) results from donor organ ischemia either prior to vascular anastomosis or secondary to perioperative hypotension. It is most common in the early postoperative period and is the major cause of delayed graft function (defined as the need for dialysis within the first week of transplantation).[38,44] In those patients requiring dialysis, recovery is usually in the first 2 weeks of transplantation, but may be delayed by up to 3 months. ATN occurs in most cadaveric grafts, and is observed infrequently in living related renal transplants due to the relatively short cold ischemic time of the donor kidney.[37]

Transplants affected by **hyperacute rejection** are rarely imaged because graft failure occurs immediately at the vascular anastomosis during surgery.[38] **Acute rejection** occurs in up to 40% of patients in the early transplant period, peaking between 1 and 3 weeks postsurgery, and is an adverse long-term prognostic indicator. While most patients with acute rejection are asymptomatic, a small proportion of patients may present with flulike symptoms, malaise, fever, and graft tenderness. Provided that the diagnosis can be rapidly established, acute rejection usually can be promptly reversed with high-dose steroids or antibiotic therapy.[37,45]

The imaging features of ATN and acute rejection are almost identical on gray-scale and Doppler ultrasound. Both conditions can produce increases in length and cross-sectional areas of the allograft. However, precise volumetric comparisons between interval studies can prove difficult, and so, subtle changes in measurements have not been adopted as a strong clinical sign of potential dysfunction. Other **gray-scale** findings include increased cortical thickness, increased or decreased cortical echogenicity, reduction of the corticomedullary differentiation, loss of the renal sinus echoes, and prominence of the pyramids (Fig. 19-30).

Color Doppler assessment may be normal or may occasionally show diffuse decreased blood flow. The **resistive index** of the intraparenchymal arteries is also nonspecific in these conditions, and may be normal or elevated. In severe cases, there may be a complete lack of flow in diastole or a reversal of diastolic flow (Fig. 19-31).[37]

Despite the lack of specificity of gray-scale and Doppler ultrasound in these acute conditions, serial spectral Doppler measurements, in combination with clinical assessments and biochemical findings, provide a useful guide to the clinician in terms of monitoring the allograft function and in determining the need for percutaneous biopsy.

Chronic Rejection

Chronic rejection is defined as a reduction in allograft function starting at least 3 months post-transplantation

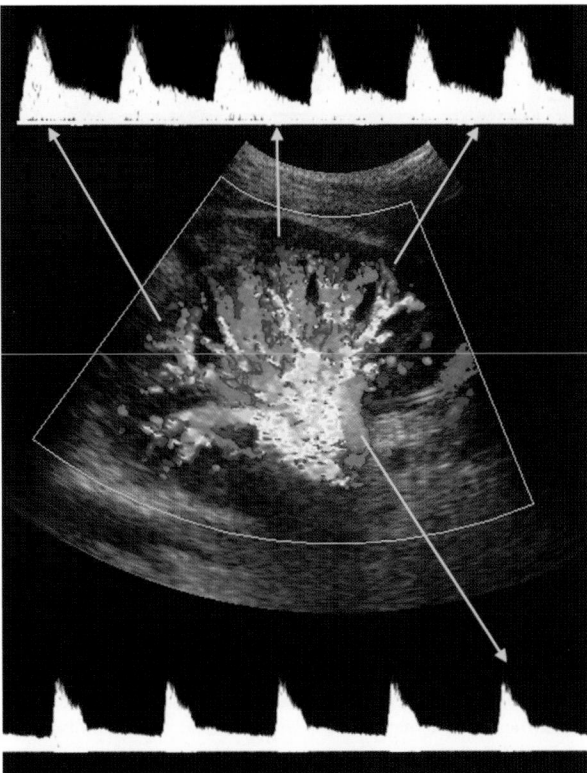

FIGURE 19-29. Normal renal transplant Doppler. Color Doppler shows flow throughout kidney (*top*). Intrarenal spectral traces of upper, mid- and lower poles show a resistive index of less than 0.8 and continuous flow throughout diastole. The main renal artery shows continuous flow with peak velocities less than 200 cm/sec (*bottom*).

the cardiac cycle. There are no accepted normal peak velocity values for these vessels. Documentation of the presence or absence of flow within the transplant and main renal vein, with an appropriate velocity gradient across the venous anastomosis, is of prime importance in the management of these patients.

Abnormal Renal Transplant

Renal transplants are routinely evaluated with sonography as either a component of a screening protocol, or as a work-up for renal dysfunction based on a rising serum creatinine level or a decreased urine output. When encountered with a graft with a clinical suspicion of dysfunction, the sonographer should approach the possible etiologies in terms of (1) parenchymal pathology, (2) prerenal causes, and (3) postrenal complications. **Parenchymal transplant pathology** includes acute tubular necrosis, acute and chronic rejection, and infection. **Prerenal problems** include all factors affecting either blood flow to the kidney or venous drainage from the graft. **Postrenal complications** include intrinsic or extrinsic lesions that can obstruct either a component of the calyceal system or the transplanted ureter.

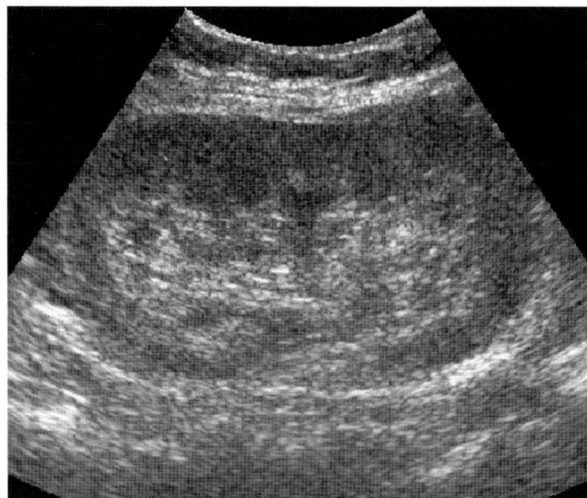

FIGURE 19-30. Acute renal failure. Sagittal scan shows increased cortical echogenicity and loss of the normal corticomedullary differentiation.

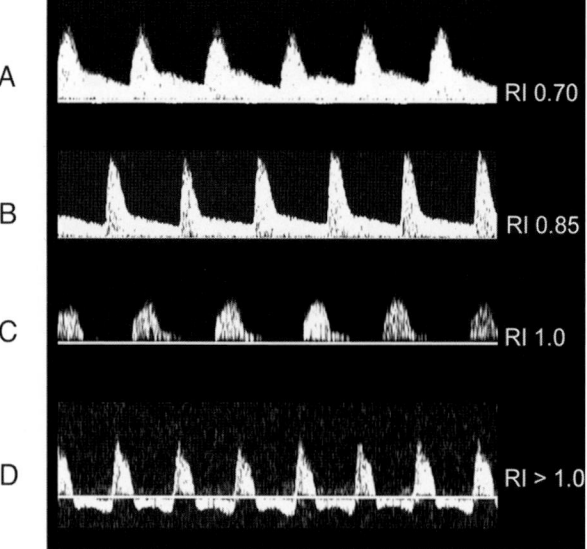

FIGURE 19-31. Intrarenal spectral waveforms in four patients. A, Normal, shows resistive index (RI) of 0.70. **B,** RI in a gray-zone (0.85). **C,** RI elevated with no flow in diastole (1.0) and **D,** elevated with reversal of flow in diastole (RI > 1.0). This is seen with severe increased vascular resistance in the kidney from hyperacute rejection or renal vein thrombosis.

in association with fibrous intimal thickening, interstitial fibrosis, and tubular atrophy on histology. It is the most common cause of late graft loss. The most frequent predisposing risk factor for development of chronic rejection is recurrent previous episodes of acute rejection.[37,38]

On **ultrasound**, there is progressive thinning of the renal cortex, prominence of the central renal sinus fat, and a reduction in the overall size of the transplant. Dystrophic calcifications may be seen scattered throughout the residual parenchyma. In the end-stage renal transplant, the entire renal cortex can become calcified, appearing as a sharp echogenic interface associated with clean distal shadowing (Fig. 19-32).

Infection

Transplant pyelonephritis can result from an ascending infection, hematologic seeding, or contiguous spread from an adjacent infected fluid collection. **Ultrasound findings** include a focal or diffusely granular, echogenic renal cortex associated with loss of the corticomedullary junction, increased echogenicity, and thickening of the perirenal fat secondary to extension of inflammation or infection into the surrounding tissue, and uroepithelial thickening (Figs. 19-33 and 19-34).

Air can be observed within the collecting system in **emphysematous pyelonephritis** appearing as a bright echogenic focus with distal dirty shadowing. Milk of calcium cysts can produce dirty shadowing, mimicking an intrarenal abscess. Scanning the patient in a decubitus position allows for differentiation, as air rises to the nondependent portion of the lumen, whereas milk of calcium does not (Fig. 19-35).

Pyonephrosis may occur occasionally in a chronically obstructed transplanted kidney. In the early stages, the lumen of the dilated collecting system appears anechoic. Once the lumen becomes filled with purulent material, low level echoes develop within the calyceal system and ureter, sometimes associated with fluid-debris levels. Echogenic material within the collecting system may also be caused by intraluminal blood, other filling defects, or may be artifactual due to scatter or side-lobe artifact.

Abscesses can arise from infection of a previously sterile collection. On ultrasound, they appear as a complex cystic structure, and may be associated with fluid-to-fluid levels or intraluminal air.

Prerenal Vascular Complications

Arterial Thrombosis

Renal artery **thrombosis** occurs in less than 1% of transplants, usually within the first month of surgery, and is often initially asymptomatic.[46] The most common cause is hyperacute or acute **rejection**, which results in occlusion of the intraparenchymal arterioles with retrograde main renal artery thrombosis. Other predisposing factors include a young pediatric donor kidney, atherosclerotic emboli, acquired renal artery stenosis, hypotension, vascular kinking, cyclosporine, hypercoagulable states, intraoperative vascular trauma, and poor intimal anastomosis.[46]

In occlusive main renal artery thrombosis, color and spectral Doppler will detect a complete absence of arterial and venous flow distal to the occlusion, within both the renal artery and the intraparenchymal vessels.

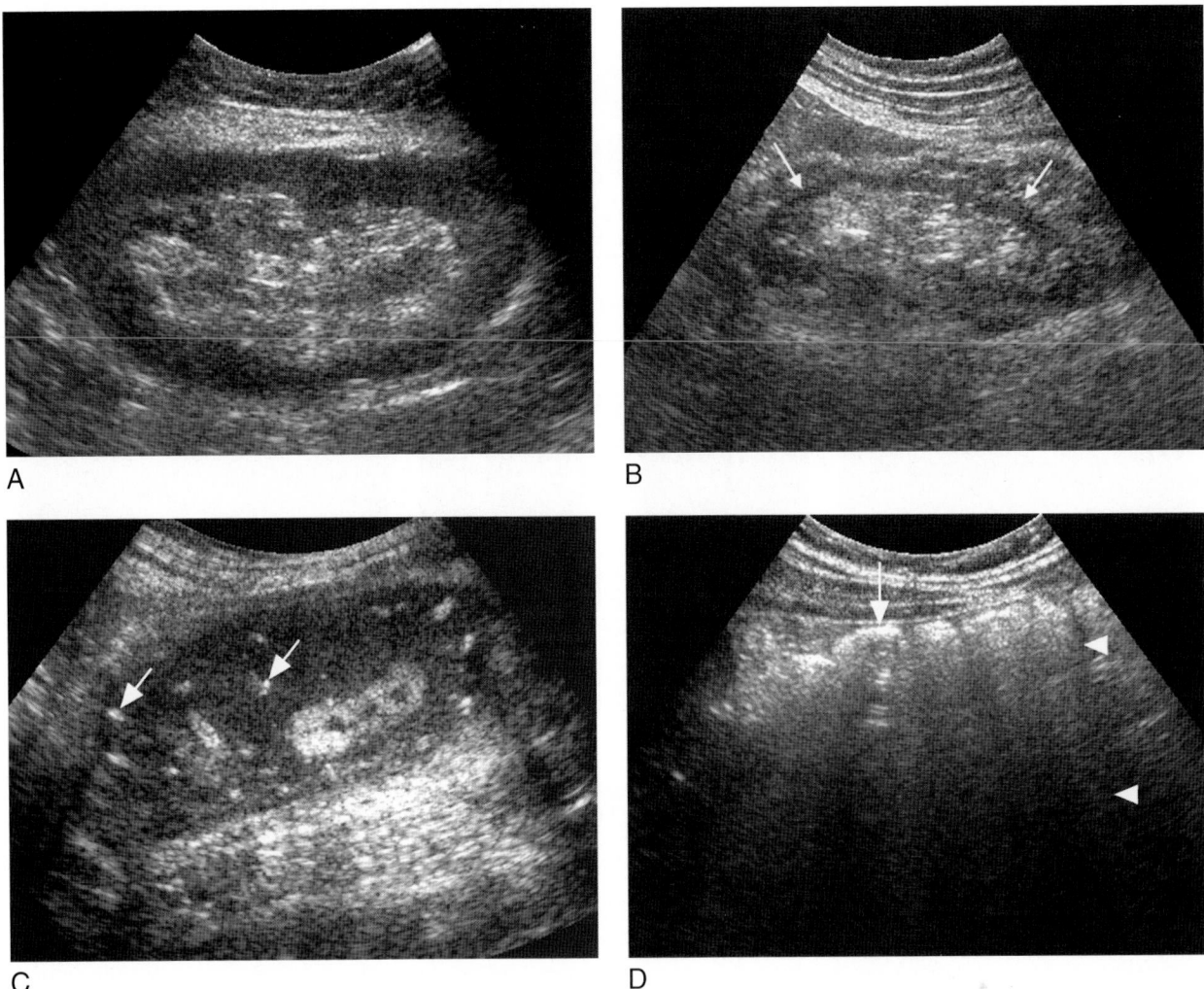

FIGURE 19-32. Chronic renal failure in four patients. A, Sagittal scan shows moderate cortical thinning with abundant renal sinus fat. **B,** With progression, the kidney becomes smaller and the cortex thinner (*arrows*). **C,** Dystrophic cortical calcifications (*arrows*) may also be observed. **D,** The end-stage kidney becomes calcified, appearing as an echogenic interface (*arrow*) associated with dirty shadowing (*arrowheads*). The kidney is frequently not identified on sonography at this stage.

In allografts with multiple renal arteries, in which only a single artery is thrombosed, segmental infarction can occur in the presence of preserved renal function (Fig. 19-36).

The absence of blood flow on Doppler interrogation in the kidney parenchyma may be observed in conditions other than arterial thrombosis. These conditions include hyperacute rejection and renal vein thrombosis. However, in these situations, the main renal artery is patent on spectral Doppler and may exhibit reversal of diastolic flow.[37]

Renal Artery Stenosis

Renal artery stenosis, the most common vascular complication of transplantation, occurs in up to 10% of patients within the first year and should be suspected in cases of severe hypertension refractory to medical therapy. Stenosis may occur in one of **three regions** of the transplanted artery: the **donor** portion, most frequently observed in end-to-side anastomoses and thought to arise from either rejection or difficult surgical technique; the **recipient** portion, which is more uncommon and usually the result of intraoperative clamp injury or intrinsic atherosclerotic disease; and at the **anastomosis**, which is more frequent in end-to-end anastomoses and is directly related to surgical technique or may be secondary to rejection.[46-48]

Initially, **color Doppler** should be used to detect the precise location of the anastomosis, as well as to document focal regions of aliasing, which would indicate the presence of high velocity turbulent flow and serve as a guide for meticulous spectral interrogation. **Peak systolic velocities** greater than 200 cm/sec, in the presence of distant turbulent flow, are suggestive of a stenotic region (Fig. 19-37). If no flow abnormality is

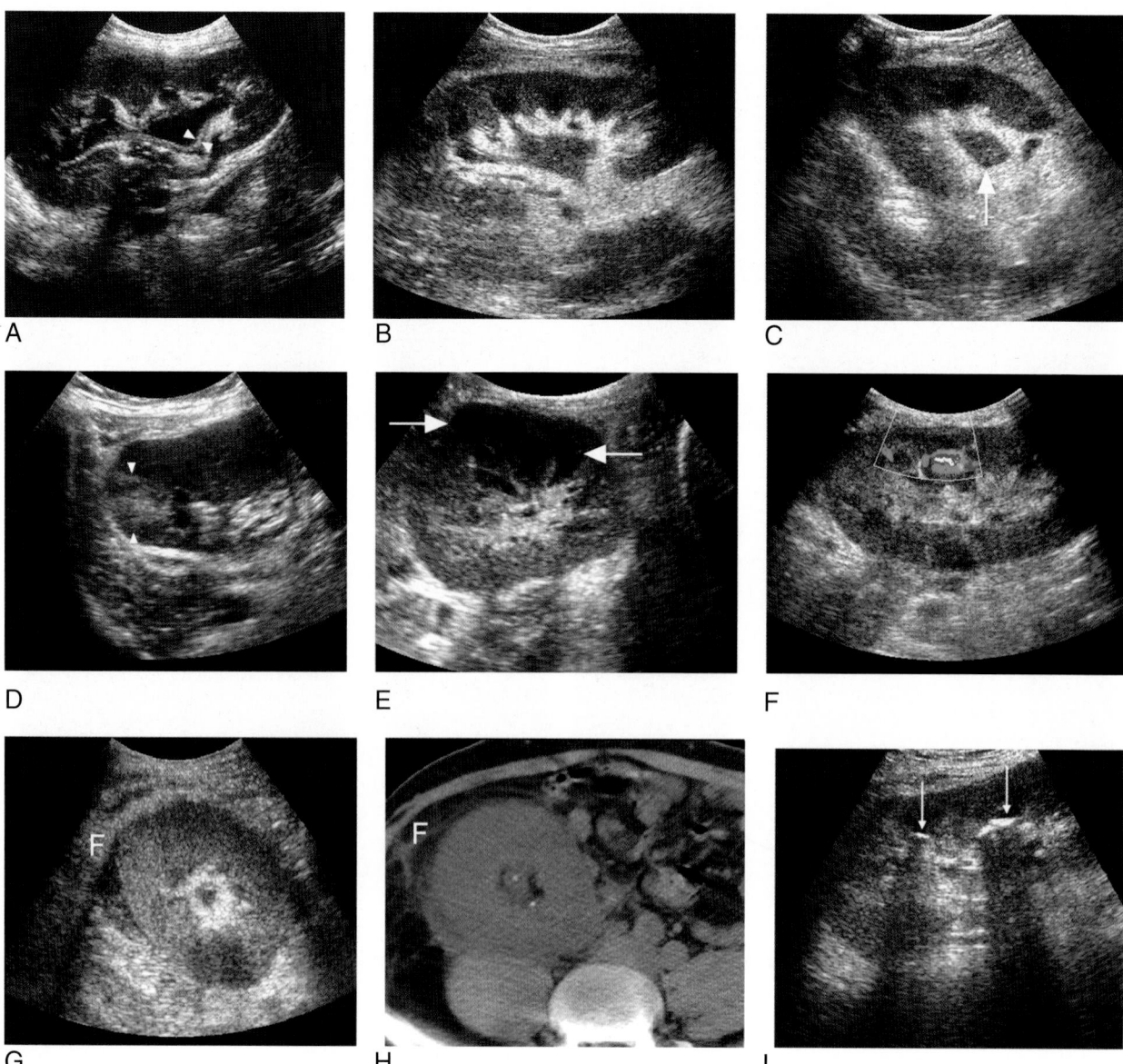

FIGURE 19-33. Renal transplant related infections: Uroepithelial thickening. **A,** Sagittal sonogram shows mild uroepithelial thickening (*arrowheads*). **B,** Sagittal and **C,** transverse sonograms show moderate-to-severe uroepithelial thickening (*arrow*), which can potentially be misinterpreted as a mass in the renal pelvis. **Focal pyelonephritis. D,** Sagittal sonogram shows subtle focal echogenic region in the upper pole cortex (*arrowheads*). **E,** Intraparenchymal phlegmon appearing as a hypoechoic mass within the renal cortex (*arrows*). **F,** On color Doppler, the phlegmon seen in image (**E**) is vascular. **Diffuse pyelonephritis. G,** Transverse sonogram shows a generous kidney with echogenic granular renal cortex, surrounded by inflamed echogenic perinephric fat (F). **H,** Corresponding CT scan shows inflamed fat (F) as perinephric streaking. **Emphysematous pyelonephritis. I,** Sagittal sonogram shows air (*arrows*) within collecting system which shows as bright echogenic linear foci with distal dirty shadowing.

detected within the main renal artery after color and spectral interrogation, significant stenosis can be excluded.[49]

Intraparenchymal arterial stenosis may be observed in chronic rejection as a result of scarring in the tissues surrounding the involved vessels. On spectral Doppler, a prolonged acceleration time may be observed in the segmental and interlobar arteries, with a normal main renal artery waveform.[38]

A false-positive Doppler diagnosis of renal artery stenosis may occur if there is an abrupt turn in the main renal artery, or if the artery is severely tortuous (Fig. 19-38). Inadvertent compression of the main renal artery by the sonographer while performing spectral interrogation may also produce transient narrowing of the artery and elevated peak systolic velocity readings.

Venous Thrombosis

Occlusive renal vein thrombosis is slightly more common than arterial thrombosis, occurring in up to 4% of transplants, and is associated with acute pain,

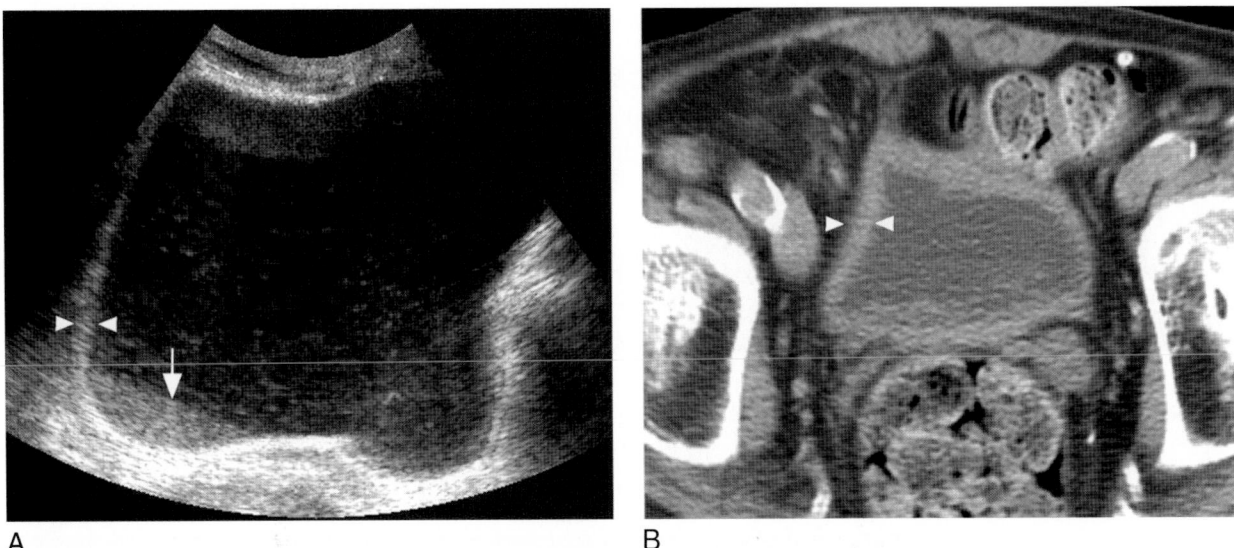

FIGURE 19-34. Renal transplant related infections: cystitis. A, Transverse sonogram shows internal echoes and fluid-debris level (*arrow*) in urinary bladder, secondary to cystitis. Bladder wall thickening (*arrowheads*) is identified on both ultrasound and **B,** corresponding CT scan.

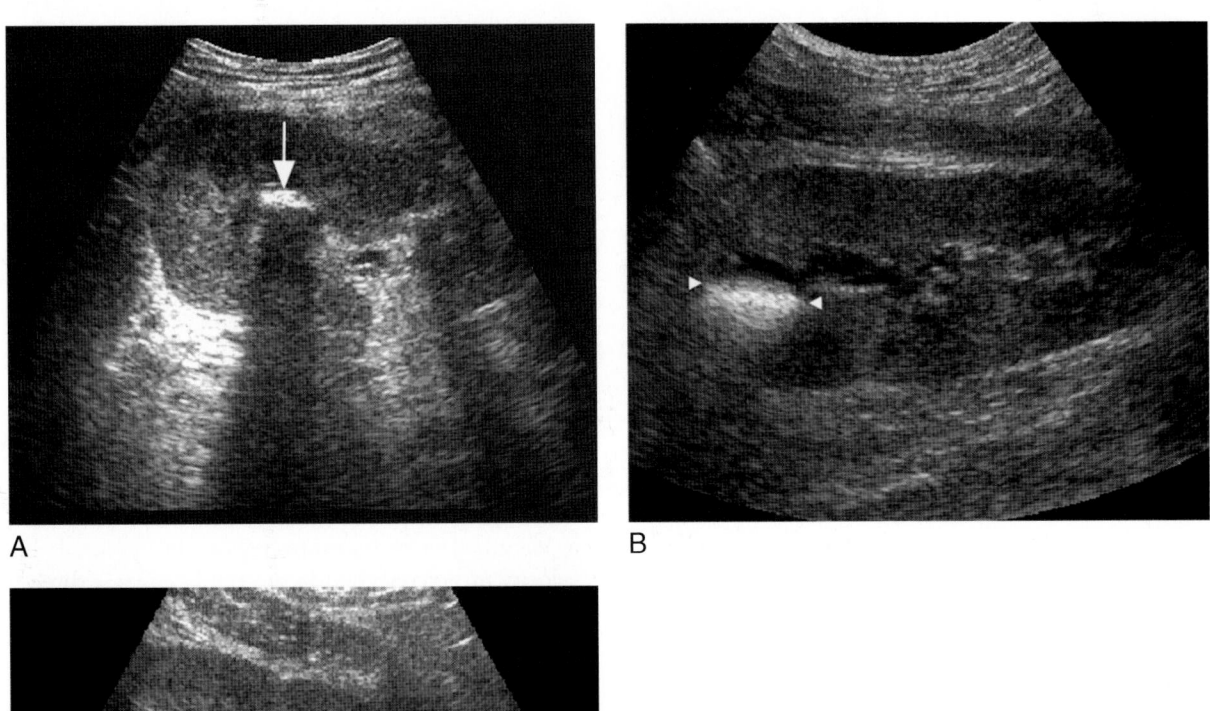

FIGURE 19-35. Mimicker of emphysematous pyelonephritis. A, Emphysematous pyelonephritis. Transverse scan shows air in collecting system (*arrow*). **B,** Milk of calcium cyst (*arrowheads*); supine sonogram shows layering of the calcification in the cyst, producing dirty shadowing. **C,** Scanning this patient in a decubitus position changes the orientation of the layering of calcium to the most dependent portion of the cyst, allowing for differentiation from an air-filled collection.

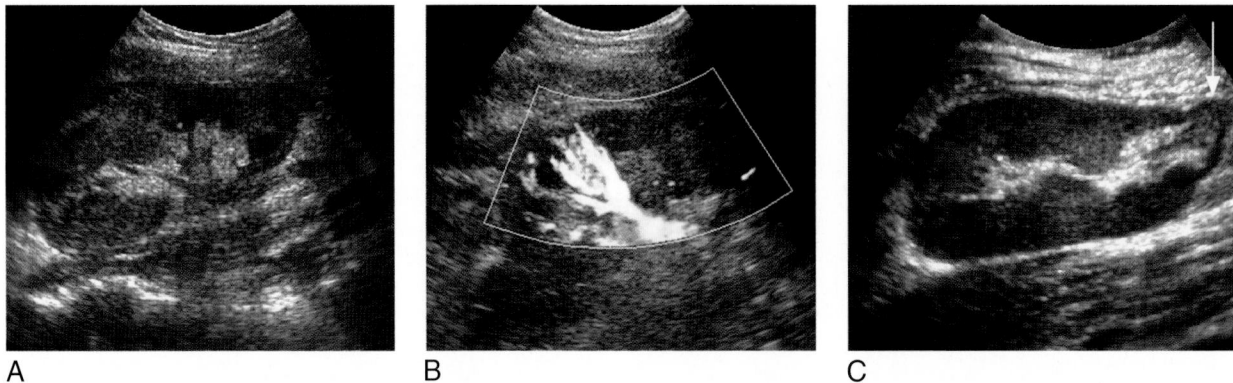

FIGURE 19-36. Renal artery thrombosis. A, Sagittal sonogram shows normal gray-scale ultrasound on postoperative day 1. **B**, However, power Doppler shows no flow in the lower pole due to thrombosis of a segmental artery. **C**, Three months later there is secondary scarring of the entire lower pole (*arrow*).

FIGURE 19-37. Renal artery stenosis. A, Color Doppler of renal artery anastomosis shows focal area of aliasing (*arrow*). **B**, Power Doppler shows area of narrowing in this region (*arrow*). **C**, Spectral Doppler shows elevated angle-corrected velocities at the site of the arrow, greater than 400 cm/sec.

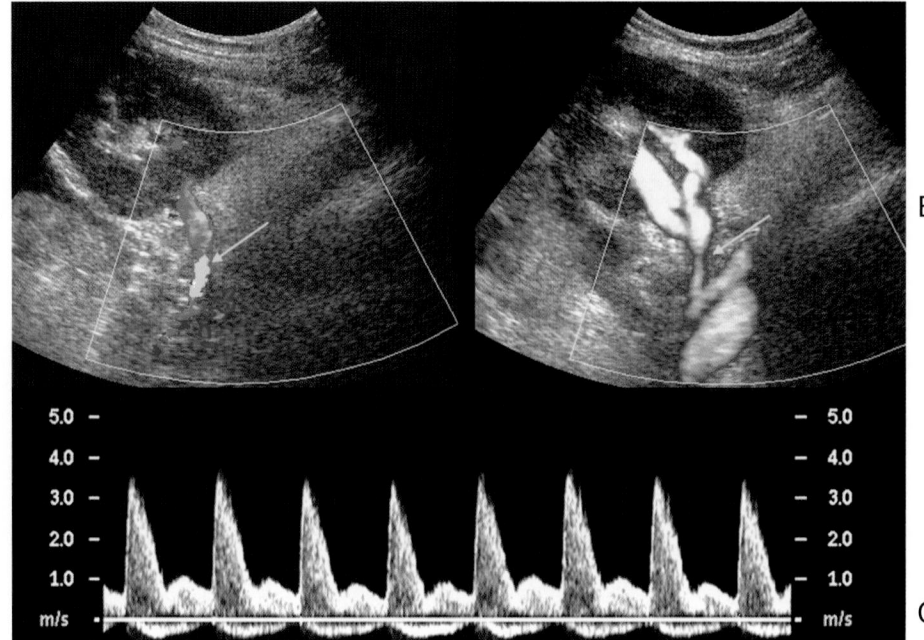

swelling of the allograft, and an abrupt cessation of renal function between the third and eighth postoperative day. Risk factors include technical difficulties at surgery, hypovolemia, propagation of femoral or iliac thrombosis, and compression by fluid collections.[46,50]

On **ultrasound**, intraluminal thrombus may rarely be detected in a dilated main renal vein or within the intraparenchymal venous system. More consistently, spectral and color Doppler show absence of flow in the main renal vein, and reversal of diastolic flow in the main renal artery (Fig. 19-39).[51,52]

Renal Vein Stenosis

Renal vein stenosis most commonly occurs from either perivascular fibrosis or external compression by adjacent fluid collections. The renal cortex appears either normal or hypoechoic, and on color Doppler, aliasing

is identified at the stenotic region due to focal, high velocity turbulent flow. On spectral Doppler, a **three- to fourfold increase in velocity** across the region of narrowing indicates a hemodynamically significant stenosis (Fig. 19-40).[49]

Postrenal Collecting System Obstruction

Collecting system obstruction is unusual in renal transplants, occurring in less than 5% of patients.[38,49] Because the allograft is denervated, the collecting system dilates without clinical signs of pain or discomfort. The diagnosis is often made as an incidental finding on routine screening sonography, or in work-up of the transplant patient for asymptomatic deterioration of renal function parameters.

The most frequent location of obstruction is at the **ureteric-vesical anastomosis**, either from a stricture

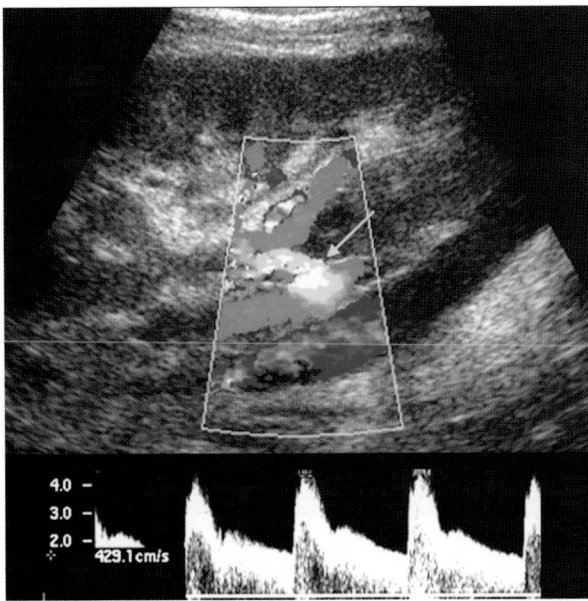

FIGURE 19-38. Mimicker of renal artery stenosis. Abrupt turn in renal artery. On color Doppler, aliasing is identified in this region (*arrow*), with peak systolic velocities of 429 cm/sec on spectral Doppler.

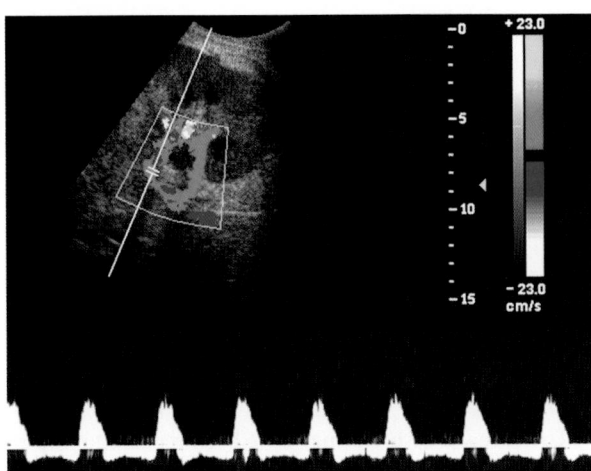

FIGURE 19-39. Renal vein thrombosis. Spectral Doppler of main renal artery shows reversal of flow in diastole. A small amount of flow is identified in the color box in the common iliac vein.

(related to ischemia or iatrogenic injury) or an intraluminal lesion, such as a stone, blood clot, or sloughed papilla. Extrinsic compression of the ureter from peritransplant collections can also result in ureteric obstruction (Fig. 19-41).

Evaluation of the collecting system with fundamental gray-scale imaging may, at times, be difficult due to side lobe and scatter artifact, which can potentially obscure optimal evaluation of the calyceal system and ureter. **Harmonic imaging,** however, utilizes a narrower ultrasound beam with smaller side lobes and is less susceptible to scatter artifact. These parameters make

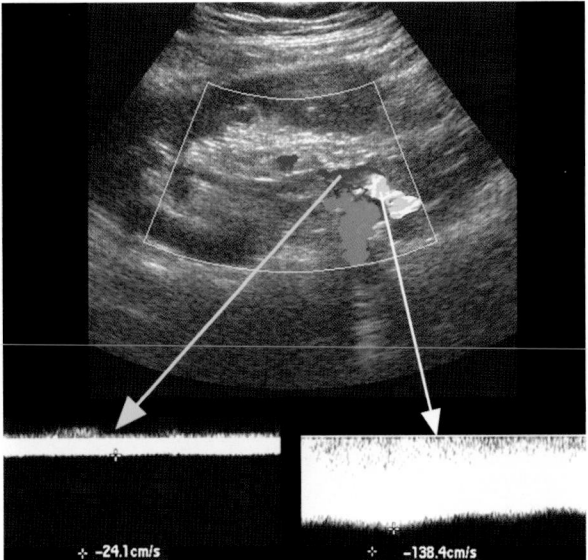

FIGURE 19-40. Renal vein stenosis. Color Doppler of renal vein anastomosis shows focal area of aliasing (*white arrow*). Spectral interrogation proximal to aliasing shows velocities of 24 cm/sec (*yellow arrow*). Spectral interrogation in region of aliasing shows velocities of 138 cm/sec, indicating a hemodynamically significant stenosis of the renal vein.

harmonic imaging ideal for evaluating anechoic structures, such as the renal collecting system for regions of subtle dilation, and the presence of small intraluminal stones (Fig. 19-42).

Mild pelvocaliectasis may be secondary to nonobstructive causes such as overhydration, decreased ureteric tone (from denervation of the transplant), ureteric-vesical reflux, or can occur transiently in the immediate postoperative period from perianastomotic edema.[38,53] In addition, multiple parapelvic cysts can mimic a dilated collecting system (Fig. 19-43).

Arteriovenous Malformations and Pseudoaneurysms

Intraparenchymal arteriovenous malformations (AVMs) result from vascular trauma to both artery and vein during percutaneous biopsies, and are usually asymptomatic with little clinical significance. Because most of these malformations are small and resolve spontaneously, the precise incidence of post-transplant AVMs is unknown, although rates of 1% to 18% have been reported. In rare instances, large AVMs may present with bleeding, high output cardiac failure, or decreased renal perfusion caused by the large shunt. In these instances, treatment usually involves percutaneous embolization therapy.[37,54]

Gray-scale ultrasound may not reveal small AVMs. **Color Doppler** shows a focal region of aliasing with a myriad of intense colors, often associated with a prominent feeding artery or draining vein. Turbulent flow within the vascular malformation produces vibration of the perivascular tissues, resulting in these tissues

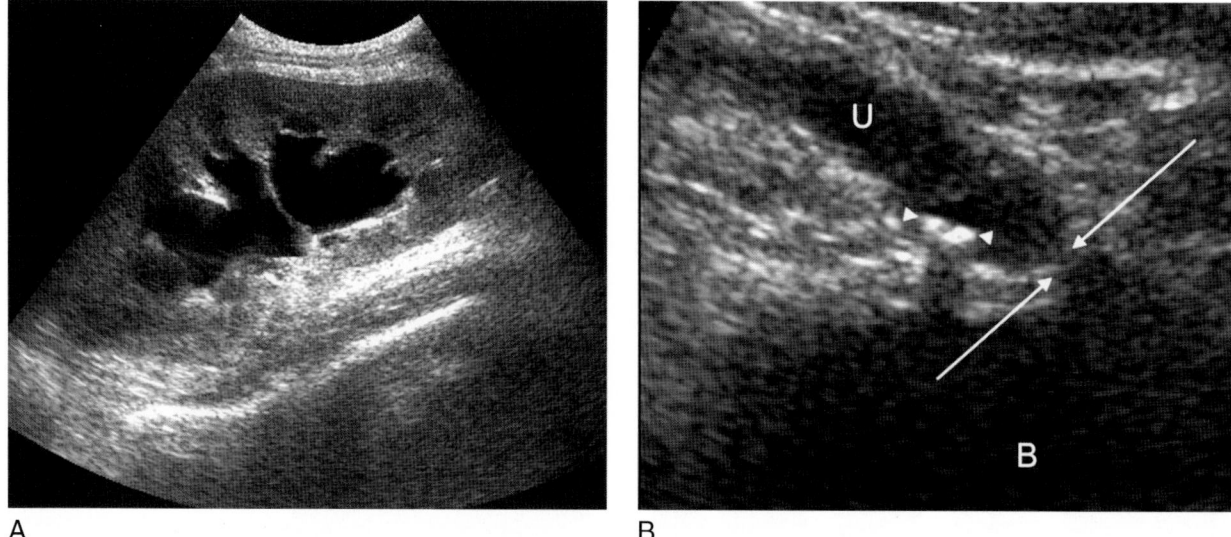

FIGURE 19-41. Uterovesical junction obstruction. A, Sagittal sonogram shows grade 3 pelvocaliectasis. **B**, This is produced by a stricture at the uterovesical junction (*arrows*). *Arrowheads* show a tiny nonobstructing stone. (B — bladder, U — ureter.)

being assigned a color signal outside of the borders of the renal vasculature. **Spectral Doppler** is typical of all AVMs in that there is low resistance, high velocity flow with difficulty differentiating between artery and vein within the malformation. If a dominant draining vein is detected, the waveform may be pulsatile or arterialized (Fig. 19-44).[46,53,55,56]

On color Doppler, focal regions of **cortical dystrophic calcifications** or **small stones** can mimic an AVM by producing an intense color signal known as a **twinkling artifact.**[57] These artifacts can be differentiated from a true AVM on spectral tracing because both calcifications and stones produce characteristic linear bands on spectral interrogation. In our clinical experience, we have also observed a linear band of color posterior to these regions of calcium that extend to the limits of the color box. We have not observed this phenomenon with AVMs, and have found it a useful tool in differentiating vascular malformations from focal calcifications (Fig. 19-45).

Pseudoaneurysms occur as a result of vascular trauma to the arterial system during percutaneous biopsy or, more commonly, they occur at the site of the vascular anastomosis (Fig. 19-46). They may be intra- or extrarenal in location. On gray-scale, **pseudoaneurysms can mimic a simple or complex cyst**. On color Doppler, flow can easily be obtained in the lumen of patent pseudoaneurysms, often with a swirling pattern, whereas on spectral Doppler, a central **to-and-fro** waveform, or a disorganized arterial tracing may be obtained.[38]

Fluid Collections

Perinephric collections are demonstrated in up to 50% of transplant recipients.[58,59] The most common collec-

tions include hematoma, urinoma, lymphocele, and abscess. The ultrasound appearances of these peritransplant collections are often nonspecific, and clinical findings are warranted to determine their etiology. The size and location of each collection should be documented on baseline scans because an increase in size may indicate the need for surgical intervention.

Postoperative hematomas are variable in size, but are often small, perirenal in location, insignificant clinically, and resolve spontaneously.[53] Their ultrasound appearance is dependent on the age of the collection. Acutely, hematomas appear as an echogenic heterogeneous solid mass. With time they liquefy, becoming a complex cystic structure with internal echoes, strands, or septations. Postbiopsy hematomas have a similar morphology to their postoperative counterpart (Fig. 19-47).

Urine leaks or urinomas have been reported in up to 6% of renal transplants and occur within the first 2 weeks following surgery.[60] They are commonly secondary to either anastomotic leaks or ureteric ischemia. Rarely, urinomas can result from high-grade collecting system obstruction (Fig. 19-48). On sonography, they are well defined and anechoic and may be associated with hydronephrosis. Large urine leaks may result in widespread extravasation and gross intraperitoneal fluid.

Lymphoceles result from surgical disruption of the iliac lymphatics and occur 4 to 8 weeks' postsurgery in up to 15% of patients. While most are discovered incidentally and are asymptomatic, lymphoceles are the most common fluid collection to result in ureteric obstruction. They have the potential to obstruct venous drainage, resulting in edema of the lower limb, scrotum or labia, or become infected.[38] Symptomatic collections are drained (surgically or percutaneously) or undergo marsupialization. On sonography, they are well-defined

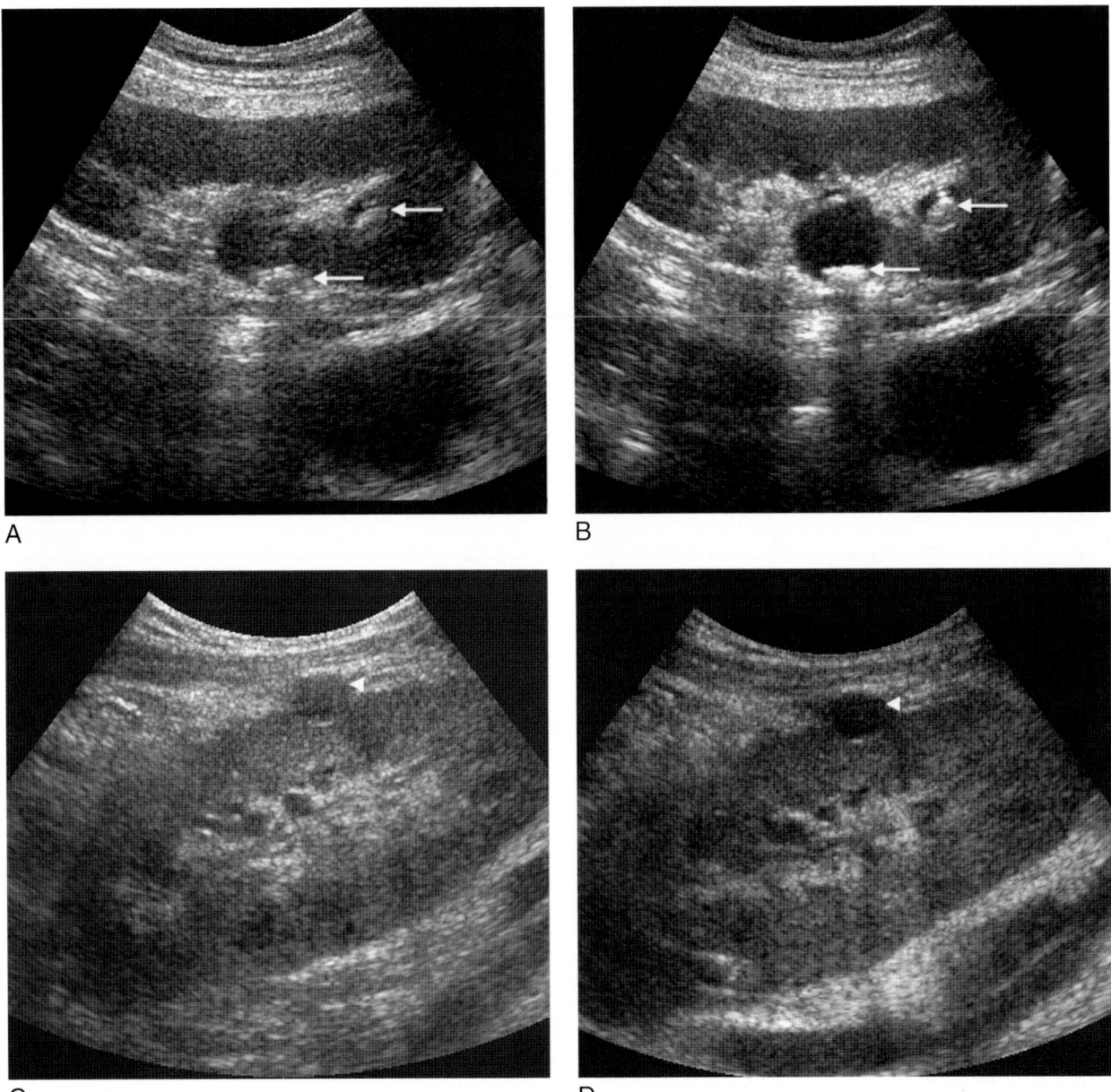

FIGURE 19-42. Harmonic imaging in two patients. A, Sagittal fundamental image shows barely detectable stones (*arrows*) and a dilated collecting system. **B**, Harmonic image shows improved resolution of stones (*arrows*) now seen associated with distal acoustic shadowing, within anechoic dilated collecting system. **C**, Fundamental image shows cortical cyst (*arrowhead*) with internal echoes and minimal through transmission. **D**, Harmonic image shows cyst to be anechoic and simple, now associated with an appropriate amount of through transmission.

collections that are either anechoic or that may contain fine internal strands (Fig. 19-49).

PANCREAS TRANSPLANTATION

Pancreatic transplantation is performed in selected patients who have major complications related to type I diabetes, and represents the only form of self-regulating endocrine replacement therapy, with over 80% of recipients becoming free of exogenous insulin require-ments within 1 year of surgery. To date, over 11,000 pancreatic transplants have been performed worldwide with a 1-year patient survival rate of greater than 90%.[5]

Surgical Technique

Since the first pancreatic transplant was performed in 1966, several surgical techniques have been described. The two most commonly utilized pancreatic transplant surgeries both involve transplantation of the entire gland, with an arterial anastomosis to the recipient common

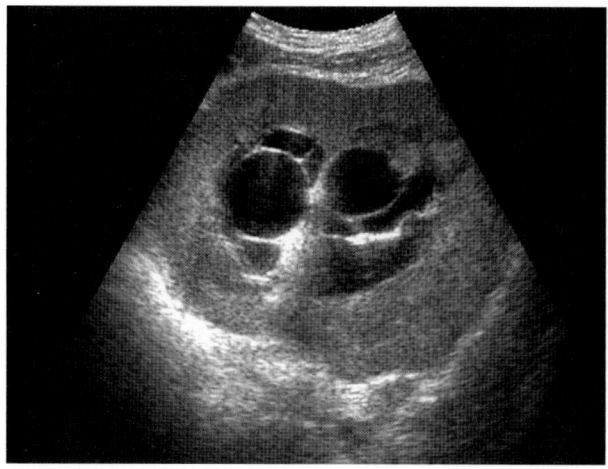
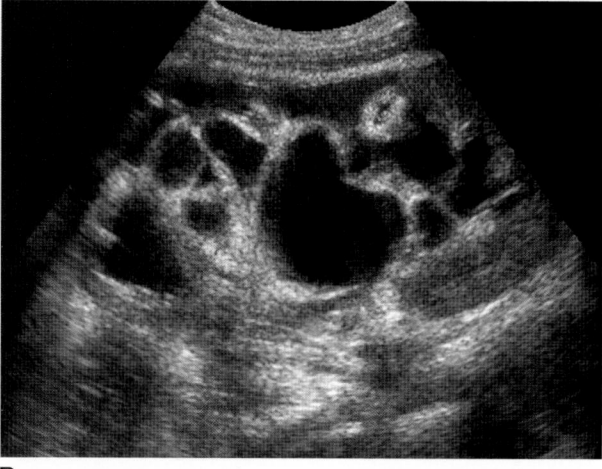

A   B

FIGURE 19-43. Parapelvic cysts. A, Transverse and **B,** sagittal sonograms show multiple parapelvic cysts mimicking pelvocaliectasis.

TABLE 19-1. SURGICAL TECHNIQUES FOR PANCREATIC TRANSPLANTATION

	Systemic Venous-Bladder Drainage	Portal Venous-Enteric Drainage
Location	Right lower quadrant	Right upper quadrant
Pancreatic orientation	Head caudad	Tail caudad
Arterial supply	Y-shaped donor arterial graft to common iliac recipient artery	Donor splenic artery to recipient common iliac artery
Venous drainage	Donor portal vein to external iliac vein	Donor portal vein to superior mesenteric vein
Endocrine drainage	Systemic venous	Portal venous
Exocrine drainage	*En-bloc* donor duodenal stump to bladder	Duodenal segment to Roux-en-Y loop of jejunum

iliac artery. However, they differ in their endocrine (i.e., portal venous) and exocrine drainage (Table 19-1).[5,61]

The more traditional surgery (**systemic venous-bladder drainage**) involves anastomosing the donor portal vein to the recipient external iliac vein (systemic venous endocrine drainage) and the donor duodenum to the urinary bladder (exocrine drainage) (Fig. 19-50).[61] The chronic loss of pancreatic secretions into the bladder can result in problems with dehydration, metabolic acidosis, local bladder irritation, and allograft pancreatitis.[5]

A more recent technique (**portal venous-enteric drainage**), which is becoming more widely utilized, involves anastomosing the donor portal vein to the recipient superior mesenteric vein (portal venous endocrine drainage), and the donor duodenum to a Roux-en-Y loop of jejunum (exocrine drainage) (Fig. 19-51). This type of surgery provides a more physiologic transplant compared to the more traditional techniques, and is not associated with dehydration or metabolic acidosis. In addition, it provides more appropriate glycemic control with lower fasting insulin levels and may be associated with a lower incidence of transplant rejection than the more traditional **systemic venous-bladder drainage** transplants.[5]

Normal Pancreas Transplant Ultrasound

In order to perform an ultrasound assessment of a transplanted pancreas, the sonographer should be aware of the surgical technique used, the position of the allograft in the abdomen at surgery, and the sites of vascular anastomosis. This often entails a detailed review of the intraoperative surgical notes or discussion with the surgeon prior to scanning the patient.

Systemic venous-bladder drainage transplants are usually located in the right lower quadrant and may show a diagonal or horizontal axis. **Portal venous-enteric drainage** transplants are usually in the right upper quadrant or right paramedian region with a vertical axis. In both instances, the allograft may be difficult to visualize because of overlying bowel gas; however, meticulous scanning with intermittent compression of the overlying intraluminal gas is frequently successful in visualizing the transplant. In our experience, although the normal pancreatic transplant may be obscured, both

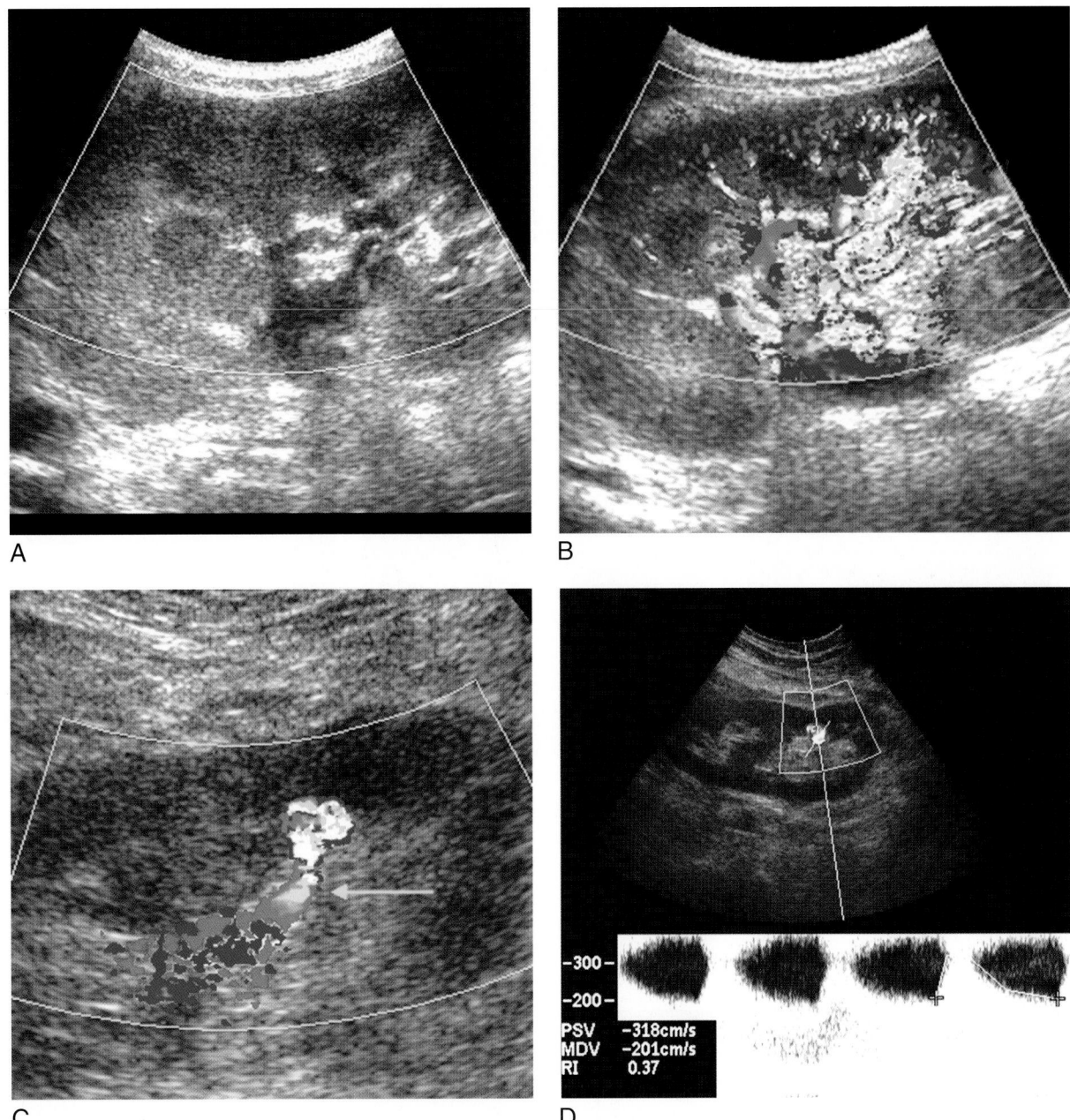

FIGURE 19-44. Arteriovenous malformations. A, Gray-scale ultrasound. Arteriovenous malformation (AVM) is not detectable. **B**, Color Doppler corresponding to gray-scale image from **A** shows large AVM. **C**, Sagittal sonogram shows AVM with feeding vessel (*arrow*). **D**, Spectral Doppler shows high-velocity, low-resistance waveform within AVM.

inflammation of the graft and perigraft fluid collections facilitate pancreatic visualization.

The normal allograft retains its normal gray-scale morphology with well-defined margins, a homogeneous echotexture, isoechoic or minimally echogenic to liver, and a thin, nondilated pancreatic duct (Fig. 19-52). The peripancreatic fat shows a normal echogenicity, and occasionally a small amount of surrounding fluid may be observed. This trace amount of peripancreatic fluid usually resolves without complication.

Color Doppler is useful for locating the mesenteric vessels, particularly in those instances where the graft

is poorly visualized because of overlying bowel gas. **Spectral** Doppler of the normal graft shows continuous monophasic venous flow and low-resistance arterial waveforms.

Abnormal Pancreas Transplant

Vascular Thrombosis

Graft thrombosis, including both venous and arterial thrombosis, occurs with a reported incidence of 2% to 19% and is the second leading cause of transplant loss,

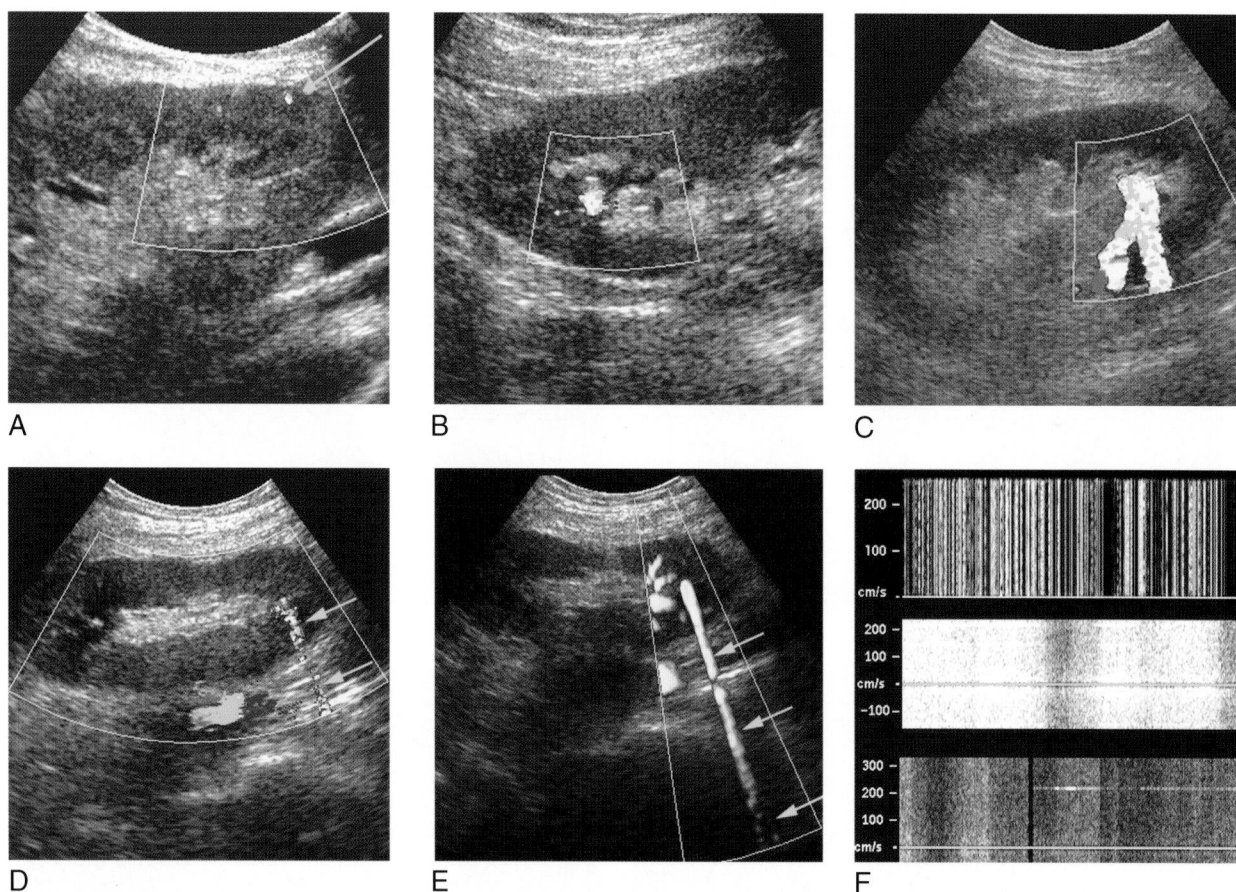

FIGURE 19-45. Arteriovenous malformation: mimicker. Sagittal sonogram shows twinkling artifact produced by **A**, lower pole dystrophic cortical calcification (*arrow*), **B**, upper pole stone and **C**, lower pole stone. Differentiation from arteriovenous malformation. On **D**, color Doppler and **E**, power Doppler, color artifact (*arrows*) may be seen posterior to the border of the kidney. The size of the twinkling artifact varies with the size of the color box. **F**, On spectral Doppler, the twinkling artifact shows linear bands as on these three spectral traces.

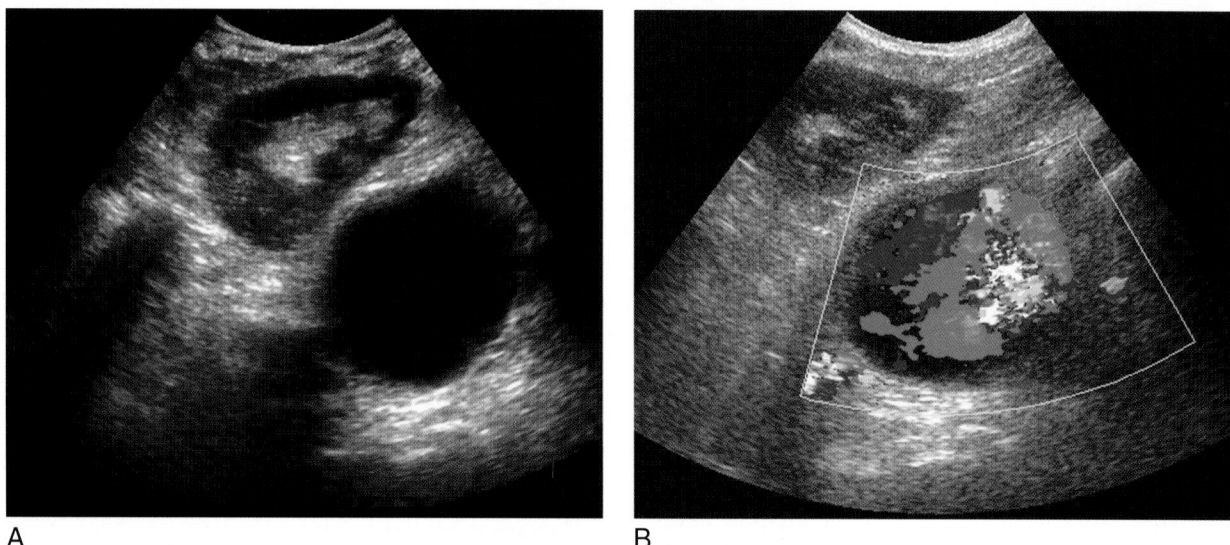

FIGURE 19-46. Renal artery pseudoaneurysm. A, Transverse sonogram shows anechoic structure adjacent to renal hilum. **B**, Color Doppler shows that this structure contains swirling flow and represents a pseudoaneurysm.

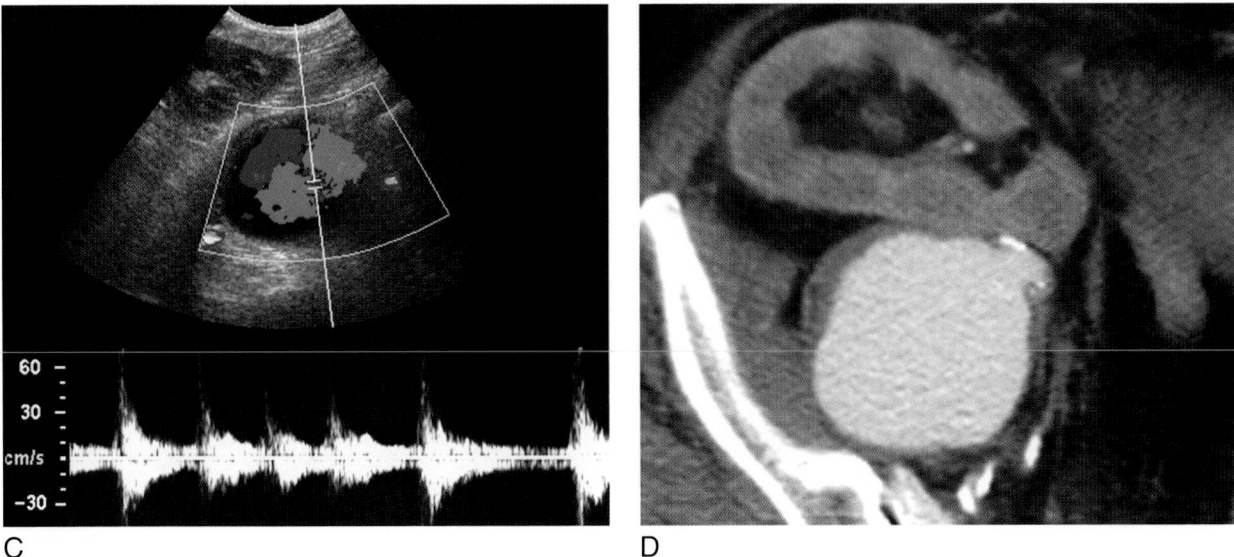

C

D

FIGURE 19-46, *cont'd*. Renal artery pseudoaneurysm. **C**, Spectral Doppler shows disorganized internal flow within pseudoaneurysm. **D**, CT scan shows pseudoaneurysm arising from site of renal artery anastomosis.

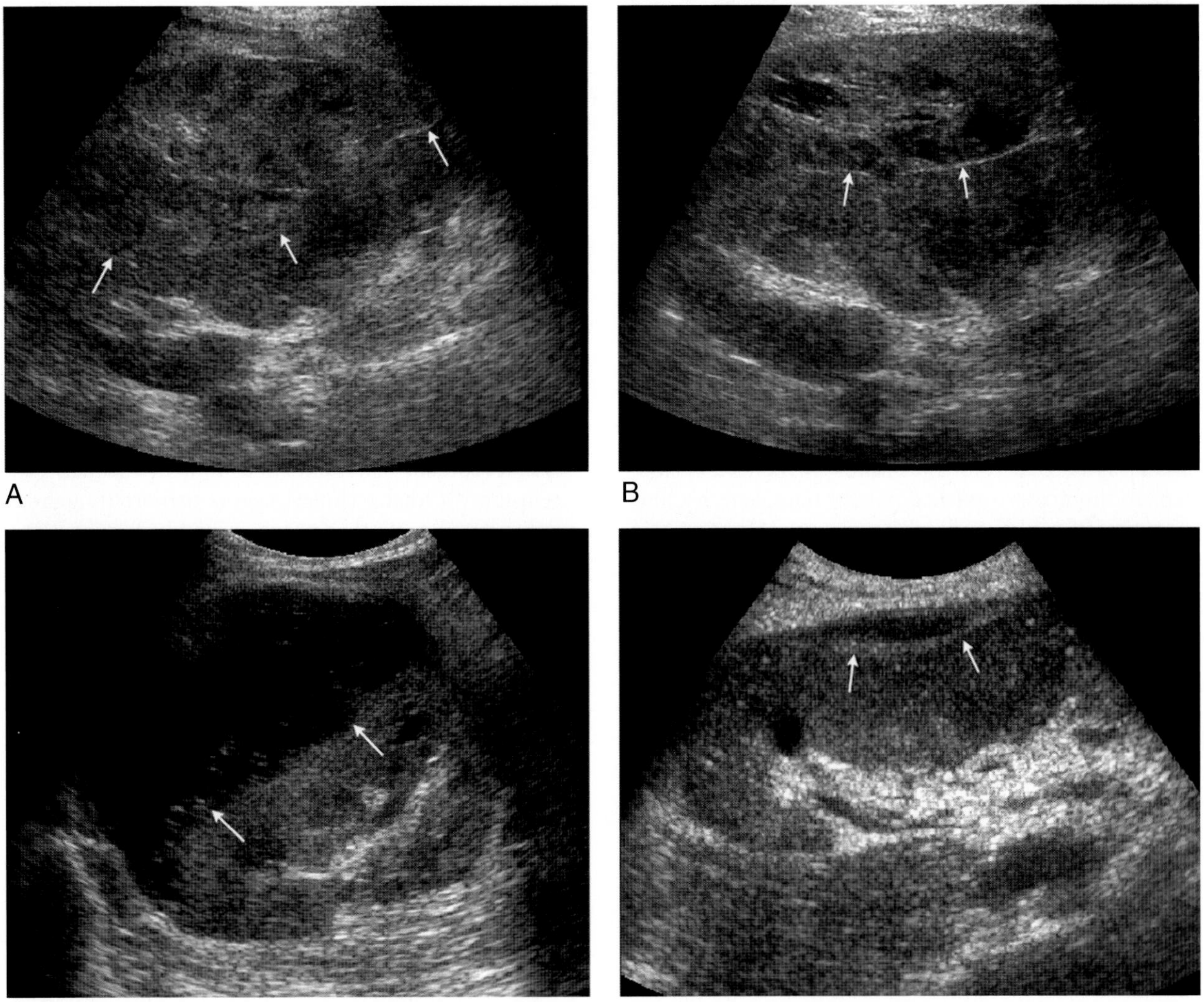

A

B

C

D

FIGURE 19-47. Subcapsular hematoma secondary to biopsy. Sagittal sonogram shows **A**, acute hematoma appearing as solid heterogeneous structure. **B**, After 1 week, cystic regions develop within the hematoma. **C**, After 1 month the hematoma liquefies and is larger due to a hyperosmolar effect and **D**, eventually decreases in size as it is reabsorbed. *Arrows* mark junction of hematoma and renal cortex.

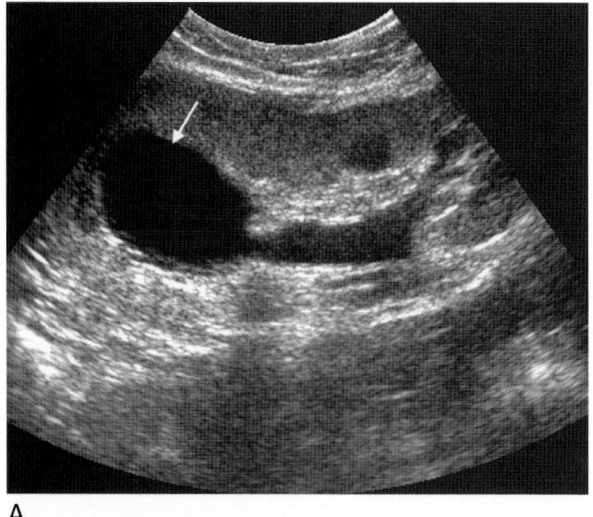

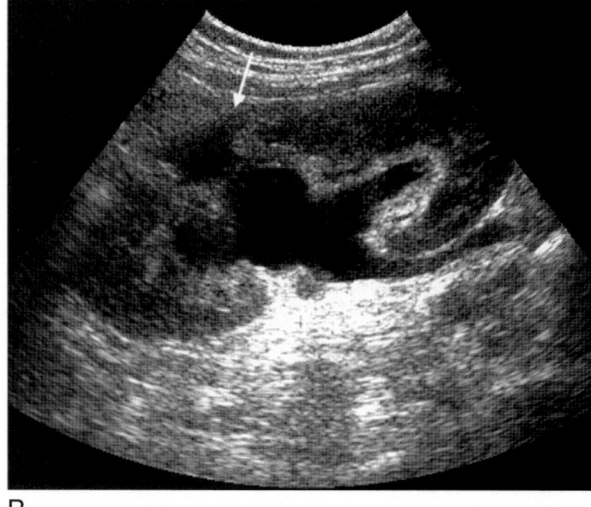

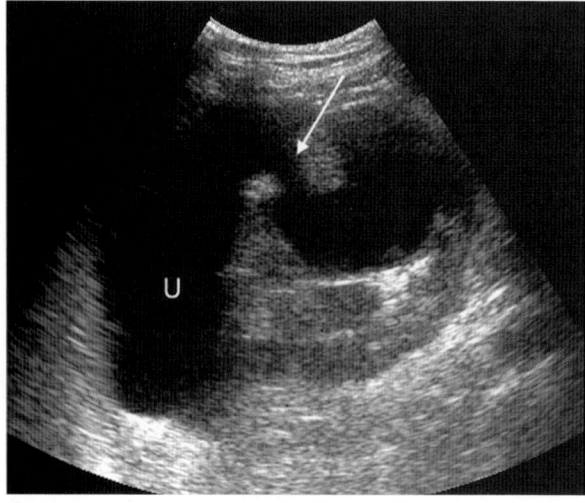

FIGURE 19-48. Urinoma secondary to high-grade uterovesical junction obstruction. A, Sagittal sonogram shows dilation of upper pole calyx (*arrow*); **B,** which eventually ruptures through the adjacent cortex (*arrow*); and **C,** forming a cortical defect (*arrow*) and subsequently a perinephric urinoma (U).

after rejection. Pancreatic transplants are more vulnerable to graft thrombosis compared to renal transplants because the rate of blood flow in the transplanted pancreas is slower compared to that in a transplanted kidney.[62,63]

Although the clinical signs and symptoms of graft thrombosis are nonspecific, detection of vascular thrombosis is imperative for both salvaging the transplant and preventing life-threatening sequelae, such as sepsis and cardiovascular collapse. Venous thrombosis, which occurs with an estimated incidence of 5%, is particularly worrisome because of the increased risk of hemorrhagic pancreatitis, tissue necrosis, infection, thrombus propagation, and pulmonary embolism.[63]

Graft thrombosis can be categorized as early or late, depending on the time of diagnosis after surgery. **Early** graft thrombosis occurs within 1 month of transplantation, and is secondary to either microvascular injury during preservation of the graft or technical error during surgery. **Late** graft thrombosis occurs 1 month after transplant surgery and is usually due to alloimmune arteritis, in which gradual occlusion of the small blood vessels eventually culminates in complete proximal vessel occlusion.[62] Other technical factors that are thought to predispose to graft thrombosis include coagulopathies, long preservation time, poor donor vessels, left-sided graft placement resulting in a deeper anastomosis, and the use of a venous extension graft.[63]

On ultrasound, **occlusive or nonocclusive thrombus** may be visualized within the lumen of the transplanted arteries or veins (Fig. 19-53). We have also observed several cases of thrombus occurring at the suture line of blind ending arteries or veins (Fig. 19-54).

On **spectral Doppler,** no arterial flow is detected in transplants with occlusive arterial thrombus. In those grafts with occlusive venous thrombus, a lack of venous flow is detected on spectral tracing, with high resistance arterial flow showing either no flow in diastole (RI = 1) or reversal of diastolic flow.[63] Surgically ligated arteries containing thrombus may show a cyclic pattern of flow adjacent to the thrombus, which we presume is secondary to local eddy currents, with a normal arterial waveform more proximally.

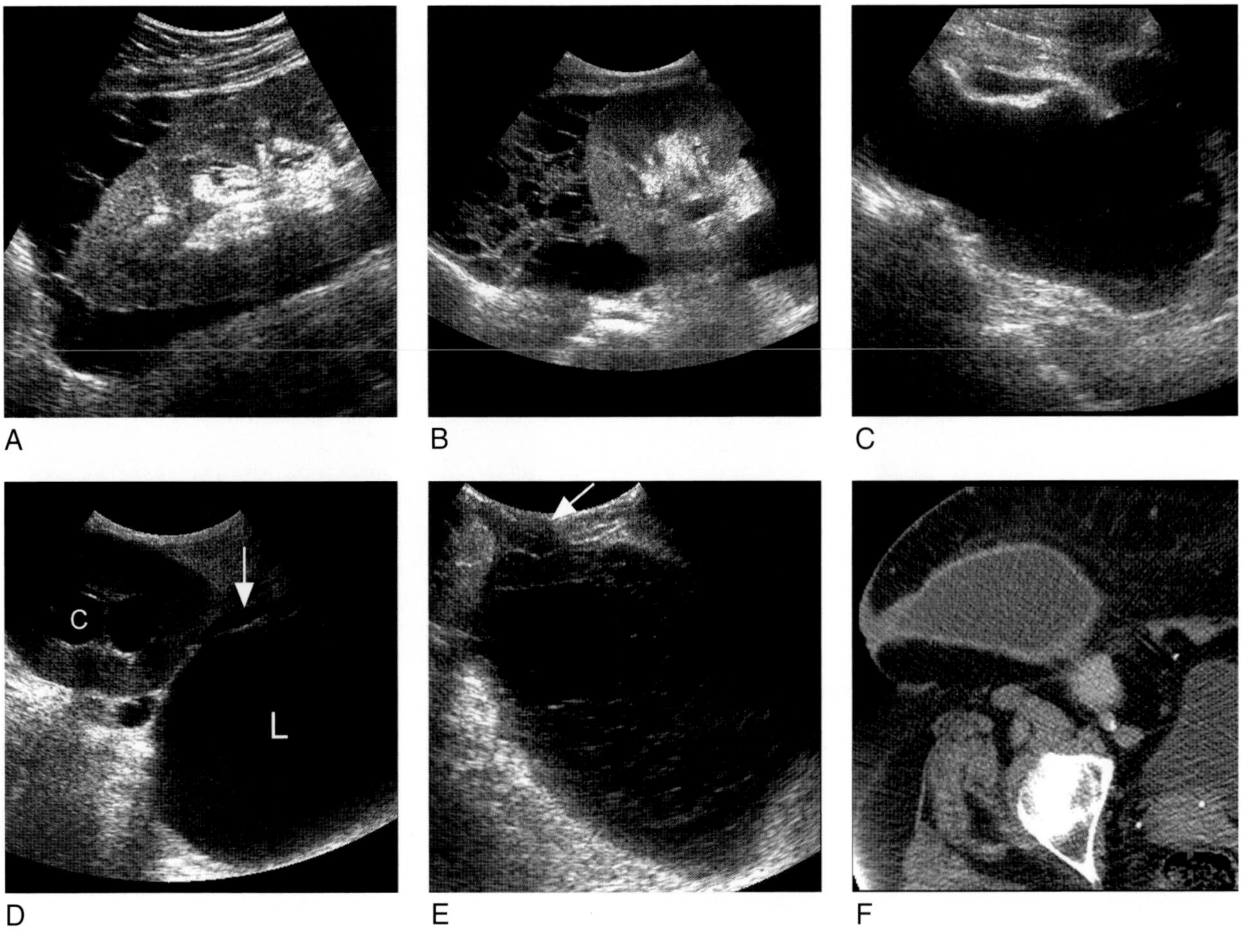

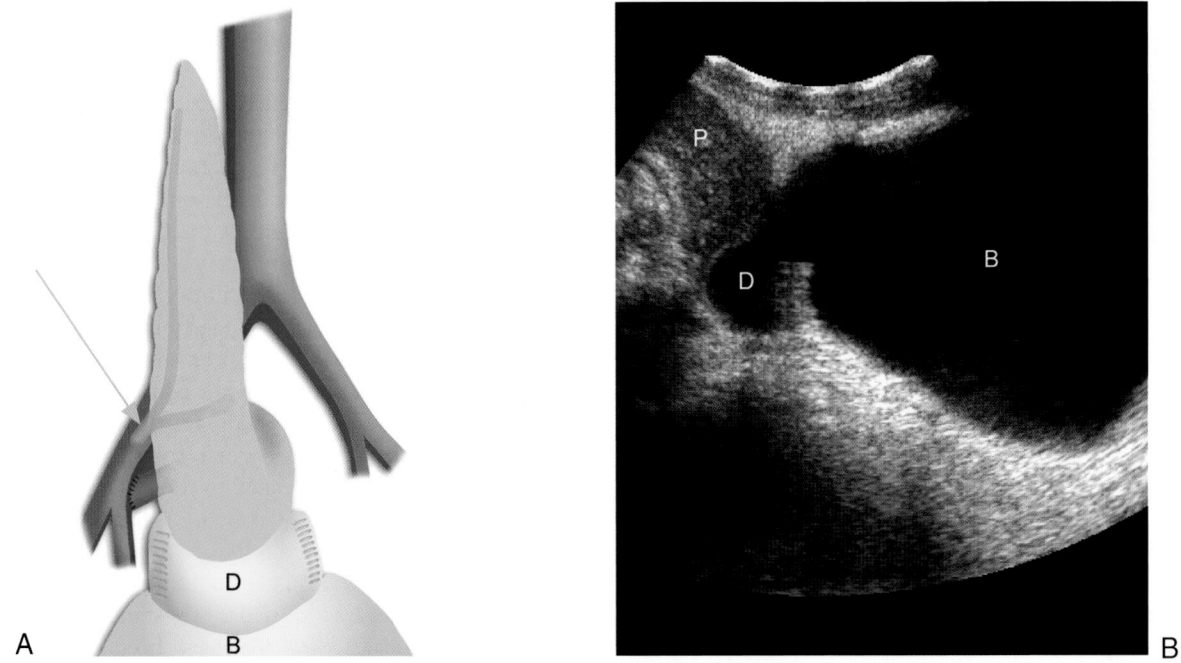

FIGURE 19-49. Lymphoceles. A, Sagittal and **B**, transverse sonograms show septated perinephric lymphoceles. **C**, Sagittal sonogram shows anechoic lymphocele, which was located above transplant kidney (*not shown*). **D**, Anechoic lymphocele (L) causing obstruction of the mid-ureter (*arrow*) and dilation of the calyceal system (C). **E**, Sagittal sonogram and **F**, correlative CT scan show infected lymphocele with internal strands, draining to the skin via a cutaneous fistula (*arrow*).

FIGURE 19-50. Systemic venous-bladder drainage (traditional surgery). A, The donor portal vein (*purple*) is anastomosed to the external iliac vein, and the donor artery Y graft (*coral arrow*) to the external iliac artery. The duodenal stump (D) is anastomosed to the bladder (B). **B**, Sagittal sonogram shows duodenal stump anastomosed to the bladder (B). (D, duodenal stump; P, pancreas.)

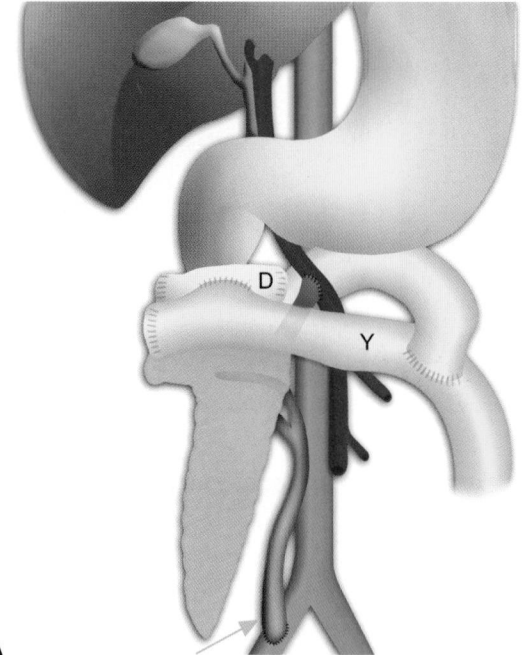

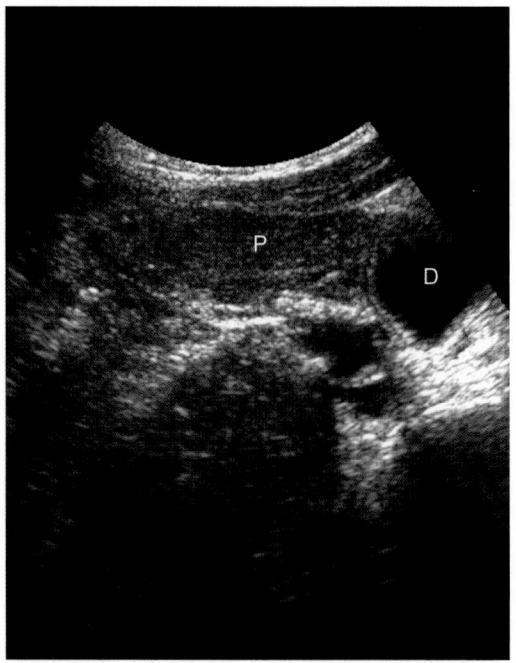

FIGURE 19-51. Portal venous-enteric drainage (new technique). A, The donor portal vein (*purple*) is anastomosed to the superior mesenteric vein (*blue*), and the donor artery (*coral arrow*) to the common iliac artery. The duodenal stump (D) is anastomosed to a Roux-en-Y (Y). **B,** Transverse sonogram shows pancreas transplant (P) with fluid-filled duodenal stump (D).

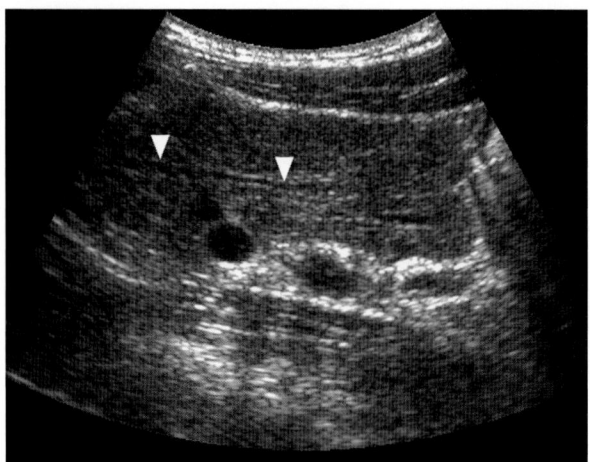

FIGURE 19-52. Normal pancreas transplant. Gray-scale ultrasound of pancreas transplant shows normal echogenicity and echotexture of allograft, with nondilated pancreatic duct (*arrowheads*).

Arteriovenous Fistula

Arteriovenous fistulas are a rare complication of pancreatic transplants. As with other arterial malformations, the lesion may not be detectable on gray-scale ultrasound. On color Doppler, however, a mosaic of intense colors may be identified that is produced by the tangle of vessels within the fistula and adjacent tissue vibration.

Spectral Doppler reveals high-velocity, low-resistance flow within the lesion, which is typical of arteriovenous shunting (Fig. 19-55).

Rejection

Rejection is the **most common cause of pancreatic graft loss post-transplantation**. Early recognition of transplant rejection remains a challenge because clinical parameters used to evaluate pancreas graft dysfunction have low sensitivity and specificity in its detection of rejection.

On **gray-scale** ultrasound, the allograft may appear hypoechoic or contain multiple anechoic regions, and the parenchymal echotexture may be patchy and heterogeneous (Fig. 19-56).[64,65] The utility of **arterial resistive indices** as an indicator of rejection appears to be somewhat controversial. It has been shown that resistive indices of the arteries supplying the pancreatic transplant cannot differentiate those allografts with mild or moderate rejection from normal transplants without rejection.[66] This may be related to the fact that the pancreatic transplant does not contain a discrete investing capsule, and therefore, swelling from transplant rejection may not necessarily result in increased parenchymal pressures or elevated vascular resistance.[67] Grossly elevated RIs greater than 0.8 have been observed in pancreatic allografts with biopsy-proven acute severe

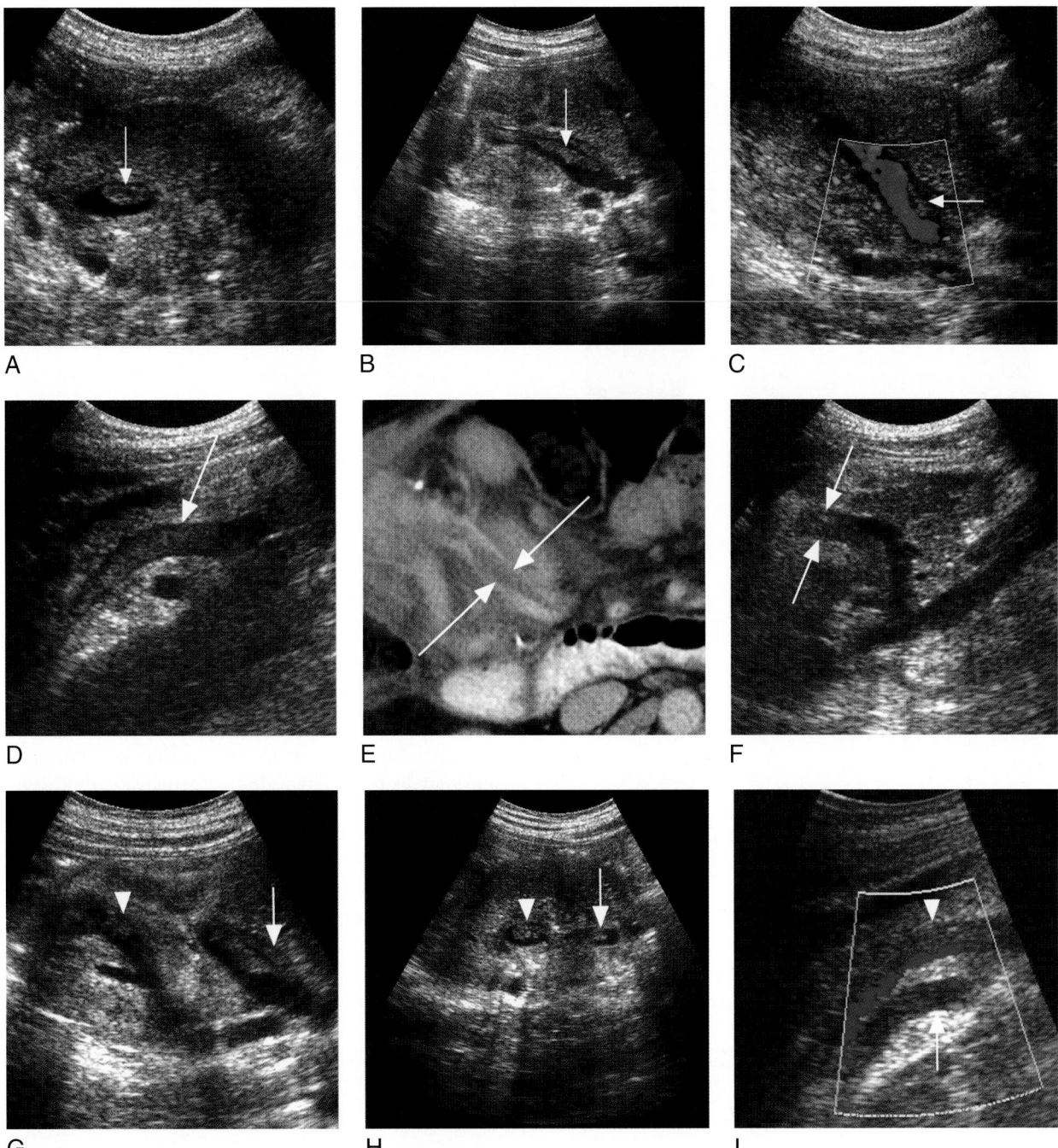

FIGURE 19-53. Graft thrombosis in different patients. A, Transverse and **B**, sagittal sonograms and **C**, color Doppler show nonocclusive venous thrombus (*arrows*). **D**, Gray-scale ultrasound (*arrow*) and **E**, correlative CT (*arrows*) show nonocclusive venous thrombus. **F**, Sagittal sonogram shows occlusive arterial thrombus (*arrows*). **G**, Sagittal sonogram, **H**, transverse sonogram and **I**, color Doppler show nonocclusive venous (*arrowhead*) and arterial (*arrow*) thrombus in the same transplant.

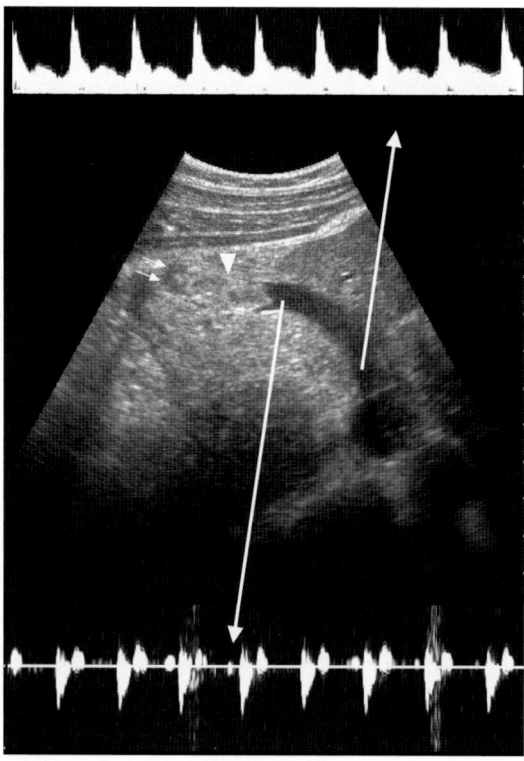

FIGURE 19-54. Thrombus adjacent to suture line. Echogenic thrombus (*arrowhead*) at suture line (*small arrows*) of blind ending ligated artery. Spectral trace adjacent to thrombus shows to-and-fro waveform (*bottom*), while spectral trace (*top*) more distally is normal.

rejection. Although these elevated RIs may be sensitive, they are not specific in the detection of severe pancreatic transplant rejection.[66]

Pancreatitis

Almost all patients develop symptoms of pancreatitis immediately after surgery, which is presumably second-

ary to preservation injury and ischemia.[67] Other causes of pancreatitis include partial or compete occlusion of the pancreatic duct, poor perfusion of the allograft, and in those patients with **systemic venous-bladder drainage**, reflux-related pancreatitis.[64,67]

The **ultrasound appearance** of pancreatitis in the allograft is **similar to that of pancreatitis in the native gland** (Fig. 19-57). Gray-scale findings include a normal-sized or bulky edematous pancreas, ill-defined margins, increased echogenicity of the peripancreatic fat secondary to surrounding inflammation, peripancreatic fluid, and thickening of the adjacent gut wall. In cases of pancreatitis resulting from ductal obstruction, a dilated pancreatic duct may be observed.[64,67] In nonacute cases of pancreatitis, pseudocysts adjacent to, or distal from the transplant may be identified usually appearing as a complex cystic structure.

Fluid Collections

Peripancreatic transplant-related fluid collections may be associated with an increased likelihood of loss of allograft function and overall increased mortality and morbidity in the recipient. Early diagnosis and characterization of these collections are imperative because treatment in the acute stages has been associated with improved graft function and decreased recipient morbidity.[68]

In the immediate postoperative period, peritransplant fluid may be caused by leakage of pancreatic fluid from transected ductules and lymphatics, an inflammatory exudate, blood, or urine (Fig. 19-58). These collections may require either close serial imaging follow-up or drainage, depending on the clinical status of the patient.

Duodenal leaks in **systemic venous-bladder drainage** transplants occur from dehiscence of the duodenal-bladder anastomosis and result in the formation of urinomas, frequently at the medial aspect of the

FIGURE 19-55. Pancreas transplant arteriovenous malformation (AVM). A, Transverse gray-scale ultrasound shows no abnormality. However, color Doppler (**B**) shows an intense mosaic of color within the pancreas, secondary to a parenchymal AVM.

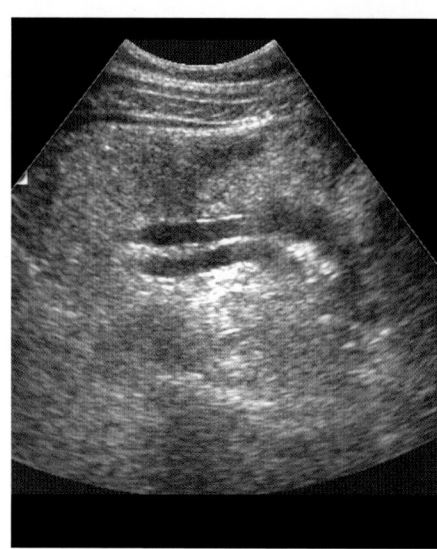

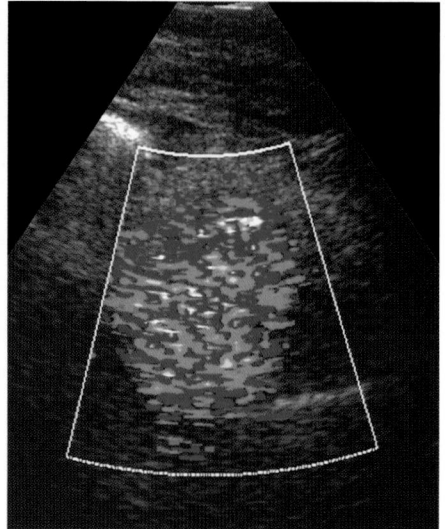

A   B

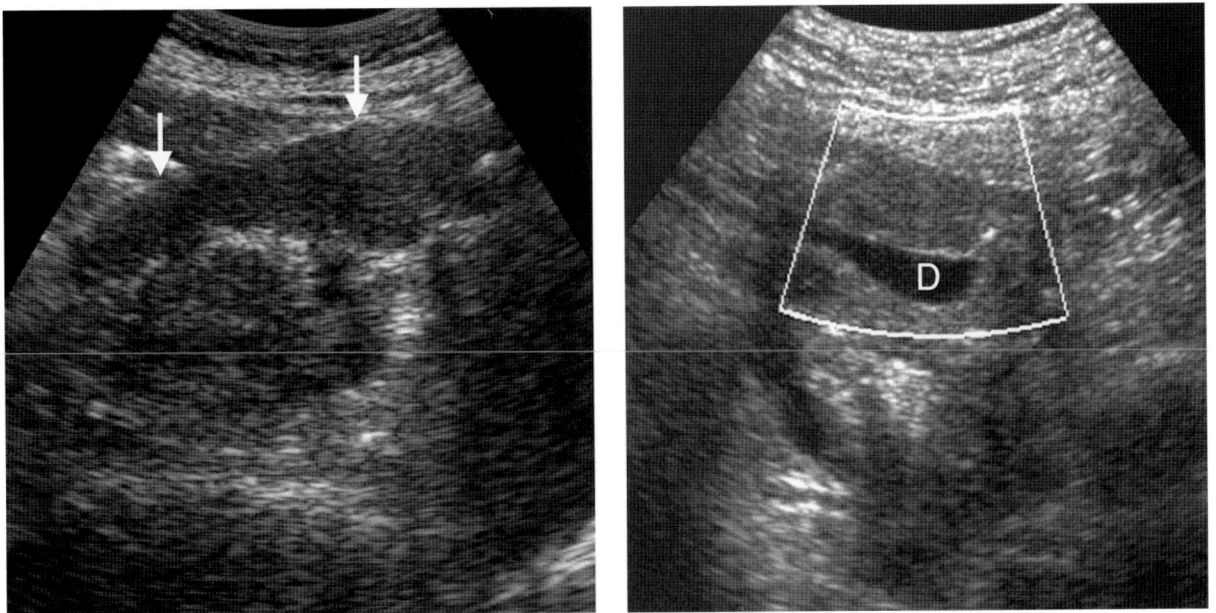

FIGURE 19-56. Pancreas transplant rejection. A, Transverse sonogram shows hypoechoic pancreas (*arrows*). The pancreatic parenchyma is also atrophied. **B,** Oblique sonogram shows dilated pancreatic duct (D) secondary to surrounding parenchymal atrophy.

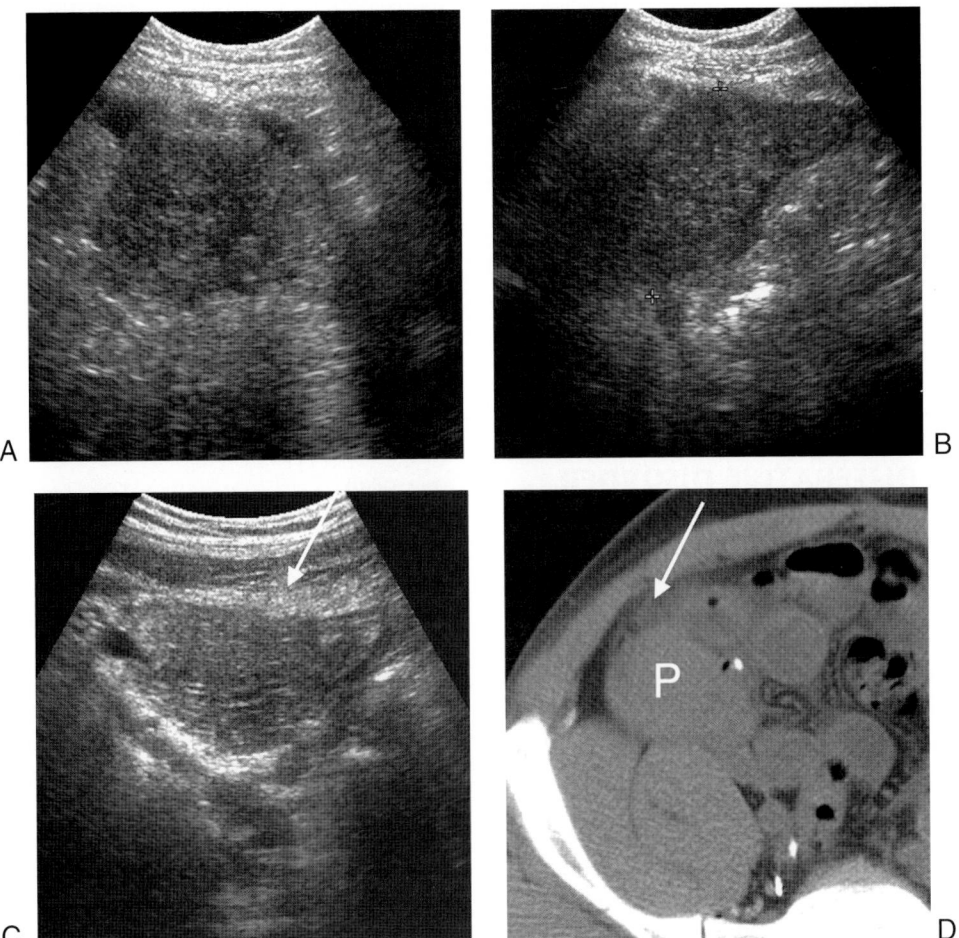

FIGURE 19-57. Pancreatitis. A, Transverse and **B,** oblique images show bulky edematous allograft. **C,** Oblique ultrasound shows echogenic inflamed peripancreatic fat (*arrow*). **D,** This appears as stranding in the peripancreatic fat on CT (*arrow*). (P, pancreas transplant.)

transplant. Urinomas may also occur as a result of infection or necrosis of the graft.[68]

Duodenal leaks in **portal venous-enteric drainage** transplants occur at either the blind end of the donor duodenum, or from the anastomosis with the recipient Roux-en-Y loop. On ultrasound, gross ascites, duodenal wall thickening, or free intraperitoneal air may be observed in patients with breakdown of the duodenal anastomoses. These leaks can be life threatening in that they may result in overwhelming sepsis. Furthermore, the presence of digestive enzymes in contact with the graft may lead to significant tissue necrosis.[67]

Patients with pancreatic transplants are also susceptible to infection due to their immunosuppressive therapy, as well as their underlying diabetes mellitus. **Abscesses** are occasionally identified and are often associated with hematomas, urinary tract infections, and pancreatitis. Although gas within a fluid collection may indicate the presence of a gas-forming organism, bubbles of air within a collection may also result from the presence of a fistula or tissue necrosis in cases of vascular thrombosis.[68]

In the post-transplant period, the development of a new collection or change in the sonographic morphology of the collection may result from a variety of etiologies, including infection, malfunction of the pancreatic duct, stent, or external drain, hemorrhage, or associated tissue infarction.[68]

Miscellaneous Complications

Other complications of pancreatic transplants include intussusception of the Roux-en-Y loop, small bowel obstruction from adhesions or adjacent graft pancreatitis, and panniculitis.

POST-TRANSPLANT LYMPHOPROLIFERATIVE DISORDER

Lymphoproliferative disorders represent a range of conditions that can occur in any patient with an underlying primary or secondary immunodeficiency. Because patients with solid organ transplants are chronically immunosuppressed, they are at risk for developing PTLD. Regardless of the type of lymphoproliferative disorder the patient is afflicted with, the pathogenesis of the condition is the same in all cases.[69]

Most patients with PTLD are actively infected with the **Epstein-Barr virus**, which induces proliferation of B lymphocytes. In the immunocompetent host, this B cell proliferation is regulated by multiple mechanisms, many of which are T cell mediated. However, if the host is immunosuppressed, with a deficiency in the T cell defenses, proliferation of B cells may continue to produce a polyclonal or monoclonal lymphoproliferative disorder.[69,70]

Post-transplant lymphoproliferative disorder accounts for up to 20% of tumors in solid organ transplantation.[71] The risk of development of PTLD, as well as the patient's prognosis, is determined by the degree of immunosuppressive therapy as opposed to the type of drug utilized. The aggressive immunosuppressive therapy required to prevent heart-lung transplant rejection has resulted in a reported incidence of PTLD as high as 4.6% in these patients. However, the gentler immunosuppression used in patients with liver or renal transplants has resulted in a lower incidence of lymphoproliferative disease, being reported as 2.2% and 1%, respectively.[70,72]

While PTLD may occur as early as 1 month after transplantation, the **type of immunosuppression** used appears to have some relationship to the onset of the disease. If cyclosporine is the medication that is used, the average length of time for development of PTLD is 15 months, whereas for azathioprine, the average length of time is 48 months.[72,73]

The disease has been described to involve almost all organ systems, with extranodal disease (81%) being more common than lymphadenopathy (22%). The most frequent areas of involvement include the abdomen, thorax, cervical lymph nodes, and the lymphatic tissue of the oropharynx. Therefore, PTLD can occur as a solitary mass or multiple masses within any organ system or as localized or distant lymphadenopathy.[69,72,74]

There is a predilection for lymphoproliferative disorders to develop in the allograft organ. It is presumed that this is related to chronic antigenic stimulation from the graft tissue, which may attract the proliferating B lymphocytes to the region of the transplant. The disorder may also show a tendency to arise in the lymphatic tissue in the periportal regions and around the anastomotic sites occurring as masses that engulf and surround the hilar vessels in both liver and kidney transplants.[69,72]

On ultrasound, the masses produced by PTLD are usually hypoechoic or are of mixed echogenicity, with sizes that range from 3 to 6 cm at the time of diagnosis.[72] Calcifications can be seen in the mass secondary to tumor necrosis or as a result of treatment. Masses that develop around the anastomotic site have the potential to encase the hilar vessels and extrinsically compress the transplanted artery and/or vein. Renal hilar masses may also obstruct the ureter causing postrenal obstruction and necessitating the placement of a drainage catheter.[72] The involved lymph nodes have an abnormal appearance showing a hypoechoic, thickened cortex with either an absent or flattened fatty hilum (Figs. 19-59 and 19-60). Pancreatic PTLD tends to produce diffuse glandular enlargement with an appearance that is indistinguishable from pancreatitis or rejection.[75]

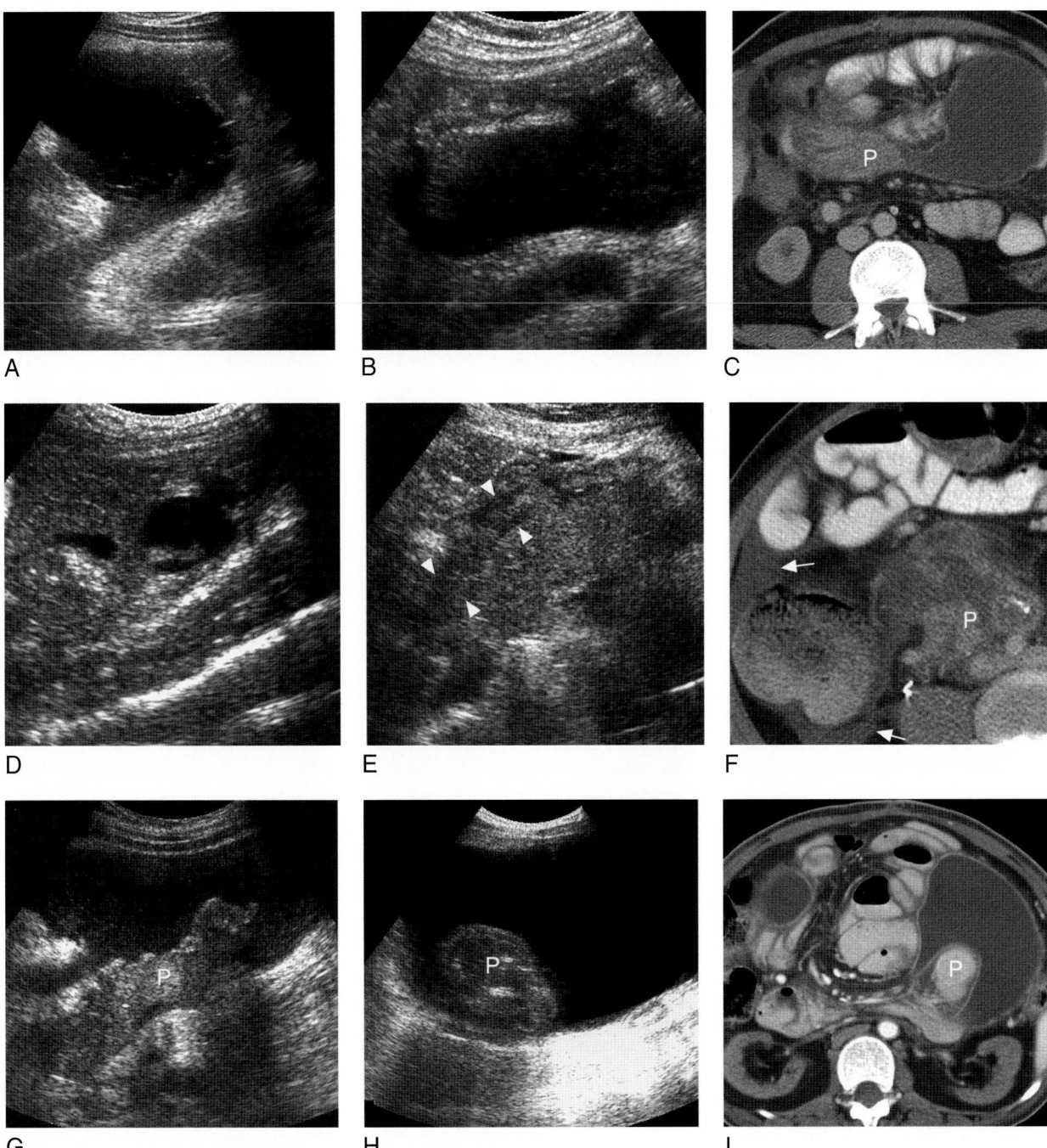

FIGURE 19-58. Fluid collections. Hematoma. A, Sagittal and **B,** transverse sonogram show complex collection with internal echoes and strands. **C,** Correlative CT scan shows hematoma in left upper quadrant that extends to pancreas (P). **Pseudocysts** in three patients: Patient 1. **D,** Sagittal sonogram shows complex epigastric cyst with internal septation. Patient 2. **E,** Sagittal sonogram shows complex collection adjacent to pancreas (*arrowheads*). **F,** Correlative CT scan shows collection extending into pancreatic head (P) and associated with free fluid (*arrows*). Patient 3. **G,** Sagittal sonogram shows large pseudocyst with internal echoes surrounding pancreatic tail (P). **Seroma. H,** Transverse sonogram and **I,** correlative CT scan show large anechoic cystic structure surrounding pancreatic body (P). The wall enhances on CT scan. The collection was sterile on aspiration.

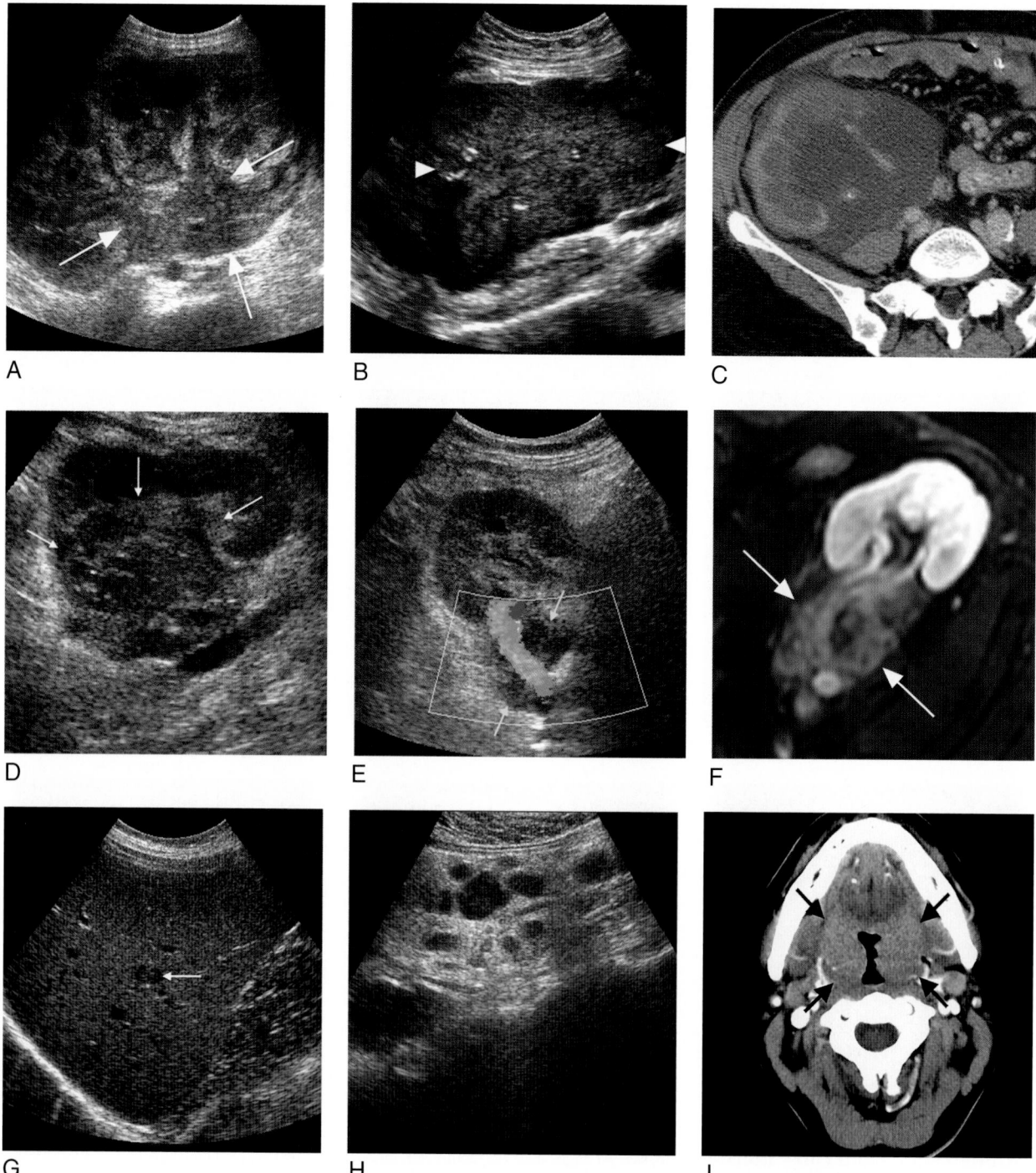

FIGURE 19-59. Renal post-transplant lymphoproliferative disease (PTLD) in two patients. Case 1. Sagittal sonogram shows **A**, infiltrative mass (*arrows*) in renal hilum. **B**, Six months later the mass (*arrowheads*) has infiltrated into the renal cortex. **C**, Correlative CT scan shows hilar mass infiltrating into renal cortex. Case 2. **D**, Sagittal sonogram shows hilar mass (*arrows*). **E**, Transverse sonogram shows that mass (*arrows*) encases transplanted renal artery. **F**, Correlative MRI shows hilar mass (*arrows*) encasing renal vessels. **G**, Transverse sonogram shows malignant-appearing hepatic nodule (*arrow*). **H**, Sagittal sonogram shows malignant lymphadenopathy. **I**, CT scan shows tonsillar adenopathy in Walder's ring (*arrows*) secondary to PTLD.

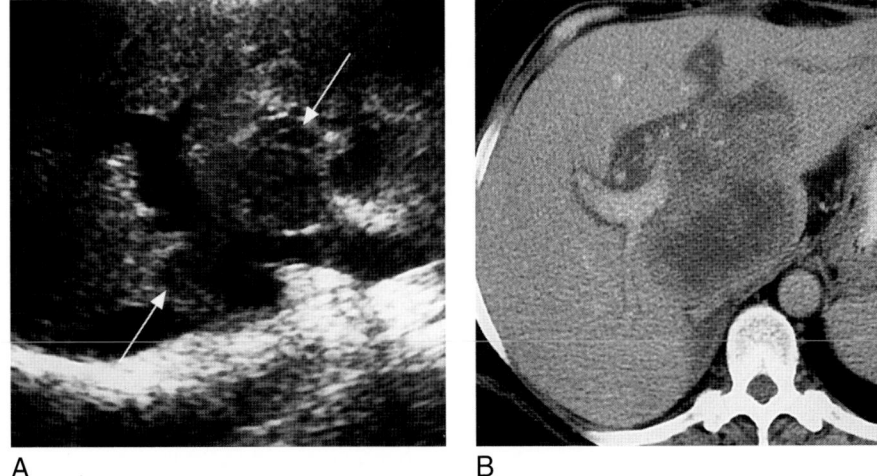

FIGURE 19-60. Hepatic post-transplant lymphoproliferative disease. A, Oblique sonogram shows malignant mass (*arrows*) encasing and narrowing main portal vein. **B,** Correlative CT scan shows mass infiltrating liver.

The initial therapy for lymphoproliferative disorders is a reduction of immunosuppressive therapy. This is often successful for cases of polyclonal lymphoproliferative disorder, and in some cases of monoclonal lymphoproliferative disorder. If this treatment option fails, chemotherapy is instituted.[69,70]

References

1. Takemoto S, Terasaki PI, Cecka JM, et al: Survival of nationally shared HLA-matched kidney transplants from cadaveric donors. New Engl J Med 1992;327:834-839.
2. The Canadian Multicentre Transplant Study Group: A randomized clinical trial of cyclosporine in cadaveric renal transplantation: Analysis at three years. N Engl J Med 1986;314:1219-1920.
3. Berthoux FC, Jones EH, Mehls O, et al: Transplantation report: Report on Management of Renal Failure in Europe, XXV, 1994. Nephrol Dial Transplant 1996;11:37-40.
4. Wozney P, Zajko AB, Bron KM, et al: Vascular complications after liver transplantation: A 5-year experience. AJR 1986;147:657-663.
5. Cattral MS, Bigam DL, Hemming AW, et al: Portal venous and enteric exocrine drainage versus systemic venous and bladder exocrine drainage of pancreas grafts. Clinical outcome of 40 consecutive transplant recipients. Ann Surg 2000;232(5):688-695.
6. Crossin J, Muradali D, Wilson SR: US of liver transplants: Normal and abnormal. Radiographics 2003; 23(5):1093-1114.
7. Mazzaferro V, Regalia E, Doci R, et al: Liver transplantation for the treatment of small hepatocellular carcinomas in patients with cirrhosis. N Engl J Med 1996;334:693-699.
8. Keeffe EB: Selection of patients for liver transplantation. In Maddrey WC, Schiff ER, Sorrell MF: Transplantation of the Liver, 3rd ed. Philadelphia, Lippincott Williams and Wilkins, 2001, pp 5-34.
9. Quiroga S, Sebastia C, Margarit C, et al: Complications of orthotopic liver transplantation: Spectrum of findings with helical CT. Radiographics 2001;21:1085-1102.
10. Nghiem HV: Imaging of hepatic transplantation. Radiol Clin North Am 1998;36(2):429-443.
11. Kamel IR, Kruskal JB, Raptopoulos V: Imaging for right lobe living donor liver transplantation. Semin Liver Dis 2001;21(2):271-282.
12. Wolfsen HC, Porayko MK, Hughes RH, et al: Role of endoscopic retrograde cholangiopancreatography after orthotopic liver transplantation. Am J Gastroenterol 1992;87:955-960.
13. Keogan MT, McDermott VG, Price SK, et al: The role of imaging in the diagnosis and management of biliary complications after liver transplantation. AJR 1999;173:215-219.
14. Letourneau JG, Castaneda-Zuniga WR: The role of radiology in the diagnosis and treatment of biliary complications after liver transplantation. Cardiovasc Intervent Radiol 1990;13:278-282.
15. Barton P, Maier A, Steininger R, et al: Biliary sludge after liver transplantation: 1. Imaging findings and efficacy of various imaging procedures. AJR 1995;164:859-864.
16. Miller WJ, Campbell WL, Zajko AB, et al: Obstructive dilatation of extrahepatic recipient and donor bile ducts complicating orthotopic liver transplantation: Imaging and laboratory findings. AJR 1991;157:29-32.
17. Zajko AB, Campbell WL, Bron KM, et al: Cholangiography and interventional biliary radiology in adult liver transplantation. AJR 1985;144:127-133.
18. Sheng R, Zajko AB, Campbell WL, et al: Biliary strictures in hepatic transplants: Prevalence and types in patients with primary sclerosing cholangitis vs. those with other liver diseases. AJR 1993;161:297-300.
19. Ward EM, Wiesner RH, Hughes RW, et al: Persistent bile leak after liver transplantation: Biloma drainage and endoscopic retrograde cholangiopancreatographic sphincterotomy. Radiology 1991:179:719-720.
20. McDonald V, Matalon TAS, Patel SK, et al: Biliary strictures in hepatic transplantation. J Vasc Interv Radiol 1991;2:533-538.
21. Gow PJ, Chapman RW: Liver transplantation for primary sclerosing cholangitis. Liver 2000;20(2):97-103.
22. Chen LY, Goldberg HI: Sclerosing cholangitis: Broad spectrum of radiographic features. Gastrointest Radiol 1984;9:39-47.
23. Ciaccia D, Branch MS: Disorders of the biliary tree related to liver transplantation. In DiMarino AJ, Benjamin SB (eds): Gastrointestinal Disease: An Endoscopic Approach. Boston, Blackwell Scientific, 1997, pp 918-927.

24. Zajko AB, Campbell WL, Bron KM, et al: Diagnostic and interventional radiology in liver transplantation. Gastroenterol Clin North Am 1988;17:105-143.

25. Starzl TE, Putnam CW, Hansbrough JF, et al: Biliary complications after liver transplantation: with special reference to the biliary cast syndrome and techniques of secondary duct repair. Surgery 1977;81:212-221.

26. Ito K, Siegleman ES, Stolpen AH, et al: MR imaging of complications after liver transplantation. AJR 2000;175:1145-1149.

27. Dodd GD, 3rd, Memel DS, Zajko AB, et al: Hepatic artery stenosis and thrombosis in transplant recipients: Doppler diagnosis with resistive index and systolic acceleration time. Radiology 1994;192:657-661.

28. Flint EW, Sumkin JH, Zajko AB, et al: Duplex sonography of hepatic artery thrombosis after liver transplantation. AJR 1988;151:481-483.

29. Shaw BW, Jr, Gordon RD, Iwatsuki S, et al: Hepatic retransplantation. Transplant Proc 1985;17:264-271.

30. Dravid VS, Shapiro MJ, Needleman L, et al: Arterial abnormalities following orthotopic liver transplantation: Arteriographic findings and correlation with Doppler sonographic findings. AJR 1994;163:585-589.

31. Fukuzawa K, Schwartz ME, Katz E, et al: The arcuate ligament syndrome in liver transplantation. Transplantation 1993;56(1):223-224.

32. Langnas A, Marujo W, Stratta R, et al: Hepatic allograft rescue following arterial thrombosis: Role of urgent revascularization. Transplantation 1991;51:86-90.

33. Raby N, Karani J, Thomas S, et al: Stenoses of vascular anastomoses after hepatic transplantation: Treatment with balloon angioplasty. AJR 1990;157:167-171.

34. Skolnick ML, Dodd GD: Doppler sonography in liver transplantation pre- and post-transplant evaluation. In Thrall JH (ed): Current Practice in Radiology. Philadelphia, Decker, 1993, pp 161-172.

35. Pfammatter T, Williams DM, Lane KL, et al: Suprahepatic caval anastomotic stenosis complicating orthotopic liver transplantation: Treatment with percutaneous transluminal angioplasty, wall stent placement or both. AJR 1997;168:477-480.

36. Ferris JV, Baron RL, Marsh JWJ, et al: Recurrent hepatocellular carcinoma after liver transplantation: Spectrum of CT findings and recurrence patterns. Radiology 1996;198:233-238.

37. Baxter GM: Ultrasound of renal transplantation. Clin Radiol 2001;56:802-818.

38. Brown ED, Chen MYM, Wolfman NT, et al: Complications of renal transplantation: Evaluation with US and radionuclide imaging. Radiographics 2000;20:607-622.

39. Memel DS, Gerald DD, Shah AN, et al: Imaging of en bloc renal transplants: Normal and abnormal postoperative findings. AJR 1993;160:75-81.

40. O'Neill WC, Baumgarten AB: Ultrasonography in renal transplantation. Am J Kidney Dis 2002;39(4):663-678.

41. Lachance SL, Adamson D, Barry JM: Ultrasonically determined kidney transplant hypertrophy. J Urol 1988;139:497.

42. Babcock DS, Slovis TL, Han BK, et al: Renal transplants in children: Long term follow-up using sonography. Radiology 1985;156:165.

43. Absy M, Metreweli C, Matthews DCR, et al: Changes in transplanted kidney volume measured by ultrasound. Br J Radiol 1987;60:525-529.

44. Rigg KM: Renal transplantation: Current status, complications and prevention. J Antimicrob Chemother 1995;36 (suppl B):51-57.

45. Pirsch JD, Ploeg RJ, Gange S, et al: Determinants of graft survival after renal transplantation. Transplant 1996;61:1581-1585.

46. Dodd GD, Tublin ME, Shah, Zajko AB: Imaging vascular complications associated with renal transplants. AJR 1991;157:449-459.

47. Jordan ML, Cook GT, Cardell CJ: Ten years of experience with vascular complications in renal transplantation. J Urol 1982;128:689-692.

48. Honto D, Simmons R: Renal transplantation: Clinical considerations in organ transplantation. Radiol Clin North Am 1987;25:239-248.

49. Tublin ME, Dodd GD, 3rd: Sonography of renal transplantation. Radiol Clin North Am 1995;33:447-459.

50. Penny MJ, Nankivell BJ, Disney APS, et al: Renal vein thrombosis: A survey of 134 consecutive cases. Transplant 1994;58:565-569.

51. Baxter GM, Morley P, Dall B: Acute renal vein thrombosis in renal allografts: New Doppler ultrasonic findings. Clin Radiol 1991;43:125-127.

52. Ruether G, Wanjura D, Bauer H: Acute renal vein thrombosis in renal allografts: Detection with duplex Doppler ultrasound. Radiology 1989;170:557-558.

53. Pozniak MA, Dodd GD, Kelcz F: Ultrasonographic evaluation of renal transplantation. Radiol Clin North Am 1992;30:1053-1066.

54. Ahari HK, Antonacci VP, Davison BD, et al: Vascular and interventional case of the day. AJR 1999;173:829-836.

55. Middleton WD, Kellman GM, Melson GL, et al: Post biopsy renal transplant arteriovenous fistulas: Color Doppler US characteristics. Radiology 1989;171:253-257.

56. Huang M, Muradali D, Thurston WA, et al: Uterine arteriovenous malformations (AVMs): Ultrasound and MR features. Radiology 1998;206:115-123.

57. Rahmouni A, Bargoin R, Herment A, et al: Color Doppler twinkling artifact in hyperechoic regions. Radiology 1996;199:269-271.

58. Letourneau JG, Day DL, Ascher NL, et al: Imaging of renal transplants. AJR 1988;150:833-838.

59. Silver TM, Campbell D, Wicks JD, et al: Peritransplant fluid collections. Radiology 1981;138:145-151.

60. Nargund VH, Cranston D: Urological complications after renal transplantation. Transplant Rev 1996;10:24-33.

61. Pozniak MA, Propeck PA, Kelcz F, et al: Imaging of pancreas transplants. Radiol Clin North Am 1995;33:581-594.

62. Krebs TL, Daly B, Wong JJ, et al: Vascular complications of pancreatic transplantation: MR evaluation. Radiology 1995;196(3):793-798.

63. Foshager MC, Hedlund LJ, Troppmann C, et al: Venous thrombosis of pancreatic transplants: Diagnosis by duplex sonography. AJR 1997;169:1269-1273.

64. Patel B, Markivee CR, Mahanta B, et al: Pancreatic transplantation: Scintigraphy, US and CT. Radiology 1988;167:685-687.

65. Yuh WTC, Wiese JA, Monzer MA, et al: Pancreatic transplant imaging. Radiology 1988;167:679-683.

66. Aideyan OA, Foshager MC, Benedetti E, et al: Correlation of the arterial resistive index in pancreas transplants of patients with transplant rejection. AJR 1997;168:1445-1447.

67. Heyneman LE, Keogan MT, Tuttle-Newhall JE, et al: Pancreatic transplantation using portal venous and enteric drainage: The postoperative appearance of a new surgical procedure. J Comput Assist Tomogr 1999;23(2):283-290.

68. Patel B, Garvin P, Aridge DL, et al: Fluid collections developing after pancreatic transplantation: Radiologic evaluation and intervention. Radiology 1991;181:215-220.

69. Donnelly LF, Frush DP, Marshall KW, et al: Lymphoproliferative disorders: CT findings in immunocompromised children. AJR 1998;171:725-731.

70. Nalesnik MA, Makowka L, Starzl TE: The diagnosis and treatment of posttransplant lymphoproliferative disorders. Curr Probl Surg1988;25:367-472.

71. Penn I: Cancers complicating organ transplantation (editorial). NEJM 1990;323:1767-1769.

72. Vrachliotis TG, Vaswani KK, Davies EA, et al: CT findings in posttransplantation lymphoproliferative disorder of renal transplants. AJR 2000;175:183-188.

73. Dodd GD 3rd, Greenler DP, Confer SR: Thoracic and abdominal manifestations of lymphoma occurring in the immunocompromised patient. Radiol Clin North Am 1992;30:597-610.

74. Pickhardt PJ, Siegel MJ: Abdominal manifestations of posttransplantation lymphoproliferative disorder. AJR 1998;171:1007-1013.

75. Meador TL, Krebs TL, Wong Y, et al: Imaging features of posttransplantation lymphoproliferative disorder in pancreas transplant recipients. AJR 2000;174:121-124.

III

Intraoperative Sonography

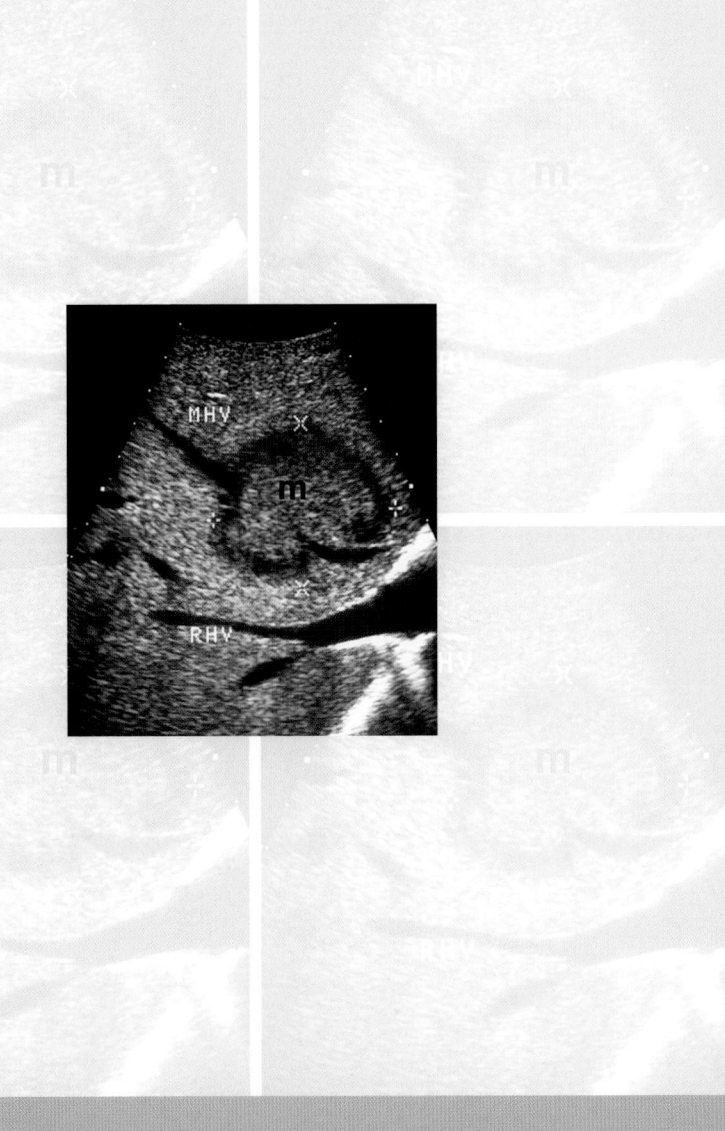

20

INTRAOPERATIVE AND LAPAROSCOPIC SONOGRAPHY OF THE ABDOMEN

Robert A. Lee / Robert A. Kane / J. William Charboneau

Chapter Outline

*I*ntraoperative sonography (IOS) is a dynamic and growing imaging technique providing important real-time diagnostic information to the radiologist and the surgeon. It identifies and characterizes lesions seen on preoperative imaging and discovers new lesions not detected by preoperative imaging or surgical inspection and palpation.[1,2] The ultimate goal is to correlate preoperative images, surgical inspection and palpation, and IOS findings to determine the most appropriate surgical procedure.[3,4] Continued growth of IOS is expected as more surgeons and radiologists become aware of its usefulness and as laparoscopic ultrasound (LUS) techniques and IOS-guided tumor ablation techniques are improved.

A-mode IOS was first used in the early 1960s for evaluating the biliary system for calculi.[5,6] Image quality was not ideal and interpretation was difficult. A number of technical advances have made IOS both practical and useful, however. Over the past 20 years there has been a resurgence in the use of IOS because equipment advances have allowed high-quality real-time imaging in the operating room. Smaller, dedicated IOS probes have also been developed that make the routine use of sonography in the operating room easier. Although IOS accounts for a small percentage of ultrasound examinations in our practices, its rate of growth has been rapid.

Many of the technical problems and limitations in routine abdominal sonography are not present in the operating room during laparotomy. Shadowing from bony structures, such as the ribs, and sound attenuation in the body wall are no longer present. All bowel can easily be moved out of the way to scan a particular solid organ or vascular structure. This allows high-frequency, high-resolution ultrasound probes to be used directly on the surface of the organ being examined. High-resolution images are routinely obtained, allowing superb lesion detection, localization, and characterization.

For the radiologist, the most important and significant drawback of IOS is the time away from the radiology department. Because of this requirement, many radiologists have been reluctant to become involved with IOS. Depending on the complexity of the case, the radiologists and the ultrasound equipment can be out of the department for 30 minutes to one hour or longer. Therefore, IOS cases should be prescheduled the day before surgery so that proper equipment and personnel are available. The surgeon should notify the radiologist

20 to 30 minutes before the actual scanning is to be done to allow sufficient time for equipment transportation and preparation. Time invested in the operating room is well spent because IOS helps to ensure the appropriate surgical procedure is performed.

EQUIPMENT

Standard ultrasound equipment used for general sonography can be used in the operating room as well. Standard curvilinear and linear array transducers of various frequencies are widely available. The curved array transducers have a large field of view that can detect masses and display their relationship to important vessels. The entire organ can be rapidly surveyed with the large field of view of curved array transducers. However, because of the larger size of these transducers, some small peritoneal spaces are inaccessible. In addition, the near field of view and resolution are inferior to the dedicated high-frequency intraoperative transducers.

Dedicated intraoperative transducers are small and of high frequency. Their small size allows the transducer to be cradled in the examiner's hand and easily maneuvered into small peritoneal spaces.[7-9] Linear array high-frequency (7 to 15 MHz) intraoperative transducers have a clear near field of view and can be used on all intra-abdominal organs. Using a combination of transducers, they can usually provide adequate penetration and have excellent spatial and contrast resolution. A disadvantage of these dedicated intraoperative linear array transducers is the small rectangular field of view.

This can make orientation difficult, particularly during scanning of a large organ, such as the liver. The combination of standard curvilinear and dedicated IOS transducers may be used when a large organ, such as the liver, is scanned (Fig. 20-1). The curvilinear transducer demonstrates a global perspective of relationships of large tumors and key structures.[9] The dedicated IOS transducer can then be used to detect and characterize small, occult masses. With experience, the familiar vascular landmarks within the liver are easily recognized.[9] Knowledge of portal and hepatic venous anatomy is essential to plan a complete and safe surgical resection.

The ultrasound transducers used in the operating room must have sterile surfaces. Some ultrasound transducers can be **gas sterilized** (ethylene oxide). However, the high temperatures used can potentially damage the transducer; therefore, some manufacturers do not recommend this technique. The manufacturers that allow gas sterilization are usually very specific in their recommendations. Sterilization with low-concentration ethylene oxide typically requires 4 hours and is followed by 18 hours of rest and aeration. Consequently, the transducer can be used only once a day.[9,10] Transducers can also be **sterilized by immersion in liquid** (glutaraldehyde), which also requires a significant delay before the ultrasound transducer can be used again.[9] This can become a problem if the transducer must be used in consecutive intraoperative cases. In addition, some surgeons do not allow any glutaraldehyde to come in contact with visceral surfaces or in the peritoneal cavity. Therefore, the sterilization method must be chosen in consultation with the surgeon.[9] In many practices the ultrasound transducer

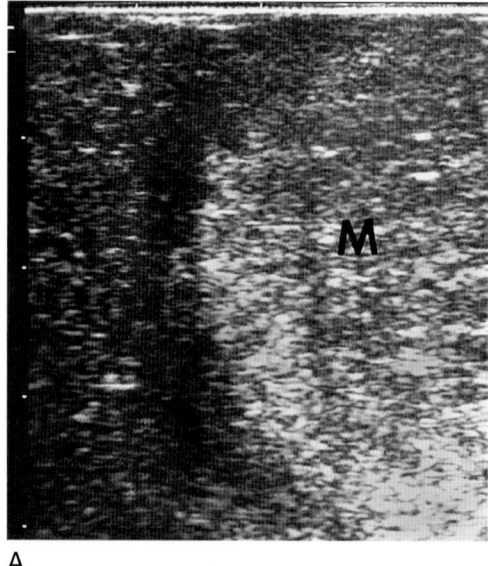
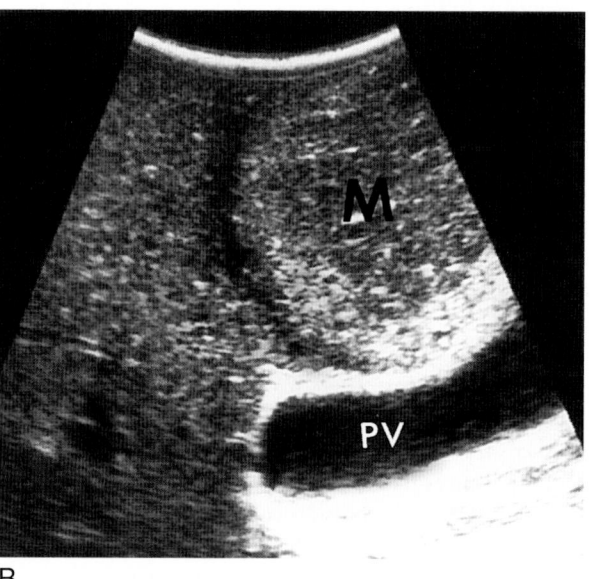

A   B

FIGURE 20-1. Comparison of linear and curved array transducers. A, Dedicated, linear array intraoperative sonography transducer has a relatively small field of view, which demonstrates only a portion of a large hepatic metastasis (M). **B**, Larger, standard curvilinear transducer better demonstrates the relationship of the large metastasis (M) to the portal vein (PV).

and cable are **covered by a sterile latex or plastic sleeve**. Gel must be applied into the sleeve to couple the transducer to the sleeve. Great care must be taken to be certain no air bubbles are present between the head of the transducer and the sterile sleeve covering it.[10] This method allows several uses of the same intraoperative probe on the same day. However, the sleeve-draped transducer is slightly more cumbersome to use than a sterilized transducer without a sleeve. Specifically designed covers are available that fit more tightly on the transducer. This decreases the chance of artifacts due to air pockets between the transducer and the cover.

TECHNIQUE

Intraoperative sonography often provides important clinical information that cannot be obtained by any other means and should be performed by a physician experienced in sonography. The time required away from the radiology department causes many radiologists to be reluctant to perform IOS. As a result, surgeons often perform IOS without a consulting radiologist. Surgeons experienced in IOS can learn to scan and interpret ultrasound images. However, less experienced IOS users may scan less thoroughly, detect fewer lesions, and be less able to interpret images. In some centers where the surgeons perform IOS, the radiologist is called to the operating room only to help interpret difficult ultrasound findings. Alternatively, a telecommunication link to the operating room may provide better access to US expertise during the critical stages of surgery.[11] Intraoperative cases should be prescheduled to allow the proper equipment and personnel to be available. Ideally, a radiologist reviews preoperative images before surgery. This sometimes is not possible, but the pertinent images should be available in the operating room and can be reviewed by the radiologist there. After reviewing the images, the radiologist knows the location of the suspected malignant masses and indeterminate lesions that need further characterization. To avoid confusion, always try to scan from the patient's right side as if performing a routine ultrasound examination. The normal moisture on the surface of the organ to be evaluated can provide acoustic coupling. Warm saline is frequently poured into the peritoneal cavity to enhance acoustic coupling. The saline can also be used as a standoff agent during a search for surface lesions. Surface lesions can be difficult to detect if the transducer is directly in contact with the mass. The contrast between the surface lesion and the normal organ parenchyma often becomes much more apparent if a standoff agent such as sterile saline is used. In most cases, the organ to be evaluated has been exposed and mobilized before scanning. The entire organ should be scanned along with the adjacent structures, such as regional lymph nodes.

When a mass is localized, it should be characterized and its relationship to vascular structures carefully delineated.

HEPATOBILIARY SYSTEM

Liver

Indications and Applications. Examination of the liver is commonly done to evaluate for colorectal metastasis.[10] The presence and extent of colorectal liver metastasis are important factors for long-term survival. Liver failure due to extensive hepatic metastatic disease accounts for 60% to 70% of the deaths in patients with colorectal cancer.[12] The 5-year survival rate for patients undergoing surgical resection for hepatic colorectal metastasis is 20% to 30%.[13] In contrast, the average survival rate in patients with liver metastasis without surgery is approximately 8 to 9 months, with no patients surviving longer than 5 years.[14] Therefore, the surgical resectability of hepatic colorectal metastasis has a major impact on long-term survival. In addition to its use for hepatic metastasis, IOS can be used for evaluation of primary hepatic malignant lesions such as hepatocellular carcinoma and cholangiocarcinoma and to guide radiofrequency[15] and cryoablation in the operating room.[16,17]

Detection of Occult Masses. Detection of occult hepatic masses is an important application for IOS (Fig. 20-2).[18] Malignant lesions in patients with otherwise normal hepatic parenchyma can be nonpalpable if they are small or located deep in the hepatic parenchyma.[19] The detection rate of hepatic lesions with preoperative imaging depends on the type and quality of imaging technique. Preoperative computed tomography (CT), magnetic resonance imaging (MRI), or sonography typically detect only 60% to 80% of hepatic masses.[19-22] With IOS, it has been estimated that 93% to 98% of the hepatic lesions are detected.[23-26] In a study by Kane et al.,[3] preoperative imaging detected 67% of the hepatic lesions; 78% of the hepatic lesions were detected when preoperative imaging was combined with surgical inspection and palpation. However, 97% of the hepatic

---

FIVE MAIN APPLICATIONS OF INTRAOPERATIVE LIVER SONOGRAPHY

Detection of occult and nonpalpable masses
Determination of the relationship of the mass to vessels
Definition of lobar and segmental liver anatomy
Characterization of small hepatic masses (e.g., cystic or solid)
Guidance for cryoablation, biopsy, or drainage

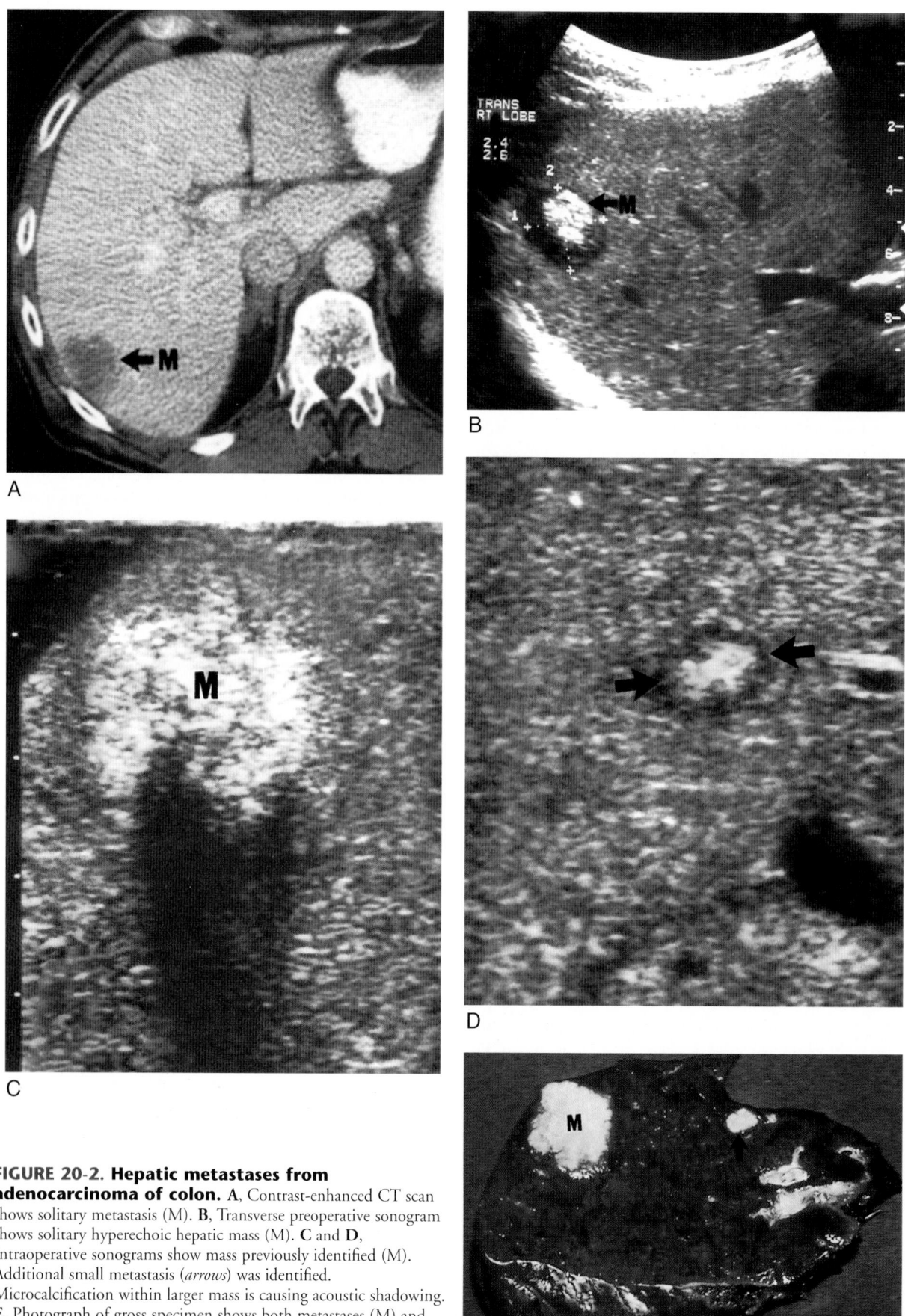

FIGURE 20-2. Hepatic metastases from adenocarcinoma of colon. A, Contrast-enhanced CT scan shows solitary metastasis (M). **B,** Transverse preoperative sonogram shows solitary hyperechoic hepatic mass (M). **C** and **D,** Intraoperative sonograms show mass previously identified (M). Additional small metastasis (*arrows*) was identified. Microcalcification within larger mass is causing acoustic shadowing. **E,** Photograph of gross specimen shows both metastases (M) and additional small metastasis (*arrow*).

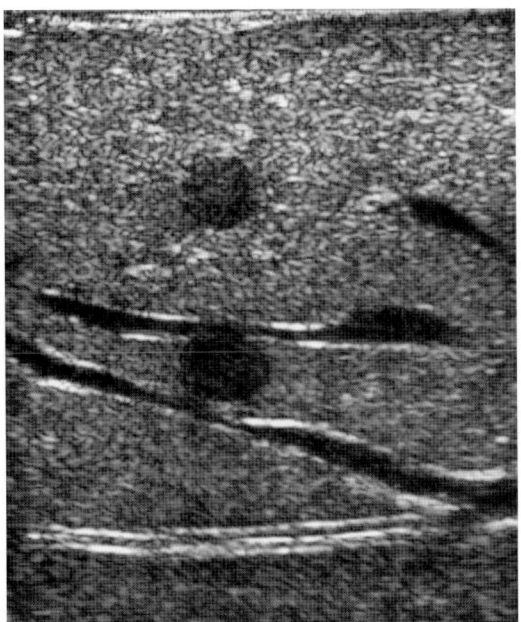

FIGURE 20-3. Small, nonpalpable hepatic metastasis. Intraoperative sonography shows two, small hepatic metastases that measure 5 mm.

masses were identified with IOS. In a recent study by Bloed et al.,[27] IOS yielded additional information compared to triphasic spiral computed tomography (CT) in 13 of 26 patients. This led to a change in the surgical procedure in four patients (15%). If additional hepatic malignant lesions are detected with IOS and then surgically removed, the 5-year survival rate in this subgroup of patients may improve. Lesions as small as 3 to 5 mm can be detected at the time of IOS (Fig. 20-3).

Intraoperative sonography is of value in the detection of occult, nonpalpable **hepatocellular carcinoma** in a cirrhotic liver. This is because both the cirrhotic liver and the hepatocellular carcinoma are firm. In a series reported by Sheu et al.,[28] 49% of hepatocellular carcinomas less than 3 cm in diameter could not be localized with inspection or palpation. In a series reported by Jin-Chuan et al.,[29] 46% of hepatocellular carcinomas could not be localized by palpation or visual inspection. In these patients, IOS is of great value in localizing the mass so that it can be resected with adequate surgical margins (Fig. 20-4).

Determination of Relationships and Vascular Abnormalities. IOS also has a role in surgical planning for known, palpable hepatic masses. Intraoperative sonography is uniquely suited to **demonstrate the relationship** of known hepatic masses to the hepatic vascularity and the biliary system (Figs. 20-5 to 20-7). Additional information obtained by IOS sometimes changes the planned surgical procedure. At the Mayo Clinic, we reviewed 150 operations for hepatic malignant disease (103 metastatic and 47 primary hepatic tumors). Fourteen percent of the operations were either extended (11%) or aborted (3%) on the basis of information provided only by IOS.[10] Several other studies have shown a significantly greater effect on operative decision making. For example, in a study by Parker et al.,[20] IOS

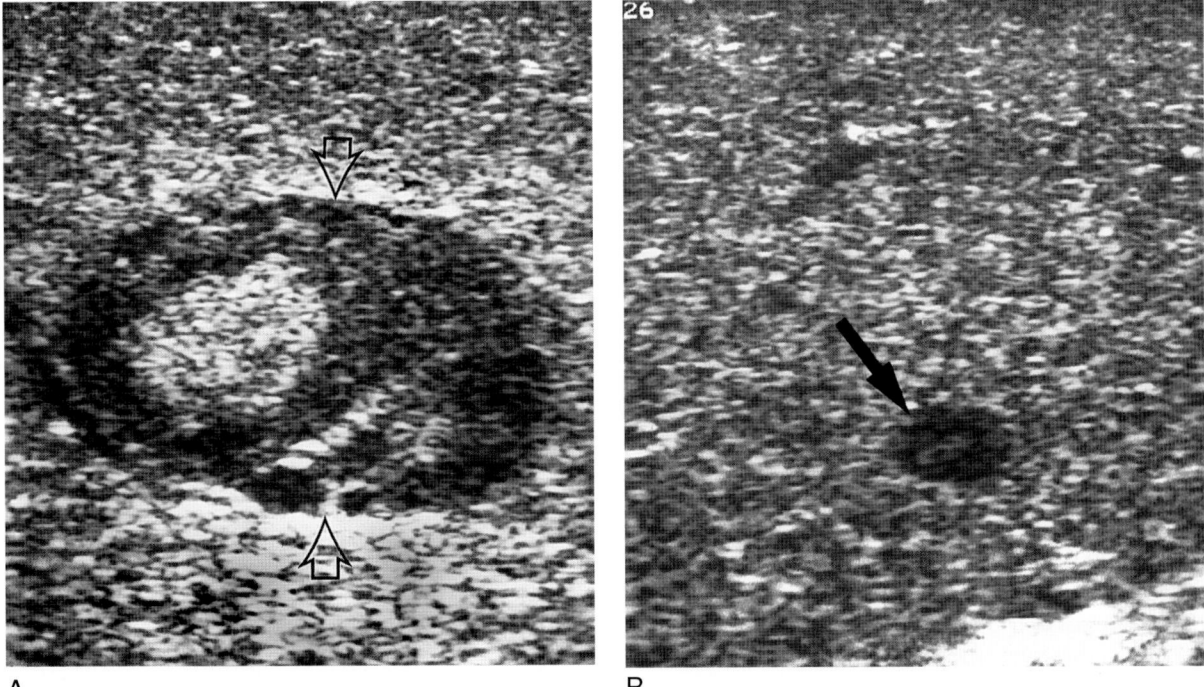

A   B

FIGURE 20-4. Nonpalpable hepatocellular carcinoma. A, Intraoperative sonography localizes a nonpalpable carcinoma (*open arrows*). **B,** Second, small, nonpalpable carcinoma (*arrow*) was also localized with IOS.

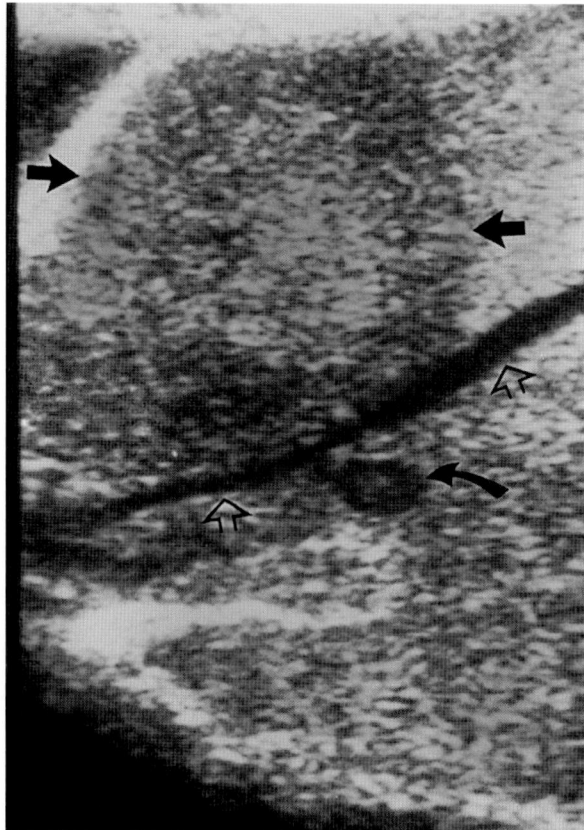

A

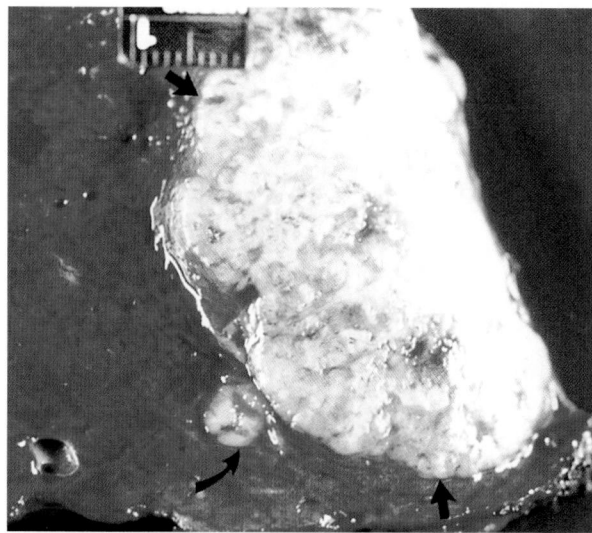

B

FIGURE 20-5. Extent of hepatic metastasis provided by operative sonography. A, Oblique longitudinal intraoperative scan in patient with metastatic adenocarcinoma of colon shows large metastasis (*black arrows*) adjacent to left hepatic vein (*open arrows*). This mass was identified on preoperative imaging. Second satellite metastasis (*curved arrow*) is identified posterior to hepatic vein. Because of tumor spread beyond left hepatic vein, a more extensive hepatic resection was required. **B,** Photograph of gross specimen demonstrating both metastases. Large metastases (*straight arrow*); satellite metastases (*curved arrow*).

of the liver was 98% sensitive for lesion detection, compared with 77% for preoperative CT. IOS affected operative management in 49% of the patients, either by allowing a lesser procedure than expected or by facilitating a more extensive resection. In another study, Kane et al.[3] found that in 19 of 46 patients (41%), the surgical procedures were altered because of IOS. In some cases, IOS demonstrates that the lesion cannot be resected because of invasion into the main bile duct or into vessels.

Intraoperative sonography is also being used to reduce vascular complications of liver transplantation.[30] In a study by Cheng et al.,[31] Doppler ultrasound was used in 24 patients (19 pediatric and 5 adult patients) to assess for vascular complications. Unsatisfactory hemodynamics was identified in nine patients (37.5%). The vascular abnormalities were all successfully reconstructed in the operating room, and a graft survival rate of 100% was achieved.[31]

Characterization of Masses. Intraoperative sonography is also invaluable in **characterizing** small, indeterminate hepatic lesions seen on preoperative radiologic studies or detected by surgical palpation. Small cysts can be difficult to differentiate from small metastatic lesions with CT because of partial volume-averaging effects. With IOS, small cysts can be easily identified and

characterized as benign (Fig. 20-8). Small hemangiomas typically appear as small, uniformly hyperechoic nodules without a peripheral halo (Fig. 20-9).

Guidance for Intervention. Some hepatic lesions are indeterminate by ultrasound criteria and may require biopsy for accurate diagnosis. This can be safely and easily accomplished in the operating room with ultrasound guidance (Fig. 20-10).

Gallbladder and Bile Ducts

The gallbladder and bile ducts can be evaluated for **calculi** with IOS.[32-36] Although gallstones are usually detected by preoperative sonography, they are occasionally noted incidentally at the time of IOS of the liver

INDICATIONS FOR INTRAOPERATIVE BILIARY SONOGRAPHY

Identification of biliary calculi
Identification of biliary neoplasms
Localization of the common bile duct and its
    relationship to other structures

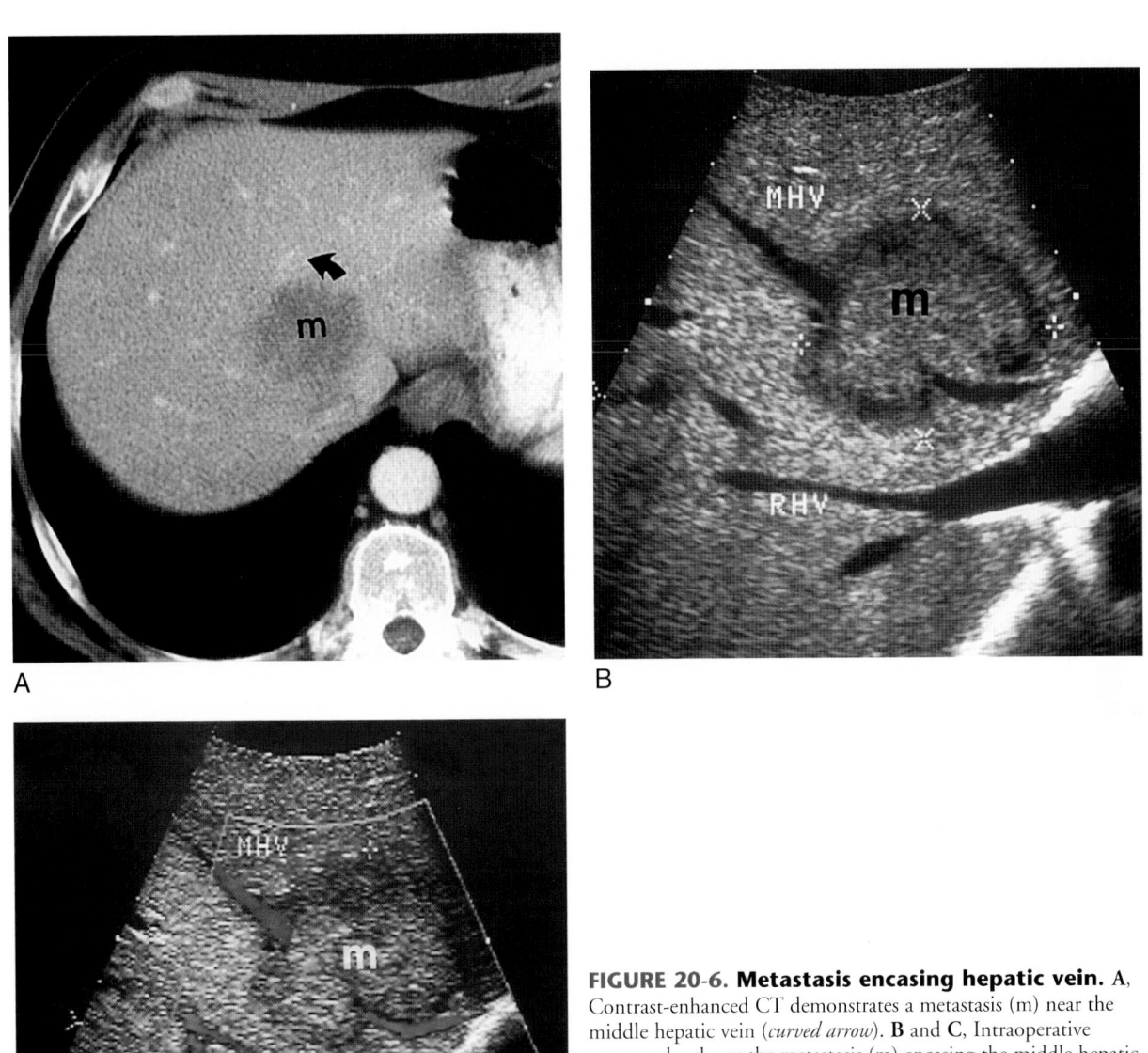

FIGURE 20-6. Metastasis encasing hepatic vein. A,
Contrast-enhanced CT demonstrates a metastasis (m) near the
middle hepatic vein (*curved arrow*). **B** and **C,** Intraoperative
sonography shows the metastasis (m) encasing the middle hepatic
vein (MHV). RHV, Right hepatic vein. IVC, Inferior vena cava.

(Fig. 20-11). Cholelithiasis affects 10% to 20% of the
U.S. population, with an increased prevalence in obese
patients (up to 45%). Therefore, preoperative gallbladder sonography is necessary when bariatric surgery
is planned. Preoperative gallbladder ultrasound is very
accurate even in obese patients with discrepancies
between radiologic and pathologic findings in 1.1%
of patients.[37] Intraoperative sonography is also used to
screen the common bile duct for stones during cholecystectomy. In a series of 449 patients who underwent both

intraoperative cholangiography and IOS, the accuracy
was 98% for IOS and 94% for cholangiography.[32] In
another series, a correct diagnosis of choledocholithiasis
was made in 85.7% of the cases, and common duct
stones were excluded correctly in 100% of the case.[38]

Primary and secondary neoplasms of the
gallbladder and bile ducts may cause a focal mass or wall
thickening (Fig. 20-12). IOS can localize the mass and
define its extent.[39] In one study by Azuma et al.,[40] IOS
was 73.9% accurate in diagnosing the depth of invasion

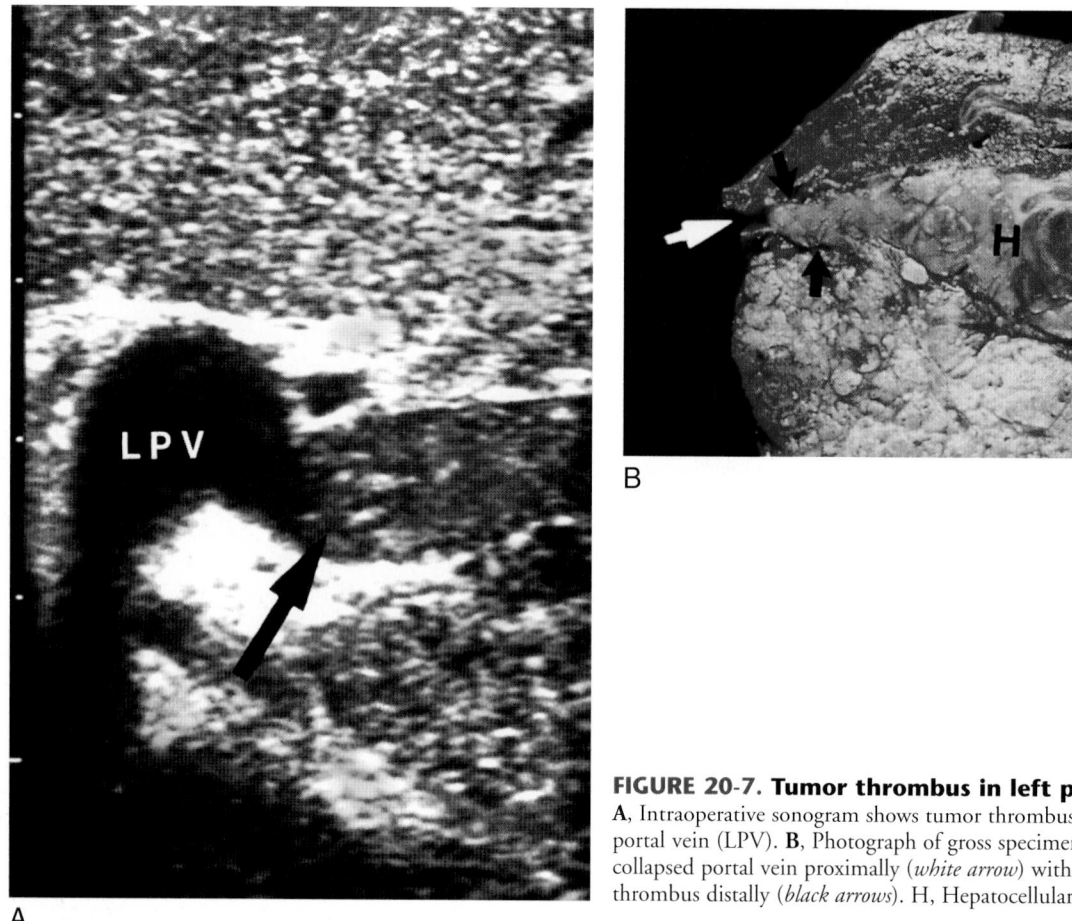

FIGURE 20-7. Tumor thrombus in left portal vein.
A, Intraoperative sonogram shows tumor thrombus (*arrow*) in left portal vein (LPV). **B,** Photograph of gross specimen shows collapsed portal vein proximally (*white arrow*) with tumor thrombus distally (*black arrows*). H, Hepatocellular carcinoma.

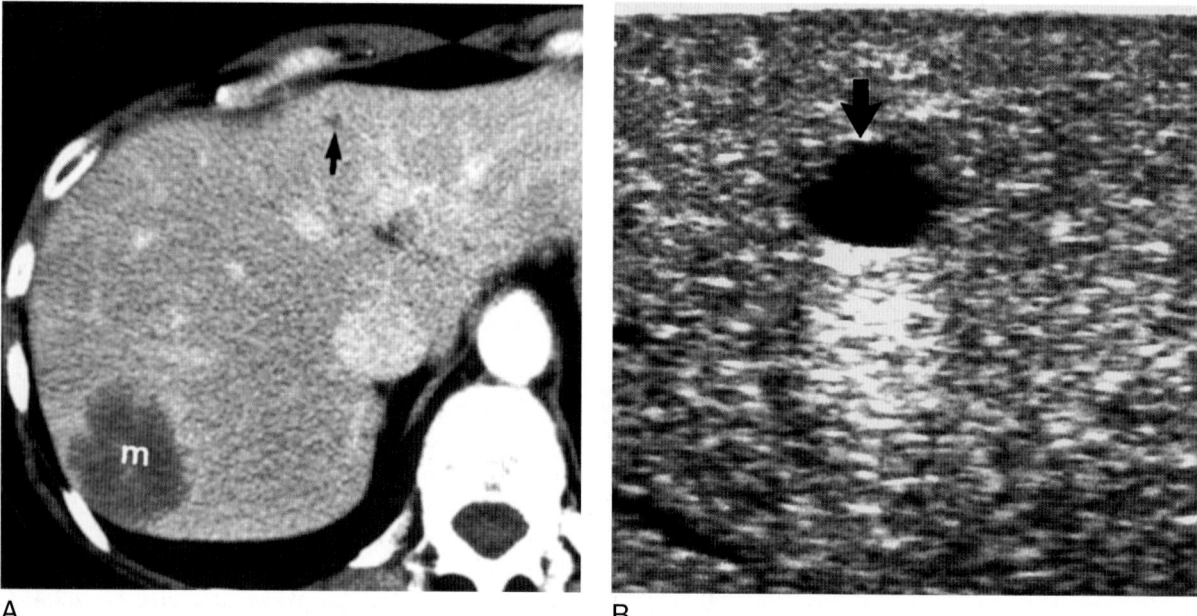

FIGURE 20-8. Small hepatic cysts. A, Preoperative contrast-enhanced CT shows a metastasis (m) in the right lobe and a small indeterminate lesion in the left lobe (*arrow*). **B,** Intraoperative sonogram shows a 0.6 cm hepatic cyst (*arrow*) in the left lobe.

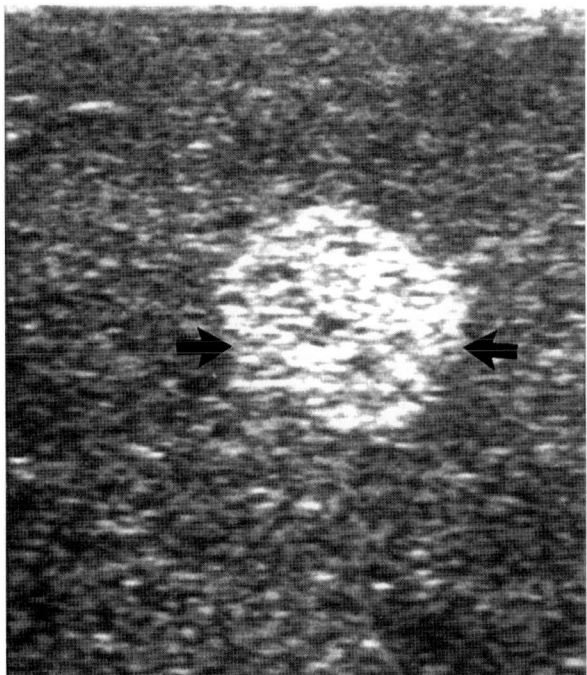

FIGURE 20-9. Incidental hemangioma. Small echogenic hemangioma (*arrows*) with a scalloped margin and tiny cystic spaces. Note there is no peripheral halo around the hemangioma.

of the nonpedunculated gallbladder cancers. In the same study, frozen section was only slightly more accurate in diagnosing depth of invasion (85.7% accuracy).[40] Adjacent normal structures and lymph nodes can also be surveyed with IOS.

Localizing a normal common bile duct (CBD) can also be important if it is to be preserved during surgery. Intraoperative sonography accurately localizes the CBD and demonstrates its relationship to adjacent masses and fluid collection. This helps plan surgery and hopefully avoids damage to the CBD (Fig. 20-13).

PANCREAS

Carcinoma

The most common pancreatic malignant lesion is **ductal adenocarcinoma**. Few patients with this tumor are surgical candidates at presentation because of vascular encasement or metastatic disease. Patients with small tumors (less than 2 cm) that have no vascular invasion or lymph node metastasis have the best prognosis.[41-44] The 5-year survival rate after pancreatoduodenectomy is between 18% and 33%.[41-45]

Multiple preoperative imaging studies can be obtained to diagnose pancreatic ductal adenocarcinoma; they include CT, sonography, endoscopic retrograde cholangio-pancreatography (ERCP), MRI, and endoscopic sonography. Intraoperative sonography is rarely used at our institution in patients with pancreatic ductal adenocarcinoma, because most of these cancers are easily palpable and cannot be resected, which is made apparent by inspection and palpation. Intraoperative sonography can be used to detect and determine the extent of a small, nonpalpable pancreatic mass.[46-48] Pancreatic ductal adenocarcinoma is usually a hypoechoic, solid mass with

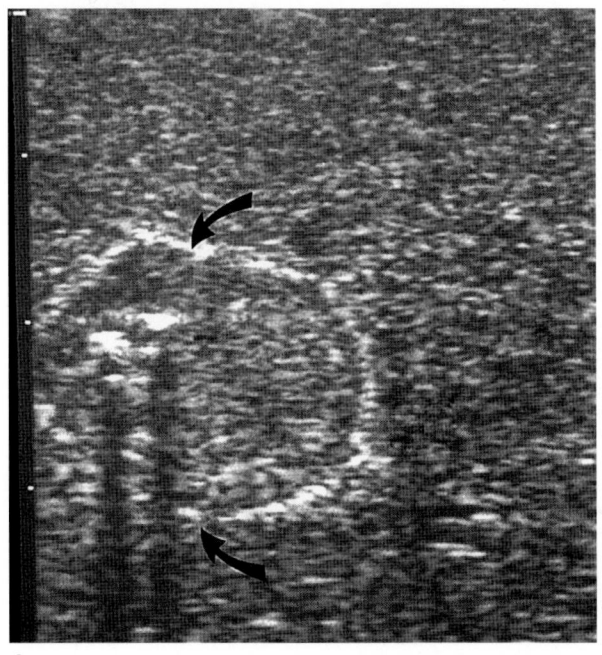

A

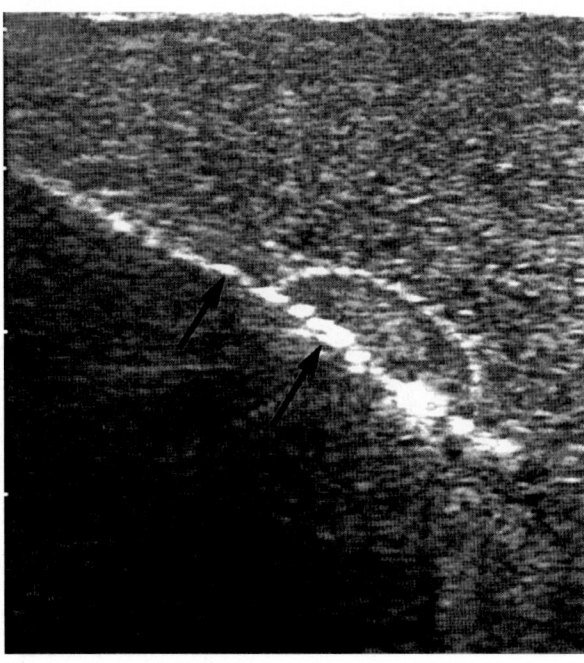

B

FIGURE 20-10. IOS—guided liver biopsy. A, Nearly isoechoic mass (*arrows*) with tiny calcifications. **B,** IOS-guided biopsy needle (*straight arrows*) within the mass, which was an atypical hemangioma.

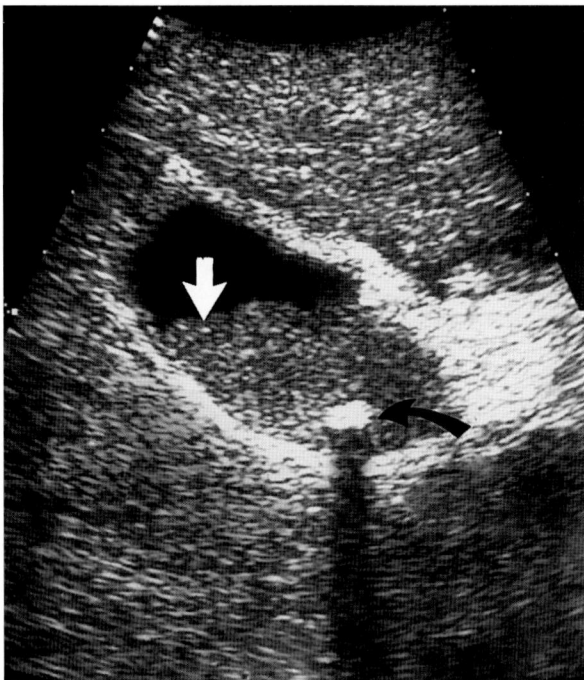

FIGURE 20-11. Incidental gallstone. Incidental gallstone (*curved arrow*) and biliary sludge (*straight arrow*).

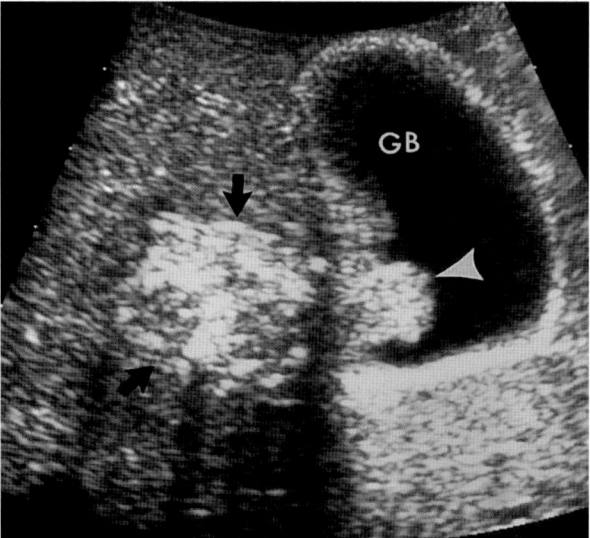

FIGURE 20-12. Colorectal liver metastasis invading gallbladder. Intraoperative sonography shows a colorectal metastasis (*arrows*) with microcalcifications invading (*arrowhead*) the gallbladder (GB).

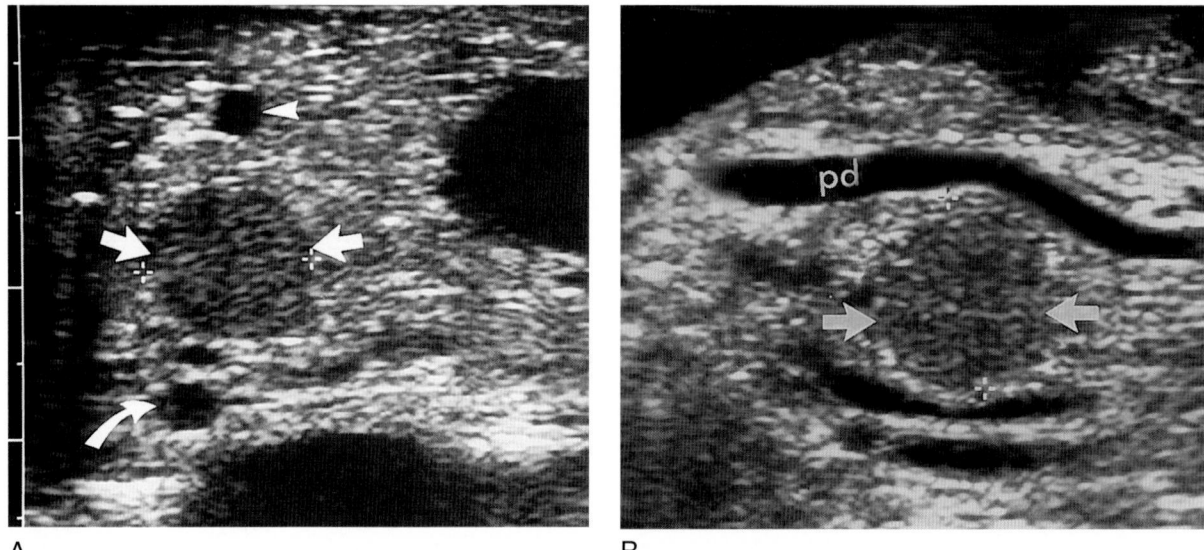

A   B

FIGURE 20-13. Insulinoma near common bile duct. A, Transverse and **B,** oblique images demonstrate a small, discrete, hypoechoic insulinoma (*white arrows*). **B,** Pancreatic duct (pd) and **A** (*white arrowhead*) and common bile duct (*curved arrow*) are in close proximity to the insulinoma.

irregular margins (Fig. 20-14). It frequently obstructs the pancreatic duct and common bile duct and causes ductal dilation up to the level of the mass. IOS can also be used to detect abnormal regional lymph nodes, vascular encasement by neoplasm, and liver metastatic lesions.[48] Demonstrating occult liver metastatic lesions with IOS can prevent an unnecessary attempt at surgical resection.[48]

Pancreatitis

Intraoperative sonography may be used to evaluate the multiple complications associated with chronic pancreatitis, including pseudocyst, abscess, and secondary involvement of the gastrointestinal tract, biliary tract, or abdominal vessels by the inflammatory process.

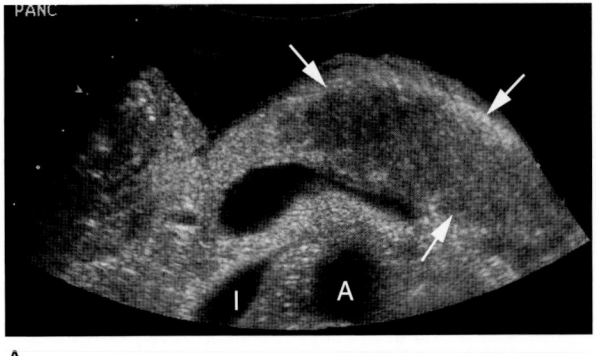

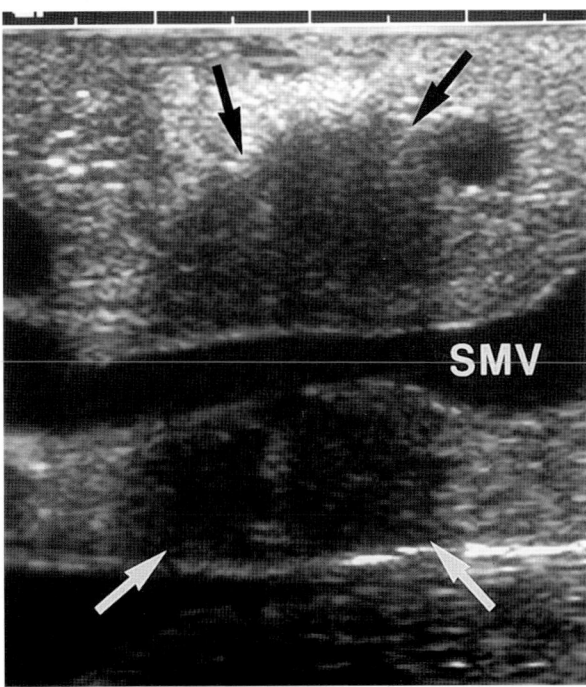

FIGURE 20-14. Pancreatic ductal adenocarcinomas.
A, Transverse IOS of the body of the pancreas demonstrates an oval, poorly marginated hypoechoic mass (*arrows*) in the body and tail of the pancreas. A, aorta; I, inferior vena cava. **B,** longitudinal IOS of another patient demonstrates a small hypoechoic carcinoma (*arrows*) surrounding the superior mesenteric vein, SMV.

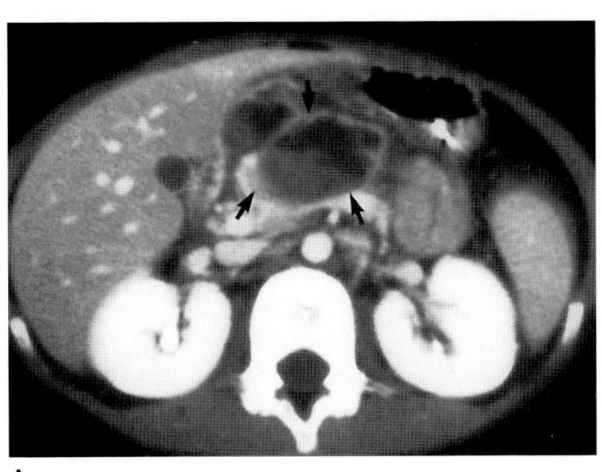

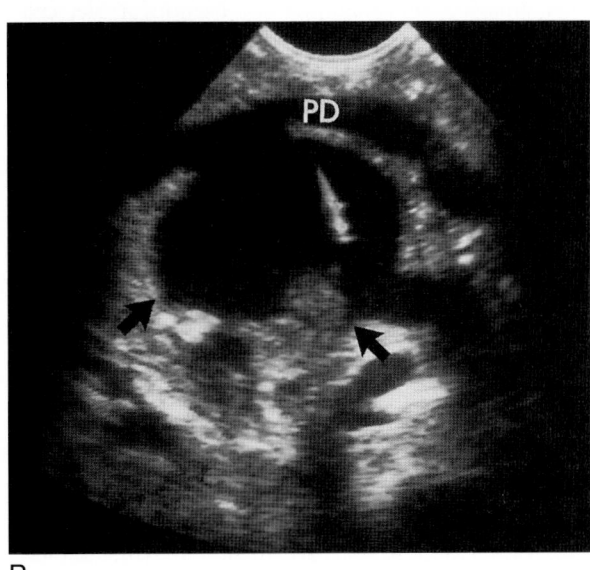

FIGURE 20-15. Drainage of pseudocyst. A, Preoperative contrast-enhanced CT shows pseudocyst (*arrows*) with dependent debris. **B,** Intraoperative sonogram shows pseudocyst (*arrows*) communicating with pancreatic duct (PD). Under ultrasound guidance, a needle was placed (*bright linear echoes*) into pancreatic pseudocyst.

Although most pseudocysts and abscesses can be readily identified with preoperative imaging, IOS can help localize and drain these fluid collections and their extensions (Fig. 20-15). Occasionally, previously unrecognized fluid collections can be identified with IOS.[47,49-51] The pancreatic duct and intraductal calcifications are easily identified with IOS (Fig. 20-16). IOS can also differentiate inflamed pancreatic parenchyma from the pseudocyst and thus save the parenchyma from unnecessary surgical removal.

In some patients, distinguishing between **chronic pancreatitis** and **pancreatic cancer** is difficult with imaging studies and clinical history.[48] In addition, small ductal adenocarcinomas can obstruct the pancreatic duct and cause secondary pancreatitis that may obscure the primary neoplasm. Ultrasound guidance may be used to biopsy an indeterminate mass within the pancreas to determine whether it is inflammatory or malignant.[48] This may be done percutaneously or in the operating room during laparotomy.

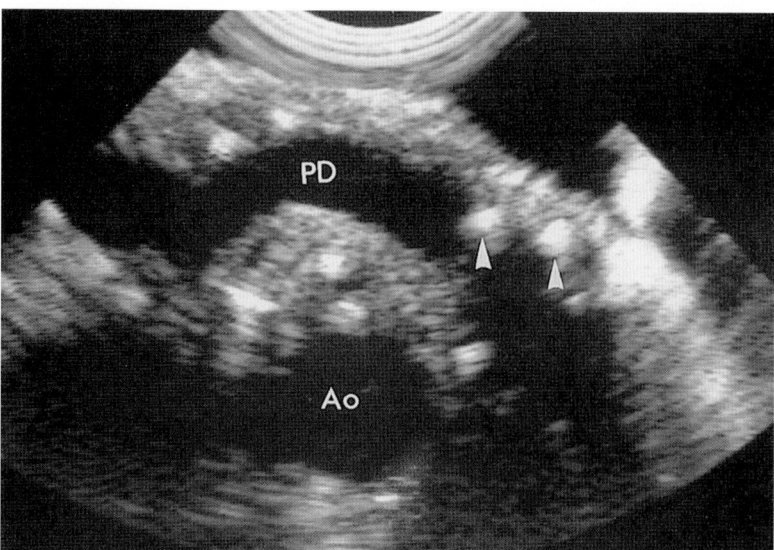

FIGURE 20-16. Chronic pancreatitis. Transverse IOS shows a dilated pancreatic duct (PD) with ductal calcifications (*arrowheads*). Ao, Aorta.

Islet Cell Neoplasm

Insulinoma. A highly valuable application for IOS is the localization of an islet cell neoplasm, such as insulinoma. Imaging and attempted localization of islet cell neoplasms can be frustrating to the radiologist, clinician, surgeon, and patient. Islet cell neoplasms often produce excessive hormone, so the clinician can make a firm clinical diagnosis. Afterward, the patient is often referred to the radiologist for localization of the neoplasm producing the excessive hormone. Various preoperative imaging studies, including sonography, CT, MRI, angiography, venous sampling, and radionuclide scanning, are used to localize islet cell neoplasms with variable results. However, islet cell neoplasms are frequently small and difficult to localize preoperatively.

A common application for IOS is to localize a small insulinoma. Insulinomas are usually small and solitary.[52,53] The insulinoma produces excessive insulin, which causes hypoglycemia. Once the laboratory evidence establishes that the patient has an insulinoma, surgical intervention is needed to prevent a neurologic catastrophe caused by severe hypoglycemia. Experienced pancreatic surgeons working with experienced sonographers can localize nearly all insulinomas during surgery by using a combination of inspection, palpation, and IOS.[52-58] Because of this capability, the number of preoperative examinations for localization can be minimized.

High-frequency (7 to 15 MHz) transducers are essential in searching for an insulinoma. Warm, sterile saline is poured into the abdomen to provide acoustic coupling and a standoff medium. Identifying small insulinomas on the surface of the pancreas can be difficult if the transducer is placed directly on the tumor. Scanning slightly off the surface using the saline as a standoff medium makes detection of surface lesions easier. The

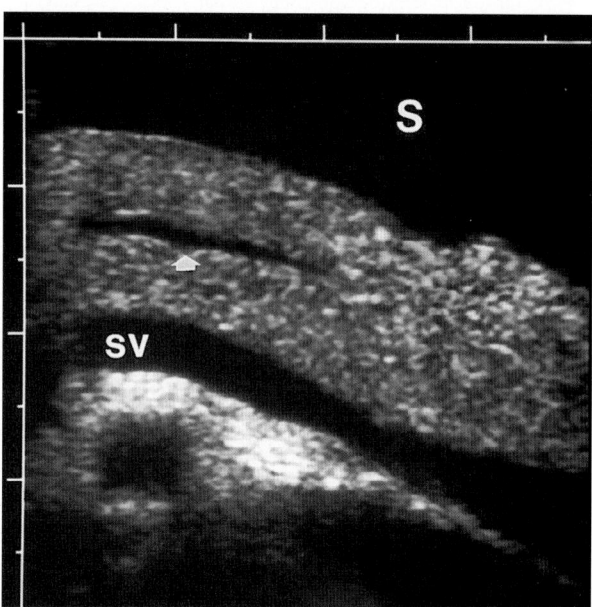

FIGURE 20-17. Normal pancreas. Saline (S), anterior to the pancreas, improves visualization of the anterior surface of the pancreas. Pancreatic duct (*arrow*). SV, Splenic vein.

normal pancreas has a uniform, coarse, hyperechoic echotexture (Fig. 20-17). Ninety percent of **insulinomas** are **discrete, small, well-defined hypoechoic nodules** (Fig. 20-18).[57] In addition to detecting the tumor, IOS should demonstrate the relationship of the insulinoma to the pancreatic duct. If the insulinoma is located a safe distance away from and superficial to the pancreatic duct, enucleation is performed. However, if the insulinoma is deeply situated or very near the pancreatic duct, safe enucleation is not possible without transecting the pancreatic duct (see Fig. 20-13). Instead, pancreatic resection may be necessary. If the insulinoma

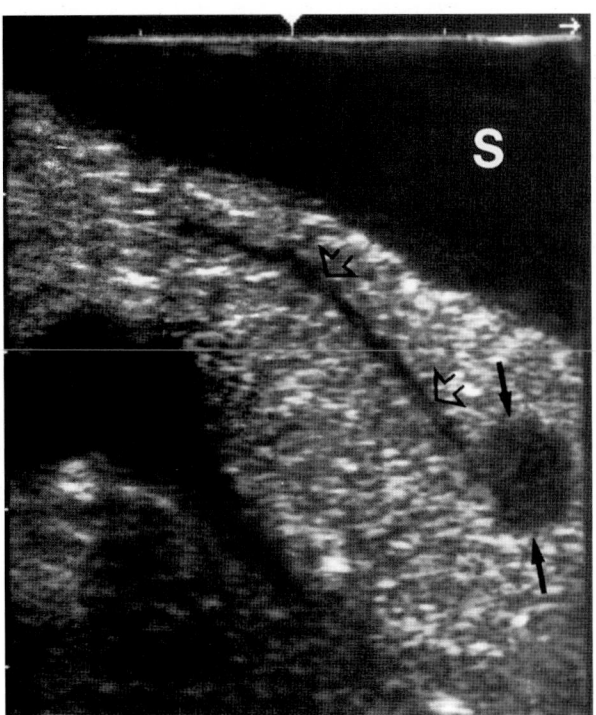

FIGURE 20-18. Solitary pancreatic insulinoma.
Transverse IOS shows 0.8 cm hypoechoic mass (*black arrows*) in pancreatic tail adjacent to pancreatic duct (*open arrows*). S, saline.

is nonpalpable, a localizing needle can be placed near it (Fig. 20-19).

Ten percent of insulinomas are hyperechoic or isoechoic relative to the pancreas.[57] Insulinomas in young patients are more difficult to detect, probably because the pancreatic parenchyma is less echogenic and can be isoechoic with the insulinoma. In these cases, the insulinoma can be detected if the edge effect from its smooth margin is detected or the fine echotexture of the insulinoma is detected in contrast to the coarse echotexture of the pancreatic parenchyma.[57] Insulinomas are **hypervascular**; therefore, color and power Doppler can aid in the localization of isoechoic insulinomas.

Gastrinoma. Gastrinoma is the second most common functioning neuroendocrine tumor. Gastrinomas produce gastrin, which causes excess secretion of gastric acid and leads to severe diarrhea and gastric ulcers (e.g., Zollinger-Ellison syndrome). Gastrinomas are often difficult to localize. Gastrinomas are multiple in 20% to 40%, and malignant in 60% to 90%.[59] Gastrinomas are extrapancreatic in 20% to 40% of patients[59] and are often located in the wall of the duodenum (Fig. 20-20). Ninety percent of gastrinomas lie in a region known as the "gastrinoma triangle.[52,60] The boundaries of the gastrinoma triangle are the second and third portions of the duodenum inferiorly, the junction of the cystic and common bile ducts superiorly, and the junction of the head and neck of the pancreas medially.[52,60] This area should be carefully scanned during IOS. Unfortunately, some gastrinomas cannot be found, despite careful preoperative imaging, laparotomy, careful surgical inspection and palpation, and IOS. However, in a study by Kisker et al.[61] of 25 patients with Zollinger-Ellison syndrome, 15 gastrinomas (60%) were identified with preoperative imaging. Using thorough surgical exploration and IOS, 24 of the 25 primary gastrinomas were localized (96%).

Multiple Endocrine Neoplasia. Multiple endocrine neoplasia, type I (MEN I) is associated with tumors of the pancreas, parathyroid glands, pituitary gland,

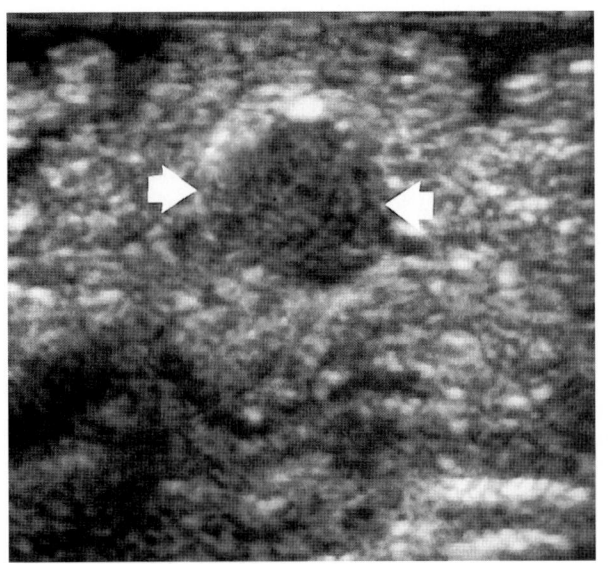

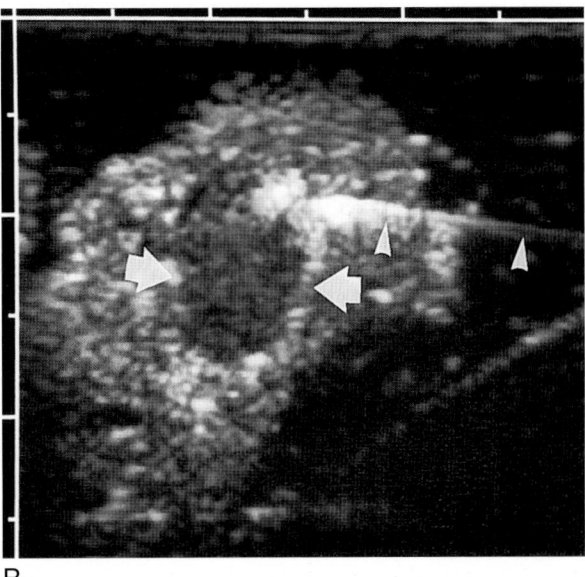

A   B

FIGURE 20-19. Nonpalpable insulinoma. A, Nonpalpable, 1 cm insulinoma (*arrows*) identified with IOS. **B,** Under IOS guidance, a localizing needle (*arrowheads*) was placed next to the insulinoma (*arrows*).

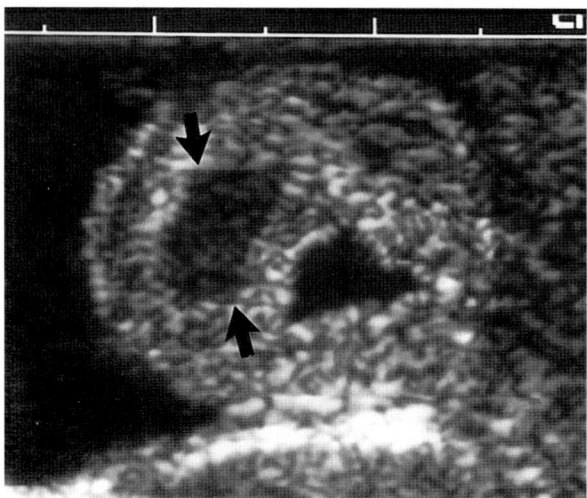

FIGURE 20-20. Gastrinoma. This gastrinoma (*arrows*) is located in the wall of the duodenum.

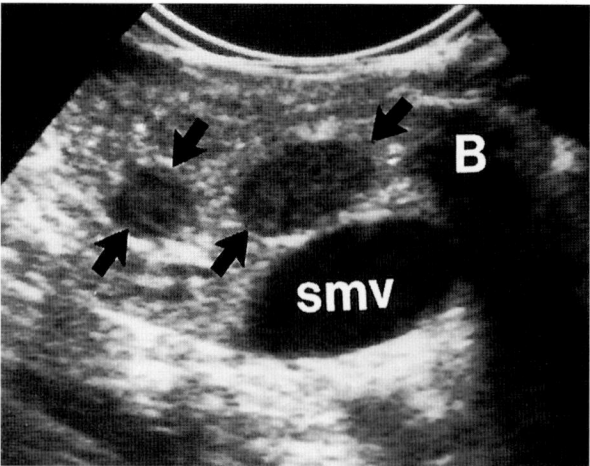

FIGURE 20-21. MEN syndrome. Multiple pancreatic insulinomas. Transverse scan in patient with multiple endocrine neoplasia syndrome, type I, shows two hypoechoic insulinomas (*arrows*) within pancreatic head. Superior mesenteric vein, smv. bowel, B.

adrenal cortex, and thyroid. MEN I is an autosomal-dominant trait with high penetrance. Pancreatic tumors are usually multifocal and account for most of the morbidity and mortality in patients with MEN I. Patients with MEN I often have several adenomas less than 1 cm in diameter and require near-total pancreatectomy for cure (Fig. 20-21).[57,62] The head of the pancreas must be carefully scanned and palpated because residual adenomas may cause the patient's symptoms to persist postoperatively.

KIDNEY

Masses

Intraoperative sonography can be of value in kidney-sparing surgery. Partial nephrectomy for renal malignant disease should be considered in patients with bilateral renal malignant lesions, a mass in a solitary kidney, renal insufficiency, or significant abnormalities in the contralateral kidney.[63-67] The goal is to preserve renal parenchyma to avoid dialysis. Some authors have recommended partial nephrectomy for small, localized renal cell carcinomas in patients with a normal contralateral kidney.[65-67] Local recurrence affects 3% to 13% of patients after partial nephrectomy.[68-73] To prevent recurrence, the entire malignant tumor must be removed with adequate surgical margins. Simple enucleation of renal cell carcinomas frequently results in incomplete tumor excision.[74,75] Mukamel et al.[76] reported that 20% of kidneys with a dominant renal cell carcinoma also had separate adenocarcinomas in another area of the renal parenchyma. Gilbert et al.[77] were the first group to use IOS in patients who were candidates for partial nephrectomy. Since then, several groups have shown that IOS is useful in surgical procedures that spare the renal paren-

chyma.[56,57,71-74,78] Sonography is useful to **locate occult, nonpalpable tumors**, to **delineate the boundaries of the renal mass**, and to **guide partial nephrectomy** (Fig. 20-22). Intraoperative sonography is especially valuable if a lesion is deeply located and difficult to palpate. Some renal masses are nearly isoechoic to the renal parenchyma. In such cases, detecting margins of the lesion or alterations in the vascularity of the lesion is important. Great care must also be taken not to mistake a hypoechoic medullary pyramid for a small renal mass.

Intraoperative sonography can also be useful in **characterizing indeterminate renal masses** (Figs. 20-23 to 20-25). Depending on CT slice thickness and the size of the renal lesion, it may be difficult to determine whether a small renal lesion is cystic or solid. IOS can readily characterize small cystic lesions and, thus, prevent unnecessary resection. IOS can also be used to guide biopsy of an indeterminate renal mass. For example, a small renal cell carcinoma may appear hyperechoic and indistinguishable from a small angiolipoma (Fig. 20-26).

Vascular

Technical problems encountered by the surgeon during renal revascularization procedures have traditionally been difficult to accurately assess. A variety of methods have been used, including palpation, continuous wave Doppler analysis, and arteriography, but each has limitations. Sonography has been increasingly used intraoperatively to evaluate the main renal arteries occasionally before, but more often following, the surgical procedure. Most patients evaluated are undergoing transaortic **renal artery endarterectomy** or **renal artery**

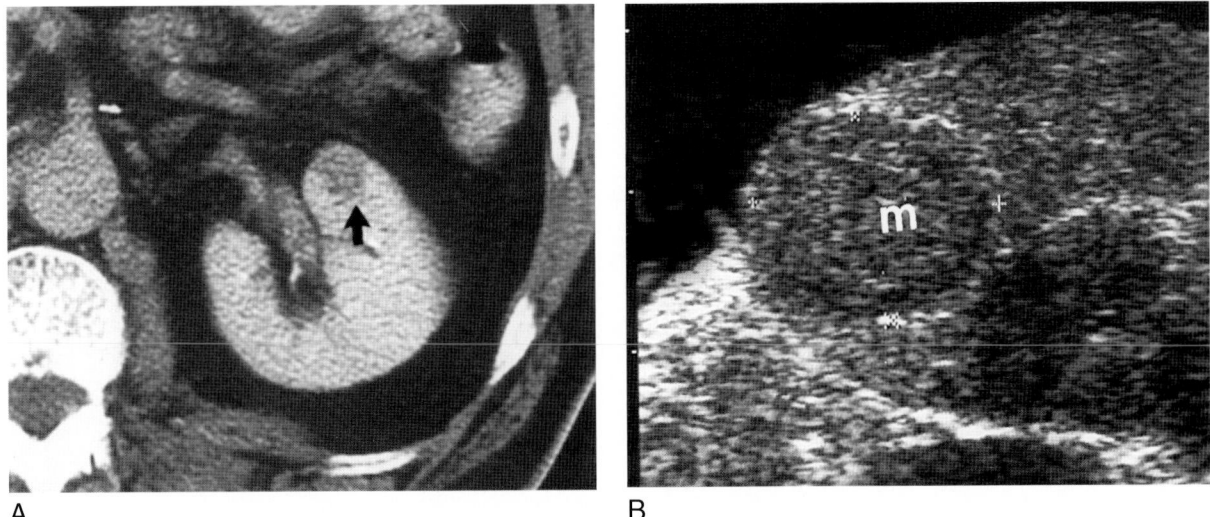

FIGURE 20-22. Small oncocytoma. A, Contrast-enhanced CT shows a small, indeterminate, left renal mass (*arrow*). **B,** IOS demonstrates small, solid, renal mass (m), which is nearly isoechoic with adjacent renal parenchyma. This mass was not palpable.

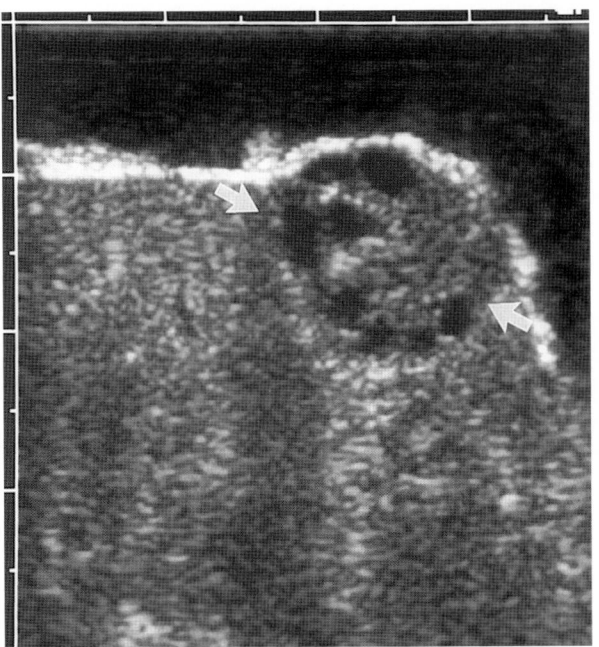

FIGURE 20-23. Small renal cell carcinoma. Intraoperative sonography demonstrates a 1.5 cm, mixed solid and cystic mass (*arrows*) in the cortex of the kidney.

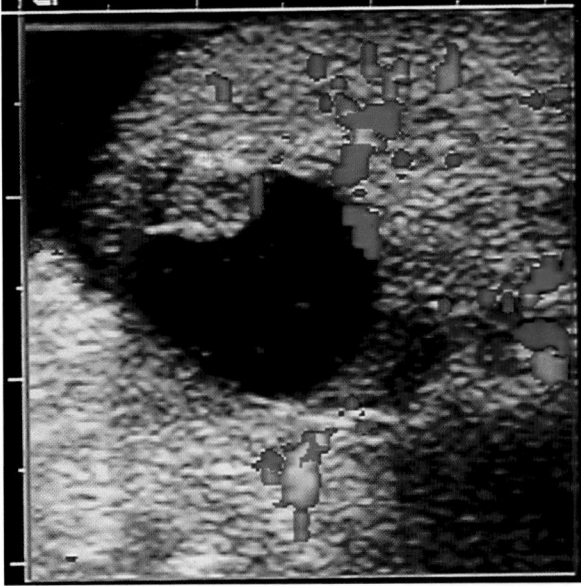

FIGURE 20-24. Small renal cell carcinoma in wall of cyst. Transverse image demonstrates a 1.5 cm cyst with a 0.5 cm mural nodule, which was a low-grade, nonpalpable, renal cell carcinoma in a patient with Hippel-Lindau syndrome.

bypass grafting to treat renal artery stenosis that has led to hypertension and/or renal insufficiency. Gray-scale, spectral, and color flow Doppler sonography allow detection of abnormalities at the time of the operation, thereby improving the chance for a successful outcome. In our experience, abnormalities requiring surgical revision have been detected in 9% to 11% of reconstructed main renal arteries scanned intraoperatively.[79,80] Data suggest that clinical outcomes of patients requiring intraoperative revision are favorable and similar to those

with normal IOS studies. A recent study concluded that the B-mode imaging was more important than hemodynamic duplex data in discriminating normal from abnormal reconstructions.[81]

Scanning is performed through the operative incision using a high-frequency transducer covered with a sterile plastic sheath. The surgeon provides exposure as needed, and the wound is filled with saline or water, which provides the acoustic window. Gray-scale, spectral, and color wave Doppler analysis complement each other in

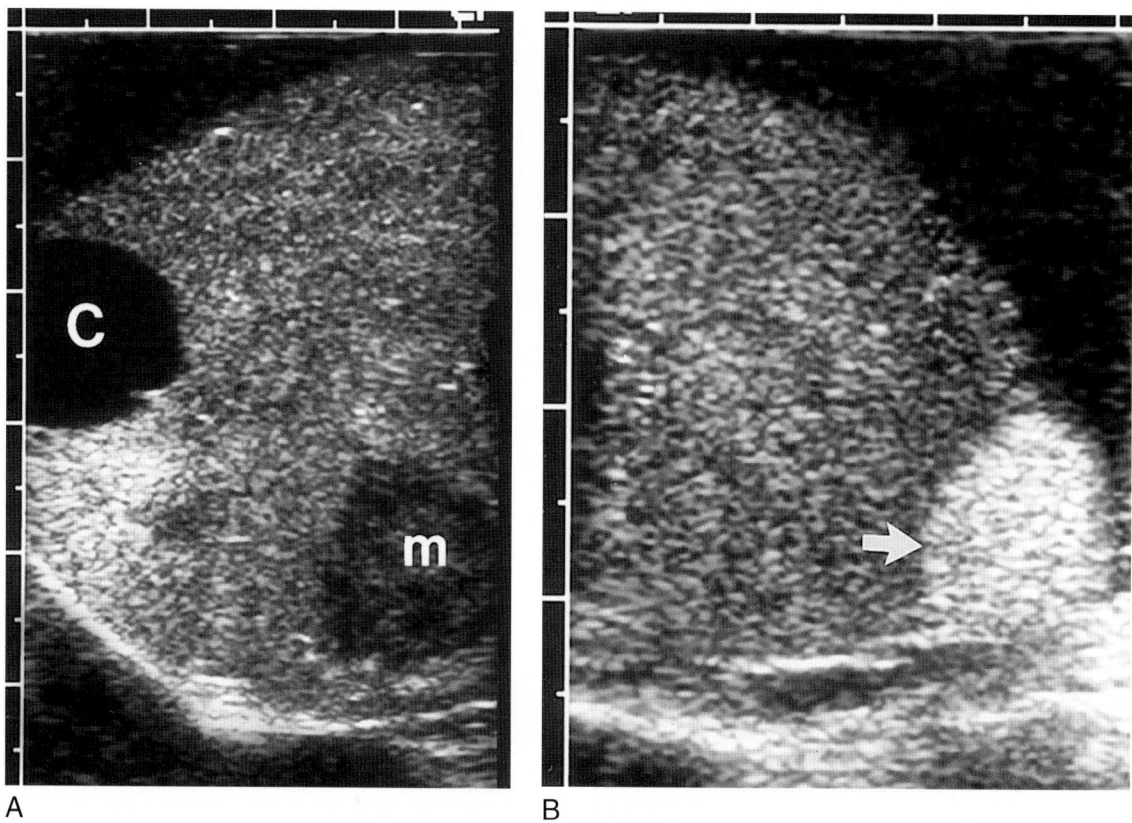

FIGURE 20-25. Cyst, angiomyolipoma, and adenoma in same kidney. A, Transverse IOS image of kidney shows a benign cyst (C) and a hypoechoic solid mass (M) which proved to be an adenoma. **B,** At a different level, a small, hyperechoic angiomyolipoma (*arrow*) was seen.

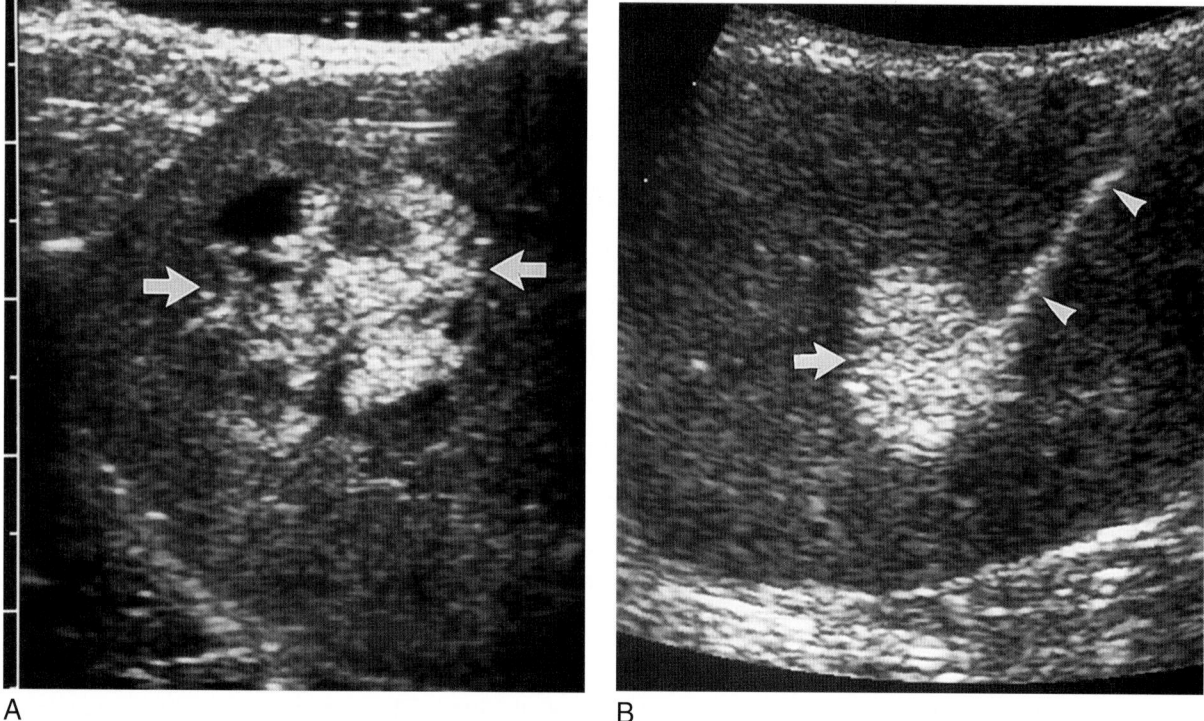

FIGURE 20-26. Incidentally detected low-grade renal cell carcinoma. A, IOS of the liver in a patient with a hepatocellular carcinoma discovered an incidental, echogenic, right renal mass (*arrows*). **B,** Under IOS guidance, a biopsy needle (*arrowheads*) was placed into the mass (*arrow*), which proved to be a low-grade renal cell carcinoma.

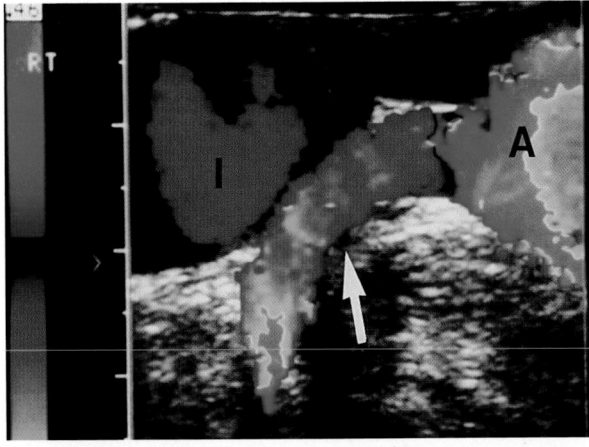

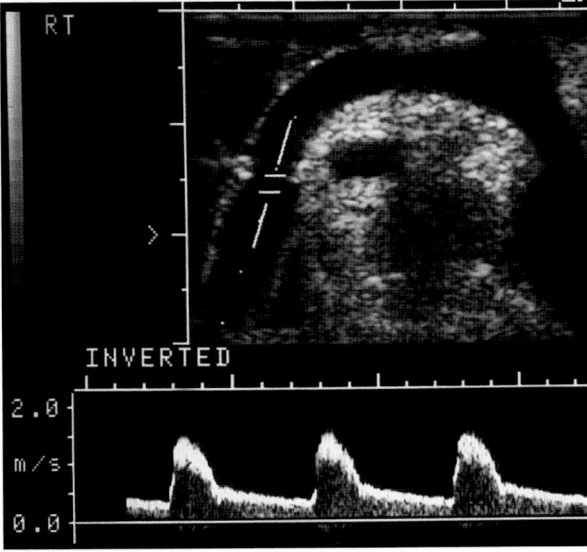

FIGURE 20-27. Normal right renal artery postendarterectomy. A, Transverse scan shows right renal artery (*arrow*) arising from the aorta (A), and passing behind the inferior vena cava (I). **B,** Right renal artery bypass graft. Spectral Doppler scan shows a normal, low-resistance waveform.

evaluation of the renal arteries. A smooth lumen and uniform flow with prompt systolic upstroke and a low resistance pattern are typical of normal renal arteries (Fig. 20-27).

RENOVASCULAR ABNORMALITIES DETECTED SONOGRAPHICALLY

Residual renal artery or anastomotic stenosis (Fig. 20-28)
Thrombosis/occlusion of the graft or renal artery (Fig. 20-29)
Intimal flap or dissection (Figs. 20-30 and 20-31)
Extrinsic compression or kinking of the graft or renal artery

LAPAROSCOPIC SONOGRAPHY

The latest development in IOS has been the application of ultrasound techniques using especially designed probes that can be inserted through standard laparoscopic ports that are typically no more than 10 to 11 mm in size. Because these laparoscopic ports are at some distance from the intra-abdominal organs, the LUS probes must be mounted on a long, thin shaft. The earliest reports of LUS utilized A mode sonography for diagnosis of intra-abdominal pathology, although this was of limited usefulness.[82,83] Miniaturization techniques were then applied to conventional gray-scale scanners, both mechanical and electronic types, allowing for a substantial decrease in probe size, thus making laparoscopic real-time ultrasound feasible.[84-86] The ultimate in miniaturization has been the catheter-based transducers, which were originally developed for intravascular ultrasound, but which have also been used laparoscopically.[87] The extremely small size of catheter-mounted transducers makes the field of view so small as to limit practical usefulness in the abdomen.

Currently, a number of commercial ultrasound manufacturers produce LUS probes, most of which share the following features in common:

- Broad-band or multiple frequency transducer with center frequency ranging from 5 to 7.5 MHz;
- Long rigid shaft of at least 15 to 20 cm length;
- Real-time gray-scale, as well as Doppler and color flow capability;
- Linear array, or curvilinear array, transducers with crystal length ranging from approximately 1 to 3 cm;
- Sterile sheaths, specifically designed for each individual probe.

Technique

Most of the available equipment also features a flexible tip including the imaging crystal and continues some distance up the shaft. Some systems will flex and extend in one plane, whereas other systems can steer to the right and left as well as offering flexion and extension capability. Movement of the flexible portion of the probe is controlled by the operator using mechanisms that are similar to controls for flexible endoscopes. The ability to flex or extend the probe is of critical importance in maintaining contact with organs having curved surfaces, such as the liver. A strictly rigid system often loses acoustic coupling due to its inability to maintain direct contact with the organ surface. An alternative approach for a nonflexible system is to fill the abdominal cavity with fluid and scan through the fluid as an acoustic

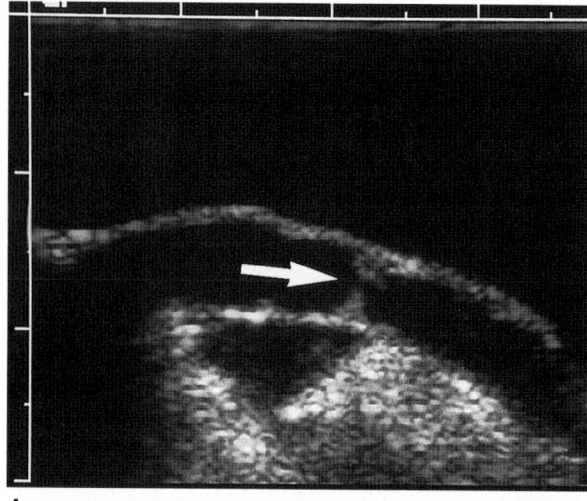

A

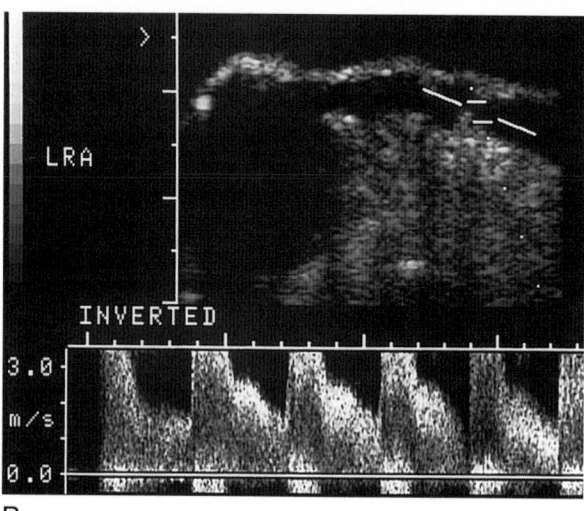

B

FIGURE 20-28. Residual stenosis after endarterectomy. A, Longitudinal image of the left renal artery shows residual plaque (*arrow*). **B,** Spectral Doppler examination shows elevated flow velocities and turbulence, indicating significant stenosis. This was surgically revised.

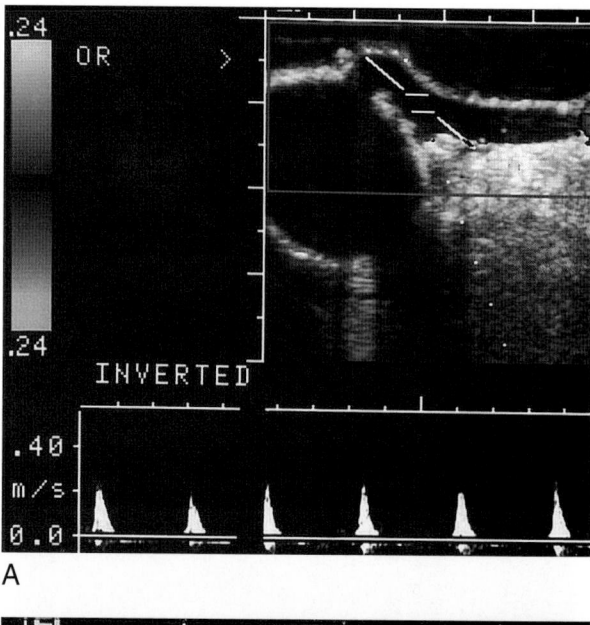

A

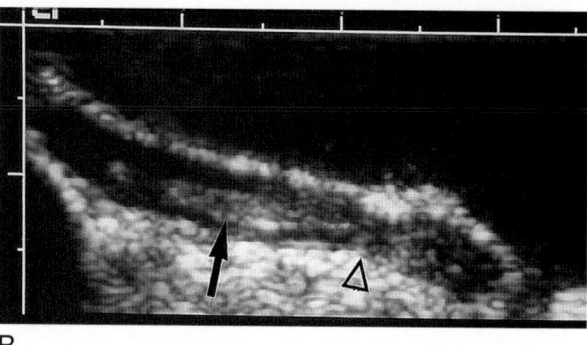

B

FIGURE 20-29. Left renal artery thrombosis. A, Transverse duplex scan following left renal artery bypass using saphenous vein graft shows low-velocity, high-resistance waveform in proximal left renal artery, suggesting obstruction distally. **B,** Gray-scale image more distally demonstrates mild narrowing at distal anastomosis (*arrowhead*) with partial thrombosis of renal artery lumen (*arrow*).(From Lantz EJ, Charboneau JW, Hallett JW, et al: Intraoperative color Doppler sonography during renal artery revascularization. AJR 1994;162:859-863.)

medium. This may work reasonably well for assessing the pancreas but is extremely awkward because the abdomen is already markedly distended with CO_2 in order to facilitate the laparoscopy.

There is usually sufficient natural moisture to allow good acoustic contact with the target organs, but sterile saline may be used to moisten surfaces, if necessary. Acoustic coupling must be maintained within the sterile probe cover as well, either by using sterile gel or sterile water inside the sheath to provide an acoustic coupling medium for the imaging array. In addition to the sterile sheath covering the probe and shaft, a larger sterile cover is also used to cover the handle of the probe, its control mechanisms, and the electrical cord.[88]

It is important that the probe frequency be sufficient to image the entire organ being studied. While 7 MHz frequency may be entirely adequate for assessment of the pancreas, bile duct, and gallbladder, the attenuation of a 7 MHz beam in the liver would allow for only a 6 to 7 cm penetration. Consequently, 5 MHz frequency is preferred for the liver, which would allow penetration to a depth of 10 to 12 cm. Most livers, therefore, could be scanned from the anterior surface, which is smooth and well suited for laparoscopic scanning. Attempts to scan the undersurface of the liver are fraught with difficulty due to the very uneven surfaces, as well as ligamentous attachments, intervening organs, such as the gallbladder and duodenum, and other impediments to effective scanning.

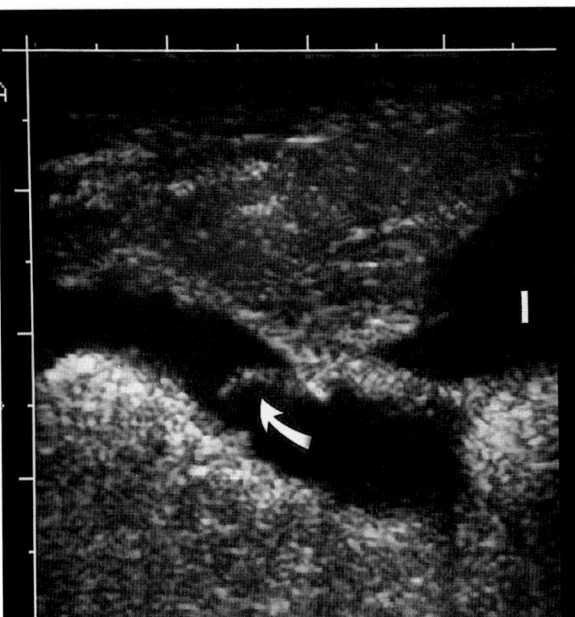

FIGURE 20-30. Intimal flap. Transverse scan of right renal artery following endarterectomy shows intimal flap (*arrow*) in vessel lumen. Vessel was opened and flap was repaired. I, inferior vena cava.

Because the probe sizes are necessarily small, the amount of time required to completely image an organ is substantially longer than imaging with standard IOS probes. A complete scan requires overlapping images through the entire organ. Intraoperative sonography probes are 2 to 4 times as large as laparoscopic probes, and consequently the time of examination is substantially longer using the laparoscopic approach. For instance, complete assessment of the liver might take 5 minutes using intraoperative probes but would take 15 to 20 minutes with a LUS examination.

Another limitation of LUS is the fact that the probe is pivoting on a single point in space, that is, the entry laparoscopic port. This limits the freedom of motion of the scan head, such that it is impossible to maintain the probe in standard transverse or longitudinal orientations. Because the probe is pivoting, the resultant image planes are most often at some obliquity to either a transverse or longitudinal image plane. This can cause disorientation and also some difficulty in ensuring that the image planes overlap one another. In liver imaging, although the right subcostal port may be sufficient for imaging the right lobe, at times the left lobe, and particularly the lateral segment and caudate lobe, cannot be adequately imaged from this site. If this is the case, the probe must be moved to another port, usually in the periumbilical, left subcostal, or epigastric region in order to complete the assessment of the left lobe.

It is important to observe the insertion of the LUS probe under direct visualization using the fiberoptic laparoscope. There is very little, if any, sense of feel as to where the probe tip is located and, in order to avoid inadvertent injury to tissues and vessels, the probe placement should be observed continuously on the TV monitor. Split-screen presentation of both the laparoscopic and real-time ultrasound images on the same monitor is most convenient and requires only a relatively inexpensive beam-splitter.

Liver

An organized, systematic approach to laparoscopic sonography of the liver is of paramount importance, keeping in mind that the imaging fields should overlap one another for complete assessment of the liver parenchyma. A center frequency of 5 MHz is optimal for imaging the entire liver from front to back as mentioned earlier. The right subcostal laparoscope port is best suited for imaging the right lobe and medial left lobe of the liver, but the left lateral segment may require repositioning of the probe into a second port in the epigastrium or midabdomen. This is easily accomplished by exchanging the LUS probe and the viewing laparoscope.

We prefer to begin at the dome of the liver, scanning across the dome, and then repositioning the probe slightly more caudal in position but no more than the length of the imaging crystal. After repositioning, a second sweep across the liver is performed, the probe is then moved further caudally and another sweep is obtained; this sequence is performed until the entire liver is scanned. It is most important to remember that the fields must overlap in order to avoid the potential for missing lesions in unscanned areas of the liver. Some laparoscopic systems present a sector format image, and this can be misleading in giving the false assurance that a large portion of the liver is imaged with each sweep. Although this is true in the far field, the extreme near field is only as wide as the length of the imaging crystal.

If the falciform ligament is well developed and obstructs access to the left lobe, the probe is then repositioned in a different port, and more scans are obtained from dome to free edge of the left lateral segment and caudate lobe. Because of the relatively small size of the imaging crystals on currently available LUS equipment, the time required for a complete scan of the liver is substantially longer than with open IOS probes. The indications and capabilities of LUS are very similar to IOS of the liver and include the following:

- to detect all possible liver lesions;
- to accurately localize these lesions to lobes and segments;
- to assess the relationship of tumors to vascular and biliary structures and to assess for invasion;

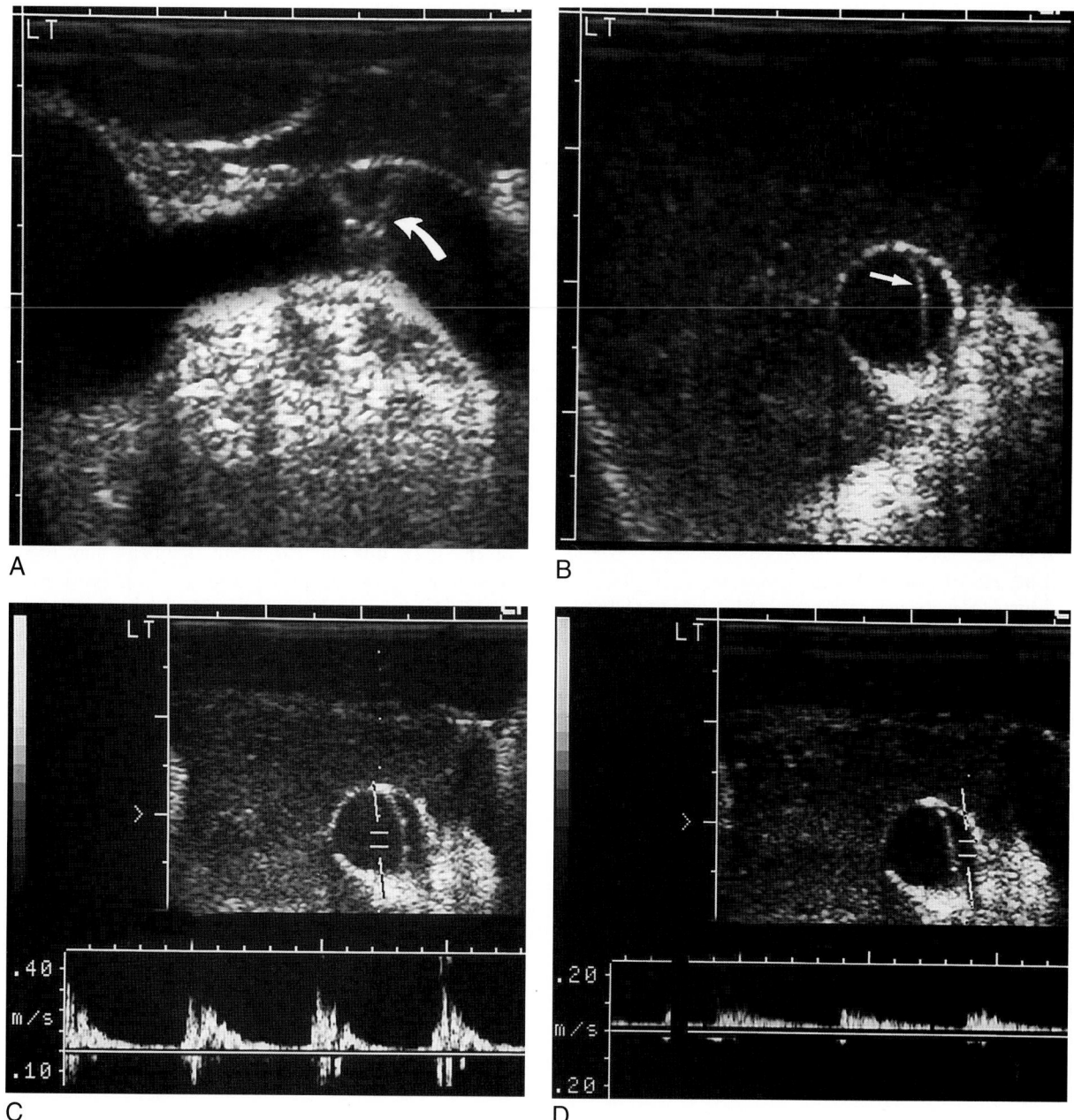

FIGURE 20-31. Dissection. A and **B**, Longitudinal and transverse images of the left renal artery following endarterectomy show an intimal dissection (*arrow*). **C** and **D**, Spectral Doppler scan shows the two lumens have different waveforms.(From Lantz EJ, Charboneau JW, Hallett JW, et al: Intraoperative color Doppler sonography during renal artery revascularization. AJR 1994;162:859-863.)

- to guide biopsy and aspirations under real-time visualization;
- to guide minimally invasive ablative techniques.

It is well known that many patients with primary or metastatic hepatic tumors are found to be unresectable at the time of laparotomy, despite multiple preoperative imaging studies. This may be due to the presence of tumor in lymph nodes or tumor deposits in the mesentery and on the peritoneal surfaces. In one prospective study of 29 patients with hepatic malignancy, all judged resectable by preoperative imaging studies, 48% were deemed unresectable due to laparoscopic findings, which included peritoneal seeding, satellite liver lesions, and unsuspected cirrhosis.[89] However, another 20% had unresectable disease not identified at laparoscopy. This is where LUS may play a key role.

Prior studies have established that IOS consistently detected 20% to -30% more liver lesions than were shown on preoperative imaging studies,[90] although this

GOALS OF LAPAROSCOPIC SONOGRAPHY

To detect and characterize all possible liver lesions
To accurately localize these lesions to lobes and segments
To assess the relationship of tumors to vascular and biliary structures
To assess for invasion
To guide biopsy and aspirations under real-time visualization
To guide minimally invasive ablative techniques

additional lesion detection rate is probably lower with current state-of-the-art multidetector CT scanning and fast MR liver imaging protocols. A more up-to-date prospective comparison study has yet to be published using state-of-the-art equipment. LUS shares this same enhanced capacity for detection of tiny liver lesions (Fig. 20-32). In one small series of 11 patients, significant additional findings were obtained at LUS, including additional masses, metastatic lymphadeno-pathy, or vascular involvement, thereby influencing surgical decision making. In five cases, LUS-guided biopsies were successfully performed.[91] In another, larger study of 50 patients, 43 of whom had successful laparo-scopic sonography, LUS depicted 33% more liver lesions than were visible through the laparoscope and added additional staging information in 42%. This resulted in a resectability rate of 93% among patients who had laparoscopy and LUS, compared with only 48% successful resections in patients without laparoscopy.[92] Improved staging of liver tumors via laparoscopy and LUS has continued to be reported in the more recent literature,[93,94] although most of these studies do not appear to have utilized the most optimal preoperative imaging.

The majority of additional liver lesions detected by LUS are very small, typically 1 cm or less in size and are, therefore, below resolution limits for conventional imaging (Fig. 20-33). This is identical to the experience with open IOS. Not all nodules detected proved to be cancer, however, and biopsy may be important to assess unsuspected lesions demonstrated only by LUS (Fig. 20-34). In a prospective study of 76 patients, Hartley et al.[95] found additional nodules in nine patients, but four of these proved to be benign. Biopsy of large or fairly superficial lesions can be accomplished quite readily by use of extra long biopsy needles punc-turing through the anterior abdominal wall and entering the liver immediately adjacent to the laparoscopic probe, which is positioned directly over the lesion. However, small and deeply seated lesions are more difficult to biopsy and some type of real-time biopsy guide, similar to those available on conventional ultrasound probes,

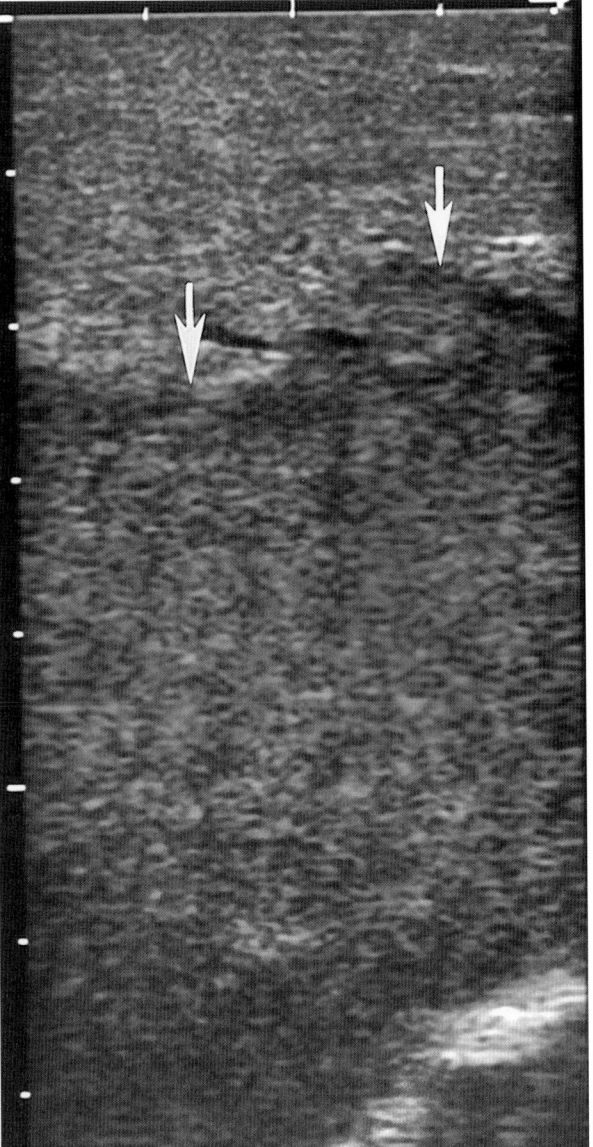

A

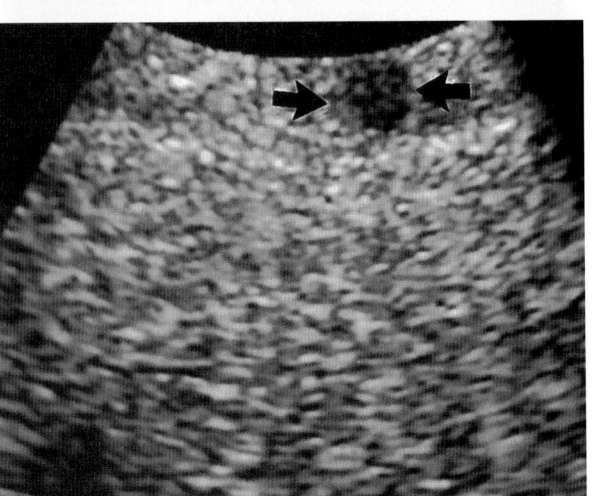

B

FIGURE 20-32. Laparoscopic ultrasound—colorectal metastases. A, Large left lobe metastasis (*white arrows*). **B,** Superficial 5 mm right lobe metastasis (*black arrows*) not visible via the laparoscope and not seen on preoperative imaging studies.

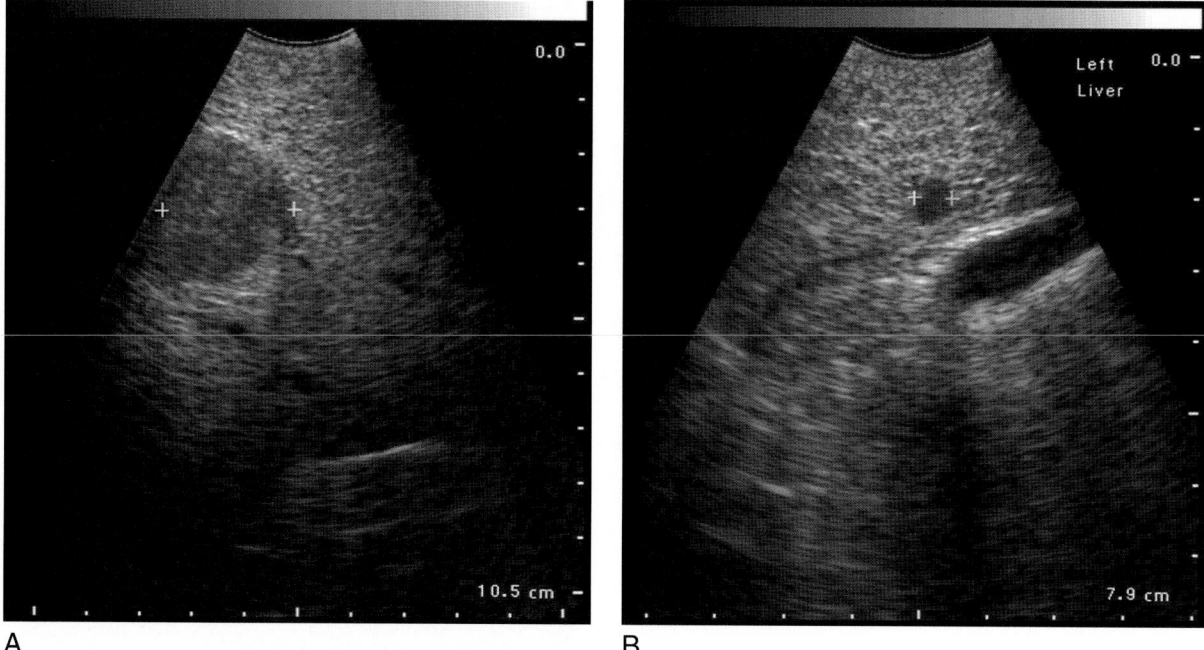

FIGURE 20-33. Laparoscopic ultrasound (LUS)—hepatocellular carcinoma (HCC). **A**, 2.5 cm hypoechoic mass in segment VI. **B**, 5 mm hypoechoic HCC nodule in segment IV (*calipers*) only detectable by LUS and rendering the patient unresectable.

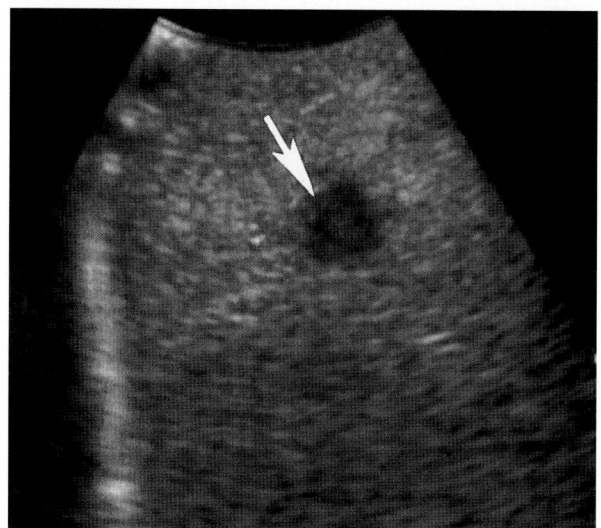

FIGURE 20-34. Laparoscopic ultrasound—focal nodular hyperplasia. Right lobe nodule, 8 mm, (*arrow*) simulating a colorectal metastasis.

would prove very useful. Most commercially available LUS systems do not provide adequate real-time biopsy guidance, although some manufacturers are now providing such systems. They are somewhat awkward at present, but further progress and development in this area are expected.

Invasion or obstruction of bile ducts can be readily demonstrated, as well as vascular invasion into the portal or hepatic veins, which is seen most often in hepatocellular carcinoma. Assessment of aberrant vascular supply to the liver may also be very important in influencing the type of resection performed, particularly in patients with replaced or accessory left hepatic or right hepatic arteries (Fig. 20-35). Accessory hepatic venous drainage, particularly in the inferior right lobe, is not infrequently seen, and an awareness of this is important for the surgeon in order to avoid unnecessary traction and trauma to this accessory vein, which could lead to substantial and even life-threatening hemorrhage. Color flow LUS imaging can be very important in defining the hepatic vasculature beneath the liver capsule, in order to define safe avascular planes for biopsy, hepatotomy, hepatic cyst fenestration, and other interventional procedures (Fig. 20-36).

Gallbladder and Biliary Tract

Initially there was great expectation for the use of LUS techniques in assessing patients who were undergoing laparoscopic cholecystectomy. In particular, LUS was felt to be at least equivalent to, if not superior to, laparoscopic intraoperative cholangiography, which can be a difficult and technically challenging study to perform. In a study by Liu et al.,[91] one out of seven patients undergoing laparoscopic cholecystectomy had **common duct stones** identified by LUS leading to an open surgical approach with removal of multiple intrahepatic and common bile duct stones. However, in a larger study of 150 patients, in whom 129 successful LUS examinations were obtained, although visualization of the common duct was good in most cases, unexpected

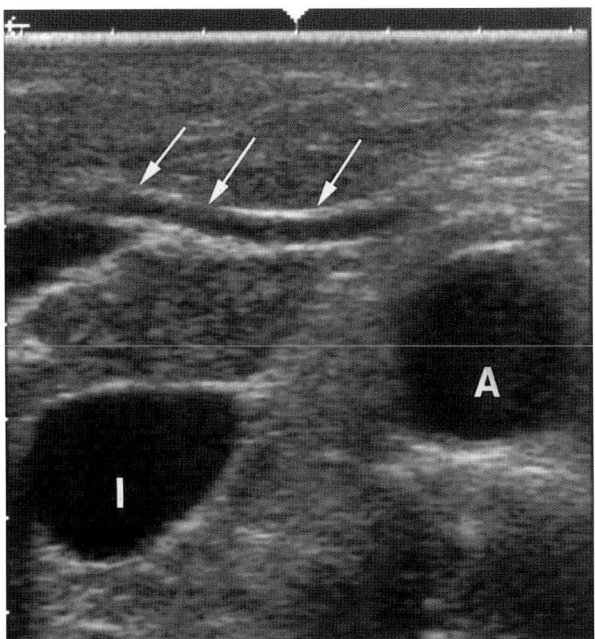

FIGURE 20-35. Laparoscopic ultrasound. Replaced left hepatic artery (*arrows*) arising from the left gastric artery. A, aorta; I, inferior vena cava.

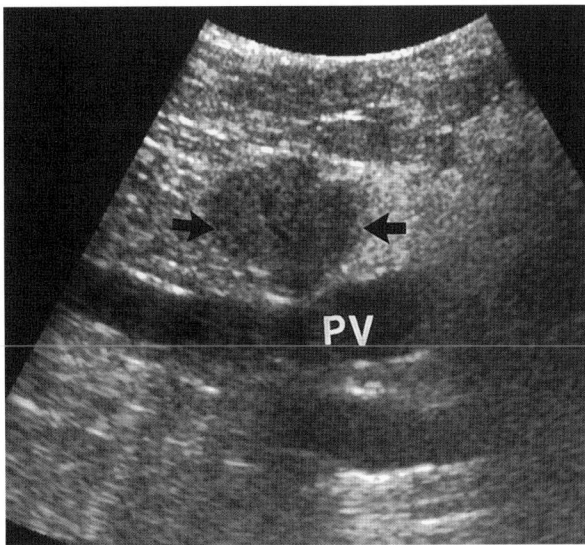

FIGURE 20-37. Laparoscopic ultrasound— lymphadenopathy. Scan in the porta hepatis demonstrates metastatic lymphadenopathy (*arrows*) anterior to the portal vein (PV) in a patient with gallbladder carcinoma.

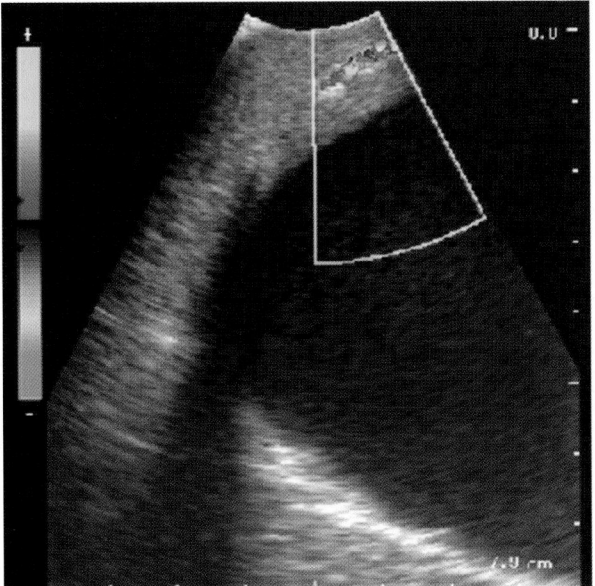

FIGURE 20-36. Laparoscopic ultrasound—giant hepatic cyst. Color flow laparoscopic ultrasound (LUS) is utilized to depict major hepatic vasculature and to find an avascular plane through which the surgeon can safely perform a cyst fenestration.

common bile duct pathology was detected in only five (approximately 3%).[96] In our experience, if there are any clinical, laboratory, or imaging findings suspicious for common bile duct pathology during the preoperative work-up of patients with gallstones, these patients are referred immediately for ERCP prior to laparoscopic cholecystectomy. If stones are demonstrated on the ERCP study, sphincterotomy and stone extraction techniques are performed and, in most cases, the patient may still undergo successful laparoscopic cholecystectomy.[97]

LUS may play a role in other types of biliary pathology. Because long-term survival is so poor in patients with **gallbladder carcinoma**, it would be appropriate to perform laparoscopic assessment for metastatic disease in the liver, adjacent lymph nodes, or peritoneal surfaces in order to avoid unnecessary and unsuccessful laparotomy (Fig. 20-37). Tumors of the biliary tract, such as **cholangiocarcinoma,** and inflammatory conditions, such as **sclerosing cholangitis** (Fig. 20-38), and **oriental cholangiohepatitis** may also benefit from LUS evaluation to assess for extent of tumor, site of intrahepatic bile duct dilation, potential for surgical bypass procedures and location of obstructed ducts, stones, and periductal infected collections for drainage. Van Delden et al.[98] found that LUS led to a change in diagnosis of tumor stage in 23% of patients with proximal bile duct tumors and to avoidance of laparotomy in 9% of patients. However, Tilleman et al.[99] felt that most of the benefit was attributed to laparoscopy with only a limited additional benefit from LUS.

Pancreas

LUS has been advocated for evaluation and staging of cancer of the pancreas and periampullary region. In one series of 70 patients with presumed stage 1 cancer of the head of the pancreas, 21 of this group proved to have distant metastases, and 16 of the 21 were detected by

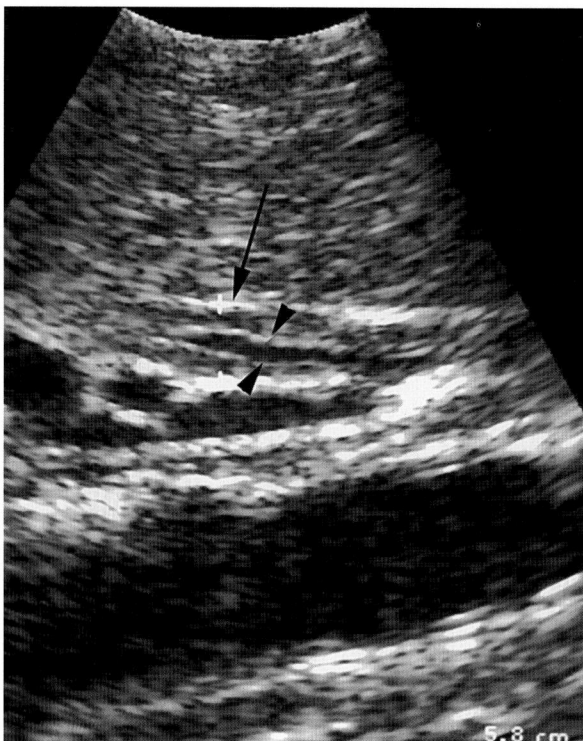

FIGURE 20-38. Laparoscopic ultrasound—sclerosing cholangitis. Scan demonstrates diffuse wall thickening of the common bile duct (*arrow*) with a barely visible narrowed lumen (*arrowheads*).

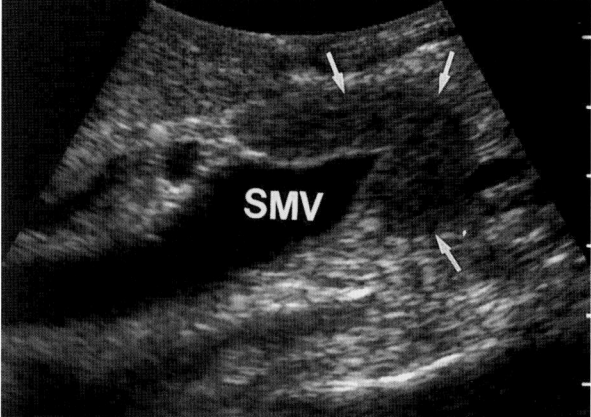

FIGURE 20-39. Laparoscopic ultrasound—unresectable pancreatic carcinoma (arrows). Sagittal scan shows encasement of the superior mesenteric vein (SMV) just distal to the confluence, an indication of unresectability.

laparoscopy and LUS. Three patients of this group had liver metastases missed at the dome of the liver, all of which were less than 5 mm in size, and two patients had lymph node metastases at the celiac axis that were missed by LUS. The authors also noted a 93% positive predictive value for vascular invasion by LUS but a sensitivity of only 59%. In this series, preoperative stage was upgraded in 41% and laparotomy was avoided in 19%.[100] A second study of 40 patients with cancer of the pancreatic head or periampullary region showed similar findings in which laparoscopy with LUS demonstrated occult metastatic disease in 35%. The addition of sonography to laparoscopy increased specificity for predicting tumor resectability.[101]

LUS may detect unresectability due to liver metastases, lymph node metastases, and direct vascular invasion of the portal vein or the superior mesenteric vein (Fig. 20-39). While these findings can be assessed by preoperative ultrasound and other imaging studies, the increased resolution available by LUS techniques can undoubtedly increase the detection rate for small liver metastases. Whether the accuracy for detection of lymphadenopathy is increased remains a subject of dispute because there are no conclusive documentation studies. One prospective study of 50 patients by Pietrabissa et al.[102] found that laparoscopy alone prevented unnecessary laparotomy in 20% of cases and

that LUS was slightly better at assessing inoperability due to critical vascular invasion when compared to preoperative CT. LUS also detected liver nodules in four patients, not seen on preoperative CT, but these proved subsequently to be due to benign conditions. There were also incomplete studies in 6% of patients due to technical difficulties from adhesions or intraperitoneal spread of tumor. These authors conclude that LUS may be useful, but only when there remains uncertainty about vascular invasion. Further studies will hopefully better define the precise role of laparoscopy and ultrasound in evaluation of patients with cancer of the pancreas.

Thus far, there has been very little, if any, experience with the use of LUS in patients with nonmalignant pancreatic disease. But LUS guidance for minimally invasive approaches to pseudocyst drainage might prove useful.

Other Uses

There are some reports in the literature of LUS for **staging of hollow viscous tumors**. One report of 56 patients with carcinoma of the esophagus and cardia, who were undergoing laparoscopy for assessment of peritoneal metastases, also had LUS of the liver and celiac lymph nodes. In 5% of patients, the laparotomy was canceled secondary to metastatic disease, and an additional 5% of patients with metastases were suspected but required laparotomy to confirm with biopsy. In one patient, LUS missed a liver metastasis in segment 7. Out of this combined group, the preoperative stage was changed, and metastases were detected primarily in patients with cancer of the stomach and rarely in patients with esophageal cancer.[103] In another report of a mixed group of 40 patients with upper gastrointestinal tumors, laparoscopy added information in 40%, including finding peritoneal, liver, and nodal metastases.[104] In a subgroup of 20 of these patients, LUS led to a stage change in seven (35%) by detecting liver metastases in three and lymph node metastases in four. In another report by Gouma et al.,[105] while the preoperative stage was changed in 17% of 56 patients, a formal laparotomy could only be avoided in 5%, making this of limited use. Part of the problem was the inability to confirm by biopsy the nature of the lesions detected by laparoscopy and LUS, which could be diagnosed only as metastases by biopsy during an open procedure.

A report was also published on the use of LUS to **localize stones** in a patient undergoing laparoscopic nephrolithotomy. Color flow Doppler via the LUS device was also useful for identifying an area of minimal vascularity to select for the cortical incision site, thereby hopefully minimizing renal cortical tissue damage.[106] LUS has also been described for use in gynecologic surgical procedures, particularly in evaluation of **hydrosalpinx**.[91]

The precise role and utility of laparoscopic sonography is not yet fully determined. Clearly, it is most promising in liver and pancreatic imaging. Demand for LUS is growing as more surgeons are performing minimally invasive procedures. Further technologic improvement in ultrasound equipment is expected. Larger crystal size or length would facilitate imaging larger areas of anatomy with each sweep and thereby shorten the rather lengthy examination times, which should lead to a more effective examination. Some new work integrating a virtual CT image with laparoscopic real-time ultrasound shows considerable promise in improving the orientation of the surgeon or sonographer to fixed landmarks in the pancreas. This is in the early developmental stages and shows considerable promise.[107] Real-time biopsy guides affixed to the transducer would be a notable advance because many lesions are now difficult, if not impossible, to biopsy freehand because of the great distances involved. Accurate real-time image guidance may allow effective biopsies and minimally invasive ablation techniques to be offered more often via the laparoscope. The ultimate role of LUS will depend on these technical innovations.

References

Hepatobiliary System

1. Luck AJ, Maddern GJ: Intraoperative abdominal sonography. Br J Surg 1999;86(1):5-16.
2. Machi J: Intraoperative and laparoscopic ultrasound. Surg Oncol Clin N Am 1999;8(1):205-226.
3. Kane RA, Hughes LA, Cua EJ, et al: The impact of intraoperative sonography on surgery for liver neoplasms. J Ultrasound Med 1994;13:1-6.
4. Boldrini G, DeGaetano AM, Giovanni I, et al: The systematic use of operative ultrasound for detection of liver metastasis during colorectal surgery. World J Surg 1987;11:622-627.
5. Eiseman B, Greenlaw RH, Gallagher JQ: Localization of common duct stones by ultrasound. Arch Surg 1965;91:195-199.
6. Knight PR, Newell JA: Operative use of ultrasonics in cholelithiasis. Lancet 1963;1:1023-1025.
7. Mack LA, Lee RA, Nyberg DA: Intraoperative sonography of the abdomen. In Rumack CM, Wilson SR, Charboneau JW (eds): Diagnostic Ultrasound, St Louis, Mosby-Year Book, 1991, pp 492-504.
8. Kane RA: Intraoperative ultrasound. In Wilson SR, Charboneau JW, Leopold GR (eds): Ultrasound: Categorical Course Syllabus. Presented at the American Roentgen Ray Society 93rd Annual Meeting, 1993, San Francisco.
9. Kruskal JB, Kane RA: Intraoperative sonography of the liver. Crit Rev Diagn Imaging 1995;36(3):175-226.
10. Reading CC: Intraoperative sonography. Abdom Imaging 1996;21:21-29.
11. Angelini L, Papaspyropoulos V: Robotics and telecommunication systems to provide better access to ultrasound expertise in the OR. Min Invas Ther 2000;9(3-4):219-224.
12. Foster JH, Ensminger WF: Treatment of metastatic cancer to liver. In Devita VT, Hellman S, Rosenberg SA (eds): Cancer: Principles and Practice of Oncology. Lippincott, Philadelphia, 1985, p 2117.
13. Hughes K, Scheele J, Sugarbaker PH: Surgery for colorectal cancer metastatic to the liver: Optimizing the results of treatment. Surg Clin North Am 1989;69:339-359.
14. Bengmark S, Hafstrom L: The natural course of liver cancer. Prog Clin Cancer 1978;7:195-200.
15. Machi JS, Uchi K, Sumida WM, et al: Ultrasound-guided radiofrequency thermal ablation of liver tumors: Percutaneous, laparoscopic, and open surgical approaches. J Gastro Surg 2001;5(5):477-489.
16. Gaitini D, Kopelman D, Soudak M, et al: Impact of intraoperative sonography on resection and cryoablation of liver tumors. J Clin Ultrasound 2001;29(5):265-272.
17. Pearson AS, Izzo F, Fleming RYD, et al: Intraoperative radiofrequency ablation or cryoablation for hepatic malignancies. Am J Surg 1999;178(6):592-598.
18. Ozsunar Y, Skjoldbye B, Court-Payen M, et al: Impact of intraoperative sonography on surgical treatment of liver tumours. Acta Radiologica 2000;41(1):97-101.
19. Clarke MP, Kane RA, Steele GD, et al: Prospective comparison of preoperative imaging and intraoperative sonography in the detection of liver tumors. Surgery 1989;106:849-855.
20. Parker GA, Lawrence W, Horsley JS, et al: Intraoperative ultrasound of the liver affects operative decision making. Ann Surg 1989;209:569-588.
21. Wernecke K, Rummeny E, Bongartz G, et al: Detection of hepatic masses in patients with carcinoma: Comparative sensitivities of sonography, CT, and MR imaging. AJR 1991;157:731-739.
22. Sitzmann JV, Coleman J, Pitt HA, et al: Preoperative assessment of malignant hepatic tumors. Am J Surg 1990;159:137-143.
23. Machi J, Isomoto H, Kurohiji T, et al: Accuracy of intraoperative sonography in diagnosing liver metastasis from colorectal cancer: Evaluation with postoperative follow-up results. World J Surg 1991;15:551-557.
24. Igawa S, Sakai K, Kinoshita H, et al: Intraoperative sonography: Clinical usefulness in liver surgery. Radiology 1985;156:473.
25. Gozzetti G, Mazziotti A, Bolondi L, et al: Intraoperative sonography in surgery for liver tumors. Surgery 1986;99:523.

26. Cervone A, Sardi A, Conaway GL: Intraoperative ultrasound (IOUS) is essential in the management of metastatic colorectal liver lesions. Am Surg 2000;66(7):611-615.

27. Bloed W, Van Leeuwen MS, Borel Rinkes IH: Role of intraoperative ultrasound of the liver with improved preoperative hepatic imaging. Eur J Surg 2000;166(9):691-695.

28. Sheu JC, Lee CS, Sung JL, et al: Intraoperative hepatic sonography: An indispensable procedure in resection of small hepatocellular carcinoma. Surgery 1985;97:97-193.

29. Jin-Chuan, Chue-Shue L, Jeui-Low S, et al: Hepatic sonography: An indispensable procedure in resection of small hepatocellular carcinomas. Surgery 1987; 97-103.

30. Waldman DL, Lee DE, Bronsther O, et al: Use of intraoperative sonography during hepatic transplantation. J Ultrasound Med 1998;17(1):1-8.

31. Cheng YF, Huang TL, Chen CL: Intraoperative Doppler ultrasound in liver transplantation. Clin Trans 1998;12(4):292-299.

32. Jakimowicz JJ, Rutten H, Jurgens PJ, et al: Comparison of operative sonography and radiography in screening of the common bile duct for calculi. World J Surg 1987;11:628-634.

33. Dunnington GL: Intraoperative sonography in abdominal surgery. Surg Ann 1993;24:101-125.

34. Sigel B, Machi J, Anderson KW, et al: Operative sonography of the biliary tree and pancreas. Semin Ultrasound CT MRI 1985;6:2-4.

35. Mack LA, Nyberg DA: Intraoperative sonography of the gallbladder and biliary act. In Rifkin MD (ed): Intraoperative and Endoscopic Sonography. New York, Churchill Livingstone, 1987, pp 105-120.

36. Herbst CA, Mittlestaedt CA, Staab EV, et al: Intraoperative sonography evaluation of the gallbladder in morbidly obese patients. Ann Surg 1984;200:691-692.

37. Oria HE: Pitfalls in the diagnosis of gallbladder disease in clinically severe obesity. Obes Surg 1998;8(4):444-451.

38. Shaikh I, Iqbal P, Mohammad S: Intraoperative sonography at open cholecystectomy to assess common bile duct for stones. J Col Phy & Surg Pakistan 2000;10(5):173-174.

39. Kusano T, Shimabukuro M, Tamai O, et al: The use of intraoperative sonography for detecting tumor extension in bile duct carcinoma. Int Surg 1997;82(1):44-48.

40. Azuma T, Yoshikawa T, Araida T, et al: Intraoperative evaluation of the depth of invasion of gallbladder cancer. Am J Surg 1999;178(5):381-384.

41. Charnsangavej C: Pancreatic duct adenocarcinoma: Diagnosis and staging by CT and MR imaging. In Freeny PC: Radiology of the liver, biliary tract, and pancreas. Categorical course syllabus. American Roentgen Ray Society, 1996, pp 165-171.

42. Trede M, Schwall G, Saeger HD: Survival after pancreatoduodenectomy. Ann Surg 1990;211:447-458.

43. Cameron JL, Crist DW, Sitzman, JV, et al: Factors influencing survival after pancreatoduodenectomy for pancreatic cancer. Am J Surg 1991;165:68-73.

44. Geer RJ, Brennan MF: Prognostic indicators for survival after resection of pancreatic adenocarcinoma. Am J Surg 1993;165:68-73.

45. Douglass HO, Jr, Tepper J, Leichman L: Neoplasms of the exocrine pancreas. In Holland JF, Frei E, 3rd, Bast RC, Jr, et al: (eds): Cancer Medicine. Philadelphia, Lea & Febiger, 1993, pp 1466-1484.

46. Rifkin MD, Weiss SM: Intraoperative sonographic identification of nonpalpable pancreatic masses. J Ultrasound Med 1984;3:409-411.

47. Sigel B, Machi J, Ramos JR, et al: The role of imaging ultrasound during pancreatic surgery. Ann Surg 1984;200(4):486-493.

48. Serio G, Fugazzola C, Iacono C, et al: Intraoperative sonography in pancreatic cancer. Int J Pancreatol 1992;11(1):31-41.

49. Freeny P: Radiologic imaging of chronic pancreatitis. In Freeny PC (ed.): Radiology of the liver, biliary tract, and pancreas. Categorical course syllabus. American Roentgen Ray Society, 1996, pp 157-163.

50. Printz H, Klotter JH, Nies C, et al: Intraoperative sonography in surgery for chronic pancreatitis. Int J Pancreatol 1992;12(3):233-237.

51. Back MR, Sandra M, Dempsey ME, et al: Intraoperative ultrasound assessment in management of complex pancreatic pseudocysts. Surg Endosc 1997;11(11):1126-1128.

52. Gorman B, Reading C: Imaging of gastrointestinal neuroendocrine tumors. In Freeny PC (ed.): Radiology of the liver, biliary tract, and pancreas. Categorical course syllabus. American Roentgen Ray Society, 1996, pp 191-198.

53. Gorman B, Charboneau JW, James EM, et al: Benign pancreatic insulinomas: Preoperative and intraoperative sonographic localization. AJR 1986;147:929-934.

54. Zeiger MA, Shawker TH, Norton JA: Use of intraoperative sonography to localize islet cell tumors. World J Surg 1993;174:448-454.

55. Bottger TC, Junginger T: Is preoperative radiographic localization of islet cell tumors in patients with insulinoma necessary? World J Surg 1993;17:427-432.

56. VanHeerden JA, Grant CS, Czako PF, et al: Occult functioning insulinomas: Which localizing studies are indicated? Surgery 1992;112(6):1010-1014.

57. Charboneau JW, Gorman B, Reading CC, et al: Intraoperative sonography of pancreatic endocrine tumors. Clinics in Diagnostic Ultrasound—Intraoperative and Endoscopic Ultrasound. 7(22):123-134, 1987.

58. Huai JC, Zhang W, Niu HO, et al: Localization and surgical treatment of pancreatic insulinomas guided by intraoperative ultrasound. Am J Surg 1998;175(1):18-21.

59. Sugg SL, Norton SL, Fraker DL, et al: A prospective study of intraoperative methods to diagnose and resect duodenal gastrinomas. Ann Surg 1993;218(2):138-144.

60. Stabile BE, Morrow DJ, Passaro E, Jr: The gastrinoma triangle: Operative implications. Am J Surg 1984;147:25-31.

61. Kisker O, Bastian D, Bartsch D, et al: Localization, malignant potential, and surgical management of gastrinomas. World J Surg 1998;22(7):651-658.

62. Davies PF, Shevland JE, Shepherd JJ: Sonography of the pancreas in patients with MEN I. J Ultrasound Med 1993;12(2):67-72.

Renal

63. Polascik TJ, Meng MV, Epstein JI, et al: Intraoperative sonography for the evaluation and management of renal tumors: Experience with 100 patients. J Urol 1995;154:1676-1680.

64. Walther MM, Choyke PL, Hayes W, et al: Evaluation of color Doppler intraoperative ultrasound in parenchymal sparing renal surgery. J Urol 1994;152:1984-1987.

65. Morgan WR, Zincke H: Progression and survival after renal-conserving surgery for renal cell carcinoma:

Experience in 104 patients and extended followup. J Urol 1990;144:852-858.

66. Steinbach F, Stöckle M, Müller SC, et al: Conservative surgery of renal cell tumors in 140 patients: 21 Years of experience. J Urol 1992;148:24-30.

67. Campbell SC, Novick AC, Streem SB, et al: Complications of nephron sparing surgery for renal tumors. J Urol 1994;151:1177.

68. Carini M, Selli C, Barbanti G, et al: Conservative surgical treatment of renal cell carcinoma: Clinical experience and reappraisal of indications. J Urol 1988;140:725-731.

69. Novick AC, Streem S, Montie JE, et al: Conservative surgery for renal cell carcinoma: A single-center experience with 100 patients. J Urol 1989;141:835-839.

70. Zincke H, Engen DE, Henning KM, et al: Treatment of renal cell carcinoma by in situ partial nephrectomy and extracorporeal operation with autotransplantation. Mayo Clin Proc 1985;60:651-662.

71. Novick AC, Zincke H, Neves RJ, et al: Surgical enucleation for renal cell carcinoma. J Urol 1986;135:235-238.

72. Smith RB, DeKernian JB, Ehrlich RM, et al: Bilateral renal cell carcinoma and renal cell carcinoma in the solitary kidney. J Urol 1984;132:450-454.

73. Topley M, Novick AC, Montie JE: Long-term results following partial nephrectomy for localized renal adenocarcinoma. J Urol 1984;131:1050-1052.

74. Blackley SK, Ladaga L, Woolfitt RA, et al: Ex situ study of the effectiveness of enucleation in patients with renal cell carcinoma. J Urol 1988;140:6-10.

75. Marshall FF, Taxy JB, Fishman EK, et al: The feasibility of surgical enucleation for renal cell carcinoma. J Urol 1986;135:231-234.

76. Mukamel E, Konichezky M, Engelstein D, et al: Incidental small renal tumors accompanying clinically overt renal cell carcinoma. J Urol 1988;140:22-24.

77. Gilbert BR, Russo P, Zirinsky K, et al: Intraoperative sonography: Application in renal cell carcinoma. J Urol 1988;139:582-584.

78. Choyke PL, Pavlovich CP, Daryanani KD, et al: Intraoperative ultrasound during renal parenchymal sparing surgery for hereditary renal cancers: A 10-year experience. J Urol 2001;165(2):397-400.

79. Dougherty MJ, Hallett JW, Naessens JM, et al: Optimizing technical success of renal revascularization: The impact of intraoperative color flow duplex sonography. J Vasc Surg 1993;7:849-857.

80. Lantz EJ, Charboneau JW, Hallett JW, et al: Intraoperative color Doppler sonography during renal artery revascularization. AJR 1994;162:859-863.

81. Van Weel V, Van Bockel JH, Van Wissen, et al: Intraoperative renal duplex sonography: A valuable method for evaluating renal artery reconstructions. Eur J Vasc & Endovasc Surg 2000;20(3):268-272.

82. Yamakawa K, Naito S, Azuma K, et al: Laparoscopic diagnosis of the intra-abdominal organs. Jpn J Gastroenterol 1958;55:741-747.

Laparoscopic Sonography

83. Yamakawa K, Yoshioka A, Shimizu K, et al: Laparoechography: An ultrasonic diagnosis under laparoscopic observation. Jpn Med Ultrasonics 1964; 2:26.

84. Fukuda M, Mima S, Tanabe T, et al: Endoscopic sonography of the liver: Diagnostic application of the echolaparoscope to localize intrahepatic lesions. Scand J Gastroenterol Suppl 1984;102:24-38.

85. Frank K, Bliesze H, Honhof JA, et al: Laparoscopic sonography: A new approach to intra-abdominal disease. J Clin Ultrasound 1985;13:60-65.

86. Fornari F, Civardi G, Cavanna L, et al: Laparoscopic sonography in the study of liver diseases. Surg Endosc 1989;3:33-37.

87. Goldberg BB, Liu JB, Merton DA, et al: Sonographically guided laparoscopy and mediastinoscopy using miniature catheter-based transducers. J Ultrasound Med 1993;12:49-54.

88. Sammons LG, Kane RA: Technical aspects of intraoperative ultrasound. In Kane RA (ed): Intraoperative, Laparoscopic, and Endoluminal Ultrasound. Philadelphia, Churchill Livingstone, WB Saunders, 1999, pp 1-11.

89. Babineau TJ, Lewis WD, Jenkins RJ, et al: Role of staging laparoscopy in the treatment of hepatic malignancy. Am J Surg 1994;167:151-155.

90. Kane RA, Hughes LA, Cua EJ, et al: The impact of intraoperative sonography on surgery for liver neoplasms. J Ultrasound Med 1994;13:1-6.

91. Liu JB, Feld RI, Goldberg BB, et al: Laparoscopic gray-scale and color Doppler US: Preliminary animal and clinical studies. Radiology 1995;194:851-857.

92. John TG, Greig JD, Crosbie JL, et al: Superior staging of liver tumors with laparoscopy and laparoscopic ultrasound. Ann Surg 1994;220:711-719.

93. Barbot DJ, Marks JH, Feld RI, et al: Improved staging of liver tumors using laparoscopic intraoperative ultrasound. J Surg Oncol 1997;64:63-67.

94. Catheline J-M, Turner R, Champault G: Laparoscopic ultrasound of the liver. Eur J Ultrasound 2000;12:169-177.

95. Hartley JE, Kumar H, Drew PJ, et al: Laparoscopic ultrasound for the detection of hepatic metastases during laparoscopic colorectal cancer surgery. Dis Colon Rectum 2000;43:320-324.

96. Jakimowicz J: Technical and clinical aspects of intraoperative ultrasound applicable to laparoscopic ultrasound. Endosc Surg Allied Technol 1994; 2:119-126.

97. Kane RA: Laparoscopic Ultrasound. In Kane RA (ed): Intraoperative, Laparoscopic, and Endoluminal Ultrasound. Philadelphia, Churchill Livingstone, 1999, pp 90-105.

98. Van Delden OM, De Wit LT, Nieveen Van Dijkum EJ, et al: Value of laparoscopic sonography in staging of proximal bile duct tumors. J Ultrasound Med 1997;16:7-12.

99. Tilleman E, DeCastro S, Busch O, TM, et al: Diagnostic laparoscopy and laparoscopic ultrasound for staging of patients with malignant proximal bile duct obstruction. J Gastrointest Surg 2002;6:426-430.

100. Bemelman WA, DeWit LT, Van Delden OM, et al: Diagnostic laparoscopy combined with laparoscopic sonography in staging of cancer of the pancreatic head region. Br J Surg 1995;82:820-824.

101. John TG, Greig JD, Carter DC, Garden OJ: Carcinoma of the pancreatic head and periampullary region: Tumor staging with laparoscopy and laparoscopic sonography. Ann Surg 1995;22:156-164.

102. Pietrabissa A, Caramella D, Di Candio G, et al: Laparoscopy and laparoscopic sonography for staging pancreatic cancer: Critical appraisal. World J Surg 1999;23:998-1002.

103. Bemelman WA, Van Delden OM, Van Lanschot JJB, et al: Laparoscopy and laparoscopic sonography in staging of carcinoma of the esophagus and gastric cardia. J Am Coll Surg 1995;181:421-425.

104. Hünerbein M, Rau B, Schlag PM: Laparoscopy and laparoscopic ultrasound for staging of upper gastrointestinal tumours. Eur J Surg Oncol 1995;21:50-55.

105. Gouma DJ, De Wit T, Van Dijkum EN, et al: Laparoscopic sonography for staging of gastrointestinal malignancy. Scan J Gastroenterol Suppl 1996;218:43-49.

106. Van Cangh P, Abi Aad AS, Lorge F, et al: Laparoscopic nephrolithotomy: The value of intracorporeal sonography and color doppler. Urology 1995;45:516-519.

107. Ellsmere J, Stoll J, Rattner D, et al: Integrating preoperative CT data with laparoscopic ultrasound images facilitates interpretation. Surg Endosc 2002, in press.

IV

SMALL PARTS, CAROTID ARTERY, AND PERIPHERAL VESSEL SONOGRAPHY

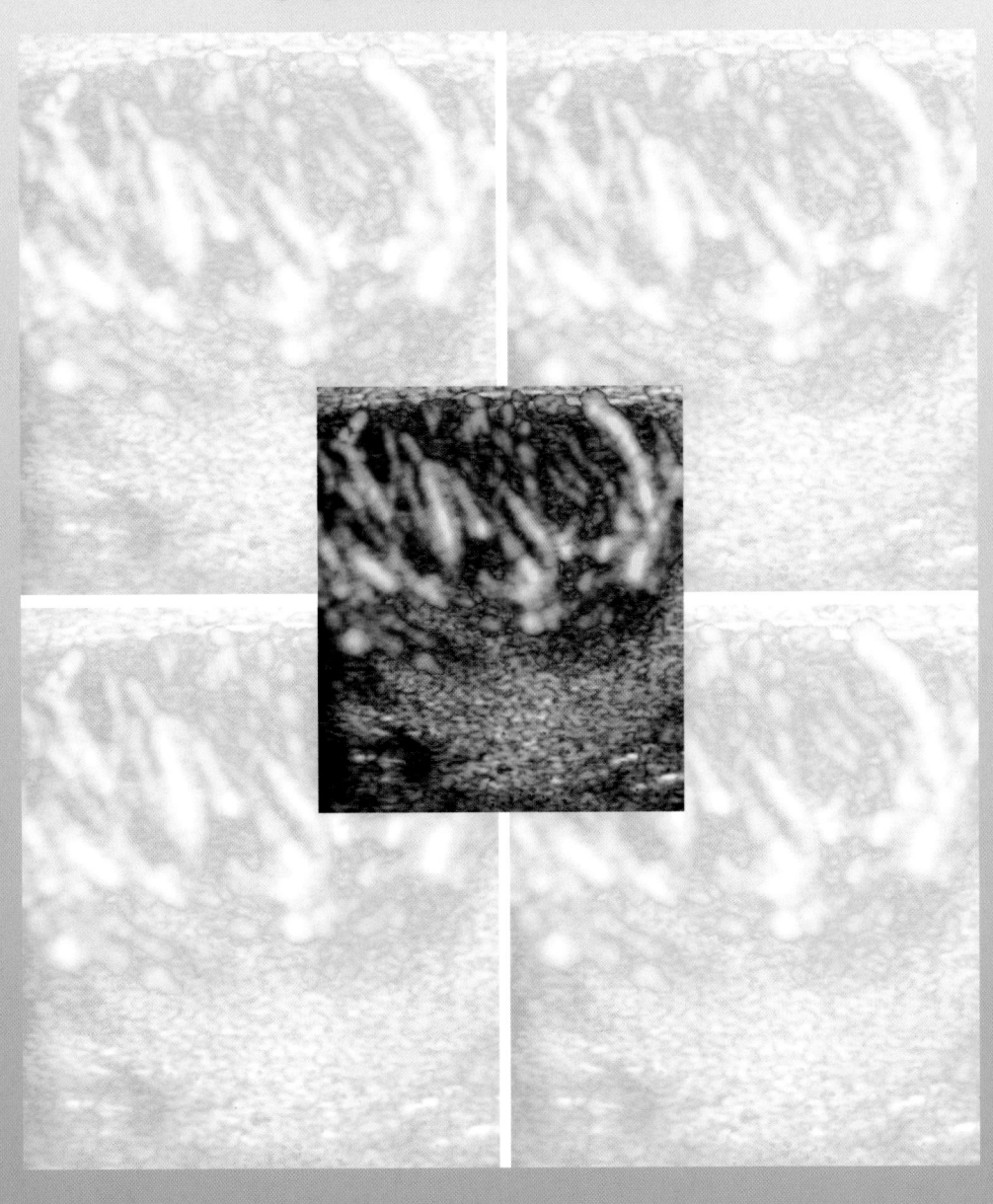

21

THE THYROID GLAND

Luigi Solbiati / J. William Charboneau / Valeria Osti /
E. Meredith James / Ian D. Hay

Chapter Outline

*B*ecause of the superficial location of the thyroid gland, high-resolution real-time gray-scale and color Doppler sonography can demonstrate normal thyroid anatomy and pathologic conditions with remarkable clarity. As a result, this technique has come to play an increasingly important role in the diagnostic evaluation of thyroid diseases. Sonography, however, is only one of several diagnostic methods currently available for use in evaluation of the thyroid. To use it effectively and economically, it is important to understand its current capabilities and limitations.

INSTRUMENTATION AND TECHNIQUE

High-frequency transducers (7.5 to 15.0 MHz) currently provide both deep ultrasound penetration—up to 5 cm—and high-definition images, with a resolution of 0.7 to 1.0 mm. No other imaging method can achieve this degree of spatial resolution. Linear-array transducers are preferred to sector transducers because of the wider near field of view and the ability to combine high-frequency gray-scale and color Doppler images. The

thyroid gland is one of the most vascular organs of the body. As a result, Doppler examination may provide useful diagnostic information in some thyroid diseases. Quite recently, contrast medium–enhanced sonography using second-generation contrast agents (microbubbles containing gas different from air) and gray-scale sonography with nondisruptive imaging (very low mechanical index) is showing promising results for the diagnosis of selected cases of nodular diseases and for the guidance and control of therapeutic ultrasound-guided procedures of the thyroid gland.

The patient is typically examined in the supine position, with the neck extended. A small pad may be placed under the shoulders to provide better exposure of the neck, particularly in patients with a short, stocky habitus. The thyroid gland must be examined thoroughly in both transverse and longitudinal planes. Imaging of the lower poles can be enhanced by asking the patient to swallow, which momentarily raises the thyroid gland in the neck. The entire gland, including the isthmus, must be examined. The examination should also be extended laterally to include the region of the carotid artery and jugular vein to identify enlarged

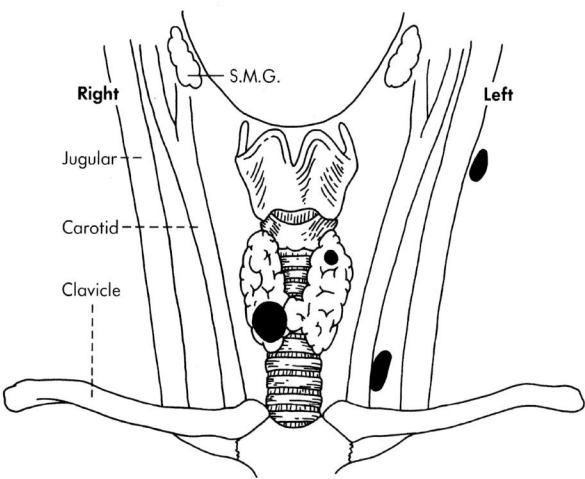

FIGURE 21-1. Cervical "map." A diagram like this helps communicate relationships of pathology to clinicians and serves as a reference for follow-up examinations. S.M.G., submandibular gland.

jugular chain lymph nodes, superiorly to visualize submandibular adenopathy, and inferiorly to define any pathologic supraclavicular lymph nodes.

In addition to the images recorded during the examination, some examiners include in the permanent record a diagrammatic representation of the neck showing the location(s) of any abnormal findings (Fig. 21-1). This cervical "map" helps to communicate the anatomic relationships of the pathology more clearly to the referring clinician and the patient. It also serves as a useful reference for the radiologist and sonographer for follow-up examinations.

ANATOMY

The thyroid gland is located in the anteroinferior part of the neck (infrahyoid compartment) in a space outlined by muscle, trachea, esophagus, carotid arteries, and jugular veins (Fig. 21-2). The thyroid gland is made up of two lobes located along either side of the trachea and connected across the midline by the isthmus, a thin structure draping over the anterior tracheal wall at the level of the junction of the middle and lower thirds of the thyroid gland. From 10% to 40% of normal patients have a small thyroid (pyramidal) lobe arising superiorly from the isthmus and lying in front of the thyroid cartilage.[1] It can be regularly visualized in younger patients, but it undergoes progressive atrophy in adulthood and becomes invisible. The size and shape of the thyroid lobes vary widely in normal patients. In tall individuals the lateral lobes have a longitudinally elongated shape on the sagittal scans, whereas in shorter individuals the gland is more oval. As a result, the normal dimensions of the lobes have a wide range of variability. In the newborn, the gland is 18 to 20 mm long, with an anteroposterior diameter of 8 to 9 mm. By 1 year of age, the mean length is 25 mm and the anteroposterior diameter is 12 to 15 mm.[2] In adults, the mean length is 40 to 60 mm and the mean anteroposterior diameter is 13 to 18 mm. The mean thickness of the isthmus is 4 to 6 mm.[3]

Sonography is an accurate method to use in calculating **thyroid volume.** In approximately one third of cases, the sonographic measurement of volume differs

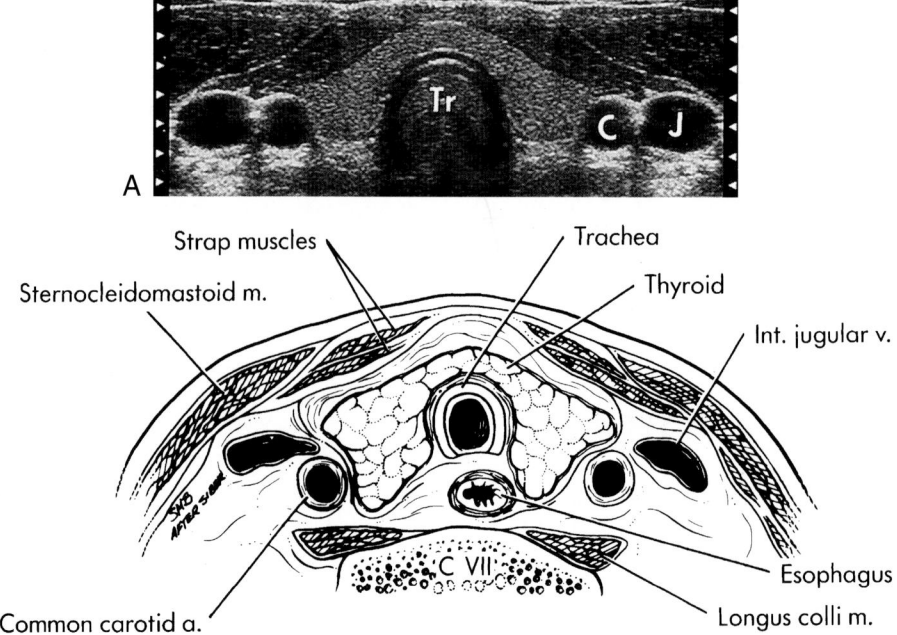

FIGURE 21-2. Normal thyroid gland. A, Transverse sonogram made with 7.5-MHz linear array transducer. **B,** Corresponding anatomic drawing. Tr, tracheal air shadow; C, common carotid artery; J, jugular vein. (From James EM, Charboneau JW: High-frequency (10 MHz) thyroid ultrasonography. Semin Ultrasound, CT, MR 1985;6:294-309.)

from the physical size estimate derived from examination.[4] Thyroid volume measurements may be useful for goiter size determination to assess the need for surgery, to permit calculation of the dose of iodine-131 needed for treating thyrotoxicosis, and to evaluate the response to suppression treatments.[5] Thyroid volume can be calculated with linear parameters or more precisely with mathematical formulas. Among the linear parameters, the anteroposterior diameter is the most precise, because it is relatively independent of possible dimensional asymmetry between the two lobes. When the anteroposterior diameter is more than 2 cm, the thyroid gland may be considered enlarged.

The most common mathematical method to calculate thyroid volume is based on the ellipsoid formula with a correction factor (length × width × thickness × 0.52 for each lobe) (Fig. 21-3). When this method is used the mean estimated error is approximately 15%. The most precise mathematical method is the integration of the cross-sectional areas of the thyroid gland achieved through evenly spaced sonographic scans[6]; with this

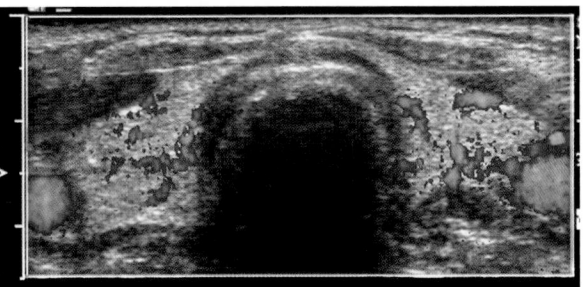

FIGURE 21-4. Normal thyroid vascularity on power Doppler ultrasound.

method the mean estimated error is 5% to 10%.[7] Modern three-dimensional ultrasound technology permits the simultaneous measurement of the three orthogonal planes of thyroid lobes, thus allowing the calculation of the volume either automatically or manually.[8]

The normal mean thyroid volume is 18.6 ± 4.5 mL (± SD), and this converts to an 18.6-g gland.[6] There is a significant difference in volume between males (19.6 ± 4.7 mL) and females (17.5 ± 4.2 mL). Thyroid volume is generally larger in patients living in regions with iodine deficiency and in patients who have acute hepatitis or chronic renal failure; it is smaller in patients who have chronic hepatitis or have been treated with thyroxine or radioactive iodine.[5,6]

Normal thyroid parenchyma has a homogeneous medium- to high-level echogenicity that makes detection of focal cystic or hypoechoic thyroid lesions relatively easy in most cases (see Fig. 21-2). The thin hyperechoic line that bounds the thyroid lobes is the capsule, which is often identifiable by ultrasound. It may become calcified in patients who have uremia or disorders of calcium metabolism. With currently available high-sensitivity Doppler instruments, the rich vascularity of the gland can be seen (Fig. 21-4). The **superior thyroid artery and vein** are found at the upper pole of each lobe. The **inferior thyroid vein** is found at the lower pole, and the **inferior thyroid artery** is located posterior to the lower third of each lobe (Fig. 21-5). The mean diameter of the arteries is 1 to 2 mm, whereas the lower veins can be up to 8 mm in diameter. Normally, peak systolic velocities reach 20 to 40 cm/sec in the major thyroid arteries and 15 to 30 cm/sec in intraparenchymal arteries. It should be noted that these are the highest velocities found in blood vessels supplying superficial organs.

The **sternohyoid** and **omohyoid muscles** are seen as thin, hypoechoic bands anterior to the thyroid gland (see Fig. 21-2). The **sternocleidomastoid muscle** is seen as a larger oval band that lies lateral to the thyroid gland. An important anatomic landmark is the **longus colli muscle** that is located posterior to each thyroid lobe, in close contact with the prevertebral space.

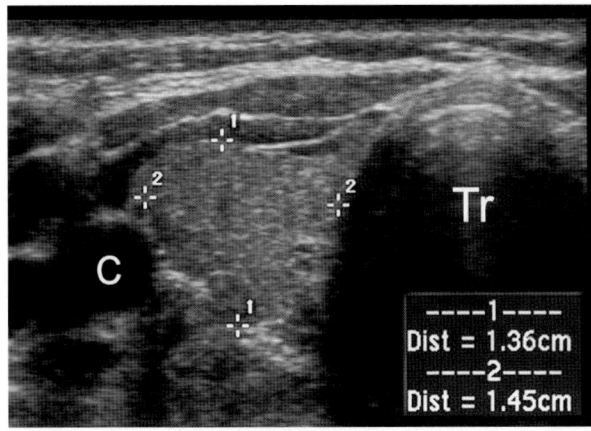

A

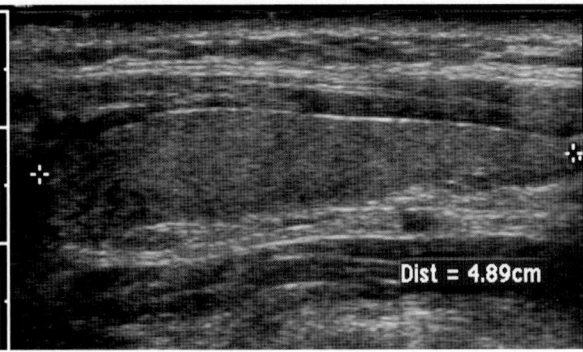

B

FIGURE 21-3. Volume measurement of thyroid gland. Transverse (**A**) and longitudinal (**B**) images show calipers at the boundaries of the gland. Tr, tracheal air shadow; C, carotid artery. The calculated thyroid volume is based on the ellipsoid formula with a correction factor (length × width × thickness × 0.52 for each lobe). In this case, the volume is 10 mL (or grams), which is within normal limits for this female.

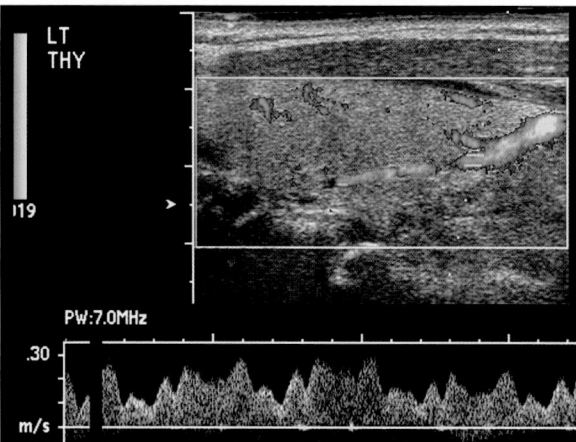

FIGURE 21-5. Normal inferior thyroid vein.
Longitudinal power Doppler image shows a large inferior thyroid vein with associated normal venous spectral waveform.

The **recurrent laryngeal nerve** and the **inferior thyroid artery pass** in the angle between the trachea, esophagus, and thyroid lobe. On longitudinal scans, the recurrent laryngeal nerve and inferior thyroid artery may be seen between the thyroid lobe and esophagus on the left and the thyroid lobe and longus colli muscle on the right. The **esophagus,** primarily a midline structure, may be found laterally and is usually on the left side. It is clearly identified by the target appearance of bowel in the transverse plane and by its peristaltic movements when the patient swallows.

CONGENITAL THYROID ABNORMALITIES

Congenital conditions of the thyroid gland include **agenesis** of one lobe or the whole gland, varying degrees of **hypoplasia,** and ectopia. Sonography can be used to help establish the diagnosis of hypoplasia by demonstrating a diminutively sized gland. High-frequency ultrasound can also be used in the study of **congenital hypothyroidism.**[9] Measurement of thyroid lobes can be used to differentiate agenesis (absent gland) from goitrous hypothyroidism (gland enlargement). Radionuclide scans are more commonly used to detect ectopic thyroid tissue (e.g., in a lingual or suprahyoid position).

NODULAR THYROID DISEASE

Many thyroid diseases can present clinically with one or more thyroid nodules. Such nodules represent common and controversial clinical problems. Epidemiologic studies estimate that between 4% and 7% of the adult population in the United States have palpable thyroid nodules, with women being more frequently affected

than men.[10,11] Exposure to ionizing radiation increases the incidence of benign and malignant nodules, with 20% to 30% of a radiation-exposed population having palpable thyroid disease.[12,13]

Although nodular thyroid disease is relatively common, thyroid cancer is rare and accounts for less than 1% of all malignant neoplasms.[14] In fact, the overwhelming majority of thyroid nodules are benign. The clinical challenge is to distinguish the few clinically significant malignant nodules from the many benign ones and, thus, to identify those patients for whom surgical excision is genuinely indicated. This task is complicated by the fact that much of the nodular disease of the thyroid gland is clinically occult (less than 10 to 15 mm) but can be readily detected by high-resolution sonography. The question of how to manage these small nodules discovered incidentally by sonography is an important one and is addressed later in this chapter.

Pathologic Features and Sonographic Correlates

Hyperplasia and Goiter

Approximately 80% of nodular thyroid disease is due to **hyperplasia** of the gland, and it occurs in up to 5% of any population.[15] Its etiology includes **iodine deficiency** (endemic), **disorders of hormonogenesis** (hereditary familial forms), and **poor utilization of iodine** as a result of medication. When hyperplasia leads to an overall increase in size or volume of the gland, the term *goiter* is used. The peak age of patients with goiter is between 35 and 50 years, and women are three times more likely than men to have the disease.

Histologically, the initial stage is cellular hyperplasia of the thyroid acini, which is followed by micronodule and macronodule formation. Hyperplastic nodules often undergo liquefactive degeneration with the accumulation of blood, serous fluid, and colloid substance. Pathologically, they are often referred to as **hyperplastic, adenomatous, or colloid nodules.** Many (if not all) cystic thyroid lesions are hyperplastic nodules that have undergone extensive liquefactive degeneration. Pathologically, true epithelial-lined cysts of the thyroid gland are rare. In the course of this cystic degenerative process, calcification, which is often coarse and perinodular, may occur.[5,16] Hyperplastic nodule function may be decreased, normal, or increased (toxic nodules).

Sonographically, most hyperplastic or adenomatous nodules are **isoechoic** compared with normal thyroid tissue (Fig. 21-6). As the size of the mass increases, it may become hyperechoic, owing to the numerous interfaces between cells and colloid substance.[5,17] Less frequently, a hypoechoic spongelike or **honeycomb pattern** is seen (Fig. 21-7). When the nodule is isoechoic or hyperechoic, a thin peripheral **hypoechoic halo** is

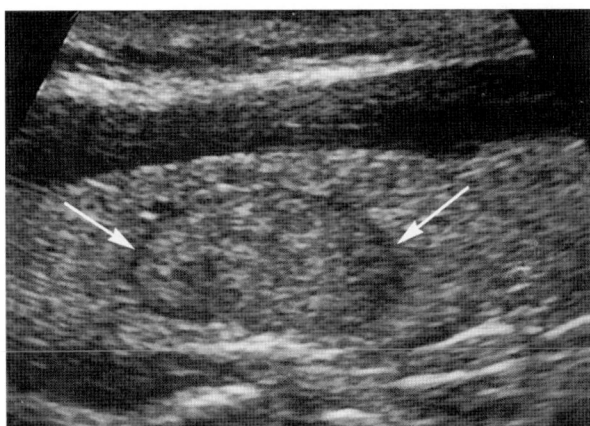

FIGURE 21-6. Hyperplastic (adenomatous) nodule. Oval homogeneous isoechoic nodule *(arrows)* with thin and uniform halo.

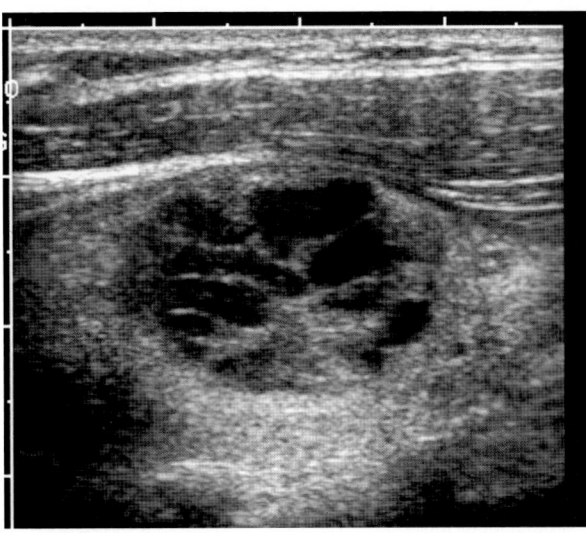

A

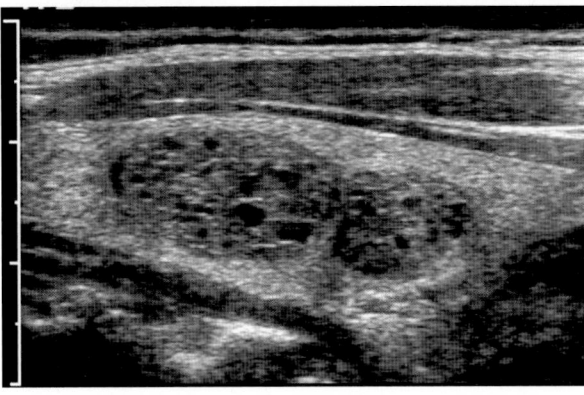

B

FIGURE 21-7. Benign nodule feature. A and **B,** Large amounts of honeycomb appearance or cystic change. These features indicate a very high probability of a benign process. Longitudinal images show a "honeycomb" cystic appearance with larger cystic spaces seen in **A** and smaller cystic spaces seen in the nodules shown in **B.**

common (see Fig. 21-6); it is most likely due to perinodular blood vessels and mild edema or compression of the adjacent normal parenchyma. Perinodular blood vessels are typically detected with the use of color Doppler sonography, but with current high-sensitivity Doppler technology intranodular vascularity can also be seen.[5,18,19] Hyperfunctioning (autonomous) nodules usually exhibit an abundant perinodular and intranodular vascularity.[18,19]

The degenerative changes of goitrous nodules correspond to their sonographic appearances (Fig. 21-8). Purely anechoic areas are caused by **serous or colloid fluid.** Echogenic fluid or moving fluid-fluid levels correspond to **hemorrhage.**[20] Bright echogenic foci with comet-tail artifacts are likely due to the presence of **microcrystals.**[21] Intracystic, **thin septations** probably correspond to attenuated strands of thyroid tissue and appear completely avascular on Doppler analysis. These degenerative processes may also lead to the formation of **calcification,** which may be either thin peripheral shells (**eggshell**) or **coarse,** highly reflective foci with associated acoustic shadows, scattered throughout the gland (Fig. 21-9).[7]

Intracystic solid projections, or papillae, usually containing color Doppler signals, may be encountered, and this appearance can be similar to that of the rare cystic papillary thyroid carcinoma.[18,19] Sometimes sonography and color Doppler imaging cannot differentiate the septations of colloid hyperplastic nodules from the vegetations seen in papillary carcinomas; before moving to aspiration cytology studies, contrast medium–enhanced sonography with second-generation microbubbles and nondisruptive imaging can be used. Benign septa do not show enhancement (and "disappear" in harmonic mode), whereas malignant vegetations show intense enhancement in arterial phase with relatively fast washout.

Adenoma

Adenomas represent only 5% to 10% of all nodular disease of the thyroid and are seven times more common in females than in males.[5] Most result in no thyroid dysfunction; a minority (probably <10%) hyperfunction, develop autonomy, and may cause thyrotoxicosis. Most adenomas are solitary, but they may also develop as part of a multinodular process.

The **benign follicular adenoma** is a true thyroid neoplasm that is characterized by compression of adjacent tissues and fibrous encapsulation. Various subtypes of follicular adenoma include the fetal adenoma, Hürthle cell adenoma, and embryonal adenoma, each distinguished according to the character and pattern of cell proliferation. The cytologic features of follicular adenomas are generally indistinguishable from those of follicular carcinoma. Vascular and capsular invasion

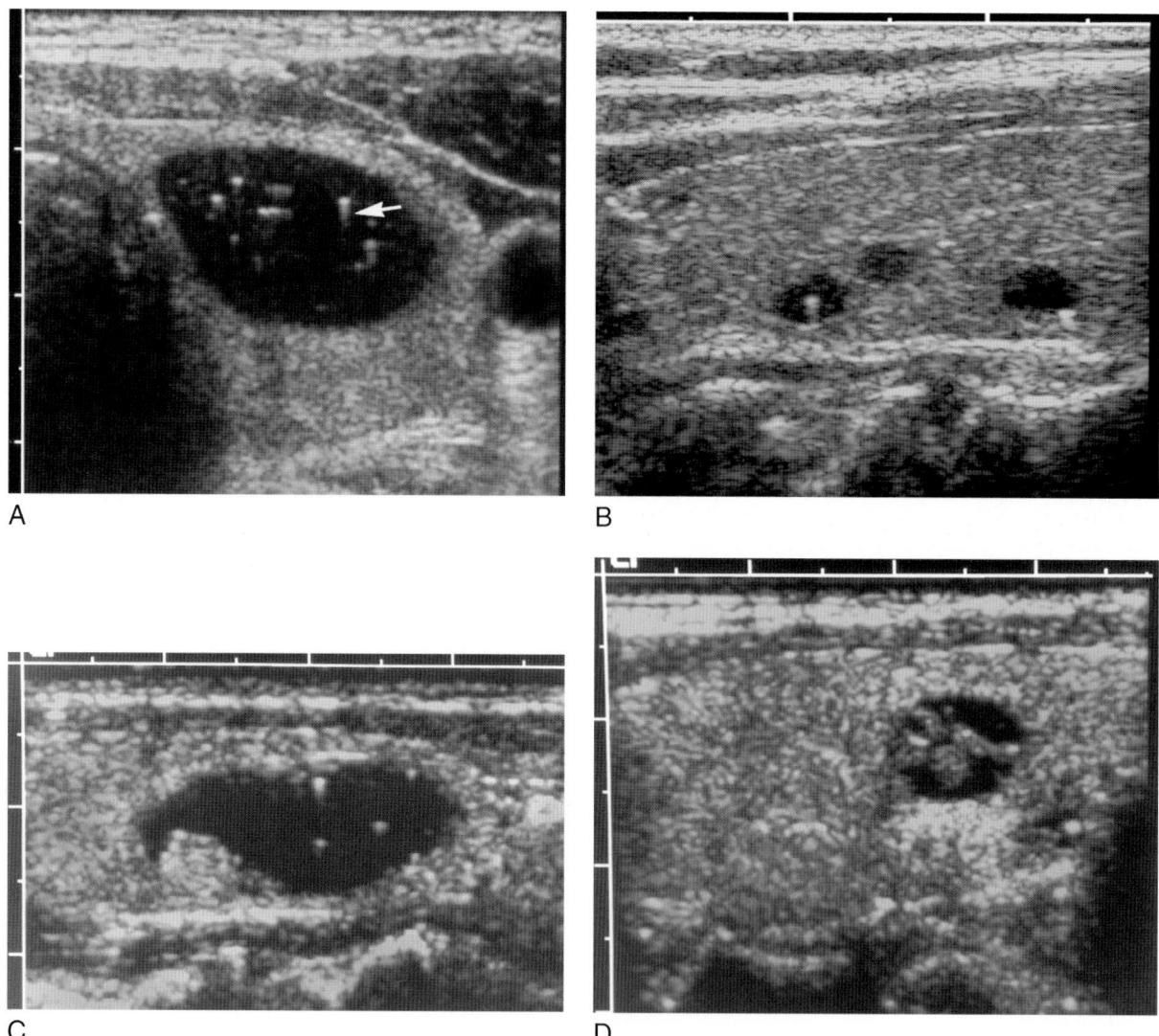

FIGURE 21-8. Colloid cysts. Transverse (**A**) and longitudinal (**B** to **D**) images of four patients show the typical appearance of colloid cysts. Some of the nodules have tiny echogenic foci that are thought to be microcrystals. A few of these foci are associated with comet-tail artifacts *(arrow in A)* posteriorly. Nodules that are mostly cystic such as these are considered benign. Colloid cysts often contain internal echoes.

are the hallmarks of **follicular carcinoma,** and these features are identified by histologic, rather than cytologic, analysis. Needle biopsy is therefore not a reliable method to distinguish between follicular carcinoma and cellular adenoma. Therefore, such tumors are usually surgically removed.

Sonographically, adenomas are commonly solid masses that may be hyperechoic, isoechoic, or hypoechoic (Fig. 21-10). They often have a peripheral hypoechoic halo that is thick and smooth. This halo is due to the fibrous capsule and blood vessels, which can be readily seen by color Doppler imaging. Often, vessels pass from the periphery to the central regions of the nodule, creating a "spoke-and-wheel-like" appearance. Hyperfunctioning (autonomous) adenomas often exhibit abundant peripheral and intralesional hypervascularity.

Carcinoma

Most primary thyroid cancers are of epithelial origin and are derived from either the follicular or the parafollicular cells.[14] Malignant thyroid tumors of mesenchymal origin are exceedingly rare, as are metastases to the thyroid. Most thyroid cancers are well differentiated, and papillary carcinoma (including so-called mixed papillary and follicular carcinoma) accounts for 75% to 90% of all cases.[14,22] In contrast, medullary, follicular, and anaplastic carcinomas, combined, represent only 10% to 25% of all thyroid carcinomas currently diagnosed in North America.

Although it can occur in patients of any age, **papillary cancer** has two peaks of prevalence: in the third and seventh decades of life.[14] Women are affected more often

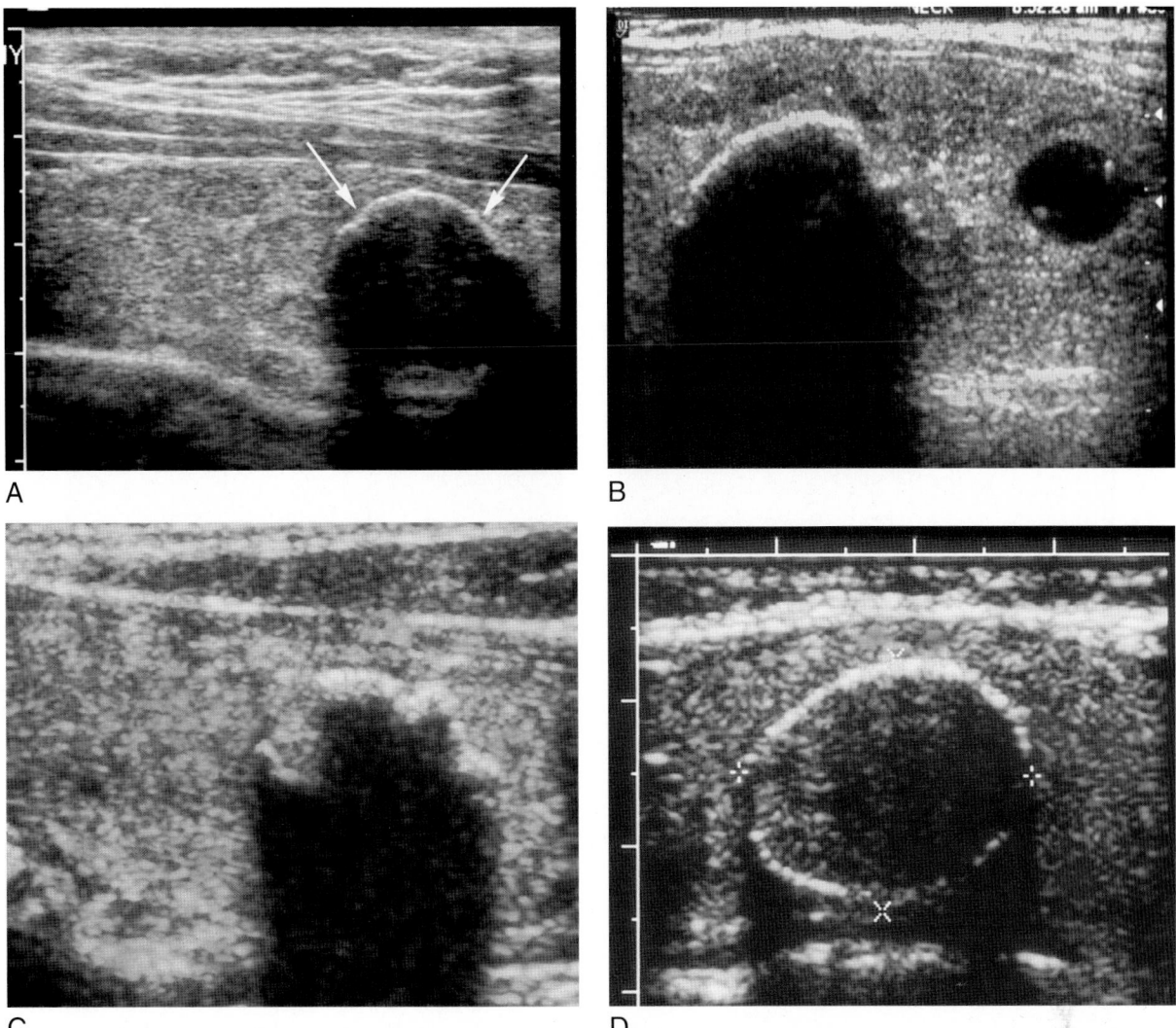

FIGURE 21-9. Peripheral "eggshell" calcification. This feature indicates a very high probability of a benign nodule.
A, Longitudinal image shows coarse peripheral, "eggshell" calcification *(arrows).* The calcification casts a large acoustic shadow.
B, Longitudinal image of another patient shows an eggshell calcification and a typical appearance of colloid cyst on the right side.
C, Longitudinal image of coarse peripheral calcification. **D,** Longitudinal image shows "eggshell" calcification.

than men. On microscopic examination, the tumor is multicentric within the thyroid gland in at least 20% of cases.[23] Round, laminated calcifications (psammoma bodies) in the cytoplasm of papillary cancer cells are seen in approximately 35% of cases. The major route of spread of papillary carcinoma is through the lymphatics to nearby cervical lymph nodes. In fact, it is not uncommon for a patient with papillary thyroid cancer to present with enlarged cervical nodes and a palpably normal thyroid gland.[24,25] Interestingly, the presence of nodal metastasis in the neck does not, in general, appear to adversely alter the prognosis for this malignancy. Distant metastases are very rare (2% to 3% of cases) and occur mostly in the mediastinum and lung. After 20 years, the cumulative mortality from papillary thyroid cancer is typically only 4% to 8%.[24]

Papillary carcinoma has peculiar histologic (fibrous capsule, microcalcifications) and cytologic features ("ground glass" nuclei, cytoplasmic inclusions in the nucleus, and indentations of the nuclear membrane) that often allow a relatively easy pathologic diagnosis.[26] In particular, microcalcifications, which result from the deposition of calcium salts in the **psammoma bodies,** can be present in both the primary tumor and the cervical lymph node metastases (Fig. 21-11).[25,27]

Similar to the pathologic features, **sonographic characteristics of typical papillary carcinoma** are relatively distinctive in most cases (Fig. 21-12):

- Hypoechogenicity (in 90% of cases) due to closely packed cell content, with minimal colloid substance

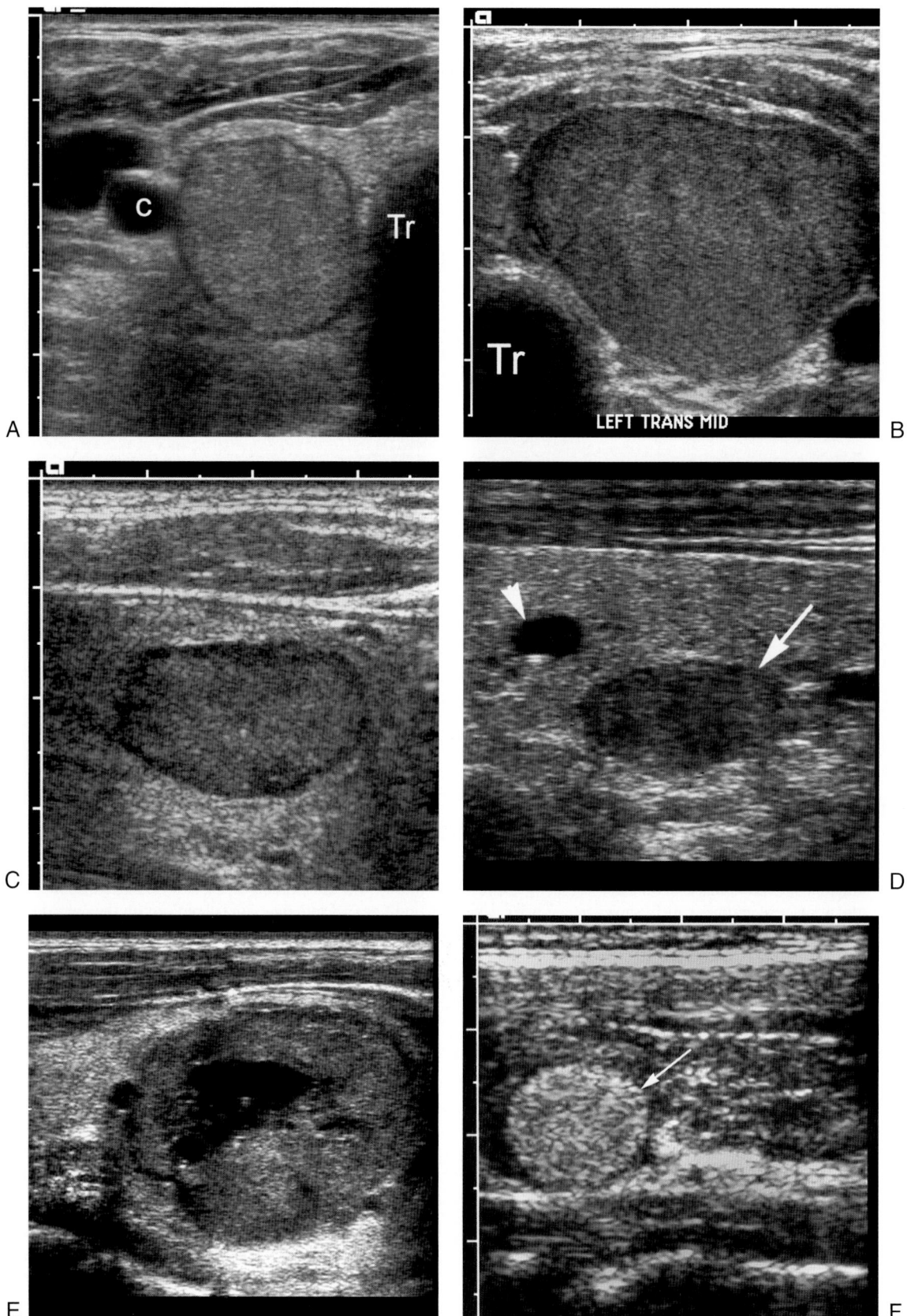

FIGURE 21-10. Benign follicular adenoma: spectrum of appearances. Transverse images of the right (**A**) and left (**B**) lobes and longitudinal image (**C**) of the thyroid glands of three patients show homogeneous, hypoechoic round to oval masses with a thin halo surrounding the mass. This halo is the capsule of the adenoma. Tr, tracheal air shadow; C, carotid artery. **D,** Longitudinal image shows oval hypoechoic adenoma *(arrow)* without a halo and a colloid cyst *(arrowhead).* **E,** Longitudinal image shows oval mass with internal cystic component. **F,** Longitudinal image shows hyperechoic round homogeneous mass *(arrow)* in a patient with Hashimoto's thyroiditis.

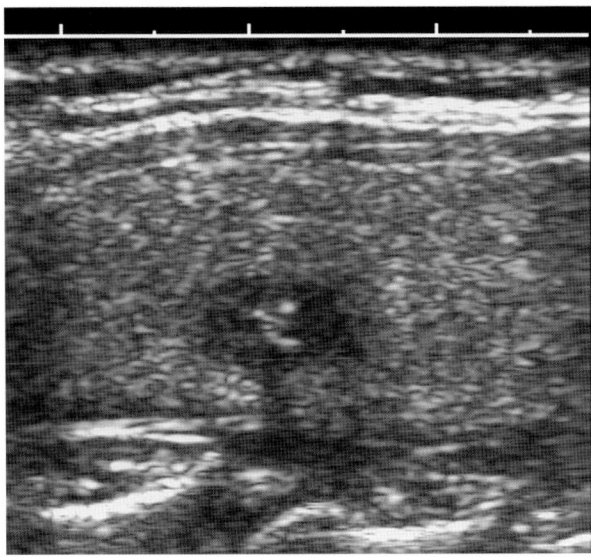

A

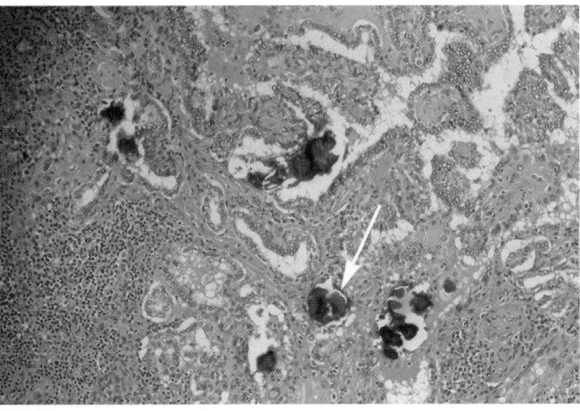

B

FIGURE 21-11. Papillary carcinoma: small cancer with microscopic correlation. A, Longitudinal image demonstrates a 7-mm solid hypoechoic nodule that contains microcalcifications. **B,** Microscopic pathologic image shows microcalcifications or "psammoma bodies" *(arrow).*

- Microcalcifications that appear as tiny, punctate hyperechoic foci, either with or without acoustic shadows (see Figs. 21-11 and 21-12)[16,19,28,29]
- Hypervascularity (in 90% of cases) with disorganized vascularity, mostly in well-encapsulated forms (Fig. 21-13)[30]
- Cervical lymph node metastases, which may contain tiny, punctate echogenic foci due to microcalcifications (Fig. 21-14E, F, G, and I). These are mostly located in the caudal half of the deep jugular chain. Occasionally, metastatic nodes may be cystic as a result of extensive degeneration (see Fig. 21-14H)

In most cases, cystic nodal metastases show a thickened outer wall, internal nodularity, and septations, whereas in younger patients they may appear purely cystic.[25] Cystic lymph node metastases in the neck occur almost exclusively in association with papillary thyroid carcinoma but occasionally may occur in nasopharyngeal carcinomas.[39] On power Doppler sonography, noncystic nodes often show diffuse hypervascularity with tortuous vessels, arteriovenous shunts, and high vascular resistance (RI > 0.8), but in some instances they can demonstrate just prominent hilar vascularity similar to that of reactive nodes and low resistive indexes.[29]

It is exceedingly rare for papillary carcinoma to exhibit a large amount of cystic change (Fig. 21-15). In our experience, this occurs in less than 5% of cases of carcinoma. The overwhelming majority of papillary carcinomas appear as a predominately solid mass. Invasion of adjacent muscles is uncommonly visualized by ultrasound imaging but when seen indicates that the mass is malignant (Fig. 21-16). A **follicular variant of papillary carcinoma** is uncommon, accounting for 10% of cases of papillary carcinoma. This lesion looks similar to a follicular neoplasm on gross pathologic inspection and by ultrasound imaging (Fig. 21-17). On high-power microscopic studies, the nuclear features are those of papillary carcinoma, and it is classified as a follicular variant of papillary carcinoma. The clinical course and treatment are the same as that of typical papillary thyroid carcinoma (see Fig. 21-11). Papillary "microcarcinoma" is a rare nonencapsulated sclerosing tumor measuring 1 cm or less in diameter (Fig. 21-18). In 80% of cases, the patient presents with enlarged cervical nodes and a palpably normal thyroid gland.[24,26] Papillary microcarcinoma can be imaged by high-frequency ultrasound in approximately 70% of cases either as a small hyperechoic patch (fibroticlike) under the capsule with thickening and retraction of the capsule or as a minute hypoechoic nodule with blurred irregular outline with no visible microcalcifications, but often with intense vascular signals within and around the lesion.

Follicular carcinoma is the second subtype of well-differentiated thyroid cancer. It accounts for 5% to 15% of all cases of thyroid cancer, affecting females more often than males.[14] There are two variants of follicular carcinoma, and they differ greatly in histology and clinical course.[22,26] The **minimally invasive** follicular carcinomas are encapsulated, and only the histologic demonstration of focal invasion of capsular blood vessels of the fibrous capsule itself permits differentiation from follicular adenoma. The **widely invasive** follicular carcinomas are not well encapsulated, and invasion of the vessels and the adjacent thyroid is more easily demonstrated. Both variants of follicular carcinoma tend to spread via the bloodstream rather than via lymphatics, and distant metastases to bone, lung, brain, and liver are more likely than metastases to cervical lymph nodes. The widely invasive variant metastasizes in about 20% to 40% of cases, and the minimally invasive metastasizes in

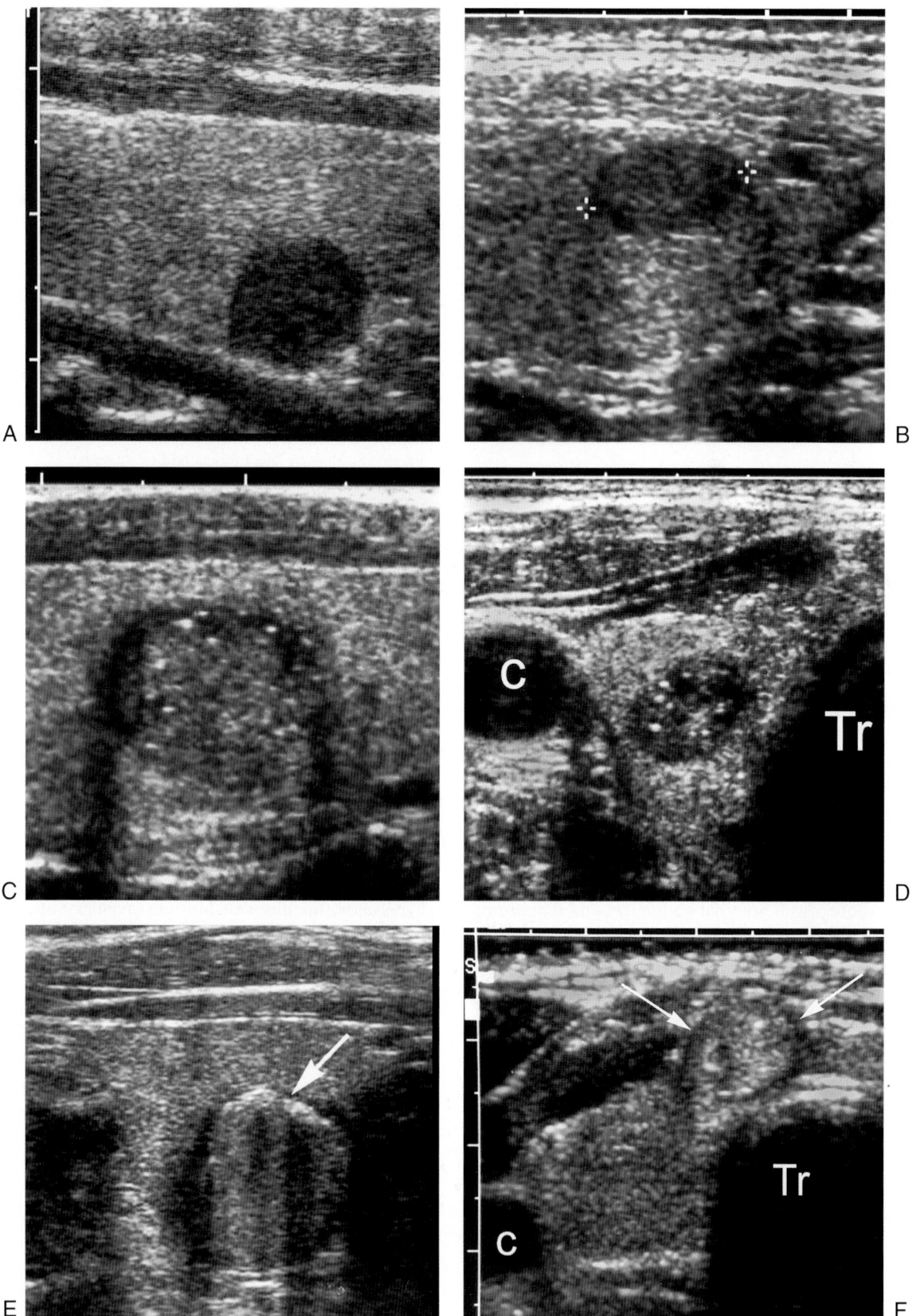

FIGURE 21-12. Papillary thyroid carcinoma: spectrum of typical appearances. A and **B,** Longitudinal images demonstrate hypoechoic solid nodules without evidence of calcification. Longitudinal (**C**) and transverse (**D**) images show hypoechoic nodules that contain echogenic foci due to microcalcification. Tr, tracheal air shadow; C, carotid artery. **E,** Longitudinal image shows hypoechoic solid nodule with irregular thick halo and linear calcification at anterior margin *(arrow).* **F,** Transverse image shows heterogeneous but isoechoic mass in the isthmus *(arrows).* The mass contains microcalcifications and has an irregular thick halo. Tr, tracheal air shadow; C, carotid artery.

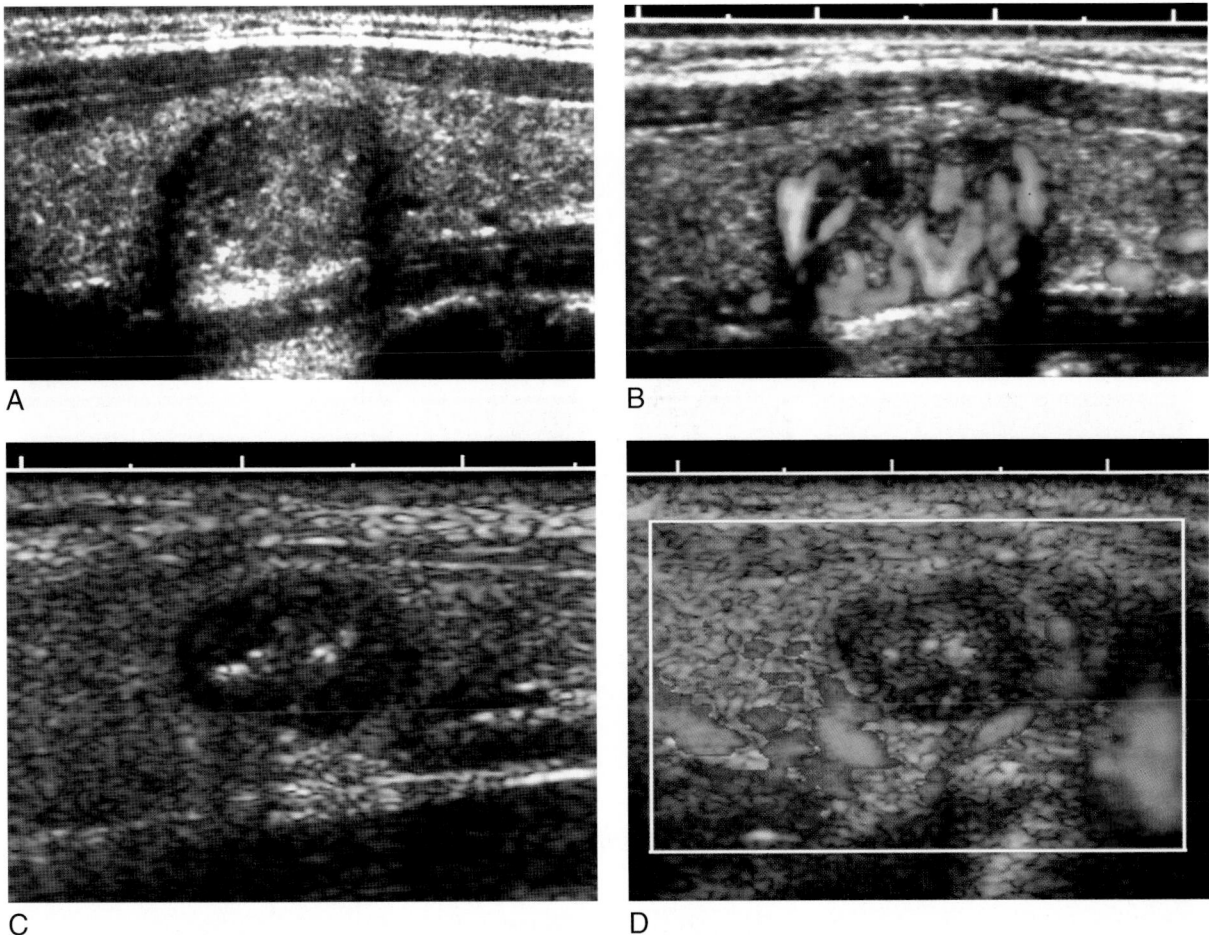

FIGURE 21-13. Papillary carcinoma: power Doppler appearances. Blood flow within cancer is often, but not always, increased. **A,** Longitudinal image shows a 1.5-cm nodule with a thick irregular halo. **B,** Power Doppler image of the nodule shows that it is hypervascular and has flow in the center and at the periphery. **C,** Longitudinal image shows hypoechoic nodule with microcalcifications. **D,** Power Doppler image shows no blood flow within the cancer.

only 5% to 10% of cases. Mortality due to follicular carcinoma is 20% to 30% at 20 postoperative years.[14,24]

There are no unique sonographic features that allow differentiation of follicular carcinoma from adenoma, which is not surprising, given the cytologic and histologic similarities of these two tumors (Figs. 21-19 and 21-20). Similarly, fine-needle aspiration (FNA) is not reliable in differentiating benign from malignant follicular neoplasms because the pathologic diagnosis is not based on cellular appearance but, rather, on capsular and vascular invasion. Therefore, most follicular nodules must be surgically removed for accurate pathologic diagnosis. Features that suggest follicular carcinoma are rarely seen but include irregular tumor margins, a thick, irregular halo, and a tortuous or chaotic arrangement of internal blood vessels on color Doppler imaging.[18,31]

Medullary carcinoma accounts for only about 5% of all malignant thyroid disease. It is derived from the parafollicular cells, or C cells, and typically secretes the hormone calcitonin, which can be a useful serum marker. This cancer is frequently familial (20%) and is an essential component of the **multiple endocrine neoplasia (MEN) type II syndromes.**[32] The disease is multicentric and/or bilateral in about 90% of the familial cases (Fig. 21-21).[14] There is a high incidence of metastatic involvement of lymph nodes, and the prognosis for patients with medullary cancer is considered to be somewhat worse than that for follicular cancer.

The sonographic appearance of medullary carcinoma is usually similar to that of papillary carcinoma and is seen most often as a hypoechoic solid mass. There are often calcifications, and they tend to be more coarse than the calcifications of typical papillary carcinoma (Fig. 21-22).[33] Calcifications can be seen not only in the primary tumor but also in lymph node metastases and even in hepatic metastases.

Anaplastic thyroid carcinoma is typically a disease of the elderly; it represents one of the most lethal of solid tumors. Although it accounts for less than 2% of all thyroid cancers, it carries the worst prognosis, with a 5-year mortality rate of more than 95%.[34] The tumor typically presents as a rapidly enlarging mass extending

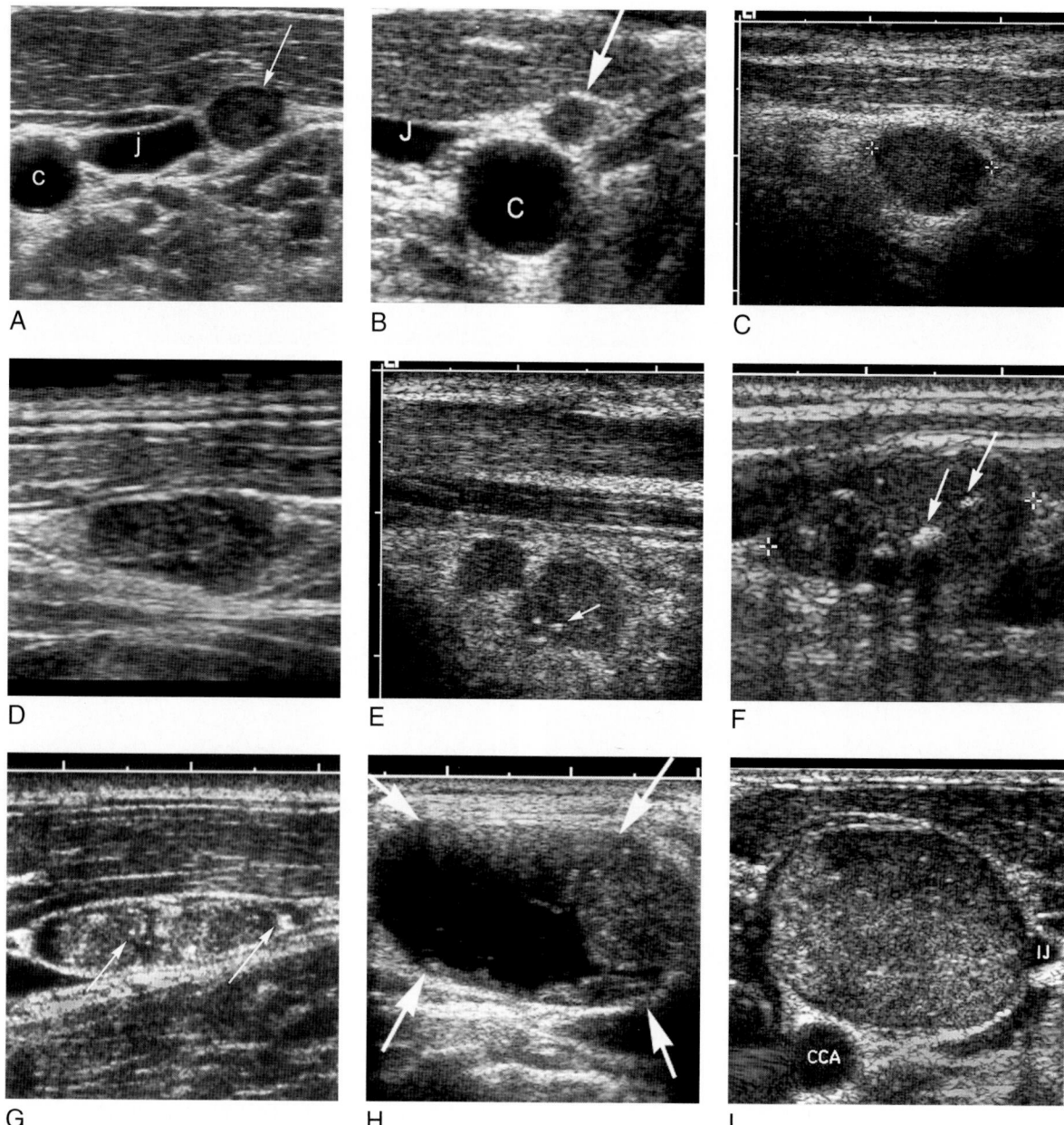

FIGURE 21-14. Metastases involving cervical lymph nodes: spectrum of appearances. **A** and **B,** Transverse images near the carotid artery (C) and jugular vein (J) show small hypoechoic round lymph nodes *(arrows)*. In spite of their small size (approximately 4 mm), the round shape and the hypoechoic appearance are highly indicative of metastasis. **C** and **D,** Longitudinal images demonstrate oval hypoechoic nodes. **E,** Longitudinal image of the thyroid bed after thyroidectomy shows two abnormal lymph nodes, one of which contains microcalcifications *(arrow)*. **F** and **G,** Longitudinal images show heterogeneous lymph nodes containing calcifications *(arrows)*. **H,** Longitudinal image shows large lymph node *(arrows)* containing cystic change. Cystic change in a cervical lymph node is almost always due to metastatic papillary carcinoma. **I,** Transverse image shows a large round lymph node between the internal jugular vein (IJ) and the common carotid artery (CCA).

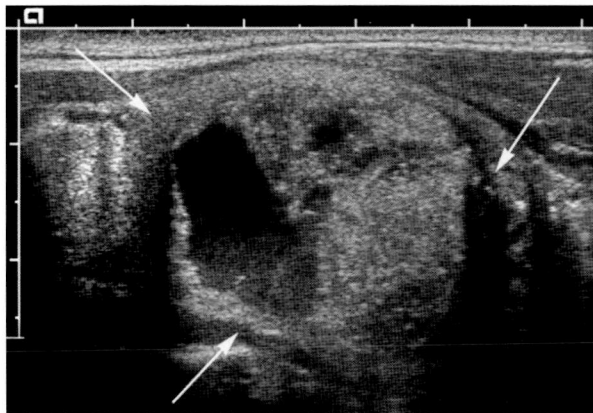

FIGURE 21-15. Papillary thyroid carcinoma: atypical. Three examples of moderate to marked cystic degeneration of papillary carcinoma. In the authors' experience, less than 5% of papillary carcinoma has this appearance of a large amount of cystic change. Over 90% of papillary thyroid carcinomas are uniformly solid masses. **A** to **C,** Longitudinal images show three large nodules *(arrows, cursors)* that have a large amount of cystic change.

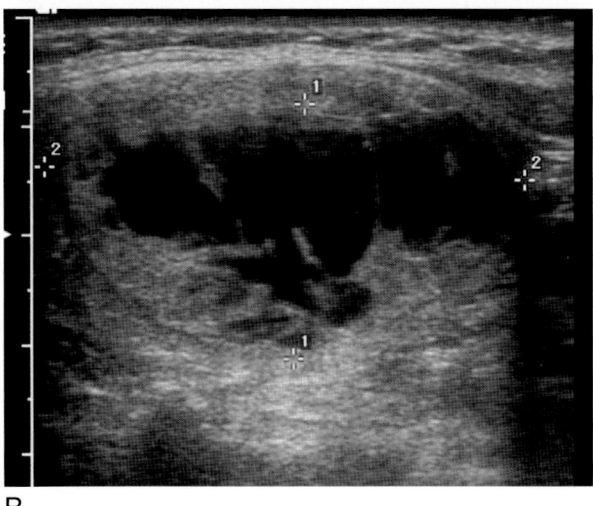

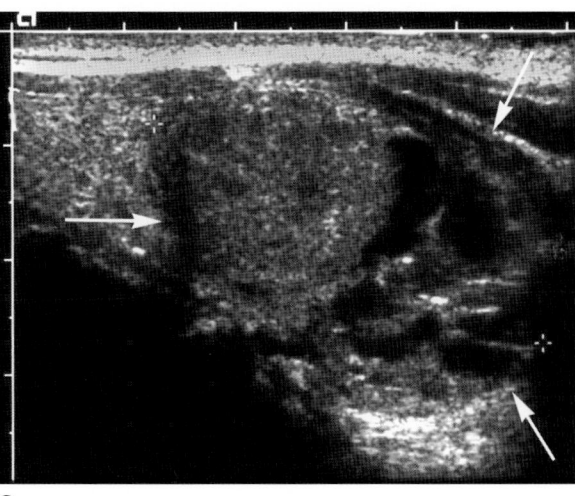

beyond the gland and invading adjacent structures. It is often inoperable at the time of presentation.

Anaplastic carcinomas may often be associated with papillary or follicular carcinomas, presumably representing a dedifferentiation of the neoplasm. They tend not to spread via the lymphatics but instead are prone to aggressive local invasion of muscles and vessels.[26] Sonographically these carcinomas are usually hypoechoic and often encase or invade blood vessels and neck muscles (Fig. 21-23). Often these tumors cannot be adequately examined by ultrasound because of their large size. Instead, CT or MRI of the neck usually demonstrates more accurately the extent of the disease.

Lymphoma

Lymphoma accounts for approximately 4% of all thyroid malignancies. It is mostly of the non-Hodgkin's type and usually affects older women. The typical clinical sign is a rapidly growing mass that may cause symptoms of obstruction, such as dyspnea and dysphagia.[35] In 70% to 80% of cases, lymphoma arises from a preexisting chronic lymphocytic thyroiditis (Hashimoto's thyroiditis) with subclinical or overt hypothyroidism. The prognosis is highly variable and depends on the stage of the disease. The 5-year survival rate may range from nearly 90% in early-stage cases to less than 5% in advanced, disseminated disease.

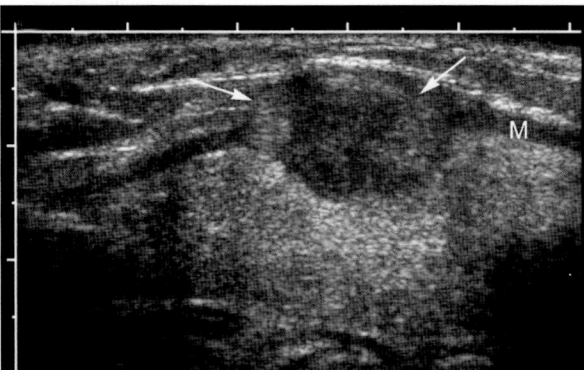

FIGURE 21-16. Papillary carcinoma invades muscle. Longitudinal image shows hypoechoic mass arising from the anterior surface of the thyroid. This mass invades *(arrows)* adjacent strap muscle (M). Muscular invasion is very rare.

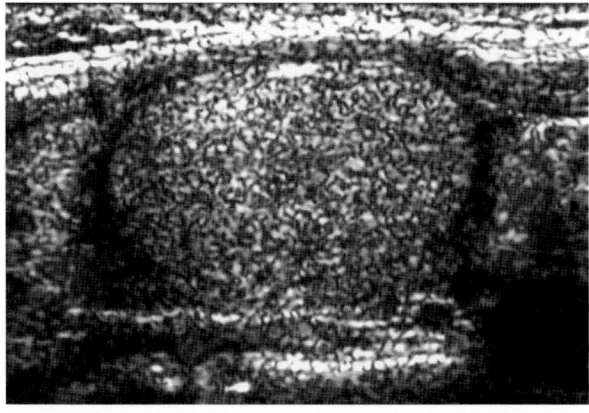

A

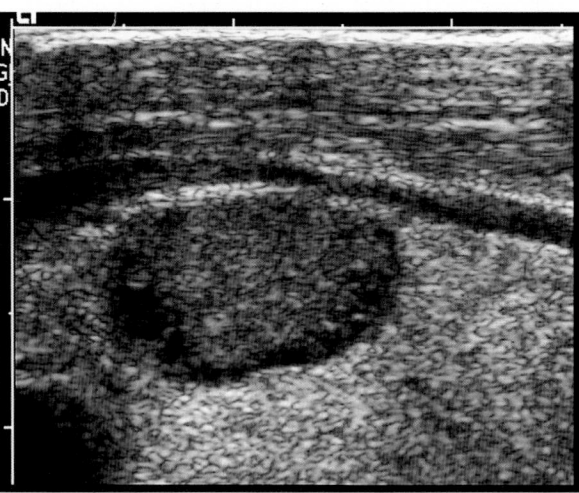

B

FIGURE 21-17. Atypical papillary thyroid carcinoma. Two examples of follicular variant of papillary thyroid carcinoma. Longitudinal images show an oval isoechoic (**A**) and hypoechoic (**B**) mass that looks similar to the typical ultrasound appearance of a follicular neoplasm. This follicular variant is uncommon, accounting for 10% of cases of papillary carcinoma. The clinical course and treatment are the same as that of typical papillary thyroid carcinoma.

Sonographically, lymphoma of the thyroid appears as a markedly hypoechoic and lobulated mass. Large areas of cystic necrosis may occur, as well as encasement of adjacent neck vessels (Fig. 21-24).[36] On color Doppler imaging both nodular and diffuse thyroid lymphomas may appear mostly hypovascular or show blood vessels with chaotic distribution and arteriovenous shunts. The adjacent thyroid parenchyma may be heterogeneous owing to associated chronic lymphocytic thyroiditis.[37]

Metastases

Metastases to the thyroid are infrequent, occurring late in the course of neoplastic diseases as the result of spread by hematogenous or, less frequently, lymphatic route. Commonly, metastases are from melanoma (39%), breast (21%), and renal cell carcinoma (10%). Metastases

may appear as solitary, well-circumscribed nodules or as diffuse involvement of the gland. On sonography, they are solid, homogeneously hypoechoic masses, without calcifications (Fig. 21-25).[38]

Clinical Work-Up

Once a thyroid nodule has been detected, the fundamental problem is to determine if it is benign or malignant. Short of surgical excision, several methods for nodule characterization are in common use, including radionuclide imaging, sonography, and FNA biopsy. Each of these techniques has advantages and limitations,

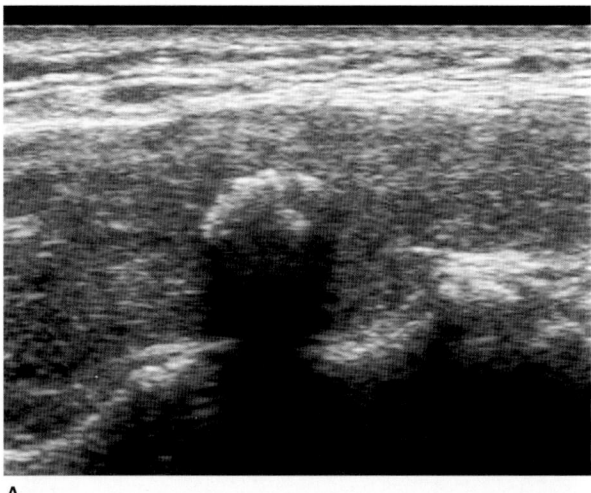

A

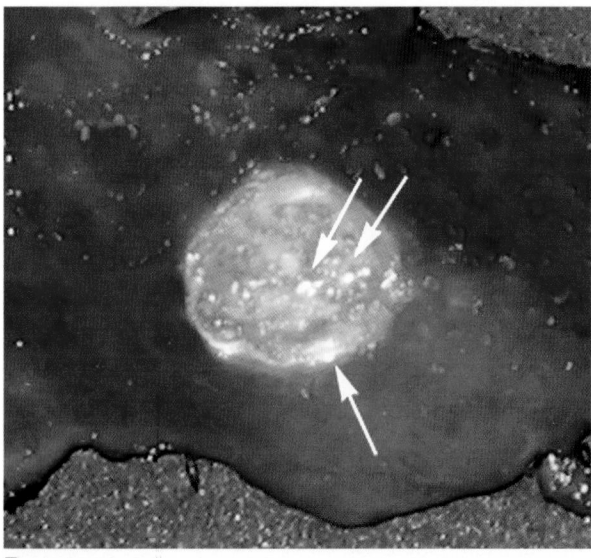

B

FIGURE 21-18. Atypical papillary carcinoma. A, Longitudinal image shows coarse calcifications without mass effect. The calcification is seen at the periphery and internally. **B,** Gross pathologic specimen of the same patient shows the round nodule that contains multiple areas of grossly visible calcifications *(arrows)*. This is a rare sclerosing form of papillary carcinoma that contains a large amount of fibrosis and calcification.

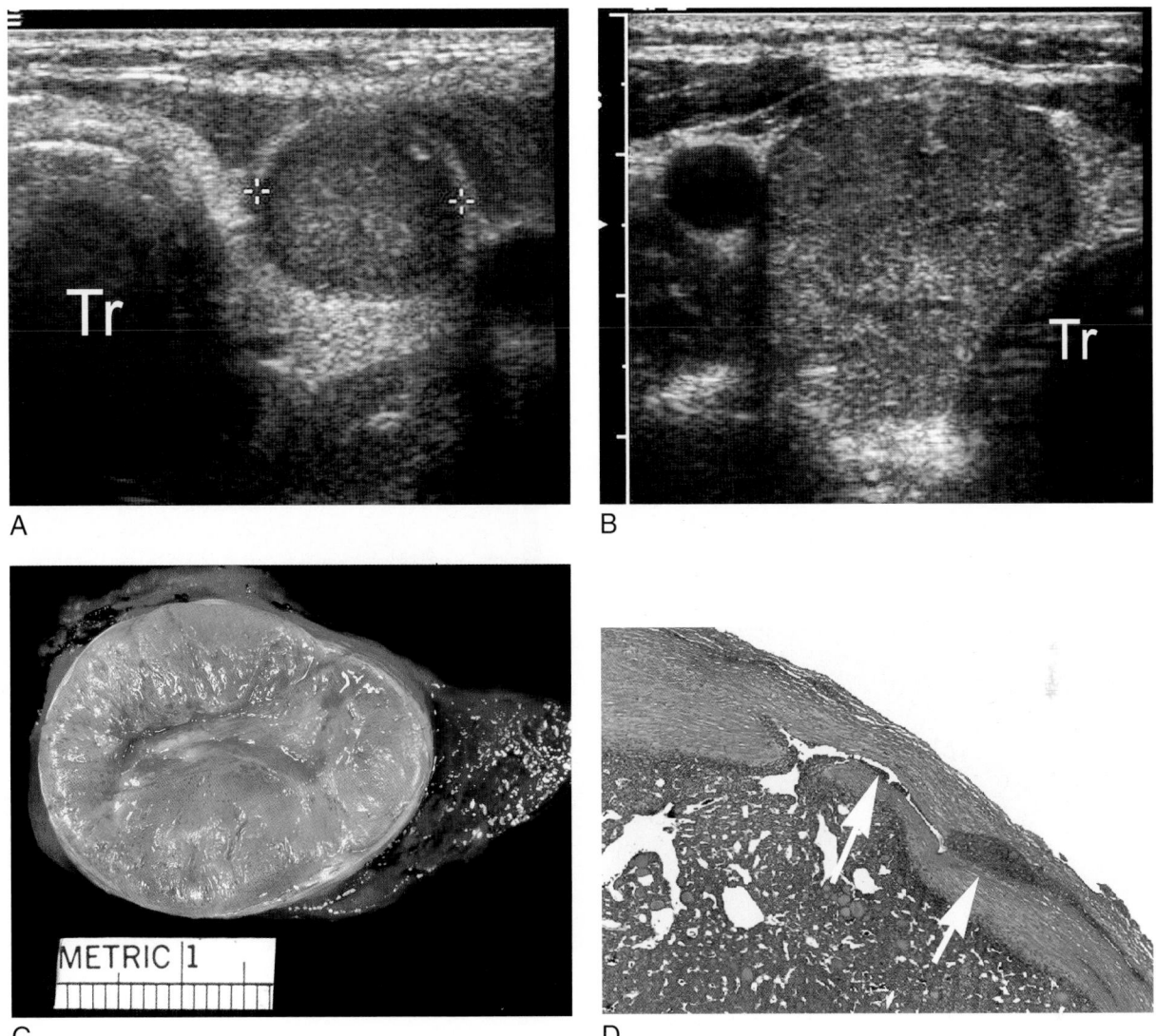

FIGURE 21-19. Follicular neoplasms: benign and malignant in same patient. Transverse image of the left (**A**) and right (**B**) lobes of the thyroid show round homogeneous hypoechoic masses that appear identical except for size differences. The smaller mass was malignant and the larger mass benign. Tr, tracheal air shadow. **C,** Gross pathologic specimen of follicular neoplasm shows a homogeneous tumor with a thin capsule. This capsule is present in both benign and malignant follicular neoplasms and it is often seen on ultrasound. **D,** Microscopic appearance of the capsule shows invasion of the follicular cells into the capsule *(arrows)*. This is one of the microscopic features that allows a pathologic diagnosis of malignancy but is not visible by ultrasound. It is not possible to differentiate benign from malignant follicular neoplasms by ultrasound imaging. Similarly, fine-needle aspiration is not reliable in differentiating benign from malignant follicular neoplasms because it cannot show capsular and vascular invasion and requires surgical removal for accurate pathologic diagnosis.

and the one(s) chosen in any specific clinical setting depends to a large extent on available instrumentation and expertise.

It is generally recognized that **FNA biopsy** is the most effective method for diagnosing malignancy in a thyroid nodule.[39-41] In many clinical practices, FNA under direct palpation is the first diagnostic examination performed on any clinically palpable nodule. Neither isotope nor sonographic imaging is used routinely. Instead, they are reserved for special situations or difficult cases. FNA has had a substantial impact on the management of thyroid nodules because it provides more direct information

than any other available diagnostic technique. It is safe, is inexpensive, and results in better selection of patients for surgery. The successful use of FNA in clinical practice, however, depends heavily on the presence of an experienced aspirationist and an expert cytopathologist.

Fine-needle thyroid aspirates are classified by the cytopathologist into one of four categories:

- Negative (no malignant cells)
- Positive for malignancy
- Suggestive of malignancy
- Nondiagnostic

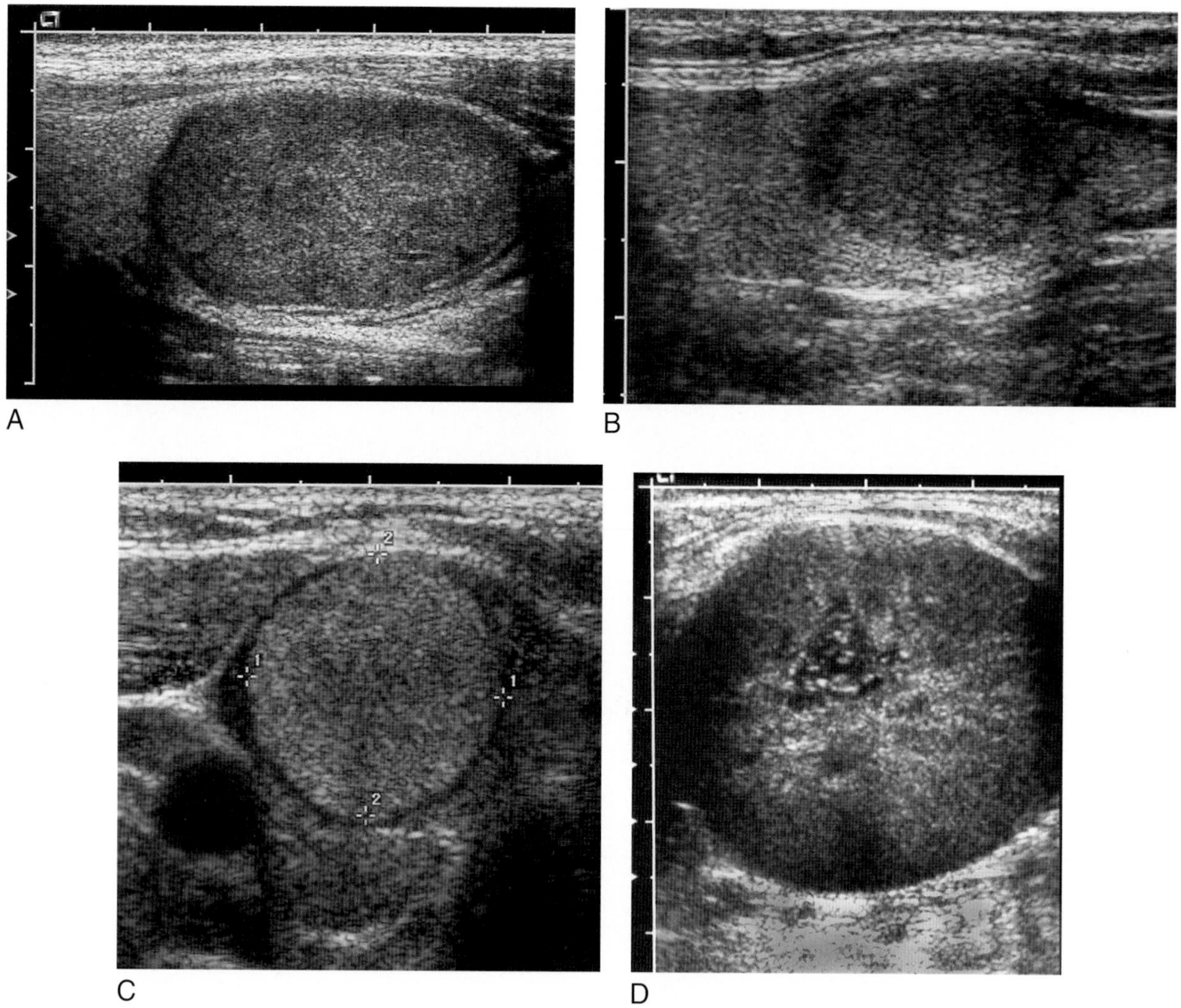

FIGURE 21-20. Malignant follicular neoplasms. A and **B,** Longitudinal images of two patients with homogeneous, oval hypoechoic masses. **C** and **D,** Transverse images of two other patients with homogeneous round masses. These four carcinomas appear identical to the benign follicular neoplasms (see Fig. 21-10), and surgical removal is required to exclude or establish malignancy of most follicular tumors.

If a nodule is classified in either of the first two categories, the results are highly sensitive and specific.[42] The major limitation of the technique is the lack of specificity in the group whose results are suggestive of malignancy, primarily because of the inability to dis-

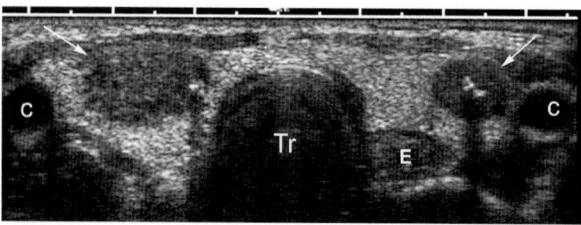

FIGURE 21-21. Multicentric medullary thyroid carcinoma. Patient has multiple endocrine neoplasia type II (MEN II). Transverse dual image shows bilateral hypoechoic masses *(arrows)* that contain areas of coarse calcification. C, carotid arteries; Tr, trachea; E, esophagus.

tinguish follicular or Hürthle cell adenomas from their malignant counterparts. In these cases, surgical excision is required for diagnosis. In addition, up to 20% of aspirates may be nondiagnostic, approximately half of which are so because of cystic lesions from which an adequate cell sample was not obtained. In these cases, repeat FNA under sonographic guidance can be performed with the goal of selectively sampling the solid elements of the mass. In the world literature, FNA of thyroid nodules has a sensitivity range of 65% to 98% and a specificity of 72% to 100%, with a false-negative rate of 1% to 11% and a false-positive rate of 1% to 8% (Table 21-1).[43-48]

In our practices, the overall accuracy of FNA exceeds 95%, and therefore it is currently the most accurate and cost-effective method for initial evaluation of patients with nodular thyroid disease. Since the introduction of FNA into routine clinical practice, the percentage of patients undergoing thyroidectomy has significantly

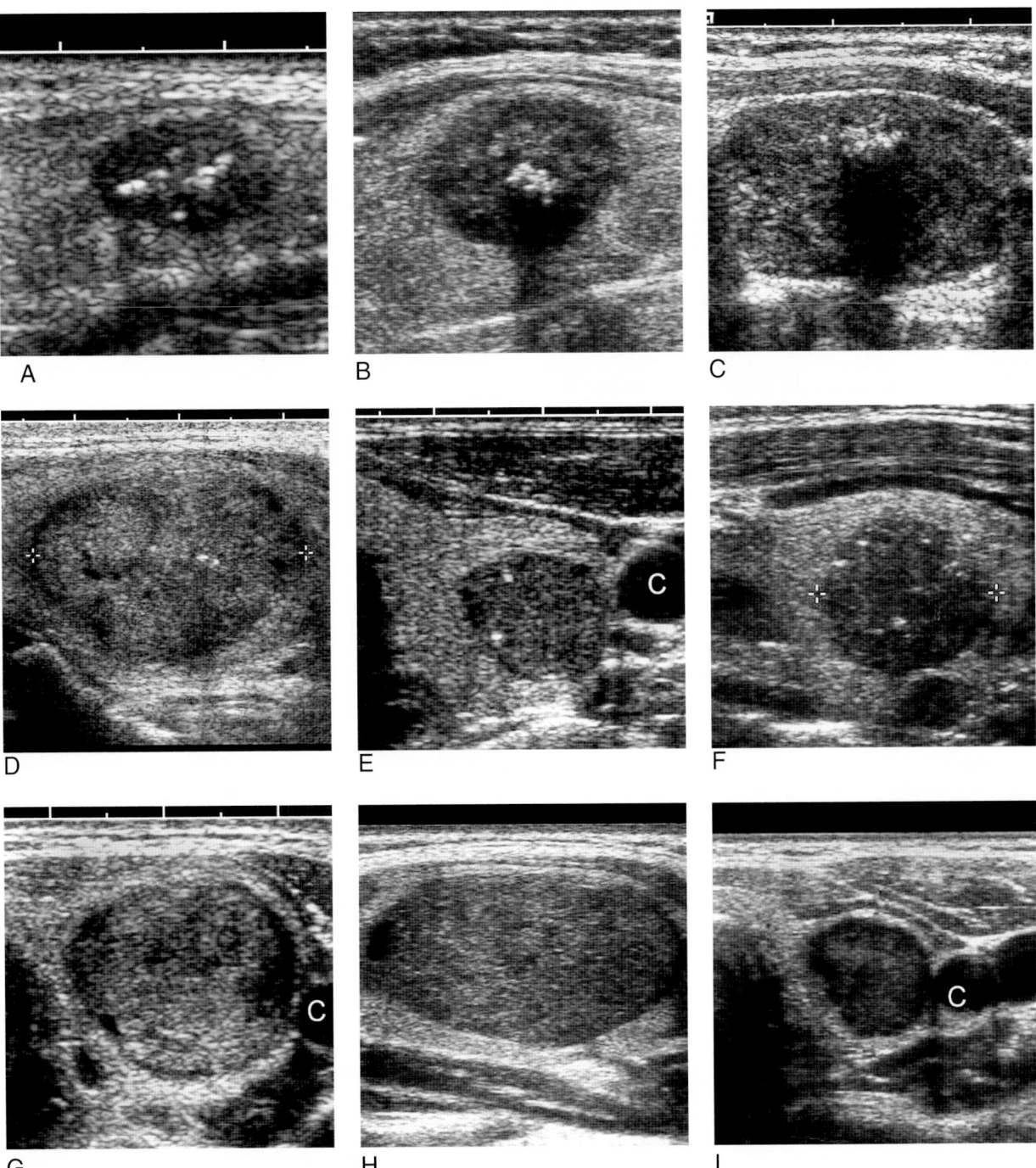

FIGURE 21-22. Medullary thyroid carcinoma: spectrum of appearances. A to **C,** Hypoechoic solid nodules with coarse internal calcifications. **D** to **F,** Hypoechoic solid nodules with fine internal calcifications. **G** to **I,** Hypoechoic solid nodules without calcification and having an appearance similar to follicular neoplasms. C, carotid artery.

decreased (to approximately 25%) and the cost of thyroid nodule care has decreased by 25%.[43]

The evaluation of thyroid nodules primarily by FNA is common in North America and northern Europe. In other European countries and Japan where goiter has a very high prevalence, the initial evaluation often relies on radionuclide and sonographic imaging, owing to the need to "select" those nodules that must undergo FNA.

Sonographic Applications

Although FNA is the most reliable diagnostic method for evaluating clinically palpable thyroid nodules, high-resolution sonography has four primary clinical applications[49-51]:

- Detection of thyroid and other cervical masses before and after thyroidectomy

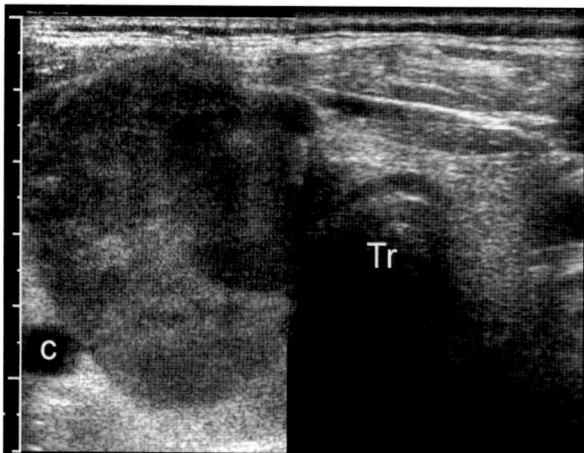

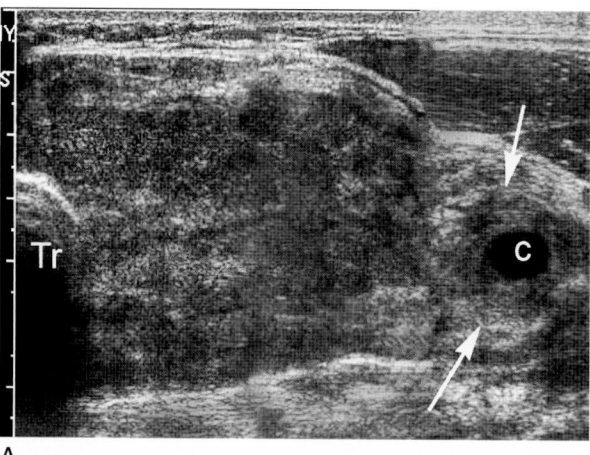

FIGURE 21-23. Anaplastic carcinoma. Transverse dual image demonstrates a large hypoechoic solid mass arising from the right thyroid lobe. Tr, tracheal air shadow; c, carotid artery.

- Differentiation of benign from malignant masses on the basis of their sonographic appearance
- Guidance for FNA/biopsy
- Guidance for the percutaneous treatment of nonfunctional and hyperfunctioning benign thyroid nodules and of lymph node metastases from papillary carcinoma

Detection

A basic and practical use of sonography is to establish the precise anatomic location of a palpable cervical mass. The determination of whether such a mass is within or adjacent to the thyroid cannot always be made on the basis of the physical examination alone. Sonography can readily differentiate thyroid nodules from other cervical

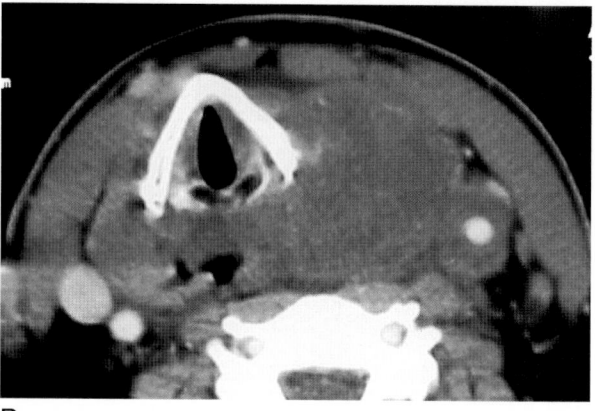

FIGURE 21-24. Lymphoma. A, Transverse image of the left lobe demonstrates a diffuse mass enlarging the lobe and extending into the soft tissues *(arrows)* surrounding the common carotid artery (c). Tr, tracheal air shadow. **B,** Contrast medium–enhanced CT scan shows a hypovascular mass in the left thyroid lobe and soft tissue encasement of the carotid artery.

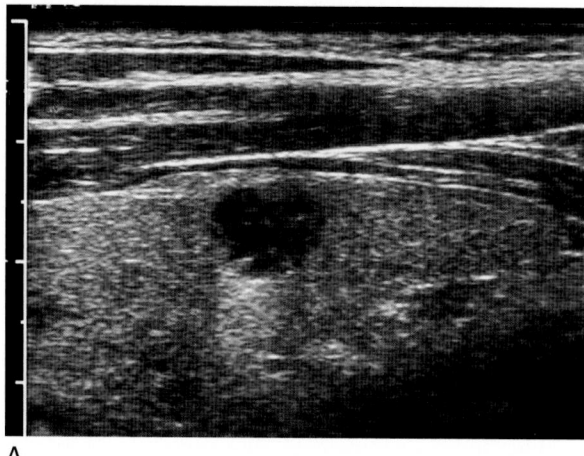

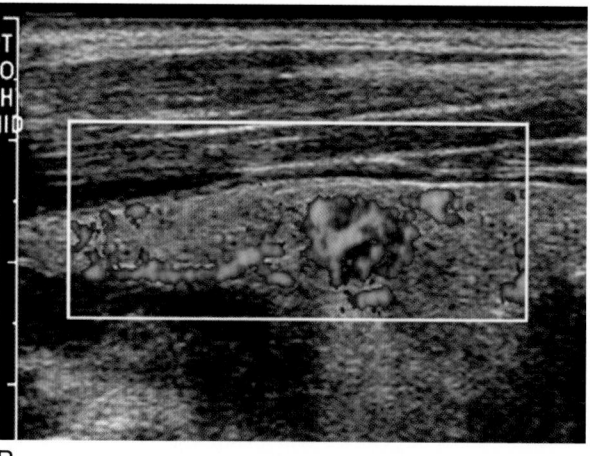

FIGURE 21-25. Thyroid metastasis. Longitudinal (gray scale) **(A)** and power Doppler **(B)** images show a 1-cm solid vascular mass that was metastatic renal cell carcinoma.

TABLE 21-1. DIAGNOSTIC YIELD OF THYROID FINE-NEEDLE ASPIRATION

Series	No. of Cases	False-Negative Rate (%)	False-Positive Rate (%)	Sensitivity (%)	Specificity (%)
Hawkins, et al.[44]	1,399	2.4	4.6	86	95
Khafagi, et al.[45]	618	4.1	7.7	87	72
Hall, et al.[46]	795	1.3	3.0	84	90
Altavilla, et al.[47]	2,433	6.0	0.0	71	100
Gharib, et al.[43]	10,971	2.0	0.7	98	99
Ravetto, et al.[48]	2,014	11.2	0.7	89	99

masses, such as cystic hygromas, thyroglossal duct cysts, or enlarged lymph nodes. Alternatively, sonography may help to confirm the presence of a thyroid nodule when the findings on physical examination are equivocal.

Sonography may be used to detect occult thyroid nodules in patients who have a **history of head and neck irradiation** during childhood as well as for those with a **family history of multiple endocrine neoplasia (MEN) type II syndrome** because both groups have a known increased risk for development of thyroid malignancy. If a nodule is discovered, a biopsy can be performed under sonographic guidance. It is unknown, however, whether the detection of a thyroid cancer before it becomes clinically palpable will change the ultimate clinical outcome for a given patient.

In the past, when thyroid nodules were evaluated primarily with isotope scintigraphy, it was generally accepted that a "solitary cold" nodule carried a probability of malignancy of between 15% and 25% whereas a "cold" nodule in a multinodular gland was malignant in less than 1% of cases.[52] However, benign goiter is multinodular in 70% to 80% of cases, and it has been demonstrated that 70% of nodules considered solitary on scintigraphy or physical examination are actually multiple when assessed with high-frequency ultrasound (Fig. 21-26).[20,53]

It has been suggested, therefore, that sonography may be used to detect additional occult nodules in patients with clinically solitary lesions, thereby implying that the dominant palpable mass is benign. Such a conclusion is unwarranted, however, in view of the fact that, pathologically, benign nodules often coexist with malignant nodules. In a series of 1500 consecutive patients operated on for papillary carcinoma, 33% had coexistent benign nodules at the time of surgery.[54] In addition, papillary thyroid cancer is recognized to be multicentric in at least 20% of cases and occult (i.e., less than 1.5 cm in diameter) in up to 48% of cases.[23,54] In a previous study, almost two thirds (64%) of patients with thyroid cancer had at least one nodule in addition to the dominant nodule that was detected sonographically.[55] Pathologically, these extra nodules can be either benign or malignant. Therefore, in patients with a clinically solitary nodule, the sonographic detection of a few additional nodules is not a reliable sign for excluding malignancy.

An ultrasound-guided FNA is performed for patients with **multinodular goiter** when there is a dominant nodule. A dominant nodule is one which is the largest or has ultrasound features that are different from the other nodules or has features that are suggestive of carcinoma as described earlier.

In patients with known thyroid cancer, sonography can be useful to **determine the extent of disease,** both preoperatively and postoperatively. In most instances a sonographic examination is not performed routinely before thyroidectomy, but it can be useful in patients with large cervical masses for evaluation of nearby structures, such as the carotid artery and internal jugular vein for evidence of direct invasion or encasement by the tumor. Alternatively, in patients who present with cervical lymphadenopathy caused by papillary thyroid cancer but in whom the thyroid gland is palpably normal, sonography may be used preoperatively to detect an occult, nonpalpable primary focus within the gland.

After partial or near-total thyroidectomy for carcinoma, sonography is the preferred method for follow-up, by **detecting residual, recurrent, or metastatic disease in the neck.**[56] In patients who have had subtotal thyroidectomy, the sonographic appearance of the remaining thyroid tissue may serve as an important factor in deciding whether complete thyroidectomy is recommended. If a mass is identified, its nature can be determined by ultrasound-guided FNA (Fig. 21-27). If no masses are seen, the clinician may choose to follow the patient with periodic sonographic studies. For patients who have had total or near-total thyroidectomy, sonography has proven to be more sensitive than physical examination in detecting recurrent disease within the thyroid bed or metastatic disease in cervical lymph nodes.[57] Patients with a history of thyroid cancer often undergo periodic sonographic examinations of the neck to detect nonpalpable recurrent or metastatic disease. When a mass is identified, FNA under sonographic guidance can establish a diagnosis of malignancy and help in surgical planning.

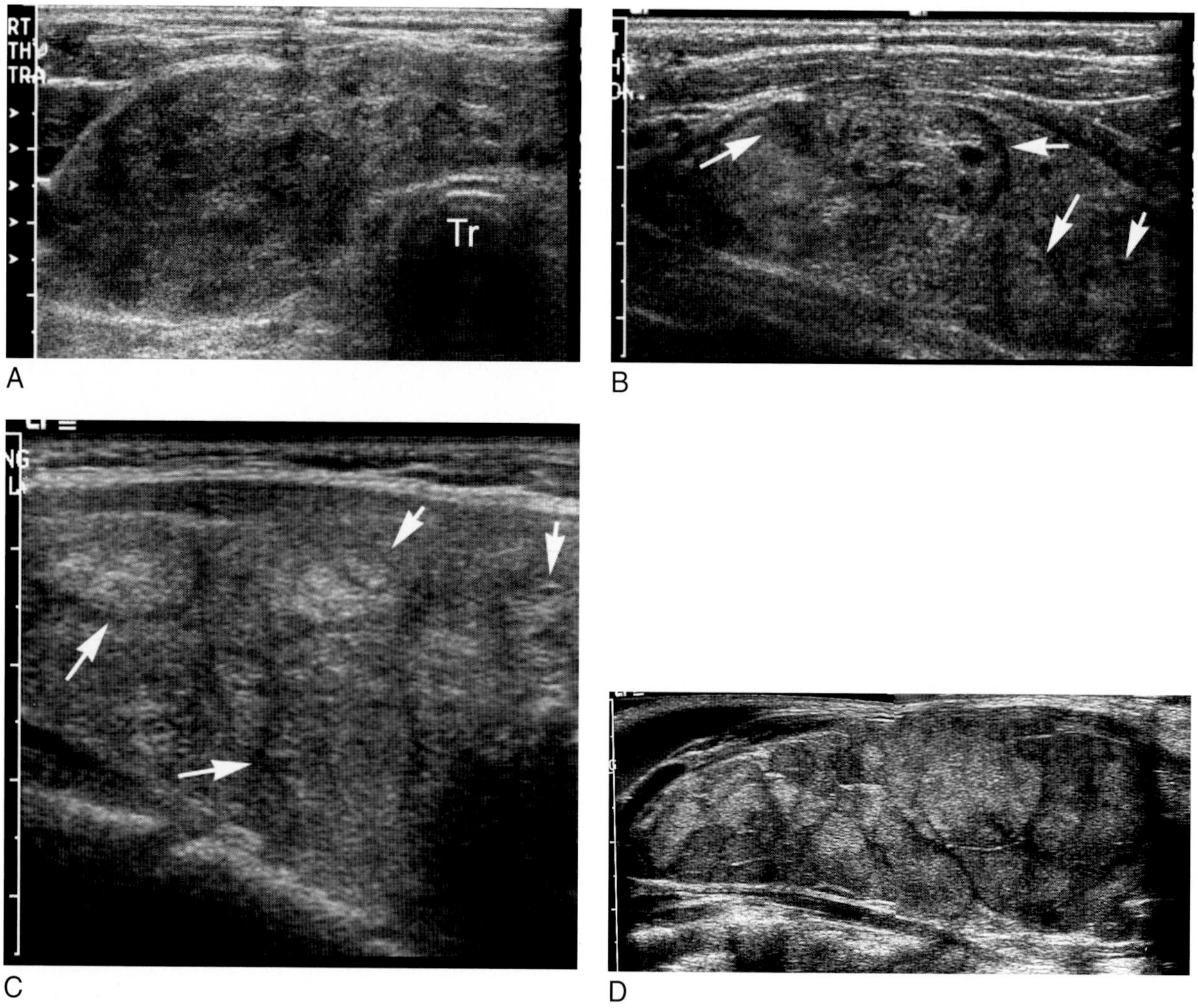

FIGURE 21-26. Multinodular goiter. A, Transverse image shows enlargement of the right lobe and isthmus by multiple confluent hypoechoic and hyperechoic nodules. Tr, tracheal air shadow. **B** and **C,** Longitudinal images show multiple confluent nodules *(arrows).* **D,** Longitudinal dual image shows enlargement of a lobe by multiple nodules.

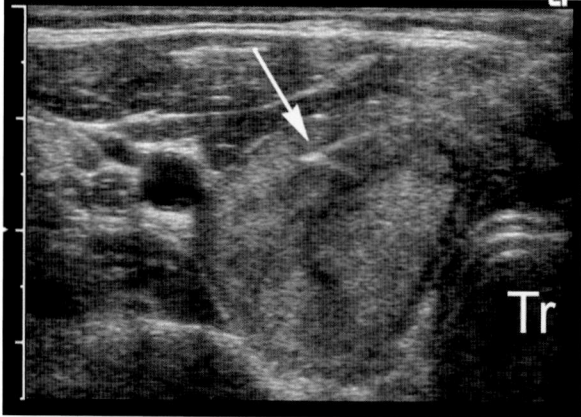

FIGURE 21-27. Fine-needle aspiration of thyroid nodule due to follicular neoplasm. Transverse image shows a large nodule replacing the right thyroid lobe. The tip of the 25 gauge needle is highly visible *(arrow),* and the shaft of the needle is faintly visible. Tr, tracheal air shadow.

Differentiation of Benign and Malignant Nodules

According to several reports, for the differentiation of benign versus malignant thyroid nodules, sonography has sensitivity rates ranging from 63% to 94%, specificity from 61% to 95%, and overall accuracy from 80% to 94%.[4,5,58-63] Currently, no single sonographic criterion distinguishes benign thyroid nodules from malignant nodules with complete reliability.[5,58-60] Nevertheless, certain sonographic features have been described that are seen more commonly with one type of histology or the other, thus establishing general diagnostic trends (Table 21-2).[31]

The fundamental anatomic features of a thyroid nodule on high-resolution sonography are:

- Internal consistency (solid, mixed solid and cystic, or purely cystic)

TABLE 21-2. RELIABILITY OF SONOGRAPHIC FEATURES IN THE DIFFERENTIATION OF BENIGN FROM MALIGNANT THYROID NODULES*

Feature	Pathologic Diagnosis	
	Benign	*Malignant*
Internal Contents		
Purely cystic content	++++	+
Cystic with thin septa	++++	+
Mixed solid and cystic	+++	++
Comet-tail artifact	+++	+
Echogenicity		
Hyperechoic	++++	+
Isoechoic	+++	++
Hypoechoic	+++	+++
Halo		
Thin halo	++++	++
Thick incomplete halo	+	+++
Margin		
Well-defined	+++	++
Poorly defined	++	+++
Calcification		
Eggshell calcification	++++	+
Coarse calcification	+++	+
Microcalcification	++	++++
Doppler		
Peripheral flow pattern	+++	++
Internal flow pattern	++	+++

+, Rare (<1%).
++, Low probability (<15%).
+++, Intermediate probability (16% to 84%).
++++, High probability (>85%).
*Based on authors' experience and literature data.

- Echogenicity relative to the adjacent thyroid parenchyma
- Margin
- Presence and pattern of calcification
- Peripheral sonolucent halo
- Presence and distribution of blood flow signals

Internal Contents. In our experience, approximately 70% of thyroid nodules are solid, whereas the remaining 30% exhibit various amounts of cystic change. A nodule that has a significant cystic component is usually a **benign adenomatous (colloid) nodule** that has undergone degeneration or hemorrhage. When detected by older, lower-resolution ultrasound machines, these lesions were called cysts because the presence of internal debris and a thick wall could not be appreciated. Pathologically, a true epithelium-lined, simple thyroid cyst is extremely rare. Virtually all cystic thyroid lesions seen with high-resolution ultrasound equipment demonstrate some wall irregularity and internal solid elements or debris caused by nodule degeneration (see Figs. 21-7 and 21-8). When high-frequency sonography and color Doppler imaging cannot differentiate debris and septa from neoplastic intracystic vegetations, contrast medium–enhanced sonography can sometimes resolve the problem through the demonstration of the arterial enhancement in tumoral projections and the complete lack of enhancement of benign septa and debris. **Comet-tail artifacts** are frequently encountered in cystic thyroid nodules, and they are likely to be related to the presence of microcrystals (see Fig. 21-8). In a published series of 100 patients presenting with this feature, FNA biopsy was benign in all cases.[21] These comet-tail artifacts can be located in the cyst walls and internal septations or in the cyst fluid. When a more densely echogenic fluid is gravitationally layered in the posterior portion of a cystic cavity, the likelihood of hemorrhagic debris is very high. Frequently, patients with hemorrhagic debris present clinically with a rapidly growing, often tender, neck mass.

Papillary carcinomas may rarely exhibit varying amounts of cystic change and appear almost indistinguishable from benign cystic nodules.[64,65] However, in cystic papillary carcinomas, the frequent sonographic detection of solid elements or projections (1 cm or more in size often with blood flow signals and/or microcalcifications) into the lumen can lead to a suspicion of malignancy (see Fig. 21-15). Cervical metastatic lymph nodes from either a solid or a cystic primary papillary cancer may also demonstrate a cystic pattern; such an occurrence, although rare, is likely to be pathognomonic of malignant adenopathy (see Fig. 21-14H).

Echogenicity. Thyroid cancers are usually hypoechoic relative to the adjacent normal thyroid parenchyma (see Fig. 21-13). Unfortunately, many benign thyroid nodules are also hypoechoic. In fact, most **hypoechoic nodules** are benign because benign nodules are so much more common than malignant nodules. A predominantly **hyperechoic nodule** is more likely to be benign.[20] The **isoechoic nodule** (visible because of a peripheral sonolucent rim that separates it from the adjacent normal parenchyma) has an intermediate risk of malignancy.

Halo. A peripheral sonolucent halo that completely or incompletely surrounds a thyroid nodule may be present in 60% to 80% of benign nodules and 15% of thyroid cancers.[20,66] Histologically, it is thought to represent the capsule of the nodule, but hyperplastic nodules that have no capsule often have this sonographic feature. The hypothesis that it represents compressed normal thyroid parenchyma seems to be quite acceptable, especially for rapidly growing thyroid cancers, which often have thick, irregular, and incomplete halos (see Fig. 21-12F) that are hypovascular or avascular on color Doppler scans. Color and power Doppler imaging have demonstrated that the thin, complete peripheral halo, which is strongly suggestive of benign nodules, represents blood vessels coursing around the periphery of the lesion (the "basket pattern").

Margin. Benign thyroid nodules tend to have sharp, well-defined margins, whereas malignant lesions tend to have irregular or poorly defined margins. For any given nodule, however, the appearance of the outer margin cannot be relied on to predict the histologic features because many exceptions to these general trends have been identified.

Calcification. Calcification can be detected in about 10% to 15% of all thyroid nodules, but the location and pattern of the calcification have a more predictive value in distinguishing benign from malignant lesions.[20] Peripheral, or eggshell-like, calcification is perhaps the most reliable feature of a benign nodule, but unfortunately it occurs in only a small percentage of benign nodules (see Fig. 21-9). Scattered echogenic foci of calcification with or without associated acoustic shadows are more common. When these calcifications are large and coarse, the nodule is more likely to be benign. When the calcifications are fine and punctate, however, malignancy is more likely. Pathologically, these fine calcifications may be caused by psammoma bodies, which are commonly seen in papillary cancers (see Figs. 21-11 and 21-12).

Medullary thyroid carcinomas often exhibit bright echogenic foci either within the primary tumor or within metastatically involved cervical lymph nodes.[33] The larger echogenic foci are usually associated with acoustic shadowing (see Fig. 21-22). Pathologically, these densities are caused by reactive fibrosis and calcification around amyloid deposits, which are characteristic of medullary carcinoma. In the appropriate clinical setting (e.g., MEN II syndrome or a patient with an increased serum calcitonin level), the finding of echogenic foci within a hypoechoic thyroid nodule or a cervical node can be highly suggestive of medullary carcinoma (see Fig. 21-21).

✳ In one study a strong association was demonstrated between sonographically detected thyroid calcifications and thyroid malignancy, particularly in young patients or with a solitary thyroid nodule. Patients younger than age 40 years with calcified nodules constitute a high-risk group, with a probability of harboring thyroid malignancies four times higher than patients of the same age but without intranodular calcifications. Similarly, the presence of calcifications within a solitary nodule increases the incidence of malignancy. Therefore, these patients must be further evaluated or followed.[67]

According to multiple studies of the various sonographic features seen in thyroid nodules, microcalcifications show the highest accuracy (76%), specificity (93%), and positive predictive value (70%) for malignancy as a single sign; however, sensitivity is low (36%) and insufficient to be reliable for detection of malignancy.[28,30,67]

Doppler Flow Pattern. It is well known from histologic studies that most hyperplastic nodules are hypovascular lesions and are less vascular than normal thyroid parenchyma. On the contrary, most **well-differentiated thyroid carcinomas** are generally hypervascular, with irregular tortuous vessels and arteriovenous shunting (see Fig. 21-13). **Poorly differentiated and anaplastic carcinomas** are often hypovascular owing to extensive necrosis associated with their rapid growth.

Because quantitative analysis of flow velocities is not accurate in differentiating benign from malignant nodules, the only Doppler feature that may be useful is the distribution of vessels. With current technology, no thyroid nodule appears totally avascular or markedly hypovascular on color and power Doppler imaging. The two main categories of vessel distribution are nodules with peripheral vascularity and nodules with internal vascularity (with or without a peripheral component).[18,19,68] In past years, it had been demonstrated that 80% to 95% of hyperplastic, goitrous, and adenomatous nodules display **peripheral vascularity** whereas 70% to 90% of thyroid malignancies display **internal vascularity, with or without a peripheral component**[5,16,68,69]; but according to other reports,[70-72] color Doppler imaging was not a reliable aid in the sonographic diagnosis of thyroid nodules. With the currently available generation of Doppler instruments, which have extremely high sensitivity to blood flow, the overlapping of the two populations of nodules significantly increased, thus causing a significant reduction of the diagnostic reliability of Doppler findings.[73]

Findings on gray scale and color Doppler ultrasound become highly predictive for malignancy only when multiple signs are simultaneously present in a nodule.[59,60] In a recent series, the combination of absent halo sign plus microcalcifications plus intranodular flow pattern achieved a 97.2% specificity for the diagnosis of thyroid malignancy.[60]

Guidance for FNA/Biopsy

Sonographically guided percutaneous needle biopsy of cervical masses has become an important technique in many clinical situations. Its main advantage is that it affords continuous real-time visualization of the needle, a crucial requirement for the biopsy of small lesions. Most physicians use a 25 gauge needle using either capillary action or minimal suction with a syringe (see Fig. 21-27). There are reports of the usefulness of large-gauge, automated, cutting needles for improved pathologic diagnosis.[74,75]

Thyroid nodules that are palpable generally undergo biopsy without imaging guidance. There are three settings, however, in which sonographically guided biopsy of a thyroid nodule is usually indicated. The first is the questionable or inconclusive physical examination when a nodule is suggested but cannot be palpated with

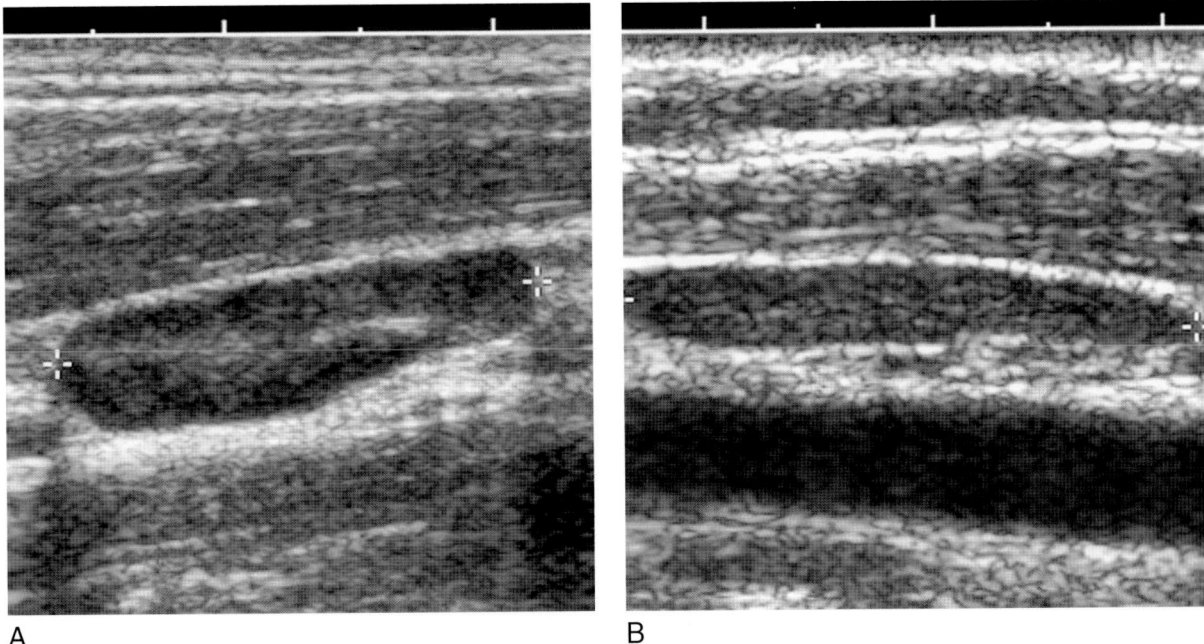

FIGURE 21-28. Normal cervical lymph nodes. Elongated shape is typical of normal cervical lymph nodes. **A,** Longitudinal image shows a slender node that is homogeneous except for central echogenic hilum. **B,** Longitudinal image demonstrates a normal homogeneous slender node near the jugular vein. This node does not have a visible hilum.

certainty. In these patients sonography is used to confirm the presence of a nodule and to provide guidance for accurate biopsy. The second setting is in the patient who is at high risk for developing thyroid cancer and who has a normal gland by physical examination but in whom sonography demonstrates a nodule. Included in this group are patients with a previous history of head and neck irradiation, those who have a positive family history for MEN II syndrome, and those who have, in the past, undergone subtotal thyroid resection for malignancy. The third group of patients includes those who have had a previous nondiagnostic or inconclusive biopsy performed under direct palpation. Usually about 20% of specimens obtained by palpation guidance are cytologically inconclusive, most often because of the aspiration of nondiagnostic fluid from cystic lesions. Sonography may be used in these cases to selectively guide the needle into a solid portion of the mass. The diagnostic accuracy of FNA is very high, with rates of sensitivity of approximately 85% and specificity of 99% in centers with a large experience with these procedures.[41-48]

In patients who have undergone a previous thyroid resection for carcinoma, sonographically guided FNA has become an important method in the early diagnosis of recurrent or metastatic disease in the neck. In patients who have undergone hemithyroidectomy for a benign nodule with the detection of one or more foci of occult malignant tumor in the surgical specimen, an ultrasound evaluation of the contralateral lobe is of value to exclude the existence of a worrisome residual nodule.

Cervical lymph nodes, both normal and abnormal, can be readily visualized by high-resolution sonography. They tend to lie along the internal jugular chain, extending from the level of the clavicles to the angle of the mandible, or to be in the region of the thyroid bed. **Benign cervical lymph nodes** usually have a slender, oval shape and often exhibit a central echogenic band that represents the fatty hilum (Fig. 21-28). **Malignant lymph nodes,** on the other hand, are usually rounder and have no echogenic hilum, presumably because of obliteration by tumor infiltration (see Fig. 21-14). Although malignant nodes are often hypoechoic, they may be diffusely echogenic, may be heterogeneous, may contain calcification, and are rarely cystic. Because these distinctions are not always clear, FNA under sonographic guidance is often used to confirm malignancy. In our experience, biopsy can be done with a high degree of accuracy in cervical nodes that are as small as 0.5 cm in diameter (Fig. 21-29).[57]

Guidance for Percutaneous Treatment

Ethanol Injection of Benign Cystic Thyroid Lesions. Lesions containing fluid (usually colloid cysts) account for 31% of thyroid nodules found on sonography, and only less than 1% of them are pure epithelial-lined cysts.[5] Management of cystic thyroid nodules relies first on fine-needle biopsy to rule out malignancy. Simple aspiration may result in permanent shrinkage of the lesion,[76] but the recurrence rate after aspiration is high (10% to 80%), depending on the number of aspirations

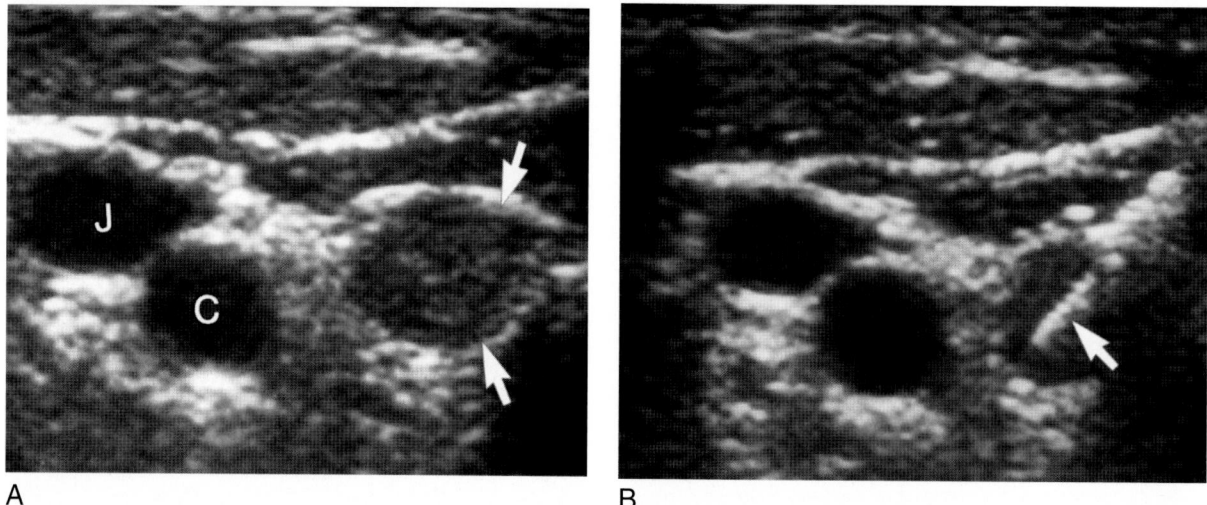

FIGURE 21-29. Biopsy of recurrent papillary carcinoma in thyroid bed after thyroidectomy. A, Transverse scan of the right side of the neck shows a 1-cm solid mass *(arrows)* medial to carotid artery (C) and jugular vein (J). **B,** Sonographically guided fine-needle aspiration with needle seen within mass *(arrow).*

and the cyst volume—the greater the volume the greater the risk of recurrence.[76]

Therefore, to avoid recurrences, intranodular injection of a sclerosing agent is needed. Ethanol has been used successfully for this therapy for the past 10 years using real-time sonographic guidance for accurate placement of the agent. Ethanol is distributed within tissues by diffusion and it induces cellular dehydration and protein denaturation, which are followed by coagulation necrosis and reactive fibrosis.

The cyst fluid is completely aspirated with a fine needle, and an amount of sterile 95% ethanol varying from 30% to 60% (according to different experiences) of the aspirated fluid is injected under ultrasound guidance (Fig. 21-30).[77,78] Subsequently, ethanol can be either reaspirated within 1 to 2 days or permanently left in place. In large cystic cavities this procedure can be repeated once or twice at intervals of several weeks. The volume reduction of the cyst is more significant if a larger amount of ethanol is injected; thus, there is a relationship between the volume of ethanol instilled and the ablative effect.

Ethanol injection is usually well tolerated by the patient. Transient mild to moderate local pain is the most common complication and occurs as a result of the leakage of ethanol into subcutaneous tissues. Rare complications of ethanol sclerotherapy are transient hyperthyroidism, hoarseness, hematoma, and dyspnea. Reported success rates (total disappearance or volume reduction greater than 70% of the initial volume) of this treatment range from 72% to 95%[77-79] and are achieved without change in thyroid function. Ethanol injection is considered the percutaneous treatment of choice for cystic lesions of the thyroid gland at some institutions.

Ethanol Injection of Autonomously Functioning Thyroid Nodules. Thyroid nodules with independent secretory and proliferative activity are defined as autonomous thyroid nodules. On radionuclide scans, these nodules appear "hot," in contrast to the low or absent extranodular uptake, likely related to the avidity of iodine trapping and the degree of thyroid hyperfunction. Patients may be toxic or nontoxic, depending on the amount of thyroid hormones secreted. The level of hyperthyroidism is usually proportional to the nodule volume. Therefore, autonomous thyroid nodules can cause a range of functional abnormalities, from euthyroidism (compensated) to subclinical hyperthyroidism (pretoxic) and clinical hyperthyroidism (toxic).

The currently available treatments of these nodules include surgery and radioactive iodine therapy. Surgery is an effective treatment, but it has the disadvantage of intrinsic anesthesiologic and surgical risks. Radioactive iodine therapy may need repeated sessions before achieving euthyroidism.

Percutaneous ethanol injection under ultrasound guidance, first proposed by Livraghi and colleagues in 1990,[80] is an alternative therapy. The diffusion of ethanol causes direct damage. Cell dehydration is followed by immediate coagulation necrosis and subsequent fibrotic changes.

Sterile 95% ethanol is injected through a 21- or 22-gauge spinal needle with closed conical tip and three terminal side holes. This allows the injection of a large amount of ethanol, reduces the total number of sessions, increases the treated volume, and minimizes the risk of laryngeal nerve damage because of the lateral diffusion of ethanol. Several treatment sessions are needed (usually four to eight), generally performed at 2-day to 2-week intervals. The total amount of ethanol delivered is usually one and one-half times the nodular volume. Color Doppler imaging and, if available, contrast medium–enhanced sonography are extremely valuable to

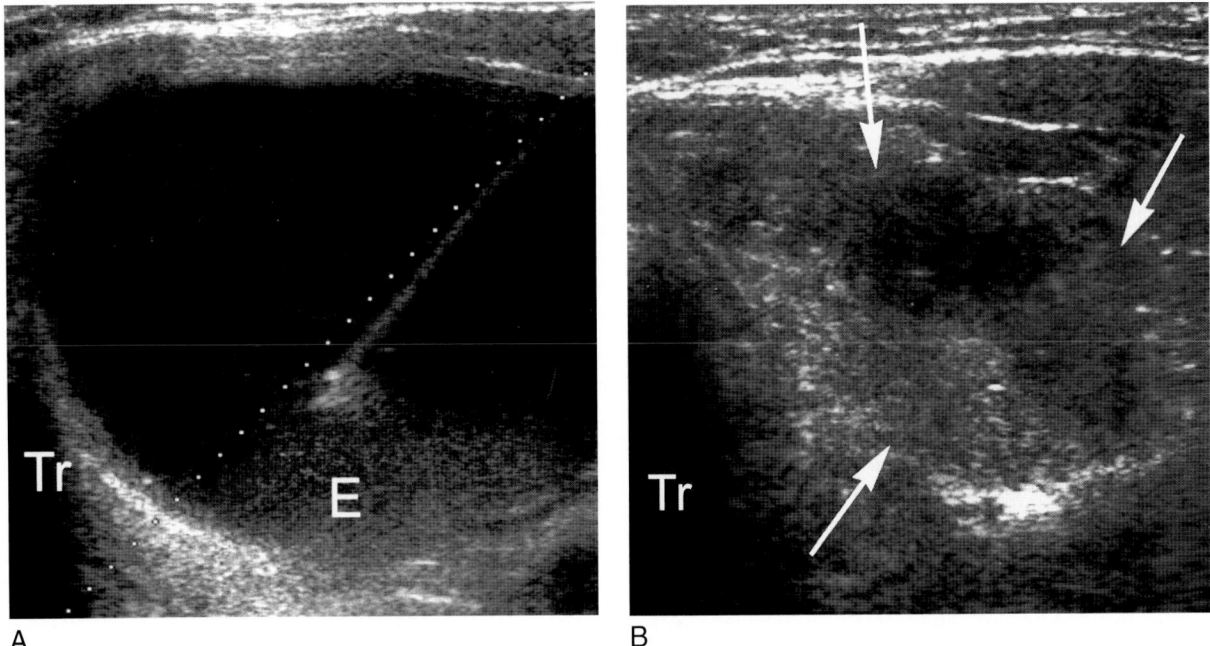

FIGURE 21-30. Ethanol treatment of large colloid cyst. A, Transverse image shows large colloid cyst with needle. Injected ethanol appears as low-level echoes (E). Tr, tracheal air shadow. **B,** Follow-up image 1 month later shows that the large cystic component has mostly resolved, leaving a slightly enlarged residual gland *(arrows)*.

assess the results of ethanol injection. The reduction (up to complete disappearance) of vascularity and contrast medium enhancement is strictly related to the necrosis induced by ethanol. In addition, residual vascularity after treatment can be targeted to achieve complete ablation.[81] Complete cure is defined as normalization of serum free thyroid hormones and serum thyrotropin and scintigraphic reactivation of extranodular tissue. Partial cure occurs when serum free thyroid hormones and thyrotropin levels are normalized but the nodule is still visible at scintigraphy.[80,82]

Percutaneous ethanol injection is generally well tolerated. The common side effect is a short-lasting burning sensation or moderate pain at the injection site, radiating to the mandibular or retroauricular regions. The slow withdrawal of the needle and the utilization of the multihole needle reduces this side effect. In some patients with larger nodules, when the amount of necrosis is high, fever lasting 2 to 3 days develops after the initial treatments. The only important complication is transient damage of the recurrent laryngeal nerve, which is reported to occur in 1% to 4% of cases.[80,82] Nerve damage is induced chemically or by compression. Full nerve recovery is likely because, in contrast to surgery, there is no anatomic nerve interruption.

Efficacy of response is inversely proportional to the nodule volume—the smaller the nodule, the more complete response is obtained. Complete cure is reported to be achieved in 68% to 100% of pretoxic nodules and in 50% to 89% of toxic nodules.[80-88] Ultrasound-guided percutaneous ethanol injection is the treatment of choice

in older patients when there are contraindications to surgery, during pregnancy, or in patients with large autonomous nodules (>40 mL) in addition to medical treatment to obtain euthyroidism more rapidly.

Percutaneous Treatment of Solitary Solid Benign "Cold" Thyroid Nodules. In patients with solitary solid, biopsy-proven benign "cold" thyroid nodules, both ethanol injection and interstitial laser photocoagulation have been proposed as ultrasound-guided percutaneous treatments, having as a major goal the achievement of a marked shrinkage of the nodule to a small fibrous-calcified mass. With percutaneous ethanol injection, a mean nodule volume reduction of 84% (range 73% to 98%) has been reported after 3 to 10 treatments.[86] With interstitial laser photocoagulation, according to preliminary experience,[87] mean thyroid nodule volumes have decreased to approximately 50% after 6 months, with improvement of clinical symptoms and no side effects.

Radiofrequency ablation has been tested for the thyroid gland in experimental studies in animals[88] and also proposed for the treatment of recurrent disease and metastatic lymph nodes in patients who have previously undergone surgery.[89]

Percutaneous Ethanol Injection of Cervical Nodal Metastases from Papillary Carcinoma. It has been shown that percutaneous ethanol injection is an effective and safe method of treatment for limited lymph node metastasis from thyroid cancer.[90] In a report from the Mayo Clinic, 14 patients who had undergone previous thyroidectomy for papillary thyroid carcinoma presented with 29 metastatic lymph nodes on follow-up sonographic imaging. Each node was treated with direct injection of ethanol using ultrasound guidance. There was a 95% decrease in size of the treated nodes on follow-up examination at 2 years. There were no major complications (e.g., recurrent laryngeal nerve palsy or bleeding) in the Mayo Clinic series or in 187 patients with papillary cancer nodes treated with percutaneous ethanol injection at the Ito Hospital in Japan.[91]

The technique is similar to the method used for percutaneous ethanol therapy of parathyroid adenomas. A 25-gauge needle is attached to a tuberculin syringe containing up to 1 mL of 95% ethanol. The needle is placed with ultrasound guidance using a free-hand technique that allows fine positioning of the needle within the node (Fig. 21-31). Each node is injected in several sites. The portion of the node that is injected becomes hyperechoic due to the formation of microbubbles of gas. After a brief time, typically less than 1 minute, the hyperechoic zone decreases. The needle is repositioned in the node, and several injections occur until the node appears adequately treated. Patients may experience mild to moderate pain at the moment of injection, but this resolves within minutes. For small nodes around 5 mm in diameter, a single injection is all that may be required. For larger nodes, a reinjection the following day is needed for complete therapy. Follow-up ultrasound examination at 3 to 6 months after injection will show a reduction in size of the node in most cases. If blood flow is visualized in the node before therapy, it will often be significantly decreased or absent on follow-up examinations. If on follow-up examinations, the size of the node has not decreased or if there is residual blood flow on power Doppler examination, a repeat injection is performed.

The Incidentally Detected Nodule

Although using high-resolution sonography to detect small, nonpalpable thyroid nodules may be beneficial in some clinical settings, it may actually introduce problems in other settings. What should one do about the many thyroid nodules detected incidentally during the course of carotid, parathyroid, or other sonographic examinations of the neck? The goal should be to avoid extensive and costly evaluations in the majority of patients with benign disease, without missing the minority of patients who have clinically significant thyroid cancer. By clinical palpation, the prevalence of thyroid nodules in the United States is 4% to 7% of the general population, but high-resolution sonography has detected thyroid nodules in approximately 40% of hypercalcemic populations.[10,92] Previous studies have shown that patients with hyperparathyroidism have statistically no more nodular thyroid disease than age-matched and sex-matched autopsy controls.[93] Of 1000

consecutive hypercalcemic patients, 410 (41%) had sonographically visible nodules, of which only 80 (8%) were clinically palpable. A similarly high prevalence of sonographically detected thyroid abnormalities was reported in Finland.[53] In this study of 101 women with no previous thyroid or parathyroid disease, 36% had one or more sonographically visible nodules. A somewhat higher prevalence of thyroid nodules has been detected at autopsy in patients who had clinically normal thyroid glands; 49.5% had one or more grossly visible nodules.[94] Thus, high-resolution sonography can detect almost as many nodules as are demonstrated by careful pathologic examination, and both studies showed a direct relationship between the prevalence of thyroid nodules and patient age (Fig. 21-32).

Although these studies have shown a high prevalence of thyroid nodules detected by autopsy and sonography, the prevalence of thyroid malignancy was only 2% and 4%, respectively, with most (90%) being occult (<1.5 cm) papillary cancers (Table 21-3).[92,94] The papillary type of thyroid cancer represents approximately 90% of all thyroid cancers diagnosed in the midwestern United States since 1970.[14,22]

The vast majority of patients with occult papillary thyroid cancer have an excellent prognosis, with essentially no reduction in life expectancy and no morbidity from appropriate surgical therapy. Further evidence that most subclinical thyroid cancers have a benign natural history is the fact that the annual incidence of clinically detected thyroid cancer is only 0.005% (5 per 100,000 persons).[14,22]

If nearly 50% of the United States population has subtle evidence of nodular thyroid disease that can be revealed by sonography, yet the annual incidence rate of clinically apparent thyroid carcinoma is only 0.005%, it is clear that only a small minority of patients with thyroid nodules have a risk of harboring clinically significant thyroid cancer (see Table 21-3). Furthermore, if 90% of those cancers are papillary and therefore eminently curable after they become clinically apparent, it seems both impractical and imprudent to pursue for diagnosis all of the small nodules detected incidentally by high-resolution sonography.

EVALUATION OF NODULES INCIDENTALLY DETECTED BY SONOGRAPHY

Nodules under 1.5 cm
  Followed by palpation at time of next physical examination
Nodules over 1.5 cm
  Evaluation (usually by FNA)
Nodules that have malignant features
  Evaluation by FNA

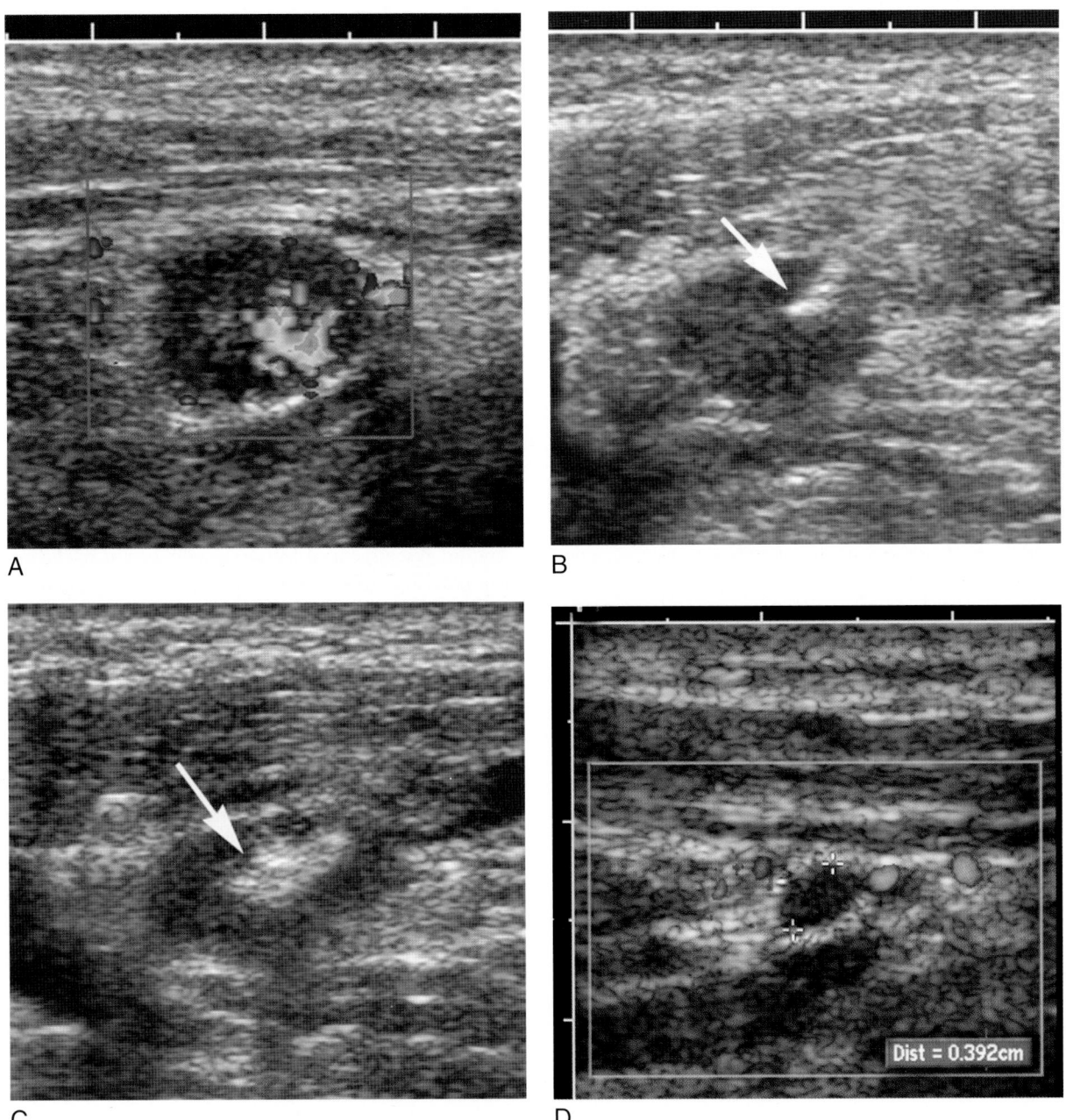

FIGURE 21-31. Ethanol treatment of thyroid metastasis in a cervical lymph node. A, Longitudinal color Doppler image shows a 1.6-cm round pathologic-appearing node with moderate vascularity. **B,** The tip of a 25-gauge needle *(arrow)* is in the lymph node. **C,** The ethanol effect is visible as a focal hyperechoic area *(arrow)* at the moment of injection and is due to microbubbles that form from the interaction of ethanol with the tissues. This hyperechoic appearance will last from several seconds to several minutes and will be followed by a normal or near-normal appearance. During the injection, the hyperechogenicity is a useful marker to identify the areas treated. **D,** Follow-up power Doppler image, 6 months after ethanol injection, shows that the lymph node has dramatically decreased in size (0.4 cm) and is no longer vascular. No further therapy is needed except to follow every 6 to 12 months to confirm lack of change.

Accordingly, for nonpalpable nodules that are incidentally detected by sonography, two imaging criteria may be used to determine the need for further diagnostic work-up.

Size

Most nodules exceeding 1.5 cm in maximum diameter should be further evaluated (usually by FNA), regardless of physical and sonographic features. Nodules under 1.5 cm may be followed by palpation at the time of the patient's next physical examination.[95]

Sonographic Appearance

Nodules that have malignant sonographic features (microcalcifications, irregular margin, thick halo, internal flow pattern) should undergo ultrasound-guided FNA (see Fig. 21-12).[96]

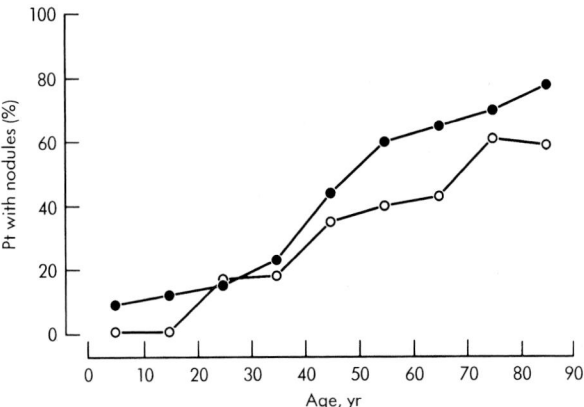

FIGURE 21-32. Comparison of prevalence of thyroid nodules detected by autopsy and sonography. Autopsy *(solid circles)* on average 49% in 1955. Sonography *(open circles)* on average 41% in 1985, as a function of patient age. (From Horlocker TT, Hay JE, James EM, et al: Prevalence of incidental nodular thyroid disease detected during high-resolution parathyroid ultrasonography. In Medeiros-Neto G, Gaitin E (eds): Frontiers in Thyroidology New York, Plenum, 1986, vol 2, pp 1309-1312.)

TABLE 21-3. PREVALENCE OF THYROID NODULES

Method of Detection	Patients (%)
Autopsy	49
Sonography	41
Palpation	7
Occult cancer (autopsy)	2
Cancer incidence (annual)	0.005

In most cases of incidentally detected nodules, we recommend the simple follow-up of neck palpation at the time of the patient's next physical examination. Follow-up sonographic examination, radionuclide imaging, FNA, or surgical excision of such incidental nodules is rarely necessary in our practice.

DIFFUSE THYROID DISEASE

Several thyroid diseases are characterized by diffuse rather than focal involvement. This usually results in generalized enlargement of the gland (goiter) and no palpable nodules. Specific conditions that commonly produce such diffuse enlargement include **chronic autoimmune lymphocytic (Hashimoto's) thyroiditis, colloid or adenomatous goiter, and Graves' disease.** Diagnosis of these conditions is usually made on the basis of clinical and laboratory findings and, on occasion, by FNA. Sonography is seldom indicated. One clinical setting in which high-resolution sonography can be helpful is when the underlying diffuse disease causes asymmetric thyroid enlargement, which raises the possibility of a mass in the larger lobe. The sonographic

finding of generalized parenchymal abnormality may alert the clinician to consider diffuse thyroid disease as the underlying cause. FNA, with sonographic guidance if necessary, can be performed if a nodule is detected. Recognition of diffuse thyroid enlargement on sonography can often be facilitated by noting the thickness of the isthmus. Normally, it is a thin bridge of tissue measuring only a few millimeters in anteroposterior dimension. With diffuse thyroid enlargement, the isthmus may be up to 1 cm or more in thickness.

There are several different types of thyroiditis including acute suppurative thyroiditis, subacute granulomatous thyroiditis (de Quervain's disease), and chronic lymphocytic thyroiditis (Hashimoto's thyroiditis).[97] Each disease has distinctive clinical and laboratory features. **Acute suppurative thyroiditis** is a rare inflammatory disease that is usually caused by bacterial infection and usually affects children. Sonography can be useful in selected cases to detect the development of a frank thyroid abscess. The infection usually begins in the perithyroidal soft tissues. On ultrasound images, an abscess is seen as an ill-defined, hypoechoic, heterogeneous mass with internal debris with or without septa and gas. Adjacent inflammatory nodes are often present. **Subacute granulomatous thyroiditis (de Quervain's disease)** is a spontaneously remitting inflammatory disease that is probably caused by viral infection. The clinical findings include fever, enlargement of the gland, and pain on palpation. Sonographically the gland may appear enlarged and hypoechoic with normal or decreased vascularity owing to diffuse edema of the gland or the process may appear as focal hypoechoic regions (Fig. 21-33).[98,99] Although usually not necessary, sonography can be used to assess evolution of the disease after medical therapy (see Fig. 21-33).

The most common type of thyroiditis is **chronic autoimmune lymphocytic thyroiditis (Hashimoto's thyroiditis).** It typically occurs clinically as a painless, diffuse enlargement of the thyroid gland in a young or middle-aged woman, often associated with hypothyroidism. It is the most common cause of hypothyroidism in North America. It is an autoimmune disease where the patient develops antibodies to their own thyroglobulin. The typical sonographic appearance of Hashimoto's thyroiditis is diffuse coarsened parenchymal echo texture, generally more hypoechoic than a normal thyroid (see Fig. 21-33).[100] In most cases the gland is enlarged. Multiple, discrete **hypoechoic micronodules** from 1 to 6 mm in diameter are strongly suggestive of chronic thyroiditis, and this appearance has been called "micronodulation" (Fig. 21-34). Micronodulation is a highly sensitive sign of chronic thyroiditis with a positive predictive value of 94.7%.[100] Histologically, they represent lobules of thyroid parenchyma that have been infiltrated by lymphocytes and plasma cells. These lobules are surrounded by multiple linear echogenic

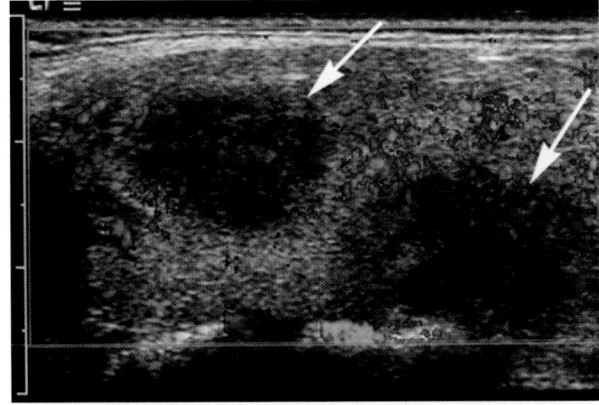

A

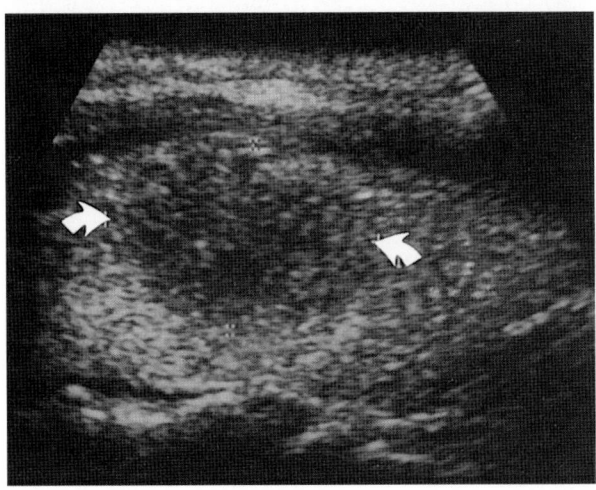

B

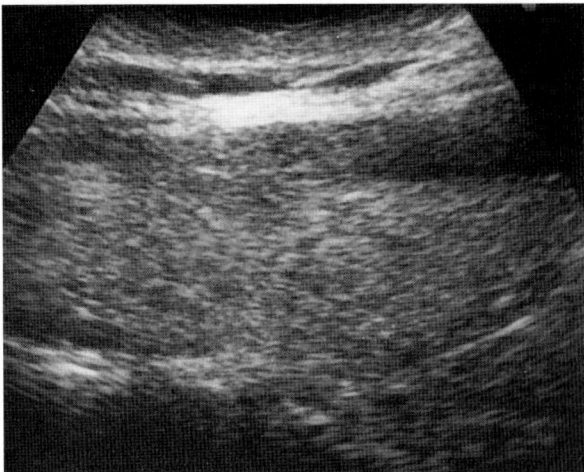

C

FIGURE 21-33. Focal areas of subacute thyroiditis. **A,** Longitudinal power Doppler image of the thyroid gland shows two ill-defined, hypoechoic areas *(arrows)* that, at fine-needle aspiration, were due to subacute thyroiditis. **B,** Longitudinal image of a different patient shows an ill-defined hypoechoic area *(arrows)* that returns to normal (**C**) on follow-up examination 4 weeks later after medical therapy.

fibrous septations (Fig. 21-35). These fibrotic septations may produce a pseudolobulated appearance of the parenchyma. Both benign and malignant thyroid nodules may coexist with chronic lymphocytic thyroiditis, and FNA is often necessary to establish the final diagnosis (Figs. 21-36 to 21-38).[101] Like other autoimmune disorders, there is an increased risk of malignancy, with a B-cell malignant lymphoma the most common to arise within the gland.

The vascularity on color Doppler imaging is normal or decreased in most patients with the diagnosis of Hashimoto's thyroiditis (see Fig. 21-35). Occasionally, hypervascularity similar to the "thyroid inferno" of Graves' disease occurs. A study suggested that hyper-

vascularity occurs when hypothyroidism develops.[102] Often, cervical lymphadenopathy is present, most evident near the lower pole of the thyroid gland (Fig. 21-39). The end stage of chronic thyroiditis is atrophy when the thyroid gland is small, with ill-defined margins and heterogeneous texture due to progressive increase of fibrosis. Blood flow signals are absent. Occasionally, discrete nodules occur, and FNA is needed to establish the diagnosis (see Fig. 21-36).[101]

Painless (silent) thyroiditis has the typical histologic and sonographic pattern of chronic autoimmune thyroiditis (hypoechogenicity, micronodulation, and fibrosis), but clinical findings resemble classical subacute thyroiditis, with the exception of node tenderness. Moderate hyperthyroidism with thyroid enlargement usually occurs in the early phase, followed sometimes by hypothyroidism of variable degrees. In postpartum thyroiditis, the progression to hypothyroidism is more frequent. In most circumstances, the disease spontaneously remits within 3 to 6 months, and the gland may return to a normal appearance.

Although the appearance of diffuse parenchymal inhomogeneity and micronodularity is quite typical of Hashimoto's thyroiditis, other diffuse thyroid diseases,

DIFFUSE THYROID DISEASE

Acute suppurative thyroiditis
Subacute granulomatous thyroiditis
Hashimoto's (chronic lymphocytic) thyroiditis
Adenomatous or colloid goiter
Painless (silent) thyroiditis
Graves' disease
Invasive fibrous thyroiditis

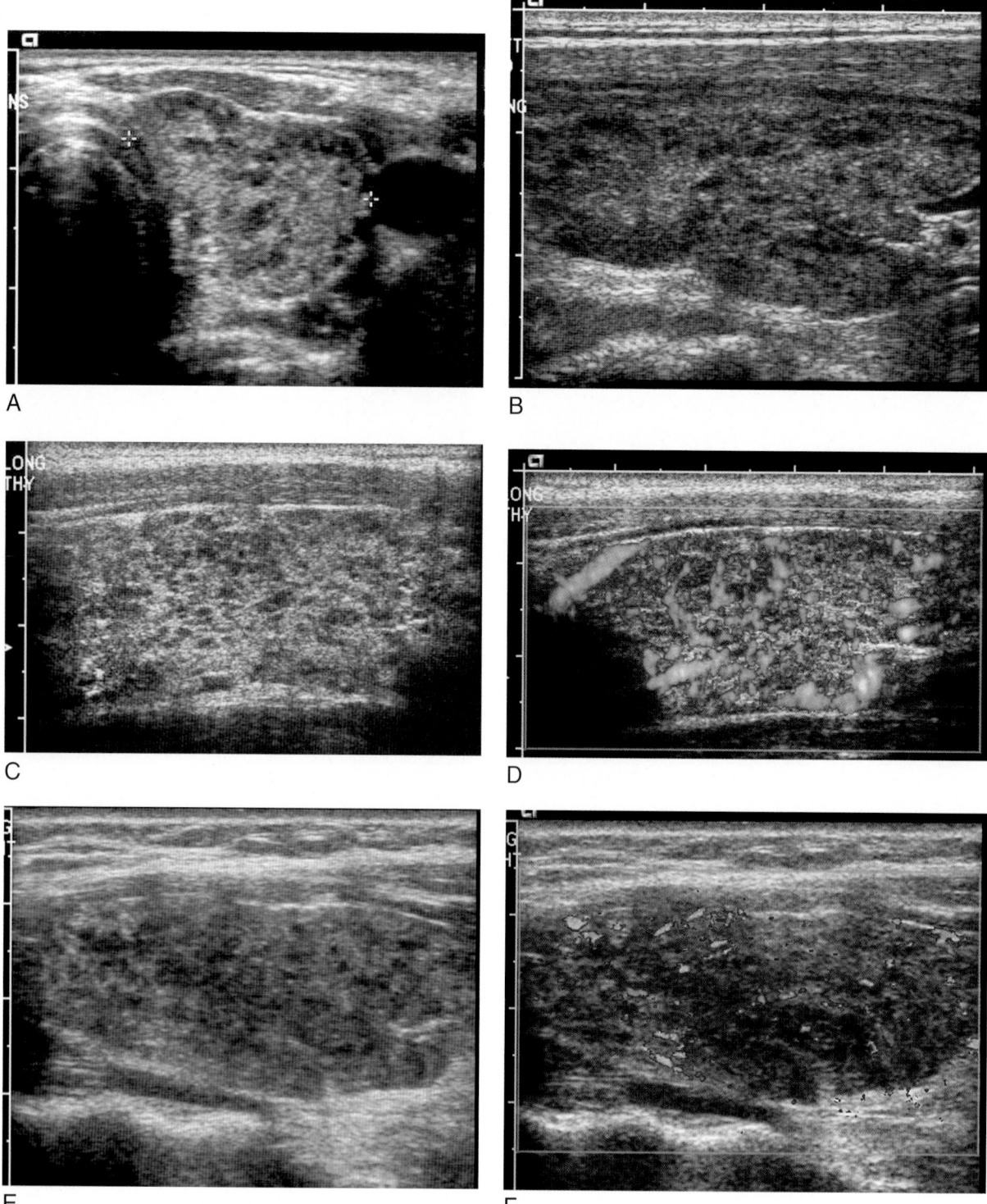

FIGURE 21-34. Hashimoto's thyroiditis: micronodularity. Transverse (**A**) and longitudinal (**B**) images of the left lobe demonstrate multiple small hypoechoic nodules that are lymphocyte infiltration of the parenchyma. **C** and **D,** Longitudinal images of another patient show multiple tiny hypoechoic nodules and increased flow on power Doppler. This increased flow may indicate an acute phase of the thyroiditis. **E** and **F,** Longitudinal images of a different patient show multiple tiny hypoechoic nodules and decreased flow on color Doppler. The blood flow is normal or diminished in most cases of Hashimoto's thyroiditis.

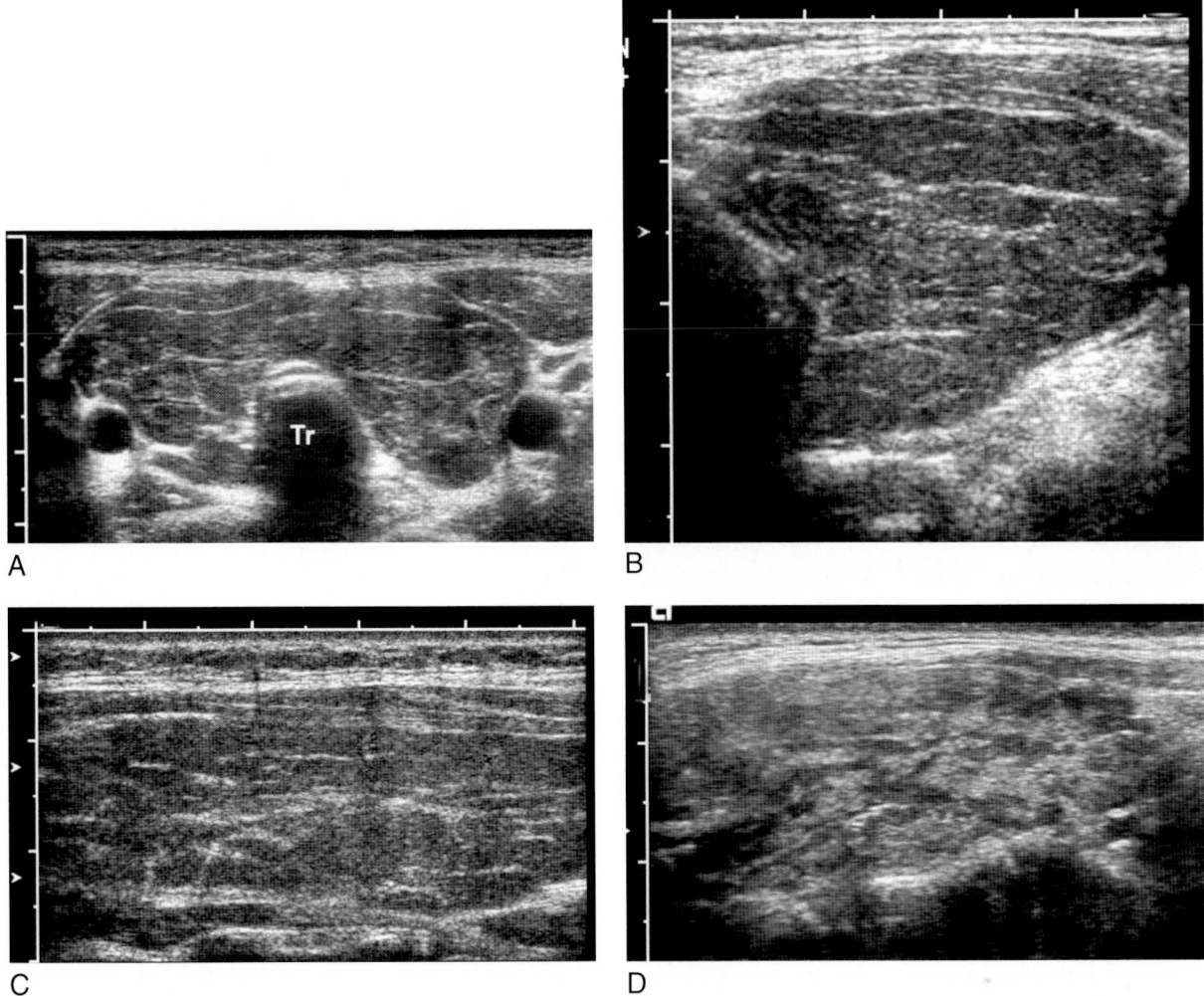

FIGURE 21-35. Hashimoto's thyroiditis: coarse septations. A, Transverse dual image of the thyroid shows marked diffuse enlargement of both lobes and the isthmus. There are multiple linear bright echoes throughout the hypoechoic parenchyma caused by lymphocytic infiltration of the gland with coarse septations from fibrous bands. Tr, tracheal air shadow. Transverse (**B**) and longitudinal (**C**) images of another patient demonstrate linear echogenic septations throughout the gland. **D,** Longitudinal image of another patient shows thicker echogenic linear areas that separate hypoechoic regions.

most commonly **multinodular or adenomatous goiter,** may have a similar sonographic appearance. Most patients with adenomatous goiter have multiple discrete nodules separated by otherwise normal-appearing thyroid parenchyma (see Fig. 21-26); others have enlargement with rounding of the poles of the gland, diffuse parenchymal inhomogeneity, and no recognizable normal tissue. Adenomatous goiter affects women three times more often than men.

Graves' disease is a common diffuse abnormality of the thyroid gland and is usually biochemically characterized by hyperfunction (thyrotoxicosis). The echo texture may be more inhomogeneous than it is in diffuse goiter, mainly because of the presence of numerous large intraparenchymal vessels. Furthermore, especially in young patients, the parenchyma may be diffusely hypoechoic because of the extensive lymphocytic infil-tration or because of the predominantly cellular content of the parenchyma, which becomes almost devoid of colloid substance. Color Doppler sonography often demonstrates a hypervascular pattern referred to as the **"thyroid inferno"** (Fig. 21-40). Spectral Doppler will often demonstrate peak systolic velocities exceeding 70 cm/sec, which is the highest velocity found in thyroid disease. There is no correlation between the degree of thyroid hyperfunction assessed by laboratory studies and the extent of hypervascularity or blood flow velocities. Previous studies have shown that Doppler analysis can be used to monitor therapeutic response in patients with Graves' disease.[103] A significant decrease in flow velocities in the superior and inferior thyroid arteries after medical treatment has been reported.

The rarest type of inflammatory thyroid disease is **invasive fibrous thyroiditis,** also called **Riedel's**

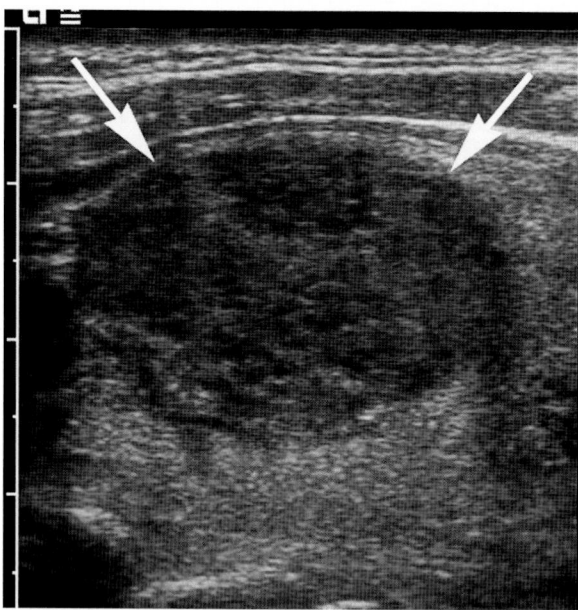

FIGURE 21-36. Hashimoto's thyroiditis: nodule.
Longitudinal image shows a discrete hypoechoic nodule *(arrows)* that at fine-needle aspiration was due to Hashimoto's thyroiditis.

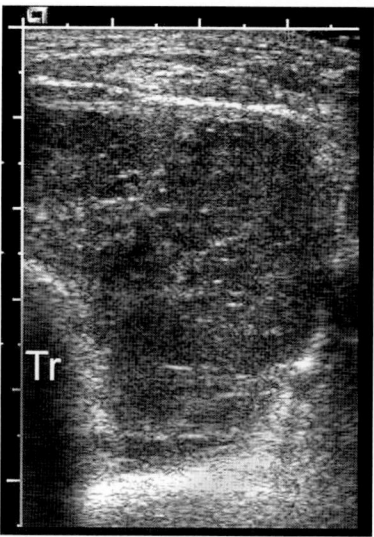

FIGURE 21-38. Lymphoma in Hashimoto's thyroiditis. Transverse image of the left lobe shows diffuse hypoechoic enlargement that was due to lymphoma in a gland with Hashimoto's thyroiditis. Tr, tracheal air shadow.

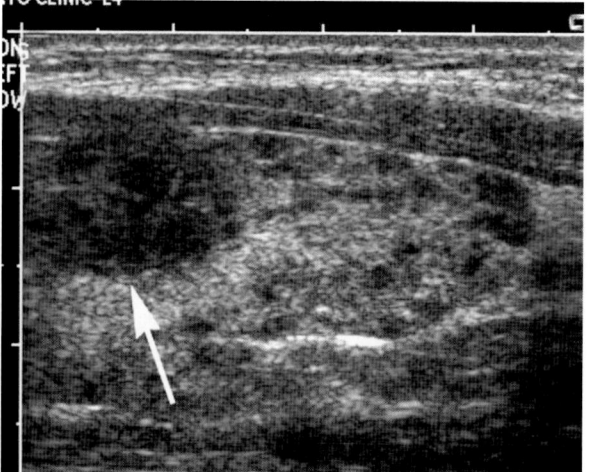

FIGURE 21-37. Hashimoto's thyroiditis with papillary thyroid cancer. Longitudinal image shows classic Hashimoto's thyroiditis (micronodularity) and a hypoechoic dominant nodule *(arrow)* in the upper pole due to papillary thyroid carcinoma. A dominant nodule in Hashimoto's thyroiditis should be considered indeterminate and fine-needle aspiration performed.

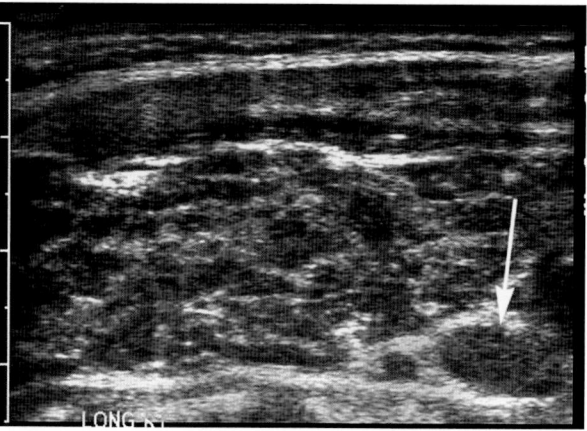

FIGURE 21-39. Hashimoto's thyroiditis with hyperplastic enlarged lymph nodes. Longitudinal image shows micronodularity of Hashimoto's thyroiditis and an enlarged lymph node *(arrow)* inferior to the lower pole.

struma.[97] This disease primarily affects women and often tends to progress inexorably to complete destruction of the gland. Some cases may be associated with mediastinal or retroperitoneal fibrosis or sclerosing cholangitis. In the few cases of invasive fibrous thyroiditis

examined sonographically, the gland was diffusely enlarged and had an inhomogeneous parenchymal echo texture. The primary reason for sonography was to check for extrathyroid extension of the inflammatory process with encasement of the adjacent vessels (Fig. 21-41). Such information can be particularly useful in surgical planning. Open biopsy is generally required to distinguish this condition from anaplastic thyroid carcinoma. The sonographic findings in these two diseases may be identical.

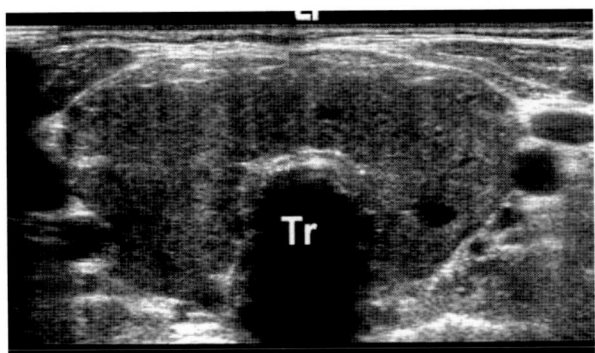

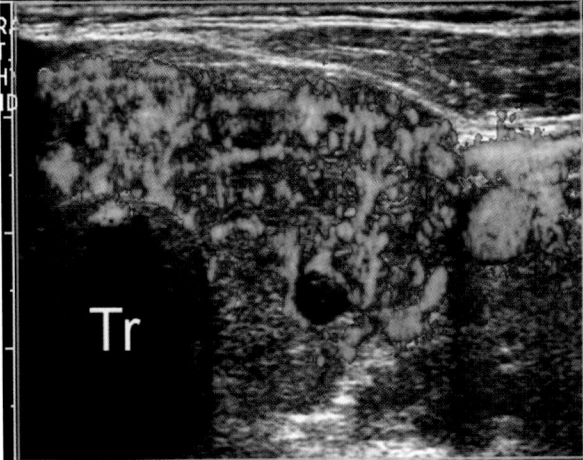

FIGURE 21-40. Hyperthyroidism: Graves' disease.
A, Transverse dual image of the thyroid gland shows marked diffuse enlargement of both lobes of the thyroid and the isthmus. The gland is diffusely hypoechoic. **B,** Transverse color Doppler image of the left lobe shows increased vascularity indicating an acute stage of the process. Tr, trachea.

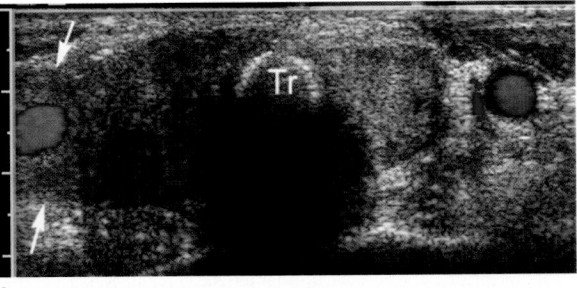

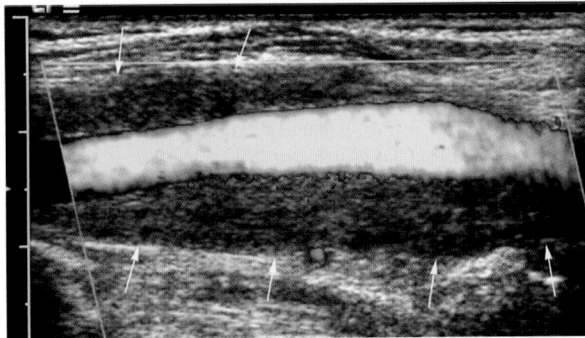

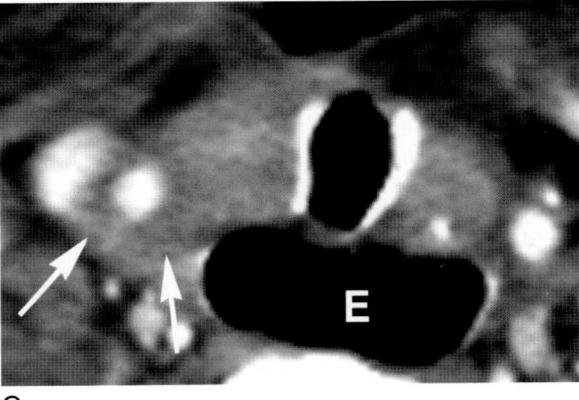

FIGURE 21-41. Reidel's struma (invasive fibrous thyroiditis). A, Transverse dual color Doppler ultrasound of the thyroid shows a diffuse hypoechoic process in the right lobe extending around the common carotid artery *(arrows)*. Tr, trachea. **B,** Longitudinal power Doppler image of the right common carotid artery shows a hypoechoic soft tissue mass *(arrows)* encasing the vessel. **C,** Contrast medium–enhanced CT scan shows mild enlargement of the right thyroid lobe and soft tissue thickening *(arrows)* around the right common carotid artery. Incidentally noted is dilatation of the air-filled esophagus (E).

References

Anatomy

1. Rogers WM: Anomalous development of the thyroid. In Werner SC, Ingbar SH (eds): The Thyroid. New York, Harper & Row, 1978, pp 416-420.
2. Toma P, Guastalla PP, Carini C, et al. Collo [The neck]. In Fariello G, Perale R, Perri G, et al (eds): Ecografia Pediatrica. Milan, Ambrosiana, 1992, pp 139-162.
3. Solbiati L: La tiroide e le paratiroidi [The thyroid and the parathyroid]. In Rizzatto G, Solbiati L (eds): Anatomia Ecografica: Quadri Normali, Varianti e Limiti con il Patologico. Milan, Masson, 1992, pp 35-45.
4. Jarlov AE, Hegedus L, Gjorup T, et al: Accuracy of the clinical assessment of thyroid size. Dan Med Bull 1991;38:87-89.
5. Kerr L: High-resolution thyroid ultrasound: The value of color Doppler. Ultrasound Q 1994;12:21-43.
6. Hegedus L, Perrild H, Poulsen LR, et al: The determination of thyroid volume by ultrasound and its relationship to body weight, age, and sex in normal subjects. J Clin Endocrinol Metab 1983;56:260-263.
7. Solbiati L, Osti V, Cova L, et al: The neck. In Meire H, Cosgrove D (eds): Abdominal and General Ultrasound. Edinburgh, Churchill Livingstone, 2001, vol 2, pp 699-737.
8. Brandl H, Gritzky A, Haizinger M. 3-D ultrasound: A dedicated system. Eur Radiol 1999;9:S331-S333.
9. Ueda D, Mitamura R, Suzuki N, et al: Sonographic imaging of the thyroid gland in congenital hypothyroidism. Pediatr Radiol 1992;22:102-105.

Nodular Thyroid Disease

10. Rojeski MT, Gharib H: Nodular thyroid disease: Evaluation and management. N Engl J Med 1985;313:428-436.

11. Van Herle AJ, Rich P, Ljung B-ME, et al: The thyroid nodule. Ann Intern Med 1992;96:221-232.

12. Favus MJ, Schneider AB, Stachura ME, et al: Thyroid cancer occurring as a late consequence of head-and-neck irradiation: Evaluation of 1056 patients. N Engl J Med 1976;294:1019-1025.

13. Degroot LJ, Reilly M, Pinnameneni K, et al: Retrospective and prospective study of radiation-induced thyroid disease. Am J Med 1983;74:852-862.

14. Grebe SKG, Hay ID: Follicular cell-derived thyroid carcinoma. Cancer Treat Res 1997;89:91-140.

15. Hennemann G: Non-toxic goitre. Clin Endocrinol Metab 1979;8:167-179.

16. Solbiati L, Cioffi V, Ballarati E: Ultrasonography of the neck. Radiol Clin North Am 1992;30:941-954.

17. Muller HW, Schroder S, Schneider C, et al: Sonographic tissue characterization in thyroid gland diagnosis. Klin Wochenschr 1985;63:706-710.

18. Lagalla R, Caruso G, Midiri M, et al: Echo Doppler: Couleur et pathologie thyroidienne. JEMU 1992;13:44-47.

19. Solbiati L, Ballarati E, Cioffi V: Contribution of color-flow mapping to the differential diagnosis of the thyroid nodules [abstract]. Presented at Radiological Society of North America Meeting, 1991.

20. Solbiati L, Volterrani L, Rizzatto G, et al: The thyroid gland with low uptake lesions: Evaluation by ultrasound. Radiology 1985;155:187-191.

21. Ahuja A, Chick W, King W, et al: Clinical significance of the comet-tail artifact in thyroid ultrasound. J Clin Ultrasound 1996;24:129-133.

22. Schlumberger M-J, Filetti S, Hay ID: Nontoxic goiter and thyroid neoplasia. In Larsen PR, Kronenberg HM, Melmed S, et al (eds): Williams Textbook of Endocrinology, 10th ed. Philadelphia, WB Saunders, 2003, pp 457-490.

23. Black BM, Kirk TA Jr, Woolner LB: Multicentricity of papillary adenocarcinoma of the thyroid: Influence on treatment. J Clin Endocrinol Metab 1960;20:130-135.

24. Hay ID, McConahey WM, Goellner JR: Managing patients with papillary thyroid carcinoma: Insights gained from the Mayo Clinic's experience of treating 2,512 consecutive patients during 1940 through 2000. Trans Am Clin Climatol Assoc 2002;113:241-260.

25. Wunderbaldinger P, Harisinghani MG, Hahn PF, et al: Cystic lymph node metastases in papillary thyroid carcinoma. AJR Am J Roentgenol 2002;178:693-697.

26. Pilotti S, Pierotti MA: Classificazione istologica e caratterizzazione molecolare dei tumori dell'epitelio follicolare della tiroide. Argomenti di Oncologia 1992;13:365-380.

27. Holtz S, Powers WE: Calcification in papillary carcinoma of the thyroid. Radiology 1958;80:997-1000.

28. Brkljacic B, Cuk V, Tomic-Brzac H, et al: Ultrasonic evaluation of benign and malignant nodules in echographically multinodular thyroids. J Clin Ultrasound 1994;22:71-76.

29. Ahuja AT, Ying M, Yuen HY, et al: Power Doppler sonography of metastatic nodes from papillary carcinoma of the thyroid. Clin Radiol 2001;56:284-288.

30. Solbiati L, Ierace T, Lagalla R, et al: Reliability of high-frequency US and color Doppler US of thyroid nodules: Italian multicenter study of 1,042 pathologically confirmed cases. Which role for scintigraphy and biopsy? [abstract] Presented at Radiological Society of North America Meeting, 1995.

31. Solbiati L, Livraghi T, Ballarati E, et al: Thyroid gland. In Solbiati L, Rizzatto G (eds): Ultrasound of Superficial Structures. Edinburgh, Churchill Livingstone, 1995, pp 49-85.

32. Chong GC, Beahrs OH, Sizemore GW, et al: Medullary carcinoma of the thyroid gland. Cancer 1975; 35:695-704.

33. Gorman B, Charboneau JW, James EM, et al: Medullary thyroid carcinoma: Role of high-resolution ultrasound. Radiology 1987;162:147-150.

34. Nel CJC, van Heerden JA, Goellner JR, et al: Anaplastic carcinoma of the thyroid: A clinicopathologic study of 82 cases. Mayo Clin Proc 1985;60:51-58.

35. Hamburger JI, Miller JM, Kini SR: Lymphoma of the thyroid. Ann Intern Med 1983;99:685-693.

36. Kasagi K, Hatabu H, Tokuda Y, et al: Lymphoproliferative disorders of the thyroid gland: Radiological appearances. Br J Radiol 1991;64:569-575.

37. Takashima S, Morimoto S, Ikezoe, et al: Primary thyroid lymphoma: Comparison of CT and US assessment. Radiology 1989;171:439-443.

38. Ahuja A, Evans R: The thyroid and parathyroid. In Practical Head and Neck Ultrasound. London, GMM, 2000.

39. Feld S, Barcia M, Baskic HJ, et al: AACE clinical practice guidelines for the diagnosis and management of thyroid nodules. Endocr Pract 1996;2:78-84.

40. Miller JM: Evaluation of thyroid nodules: Accent on needle biopsy. Med Clin North Am 1985;69:1063-1077.

41. Hamberger B, Gharib H, Melton LJ III, et al: Fine-needle aspiration biopsy of thyroid nodules: Impact on thyroid practice and cost of care. Am J Med 1982;73:381-384.

42. Goellner JR, Gharib H, Grant CS, et al: Fine-needle aspiration cytology of the thyroid, 1980 to 1986. Acta Cytol 1987;31:587-590.

43. Gharib H, Goellner JR: Fine-needle aspiration biopsy of the thyroid: An appraisal. Ann Intern Med 1993; 118:282-289.

44. Hawkins F, Bellido D, Bernai C, et al: Fine-needle aspiration biopsy in the diagnosis of thyroid cancer and thyroid disease. Cancer 1987;59:1206-1209.

45. Khafagi F, Wright G, Castles H, et al: Screening for thyroid malignancy: The role of fine-needle biopsy. Med J Aust 1988;149:302-303, 306-307.

46. Hall TL, Layfield LJ, Philippe A, et al: Sources of diagnostic error in fine-needle aspiration of the thyroid. Cancer 1989;63:718-725.

47. Altavilla A, Pascale M, Nenci I: Fine-needle aspiration cytology of thyroid gland diseases. Acta Cytol 1990;34:251-256.

48. Ravetto C, Spreafico GL, Colombo L: L'esame citologico con agoaspirato nella diagnosi precoce delle neoplasie tiroidee. Rec Progr Med 1977;63:258-267.

49. James EM, Charboneau JW: High-frequency (10 MHz) thyroid ultrasonography. Semin Ultrasound CT MR 1985;6:294-309.

50. Scheible W, Leopold GR, Woo VL, et al: High-resolution real-time ultrasonography of thyroid nodules. Radiology 1979;133:413-417.

51. Simeone JF, Daniels GH, Mueller PR, et al: High-resolution real-time sonography of the thyroid. Radiology 1982;145:431-435.

52. Brown CL: Pathology of the cold nodule. Clin Endocrinol Metab 1981;10:235-245.

53. Brander A, Viikinkoski P, Nickels J, et al: Thyroid gland: US screening in middle-aged women with no previous thyroid disease. Radiology 1989;173:507-510.

54. Hay ID. Papillary thyroid carcinoma. Endocrinol Metab Clin North Am 1990;19:545-576.

55. Hay ID, Reading CC, Weiland LH, et al: Clinico-pathologic and high-resolution ultrasonographic evaluation of clinically suspicious or malignant thyroid disease. In Medeiros-Neto G, Gaitan E (eds): Frontiers in Thyroidology. New York, Plenum, 1986, vol 2.

56. Simeone JF, Daniels GH, Hall DA, et al: Sonography in the follow-up of 100 patients with thyroid carcinoma. AJR Am J Roentgenol 1987;148:45-49.

57. Sutton RT, Reading CC, Charboneau JW, et al: Ultrasound-guided biopsy of neck masses in postoperative management of patients with thyroid cancer. Radiology 1988;168:769-772.

58. Kim EK, Park CS, Chung WY, et al: New sonographic criteria for recommending fine-needle aspiration biopsy of nonpalpable solid nodules of the thyroid. AJR Am J Roentgenol 2002;178:687-691.

59. Koike E, Noguchi S, Yamashita H, et al: Ultrasonographic characteristics of thyroid nodules: Prediction of malignancy. Arch Surg 2001;136:334-337.

60. Rago T, Vitti P, Chiovato L, et al: Role of conventional ultrasonography and color flow Doppler sonography in predicting malignancy in "cold" thyroid nodules. Eur J Endocrinol 1998;138:41-46.

61. Watters DAK, Ahuja AT, Evans RM, et al: Role of ultrasound in the management of thyroid nodules. Am J Surg 1992;164:654-657.

62. Okamoto T, Yamashita T, Harasawa A, et al: Test performances of three diagnostic procedures in evaluating thyroid nodules: Physical examination, ultrasonography and fine-needle aspiration cytology. Endocr J 1994;41:243-247.

63. Leenhardt L, Tramalloni J, Aurengo H, et al: Echographie des nodules thyroidiens: l'Echographiste face aux exigences du clinicien. Presse-Med 1994;23:1389-1392.

64. Hammer M, Wortsman J, Folse R: Cancer in cystic lesions of the thyroid. Arch Surg 1982;117:1020-1023.

65. Livolsi A: Pathology of thyroid disease. In Falj SA (ed): Thyroid Disease: Endocrinology, Surgery, Nuclear Medicine and Radiotherapy. Philadelphia, Lippincott-Raven, 1997, pp 65-104.

66. Propper RA, Skolnick ML, Weinstein BJ, et al: The nonspecificity of the thyroid halo sign. J Clin Ultrasound 1980;8:129-132.

67. Kakkos SK, Scopa CD, Chalmoukis AK, et al: Relative risk of cancer in sonographically detected thyroid nodules with calcifications. J Clin Ultrasound 2000;7:347-352.

68. Fobbe F, Finke R, Reichenstein E, et al: Appearance of thyroid diseases using colour-coded duplex sonography. Eur J Radiol 1989;9:29-31.

69. Argalia G, D'Ambrosio F, Lucarelli F, et al: L'eco color Doppler nella caratterizzazione della patologia nodulare tiroidea. Radiol Med 1995;89:651-657.

70. Spiezia S, Colao A, Assanti AP, et al: Utilita' dell'eco color Doppler con power Doppler nella diagnostica dei noduli tiroidei ipoecogeni: Work in progress. Radiol Med 1996;91:616-621.

71. Clark KJ, Cronan JJ, Scola FH: Color Doppler sonography: Anatomic and physiologic assessment of the thyroid. J Clin Ultrasound 1995;23:215-223.

72. Shimamoto K, Endo T, Ishigaki T, et al: Thyroid nodules: Evaluation with color Doppler ultrasonography. J Ultrasound Med 1993;11:673-678.

73. Frates MC, Benson CB, Doubilet PM, et al: Can color Doppler sonography aid in the prediction of malignancy of thyroid nodules? J Ultrasound Med 2003;22:127-131.

74. Quinn SF, Nelson HA, Demlow TA: Thyroid biopsies: Fine-needle aspiration biopsy versus spring-activated core biopsy needle in 102 patients. JVIR 1994;5:619-623.

75. Taki S, Kakuda K, Kakuma K, et al: Thyroid nodules: Evaluation with US-guided core biopsy with an automated biopsy gun. Radiology 1997;202:874-877.

76. Miller JM, Hamburger JI, Taylor CI: Is needle aspiration of the cystic thyroid nodule effective and safe treatment? In Hamburger JI, Miller JM (eds): Controversies in Clinical Thyroidology. New York, Springer-Verlag, 1981.

77. Verde G, Papini E, Pacella CM, et al: Ultrasound guided percutaneous ethanol injection in the treatment of cystic thyroid nodules. Clin Endocrinol 1994;41:719-724.

78. Yasuda K, Ozaki O, Sugino K, et al: Treatment of cystic lesions of the thyroid by ethanol instillation. World J Surg 1992;16:958-963.

79. Antonelli A, Campatelli A, Di Vito A, et al: Comparison between ethanol sclerotherapy and emptying with injection of saline in treatment of thyroid cysts. Clin Invest 1994;72:971-974.

80. Livraghi T, Paracchi A, Ferrari C, et al: Treatment of autonomous thyroid nodules with percutaneous ethanol injection: Preliminary results. Radiology 1990; 175:827-829.

81. Cerbone G, Spiezia S, Colao A, et al: Percutaneous ethanol injection under Power Doppler ultrasound assistance in the treatment of autonomously functioning thyroid nodules. J Endocrinol Invest 1999;22:752-759.

82. Goletti O, Monzani F, Caraccio N, et al: Percutaneous ethanol injection treatment of autonomously functioning single thyroid nodules: Optimization of treatment and short term outcome. World J Surg 1992;16:784-790.

83. Livraghi T, Paracchi A, Ferrari C, et al: Treatment of autonomous thyroid nodules by percutaneous ethanol injection: 4-year experience. Radiology 1994;190:529-534.

84. Ozdemir H, Ilgit ET, Yucel C, et al: Treatment of autonomous thyroid nodules: Safety and efficacy of sonographically guided percutaneous injection of ethanol. AJR Am J Roentgenol 1994;163:929-932.

85. Pacella CM, Papini E, Bizzarri G, et al: Assessment of the effect of percutaneous ethanol injection in autonomously functioning thyroid nodules by colour-coded duplex sonography. Eur J Radiol 1995;5:395-400.

86. Goletti O, Monzani F, Lenziardi M, et al: Cold thyroid nodules: A new application of percutaneous ethanol injection treatment. J Clin Ultrasound 1994;22:175-178.

87. Dossing H, Bennedbaek FN, Karstrup S, et al: Benign solitary cold thyroid nodules: US-guided interstitial laser photocoagulation: Initial experience. Radiology 2002;225:53-57.

88. Kanauchi H, Mimura Y, Kaminishi M: Percutaneous radiofrequency ablation of the thyroid guided by ultrasonography. Eur J Surg 2001;167:305-307.

89. Dupuy ED, Monchik JM, Decrea C, et al: Radiofrequency ablation of regional recurrence from well differentiated thyroid malignancy. Surgery 2001;130:971-977.

90. Lewis BD, Hay ID, Charboneau JW, et al: Percutaneous ethanol injection for treatment of cervical lymph node metastases in patients with papillary thyroid carcinoma. AJR Am J Roentgenol 2002;178:699-704.

91. Fukunari N: PEI therapy for thyroid lesions. Biomed Pharmacother 2002;56:79-82.

92. Horlocker TT, Hay JE, James EM, et al: Prevalence of incidental nodular thyroid disease detected during high-

resolution parathyroid ultrasonography. In Medeiros-Neto G, Gaitan E (eds): Frontiers in Thyroidology. New York, Plenum, 1986, vol 2, pp 1309-1312.

93. Lever EG, Refetoff S, Straus FH II, et al: Coexisting thyroid and parathyroid disease: Are they related? Surgery 1983;94:893-900.

94. Mortensen JD, Woolner LB, Bennett WA: Gross and microscopic findings in clinically normal thyroid glands. J Clin Endocrinol Metab 1955;15:1270-1280.

95. Giuffrida D, Gharib H: Controversies in the management of cold, hot, and occult thyroid nodules. Am J Med 1995;99:642-650.

96. Tan GH, Gharib H, Reading CC: Solitary thyroid nodule: Comparison between palpation and ultrasonography. Arch Intern Med 1995;155:2418-2423.

Diffuse Thyroid Disease

97. Hay ID: Thyroiditis: A clinical update. Mayo Clin Proc 1985;60:836-843.

98. Adams H, Jones NC: Ultrasound appearances of de Quervain's thyroiditis. Clin Radiol 1990;42:217-218.

99. Birchall IWJ, Chow CC, Metreweli C: Ultrasound appearances of de Quervain's thyroiditis. Clin Radiol 1990;41:57-59.

100. Yeh HC, Futterweit W, Gilbert P: Micronodulation: Ultrasonographic sign of Hashimoto's thyroiditis. J Ultrasound Med 1996;15:813-819.

101. Takashima S, Matsuzuka F, Nagareda T, et al: Thyroid nodules associated with Hashimoto's thyroiditis: Assessment with US. Radiology 1992;185:125-130.

102. Lagalla R, Caruso G, Benza I, et al: Echo-color Doppler in the study of hypothyroidism in the adult [Italian]. Radiol Med 1993;86:281-283.

103. Castagnone D, Rivolta R, Rescalli S, et al: Color Doppler sonography in Graves' disease: Value in assessing activity of disease and predicting outcome. AJR Am J Roentgenol 1996;66:203-207.

22

THE PARATHYROID GLANDS

Bonnie J. Huppert / Carl C. Reading

Chapter Outline

High-frequency sonography is a well-established, noninvasive imaging method used in the evaluation and treatment of patients with parathyroid disease. Sonography is most commonly used for the preoperative localization of enlarged parathyroid glands or adenomas in patients with hyperparathyroidism. It is also used to guide the percutaneous biopsy of suspected parathyroid adenomas, particularly in the setting of persistent or recurrent hyperparathyroidism, and for the intraoperative localization of abnormal parathyroid glands. In selected patients, sonography can be used to guide the percutaneous ethanol ablation of parathyroid adenomas as an alternative to surgical treatment.

EMBRYOLOGY AND ANATOMY

The paired superior and inferior parathyroid glands have different embryologic origins, and a knowledge of their development aids in understanding their ultimate anatomic locations.[1-3] The **superior parathyroid glands** arise from the fourth branchial cleft pouch. Minimal migration occurs during fetal development, and the superior parathyroids associate with the posterior aspect of the mid to upper portion of the thyroid gland. The majority of superior parathyroid glands (80%) are found at autopsy within a 2 cm area located just superior to the crossing of the recurrent laryngeal nerve and the inferior thyroid artery.[4] The **inferior parathyroid glands** arise from the third branchial cleft pouch, along with the thymus.[2] During fetal development, these "parathymus glands" migrate caudally along with the thymus in a more anterior plane than their superior counterparts, bypassing the superior glands to become the inferior parathyroid glands.[3] The inferior glands are more variable in location than the superior parathyroids but usually—over 60%—come to rest at or just inferior to the posterior aspect of the lower pole of the thyroid (Fig. 22-1).[4] About 25% of the inferior glands fail to dissociate from the thymus and continue to migrate lower in the neck tissues or into the anterosuperior mediastinum, usually within the thyrothymic ligament.

Ectopic Parathyroid Glands

A significant percentage of parathyroid glands lie in relatively or frankly ectopic locations in the neck or mediastinum. The inferior parathyroid gland is more

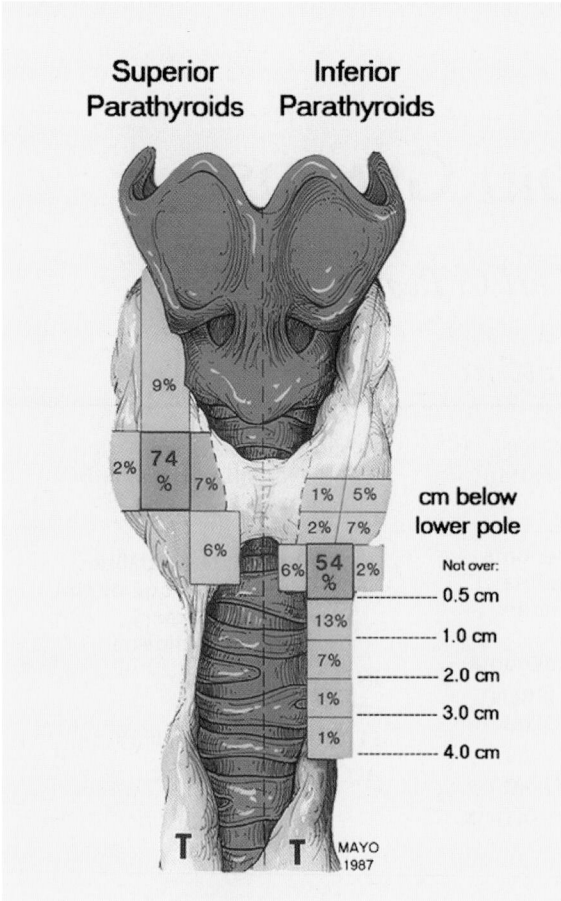

FIGURE 22-1. Frequency of the location of normal superior and inferior parathyroid glands. Anatomic drawing from 527 autopsies. T, Thymus. (Adapted with permission from Gilmour JR: The gross anatomy of the parathyroid glands. J Pathol 1938;46:133-148.)

frequently ectopic than its superior counterpart. Symmetry to fixed landmarks occurs in 70% to 80%, so side-to-side comparisons usually can be made.[3,4] The ectopic superior parathyroid gland usually lies far posteriorly in the tracheoesophageal groove or has enlarged and has continued its descent from the posterior neck into the posterosuperior mediastinum.[5,6] Superior glands are found less commonly higher in the neck, near the superior extent of the thyroid lobe, or, rarely, surrounded by thyroid tissue within the thyroid capsule.[4] The ectopic inferior parathyroid gland usually has continued to migrate in an anterocaudal direction and is found in the low neck or anterosuperior mediastinum, associated with the thymus. Less common ectopic positions of the inferior parathyroid glands include an undescended position high in the neck with a remnant of thymus near the carotid bifurcation, or lower in the neck along the carotid sheath.[7] In other rare cases, ectopic glands have been reported low in the mediastinum in the aortopulmonic window, posterior to the carina or esophagus, and within the pericardium. Rarely,

inferior glands may also be found far laterally within the posterior triangle of the neck or in an intrathyroidal location.

Most adults have four parathyroid glands (two superior and two inferior), each measuring about 5 mm by 3 mm by 1 mm and weighing on average 35 to 40 mg (range 10 to 78 mg).[3,8] Supernumerary "fifth" glands are present in up to 13% of the population[3] and may result from the separation of parathyroid anlage when the glands pull away from the pouch structures during the embryologic branchial complex phase.[9,10] These supernumerary glands are often associated with the thymus in the anterior mediastinum, suggesting a relationship in their development with the inferior parathyroid glands.[11]

Normal parathyroid glands vary from a yellow to a red-brown color, depending on the amount of yellow parenchymal fat and chief cell content. The chief cells are the primary source for the production of parathyroid hormone. The glands are generally oval or bean-shaped, but may be spherical, elongated, or lobulated. Normal glands can be seen occasionally with high-frequency ultrasound, especially in young patients, but sonographic visualization of a normal parathyroid gland in a patient without hyperparathyroidism is not an indication for surgery.[12]

PRIMARY HYPERPARATHYROIDISM

Prevalence

Primary hyperparathyroidism is now recognized as a common endocrine disease, with a prevalence in the United States of 1 to 2 per 1000 population.[13] Women are affected two to three times more frequently than are men, particularly after menopause. More than half of the patients with this disease are older than 50 years of age, and cases are rare before 20 years of age.

Diagnosis

Hyperparathyroidism is usually suspected because an increased serum calcium level is detected on routine biochemical screening. Elevated ionized serum calcium level, hypophosphatasia, and hypercalciuria may be further biochemical clues to the disease. A serum parathyroid hormone (PTH) level that is inappropriately high for the corresponding serum calcium level confirms the diagnosis. Even when the PTH level is within the upper limits of the normal range in a hypercalcemic patient, the diagnosis of primary hyperparathyroidism should still be suspected because hypercalcemia from other nonparathyroid causes (including malignancy) should suppress the glandular function and decrease the serum PTH level. Due to earlier detection by increasingly routine laboratory examinations, the later classic signs of hyperparathyroidism, such as "painful bones, renal stones, abdominal groans, and psychic moans" are often not present. Few patients currently present with the severe manifestations of hyperparathyroidism, such as **nephrolithiasis, osteopenia, subperiosteal resorption, and osteitis fibrosis cystica**. In general, patients rarely have obvious symptoms unless their serum calcium level exceeds 12 mg/dL. However, subtle nonspecific symptoms, such as muscle weakness, malaise, constipation, dyspepsia, polydipsia, and polyuria, may be elicited from these otherwise asymptomatic patients by more specific questioning.

Pathology

Primary hyperparathyroidism is caused by a single adenoma in 80% to 90% of cases, by multiple gland enlargement in 10% to 20%, and by carcinoma in less than 1% (see box).[14,15]A solitary adenoma may involve any one of the four glands with equal frequency.[16] Multiple gland enlargement is most commonly due to primary parathyroid hyperplasia and less commonly to multiple adenomas. Hyperplasia usually involves all four glands asymmetrically, whereas multiple adenomas may involve two or possibly three glands. Because of this inconsistent pattern of gland involvement and the fact that distinguishing hyperplasia from multiple adenomas is difficult pathologically, these two entities are often histologically considered together as **multiple gland disease**.[17] Thus, there is a spectrum between the concepts of the single adenoma and four-gland hyperplasia.

Most cases of primary hyperparathyroidism are sporadic. However, **prior external neck irradiation** has been associated with the development of hyperparathyroidism in a small percentage of cases. Patients on **long-term lithium therapy** may also present with the disease. Up to 10% of primary hyperparathyroid cases may occur on a hereditary basis, most commonly due to **multiple endocrine neoplasia syndrome**, type I (MEN I). This condition is an uncommon disorder that follows an autosomal-dominant pattern of inheritance and has a high penetrance, resulting in adenomatous parathyroid hyperplasia. Multiple parathyroid gland enlargement occurs in more than 90% of patients with MEN I.[18,19] Most MEN I patients present with hypercalcemia before their third or fourth decade of life. Though not all of the parathyroid glands may be grossly enlarged at the time of these patients' initial operation, it is likely that all of them will ultimately be involved with hyperplasia. Patients with the MEN II syndrome less commonly develop parathyroid hyperplasia.

Parathyroid carcinoma is a rare cause of primary hyperparathyroidism. The histologic distinction from adenoma is difficult to establish with certainty because both carcinomas and atypical adenomas can exhibit increased mitotic activity and cellular atypia.[20] These patients usually present with a very high serum calcium level (>14 mg/dL). The diagnosis is often made at operation when the surgeon discovers an enlarged, firm gland that is adherent to the surrounding tissues due to local invasion.[21-24] A thick, fibrotic capsule is often present. Treatment consists of *en bloc* resection without entering the capsule in order to prevent seeding. In many cases, cure may not be possible because of the invasive and metastatic nature of the disease. Generally, death occurs, not from tumor spread, but from complications associated with unrelenting hyperparathyroidism.[16]

Treatment

In symptomatic patients with primary hyperparathyroidism, the treatment of choice is surgical excision of the involved parathyroid gland or glands. However, now that many cases are discovered in the early stages of the disease, some controversy exists as to whether asymptomatic patients with minimal hypercalcemia should be treated surgically or followed medically with frequent measurements of bone density, serum calcium levels, and urinary calcium excretion. In one prospective study, clinical follow-up of 147 asymptomatic patients with a provisional diagnosis of hyperparathyroidism and serum calcium levels less than 11 mg/dL revealed that 20% of the patients needed surgery within 5 years due to progression of their disease.[25,26] More recently, a prospective 10-year clinical follow-up study reported that of 52 asymptomatic patients with primary hyperparathyroidism with calcium levels less than 11 mg/dL, 73% did well with no evidence of disease progression. However, 27% had evidence of progression based on the new development of one or more indications for surgery.[27]

No effective definitive medical therapies are available for the treatment of primary hyperparathyroidism. Short-term hypocalcemic agents include calcitonin and the bisphosphonates. Estrogen replacement therapy has been used in postmenopausal women to decrease bone resorption and reduce serum calcium levels. Calcimimetics (calcium-sensing receptor agonists) are not yet widely studied or available. Studies demonstrate that surgical cure rates by an experienced surgeon are greater than 95%, and the morbidity and mortality rates are extremely low.[16,28] Therefore, surgery remains the most definitive treatment of hyperparathyroidism for both

---

CAUSES OF PRIMARY HYPERPARATHYROIDISM

Single adenoma 80% to 90%
Multiple gland enlargement 10% to 20%
Carcinoma 1%

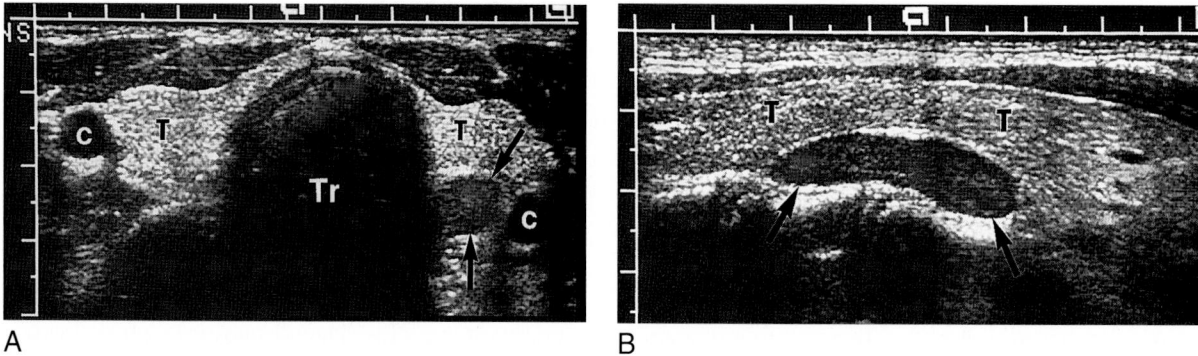

FIGURE 22-2. Typical parathyroid adenoma. A, Transverse and, B, longitudinal sonograms of a typical adenoma (*arrows*) located adjacent to the posterior aspect of the thyroid (T). Tr, Trachea. C, common carotid artery.

asymptomatic and symptomatic patients.[29,30] Recommendations for the management of asymptomatic primary hyperparathyroidism have been outlined in various articles, many of which are still based on the National Institutes of Health Consensus Development Conference.[31-32]

SONOGRAPHIC APPEARANCE

Shape

Parathyroid adenomas are most commonly oval (Fig. 22-2). As parathyroid glands enlarge, they dissect between longitudinally oriented tissue planes in the neck and acquire a characteristic oblong shape. If this process is exaggerated, they can become tubelike or even bilobar. There is often asymmetry in the enlargement, and the cephalic or caudal end can be more bulbous, producing a triangular, tapering, or teardrop shape.[16,34-36]

Echogenicity

The characteristic hypoechoic echogenicity of parathyroid adenomas is due to the uniform hypercellularity of the gland, which leaves few interfaces for reflecting sound. The echogenicity of most parathyroid adenomas is substantially less than thyroid tissue (Fig. 22-3). Cases of rare functioning parathyroid lipoadenoma have been reported, which are more echogenic than the adjacent thyroid gland due to their high fat content (see Fig. 22-3).[37]

Internal Architecture

The vast majority of parathyroid adenomas are **homogeneously solid**. About 2% have internal cystic components that are due to **cystic degeneration** (most commonly) or true simple cysts (less commonly) (see Fig. 22-3).[36,38-40] Rare adenomas may contain **focal internal calcification**. Color flow Doppler sonography of an enlarged parathyroid gland may demonstrate a

hypervascular pattern with prominent diastolic flow (Fig. 22-4). An enlarged extrathyroidal feeding artery supplying the adenoma may be recognized, often originating from branches of the inferior thyroidal artery.[41] A typical finding described in parathyroid adenomas is a **vascular arc,** which arises from thyroidal artery branches and envelops between 90 and 270 degrees of the mass.[42] While this arc of flow has not been shown to increase the sensitivity of initial detection of parathyroid adenomas, it may allow for differentiation from lymph nodes, which have a central hilar flow pattern.[42-44]

Size

Most parathyroid adenomas are 0.8 to 1.5 cm long and weigh 500 to 1000 mg. The smallest adenomas can be minimally enlarged glands that appear virtually normal during surgery but are found to be hypercellular on pathologic examination. The largest adenomas can be 5 cm or more in length and weigh more than 10 g. Preoperative serum calcium levels are usually higher in patients with larger adenomas (Fig. 22-5).[25,36]

Multiple Gland Disease

Multiple gland disease can be due to hyperplasia or to multiple adenomas. Individually, these enlarged glands have the same sonographic and gross appearance as other parathyroid adenomas (Fig. 22-6).[16] However, the glands may be inconsistently and asymmetrically enlarged, and the diagnosis of multiple gland disease is often difficult to make sonographically. The appearance may be misinterpreted as solitary adenomatous disease, or the diagnosis may be missed altogether if the glandular enlargement is minimal.

Carcinoma

Carcinomas are usually larger than adenomas. The average carcinoma measures more than 2 cm, in contrast

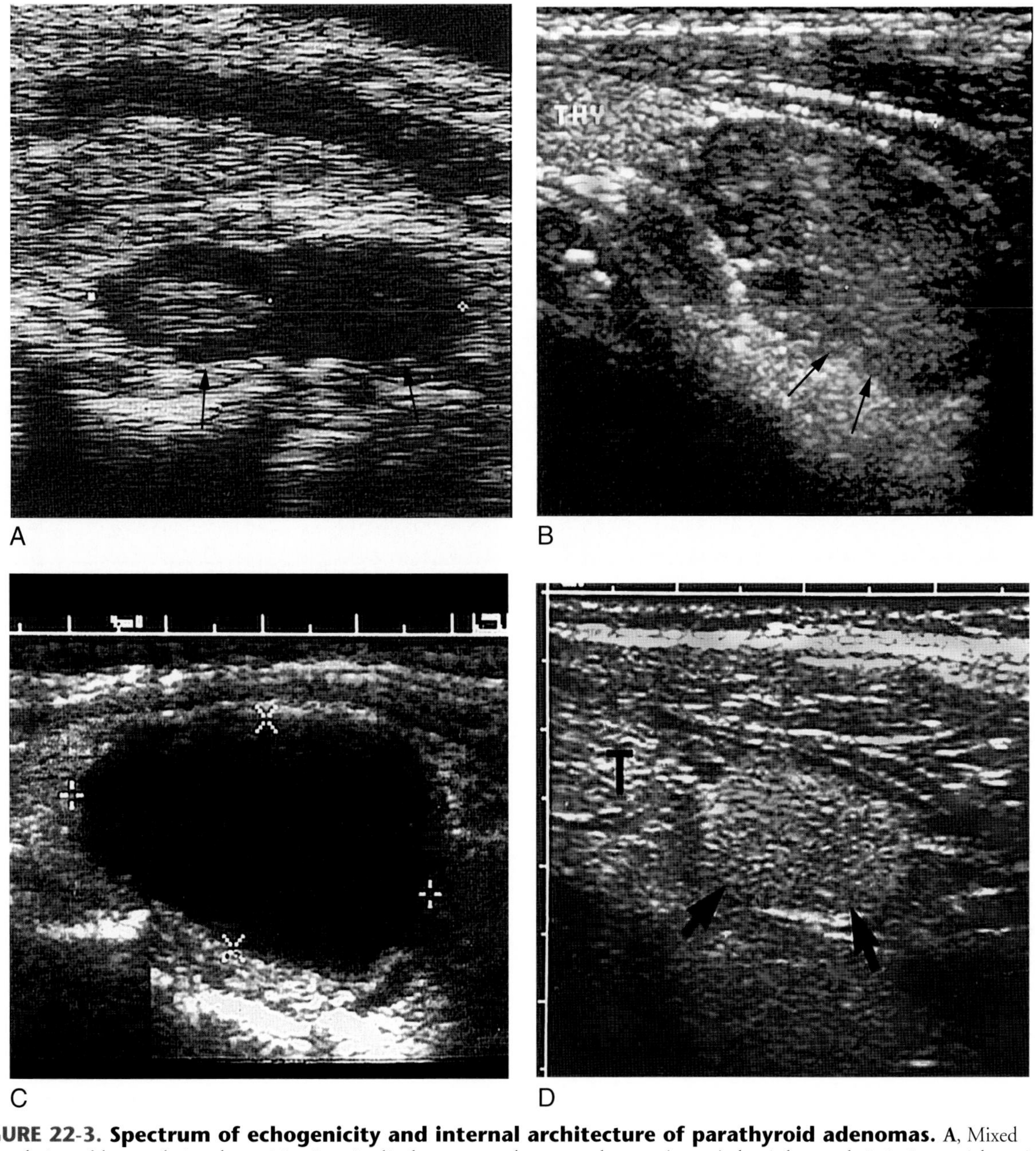

FIGURE 22-3. Spectrum of echogenicity and internal architecture of parathyroid adenomas. A, Mixed hypoechoic and hyperechoic echogenicity. Longitudinal sonogram shows an adenoma (*arrows*) that is hyperechoic in its cranial portion and hypoechoic in its caudal portion. **B,** Heterogeneous echogenicity. Longitudinal sonogram shows an adenoma (*arrows*) that is diffusely heterogeneous. **C,** Cystic change. Longitudinal sonogram shows a 4 cm adenoma that is predominantly cystic. **D,** Lipoadenoma. Longitudinal sonogram demonstrates a lipoadenoma (*arrows*) that is more echogenic than the adjacent thyroid tissue (T).

to about 1 cm for adenomas (Fig. 22-7). Sonographically, carcinomas also frequently have a lobular contour, heterogeneous internal architecture, and internal cystic components. However, large adenomas may also have these features.[45] In most cases, prospective carcinomas are indistinguishable sonographically from large benign adenomas.[46] Some authors have reported that a depth-width ratio greater than or equal to 1 is a sonographic feature more associated with carcinoma rather than adenoma, having a sensitivity and specificity of 94% and 95%, respectively.[47] Gross evidence of invasion of adjacent structures, such as vessels or muscles, is the only reliable preoperative sonographic criterion for the diagnosis of malignancy, but this is an uncommon finding.

ADENOMA LOCALIZATION

Sonographic Examination

The sonographic examination of the neck for parathyroid adenoma localization is performed with the patient in a supine position. The patient's neck is

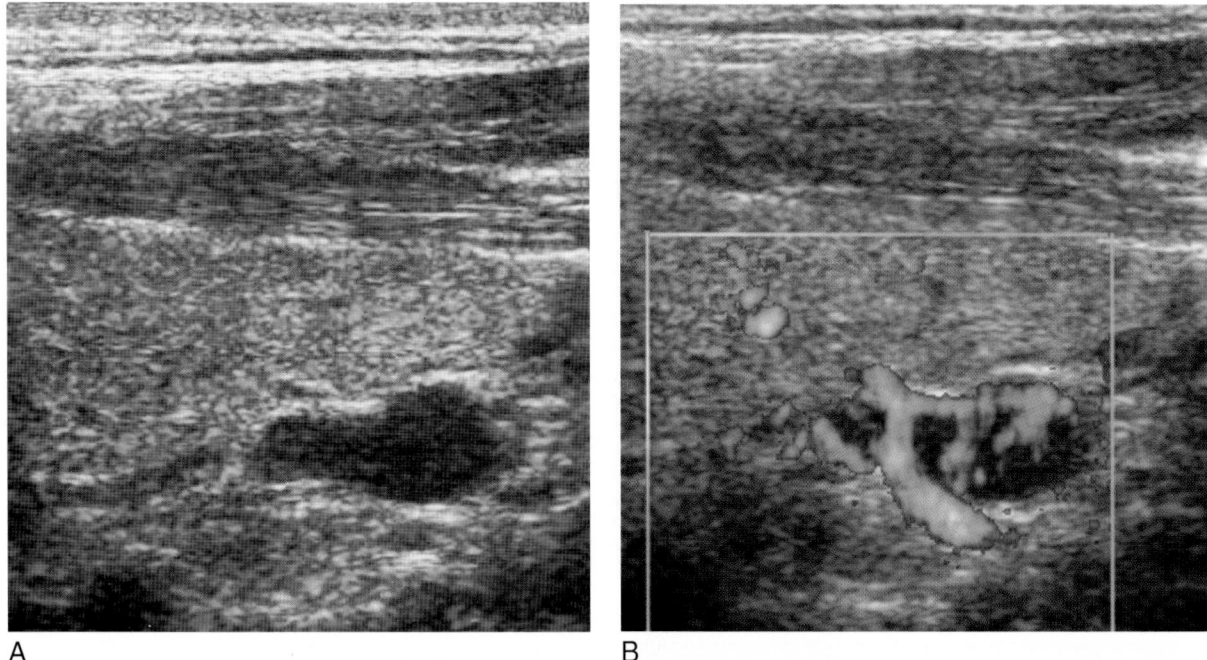

FIGURE 22-4. Typical hypervascularity of parathyroid adenoma. A and **B**, Longitudinal gray-scale and color Doppler images show hypervascularity of the parathyroid adenoma and prominent peripheral vascular arcs.

hyperextended by a pad centered under the scapulae, and the examiner usually sits at the patient's head. High-frequency (7.5 to 15 MHz) transducers are used to provide optimal spatial resolution and visualization in most patients. In obese patients with thick necks or with large multinodular thyroid goiters, use of a 5-MHz transducer may be necessary to obtain adequate depth of penetration.

Typical Locations

The pattern of the sonographic survey of the neck for adenoma localization can be considered in terms of the pattern of dissection and visualization that the surgeon uses in a thorough neck exploration. The examination is initiated on one side of the neck in the region of the thyroid gland. The typical **superior parathyroid adenoma** is usually adjacent to the posterior aspect of the midportion of the thyroid (Fig. 22-8). The location of the typical **inferior parathyroid adenoma** is more variable, but it usually lies close to the lower pole of the thyroid (Fig. 22-9). Most of these inferior adenomas are adjacent to the posterior aspect of the thyroid, and the rest are in the soft tissues 1 to 2 cm inferior to the thyroid. After one side of the neck has been examined, a similar survey is conducted of the opposite side. However, 1% to 3% of parathyroid adenomas are ectopic and will not be found in typical locations adjacent to the thyroid. The four most common ectopic locations will be considered separately.

Ectopic Locations

Retrotracheal Adenoma. The most common location of an ectopic superior adenoma is deep in the neck, posterior or posterolateral to the trachea (Fig. 22-10). Superior adenomas tend to enlarge between tissue planes that extend toward the posterior mediastinum. Acoustic shadowing from air in the trachea can make evaluation of this area difficult. The transducer should be angled medially to visualize the tissues posterior to the trachea. Often the adenoma protrudes slightly from behind the trachea, and only a portion of the mass will be visible. **Turning the patient's head to the opposite side** will accentuate the protrusion and provide better accessibility to the retrotracheal area. This process is then repeated from the other side of the neck to visualize the contralateral aspect of the retrotracheal area. This process is analogous to the maneuver that a surgeon uses to run a fingertip behind the trachea in an attempt to palpate a retrotracheal adenoma. Maximal turning of the head also often causes the esophagus to move to the opposite side of the trachea as it becomes compressed between the trachea and the cervical spine. If the radiologist sees the esophagus move completely from behind one side of the trachea to the opposite side during maximal head turning, the esophagus has effectively "swept" the retrotracheal space and will have pushed any parathyroid adenoma in this location out from behind the trachea.

Mediastinal Adenoma. The most common location for ectopic inferior parathyroid adenomas is low within the

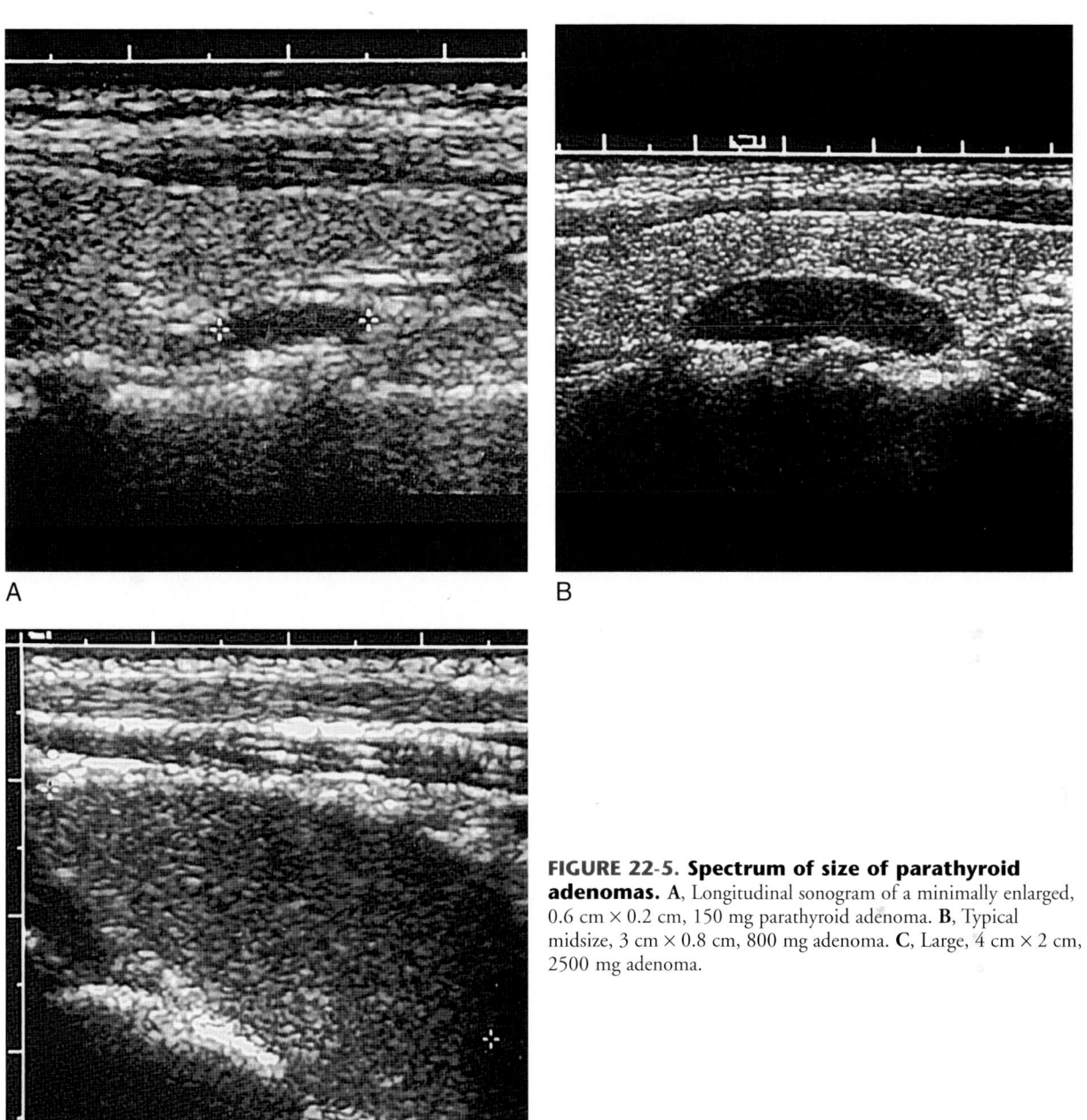

A

B

C

FIGURE 22-5. Spectrum of size of parathyroid adenomas. **A**, Longitudinal sonogram of a minimally enlarged, 0.6 cm × 0.2 cm, 150 mg parathyroid adenoma. **B**, Typical midsize, 3 cm × 0.8 cm, 800 mg adenoma. **C**, Large, 4 cm × 2 cm, 2500 mg adenoma.

neck or in the anterosuperior mediastinum (Fig. 22-11).[48] Parathyroid adenomas are sufficiently hypoechoic that they usually can be visualized as discrete structures separate from the thymus and surrounding tissues. To visualize this area optimally, **the patient's neck is hyperextended maximally**. With this technique and the transducer angled posterior and caudal to the clavicular heads, sonographic visualization is often possible to the level of the brachiocephalic veins. If the adenoma lies caudal to this level or far anterior, just deep to the sternum, it cannot be visualized sonographically.

Ectopic superior adenomas located in the mediastinum tend to stay in a more posterior plane than their ectopic inferior counterparts. They often lie deep in the low neck or posterosuperior mediastinum, requiring use of a 5-MHz transducer for maximal penetration. These adenomas may be intimately associated with the posterior aspect of the trachea, and the head-turning maneuver described for retrotracheal adenomas in the neck can be applied here as well. With the patient's neck hyperextended and the transducer angled caudally, the posterior mediastinum may sometimes be visualized to

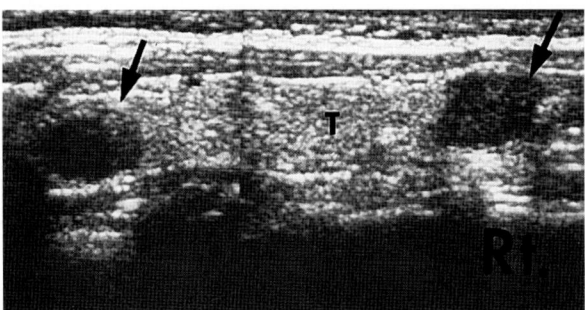

FIGURE 22-6. Multiple gland disease. Longitudinal sonogram of the right neck shows superior and inferior parathyroid gland enlargement due to hyperplasia (*arrows*), which can be difficult to distinguish from multiple adenomas. T, Thyroid.

the level of the apex of the aortic arch. Adenomas lying caudal to this level cannot be visualized sonographically. **Intrathyroid Adenoma.** Intrathyroid adenomas are uncommon and may represent either superior or inferior gland adenomas.[4,49-51] Most intrathyroid adenomas are in the posterior half of the mid to lower thyroid, are completely surrounded by thyroid tissue, and are oriented with their greatest dimension in the cephalocaudal direction (Fig. 22-12). Intrathyroid adenomas may be overlooked at the time of operation because they are soft and are similar to the surrounding thyroid tissue on palpation. A thyroidotomy or subtotal lobectomy may be needed to find an intrathyroid adenoma. Sonographically, however, parathyroid adenomas usually are well visualized because they are **hypoechoic, in contrast to the echogenic thyroid parenchyma.** The internal architecture and appearance of these adenomas are the same as those of adenomas elsewhere in the neck. Sonographically, intrathyroid parathyroid adenomas can be similar to thyroid nodules in appearance, and percutaneous biopsy is often necessary to distinguish between these entities.

Some adenomas may lie under the pseudocapsule or sheath that covers the thyroid gland or within a sulcus of the thyroid, but these are not usually considered to be true intrathyroid adenomas. These adenomas may be difficult for the surgeon to visualize at the time of surgery unless this sheath is opened.[8,49] Sonographically, these adenomas appear the same as other parathyroid adenomas that lie immediately adjacent to the thyroid. **Carotid Sheath or Undescended Adenoma.** Rare ectopic adenomas can lie in a high position superior and lateral in the neck, near the carotid bifurcation at the level of the hyoid bone or attached to the carotid sheath along the course of the common carotid artery (Fig. 22-13).[52-54] These adenomas likely arise from inferior glands that are embryologically undescended, or partially descended, having come to reside within or adjacent to the carotid sheath that surrounds the carotid artery, jugular vein,

and vagus nerve. These adenomas are frequently overlooked during surgery unless the surgeon specifically opens the carotid sheath and dissects within it.[6,7,55] Sonographically, these masses can appear similar to mildly enlarged lymph nodes in the jugular chain, and percutaneous biopsy is often necessary for confirmation.

PERSISTENT OR RECURRENT HYPERPARATHYROIDISM

Persistent hyperparathyroidism is the persistence of hypercalcemia after earlier failed parathyroid surgery. This is frequently due to an undiscovered ectopic parathyroid adenoma or unrecognized multiple gland disease with failure to resect all of the hyperfunctioning tissue during surgery. Persistent postoperative hypercalcemia has been reported in the range of 3% to 10% in some series.[56] Recurrent hyperparathyroidism is defined as hypercalcemia occurring after a 6-month interval of normocalcemia, resulting from the new development of hyperfunctioning parathyroid tissue from previously normal glands.[57] Recurrent hyperparathyroidism is often seen in patients with unrecognized MEN I.

In reoperated patients, the surgical cure rate is approximately 10% to 30% lower than initial surgery. Because of scarring and fibrosis from the previous operation, the morbidity of severe postoperative hypocalcemia and recurrent laryngeal nerve damage is up to 20 times higher.[58-65] During sonographic evaluation of reoperated patients, specific attention is paid to the most likely ectopic parathyroid locations—those associated with a gland that was not discovered at the initial neck dissection.

Imaging prior to reoperation is particularly beneficial, and most care strategies recommend liberal use of studies in this situation.[16,65-67] For some surgeons, the preferred approach prior to reoperation is to use the simplest and least expensive imaging modality used in the preoperative setting, that of ultrasound, as the first-line imaging strategy. Sonography has demonstrated some of the highest sensitivities and accuracies of all modalities for adenoma detection in the reoperative setting, especially when combined with ultrasound-guided fine-needle aspiration biopsy (FNAB) of a suspected parathyroid adenoma.[65,66,68] Ultrasound imaging may be complemented by scintigraphy or magnetic resonance imaging (MRI) when sonographic findings are ambiguous or the operative risk is high.[67,69] This approach has been shown to turn the nonimaged reoperation procedure with only a 62% success rate into a significantly shorter and less expensive procedure with a success rate of near 90%.[65,66]

A small subgroup of patients in whom recurrent hyperparathyroidism develops postoperatively has undergone previous autotransplantation of parathyroid

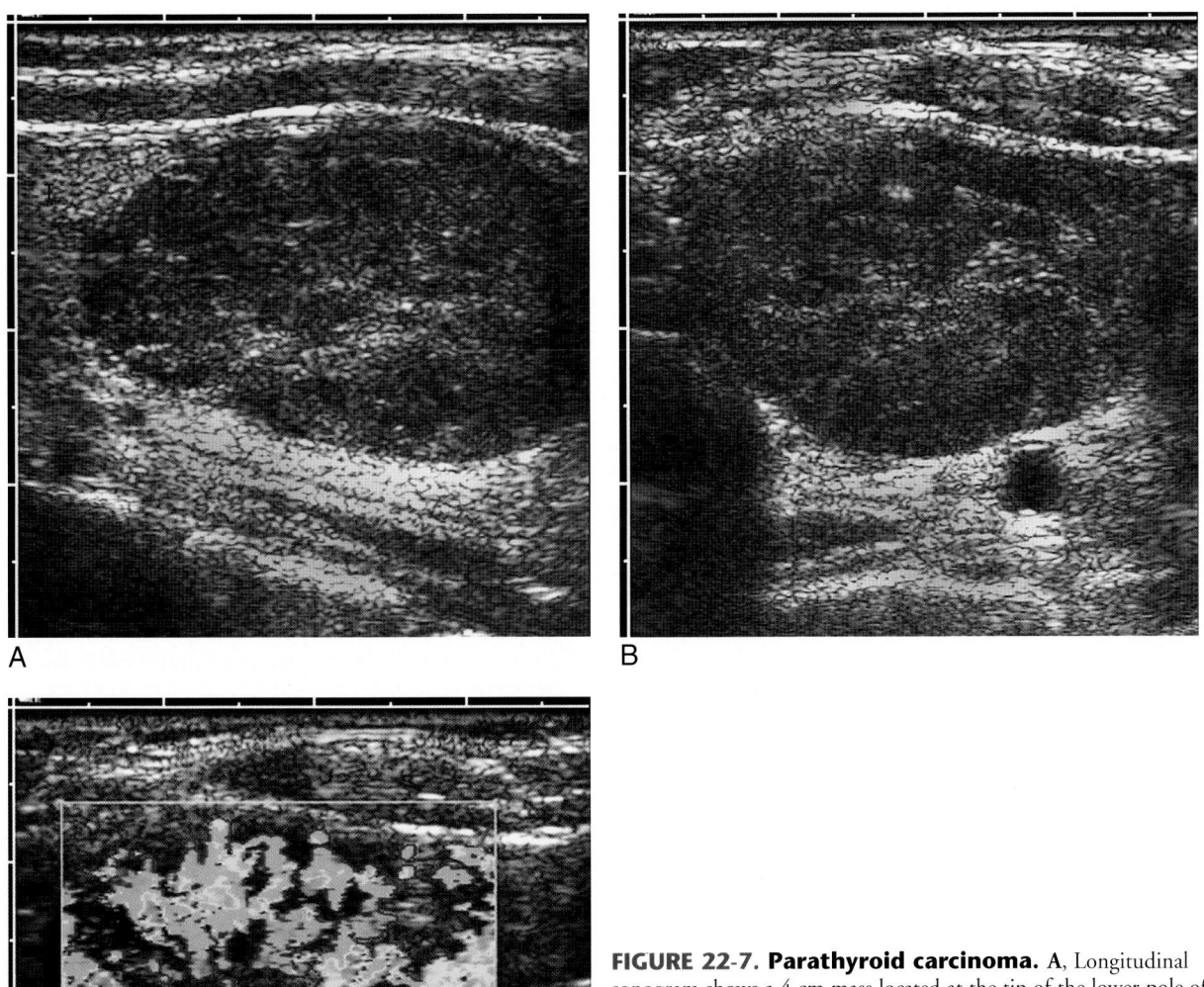

A

B

C

FIGURE 22-7. Parathyroid carcinoma. A, Longitudinal sonogram shows a 4 cm mass located at the tip of the lower pole of the left thyroid lobe (T). **B,** Transverse sonogram demonstrates the carcinoma anterior to the left common carotid artery. **C,** Transverse sonogram with color flow Doppler demonstrates prominent internal vascularity of the carcinoma. C, common carotid artery.

tissue in conjunction with previous total parathyroidectomy, usually for complications of chronic renal failure.[70,71] In this procedure, a parathyroid gland is sliced into fragments that are inserted into surgically prepared intramuscular pockets in the forearm or sternocleidomastoid muscle. Up to 20% to 33% of patients with parathyroid autotransplantation will develop graft-dependent hypercalcemia.[71,72] Usually these auto-transplanted fragments are too small and similar in echotexture to the surrounding muscle to be adequately visualized sonographically, but occasionally they can be

identified. Graft-dependent recurrent hyperparathyroidism appears as oval, sharply marginated, hypoechoic tissue nodules, measuring 5 to 11 mm—similar in appearance to adenomas arising in the neck (Fig. 22-14).[72,73] Regardless of the success of preoperative localization studies, the autotransplanted fragments usually are readily found by the surgeon while the patient is under local anesthesia, and a portion of the grafted tissue can be excised to cure the hypercalcemia. Occasionally, for patients who are not reoperative candidates, ultrasound-guided percutaneous ethanol injection (see "Alcohol

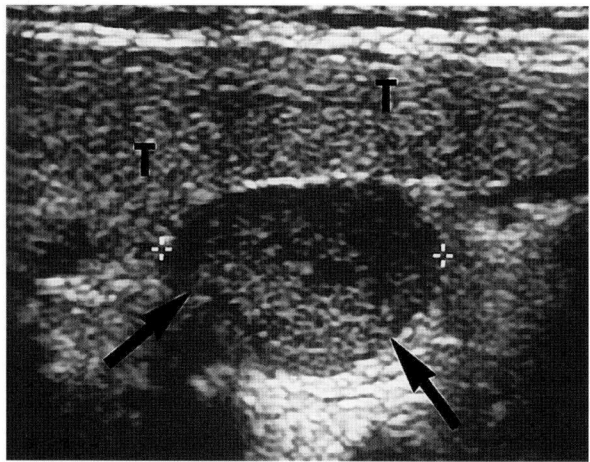

A

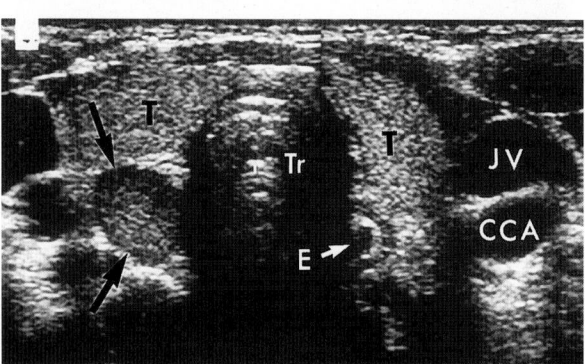

B

FIGURE 22-8. Superior parathyroid adenoma. A,
Longitudinal and, **B,** transverse sonograms show an adenoma
(*arrows*) adjacent to the posterior aspect of the midportion of the
right lobe of the thyroid (T). CCA, Common carotid artery; E,
esophagus; JV, internal jugular vein; Tr, trachea.

Ablation" section) may be used for ablation of residual
adenomatous disease in the neck or at a graft site.

SECONDARY HYPERPARATHYROIDISM

Secondary hyperparathyroidism is characteristically
found in patients with chronic renal failure. In these
patients chronic hypocalcemia is the result of multiple
complex factors, including decreased synthesis of the
active form of vitamin D with poor calcium absorption,
persistent hyperphosphatemia, and skeletal resistance
to the actions of parathyroid hormone. These factors
contribute to parathyroid hyperplasia. If untreated,
secondary hyperparathyroidism can result in bone
demineralization, soft tissue calcification, and acceleration of vascular calcification. Surgical treatment for
secondary hyperparathyroidism is uncommon because
of the success of dialysis therapy; however, in symptomatic patients who are refractory to dialysis and medical

therapy, subtotal parathyroidectomy or total parathyroidectomy with autotransplantation is indicated.[74-77]

Patients with secondary hyperparathyroidism have
multiple enlarged glands. Individually, these glands
have the same sonographic appearance as other parathyroid adenomas (see Fig. 22-6). The glands may be
asymmetrically enlarged. Although imaging is not
usually necessary, sonography can be used in screening
for the evaluation of the severity of parathyroid hyperplasia by assessing gland enlargement.[78] Patients with
sonographically enlarged glands tend to have significantly worse symptoms, laboratory values, and radiographic signs of secondary hyperparathyroidism than
patients without gland enlargement. Sonography can
also be used to aid in localization of the enlarged
parathyroid glands prior to surgical resection for
secondary hyperparathyroidism.[79] Ultrasound-guided
percutaneous ethanol injection (see "Alcohol Ablation"
section) is also a treatment option for ablation of hyperplastic parathyroid glands in patients with secondary
hyperparathyroidism who are not surgical candidates.

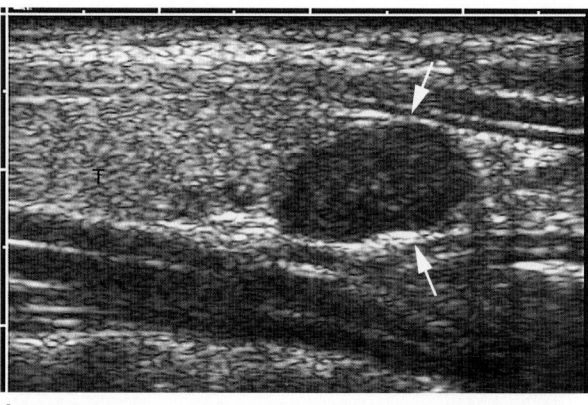

A

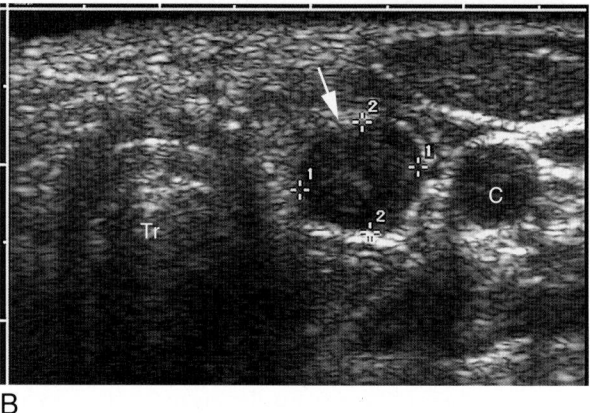

B

FIGURE 22-9. Inferior parathyroid adenoma. A,
Longitudinal and, **B,** transverse sonograms show an adenoma
(*arrows*) inferior to the tip of the lower pole of the left lobe of
the thyroid (T). C, Common carotid artery; Tr, trachea.

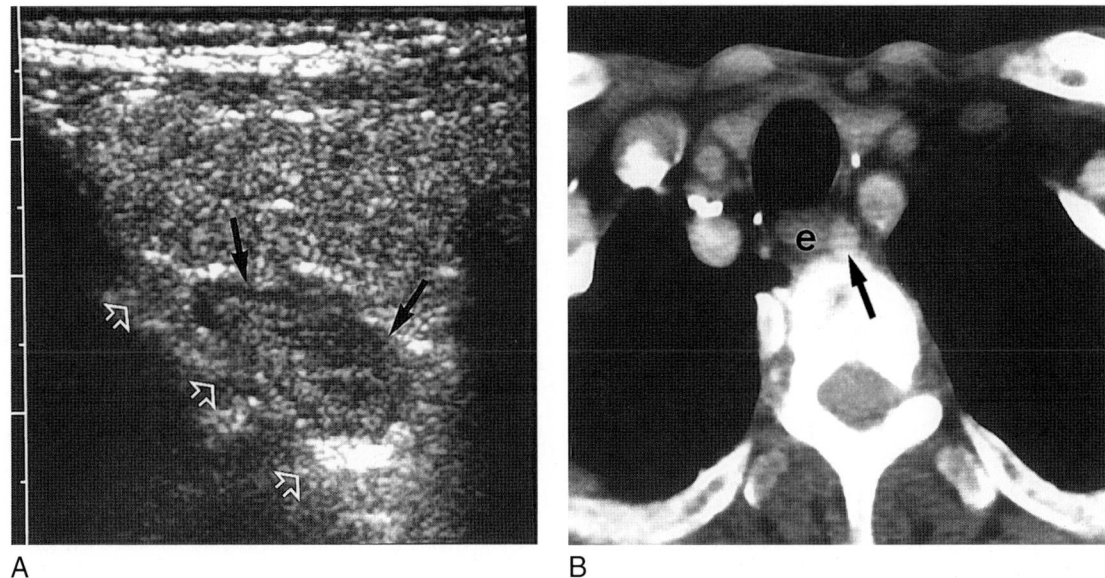

FIGURE 22-10. Ectopic adenoma—tracheoesophageal groove. A, Angled parasagittal sonogram shows 2 cm ectopic superior parathyroid adenoma (*arrows*) deep in the low neck/upper mediastinum adjacent to the cervical spine (*open arrowheads*). **B**, CT scan of the low neck/upper mediastinum shows ectopic adenoma (*arrow*) in the left tracheoesophageal groove adjacent to the esophagus (e).

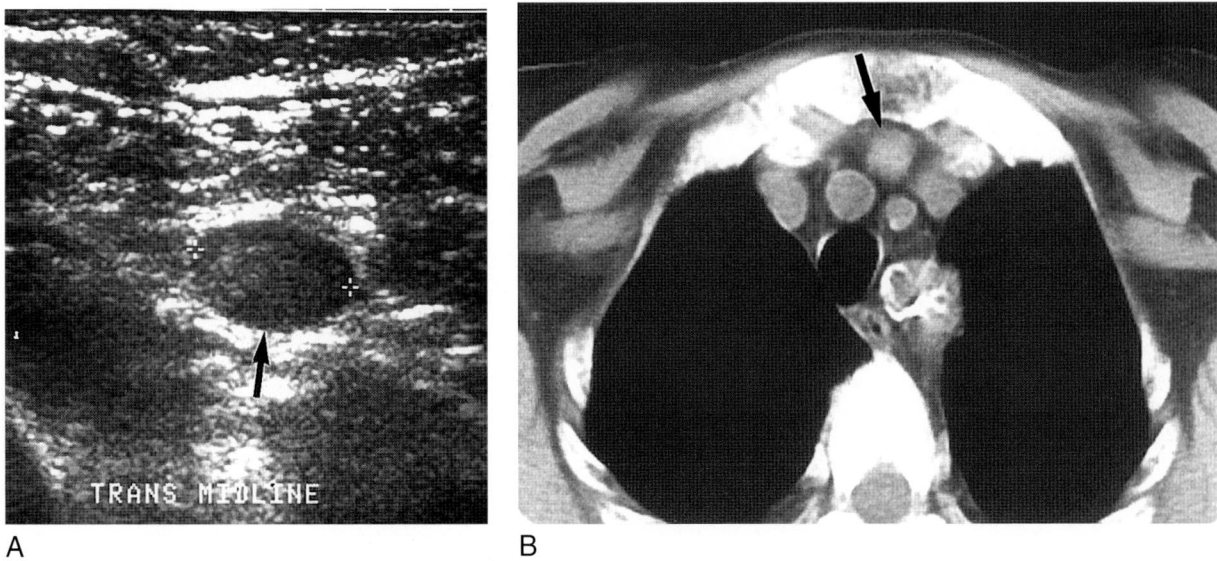

FIGURE 22-11. Ectopic adenoma—anterosuperior mediastinum. A, Transverse sonogram angled caudal to the clavicles shows 1 cm ectopic inferior oval parathyroid adenoma (*arrow*) in the soft tissues of the anterosuperior mediastinum. **B**, CT scan of the upper mediastinum shows the ectopic adenoma (*arrow*) in the anterosuperior mediastinum, deep to the manubrium and adjacent to the great vessels.

PITFALLS IN INTERPRETATION

False-Positive Examination

Normal and pathologic cervical structures, such as lymph nodes, small veins adjacent to the thyroid, the esophagus, the longus colli muscles, and thyroid nodules, can simulate parathyroid adenomas, producing false-positive results during neck sonography (see box).

PARATHYROID ADENOMA: CAUSES OF FALSE-POSITIVE EXAMINATION

Cervical lymph node
Prominent blood vessel
Esophagus
Longus colli muscle
Thyroid nodule

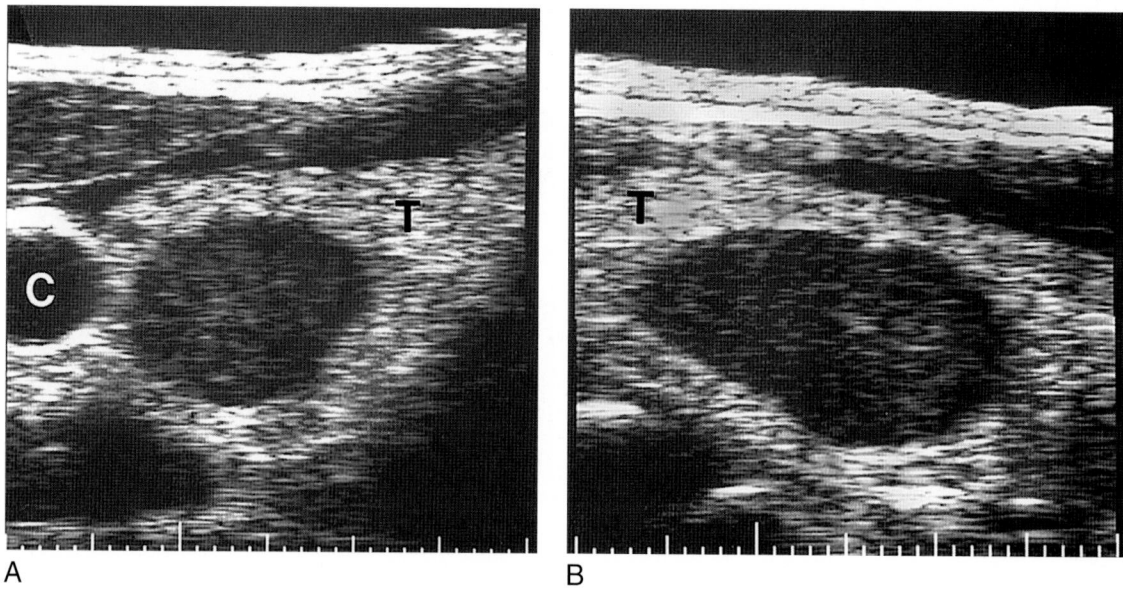

FIGURE 22-12. Ectopic adenoma—intrathyroidal. A, Transverse and, **B,** longitudinal sonograms of the right neck show a hypoechoic intrathyroid parathyroid adenoma completely surrounded by thyroid tissue. This occult adenoma was not palpable at the time of two failed neck operations. C, Common carotid artery; T, thyroid.

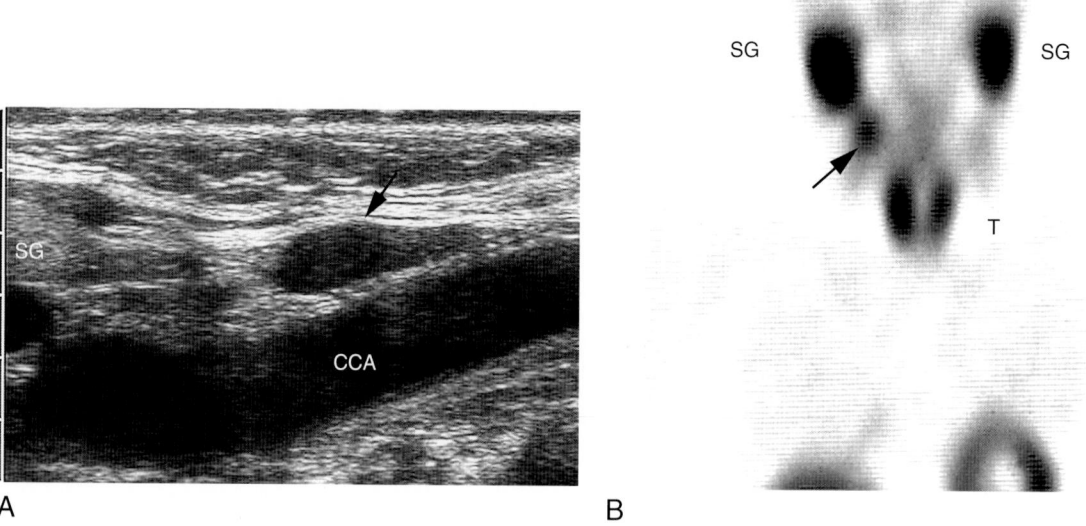

FIGURE 22-13. Ectopic adenoma—carotid sheath. A, Longitudinal sonogram of the right side of the neck shows an ectopic parathyroid adenoma (*arrow*) anterior to the common carotid artery (CCA). SG, Salivary gland. **B,** Scintigraphy using technetium-99m sestamibi and coronal SPECT imaging shows a focal area of increased activity in right lateral neck (*arrow*), which corresponds to the ectopic adenoma. SG, Salivary gland; T, thyroid.

One common source for a false-positive ultrasound study is confusion of **cervical lymph nodes** for a parathyroid adenoma.[36] Sonographically visible cervical lymph nodes usually lie in the lateral neck adjacent to the jugular vein and away from the thyroid. However, lymph nodes may occasionally be found near the inferior pole of the thyroid, simulating an ectopic parathyroid adenoma. Lymph nodes are commonly found adjacent to the carotid artery, and these may simulate an ectopic gland or adenoma located in the carotid sheath. Enlarged cervical lymph nodes may have an oval, hypoechoic appearance like parathyroid adenomas, but they often also have a central echogenic band or hilum composed of fat, vessels, and fibrous tissue, which is a feature that distinguishes them from parathyroid adenomas.[80] Most lymph nodes are negative on

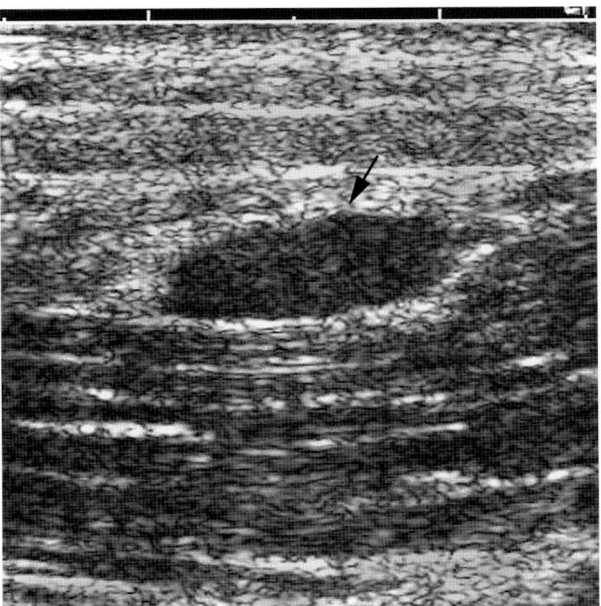

FIGURE 22-14. Graft-dependent hyperparathyroidism. Longitudinal sonogram of left forearm shows a 2 cm oval hypoechoic nodule (*arrow*) due to hyperplasia of autotransplanted parathyroid tissue.

sestamibi scintigraphy. Nonetheless, ultrasound-guided FNAB may be necessary to distinguish a potential parathyroid adenoma from an abnormal lymph node, particularly in the reoperative setting. At least two cases of enlarged lymph nodes containing **sarcoid granulomas** causing hypercalcemia and false-positive scintigraphic and sonographic examinations have been described.[81]

Many **small veins** lie immediately adjacent to the posterior and lateral aspects of both lobes of the thyroid, and when one is tortuous or segmentally dilated, it can simulate a small parathyroid adenoma. Scanning maneuvers that help to establish if the structure in question is a vein, and not an adenoma, include the use of the following: (1) real-time imaging in multiple planes to show the tubular nature of the vein; (2) a Valsalva maneuver by the patient, which may cause transient engorgement of the vein; and (3) spectral or color Doppler imaging to show flow within the vein.

The **esophagus** may partially protrude from behind the posterolateral aspect of the trachea and simulate a large parathyroid adenoma (see Fig. 22-8B).[82] Turning the patient's head to the opposite side will accentuate the protrusion. Careful inspection of this structure in the transverse plane will show that it has the typical concentric ring appearance of bowel, with a peripheral hypoechoic muscular layer and the central echogenic appearance of the mucosa and intraluminal contents. Using a longitudinal scan plane helps to demonstrate the tubular nature of this structure. Real-time imaging while the patient swallows will cause a stream of brightly echogenic mucus and microbubbles to flow through the

lumen, which confirms that the structure is the esophagus.

The **longus colli muscle** lies adjacent to the anterolateral aspect of the cervical spine. If viewed in the transverse plane, it appears as a hypoechoic triangular mass that can simulate a large parathyroid adenoma located posterior to the thyroid gland. However, scanning in the longitudinal plane will show that this structure is long and flat and contains longitudinal echogenic striations typical of skeletal muscle. Real-time imaging while the patient swallows can be useful because swallowing will cause movement of the thyroid gland and perithyroid structures, such as a parathyroid adenoma, but the longus colli muscle, which is attached to the spine, will remain stationary. Finally, comparison with the opposite side of the neck will demonstrate similar symmetrical findings because the longus colli muscles are paired structures located on both sides of the cervical spine.

Thyroid nodules are also potential causes of false-positive ultrasound and scintigraphic imaging.[83,84] Thyroid nodules can be visualized in up to 40% of patients undergoing sonographic examination of the neck for parathyroid disease.[85] If a thyroid nodule protrudes from the posterior aspect of the thyroid, it can simulate a mass in the location of a parathyroid adenoma. One sign that can be useful in this situation is a thin echogenic line that separates the parathyroid adenoma (which usually arises outside of the thyroid gland) from the thyroid gland itself. Thyroid nodules, which arise within the thyroid gland, do not show this tissue plane of separation.[86] Morphologically, thyroid nodules, unlike parathyroid adenomas, are often partially cystic and some are calcified. Also, thyroid nodules often are of a heterogeneous, mixed echogenicity, whereas parathyroid adenomas are of a homogeneous, hypoechoic echogenicity (Fig. 22-15).[12] When a parathyroid adenoma cannot be distinguished from a thyroid nodule by imaging criteria, ultrasound-guided percutaneous biopsy may be necessary.

False-Negative Examination

The three major situations in which examinations give false-negative results are minimally enlarged adenomas, adenomas displaced posteriorly and obscured by a markedly enlarged thyroid goiter, and ectopic adenomas (see box).

Minimally enlarged adenomas are a common cause of error because these small masses can be difficult to distinguish from the thyroid and adjacent soft tissues. **Multinodular thyroid goiters** interfere with parathyroid adenoma detection in two ways. First, the thyroid gland enlargement displaces structures located adjacent to the posterior thyroid, away from the transducer. This can necessitate the use of 5-MHz transducers rather than

PARATHYROID ADENOMA: CAUSES OF FALSE-NEGATIVE EXAMINATION

Minimally enlarged adenoma
Multinodular thyroid goiter
Ectopic parathyroid adenoma

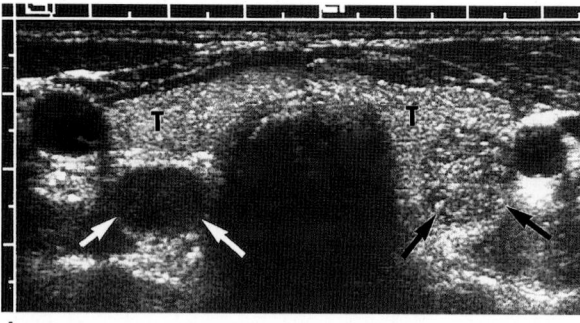

A

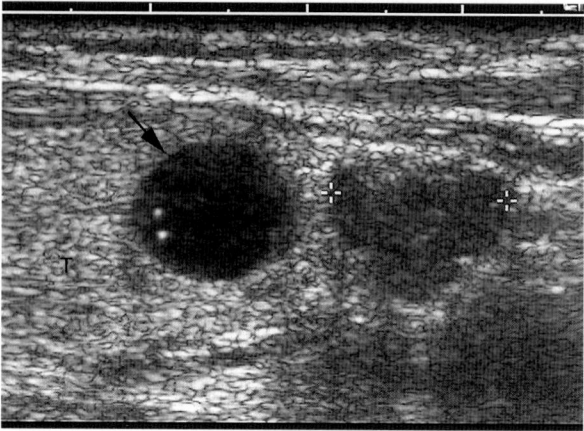

B

FIGURE 22-15. Thyroid nodules may simulate a parathyroid adenoma. A, Transverse view of neck shows a 1.5 cm heterogeneous thyroid nodule (*black arrows*) arising within the posterior aspect, left lobe of the thyroid (T). This could be a parathyroid adenoma. Compare this mass to the 1 cm homogeneous hypoechoic true parathyroid adenoma (*white arrows*) arising in the soft tissues posterior to the right lobe of the thyroid. **B,** Longitudinal sonogram shows a hypoechoic parathyroid adenoma (*cursors*) at the inferior tip of the left lobe of the thyroid. An adjacent intrathyroidal colloid cyst (*arrow*) is also present in the lower pole of the thyroid (T).(**A,** reproduced with permission from Hopkins CR, Reading CC: Thyroid and parathyroid imaging. Semin Ultrasound CT MR 1995;16:279-295.)

higher frequency transducers to obtain the necessary penetration, which decreases spatial resolution. Second, thyroid goiters have a multinodular contour and irregular echotexture, which hinders the detection of adjacent parathyroid gland enlargement. Some **ectopic adenomas**, such as retrotracheal adenomas or adenomas located deep in the mediastinum, will be inaccessible

and nonvisible due to acoustic shadowing from the overlying air and bone.

ACCURACY

Sonography

Ultrasound imaging provides a noninvasive and economical means to localize parathyroid adenomas in the preoperative setting of primary hyperparathyroidism. However, the success of sonographic parathyroid imaging is highly dependent on operator experience and the use of newer high-resolution technology. The sensitivity of sonographic parathyroid adenoma localization in primary hyperparathyroidism varies by institution, but most reports range between 70% and 90%.[36,67,86-104] The positive predictive value and the specificity for ultrasound in detecting adenomatous disease have been reported between 88% and 100%. Sensitivity improves with the use of higher resolution sonography and in the hands of an experienced examiner. However, the sensitivity of ultrasound to detect ectopic mediastinal adenomas is predictably much lower, and the accuracy decreases in the presence of concomitant multinodular thyroid. As described in detail later (see "Percutaneous Biopsy" section), FNAB is a valuable adjunct to ultrasound examination and can be used to improve the accuracy, specificity, and sensitivity of the examination. For a suspected adenoma mass, aspirate specimens should be sent for cytologic analysis as well as PTH assay.[65,67,105-109]

In persistent or recurrent hyperparathyroidism, the sensitivity of sonography in adenoma localization has been reported to be between 36% and 75%.[65,67,69,110-114] Ultrasound augmented by FNAB and PTH assay can lead to a specificity approaching 100% and a sensitivity and accuracy of 90% and 82%, respectively.[65,114] It is important to understand that in most large clinical series of patients undergoing reoperation for hyperparathyroidism, 70% to 80% of parathyroid adenomas are found in the neck or are accessible through a neck incision.[60,62,63] Therefore, a thorough ultrasound examination of the neck is important in these reoperative patients. If the adenoma is not visible sonographically, an ectopic mediastinal location should be considered.[67,114,115]

Other Imaging Modalities

Other methods that have been used commonly for parathyroid adenoma localization are MRI[116-119] and scintigraphy using technetium-99m sestamibi.[84,101,120-126] Technetium-99m sestamibi scintigraphy combined with SPECT imaging has sensitivities of 75% to 90%, similar to that of ultrasound.[68,84,96,127,128] Scintigraphy, like ultrasound, appears to be less accurate in the setting of multiglandular parathyroid disease and in the presence of multinodular thyroid disease. Less commonly used methods include computed tomography (CT), angiography, and venous sampling.[129-134] Initial studies to evaluate both transesophageal ultrasound[135] and positron emission tomography[136,137] have shown success in some patients. In the patient being considered for repeat surgery, sestamibi scintigraphy or MRI may be useful if sonography is negative, particularly for evaluation of the portion of the mediastinum and retrotracheal areas that are not well seen by sonography. Angiography and venous sampling are more invasive, expensive, and technically demanding than the imaging modalities mentioned above and are being used in few centers. Studies evaluating the combined sensitivities of multiple preoperative imaging examinations describe improved overall accuracy when compared to single modality evaluation.[91,128] Recently, several authors have reported that combined imaging with ultrasound and sestamibi scintigraphy increases the sensitivity for the preoperative diagnosis of parathyroid disease (Fig. 22-16).[101,127,128,138] When multiple studies are used, ultrasound is a good choice as the initial imaging examination for preoperative imaging because of its noninvasiveness, low cost, and competitive sensitivity and accuracy.

Discussion: To Image or Not to Image in Primary Hyperparathyroidism

The indications for preoperative imaging of the parathyroid glands in patients with primary hyperparathyroidism vary by institution and surgeon preference. In some medical centers where an experienced surgeon is available, routine preoperative parathyroid imaging is not performed.[139] This is because normocalcemia is restored postoperatively in 95% to 98% of patients and because morbidity is rare when parathyroidectomy is performed by an experienced surgeon.[66,140,141] Except in diagnostically difficult cases or the high-risk patient, it is unlikely that preoperative imaging in primary hyperparathyroidism is cost effective enough to significantly improve the high reported rate of surgical success when standard bilateral neck dissection is performed.[139,140]

However, there is now support from many investigators for preoperative imaging in primary hyperparathyroidism. **Unilateral neck exploration** and, more recently, **minimally invasive surgical techniques** have been described and are becoming increasingly popular for first-time surgery in primary hyperparathyroidism.[56,115,142-148] In the latter, the surgeon selectively removes the abnormal gland or adenoma through a small (2 cm) incision in the neck, thereby potentially improving cosmesis, reducing complication risks, and decreasing operative time and hospital stays—all without sacrificing operative efficacy (Fig. 22-17). Moreover, postsurgical fibrosis is limited to a smaller area, thus

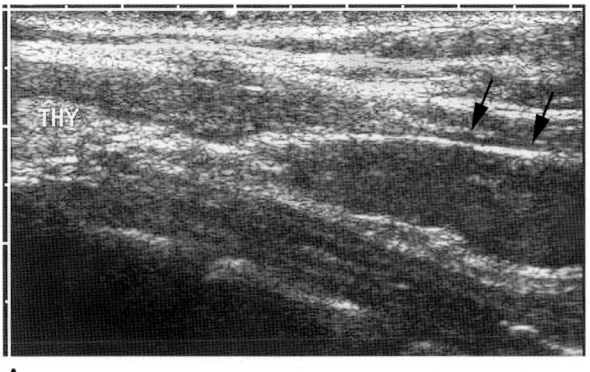

A

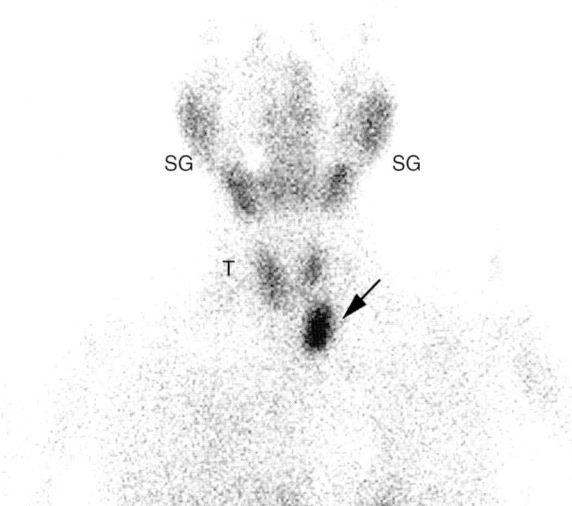

B

FIGURE 22-16. Correlation of ultrasound and scintigraphic imaging of a parathyroid adenoma. **A,** Longitudinal sonogram shows a hypoechoic 3 cm adenoma (*arrows*) located inferior to the tip of the lower pole of the left thyroid lobe (THY). **B,** Planar imaging with technetium-99m sestamibi shows increased focal activity in the inferior left neck corresponding to the adenoma (*arrow*), well below the level of the thyroid (T) and salivary glands (SG).

facilitating any necessary repeat surgery in the future. The successful institution of these minimally invasive techniques is predicated on two things. First, the availability of rapid (10- to 15-minute) **intraoperative parathyroid hormone (IOPTH) monitoring**, and second, the availability of **accurate preoperative imaging techniques** that allow a focused surgical approach.

Investigators contend that, in selected first-time surgical patients, focused surgical techniques with preoperative imaging guidance have a cure rate comparable to conventional bilateral neck dissection.[115,142-148] A higher rate of persistent hypercalcemia is potentially possible with unilateral parathyroidectomy, if preoperative imaging misses a contralateral second adenoma. However, double and triple adenomas have an incidence of much less than 5%, with some studies quoting inci-

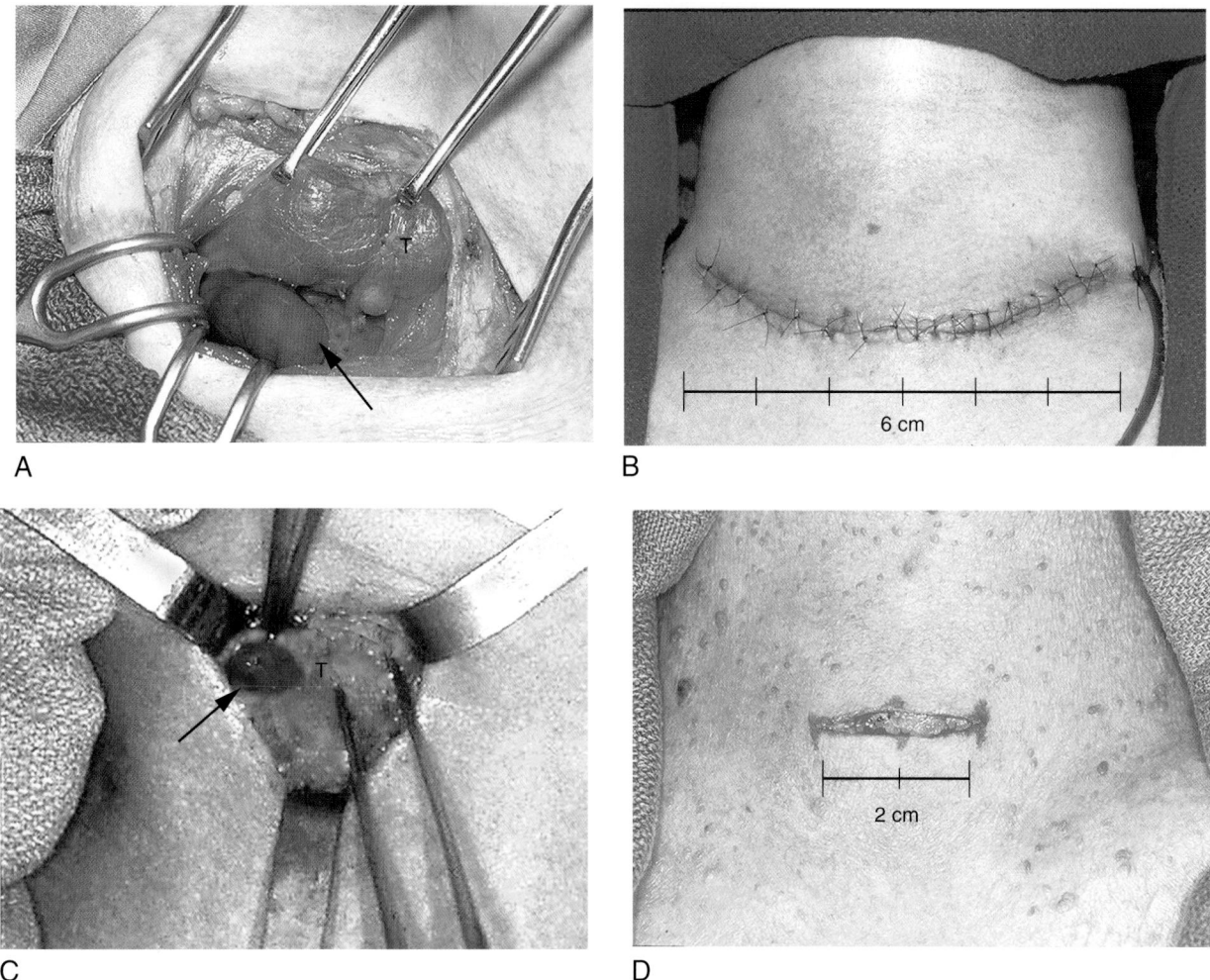

FIGURE 22-17. Comparison of operative procedures for removal of parathyroid adenoma. A, Intraoperative photograph during conventional neck dissection for parathyroidectomy. The thyroid gland (T) is retracted back and a parathyroid adenoma (*arrow*) is exposed. **B**, The corresponding 6 cm "collar" incision with a surgical drain. **C**, Intraoperative photograph during minimally invasive surgery uses a smaller incision. The parathyroid adenoma (*arrow*) is exposed adjacent to the thyroid (T). **D**, The corresponding incision measures approximately 2 cm. (Photographs courtesy of Geoffrey B. Thompson, MD; Mayo Clinic, Rochester, Minnesota.)

dences of less than 1%.[16,115] Many investigators promote the use of dual-modality imaging (e.g., ultrasound and sestamibi scintigraphy or ultrasound and CT) to increase the preoperative predictivity of unilateral disease and aid in excluding multigland disease.[145,147-150] In addition, the use of IOPTH monitoring allows the surgeon to quickly assess the success of a unilateral approach. If intraoperative PTH levels fail to decrease appropriately, multigland disease should be suspected and the procedure must then be converted to a bilateral dissection.

Proponents of preoperative imaging in primary hyperparathyroidism also note that some adenomas are found low in the mediastinum and that the initial operative approach may be changed or optimized if imaging shows parathyroid disease near the thymus.[56] Accurate preoperative localization decreases surgical morbidity in high-risk patients, including those with severe cardiac or pulmonary disease.[151-154] Sonography

can also shorten the evaluation necessary prior to urgent surgery in a patient with a life-threatening hypercalcemic crisis.[154]

In persistent or recurrent hyperparathyroidism, localization studies are clearly indicated and liberally used because of the lower surgical success rate and the higher morbidity of reoperations. Preoperative localization studies in recurrent hyperparathyroidism contribute to both the success and speed of the repeat operation. In two separate series of 157 and 124 patients who had undergone re-exploration for persistent or recurrent hyperparathyroidism, the surgical cure rate was 88% to 89%, and it was thought that prospective localization studies contributed to this high rate of success.[65,66] When the adenoma was localized preoperatively, the time of operation was decreased. Because most persistent and recurrent parathyroid adenomas are accessible in the neck or the upper mediastinum via a cervical incision versus a sternotomy, sonography and sestamibi scintigraphy may be the localizing procedures of choice in the setting of recurrent or persistent hyperparathyroidism.[65,112,124,155]

INTRAOPERATIVE SONOGRAPHY

Intraoperative sonography occasionally can be a useful adjunct in the surgical detection of parathyroid adenomas, particularly in the reoperative setting.[156,157] Intraoperative scanning can be performed with a conventional, high-frequency (7.5 to 15 MHz) transducer draped with a sterile plastic sheath or with a dedicated sterilized intraoperative transducer. Intraoperative sonography appears to be best suited for the localization of inferior and intrathyroid abnormal parathyroid glands. Superior abnormal glands are more difficult to detect.[157] If intraoperative sonography detects an abnormal parathyroid gland, operative time can be shortened. In most studies, however, intraoperative sonography has not affected the outcome of the operation.

PERCUTANEOUS BIOPSY

Sonographically guided percutaneous FNAB is being used with increasing frequency for preoperative confirmation of suspected abnormal parathyroid glands, particularly in the patient who is a candidate for reoperation.[65,105-108,158-164] This technique can decrease the false positive rate and increase the specificity of sonography by permitting the reliable differentiation of parathyroid adenomas from other pathologic structures, such as thyroid nodules and cervical lymph nodes. In addition to its value to the surgeon, a positive biopsy may reassure the reluctant reoperative patient. FNAB is also generally obtained for diagnostic confirmation prior to percutaneously injected ethanol ablation of a suspected abnormal gland.

If the suspected parathyroid adenoma is in a location remote from the thyroid gland, the main differential diagnostic consideration is a lymph node. Percutaneous biopsy is performed by using a small-caliber, noncutting needle, such as a 25 gauge standard injection needle, to obtain aspirates that show either parathyroid cells or lymphocytes (Fig. 22-18).[161] The aspirate should also be analyzed for parathyroid hormone content.[109,165] A clearly detectable concentration of PTH in the aspirate, even if it does not exceed that of the serum level, indicates the presence of parathyroid tissue. Three to four aspirates can be diluted with 1 mL of saline. If the suspected parathyroid adenoma lies adjacent to the thyroid gland, a larger specimen (histologic, rather than cytologic, specimen) may be necessary to differentiate

parathyroid tissue from thyroid tissue.[162] A histologic specimen can be obtained with a small caliber (20 to 25 gauge) cutting needle. There have been few reported complications of FNAB of suspected parathyroid adenomas. However, there has been at least one report of a serious postprocedure hematoma requiring emergent surgery.[166]

The accuracy of percutaneous biopsy in the differentiation of parathyroid gland from other structures was 87% in one series of 52 cases.[159] Biopsy failures were due to inadequate recovery of parathyroid tissue. The addition of PTH assay to the analysis of the aspirate reduces the number of false positive cytology results, thereby potentially increasing the overall procedural specificity. Although a theoretical consideration, parathymosis (the implantation of hyperfunctioning parathyroid tissue in the neck or mediastinum resulting in hypercalcemia) does not appear to be a complication of FNAB.[167]

ALCOHOL ABLATION

Sonography has been used to guide percutaneous injection of ethanol into abnormally enlarged parathyroid glands for chemical ablation.[165,166,168-178] Alcohol ablation is most commonly used in postoperative patients with recurrent or persistent hyperparathyroidism who have a sonographically visible, biopsy-proven parathyroid adenoma, but who are poor surgical candidates.[165,177,179] Some dialysis patients with secondary hyperparathyroidism, or patients with a history of multigland disease with recurrent hyperparathyroidism

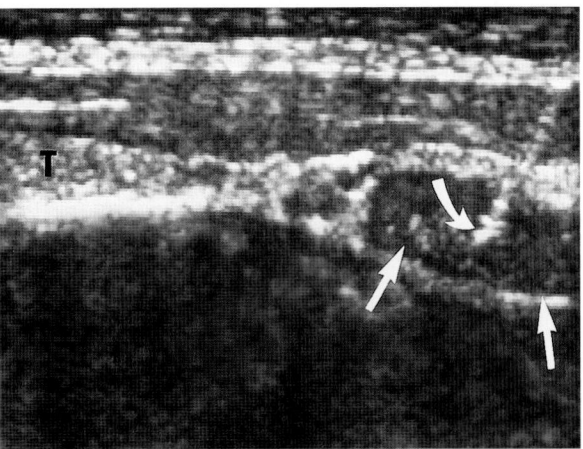

FIGURE 22-18. Percutaneous needle biopsy of parathyroid adenoma. Longitudinal sonogram shows a 1.5 cm oval hypoechoic parathyroid adenoma (*straight arrows*) in the low neck in a patient with recurrent hyperparathyroidism. Needle (*curved arrow*) biopsy obtained parathyroid cells and an aspirate positive for PTH, confirming that this mass was a parathyroid adenoma. T, Thyroid.

after previous subtotal surgery that is resistant to calcitriol therapy, may also be candidates.[165,171,178,180-183] Subtotal alcohol ablation is also occasionally utilized in autograft patients with recurrent graft-dependent hyperparathyroidism (Fig. 22-19). Adenomatous hyperplasia with autonomously functioning glands (tertiary hyperparathyroidism) has also been treated with ultrasound-guided alcohol injection to reduce gland mass, but with unpredictable results.[184,185]

Alcohol ablation is generally performed under local anesthesia, usually after a percutaneous biopsy has confirmed the presence of parathyroid tissue or PTH content in the tissue. A small (22 to 25 gauge) needle is inserted into multiple regions of the mass, and 95%

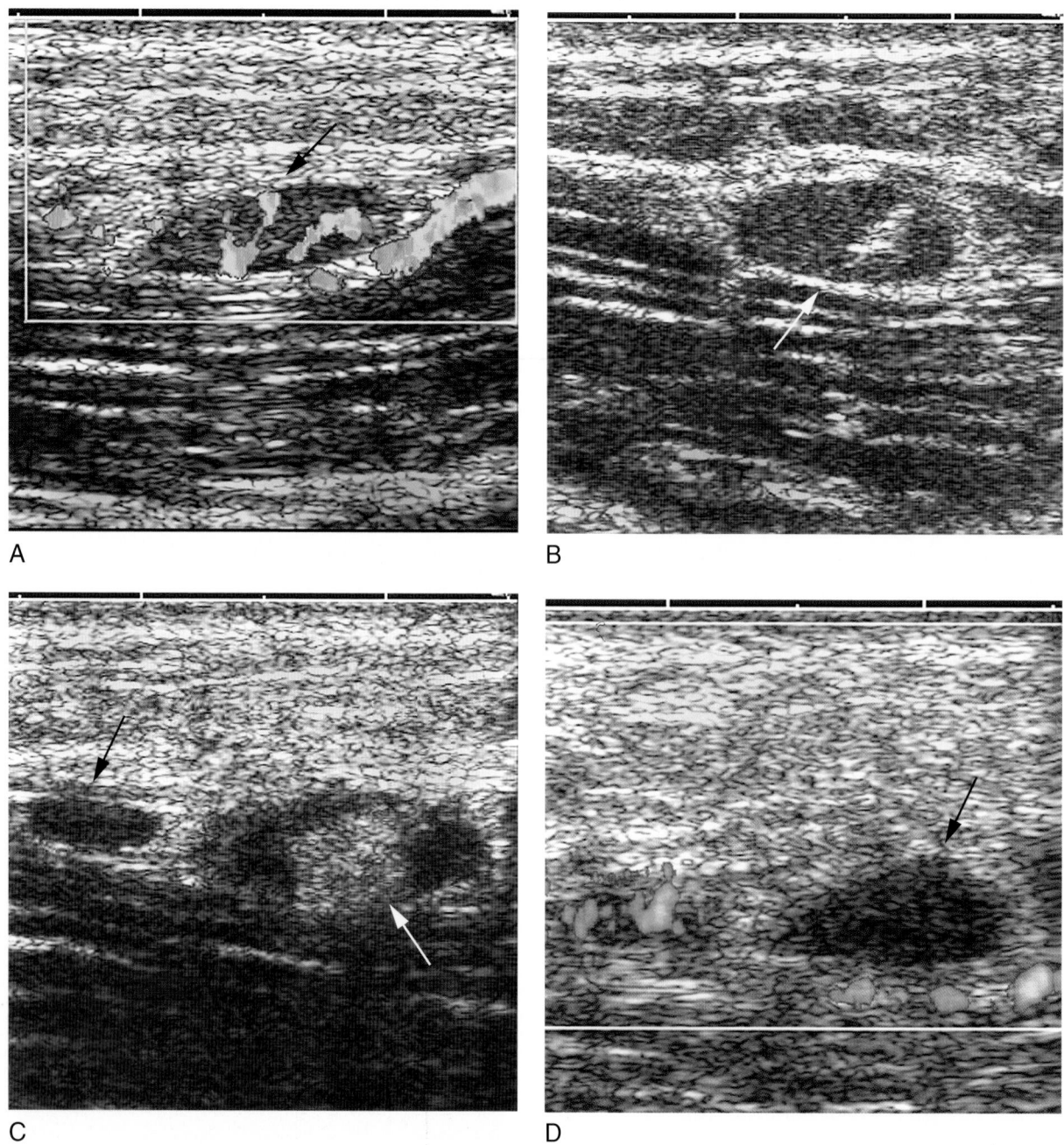

FIGURE 22-19. Alcohol ablation of hyperplastic autotransplanted parathyroid tissue. A, Color flow Doppler sonogram of the superficial forearm tissues shows a dominant vascular nodule that represents hyperfunctioning parathyroid tissue (*arrow*) in a patient with recurrent graft-dependent hyperparathyroidism. **B,** Under sonographic guidance, a needle tip (*arrow*) is placed within the nodule and **C,** ethanol is injected into portions of the adenoma, which causes the tissues adjacent to the needle tip to become transiently, brightly echogenic (*white arrow*). A smaller adjacent nodule of parathyroid tissue (*black arrow*) is not injected in order to maintain baseline graft function. **D,** After alcohol ablation, color Doppler sonogram shows minimal residual vascularity in the injected nodule (*arrow*)

ethanol is injected in a volume equal to approximately one half the volume of the mass. Under real-time visualization, the tissue becomes highly echogenic at the moment of injection. This echogenicity slowly disappears over a period of approximately 1 minute. There is also a marked decrease in vascularity of the parathyroid adenoma after alcohol injection, presumably secondary to thrombosis and occlusion of the parathyroid vessels (see Fig. 22-19). The injections are repeated every day or every other day until the serum calcium level reaches the normal range. In some cases, three to five injections are necessary. All patients undergoing parathyroid alcohol ablation require long-term close follow-up of serum calcium levels to detect subsequent hypoparathyroidism or, more commonly, recurrent hyperparathyroidism.

The results of alcohol injection as a treatment for hyperparathyroidism remain promising, although mixed. Certainly, the long-term efficacy of alcohol ablation does not approach that of surgery for patients presenting with primary hyperparathyroidism.[165,166,176,177] In addition, postablation periglandular fibrosis often makes future surgical and ablation procedures increasingly difficult. In a series of 36 patients with primary hyperparathyroidism, 89% of patients had a partial or complete biochemical improvement, whereas 33% remained completely eucalcemic over a median follow-up period of 16 months.[165] In another series of 27 patients with primary hyperparathyroidism, more than 90% of patients had at least partial biochemical response to treatment, whereas 56% had complete normalization in the first 3 months.[166] In a series of 46 chronic dialysis patients with recalcitrant secondary hyperparathyroidism, 80% achieved successful maintenance of parathyroid function within a target range aided by alcohol ablation of glandular hyperplasia and 100% avoided surgery.[178]

Some treatments fail because the gland is not completely ablated and hyperfunctioning parathyroid tissue remains. Other treatments fail simply because the correct gland is not identified and injected. This can usually be avoided with preprocedure FNAB of the suspect gland. Even with preprocedural FNAB confirmation of parathyroid disease, occult multiglandular disease remains a possibility. In such a setting, alcohol ablation outcomes are predictably less effective when only a single site is treated.

The reported adverse effects from ethanol ablation of parathyroid adenomas have been limited to moderate to severe jaw pain during the procedure and dysphonia from vocal cord paralysis. The latter is due to recurrent laryngeal nerve palsy, which is typically transient, although there has been at least one report describing permanent vocal cord paralysis.[176] Patients who have had prior subtotal parathyroid surgery are also theoretically at increased risk for postablation hypoparathyroidism and a conservative, subtotal approach may be prudent.

There has been at least one report of successful treatment of a parathyroid adenoma using ultrasound-guided thermal ablation with interstitial laser photocoagulation.[186] In the future, this may prove to be a useful ablation technique in which the tissue destruction is better controlled, potentially avoiding the fibrosis associated with chemical ablation techniques.

References

Embryology and Anatomy

1. Gilmour JR: The gross anatomy of the parathyroid glands. J Pathol 1938;46:133-148.
2. Weller GL, Jr: Development of the thyroid, parathyroid and thymus glands in man. Carnegie Institution of Washington: Contributions to Embryology 1933;24(141):93-139.
3. Mansberger AR, Wei JP: Surgical embryology and anatomy of the thyroid and parathyroid glands. Surg Clin North Am 1993;73:727-746.
4. Akerstrom G, Malmaeus J, Bergstrom R: Surgical anatomy of human parathyroid glands. Surgery 1984;95:14-21.
5. Edis AJ: Surgical anatomy and technique of neck exploration for primary hyperparathyroidism. Surg Clin North Am 1977;57:495-504.
6. Thompson NW, Eckhauser FE, Harness JK: The anatomy of primary hyperparathyroidism. Surgery 1982;92:814-821.
7. Edis AJ, Purnell DC, Van Heerden JA: The undescended "parathymus." An occasional cause of failed neck exploration for hyperparathyroidism. Ann Surg 1979;190:64-68.
8. Wang C-A: The anatomic basis of parathyroid surgery. Ann Surg 1976;183:271-275.
9. Norris EH: The parathyroid glands and the lateral thyroid in man: Their morphogenesis, histogenesis, topographic anatomy and prenatal growth. Carnegie Institution of Washington: Contributions to Embryology 1937;26(159):247-294.
10. Castleman B, Roth SI: Tumors of the parathyroid glands. In Atlas of Tumor Pathology. Fascicle 14, 2nd series. Washington, DC, Armed Forces Institute of Pathology;1978.
11. Russell CF, Grant CS, Van Heerden JA: Hyperfunctioning supernumerary parathyroid glands: An occasional cause of hyperparathyroidism. Mayo Clin Proc 1982;57:121-124.
12. Hopkins CR, Reading CC: Thyroid and parathyroid imaging. Semin Ultrasound CT MR 1995;16:279-295.

Primary Hyperparathyroidism

13. Heath H, 3rd, Hodgson SF, Kennedy MA: Primary hyperparathyroidism: Incidence, morbidity, and potential economic impact in a community. N Engl J Med 1980;302:189-193.
14. Van Heerden JA, Beahrs OH, Woolner LB: The pathology and surgical management of primary hyperparathyroidism. Surg Clin North Am 1977;57:557-563.
15. Wang CA: Surgery of the parathyroid glands. Adv Surg 1966;5:109-127.
16. Kaplan EL, Yashiro T, Salti G: Primary hyperthyroidism in the 1990s. Choice of surgical procedures for this disease. Ann Surg 1992;215:300-317.
17. Black WC, 3rd, Utley JR: The differential diagnosis of parathyroid adenoma and chief cell hyperplasia. Am J Clin Pathol 1968;49:761-775.

18. Prinz RA, Gamvros OI, Sellu D, et al: Subtotal parathyroidectomy for primary chief cell hyperplasia of the multiple endocrine neoplasia type I syndrome. Ann Surg 1981;193:26-29.

19. Van Heerden JA, Kent RB III, Sizemore GW, et al: Primary hyperparathyroidism in patients with multiple endocrine neoplasia syndromes. Arch Surg 1983;118:533-535.

20. Weiland LH: Practical endocrine surgical pathology. In Van Heerden JA (ed): Common Problems in Endocrine Surgery. Chicago, Year Book Medical Publishers, 1989.

21. Schantz A, Castleman B: Parathyroid carcinoma: A study of 70 cases. Cancer 1973;31:600-605.

22. Delallis RA: Tumors of the parathyroid gland. In Atlas of Tumor Pathology. Fascicle 6, 3rd series. Washington, DC, Armed Forces Institute of Pathology, 1993.

23. Shane E, Bilezikian JP: Parathyroid carcinoma: A review of 62 patients. Endocrinol Rev 1982;3:218-226.

24. Holmes EC, Morton DL, Ketcham AS: Parathyroid carcinoma: A collective review. Ann Surg 1969;169:631-640.

25. Purnell DC, Smith LH, Scholz DA, et al: Primary hyperparathyroidism: A prospective clinical study. Am J Med 1971;50:670-678.

26. Purnell DC, Scholz DA, Smith LH, et al: Treatment of primary hyperparathyroidism. Am J Med 1974;56:800-809.

27. Silverberg SJ, Shane E, Jacobs TP, et al: A 10-year prospective study of primary hyperparathyroidism with or without parathyroid surgery. N Engl J Med 1999;341:1249-1255.

28. Clark OH, Duh QY: Primary hyperparathyroidism: A surgical perspective. Endocrinol Metab Clin North Am 1989;18:701-714.

29. Kaplan RA, Snyder WH, Stewart A, et al: Metabolic effects of parathyroidectomy in asymptomatic primary hyperparathyroidism. J Clin Endocrinol Metab 1976;42:415-426.

30. Gaz RD, Wang CA: Management of asymptomatic hyperparathyroidism. Am J Surg 1984;147:498-501.

31. NIH Consensus Development Conference Panel. Diagnosis and management of asymptomatic primary hyperparathyroidism: Consensus development conference statement. Ann Intern Med 1991;114:593-597.

32. Irvin GL, Carneiro DM: Management changes in primary hyperparathyroidism. JAMA 2000;284:934-936.

33. Kearns AE, Thompson GB: Medical and surgical management of hyperparathyroidism. Mayo Clin Proc 2002;77:87-91.

Sonographic Appearance

34. Graif M, Itzchak Y, Strauss S, et al: Parathyroid sonography: Diagnostic accuracy related to shape, location and texture of the gland. Br J Radiol 1987;60:439-443.

35. Randel SB, Gooding GAW, Clark OH, et al: Parathyroid variants: Ultrasound evaluation. Radiology 1987;165:191-194.

36. Reading CC, Charboneau JW, James EM, et al: High-resolution parathyroid sonography. AJR 1982;139:539-546.

37. Obara T, Fujimoto Y, Ito Y, et al: Functioning parathyroid lipoadenoma—report of four cases: Clinicopathological and ultrasonographic features. Endocrinol Jpn 1989;36:135-145.

38. Lack EF, Clark MA, Buck DR, et al: Cysts of the parathyroid gland: Report of two cases and review of the literature. Am Surg 1978;44:376-381.

39. Krudy AG, Doppman JL, Shawker TH, et al: Hyperfunctioning cystic parathyroid glands: Computed tomography and sonographic findings. AJR 1984;142:175-178.

40. Sistrom CL, Hanks JB, Feldman PS: Supraclavicular mass in a woman with hyperparathyroidism. Invest Radiol 1994;2:244-247.

41. Lane MJ, Desser TS, Weigel RJ, et al: Use of color and power Doppler sonography to identify feeding arteries associated with parathyroid adenomas. AJR 1998;171:819-823.

42. Wolf RJ, Cronan JJ, Monchik JM: Color Doppler sonography: An adjunctive technique in assessment of parathyroid adenomas. J Ultrasound Med 1994;13:303-308.

43. Calliada F, Bergonzi M, Passamonti C, et al: [Doppler color in the echographic study of hyperplastic parathyroid glands]. Radiol Med (Torino) 1989;78(6):607-611.

44. Gooding GAW, Clark OH: Use of color Doppler imaging in the distinction between thyroid and parathyroid lesions. Am J Surg 1992;164:51-56.

45. Daly BD, Coffey SL, Behan M: Ultrasonographic appearances of parathyroid carcinoma. Br J Radiol 1989;62:1017-1019.

46. Edmonson GR, Charboneau JW, James EM, et al: Parathyroid carcinoma: High-frequency sonographic features. Radiology 1986;161:65-67.

47. Hara H, Igarashi A, Yano Y, et al: Ultrasonographic features of parathyroid carcinoma. Endocr J 2001;48:213-217.

Adenoma Localization

48. Clark OH: Mediastinal parathyroid tumors. Arch Surg 1988;123:1096-1099.

49. Thompson NW: The techniques of initial parathyroid exploration and re-operative parathyroidectomy. In Thompson NW, Vinik AI (eds): Endocrine Surgery Update. New York, Grune & Stratton, 1983.

50. Al-Suhaili AR, Lynn J, Lavender JP: Intrathyroidal parathyroid adenoma: Preoperative identification and localization by parathyroid imaging. Clin Nucl Med 1988;13:512-514.

51. Spiegel AM, Marx SJ, Doppman JL, et al: Intrathyroidal parathyroid adenoma or hyperplasia; An occasionally overlooked cause of surgical failure in primary hyperparathyroidism. JAMA 1975;234:1029-1033.

52. Fraker DL, Doppman JL, Shawker TH, et al: Undescended parathyroid adenoma: An important etiology for failed operations for primary hyperparathyroidism. World J Surg 1990;14:342-348.

53. Doppman JL, Shawker TH, Krudy AG, et al: Parathymic parathyroid: Computed tomography, ultrasound and angiographic findings. Radiology 1985;157:419-423.

54. Doppman JL, Shawker TH, Fraker DL, et al: Parathyroid adenoma within the vagus nerve. AJR 1994; 163:943-945.

55. Kurtay M, Crile G, Jr: Aberrant parathyroid gland in relationship to the thymus. Am J Surg 1969;117:705.

Persistent or Recurrent Hyperparathyroidism

56. Irvin GL, Prudhomme DL, Deriso GT, et al: A new approach to parathyroidectomy. Ann Surg 1994;219:574-581.

57. Clark OH, Way LW, Hunt TK: Recurrent hyperparathyroidism. Ann Surg 1976;184:391-399.

58. Levin KE, Clark OH: The reasons for failure in parathyroid operations. Arch Surg 1989;124:911-914.

59. Cheung PSY, Borgstrom A, Thompson NW: Strategy in re-operative surgery for hyperparathyroidism. Arch Surg 1989;124:676-680.

60. Palmer JA, Rosen IB: Re-operative surgery for hyperparathyroidism. Am J Surg 1982;144:406-410.

61. Prinz RA, Gamvros OI, Allison DJ, et al: Re-operations for hyperparathyroidism. Surg Gynecol Obstet 1981;152:760-764.

62. Grant CS, Charboneau JW, James EM, et al: Re-operative parathyroid surgery. Wien Klin Wochenschr 1988;100:360-363.

63. Wells SA: Advances in the operative management of persistent hyperparathyroidism. Mayo Clin Proc 1991;66:1175-1177.

64. Brennan MF, Marx SJ, Doppman J, et al: Results of re-operation for persistent and recurrent hyperparathyroidism. Ann Surg 1981;194:671-676.

65. Thompson GB, Grant CS, Perrier ND, et al: Reoperative parathyroid surgery in the era of sestamibi scanning and intraoperative parathyroid hormone monitoring. Arch Surg 1999;134:699-705.

66. Grant CS, Van Heerden JA, Charboneau JW, et al: Clinical management of persistent and/or recurrent primary hyperparathyroidism. World J Surg 1986;10:555-565.

67. Rodriquez JM, Tezelman S, Siperstein AE, et al: Localization procedures in patients with persistent or recurrent hyperparathyroidism. Arch Surg 1994;129:870-875.

68. Feingold DL, Alexander HR, Chen CC, et al: Ultrasound and sestamibi scan as the only preoperative imaging tests in the reoperation for parathyroid adenomas. Surgery 2000;128:1103-1110.

69. Higgins CB: Role of magnetic resonance imaging in hyperparathyroidism. Radiol Clin North Am 1993;31:1017-1028.

70. Brunt LM, Sicard GA: Current status of parathyroid autotransplantation. Sem Surg Oncol 1990;6:115-121.

71. Brunt LM, Wells SA, Jr: Parathyroid transplantation: Indications and results. In Van Herrden JA (ed): Common Problems in Endocrine Surgery. Chicago, Year Book Medical Publishers, 1989.

72. Winkelbauer F, Ammann ME, Langle F, et al: Diagnosis of hyperparathyroidism with US after autotransplantation: Results of a prospective study. Radiology 1993;186:255-257.

73. Hergan K, Neyer U, Doringer W, et al: MR imaging in graft-dependent recurrent hyperparathyroidism after parathyroidectomy and autotransplantation. J Magn Reson Imaging 1995;5:541-544.

Secondary Hyperparathyroidism

74. Wilson RE, Hampers CL, Bernstein DS, et al: Subtotal parathyroidectomy in chronic renal failure: A seven-year experience in a dialysis and transplant program. Ann Surg 1971;174:640-652.

75. Diethelm AG, Adams PL, Murad TM, et al: Treatment of secondary hyperparathyroidism in patients with chronic renal failure by total parathyroidectomy and parathyroid autograft. Ann Surg 1981;193:777-791.

76. Reid DJ: Surgical treatment of secondary and tertiary hyperparathyroidism. Br J Clin Pract 1989;43:68-70.

77. Leapman SB, Filo RS, Thomalla JV, et al: Secondary hyperparathyroidism: The role of surgery. Am Surg 1989;55:359-365.

78. Gladziwa U, Ittel TH, Dakshinamurty KV, et al: Secondary hyperparathyroidism and sonographic evaluation of parathyroid gland hyperplasia in dialysis patients. Clin Nephrol 1992:38;162-166.

79. Takebayashi S, Matsui K, Onohara Y, et al: Sonography for early diagnosis of enlarged parathyroid glands in patients with secondary hyperparathyroidism. AJR 1987;148:911-914.

Pitfalls in Interpretation

80. Sutton RT, Reading CC, Charboneau JW, et al: US-guided biopsy of neck masses in postoperative management of patients with thyroid cancer. Radiology 1988;168:769-772.

81. Nabriski D, Bendahan J, Shapiro MS, et al: Sarcoidosis masquerading as a parathyroid adenoma. Head Neck 1992;14:384-386.

82. Ngo C, Sarti DA: Simulation of the normal esophagus by a parathyroid adenoma. J Clin Ultrasound 1987;15:421-424.

83. Karstrup S, Hegedus L: Concomitant thyroid disease in hyperparathyroidism: Reasons for unsatisfactory ultrasonographical localization of parathyroid glands. Eur J Radiol 1986;6:149-152.

84. Mazzeo S, Caramella D, Lencioni R, et al: Comparison among sonography double-tracer subtraction scintigraphy, and double-phase scintigraphy in the detection of parathyroid lesions. AJR 1996;166:1465-1470.

85. Funari M, Campos Z, Gooding GAW, et al: MRI and ultrasound detection of asymptomatic thyroid nodules in hyperparathyroidism. J Comput Assist Tomogr 1992;16:615-619.

86. Scheible W, Deutsch AL, Leopold GR: Parathyroid adenoma: Accuracy of preoperative localization by high-resolution real-time sonography. J Clin Ultrasound 1981;9:325-330.

87. Simeone JF, Mueller PR, Ferrucci JT, Jr, et al: High-resolution real-time sonography of the parathyroid. Radiology 1981;141:745-751.

88. Kobayashi S, Miyakawa M, Kasuga Y, et al: Parathyroid imaging comparison of 201 TI-99mTc subtraction scintigraphy, computed tomography, and ultrasonography. Jpn J Surg 1987;17:9-13.

89. Buchwach KA, Mangum WB, Hahn FW, Jr: Preoperative localization of parathyroid adenomas. Laryngoscope 1987;97:13-15.

90. Attie JN, Khan A, Rumancik WM, et al: Preoperative localization of parathyroid adenomas. Am J Surg 1988;156:323-326.

91. Erdman WA, Breslau NA, Weinreb JC, et al: Noninvasive localization of parathyroid adenomas: A comparison of x-ray, computed tomography, ultrasound, scintigraphy and magnetic resonance imaging. J Magn Reson Imaging 1989;7:187-194.

92. Summers GW, Dodge DL, Kammer H: Accuracy and cost-effectiveness of preoperative isotope and ultrasound imaging in primary hyperparathyroidism. Otolaryngol Head Neck Surg 1989;100:210-217.

93. Kohri K, Ishikawa Y, Kodama M, et al: Comparison of imaging methods for localization of parathyroid tumors. Am J Surg 1992;164:140-145.

94. Gooding GA: Sonography of the thyroid and parathyroid. Radiol Clin North Am 1993;31:967-989.

95. Weinberger MS, Robbins KT: Diagnostic localization studies for primary hyperparathyroidism: A suggested algorithm. Arch Otolaryngol Head Neck Surg 1994;120:1187-1189.

96. Chapuis Y, Fulla Y, Bonnichon P, et al: Values of ultrasonography, sestamibi scintigraphy and intraoperative measurement of 1-84 PTH for unilateral neck exploration

of primary hyperparathyroidism. World J Surg 1996;20:835-840.

97. Koslin DB, Adams J, Andersen P, et al: Preoperative evaluation of patients with primary hyperparathyroidism: Role of high-resolution ultrasound. Laryngoscope 1997;107:1249-1253.

98. Gofrit ON, Lebensart PD, Pikarsky A, et al: High-resolution ultrasonography: Highly sensitive, specific technique for preoperative localization of parathyroid adenoma in the absence of multinodular thyroid disease. World J Surg 1997;21:287-291.

99. Preventza OA, Yang S, Karo JJ, et al: Pre-operative ultrasonography guiding minimal, selective surgical approach in primary hyperparathyroidism. Int Surgery 2000;85:99-104.

100. Shawker TH, Avila NA, Premkumar A, et al: Ultrasound evaluation of primary hyperparathyroidism. Ultrasound Quart 2000;16:73-87.

101. De Feo ML, Colagrande S, Biagini C, et al: Parathyroid glands: Combination of 99mTc MIBI scintigraphy and US for demonstration of parathyroid glands and nodules. Radiology 2000;214:393-402.

102. Gritzmann N, Koischwitz D, Rettenbacher T: Sonography of the thyroid and parathyroid glands. Radiol Clin North Am 2000;38(5):1131-1145.

103. James C, Starks M, MacGillivray DC, et al: The use of imaging studies in the diagnosis and management of thyroid cancer and hyperparathyroidism. Surg Oncol Clin North Am 1999;8(1):145-169.

104. Gotway MB, Leung JW, Gooding GA, et al: Hyperfunctioning parathyroid tissue: Spectrum of appearances on noninvasive imaging. AJR 2002; 179:495-502.

105. Bergenfelz A, Forsberg L, Hederstrom E, et al: Preoperative localization of enlarged parathyroid glands with ultrasonically guided fine needle aspiration for parathyroid hormone assay. Acta Radiol 1991; 32:403-405.

106. Sacks BA, Pallotta JA, Cole A, et al: Diagnosis of parathyroid adenomas: Efficacy of measuring parathormone levels in needle aspirates of cervical masses. AJR 1994;163:1223-1226.

107. MacFarlane MP, Fraker DL, Shawker TH, et al: Use of preoperative fine-needle aspiration in patients undergoing re-operation for primary hyperparathyroidism. Surgery 1994;116:959-965.

108. Sardi A, Bolton JS, Mitchell WT, et al: Immunoperoxidase confirmation of ultrasonically guided fine needle aspirates in patients with recurrent hyperparathyroidism. Surg Gynecol Obstet 1992;175:563-568.

109. Marcocci C, Mazzeo S, Bruno-Bossio G, et al: Preoperative localization of suspicious parathyroid adenomas by assay of parathyroid hormone in needle aspirates. Eur J Endocrinol 1998;139:72-77.

110. Levin KE, Gooding GAW, Okerlund M, et al: Localizing studies in patients with persistent or recurrent hyperparathyroidism. Surgery 1988;102:917-924.

111. Miller DL, Doppman JL, Shawker TH, et al: Localization of parathyroid adenomas in patients who have undergone surgery. PI. Noninvasive imaging methods. Radiology 1987;162:133-137.

112. Reading CC, Charboneau JW, James EM, et al: Postoperative parathyroid high-frequency sonography: Evaluation of persistent or recurrent hyperparathyroidism. AJR 1985;144:399-402.

113. Grant CS, Van Heerden JA, Charboneau JW, et al: Clinical management of persistent and/or recurrent

primary hyperparathyroidism. World J Surg 1986;10:555-565.

114. Kairaluoma MV, Kellosalo J, Makarainen H, et al: Parathyroid re-exploration in patients with primary hyperparathyroidism. Ann Chir Gynaecol 1994;83:202-206.

115. Pearl AJ, Chapnik JS, Freeman JL, et al: Pre-operative localization of 25 consecutive parathyroid adenomas: A prospective imaging/surgical correlative study. J Otolaryngol 1993;22:301-306.

Other Imaging Methods

116. Yao M, Jamieson C, Blend R: Magnetic resonance imaging in preoperative localization of diseased parathyroid glands: A comparison with isotope scanning and ultrasonography. Can J Surg 1993;36:241-244.

117. Stevens SK, Chang J, Clark OH, et al: Detection of abnormal parathyroid glands in postoperative patients with recurrent hyperparathyroidism: Sensitivity of MR imaging. AJR 1993;160:607-612.

118. Kang YS, Rosen K, Clark OH, et al: Localization of abnormal parathyroid glands of the mediastinum with MR imaging. Radiology 1993;189:137-141.

119. Wright AR, Goddard PR, Nicholson S, et al: Fat-suppression magnetic resonance imaging in the preoperative localization of parathyroid adenomas. Clin Radiol 1992;46:324-328.

120. Lee VS, Wilkinson RH, Leight GS, et al: Hyperparathyroidism in high-risk surgical patients: Evaluation with double-phase technetium-99m sestamibi imaging. Radiology 1995;195:624-633.

121. Billy HT, Rimkus DR, Hartzman S, et al: Technetium-99m sestamibi single agent localization versus high-resolution ultrasonography for the preoperative localization of parathyroid glands in patients with hyperparathyroidism. Am Surg 1995;61:882-888.

122. Schurrer ME, Seabold JE, Gurll NJ, et al: Sestamibi SPECT scintigraphy for detection of postoperative hyperfunctioning parathyroid gland. AJR 1996;166:1471-1474.

123. Burke GJ, Wei JP, Binet EF: Parathyroid scintigraphy with iodine-123 and 99mTc-sestamibi: imaging findings. AJR 1993;161:1265-1268.

124. Thompson GB, Mullan BP, Grant CS, et al: Parathyroid imaging with technetium-99m sestamibi: An initial institutional experience. Surgery 1994;116:966-973.

125. Oates E: Improved parathyroid scintigraphy with Tc-99m MIBI, a superior radiotracer. Appl Radiol March 1994:37-40.

126. Gordon BM, Gordon L, Hoang K, et al: Parathyroid imaging with 99mTc sestamibi. AJR 1996;167:1563-1568.

127. Lumachi F, Marzola MC, Angelini F, et al: Advantages of combined technetium-99m sestamibi scintigraphy and high-resolution ultrasonography in parathyroid localization: comparative study in 91 patients with primary hyperparathyroidism. European J Endocrinol 2000;143:755-760.

128. Lumachi F, Ermani M, Zucchetta P, et al: Localization of parathyroid tumours in the minimally invasive era: Which technique should be chosen? Population-based analysis of 253 patients undergoing parathyroidectomy and factors affecting parathyroid gland detection. Endocrine-Related Cancer 2001;8:63-69.

129. Sommer B, Welter HF, Spelsberg F, et al: Computed tomography for localizing enlarged parathyroid glands in primary hyperparathyroidism. J Comput Assist Tomogr 1982;6:521-526.

130. Stark DD, Gooding GAW, Moss AA, et al: Parathyroid imaging: Comparison of high-resolution computed tomography and high-resolution sonography. AJR 1983;141:633-638.

131. Okerlund MD, Sheldon K, Corpuz S, et al: A new method with high sensitivity and specificity for localization of abnormal parathyroid glands. Ann Surg 1984;200:381-387.

132. Ferlin G, Borsato N, Camerani M, et al: New perspectives in localizing enlarged parathyroids by technetium-thallium subtraction scan. J Nucl Med 1983;24:438-441.

133. Krudy AG, Doppman JL, Miller DL, et al: Work in progress: Abnormal parathyroid glands: Comparison of nonselective arterial digital arteriography, selective parathyroid angiography, and venous digital arteriography as methods of detection. Radiology 1983;148:23-29.

134. Krudy AG, Doppman JL, Miller DL, et al: Detection of mediastinal parathyroid glands by nonselective digital arteriography. AJR 1984;142:693-695.

135. Henry J, Audiffret J, Denizot A, et al: Endosonography in the localization of parathyroid tumors: A preliminary study. Surgery 1990;108:1021-1025.

136. Hellman P, Ahlstrom H, Bergstrom M, et al: Positron emission tomography with ^{11}C-methionine in hyperparathyroidism. Surgery 1994;116:974-981.

137. Sundin A, Johansson C, Hellman P, et al: PET and parathyroid L-[carbon-11] methionine accumulation in hyperparathyroidism. J Nucl Med 1996;37:1766-1770.

138. Krausz Y, Lebensart PD, Klein M, et al: Preoperative localization of parathyroid adenoma in patients with concomitant thyroid nodular disease. World J Surg 2000;24:1573-1578.

Discussion: To Image or Not to Image in Primary Hyperparathyroidism

139. Wei JP, Burke GJ, Mansberger AR: Preoperative imaging of abnormal parathyroid glands in patients with hyperparathyroid disease using combination Tc-99m-pertechnetate and Tc-99m-sestamibi radionuclide scans. Ann Surg 1994;219:568-573.

140. Roe SM, Burns RP, Graham LD, et al: Cost-effectiveness of preoperative localization studies in primary hyperparathyroid disease. Ann Surg 1994;219:582-586.

141. Shaha AR, La Rosa CA, Jaffe BM: Parathyroid localization prior to primary exploration. Am J Surg 1993;166:289-293.

142. Miccoli P, Pinchera A, Cecchini G, et al: Minimally invasive, video-assisted parathyroid surgery for primary hyperparathyroidism. J Endocrinol Investig 1997;20:429-430.

143. Miccoli P, Bendinelli C, Vignali E, et al: Endoscopic parathyroidectomy: Report of an initial experience. Surgery 1998;124:1077-1080.

144. Vogel LM, Lucas R, Czako P: Unilateral parathyroid exploration. Am Surg 1998;64:693-696.

145. Dralle H, Lorenz K, Nguyen-Thanh P: Minimally invasive video-assisted parathyroidectomy—selective approach to localized single gland adenoma. Langenbeck's Arch Surg 1999;384:556-562.

146. Lorenz K, Nguyen-Thanh P, Dralle H: Unilateral open and minimally-invasive procedures for primary hyperparathyroidism: A review of selective approaches. Langenbeck's Arch Surg 2000;385:106-117.

147. Hallfeldt KK, Trupka A, Gallwas J, et al: Minimally invasive video-assisted parathyroidectomy: Early experience using an anterior approach. Surg Endosc 2001;15:409-412.

148. Van Dalen A, Smit CP, Van Vroonhoven TJ, et al: Minimally invasive surgery for solitary parathyroid adenomas in patients with primary hyperparathyroidism: Role of US with supplemental CT. Radiology 2001;220:631-639.

149. Arkles LB, Jones T, Hicks RJ, et al: Impact of complementary parathyroid scintigraphy and ultrasonography on the surgical management of hyperparathyroidism. Surgery 1996;120:845-851.

150. Purcell GP, Dirbas FM, Jeffrey RB, et al: Parathyroid localization with high-resolution ultrasound and technetium Tc99m sestamibi. Arch Surg 1999;134:824-828.

151. Wu DTD, Shaw JHF: The use of pre-operative scan prior to neck exploration for primary hyperparathyroidism. Aust NZ J Surg 1988;58:35-38.

152. Brewer WH, Walsh JW, Newsome HH, Jr: Impact of sonography on surgery for primary hyperparathyroidism. Am J Surg 1983;145:270-272.

153. Russell CFJ, Laird JD, Ferguson WR: Scan-directed unilateral cervical exploration for parathyroid adenoma: A legitimate approach? World J Surg 1990;14:406-409.

154. Windeck R, Olbricht TH, Littmann K, et al: Halessonographie in der hypercalamischen Krise. Dtsch Med Wochenschr 1985;110:368-370.

155. Wang CA: Parathyroid re-exploration: A clinical and pathological study of 112 cases. Ann Surg 1977;186:140-145.

Intraoperative Sonography

156. Kern KA, Shawker TH, Doppman JL, et al: The use of high-resolution ultrasound to locate parathyroid tumors during re-operations for primary hyperparathyroidism. World J Surg 1987;11:579-585.

157. Norton JA, Shawker TH, Jones BL, et al: Intraoperative ultrasound and reoperative parathyroid surgery: An initial evaluation. World J Surg 1986;10:631-638.

Percutaneous Biopsy

158. Gooding GAW, Clark OH, Stark DD, et al: Parathyroid aspiration biopsy under ultrasound guidance in the postoperative hyperparathyroid patient. Radiology 1985;155:193-196.

159. Solbiati L, Montali G, Croce F, et al: Parathyroid tumors detected by fine-needle aspiration biopsy under ultrasonic guidance. Radiology 1983;148:793-797.

160. Charboneau JW, Grant CS, James EM, et al: High-resolution ultrasound-guided percutaneous needle biopsy and intraoperative ultrasonography of a cervical parathyroid adenoma in a patient with persistent hyperparathyroidism. Mayo Clin Proc 1983;58:497-500.

161. Glenthoj A, Karstrup S: Parathyroid identification by ultrasonically guided aspiration cytology. Is correct cytological identification possible? APMIS 1989;97:497-502.

162. Karstrup S, Glenthoj A, Hainau B, et al: Ultrasound-guided, histological, fine-needle biopsy from suspect parathyroid tumors: Success-rate and reliability of histological diagnosis. Br J Radiol 1989;62:981-985.

163. Doppman JL, Krudy AG, Marx SJ, et al: Aspiration of enlarged parathyroid glands for parathyroid hormone assay. Radiology 1983;148:31-35.

164. Winkler B, Gooding GAW, Montgomery CK, et al: Immunoperoxidase confirmation of parathyroid origin of ultrasound-guided fine needle aspirates of the parathyroid glands. Acta Cytologica 1987;31:40-44.

165. Harman CR, Grant CS, Hay ID, et al: Indications, technique, and efficacy of alcohol injection of enlarged parathyroid glands in patients with primary hyperparathyroidism. Surgery 1998;124:1011-1020.

166. Cercueil JP, Jacob D, Verges B, et al: Percutaneous ethanol injection into parathyroid adenomas: Mid- and long-term results. Eur Radiol 1998;8:1565-1569.

167. Kendrick ML, Charboneau JW, Curlee KJ, et al: Risk of parathymosis after fine-needle aspiration. Am Surg 2001;67:290-294.

Alcohol Ablation

168. Charboneau JW, Hay ID, Van Heerden JA: Persistent primary hyperparathyroidism: Successful ultrasound-guided percutaneous ethanol ablation of an occult adenoma. Mayo Clin Proc 1988;63:913-917.

169. Karstrup S, Holm HH, Glenthoj A, et al: Nonsurgical treatment of primary hyperparathyroidism with sonographically guided percutaneous injection of ethanol: Results in a selected series of patients. AJR 1990;154:1087-1090.

170. Karstrup S, Transbol I, Holm HH, et al: Ultrasound-guided chemical parathyroidectomy in patients with primary hyperparathyroidism: A prospective study. Br J Radiol 1989;62:1037-1042.

171. Solbiati L, Giangrande A, DePra L, et al: Percutaneous ethanol injection of parathyroid tumors under ultrasound guidance: Treatment for secondary hyperparathyroidism. Radiology 1985;155:607-610.

172. Verges BL, Cercueil JP, Jacob D, et al: Results of ultrasonically guided percutaneous ethanol injection into parathyroid adenomas in primary hyperparathyroidism. Acta Endocrinol 1993;129:381-387.

173. Karstrup S, Hegedus L, Holm HH: Acute change in parathyroid function in primary hyperparathyroidism following ultrasonically guided ethanol injection into solitary parathyroid adenomas. ACTA Endocrinol 1993;129:377-380.

174. Karstrup S: Ultrasonically guided localization, tissue verification, and percutaneous treatment of parathyroid tumors. Dan Med Bull 1995;42:175-191.

175. Reading CC: Ultrasound-guided percutaneous ethanol ablation of solid and cystic masses of the liver, kidney, thyroid, and parathyroid. Ultrasound Q 1994;12:67-68.

176. Karstrup S, Hegedus L, Holm HH: Ultrasonically guided chemical parathyroidectomy in patients with primary hyperparathyroidism: A follow-up study. Clin Endocrinol 1993;38:523-530.

177. Bennedbaek FN, Karstrup S, Hegedus L: Percutaneous ethanol injection therapy in the treatment of thyroid and parathyroid lesions. Eur J Endocrinol 1997;136:240-250.

178. Kakuta T, Fukagawa M, Fujisaki T, et al: Prognosis of parathyroid function after successful percutaneous ethanol injection therapy guided by color Doppler flow mapping in chronic dialysis patients. Am J Kidney Dis 1999;33:1091-1099.

179. Karstrup S, Lohela P, Apaja-Sarkkinen M, et al: Non-operative hypercalcemic crisis. Acta Med Scand 1988;224:187-188.

180. Takeda S, Michigishi T, Takazakura E: Ultrasonically guided percutaneous ethanol injection to parathyroid autografts for recurrent hyperparathyroidism. Nephron 1993;65:651-652.

181. Takeda S, Michigishi T, Takazakura E: Successful ultrasonically guided percutaneous ethanol injection for secondary hyperparathyroidism. Nephron 1992;62:100-103.

182. Kitaoka M, Fukagawa M, Ogata E, et al: Reduction of functioning parathyroid cell mass by ethanol injection in chronic dialysis patients. Kidney Int 1994;46:1110-1117.

183. Giangrande A, Castiglioni A, Solbiati L, et al: Ultrasound-guided percutaneous fine-needle ethanol injection into parathyroid glands in secondary hyperparathyroidism. Nephrol Dial Transplant 1992;7:412-421.

184. Cintin C, Karstrup S, Ladefoged S, et al: Tertiary hyperparathyroidism treated by ultrasonically guided percutaneous fine-needle ethanol injection. Nephron 1994;68:217-220.

185. Fletcher S, Kanagasundarem NS, Rayner HC, et al: Assessment of ultrasound guided percutaneous ethanol injection and parathyroidectomy in patients with tertiary hyperparathyroidism. Nephrol Dial Transplant 1998;13:3111-3117.

186. Bennedbaek FN, Karstrup S, Hegedus L: Ultrasound guided laser ablation of a parathyroid adenoma. Brit J Radiol 2001;74:905-907.

THE BREAST

A. Thomas Stavros

Chapter Outline

There are three roles for sonography in breast imaging: (1) primary screening; (2) secondary screening (following mammography); and (3) diagnosis. Sonography currently does not have a proven role in primary breast cancer screening, but the role of sonography in secondary screening (after mammography) is still being actively investigated. Kolb et al. (two studies), Buchberger et al., and Kaplan have all recently shown very promising results for sonography as a secondary breast cancer screening examination when used after primary screening mammography in patients who have dense breasts on mammography. In all four studies, sonography detected approximately three carcinomas that were missed by primary screening mammography per 1000 patients. The lesions were missed on mammography because they did not contain calcifications and were obscured by surrounding or superimposed dense tissues on the mammogram. Three per thousand patients is the mammographic detection rate expected for interval cancers in previously screened mammography patients and suggests that sonography might be very useful as a secondary screening role in patients who have dense breasts on mammograph. Additionally, the maximum diameters and prognoses of lesions detected only by ultrasound are similar to lesions found by mammographic screening and the cost per cancer detected is similar to the cost per cancer detected on a mammogram.

It seems likely that the value of **secondary screening ultrasound** will eventually be proved in prospective randomized multicenter trials. There are problems with secondary screening sonography other than reimbursement, particularly because sonography is operator dependent. The proven and approved role for breast ultrasound is diagnosis. This is usually performed in a targeted fashion following mammography and clinical examination alone to provide a more specific diagnosis. Specific goals of targeted diagnostic sonography are to prevent biopsies and short interval follow-up mammography of benign lesions, to guide interventions of all types, to give feedback that improves clinical and mammographic skills, and to find malignancies that are missed by mammography.

EQUIPMENT

Breast ultrasound requires high frequency transducers that are optimized for near-field imaging. Transducers used for breast sonography are usually electronically

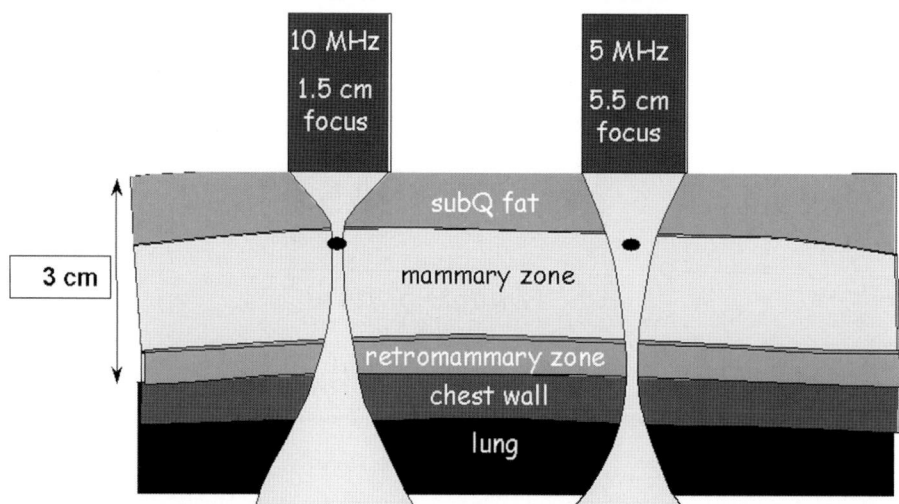

FIGURE 23-1. Short axis (elevation axis) of typical 10-MHz and 5-MHz transducers. Conventional transducers cannot be electronically focused in the short axis and include a fixed acoustic lens. When scanned in recumbent positions with the ipsilateral hand behind the head and with use of compression, the thickness of the breast in most patients is less than 3 cm. The optimal short axis focal length of the 5-MHz transducer lies within the chest wall behind the breast tissue where most lesions occur. A small lesion that lies at a depth of 1.5 cm will be subject to volume averaging with surrounding tissues when scanned with a 5-MHz transducer, causing cysts to appear solid and some solid lesions to be isoechoic with surrounding tissues, and therefore, undetectable. Most 10- to 12-MHz transducers have short axis acoustic lenses that are focused at depths between 1.5 and 2.0 cm, ideal for breast ultrasound. The same small lesion will be larger than the 10 MHz beam width, and therefore, not subject to volume averaging.

focused linear arrays. All of the organizations involved in accreditation of breast sonography (American Cancer Society (ACS), American College of Radiology (ACR), and American Institute of Ultrasound in Medicine (AIUM)) require a minimum transducer frequency of 7 MHz. These linear arrays can be electronically focused along the long axis of the transducer, but not along the short axis (unless they are of 1.5 dimensional array). Focusing in the short axis requires that a fixed acoustic lens be placed when the transducer is constructed. The focal length of the short axis lens varies with transducer frequency and the application for which the transducer will typically be used, being deeper for lower frequencies and shallower for higher frequencies. Transducers of 5 MHz typically are used for peripheral vascular ultrasound, not near-field imaging, and are focused too deeply (3.5 to 4.0 cm, usually within the chest wall) for breast ultrasound. When the focal length of the transducer is in the chest wall, small lesions in the middle and near portions of the breast may be subject to volume averaging. Volume averaging can alter the echogenicity so much that cystic lesions falsely appear solid and hypoechoic solid lesions become isoechoic and inconspicuous. The 7.5 to 12 MHz transducers that are usually employed in breast ultrasound are focused at 1.5 to 2.0 cm, an ideal focal length for breast ultrasound, minimizing volume averaging (Fig. 23-1). However, even transducers that are focused in the mid-breast in the short axis can result in volume averaging for very superficially located small lesions, unless a thin acoustic standoff pad or a standoff of gel is used (Fig. 23-2).

A good general rule for breast ultrasound is that lesions that appear to be just under the skin on the mammogram or that are palpable and pea-sized or smaller are those that are most prone to volume averaging and should routinely be imaged through an acoustic standoff. In some cases, simply scanning with lighter compression can alter the position of the short axis focal zone enough to obviate the need for a standoff. A 1.5-dimensional array transducer can be focused electronically in the short axis as well as in the long axis and can reduce, but not totally eliminate, difficulties with near-field volume averaging.

Split screen imaging capability is invaluable in breast imaging. Split screen images are most frequently used to compare mirror image locations in the right and left breasts to document that **asymmetrical fibroglandular tissue** causes either a mammographic asymmetry or a palpable lump (Fig. 23-3). Split-screen imaging can be used to document dynamic events, such as compressibility and mobility, on a single freeze frame image and in simultaneous mode to show both the gray-scale image on one side and the color or power Doppler image on the other.

Large lesions or multifocal or multicentric disease can require special techniques for demonstration. There are several different methods of demonstrating larger fields of view. One can utilize combined split screen images, virtual convex imaging, or extended field of view imaging (Fig. 23-4). Picture archiving and communication systems (PACS) can be useful not only for filmless interpretation and archiving images, but also for digitally

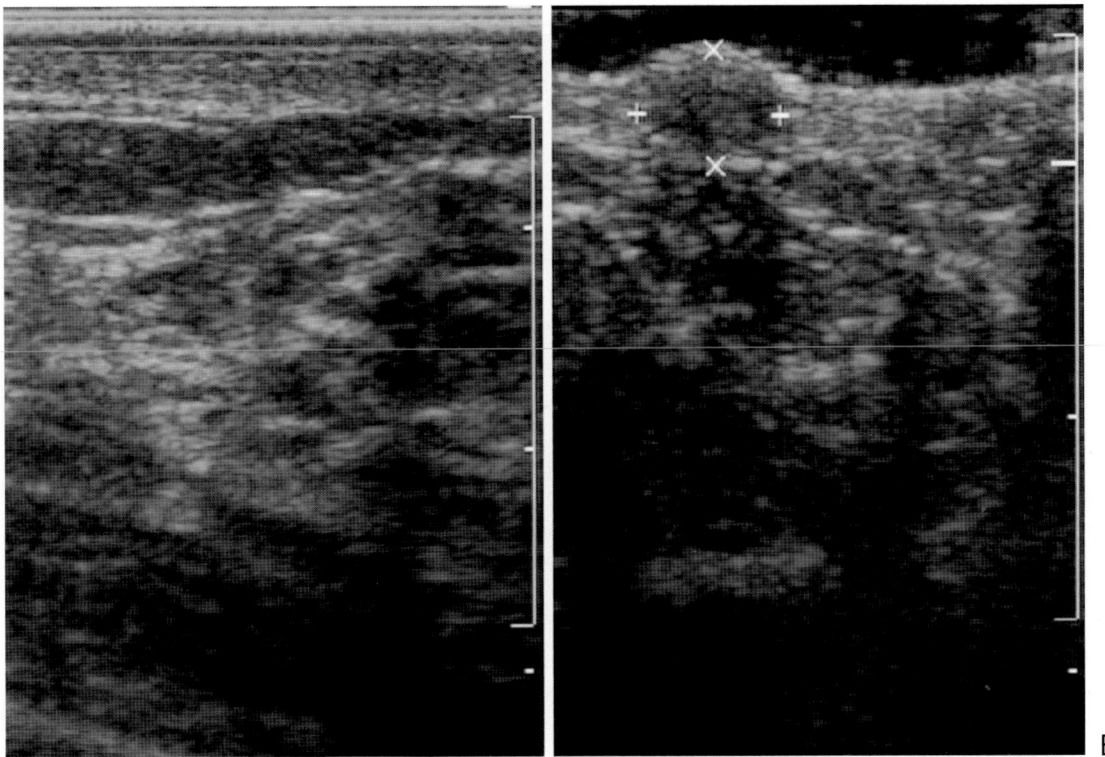

A   B

FIGURE. 23-2. Value of standoff pad. Even with adequate high frequency near-field imaging transducers that have appropriate short-axis acoustic lens focal lengths of 1.5 cm, in very superficial lesions, an acoustic standoff may be necessary. **A**, Sebaceous cyst presented as BB-sized palpable lump. It is not visible without an acoustic standoff. **B**, With a thick layer of acoustic gel as a standoff, the lesion can be clearly seen to originate from the skin.

storing video loops, the most efficient and esthetically pleasing method of documenting dynamic events.

ANATOMY

The breast is a modified sweat gland that is composed of 15 to 20 lobes that are not well delineated from each other, that overlap, and that vary greatly in size and distribution. Each lobe consists of parenchymal elements (lobar duct, smaller branch ducts, and lobules) and supporting stromal tissues (compact interlobular stromal fibrous tissue, loose periductal and intralobular stromal fibrous tissue, and fat). The functional unit of the breast is the **terminal ductolobular unit** (TDLU), which consists of a lobule and its extralobular terminal duct. Each lobule consists of the intralobular segment of the terminal duct, ductules, and intralobular stromal fibrous tissue. TDLUs are important because they are the site of origin of most breast pathology and of **aberrations of normal development and involution** (ANDI).

Most breast carcinomas are thought to arise in the terminal duct near the junction of the intralobular and extralobular segments. Lobar ducts give rise to much less pathology than do TDLUs—mainly large **duct papillomas** and the **duct ectasia/periductal mastitis**

complex. However, most **invasive ductal carcinomas** have ductal carcinoma in situ (DCIS) components that can use the lobar ducts as conduits for growth into other parts of the breast. Teboul has shown that each lobar duct has several rows of TDLUs arising from it. Anterior TDLUs tend to have long extralobular terminal ducts, whereas posterior TDLUs tend to have shorter extralobular terminal ducts. Some TDLUs lie at the distal end of the ductal system and are horizontally oriented. Anterior TDLUs are more numerous than posterior and terminal TDLUs, and over time, the posterior TDLUs tend to regress, leaving a progressively larger percentage of anterior TDLUs. Because anterior TDLUs greatly outnumber posterior TDLUs, most breast pathology that arises from TDLUs occurs in the superficial half of the mammary zone, just deep to the anterior mammary fascia.

The breast can be divided into three zones from superficial to deep—the premammary zone, the mammary zone, and the retromammary zone (Fig. 23-5). The most superficial zone is the **premammary** or **subcutaneous zone** that lies between the skin and the anterior mammary fascia. The premammary zone is really part of the integument, and processes that arise primarily within the premammary zone are usually not true breast lesions. Rather, they are lesions of the skin and/or subcutaneous

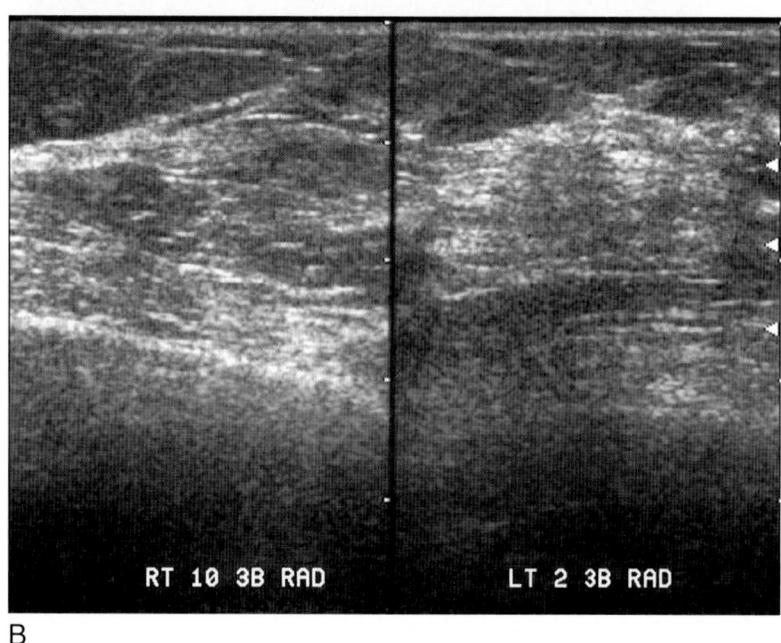

FIGURE 23-3. Value of split-screen mirror ultrasound image. A, Mammography of both breasts showed a nodule in the left breast, upper outer quadrant on the cranial caudal (CC) view (*arrow*). **B,** Split-screen mirror image ultrasounds show focal fibroglandular tissue in the upper outer quadrant of the left breast that is markedly asymmetrical with the thickness of tissue in the mirror image upper outer quadrant location of the right breast causing a focal, palpable, and mammographic abnormality.

tissues that are identical to those that arise from skin and subcutaneous tissues that cover any other part of the body. The **mammary zone** is the middle zone and lies between the anterior mammary fascia and the posterior mammary fascia. It contains the lobar ducts, their branches, most of the TDLUs, and most of the fibrous stromal elements of the breast. The deepest of the zones is the **retromammary zone**. It contains mainly fat, blood vessels, and lymphatics and is usually much less apparent on sonograms than on mammograms because sonographic compression compresses it against the chest wall. This differs greatly from mammography, where mammographic compression pulls the retromammary fat away from the chest wall and expands it in the anteroposterior (AP) direction. Because most breast pathology arises from TDLUs and, to a lesser extent, from the mammary ducts, and because most of the ducts and lobules lie within the mammary zone, most true breast pathology arises from the mammary zone. Although lesions that arise within the premammary or retromammary zone are usually not true breast lesions, true breast lesions that arise within the mammary zone can secondarily involve the premammary and retromammary tissues.

The **mammary fascia** that envelops the mammary zone is tough and is relatively more resistant to invasive

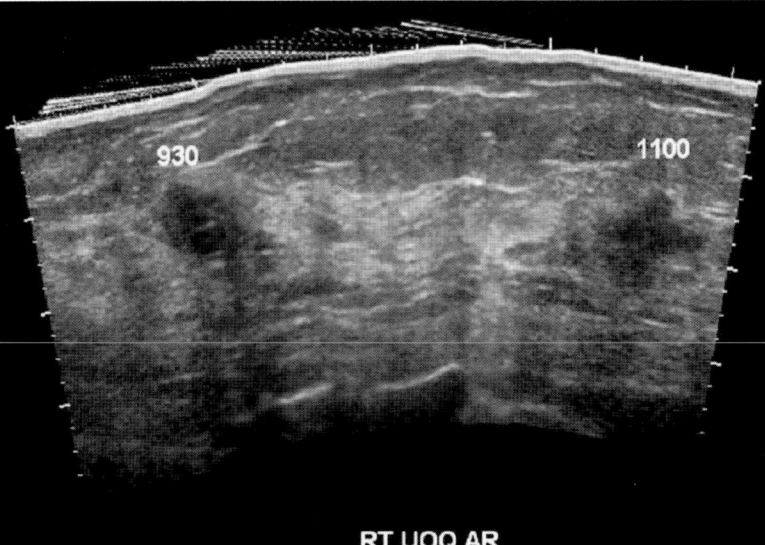

FIGURE 23-4. Extended field-of-view images. These images can be helpful in demonstrating very large lesions, multicentric disease, or—as in this case—multifocal malignant disease (located at 9:30 and 11:00 o'clock positions).

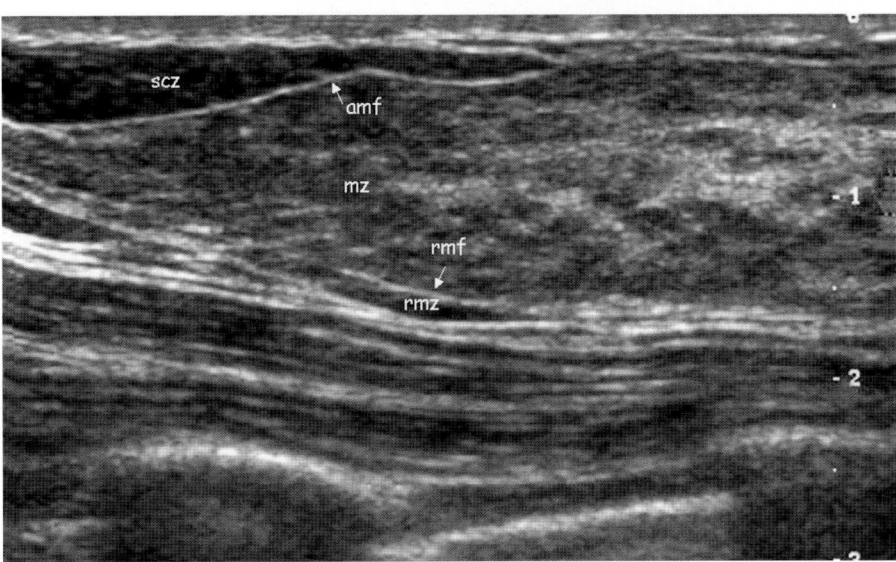

FIGURE 23-5. Three zones of the breast. The **premammary** or **subcutaneous zone** (scz), the **mammary zone** (mz), and the **retromammary zone** (rmz). The mammary zone is where most of the ducts and lobules of the breast that give rise to breast pathology lie. The retromammary zone is compressed during real-time sonography in the recumbent position and is relatively small and inapparent in comparison to its appearance on mammography. The mammary zone is enveloped in thick, tough fascia. Anteriorly it is delineated from the subcutaneous fat by the premammary or anterior mammary fascia (amf) and posteriorly from the retromammary fat by the posterior or retromammary fascia (rmf). The anterior mammary fascia is continuous with Cooper's ligaments, with each ligament being formed by two apposed layers of anterior mammary fascia.

malignancy than are loose stroma fibrous tissues. The anterior mammary fascia is continuous with Cooper's ligaments. At the points where it is continuous with a ligament, the anterior mammary fascia continues superficially obliquely through the subcutaneous fat, attaches to the skin, and then courses back down through the subcutaneous fat where it continues as anterior mammary fascia. Each **Cooper's ligament** is composed of two closely applied layers of anterior mammary fascia with a potential space inferiorly, where the two layers separate and course away from each other as anterior

mammary fascia. This affects the sonographic appearance of invasive malignancies and will be discussed in the section on sonographic assessment of solid breast nodules.

The normal anatomic structures of the breast span a spectrum of echogenicities from midlevel gray to intensely hyperechoic. Hyperechoic normal structures include compact interlobular stromal fibrous tissue, anterior and posterior mammary fascia, Cooper's ligaments, and skin. Duct walls, when visible, also appear hyperechoic. Normal structures that have midlevel echogenicity (isoechoic) include fat, epithelial tissues in ducts and lobules, and loose intralobular and periductal stromal fibrous tissue. Water density tissue on mammography corresponds to a variety of different normal tissues that can be shown sonographically. Dense interlobular stromal fibrous tissue, loose periductal or intralobular stromal fibrous tissue, and epithelial elements in ducts and lobules all appear to be of equal density mammographically. **Mammographically dense tissue** can correspond to purely hyperechoic, purely isoechoic, or mixed hyperechoic and isoechoic tissues

on sonography (Fig. 23-6). Most contain mixtures of fibrous and glandular elements interspersed with variable amounts of fat (Fig. 23-7). Over time, atrophy tends to occur more rapidly in the areas of the mammary zone that lie between Cooper's ligaments, leaving progressively more of the residual fibroglandular elements within Cooper's ligaments (Fig. 23-8).

Normal mammary ducts that are not ectatic can appear two different ways sonographically. A mammary duct can appear to be purely isoechoic when the centrally located hyperechoic duct wall cannot be

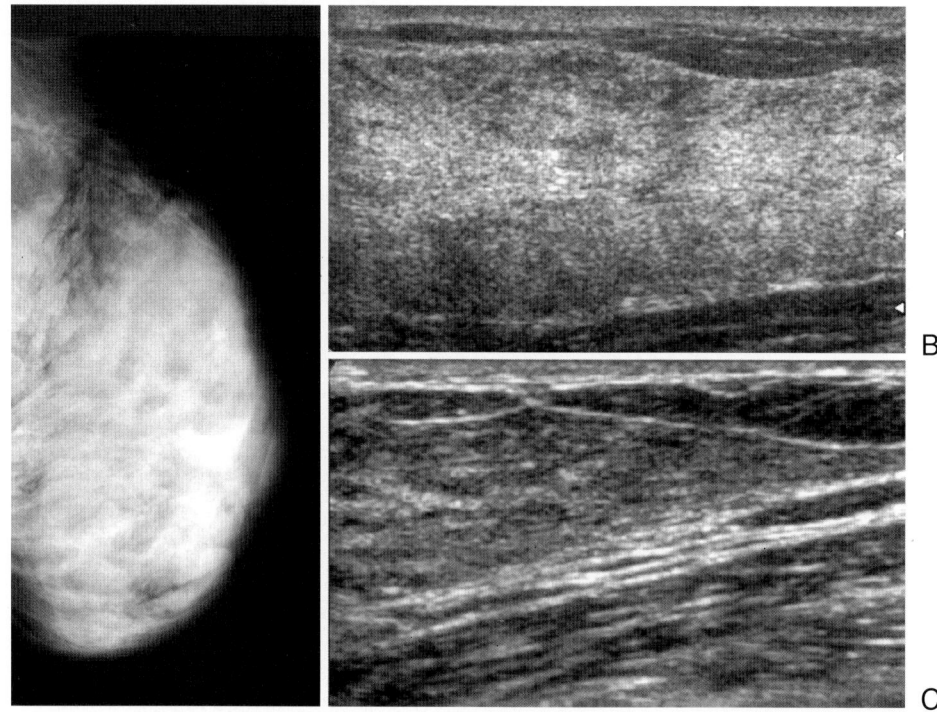

FIGURE 23-6. Radiographically dense tissue. Radiographically dense (water density) tissue on mammograms (**A**) can correspond to two different types of tissue on sonograph. **B**, Intensely hyperechoic interlobular stromal fibrous tissue and **C**, nearly isoechoic glandular tissue.

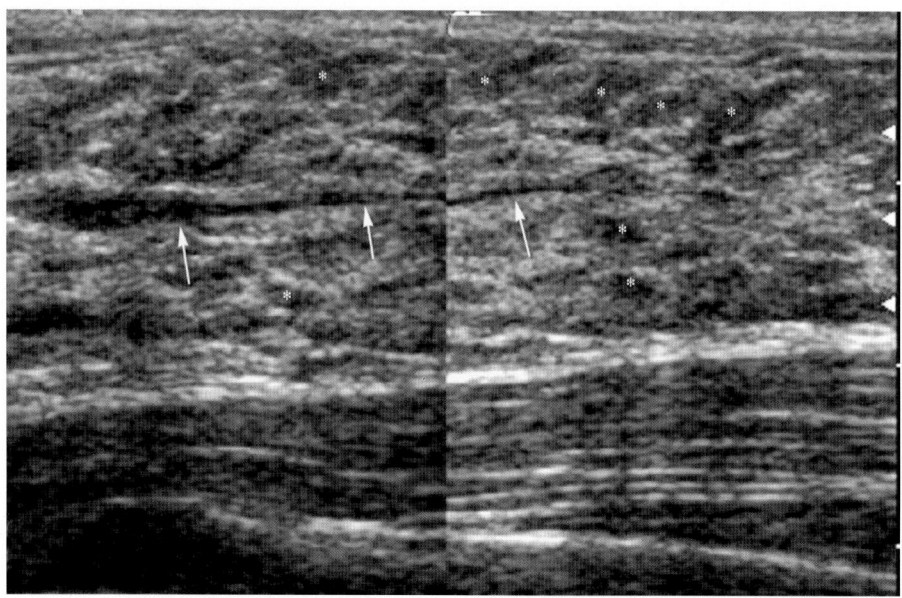

FIGURE 23-7. Water density tissue. Most water density tissue on mammography is not pure fibrous or glandular tissue, but a mixture of hyperechoic interlobular stromal fibrous tissue and isoechoic glandular or loose periductal and intralobular stromal tissue. Note that the lobar duct is mildly ectatic (*arrows*). The taller-than-wide isoechoic elements (*) within the superficial aspect of the mammary zone represent epithelial and loose stromal tissues within lobules. Note that they are more numerous and prominent anteriorly because terminal ductolobular units (TDLUs) are more numerous anteriorly than posteriorly.

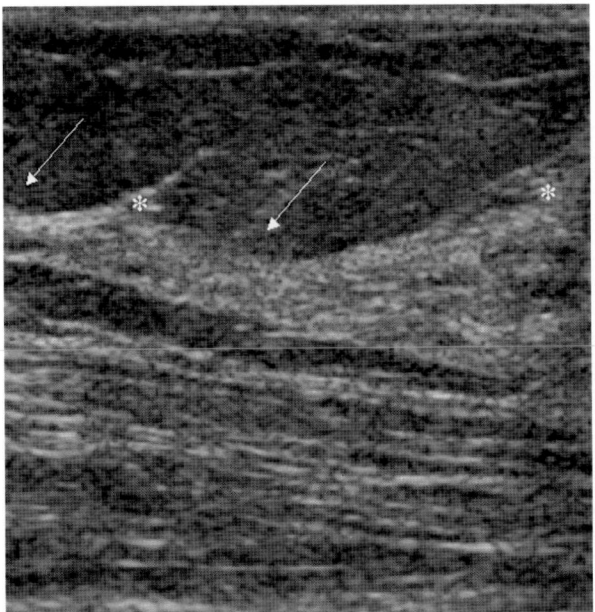

FIGURE 23-8. Breast atrophy. With advancing age, the fibroglandular elements of the breast regress more rapidly in the areas of the mammary zone (*arrows*) that lie between Cooper's ligaments than the area within the ligaments. This eventually can leave much or all of the residual breast tissue entrapped within Cooper's ligaments (*).

visualized because of poor angle of incidence and/or suboptimal transducer resolution—when only the loose periductal stromal fibrous tissue is visible. A mammary duct can also be shown as a central, bright echo surrounded by isoechoic loose stromal fibrous tissue when the apposed walls of the central duct can be optimally demonstrated (Fig. 23-9). It is common for a single duct

to have both sonographic appearances, depending on the angle of incidence with the duct walls. Variable degrees of **duct ectasia** are common and become increasingly common with age, particularly within the lactiferous sinus portion of the lobar duct in the subareolar region. In ectatic ducts, anechoic or hypoechoic fluid separates the two duct walls and compresses the loose periductal stromal tissues to variable degrees (Fig. 23-10). Duct ectasia is common, occurring in up to 50% of women over the age of 50 years, and usually is asymptomatic. However, in certain patients, duct ectasia can lead to periductal mastitis and its acute and chronic complications.

The ducts within the nipple and immediate subareolar regions are poorly seen when scanned from straight anteriorly because they course nearly parallel to the beam in those locations. However, special maneuvers designed to improve the angle of incidence enable us to adequately demonstrate the entire mammary duct throughout the subareolar region and even within the nipple when necessary. These maneuvers include the **peripheral compression technique**, **two-handed compression technique**, and **rolled nipple technique**. These maneuvers are most useful when evaluating patients with nipple discharge (Fig. 23-11) and in assessing malignant nodules for extensive intraductal involvement growing within the duct toward the nipple. The two-handed compression technique is also useful in assessing gynecomastia.

Individual TDLUs may be sonographically visible—under ideal conditions—as small isoechoic structures. Normal TDLUs are about 2 mm in diameter but may be as large as 5 mm in patients with **fibrocystic change**,

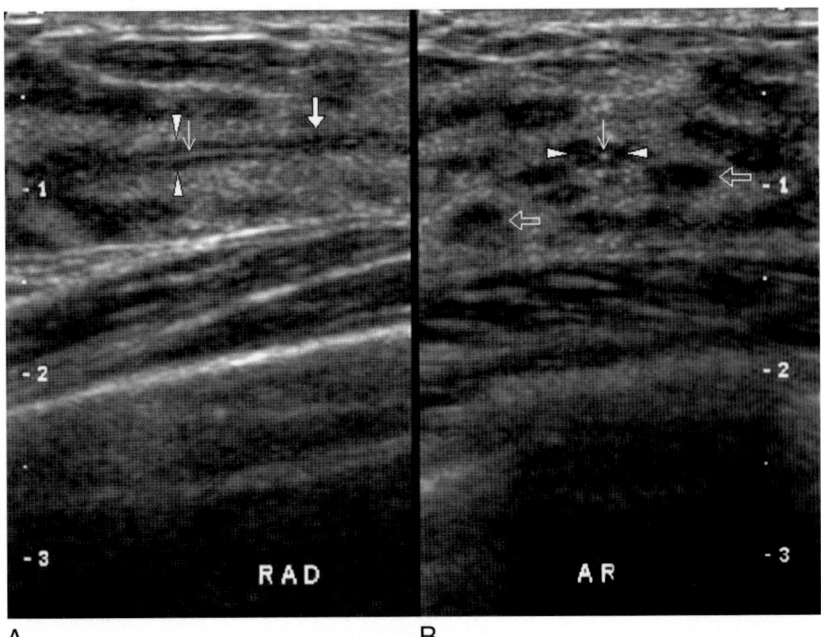

FIGURE 23-9. Normal, nonectatic mammary ducts have two sonographic appearances. A, With high spatial resolution, 90-degree angle of incidence, and perfect centering, the duct appears to be composed of a central echogenic line (*arrows*) which is the apposed walls of the collapsed mammary duct. The surrounding isoechoic tissue (*white arrowheads*) represents loose periductal stromal tissue. **B,** Only the isoechoic loose periductal stromal tissue can be demonstrated if spatial resolution is suboptimal, the scan plane is not perpendicular to the duct (*hollow white arrow*), or the beam is not well centered on the duct (*solid white arrow*).

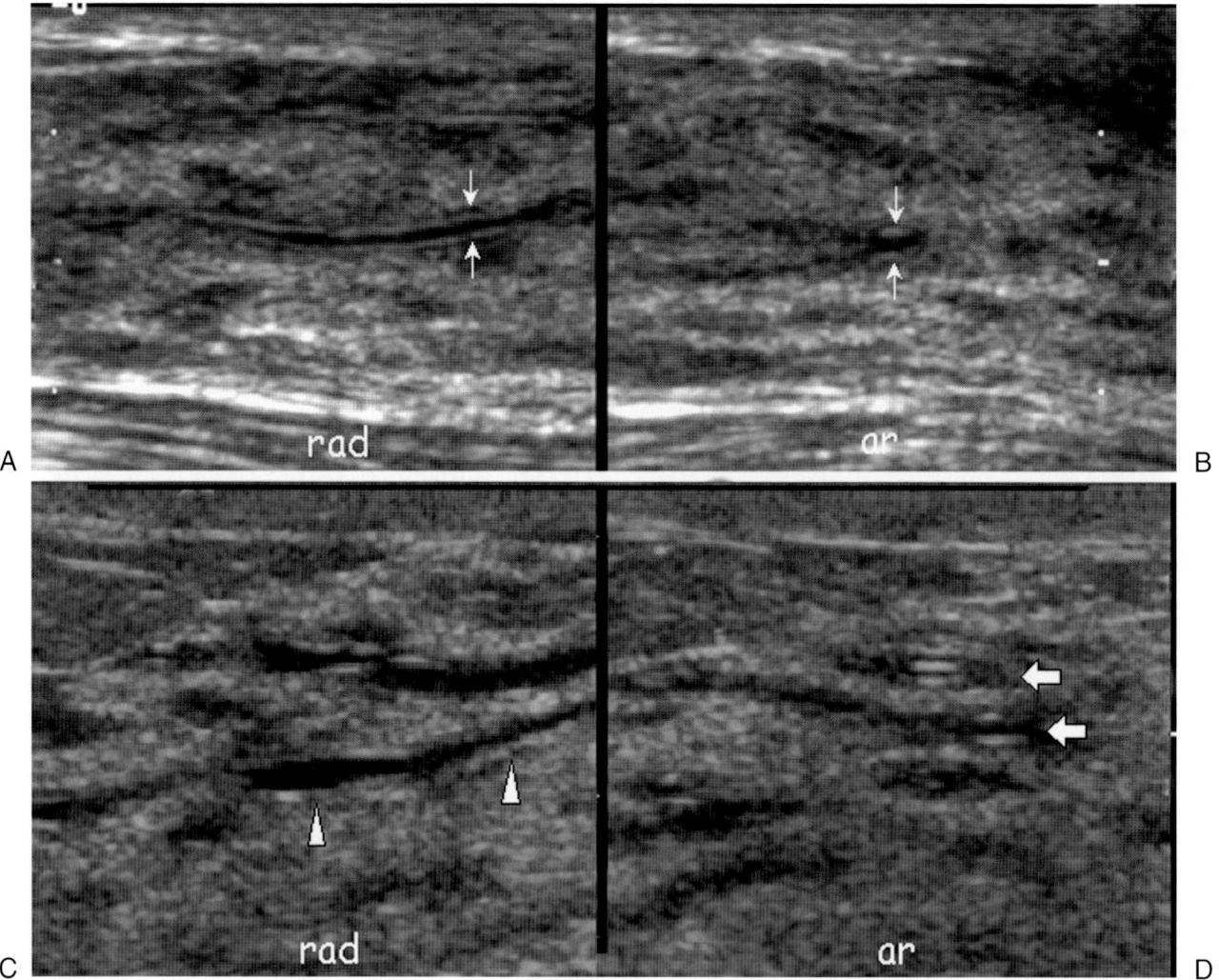

FIGURE 23-10. Duct ectasia. Echogenic duct walls are separated by secretions within the duct lumen and the isoechoic periductal loose stromal tissue becomes thinner, either by compression or because of atrophy. **A** and **B, Mild duct ectasia** in radial (rad) and antiradial (ar) views (*arrows*). **C** and **D, Moderate to severe duct ectasia**, with the degree of ectasia varying within an individual duct in the radial (rad) plane (*arrowheads*) and between ducts in the antiradial (ar) plane (*arrows*).

adenosis, or other ANDIs (Fig. 23-12). In patients who are pregnant or lactating and in patients with adenosis, not only are TDLUs enlarged, but they are also increased in number. In certain cases, TDLUs become large and numerous enough to form continuous sheets of iso-echoic tissue. The variable prominence of TDLUs creates a continuous spectrum in the appearance of breast tissue from TDLUs that are not sonographically visible in breasts that appear to be purely isoechoic (Fig. 23-13). This most commonly occurs anteriorly, where lobules are most numerous, but in certain cases can fill and distend the entire mammary zone. One of the most valuable features of high frequency coded **harmonic imaging** is that it tends to make pathologic solid nodules appear relatively more hypoechoic and conspicuous in a background of isoechoic tissues, reducing the chance that such a nodule will not be detected and distinguished from normal lobules.

Lymphatic drainage from most of the breast is from deep to superficial, toward the subdermal lymphatic network, then to the periareolar area, and finally on to the axilla. Some of the deep portions of the breast, particularly medially, preferentially drain along the chest wall to the internal mammary lymph nodes. Most of the drainage of the breast is to the axillary lymph nodes. Most lymphatic metastases from the breast are to the axilla with a minority occurring in the internal mammary lymph nodes. There are three levels of axillary lymph nodes that are determined by their location relative to the pectoralis minor muscle. Lymph nodes that lie peripheral to the inferolateral edge of the pectoralis muscle are **level 1 lymph nodes**; nodes that lie posterior to the pectoralis minor muscle are **level 2 nodes**; and nodes that lie proximal to the superomedial border of the pectoralis minor muscle are **level 3 lymph nodes** or **infraclavicular nodes**. Lymphatic drainage to

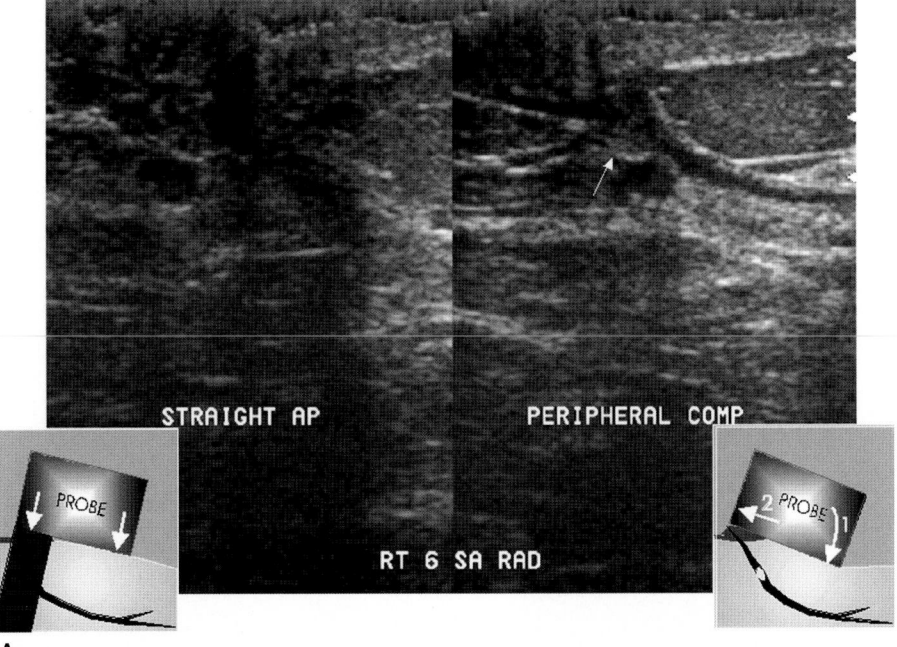

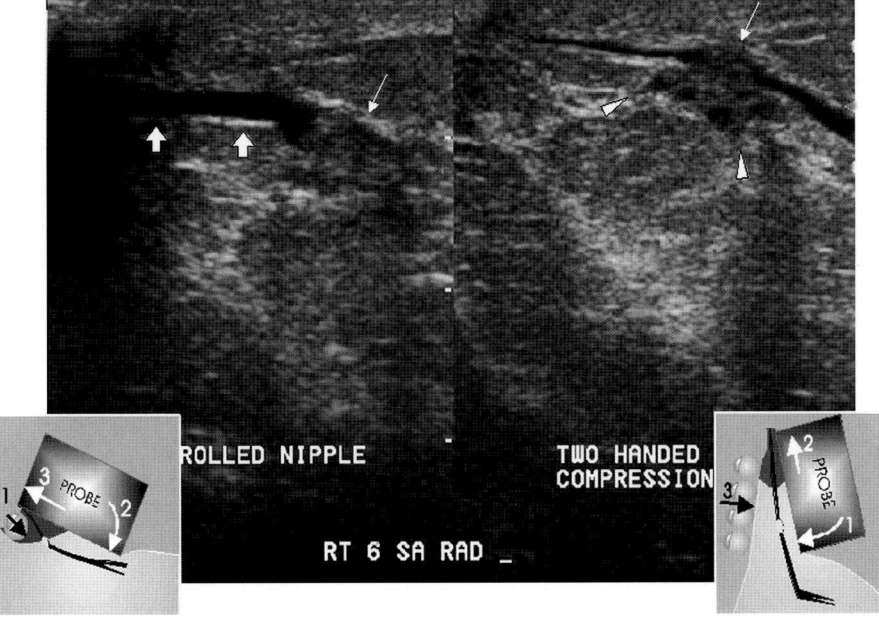

FIGURE 23-11. Importance of transducer position. A, Left image. The subareolar ducts are difficult to assess from a straight anterior approach because shadowing arises from the nipple and areola and the tissue planes of the nipple are parallel to the ultrasound beam. **A,** Right image. **Peripheral compression technique.** With vigorous compression on the peripheral end of the transducer and sliding it over the nipple to push the nipple to the side, shadowing can be minimized and the angle of incidence of the beam with the subareolar ducts can be improved. Lesions that lie in the immediate subareolar region (*arrow*) can often be demonstrated. **B, Right two-handed compression** technique further improves the angle of incidence with the subareolar ducts and helps assess the compressibility of the ducts. This can help to distinguish echogenic, inspissated secretions from intraductal papillary lesions and determine whether the lesion (*arrows*) has penetrated through the duct wall (*arrowheads*). This intraductal papillary lesion does not extend into the intranipple segment of duct (*thick white arrows*). **B,** Left image. **The rolled nipple technique** is the best way to demonstrate the ducts within the nipple, and if a lesion extends into the nipple from the subareolar ducts.

the axilla usually passes through level 1, then level 2, and finally, to level 3 lymph nodes.

Internal mammary nodes lie in a chain along the deep side of the chest wall just lateral to the edges of the sternum in parallel to the internal mammary artery and veins. Metastases most often involve internal mammary lymph nodes in the second and third interspaces. Using color Doppler to identify the internal mammary vessels can be helpful in finding abnormal internal mammary lymph nodes. Normal internal mammary lymph nodes can be identified under ideal circumstances, but not in all patients.

A significant minority of patients have lymph nodes within the breast or **intramammary lymph nodes.** These can lie anywhere within the breast, but are most common in the axillary segment just below the axilla. Intramammary lymph nodes are also relatively common in the most medial breast lying parallel to the internal mammary lymph nodes. They are actually seen quite commonly at sonography, but are seldom demonstrated mammographically because mammographic compression can seldom pull them far enough away from the chest wall for them to be visible. They are also difficult to demonstrate sonographically without the use of an

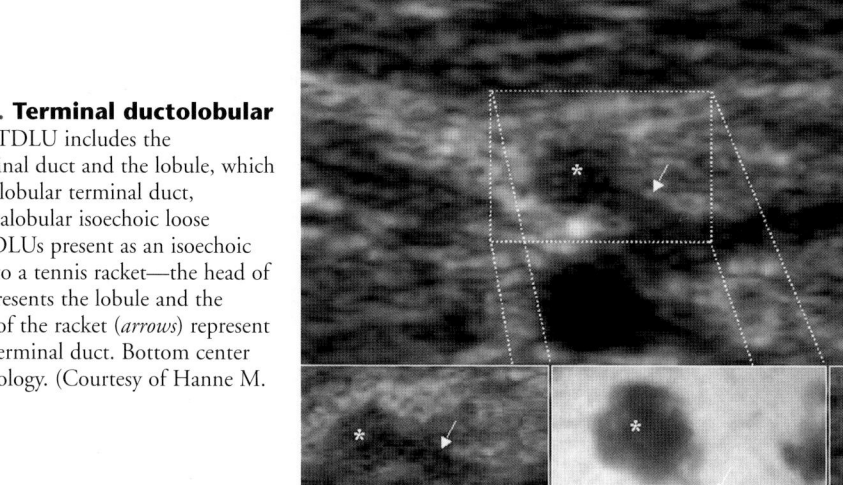

FIGURE 23-12. Terminal ductolobular unit (TDLU). TDLU includes the extralobular terminal duct and the lobule, which contains the intralobular terminal duct, ductules, and intralobular isoechoic loose stromal tissue. TDLUs present as an isoechoic structure similar to a tennis racket—the head of the racket (*) represents the lobule and the handle and neck of the racket (*arrows*) represent the extralobular terminal duct. Bottom center image is 3-D histology. (Courtesy of Hanne M. Jensen, M.D.)

acoustic standoff because of their superficial location just beneath the skin.

Breast cancer metastases can involve the **supraclavicular lymph nodes**, but such metastases are considered distant metastases for purposes of staging, because there is no direct drainage to the supraclavicular nodes. Breast cancer metastases to these nodes must first pass through levels 1, 2, and 3 axillary lymph nodes or through the internal mammary nodes before reaching the supraclavicular nodes.

The first lymph node to which lymphatic drainage flows and the first node involved by metastases has been termed the **sentinel lymph node**. The location of the sentinel node varies, depending on the location within the breast of the primary. The sentinel lymph node is usually a level 1 axillary lymph node, but in certain cases, it can be an intramammary node and can even bypass level 1 lymph nodes and go straight to a level 2 node. Occasionally, the sentinel node may lie within the internal mammary chain.

TECHNIQUE

Annotation

The organizations that accredit breast ultrasound require minimum standards for annotation of the location of a sonographic breast image. The side (left and right), clock face position, distance from the nipple, and transducer orientation must be recorded. We use 5 zones to record the distance from the nipple: SA for subareolar location, AX for axillary segment, and 1, 2, or 3 for equal width rings starting at the areolar margin and extending to the edge of the breast (with 1 being the central ring, 2 the middle ring, and 3 the outer ring). Alternatively, the distance from the nipple can be recorded in centimeters or by zones, and this method is becoming more popular because it is thought to be less subjective and less variable than the ring method. Painting centimeter markers on the transducer can facilitate recording the distance from the nipple in centimeters. The transducer orientation can be longitudinal, transverse, radial, or antiradial, which is orthogonal to the radial plane. The advantage of radial imaging is that the central ducts are radially oriented with respect to the nipple, and scanning in the plane that is parallel to the long axis of the duct has the best chance of showing ductal carcinoma in situ (DCIS) components that extend away from the tumor into surrounding ducts.

Identifying intraductal components of tumor can reduce the chances of errantly characterizing a solid nodule as benign or probably benign and also can help to better demonstrate the true extent of DCIS components of mixed invasive and intraductal malignant lesions. The farther from the nipple a lesion lies, the less likely it is that the duct will course in a plane that is truly radial with respect to the nipple because of tortuosity of the duct or because the duct of interest is a branch duct that is not oriented perfectly radially. The sonographer should think of internal radial planes versus the external true radial plane with respect to the nipple. The internal radial plane is parallel to the long axis of the ducts in the region of interest. In particular, when assessing solid nodules, we want to know if the lesion is growing into

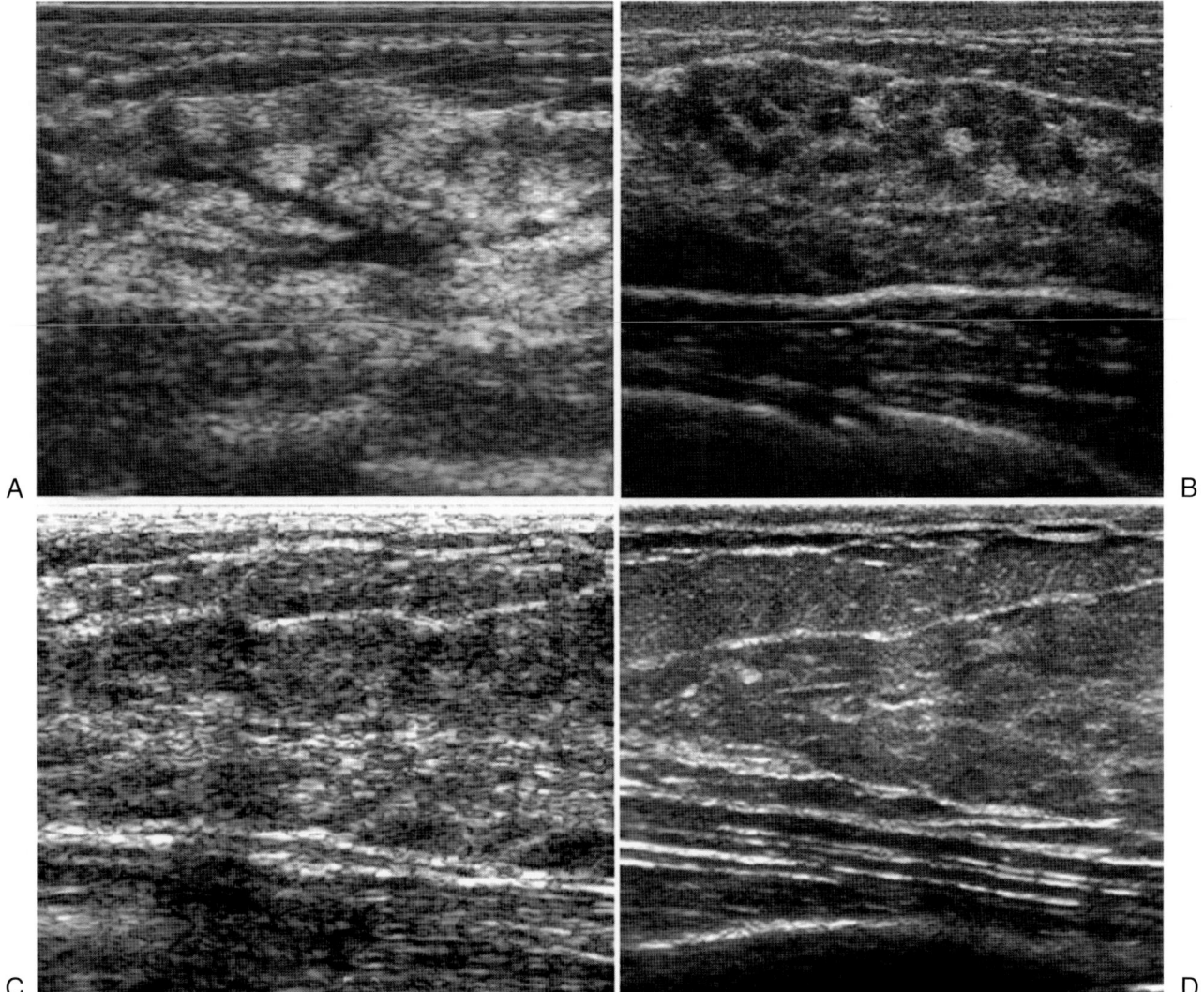

FIGURE 23-13. Prominence of TDLUs varies greatly. A, Only a few scattered TDLUs may be visible. **B,** As TDLUs become larger and more numerous in adenosis and adenosis of pregnancy, they may almost touch each other. Because anterior TDLUs are more numerous than posterior TDLUs, these changes tend to affect the superficial aspect of the mammary zone earlier and to a greater extent than they affect its deep aspect. **C,** When lobular enlargement is pronounced, the entire superficial aspect of the mammary zone may appear isoechoic with the deep half still being hyperechoic. **D,** When lobular prominence is most pronounced, both superficial and deep aspects of the mammary zone may appear nearly homogeneously isoechoic. Prominent TDLUs create an "in between" sensitivity state for sonography that lies between that of purely hyperechoic and purely isoechoic breasts.

the ducts that surround it. This can be best accomplished when the scan plane is parallel to the long axis of the ducts in the region of the solid nodule.

We elect to record the depth of a lesion in addition to the parameters discussed above, but the accrediting organizations do not require this. We use three zones: A for the superficial third, B for the middle third, and C for the deep third of the breast. Thus, a lesion at the 12:00 o'clock position of the right breast in the middle ring and middle third in depth, when scanned radially would be annotated as R 12 2B RAD. Alternatively, using the centimeters from the nipple method for a lesion 6 cm from the nipple, this would be annotated as 12:00, N + 6, B RAD. These methods of annotation are cryptic and reproducible. An icon of the right or left breast with a linear marker that demonstrates the position and orientation of the transducer is an acceptable alternative for annotation of scan location, and most ultrasound equipment manufacturers provide breast icons.

Documentation of Lesions

All lesions should be scanned in their entirety in two orthogonal planes to assess the surface and internal characteristics and shape. Hard copy images should be obtained in a minimum of two orthogonal planes. These could be longitudinal and transverse, but we prefer radial and antiradial planes. Each image plane should be recorded with and without calipers. It is important to document the maximum diameter of the lesion, an important prognostic indicator. If the maximum diameter does not lie in the longitudinal, transverse, radial, or antiradial planes, an additional oblique view parallel to the long axis of the lesion should be obtained with and without calipers. Films without calipers are especially important in small lesions where the calipers may interfere with assessment of surface characteristics.

BIRADS Nomenclature and Lexicon

An official breast imaging reporting and data system (BIRADS) ultrasound lexicon is being developed by the ACR in hopes of standardizing reporting and data. At present it is not complete, but we still believe in using BIRADS risk categories for the final assessment of every sonogram. Because most sonograms are targeted to clinical or mammographic abnormalities that require the preceding mammogram to be characterized as "BIRADS 0, incomplete, needs additional assessment," any final assessment will require sonography to assign a BIRADS category in order for a recommendation to be made. BIRADS categories are also important to assess and improve sonographic performance. If each sonographic category carries the same risk as the corresponding mammographic BIRADS category, then the rules for managing sonographic lesions can be identical to the mammographic rules for the same category. Separate rules will not need to be developed for sonography. We do not use the BIRADS 0 category after sonography except in the rare cases in which sonography is performed before mammography. In general, BIRADS categories are 1, 2, 3, 4a, 4b, and 5.

The sonographic **BIRADS 1** category corresponds to *sonographically normal tissues that cause mammographic or clinical abnormalities.* The sonographic **BIRADS 2** category corresponds to *benign entities* and includes intramammary lymph nodes, ectatic ducts, simple cysts, and definitively benign solid nodules, such as lipomas. The **BIRADS 3** category corresponds to *probably benign* lesions that have a 2% or less chance of being malignant and includes some complex cysts, small intraductal papillomas, and a subset of fibroadenomas. We divide the ACR **BIRADS 4** category that is termed *suspicious* into two subcategories because it is so large, extending from >2% risk to <90% risk of malignancy. We simply divide the ACR BIRADS 4 category at 50% or greater risk into 4a and 4b subcategories. We term the BIRADS 4a category *mildly suspicious*. It carries a risk between 3% and 49%. We term the BIRADS 4b category *moderately suspicious*. It carries a risk of 50% to 89%. These categories include lesions that do not meet strict criteria for BIRADS 3 or lower characterization. The **BIRADS 5** category is termed *malignant* and indicates a risk of

malignancy of 90% or greater. The management rules for each category have already been developed for mammography and are quite simple. BIRADS 1 and 2 characterizations enable the patient to return to routine screening follow-up. BIRADS 3 characterization presents the patient with three choices—surgical biopsy, image-guided needle biopsy, or short interval sonographic follow-up. BIRADS 4a, 4b, and 5 lesions require biopsy.

Special Breast Techniques

Breast sonographic evaluation depends heavily on special dynamic maneuvers performed during the examination. Dynamic maneuvers include **varying compression** to assess compressibility and mobility. Lesions that are more than 30% compressible are fatty with a high degree of certainty—either a normal fat lobule or a benign lipoma. Superficial venous thrombosis (Mondor's disease) requires incompressibility and lack of flow on Doppler for diagnosis. It can be helpful to demonstrate mobility of echoes with ectatic ducts or complex cysts. Varying compression can also eradicate artifactual shadowing due to critical angle shadowing off steeply oblique tissue planes. **Heeling and toeing of the transducer** can minimize critical angle shadowing arising from Cooper's ligaments and can also better demonstrate the thin, echogenic capsule on the ends of solid nodules that is an important sign of a noninvasive lesion margin. Heeling and toeing can also improve the angle of incidence with duct walls, allowing better demonstration of ductal anatomy and pathology, especially in the subareolar portions of the ducts. **Doppler assessment** of the breast depends greatly on using as little compression pressure as possible. Blood flow in breast lesion can easily be decreased or even completely ablated if compression is too vigorous. Positional changes are important in assessment of complex cysts. **Fluid-debris levels**, **milk of calcium**, and **fat-fluid levels** can all be shown to change positions between supine and upright or lateral decubitus positions. Some palpable abnormalities are clinically evident only in the upright position and, therefore, require that the scan be performed in the upright position. Even routine whole-breast scanning may require that the position of the patient be changed during the examination. Certain positions are better for evaluating one quadrant of the breast, whereas other positions may be optimal for other parts of the breast.

MAIN INDICATIONS

Most diagnostic breast ultrasound is performed in a targeted fashion to evaluate a particular palpable or mammographic abnormality.

Palpable Lumps

Sonography is very useful in evaluating palpable lumps when there is dense tissue in the area of the palpable lump on mammography. If lesions do not contain calcifications and the surrounding tissue obscures them, they can be missed on mammography. Sonography has much less to contribute to cases where there is only fatty density in the area of the palpable lump on mammography. There is very little chance that the mammogram has missed anything significant, and the palpable lump is almost certain to be either a fat lobule or a benign lipoma in such cases. The only exception to this general rule occurs in cases of pea-sized or smaller palpable lumps when the skin line is overpenetrated on the mammogram so that it cannot be appreciated, even with the use of a hot light. In such cases, there may be a tiny and very superficial lesion just under the skin that is not adequately shown on the mammogram. When the mammographic area of the palpable lump is of mixed fatty and water density, then sonographic evaluation should be aggressively performed.

The goals of targeted sonographic evaluation of palpable lumps that correspond to dense tissues mammographically are to find something benign, so biopsy can be prevented or to find a malignant lesion that has been obscured by surrounding dense tissues on the mammogram. If sonography is to be truly effective at preventing biopsy of palpable normal breast tissues or definitively benign lesions (BIRADS 1 and 2 findings), it is essential that the abnormality be palpated while being scanned and the image should be annotated with the word "palpable" (Fig. 23-14). Simply showing that normal tissues or a benign cyst exists in the same quadrant is insufficient proof that it is the cause of the palpable lump. Only by simultaneous scanning and palpating can this be accomplished. For large lesions in compressible breasts, the nonscanning index finger can usually be slid under the transducer while scanning. For smaller lesions and firmer breasts, the index finger may lift the ends of the transducer so far off the skin that the lesion cannot be scanned with the finger between the transducer and skin. In such cases, trapping the lesion between the index and middle fingers and scanning the lesion while it is trapped may be useful. For very small and superficial lesions, an opened paper clip or empty metal ballpoint pen cartridge can be used to palpate the lesion during scanning without lifting the ends of the transducer off the skin.

By aggressively scanning palpable lumps in patients who have dense tissue in the area of the palpable lumps, sonography should regularly detect malignant nodules that are missed by mammography. That sonography finds carcinomas that are missed by mammography does not reflect badly on mammography. Rather, it indicates that understanding the limitations of mammography, and proper use of sonography in those highly selected cases, can improve imaging performance in dense breasts on mammography.

Sonography can prevent biopsy by showing normal or definitively benign findings. Several studies have now shown an extremely high negative-predictive value for the combination of negative mammography and normal or benign ultrasound findings. The old common

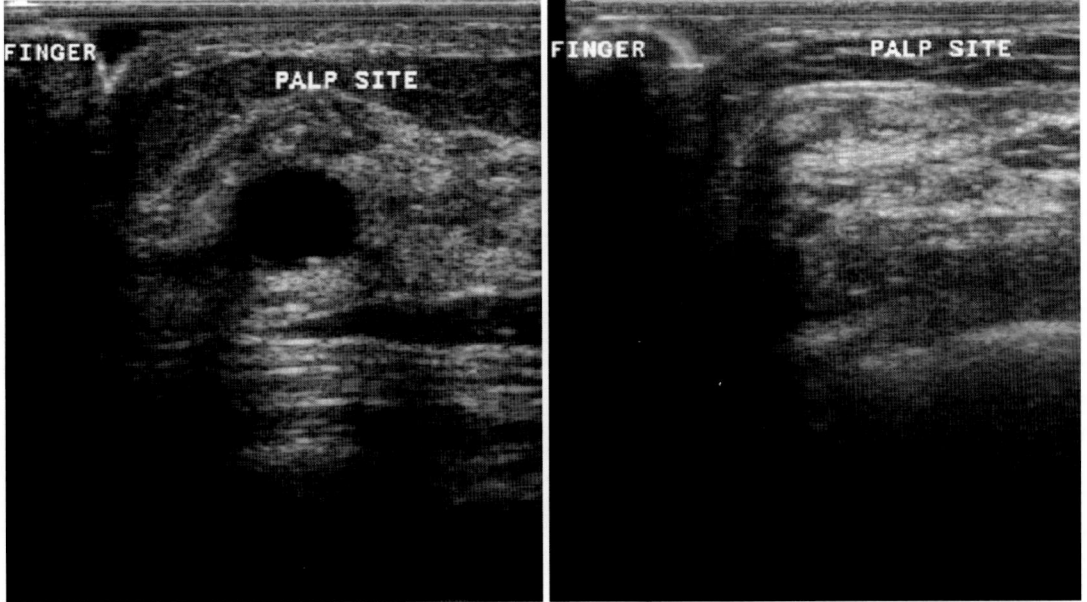

FIGURE 23-14. Palpation during sonography is critical. A, Cysts and **B,** fibroglandular ridges that protrude anteriorly into the subcutaneous fat are the two most common causes of palpable abnormalities. It is also important to annotate the images to signify that the area being scanned was palpable.

wisdom that all palpable lumps need to be biopsied is no longer true. However, palpable abnormalities span a spectrum from vague thickenings to rock-hard immovable lumps, and the latter would obviously engender greater clinical concern. But the rock hard immovable lump would virtually always be associated with suspicious sonographic findings.

The concept of a negative ultrasound report in patients with palpable breast lesions is not acceptable. Negative sonograms imply that the breast imager is detached from the interpretation of the images and may not fully understand the problem for which the patient presented. Rather, we prefer to think of all sonograms in patients with palpable lumps as being positive for an explanation. The positive finding can be palpable normal breast tissue or a palpable, clearly benign lesion, such as a simple cyst, but the finding positively and definitively explains the cause of the palpable abnormality. It is far more reassuring to the patient to be shown on the monitor that the lump that is being palpated during the scan corresponds to a positive but normal finding, such as a ridge of normal fibroglandular tissue, than it is to be told her ultrasound is negative. The positive, but normal, ultrasound engenders confidence that the breast imager truly understands her problem, whereas a negative ultrasound engenders fear that the breast imager does not understand why she presented and might have missed something more sinister.

Mammographic Densities

Sonography is the best diagnostic tool for assessing mammographic abnormalities that do not contain calcifications. These mammographic abnormalities range from discrete masses to focal asymmetrical densities. As in the case for palpable abnormalities, sonography will demonstrate either asymmetrical normal tissues or definitely benign abnormalities, such as simple cysts in most cases. In a smaller percentage of cases, sonography will show findings that are more suspect or more malignant appearing than suggested by mammography.

When sonography suggests that a benign abnormality, such as a simple cyst or asymmetrical normal breast tissue, causes the mammographic abnormality, it is important to be sure that the sonographic finding really explains the mammographic abnormality. It is important to be sure that there are not really two completely different findings—a mammographic finding and a separate incidental sonographic finding. In order to make sure that there is only a single finding and that the sonographic finding and the mammographic finding are the same, we must rigorously assure that the size, shape, location, and surrounding tissue density of the mammographic and sonographic findings are the same. Mammographic-sonographic correlation of size, shape, location, and surrounding tissue density can be best

made between the cranial-caudal (CC) mammographic view and the transverse sonographic view because there is little rotation and no obliquity of the x-ray beam on the mammographic CC view. Thus, the sonographic transverse view is obtained in the exact plane of mammographic compression. The medial-lateral-oblique (MLO) view is obtained between 30 degrees and 60 degrees of obliquity off the true mediolateral plane and also usually involves some rotation of the breast. It is difficult to obtain an oblique sonographic plane that exactly reproduces the unknown degree of obliquity used to obtain the mammographic MLO view. The sonographic plane also cannot reproduce the rotation of the breast that can occur when obtaining an MLO mammographic view. If a mammographic lesion can only be seen on the MLO view, it is usually best to obtain a true mediolateral view, taking care not to rotate the breast during compression and then obtain a true longitudinal ultrasound view to correlate with the mammographic ML view.

Size Correlation

Mammographic-sonographic correlation of size should take into account everything that is water density. Therefore, a 3 cm oval-shaped, circumscribed mass might be shown to be a cyst or solid nodule with a thin echogenic capsule, a cyst that contains a mural nodule, a 3 cm collection of fibroglandular tissue, or a smaller cyst or solid nodule surrounded by fibroglandular tissue, where the cyst or solid nodule, together with the surrounding fibrous tissue, measures 3 cm (Fig. 23-15). All six of the above sonographic structures would constitute a perfect mammographic-sonographic size match if all structures that appear as water density mammographically were appropriately taken into account. Measurements should be made outside-to-outside to include the capsule that surrounds the cyst or solid nodules because the capsule is water density and will be included in the measurement of the lesion on mammogram. Sonographic-mammographic correlation works best when the lesion is measured identically by both modalities. Mammography cannot distinguish the water density capsule from the water density lesion that it surrounds, so the capsule must be included in the measurement of the lesion. Maximum diameter is better suited for sonographic-mammographic correlation than is mean diameter. This is because many mammographic lesions are partially compressible. To obtain the three measurements necessary for calculation of mean diameter on mammograms, two views are necessary. These views are not truly orthogonal. Only the dimensions of the lesion that are perpendicular to the axis of compression can be shown, and neither view shows the compressed dimension of the lesion. The two mammographic views will yield three measurements that are all obtained perpendicular to the

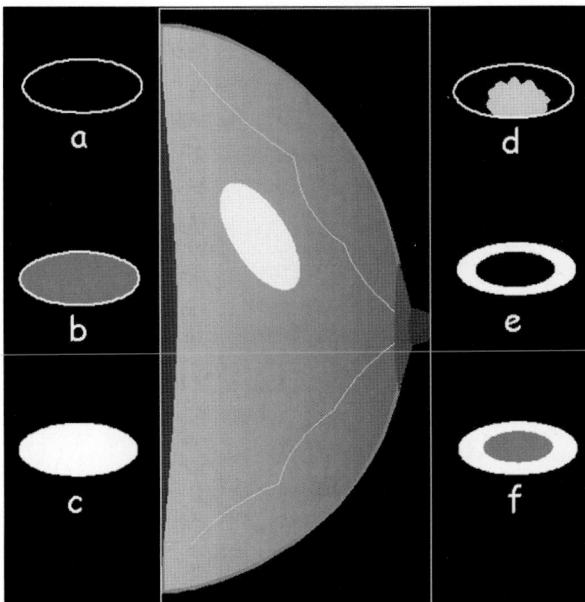

FIGURE 23-15. Importance of mammographic-sonographic correlation. Everything that is water density could contribute to the size of the mammographic lesion. Thus, a 3 cm ovoid, circumscribed mammographic mass could represent **A**, a cyst or **B**, a solid nodule that is surrounded by a thin echogenic capsule; **C**, 3 cm collection of interlobular stromal fibrous tissue, **D**, 3 cm cyst containing a mural nodule, **E**, smaller cyst or **F**, solid nodule that is surrounded by fibrous or glandular tissue.

axis of compression. Sonography also requires two views in order to obtain the three measurements necessary for calculation of mean diameter, but these views are truly orthogonal. Whereas two of the three dimensions obtained from sonography also lie perpendicular to the axis of compression, sonography can show the compressed diameter which is the third measurement. As a result, sonography shows two large diameters and one small diameter (Fig. 23-16). This causes the mean diameter of compressible lesions that is obtained from sonography to be smaller than the mean diameter of the same lesion obtained from mammography. Despite the different mean diameters obtained by mammography and sonography, the maximum diameters will be the same. Maximum diameter, not mean diameter, should be used for sonographic correlation of lesion size. Mean sonographic diameters should be used for short interval follow-up of a lesion.

Shape Correlation

Sonographic-mammographic correlation of shape must take two phenomena into account: **partial compressibility** and **rotatory forces** applied during compression. The same phenomenon that causes the mean diameter of partially compressible lesions to appear larger on mammography than it is on sonography also causes a

consistent shape difference between mammography and sonography. Partially compressible lesions that appear spherical in shape on mammography are oval-shaped on sonography because sonography is capable of showing the compressed diameter of the lesion, whereas mammography cannot. When the lesion is incompressible, the shape will be similar on mammography and sonography. Mammographic compression and sonographic compression apply different rotatory forces on lesions that are not spherical in shape (Fig. 23-17). Mammographic compression not only pulls lesions away from the chest wall, but it tends to rotate the lesion so that its long axis lies perpendicular to the chest wall. Sonographic compression will push lesions closer to the chest wall and tends to rotate the lesion's long axis parallel to the chest wall. There is typically a 90 degree difference in the orientation of the long axis of lesions between the mammogram and the sonogram. If this rotation is not taken into account, the breast imager may falsely conclude that the shape of the lesion is different on the mammographic and sonographic images.

Location or Position Correlation

Because mammographic compression pulls a lesion away from the chest wall and sonographic compression pushes the lesion closer to the chest wall, lesions usually appear much closer to the chest wall on sonography than they do on mammography. Lesions that appear to lie several centimeters from the chest wall on mammography may appear to lie very close to, adjacent to, or might even indent the chest wall musculature on sonography. Lesions that would be considered in the B zone in depth on mammograms often lie within the C zone sonographically. If this routine apparent difference in depth of lesions on mammography and sonography is not understood, one might falsely conclude that the sonographic lesion lies too deep to correspond to the mammographic lesion.

Surrounding Tissue Density Correlation

The final step in correlating the sonographic and mammographic findings is assessment of the density of surrounding tissues. A lesion that protrudes into the subcutaneous fat from the mammary zone and that is surrounded by fat superficially and water density tissue along its deep margins on the mammogram, should lie at the junction of the subcutaneous fat and mammary zone on the sonogram. It should be surrounded by subcutaneous fat along its superficial margin sonographically, and by either hyperechoic fibrous tissue or isoechoic glandular tissue along its deep border on the sonogram (Fig. 23-18).

Correlating size, shape, location, and surrounding tissue density will allow the mammographic and sono-

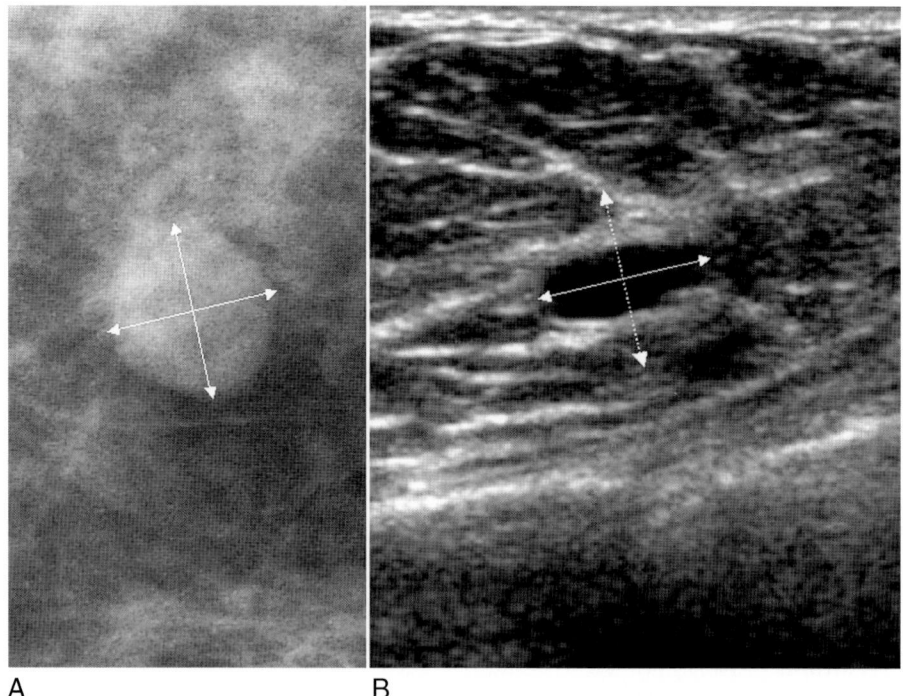

A   B

FIGURE 23-16. Lesions that appear to be spherical in shape on mammography often appear to be elliptical in shape on sonography. **A,** Circumscribed isodense mammographic nodule appeared circular in both views (spherical) because the mammogram only demonstrates the axes of the cyst that lies perpendicular to the axis of compression and not the compressed axis. Sonography does show the compressed axes. The mean diameter calculated from mammograms includes three large diameters that all lie in axes that are perpendicular to the axis of compression. **B,** The mean diameter calculated from the sonographic views includes two large diameters that lie perpendicular to the axis of compression (*solid arrows*) and one smaller diameter that lies parallel to the axis of compression (*dotted arrows*). For compressible lesions, the mean diameter obtained from sonograms is often smaller than the mean diameter obtained from mammography, but the maximum diameters will be similar.

FIGURE 23-17. Mammographic compression and sonographic compression. Mammographic compression (**A**) tends to rotate the long axis of the lesion perpendicular to the chest wall, whereas sonographic compression (**B**) tends to rotate the long axis parallel to the chest wall. The long axes of lesions on mammography and sonography often differ by nearly 90 degrees. The mammogram has been rotated 90 degrees to the right to display the pectoralis muscle (PM) deep to the lesion, as it appears on sonography. The double-headed arrow shows the long axis of the lesion.

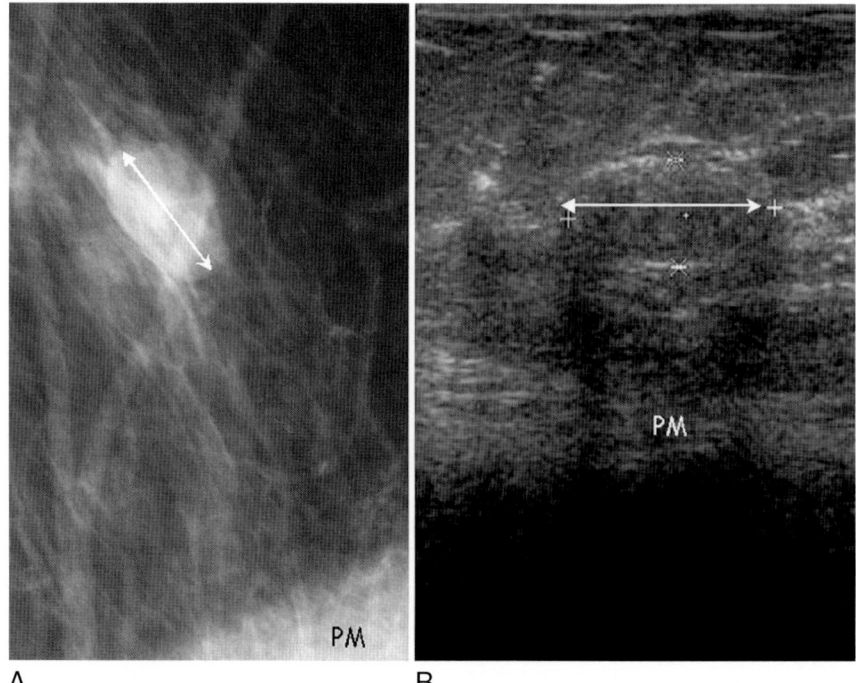

A   B

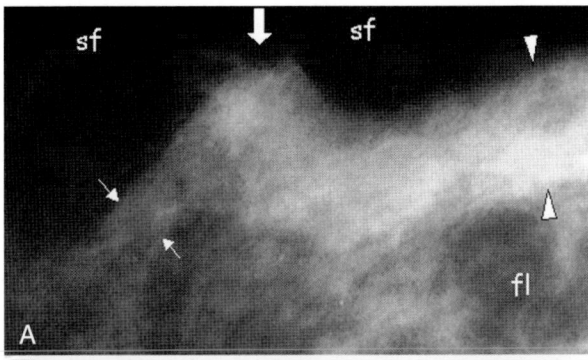

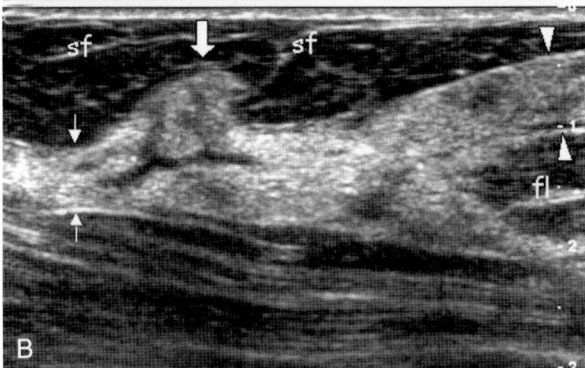

FIGURE 23-18. Importance of mammographic-sonographic correlation. Surrounding tissue densities should be compared when sonography suggests that the mammographic density corresponds to normal breast tissue or benign abnormalities such as simple cysts. **A,** Mammographically suspicious architectural distortion, an angular anterior bulge of the mammary zone into the subcutaneous fat (*thick white arrow*) corresponds on sonography (**B**) to a ridge of normal fibroglandular tissue (*thick white arrow*) that contains no isoechoic areas larger than normal ducts and TDLUs. The mammographic density is outlined by subcutaneous fat (sf) along its anterior border on both sonography and mammography. There are narrow bands of water density tissue laterally (*small arrows*) and medially (*arrowheads*) on both mammography and sonography. There is a prominent fat lobule (fl) medially on both sonography and mammography. Cranial caudal view, mammogram, rotated 90° to the right to correspond with the ultrasound.

graphic findings to be definitively correlated in most cases, but in some cases may fail. If it cannot be determined with absolute certainty that the mammographic and sonographic lesions are, indeed, the same, minimally invasive sonographic procedures can be performed to confirm the correlation. If sonography shows the suspected mammographic lesion to be cystic, sonographically guided cyst aspiration can be performed and the mammogram can be repeated to see if the mammographic lesion has disappeared. If sonography shows the suspected lesion to be solid, sonographically guided needle localization with a removable wire can be performed, and the mammogram can be repeated with the wire in place to document that the sonographic and mammographic lesion is, indeed, the same lesion.

FINDINGS

The sonographic findings that correlate with palpable or mammographic abnormalities can fall into several different categories—(1) ANDIs, (2) cysts, (3) solid nodules, and (4) indeterminate (cystic versus solid) lesions.

Normal Tissues and Aberrations of Normal Development and Involution

Normal breast tissues and variations of normal tissues that include duct ectasia, fibrocystic change, or benign proliferative disorders can cause both mammographic and sonographic abnormalities. Some have termed these changes as ANDIs, aberrations of normal development, and involution. ANDIs can present not only as normal tissues but as cysts and solid nodules as well, accounting for some false positives at biopsy. As noted earlier, because normal tissue and ANDIs can cause both palpable and mammographic abnormalities, it is best to discard the concept of a "negative ultrasound" when evaluating clinical or mammographic abnormalities. It is better to think of all sonograms as positive—positive for a definitive explanation of the clinical or mammographic abnormality. That positive finding, however, may be a ridge of palpable fibroglandular tissues or a collection of asymmetric fibroglandular tissues that cause an asymmetric mammographic density. Most sonographically normal tissues can be characterized as BIRADS 1. ANDIs cause a spectrum of abnormalities that can be characterized as BIRADS 2, 3, or 4.

Simple Cysts

The initial role of diagnostic breast sonography was to distinguish between cysts and solid nodules. Today, that remains a key role for sonography, but certainly not its only role. Demonstrating that a simple cyst causes a palpable lump or mammographic nodule is by far the most valuable finding that we can demonstrate sonographically because simple cysts are as definitively benign as anything we can identify by any modality in diagnostic imaging. Furthermore, the negative-predictive value of a simple cyst is 100%, higher than the 99+% negative-predictive value of sonographic demonstration of normal breast tissues causing mammographic or palpable abnormalities. If strict criteria for a simple cyst are met, the lesion is BIRADS 2, and no biopsy, aspiration, or follow-up is necessary. In general, we only aspirate simple cysts in cases where they are so tense that they cause severe pain. The negative-predictive value of demonstrating that a simple cyst causes a palpable or mammographic abnormality is higher than if we demonstrate normal tissue or ANDIs as the cause. Complex and complicated cysts create a spectrum of lesions that can be characterized as BIRADS 2, 3, or 4.

Solid Nodules

Because the initial role of sonography in breast diagnosis was to distinguish between cysts and solid nodules, demonstration of a solid nodule initially was an automatic indication for biopsy. Several of the early sonographic studies in which characterization of solid nodules was attempted reported too much overlap between the features of benign and malignant solid nodules to allow distinction between all solid malignant and all solid benign nodules. These studies were performed with older, lower frequency, lower resolution equipment, and generally assessed only single sonographic findings. Since then, the approach to characterizing solid nodules has evolved.

The key to developing a successful algorithm for characterizing solid nodules is having a realistic goal. The goal of distinguishing all benign from all malignant solid nodules was overly ambitious and not achievable. A more realistic goal is to identify a subpopulation of all solid nodules that is so likely to be benign that the patient can be offered the option of follow-up in addition to the option of biopsy. The precedent for this has been established in the mammographic literature. BIRADS 3 lesions, as they are currently defined in the mammographic literature, must have a 2% or lower risk of being malignant. To be prudent and conservative, any algorithm developed to identify the BIRADS 3 solid nodule subgroup sonographically must adhere to criteria that are identical to those accepted as the standard of care in the mammographic literature.

Figure 23-19 illustrates the heterogeneity of breast cancer, which can be thought of as spanning a spectrum from spiculated to circumscribed lesions. Not only is breast cancer heterogeneous from one nodule to another, it can also be heterogeneous within an individual nodule, so any sonographic algorithm designed to identify a BIRADS 3 subgroup must take this into account. The histologic and gross morphologic features of the spiculated and circumscribed ends of the malignant spectrum differ greatly from each other in several ways: cellularity, constituents of the extracellular matrix, host reaction to the tumor, and water content. The classic **spiculated breast carcinoma** is composed of tumor cells, extracellular matrix, and desmoplastic host response to the lesion. Compared to circumscribed carcinomas, spiculated carcinomas are paucicellular—a small percentage of the total volume of the lesion is composed of tumor cells.

Circumscribed carcinomas are highly cellular. The algorithm that we use to evaluate lesions must account for internal heterogeneity by (1) assessing the surface, shape, and volume of the lesion for suspicious findings completely in two orthogonal planes (preferably radial and antiradial); and (2) ignoring benign or nonsuspicious findings in lesions that have a mixture of suspicious and nonsuspicious findings. The entire lesion must always be characterized by its most suspicious features.

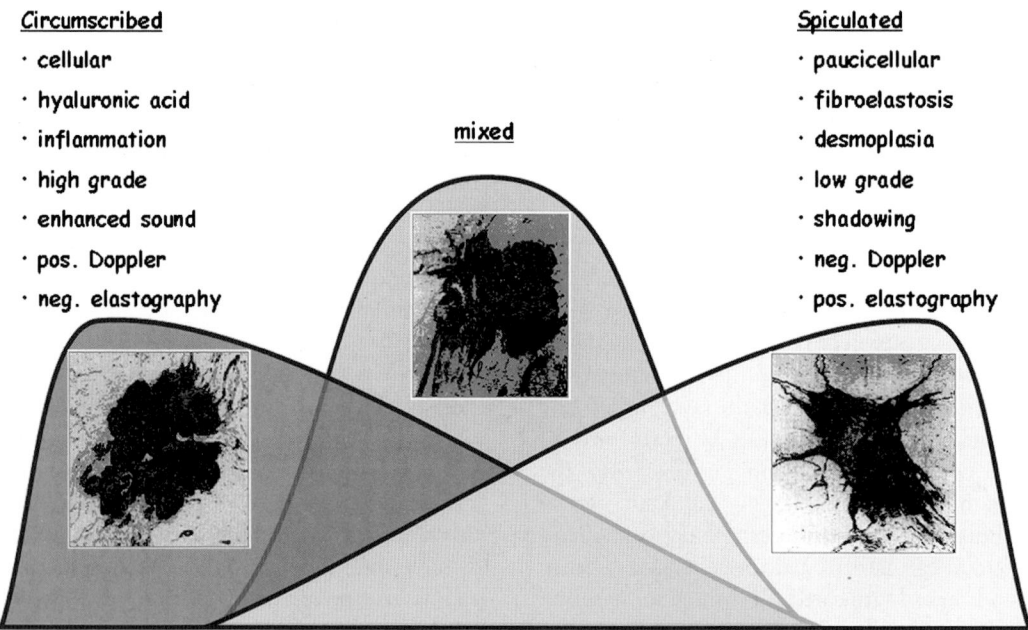

FIGURE 23-19. Malignant masses—spectrum of appearances. The appearance of breast cancer varies from classic crablike spiculated lesions to circumscribed carcinomas. Sonographic findings can be nearly opposite. Only by using multiple findings that are capable of identifying lesions at both ends of the spectrum can we identify carcinomas with adequate sensitivity.

TABLE 23-1. SONOGRAPHIC FINDINGS IN SOLID BREAST NODULES COMPARED TO SUSPICIOUS MAMMOGRAPHIC FINDINGS	
Suspicious Mammographic Findings	**Suspicious Sonographic Findings**
Spiculation	Spiculation (thick, echogenic halo)
Irregular or ill-defined margins	Angular margins
Microlobulation	Microlobulation
Calcifications	Calcifications
Linear calcification pattern	Duct extension
Branching calcification pattern	Branch pattern
Mass or nodule	**Taller-than-wide**
Asymmetrical density	**Acoustic shadowing**
Developing density	**Hypoechogenicity**

TABLE 23-2. SONOGRAPHIC-PATHOLOGIC FEATURES OF SUSPICIOUS FINDINGS	
Morphologic Categories	**Histopathologic Categories**
Surface Characteristics	**"Hard" Findings**
Spiculation	Spiculation
Angular margins	Angular margins
Microlobulation	Acoustic shadowing
Shapes	Hypoechogenicity
Taller-than-wide	**Mixed Findings**
Duct extension	Taller-than-wide
Branch pattern	Microlobulation
Internal Characteristics	**"Soft" Findings**
Acoustic shadowing	Duct extension
Calcifications	Branch pattern
Hypoechogenicity	Calcifications

Table 23-1 shows the suspicious sonographic findings in solid breast nodules and compares them to suspicious mammographic findings. Note that six of the nine suspicious sonographic findings are suspicious mammographic findings that we have applied directly to sonography. Of the nine findings, only **taller than wide, acoustic shadowing**, and **hypoechogenicity** are unique to sonography.

The suspicious sonographic findings can be classified into 3 subgroups by morphologic features or by histopathologic features (Table 23-2). The morphologic features include surface characteristics (spiculation, angular margins, and microlobulations), shapes (taller than wide, duct extension, and branch pattern), and internal characteristics (acoustic shadowing, hypoechoic echotexture, and calcifications). Morphologic classification is less useful than histopathologic classification. Histopathologic categories are hard findings (indicating invasion of surrounding tissues), soft findings (indicating DCIS components of tumor), and mixed findings (indicating either invasive or DCIS components of tumor).

Including soft findings is important because the most common breast carcinoma, invasive duct carcinoma—invasive not otherwise specific (NOS) or no specific type (NST) carcinoma—usually contains DCIS components. Soft suspicious findings help us in two ways. First, soft findings can help us to detect pure DCIS, which rarely develops hard suspicious findings. Second, including soft findings can help to detect and characterize the invasive duct carcinomas that contain both invasive and DCIS components. Soft findings increase the sensitivity of the sonographic algorithm for detecting malignant disease, but increase the false-positive rate, especially for lesions that contain only soft findings. Lesions that demonstrate only soft findings are most likely to be benign—papillomas and fibrocystic change

SONOGRAPHIC FINDINGS SUSPICIOUS FOR CANCER

Spiculation or thick, echogenic halo
Angular margin
Microlobulations
Shape taller than wide
Duct extension and branch pattern
Acoustic shadowing
Calcification
Hypoechogenicity

(FCC). However, the risk of malignancy for solid nodules that demonstrate only soft suspicious findings is greater than 2%, requiring that such lesions be characterized as mildly suspicious (BIRADS 4a) and biopsied. Each individual suspicious sonographic finding has a solid histopathologic basis.

Spiculation or Thick, Echogenic Halo

Spiculation is a hard sonographic finding that corresponds to invasion of surrounding tissues and a desmoplastic host response to the lesion. Spiculation is a mammographic finding that can be directly applied to sonography. Spiculations may manifest as alternating hypoechoic and hyperechoic lines that radiate perpendicular to the surface of the nodule, where the hypoechoic components represent either fingers of invasive tumor or DCIS components of tumor extending into the surrounding tissues and the hyperechoic components represent the interfaces between the spicules and surrounding breast tissues. In most cases, however, spicules appear as purely hyperechoic or purely hypoechoic depending on echogenicity of the tissue within which the lesion lies.

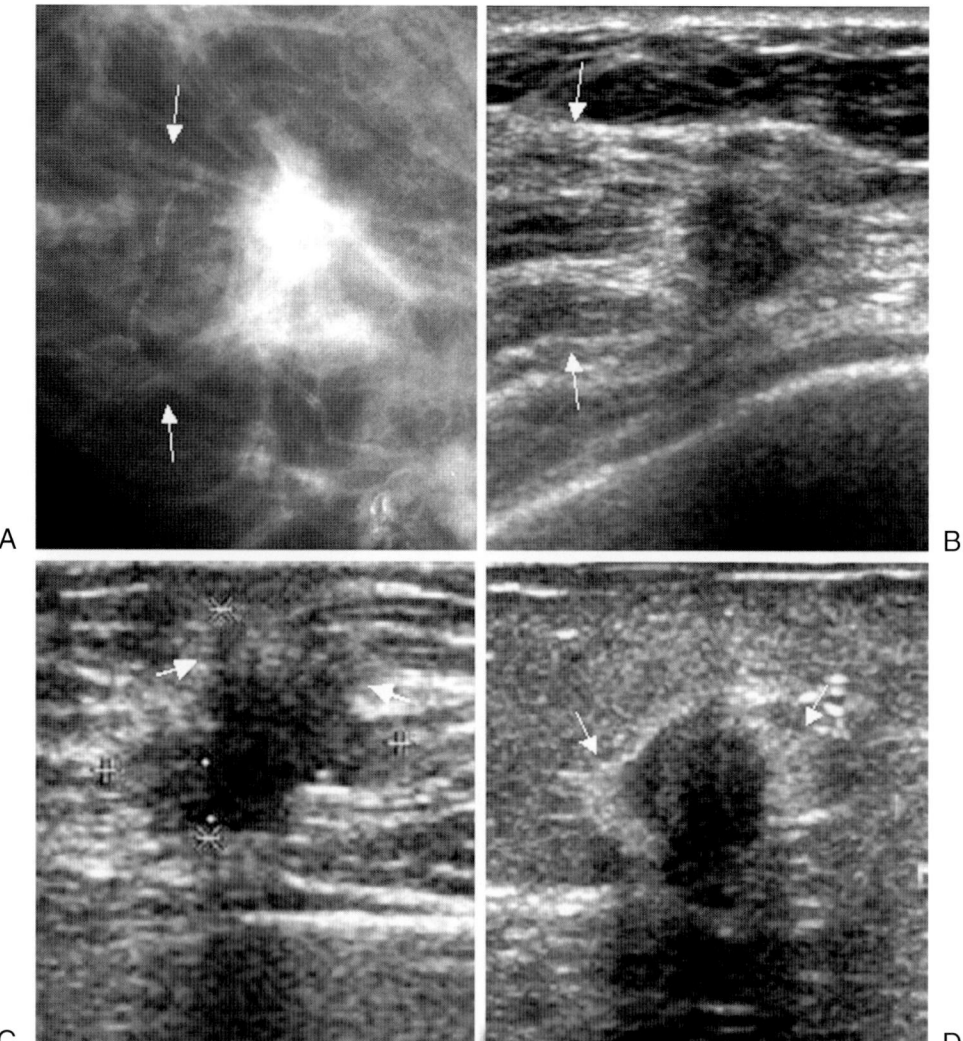

FIGURE 23-20. Spiculation. A, Mammogram and **B,** ultrasound. Spiculation (*arrows*) is a hard mammographic finding that indicates invasion. The spicules in fat-surrounded lesions appear hyperechoic. **C,** Spiculated lesions that are surrounded by fibroglandular tissues may not be visible mammographically and appear hypoechoic (*arrows*) sonographically. The hypoechoic spiculations involve only the anterior surface of this nodule. The lesion is more circumscribed than spiculated along its posterior right border. **D, Thick, echogenic halo** that surrounds this cancer represents spiculations that are too small to resolve. The halo is thicker and brighter along the lateral edges of the nodules because the spicules are oriented perpendicular to the ultrasound beam along the edges and make brighter specular reflectors. The halo is poorly demonstrated along the anterior and posterior surfaces of the nodule where the spicules are parallel to the beam and make weak specular reflectors.

The spicules in malignant nodules that are surrounded by hyperechoic fibrous tissues appear hypoechoic (Fig. 23-20A, B), whereas spicules in malignant nodules that are surrounded by fat appear hyperechoic (see Fig. 23-20C). The role of sonography in fat-surrounded lesions is usually to guide interventional procedures or to determine extent of disease, whereas its role in fibrous-surrounded lesions may be diagnostic because such lesions can be completely obscured by surrounding dense tissues on the mammogram. The thick, echogenic halo that surrounds some malignant solid nodules represents spiculations that are too small to demonstrate sonographically. For this reason, either frank spiculations or the presence of a thick, echogenic halo should be considered to be spiculations. The classic thick, echogenic halo appears thicker along the edges of the nodule than on its anterior and posterior surfaces (see Fig. 23-20D). This is because the spicules are perpendicular to the beam along the edges of the nodule, forming strong specular reflectors. The spicules that lie along the anterior and posterior surfaces of the nodule lie nearly parallel to the sonographic beam, and therefore, are very weak specular reflectors. Considering the thick, echogenic halo to be a variant of frank speculations approximately doubles the sensitivity of spiculation for malignant nodules from 36% to 70%.

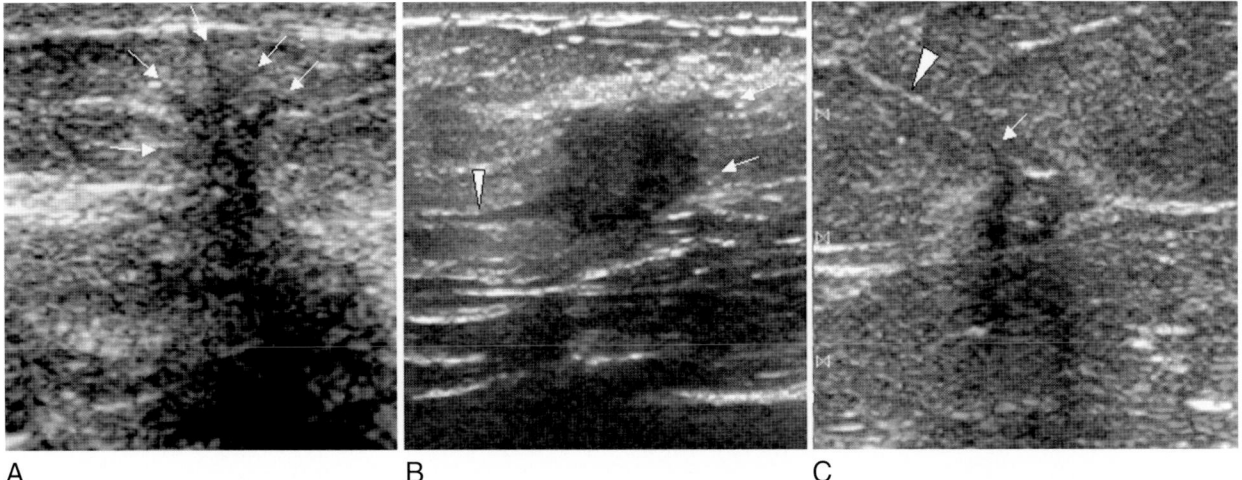

FIGURE 23-21. Angular margins represent invasion of carcinoma into pathways that have low resistance to invasion. A, Fat offers little resistance to invasion, so fat-surrounded malignant nodules can develop angles along any surface (*arrows*). **B,** In lesions that are surrounded by hyperechoic fibrous tissues, paths of low resistance are along the periductal tissues (*arrowhead*) and horizontally along the tissue planes within the fibrous tissue (*arrows*). **C,** Following Cooper's ligaments (*arrowhead*) down to their base where they intersect the surface of the nodule is the best way to detect angles (*arrow*) on the surface of malignant solid nodules.

Angular Margin

Angular margins are identical to the jagged or irregular margins discussed in the mammography and breast ultrasound literature. Angular margin represents a hard sonographic finding indicative of invasion and is a mammographic finding that has been applied directly to sonography. The angles of the lesion margins can be acute, right angle, or obtuse. A single angle of any type on the surface of the lesion should be considered suspicious and should exclude the lesion from the probably benign, BIRADS 3, category. Angles on the surface of the nodule occur in regions of low resistance to invasion. In lesions that are surrounded by fat, they can occur on any surface of the nodule (Fig. 23-21). In fibrous-surrounded lesions, they tend to occur on the edges of the lesion, within loose periductal stromal tissues and between tissue planes within the fibrous tissue (see Fig. 23-21B). In the approximately two thirds of malignant nodules that arise within anteriorly located TDLUs that abut the anterior mammary fascia, angulations tend to occur at points where Cooper's ligaments intersect the surface of the nodule (see Fig. 23-21C). Angular margins have the second best sensitivity of all of the individual suspicious findings (90%), but have the best combination of sensitivity and positive-predictive value of any of the findings.

Microlobulations

Microlobulations are 1 to 2 mm lobulations that vary in number and distribution along the surface and within the substance of a nodule. Microlobulation is a mixed finding that can be seen with both invasive and DCIS components of tumor. It is a mammographic finding that applies directly to sonography. When microlobulations are angular and are associated with either spiculations or a thick, echogenic halo, they usually correspond to fingers of invasive carcinoma (Fig. 23-22A). When the microlobulations are rounded and associated with a thin, echogenic capsule, they usually represent DCIS components of tumors. DCIS components can manifest as microlobulations in two different ways: (1) ductules or ducts that are distended with tumor and/or necrosis (see Figure 23-22B), or (2) cancerized lobules (see Fig. 23-22C). The size of microlobulations correlates with the histologic grade of the tumor. High-grade lesions tend to have large microlobulations, whereas low-grade lesions tend to have very small microlobulations, and intermediate-grade lesions tend to have intermediate-sized microlobulations.

Shape Taller Than Wide

Lesions that are larger in the anteroposterior dimension than in any horizontal dimension are suspicious for malignancy. This is a mixed finding that can be seen with both invasive and DCIS lesions (Fig. 23-23). It is a finding unique to sonography. Taller-than-wide shape was originally described in the Japanese literature. Later, Fornage found that taller than wide (not parallel) is primarily a feature of small, malignant solid nodules that have a volume of 1 cc or less. Our data confirm this. As lesions enlarge, they tend to become wider than tall (parallel). There are several possible explanations for this finding, but we believe that the best explanation is that

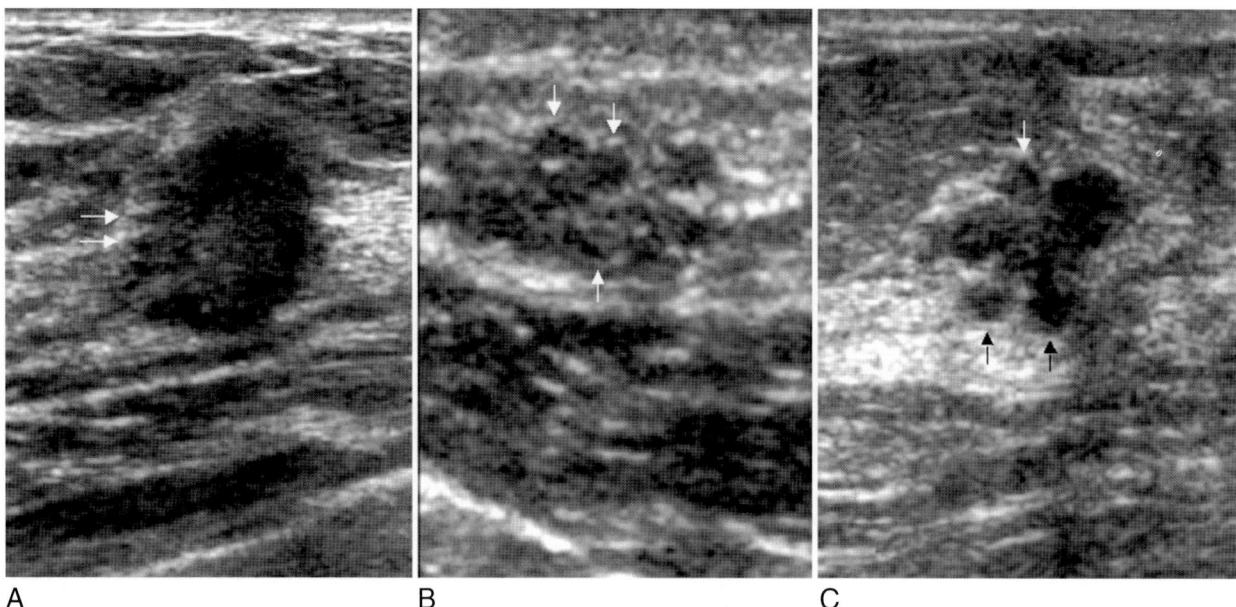

FIGURE 23-22. Microlobulations. These can represent either fingers of invasive tumor or DCIS components of the lesion. **A**, When the microlobulations are pointed or angular and associated with spiculations or thick, echogenic halo, they represent fingers of invasive tumor (*arrows*). **B**, When the microlobulations are round and have a thin, echogenic capsule, they usually represent ducts or ductules grossly distended with DCIS (*arrows*). **C**, When the microlobulations extend away from the main tumor nodule into surrounding tissues and have the shape of TDLUs, they usually represent cancerized lobules (*arrows*). DCIS, Ductal carcinoma in situ; TDLU, terminal ductolobular unit.

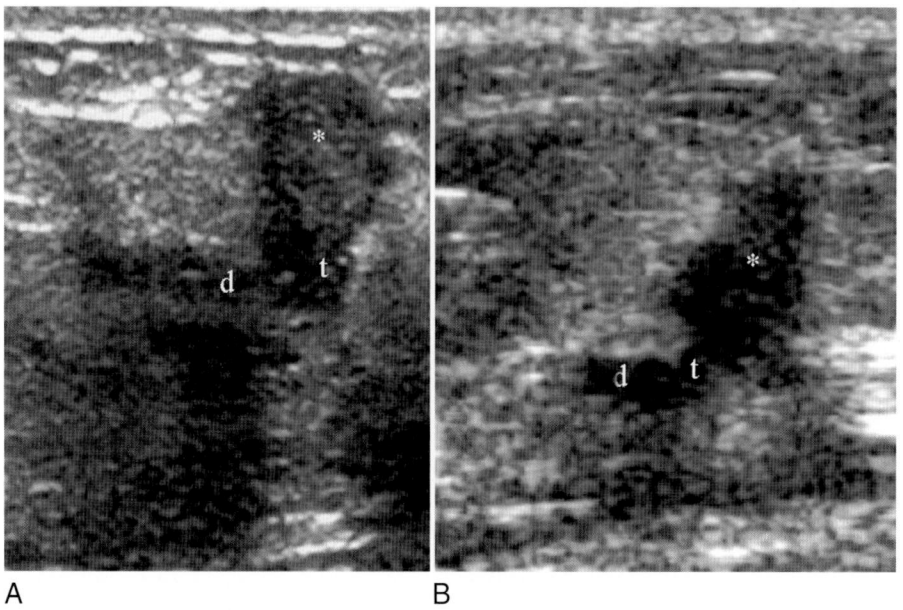

FIGURE 23-23. Ductal carcinoma in situ: Taller than wide. A, High nuclear-grade DCIS and **B**, small intermediate-grade invasive ductal carcinoma with DCIS components are both taller than wide because they affect primarily a single anterior TDLU whose long axis is oriented in the anteroposterior direction. (*—tumor distended lobule; t—tumor distended extralobular terminal duct; and d—tumor distended lobar duct). The pure DCIS manifests nonspecific (taller than wide and microlobulations) and soft findings (calcifications and duct extension). The invasive carcinoma manifests nonspecific (taller than wide), hard (angular margins and thick echogenic halo), and soft findings (duct extension). DCIS, Ductal carcinoma in situ; TDLU, terminal ductolobular unit.

the shape of small carcinomas merely reflects the shape of the TDLUs within which the carcinoma arose. Most TDLUs lie in the anterior aspect of the mammary zone and are oriented in the AP dimension. The percentage of all TDLUs that lie anteriorly tends to increase with age, because posterior lobules tend to atrophy and regress more rapidly than do anterior lobules. As malignant lesions expand into the lobar ductal system, which is oriented horizontally within the breast, they have a tendency to rapidly become wider than tall (Fig. 23-24).

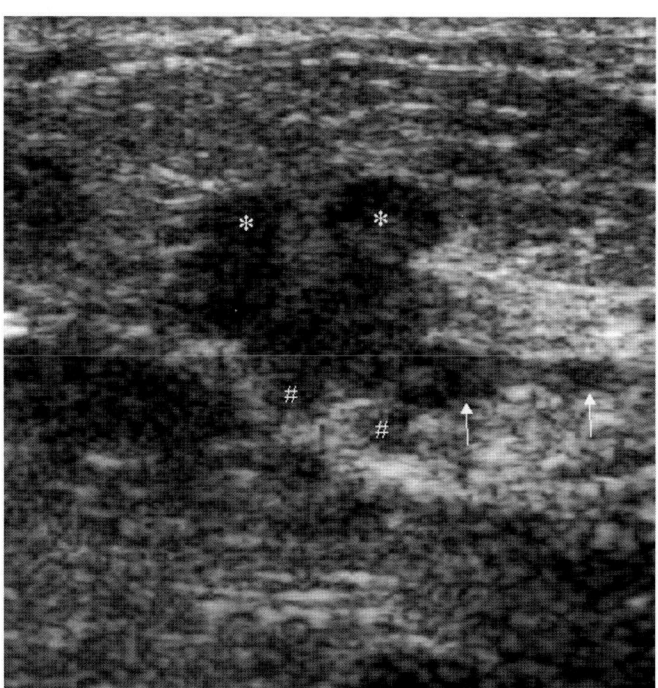

FIGURE 23-24. Growth of ductal carcinoma in situ changes shape to wider than tall. As malignant solid nodules enlarge, DCIS components grow down the lobar duct toward the nipple and invade lobules, changing the shape from taller than wide to wider than tall. Tumor distended anterior lobules (*), tumor distended but smaller posterior lobules (#), and tumor distended lobar duct (*arrows*). DCIS, Ductal carcinoma in situ.

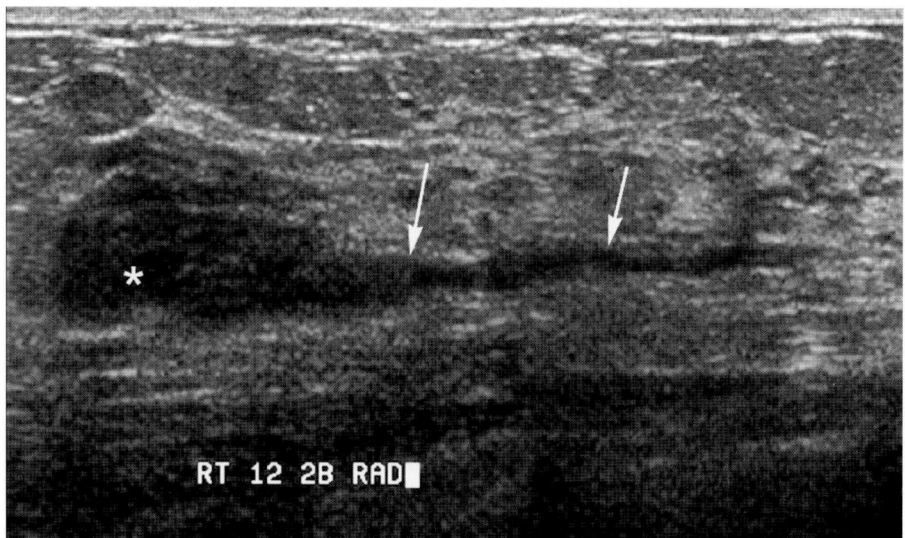

FIGURE 23-25. Invasive duct carcinoma, duct extension of invasive NOS carcinoma. Most invasive duct carcinomas contain DCIS components that may extend away from the invasive tumor (*) within surrounding lobar ducts (*arrows*) and grow toward the nipple to create duct extensions. If such duct extensions are not recognized sonographically, they might be transected at surgery, leading to positive margins and the need for re-resection. If the positive margins are not recognized, unresected duct extensions can lead to local recurrences. DCIS, Ductal carcinoma in situ; NOS, not otherwise specific.

About 70% of malignant nodules with maximum diameters under 10 mm are taller than wide. Only 20% of malignant nodules over 2.0 cm in maximum diameter are taller than wide.

Duct Extension and Branch Pattern

Duct extension and branch pattern are soft-shape findings that correlate with the presence of DCIS components of tumor. Duct extension and branch pattern are mammographic calcification findings that we have applied to components of solid nodules, which can best be demonstrated when the scan plane is oriented parallel to the long axis of the mammary ducts in the region of the nodule. Duct extension usually manifests as a single projection of solid growth toward the nipple from the main nodule (Fig. 23-25). Because the duct extension often involves the highly distensible lactiferous sinus portion of the major lobar duct, it can be quite large, up to 5 mm in diameter. Branch pattern manifests as projection of the solid nodule into multiple small ducts away from the nipple (Fig. 23-26). Because these are small ducts, branch-pattern involvement is generally smaller than duct extension.

The size of the branch pattern correlates with the histologic grade of the lesion. High-grade lesions tend to have large branch patterns; low-grade lesions tend to have small branch patterns; and intermediate-grade

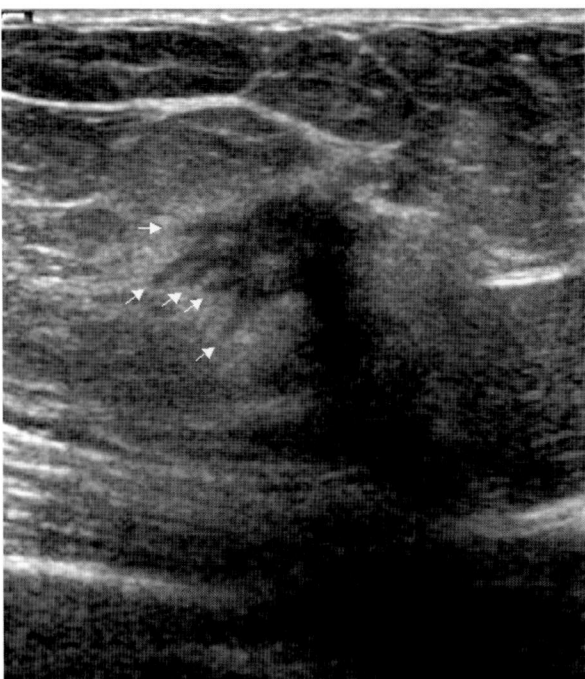

FIGURE 23-26. Carcinoma involving branch ducts.
This creates a branch pattern due to DCIS that involves multiple small ducts peripheral to the nodule. They are often shorter than duct extensions and their size varies with the grade of the lesion. High-grade invasive ductal carcinomas tend to have high nuclear-grade DCIS components that cause large branch ducts; low-grade lesions tend to cause small branch patterns that can be difficult to distinguish from hypoechoic spiculations; and intermediate-grade lesions tend to cause intermediate-sized branch patterns (*arrows*). DCIS, Ductal carcinoma in situ.

lesions tend to have intermediate-sized branches. The presence of duct extension and/or branch pattern is not a specific sign of malignancy, but rather suggests an intraductal growth pattern. Benign intraductal lesions such as papillomas and periductal fibrosis can also demonstrate duct extension or branch pattern. In fact, when only duct extension and/or branch pattern are present, the lesion is a benign papilloma 87% of the time. However, 6% of such lesions represent DCIS and another 7% represent papillomas that have atypia within the surface epithelium. Even in the absence of other suspicious findings, the risk of malignancy in nodules that have duct extension and/or branch pattern as their only suspicious findings is greater than 2% for lesions, and such lesions must be excluded from the BIRADS 3 category. It is important to recognize duct extension and branch pattern for two reasons: (1) to minimize false-negative characterization of pure DCIS, and (2) to identify extensive intraductal components of tumor. Solid nodules that have long duct extensions or extensive branch patterns tend to have extensive intraductal (DCIS) components (EIC) that increase the likelihood of local recurrence.

Acoustic Shadowing

Acoustic shadowing is a hard suspicious finding that suggests the presence of invasive malignancy. Acoustic shadowing tends to occur in solid nodules that lie on the spiculated end of the malignant spectrum and represent about one third of all solid malignant nodules. The desmoplastic components of the tumor substance and spiculations cause the shadowing (Fig. 23-27A). Because breast carcinomas can be internally heterogeneous, only part of a solid malignant nodule might give rise to acoustic shadowing (see Fig. 23-27B). High-grade invasive ductal carcinomas, the most frequent nodules that lie within the circumscribed end of the malignant spectrum, do not cause shadowing, and in fact, usually result in **enhanced sound transmission** (Fig. 23-28A), and many intermediate-grade lesions demonstrate normal sound transmission (see Fig. 23-28B). Other parts of the lesion might be associated with normal or enhanced sound transmission. Even pure DCIS that is high nuclear grade may be associated with enhanced through transmission. Special type tumors and invasive lobular carcinomas also tend to cause either acoustic shadowing or enhanced sound transmission. Most invasive lobular carcinomas and all tubulolobular carcinomas cause acoustic shadowing. Some tubular carcinomas that are less than 1.5 cm in diameter and all tubular carcinomas 1.5 cm or larger in maximum diameter cause acoustic shadowing. The differential diagnosis for malignant nodules that cause acoustic shadowing in order of frequency is: (1) low- to intermediate-grade invasive ductal carcinoma; (2) invasive lobular carcinoma; (3) tubulolobular carcinoma; and (4) tubular carcinomas. Special type tumors that are associated with enhanced through transmission include colloid (mucinous) carcinomas 1.5 cm or larger in diameter, medullary carcinomas, and invasive lobular carcinomas. The differential diagnosis for malignant nodules that are associated with enhanced through transmission in order of frequency is (1) high-grade invasive ductal carcinomas; (2) high nuclear-grade DCIS; (3) colloid carcinomas 1.5 cm in diameter or larger; (4) medullary carcinomas; and (5) invasive papillary carcinomas.

Calcifications

Calcifications are mammographic suspicious findings that have been applied directly to sonography. Calcifications within solid nodules are soft suspicious sonographic findings that suggest the presence of DCIS components. The calcifications occur in necrotic debris within the center of the lumen of DCIS-distended ductules or ducts and are usually associated with other soft suspicious findings, occurring within the center of microlobulations, duct extensions, or branch patterns (Fig. 23-29). The calcifications shown sonographically

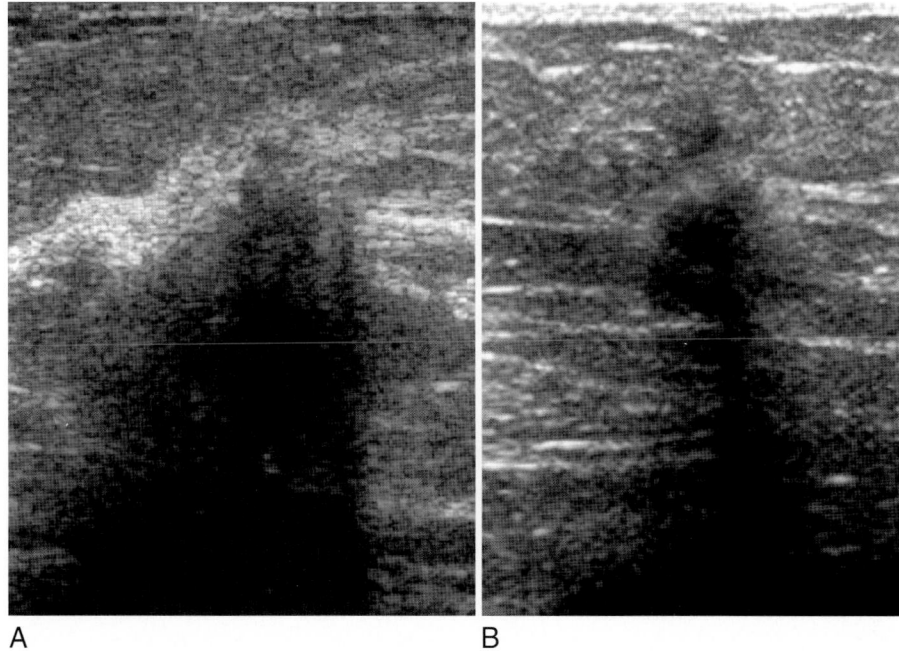

A   B

FIGURE 23-27. Cancer causing acoustic shadowing. Acoustic shadowing is a "hard" finding that suggests the presence of desmoplastic invasive tumor. Any acoustic shadowing should be considered suspicious—whether **A**, complete or **B**, partial. Tumors that are becoming progressively more de-differentiated and that contain mixtures of low- and intermediate- or high-grade components tend to create partial shadows.

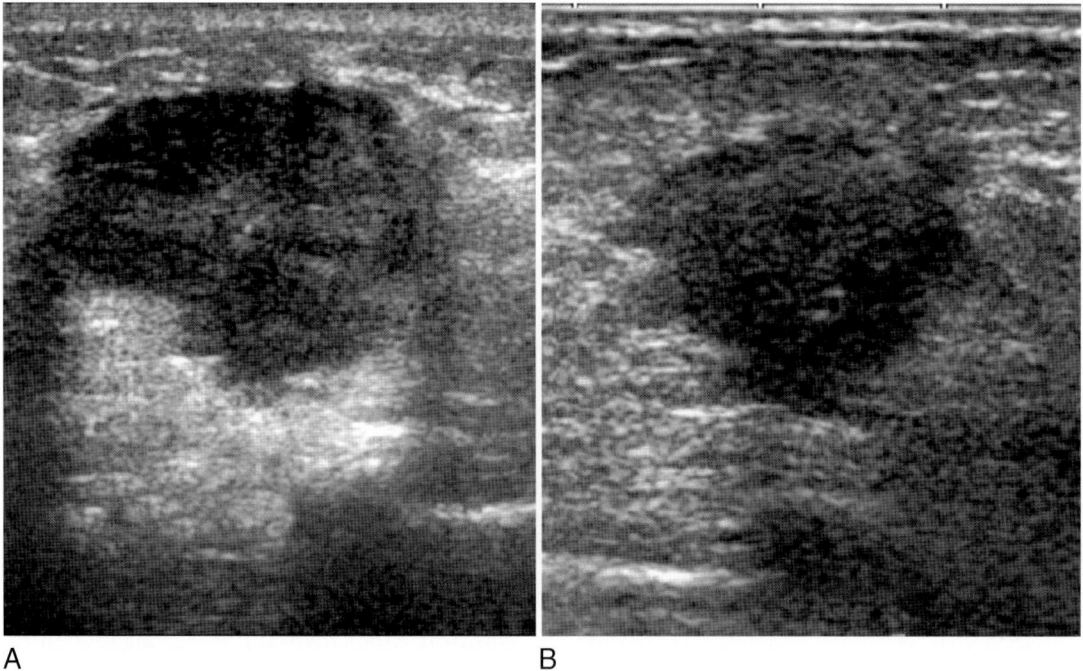

A   B

FIGURE 23-28. Variable sound transmission deep to carcinomas. About one third of malignant nodules cause acoustic shadowing, but one third have normal sound transmission and one third cause enhanced sound transmission. High-grade invasive ductal carcinomas tend to be associated with **A**, enhanced sound transmission, and intermediate-grade invasive duct carcinomas tend to be associated with **B**, normal or mixed sound transmission.

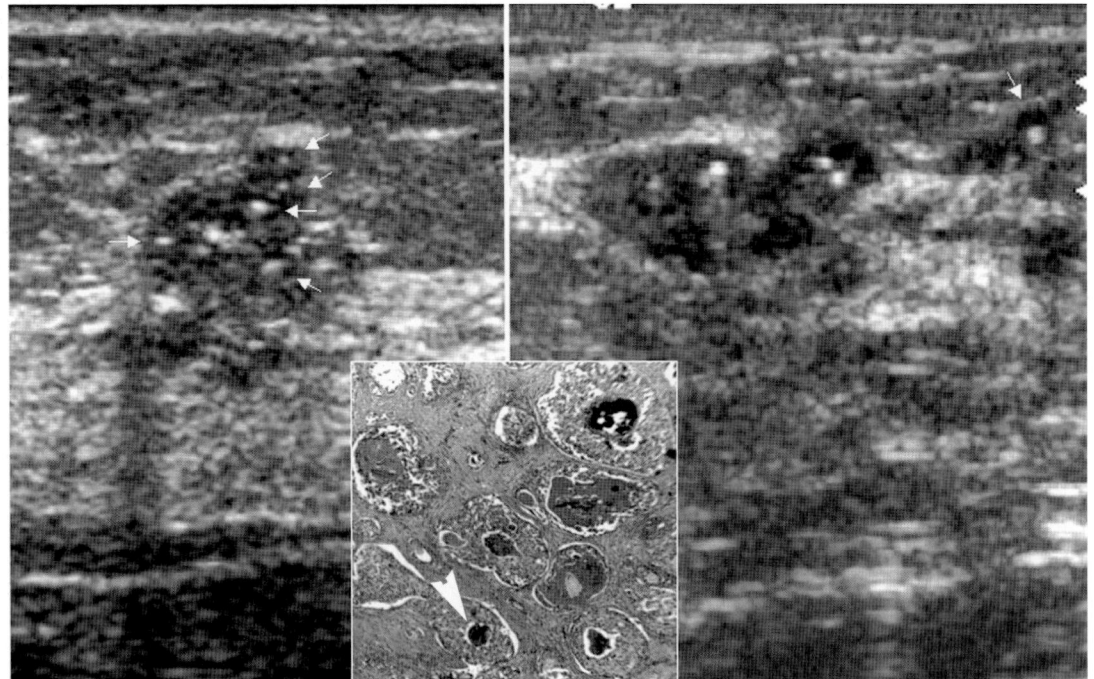

FIGURE 23-29. Calcifications. Calcifications appear as bright echoes without acoustic shadows. They are soft findings that suggest the presence of DCIS elements and are usually associated with other soft findings occurring **A,** within microlobulations (*arrows*) and **B,** duct extensions or branch patterns (*arrow*). Inset box shows histologic appearance of microcalcification (*arrowhead*) within small ducts. DCIS, Ductal carcinoma in situ.

are smaller than the beam width; therefore, they are subject to volume averaging and do not cast acoustic shadows. They appear as bright echoes that seem larger than their true size when sonographically visible. Most **benign calcifications** lie within a fairly echogenic background, so that when volume is averaged with the surrounding tissues, they are no longer bright enough to be identified sonographically. **Malignant calcifications** lie within rather homogeneously hypoechoic tumor substance and remain visible even though they are subject to volume averaging with surrounding tissues. Sonography can generally demonstrate a higher percentage of malignant than benign calcifications.

Hypoechogenicity

Marked hypoechogenicity of the substance of a solid nodule (compared to fat) is a mixed suspicious sonographic finding for malignancy. It can be the result of several different tumor characteristics. High-grade invasive ductal carcinomas that contain abundant hyaluronic acid within the extracellular matrix may appear hypoechoic because of the high water content. Pure DCIS may appear hypoechoic because of comedonecrosis and secretion within the lumens of tumor filled ductules, and low-grade invasive ductal carcinomas may appear markedly hypoechoic because of acoustic shadowing (Fig. 23-30). In recent years, as we have pushed the transducer frequency, bandwidth, and system dynamic

range to their limits, the percentage of malignant nodules that appears markedly hypoechoic has decreased from about 70% to 50%. Relatively recent technical development, coded harmonic ultrasound, has made a larger percentage of all nodules appear markedly hypoechoic (Fig. 23-31).

None of the individual findings achieve a sensitivity of 98% or better because breast carcinoma is too heterogeneous to be detected with high sensitivity using a single finding. Remember that single findings can detect only one end of the malignant spectrum and some of the mixed cases, but not cases at the other end of the spectrum. Because the average breast carcinoma has five or six of the suspicious findings, the overall sensitivity for breast cancer of the algorithm using multiple findings easily exceeds our goal of 98% or greater.

Only if no suspicious findings are present should one of three benign findings be sought. These findings are (1) **pure and marked hypoechogenicity**—which represents interlobular stromal fibrous tissue; (2) an **elliptical wider-than-tall lesion shape** with the lesion completely encompassed by a thin, echogenic capsule; and (3) a **gently lobulated wider-than-tall shape with three or fewer lobulations** and with the lesion completely encompassed by a thin, echogenic capsule.

Purely hyperechoic tissue is normal interlobular stromal fibrous tissue, which can result in either palpable or mammographic abnormalities (Fig. 23-32A, B). To be considered benign, the hyperechoic tissue may contain

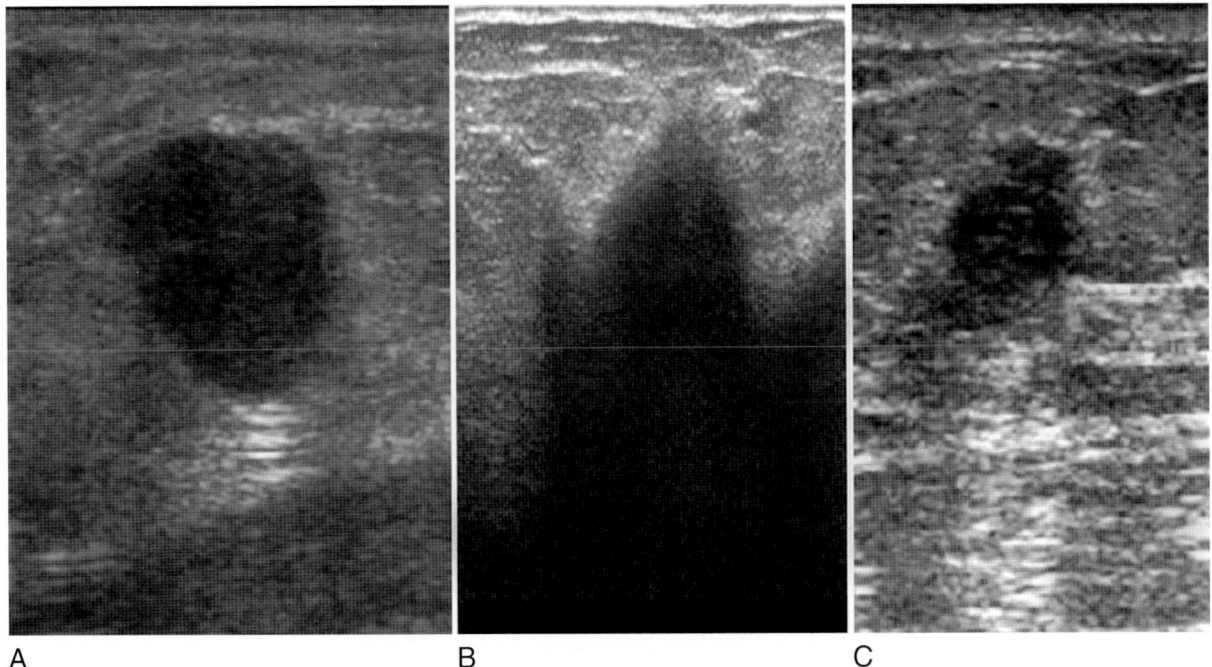

A   B   C

FIGURE 23-30. Hypoechoic carcinomas. Malignant nodules are often markedly hypoechoic in comparison to fat. Hypoechogenicity can be the result of high **A**, cellularity and high content of hyaluronic acid within the extracellular matrix or **B**, from intense acoustic shadowing associated with invasive carcinomas. **C**, Necrosis within the lumen of tumor containing ductules can cause marked hypoechogenicity in lesions composed of pure ductal carcinoma in situ (DCIS).

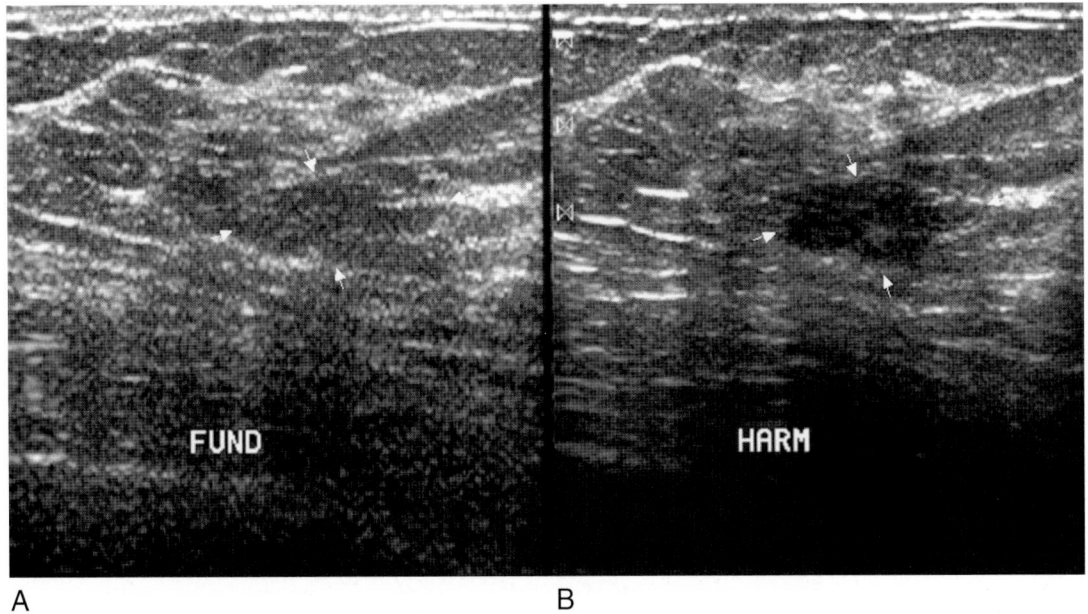

A   B

FIGURE 23-31. Harmonic imaging improves mass visibility. A, Nodules that are isoechoic with surrounding tissues and difficult to identify with fundamental imaging (*arrows*) often appear **B**, markedly hypoechoic and more conspicuous (*arrows*) when viewed with harmonics.

normal-sized ducts or TDLUs, but should contain no isoechoic or hypoechoic structures larger than normal ducts or lobules. Purely hyperechoic carcinomas are exceedingly rare, but occasionally, a carcinoma may have a very small hypoechoic central nidus and a very thick, echogenic halo, and technical errors such as volume averaging or tangential imaging through the halo can make the lesion falsely appear to be purely hyperechoic (see Fig. 23-32C).

An elliptical wider-than-tall shape is the classic shape of fibroadenomas. However, we require that this shape also be encompassed completely by a thin, echogenic

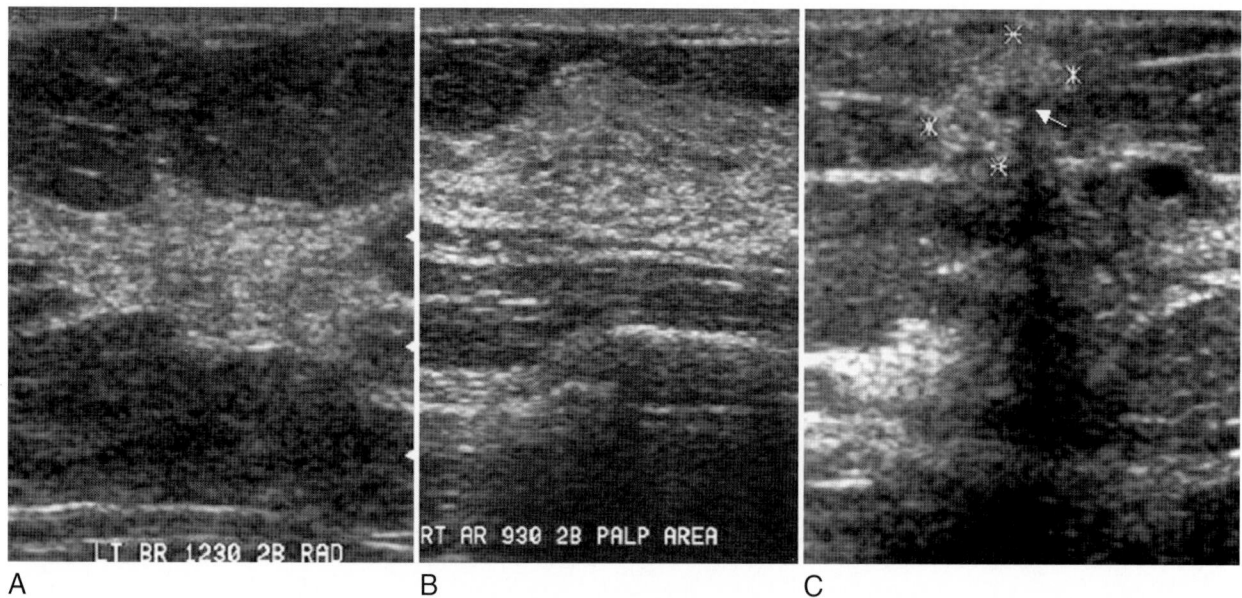

FIGURE 23-32. Normal interlobular stromal fibrous tissue. Patients can present with purely and intensely hyperechoic breast tissue. Isolated collections of hyperechoic fibrous tissue can cause **A**, mammographic nodules and masses or **B**, palpable ridges. The negative-predictive value of purely and intensely hyperechoic tissue is essentially 100%. However, collections of hyperechoic tissue should not contain any hypoechoic or isoechoic areas that are larger than normal ducts or TDLUs. **C**, Certain small invasive carcinomas can occur with very small hypoechoic foci (*arrow*) that are surrounded by very thick, echogenic halos (*caliper markers*). Near-field volume averaging or tangential imaging through the thick, echogenic halo of such lesions can make them falsely appear to be purely hyperechoic. TDLUs, Terminal ductolobular units.

FIGURE 23-33.
Fibroadenoma. A, The classic shape of benign fibroadenomas is elliptical. Such lesions are wider than tall and completely encompassed by a thin, echogenic capsule. **B**, The second most common shape of benign fibroadenomas is gently lobulated. Classic lobulated fibroadenomas have three or fewer lobulations, are wider than tall, and are completely encompassed by a thin, echogenic capsule.

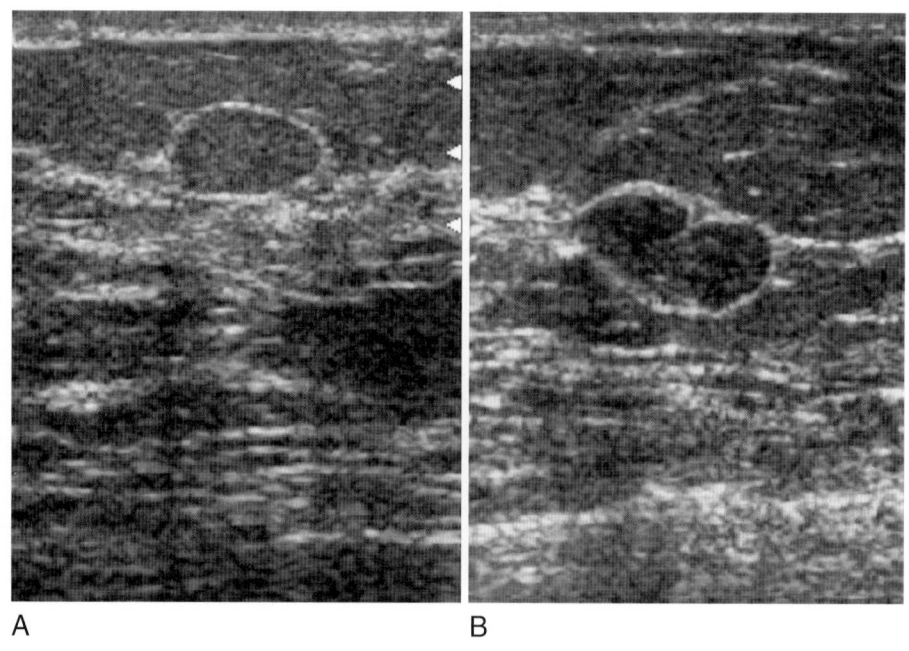

capsule to meet strict criteria for BIRADS 3 classification (Fig. 23-33A).

A gently lobulated wider-than-tall shape that contains three or fewer lobulations is the second most common shape of fibroadenomas. As is the case for elliptical lesions, there must be a demonstrable thin, echogenic capsule surrounding the entire lesion before it can be characterized as BIRADS 3. Nodules that appear to be

elliptical in one view and gently lobulated in the orthogonal view are common (see Fig. 23-33B). The negative-predictive value of the elliptical shape is 97%, and the negative-predictive value of the gently lobulated shape is 99% in a population of nodules where 33% of the nodules are malignant.

It is important to combine the elliptical or gently lobulated shapes with the presence of a complete, thin, echogenic capsule in order to minimize false negatives in circumscribed carcinomas (which may be surrounded by a thin, echogenic pseudocapsule) and in pure DCIS (which is surrounded by the intact thin, echogenic duct wall). Circumscribed carcinomas or pure DCIS nodules that are surrounded by thin, echogenic capsules are almost never elliptical or gently lobulated in shape. They are usually associated with other suspicious findings, such as angular margins, taller-than-wide shape, micro-lobulation, duct extension, or branch pattern. The thin, echogenic pseudocapsule that can be seen around circumscribed carcinomas is often absent along part of the surface of the nodule. By combining the presence of a **complete thin**, **echogenic capsule** with the elliptical or gently lobulated shape, the negative-predictive value is increased to greater than 99%.

Rocking the transducer in its short axis and heeling and toeing the transducer along its long axis are often necessary in order to demonstrate the presence of a thin, echogenic capsule along the edges of the nodule. Using less compression often helps to demonstrate the thin, echogenic capsule in benign nodules that are surrounded by hyperechoic fibrous tissue.

The sensitivity for carcinoma in the entire population of solid nodules and the negative-predictive value for nodules meeting strict criteria for BIRADS 3 both exceed 98%. Thus, by using multiple findings in a strict algorithmic approach, we are able to identify a subgroup of solid nodules that meets the mammographic definition for BIRADS 3—a 2% or lower risk of being malignant (Table 23-3). Table 23-4 shows the results of sonographic characterization into BIRADS categories. Note that the actual percentage of malignant nodules within each BIRADS category falls within the predicted risk for that specific category.

Complex and Complicated Cysts

Simple cysts are anechoic, are surrounded completely by a thin, echogenic capsule, have enhanced sound transmission and thin edge shadows (Fig. 23-34). Cysts that meet strict criteria for being simple are definitively benign and do not require further diagnosis. Biopsy, aspiration, and even follow-up are not necessary. Aspiration is generally reserved for relief of pain and tenderness in very tense simple cysts.

Traditionally, any cyst that did not meet the strict criteria for a simple cyst was characterized as complex. Recently, a further distinction has been made. Cysts that have thick walls, thick septations, or mural nodules have

TABLE 23-3. CURRENT STUDY—CHARACTERIZATION OF SOLID BREAST NODULES

	Benign Histology	Malignant Histology	Totals
Negative US (BIRADS 2,3)	245(TN)	1 (FN)	246
Positive US (BIRADS 4a,4b,5)	559 (FP)	406 (TP)	965
Total	804	407	1211

Sensitivity-406/ 07 = 99.8%
Negative predictive value-245/246 = 99.6%
Specificity-245/804 = 30.5%
Positive predictive value-406/965 = 42.1%
Accuracy—(245 + 406)/1211 = 53.8%
TN—True negative
FP—False positive
FN—False negative
TP—True positive

TABLE 23-4. PROSPECTIVE CHARACTERIZATION OF 1211 SOLID NODULES INTO BIRADS CATEGORIES*

BIRADS Category	No. of Nodules Biopsied	No. of Malignant Nodules	Expected Risk of CA	Actual Risk of CA
2	15	0	0%	0%
3	231	1	<2%	0.4%
4a	515	52	3%-49%	10%
4b	191	118	50%-89%	62%
5	259	236	>90%	91%
TOTALS	1211	407		34%

All 1211 nodules have undergone biopsy.

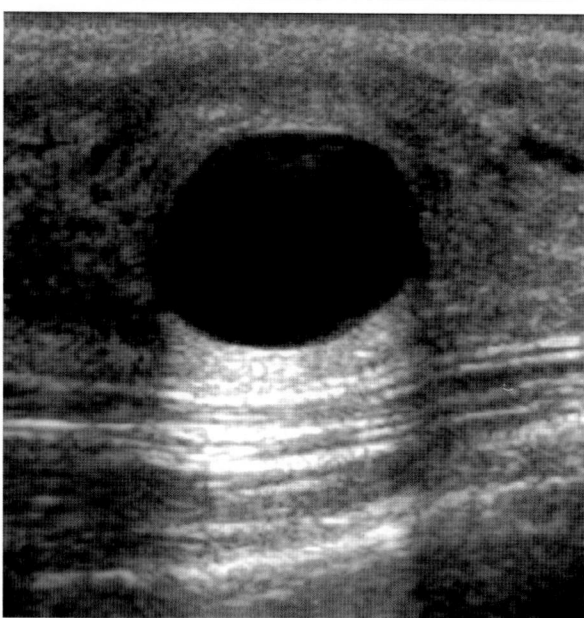

FIGURE 23-34. Cysts. Cysts that are anechoic, have enhanced sound transmission, well-circumscribed borders, thin edge shadows, and thin echogenic walls are simple cysts. They are benign (BIRADS 2) and do not need to be aspirated or even followed.

been classified as **complex**, whereas those containing echogenic fluid or debris have been considered **complicated**. We prefer the older, more traditional approach.

We all generally worry too much about complex cysts. A good general rule is that most complex cysts fall within the broad spectrum of fibrocystic change and malignant cysts are rare. However, general rules are never comforting to a patient. A systematic method for evaluating complex breast cysts is needed. The greatest difficulty in developing an algorithm for evaluating complex cysts is that the standards for cysts (aspiration with fluid cytology and follow-up) are much less reliable than the histologic standard used for solid nodules. It takes many more cases over a much longer period of time to develop an algorithm for complex cysts than it does for developing a solid nodule algorithm. The algorithm that we use for evaluation of complex cysts has been derived from the mammographic and solid nodule algorithms. Like the mammographic and sonographic solid nodule algorithms, it contains multiple suspicious and benign findings, requires looking for suspicious findings first, and looking for benign findings only in cases where no suspicious findings are present. The presence of even a single suspicious finding requires exclusion from BIRADS 2 category, and in most instances exclusion from the BIRADS 3 category as well.

Strict criteria must be met for characterization as BIRADS 2. BIRADS 3 lesions must undergo short interval follow-up. If strict criteria for BIRADS 2 or 3 cannot be met, the lesion must be characterized as

BIRADS 4a by default. We believe strongly that complex cysts that are classified as BIRADS 4a should not be assessed with fluid cytology, but should be evaluated histologically either by ultrasound-guided needle localization excisional biopsy, or more often, with ultrasound-guided 11 gauge directional vacuum-assisted biopsy (DVAB). In cases undergoing ultrasound-guided DVAB, a marker should always be deployed in case the histology reveals malignancy or atypia.

There are two levels of suspicion for complex cysts. The first is suspicion of a true intracystic papillary lesion such as **intracystic papilloma or carcinoma**, and the second is **for acute inflammation or infection**. Sonography is not as effective at distinguishing benign intracystic papilloma from carcinoma as it is in characterizing solid nodules because of the direction of invasion. Invasion arising from solid nodules is outwardly directed, greatly affecting the shape and the surface characteristics of the lesion that we greatly rely on. However, invasion arising from intracystic lesions is inwardly directed, extending into the fibrovascular stalk of the lesion. It does not affect the surface characteristics and shape that we depend on for sonographic characterization of solid nodules. Any intracystic papillary lesion should be characterized as BIRADS 4a or higher and undergo histologic evaluation. Acutely inflamed or infected cysts can be characterized as BIRADS 3 and can undergo ultrasound-guided aspiration.

Findings that are suspicious for true intracystic papillary lesions include thick isoechoic septations, certain mural nodules, the presence of a Doppler demonstrable vascular stalk within a thick septation, mural nodule, or clustered complex microcysts. Thick, isoechoic septations are suspicious for **intracystic papilloma or intracystic carcinoma** (Fig. 23-35A), whereas thin echogenic septations merely represent **fibrocystic change** and the intact walls between multiple severely cystically dilated ductules within an individual TDLU (see Fig. 23-35B). Most **mural nodules** are caused by papillary apocrine metaplasia (PAM), which is part of the fibrocystic spectrum, or are pseudonodules caused by tumefactive sludge or lipid layers in cysts that contain fat-fluid levels rather than papillomas or intracystic papillary carcinomas. Mural nodules that are suspicious demonstrate loss of the thin, echogenic outer cyst wall along their points of attachment, extension beyond the circular or oval shape of the cyst into surrounding ducts, (Fig. 23-36A) or angular margins at the point of attachment. Mural nodules that are caused by PAM remain confined within the circular or round shape of the cyst in which they lie and do not disrupt the thin, echogenic outer cyst wall (see Fig. 23-36B).

Papillomas and intracystic carcinomas are generally vascular and tend to develop easily demonstrable and prominent vascular stalks (Fig. 23-37A), whereas mural

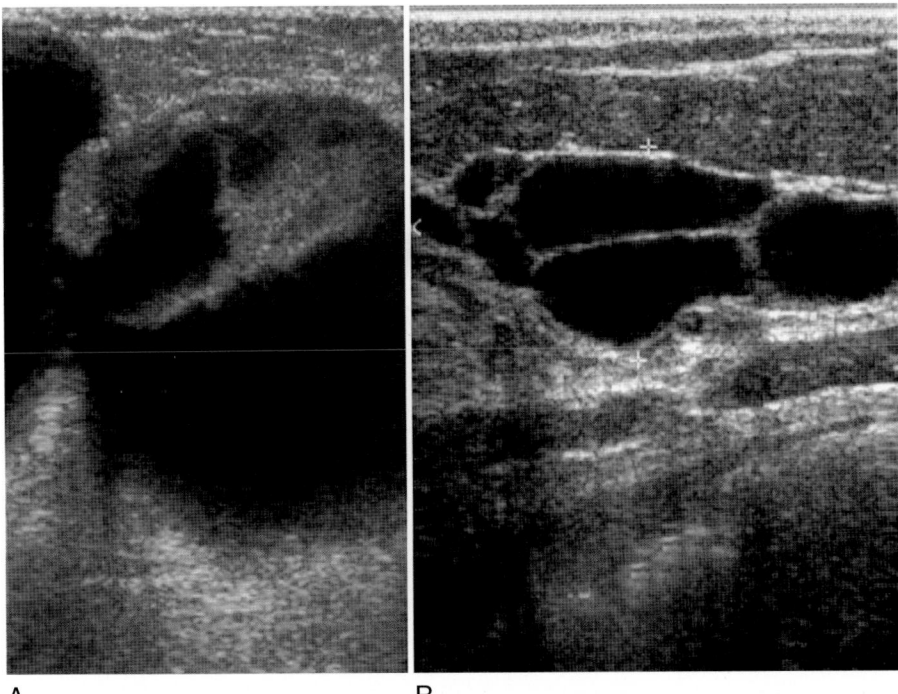

A

B

FIGURE 23-35. Septations within cystic masses. A, Thick, isoechoic septations within complex cysts are suspicious for intracystic papilloma or intracystic papillary carcinoma. **B,** Thin, echogenic septations within complex cysts are not suspicious. Such septations represent residual walls of cystically dilated ductules and are clusters of simple cysts.

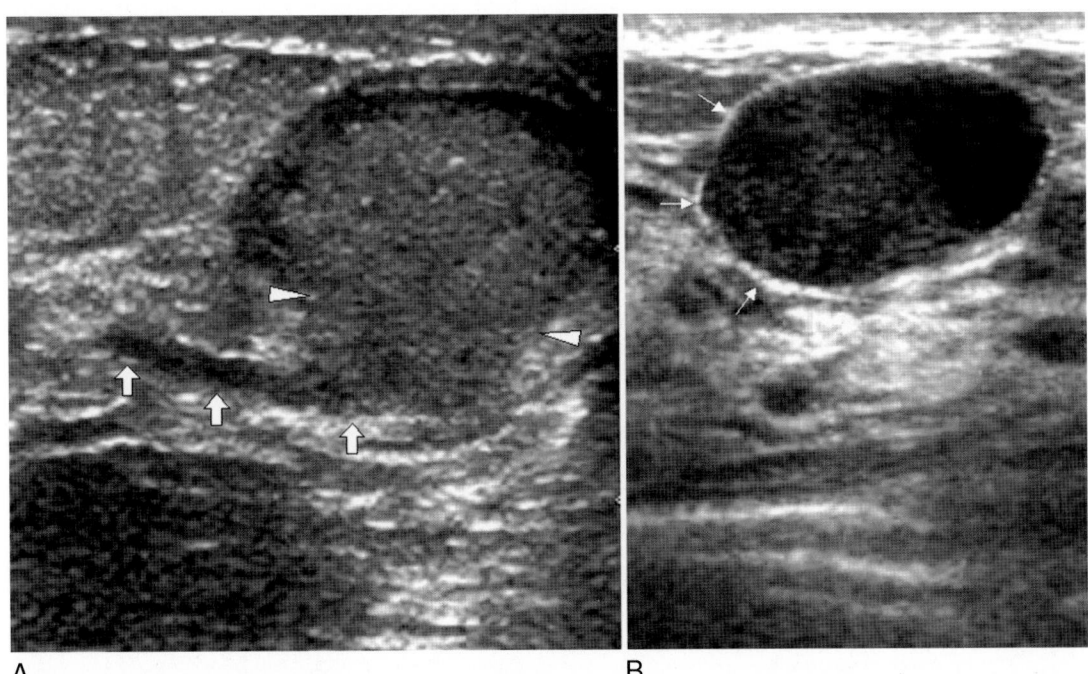

A

B

FIGURE 23-36. Mural nodules. A, Mural nodules that protrude beyond a circular or elliptical shape (*arrowheads*), lack a thin, echogenic capsule at the point of attachment to the cyst wall, are angular at the point of attachment, or extend into surrounding ducts (*arrows*) are suspicious for intracystic papilloma or intracystic papillary carcinoma. **B,** Mural nodules that are caused by papillary apocrine metaplasia remain confined within the circular or elliptical shape of the cyst. The thin, echogenic outer wall of the cyst is intact all along the attached surface of the mural nodule (*arrows*).

nodules and thick internal septations caused by florid PAM rarely develop vascular stalks (see Fig. 23-37B). Clustered complex microcysts most frequently merely represent fibrocystic change (FCC) (Fig. 23-38A), but high nuclear-grade DCIS with extensive comedonecrosis can also appear as complex clustered microcysts (see Fig. 23-38B). High nuclear-grade DCIS is usually vascular on color Doppler, whereas fibrocystic change is usually avascular on color Doppler assessment. Papillomas and intracystic carcinomas frequently undergo

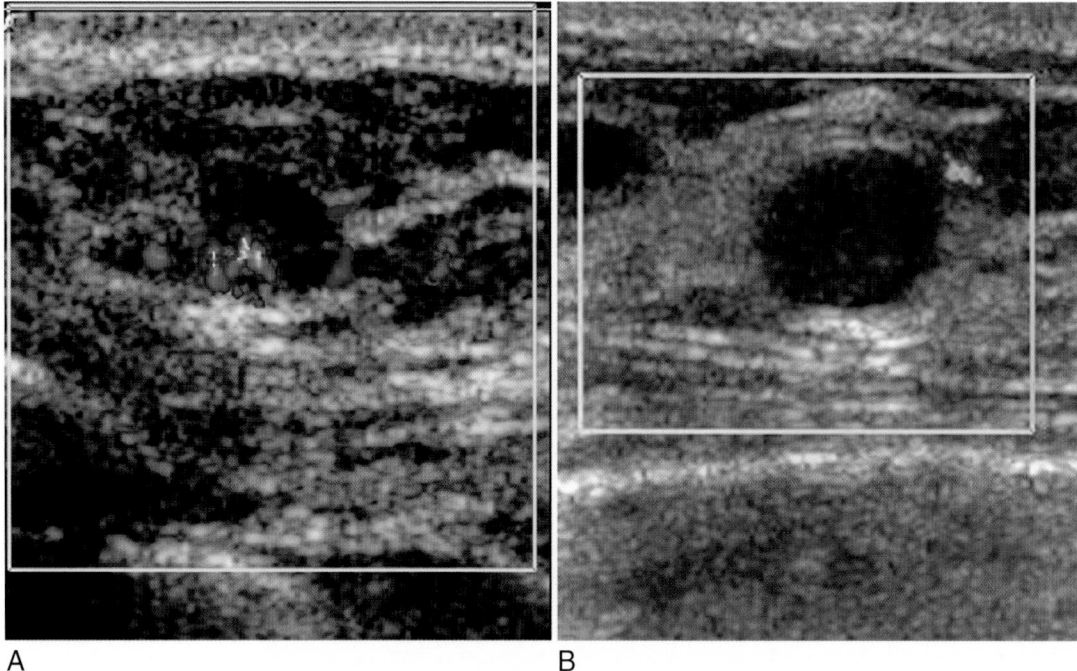

FIGURE 23-37. Use of color Doppler for mural nodules. Mural nodules caused by papilloma or papillary carcinoma frequently have very prominent vascular stalks. **A,** Mural nodules caused by intracystic carcinoma tend to be fed by multiple vessels, whereas benign papillomas tend to be fed by a single vessel. **B,** Papillary apocrine metaplasia rarely develops a fibrovascular stalk and their mural nodules do not have demonstrable flow with color Doppler.

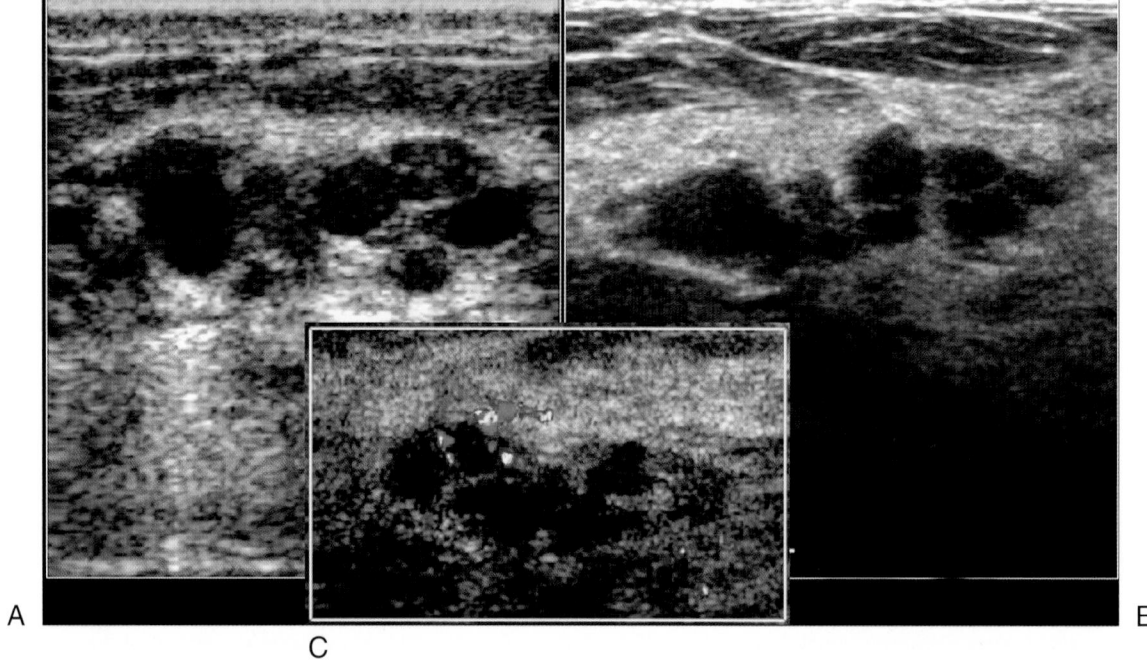

FIGURE 23-38. Clustered microcysts. Complex clustered microcysts can represent **A,** garden-variety fibrocystic change or **B,** high nuclear-grade DCIS with extensive cystic change or necrosis within tumor-filled ductules. Unfortunately, the gray-scale appearances of FCC and DCIS may be indistinguishable. **C,** Complex clustered microcysts caused by DCIS frequently show internal blood flow on color or power Doppler, whereas clustered microcysts caused by FCC usually do not have demonstrable internal flow. DCIS, Ductal carcinoma in situ; FCC, fibrocystic change.

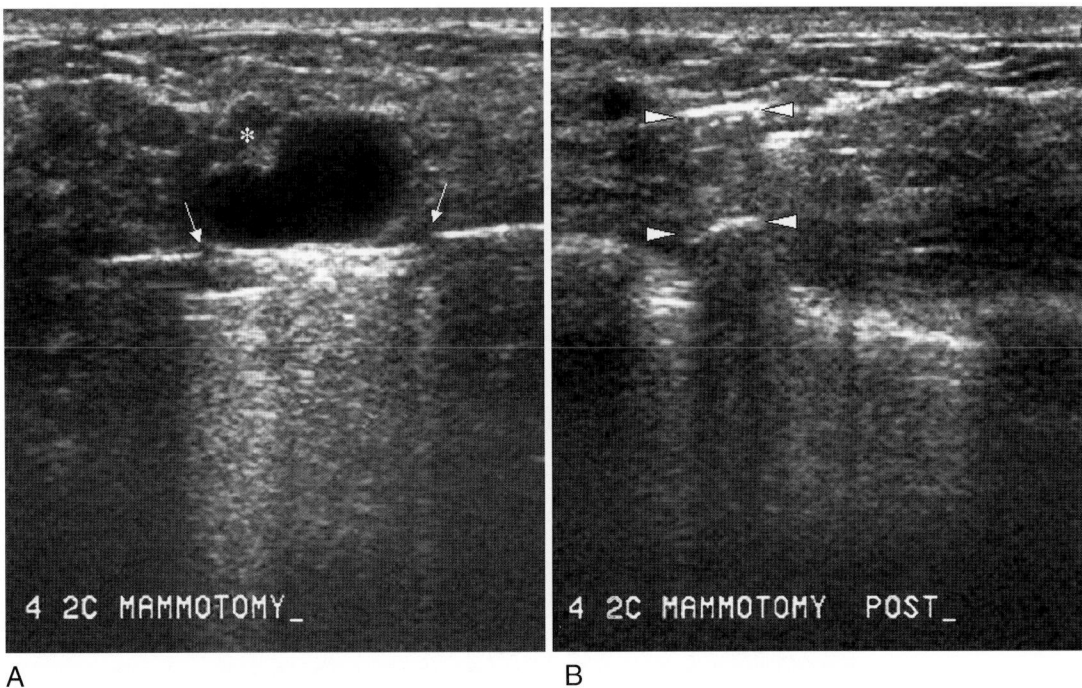

A   B

FIGURE 23-39. Complex cyst biopsy. Aspiration of complex cysts that have suspicious features is inadequate for diagnosis because cyst fluid cytology has too many false negatives and false positives. Furthermore, aspiration of the fluid may make the mural nodule or thick septation difficult to find later should the cytology be malignant or atypical. Instead, these lesions require histologic evaluation. Our preference is to perform ultrasound-guided 11 gauge directional vacuum-assisted biopsy (DVAB) and to deploy a marker at the biopsy site. **A,** This complex cyst contains a mural nodule (*). The DVAB probe has been put in position just deep to the nodule. The aperture (*arrows*) and the ringdown artifact from the vacuum holes are easily visible. **B,** After the DVAB there is no sonographically visible residual cystic or solid lesion. There is some air within the DVAB cavity (*arrowheads*).

hemorrhagic infarction that can prevent demonstration of vascularity. Most benign intracystic papillomas have a single feeding vessel, whereas malignant intracystic papillary lesions tend to incite the formation of multiple feeding vessels. As is always the case with Doppler, a positive Doppler assessment is always a better positive predictor than is a negative Doppler assessment a negative predictor. If even one of these suspicious findings is present, the cystic lesion should be characterized as BIRADS 4a or higher and should be evaluated histologically (Fig. 23-39).

The findings that are suspicious for **acute inflammation or infection** are: (1) uniform isoechoic thickening of the cyst wall; (2) fluid-debris levels (especially tumefactive sludge); and (3) inflammatory hyperemia of cyst wall. Usually all three findings coexist (Fig. 23-40A). Uniform isoechoic thickening is typical of inflammation, not tumor, so this finding does not raise concern about malignancy. Debris levels can be shown to shift to the dependent portion of the complex cyst when the patient is placed in lateral decubitus or upright positions (see Fig. 23-40B, C), but tumefactive sludge may be so viscous that 5 or more minutes are necessary for the shift to the new dependent position to occur. The hyperemic vessels in the wall of inflamed cysts course in a direction that is parallel to the cyst wall, as opposed to vessels

that feed intracystic malignancies, which tend to course perpendicular to the cyst wall. Uniform wall thickening can be seen in cysts with fibrotic walls, but in such cases, there is no hyperemia of the thickened wall. That cysts with fibrotic walls simulate the sonographic appearance of acutely inflamed cysts should not be surprising because cysts with fibrotic walls represent the healed phase of acute inflammation.

These findings indicate acute inflammation, which is common in FCC, but they do not necessarily indicate infection. However, sonographically, even after aspirating pus under ultrasound guidance, there is no way to distinguish acute bland inflammation from infection. The fluid contents and the debris layer within acutely inflamed cysts can be completely aspirated in most cases, but the residually thickened cyst wall will persist. Because the sonographic appearances of acute inflammation are so characteristic and do not raise questions about neoplasm, we usually do not perform cytologic evaluation of the aspirated cyst fluid. Rather, we obtain gram stain and culture, and in most cases cover the patient with a 72-hour prescription of antibiotics that cover *Staphylococcus* while we await culture results.

Only when there are no findings suspicious for true intracystic papillary lesions or acute inflammation do we look for definitively benign (BIRADS 2) findings. Many

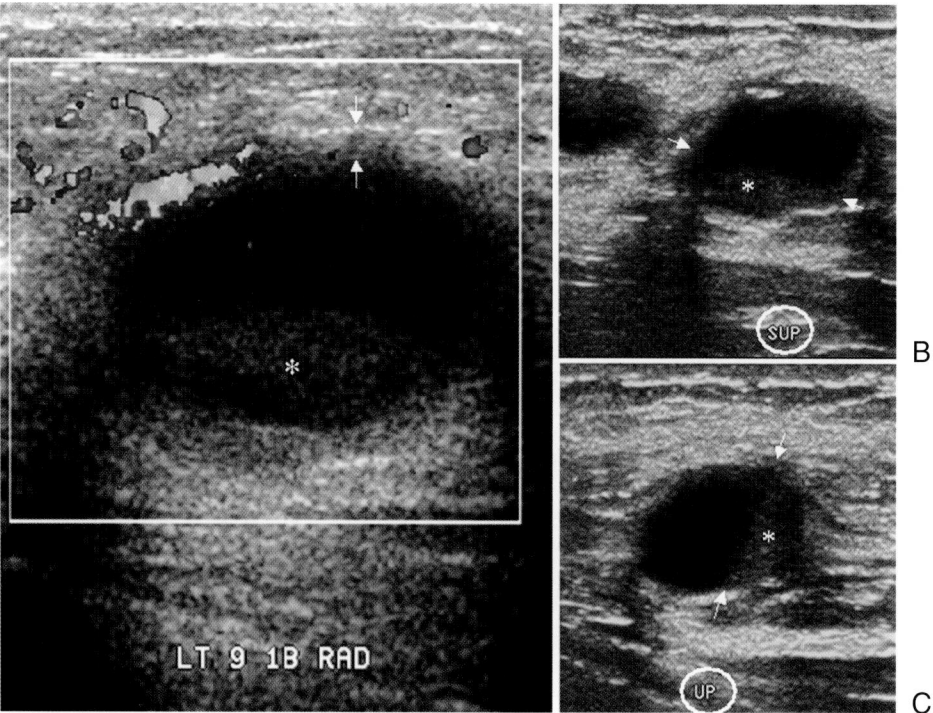

FIGURE 23-40. Inflamed or infected cyst. A, Acutely inflamed or infected cysts demonstrate abnormal uniform isoechoic wall thickening (between arrows), fluid debris levels, and hyperemia of the thickened wall. **B,** Supine and **C,** upright images show the debris level, like sludge within a gallbladder, will shift to the dependent part of the cyst when the position of the patient is changed from supine to upright or lateral decubitus (*—dependent debris, *arrows*—thick, isoechoic wall).

types of complex cysts can be characterized as BIRADS 2. These include: (1) cysts with mobile cholesterol crystals; (2) cysts with milk of calcium; (3) cysts with fat-fluid levels; (4) lipid cysts; (5) cysts with calcified walls; (6) cysts with thin, echogenic septations; and (7) cysts of skin origin.

Cysts can contain particles suspended in fluid that are so light that they can be moved with the energy of the B-mode imaging beam or with color or power Doppler. Such particles are subcellular in size and are commonly seen with uncomplicated FCC. Generally, high transmit power settings are necessary to cause such particles to move during real-time B-mode imaging. However, the energy of the color or power Doppler beam is high enough to cause these particles to move at even default low-power settings, creating what has been termed "color streaking." Particles are forced posteriorly by the energy of the Doppler beam, creating vertically oriented color streaks within the cyst as they move. The particles that cause color streaking appear to be cholesterol crystals that can be seen on cytologic evaluation only when viewed with polarized light.

Milk of calcium is a BIRADS 2 mammographic finding that has been directly applied to sonography. Milk of calcium is not really milk, but a collection of tiny calculi within the lumen of a cyst. Such calcifications are extremely common in FCC and can be demonstrated definitively on horizontal beam mammographic films. Sonography can prove the presence of milk of calcium by demonstrating that the calcifications move within the cyst to new dependent positions created by

lateral decubitus or upright positioning of the patient (Fig. 23-41). Although mammography can generally show smaller and more numerous calcifications than can sonography, sonography actually has one advantage over mammography in demonstrating milk of calcium. Mammography requires dozens of small calcifications before the classic "teacup" appearance can be shown on horizontal beam films, whereas sonography can definitively demonstrate milk of calcium, even when there is only a single mobile calculus within a cyst.

Fat-fluid levels within cysts are definitively benign mammographic findings that have been directly applied to ultrasound. Fat-fluid levels are rarely demonstrated mammographically, usually within classic galactoceles. Fat-fluid levels are more frequently demonstrated sonographically than they are mammographically. The lipid layer appears echogenic compared to cyst fluid and floats on the fluid in the nondependent portion of the cyst. The lipid layer can be forced to move within the cyst to a new nondependent position within the cyst by changing the patient's position from supine to lateral decubitus or upright (Fig. 23-42). Like tumefactive sludge, lipid layers tend to shift very slowly within a cyst when the patient's position is changed. It may take as long as 5 minutes to document the shift of a fat-fluid level after the patient's position is changed. During the shift in position, the shape of the interface between the lipid and fluid layers changes and is usually obliquely oriented with respect to the tabletop and has a sigmoid shape. The oblique orientation of the interface in combination with the sigmoid shape are characteristic of

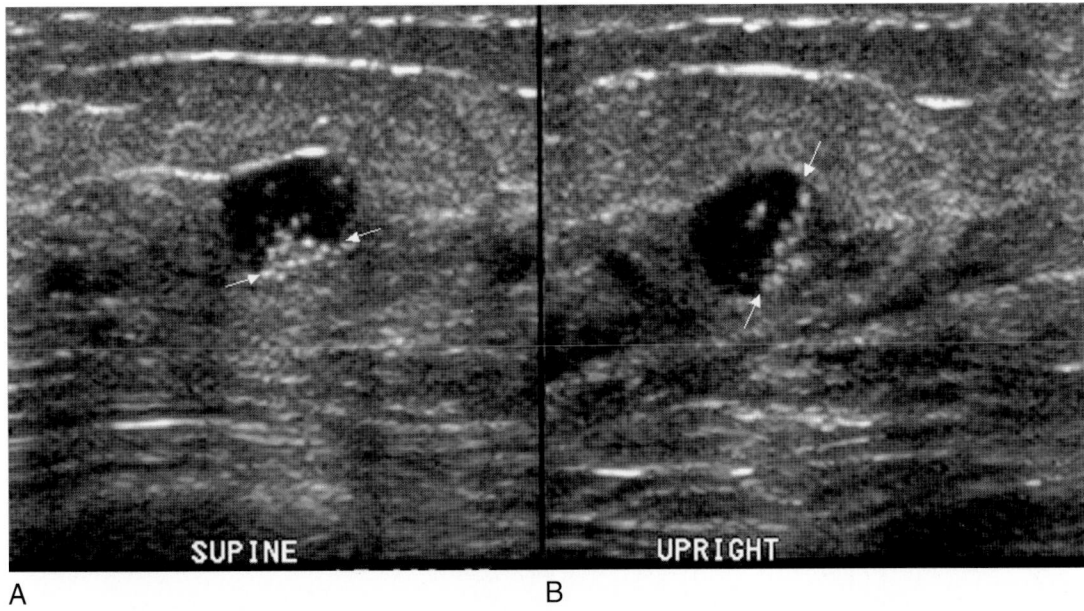

FIGURE 23-41. Milk of calcium. This is composed of tiny calculi (between arrows) within the breast cyst lumen that move to the dependent portion of the cyst when the patient changes position. **A,** They lie along the dependent posterior wall in the supine position and **B,** fall to the dependent inferior position in the upright position.

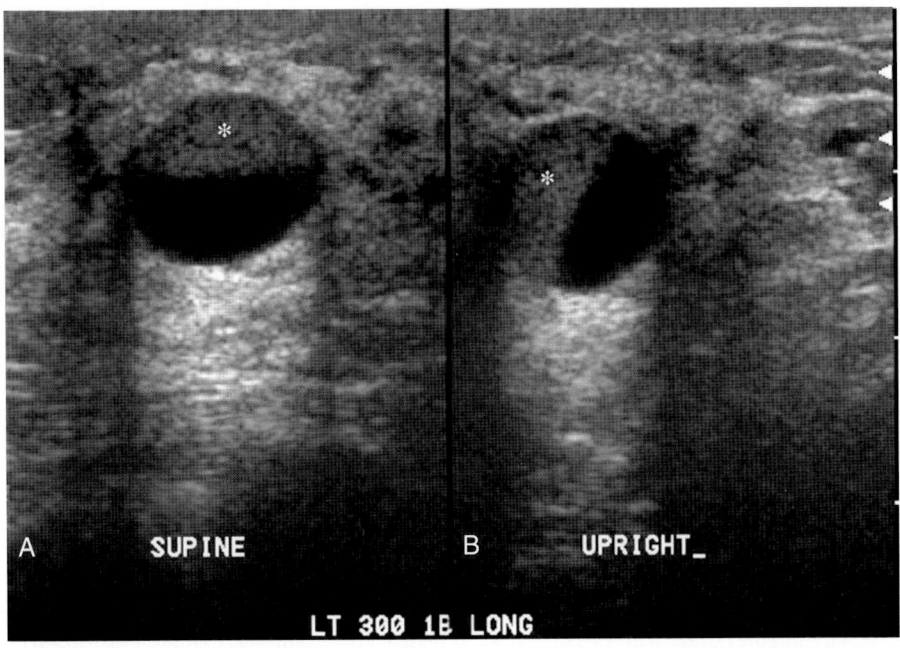

FIGURE 23-42. Fat-fluid level. The lipid layer is echogenic compared to cyst fluid and moves within the cyst to the nondependent part of the cyst when the patient changes position. **A,** Shows the echogenic lipid layer floating to the nondependent anterior wall when the patient is scanned in the supine position. **B,** Shows that the echogenic lipid layer has floated to the newly nondependent superior wall with the patient in the upright position.

a fat-fluid level in the process of equilibrating to a new position and may, in fact, represent a short cut to waiting 5 minutes or more for the fat fluid level to shift.

Lipid cysts are definitively benign mammographic findings that can be applied directly to ultrasound. Unfortunately, lipid cysts usually appear more definitively benign mammographically than they do sonographically.

Most lipid cysts have some suspicious features on sonography, such as (1) mural nodules; (2) thick septations; (3) thick walls; and (4) fluid debris levels (Fig. 23-43). This should not be surprising because it is thought that most lipid cysts originate in chronic seromas/hematomas, which often manifest such findings. The suspicious sonographic findings in lipid cysts, unlike those in cysts

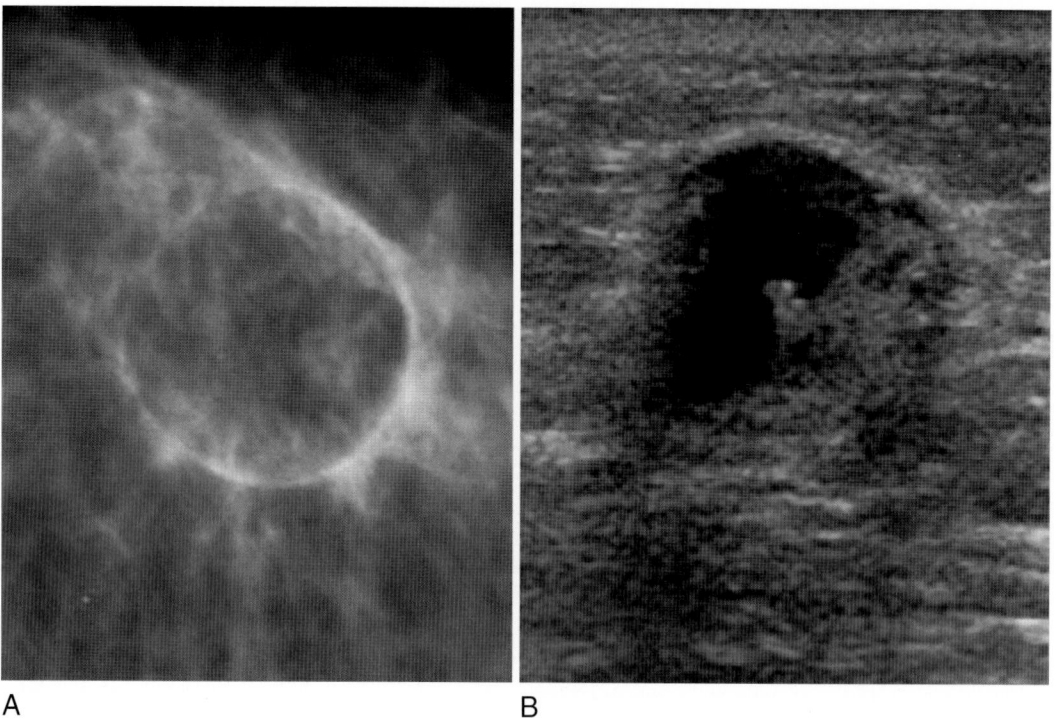

A   B

FIGURE 23-43. Lipid cyst. Mammographic spot compression views can more accurately characterize lipid cysts than can sonography. **A,** Lesions that appear to be classic, benign lipid cysts on mammography typically have suspicious features such as **B,** thick wall, thick isoechoic septations, and mural nodules on ultrasound images. These sonographic suspicious features are features of chronic hematomas from which most lipid cysts evolve.

containing true papillary lesions, do not have associated vascularity. Most lipid cysts are part of the fat necrosis spectrum, which is avascular by its nature. Nevertheless, sonography can be worrisome in patients with lipid cysts compared to spot compression mammograms. In the post lumpectomy patient or post reduction mammoplasty patients, when sonographic findings are more worrisome than mammographic findings, we rely more heavily on the mammographic findings unless there is vascularity within the lesion demonstrated on Doppler.

Eggshell calcifications are benign findings that have been applied directly to sonography. In general, eggshell calcifications are so definitively benign mammographically that they do not require sonographic assessment (Fig. 23-44A, B). Occasionally they will be seen on sonography in a patient who has not had mammography or in whom the mammograms are not available. Punctate calcifications that occur within the normal thin, echogenic cyst wall can be thought of as incomplete eggshell calcifications, and therefore, can also be considered to be BIRADS 2 sonographic findings (see Fig. 23-44C). In such cases, the sonographic findings are more definitively benign than are the mammographic findings. Calcifications that are suspended within the lumen of a cyst cannot be characterized as BIRADS 2. In most instances, they occur with papillary apocrine metaplasia (PAM), but they can also occur in DCIS.

Clusters of simple macrocysts are benign. They are the same as thinly septated cysts. Clusters of simple cysts, like individual simple cysts, are benign. Clustered macrocysts are identical to thinly septated cysts discussed and illustrated above (see Fig. 23-35B). The septations actually represent the residual walls of individual cystically dilated ductules within an individual TDLU. Each cystically dilated ductule can be thought of as a simple cyst; a thinly septated cyst is actually a cluster of simple cysts, each having BIRADS 2 characteristics.

Complex **cysts of skin origin** are benign and usually represent sebaceous cysts. Occasionally, a cyst of skin origin can represent **an epidermal inclusion cyst**. There are three typical appearances of **sebaceous cysts**. The first appearance is that of a complex or solid-appearing lesion that lies entirely within the skin (Fig. 23-45A). The second appearance is that of a complex cyst that lies mainly within the subcutaneous tissues but has clawlike hyperechoic skin wrapped around it (see Fig. 23-45B). The third appearance is that of a lesion that lies entirely within the subcutaneous fat but that has an abnormally hypoechoic, thickened inflamed hair follicle associated with it (see Fig. 23-45C). The hair follicle, which resembles a gland neck, is obliquely oriented and is often better demonstrated by heeling or toeing the transducer in order to change the angle of incidence. Because cysts of skin origin are so superficial in location that they

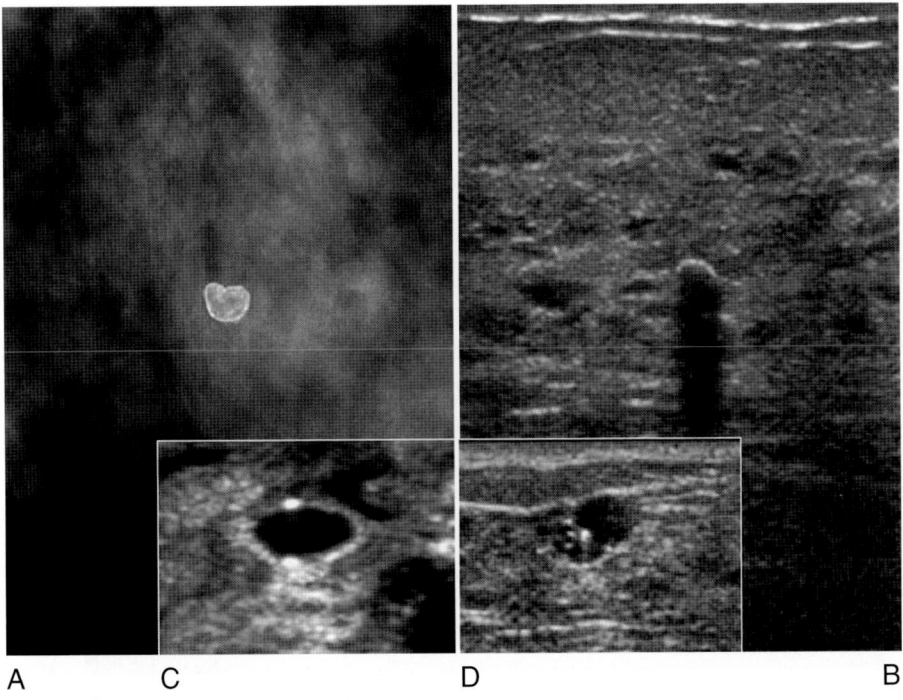

FIGURE 23-44. Eggshell calcification. A, Eggshell calcifications are mammographic findings that are definitively benign. **B,** On sonography. **C,** Punctate calcifications confined to the thin echogenic wall around cysts can be thought of as incomplete eggshell calcifications, and therefore, are benign. **D,** Immobile punctate calcifications within the interior of the cyst can be associated with papillary apocrine metaplasia or ductal carcinoma in situ.

A   C   D   B

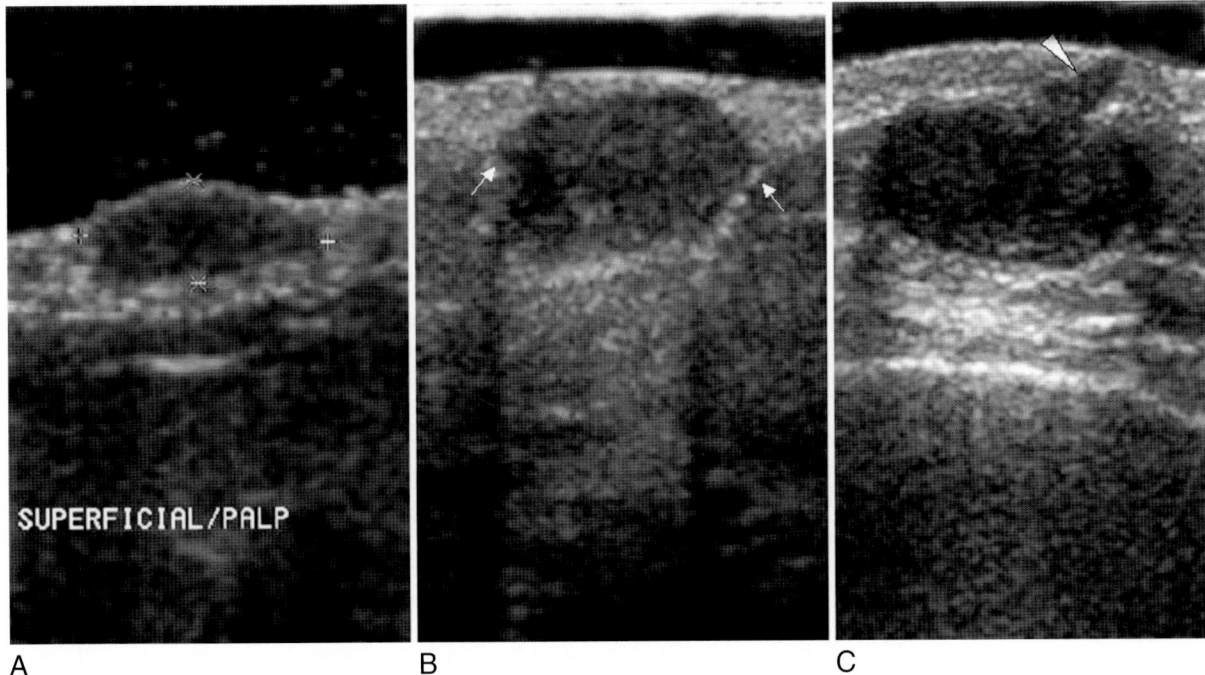

A   B   C

FIGURE 23-45. Sebaceous skin cysts. These are usually benign. **A,** Sebaceous cyst entirely within the skin (*caliper markers*). **B,** Primarily within the subcutaneous fat, but a thin claw sign of echogenic skin (*arrows*) can be shown to wrap around the cyst, confirming that it originates within the skin. **C,** Entirely within the subcutaneous fat, but an enlarged inflamed hair follicle into which the sebaceous cyst drains can be seen (*arrowhead*). A standoff of acoustic gel is necessary to see these lesions. To show the obliquely oriented hair follicle, heeling or toeing of the transducer may be necessary.

are subject to severe volume-averaging artifact, optimal demonstration of one of these three patterns usually requires that an acoustic standoff be used.

If BIRADS 2 findings cannot be demonstrated one of two BIRADS 3 appearances can be sought: (1) the "foam cyst" appearance, or (2) the "acorn cyst" appearance.

Foam cysts are cysts whose lumens are completely filled with low-level echoes (Fig. 23-46A). They have been given many different names in the literature, including: foam cysts, gel cysts, inspissated cysts, and mucoceles. In fact, foam cysts actually represent a spectrum of lesions from those that are completely filled with papillary

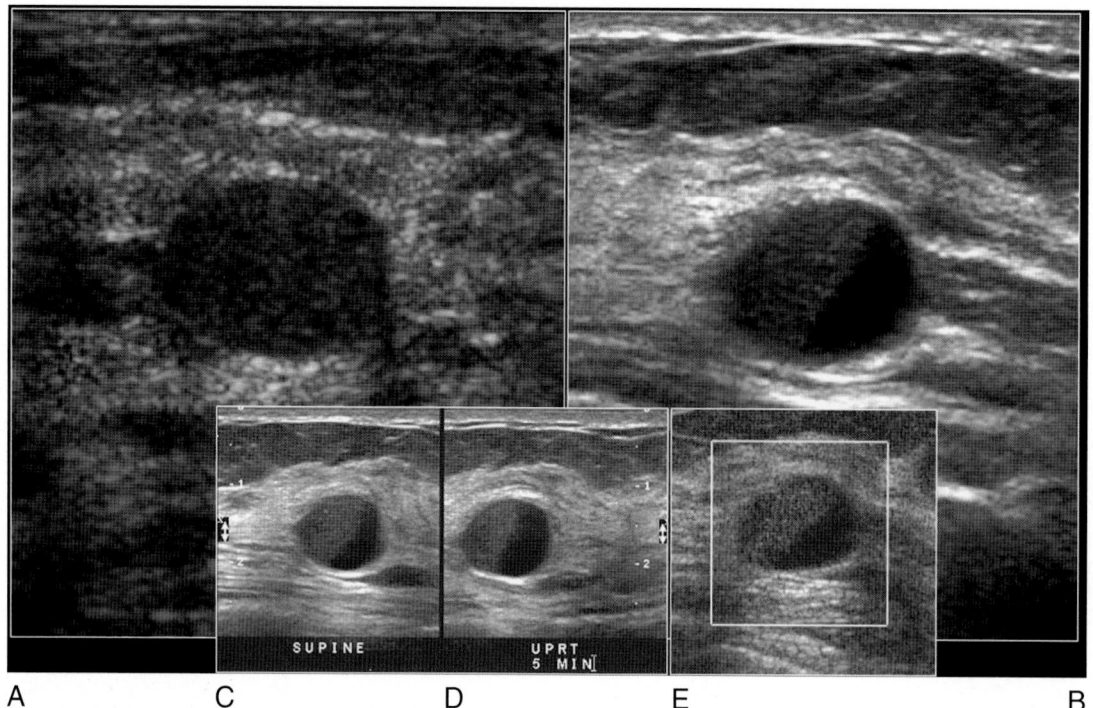

FIGURE 23-46. Foam cysts. A, Foam cysts are filled with diffuse low-level echoes, and in certain cases, can be difficult to distinguish from solid nodules and have been called inspissated cysts, gel cysts, and mucoceles in the literature. **B,** Acorn cysts have an echogenic concave rim of papillary apocrine metaplasia (PAM) that appears similar to the cap on an acorn. Unlike similar-appearing lipid layers within cysts that have fat fluid levels, the position of the PAM does not change from the **C,** supine to the **D,** upright or left lateral decubitus positions. **E,** Color Doppler image shows that, unlike intracystic papillomas or carcinomas, PAM rarely has a demonstrable vascular stalk.

apocrine metaplasia (PAM) to those that contain only echogenic proteinaceous debris or lipid material. Others may contain mixtures of PAM and proteinaceous or fatty debris. Such lesions have sonographic features that overlap with those of fibroadenomas, and in some cases (about 3%), it may not be possible to determine with certainty whether the lesion is cystic or solid. In such cases, one must assume either that the lesion is a solid nodule and characterize it or attempt to aspirate it. When these lesions are assumed to be solid nodules, they usually have characteristics that allow them to be characterized as BIRADS 3. If aspiration is attempted, it cannot be determined in advance whether the cyst can be aspirated. When the internal echoes are all caused by PAM, the lesion cannot be aspirated. When the lesion is filled with proteinaceous and/or fatty debris, it can be completely aspirated. If partially filled with PAM, the lesion will be only partially aspirated. Cytologic evaluation of aspirate of such lesions often shows apocrine snouts diagnostic of benign FCC.

Acorn cysts have either a mural nodule or a crescentic, eccentrically thickened wall caused by PAM that does not completely fill the cyst (see Fig. 23-46B). Unlike the echogenic crescent within cysts that contain fat-fluid levels, the echogenic crescent caused by PAM

does not shift within the cyst when the patient changes position (see Fig. 23-46C, D). In these cases, the normal, thin echogenic outer cyst wall is preserved along the entire thickened wall and there is no vascular stalk (see Fig. 23-46E).

Acorn cysts and foam cysts that are characterized as BIRADS 3 should undergo short interval follow-up. If it cannot be determined whether a lesion is cystic or solid, and if it can be characterized as BIRADS 3, the patient should be offered the options of attempted aspiration, biopsy, or short interval follow-up. If a complex cyst cannot be characterized as BIRADS 2 or 3, it must be characterized as BIRADS 4a and evaluated histologically. The algorithm for complex cysts is necessarily elaborate because of their huge histopathologic variability.

NICHE APPLICATIONS FOR BREAST ULTRASOUND

There are several niche indications for breast ultrasound that occur much less frequently than do palpable and mammographic abnormalities. Among these are assessment of: (1) nipple discharge; (2) mastitis; and (3) implants.

Nipple Discharge

This is an important niche application for breast ultrasound. Nipple discharge can be caused by large duct papillomas, carcinoma, duct ectasia, fibrocystic change with communicating cysts, and hyperprolactinemia, and may be idiopathic.

Galactography is considered the procedure of choice for evaluating nipple discharge, but the role of ultrasound is expanding and becoming more important. Sonography can be used in cases where galactography fails for technical reasons or because the patient's intermittent discharge has stopped. However, it can also be used together with galactography, and, in many cases, it can obviate both diagnostic and localizing galactography and surgery. Sonography can also be used for low-risk nipple discharge, whereas galactography can be reserved for high-risk discharge. High-risk discharge is unilateral, spontaneous, from a single duct orifice, and clear, serous, serosanguineous, or frankly bloody. It is high risk because it is often caused by papillomas or carcinoma. Low-risk discharge is bilateral, from multiple duct orifices, may be expressible rather than spontaneous, and milky or greenish in color. It is considered low risk because it is usually caused by fibrocystic change or duct ectasia. However, in our experience, even low-risk secretions can also be caused by intraductal papillary lesions.

Most **intraductal papillary** lesions that cause nipple discharge lie in the large mammary ducts under or near the areola. Such ducts are readily demonstrated sonographically, especially when distended with secretions, if appropriate scan planes and maneuvers are used. The central ducts are generally radially oriented, so radial scans are essential to show the ducts in their long axes. Warm room temperature, warm acoustic gel, and special maneuvers, such as the two-handed compression maneuver and the rolled nipple technique, help minimize shadowing that can arise in the nipple and areola.

Large **duct papillomas** appear to be isoechoic nodules (less echogenic than the duct wall) within ectatic fluid-filled ducts. The appearance of papillomas varies with the degree and distribution of duct dilation, with the diameter and length of the lesion, and with involvement of branch ducts and TDLUs. Small ovoid lesions less than 1 cm in length that do not expand the duct lumen are benign in more than 98% of cases and qualify for BIRADS 3 characterization (Fig. 23-47). However, because they cause the symptoms for which the patient presented, they usually require removal and histologic evaluation. Intraductal papillary lesions that expand the duct, that are longer than 1.5 cm, or that involve branch ducts or TDLUs have greater than a 2% risk of being malignant and should be characterized as BIRADS 4a or higher (Fig. 23-48).

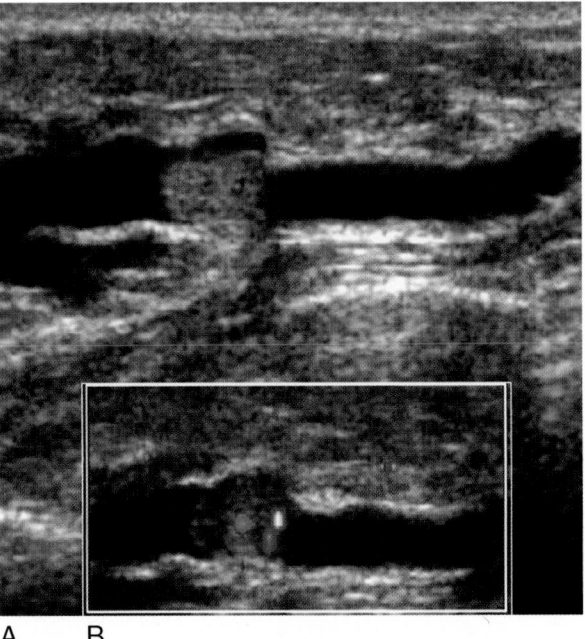

A   B

FIGURE 23-47. Intraductal papillary lesion. A, Small ovoid intraductal papillary lesions that do not expand the duct represent benign large duct papillomas in more than 98% of cases. **B,** Even small intraductal papillomas have a readily demonstrable vascular stalk in most cases.

Sonography can show causes of nipple discharge other than large duct papilloma, such as **carcinoma, duct ectasia, communicating cysts,** and **hyperprolactinemia** (Fig. 23-49). Galactography is probably superior to sonography for demonstrating causes of nipple discharge other than papilloma. Our current practice is to schedule patients who present with nipple discharge for both sonography and galactography. The sonogram is performed first, and if an intraductal papillary lesion can be identified as the cause of nipple discharge, the galactogram is canceled. The patient then undergoes ultrasound-guided 11 gauge DVAB. If a definitive cause for nipple discharge cannot be identified sonographically, galactography is performed.

When ultrasound-guided DVAB is used to biopsy intraductal papillary lesions, a marker is deployed when all imaging evidence of the lesion is removed to facilitate image-guided excisional biopsy, in case the histology is atypical or malignant. In 90% of the cases where all imaging evidence of the lesion is removed, the nipple discharge stops for a minimum of 2 years.

Infection

The main use of sonography in patients who present with mastitis is to determine whether there is an abscess and to guide aspiration of, or drain placement into, the abscess. The appearance of abscesses varies, depending on whether the mastitis is puerperal or nonpuerperal and whether it is centrally or peripherally located. **Peripheral**

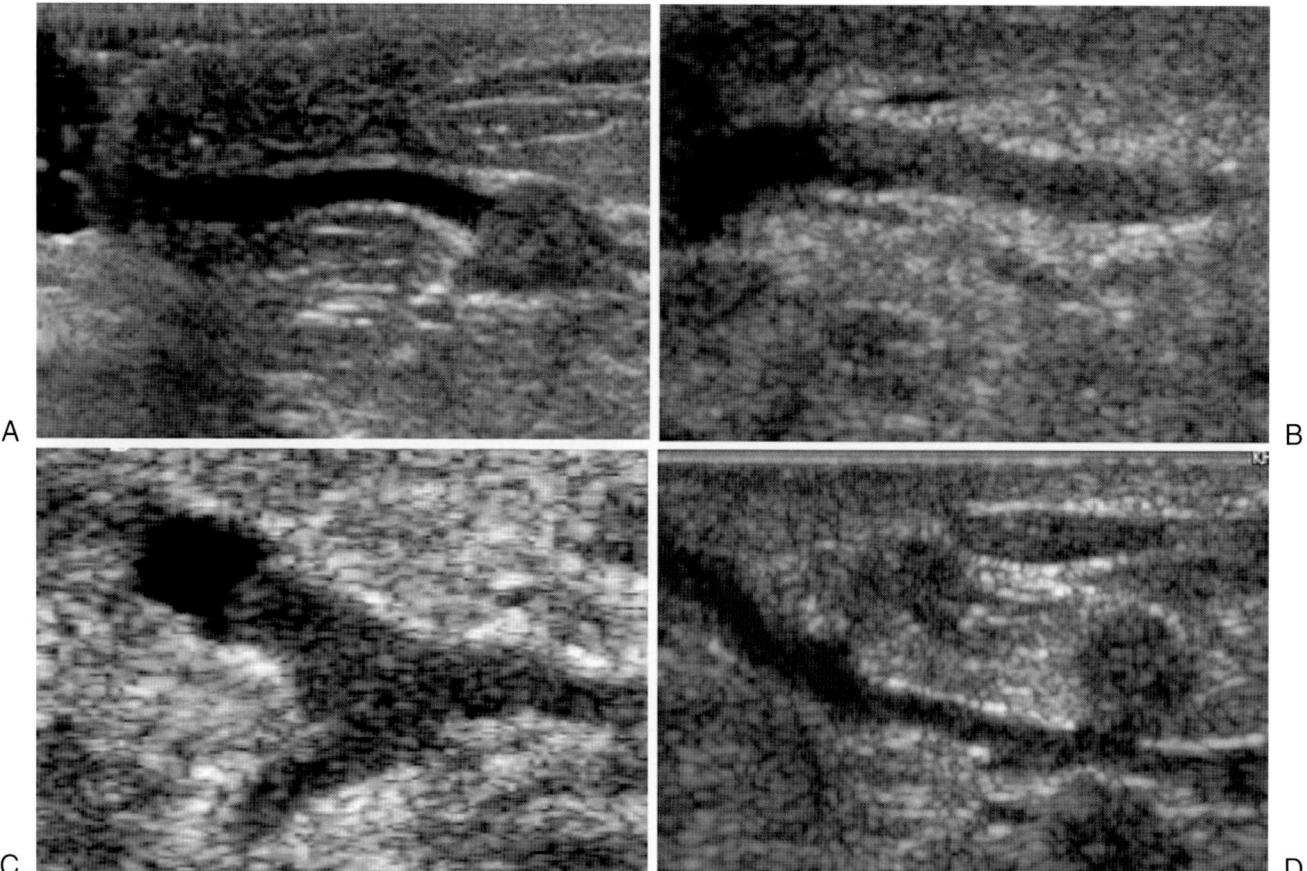

FIGURE 23-48. Intraductal papillary lesions. Intraductal papillary lesions that have greater than a 2% risk of being malignant and that should be characterized as BIRADS 4 and undergo biopsy include **A**, lesions that expand the duct or breach its wall, **B**, that are longer than 1.5 cm, **C**, that involve multiple peripheral branch ducts, or **D**, that involve TDLUs (peripheral papillomas). TDLUs, Terminal ductolobular units.

abscesses in puerperal mastitis usually arise in pre-existing galactoceles (Fig. 23-50) whereas peripheral abscesses in nonpuerperal mastitis often arise within inflamed cysts. **Central abscesses,** whether arising from puerperal or nonpuerperal mastitis (Fig. 23-51), usually result from rupture of an inflamed or infected duct and tend to be elongated in a plane that is parallel to the inflamed duct. Unilocular cysts can be treated with ultrasound-guided aspirations as needed. Loculated abscesses may require placement of a drain or surgical drainage.

Implants

MRI is generally considered the modality of choice for evaluating mammary implants. However, patients who have implants that are at risk for **rupture** are within the mammographic screening population. Such patients present with palpable lumps and mammographic densities that require sonographic evaluation more often than they present for MRI with concerns about their implants. Breast sonography has and will continue to see more implants than will ever be seen on MRI.

Sonographers must understand the wide variations of normal in implants and must be able to identify intracapsular and extracapsular rupture, silicone granulomas, herniation, and capsular infection. Implant abnormalities can cause palpable lumps or mammographic abnormalities or may be detected as incidental abnormalities in the course of evaluating other pathology.

Sonography can identify the type of implant, its implantation site, and many of the complications that affect implants. The capsule that surrounds the implant is fibrous and is a normal foreign body reaction to the implant. It is abnormal only when it becomes too thick and causes capsular contracture, when it develops a tear through which the implant can herniate, or when it becomes inflamed or infected. The implant is filled with saline or silicone gel and is surrounded by a silicone elastomer shell. The shell, a part of the implant, must be distinguished from the capsule, which is living tissue formed by the patient in response to the implant.

Normal implants can give rise to palpable abnormalities in certain cases. **Radial folds** can be palpable when the patient is in certain positions. It is important to scan the patient when she is in the position where

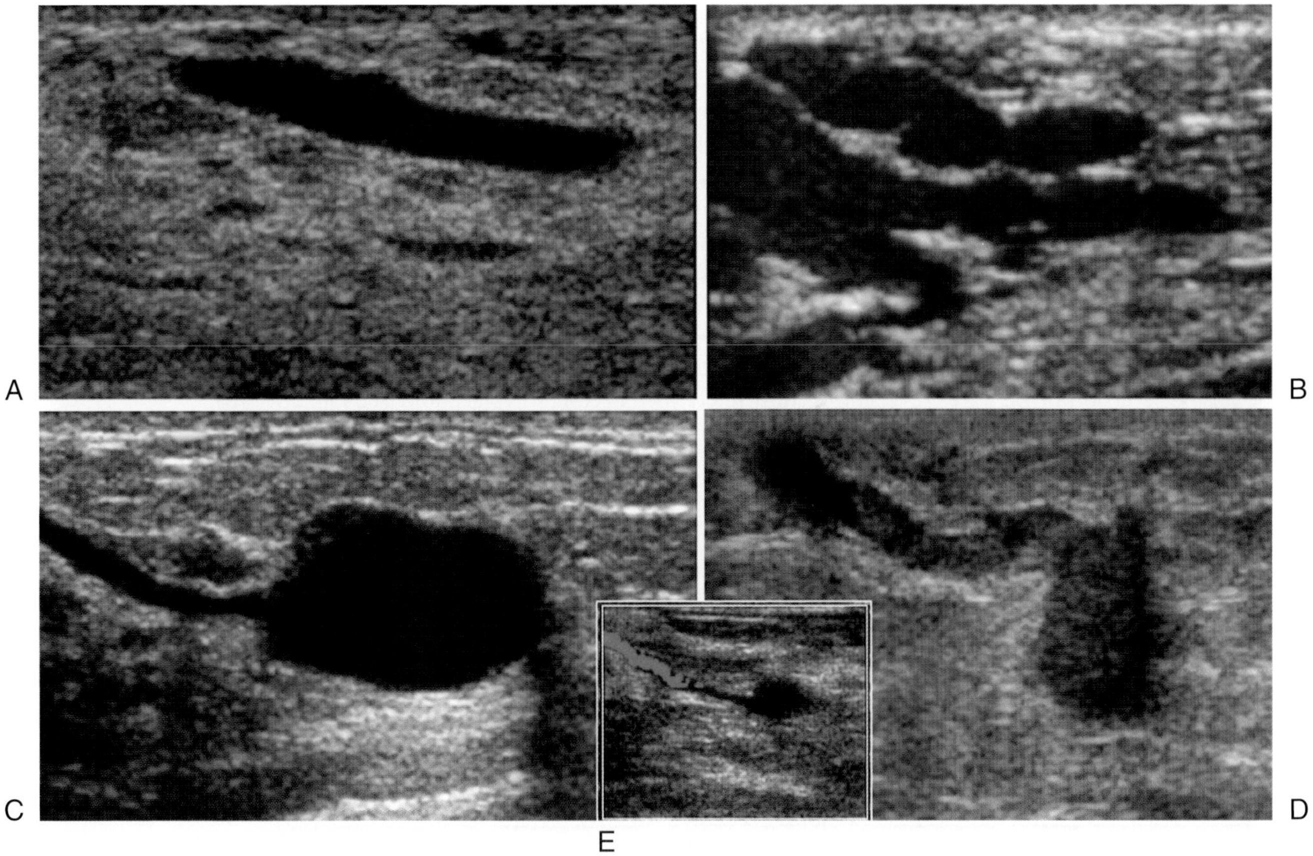

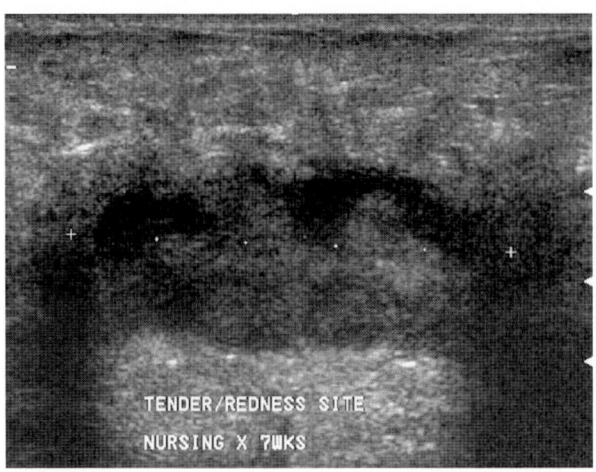
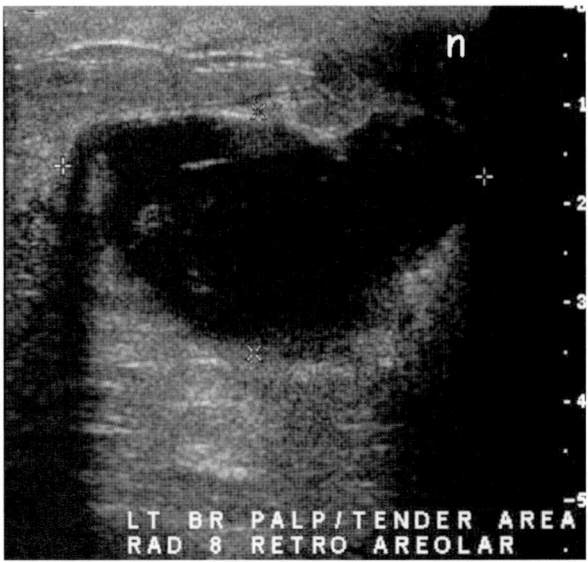

A

B

C

E

D

FIGURE 23-49. Lesions causing nipple discharge. Duct ectasia usually involves one lobar ductal system at a time. **A,** Early in its course, only a single duct might be involved. **B,** Over time, additional lobar ducts can become involved, leading to multiple dilated ducts. When all the ducts are severely involved, one must consider hyperprolactinemia as an underlying factor. **C, Communicating cysts. D,** That the cyst truly communicates with the ductal system can be confirmed by showing a "color-swoosh" with the communicating duct when the cyst undergoes ballottement with the transducer. **E, Pure DCIS** and invasive duct carcinomas that have DCIS components can also give rise to nipple discharge. DCIS, Ductal carcinoma in situ.

FIGURE 23-50. Peripheral abscess. Peripheral puerperal abscesses (*caliper markers*) often arise within preexisting galactoceles and have very irregular walls and mixtures of fluid and echogenic debris.

FIGURE 23-51. Central periareolar abscess. Periareolar abscesses (*caliper markers*), whether puerperal or nonpuerperal, usually arise when an inflamed or infected duct ruptures, spilling its contents into the periductal tissues (n—nipple).

she feels the lump, because radial folds are dynamic and might only be present in certain positions. Only anteriorly located radial folds will be palpable. Radial folds on the posterior surface of the implant are never palpable. In patients with saline implants, the fill valve can cause palpable abnormalities. **Fill valves** are generally placed behind the nipple. However, in certain cases, the valve either may not be placed directly behind the nipple or the implant may have rotated after placement. In such cases, the valve can be palpable if there is very little overlying breast tissue. In other cases, valves become palpable years after the implant is placed because of eversion of the valve. Eversion is most likely to occur in implants that are under chronic pressure owing to capsular contracture.

In **intracapsular rupture**, the shell develops a tear through which silicone gel extravasates into the space between the shell and the capsule, but the capsule remains intact. In **extracapsular rupture**, there is a tear in the capsule as well as in the shell and silicone gel extravasates into the breast tissues outside the capsule. By definition, all cases of extracapsular rupture must be preceded by intracapsular rupture, but in many cases, the intracapsular component is difficult to demonstrate sonographically.

The classic findings of intracapsular rupture are the **stepladder sign** ("linguini" sign in MRI literature) and abnormally increased echogenicity in the extravasated gel that lies within the intracapsular extra-shell space (Fig. 23-52). Unfortunately, these signs have low sensitivity for intracapsular rupture because they are only present in cases where nearly all the silicone gel has

extravasated from the shell and the shell is completely collapsed. In cases of intracapsular rupture, lesser degrees of collapse merely lead to abnormal sheetlike separation of the shell inwardly away from the capsule (Fig. 23-53A). There is a continuous spectrum of collapse from radial fold to complete collapse. Radial folds are quite dynamic, forming when the patient is in one position, and then disappearing when the patient assumes another position. For this reason, the apex of radial folds is prone to fatigue fractures. For any individual radial fold it is impossible to know whether there is a fatigue fracture at the apex of the fold unless the fluid within the fold becomes hyperechoic (see Fig. 23-53B).

Radial folds should be considered normal unless they contain hyperechoic contents (snowstorm appearance). Intracapsular ruptures with only minimal collapse can be distinguished from radial folds by shape that can be evaluated with orthogonal views that are oriented parallel and perpendicular to the long axis of the fold. Radial folds are one-dimensional, showing a long separation between the capsule and shell parallel to the long axis of the fold, but a very short separation when the fold is imaged perpendicular to the long axis. Intra-capsular ruptures are two-dimensional, showing long capsular-shell separations in both views.

Extracapsular rupture indicates that silicone gel has extravasated not only from the implant shell, but also through the capsule into surrounding tissues. The classical finding is the **silicone granuloma** with a **snowstorm** appearance. Such granulomas are markedly hyperechoic and well circumscribed anteriorly, but have an incoherent dirty appearing retrogranuloma shadow.

FIGURE 23-52. Breast implant rupture. A, The classic findings of intracapsular rupture of a single-lumen silicone gel implant are the "stepladder" sign and hyperechoic silicone gel in the right breast. Several linear horizontally oriented echoes represent folds in a collapsed shell. Several of these are double echogenic lines that represent the inner and outer surfaces of each fold of the shell (*arrows*). The extravasated gel that lies outside the implant shell has become hyperechoic (*). Note only a single echogenic line that represents the peri-implant capsule can be seen on the right (*gray arrowhead*). **B, Normal left breast implant**. Note that the superficial aspect of the unruptured left implant shows the double echogenic line (*white arrowhead*) of the shell at the anterior aspect of the silicone gel.

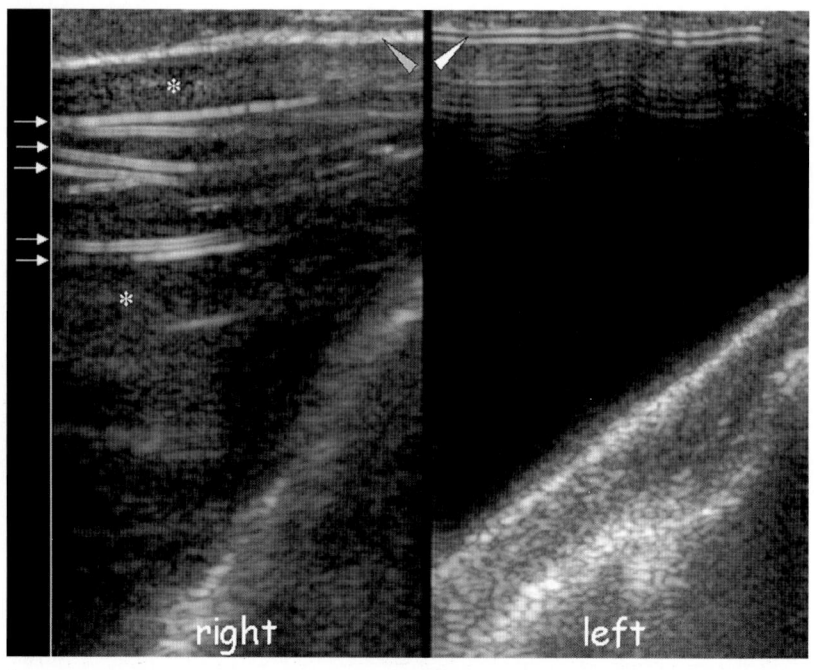

A   B

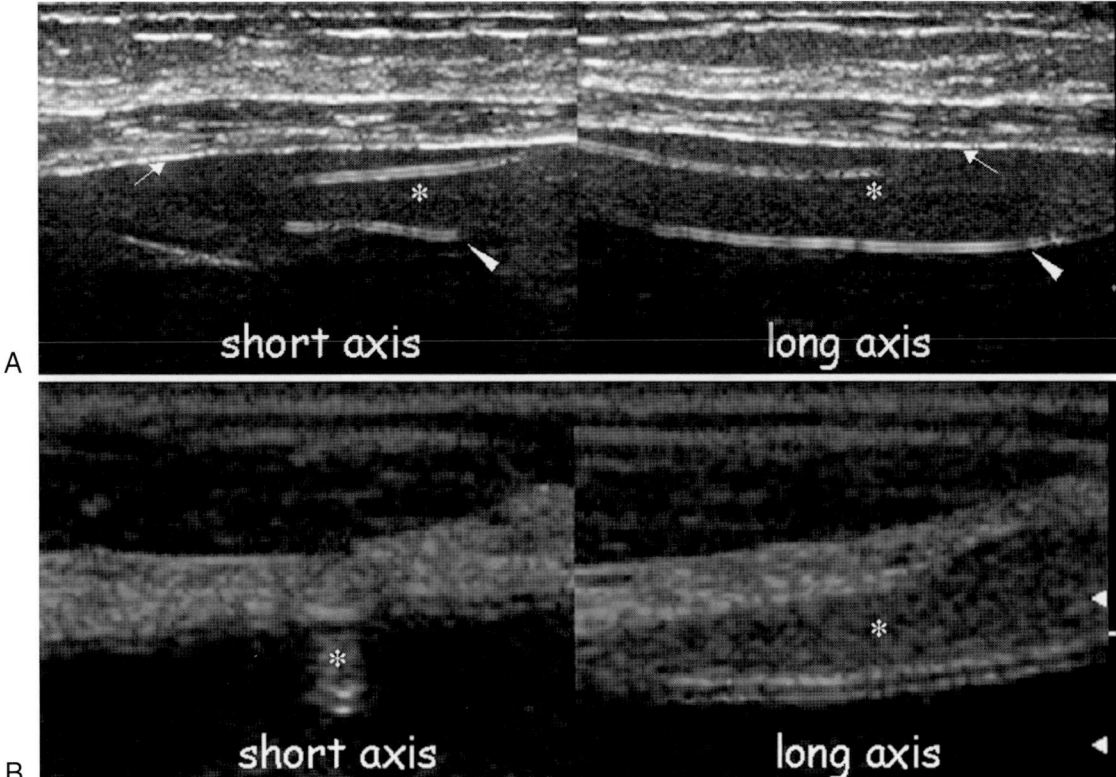

FIGURE 23-53. Breast implant partial rupture. In cases of intracapsular rupture, where collapse is incomplete, the classic finding of the "stepladder sign" may be absent. **A,** In partial collapse, there will be abnormal sheetlike separation between the capsule (*arrow*) and the shell (*arrowheads*). **B,** The extravasated gel that has extruded into the abnormal space between the capsule and the shell tends to become hyperechoic over time (*). In many cases, the earliest leakage of silicone gel arises from the apex of radial folds, where fatigue fractures of the shell are common. Only if the fluid within the radial fold becomes hyperechoic can we be sure that the fold is the site of intracapsular rupture and not merely a variation of normal.

Silicone granulomas can occur superficial to implants (Fig. 23-54A), but most commonly occur at the edges of the implant, where the shell is thinnest and where fatigue fractures are more likely to occur (see Fig. 23-54B). In certain cases, extravasated silicone gel forms a thin sheet over the outer surface of the implant rather than a discrete mass (see Fig. 23-54C). In other cases, extravasated silicone gel can migrate away from the edge of the implant to the axilla, chest wall, back, or abdominal wall (see Fig. 23-54D). In some cases, extravasated silicone gel can be carried by lymphatic vessels to axillary lymph nodes where it accumulates within the medullary sinuses of lymph nodes. The silicone gel accumulates from the mediastinum of the lymph node outward. Early accumulation **of silicone gel within lymph nodes** can be difficult to detect because the hyperechoic silicone gel is difficult to distinguish from the normal hyperechogenicity of the lymph node mediastinum. However, silicone gel within the mediastinum of a lymph node will cause a subtle, incoherent dirty shadow, which originates within the mediastinum, that will allow it to be detected. As more silicone gel accumulates within the lymph node, the diagnosis of silicone gel accumulation within the lymph node becomes more obvious. Silicone gel fills the cortical sinusoids as well as the medullary sinusoids, the cortex of the lymph node becomes hyperechoic, and dirty shadowing arises from the entire lymph node (see Fig. 23-54E).

Not all silicone granulomas have the classic snowstorm appearance. There is a spectrum of appearances. Large acute accumulations of extracapsular silicone gel may appear complex and cystic (Fig. 23-55A). Over time, these may become solid appearing and isoechoic (see Fig. 23-55B). The classic snowstorm appearance develops from the solid, isoechoic phase. In some cases, the hyperechoic granuloma can become hypoechoic, cause architectural distortion, and can develop clean acoustic shadowing (see Fig. 23-55C). This appearance can be difficult to distinguish from that of spiculated malignant nodules. The sensitivity of ultrasound for extracapsular rupture will be enhanced if the sonographer appreciates that not all silicone granulomas have the classic snowstorm appearance.

The presence of implants should not discourage necessary ultrasound-guided procedures. With ultrasound guidance, an angle of approach that is nearly parallel to the surface of the implant can be used, and a large amount of local anesthetic can be injected between

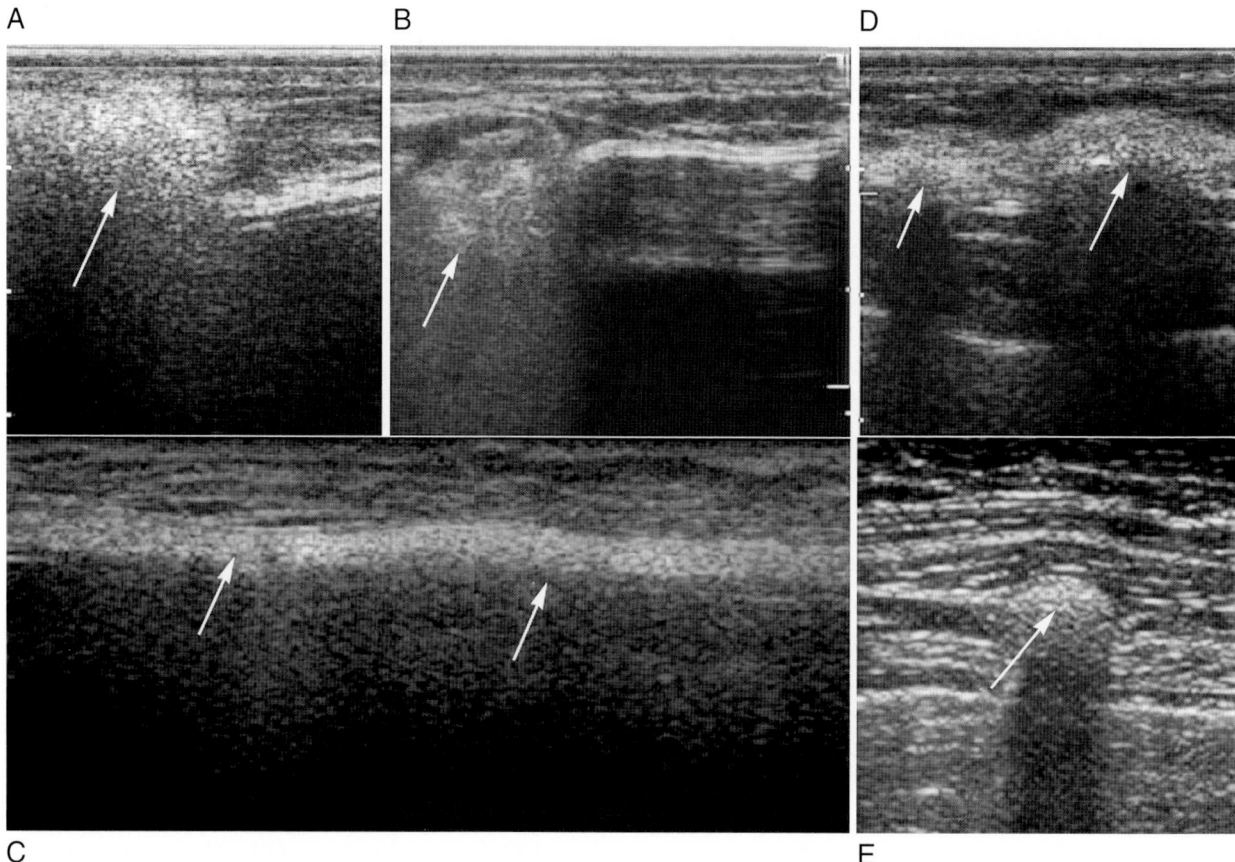

FIGURE 23-54. Silicone granulomas—typical. Extracapsular rupture "snowstorm" sign. Silicone granulomas that manifest the snowstorm sign are hyperechoic, have a well-circumscribed superficial border, and a posterior border that is obscured by dirty, incoherent shadowing. **A**, Silicone granulomas can occur anterior to the implant (*arrow*), but most occur along the edges of the implant where the shell is thinner (*arrow*) as in image **B**. **C**, Silicone granulomas can spread over the surface of the implant in a thin sheet (*arrows*) rather than forming a discrete mass. **D**, Silicone granulomas can migrate away from the edge of the implant to lie on the chest or abdominal wall or in the axilla (*arrows*). **E**, Extravasated silicone can be carried by lymphatics to regional lymph nodes (*arrow*) where they fill the lymph nodes with hyperechoic gel, giving a snowstorm appearance (*arrow*), from the medulla outward, as with this Rotter node that lies between the pectoralis major and pectoralis minor.

the lesion and the implant to hydrodissect the lesion away from the implant and create a safe working space.

It is important to remember that patients with implants are subject to all the same disease processes as are patients who do not have implants. Most patients are happy with their implants, and in most cases, the implants are not causing clinical problems. The greatest danger presented to the sonographer by implants is that they are distracting. One may spend so much time and effort assessing implants that one misses the real reason for presentation, a breast cancer. In order to minimize the chance of missing a breast cancer, it is important to evaluate breast tissues overlying the implant before turning attention to the implants.

Doppler

The original and most important **use of Doppler in the breast** has been for characterization of solid breast nodules. Once a breast malignancy reaches a certain size,

it must stimulate neovascularity in order to continue to grow. To accomplish this, tumors elaborate a variety of angiogenesis factors. A net of peripheral neovessels forms to nourish the rapidly proliferating periphery of the tumor. Much attention has been paid to detecting this neovascularity with Doppler, with and without ultrasound contrast agents. Many different parameters have been evaluated. Subjective findings, such as presence or absence of flow, and the distribution and pattern of vessels have been evaluated. Semiquantitative criteria such as vessel density, peak systolic velocity, pulsatility indices, resistivity indices, and systolic-to-diastolic velocities have been evaluated. However, all of these subjective and semiquantitative criteria can easily be altered by compression of the pressure during scanning. Only a few authors have appropriately emphasized how critical it is to use exceedingly light compression when assessing blood flow in the breast. The transducer is hard, the chest wall is firm, and even the weight of the sonographer's arm on the transducer can compress a

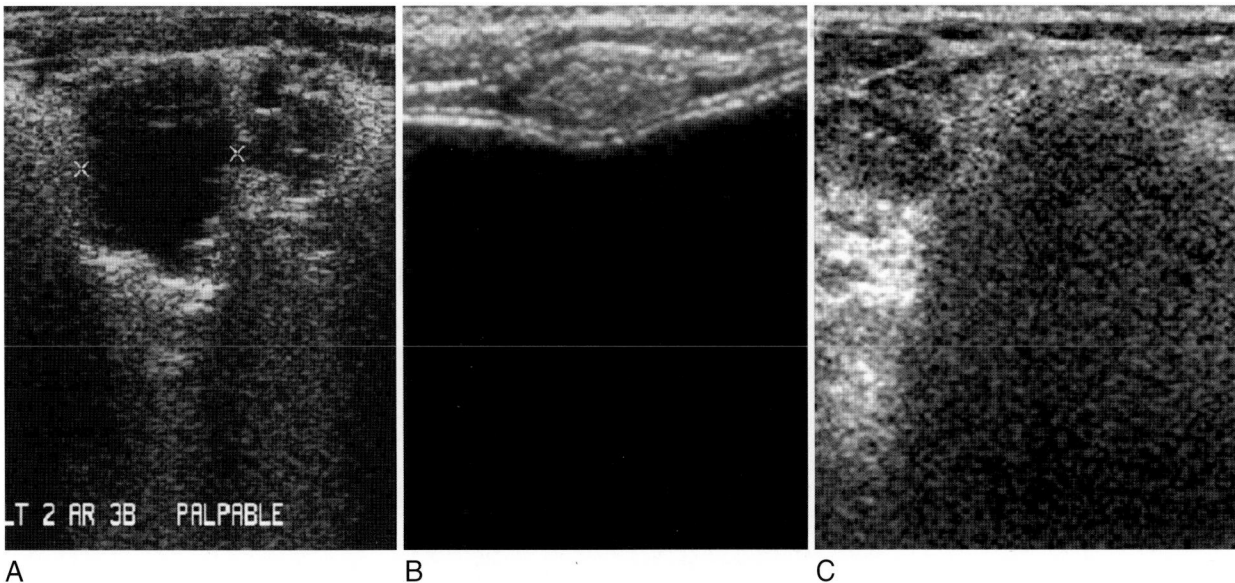

FIGURE 23-55. Silicone granulomas—atypical. A, Large collections of acutely extravasated silicone gel can have a complex cystic appearance. **B,** Silicone granulomas of a few weeks to a few months' duration can appear isoechoic. These usually progress to the "snowstorm appearance" over a matter of months. **C,** Silicone granulomas that are many years old can create intensely shadowing masses that simulate malignancy. Note also that, although most silicone granulomas result from extracapsular rupture, they can form between the capsule and the shell in certain patients as in image **B.**

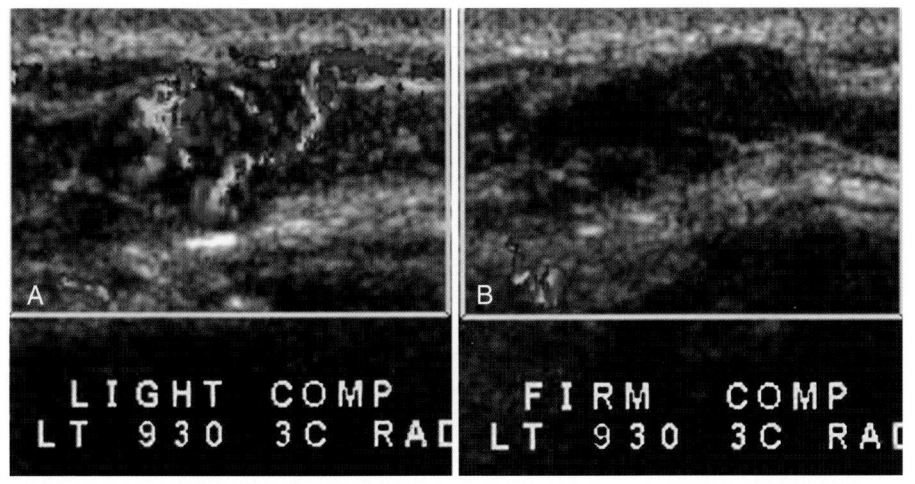

FIGURE 23-56. Importance of light pressure for color Doppler examination. A, This abundantly vascular malignant breast nodule, when scanned with light pressure, **B,** appears avascular when just the weight of one's scanning arm is allowed to rest on the transducer while scanning.

lesion enough to decrease or even completely ablate flow to certain lesions (Fig. 23-56). Not only can the presence or absence of flow be affected, but semiquantitative criteria can also be altered. It is critical if Doppler is to be used for characterizing breast lesions; it must be performed with such light scan pressure that the transducer barely contacts the skin. In some cases, using a standoff of acoustic gel may be necessary so that Doppler detectable blood flow will not be affected.

The most useful finding has been to compare the pulsed Doppler spectral waveform in the periphery of the lesion with that in the center of the lesion. The waveform pattern in malignant nodules tends to differ from that of benign lesions. In **benign lesions**, the waveforms obtained from the center and periphery of the lesions are similar—low impedance flow with relatively low systolic velocities and rounded systolic peaks. **Malignant lesions** tend to have waveform patterns in the center of the lesion that differ from those in the periphery. The waveforms obtained from the periphery of malignant lesions are similar to those obtained from benign lesions—low impedance with rounded systolic peaks. The waveforms obtained from the center of malignant lesions demonstrate higher impedance, higher systolic velocities, and sharp systolic peaks (Fig. 23-57). These intratumoral waveforms are probably a manifestation of increased pressures within the extracellular matrix of tumors that extrinsically

FIGURE 23-57. Central and peripheral Doppler signals. A, Pulsed Doppler spectral waveforms obtained from the center of malignant solid nodule tend to have high peak-systolic velocities and relatively high resistivity indices. **B,** Waveforms obtained from the periphery of a malignant solid breast nodule tend to have lower peak-systolic velocities, more rounded systolic peaks, and lower resistivity indices (*right image*). Benign solid nodules differ in that they tend to have low peak systolic velocities, rounded systolic peaks, and relatively low resistivity indices in both the interior and the periphery of the nodule.

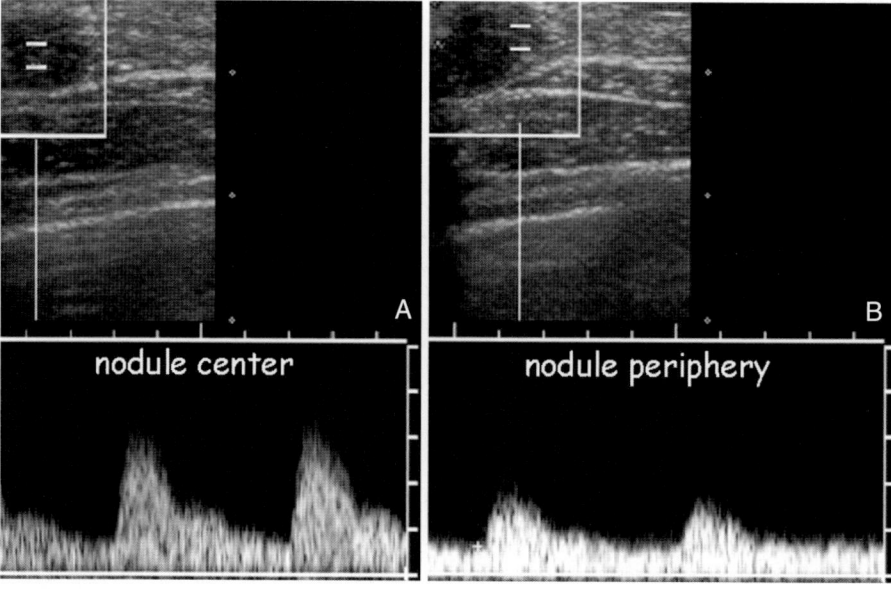

compresses the thin-walled sinusoidal vessels within the center of the tumor.

Although the main published use for Doppler sonography has been for characterizing solid breast nodules, we have found the gray-scale image characteristics much more powerful and accurate in characterizing most solid nodules. In only a small percentage of cases has Doppler added useful information to the gray-scale imaging in characterizing solid breast nodules. This is most likely to occur in small, high-grade invasive carcinomas that are about 5 mm in diameter. Such lesions are typically circumscribed and are the lesions most likely to be mischaracterized as BIRADS 3 by image alone. Despite their small size, such lesions are frequently quite vascular in comparison to benign lesions of the same size. We believe the gray-scale image will continue to be better for characterizing breast lesions than Doppler in most cases, even with the use of contrast agents. Doppler is very useful, however, in assessing the aggressiveness of lesions. Increased vascularity on Doppler is a manifestation of biologically aggressive (high histologic grade) lesions that are most likely to spread distantly hematogenously. Patients with such lesions are those who are most likely to benefit from aggressive adjuvant therapy with chemotherapeutic or immunotherapeutic agents, and anti-angiogenesis drugs. The main use of Doppler will be for assessing prognosis and guiding treatment rather than distinguishing between benign and malignant nodules.

Doppler ultrasound does not characterize solid breast nodules as well as the image, but Doppler capabilities are essential in breast imaging. The niche applications for which we find Doppler invaluable are myriad. Doppler is useful for assessing internal echoes within cysts and ectatic ducts, diagnosing acute inflammation or infection, and avoiding large vessels, particularly arteries,

during interventional procedures. It is essential to diagnose vascular conditions such as **arteriovenous malformations**, **arteriovenous fistulas**, **venous malformations**, and **superficial venous thrombosis (Mondor's disease)**. Doppler ultrasound is valuable in distinguishing between reactive or inflamed lymph nodes and metastasis-bearing nodes in certain cases.

Real, rather than artifactual, internal echoes frequently complicate breast cysts. Such echoes can result from a variety of cellular and acellular particles within the cyst. It can be difficult with images alone to distinguish between the different causes of internal echoes. Additionally, some markedly hypoechoic solid nodules can have a pseudocystic appearance. In some cases, it can be difficult to determine whether a lesion is a solid nodule or a complex cyst that is filled with diffuse low-level internal echoes. Demonstrating an internal vessel on color Doppler indicates that the lesion is either solid or a cyst that is completely filled by a papillary lesion (Fig. 23-58). As is always the case with Doppler, a positive study is more valuable than a negative study because, in certain solid nodules, a central vessel will not be demonstrable. In other cases, the energy of the Doppler beam will displace particles within the cyst to move posteriorly—so called **color streaking**. Particles that can be moved solely by the energy of the Doppler beam are tiny, subcellular in size, and are usually cholesterol crystals that are part of the benign fibrocystic spectrum. Color Doppler can be useful in distinguishing between an echogenic lipid layer or tumefactive sludge within a cyst and a true intracystic papillary lesion. Intracystic papillary lesions, whether benign or malignant, are among the most vascular lesions of the breast and usually have a prominent vascular stalk that is demonstrable with color or power Doppler (Fig. 23-59).

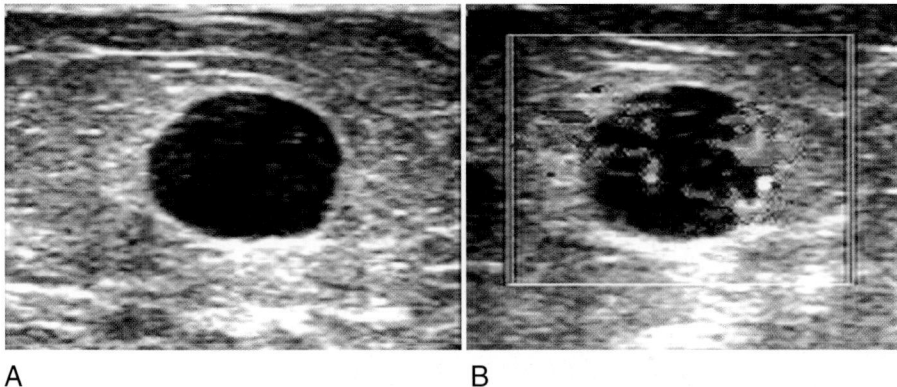

FIGURE 23-58. Complex cysts and solid nodules. Color Doppler can be helpful in distinguishing between complex cysts and solid nodules when the distinction is uncertain based on the image alone. **A,** Metastatic leiomyosarcoma of the breast had a pseudocystic appearance on the sonogram. **B,** Color Doppler showed abundant internal flow, indicating that the lesion was solid.

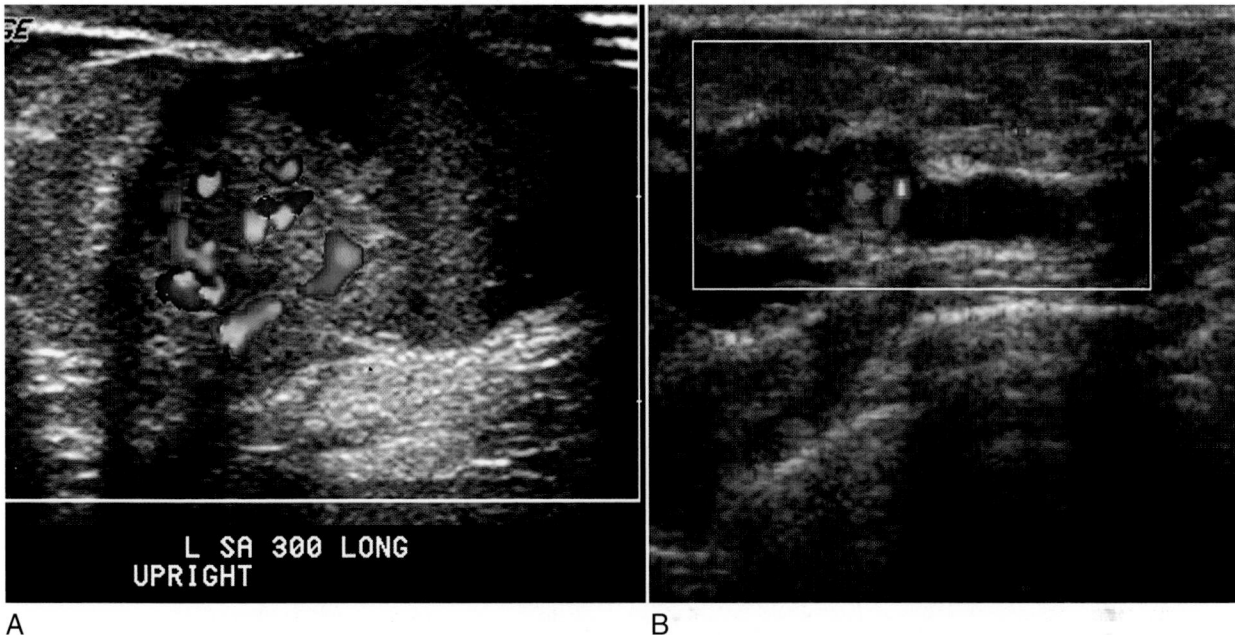

FIGURE 23-59. A, Intracystic papillary lesions and intraductal papillomas. Intracystic papillary lesions, whether benign or malignant, are among the most vascular lesions in the breast. One or more vascular stalks and internal vascularity are usually readily demonstrable with color or power Doppler. Malignant lesions tend to be fed by multiple vessels, while benign intracystic papillomas usually have a single feeding vessel. **B,** Even very small intraductal papillomas usually have a vascular stalk that can be demonstrated with color or power Doppler.

Demonstration of a vessel within such an intracystic area of increased echogenicity indicates the presence of an intracystic papilloma or carcinoma. Benign intracystic papillomas tend to have a single large feeding vessel within the vascular stalk, whereas malignant intracystic papillary lesions tend to be fed by multiple feeding vessels.

Ectatic ducts, like cysts, often contain echogenic secretions or blood that can be difficult to distinguish from intraductal papillomas or DCIS by gray-scale imaging alone. Ballottement of ectatic ducts that contain diffuse low-level echoes can cause the echoes to slosh back and forth within the duct. This can be appreciated on the gray-scale image in certain cases and can be documented on a single hard copy image by using color Doppler. The secretions are echogenic enough to create a color signal when moving within the duct. They tend to move posteriorly during compression and anteriorly during compression release, creating color signals of opposite color. Demonstrating such a "color-swoosh" documents that the internal echoes are caused by inspissated echogenic secretions or blood rather than tumor. It is important that the color signal fill the duct, because in some cases, echogenic blood resulting from an intraductal papillary lesion can lead to a color swoosh, but the underlying papillary lesion will cause a defect in the color signal. As is the case with intracystic papillary lesions, intraductal papillary lesions are often vascular enough to have a demonstrable vascular stalk on color Doppler (see Fig. 23-59). This helps identify intraductal papillary lesions and helps to distinguish them from echogenic lipid or debris layers within the duct.

Acute pain is a frequent indication for breast ultrasound. In most cases, the cause for pain is unclear. In some cases, however, sonography with Doppler may show an acute inflammatory etiology for pain. Acutely inflamed cysts and acute periductal mastitis are the most common causes for this pain. The normally thin, echogenic wall of acutely inflamed cysts or ducts becomes thick and isoechoic and also becomes hyperemic. The walls of noninflamed cysts and ducts have no demonstrable flow on color Doppler. The thickened walls of acutely inflamed cysts and ducts are easily demonstrated as inflammatory hyperemia on color or power Doppler. Interestingly, the direction in which the vessels course within the walls of inflamed cysts and ducts differs from the orientation of vessels that feed intracystic or intraductal papillary lesions. Vessels in the walls of inflamed ducts course parallel to the duct wall because they are feeding and draining the duct wall. Vessels that feed intraductal papillary lesions are oriented perpendicular to the axis of the duct wall, because the vessels are merely passing through the wall to feed a lesion inside the duct. Doppler and imaging findings in acutely inflamed or infected peri-implant capsules are similar to those in acutely inflamed cysts or ducts. Acute superficial venous thrombosis of the breast can also be a cause of acute pain. Compression gray-scale sonography and color Doppler are essential in making the diagnosis, just as they are in lower extremity DVT.

Doppler can be helpful in assessing **lymph nodes** that are not normal, but have nonspecific imaging findings that prevent us from determining whether the node is merely reactive or inflamed, or whether it contains metastasis. The histologic and biologic behavior of lymph node metastases is usually identical to that of the primary. A vascular primary tumor will tend to have a vascular lymph node metastasis. If the spectral waveforms obtained from the center of the primary are high impedance and have high and sharp systolic peaks, then the waveforms obtained from lymph node metastases from that primary will have similar waveforms. Conversely, inflamed or reactive lymph nodes will usually have low impedance waveforms with low rounded systolic peaks. The pattern of blood vessels within lymph nodes can also be helpful. Inflamed or reactive lymph nodes tend to be fed by a single hilar artery that arborizes to various extents within the mediastinum of the lymph nodes (Fig. 23-60A). Well-differentiated and low-grade lymphomas tend to have a similar pattern. Metastases to lymph nodes can stimulate development of transcapsular tumor neovascularity (Fig. 23-60B). The afferent lymphatics enter the lymph node through the capsule of the lymph node and exit as efferent lymphatics through the hilar notch. Metastases tend to implant in the subcapsular and cortical sinusoids. With Doppler, the presence of transcapsular feeding arteries is a better positive predictor of metastasis than is absence of trans-

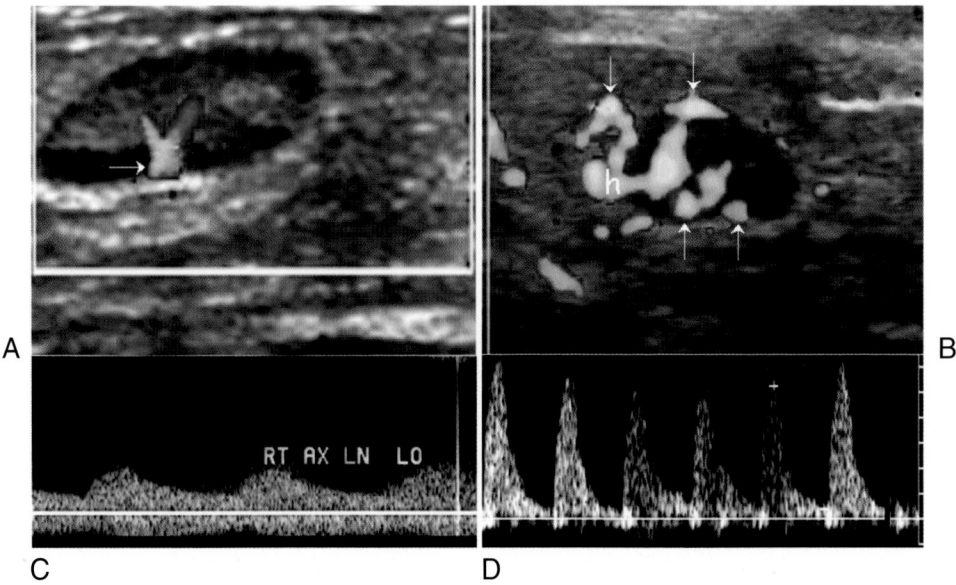

FIGURE 23-60. The pattern of flow on color Doppler can help distinguish between metastatic and inflammatory etiologies of mild lymphadenopathy. A, Inflamed or reactive nodes, like normal nodes, are usually fed by a single hilar artery (*arrow*). **B,** Lymph nodes that bear metastases, however, often develop tumor vessels that feed subcapsular metastatic implants from the periphery (*arrows*), in addition to the normal hilar vessel (h). **C,** The pulsed Doppler spectral waveforms obtained from inflamed or reactive nodes tend to be low resistance and to have low peak systolic velocities with rounded systolic peaks. **D,** Waveforms obtained from metastasis-bearing lymph nodes tend to have high resistivity indices, high peak systolic velocities, and sharp systolic peaks.

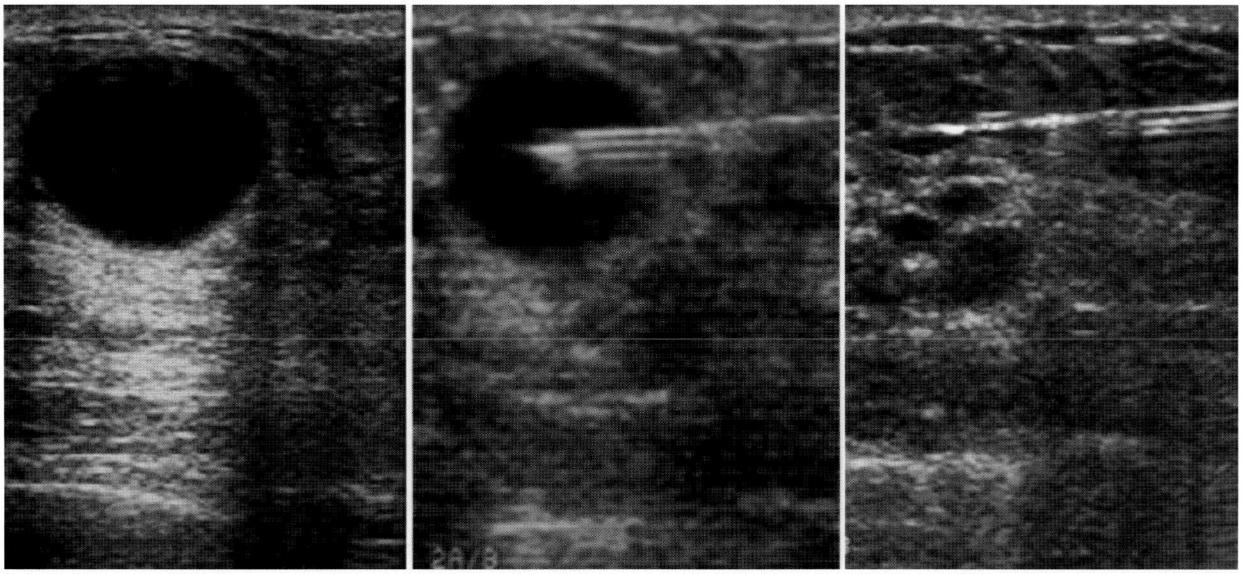

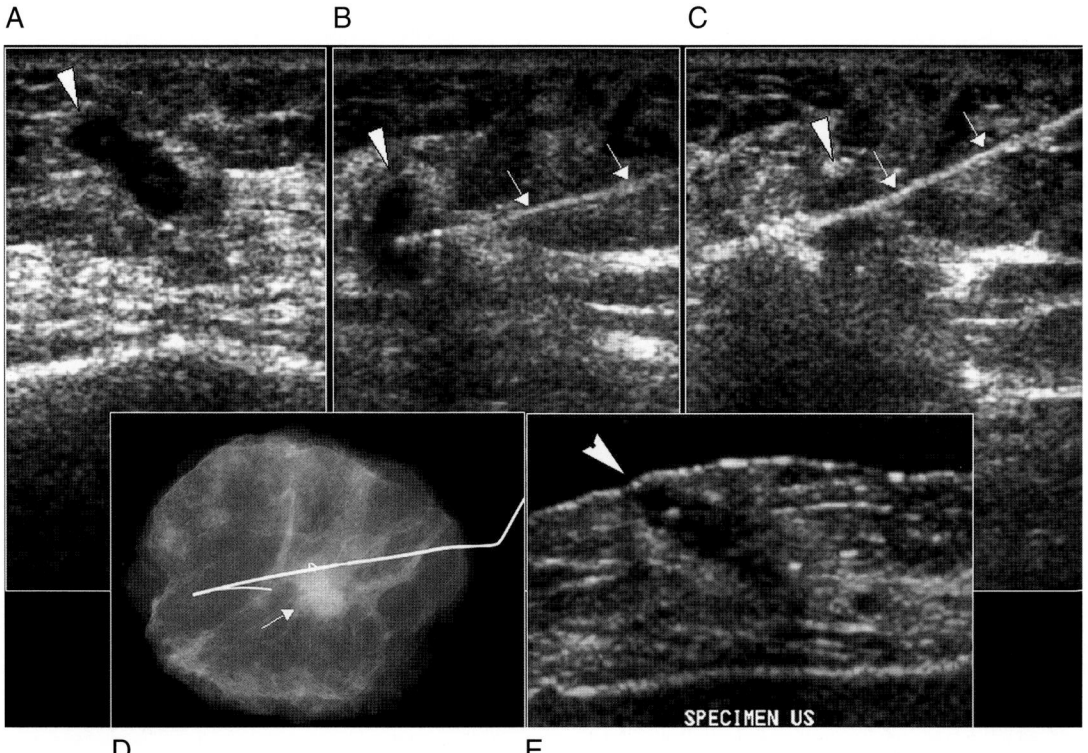

FIGURE 23-61. Technique of needle aspiration and biopsy. Ultrasound-guided interventional procedures of the breast are performed with the needle oriented along the long axis of the transducer and with angulation of the needle and appropriate heeling or toeing of the transducer in order to place the needle nearly parallel to the transducer face and perpendicular to the ultrasound beam. These images show aspiration of a tender, simple tension cyst. **A,** preaspiration; **B,** during aspiration; **C,** postaspiration.

FIGURE 23-62. Ultrasound-guided wire localization for excisional biopsy. A, Shows the nodule (*arrowhead*) preprocedure. **B,** Shows the nodule (*arrowhead*) with the localization needle (*arrows*) in place. **C,** Shows the localization wire (*arrows*) in place after the needle is removed (nodule—*arrowhead*). **D,** The specimen radiograph shows the nodule (*arrow*) in the center of the specimen. **E,** The specimen sonogram, however, shows the nodule extending to the superficial margin of the specimen (*arrowhead*).

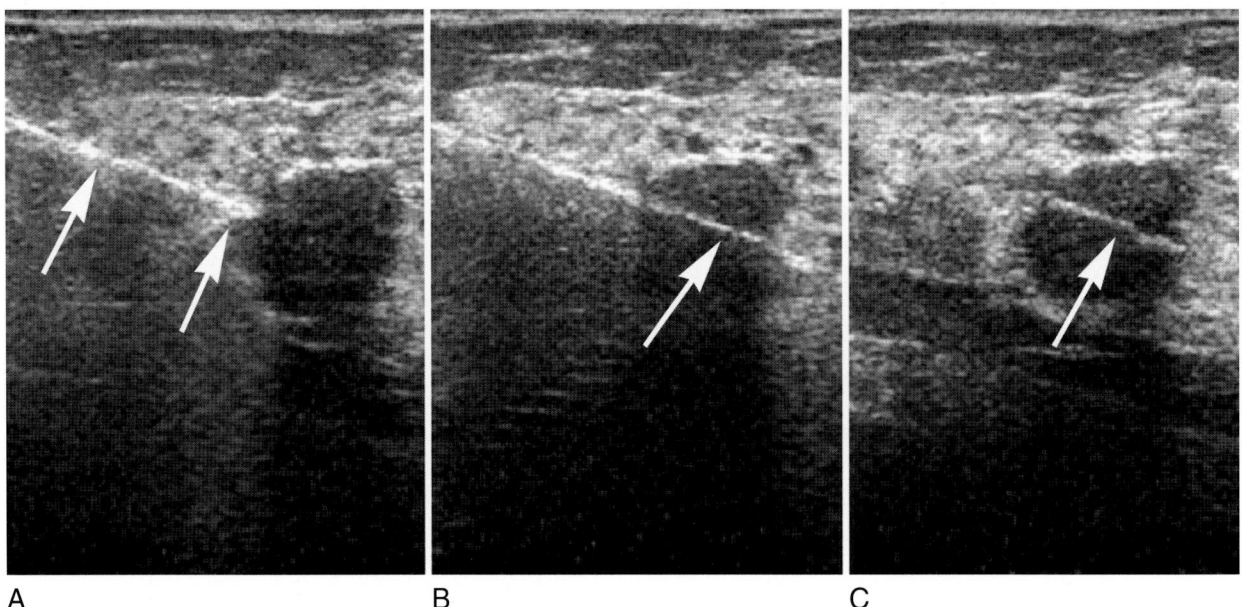

A   B   C

FIGURE 23-63. Ultrasound-guided needle biopsy with a 14 gauge Tru-Cut needle. A, Needle (*arrows*) has been advanced to the edge of the nodule in the prefire position. **B,** Needle (*arrow*) has been fired through the nodule and now is in the postfire position. **C,** Needle has been withdrawn, but a vapor trail of microbubbles (*arrow*) can still be seen within the needle tract, which documents that the needle did, indeed, pass through the target nodule.

capsular vessels an indicator of inflammation. Not all lymph node metastases stimulate formation of transcapsular neovessels.

INTERVENTION

The use of sonography for guiding interventional procedures is limited only by the imagination. Any type of interventional procedure for a lesion that is visible by sonography can be guided by sonography. Sonographic guidance is usually quicker, more precise, and less expensive than mammographic free hand, grid-guided, mammographic stereotaxic, or MRI guidance.

Our strong preference is to place the **needle along the long axis of the transducer,** enabling the needle to be visualized along its entire course in real time throughout the entire procedure. A short-axis approach allows visualization of the needle only when it is within the short axis of the ultrasound beam and requires a much steeper approach. This is especially problematic for deeply located lesions and in patients with implants. The main difficulty encountered during a long axis approach is in keeping the needle and the long axis of the transducer exactly parallel to each other. Watching the ultrasound monitor before the needle has passed far enough into the breast to be within the ultrasound beam is the main cause of misalignment. It is best to watch one's hands until the needle is deep enough within the breast to be within the ultrasound beam before moving the eyes to the ultrasound monitor. Once the needle is

within the beam, it is relatively easy to keep it precisely parallel to the beam.

Ultrasound can be used to guide cyst aspiration (Fig. 23-61), needle localization for surgical biopsy with specimen sonography (Fig. 23-62), sentinel node injection, sentinel node localization, abscess drainage, percutaneous ductography, foreign body removal (broken localization wires), and biopsy using fine needles, large Tru-Cut needles (Fig. 23-63), vacuum-assisted biopsy, and en-bloc removal. It can be used to locate and orient the lumpectomy cavity for booster doses of external radiation and to guide placement of brachytherapy needles. It can also be used to guide lesion ablation using laser, radiofrequency, and cryotherapy.

Recommended Reading

General

Berg WA, Campassi C, Lanenberg P, et al: Breast imaging and reporting data system: Inter- and intraobserver variability in feature analysis and final assessment. AJR 2000; 174:1769-1777.

Farria DM, Mund DF, Bassett LW: Evaluation of missed cancers using screening mammography (abstr). AJR 1995; 126:1645.

Ma L, Fishell E, Wright B, et al: Case-control study of factors associated with failure to detect breast cancer by mammography. J Natl Cancer Inst 1992;84:781-785.

Secondary Screening with Ultrasound

Buchberger W, DeKoekkoek-Doll P, Springer P, et al: Incidental findings on sonography of the breast: Clinical significance and diagnostic workup. AJR 1999;173:921-927.

Kaplan SS: Clinical utility of bilateral whole breast-breast US in the evaluation of women with dense breast tissue. Radiology 2001;221:641-649.

Kolb TM, Lichy J, Newhouse JH: Comparison of the performance of screening mammography, physical examination, and breast US and evaluation of the factors that influence them: An analysis of 27,825 patients. Radiology 2000;225:165-175.

Kolb TM, Lichy J, Newhouse JH: Occult cancer in women with dense breasts: Detection with screening US—diagnostic yield and tumor characteristics. Radiology 1998;207:191-199.

Equipment and Physics

Kremkau FW: Multiple-element transducers. Radiographics 1993;13:1163-1176.

Ritchie WGM: Axial Resolution. Ultrasound Quarterly 1992;10(2):80-100.

Smith SW, Trahey GE, von Ramm OT: Two-dimensional arrays for medical ultrasound. Ultrason Imaging 1992;14(3):213-233.

Breast Anatomy and Technique

Blend R, Rideout DF, Kaizer L, et al: Parenchymal patterns of the breast defined by real time ultrasound. Eur J Cancer Prev 1995;4(4):293-298.

Moy L, Slanetz PJ, Moore R, et al: Specificity of mammography and US in the evaluation of a palpable abnormality: Retrospective review. Radiology 2002;225:176-181.

Richter K: Technique for detecting and evaluating breast lesions. J Ultrasound Med 1994;13(10):797-802.

Stavros AT: An introduction to breast ultrasound. In Parker SH, Jobe WE (eds): Percutaneous Breast Biopsy. New York, Raven Press, 1993, pp 95-110.

Teboul M, Halliwell M: Atlas of Ultrasound of Ductal Echography of the Breast. Cambridge, Mass. Blackwell Science, 1995.

Yang WT, Ahuja A, Tang A, et al: Ultrasonographic demonstration of normal axillary lymph nodes: A learning curve. J Ultrasound Med 1995;14:823-827.

Targeted Indications

Dennis MA, Parker SH, Klaus AJ, et al: Breast biopsy avoidance: The value of normal mammograms and normal sonograms in the setting of a palpable lump. Radiology 2001;219:186-191.

Langer TG, Shaw de Paredes E: Evaluation of nonpalpable mammographic nodules. Applied Rad 1991;4:19-28.

Leung JWT, Kornguth PJ, Gotway MB: Utility of targeted sonography in evaluation of focal breast pain. J Ultrasound Med 2002;21:521-526.

Lunt LG, Peakman DJ, Young JR: Mammographically guided ultrasound: A new technique for assessment of impalpable breast lesions. Clin Radiol 1991;44(2):85-88.

McNicholas MM, Mercer PM, Miller JC, et al: Color Doppler sonography in the evaluation of palpable breast masses. Am J Roentgenol 1993;161(4):765-771.

Perre CI, Koot VC, de Hooge P, et al: The value of ultrasound in the evaluation of palpable breast tumours: A prospective study of 400 cases. Eur J Surg Oncol 1994;20(6):637-640.

Weinstein SP, Conant EF, Orel SG, et al. Retrospective review of palpable breast lesions after negative mammography and sonography. J Women's Imaging 2000;2:15-18.

Solid Nodules

Baker JA, Kornguth PJ, Soo MS, et al: Sonography of solid breast lesions: Observer variability of lesion description and assessment. Am J Roentgenol 1999;172:1621-1625.

Butler RS, Venta LA, Wiley EL, et al: Sonographic evaluation of infiltrating lobular carcinoma. Am J Roentgenol 1999;172(2):325-330.

Chao TC, Lo YF, Chen SC, et al: Prospective sonographic study of 3093 breast tumors. J Ultrasound Med 1999;18:363-370.

Cohen MA, Sferlazza SJ. Role of sonography in evaluation of radial scars of the breast. Am J Roentgenol 2000;174(4):1075-1078.

Conant EF, Dillon RL, Palazzo J, et al: Imaging findings in mucin-containing carcinomas of the breast: Correlation with pathologic features. Am J Roentgenol 1994;163:821-824.

Ellis RL: Differentiation of benign versus malignant breast disease. Radiology 1999;210:878-880.

Finlay ME, Liston JE, Lunt LG, et al: Assessment of the role of ultrasound in the differentiation of radial scars and stellate carcinoma of the breast. Clin Radiol 1994;49(1):52-55.

Fornage BD, Lorigan JB, Andry E: Fibroadenoma of the breast: Sonographic appearance. Radiology 1989;172:671-675.

Fornage BD, Sneige N, Faroux MJ, et al: Sonographic appearance and ultrasound-guided fine-needle aspiration biopsy of breast carcinomas smaller than 1 cm3. J Ultrasound Med 1990;9:559-568.

Franquet T, De Miguel C, Cozculluela R, et al: Spiculated lesions of the breast: Mammographic-pathologic correlations. Radiographics 1993;13(4):841-852.

Hall FM: Sonography of the breast: Controversies and opinions. Am J Roentgenol 1997;169(6):1635-1636.

Jackson VP: Management of solid breast nodules: What is the role of sonography? Radiology 1995;196(1):14-15.

Kobayashi T, Shinozaki H, Yomon M, et al. Hyperechoic pattern in breast cancer—Its bio-acoustic genesis and tissue characterization. J UOEH 1989;11(2):181-187.

Kornguth PJ, Bentley RC: Mammographic-pathologic correlation: Part 1, Benign breast lesions. J Women's Imaging 2001;3:29-37.

Kossoff G: Causes of shadowing in breast sonography. Ultrasound Med Biol 1988;14 Supp: 211-215.

Leucht WJ, Rabe DR, Humbert KD: Diagnostic value of different interpretive criteria in real-time sonography of the breast. Ultrasound Med Biol 14 Supp 1988;1:59-73.

Liberman L, Bonaccio E, Hamele-Bena D, et al: Benign and malignant phyllodes tumors: Mammographic and sonographic findings. Radiology 1996;198(1):121-124.

Meyer JE, Amin E, Lindfors KK, et al: Medullary carcinoma of the breast: Mammographic and US appearance. Radiology 1989;170:79-82.

Moon WK, Im JG, Koh YH, et al: US of mammographically detected clustered microcalcifications. Radiology 2000;217(3):849-854.

Moss HA, Britton PD, Flower CD, et al: How reliable is modern breast imaging in differentiating benign from malignant breast lesions in the symptomatic population? Clin Radiol 1999;54(1):676-682.

Rahbar G, Sie AC, Hansen G, et al: Benign versus malignant solid breast masses: Differentiation. Radiology 1999;213:889-894.

Richter K, Willrodt RG, Opri F, et al: Differentiation of breast lesions by measurements under craniocaudal and lateromedial compression using a new sonographic method. Invest Radiol 1996:401-414.

Rizzato G, Chersevani R, Abbona M, et al: High-resolution sonography of breast carcinoma. Eur J Radiol 1997; 24(1):11-19.

Rubin E: Cutting-edge sonography obviates breast biopsy. Diagn Imaging 1996;Supp:AU14-16, AU32.

Schepps B, Scola FH, Frates RE: Benign circumscribed breast masses. Mammographic and sonographic appearance. Obstet Gynecol Clin North Am 1994;21(3):519-537.

Schoonjans JM, Brem RF: Sonographic appearance of ductal carcinoma in situ diagnosed with ultrasonographically guided large core needle biopsy: Correlation with mammographic and pathologic findings. J Ultrasound Med 2000;19(7):449-457.

Shimato SH, Sawaki A, Niimi R, et al: Role of ultrasonography in the detection of intraductal spread of breast cancer: Correlation with pathologic findings, mammography, and MR imaging. Eur Radiol 2000;10(11):1726-1732.

Skaane P, Engedal K: Analysis of sonographic features in the differentiation of fibroadenoma and invasive ductal carcinoma. Am J Roentgenol 1998;170(1):109-114.

Skaane P, Skjorten F: Ultrasonographic evaluation of invasive lobular carcinoma. Acta Radiol 1999;40(4):369-375.

Stavros AT: Ultrasound of breast pathology. In Parker SH: Percutaneous Breast Biopsy. New York, Raven Press, 1993, pp 111-127.

Stavros AT: Ultrasound of DCIS. In Silverstein JM (ed): Ductal Carcinoma in situ: A diagnostic and Therapeutic Dilemma. Baltimore, Williams and Wilkins, 1997, pp 135-177.

Stavros AT: Ultrasound of DCIS. In Silverstein JM (ed): Ductal Carcinoma in situ: A diagnostic and Therapeutic Dilemma. 2nd ed. Baltimore, Williams and Wilkins, 2002, pp 128-167; 135-177.

Stavros AT, Thickman D, Rapp CL, et al: Solid breast nodules: Use of sonography to distinguish between benign and malignant nodules. Radiology 1995;196:123-134.

Teboul M, Halliwell M: Atlas of Ultrasound and Ductal Echography of the Breast: The Introduction of Anatomic Intelligence into Breast Imaging. London, Blackwell Science, 1995.

Vignal P, Meslet MR, Romeo JM, et al: Sonographic morphology of infiltrating breast carcinoma: Relationship with the shape of the hyaluronic extracellular matrix. J Ultrasound Med 2002;21:531-538.

Williams JC: US of solid breast nodules. Radiology 1996;198(2):123-134.

Sonography of Cystic Lesions

Bargum K, Nielsen SM: Case report: Fat necrosis of the breast appearing as oil cysts with fat-fluid levels. Br J Radiol 1993;66(788):718-720.

Chatterton BE, Spyropoulos P: Colour Doppler induced streaming: An indicator of the liquid nature of lesions. Br J Radiol 1998;71(852):1310-1312.

Karstrup S, Solvig J, Nolsoe CP, et al: Acute puerperal breast abscesses: US-guided drainage. Radiology 1993;188(3):807-809.

Liberman L, Feng T, Susnik B: Case 35: Intracystic papillary carcinoma with invasion. Radiology 2001;219:781-784.

Loyer IM, Harmeet K, David CL, et al: Importance of dynamic assessment of the soft tissues in the sonographic diagnosis of echogenic superficial abscesses. J Ultrasound Med 1995;14:669-671.

Maier WP, Au FC, Tang CK: Nonlactational breast abscess. Am Surg 1994;60(4):247-250.

Nightingale KR, Korguth PJ, Walker WF, et al: A novel ultrasonic technique for differentiating cysts from solid lesions: Preliminary results in the breast. Ultrasound Med Biol 1995;21(6):745-751.

Stavros AT: Ultrasound of Breast Pathology. In Parker SH: Percutaneous Breast Biopsy. New York, Raven Press, 1993, pp 111-127.

US of Nipple Discharge and Intraductal Papillary Lesions

Cilotti A, Bagnolesi P, Napoli V, et al: Solitary intraductal papilloma of the breast. An echographic study of 12 cases. Radiol Med (Torino) 1991;82(5):617-620.

Dennis MA, Parker S, Kaske TI, et al: Incidental treatment of nipple discharge caused by benign intraductal papilloma through diagnostic Mammotome biopsy. Am J Roentgenol 2000,174:1263-1268.

Rissanen T, Typpo T, Tikkakoski T, et al: Ultrasound-guided percutaneous galactography. J Clin Ultrasound 1993;21(8):497-502.

US of Mammary Implants

Ahn CY, De Bruhl Nd, Gorczyca DP, et al: Comparative silicone breast implant evaluation using mammography, sonography, and magnetic resonance imaging: Experience with 59 implants. Plast Reconstr Surg 1994;94(5):620-627.

Berg WA, Caskey CI, Hamper UM, et al: Diagnosing breast implant rupture with MR imaging, US, and mammography. Radiographics 1993;13(6):1323-1336.

Caskey CI, Berg WA, Anderson ND, et al: Breast implant rupture: Diagnosis with US. Radiology 1994;190(3):819-823.

Chung KC, Wilkins EG, Beil RJ, Jr, et al: Diagnosis of silicone gel breast implant rupture by ultrasonography. Plast Reconstr Surg 1996;97(1):104-109.

De Bruhl ND, Gorczyca DP, Ahn CY, et al: Silicone breast implants: US evaluation. Radiology 1993;189(1):95-98.

Everson LI, Parantainen H, Detlie T, et al: Diagnosis of breast implant rupture: Imaging findings and relative efficacies of imaging techniques. AJR Am J Roentgenol 1994;163(1):57-60.

Harris KM, Ganott MA, Shestak KC, et al: Silicone implant rupture: Detection with US. Radiology 1993;187(3):761-768.

Leibman AJ: Imaging of the breast after cosmetic surgery. Applied Radiology 1993;(4):45-48.

Leibman AJ: Imaging of complications of augmentation mammaplasty. Plast Reconstr Surg 1994;93(6):1134-1140.

Leibman AJ, Kruse B: Breast cancer: Mammographic and sonographic findings after augmentation mammoplasty. Radiology 1990;174(1):195-198.

Leibman AJ, Sybers R: Mammographic and sonographic findings after silicone injection. Ann Plast Surg 1994;33(4):412-414.

Levine RA, Collins TL: Definitive diagnosis of breast implant rupture by ultrasonography. Plast Reconstr Surg 1991;87(6):1126-1128.

Peters W, Pugash R: Ultrasound analysis of 150 patients with silicone gel breast implants. Ann Plast Surg 1993;31(1):7-9.

Petro JA, Klein SA, Niazi Z, et al: Evaluation of ultrasound as a tool in the follow-up of patients with breast implants: A preliminary, prospective study. Ann Plast Surg 1994;32(6): 580-587.

Reynolds HE, Buckwalter KA, Jackson VP, et al: Comparison of mammography, sonography, and magnetic resonance imaging in the detection of silicone-gel breast implant rupture. Ann Plast Surg 1994;33(3):247-255.

Rivero MA, Schwartz DS, Mies C: Silicone lymphadenopathy involving intramammary lymph nodes: A new complication of silicone mammaplasty. Am J Roentgenol 1994;162(5): 1089-1090.

Rosculet KA, Ikeda DM, Forrest ME, et al: Ruptured gel-filled silicone breast implants: Sonographic findings in 19 cases. Am J Roentgenol 1992;159(4):711-716.

Shestak KC, Ganott MA, Harris KM, Losken HW: Breast masses in the augmentation mammaplasty patient: The role of ultrasound. Plast Reconstr Surg 1993;92(2):209-216.

Inflammation/Infection of the Breast

Crowe DJ, Helvie MA, Wilson TE: Breast infection. Mammographic and sonographic findings with clinical correlation. Invest Radiol 1995;30(10):582-587.

Hayes R, Michell M, Nunnerley HB: Acute inflammation of the breast—The role of breast ultrasound in diagnosis and management. Clin Radiol 1991;44(4):253-256.

Hughes LE: The duct ectasia/periductal mastitis complex. In

Hughes LE, Mansel RE, Webster DJT (eds): Benign Disorders and Diseases of the Breast: Concepts and Clinical Management, 2nd ed. London, WB Saunders, 2000, pp 143-165.

Doppler of the Breast

Cosgrove DO, Kedar RP, Bamber JC, et al: Breast diseases: Color Doppler US in differential diagnosis. Radiology 1993;189:99-104.

Dock W: Duplex sonography of mammary tumors: A prospective study of 75 patients. J Ultrasound Med 1993;12:79-82.

Fornage BD: Role of color Doppler imaging in differentiating between pseudocystic malignant tumors and fluid collections. J Ultrasound Med 1995;14:125-128.

Hayes R, Michell M, Nunnerley HB: Acute inflammation of the breast—The role of breast ultrasound in diagnosis and management. Clin Radiol 1991;44(4):253-256.

Kubek KA, Chan L, Frazier TG: Color Doppler flow as an indicator of nodal metastasis in solid breast masses. J Ultrasound Med 1996;15(12):835-841.

Madjar H, Prompeler HJ, Sauerbrei W, et al: Color Doppler flow criteria of breast lesions. Ultrasound Med Biol 1994;20:849-858.

Mehta TS, Raza S: Power Doppler sonography of breast cancer: Does vascularity correlate with node status or lymphatic invasion? Am J Roentgenol 1999;173:303-307.

Ozdemir A, Ozdemir H, Maral I, et al: Differential diagnosis of solid breast nodules: Contribution of Doppler studies to mammography and gray scale. J Ultrasound Med 2001;20:1091-1101.

Walsh JS, Dixon JM, Chetty U, et al: Colour Doppler studies of axillary node metastases in breast carcinoma. Clin Radiol 1994;49:189-191.

Yang WT, Metreweli C: Colour Doppler flow in normal axillary lymph nodes. Br J Radiol 1998;71(844):381-383.

24

THE SCROTUM

Brian Gorman / Barbara A. Carroll

Chapter Outline

$\mathcal{D}$iagnostic ultrasound is the most common imaging technique used to supplement the physical examination of the scrotum and is an accurate means of evaluating many scrotal diseases. Technical advancements in high-resolution real-time and color flow Doppler sonography have led to an increase in the clinical applications of scrotal sonography.

IMAGING TECHNIQUE

It is helpful if patients can localize palpable nodules within the scrotum, which may then be palpated by the sonographer during the examination. The patient is examined in the supine position. The scrotum is elevated with a towel draped over the thighs, and the penis is placed on the patient's abdomen and covered with a towel. Alternatively, the scrotal sac may be supported by the examiner's hand. A high-frequency (7.5- to 15-MHz) linear-array transducer is commonly used because it provides increased resolution of the scrotal contents. If greater penetration is needed because of scrotal swelling, a 6-MHz or lower frequency transducer may be used. A direct-contact scan is most commonly performed using

any acoustic coupling gel. Images of both testes are obtained in transverse and sagittal planes. If possible, a transverse scan showing both testes for comparison is obtained using a dual imaging technique, a larger foot-print transducer, or extended-field-of-view imaging. Additional views may be obtained in the coronal or oblique planes, with the patient upright or performing the Valsalva maneuver when necessary. Color flow and power mode Doppler examinations are also performed to evaluate testicular blood flow in normal and pathologic states.

ANATOMY

The adult testes are ovoid glands measuring 3 to 5 cm in length, 2 to 4 cm in width, and 3 cm in antero-posterior dimension. Each testis weighs from 12.5 to 19 g. Testicular size and weight decrease with age.[1,2,3] The testes are surrounded by a dense white fibrous capsule, the **tunica albuginea**. Multiple thin septations (septula) arise from the innermost aspect of the **tunica albuginea** and converge posteriorly to form the **mediastinum testis** (Fig. 24-1). The mediastinum testis forms the

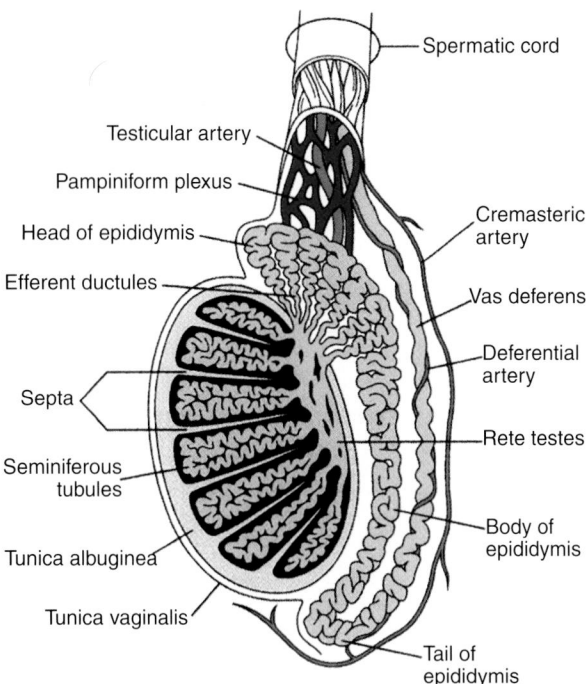

FIGURE 24-1. Normal intrascrotal anatomy. (From Sudakoff GS, Quiroz F, Kaarcaaltincaba M, Foley WD: Scrotal ultrasonography with emphasis on the extratesticular space: Anatomy, embryology and pathology. Ultrasound Quarterly 2002;18:255–273.)

support for the entering and exiting testicular vessels and ducts. As the septula proceed posteriorly from the tunica albuginea, they form 250 to 400 wedge-shaped lobuli that contain the seminiferous tubules. There are approximately 840 tubules per testis. As the tubules course centrally, they join other seminiferous tubules to form 20 to 30 larger ducts, known as the **tubuli recti**. The tubuli recti enter the mediastinum testis, forming a network of channels within the testicular stroma, called

SCROTAL SONOGRAPHY: CURRENT USES*

Evaluation of the location and characteristics of scrotal masses
Detection of an occult primary tumor in patients with known metastatic disease
Follow-up of patients with testicular microlithiasis
Follow-up of patients with previous testicular neoplasms, leukemia, or lymphoma
Evaluation of extratesticular pathologic lesions
Evaluation of acute scrotal pain
Evaluation of scrotal trauma
Localization of the undescended testis
Detection of varicoceles in infertile men
Evaluation of testicular ischemia with color flow and power mode Doppler sonography

*From references 1,7,9,12,14,118,204.

the **rete testis**. The rete terminate in 10 to 15 efferent ductules at the superior portion of the mediastinum, which carry the seminal fluid from the testis to the epididymis.

Sonographically the **normal testis** has a homogeneous granular echo texture composed of uniformly distributed medium-level echoes, similar to that of the thyroid (Fig. 24-2A). The **septula testis** may be seen as linear echogenic or hypoechoic structures (see Fig. 24-2B). The mediastinum testis is sometimes seen as a linear echogenic band extending craniocaudally within the testis (see Fig. 24-2C). Its appearance varies according to the amount of fibrous and fatty tissue present. It is best visualized between the ages of 15 and 60 years.[3] The tunica albuginea is not normally visualized as a separate structure.

The **epididymis** is a curved structure measuring 6 to 7 cm in length and lying posterolateral to the testis. It is composed of a head, a body, and a tail. The head of the epididymis, also known as the **globus major**, is located adjacent to the superior pole of the testis and is the largest portion of the epididymis. It is formed by 10 to 15 efferent ductules from the rete testis joining together to form a single convoluted duct, the **ductus epididymis**. This duct forms the body and the majority of the tail of the epididymis. It measures approximately 600 cm in length and follows a very convoluted course from the head to the tail of the epididymis. The body or corpus of the epididymis lies adjacent to the posterolateral margin of the testis. The **tail** or **globus minor** is loosely attached to the lower pole of the testis by areolar tissue. The ductus epididymis forms an acute angle at the inferior aspect of the globus minor and courses cephalad on the medial aspect of the epididymis to the spermatic cord. Sonographically the epididymis is normally iso-echogenic or slightly more echogenic than the testis, and its echo texture may be coarser. The globus major normally measures 10 to 12 mm in diameter and lies lateral to the superior pole of the testis (see Fig. 24-2D). The **body** tends to be isoechoic or slightly less echogenic than the globus major and testis. The normal body measures less than 4 mm in diameter, averaging 1 to 2 mm.

The **appendix testis**, a remnant of the upper end of the paramesonephric (müllerian) duct, is a small ovoid structure located most commonly on the superior pole of the testis or in the groove between the testis and the head of the epididymis. The appendix testis is identified sonographically in 80% of testes and is more readily visible when a hydrocele is present (see Fig. 24-2E).[4] The appendices of the head and tail of the epididymis are blind-ending tubules (**vasa aberrantia**) derived from the mesonephric (wolffian) duct; they form small stalks, which may be duplicated, and project from the epididymis (see Fig. 24-2F).[5] Rarely, other appendages, the paradidymis (organ of Giraldés) and the superior and inferior vas aberrans of Haller, may be seen.[6] The appendages of the epididymis are most often identified

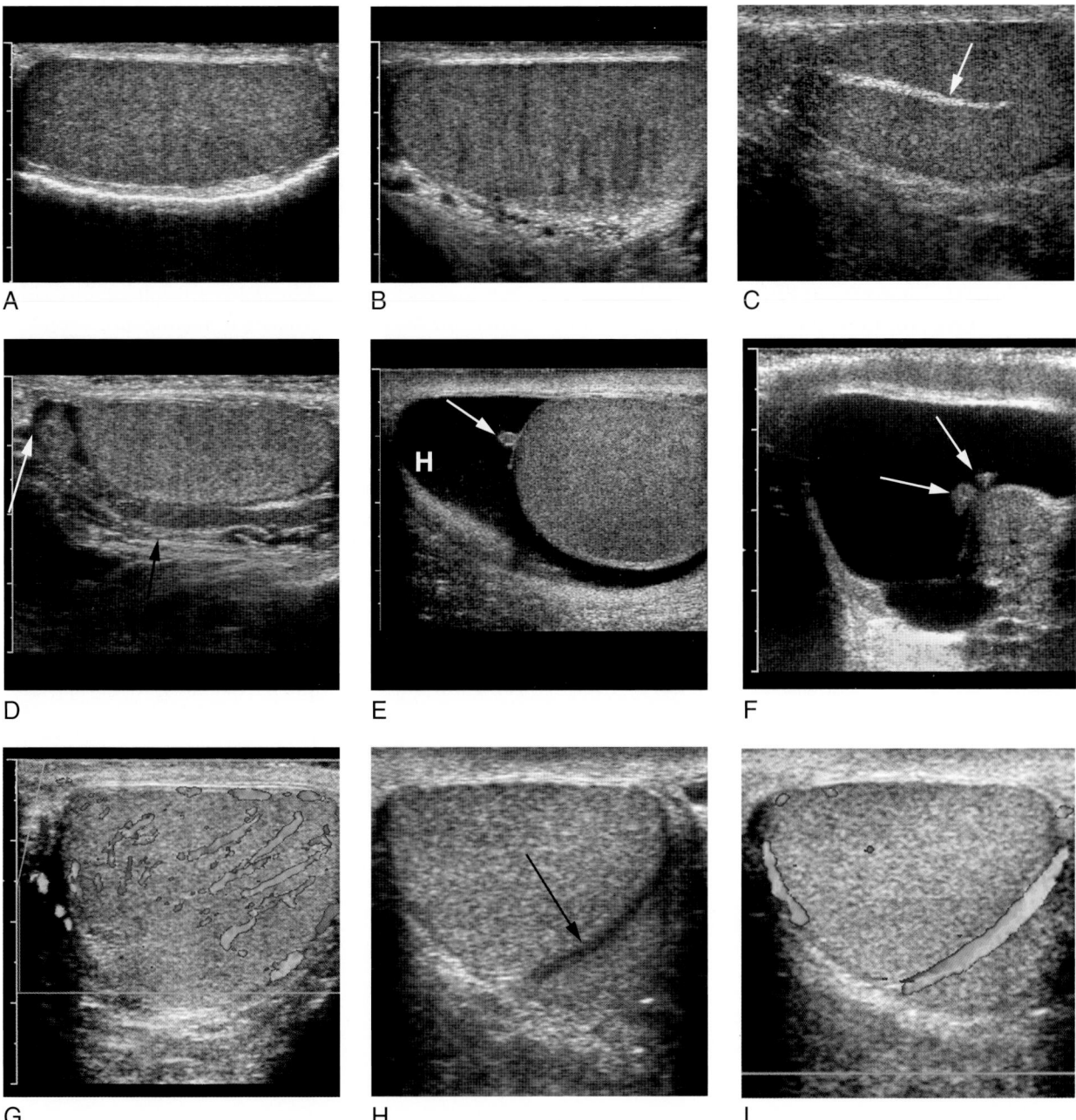

FIGURE 24-2. Normal scrotal contents. Longitudinal scans showing normal intrascrotal anatomy. **A**, Normal homogeneous echotexture of the testis. **B**, Striated appearance of the septula testis. **C**, Mediastinum testis (*arrow*) as a linear echogenic band of fibrofatty tissue. **D**, Head (*white arrow*) and body (*black arrow*) of epididymis. **E**, Hydrocele (H) showing appendix testis (*arrow*). **F**, Appendages of epididymis (*arrows*). **G**, Color Doppler scan shows normal testicular arteries. Transverse scans show normal intrascrotal anatomy. **H**, Hypoechoic band of transmediastinal artery (*arrow*). **I**, Color Doppler scan showing transmediastinal artery.

sonographically as separate structures when a hydrocele is present.

Knowledge of the arterial supply of the testis is important for interpretation of color flow Doppler sonography of the testis. **Testicular blood flow** is supplied primarily by the deferential, cremasteric (external spermatic), and testicular arteries. The **deferential artery** originates from the inferior vesical artery and courses to the tail of the epididymis, where it divides and forms a capillary

network. The **cremasteric artery** arises from the inferior epigastric artery. It courses with the remainder of the structures of the spermatic cord through the inguinal ring, continuing to the surface of the tunica vaginalis, where it anastomoses with capillaries of the testicular and deferential arteries. The **testicular arteries** arise from the anterior aspect of the aorta immediately below the origin of the renal arteries. They course through the inguinal canal with the spermatic cord to the posterosuperior aspect of the testis. Upon reaching the testis, the testicular artery divides into branches that pierce the tunica albuginea and arborize over the surface of the testis in a layer known as the **tunica vasculosa**. Centripetal branches arise from these capsular arteries; these branches course along the septula to converge on the mediastinum. From the mediastinum, these branches form recurrent rami that course centrifugally within the testicular parenchyma, where they branch into arterioles and capillaries (see Fig. 24-2G).[7] In roughly half of normal testes a transmediastinal artery supplies the testis, entering through the mediastinum and coursing toward the periphery of the gland. These arteries may be unilateral or bilateral and single or multiple, and they are frequently seen as a hypoechoic band in the mid testis (see Figs. 24-2H and 24-2I).[7,8]

The **velocity waveforms of the normal capsular and intratesticular arteries** show high levels of antegrade diastolic flow throughout the cardiac cycle, reflecting the low vascular resistance of the testis (Fig. 24-3A).[9] Supratesticular arterial waveforms vary in appearance. Two main types of waveforms exist: a low-resistance waveform such as the capsular and intratesticular arteries and a high-resistance waveform with sharp, narrow systolic peaks and little or no diastolic flow (see Fig. 24-3B).[9]

This high-resistance waveform is believed to reflect the high vascular resistance of the extratesticular tissues. The deferential and cremasteric arteries within the spermatic cord primarily supply the epididymis and extratesticular tissues, but they also supply the testis through anastomoses with the testicular artery.

The **spermatic cord** consists of the vas deferens; the cremasteric, deferential, and testicular arteries; a pampiniform plexus of veins; the lymphatics; and the nerves of the testis. Sonographically the normal spermatic cord lies just beneath the skin and is difficult to distinguish from the adjacent soft tissues of the inguinal canal.[10] It may be visualized within the scrotum when a hydrocele is present or with the use of color flow Doppler sonography.

The **dartos**, a layer of muscle fibers lying beneath the scrotal skin, is continuous with the scrotal septum, which divides the scrotum into two chambers. The walls of the chambers are formed by the fusion of the three fascial layers.

The **tunica vaginalis** is the space between these scrotal fascial layers and the tunica albuginea of the testis. During embryologic development, the tunica vaginalis arises from the **processus vaginalis**, an outpouching of fetal peritoneum that accompanies the

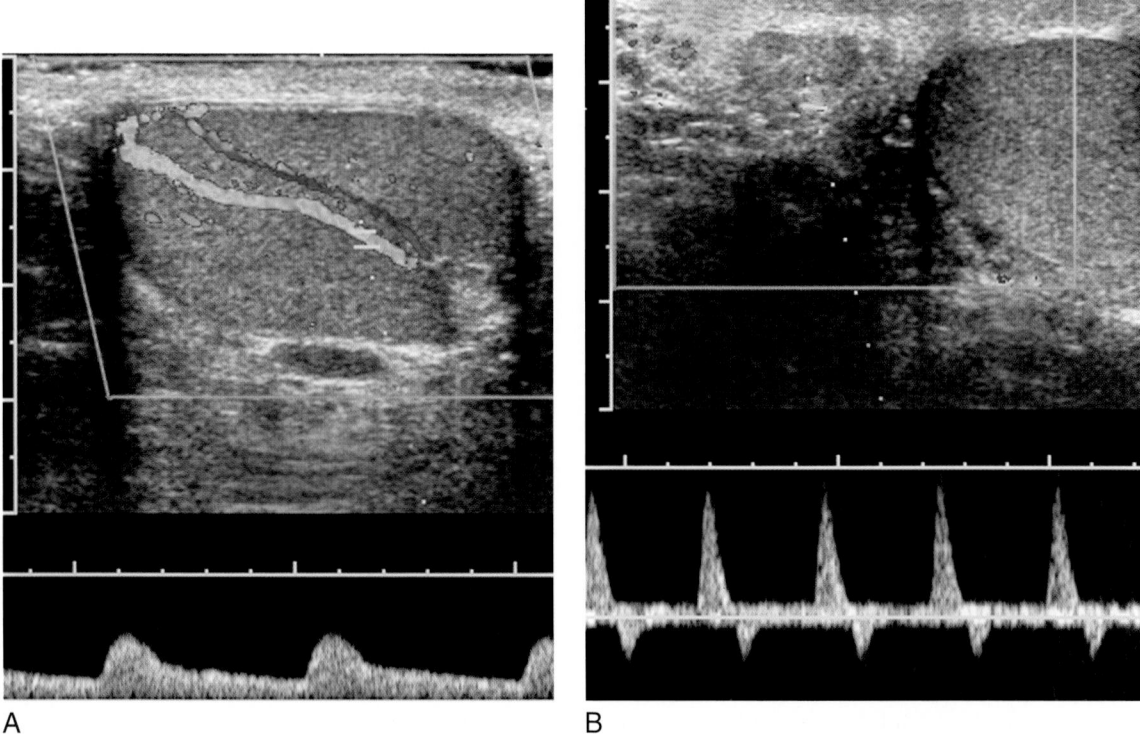

A   B

FIGURE 24-3. Spectral Doppler of normal intratesticular and extratesticular arterial flow. A, Spectral Doppler of the intratesticular artery shows a low-impedance waveform with large amount of end-diastolic flow. **B,** Spectral Doppler of the extratesticular scrotal arterial supply (cremasteric and deferential arteries) shows high-impedance waveform with reversed flow in diastole.

testis in its descent into the scrotum. The upper portion of the processus vaginalis, extending from the internal inguinal ring to the upper pole of the testis, is normally obliterated. The lower portion, the tunica vaginalis, remains as a closed pouch folded around the testis. Only the posterior aspect of the testis, the site of attachment of the testis and epididymis, is not in continuity with the tunica vaginalis. The inner or visceral layer of the tunica vaginalis covers the testis, epididymis, and lower portion of the spermatic cord. The outer or parietal layer of the tunica vaginalis lines the walls of the scrotal pouch and is attached to the fascial coverings of the testis. A small amount of fluid is normally present between these two layers, especially in the polar regions and between the testicle and epididymis.

The scrotal covering layers are normally indistinguishable by sonography and are visualized as a single echogenic stripe. If any type of fluid is present in the scrotal wall, the tunica vaginalis may be identified as a separate structure.[1]

SCROTAL MASSES

With ultrasonographic examination intrascrotal masses can be detected with a sensitivity of nearly 100%.[11] Sonography is important in the evaluation of scrotal masses because its accuracy is 98% to 100% in distinguishing intratesticular and extratesticular pathologic features.[12,13] This distinction is important in disease management because most extratesticular masses are benign, but the majority of intratesticular lesions are malignant.[3,14] Virtually all intratesticular masses should be considered malignant until proved otherwise.[1]

Most malignant testicular neoplasms are more hypoechoic than normal testicular parenchyma; however, hemorrhage, necrosis, calcification, or fatty changes can produce areas of increased echogenicity within tumors.

Testicular neoplasms account for 1% to 2% of all malignant neoplasms in men and are the fifth most frequent cause of death in men aged 15 to 34 years.[15] Approximately 65% to 94% of patients with testicular neoplasms present with painless unilateral testicular masses or diffuse testicular enlargement, and 4% to 14% present with symptoms of metastatic disease.[1,16,17] Most primary testicular tumors are of germ cell origin and are generally highly malignant.[18] Only 60% of testicular germ cell tumors are of one histologic subtype, and the remainder are of two or more histologic subtypes. Although there are potentially several histologic subtypes of germ cell tumor, clinically it is important to recognize only two basic tumor types: **seminomas** and **nonseminomatous germ cell tumors (NSGCT)**. This is because seminomas and NSGCT behave differently biologically and, therefore, have different therapeutic

and prognostic implications.[19] Seminomas are more radiosensitive and usually have a better prognosis.

Gonadal stromal tumors, arising from Sertoli or Leydig cells, account for 3% to 6% of testicular masses,[1,3,17] and the majority of these mesenchymal neoplasms are benign (see box.)

Malignant Tumors

Germ Cell Tumors. Seminoma is the most common single-cell type of testicular tumor in adults, accounting for 40% to 50% of all germ cell neoplasms. It is also a common component of mixed germ cell tumors,

---

PATHOLOGIC CLASSIFICATION OF TESTICULAR TUMORS*

GERM CELL TUMORS

Seminoma
  Classic
  Spermatocytic
Nonseminomatous germ cell tumors
  Mixed malignant germ cell
  Embryonal cell carcinoma
  Yolk sac (endodermal sinus tumor)
  Teratoma
  Choriocarcinoma

STROMAL TUMORS

Leydig cell (interstitial)
Sertoli cell
Granulosa cell
Mixed undifferentiated sex cord

MIXED GERM CELL-STROMAL TUMORS

Gonadoblastoma
Germ cell-stromal-sex cord

METASTATIC NEOPLASMS

Lymphoma
Leukemia
Myeloma
Carcinoma

RARE TUMORS AND NON-NEOPLASTIC TUMOROUS CONDITIONS

Adrenal rests
Epidermoid cyst
Malacoplakia
Carcinoid
Mesenchymal

*From Mostofi FK, Sobin LH: International histological classification of tumors of the testes No. 16, WHO, Geneva 1977.

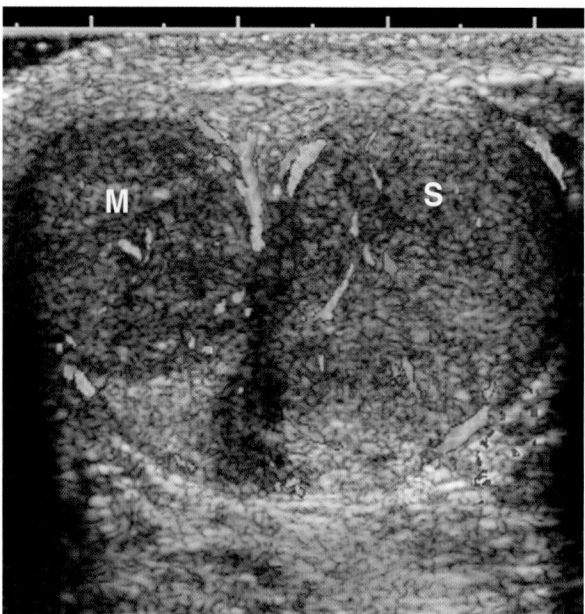

FIGURE 24-4. Coexistent mixed germ cell tumor and seminoma. Transverse scan shows mixed germ cell tumor (M) and seminoma (S).

occurring in 30% of these tumors. Seminomas occur in slightly older patients than do other testicular neoplasms, with a peak incidence in the fourth and fifth decades.[1,11,21-23] They rarely occur before puberty. They are less aggressive than other testicular tumors and are commonly confined within the tunica albuginea at presentation with only 25% of patients having metastases at diagnosis. As a result of the radiosensitivity and chemosensitivity of the primary tumor and its metastases, seminomas have the most favorable prognosis of the malignant testicular tumors. A second primary synchronous or metachronous germ cell tumor occurs in 1% to 2.5% of patients with seminomas (Fig. 24-4).

Seminoma is the most common tumor type in **cryptorchid testes**. Between 8% and 30% of patients with seminoma have a history of undescended testes.[17,22,23] The risk of a seminoma developing is substantially increased in an undescended testis, even after orchiopexy. There is also an increased risk of malignancy developing in the contralateral, normally located testis; therefore, sonography is often used to screen for an occult tumor in the remaining testis after orchiectomy.

Macroscopically, seminoma is a homogeneously solid, firm, round or oval tumor that varies in size from a small nodule in a normal-size testis to a large mass causing diffuse testicular enlargement.[15] The sonographic features of pure seminoma parallel this homogeneous macroscopic appearance (Fig. 24-5). Pure seminomas usually have predominantly uniform, low-level echoes without calcification, and they appear hypoechoic compared with normally echogenic testicular parenchyma.[24] With high-resolution sonography, some seminomas may

have a more heterogeneous echotexture (see Fig. 24-5E). Very rarely seminomas become necrotic and appear partly cystic on sonography (see Fig. 24-5I).

Non-Seminomatous Germ Cell Tumors. NSGCT include **embryonal carcinomas, teratomas, yolk sac tumors, choriocarcinomas, and mixed germ cell tumors.** These tumors occur more often in younger patients than do seminomas, with a peak incidence during the latter part of the second decade and the third decade. They are uncommon before puberty and after the age of 50 years. These malignancies are more aggressive than seminomas, frequently invading the tunica albuginea and resulting in distortion of the testicular contour (Fig. 24-6). They frequently cause visceral metastases.[1,23] The sonographic appearance of NSGCT reflects the histologic features. Typically these tumors are more heterogeneous than seminoma and may have both solid and cystic components (see Fig. 24-6). Coarse calcifications are common. It is not possible to distinguish the various subtypes of NSGCT by sonography.

Mixed germ cell tumors are the most common NSGCT. They contain non-seminomatous germ cell elements in various combinations. Seminomatous elements may also be present but do not influence prognosis.[19] The most common combination, previously called teratocarcinoma, is that of teratoma and embryonal cell carcinoma. Mixed germ cell tumors are the second most common primary testicular malignancy after seminoma, constituting 40% of all germ cell tumors.

Pure **embryonal cell carcinoma** is a rare tumor accounting for only 2% to 3% of testicular germ cell neoplasms.[25] It often occurs in combination with other neoplastic germ cell elements, particularly yolk sac tumor and teratoma. Like other NSGCT, these tumors occur in younger patients than do seminomas, with a peak incidence during the latter part of the second and third decades. The infantile form, **endodermal sinus** or **yolk sac tumor**, is the most common germ cell tumor in infants younger than two years, accounting for 60% of testicular neoplasms in this age group. Yolk sac tumor is associated with elevated levels of α-fetoprotein in 95% of infants. Both embryonal cell carcinoma and yolk sac tumor are less radiosensitive and chemosensitive than seminomas, and patients with these tumors have a five-year survival rate of 25% to 35%.[23] The sonographic features of pure embryonal cell carcinoma are similar to those of mixed NSGCT (see Fig. 24-6A-C). Cystic areas are present in one third of tumors,[11] and echogenic foci, with or without acoustic shadowing, are not uncommon.

Teratomas constitute approximately 5% to 10% of primary testicular neoplasms.[23] They are defined according to the World Health Organization classification on the basis of the presence of derivatives of the different germinal layers (endoderm, mesoderm, and ectoderm). There are three categories of teratomas according to this

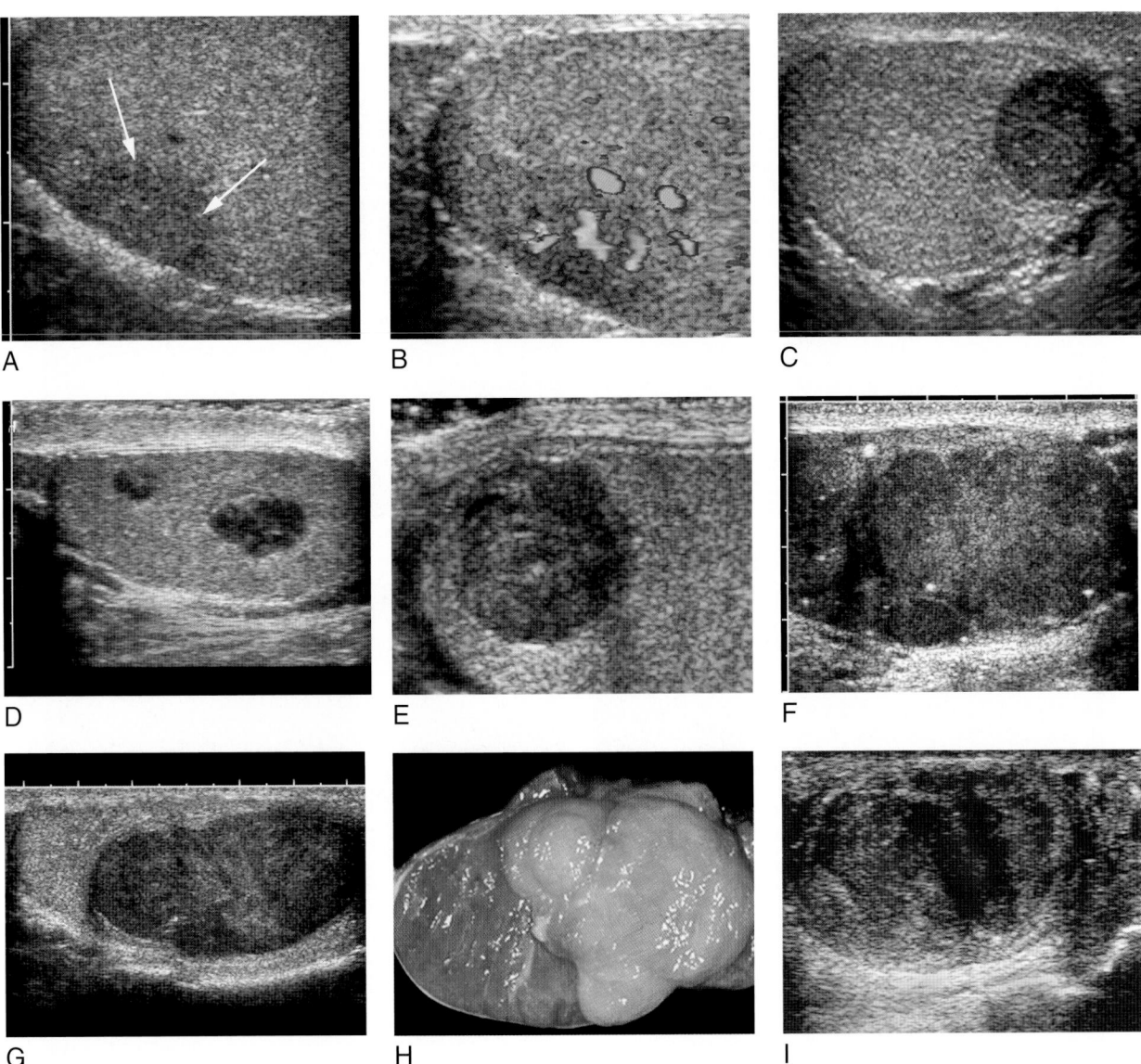

FIGURE 24-5. Seminoma—spectrum of appearances. Longitudinal scans show (**A**) and (**B**) subtle hypoechoic seminoma (*arrows*), with increased flow. **C**, Typical homogeneous hypoechoic seminoma. **D**, Two small foci of seminoma. **E**, Slightly heterogeneous seminoma. **F**, Seminoma associated with microlithiasis and coarser calcifications. **G**, Seminoma occupying most of testis. **H**, Gross specimen of seminoma in **G**. Typical homogeneous hypoechoic sonographic appearance. **I**, Necrotic seminoma replacing testicle.

classification: mature, immature, and teratoma with malignant transformation.[17] One third of teratomas metastasize, usually by a lymphatic route, within 5 years.[1,23] The reported 5-year survival rate is 70%. The peak incidence is in infancy and early childhood, with another peak in the third decade of life. In infants and young children, teratomas are the second most common testicular tumor and are most commonly mature, well differentiated, and benign. Occasional cases may contain immature elements, but metastases are rare.[22] After puberty, teratomas commonly contain immature and mature elements admixed with other germ cell types. Teratomas in adults are usually malignant. Elevated levels of α-fetoprotein or human chorionic gonadotropin may be found and are suggestive of malignancy.[19]

Sonographically the **teratoma** is commonly a well-defined, markedly inhomogeneous mass containing cystic and solid areas of various sizes and appears similar to other NSGCT. Dense echogenic foci causing acoustic shadowing are common, resulting from focal calcification, cartilage, immature bone, fibrosis, and noncalcific scarring (see Fig. 24-6D,E).[24]

Pure **choriocarcinoma** is the rarest type of germ cell tumor, accounting for less than 0.5% of malignant primary testicular tumors.[25] Only 18 cases were encountered among more than 6000 testicular tumors registered at the Armed Forces Institute of Pathology.[26] Approximately 23% of mixed germ cell tumors contain a component of choriocarcinoma.[22] The peak incidence is in the second and third decades. These tumors are

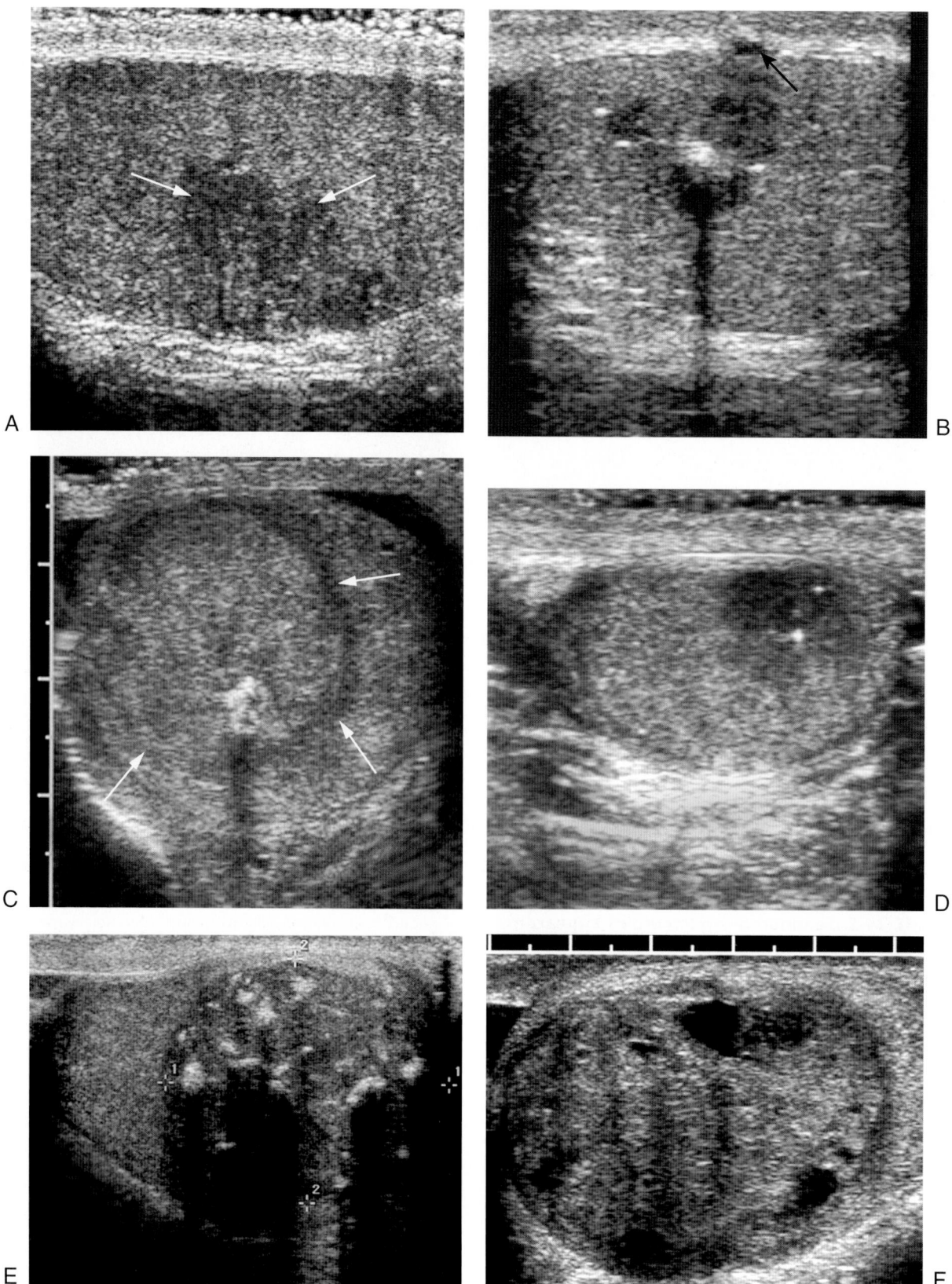

FIGURE 24-6. Non-seminomatous germ cell tumors—spectrum of appearances. A, Embryonal carcinoma. Longitudinal scan shows relatively homogeneous tumor (*arrows*). **B, Embryonal carcinoma.** Longitudinal scan shows partly cystic calcified mass invading the tunica (*arrow*). **C, Embryonal carcinoma.** Transverse scan shows tumor (*arrows*) with coarse calcification. **D, Teratoma.** Longitudinal scan shows cystic change and calcification. **E, Teratoma.** Longitudinal scan shows extensive calcification. **F, Mixed germ cell tumor.** Longitudinal scan shows a large tumor with cystic change occupying most of the testis.

highly malignant and metastasize early by hematogenous and lymphatic routes. Often patients have symptoms resulting from hemorrhagic metastases: hemoptysis, hematemesis, and symptoms related to the central nervous system. Gynecomastia is common because of the high levels of circulating chorionic gonadotropins produced by all these tumors.[17] Metastases may be present without any evidence of choriocarcinoma in the testicle. Hemorrhage with focal necrosis of tumor is an almost invariable feature, and calcification may be present, giving a sonographic appearance similar to the other NSGCT (see Fig. 24-6F).

Stromal Tumors

Gonadal stromal tumors account for 3% to 6% of all testicular neoplasms. Approximately 20% of these tumors occur in children.[15] The term *gonadal stromal tumor* refers to a neoplasm containing Leydig, Sertoli, thecal, granulosa, or lutein cells and fibroblasts in various degrees of differentiation. These tumors may contain single or multiple cell types because of the totipotentiality of the gonadal stroma.[17] Gonadal stromal tumors in conjunction with germ cell tumors are called **gonadoblastomas**. The majority of gonadoblastomas occur in males with cryptorchidism, hypospadias, and female internal secondary sex organs.[22]

The majority of stromal tumors are **Leydig cell tumors**. They account for 1% to 3% of all testicular neoplasms and occur predominantly in patients between the ages of 20 and 50 years.[21,22,27] Patients most commonly present with painless testicular enlargement or a palpable mass. Approximately 15% to 30% of patients present with gynecomastia resulting from the secretion of androgens or estrogens or both. Impotence, loss of libido, or precocious virilization may also occur in young men. The tumor is bilateral in 3% of cases. From 10% to 15% of the tumors are malignant, having invaded the tunica at diagnosis. Leydig cell tumors are homogeneous, but foci of hemorrhage and necrosis are present in 25% of the tumors.[21,27] These gonadal tumors are usually small, solid, and hypoechoic on sonography (Fig. 24-7A-C). Cystic spaces resulting from hemorrhage and necrosis are occasionally seen in larger lesions.[28]

Sertoli cell tumors are rare and account for less than 1% of all testicular tumors; they occur with equal frequency in all age groups.[29] The most common presentation is with a painless testicular mass. Feminization with gynecomastia may occur, especially with malignant Sertoli cell tumors or with the large cell calcifying variant. Sertoli cell tumors may occur in undescended testes, in patients with testicular feminization, Klinefelter's syndrome, and Peutz-Jeghers syndrome.[30] Sertoli cell tumors are usually small and homogeneous, and this is reflected in the sonographic appearance, which shows a small hypoechoic mass similar to a Leydig cell tumor.

Occasionally hemorrhage or necrosis may occur giving a more heterogeneous appearance on sonography. The large, cell-calcifying Sertoli cell tumor is a subtype with distinctive clinical, histologic, and sonographic features.[30] These tumors are often bilateral and multifocal and may be almost completely calcified (see Fig. 24-7D).

Occult Primary Tumors. Sonography is an important diagnostic tool for patients who present with mediastinal, retroperitoneal, or supraclavicular metastases from metastatic testicular carcinoma but have a normal physical examination of the testes (Fig. 24-8).[32-34] The detection of the occult primary tumor is important in disease management because if the tumor is not removed, metastasis will continue. Sonography can detect nonpalpable testicular neoplasms. The primary testicular tumor may regress, despite widespread advancing metastatic disease, resulting in an echogenic fibrous and, possibly, calcific scar. A hypothesis is that regression is due to the high metabolic rate of the tumor and vascular compromise from the tumor outgrowing its blood supply. Usually no viable tumor cells are identifiable on histologic section in these cases.[15,16] The size of the affected testis is often normal or small. The sonographic finding of an echogenic focus with or without posterior acoustic shadowing is not specific for a **"burned-out" tumor**, but it is strongly suggestive of this diagnosis in the context of histologically proven testicular metastases (Fig. 24-9).[35]

Approximately 95% of primary testicular neoplasms larger than 1.6 cm in diameter show increased vascularity on color flow Doppler sonographic examinations. Color flow Doppler findings do not appear to be important, however, in the evaluation of adult testicular tumors.[36] Color flow may help to identify tumors that are relatively isoechoic with testicular parenchyma,[37] but focal or diffuse inflammatory lesions cannot be distinguished from neoplasms on the basis of color flow Doppler or pulsed Doppler findings.

Nonpalpable testicular tumors have also been detected in patients presenting with infertility.[18] Incidentally discovered nonpalpable lesions are usually benign.[38] Many believe that if tumor markers and the chest radiograph are normal, patients can undergo an excisional testicular biopsy using an inguinal, organ-sparing approach. In these cases, intraoperative sonography may facilitate resection of the testicular mass. If the frozen section shows a benign lesion, the testis can be spared. Sonographic follow-up of an incidentally detected lesion is only recommended if there is a strong clinical suggestion that the lesion is non-neoplastic (i.e., a recent history of trauma or infection).

Testicular Metastases

Metastases, Lymphoma, and Leukemia. Lymphoma and leukemia are the most common metastatic tes-

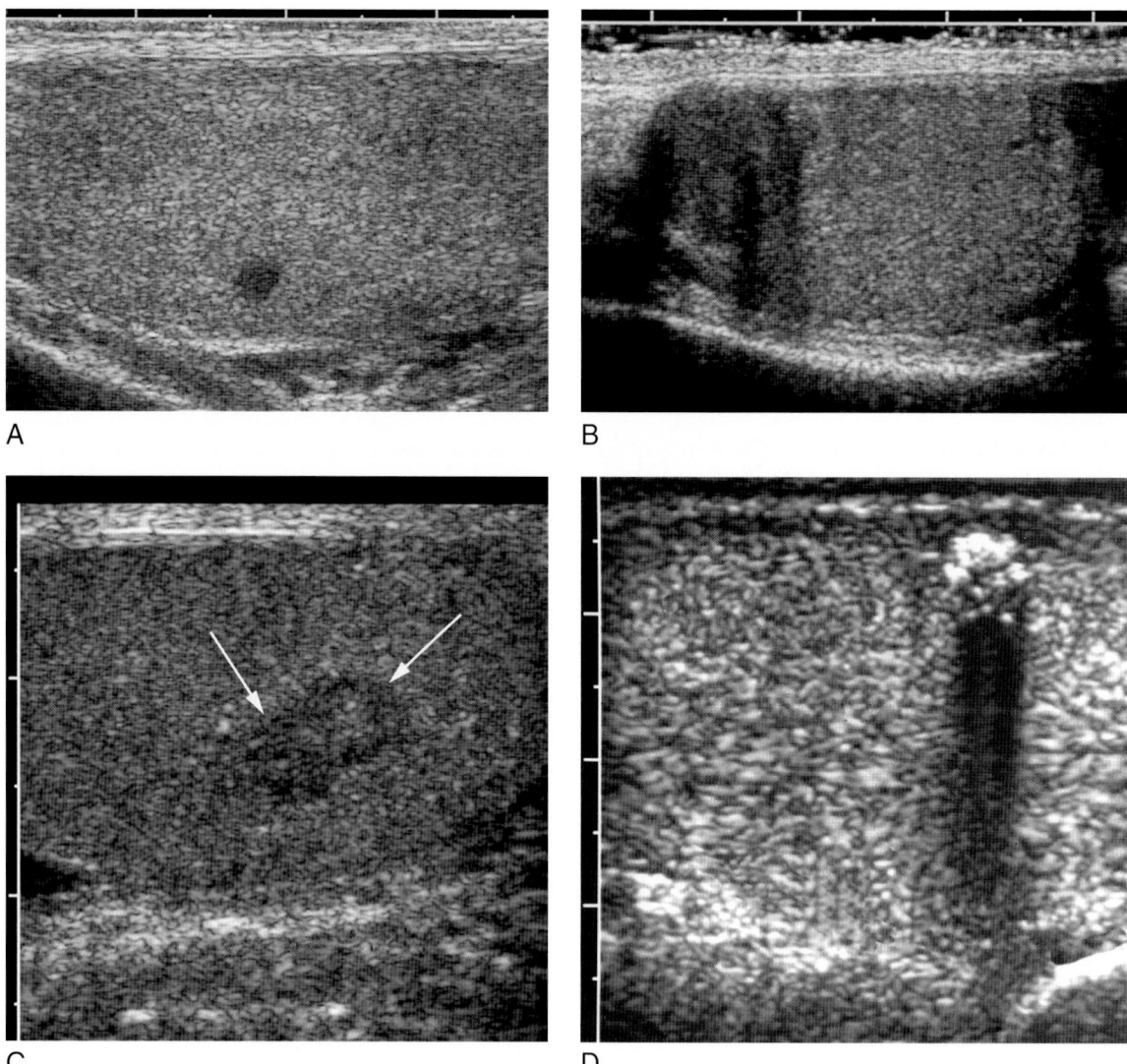

FIGURE 24-7. Stromal tumors—spectrum of appearances. A–C. Longitudinal scans of **Leydig cell tumor. A,** Small hypoechoic solid mass in the midtestis. **B,** Hypoechoic solid mass at the upper pole of the testis. **C,** Subtle hypoechoic mass (*arrows*) in the midtestis. The patient had bilateral stromal tumors. Transverse scan. **D,** Large cell calcifying **Sertoli tumor.**

ticular tumors. **Malignant lymphoma** is the most common secondary testicular neoplasm. Lymphoma accounts for 1% to 8% of all testicular tumors and is the most common testicular tumor in men older than 60 years. However, testicular involvement occurs in only 0.3% of patients with lymphoma.[17,39] The peak age at diagnosis of lymphoma is between 60 and 70 years; 80% of the patients are older than 50 years at diagnosis. Malignant lymphoma is the most common bilateral testicular tumor, occurring bilaterally either in a synchronous or, more commonly, metachronous manner in 6% to 38% of cases. One half of bilateral testicular neoplasms are malignant lymphomas.[17,21] Most malignant lymphomas of the testicle are of the non-Hodgkin's type. As categorized with the Rappaport classification, diffuse histiocytic lymphoma is the most common type of testicular lymphoma, followed by poorly differentiated lymphocytic lymphoma.[17] Hodgkin's lymphoma is extremely rare.[40]

Testicular lymphoma most commonly occurs in association with disseminated disease or as the initial manifestation of occult nodal disease. Approximately 10% of the patients with lymphoma present with a testicular mass and appear to have a relatively good prognosis, although meticulous examination usually reveals lymph node involvement.[17,39] True primary lymphoma of the testis has not been conclusively documented.[19] The other patients with diffuse testicular involvement have a poor prognosis. The 5-year survival rate is 5% to 20%. Median survival is 9.5 to 12 months.[41,42]

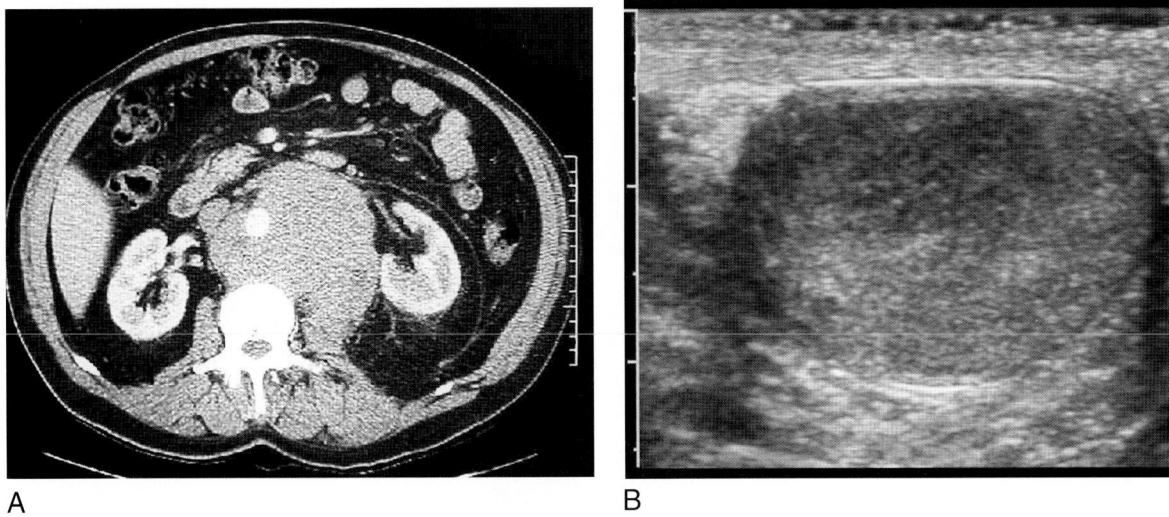

FIGURE 24-8. Occult testicular seminoma with retroperitoneal metastases. A, Contrast-enhanced CT scan showing extensive retroperitoneal adenopathy from seminoma. **B**, Longitudinal sonographic scan shows occult homogeneous hypoechoic seminoma. The physical examination of the testis was negative.

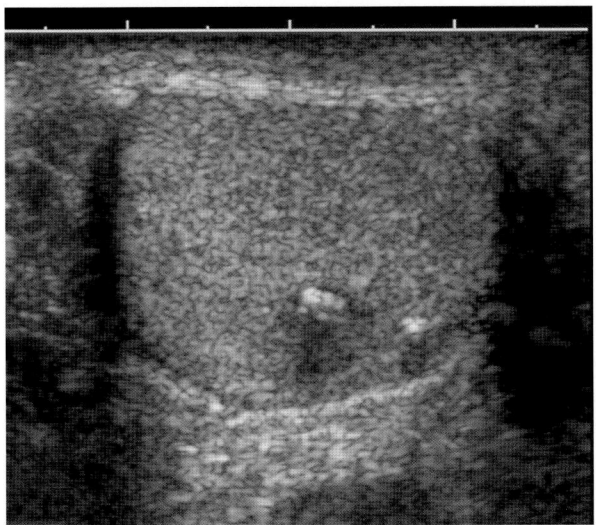

FIGURE 24-9. "Burned-out" germ cell tumor.
Longitudinal scan shows a partly calcified nonviable germ cell tumor in a patient with retroperitoneal metastases. Notice the hypoechoic mass around the focus of calcification.

Most patients with malignant lymphoma of the testis have a painless testicular mass or diffuse testicular enlargement. Approximately 25% of the patients have constitutional symptoms of lymphoma, such as fever, weakness, anorexia, or weight loss.[39]

Lymphoma of the testis is often large at diagnosis. The tunica vaginalis is usually intact, but unlike germ cell tumors, extension into the epididymis and spermatic cord is common, occurring in up to 50% of cases.[20] The scrotal skin is rarely involved. Grossly, the tumor is not encapsulated but compresses the parenchyma to the periphery. The sonographic appearance of lymphoma is nonspecific and similar to that of seminoma. Most malignant lymphomas are homogeneous and hypoechoic, and they diffusely replace the testis.[17,39] Focal hypoechoic lesions can occur, however (Fig. 24-10). Hemorrhage and necrosis are rare.

Color flow Doppler imaging shows increased vascularity in testicular lymphoma, and the appearance may resemble diffuse inflammation (see Fig. 24-10).[43] Unlike inflammation, lymphoma is usually painless and the testes are not tender to palpation.

Leukemia is the second most common metastatic testicular neoplasm. Primary testicular leukemia is rare, but leukemic infiltration of the testicle during bone marrow remission is common in children.[17,44] The testis appears to act as a sanctuary site for leukemic cells during chemotherapy because of the **blood-testis barrier** that inhibits concentration of chemotherapeutic agents.[44] The highest frequency of testicular involvement is found in patients with acute leukemia (64%). Approximately 25% of patients with chronic leukemia have testicular involvement.[45] Most cases of testicular involvement occur within one year of the discontinuation of long-term remission maintenance chemotherapy. The rate of relapse in this setting is nearly 13%.[44]

The sonographic appearance of leukemia is nonspecific and similar to lymphoma. Patients most frequently present with diffuse infiltration, which produces diffusely enlarged, hypoechoic testes (see Fig. 24-10). Focal, sharply marginated, anechoic masses with through-sound transmission and occasional low-level internal echoes have been described in chronic lymphocytic leukemia.[45]

Myeloma. Involvement of the testis is usually a manifestation of diffuse myeloma, although rarely the testis may be the site of primary focal myeloma (plasmacytoma).[46] The testis may have single or multiple

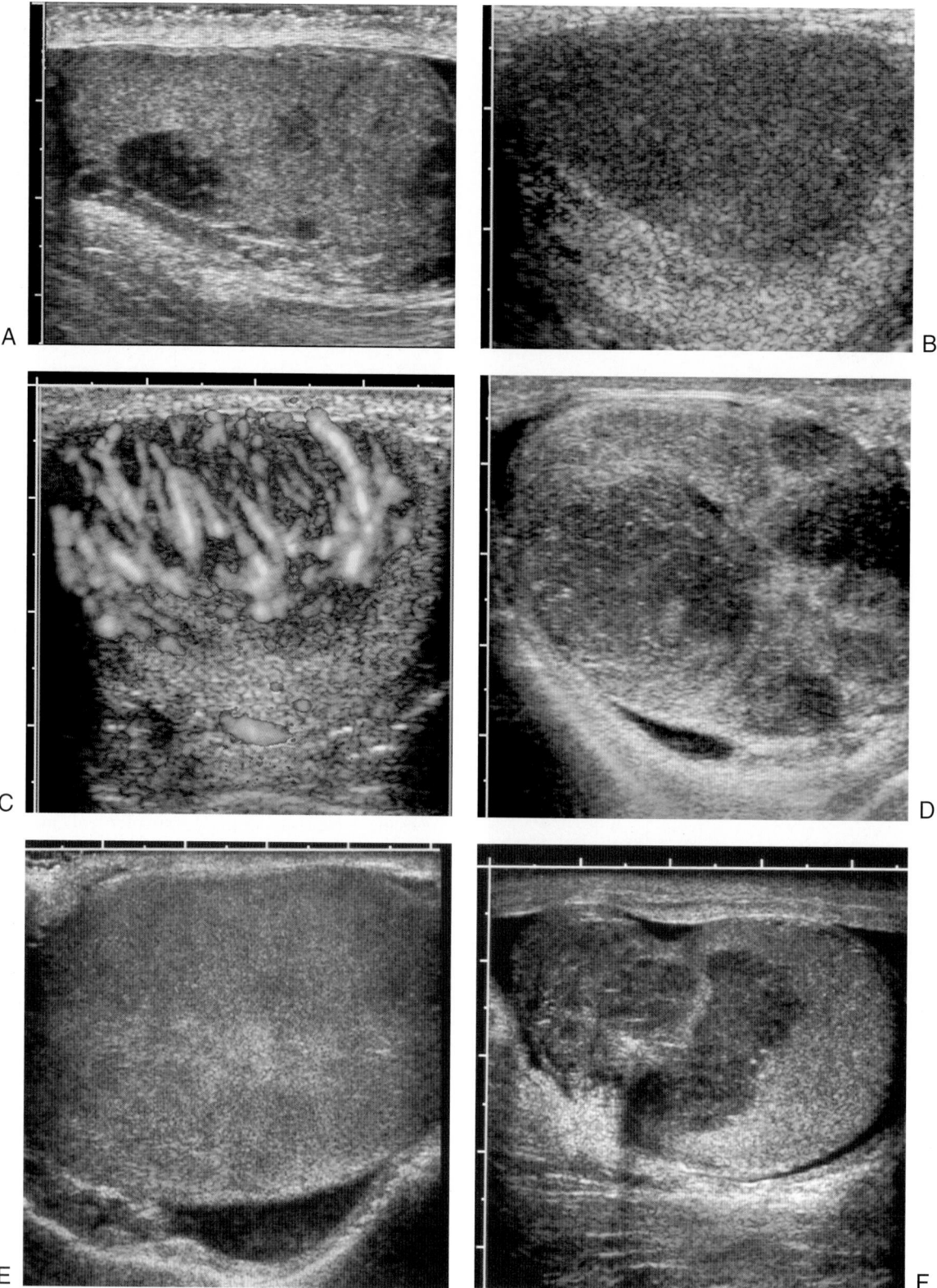

FIGURE 24-10. Lymphoma, leukemia, and metastases. A, Lymphoma. Longitudinal scan shows two subtle hypoechoic foci of lymphoma. **B, Lymphoma.** Longitudinal scan shows diffuse, homogeneous hypoechoic involvement of the testis. **C, Lymphoma.** Longitudinal power Doppler of **B** shows marked vascularity of lymphoma. **D,** Corresponding longitudinal scan. **E, Leukemia.** Longitudinal scan shows diffuse hypoechoic involvement. **F, Melanoma metastasis.** Longitudinal scan shows a hypoechoic mass in the upper pole of the testis and epididymis.

nodules that appear hypoechoic and homogeneous on sonographic examination. Bilateral involvement occurs in approximately 20% of cases.[19]

Other Metastases. Nonlymphomatous metastases to the testes are uncommon, representing only 0.02% to 5% of all testicular neoplasms.[47,48] The most frequent primary sites are the **lung** and **prostate**.[21] Other frequent primary sites for metastatic neoplasms include **melanoma, kidney, colon, stomach**, and **pancreas**.[47,49] Most metastases are clinically silent, being discovered incidentally at autopsy or after orchiectomy for prostatic carcinoma. Testicular metastases are most common in patients during the sixth and seventh decades and are more frequent than primary germ cell tumors in patients older than 50 years.[1,42] They are commonly multiple and are bilateral in 15% of cases.[21] Because primary germ cell tumors may also be multicentric and bilateral, these features are not helpful in distinguishing primary from metastatic testicular neoplasms. Widespread systemic metastases are usually present in patients with testicular metastases.[42] Possible routes of metastases to the testis include retrograde venous, hematogenous, retrograde lymphatic, and direct tumor invasion.[39,41] Metastases in sites remote from the testis, such as the lung and skin, most likely spread hematogenously. Retrograde venous extension through the spermatic vein occurs in renal cell carcinoma and may also occur in bladder and prostate tumors.[50] Neoplasms with metastases to the periaortic lymph nodes may involve the testis through retrograde lymphatic extension. Colorectal carcinoma may directly invade the testes. Sonographic features of nonlymphomatous testicular metastases vary. The appearance is often hypoechoic but may be echogenic or complex (see Fig. 24-10F).[1]

Other rare tumors of the testis include hamartoma (Fig. 24-11), dermoid, hemangioma, intratesticular adenomatoid tumor, carcinoid, carcinoma of the mediastinum testis, neuroectodermal tumor, Brenner tumor, fibroma, fibrosarcoma, osteosarcoma, chondrosarcoma, and undifferentiated sarcoma.

Benign Intratesticular Lesions

Cysts. Testicular cysts are discovered incidentally on sonography in 8% to 10% of the population.[51,52] Cystic testicular lesions are not always benign because testicular tumors (especially NSGCT) may undergo cystic degeneration due to hemorrhage or necrosis. The distinction between a benign cyst and a cystic neoplasm is of utmost clinical importance. Of the 34 cystic testicular masses discovered with sonography by Hamm et al.,[51] 16 were neoplastic and all of these had sonographic features of complicated cysts. NCGCTs, especially those with teratoma elements, are the most common tumors to contain both cystic and solid components.

Cysts of the tunica albuginea are located within the tunica, which surrounds the testis. They vary in size

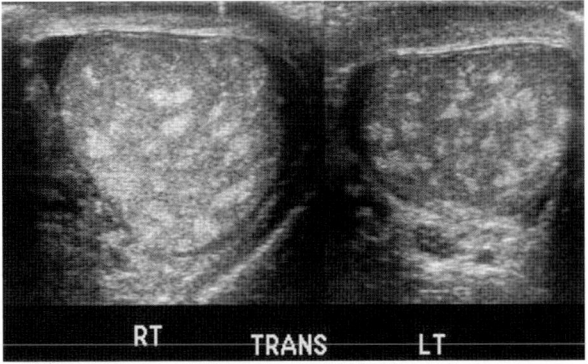

FIGURE 24-11. Dual transverse image shows multiple bilateral hamartomas. The patient had Cowden disease, an inherited autosomal dominant disorder, which causes multiple hamartomas in the gastrointestinal tract.

from 2 to 30 mm and are well defined. They are usually solitary and unilocular but may be multiple or multilocular (Fig. 24-12A).[51,53] The mean age at presentation is 40 years but patients can also have cysts in the fifth and sixth decades.[54] The cysts may be asymptomatic, but patients frequently present with cysts that are clinically palpable, firm scrotal nodules. Histologically, they are simple cysts lined with cuboid or low columnar cells and filled with serous fluid.[55-57] Complex tunica albuginea cysts may simulate a testicular neoplasm.[58] Careful scanning in multiple planes may help identify the benign nature of a tunica albuginea cyst.

Cysts of the tunica vaginalis are rare and arise from the visceral or parietal layer of the tunica vaginalis. They may be single or multiple. Sonographically they usually appear anechoic but may have septations or may contain echoes due to hemorrhage.[59]

Intratesticular cysts are simple cysts filled with clear serous fluid; they vary in size from 2 to 18 mm.[60,61] Sonographically they are well-defined, anechoic lesions with thin, smooth walls and posterior acoustic enhancement. Hamm et al.[51] reported that in all 13 of their

TESTICULAR METASTASES

LYMPHOMA

Mostly non-Hodgkin's

LEUKEMIA

Second most common
64% acute leukemia
Sanctuary site

NONLYMPHOMA METASTASES

Lung and prostate most common
Kidney, stomach, colon, pancreas, melanoma

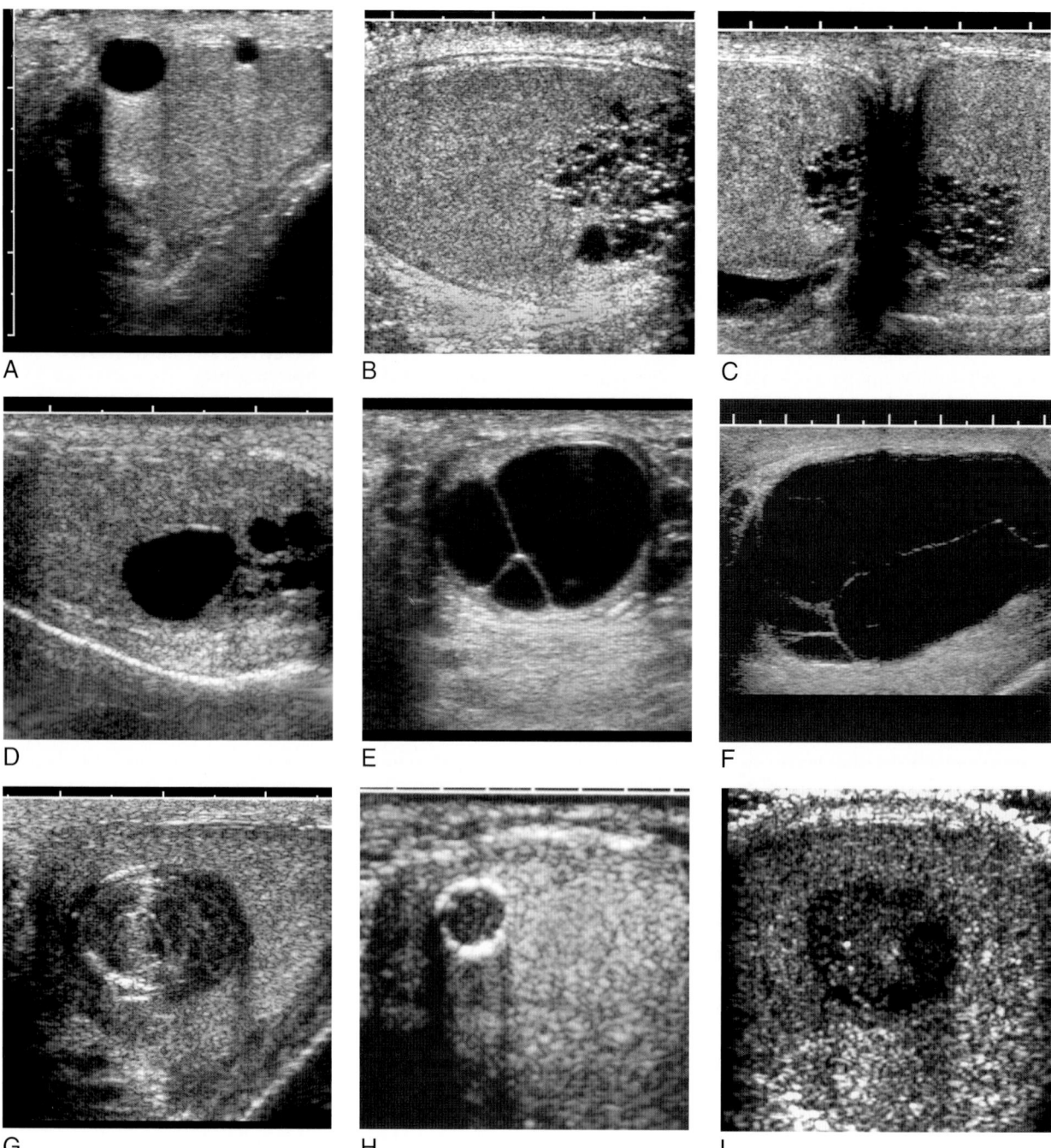

FIGURE 24-12. Benign cystic lesions of the testis. A, Tunica albuginea cysts. Longitudinal scan shows two cysts arising from the tunica. These cysts are usually palpable. **B** and **C, Cystic dilation rete testis.** Longitudinal and transverse scans show dilated tubules of the rete testis in both testes. **D, Benign intratesticular cyst** associated with dilated rete testis on longitudinal scan. **E** and **F,** Transverse longitudinal. **Benign intratesticular cyst with multiple septations. G, Epidermoid cyst (benign).** Typical whorled appearance. **H, Epidermoid cyst.** Typical peripheral calcification. **I, Epidermoid cyst.** Transverse scan shows hypoechoic mass with central calcifications similar to other tumors on gray-scale, but it was avascular on Doppler examination. (**H,** Courtesy of Ben Hollenberg, M.D., Presbyterian Hospital, Charlotte, NC.)

cases, the cysts were located near the mediastinum testis, supporting the theory that they originate from the rete testis, possibly secondary to posttraumatic or post-inflammatory stricture formation (see Fig. 24-12D-F).[51,55]
Tubular Ectasia of the Rete Testis. Tubular ectasia of the rete testis can be mistaken for a testicular

neoplasm.[62-67] This tubular ectasia is usually associated with epididymal obstruction due to inflammation or trauma. Variably sized cystic lesions are seen in the region of the mediastinum testis with no associated soft tissue abnormality, and no flow on color flow Doppler imaging is seen (see Fig. 24-12B-D). Most of these lesions are bilateral and asymmetrical. There is frequently an associated spermatocele. The characteristic sonographic appearance and location should make it possible to distinguish this benign condition from a malignancy, thus avoiding an orchiectomy. Characteristic findings on magnetic resonance imaging (MRI) include intratesticular abnormal signal intensity similar to that of water in the region of the mediastinum testis.[64]

Cystic Dysplasia. Cystic dysplasia is a very rare congenital malformation, usually occurring in infants and young children, although one case was reported in a 30-year-old man.[68,69] This lesion is thought to result from an embryologic defect that prevents connection of the tubules of the rete testis and the efferent ductules. Pathologically, the lesion consists of multiple, interconnecting cysts of various sizes and shapes, separated by fibrous septae.[69] This lesion originates in the rete testis and extends into the adjacent parenchyma, resulting in pressure atrophy of the adjacent testicular parenchyma. The cysts are lined by a single layer of flat or cuboidal epithelium. Sonographically, the appearance is similar to acquired cystic dilation of the rete testis. Renal agenesis or dysplasia frequently coexists with testicular cystic dysplasia.[69]

Epidermoid Cysts. The epidermoid cyst is a benign, generally well-circumscribed tumor of germ cell origin, representing approximately 1% of all testicular tumors. These tumors occur at any age, but they are most common during the second to fourth decades.[21,70,71] Usually patients present with a painless testicular nodule; one-third of the tumors are discovered incidentally on physical examination. Diffuse, painless testicular enlargement occurs in 10% of the cases.[70,72] Pathologically the tumor wall is composed of fibrous tissue with an inner lining of squamous epithelium. The cyst is filled with flaky, cheesy, white keratin.

The histogenesis of epidermoid cysts is controversial. The most favored current opinion is that most epidermoid cysts are derived from epithelial rests or inclusions and have no malignant potential.[73] It has also been postulated that epidermoid cysts may represent monomorphic or monodermal development of a teratoma along the line of ectodermal cell differentiation.[70,72,74] These benign lesions can be differentiated from premalignant teratomas only through histologic examination. Sonographically, epidermoid cysts are generally well defined, avascular masses that may be multiple or bilateral. They may have various sonographic appearances.[73] A characteristic whorled appearance, like the layers of an onion skin, corresponds to the alternating layers of compacted keratin and desquamated squamous cells seen histologically (see Fig. 24-12G).[75-77] Another typical appearance of epidermoid cyst is a well-defined hypoechoic mass with an echogenic capsule that may be calcified (see Fig. 24-12H).[71,72] There may be central calcification giving a *bull's eye* or *target* appearance (see

Fig. 24-12I).[73] Epidermoid cysts may also have the nonspecific appearance of a hypoechoic mass with or without calcifications and may resemble germ cell tumors. Avascularity is a clue to the diagnosis.[77] When the sonographic appearance is characteristic, histologic confirmation is still obtained by a conservative testicle-sparing approach with local excision (enucleation).[70,78] MR imaging has been used to support the sonographic diagnosis of epidermoid cysts if further confirmation is desired prior to testis-sparing surgery.[79,80] Distinguishing an epidermoid cyst from a teratoma requires careful pathologic examination of the cyst wall and adjacent testis.[70]

Abscess. Testicular abscesses are usually a complication of epididymo-orchitis; they may also result from an undiagnosed testicular torsion, a gangrenous or infected tumor, or a primary pyogenic orchitis. Common infectious causes of abscess formation are **mumps, smallpox, scarlet fever, influenza, typhoid, sinusitis, osteomyelitis,** and **appendicitis.**[81] A testicular abscess may rupture through the tunica vaginalis, resulting in formation of a pyocele or a fistula to the skin.

Most commonly, sonography shows an enlarged testicle containing a predominantly fluid-filled mass with hypoechoic or mixed echogenic areas (Fig. 24-13). An atypical appearance has been described in which the testicular architecture was disrupted with hyperechoic striations separating hypoechoic spaces (see Fig. 24-13).[82] The striations were thought to be fibrous septa in the hypoechoic, necrotic testicular parenchyma. Testicular abscesses have no diagnostic sonographic features, but they can often be distinguished from tumors on the basis of clinical symptoms.

In patients with acquired immunodeficiency syndrome, distinguishing an abscess from a neoplastic process may be difficult on sonographic examination. Clinical find-

TESTICULAR CYSTIC LESIONS

BENIGN

Tunica albuginea cysts
Tunica vaginalis cysts
Intratesticular cysts
Tubular ectasia of rete testis
Cystic dysplasia
Epidermoid cysts
Abscess

MALIGNANT

Non-seminomatous germ cell tumor
Necrosis or hemorrhage in tumor
Tubular obstruction by tumor
Lymphoma

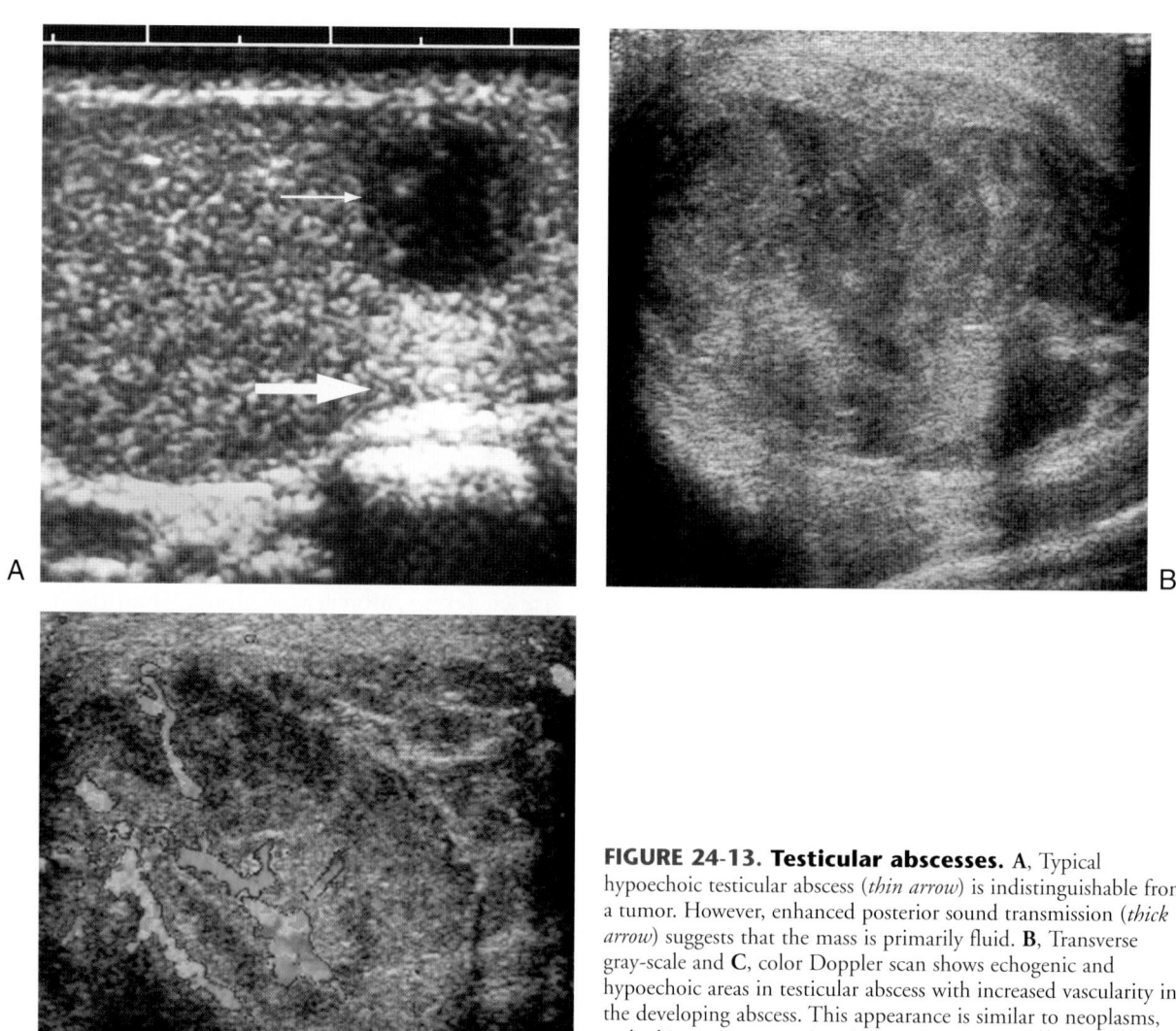

FIGURE 24-13. Testicular abscesses. A, Typical hypoechoic testicular abscess (*thin arrow*) is indistinguishable from a tumor. However, enhanced posterior sound transmission (*thick arrow*) suggests that the mass is primarily fluid. **B,** Transverse gray-scale and **C,** color Doppler scan shows echogenic and hypoechoic areas in testicular abscess with increased vascularity in the developing abscess. This appearance is similar to neoplasms, and a history is required to distinguish them.

ings may be helpful; however, orchiectomy is frequently necessary to obtain a histologic diagnosis.[83,84]

Infarction. Testicular infarction may occur after **torsion, trauma, bacterial endocarditis, vasculitis, leukemia,** and **hypercoagulable states**.[85-87] Spontaneous infarction of the testis is rare. The sonographic appearance depends on the age of the infarction. Initially, an infarct is seen as a focal, hypoechoic mass or as a diffusely hypoechoic testicle of normal size. The focal hypoechoic mass cannot be distinguished from a neoplasm on the basis of its appearance.[88,89] These lesions should be largely avascular, depending on the age of the infarction. If a well-circumscribed, nonpalpable, relatively peripheral, hypoechoic mass shows a complete lack of vascularity on

power mode Doppler imaging or after the administration of sonographic contrast agent, it may be possible to distinguish such benign infarctions from neoplasm (Fig. 24-14).[90,91] With time, the hypoechoic mass or the entire testicle often decreases in size and develops areas of increased echogenicity because of fibrosis or dystrophic calcification.[3,82,86] The early sonographic appearance may be difficult to distinguish from a testicular neoplasm, but infarcts decrease substantially in size, whereas tumors characteristically enlarge with time.[1,89]

Sarcoidosis. Sarcoidosis may involve the epididymis or the testis.[92-94] Genital involvement occurs in less than 1% of patients with systemic sarcoidosis.[1,3] The clinical presentation is one of acute or recurrent epididymitis or

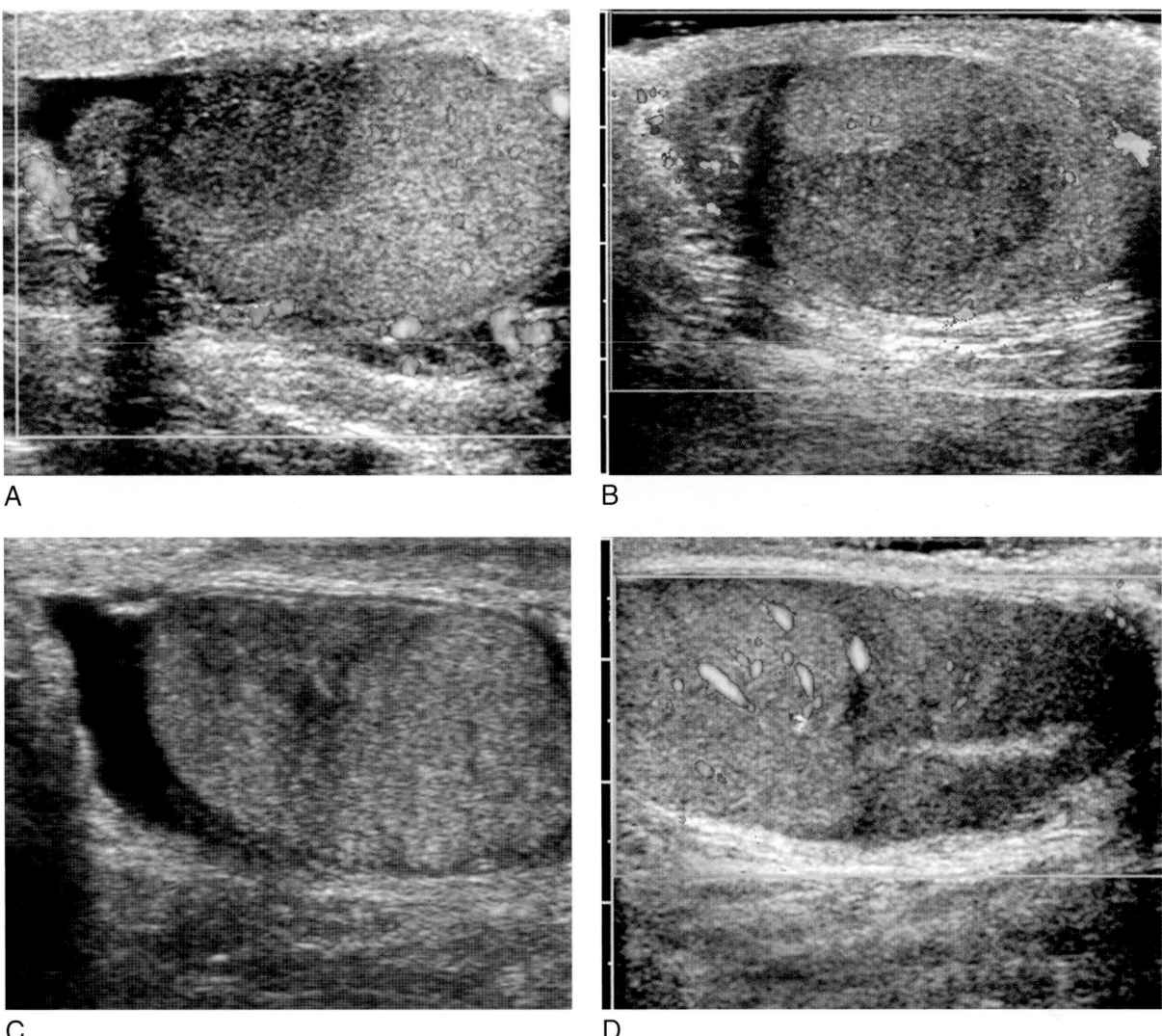

FIGURE 24-14. Testicular infarcts—spectrum of appearances. A, **Acute infarct**. Longitudinal power Doppler shows an avascular area at the upper pole from partial torsion. **B**, **Acute infarct**. Longitudinal color Doppler scan shows an avascular area in the midtestis caused by vasculitis. **C**, **Chronic infarct**. Longitudinal scan shows a peripheral wedge-shaped hypoechoic area due to prior mumps orchitis. **D**, **Chronic infarct**. Longitudinal power Doppler scan shows lack of vascularity in the lower pole.

of painless enlargement of the testis or epididymis. Sonographically, sarcoid lesions are irregular, hypoechoic solid masses in the testis or epididymis (Fig. 24-15).[12,95] Occasionally, hyperechoic, calcific foci with acoustic shadowing may be seen.[9] Distinguishing sarcoidosis from an inflammatory process or a neoplasm is difficult on sonography alone. Resection or orchiectomy may be necessary for definitive diagnosis.

Adrenal Rests. Congenital adrenal hyperplasia is an autosomal recessive disease involving an adrenal cortical enzyme defect. This disease may become clinically obvious early in life or in early adulthood. Often patients present with a testicular mass or enlargement, and with precocious puberty with or without salt-depletion syndrome. Adrenal rests arise from aberrant adrenal cortical cells that migrate with gonadal tissues in the fetus. They can form tumor-like masses in response to elevated levels of circulating corticotropin in congenital adrenal hyperplasia and Cushing syndrome and rarely may undergo malignant transformation. On sonography, these lesions are multifocal hypoechoic lesions. Occasionally, posterior acoustic shadowing has been described. Many adrenal rests demonstrate spokelike vascularity with multiple peripheral vessels radiating toward a central point within the mass. In most instances, if the patient has the appropriate hormonal abnormalities associated with congenital adrenal hyperplasia and if sonography shows the appropriate findings, no further work-up is necessary.[96,97]

Scrotal Calcifications. Scrotal calcifications may be seen within the parenchyma of the testicle, on the surface of the testicle, or freely located in the fluid between the

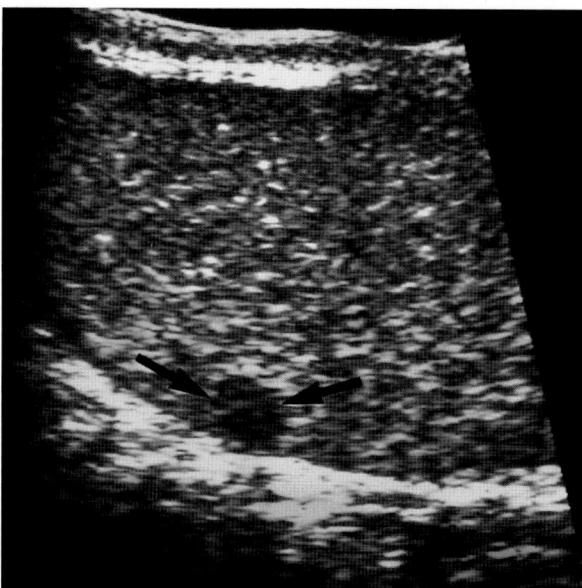

FIGURE 24-15. Testicular sarcoid. Longitudinal scan of the testis shows the small, hypoechoic, solid mass (*arrows*) that is sarcoid.

layers of the tunica vaginalis. Large, smooth, curvilinear calcifications without an associated soft-tissue mass are very characteristic of a large cell, calcifying, **Sertoli cell tumor**, although occasionally **burned-out germ cell tumors** may have a similar appearance.[31] Scattered calcifications may be found in **tuberculosis, filariasis,** and scarring from regressed **germ cell tumor or trauma.**

Testicular microlithiasis is a condition in which calcifications are present within the seminiferous tubules of the testis either unilaterally or bilaterally.[3] It is postulated that microlithiasis is due to defective Sertoli cell phagocytosis of degenerating tubular cells, which then calcify within the seminiferous tubules.[98,99] Microlithiasis has been classified as **diffuse** and **limited.**[100] In the **diffuse** form, innumerable small, hyperechoic foci are diffusely scattered throughout the testicular parenchyma. These tiny (1-3 mm) foci rarely show a shadow and occasionally show a comet-tail appearance (Fig. 24-16). In the **limited** form, previously thought to be insignificant, less than five hyperechoic foci are seen per image of the testis (see Fig. 24-16B).

Microlithiasis is seen in 1% to 2% of the patients referred for testicular sonography and has been associated with **cryptorchidism, Klinefelter's syndrome, Down's syndrome, pulmonary alveolar microlithiasis, previous radiotherapy,** and **subfertility.**[98,101-103] Most importantly, many reports associate microlithiasis with **testicular germ cell neoplasms** (seminoma or non-seminoma), **intratubular germ cell neoplasia,** and **extratesticular germ cell tumor.**[100,104-113] There is general agreement that an **association with malignancy** exists, but there is controversy about the strength of this association and the significance of limited microlithiasis. In part, this

is because no large study has shown the prevalence of microlithiasis in an asymptomatic population. Prospective data show that coexisting testicular tumors occur more frequently in patients who have both diffuse and limited microlithiasis, occurring in 5% to 10% of patients.[100] Despite case reports, it is not yet clear, however, whether the incidence of de novo testicular tumors is significantly increased in patients with preexisting microlithiasis.[112] Therefore, there is no consensus on the appropriate follow-up (clinical or radiologic) for patients with testicular microlithiasis. Most commonly, annual sonography is recommended, although some authors suggest annual physical and periodic self-examination instead.[100]

Extratesticular scrotal calculi arise from the surface of the tunica vaginalis and may break loose to migrate between the two layers of the tunica (Fig. 24-17). They have been called fibrinoid loose bodies or **"scrotal pearls"** because of their macroscopic appearance, which is usually round, pearly white, and rubbery. Histologically they consist of fibrinoid material deposited around a central nucleus of hydroxyapatite.[114] They may result from inflammation of the tunica vaginalis or torsion of the appendix testis or epididymis. Hydroceles facilitate the sonographic diagnosis of scrotal calculi (see Fig. 24-17).

Extratesticular Pathologic Lesions

Hydrocele, Hematocele, and Pyocele. Serous fluid, blood, pus, or urine may accumulate in the space between the parietal and visceral layers of the tunica vaginalis lining the scrotum. These fluid collections are confined to the anterolateral portions of the scrotum because of the attachment of the testis to the epididymis

---

SCROTAL CALCIFICATIONS

TESTICULAR

Solitary, postinflammatory granulomatous, vascular
Microlithiasis
"Burned-out" germ cell tumor
Large cell calcifying Sertoli cell tumor
Teratoma
Mixed germ cell tumor
Sarcoid
Tuberculosis
Chronic infarct

EXTRATESTICULAR

Tunica vaginalis "scrotal pearls"
Chronic epididymitis
Schistosomiasis

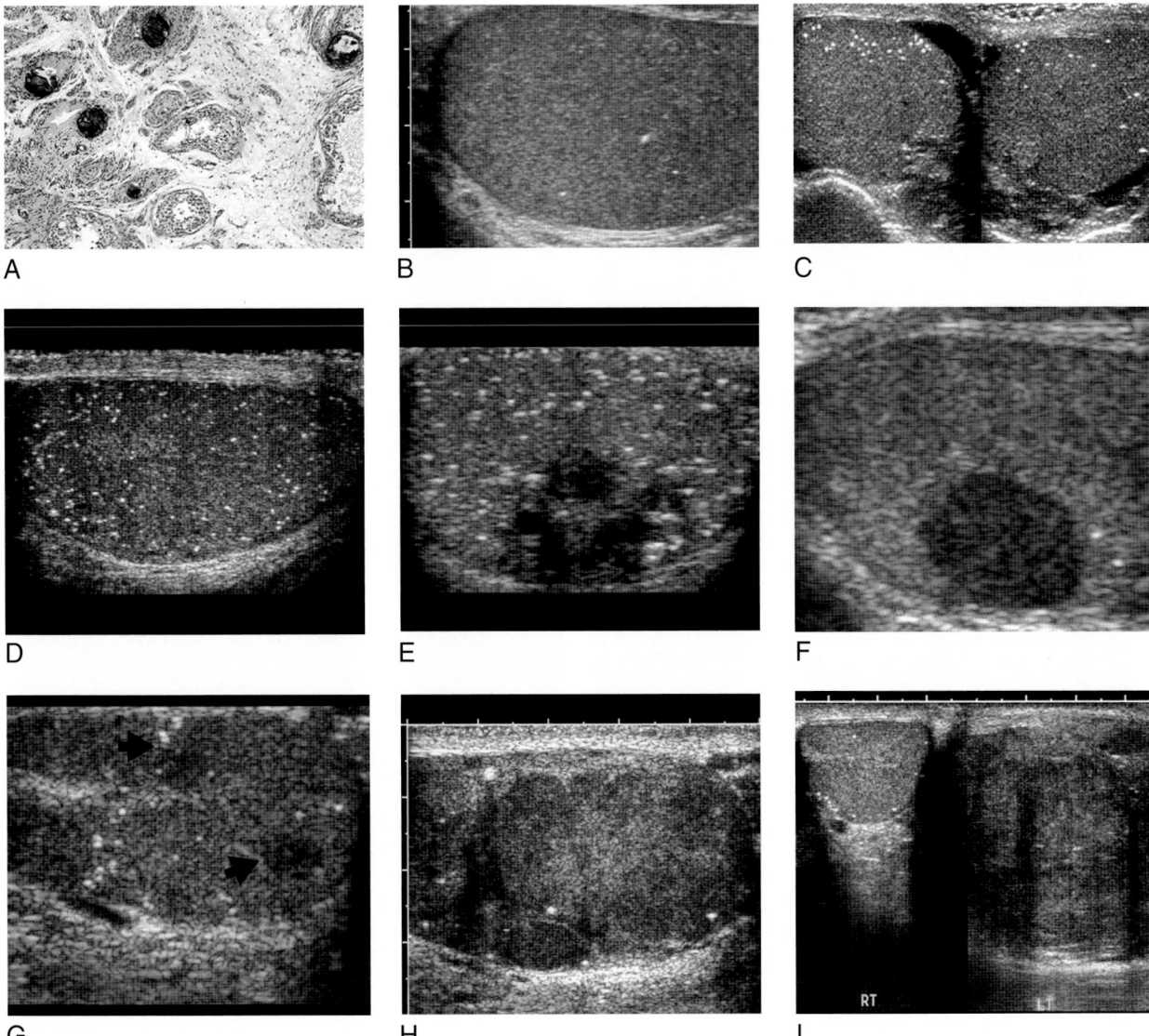

FIGURE 24-16. Microlithiasis and associated testicular tumors—spectrum of appearances. A, Microlithiasis. Light microscopy examination shows multiple intratubular calcifications (*dark areas*). **B, Limited microlithiasis.** Longitudinal scan shows a few tiny calcifications. **C** and **D, Diffuse microlithiasis. E, Microlithiasis with mixed germ cell tumor.** Transverse scan of testis shows microlithiasis and partially cystic mass due to mixed germ cell tumor. **F, Limited microlithiasis with seminoma.** Longitudinal scan shows a few tiny calcifications and a homogeneous hypoechoic mass. **G, Microlithiasis and two foci of seminoma.** Longitudinal scan shows multiple tiny calcifications and two hypoechoic homogeneous masses (*arrows*). **H, Microlithiasis and seminoma.** Longitudinal scan shows large hypoechoic mass with multiple small and coarser calcifications. **I, Microlithiasis and seminoma.** Dual transverse image shows large hypoechoic left testicular mass and microcalcifications in the right testis.

and scrotal wall posteriorly (the bare area) (Fig. 24-18).[5] The normal scrotum contains a few milliliters of serous fluid between the layers of the tunica vaginalis and this is usually visible on sonographic examination.[115]

Hydrocele is an abnormal accumulation of serous fluid between the layers of the tunica vaginalis. Rarely, hydrocele may be loculated around the spermatic cord above the testis and epididymis (see Fig. 24-18A-C).[116] Hydrocele is the most common cause of painless scrotal swelling[9] and may be congenital or acquired. The **congenital type** results from incomplete closure of the processus vaginalis, with persistent open communication between the scrotal sac and the peritoneum, usually resolving by 18 months of age.

Acquired hydroceles are the result of trauma in 25% to 50% of the cases. Hydroceles associated with testicular tumors are usually small and occur in about 10% of the patients.[1,117-119] Other causes of secondary hydroceles include epididymitis, epididymo-orchitis, and torsion.[3,23]

Sonography is useful in detecting a potential cause of the hydrocele by allowing evaluation of the testicle when a large hydrocele hampers palpation. Hydroceles are characteristically anechoic collections with good sound

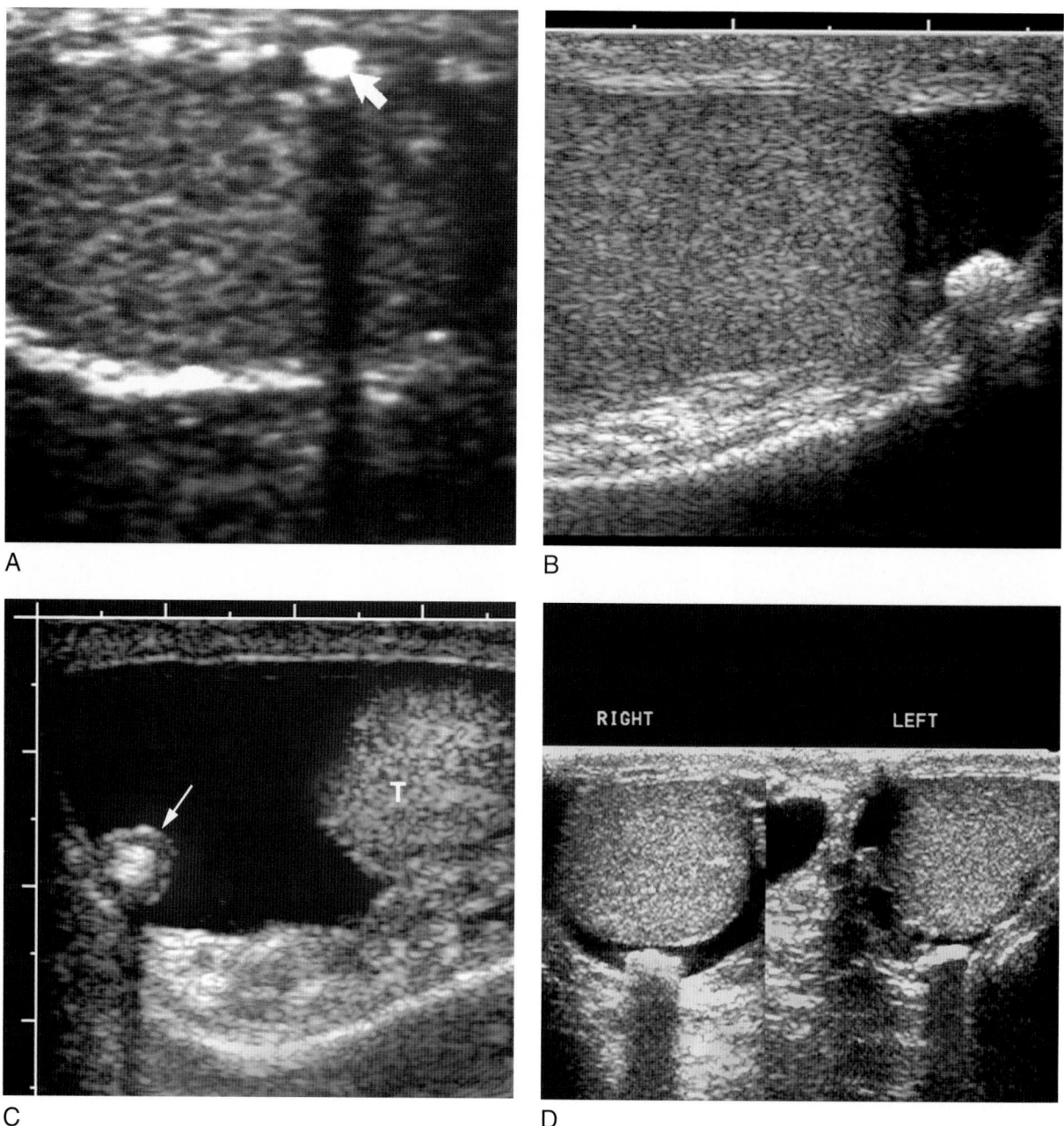

FIGURE 24-17. Benign intrascrotal calcification. **A,** **Calcified tunica plaque** on the tunica vaginalis. **B,** **"Scrotal pearl."** Mobile scrotal calcification in a small hydrocele. **C,** **Scrotal pearl.** Longitudinal scan shows a mostly calcified scrotal pearl (*arrow*) in a hydrocele. T, Testis. **D,** **Bilateral scrotal pearls.**

transmission surrounding the anterolateral aspects of the testis. Low-level to medium-level echoes from fibrin bodies or cholesterol crystals may occasionally be visualized moving freely within a hydrocele.[11,118,120] Rarely a large hydrocele may impede testicular venous drainage and cause absence of antegrade arterial diastolic flow.[117]

Hematoceles and **pyoceles** are less common than simple hydroceles. Hematoceles result from trauma, surgery, diabetes, neoplasms, torsion, or atherosclerotic disease.[121] Pyoceles result from rupture of an abscess into an existing hydrocele or directly into the space between the layers of the tunica vaginalis. Both hematoceles and pyoceles contain internal septations and loculations (see Fig. 24-18D-F). Thickening of the scrotal skin and calcifications may be seen in chronic cases.

Varicocele. A varicocele is a collection of abnormally dilated, tortuous, and elongated veins of the pampiniform plexus located posterior to the testis, accompanying the epididymis and vas deferens within the spermatic cord (Fig. 24-19).[3,9,118,122] The veins of the pampiniform plexus normally range from 0.5 to 1.5 mm in diameter, with a main draining vein up to 2 mm in diameter.

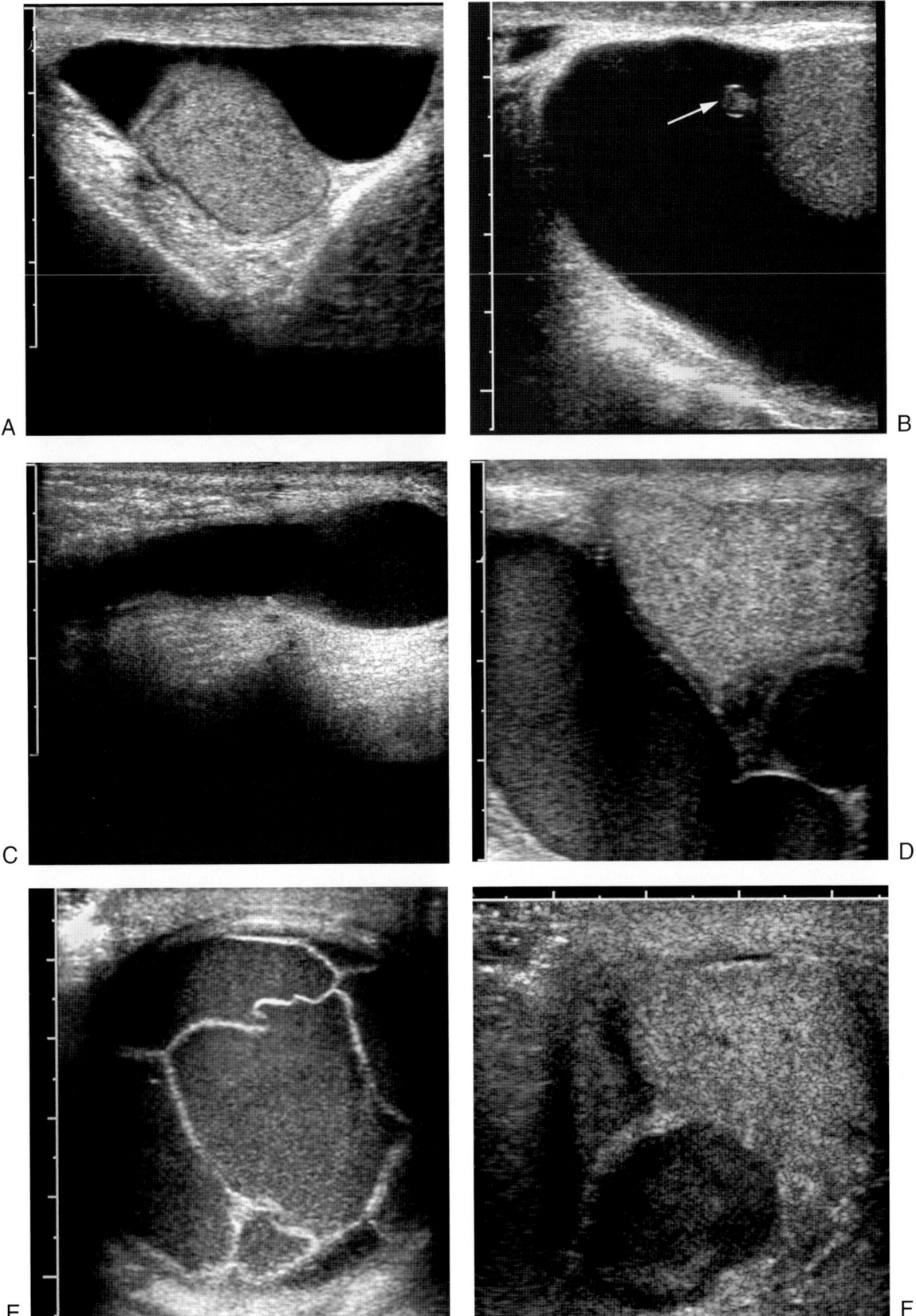

FIGURE 24-18. Scrotal fluid collections—spectrum of appearances. A, Hydrocele. Transverse scan shows hydrocele anterolaterally with attachment of testis to tunica vaginalis posteriorly. **B, Hydrocele.** Fluid outlines appendix testis (arrow). **C, Hydrocele of cord.** Longitudinal scan of inguinal region shows elongated fluid collection above the level of the testis and epididymis. **D, Hematocele.** Transverse scan shows loculated fluid with internal echoes. **E, Hematocele.** Transverse scan shows fluid with internal echoes and linear membranes. **F, Pyocele.** Transverse scan shows fluid collection with internal echoes.

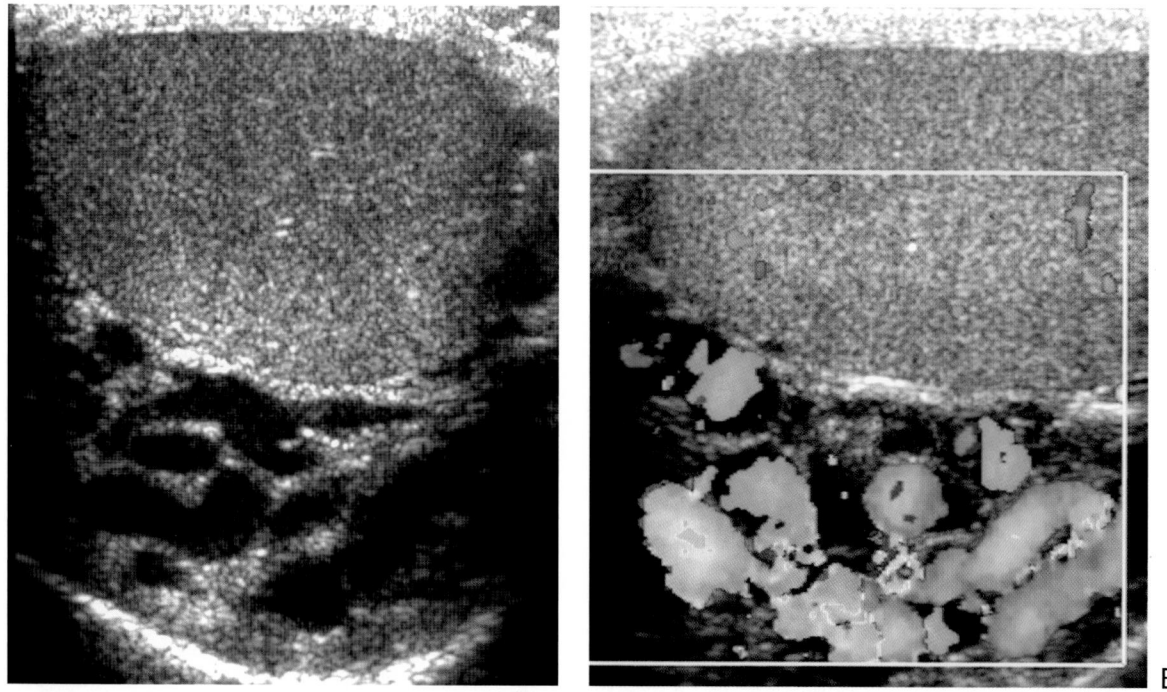

FIGURE 24-19. Varicocele. A, Longitudinal scan and **B,** color Doppler shows serpentine, hypoechoic, dilated veins posterior to the testis. The blood flow in a varicocele is slow and may be detected only with low-flow Doppler settings or the Valsalva maneuver.

There are two types of varicoceles: primary (idiopathic) and secondary. The **idiopathic varicocele** is caused by incompetent valves in the internal spermatic vein, which permit retrograde passage of blood through the spermatic cord into the pampiniform plexus. Varicocele is the most common correctable cause of male infertility, occurring in 21% to 39% of the men attending infertility clinics.[123-125] Idiopathic varicoceles occur on the left side in 98% of cases and are usually detected in men aged 15 to 25 years.[3] The left-sided predominance is thought to exist because the venous drainage on the left side is into the renal vein, as opposed to the right spermatic vein, which drains directly into the vena cava. Idiopathic varices normally distend when the patient is upright or performs the Valsalva maneuver and may decompress when the patient is supine. Primary varicoceles are bilateral in up to 70% of the cases.[126]

Secondary varicoceles result from increased pressure on the spermatic vein or its tributaries by marked hydronephrosis, an enlarged liver, abdominal neoplasms, or venous compression by a retroperitoneal mass.[22,118] Secondary varicocele may also occur in the **"nutcracker syndrome"** in which the superior mesenteric artery compresses the left renal vein.[127] A search for neoplastic obstruction of gonadal venous return must be undertaken in cases of a right-sided, nondecompressible, or newly discovered varicocele in a patient older than 40 years because these cases are rarely idiopathic (Fig. 24-20).[9] The appearance of secondary varicoceles is not affected by patient position.

In infertile men, sonography aids in the diagnosis of clinically palpable and subclinical varicoceles. There is no correlation between the size of the varicocele and the degree of testicular tissue damage leading to infertility. Therefore, early detection and treatment of subclinical varicoceles are important.[125]

Sonographically, the varicocele consists of multiple, serpentine, anechoic structures more than 2 mm in diameter, creating a tortuous multicystic collection located adjacent or proximal to the upper pole of the testis and head of the epididymis. Occasionally the varicocele may appear similar to a small, septate spermatocele. Distinguishing between a varicocele and a spermatocele may be accomplished using duplex or color flow Doppler sonography. Similarly, dilated veins in the mediastinum testes can be distinguished from tubular ectasia of the rete testes by use of color flow or pulsed wave Doppler sonography. A high-frequency transducer in conjunction with low-flow Doppler settings should be used to optimize slow-flow detection within varices. Slowly moving red blood cells may be visualized with high-frequency transducers, even when flow is too slow to be detected by Doppler imaging. Venous flow can be augmented with the patient in the upright position or during the Valsalva maneuver. In addition, varicoceles, unlike spermatoceles, follow the course of the spermatic cord into the inguinal canal and are easily compressed by the transducer.[1,23,118] Rarely varicoceles may be intratesticular, either in a subcapsular location or around the mediastinum testis (Fig. 24-21).[128]

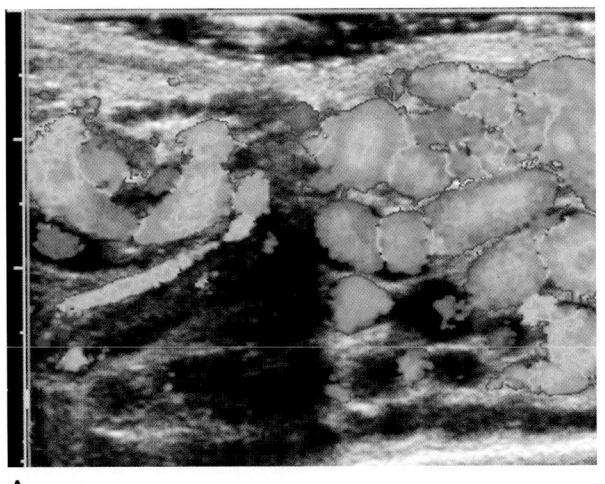

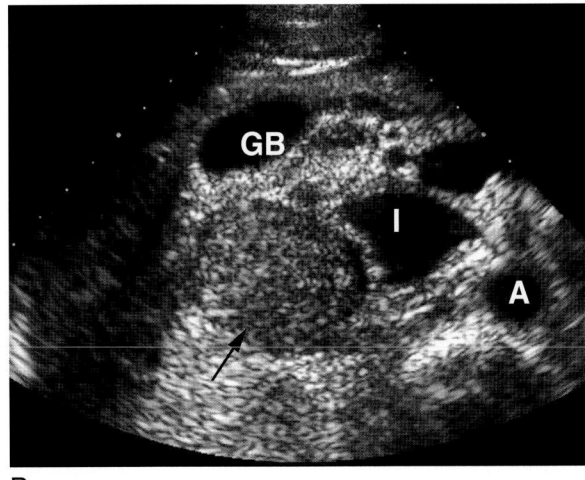

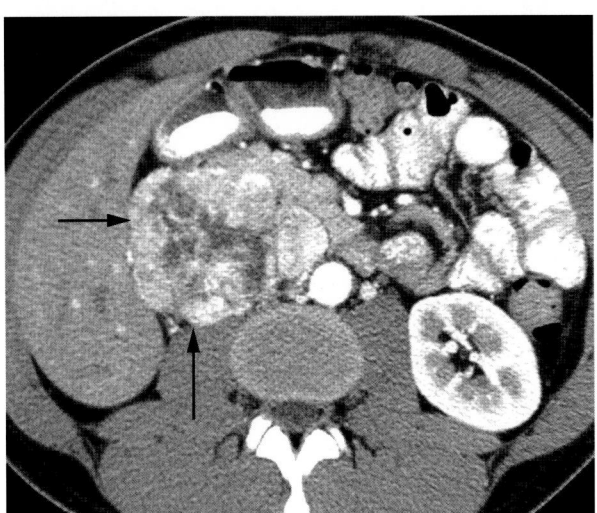

FIGURE 24-20. Varicocele due to retroperitoneal paraganglioneuroma. A, Longitudinal scan shows very dilated veins of large right varicocele. **B,** Transverse abdominal sonogram shows paraganglioneuroma (*arrow*) adjacent to the inferior vena cava (I). A, aorta. GB, gallbladder. **C,** Axial CT shows the vascular mass (*arrows*) adjacent to I.

FIGURE 24-21. Intratesticular varicocele.
Longitudinal scan shows the dilated vein.

EXTRATESTICULAR TUMORS

BENIGN

Adenomatoid tumor
Fibroma
Lipoma
Hemangioma
Leiomyoma
Neurofibroma
Cholesterol granuloma
Adrenal rest
Papillary cystadenoma

MALIGNANT

Fibrosarcoma
Liposarcoma
Rhabdosarcoma
Histiocytoma
Lymphoma
Metastases

Scrotal Hernia. A scrotal hernia is another common paratesticular mass. Although scrotal hernias are usually diagnosed on the basis of clinical history and physical examination, sonography is useful in the evaluation of atypical cases. The hernia may contain small bowel or colon, with or without omentum.[129] The presence of bowel loops within the hernia may be confirmed by the visualization of valvulae conniventes or haustrations and detection of peristalsis on real-time examination. If these features are absent, distinguishing a hernia from other extratesticular multicystic masses, such as hematoceles and pyoceles, may be difficult. The presence of highly echogenic material within the scrotum may be due to a hernia-containing omentum or other fatty masses (Fig. 24-22). Sonographic examination of the inguinal canal must also be performed to identify the extension of omentum or bowel loops from the inguinal canal into the scrotum.[23,129]

Tumors. Extratesticular scrotal neoplasms are rare and usually involve the epididymis. The most common extratesticular neoplasm is the benign **adenomatoid tumor,** representing 32% of these tumors.[16,130] It is most frequently located in the epididymis, especially in the globus minor, but may also arise in the spermatic cord or testicular tunica (Fig. 24-23D,E).[18] This neoplasm may occasionally invade adjacent testicular parenchyma. It may occur at any age, but it is most commonly found in patients aged 20 to 50 years.[1,18,131] Adenomatoid tumors are generally unilateral, solitary, well defined, and round or oval, rarely measuring more than 5 cm in diameter. Occasionally they may appear plaque-like and ill defined. Sonography usually shows a solid, well-circumscribed mass with echogenicity that is at least as great as the testis.[1] It may also be hypoechoic.

Other benign extratesticular tumors are rare and include **fibromas, hemangiomas, lipomas, leiomyomas** (Fig. 24-23G), **neurofibromas,** and **cholesterol granulomas.**[18] **Adrenal rests** may also be encountered in the spermatic cord, testis, epididymis, rete testis, and tunica albuginea in approximately 10% of infants.[18]

Papillary cystadenomas of the epididymis may be seen in patients with Hippel-Lindau disease.[95] These tumors are considered **hamartomas** and are usually found in the epididymal head.[59] Primary extratesticular scrotal malignant neoplasms include **fibrosarcoma, liposarcoma, malignant histiocytoma** and **lymphoma** in adults, and **rhabdomyosarcoma** in children (Fig. 24-23H).

Metastatic tumors to the epididymis are also rare. The most common primary sites include the testicle, stomach, kidney, prostate, colon, and, less commonly, the pancreas (see Fig. 24-23I).[95,130,132,133] Sonography shows focal, echogenic areas of thickening within the epididymis, commonly in association with a hydrocele.

Epididymal Lesions

Sperm Granuloma. Sperm granulomas are thought to arise from extravasation of spermatozoa into the soft tissues surrounding the epididymis, producing a necrotizing granulomatous response.[1,3,134,135] These lesions may be painful or asymptomatic, and they are most often found in patients after vasectomy. They may also be associated with prior epididymal infection or trauma. The typical sonographic appearance is that of a solid, hypoechoic or heterogeneous mass that is usually located within the epididymis, but it may simulate an intratesticular lesion (Fig. 24-23B).[134] Chronic sperm granuloma may contain calcification.[136]

Fibrous Pseudotumor. Fibrous Pseudotumor is a rare non-neoplastic mass of reactive fibrous tissue that may involve the tunica vaginalis or epididymis. On sonography, fibrous pseudotumors may appear as hypoechoic, hyperechoic, or heterogeneous paratesticular masses (see Fig. 24-23C).[137-139]

Cystic Lesions. Spermatoceles are more common than epididymal cysts. Both were seen in 20% to 40% of all asymptomatic patients studied by Leung, et al.[115] and 30% were multiple cysts. Both epididymal cysts and spermatoceles are thought to result from dilation of the epididymal tubules, but the contents of these masses differ.[9,95] Cysts contain clear serous fluid, whereas spermatoceles are filled with spermatozoa and sediment-containing lymphocytes, fat globules, and cellular debris, giving the fluid a thick, milky appearance.[1,95] Both lesions may result from prior episodes of epididymitis or trauma. Spermatoceles and epididymal cysts appear identical on sonography: anechoic, circumscribed masses

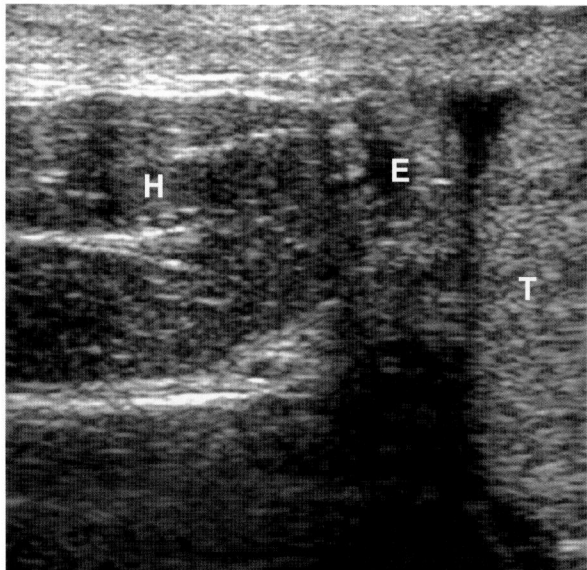

FIGURE 24-22. Herniated mesenteric fat.
Longitudinal scan shows herniated fat (H) above testis (T) and epididymis (E).

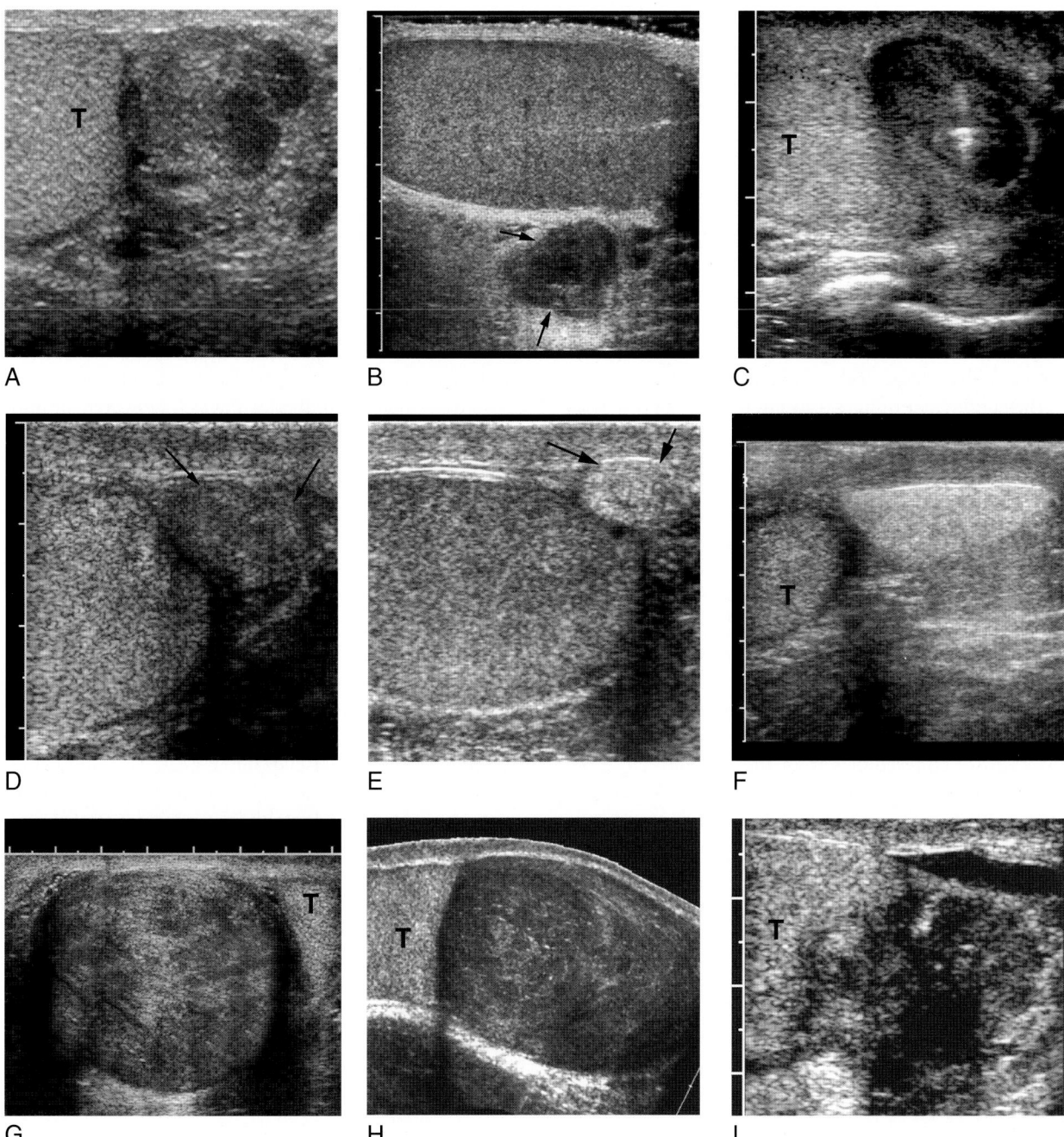

FIGURE 24-23. Extratesticular scrotal solid masses—spectrum of appearances. A, Chronic epididymitis. Longitudinal scan of the scrotum shows mass in the tail of the epididymis. T, testis. **B, Sperm granuloma.** Longitudinal scan shows hypoechoic solid mass (*arrows*) posterior to the testis in a patient with previous vasectomy. **C, Fibrous pseudotumor.** Longitudinal scan shows a mass of mixed echogenicity inferior to the testis (T). **D, Benign adenomatoid tumor of epididymis.** Longitudinal scan shows a hypoechoic mass (*arrows*) in the tail. **E, Benign adenomatoid tumor of the tunica.** Longitudinal scan shows a hyperechoic mass (*arrows*). **F, Intrascrotal lipoma.** Longitudinal scan shows a hyperechoic mass inferior to the testis (T). **G, Leiomyoma of cord.** Longitudinal scan shows a solid mass superior to the testis (T). **H, Rhabdomyosarcoma.** Longitudinal extended field-of-view scan in a 12-year-old shows a large paratesticular mass inferior to the testis (T). **I, Metastasis from lung carcinoma.** Longitudinal scan shows a mass in the tail of the epididymis. T, testis.

with no or few internal echoes (Fig. 24-24). Loculations and septations are commonly seen (see Fig. 24-24). Rarely, a spermatocele may be hyperechoic.[5] Differentiation between a spermatocele and an epididymal cyst is rarely important clinically. Spermatoceles almost always occur in the head of the epididymis, whereas epididymal cysts arise throughout the length of the epididymis.

Postvasectomy Changes in the Epididymis. Sonographic changes in the epididymis have been reported in 45% of patients after vasectomy. These findings include epididymal enlargement and inhomogeneity and the development of sperm granulomas and cysts. It is assumed that vasectomy produces increased pressure in the epididymal tubules, causing tubular rupture with subsequent formation of sperm granulomas. This tubular rupture may protect the testis from the effects of increased back pressure. These sonographic findings are nonspecific and may be seen in patients who have epididymitis.[140] Postorchiectomy sonographic findings include hematomas (Fig. 24-25), local tumor recurrence, secondary primary tumor, and the sonographic appearance of a testicular prosthesis.[141]

Chronic Epididymitis. Patients with incompletely treated acute **bacterial** epididymitis usually present with a chronically painful scrotal mass (see Fig. 24-23A). Patients with chronic granulomatous epididymitis due to spread of **tuberculosis** from the genitourinary tract complain of a hard, nontender scrotal mass.[9] Sonography most commonly shows a thickened tunica albuginea and a thickened, irregular epididymis (Fig. 24-26). Calcification may be identified within the tunica albuginea or epididymis.[1,142] Untreated granulomatous epididymitis will spread to the testes in 60% to 80% of cases.[3] Focal testicular involvement may simulate the appearance of a testicular neoplasm on sonography, whereas diffuse testicular involvement results in an enlarged, irregular testis with diffuse homogeneous hypoechogenicity.

ACUTE SCROTAL PAIN

The differential diagnosis of an acutely painful and swollen scrotum includes torsion of the spermatic cord and testis, torsion of a testicular appendage, epididymitis or orchitis, acute hydrocele, strangulated hernia, idiopathic scrotal edema, Henoch-Schönlein purpura, abscess, traumatic hemorrhage, hemorrhage into a testicular neoplasm, and scrotal fat necrosis. Torsion of the spermatic cord and acute epididymitis or epididymo-orchitis are the most common causes of acute scrotal pain. These entities cannot be distinguished by physical examination or laboratory tests in up to 50% of cases.[143] Immediate surgical exploration has been advised in boys and young men with acute scrotal pain, unless a definitive diagnosis of epididymitis or orchitis can be made. This aggressive approach has resulted in an increased testicular salvage rate from torsion but also an increase in unnecessary surgical procedures.[144] Testicular radionuclide scintigraphy, MRI, real-time sonography, and Doppler sonography have been used to increase the accuracy of distinguishing between infection and torsion.[145,146] Currently sonography, using color flow or power mode Doppler, is the imaging study of choice to diagnose the cause of acute scrotal pain.

Torsion

Torsion is more common in boys than in men, and it represents only 20% of the acute scrotal pathologic phenomena in postpubertal males.[1] However, prompt diagnosis is necessary because torsion requires immediate surgery to preserve the testis. The testicular salvage rate is 80% to 100% if surgery is performed within 5 to 6 hours of the onset of pain, 70% if surgery is performed within 6 to 12 hours, and only 20% if surgery is delayed for more than 12 hours.[147]

There are two types of testicular torsion: intravaginal and extravaginal. **Intravaginal torsion** is the more common type, occurring most frequently at puberty. It results from anomalous suspension of the testis by a long stalk of spermatic cord, resulting in complete investment of the testis and epididymis by the tunica vaginalis. It has been likened to a **bell-clapper** (Fig. 24-27). Anomalous testicular suspension is bilateral in 50% to 80% of patients.[23] There is a tenfold greater incidence of torsion in undescended testes after orchiopexy.[148]

Most commonly, **extravaginal torsion** occurs in newborns without the "bell-clapper" deformity. It is thought to be due to a poor or absent attachment of the testis to the scrotal wall, allowing rotation of the testis, epididymis, and tunica vaginalis as a unit and causing torsion of the cord at the level of the external ring (see Fig. 24-27D).[149,150]

The more compliant veins are obstructed before the arteries in both forms of torsion, resulting in early vascular engorgement and edema of the testicle.

Several gray-scale sonographic changes occur in the **acute phase of torsion**, within 1 to 6 hours.[143,151-153] Initially the testis becomes enlarged, with a normal echo-

---

ACUTE SCROTAL PAIN

Torsion of the testis
Epididymo-orchitis
Testicular appendage torsion
Strangulated hernia
Idiopathic scrotal edema
Trauma
Henoch-Schönlein purpura

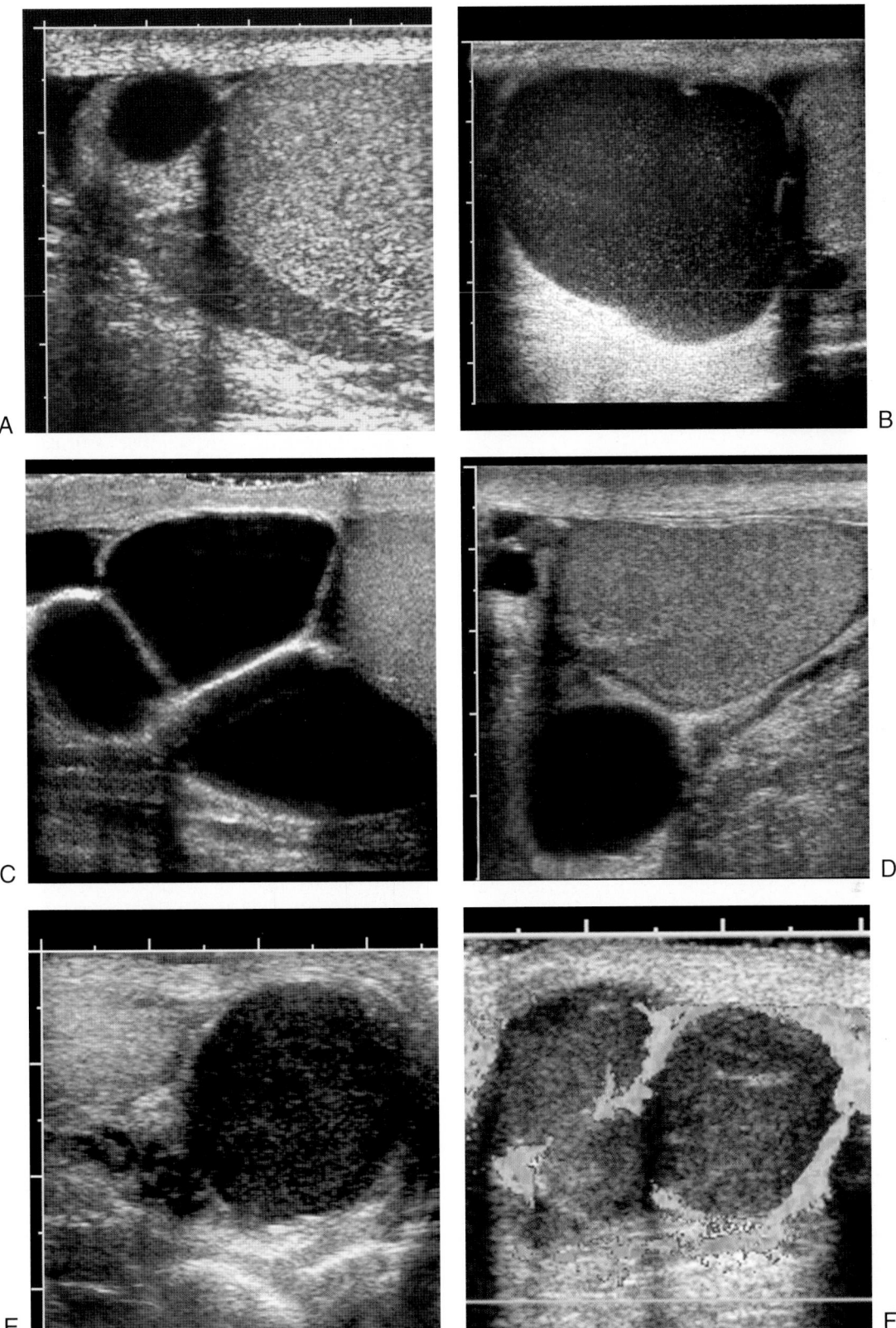

FIGURE 24-24. Extratesticular scrotal cysts—spectrum of appearances. A, Spermatocele. Longitudinal scan shows an anechoic cyst in the head of the epididymis. **B**, **Spermatocele**. Longitudinal scan shows a large cyst containing internal echoes in the head of the epididymis. **C**, **Septate spermatocele**. Longitudinal scan shows a septate cyst in the head of the epididymis. **D**, **Epididymal cyst**. Longitudinal scan shows a cyst in the body of the epididymis. **E, Cyst of vas deferens remnant**. Longitudinal scan shows a cyst with internal echoes inferior to the testis (surgically proven). **F**, **Epidermoid inclusion cyst of epididymis**. Longitudinal color Doppler scan shows bilobed cystic mass in the head of the epididymis with vessels surrounding it.

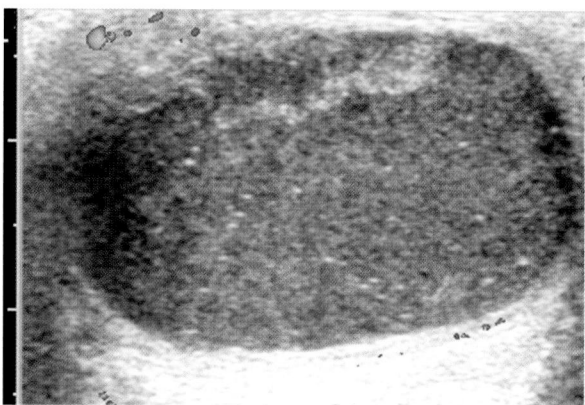

FIGURE 24-25. Hematoma after orchiectomy.
Longitudinal color Doppler image shows an avascular, debris-containing cystic mass in the scrotum where the testis was removed for embryonal cell carcinoma 3 weeks previously.

genicity, and later it becomes heterogeneous and hypoechoic as compared with the contralateral normal testis (Fig. 24-28).[154-157] A hypoechoic or heterogeneous echogenicity may indicate nonviability.[158] Generalized testicular hyperechogenicity has been reported in two cases of acute torsion in the absence of histologic changes of testicular hemorrhage or infarction.[143-145,147,148,151,154-156,159]

Torsion may change the position of the long axis of the testis (see Fig. 24-28B). Extratesticular sonographic findings commonly occur in torsion and are important to recognize. The spermatic cord immediately cranial to the testis and epididymis is twisted, causing a characteristic **"torsion knot"** or **"whirlpool"** pattern of concentric layers seen on sonography or MRI (see Fig. 24-28G).[159,160] The epididymis may be enlarged and

heterogeneous because of hemorrhage and difficult to separate from the torsion knot of the spermatic cord (see Fig. 24-28G,H). This spherical epididymis/cord complex can be mistaken for epididymitis.[152] A reactive hydrocele and scrotal skin thickening are often seen with torsion. During the **subacute phase of torsion** (1 to 10 days), the degree of testicular hypoechogenicity and enlargement increases within the first 5 days, then diminishes over the next 4 to 5 days. The epididymis remains enlarged and is often echogenic. Hydroceles are common in cases of torsion.[151] Large echogenic or complex extratesticular masses caused by hemorrhage within the tunica vaginalis or epididymis may be seen in cases of undiagnosed torsion.[159] The gray-scale findings of acute and subacute torsion are not specific and may be seen in testicular infarction due to epididymitis, epididymo-orchitis, and traumatic testicular rupture or infarction.[161,162]

Color Doppler sonography is the most useful and most rapid technique to establish the diagnosis of testicular torsion and to help distinguish torsion from epididymo-orchitis (see Fig. 24-28).[143,155,162,163] In torsion, blood flow is absent in the affected testicle or significantly less than in the normal, contralateral testicle. Meticulous scanning of the testicular parenchyma with the use of low-flow detection Doppler settings (low pulse repetition frequency, low wall filter, and high Doppler gain) is important because testicular vessels are small and have low flow velocities, especially in prepubertal boys. Color flow Doppler sonography is more sensitive for showing decreased testicular flow in incomplete torsion than is nuclear scintigraphy.[164] Power Doppler and frequency shift color Doppler are used, although

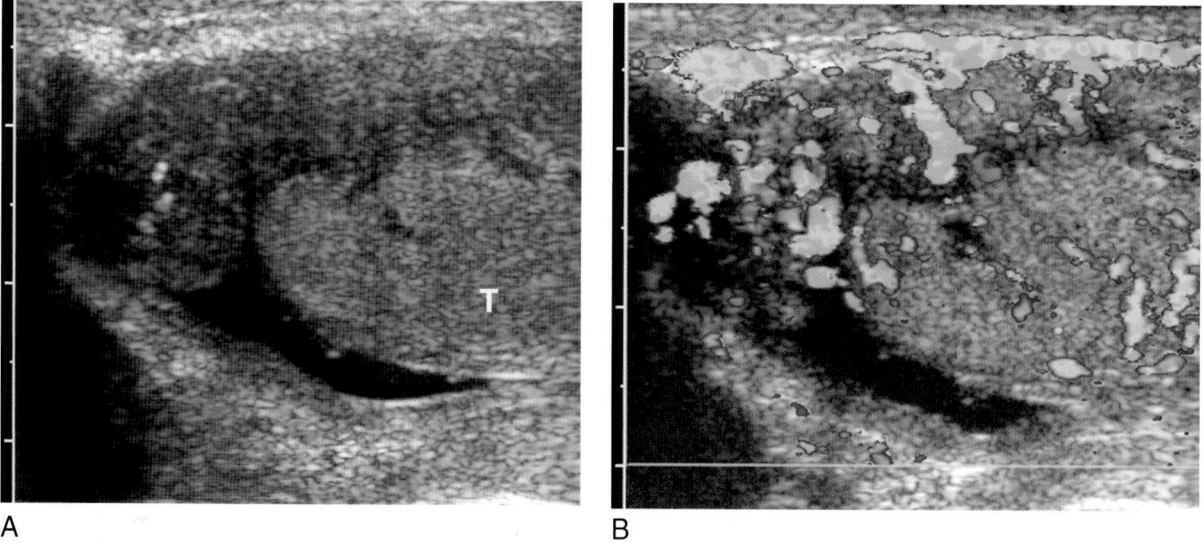

A   B

FIGURE 24-26. Tuberculous epididymo-orchitis. A, Longitudinal scan shows a heterogeneous mass with calcification involving the head and body of the epididymis and the adjacent testis (T). **B,** Longitudinal color Doppler image shows increased vascularity in the epididymis and adjacent testis.

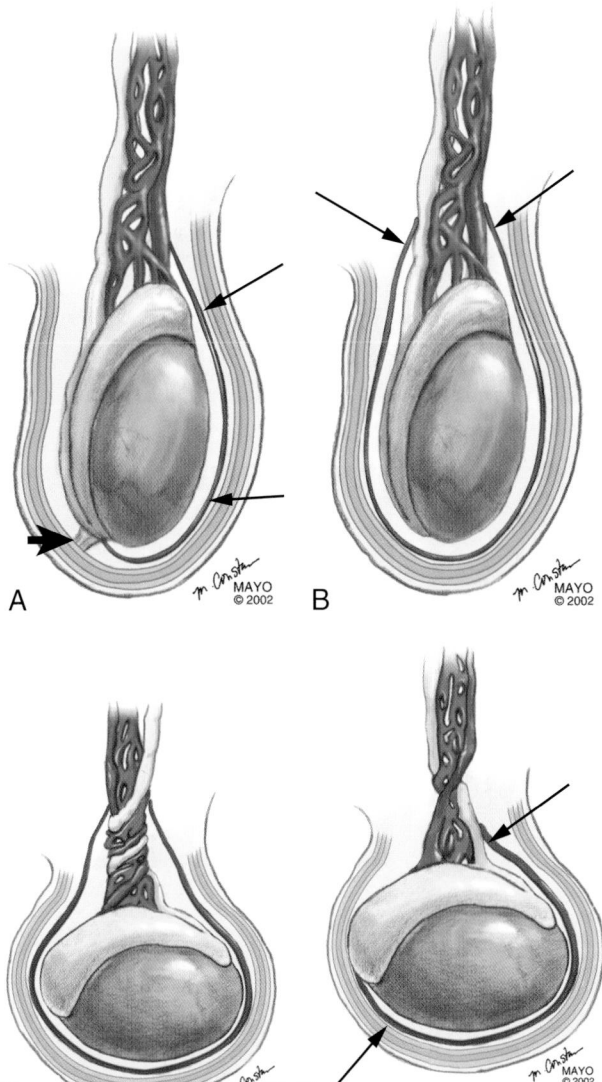

FIGURE 24-27. "Bell-clapper" anomaly, intravaginal torsion and extravaginal torsion. A, Normal anatomy. The tunica vaginalis (*arrows*) does not completely surround the testis and epididymis, which are attached to the posterior scrotal wall (*short arrow*). **B, Bell-clapper anomaly.** The tunica vaginalis (*arrows*) completely surrounds the testis, epididymis, and part of the spermatic cord, predisposing to torsion. **C, Intravaginal torsion.** Bell-clapper anomaly with complete torsion of the spermatic cord, compromising the blood supply to the testis. **D, Extravaginal torsion in a neonate.** Tunica vaginalis (*arrows*) is in normal position, but abnormal motility allows rotation of the testis, epididymis, and spermatic cord.

the techniques appear to have equivalent sensitivity in the diagnosis of torsion.[165-170] In testicular torsion, color Doppler sonography has a sensitivity of 80% to 98%, a specificity of 97% to 100%, and an accuracy rate of 97%.[152,163,171] The use of intravascular contrast agents in sonography may improve the sensitivity of detecting blood flow in the scrotum, but this has not yet been proved in a large series.[167] In pediatric patients, it may

be difficult to document flow in a normal testis, and testicular scintigraphy has been advocated to corroborate sonographic findings.[172] In practice, many surgeons elect to explore the testis surgically if clinical symptoms and signs are suggestive and results of the sonographic examination are equivocal.

Potential pitfalls in using sonography in the diagnosis of torsion are **partial torsion**, **torsion/detorsion,** and **ischemia** due to orchitis. Torsion of at least 540 degrees is necessary for complete arterial occlusion.[163,173,174] With partial torsion of 360 degrees, or less, arterial flow may still occur, but venous outflow is often obstructed causing diminished diastolic arterial flow on spectral Doppler examination (see Fig. 24-28).[175] If spontaneous detorsion occurs, flow within the affected testis may be normal or it may be increased and mimic orchitis.[176] Spontaneous detorsion rarely occurs leaving a segmental testicular infarction.[91,177] Segmental testicular infarction may also occur with Henoch-Schönlein purpura or with orchitis (see Fig. 24-14). Orchitis may also cause global ischemia of the testis and mimic torsion.[176]

In cases of subacute or chronic torsion, color flow Doppler shows no flow in the testis and increased flow in the paratesticular tissues, including the epididymis-cord complex and dartos fascia (see Fig. 24-28).

Torsion of the testicular appendage is a common cause of acute scrotal pain and may mimic testicular torsion clinically. Patients are rarely referred for imaging because the pain is usually not severe and the twisted appendage may be evident clinically as the **"blue dot" sign**.[178] The sonographic appearance of the twisted testicular appendage has been described as an avascular hypoechoic mass adjacent to a normally perfused testis and surrounded by an area of increased color flow Doppler perfusion.[163] However, the twisted appendage may appear as an echogenic extratesticular mass situated between the head of the epididymis and the upper pole of the testis.[179]

Epididymitis and Epididymo-Orchitis

Epididymitis is the most common cause of acute scrotal pain in postpubertal men, causing 75% of all acute intrascrotal inflammatory processes. It usually results from a lower urinary tract infection and is less commonly hematogenous or traumatic in origin. The common causative organisms are *Escherichia coli*, *Pseudomonas*, and *Klebsiella*.[180] Sexually transmitted organisms causing urethritis, such as gonococcus and *Chlamydia*, are common causes of epididymitis in young men. Less commonly, epididymitis may be due to tuberculosis, mumps, or syphilitic orchitis.[181,182] The age of peak incidence is 40 to 50 years. Typically, patients present with the insidious onset of pain, which increases over 1 to 2 days. Fever, dysuria, and urethral discharge may also be present.

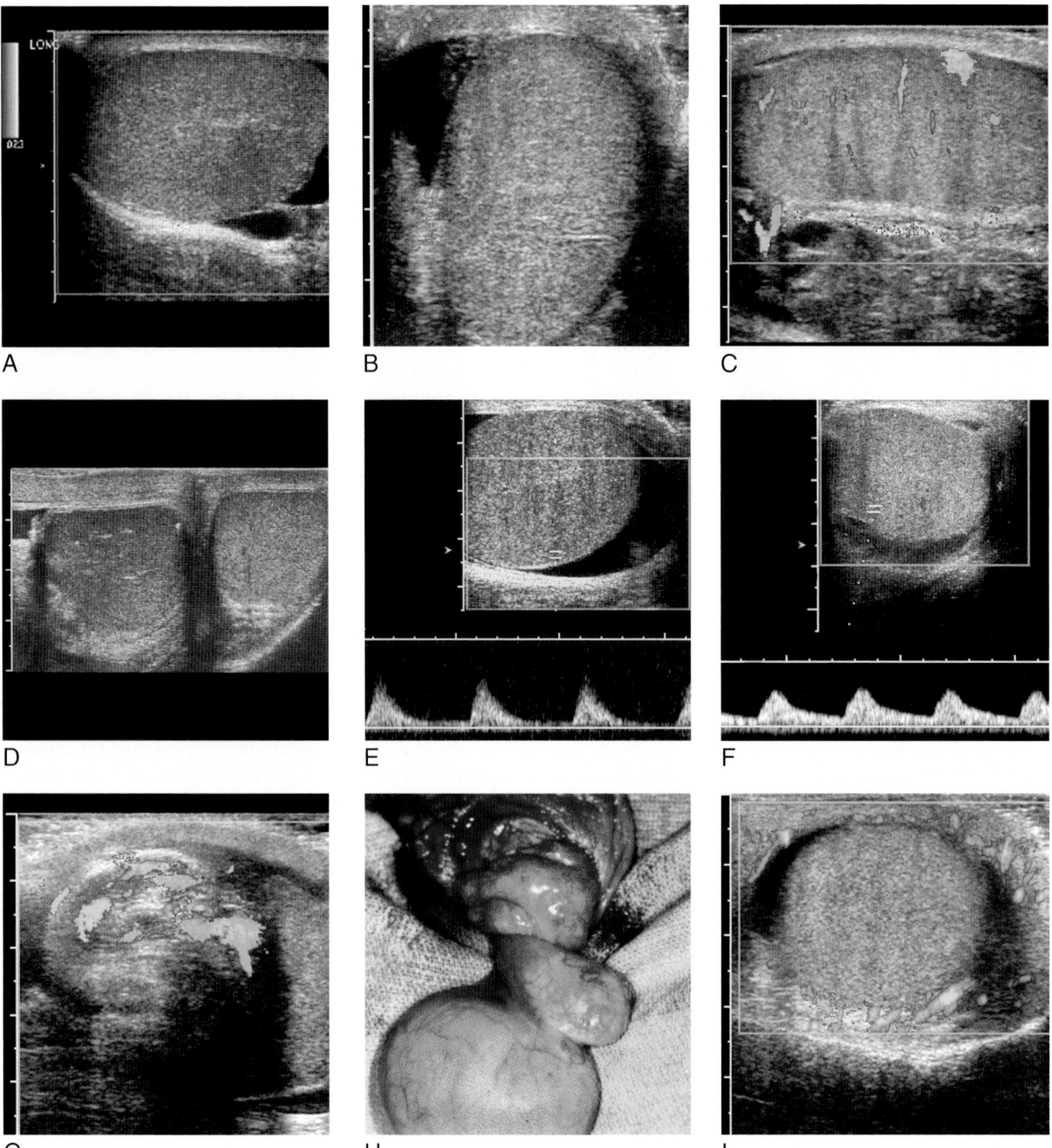

FIGURE 24-28. Torsion of the spermatic cord and testis—spectrum of appearances. A, Acute torsion. Longitudinal power Doppler scan shows no flow in the testis. **B, Acute torsion.** Longitudinal power Doppler scan shows abnormal, transverse, and vertical orientation of the testis with no flow. **C, After manual detorsion** of the same case as in **B**, a longitudinal color Doppler scan shows the normal orientation of the testis with blood flow present. The testis has a striated appearance due to the previous ischemia. **D, Acute torsion—gray-scale changes.** Dual transverse scan shows enlarged hypoechoic right testis due to torsion and skin thickening in the right hemiscrotum. **E, Partial torsion.** Longitudinal scan with spectral Doppler shows a high-resistance testicular arterial waveform with little diastolic flow because of venous occlusion. Small reactive hydrocele. **F, After spontaneous detorsion.** Same case as in **E**. Longitudinal scan with spectral Doppler shows return of diastolic flow. **G, "Torsion knot."** Longitudinal scan with acute spermatic cord torsion shows the torsion knot complex of epididymis and spermatic cord. **H, Acute torsion.** Intraoperative photograph shows the twisted spermatic cord that gives the "torsion knot" appearance on sonograph. **I, Subacute torsion** (3 days of pain). Transverse power Doppler scan shows absent flow within the testis with surrounding hyperemia. (**H,** From Winter TC: Ultrasonography of the scrotum. Appl Radiol 2002;31(3). **H** courtesy of Drs. R.E. Berger, University of Washington, Seattle, Washington, and T.C. Winter, University of Wisconsin, Madison, Wisconsin.)

In acute epididymitis, sonography characteristically shows thickening and enlargement of the epididymis, involving the tail initially and frequently spreading to involve the entire epididymis (Fig. 24-29A,B).[183] The echogenicity of the epididymis is usually decreased, and its echo texture is often coarse and heterogeneous, probably because of edema or hemorrhage, or both. Reactive hydrocele formation is common, and associated skin thickening may be seen. Color flow Doppler sonography usually shows increased blood flow in the epididymis or testis, or both, as compared with the asymptomatic side (see Fig. 24-29C).[184]

Direct extension of epididymal inflammation to the testicle, called **epididymo-orchitis**, occurs in up to 20% of patients with acute epididymitis. Isolated orchitis may also occur. In such cases, increased blood flow is localized to the testis (see Fig. 24-29D,E,H,I). Testicular involvement may be focal or diffuse. Characteristically, **focal orchitis** produces a hypoechoic area adjacent to an enlarged portion of the epididymis. Color Doppler shows increased flow in the hypoechoic area of the testis; increased flow in the tunica vasculosa may be visible as lines of color signal radiating from the mediastinum testis.[185] These lines of color correspond to septal accentuation that is visible as hypoechoic bands on gray-scale sonography (see Fig. 24-29H,I). Spectral Doppler shows increased diastolic flow in uncomplicated orchitis (Fig. 24-30A). If left untreated, the entire testicle may become involved, appearing hypoechoic and enlarged. As pressure in the testis increases from edema, venous infarction with hemorrhage may occur, appearing hyperechoic initially and hypoechoic later (see Fig. 24-29).[185] Ischemia and subsequent infarction may occur when the vascularity of the testis is compromised by venous occlusion in the epididymis and cord.[186] When vascular disruption is severe, resulting in complete **testicular infarction**, the changes are indistinguishable from those seen in testicular torsion. Color flow Doppler sonography may show focal areas of reactive hyperemia and increased blood flow associated with relatively avascular areas of infarction in both the testis and epididymis in cases of severe epididymo-orchitis. Diastolic flow reversal in the arterial waveforms of the testis is an ominous finding associated with testicular infarction in cases of severe epididymo-orchitis (see Fig. 24-30B).[187] In addition to infarction, other complications of acute epididymo-orchitis include abscess and pyocele (see Figs. 24-13 and 24-18F). Chronic changes may be seen in the epididymis or testis from clinically resolved epididymo-orchitis. Swelling of the epididymis may persist and appear as a heterogeneous mass on sonography (see Fig. 24-23A). The testis may have a persistent, striated appearance of septal accentuation from fibrosis (Figs. 24-31 and 24-32).[185,188] This striated appearance of the testis is nonspecific and may also be seen after ischemia from torsion or during a hernia repair.[185,188] A

similar heterogeneous appearance in the testis may be seen in elderly patients because of seminiferous **tubule atrophy and sclerosis**.[189] Focal areas of infarction in the testis may persist as wedge- or cone-shaped hypoechoic areas or may appear as hyperechoic scars.[185] If complete infarction of the testis has occurred because of epididymo-orchitis, the testis may become small, with a hypoechoic or heterogeneous echotexture.

TRAUMA

Prompt diagnosis of a **ruptured testis** is of utmost importance because of the direct relationship between early surgical intervention and testicular salvageability. Approximately 90% of ruptured testicles can be saved if surgery is performed within the first 72 hours, whereas only 45% may be salvaged after 72 hours.[190,191] Clinical diagnosis is often impossible because of marked scrotal pain and swelling. Jeffrey et al.[190] correctly identified 12 of 12 cases of testicular rupture by using sonography. Sonographic features include focal areas of altered testicular echogenicity, corresponding to areas of hemorrhage or infarction, and hematocele formation in 33% of patients. A discrete fracture plane was identified in only 17% of cases (Fig. 24-33). The testicular contour is often irregular. Although these features are not specific for a ruptured testicle, they may be suggestive of the diagnosis in the appropriate clinical setting, prompting immediate surgical exploration. Vascular disruption may also be apparent on color flow Doppler sonography. Care should be taken to avoid misdiagnosing a complex intrascrotal hematoma as a testicular rupture. Use of Doppler and color flow Doppler imaging may aid in distinguishing the normal vascularized testis from a complex hematoma.[192] Sonography can also be used to discern the severity of scrotal trauma due to bullet wounds. Hematomas and hematoceles can be distinguished from testicular rupture, and foreign bodies can be localized.[193] A careful gray-scale and color flow Doppler evaluation of the epididymis should be performed in all examinations done for blunt trauma. Traumatic epididymitis may be an isolated finding that should not be confused with an infectious process.[194]

CRYPTORCHIDISM

The testes normally begin their descent through the inguinal canal into the scrotal sac at approximately 36 weeks of gestation. The gubernaculum testis is a fibromuscular structure that extends from the inferior pole of the testis to the scrotum and guides the testis in its descent, which normally has been completed at birth.[3] Undescended testis is one of the most common genitourinary anomalies in male infants. At birth, 3.5% of

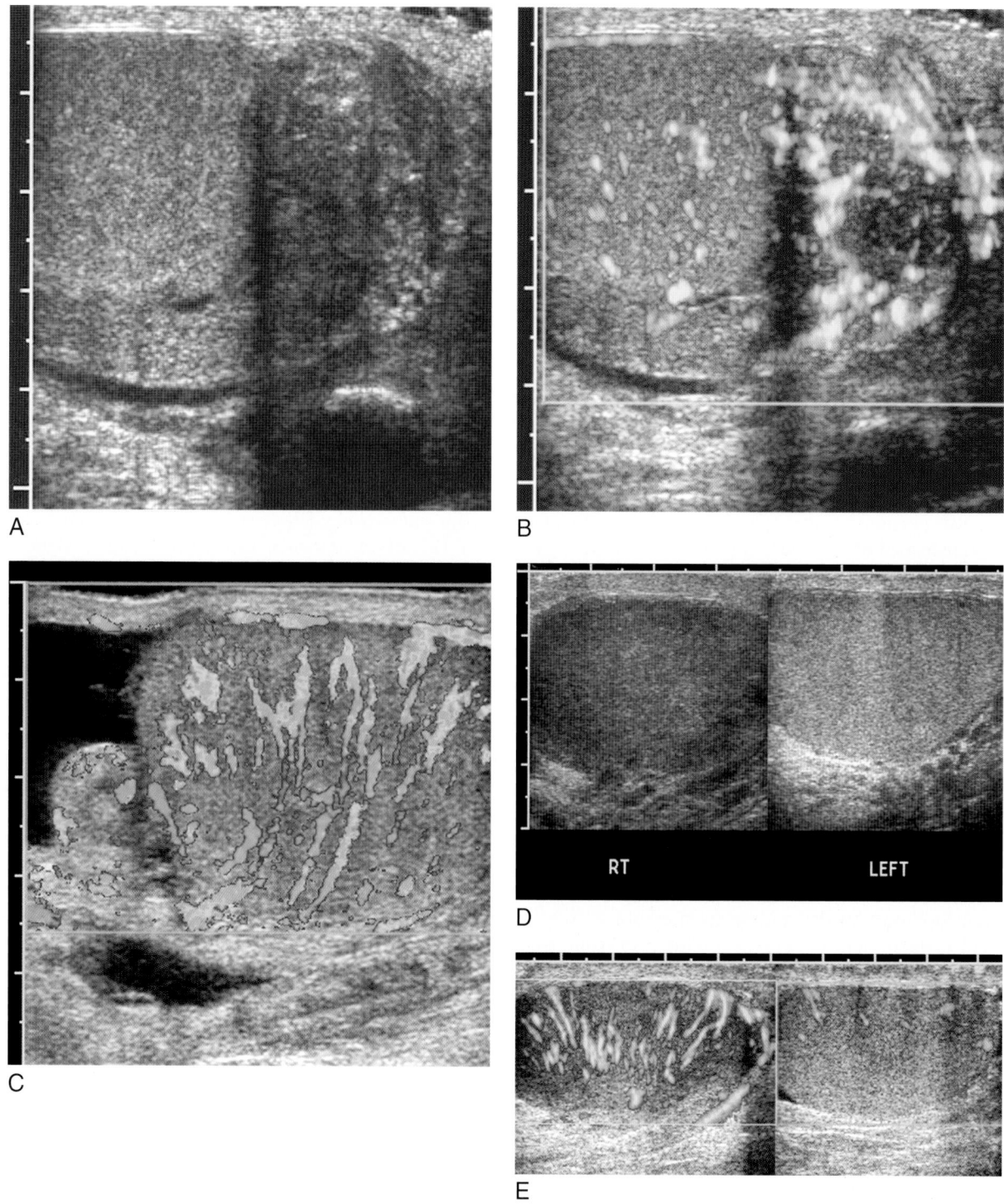

FIGURE 24-29. Epididymo-orchitis, epididymitis, and orchitis—spectrum of appearances. A and **B**, **Acute epididymitis**. Longitudinal gray-scale scan (**A**) and color Doppler (**B**) examinations show enlargement and a heterogeneous echotexture of the tail of the epididymis with marked increased flow in the tail of the epididymis and minimally increased flow in the adjacent testis. **C, Acute epididymo-orchitis**. Longitudinal color Doppler scan shows increased flow in the epididymis and testis. **D** and **E**, **Acute orchitis**. Longitudinal dual-image gray-scale (**D**) and color Doppler (**E**) images show the right testis is hypoechoic and has markedly increased flow.

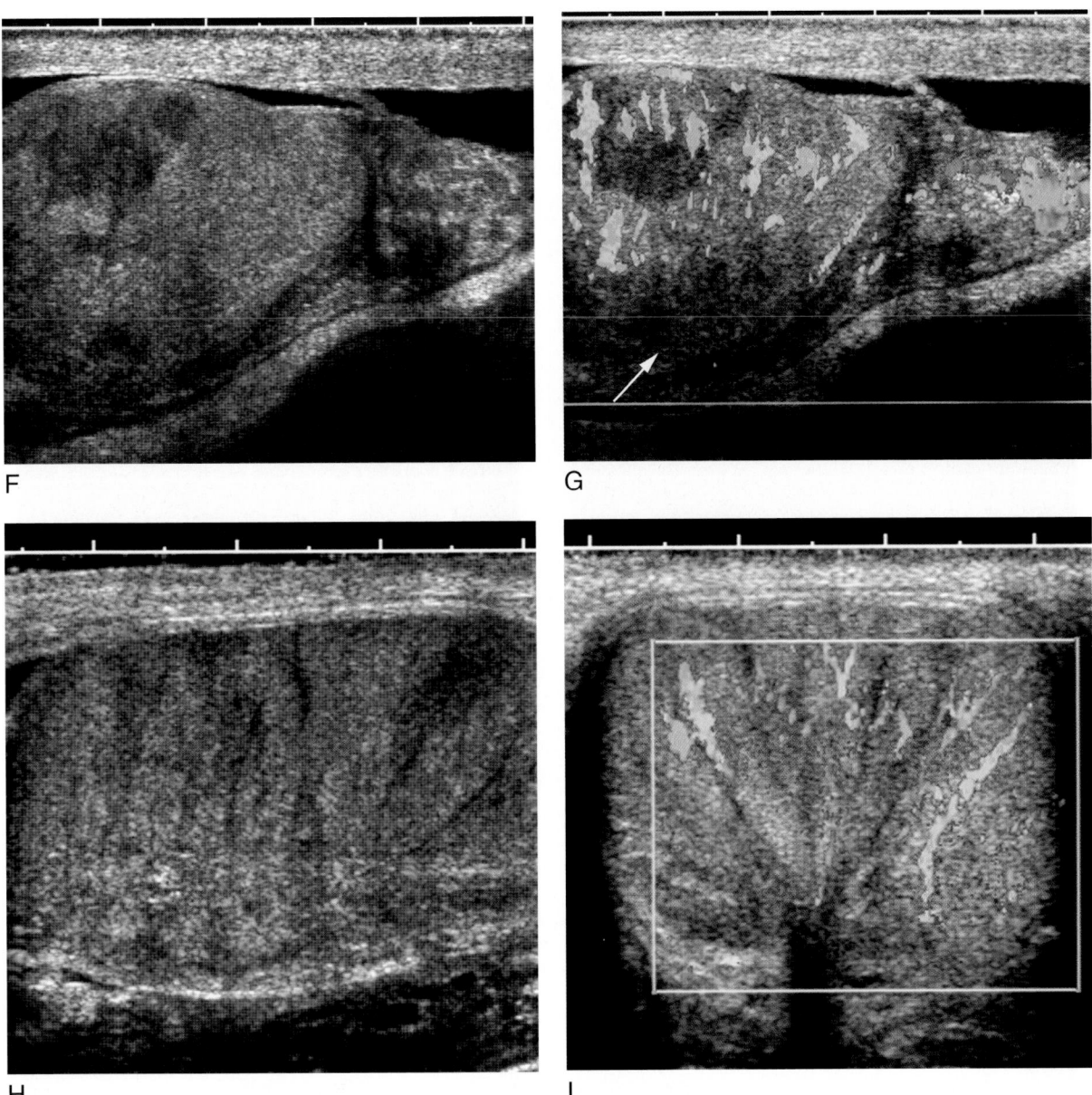

FIGURE 24-29, *cont'd*. Epididymo-orchitis, epididymitis, and orchitis—spectrum of appearances. F,
Longitudinal gray-scale scan with 3 weeks of epididymo-orchitis unresolved with antibiotic therapy shows hypoechoic areas in the testis and an enlarged heterogeneous tail of the epididymis. **G,** Color Doppler image shows increased flow in the testis and epididymis with an area of decreased flow due to ischemia (*arrow*). **H** and **I, Acute orchitis.** Longitudinal gray-scale and color Doppler images show hypoechoic bands due to septal accentuation from edema and increased vascularity of the testis.

male infants weighing more than 2500 g have an undescended testis; 10% to 25% of these cases are bilateral. This figure decreases to 0.8% by age one year because the testes descend spontaneously in most infants. The incidence of undescended testes increases to 30% in premature infants, approaching 100% in neonates who weigh less than 1 kg at birth.[195,196] Complete descent is necessary for full testicular maturation.[195,196]

Malpositioned testes may be located anywhere along the pathway of descent from the retroperitoneum to the scrotum. Most (80%) undescended testes are palpable, lying at or below the level of the inguinal canal. Anorchia

occurs in 4% of the remaining patients with impalpable testes.[196]

Localization of the undescended testis is important for the prevention of two potential **complications of cryptorchidism: infertility** and **cancer.** Infertility results from progressive pathologic changes that develop in both the undescended testis and the contralateral, normal testis after age one year.[196-198] The undescended testis is 48 times more likely to undergo malignant change than is the normally descended testis.[1] It is thought that the hormonal deficiency resulting in failure of testicular descent predisposes the patient to malig-

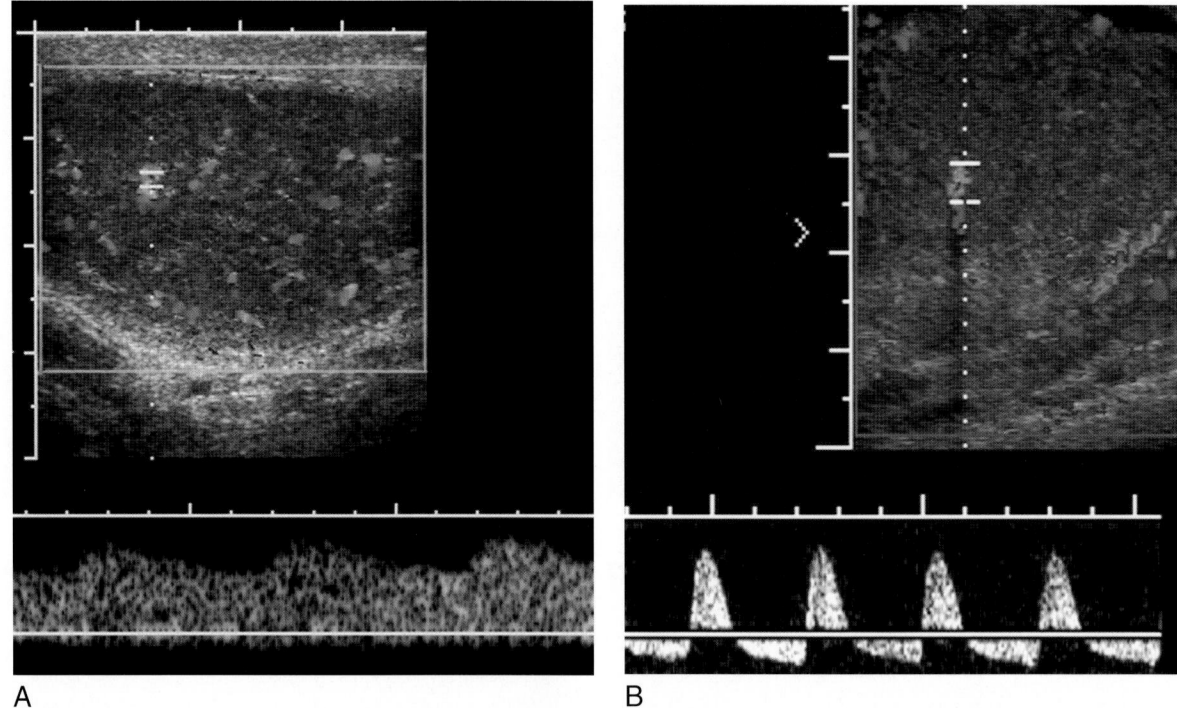

A   B

FIGURE 24-30. Spectral Doppler changes in orchitis. A, Uncomplicated orchitis. Longitudinal scan with spectral Doppler tracing shows increased diastolic flow in the testis. **B, Orchitis with venous compromise.** Longitudinal scan with spectral Doppler tracing in more severe orchitis shows reversal of flow in diastole due to edema impeding venous flow.

nancy. Each year, in approximately 0.04% of patients with an undescended testis, carcinoma develops. The lifetime risk of death from a testicular malignancy in men of any age with an undescended testis is approximately 9.7 times the risk in normal men.[197] The most common malignancy is seminoma. The risk of malignancy is increased in both the undescended testis after orchiopexy and the normally descended testis. Therefore, careful serial examinations of both testes are essential.

Because of the superficial location of the inguinal canal in children, sonography of the undescended testis should be performed with a high-frequency transducer.

Sonographically, the **undescended testis** is often smaller and slightly less echogenic than the contralateral, normally descended testis (Fig. 24-34). A large lymph node or the pars infravaginalis gubernaculi (PIG), which is the distal bulbous segment of the gubernaculum testis, can be mistaken for the testis. After completion of testicular descent, the PIG and the gubernaculum normally atrophy. If the testis remains undescended, both structures persist. The PIG is located distal to the undescended testis, usually in the scrotum, but it may be found in the inguinal cord. Sonographically, the PIG is a hypoechoic, cord-like structure of echogenicity similar to the testis, with the gubernaculum leading to it.[199]

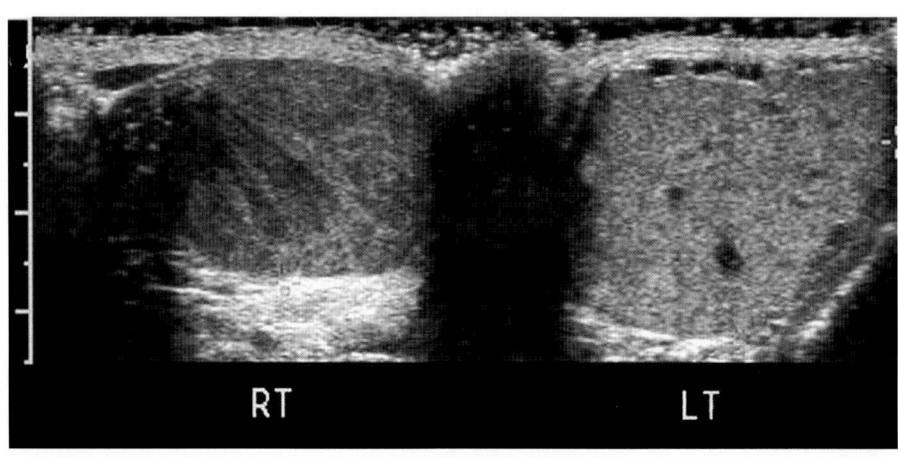

FIGURE 24-31. Heterogeneous "striped" testis. Transverse dual image shows heterogeneity in the right testis with marked septal accentuation due to previous orchitis. This appearance may also be seen after ischemia.

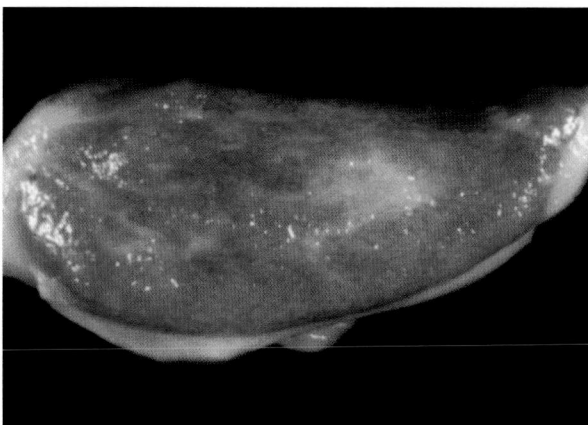

FIGURE 24-32. Fibrosis of testis after orchitis.
Pathological specimen of testis shows linear bands of fibrosis (*white areas*) due to previous severe orchitis. A similar "end-stage" testis could have this appearance due to ischemia.

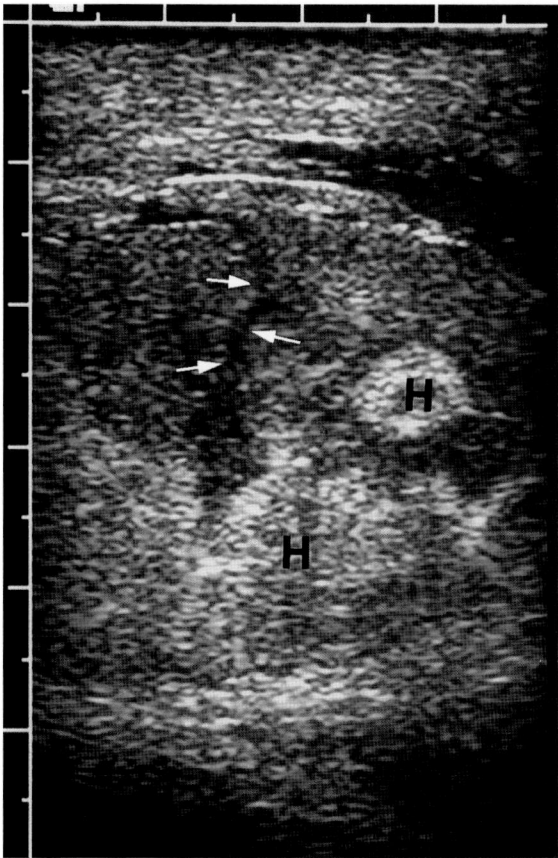

FIGURE 24-33. Fracture of testis. Transverse scan shows a heterogeneous testicle with a linear band (*arrows*) indicating a fracture. H, Testicular hematoma.

The success of sonography in the localization of undescended testes varies among series. Wolverson et al.[200] reported a sensitivity of 88%, a specificity of 100%, and an accuracy of 91% in the sonographic localization of undescended testes. In a later study, Weiss et al.[201] reported a sensitivity of 70% for palpable testes

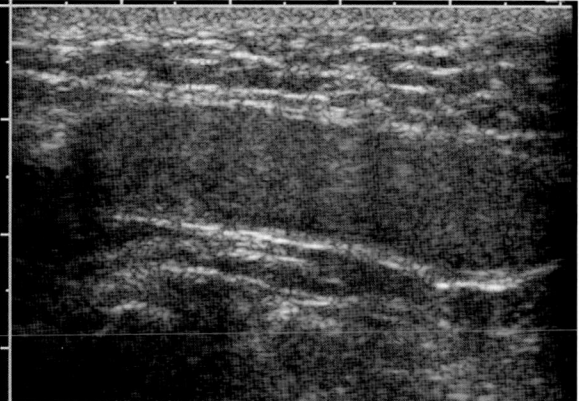

FIGURE 24-34. Testis in inguinal canal. Longitudinal scan shows an elongated, ovoid, undescended testis.

and 13% for nonpalpable testes. The sensitivity and specificity of MRI are similar to sonography in the evaluation of cryptorchidism.[202,203] MRI shares two main advantages with sonography: noninvasiveness and lack of ionizing radiation. An additional advantage of MRI is the ability to obtain multiplanar images of the retroperitoneum and inguinal region. Undescended testes are characteristically hypointense with respect to fat on short repetition time/echo time sequences, and hyperintense or isointense with respect to fat on long repetition time/echo time sequences. These signal characteristics of undescended testes are identical to those of scrotal testes. Disadvantages of MRI include cost, long scanning time, and, frequently, the need for sedation. Sonography is often used in the initial evaluation of cryptorchidism, although the value of this has been questioned because it is insensitive in detecting high intra-abdominal testes.[197] Many surgeons use the same surgical approach whether the testis is seen sonographically or not. Nonvisualization of an undescended testis on sonography or MRI does not exclude its presence, and therefore laparoscopy or surgical exploration should be performed if clinically indicated.

Acknowledgement

Frank Thornton M.D. assisted in gathering images.

References

1. Krone KD, Carroll BA: Scrotal ultrasound. Radiol Clin North Am 1985;23:121-139.
2. Trainer TD: Histology of the normal testis. Am J Surg Pathol 1987;11:797-809.
3. Rifkin MD, Foy PM, Goldberg BB: Scrotal ultrasound: Acoustic characteristics of the normal testis and epididymis defined with high resolution superficial scanners. Med Ultrasound 1984;8:91-97.
4. Johnson KA, Dewbury KC: Ultrasound imaging of the appendix testis and appendix epididymis. Clinical Radiology 1996;51:335-337.

5. Black JAR, Patel A: Sonography of the Normal Extratesticular Space. AJR 1996;167:503-506.

6. Allen TD: Disorders of the male external genitalia. In Kelalis PP, King LR (eds): Clinical Pediatric Urology. Philadelphia, WB Saunders, 1976, pp 636-668.

7. Middleton WD, Bell MW: Analysis of intratesticular arterial anatomy with emphasis on transmediastinal arteries. Radiology 1993;189:157-160.

8. Fakhry J, Khoury A, Barakat K: The hypoechoic band: A normal finding on testicular sonography. AJR 1989;153:321-323.

9. Middleton WD, Thorne DA, Melson GL: Color Doppler ultrasound of the normal testis. AJR 1989;152:293-297.

10. Gooding GAW: Sonography of the spermatic cord. AJR 1988;151:721-724.

11. Benson CB, Doubilet PM, Richie JP: Sonography of the male genital tract. AJR 1989;153:705-713.

12. Rifkin MD, Kurtz AB, Pasto ME, et al: The sonographic diagnosis of focal and infiltrating intrascrotal lesions. Urol Radiol 1984;6:20-26.

13. Rifkin MD, Kurtz AB, Pasto ME, et al: Diagnostic capabilities of high-resolution scrotal ultrasonography: Prospective evaluation. J Ultrasound Med 1985;4:13-19.

14. Carroll BA, Gross DM: High-frequency scrotal sonography. AJR 1983;140:511-515.

15. Grantham JG, Charboneau JW, James EM, et al: Testicular neoplasms: 29 tumors studied by high-resolution ultrasound. Radiology 1985;775-780.

16. Kirschling RJ, Kvols LK, Charboneau JW, et al: High-resolution ultrasonographic and pathologic abnormalities of germ cell tumors in patients with clinically normal testes. Mayo Clin Proc 1983;58:648-653.

17. Javadpour N: Principles and Management of Testicular Cancer. New York, Thieme, 1986.

18. Goldfinger SS, Rothberg R, Buckspan MB, et al: Incidental detection of impalpable testicular neoplasm by sonography. AJR 1986;146:349-350.

19. Damjanov I: Tumors of the testis and epididymis. In Murphy WM: Urological Pathology, 2nd ed. Philadelphia, WB Saunders, 1997, pp 342-400.

20. Mostofi FK, Sobin LH: International histological classification of tumors of the testes No. 16, WHO, Geneva 1977.

21. Talerman A, Roth LM: Pathology of the testis and its adnexa. New York, Churchill Livingstone, 1986.

22. Jacobsen GK, Talerman A: Atlas of germ cell tumors. Copenhagen, Munksgaard, 1989.

23. Ruzal-Shapiro C, Newhouse JH: Genitourinary Ultrasound. In Taveras JM, Ferrucci JT (eds): Radiology: Diagnosis-Imaging Intervention. Philadelphia, JB Lippincott, 1986, p 4.

24. Schwerk WB, Schwerk WNM, Rodeck G: Testicular tumors: Prospective analysis of real-time ultrasound patterns and abdominal staging. Radiology 1987; 164:369-374.

25. Ulbright TM: Germ cell neoplasms of the testis. Am J Surg Pathol 1993;17:1075.

26. Mostofi FK, Price EB, Jr: Tumors of the male genital system. In Atlas of Tumor Pathology, Fascicle 8, 2nd series. Washington, DC: Armed Forces Institute of Pathology, 1973.

27. Emory TH, Charboneau JW, Randall RV, et al: Occult testicular interstitial-cell tumor in a patient with gynecomastia: Ultrasonic detection. Radiology 1984;151:474.

28. Cunningham JJ: Echographic findings in Sertoli cell tumor of the testis. J Clin Ultrasound 1981;9:341-342.

29. Gabrilove JL, Frieberg EK, Leiter E, Nicolis GL: Feminizing and non-feminizing Sertoli cell tumors. J Urology 1980;124:757.

30. Young S, Gooneratne S, Strauss FH, et al: Feminizing Sertoli cell tumors in boys with Peutz-Jeghers syndrome. Am J Surg Pathol 1995;19:50.

31. Gierke CL, King BF, Bostwick DG, et al: Large-cell calcifying Sertoli cell tumor of the testis: Appearance at sonography. AJR 1994;163:373-375.

32. Glazer HS, Lee JKT, Melson GL, et al: Sonographic detection of occult testicular neoplasms. AJR 1981;138:673-675.

33. Bockrath JJ, Schaeffer AJ, Kies JS, et al: Ultrasound identification of impalpable testicular tumor. J Urol 1981;130:355-356.

34. Moudy PC, Makhija JS: Ultrasonic demonstration of a nonpalpable testicular tumor. J Clin Ultrasound 1983;11:54-55.

35. Shawker TH, Javadpour N, O'Leary T, et al: Ultrasonographic detection of "burned-out" primary testicular germ cell tumors in clinically normal testes. J Ultrasound Med 1983;2:477-479.

36. Horstman WG, Melson GL, Middleton WD, et al: Testicular tumors: Findings with color Doppler US. Radiology 1992;185:733-737.

37. Luker GD, Siegel MJ: Pediatric testicular tumors: Evaluation with gray-scale and color Doppler US. Radiology 1994;191:561-564.

38. Horstman WG, Haluszka MM, Burkhard TK: Management of testicular masses incidentally discovered by ultrasound. J Urol 1994;151:1263-1265.

39. Doll DC, Weiss RB: Malignant lymphoma of the testis. Am J Med 1986;81:515-523.

40. Hamlin JA, Kagan AR, Friedman NB: Lymphomas of the testicle. Cancer 1972;29:1532-1536.

41. Tepperman BS, Gospodarowicz M, Bush RS, et al: Non-Hodgkin lymphoma of the testis. Radiology 1982;142:203-208.

42. Paladugu RP, Bearman RM, Rappaport H: Malignant lymphoma with primary manifestation in the gonad: A clinicopathologic study of 38 patients. Cancer 1980;45:561-571.

43. Mazzu D, Jeffrey RB, Jr, Ralls PW: Lymphoma and leukemia involving the testicles: Findings on gray-scale and color Doppler sonography. AJR 1995;164:645-647.

44. Rayor RA, Scheible W, Brock WA, et al: High resolution ultrasonography in the diagnosis of testicular relapse in patients with lymphoblastic leukemia. J Urol 1982;128:602-603.

45. Phillips G, Kumari-Subaiya S, Sawitsky A: Ultrasonic evaluation of the scrotum in lymphoproliferative disease. J Ultrasound Med 1987;6:169-175.

46. Iizumi T, Shinohara S, Ameniya H, et al: Plasmacytoma of the testis. Urology Int 1995;55:218.

47. Dahnert WF, Rifkin MD, Kurtz AB: Ultrasound case of the day. Radiographics 1989;9:554-558.

48. Grignon DJ, Shum DT, Hayman WP: Metastatic tumors of the testes. Can J Surg 1986;29:359-361.

49. Werth V, Yu G, Marshall FF: Nonlymphomatous metastatic tumor to the testis. J Urol 1981;127:142-144.

50. Hanash KA, Carney JA, Kelalis PP: Metastatic tumors to testicles: Routes of metastasis. J Urol 1969;102:465-468.

51. Hamm B, Fobbe F, Loy V: Testicular cysts: Differentiation with ultrasound and clinical findings. Radiology 1988;168:19-23.

52. Gooding Gaw, Leonhardt W, Stein R: Testicular cysts: US findings. Radiology 1987;163:537-538.

53. Martinez-Berganza MT, Sarria L, Cozcolluela R, et al: Cysts of the tunica albuginea: Sonographic appearance. AJR 1998;170:183-185.

54. Dogra VS, Gottlieb RH, Rubens DJ, Liao L: Benign intratesticular cystic lesions: US features. Radiographics 2001;21:S273-S281.

55. Becker J, Arger PH, Wein AJ, et al: Inclusion cyst of the tunica albuginea: Demonstration by ultrasound. Urol Radiol 1983;5:127-129.

56. Turner WR, Derrick FC, Sanders P, et al: Benign lesions of the tunica albuginea. J Urol 1977;117:602-604.

57. Warner KE, Noyes DT, Ross JS: Cysts of the tunica albuginea testis: A report of 3 cases with a review of the literature. J Urol 1984;132:131-132.

58. Poster RB, Spirt BA, Tamsen A, et al: Complex tunica albuginea cyst simulating an intratesticular lesion. Urol Radiol 1991;13:129-132.

59. Sudakoff GS, Quiroz F, Karcaaltincaba M, Foley WD: Scrotal Ultrasonography with emphasis on the extratesticular space: Anatomy, embryology, and pathology. Ultrasound Quarterly 2002;18:255-273.

60. Takihari H, Valvo JR, Tokuhara M, et al: Intratesticular cysts. Urology 1982;20:80-82.

61. Rifkin MD, Jacobs JA: Simple testicular cyst diagnosed preoperatively by ultrasound. J Urol 1983;129:982-983.

62. Fisher JE, Jewett TC, Nelson SJ, et al: Ectasia of the rete testis with ipsilateral renal agenesis. J Urol 1982; 128:1040-1043.

63. Nistal M, Regadera J, Paniagua R: Cystic dysplasia of the testis. Arch Pathol Lab Med 1984;104:579-583.

64. Tartar VM, Trambert MA, Balsara ZN, et al: Tubular ectasia of the testicle: Sonographic and MR imaging appearance. AJR 1993;160:539-542.

65. Brown DL, Benson CB, Doherty FJ, et al: Cystic testicular mass caused by dilated rete testis: Sonographic findings in 31 cases. AJR 1992;158:1257-1259.

66. Weingarten BJ, Kellman GM, Middleton WD, et al: Tubular ectasia within the mediastinum testis. J Ultrasound Med 1992;11:349-353.

67. Older RA, Watson LR: Tubular ectasia of the rete testis: A benign condition with a sonographic appearance that may be misinterpreted as malignant. J Urol 1994;152:477-478.

68. Cho CS, Kosek J: Cystic dysplasia of the testis: Sonographic and pathologic findings. Radiology 1985;156:777-778.

69. Keetch DW, McAlister WH, Manley CB, et al: Cystic dysplasia of the testis-sonographic features with pathologic correlation. Pediatr Radiol 1991;21:501-503.

70. Shah KH, Maxted WC, Dhun B: Epidermoid cysts of the testis: A report of three cases and an analysis of 141 cases from the world literature. Cancer 1981;47:577-582.

71. Caravelli JF, Peters BE: Sonography of bilateral testicular epidermoid cysts. J Ultrasound Med 1984;3:273-274.

72. Buckspan MB, Skeldon SC, Klotz PG, et al: Epidermoid cysts of the testicle. J Urol 1985;134:960-961.

73. Atchley JTM, Dewbury KC: Ultrasound appearances of testicular epidermoid cysts. Clin Radiol 2000;55:493-502.

74. Malek RS, Rosen JS, Farrow GM: Epidermoid cyst of the testis: A critical analysis. Br J Urol 1986;58:55-59.

75. Sanderson AJ, Birch BR, Dewbury KC: Case report: Multiple epidermoid cysts of the testes—the ultrasound appearances. Clin Radiol 1995; 50:414-415.

76. Malvica RP: Epidermoid cyst of the testicle: An unusual sonographic finding. AJR 1993;160:1047-1048.

77. Stein MM, Stein MW, Cohen BC, et al: Unusual sonographic appearance of an epidermoid cyst of the testis. J Ultrasound Med 1999;18:723-726.

78. Eisenmenger M, Lang S, Donner CH, et al: Epidermoid cysts of the testis: Organ-preserving surgery following diagnosis by ultrasonography. Br J Urol 1993;71:955-957.

79. Cho JH, Chang JC, Park BH, et al: Sonographic and MR imaging findings of testicular epidermoid cysts. AJR 2002;178:743-748.

80. Langer JE, Ramchandani P, Siegelman ES, Banner MP: Epidermoid cysts of the testicle: Sonographic and MRI imaging features. AJR 1999;173:1295-1299.

81. Hermansen JC, Dhusid MJ, Sty MR: Bacterial epididymo-orchitis in children and adolescents. Clin Pediatr 1980;19:812-815.

82. Mevorach RA, Lerner RM, Dvoretsky PM, et al: Testicular abscess: Diagnosis by ultrasonography. J Urol 1986;136:1213-1216.

83. Korn RL, Langer JE, Nisenbaum HL, et al: Non-Hodgkin's lymphoma mimicking a scrotal abscess in a patient with AIDS. J Ultrasound Med 1994; 13:715-718.

84. Smith FJ, Bilbey JH, Filipenko JD, et al: Testicular pseudotumor in the acquired immunodeficiency syndrome. Urology 1995;45:535-537.

85. Vick CW, Bird LI, Rosenfield AT, et al: Scrotal masses with a uniformly hyperechoic pattern. Radiology 1983;148:209-211.

86. Blei L, Sihelnik S, Bloom D, et al: Ultrasonographic analysis of chronic intratesticular pathology. J Ultrasound Med 1983;2:17-23.

87. Wu VH, Dangman BC, Kaufman RP, Jr: Sonographic appearance of acute testicular venous infarction in a patient with a hypercoagulable state. J Ultrasound Med 1995;14:57-59.

88. Flanagan JJ, Fowler RC: Testicular infarction mimicking tumour on scrotal ultrasound—a potential pitfall. Clin Radiol 1995;50:49-50.

89. Einstein DM, Paushter DM, Singer AA, et al: Fibrotic lesions of the testicle: Sonographic patterns mimicking malignancy. Urol Radiol 1992;14:205-210.

90. Ledwidge ME, Lee DK, Winter TC, et al: Sonographic diagnosis of superior hemispheric testicular infarction. AJR 2002;179:775-776.

91. Sriprasad S, Kooiman GG, Muir GH, Sidhu PS: Acute segmental testicular infarction: Differentiation from tumour using high frequency colour Doppler ultrasound. Br J Radiol 2001;74:965-967.

92. Carmody JP, Sharma OP: Intrascrotal sarcoidosis: Case reports and review. Sarcoidosis Vasc Diffuse Lung Dis. 1996;13:129.

93. Winter TC, III, Keener TS, Mack LA: Sonographic appearance of testicular sarcoid. J Ultrasound Med 1995;14:153.

94. Eraso CE, Vrachliotis TG, Cunningham JJ: Sonographic findings in testicular sarcoidosis simulating malignant nodule. J Clin Ultrasound 1999;27(2):81-83.

95. Rifkin MD, Kurtz AB, Goldberg BB: Epididymis examined by ultrasound: Correlation with pathology. Radiology 1984;151:187-190.

96. Avila NA, Premkumar A, Shawker TH, et al: Testicular adrenal rest tissue in congenital adrenal hyperplasia: Findings at gray-scale and color Doppler US. Radiology 1996;198:99-104.

97. Vanzulli A, DelMaschio A, Paesano P, et al: Testicular masses in association with adrenogenital syndrome: US findings. Radiology 1992;183:425-429.

98. Vegni-Talluri M, Bigliardi E, Vanni MG, et al: Testicular microliths: Their origin and structure. J Urol 1980;124:105-107.

99. Breger RC, Passarge E, McAdams AJ: Testicular intratubular bodies. J Clin Endocrinol Metab 1965;25:1340-1346.

100. Middleton WD, Teefey SA, Santillan CS: Testicular microlithiasis: Prospective analysis of prevalence and associated tumor. Radiology 2002;224:425-428.

101. Doherty FJ, Mullins TL, Sant GR, et al: Testicular microlithiasis: A unique sonographic appearance. J Ultrasound Med 1987;6:389-392.

102. Nistal M, Paniagua R, Diez-Pardo JA: Testicular microlithiasis in 2 children with bilateral cryptorchidism. J Urol 1979;121:535-537.

103. Janzen DL, Mathieson JR, March JI, et al: Testicular microlithiasis: Sonographic and clinical features. AJR 1992;158:1057-1060.

104. Backus ML, Mack AL, Middleton WD, et al: Testicular microlithiasis: Imaging appearances and pathologic correlation. Radiology 1994;192:781-785.

105. Patel MD, Olcott EW, Kerschmann RL, et al: Sonographically detected testicular microlithiasis and testicular carcinoma. J Clin Ultrasound 1993;21:447-452.

106. Cast JE, Nelson WM, Early AS, et al: Testicular microlithiasis: Prevalence and tumor risk in a population referred for scrotal sonography. AJR 2000;175:1703-1706.

107. Bennett HF, Middleton WD, Bullock AD, Teefey SA: Testicular microlithiasis: US follow up. Radiology 2001;218:359-363.

108. Bach AM, Hann LE, Hadar O, et al: Testicular microlithiasis: What is its association with testicular cancer? Radiology 2001;220:70-75.

109. Frush DP, Kliewer MA, Madden JF: Testicular microlithiasis and subsequent development of metastatic germ cell tumor. AJR 1996;167:889-890.

110. Smith SW, Brammer HM, Henry M, Frazier H: Testicular microlithiasis: Sonographic features with pathologic correlation. AJR 1991;157:1003-1004.

111. McEniff N, Doherty F, Katz J, et al: Yolk sac tumor of the testis discovered on a routine annual sonogram in a boy with testicular microlithiasis. AJR 1995;164:971-972.

112. Miller FNAC, Sidhu PS: Does testicular microlithiasis matter? A Review. Clin Radiol 2002;57:883-890.

113. Quane LK, Kidney DD: Testicular microlithiasis in a patient with a mediastinal germ cell tumour. Clin Radiol 2000;8:642-644.

114. Linkowski GD, Avellone A, Gooding GAW: Scrotal calculi: Sonographic detection. Radiology 1985;156:484.

115. Leung ML, Gooding GAW, Williams RD: High-resolution sonography of scrotal contents in asymptomatic subjects. AJR 1984;143:161-164.

116. Rathaus V, Konen O, Shapiro M, et al: Ultrasound features of spermatic cord hydrocele in children. Br J Radiol 2001;74:818-820.

117. Nye PJ, Prati RC: Idiopathic hydrocele and absent testicular diastolic flow. J Clin Ultrasound 1997;25:43-46.

118. Hricak H, Filly RA: Sonography of the scrotum. Invest Radiol 1983;18:112-121.

119. Worthy L, Miller EI, Chin DH: Evaluation of extratesticular findings in scrotal neoplasms. J Ultrasound Med 1986;5:261-263.

120. Gooding GAW, Leonhardt WC, Marshall G, et al: Cholesterol crystals in hydroceles: Sonographic detection and possible significance. AJR 1997;169:527-529.

121. Cunningham JJ: Sonographic findings in clinically unsuspected acute and chronic scrotal hematoceles. AJR 1983;140:749-752.

122. Wolverson MK, Houttuin E, Heiberg E, et al: High-resolution real-time sonography of scrotal varicocele. AJR 1983;141:775-779.

123. Belker AM: The varicocele and male infertility. Urol Clin North Am 1981;8:41-44.

124. Gonda RL, Karo JJ, Forte RA, et al: Diagnosis of subclinical varicocele in infertility. AJR 1987;148:71-75.

125. Hamm G, Fobbe F, Sorensen R, et al: Varicoceles: Combined sonography and thermography in diagnosis and post-therapeutic intervention. Radiology 1986;160:419-424.

126. McClure RD, Hricak H: Scrotal ultrasound in the infertile man: Detection of subclinical unilateral and bilateral varicoceles. J Urol 1986;135:711-714.

127. Graif M, Hauser R, Hirshebein A, et al: Varicocele and the testicular-renal venous route; Hemodynamic Doppler sonographic investigation. J Ultrasound Med 2000;19:627-631.

128. Atasoy C, Fitoz S: Gray-scale and color Doppler sonographic findings in intratesticular varicocele. J Clin Ultrasound 2001;29:369-373.

129. Subramanyam BR, Balthazar EJ, Raghavendra BN, et al: Sonographic diagnosis of scrotal hernia. AJR 1982;139:535-538.

130. Faysal MH, Strefling A, Kosek JC: Epididymal neoplasms: A case report and review. J Urol 1983;129:843-844.

131. Pavone-Macaluso M, Smith PH, Bagshaw MA: Testicular Cancer and Other Tumors of the Genitourinary Tract. New York, Plenum, 1985.

132. Smallman LA, Odedra JK: Primary carcinoma of sigmoid colon metastasizing to epididymis. Urology 1984;23:598-599.

133. Wachtel TL, Mehan DJ: Metastatic tumors of the epididymis. J Urol 1970;103:624-626.

134. Dunner PS, Lipsit ER, Nochomovitz LE: Epididymal sperm granuloma simulating a testicular neoplasm. J Clin Ultrasound 1982;10:353-355.

135. Ramanathan K, Yaghoobian J, Pinck RL: Sperm granuloma. J Clin Ultrasound 1986;14:155-156.

136. Oh C, Nisenbaum HL, Langer J, et al: Sonographic demonstration including color Doppler imaging of recurrent sperm granuloma. J Ultrasound Med 2000;19:333-335.

137. Krainik A, Sarrazin JL, Camparo P, et al: Fibrous pseudotumor of the epididymis: Imaging and pathologic correlation. Eur Radiol 2000;10:1636-1638.

138. Al-Otaibi L, Whitman GJ, Chew FS: Fibrous pseudotumor of the epididymis. AJR 1997;168:1586.

139. Oliva E, Young RH: Paratesticular tumor-like lesions. Semin Diagn Pathol 2000;17(4):340-358.

140. Jarvis LJ, Dubbins PA: Changes in the epididymis after vasectomy: Sonographic findings. AJR 1989;152:531-534.

141. Eftekhari F, Smith JK: Sonography of the scrotum after orchiectomy: Normal and abnormal findings. AJR 1993;160:543-547.

142. Fowler RC, Chennells PM, Ewing R: Scrotal ultrasonography: A clinical evaluation. Br J Radiol 1987;60:649-654.

143. Mueller DL, Amundson GM, Rubin SZ, et al: Acute scrotal abnormalities in children: Diagnosis by combined sonography and scintigraphy. AJR 1988;150:643-646.

144. Donahue RE, Cass BP, Veeraraghavan K: Immediate exploration of the unilateral acute scrotum in young male subjects. J Urol 1978;124:829-832.

145. Chen DCP, Holder LE, Kaplan GN: Correlation of radionuclide imaging and diagnostic ultrasound in scrotal diseases. J Nucl Med 1986;27:1774-1781.

146. Watanabe Y, Dohke M, Ohkubo K: Scrotal Disorders: Evaluation of enhancement patterns at dynamic contrast-enhanced subtraction MR imaging. Radiology 2000;217:219-227.

147. Hricak H, Lue T, Filly RA, et al: Experimental study of the sonographic diagnosis of testicular torsion. J Ultrasound Med 1983;2:349-356.

148. Williamson RCN: Torsion of the testis and allied conditions. Br J Surg 1976;63:465-476.

149. Pillai SB, Besner GE: Pediatric testicular problems. Pediatr Clin North Am 1998;45:813-829.

150. Paltiel HJ: Sonography of pediatric scrotal emergencies. Ultrasound Quarterly 2000;16:53-71.

151. Finkelstein MS, Rosenberg HK, Snyder HM, et al: Ultrasound evaluation of scrotum in pediatrics. Urology 1986;27:1-9.

152. Prando D: Torsion of the spermatic cord: Sonographic diagnosis. Ultrasound Quarterly 2002;18:41-57.

153. Sidhu PS: Clinical and imaging features of testicular torsion: Role of ultrasound. Clin Radiol 1999;54:343-352.

154. Bird K, Rosenfield AI, Taylor KJW: Ultrasonography in testicular torsion. Radiology 1983;147:527-534.

155. Middleton WD, Melson GL: Testicular ischemia: Color Doppler sonographic findings in five patients. AJR 1989;152:1237-1239.

156. Chinn DH, Miller EI: Generalized testicular hyperechogenicity in acute testicular torsion. J Ultrasound Med 1985;4:495-496.

157. Winter TC: Ultrasonography of the scrotum. App Radiol 2002;31(3).

158. Middleton WD, Middleton MA, Dierks M, et al: Sonographic prediction of viability in testicular torsion: Preliminary observations. J Ultrasound Med 1997; 16:23-27.

159. Vick CW, Bird K, Rosenfield AT, et al: Extratesticular hemorrhage associated with torsion of the spermatic cord: Sonographic demonstration. Radiology 1986; 158:401-404.

160. Trambert MA, Mattrey RF, Levine D, et al: Subacute scrotal pain: Evaluation of torsion versus epididymitis with MR imaging. Radiology 1990;175:53-56.

161. Bird K, Rosenfield AT: Testicular infarction secondary to acute inflammatory disease: Demonstration by B-scan ultrasound. Radiology 1984;152:785-788.

162. Margin B, Conte J: Ultrasonography of the acute scrotum. J Clin Ultrasound 1987;15:37-44.

163. Lerner RM, Mevorach RA, Hulbert WC, et al: Color Doppler ultrasound in the evaluation of acute scrotal disease. Radiology 1990;176:355-358.

164. Fitzgerald SW, Erickson S, DeWire DM, et al: Color Doppler sonography in the evaluation of the adult acute scrotum. J Ultrasound Med 1992;11:543-548.

165. Barth RA, Shortliffe LD: Normal pediatric testis: Comparison of power Doppler and color Doppler US in the detection of blood flow. Radiology 1997;204: 2289-2393.

166. Bader TR, Kammerhuber F, Herneth AM: Testicular blood flow in boys as assessed at color Doppler and power Doppler sonography. Radiology 1997;202:559-564.

167. Oley BD, Frush DP, Babcock DS, et al: Acute testicular torsion: Comparison of unenhanced and contrast-enhanced power Doppler US, color Doppler US and radionuclide imaging. Radiology 1996;199:441-446.

168. Luker GD, Siegel MJ: Scrotal US in pediatric patients: Comparison of power and standard color Doppler US. Radiology 1996;198:381-385.

169. Albrecht T, Lotzof K, Hussain HK, et al: Power Doppler US of the normal prepubertal testis: Does it live up to its promise? Radiology 1997;203:227-231.

170. Lee FT, Winter DB, Madsen FA, et al: Conventional color Doppler velocity sonography versus color Doppler energy sonography for the diagnosis of acute experimental torsion of the spermatic cord. AJR 1996;167:785-790.

171. Burks DD, Markey BJ, Burkhard TK, et al: Suspected testicular torsion and ischemia: Evaluation with color Doppler sonography. Radiology 1990;175:815-821.

172. Atkinson GO, Jr, Patrick LE, Ball TI, Jr, et al: The normal and abnormal scrotum in children: Evaluation with color Doppler sonography. AJR 1992;158:613-617.

173. Middleton WD, Siegel BA, Melson GL, et al: Acute scrotal disorders: Prospective comparison of color Doppler US and testicular scintigraphy. Radiology 1990;177: 177-181.

174. Bude RO, Kennelly MJ, Adler RS, et al: Nonpulsatile arterial waveforms: Observations during graded testicular torsion in rats. Acad Radiol 1995;2:879-882.

175. Sanelli, PC, Burke BJ, Lee L: Color and spectral Doppler sonography of partial torsion of the spermatic cord. AJR 1999;172:49-51.

176. Alcantra AL, Sethi Y. Imaging of testicular torsion and epididymitis/orchitis: Diagnosis and pitfalls. Emerg Radiol 1998;5:394-402.

177. Ledwidge ME, Lee DK, Winter TC, 3rd, et al: Sonographic diagnosis of superior hemispheric testicular infarction. AJR 2002;179:775-776.

178. Dresner ML: Torsed appendage: Diagnosis and management. Urology 1973;1:63-66.

179. Hesser U, Rosenberg M, Gierup J, et al: Gray-scale sonography in torsion of the testicular appendages. Pediatr Radiol 1993;23:529-532.

180. Berger RE, Alexander ER, Harnisch JP, et al: Etiology, manifestations and therapy of acute epididymitis: Prospective study of 50 cases. J Urol 1979;121:750-754.

181. Chung JJ, Kim MJ, Lee T, et al: Sonographic findings in tuberculous epididymitis and epididymo-orchitis. J Clin Ultrasound 1997;25:390-394.

182. Basekim CC, Kizilkaya E, Pekkafali Z, et al: Mumps epididymo-orchitis: Sonography and color Doppler sonographic findings. Abdom Imaging 2000; 25:322-325.

183. Gondos B, Wong T-W: Non-neoplastic diseases of the testis and epididymis. In Murphy WM (ed):Urological Pathology, 2nd ed. Philadelphia, WB Saunders,1997, pp 277-341.

184. Horstman WG, Middleton WD, Melson GL: Scrotal inflammatory disease: Color Doppler US findings. Radiology 1991;179:55-59.

185. Cook JL, Dewbury K: The Changes seen on high-resolution ultrasound in orchitis. Clin Radiology 2000;55:13-18.

186. Hourihane DO'B: Infected infarcts of the testis: A study of 18 cases proceeded by pyogenic epididymo-orchitis. J Clin Pathol 1970;23:668-675.

187. Sanders LM, Haber S, Dembner A, et al: Significance of reversal of diastolic flow in the acute scrotum. J Ultrasound Med 1994;13:137-139.

188. Casalino DD, Kim R: Clinical importance of a unilateral striated pattern seen on sonography of the testicle. AJR 2002;178:927-930.

189. Harris RD, Chouteau C, Partrick M, Schned A: Prevalence and significance of heterogeneous testes revealed on sonography: Ex vivo sonographic-pathologic correlation. AJR 2000;175:347-352.

190. Jeffrey RB, Laing FC, Hricak H, et al: Sonography of testicular trauma. AJR 1983;141:993-995.

191. Lupetin AR, King W, Rich PJ, et al: The traumatized scrotum: Ultrasound evaluation. Radiology 1983;148: 203-207.

192. Cohen HL, Shapiro ML, Haller JO, et al: Sonography of intrascrotal hematomas simulating testicular rupture in adolescents. Pediatr Radiol 1992;22:296-297.

193. Learch TJ, Hansch LP, Ralls PW: Sonography in patients with gunshot wounds of the scrotum: Imaging findings and their value. AJR 1995;165:879-883.

194. Gordon LM, Stein SM, Ralls PW: Traumatic epididymitis: Evaluation with color Doppler sonography. AJR 1996;166:1323-1325.

195. Elder JS: Cryptorchidism: Isolated and associated with other genitourinary defects. Pediatr Clin North Am 1987;34:1033-1053.

196. Harrison JH, et al: Campbell's Urology, 4th ed. Philadelphia, WB Saunders, 1979.

197. Friedland GW, Chang P: The role of imaging in the management of the impalpable undescended testis. AJR 1988;151:1107-1111.

198. Kogan SJ. Cryptorchidism and infertility: An overview. Dialog Pediatr Urol 1982;4:2-3.

199. Rosenfield AT, Blair DN, McCarthy S, et al: The pars infra-vaginalis gubernaculi: Importance in the identification of the undescended testis. AJR 1989;153:775-778.

200. Wolverson MK, Houttuin E, Heiberg E, et al: Comparison of computed tomography with high-resolution real-time ultrasound in the localization of the impalpable undescended testis. Radiology 1983;146:133-136.

201. Weiss R, Carter AR, Rosenfield AT: High-resolution real-time ultrasound in the localization of the undescended testis. J Urol 1986;135:936-938.

202. Fritzsche PJ, Hricak H, Kogan BA, et al: Undescended testis: Value of magnetic resonance imaging. Radiology 1987;169:173.

203. Kier R, McCarthy S, Rosenfield AT, et al: Nonpalpable testes in young boys: Evaluation with magnetic resonance imaging. Radiology 1988;169:429-433.

204. Rifkin MD: Scrotal ultrasound. Urol Radiol 1987;9:119-126.

25

THE ROTATOR CUFF

Marnix T. van Holsbeeck

Chapter Outline

Shoulder pain has many causes. Tendinitis, cuff strain, and partial- or full-thickness tear may cause pain and weakness on elevation of the arm.[1] The pain in rotator cuff disease is often worse at night and might keep the patient awake for prolonged periods of time. Underlying these symptoms in many patients over 40 years of age is rotator cuff fiber failure.[2] The supraspinatus tendon fibers typically fail first. The subscapularis and infraspinatus tendons, two other tendons of the rotator cuff, fail when the tear extends. The teres minor, the fourth component of the **rotator cuff**, is rarely affected. Calcific tendinitis, cervical radiculopathy, and acromioclavicular arthritis may mimic rotator cuff pathology. Contrast arthrography has long been the premier radiologic examination used to diagnose full-thickness tears of the rotator cuff.[3] Two competing non-invasive imaging techniques, ultrasound and magnetic resonance imaging (MRI), are taking over the role of arthrography. High-resolution real-time ultrasound has been shown to be a cost-effective means of examining the rotator cuff.[4-8] Ultrasound is the modality of choice in our institution. In the last 10 years, we performed over 20,000 shoulder ultrasound studies.

CLINICAL CONSIDERATIONS

Rotator cuff fiber failure is the most common cause of shoulder pain and dysfunction in the patient older than age 40.[1] Epidemiologic studies by Codman, DePalma, and others have demonstrated that the frequency of rotator cuff fiber failure increases with age.[9-11] This aging of tendons has been shown in imaging studies as well.[12-15] The earliest changes are often located in the substance of the tendon, resulting in so-called *delamination* of the cuff. Fiber failure is a step-by-step process from partial-thickness tear, almost always first in the supraspinatus, to massive tears involving multiple cuff tendons.

Rotator cuff tear may occur insidiously and, in fact, may be unnoticed by the patient, a process termed by some as **"creeping tendon ruptures."**[16] Asymptomatic tears affect a fraction of the population—as large as 30% in the group over age 60.[12] When a larger group of fibers fails at one time, the shoulder demonstrates pain at rest and accentuation of pain on use of the rotator cuff (e.g., extension, abduction, or external rotation). When even greater numbers of fibers fail at one time, a process known as *acute extension* of the shoulder may demonstrate sudden onset of substantial weakness in flexion, abduction, and external rotation.

As we age, the rotator cuff becomes increasingly susceptible to tearing with less severe amounts of applied force. Thus, although a major force is required to tear the usual rotator cuff of a 40-year-old person, a relatively trivial force may result in tear of the rotator cuff of the average 60-year-old individual. This is analogous to the predisposition of older women to femoral neck fractures. Although differences of the acromial shape, abnormalities of the acromial-clavicular joint, and other factors may also affect the susceptibility of the rotator cuff to fiber failure, age-related deterioration and loading of the rotator cuff seem to be the dominant factors in determining the failure patterns of the cuff tendons.

Symptoms of rotator cuff fiber failure in the acute phase usually include pain at rest and on motion. Later, subacromial crepitance occurs when the arm is rotated in the partially flexed position, and, finally, arm weakness occurs. When the rotator cuff fails, shoulder instability can result and so-called impingement may then manifest itself. The humeral head is no longer stabilized and may impinge on the tissues in between the head and the acromion or between the head and the posterior glenoid. In cases of subacromial impingement, the process will lead to sclerosis and remodeling of the acromion, and it may result in a traction spur along the coracoacromial ligament.[17]

TECHNICAL CONSIDERATIONS

Mechanical sector scanners with frequencies between 5 and 10 MHz have been used in the shoulder successfully in the early literature of rotator cuff sonography. The use of these mechanical sector scanners is now outdated. The utility of these transducers is limited by several factors: near-field artifact, narrow superficial image field, and **tendon anisotropy**. This last-named artifact is caused by the anisotropic structure of tendons. Parallelism of collagenous structures within the cuff results in peculiar imaging characteristics: the echogenicity of the tendon depends on the angle of the transducer relative to the tendon during tendon interrogation. The curved footprint of the mechanical sector scanners will result in heterogeneous appearance of the tendons. Even with optimal perpendicular technique, the center of the image will appear hyperechoic, whereas the side lobes will be hypoechoic. This hypoechogenicity can be mistaken for pathology by the inexperienced ultrasound reader.

State-of-the-art imaging of the cuff should be done with a high-resolution linear array transducer. In patients with a normal subcutaneous layer, we now routinely use a linear array transducer with a center frequency of 12 MHz. These transducers demonstrate marked improvement in near resolution when compared with other devices. In addition, the broad superficial field of view is helpful to improve the near-field image.

TECHNIQUE

Understanding the complex three-dimensional rotator cuff anatomy during sonography is crucial to successful rotator cuff sonography. The bone might limit the examination of the inexperienced examiner. For those who start in shoulder ultrasound, but who have experience in arthrography, we would recommend performing a quick **ultrasound examination before and after each arthrogram**. This allows the examiner to test his or her diagnostic abilities instantaneously. When we started, we did the arthrograms in single contrast; this enabled us to repeat the examination and correct our mistakes in those cases in which we failed to make the diagnosis of a tear. Those who have no experience with arthrography can **scan in the operating room or in the anatomy laboratory**. Surgical exploration or dissection may teach the most valuable lessons. Those initial steps are necessary to improve knowledge of the anatomy, which is essential in mastering the technique and accelerating the learning curve. Noteworthy is that some investigators have been combining arthrographic technique with the sonographic examination—**arthrosonography** as it has been called, may be more sensitive in assessing synovial proliferation and in estimating the size of rotator cuff tears.[18] Future applications may also include the diagnosis of labral abnormalities.[19-22] As with MRI, ultrasound's display of anatomy improves when enhanced by injection of intra-articular fluid. Saline used as a contrast agent in arthrosonography is far less expensive than gadolinium, the contrast agent universally used for MR arthrography.

The bony landmarks guide the shoulder ultrasound examination (Fig. 25-1). The fingers of the examiner can palpate the acromion, the scapular spine, the coracoid, and the acromioclavicular joint. Transducer orientation relative to those landmarks will be essential in making corrections to the technique in viewing complex shoulder pathology. External bony landmarks are important in shoulder imaging when scanning a patient with significant pathology and loss of normal soft tissue landmarks.

The patient is scanned while seated on a rotating stool without armrests. The examiner sits comfortably on a stool adjusted so that the examiner rises above the shoulder level of the patient. Both shoulders, starting with the less symptomatic one, should be examined if the examiner is a beginner. The following technique is used at our institution.[8]

Transverse images through the long biceps are obtained with the arm and forearm on the patient's

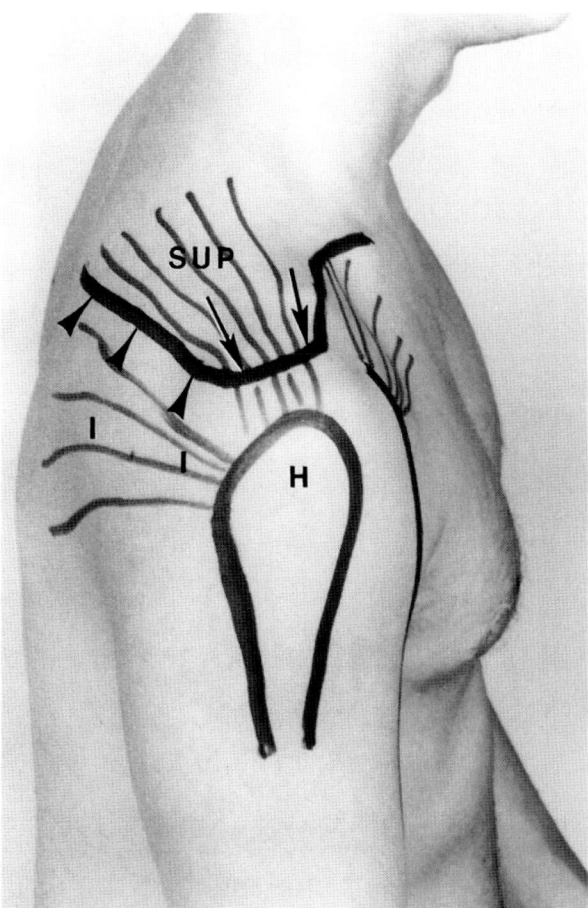

FIGURE 25-1. General anatomic landmarks. Lateral photograph shows the bony structure, which limits the acoustic window for the examination of the cuff. Acromion (*arrows*); H, humerus; I, infraspinatus muscle and tendon, scapular spine (*arrowheads*); Sup, supraspinatus muscle and tendon.

thigh, the palm supinated (Fig. 25-2). The **bicipital groove** serves as the anatomic landmark to differentiate the subscapularis tendon from the supraspinatus tendon. The groove is concave; bright echoes reflect off the bony surface of the humerus. The tendon of the long head of the biceps is visualized as a hyperechoic oval structure within the bicipital groove on the transverse images. The tendon courses through the rotator cuff interval and divides the subscapularis from the supraspinatus tendon. Scanning should begin with the proximal long biceps tendon above the biceps tendon groove. The intracapsular biceps shows more obliquely in the shoulder capsule. The biceps is then followed throughout its course in the bicipital groove; the scan should extend as far down as the musculotendinous junction. This allows detection of the smallest fluid collections in the medial triangular recess at the distal end of the tendon sheath.[23] Such small biceps sheath collections are a very sensitive indicator of joint fluid. A 90-degree rotation of the transducer into a longitudinal view will ascertain the intactness of the biceps tendon.[24] The transducer must

be carefully aligned along the biceps groove (Fig. 25-3). Gentle pressure on the distal aspect of the transducer is necessary to align the transducer parallel to the tendon to avoid artifact due to anisotropy.

The transducer position is then returned to the transverse plane and moved proximally along the humerus to visualize the subscapularis tendon, which appears as a band of medium-level echoes deep to the subdeltoid fat and bursa. The subscapularis tendon is viewed parallel to its axis (Fig. 25-4); scanning during passive and external rotation may be helpful in assessing the integrity of the **subscapularis tendon**, which may be disrupted in patients with chronic anterior shoulder dislocation. External rotation is also necessary to diagnose subluxation of the long biceps tendon, especially if only present intermittently.[25]

The normal **subdeltoid bursa** is recognized as a thin, hypoechoic layer in between the deltoid muscle on one side and the rotator cuff tendons and biceps tendon on the deep side. Hyperechoic peribursal fat surrounds the outer aspect of the synovial layer.[26]

The **supraspinatus tendon** is scanned perpendicular to its axis (transversely) by moving the transducer laterally posteriorly. The sonographic window is very narrow, and careful transducer positioning is essential (Fig. 25-5). The supraspinatus tendon is visualized as a band of medium-level echoes deep to the subdeltoid bursa and superficial to the bright echoes originating from the bone surface of the greater tuberosity.

The rest of the examination is done with the arm adducted and hyperextended and the shoulder in moderate internal rotation (Fig. 25-6).[5,7,27] This position can best be explained to the patient by asking him or her to reach to the opposite back pocket. Both longitudinal sections along the course of the supraspinatus tendon and images transverse to the tendon insertion and perpendicular to the humeral head are obtained. Correct orientation is achieved when an imaging plane shows crisp bone surface definition and sharp outline of the cartilage of the humeral head. During longitudinal scanning, the transducer overlays the acromion medially and the lateral aspect of the greater tuberosity laterally (see Fig. 25-6C). The transducer sweeps around the humeral head circumferentially; the transducer should be held perpendicular to the humeral head surface at all times. This sweeping motion through the supraspinatus tendon starts anteriorly next to the long biceps tendon; we cover an area of approximately 2.5 cm lateral to the long biceps tendon. Infraspinatus tendon is scanned beyond this point. The musculotendinous junction shows as hypoechoic muscle surrounding hyperechoic infraspinatus tendon. The transverse scan starts just lateral to the acromion and translates downward over the supraspinatus tendon and the greater tuberosity. The critical zone is that portion of the tendon that begins approximately 1 cm posterolateral to the biceps tendon.

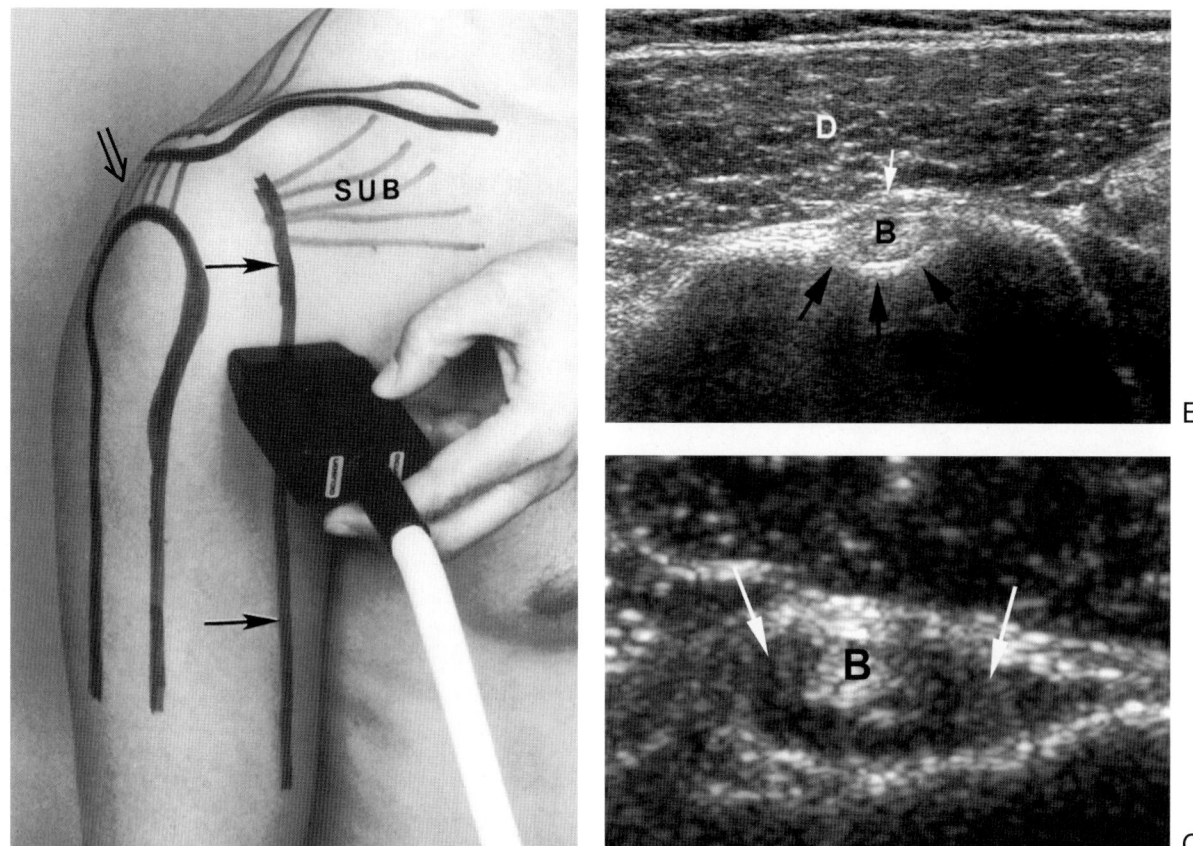

FIGURE 25-2. Biceps tendon. A, Clinical photograph. The patient rests the dorsum of the hand comfortably on his own thigh with the elbow flexed. The long biceps (*arrows*) separates the subscapularis (SUB) from the supraspinatus (*open arrow*). **B,** Normal transverse sonogram shows the biceps tendon, B, as a hyperechoic oval structure within the bicipital groove (*arrows*). Transverse ligament (*white arrow*)—a lateral extension of the subscapularis tendon—covers the anterior aspect of the long biceps tendon. Deltoid muscle (D). **C, Transverse scan in a patient with rotator cuff disease.** The long biceps tendon (B) appears enveloped in a distended hypoechoic sheath (*arrows*). The hypoechogenicity of the tendon sheath may represent fluid, synovial hypertrophy, or a combination of both.

Failure to adequately visualize this area may cause a false-negative result.[5]

Scanning of the supraspinatus tendon is followed by the visualization of the infraspinatus and teres minor tendons by moving the transducer posteriorly and in the plane parallel to the scapular spine. The **infraspinatus tendon** appears as a beak-shaped soft-tissue structure as it attaches to the posterior aspect of the greater tuberosity (Fig. 25-7).[6] Internal and external shoulder rotation may be helpful in the examination of the infraspinatus tendon. This maneuver relaxes and contracts the infraspinatus tendon in alternating fashion. At this level, a portion of the posterior glenoid labrum is seen as a hyperechoic, triangular structure. The fluid of the infraspinatus recess surrounds the labrum. Optimal image contrast for detection of intra-articular fluid will be obtained by bringing the arm in external rotation. In this position, the normal labrum will be covered by infraspinatus tendon; both structures appear hyper-echoic and they become nearly indistinguishable in a joint without effusion. In contrast, hypoechoic fluid or synovium may considerably separate these tissues in the joint with arthritis. The hypoechoic articular cartilage of the humeral head, which shows lateral to the labrum, contrasts significantly with the hyperechogenicity of the fibrocartilage. Scanning is extended medially to encompass the spinoglenoid notch and the suprascapular vessels and nerve. Visualization of the notch may be improved by bringing the transducer in the transverse plane but with the medial end of the transducer slightly more cephalad than the lateral end. If one uses the external-internal rotation dynamic during visualization of the neurovascular bundle that wraps around the spinoglenoid notch, one will perceive an abnormal bulging of the suprascapular vein during external rotation. The transversely oriented transducer is moved distally, and the teres minor is then visualized. The **teres minor** is a trapezoidal structure (Fig. 25-8).[28] It is differentiated from the infraspinatus tendon by its broader and more muscular attachment. Tears of this tendon are rare, and we have not encountered isolated teres minor tears in the 20,000 symptomatic shoulders we have scanned. Despite this, we scan this region to ensure ourselves that the infraspinatus tendon has been

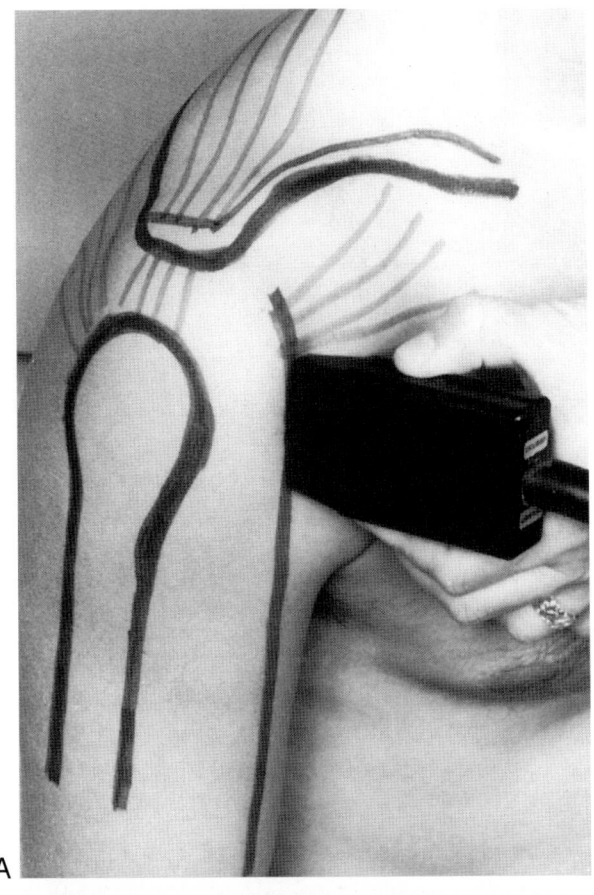

A

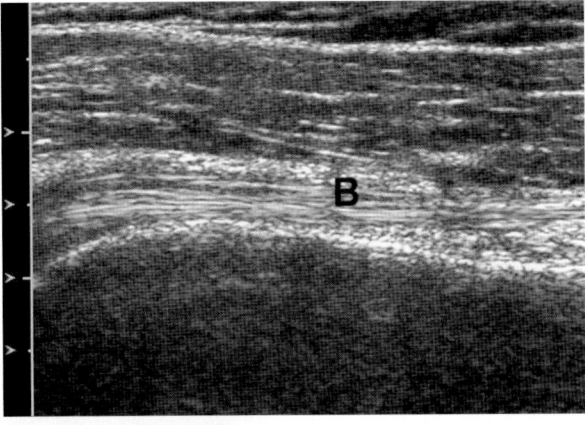

B

C

FIGURE 25-3. Biceps tendon scanning: use of anisotropy. A, Clinical photograph. **B,** Longitudinal scan shows the biceps tendon (B) with distinct fibrillar architecture. The predominant longitudinal orientation of the collagen in tendons like the biceps (B) make them strong anisotropic reflectors. **C,** Composite of images through the proximal long biceps tendon showing tendon anisotropy. The images on top result from a transverse imaging approach; images on the bottom relate to sagittal scanning through the middle of the bicipital groove. The column on the left shows correct scanning technique. **Normal tendons** appear hyperechoic only when scanned perpendicularly. The column on the right demonstrates how tendons appear hypoechoic as the angle of the transducer diverges from 90 degrees. **Visualization of this transition of tendon echogenicity from hyperechoic to hypoechoic can be used sometimes to improve tissue contrast;** it is also a useful trick to distinguish tendon from scar.

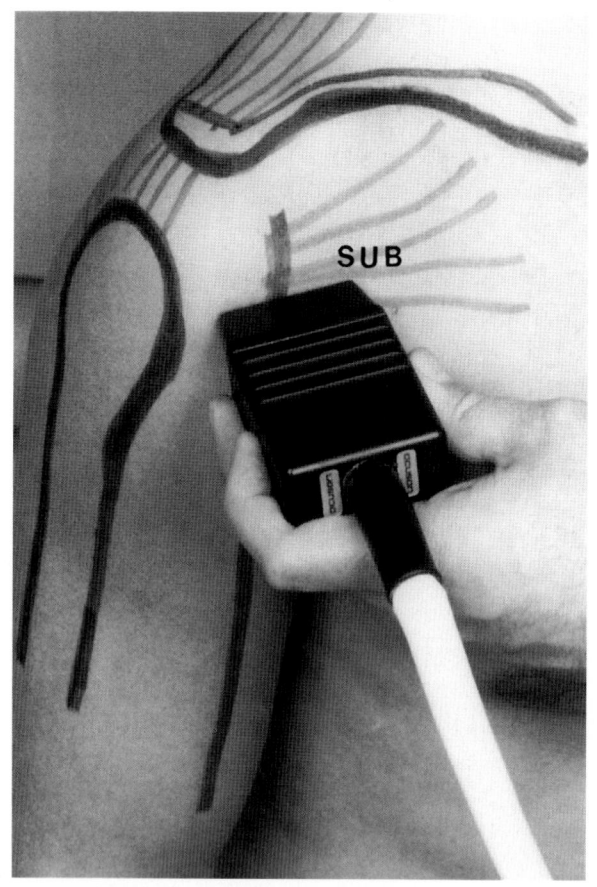

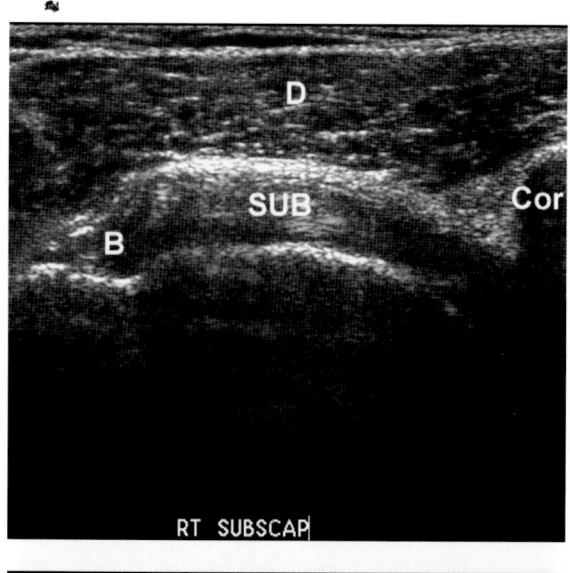

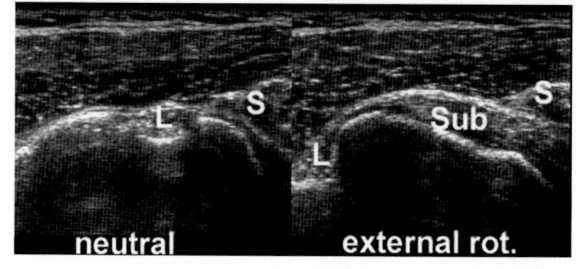

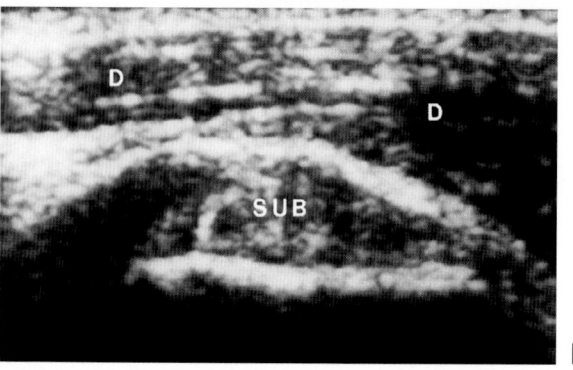

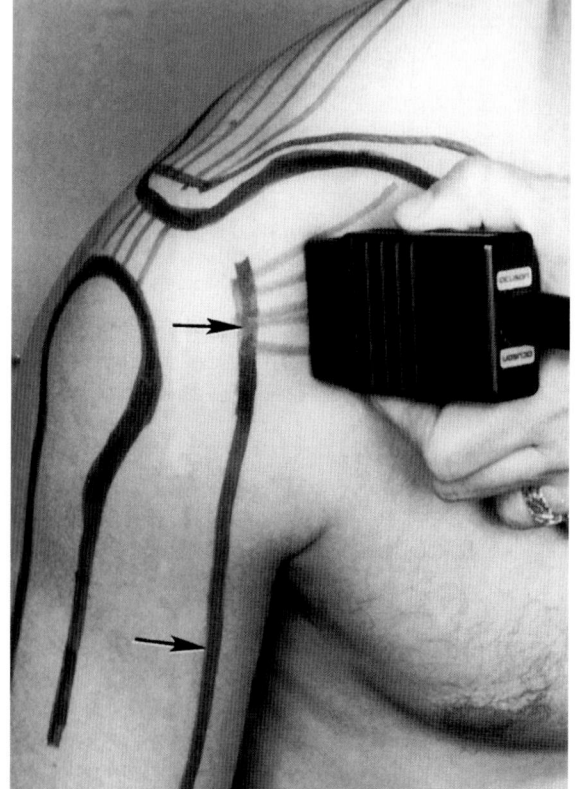

FIGURE 25-4. Subscapularis tendon. A, Clinical photograph and, **B,** longitudinal sonogram show the subscapularis tendon (SUB) parallel to its axis viewed as a band of medium-level echoes deep to the deltoid muscle (D); B, biceps tendon; Cor, coracoid. **C,** Dual image illustrates the use of external rotation in bringing out the subscapularis from under the coracoid and short head of biceps (S). In the neutral position, the long head (L) of biceps will show over the middle of the proximal anterior humerus. In external rotation, the long head of biceps (L) separates from the short head. The subscapularis tendon (SUB) shows in its full length over the anterior humeral head. **D** and **E,** Clinical photograph and scan perpendicular to the axis of the subscapularis tendon. Biceps tendon (*arrows*); SUB, subscapularis tendon; D, deltoid muscle.

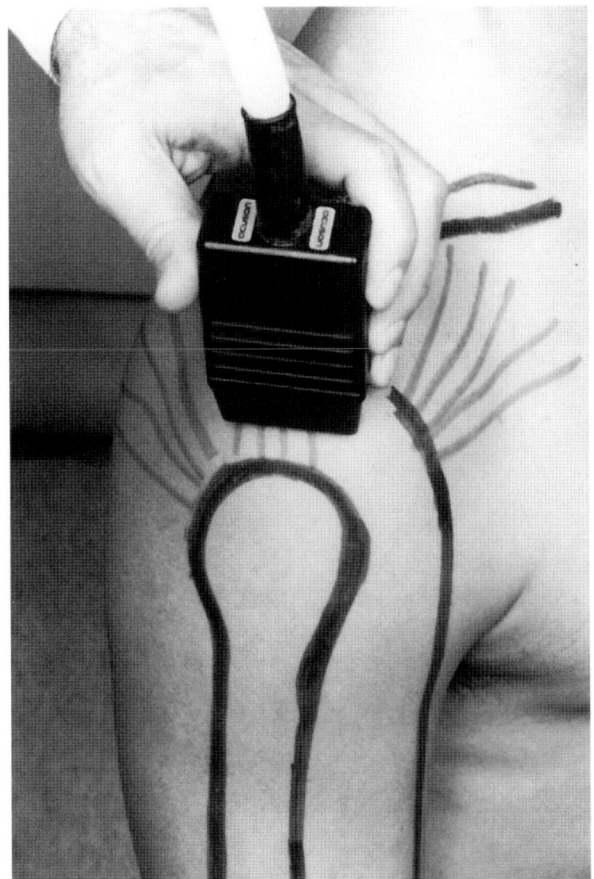

A

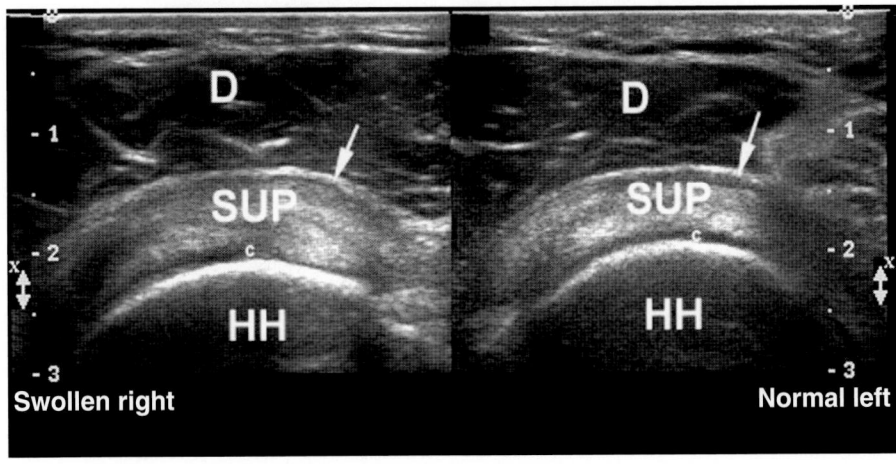

B

FIGURE 25-5. Supraspinatus tendon (transverse). **A** and **B**, Clinical photograph and scan show the supraspinatus tendon (SUP) as a band of medium-level echoes deep to the subdeltoid bursa (*arrows*) and draped over the cartilage (c) of the humeral head (HH). The swollen symptomatic tendon shows on the left side of the split-screen image; the patient's normal shoulder shows on the right. D, deltoid muscle.

scanned in its entirety. Small joint effusions will also easily show in this location.[29] Demonstration of this effusion helps distinguish articular processes, such as rheumatoid arthritis and septic arthritis, which will cause effusion. In rotator cuff disease, it is rare to find fluid in this location.

Coronal images through the acromioclavicular joints are obtained at the end of the examination. Right-left comparison can show degenerative or traumatic pathology that can mimic or cause impingement-like symptoms. The superior glenoid labrum can be shown with the transducer aligned posterior to the acromioclavicular joint and oriented perpendicular to the superior glenoid. A curved linear array transducer will be necessary if diagnosis of **superior labral detachment (SLAP lesions)** is desired.

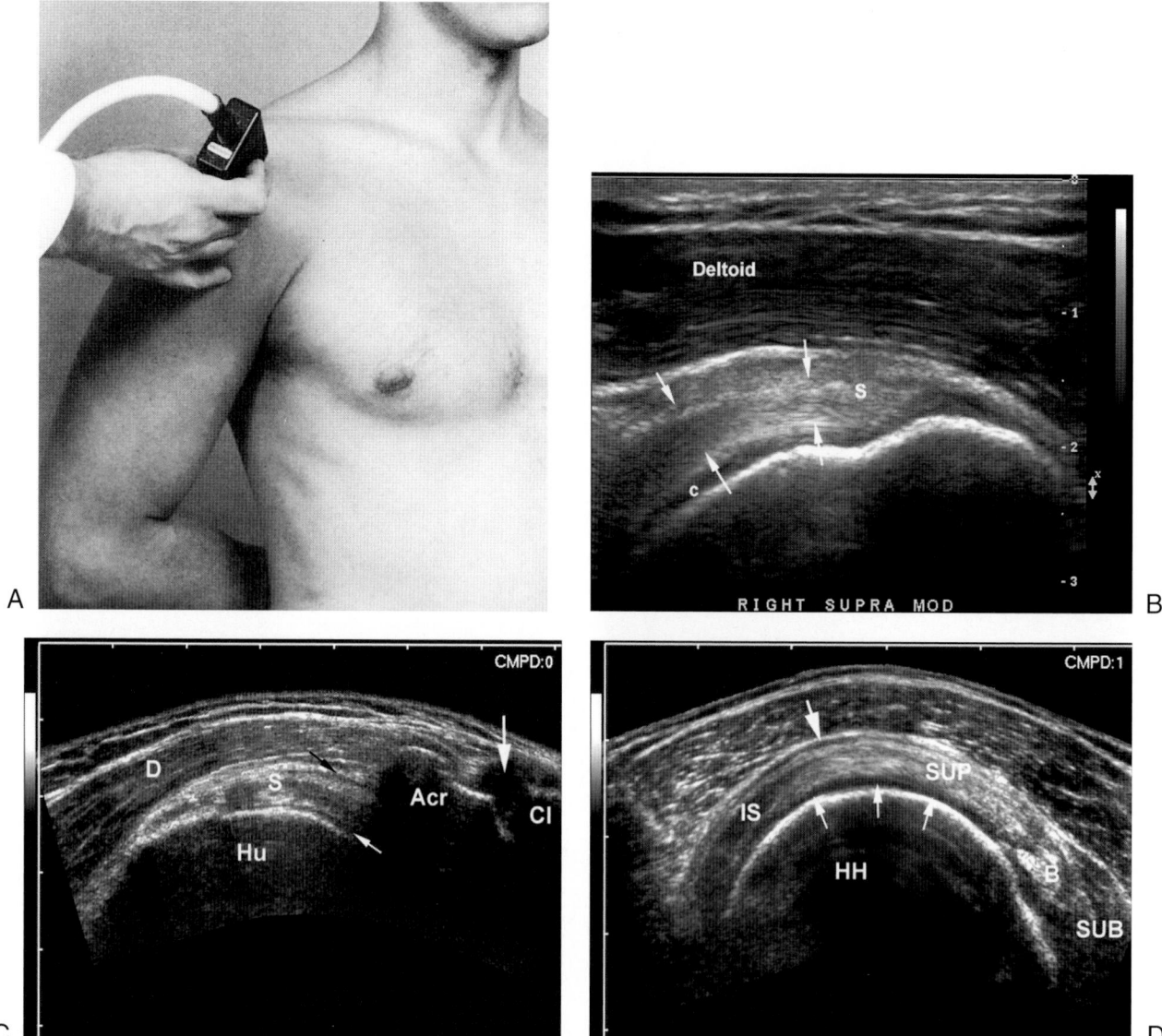

FIGURE 25-6. Supraspinatus tendon. A, Transducer position with arm in extension and internal rotation. The patient will be asked to bring the elbow as close to the body as possible to obtain maximal adduction. This view improves visualization of the supraspinatus (s). **B,** Longitudinal image. More tendon will stretch beyond the lateral and anterior aspect of the acromion than in the neutral position. Echogenicity changes within the rotator cuff relate to tendon anisotropy. The propagation of ultrasound through supraspinatus tendon appears uneven. This feature stands out more clearly in one sublayer of the supraspinatus tendon (*arrows*). The fibers in this layer have a longitudinal orientation along the long axis of the tendon. Hyaline cartilage over the humeral head (c). **C,** Panoramic overview demonstrates the anatomic relationship of the longitudinal supraspinatus tendon (s) with the acromion (Acr) and acromioclavicular joint (*large arrow*). Deltoid (D) originates from the acromion. Lateral clavicle (Cl); proximal humerus (Hu). The shape of the tendon has often been compared with a parrot's beak. Hypoechoic tissue covers the tendon on either side. Hypoechogenicity between tendon and bone represents hyaline cartilage (*white arrow*), and the thin hypoechoic layer between tendon and deltoid corresponds to subdeltoid bursa (*black arrow*). **D,** Panoramic overview of the transverse anatomy of the supraspinatus tendon (SUP) relative to the subscapularis (SUB) and the intracapsular biceps (B) in the front and the infraspinatus (IS) in the back. Again, the tendon appears sandwiched between two hypoechoic layers. Note that the normal subdeltoid bursa (*large arrow*) remains slightly thinner than the hyaline cartilage (*small arrows*) over the humeral head (HH). The supraspinatus and infraspinatus form a conjoined tendon, whereas the biceps tendon separates supraspinatus and subscapularis.

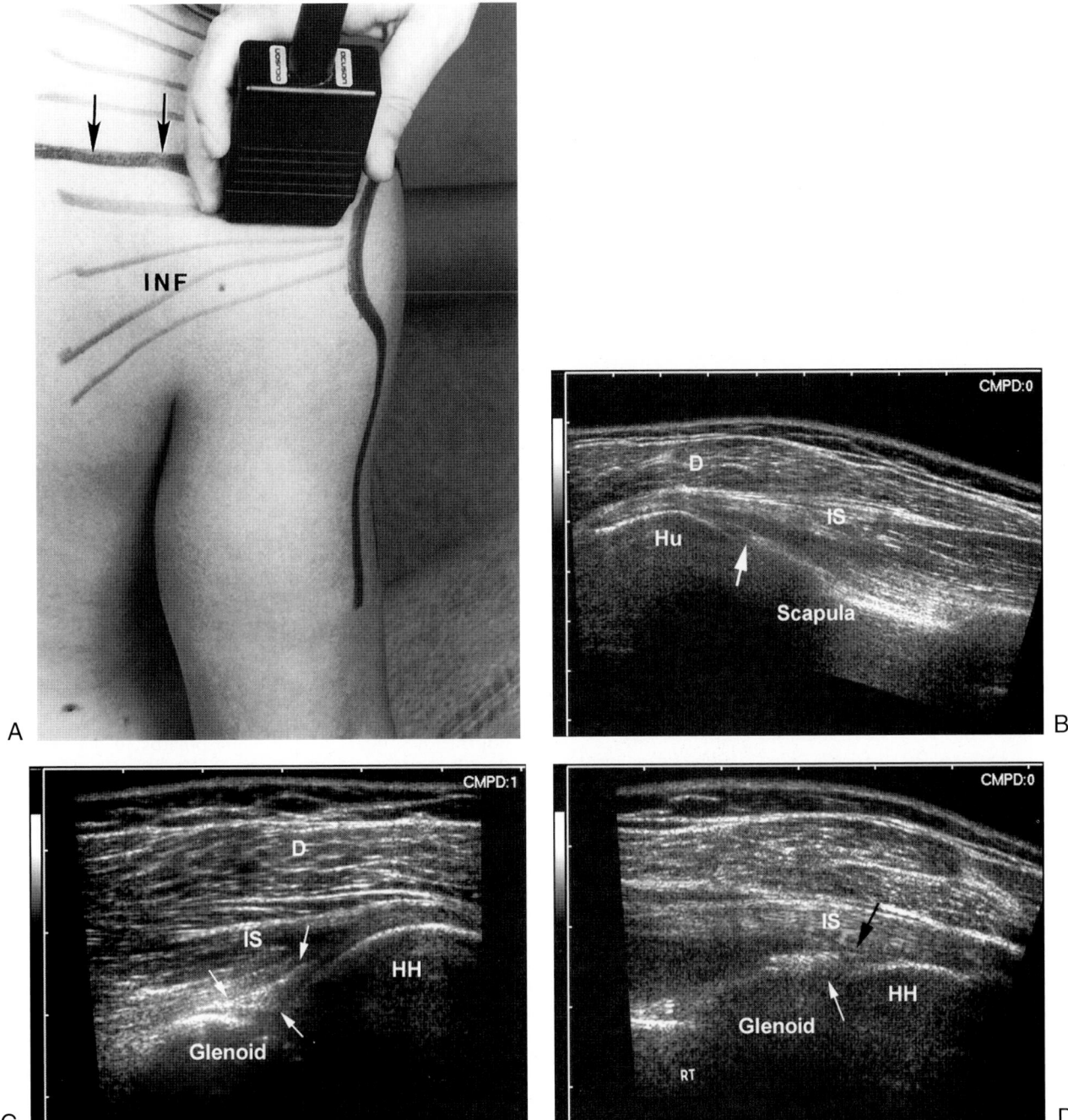

FIGURE 25-7. Infraspinatus tendon. A, Clinical photograph. **B,** Transverse panoramic overview of the soft tissue over the posterior scapula and humerus (Hu). The infraspinatus (IS) covers the posterior shoulder directly. The echogenic tendon overlies the posterior glenohumeral joint space and fibrous labral cartilage (*arrow*). Deltoid muscle (D). **C,** Transverse overview of the anatomy through the middle of the posterior glenohumeral joint—opposite shoulder to the one depicted in Fig. 25-7B. The fibrous labrum appears as a hyperechoic triangle (*arrows*). With the arm in internal rotation, as in this image, the contrast between the hypoechoic muscle and the hyperechoic labrum is accentuated. The infraspinatus muscle has a bipennate muscle structure (IS). Deltoid muscle (D); humeral head (HH). **D,** Same transducer position as in Fig. 25-7C. The arm position changed into external arm rotation. With this movement, one brings hyperechoic tendon (IS) in direct proximity to the hyperechoic posterior labrum (*white arrow*). This view allows for optimal quantification of joint fluid. As seen in this normal patient, the separation (*black arrow*) between normal tendon and labrum is barely perceptible. If one has an intra-articular effusion, hypoechoic fluid will distend the capsule in between these two structures. Humeral head, HH.

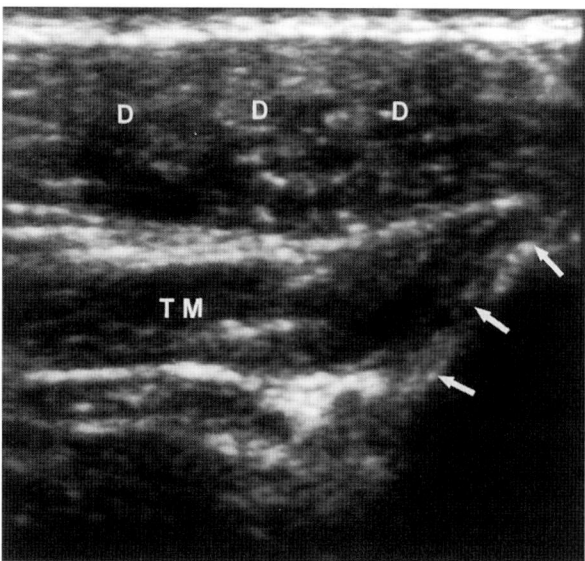

FIGURE 25-8. Teres minor. TM is visualized as a trapezoidal structure. D, deltoid muscle; humerus (*arrows*). (Reproduced with permission of Mack LA, Nyberg DA, Matsen FA: Sonographic evaluation of rotator cuff. Radiol Clin North Am 1988;25:161-177.)

THE NORMAL CUFF

The Cuff in the Adolescent

The rotator cuff tendons are hyperechoic relative to the deltoid muscle bellies (see Fig. 25-6). The cuff tendons are enveloped in a thin synovial layer that is normally thinner than 1.5 mm and appears hypoechoic relative to the tendons. The thickness of this bursal layer does not change; the **subacromial-subdeltoid bursa** is as thick over the long biceps tendon as it is over the subscapularis, supraspinatus, and infraspinatus tendons. A correctly performed examination will show a neatly defined bursa that shows as a hypoechoic stripe thinner than the thickness of the hypoechoic hyaline cartilage over the humeral head. This extra-articular bursa is a virtual space, as it contains lubricant synovial fluid; this fluid cannot be distinguished on a routine shoulder ultrasound study. The bursa is hoof-shaped in cross section, and it often extends from the coracoid anteriorly around the lateral shoulder and posteriorly past the glenoid. The pleural space and the bursal synovial space share a number of similarities, including the virtual space (which can become distended in effusions), the thin lubricating layer of fluid in their lumen, and the extensive network of capillary vessels and lymph vessels in their walls. Those vessels are not visible with color flow Doppler studies in patients with normal rotator cuff anatomy, but they have been shown in the power color flow Doppler studies of patients with inflamed cuffs.[30] The boundary between the bursa and the deltoid muscle consists of the so-called peribursal fat. This layer appears

hyperechoic, and its thickness is remarkably uniform; body habitus seems to have little influence on the thickness of this fat layer.

Rotator cuff pathology is rare in young patients. Bursal and labral pathology can occur, however. Some of these conditions can mimic tendon tears. It is important to know that the adolescent cuff consists of more muscle than the aging cuff. The relative length of tendon to muscle increases with age.[31] Hypoechoic areas in the cuff in patients under age 20 may simply represent muscle, and the finding should not easily be attributed to a tear. Meticulous right-left comparison of the thickness of the subscapular tendons in adolescents may demonstrate tears of the anterior rotator cuff due to athletic injuries. In our experience, the subscapular insertion appears the weaker link of the rotator cuff in the growing shoulder. Ultrasound has proved its usefulness in detecting subscapularis tendon tears.[32]

Age-Related Changes

The cuff in individuals under age 30 is watertight. Arthrography studies show that there should not be a communication with the subacromial-subdeltoid bursa.[18] Postmortem and cadaver studies have shown a high prevalence of rotator cuff tears in aging shoulders. Keyes[33] examined 73 unselected cadavers and found full-thickness tears of the supraspinatus in 13.4% of shoulders. Full-thickness tears were not recorded for those younger than 50 years of age; the prevalence over 50 years of age was 31%. Wilson and Duff[34] examined an unselected series of 74 bodies at postmortem and 34 dissecting-room cadavers over age 30 years. They found full-thickness tears of the supraspinatus tendon in 11% and partial-thickness tears in 10% of the shoulders. Fukuda[35] reported a 7% prevalence of complete tears and a 13% prevalence of incomplete tears in a study of cadavers that included no details on age. With such high percentages of rotator cuff tears in cadaver studies, how many of these tears would have been asymptomatic? A study we conducted showed that ultrasound can detect asymptomatic tears.

Ninety volunteer subjects (47 women and 43 men) in a population who had never sought medical attention for shoulder disease, underwent shoulder sonography; 77% (69 of 90) were white, 13% (12 of 90) were African-American, 9% (8 of 90) were Asian, and 1% (1 of 90) was Hispanic. Eighteen subjects were between the ages of 30 and 39 years; 18 were between ages 40 and 49 years; 18 were between ages 50 and 59 years; 13 were between ages 60 and 69 years; 13 were between ages 70 and 79 years; and 10 were between ages 80 and 99 years. The proportion of women to men was nearly equal for each decade.

No statistically significant differences were found in the prevalence of rotator cuff lesions in each gender for

Rotator-cuff Changes in Asymptomatic Adults
Dominant versus Non-dominant

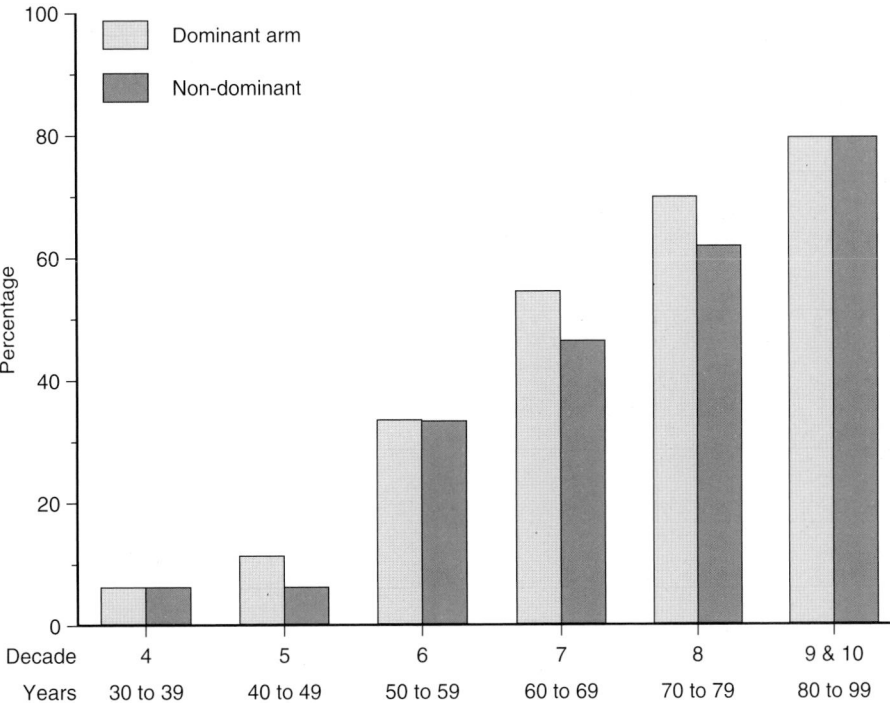

FIGURE 25-9. Asymptomatic rotator cuff tears. Percentage of shoulders with rotator cuff tears in asymptomatic adults in different age groups. Chart shows comparison between dominant and nondominant arms.

either the dominant or nondominant arm (Fig. 25-9). We found no statistically significant differences in the incidence of rotator lesions related to gender or reported level of exertional activities. But the prevalence of rotator cuff tears in both the dominant and nondominant arms showed a linear increase after the fifth decade of life. This difference was statistically very significant between the third, fourth, and fifth decades and above.[12] The cumulative percentage of partial- and full-thickness tears was approximately 33% between the ages of 50 and 59 years, 55% between 60 and 69 years, 70% between 70 and 79 years, and as high as 78% above age 80 (see Fig. 25-9; Fig. 25-10). A total of 25 full-thickness and 15 partial-thickness tears were found. Sixteen individuals or 64% of the patients with tears had bilateral rotator cuff tears. The youngest subject with a partial-thickness tear was 35 years old. The youngest subject with a full-thickness tear was 54 years old. The age range for partial-thickness tears was from 35 to 80 years of age. The age range of full-thickness tears was from 54 to 92 years of age. The average age in the partial-thickness group was 56 years. The average age in the full-thickness group was 63 years.

In 19 cases (46%) the rotator cuff tears had associated intrasynovial fluid. In 15 cases the fluid was located in the biceps tendon sheath, and in the remaining four cases it was located in the subacromial-subdeltoid bursa. There were two individuals with tears and fluid in the

biceps tendon sheath and in the bursa simultaneously. The infraspinatus recess appeared normal in all of our patients. Eleven effusions were noted in the long biceps tendon sheath in subjects who did not have tears of the cuff. There was never excess fluid in the subacromial-subdeltoid bursa in the absence of rotator cuff tear. Shallow erosion or irregularity of the bone surface under the tear was noted in 90% of tears; bone changes were present in all but four partial-thickness tears. Greater tuberosity irregularity was noted in 37 shoulders or in 21% of shoulders in this study. Twelve shoulders showed irregular greater tuberosities and no rotator cuff tear. A statistically significant correlation between asymptomatic rotator cuff tears and irregularity of the greater tuberosity was found (Fig. 25-11).

Twenty of the full-thickness tears were considered large and involved more than one tendon. Three tears were massive and over 4 cm in diameter, and three tears were small and under 2 cm in width when measured over the base of the greater tuberosity. Ten partial-thickness tears were mixed echogenicity, and five were hypoechoic. Nine mixed echogenicity lesions and two hypoechoic tears exhibited bone change in the greater tuberosity.

Our results indicate that the finding of a rotator cuff abnormality or an effusion in the biceps tendon sheath can be compatible with normal and pain-free mobility of the shoulder. Rotator cuff findings should be interpreted

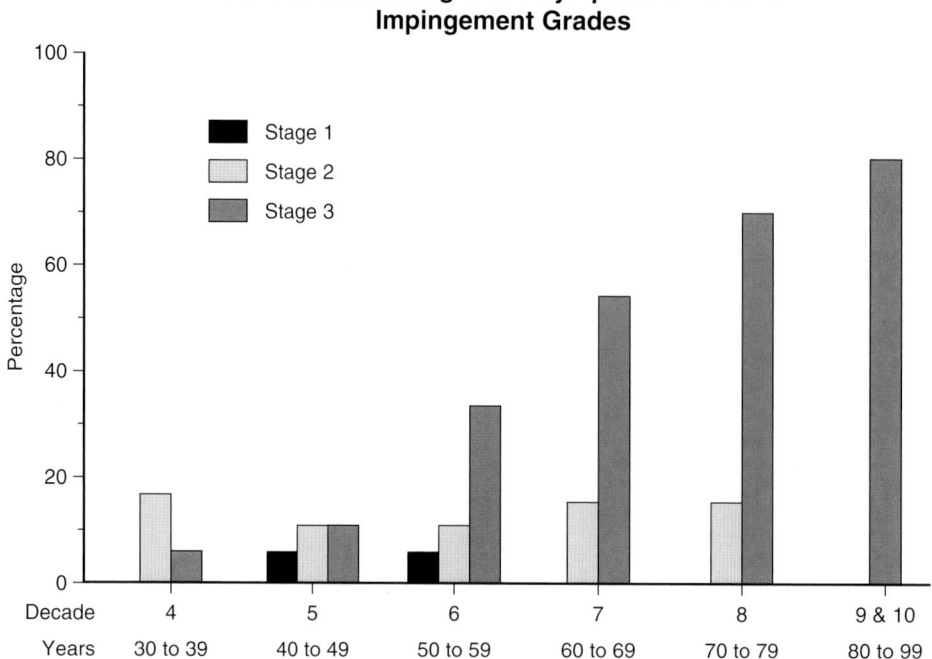

FIGURE 25-10. Prevalence of stage 1 to stage 3 impingement for dominant arm in different age groups. Abnormalities in the subacromial space were staged sonographically as follows: stage 1 if bursal thickness from 1.5 to 2 mm; stage 2 if bursal thickness over 2 mm; stage 3 if partial- or full-thickness rotator cuff tear.

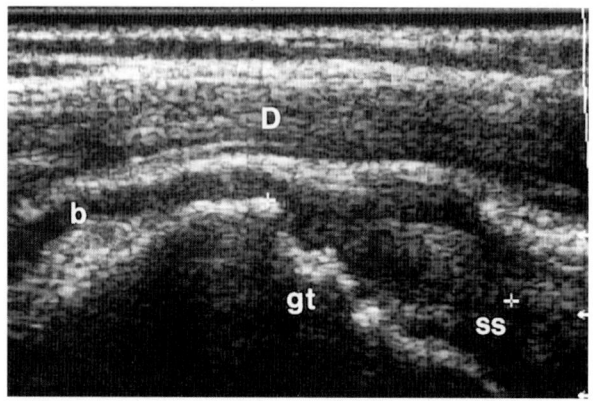

FIGURE 25-11. Asymptomatic full-thickness rotator cuff tear. The longitudinal scan through the supraspinatus tendon (ss) shows retraction of tissue (calipers). The bone surface of the uncovered greater tuberosity (gt) is irregular. The subdeltoid bursa (b) is filled with fluid. D, deltoid muscle.

with care in patients older than the age of 50. A rotator cuff tear is not necessarily the cause of the pain in an aging shoulder and can be an incidental finding. **Degenerative rotator cuff changes** may be regarded as a natural correlate of aging, with a statistically significant linear increase after the fifth decade of life. On the one hand, clinical judgment must be used to distinguish asymptomatic from symptomatic rotator cuff tears. On the other hand, finding a rotator cuff tear should not stop the clinician from searching for other causes of

shoulder pain. Our shoulder ultrasound reading is done in conjunction with the reading of the initial shoulder radiographic evaluation. It is not uncommon that we find missed primary or secondary neoplasms of bone, myeloma, or Pancoast tumors using this careful approach. Limited and painful shoulder elevation can be due to a number of diseases, of which rotator cuff disease is the most common. Simultaneous occurrence of a full-thickness tear with a tumor in or around the shoulder is not rare in our experience.

PREOPERATIVE APPEARANCES

Criteria of Rotator Cuff Tears

Previously published sonographic criteria for rotator cuff pathology can be categorized into four groups[36]: nonvisualization of the cuff, localized absence or focal nonvisualization, discontinuity, and focal abnormal echogenicity.

Nonvisualization of the Cuff. Direct contact of the humeral head with the acromion is an indication of massive cuff tear. In this situation, the ultrasound image shows deltoid muscle directly on top of the humeral head (Fig. 25-12). In some cases, thickened bursa and fat will be noted between the deltoid muscle and the surface of the humeral head. This tissue layer is more hypo-echoic and patchy in texture. The thickness of this layer will depend on the location of the tear, but generally it will be thinner and more irregular than the normal cuff

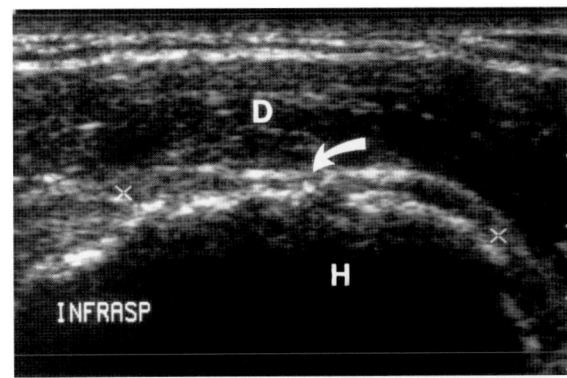

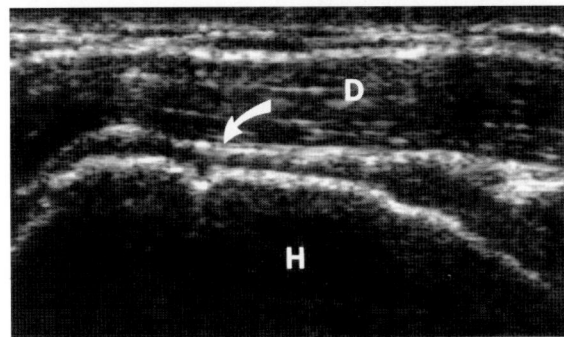

FIGURE 25-12. Nonvisualization of cuff. A,
Transverse view. The deltoid muscle (D) is in direct contact with the humeral head (H). A hyperechoic layer (*curved arrow*) of fat shows deep to the deltoid; this layer is interposed between the deltoid and the humerus. **B,** Longitudinal view through the expected location of the supraspinatus tendon. The supraspinatus tendon is absent. A hyperechoic layer of fat (*curved arrow*) is noted deep to the deltoid (D). H, Humeral head.

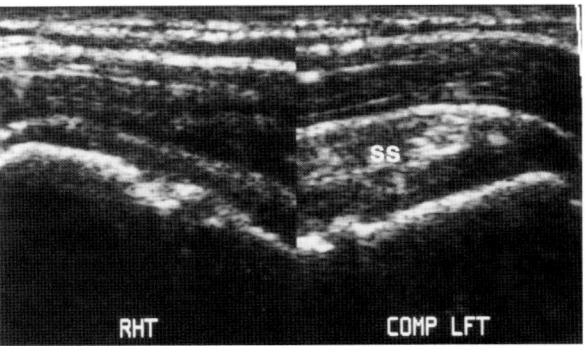

FIGURE 25-13. Irreparable rotator cuff tear.
Longitudinal right-left comparison shows a significant discrepancy in the thickness of the soft tissues. The supraspinatus tendon (ss) appears normal in the asymptomatic left shoulder (LFT). The supraspinatus tendon in the right (RHT) shoulder is retracted out of sight. The deltoid and the subdeltoid fascial layer cover the humeral head directly. Arthroscopy showed the torn edge of the supraspinatus tendon withdrawn beyond the glenoid cavity. The rotator cuff defect was deemed irreparable.

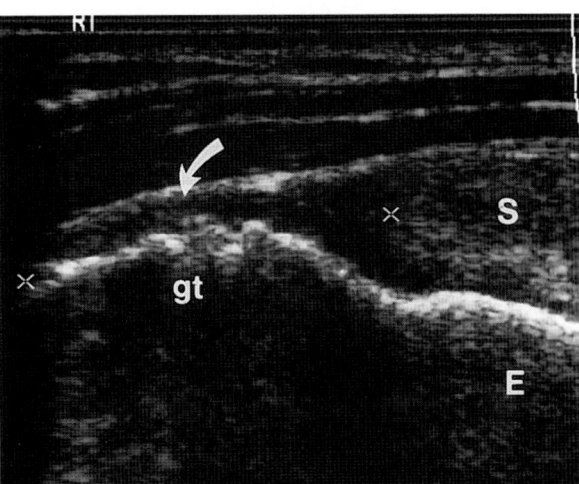

FIGURE 25-14. Horizontal full-thickness tear. The longitudinal image through the supraspinatus tendon (S) shows 2 cm retraction of the torn tendon (*distance between calipers*). Bursa and peribursal fat (*curved arrow*) rest directly on the irregular bone surface of the greater tuberosity (gt). E, humeral epiphysis.

layer. Some bursae have been noted to be up to 5 mm thick. This synovial layer has been mistaken for normal cuff by the inexperienced sonographer. With massive tears, exceeding 4 cm, the humeral head may ascend through the defect because of pulling of the deltoid muscle. The supraspinatus tendon is retracted under the acromion, and, as a rule, surgical reattachment will be impossible at this stage (Fig. 25-13). The extent of tear should be reported because multiple tendons are often involved. The diagnosis of these tears can be predicted on shoulder radiographs. Some centers use radiographs with comparison views during active shoulder abduction or anteroposterior supine views of the subacromial space to counteract the gravitational pull on the humerus.[37] The subacromial space should not be smaller than 5 mm.

Focal Nonvisualization of the Cuff. Smaller tears will appear as localized absence of supraspinatus tendon or, in rare cases, local absence of subscapularis or infraspinatus tendon. The most common tear pattern is caused by disease at the tendon-bone junction. The tendon will retract from the bone surface, leaving a bare area of bone (Fig. 25-14). This finding has been reported in the past as the **"naked tuberosity"** sign.[38] The bone surface of

the greater tuberosity and anatomic neck of the humerus are irregular in approximately 79% of this type of tears. A recent anatomic study has confirmed these bone changes. This pathologic process affects not only the surface of the bone, but also the internal structure of the greater tuberosity. The exterior changes consist of pitting of the cortex, erosion of bone, sclerosis, fragmentation of the tuberosity, and crystal deposition beyond the tidemark.[39] The changes of the architecture of the tuberosity manifest as fewer trabeculae and fewer connections between trabeculae. The vast majority of such tears will occur anteriorly in the supraspinatus tendon and in the critical zone. Characteristically, a small amount of tissue will be preserved surrounding the

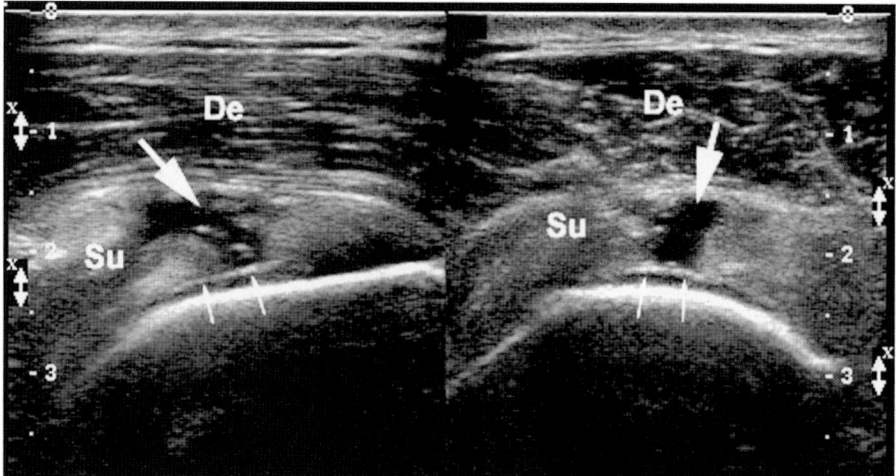

FIGURE 25-15. Vertical full-thickness tear. Images through the supraspinatus tendon (Su) show an anechoic area of discontinuity (*large arrows*) within the rotator cuff layer. The cartilage of the humeral head is surrounded by a bright interface (*small arrows*). Deltoid muscle, De. The longitudinal image shows on the left of the split screen; the transverse view shows on the right.

biceps tendon. Ideally, such tears can be confirmed in two perpendicular scan planes. Sometimes this will not be possible because the tear may show full thickness in one plane but not be identified as such in the orthogonal plane. This phenomenon has been attributed to partial-volume averaging in tears that are smaller than the footprint of the transducers. Small **horizontal tears** typically appear on longitudinal images but can be missed on transverse images.[38] A helpful finding is the "infolding" of bursal and peribursal fat tissue into the focal defect. With few exceptions, this infolding is a sign of a full-thickness tear. If the tear is larger, bursal and peribursal tissue will approximate the bone surface (see Fig. 25-14).

Focal nonvisualization should not be confused with segmental thinning of cuff after rotator cuff surgery. This thinning is normal after most tendon-bone reimplantations. In those cases, a bony trough is detected as a rounded or V-shaped defect in the humeral contour. The tendon is brought down into this narrow slit. The tendon is not repaired onto the tuberosity anatomically with a broad insertion but with a tapered end. It is well known that a number of those reconstructions fail to be watertight even after successful surgery. The rents in the capsule cause additional focal thinning. In a patient with a negative baseline study, retears can be identified by visualizing anechoic fluid leaking through a tear.

Discontinuity in the Cuff. This term has been used for tears that are located more proximally in the tendon. These tears tend to be of the **vertical type** and are more often traumatic.[38,40] The patient may have a history of prior shoulder dislocation. Discontinuity is observed when the small defects fill with joint fluid or hypoechoic reactive tissue (Fig. 25-16). Such defects are often accentuated by placing the arm in extension and internal rotation (Fig. 25-16). Often, a small amount of bursal fluid is also present. The sonographer can use this fluid as a natural contrast medium to show the tear in more detail. Manual compression of the subdeltoid bursa can

move the fluid through the tear into the joint. This maneuver will show the tear more clearly. A focally bright interface around a segment of hyaline cartilage and deep to hypoechoic tendon is considered a sign of a full-thickness tear (see Fig. 25-15). This sign has been named the **cartilage-interface sign** in an earlier report.[38]

Focal Abnormal Echogenicity. Cuff echogenicity may be diffusely or focally abnormal. Diffuse abnormalities of cuff echogenicity have proved to be unreliable sonographic signs for cuff tear. Focal abnormal echogenicity has been associated with small full- and partial-thickness tears. An area of increased echogenicity might represent a new interface within the tendon at the site of fiber failure, as has been observed in some partial-thickness tears.[8] The small linear or comma-shaped hyperechoic lesion is often surrounded by edema or fluid and appears as a hypoechoic halo (Fig. 25-17). The partial-thickness tears are similar to the **rim rents** that were first observed pathologically by Codman.[9] A slightly different type of partial-thickness tear can appear as an anechoic spot on the articular or bursal side of the tendon.[8] Careful inspection of the synovial surfaces of the tendon is necessary. Only those focal hypoechoic defects that violate the surface may be considered tears by the arthroscopist (Fig. 25-18). **Intrasubstance lesions** are the most common type of partial lesions and they account for almost 50% of the defects. We do not call them tears because they are not considered tears by the surgeons who cannot observe them by direct tendon inspection. This poses a diagnostic problem similar to that of intrasubstance lesions of the menisci seen on MRI studies. Associated bone or synovial findings may be helpful if the ultrasound findings are equivocal.

Associated Findings

Subdeltoid Bursal Effusion. Visualization of subdeltoid bursal effusion is the most reliable associated finding of rotator cuff tear (Fig. 25-19). It is found

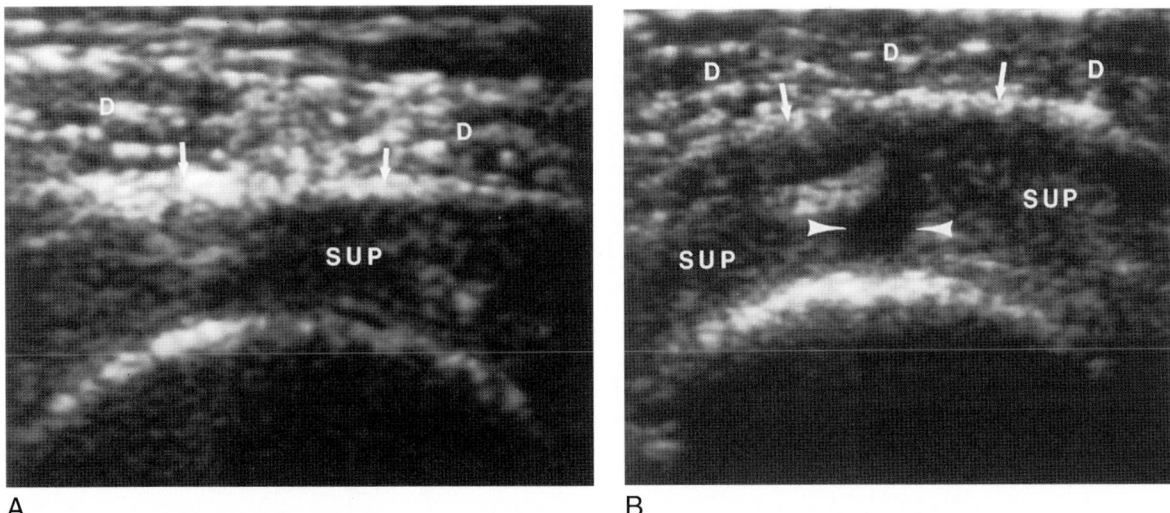

FIGURE 25-16. Discontinuity of the cuff. Transverse scans of the supraspinatus tendon (SUP) in **A**, neutral position and **B**, with the arm in extension and internal rotation show a small tear filled with fluid (*arrowheads*). Note the tear is more distinctly visible with the arm in extension. D, deltoid muscle; subdeltoid bursa (*arrows*).

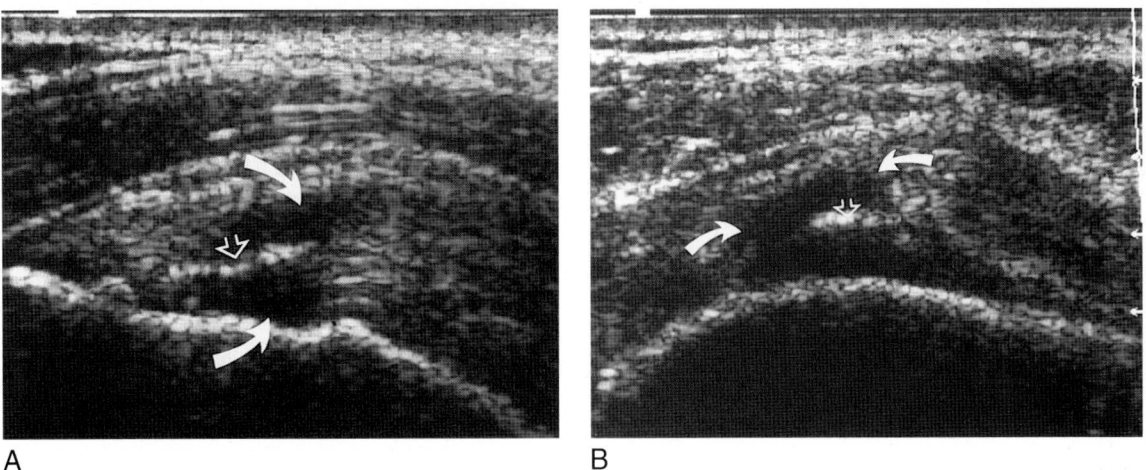

FIGURE 25-17. Focal abnormal echogenicity. A, Longitudinal supraspinatus tendon view of an articular side partial-thickness tear, the so-called *rim rent*. A linear hyperechoic lesion in the supraspinatus tendon (*open arrow*) is surrounded by hypoechoic edema (*curved arrows*). **B**, Transverse supraspinatus tendon view of same partial-thickness defect. The same hyperechoic lesion is noted.

in both full- and partial-thickness tears. Anechoic fluid differs from hypoechoic edema of the bursal synovium. Edema is a common finding in shoulder impingement but is only rarely associated with a tear. Edema and fluid can be distinguished from each other using the *transducer compression test*. A synovial recess filled with fluid will be emptied by compression; a recess with synovial edema changes little in shape. Other causes for fluid in the bursa include calcium milk with synovitis and septic bursitis. Hollister et al.[41] found the sonographic appearance of bursal fluid to have a specificity of 96% for the diagnosis of rotator cuff tears. Similar results were found by Farin et al.[42] In our prospective study of rotator cuff disease,[8] all patients with fluid in the bursa had a rotator cuff tear.

Joint Effusion. Joint fluid can be found in the joint recesses, including the infraspinatus, subcoracoid, and axillary recesses. In a patient who sits in the upright position, most fluid will accumulate in the biceps tendon sheath. Approximately half of these effusions are associated with rotator cuff tears.[6] The other half roughly will be due to a variety of articular causes of shoulder disease. When a large fluid collection is found in the infraspinatus recess without fluid in the subdeltoid bursa, inflammatory or infectious causes of joint disease should always be excluded.[29]

Concave Subdeltoid Fat Contour. In the normal patient, the bright linear echoes from the subdeltoid bursal fat are convex. Concavity of the subdeltoid contour may be noted in medium and large tears, reflecting the absence of cuff tendon. It may be possible to approximate the deltoid and the humeral surface even

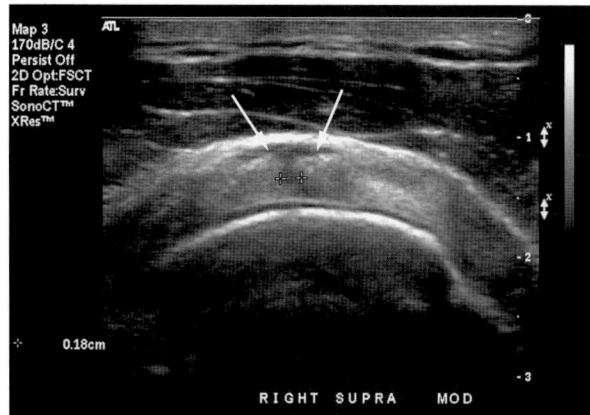

A

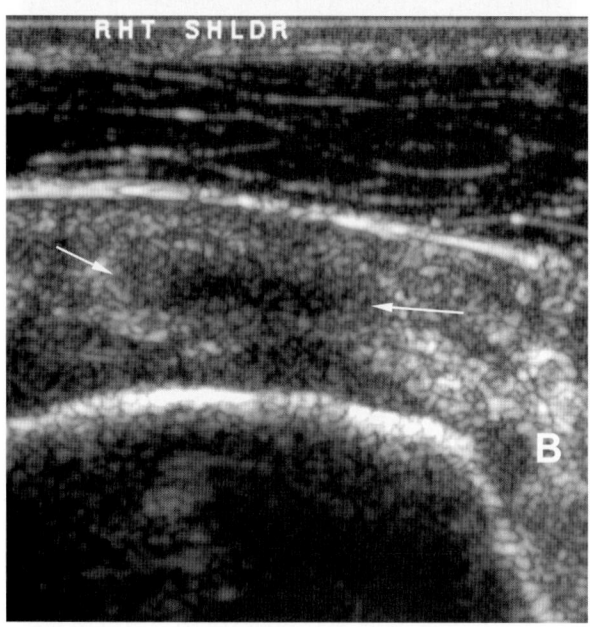

B

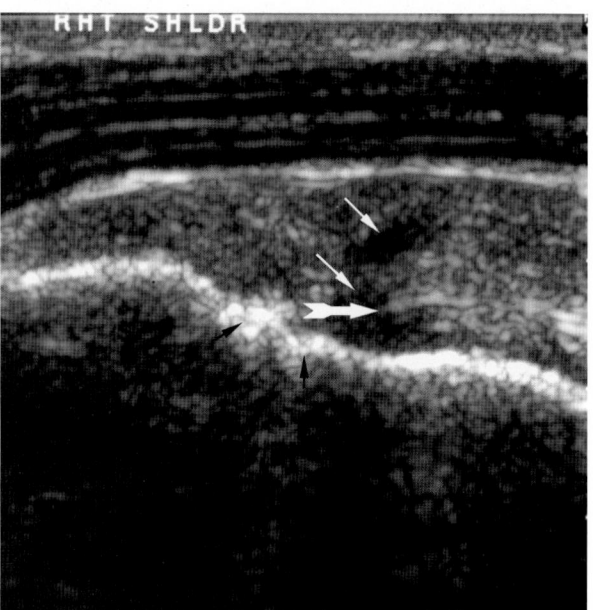

C

FIGURE 25-18. Focal abnormal echogenicity. A, Transverse supraspinatus tendon view of a bursal side partial thickness tear. The hypoechoic change violates the bursal surface (*arrows*). **B,** Transverse supraspinatus tendon view of hypoechoic change within the substance of the tendon. **C,** Longitudinal view through the same abnormality as in **B**. The hypoechoic disruption appears intrasubstance (*arrows*); intact tendon fibers (*large arrow*), which are seen curving toward the bone, still cover the articular surface of the tendon. The greater tuberosity surface is irregular (*small black arrows*). Such lesions cannot be seen by arthroscopy.

in smaller tears using transducer compression at the site of the tear.

Bone Surface Irregularity. Only recently has bone irregularity been cited in imaging literature as an important and common associated finding in rotator cuff tears.[8,39,43] The majority of partial- and full-thickness tears of the distal 1 cm of the rotator cuff are associated with small bone spurs and pits in the bone surface of the greater tuberosity. It is possible that the use of higher-frequency transducers for rotator cuff imaging has made these findings more evident. The tuberosity abnormality matches the tendon abnormality in location, size, and shape. The cause of the abnormality is unknown. Trauma due to an impaction of the tuberosity on the acromion during shoulder elevation has been considered.

POSTOPERATIVE APPEARANCES

The literature suggests that sonography can play an important role in the postoperative follow-up after rotator cuff repair.[43,44] Because surgery may distort sonographic landmarks, sonography in the postoperative patient is rendered more difficult than in the preoperative patient. It is important, therefore, to understand the surgical procedures used in acromioplasty and cuff repair.

In acromioplasty, the anterior inferior aspect of the acromion is surgically removed. Sonographically, this appears as disruption of the normal, rounded, smooth acromial contour. After surgery, the acromion appears pointed (Fig. 25-20). Because the inferior aspect of the acromion is removed, a greater extent of the supraspinatus tendon may be visualized.

Repair of a cuff tear creates unique sonographic landmarks. The cuff tendons are reimplanted into a trough made perpendicular to the axis of the supraspinatus tendon. The reimplantation trough is placed in the humerus at a site that provides optimal tendon tension. The trough appears sonographically as a defect in the humeral contour, which is best viewed with the transducer longitudinal to the supraspinatus tendon (see

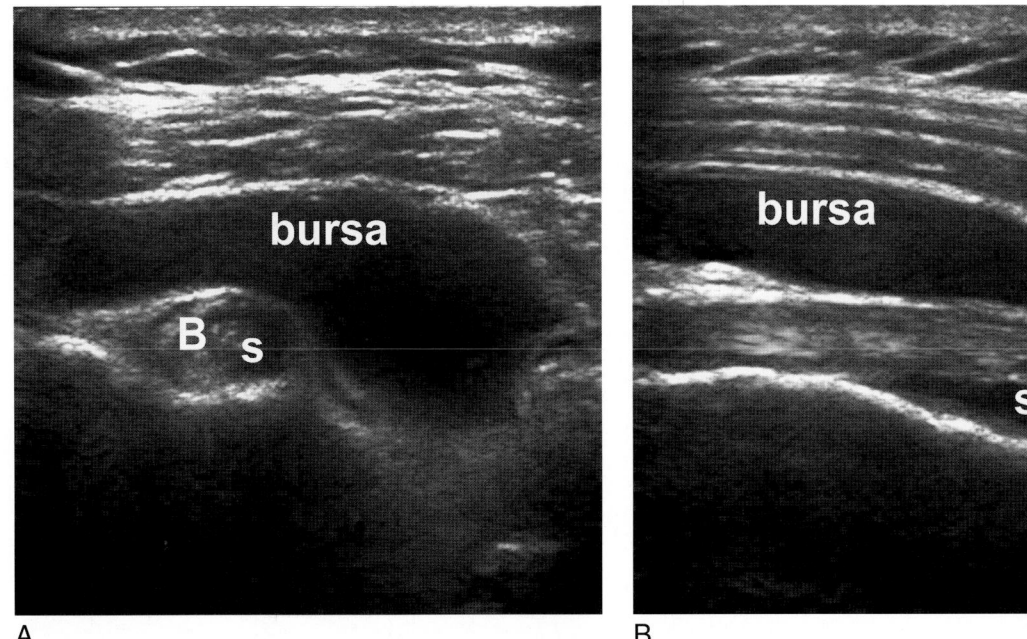

A   B

FIGURE 25-19. Subdeltoid bursal effusion. A, Transverse view over the anterior shoulder demonstrates fluid in two different synovial compartments. Synovial effusion (s) surrounds the long biceps tendon (B). This fluid does not extend beyond the biceps groove. The larger collection of fluid noted deep to the deltoid fills the subdeltoid bursa and extends both medial and lateral to the confines of the groove. **B,** Longitudinal scan of the long biceps tendon. Joint effusion (s) extends deep to the tendon. The subdeltoid bursa extends as a large sac over the anterior aspect of the shoulder. Fluid in joint and bursa signifies rotator tear in most patients.

Fig. 25-20). Suture material may be seen deep in the trough as specular echoes. Scanning the arm in extension and internal rotation may be necessary to visualize this site of tendon reimplantation, especially when it is medially placed (Fig. 25-21). Failure to scan in this position may lead to a false-positive diagnosis. Such a maneuver, however, should be used with care, especially in the immediate postoperative period, to avoid reinjury of the friable, newly reimplanted tendons.

Sonographic appearances of the cuff tendons never return to normal in the postoperative patient. Tendons, especially the supraspinatus tendon, are often echogenic and thinned when compared with the contralateral shoulder. Joint effusions are common and best visualized along the biceps tendon. Because resection of the subdeltoid bursa removes an important landmark, dynamic scanning is especially important in distinguishing a thin, hyperechoic cuff from adjacent deltoid muscle.

Recurrent Tear

Sonographically, recurrent tears most often appear as absence of the cuff. Fluid filling a defect in a rotator cuff repair and loose sutures or screws are other indications of recurrent tear (Fig. 25-22). Unless baseline scans are available in the postoperative period, it may be difficult to differentiate small recurrent tears from the appearances created when only a small amount of cuff tendon remains to be reattached. Thinning of the tendon is

useless as a criterion, and bone irregularity is the rule in the postoperative patient. Recurrent tears are common. They occur in up to 40% of patients in whom a small defect was repaired and in 80% of those patients who had large tears preoperatively.

PITFALLS IN ROTATOR CUFF SONOGRAPHY

Inadequate transducer positioning is the most common error in scanning the rotator cuff. False-positive and false-negative results may be produced in this manner. For example, scanning the supraspinatus tendon transversely with the transducer placed laterally may artifactually mimic a rotator cuff tear. An oblique transverse scan of the supraspinatus tendon can be falsely reported as thinning of the cuff. The examiner must, therefore, view the cuff in two orthogonal planes. Visualization of neatly depicted bony contour will help in avoiding these pitfalls.

A cause of tendon heterogeneity is the geometric relationship of the tendon to the transducer. As demonstrated by Crass et al.[46] and Fornage,[47] failure to orient the transducer parallel to the fibers of the tendon may result in **artifactual areas of decreased echogenicity** (Fig. 25-23). When only a small area of the tendon is parallel to the transducer, a focal area of increased echogenicity may be produced, mimicking a small

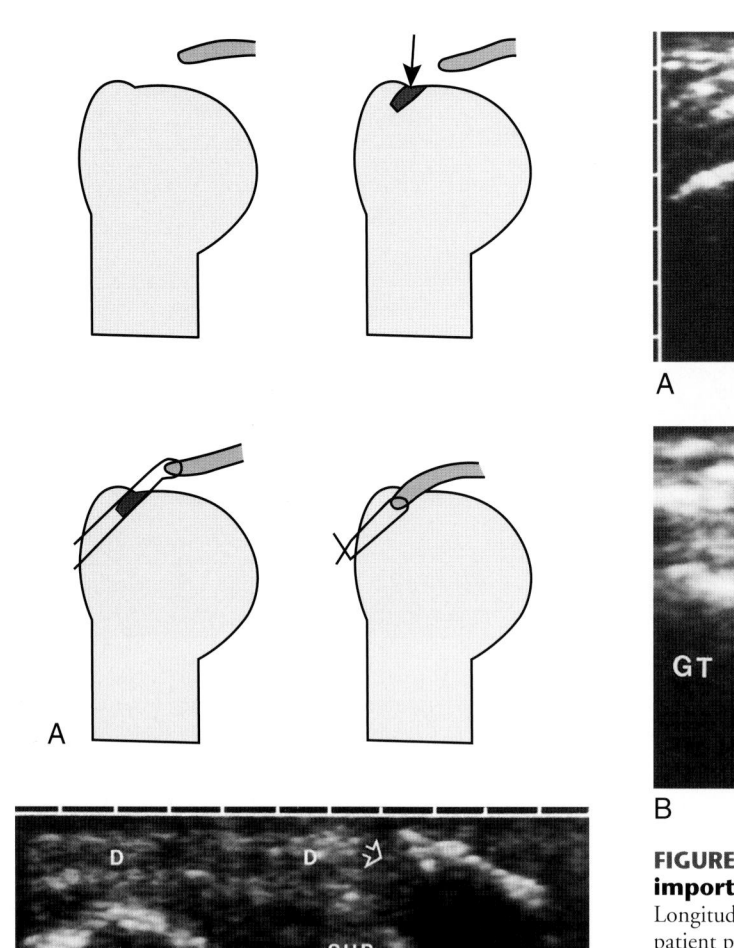

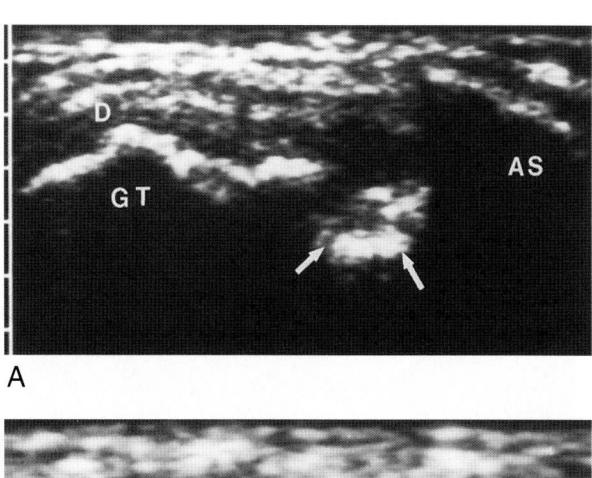

A

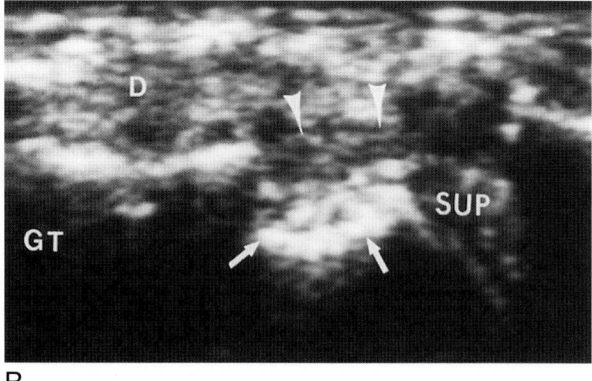

B

FIGURE 25-21. Postoperative rotator cuff—importance of examination during extension. A, Longitudinal supraspinatus tendon view in neutral position of a patient postoperative for repair of full-thickness rotator cuff tear demonstrates the reimplantation trough, but fails to reveal evidence of the supraspinatus tendon, thus suggesting recurrent injury. **B,** Scan with the arm in extension and internal rotation demonstrates that the repair is intact. The residual supraspinatus tendon (SUP), is thinned. Note absence of characteristic echoes of the subdeltoid bursa (*arrowheads*). AS, acromial shadow; D, deltoid muscle; GT, greater tuberosity; reimplantation trough (*arrows*). (Reproduced with permission of Mack LA, Nyberg DA, Matsen FA: Sonographic evaluation of rotator cuff. Radiol Clin North Am 1988;25:161-177.)

FIGURE 25-20. Rotator cuff repair. A, Drawing demonstrating the surgical technique for cuff reimplantation with creation of trough (*arrow*) in the humeral head, reimplantation of the residual tendon within that trough, and characteristic method of suture placement. **B,** Longitudinal supraspinatus tendon (SUP) image shows characteristic appearances of reimplantation trough (*arrows*). Acromioplasty defect (*open arrow*) is also visualized. D, deltoid muscle; GT, greater tuberosity; reimplantation suture (*curved arrow*). (Reproduced with permission of Mack LA, Nyberg DA, Matsen FA, III, et al: Sonography of the postoperative shoulder. AJR 1988;150:1089-1093.)

partial- or full-thickness tear. This artifact is especially pronounced with sector transducers.

ROTATOR CUFF CALCIFICATIONS

Calcifications can affect any of the four tendons of the rotator cuff. Subscapular tendon calcifications can be particularly difficult to diagnose without the aid of ultrasound. The calcium can burst out from the tendon into the subacromial-subdeltoid bursa and cause an acute and very painful inflammatory synovitis.[48] Standard texts on calcific tendonitis have distinguished a chronic phase of formation and an acute phase of resorption.[49] Ultrasound appears incapable of staging calcium according to those phases. However, ultrasound has shown great potential in demonstrating the physical form of the crystal deposition.[50] Aggregates of calcium can be solid, pastelike, or liquid. The liquid deposits appear hyperechoic without shadow; the calcium paste casts a vague shadow; and hard deposits show with distinct acoustic shadow. This unique capability of ultrasound aids in the treatment when ultrasound is used to localize and aspirate calcium.[51,52] Before the procedure, one will decide what size needle and the number of needles that will be necessary for treatment. Expectations

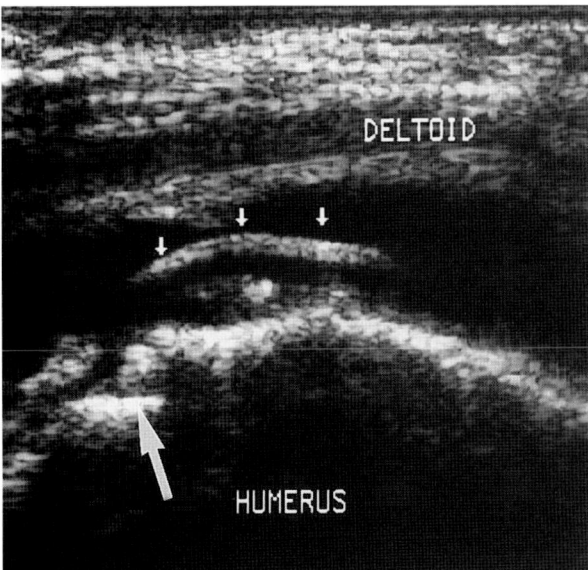

FIGURE 25-22. Recurrent tear—postoperative ultrasound exam. Longitudinal scan along the deltoid muscle in the region of the reimplantation trough (*arrow*). A loose suture (*small arrows*) is noted within a subdeltoid bursal effusion. The supraspinatus has left this subdeltoid space. The proximal humerus has an abnormal round appearance. The anatomic neck has disappeared through the process of bone remodeling.

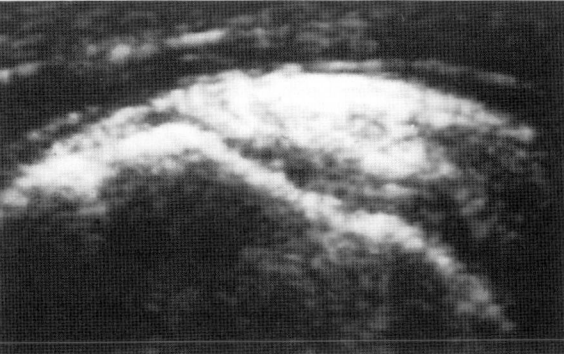

A

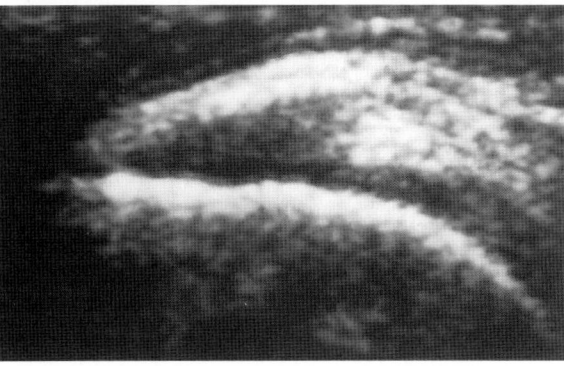

B

FIGURE 25-23. Artifactual areas of decreased tendon echogenicity. A and **B**, Two views of the same supraspinatus tendon demonstrate considerable changes in echogenicity that may be artifactually created by transducer position and orientation.

for complete recovery will have to be diminished somewhat if the pain is caused by the hard rock-type calcifications. A small amount of corticosteroid is then often added after multiple passes have been made through the calcium using 16 to 18 gauge needles.

References

1. Matsen FA, Arntz CT: Subacromial impingement. In Rockwood CA: Matsen FA II (eds): The Shoulder. Vol II. Philadelphia, WB Saunders, 1990.
2. Neviaser RJ, Neviaser TJ: Observations on impingement. Clin Orthop 1990;254:60-63.
3. Resnick D: Shoulder arthrography. Radiol Clin North Am 1981;19:243-252.
4. Mack LA, Matsen FA, Kilcoyne JF, et al: Ultrasound evaluation of the rotator cuff. Radiology 1985;157:205-209.
5. Mack LA, Gannon MK, Kilcoyne RF, et al: Sonographic evaluation of the rotator cuff. Accuracy in patients without prior surgery. Clin Orthop 1988;234:21-27.
6. Middleton WD, Reinus WR, Totty WF, et al: Ultrasonographic evaluation of the rotator and biceps tendon. J Bone Joint Surg 1986;68:440-450.
7. Crass JR, Craig EV, Feinberg SB: Ultrasonography of rotator cuff tears: A review of 500 diagnostic cuffs. J Clin Ultrasound 1988;16:313-327.
8. Van Holsbeeck MT, Kolowich PA, Eyler WR, et al: Ultrasound depiction of partial-thickness tear of the rotator cuff. Radiology 1995;197:443-446.

Clinical Considerations
9. Codman EA: The Shoulder, 2nd ed. Boston, Thomas Todd, 1934.

10. DePalma AF: Surgery of the Shoulder, 2nd ed. Philadelphia, JB Lippincott, 1973.
11. Refior HJ, Kroedel A, Melzer C: Examinations of the pathology of the rotator cuff. Arch Orthop Trauma Surg 1987;106:301-308.
12. Milgrom C, Schaffler M, Gilbert S, et al: Rotator-cuff changes in asymptomatic adults. The effect of age, hand dominance and gender. J Bone Joint Surg 1995; 77(B):296-298.
13. Sher JS, Uribe JW, Posada A, et al: Abnormal findings on magnetic resonance images of asymptomatic shoulders. J Bone Joint Surg 1995; 77(A):10-15.
14. Raven PB: Asymptomatic tears of rotator cuff are commonplace. Sports Med Diag 1995;17:11-12.
15. Miniaci A, Dowdy PA, Willits KR, et al: Magnetic resonance imaging evaluation of the rotator cuff tendons in the asymptomatic shoulder. Am J Sports Med 1995; 23:142-145.
16. Petterson G: Rupture of the tendon aponeurosis of the shoulder joint in anterior inferior dislocation. Acta Chir Scand Suppl 1942;77:1-184.
17. Neer CS: Anterior acromioplasty for the chronic impingement syndrome in the shoulder: A preliminary report. J Bone Joint Surg 1972;54A:41-51.
18. Lee HS, Joo KB, Park CK, et al: Sonography of the shoulder after arthrography. J Clin Ultrasound 2002;30:23-32.
19. Taljanovic MS, Carlson KL, Kuhn JE, et al: Sonography of the glenoid labrum: A cadaveric study with arthroscopic correlation. AJR 2000;174:1717-1722.

20. Schydlowsky P, Strandberg C, Galatius S, et al: Ultrasonographic examination of the glenoid labrum of healthy volunteers. Euro J Ultrasound 1998;8:85-89

21. Schydlowsky P, Strandberg C, Tranum-Jensen J, et al: Post-mortem ultrasonographic assessment of the anterior glenoid labrum. Euro J Ultrasound 1998;8:129-133.

22. Schydlowsky P, Strandberg C, Galbo H, et al: The value of ultrasonography in the diagnosis of labral lesions in patients with anterior shoulder dislocation. Euro J Ultrasound 1998;8:107-113.

23. Rakofsky M: Fractional Arthrography of the Shoulder. Stuttgart, Gustav Fisher, 1987.

24. Ptasznik R, Hennessy OF: Abnormalities of the biceps tendon of the shoulder: Sonographic findings. AJR 1995;164:409.

25. Farin PU, Jaroma H, Harju A, et al: Medial displacement of the biceps brachii tendon: Valuation with dynamic sonography during maximal external rotation. Radiology 1995;195:845.

26. Van Holsbeeck M, Strouse PJ: Sonography of the shoulder: Evaluation of the subacromial-subdeltoid bursa. AJR 1993;160: 561-564.

27. Crass JR, Craig EV, Feinberg SB: The hyperextended internal rotation view in rotator cuff ultrasound. J Clin Ultrasound 1987;15:416-420.

28. Mack LA, Nyberg DA, Matsen FA: Sonographic evaluation of rotator cuff. Radiol Clin North Am 1988;25:161-177.

29. Van Holsbeeck M, Introcaso J, Hoogmartens M: Sonographic detection and evaluation of shoulder joint effusion. Radiology 1990;177(P):214.

30. Newman JS, Adler RS, Bude RO, et al: Detection of soft tissue hyperemia: Value of power Doppler sonography. AJR 1994;163:385-389.

31. Petersson CJ: Ruptures of the supraspinatus tendon. Cadaver dissection. Acta Orthop Scand 1984;55:52-56.

32. Farin P, Jaroma H: Sonographic detection of tears of the anterior portion of the rotator cuff. J Ultrasound Med 1996;15:221-225.

33. Keyes EL: Observations on rupture of the supraspinatus tendon. Ann Surg 1933;97:849-856.

34. Wilson CL, Duff GL: Pathological study of degeneration and rupture of the supraspinatus tendon. Ann Surg 1943;47:121-135.

35. Fukuda H, Mikasa M, Yamanaka K: Incomplete thickness rotator cuff tears diagnosed by subacromial bursography. Clin Orthop 1987;223:51-58.

36. Middleton WD: Status of rotator cuff sonography. Radiology 1989;173:307-309.

37. Bloom RA. Active abduction view: A new maneuver in the diagnosis of rotator cuff tears. Skeletal Radiol 1991;20:255.

38. Van Holsbeeck M, Introcaso J: Ultrasound of tendons. Patterns of disease. Instruction Course Lectures 1993;47:475-481.

39. Jiang Y, Zhao J, van Holsbeeck MT, et al: Trabecular microstructure and surface changes in the greater tuberosity in rotator cuff tears. Skeletal Radiol 2002;31:522-528.

40. Teefey SA, Middleton WD, Bauer GS, et al: Sonographic differences in the appearance of acute and chronic full-thickness rotator cuff tears. J Ultrasound Med 2000; 19:377-378.

41. Hollister MS, Mack LA, Pattern RM, et al: Association of sonographically detected subacromial/subdeltoid bursal effusion and intraarticular fluid with rotator cuff tear. AJR 1995;165:605-608.

42. Farin PU, Jaroma H, Jarju A, et al: Shoulder impingement syndrome: Sonographic evaluation. Radiology 1990;176:845-849.

43. Wohlwend JR, van Holsbeeck M, Craig J, et al: The association between irregular tuberosities and rotator cuff tears: A sonographic study. AJR 1998;171:229-233.

44. Mack LA, Nyberg DA, Matsen FA, III, et al: Sonography of the postoperative shoulder. AJR 1988;150:1089-1093.

45. Crass JR, Craig EV, Feinberg SB: Sonography of the postoperative rotator cuff. AJR 1988;148:561-564.

46. Crass JB, Van de Vegte GL, Harkavy LA: Tendon echogenicity: Ex vivo study. Radiology 1988;169:791-794.

47. Fornage BD: The hypoechoic normal tendon: A pitfall. J Ultrasound Med 1987;6:19-22.

48. Resnick D, Niwayama G: Diagnosis of bone and joint disorders, 2nd ed. Philadelphia, WB Saunders, 1988.

49. Gärtner J, Simons B: Analysis of calcific deposits in calcifying tendinitis. Clin Orthop 1990;254:111-120.

50. Farin PU: Consistency of rotator-cuff calcifications. Observations on plain radiography, sonography, computed tomography, and at needle treatment. Invest Radiol 1996;31:300-304.

51. Farin PU, Jaroma H, Soimakallio S. Rotator cuff calcifications: treatment with US-guided technique. Radiology 1995;195:841-843.

52. Chiou HJ, Chou YH, Wu JJ, et al: The role of high-resolution ultrasonography in management of calcific tendinitis of the rotator cuff. Ultrasound Med Biol 2001;27:735-743.

26

THE TENDONS

Bruno D. Fornage / Didier H. Touche / Beth S. Edeiken-Monroe

Chapter Outline

The tendons of the extremities are particularly well suited for sonographic examination using high-frequency (7.5- to 15-MHz) or even very high-frequency (15- to 20-MHz) transducers because of their superficial location. Tendons are best evaluated dynamically during their gliding motion and, for that purpose, the unique real-time capability of sonography is invaluable. Sonography of the musculoskeletal system, in general, and of the tendons of the extremities, in particular, has enjoyed a growing popularity in the last decade and has become the first-line imaging modality in many centers specializing in musculoskeletal imaging and sports medicine—in spite of the availability of MRI. Indeed, in expert hands, high-frequency sonography, combined with physical examination and plain radiography, often solves the diagnostic challenges, making MRI unnecessary. The vast majority of tendon disorders are related to trauma and inflammation and are associated with athletic or occupational activities that result in overuse of the tendon, mostly through excessive tension or repetitive microtrauma.

ANATOMY

Tendons are made of dense connective tissue and are extremely resistant to traction forces.[1] The densely packed collagen fibers are separated by a small amount of ground substance with a few elongated fibroblasts and are arranged in parallel bundles. The **peritenon** is a layer of loose connective tissue that wraps around the tendon and sends intratendinous septa between the bundles of collagen fibers. In large tendons, blood and lymphatic vessels course, along with nerve endings, within these septa, whereas small tendons are almost avascular.

At the musculotendinous junction, the muscle fibers interdigitate with the collagen fibrils. The bony insertion of tendons is usually markedly calcified and characterized by the presence of cartilaginous tissue. Tendons usually attach to tuberosities, spinae, trochanters, processes, or ridges. Blood supply to tendons is poor, and nutritional exchange occurs mostly via the ground substance. With aging, the amount of ground substance and the number of fibroblasts decrease, whereas the number of fibers and the amount of fat within the tendon increase.

In certain areas of mechanical constraint, tendons are associated with additional structures that provide mechanical support, protection, or both. **Fibrous sheaths** keep certain tendons close to the bones and prevent them from "bowstringing"; examples include the flexor and extensor retinacula in the wrist, the fibrous sheaths ("pulleys") of the flexor tendons in the fingers, and the peroneal and flexor retinacula in the foot. The sesamoid bones are intended to reinforce tendon strength. **Synovial sheaths** are double-walled tubular structures that surround some tendons; the inner wall of these sheaths is in intimate contact with the tendon, and the two layers are in continuity with each other at both ends and also occasionally via a mesotenon. A minimal amount of synovial fluid allows the tendon to glide smoothly within its sheath. Large tendons (e.g., patellar and Achilles tendons) lack a synovial sheath and are surrounded instead by a sheath of loose areolar and adipose tissue known as **paratenon. Synovial bursae** are small, fluid-filled pouches that are found in specific locations and act as bolsters to facilitate the play of tendons.

INSTRUMENTATION AND EXAMINATION TECHNIQUE

Because of their wider field of view and their better resolution in the near field relative to those of other types of transducers, **linear-array electronic transducers** are the best choice for tendon sonography. Images of exquisite resolution are obtained with the broadband (e.g., 5- to 12-MHz, 7- to 15-MHz) linear-array transducers that are available on current state-of-the-art scanners (Fig. 26-1). Some mechanical transducers of up to 20 MHz are also commercially available on some scanners.

The field of view of most high-frequency broadband linear-array transducers is restricted to a width of less than 4 cm. Although most scanners allow splitting of the screen on the monitor to obtain a montage of two contiguous scans, there is always a risk of some overlapping between the two contiguous views, so measurements of lesions that straddle the two half screens may be inaccurate. An alternative would be to use a lower-frequency transducer with a wider field of view, but that reduces resolution. Recently, built-in image-processing software has been made available that allows stretching the width of the field of view up to 50 to 60 cm. By offering a **panoramic view** of the structures examined, this new technique has removed a long-standing limitation of real-time sonography, and it has been particularly welcomed in the field of musculoskeletal sonography in which long anatomic segments or lesions must be scanned (Figs. 26-2 and 26-3).[2,3]

Real-time spatial compound scanning involves the acquisition of echoes at a given point in an image using multiple different apertures generated by computed beam-steering technology. The images obtained from the multiple lines of sight (up to nine) are compounded in real-time. Real-time compound scanning has shown some success in reducing the amount of speckle in the image, making uniform tissue look more uniform and

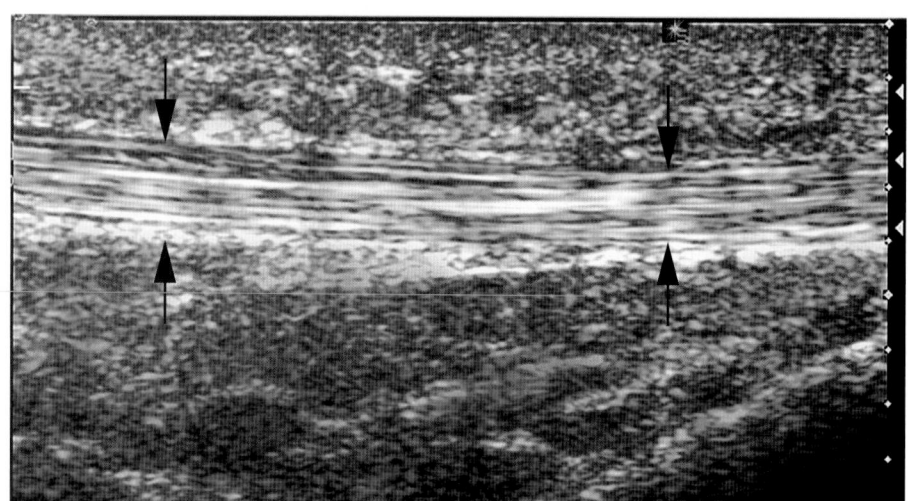

FIGURE 26-1. Normal patellar tendon.
Longitudinal sonogram of the midportion of the tendon using a broadband 5- to 13-MHz linear-array transducer shows the fibrillar echotexture of the tendon (*arrows*).

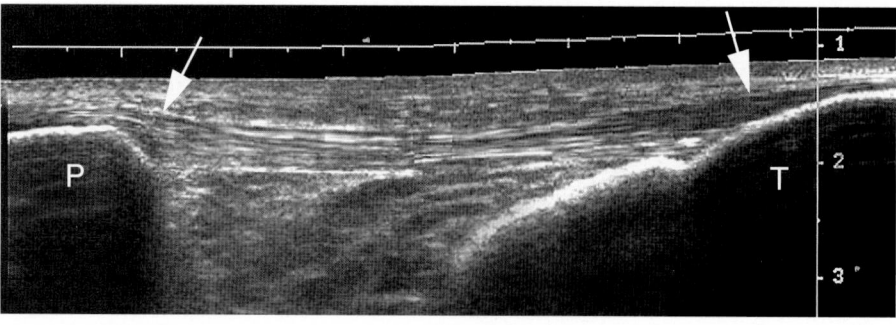

FIGURE 26-2. Normal patellar tendon.
Longitudinal extended-field-of-view sonogram shows both insertions (*arrows*) of the tendon. P, patella; T, tibia.

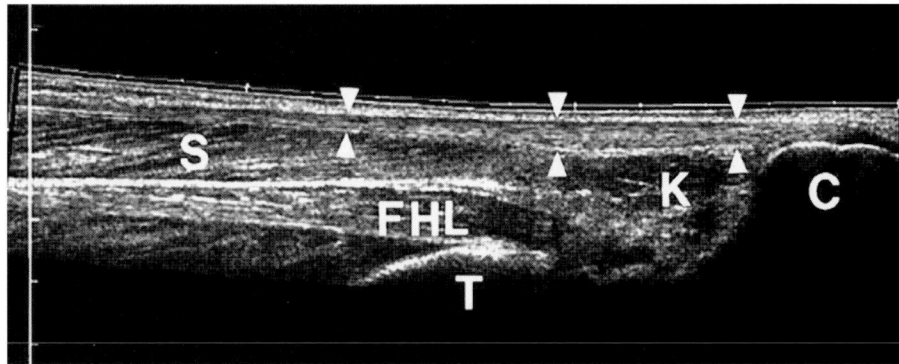

FIGURE 26-3. Normal Achilles tendon. Longitudinal extended-field-of-view sonogram shows the entire length of the Achilles tendon (*arrowheads*) from its origin to its insertion into the calcaneus (C). FHL, flexor hallucis longus muscle; K, Kager's fatty triangle; S, termination of the soleus muscle; T, tibia.

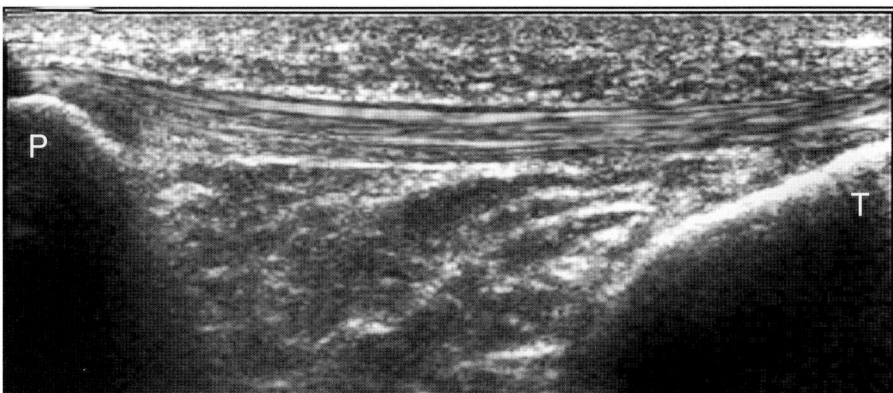

FIGURE 26-4. Compound sonogram. Real-time spatial compound longitudinal sonogram of the patellar tendon shows well the tendon margins. Note the associated blur. P, patella; T, tibia.

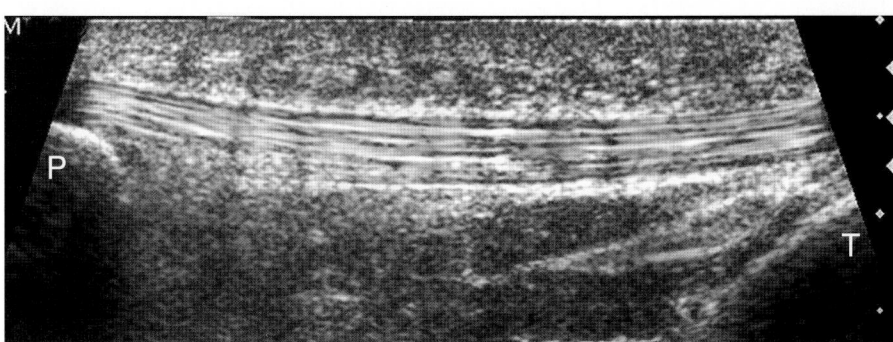

FIGURE 26-5. Electronic beam steering. Longitudinal sonogram of the patellar tendon using electronic beam steering to achieve a trapezoidal format. This allows the beam to remain perpendicular to the tendon fibers even at the patellar insertion, thereby avoiding areas of false hypoechogenicity. P, patella; T, tibia.

boundaries look more continuous (Fig. 26-4). This may appear beneficial in imaging the fibrillar texture of tendons and in reducing the anisotropy artifact, but these potential benefits must be carefully weighed against the risks that the unavoidable blurring associated with this technique may obscure minute lesions and that the reduction or disappearance of subtle useful artifacts, such as fine trails of shadowing or reverberations, may impair the detection of tiny reflectors, such as foreign bodies or microcalcifications.

Electronic beam steering is available on some high-end scanners. This may be useful when the beam from the linear-array transducer is not perpendicular to the tendon and needs to be corrected slightly to hit the fibers at a 90-degree angle.[4] This technique helps suppress the anisotropy artifact related to the obliquity or concavity

of tendons without the blurring associated with real-time spatial compound scanning (Fig. 26-5). In addition, beam steering can be used to change the image format from rectangular to trapezoidal and, thus, to increase the size of the field of view.

Tissue harmonic imaging is now available with high-frequency linear-array transducers. Because harmonic imaging boosts both spatial and contrast resolutions, it can help in confirming the anechoic appearance of minute and deep fluid collections, such as small joint effusions, ganglia, or early acute tenosynovitis, which would otherwise display spurious echoes on fundamental imaging.

Color Doppler imaging is now available, not only on high-end but also on most midrange ultrasound scanners, and it is always good practice to use it when

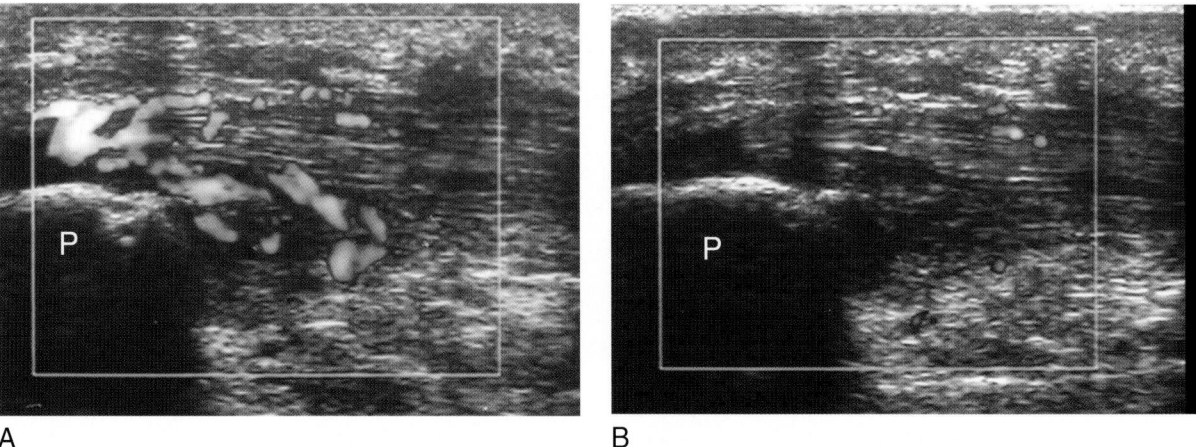

FIGURE 26-6. Effect of examination technique on power Doppler imaging findings. Patellar tendinitis. **A,** Longitudinal sonogram obtained without pressure exerted on the tendon with the transducer shows substantial hypervascularity. P, patella. **B,** Longitudinal sonogram obtained with the usual pressure applied with the transducer shows the nearly complete disappearance of the color Doppler signals. P, patella.

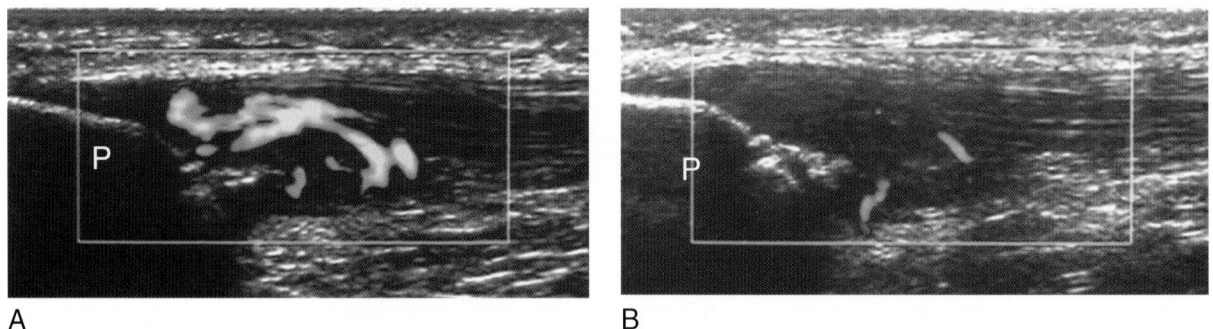

FIGURE 26-7. Effect of examination technique on power Doppler imaging findings. Patellar tendinitis. **A,** Longitudinal sonogram obtained with the knee extended shows substantial hypervascularity. P, patella. **B,** Longitudinal sonogram obtained with the knee flexed shows the nearly complete disappearance of the color Doppler signals. P, patella.

evaluating inflammatory or tumoral conditions. **Power Doppler** imaging is preferred because of its greater sensitivity in flow detection, especially in light of the low baseline vascularity of tendons. It is important to keep in mind that the color Doppler signals associated with inflammatory conditions of tendons are easily obliterated by even modest pressure exerted with the transducer or when the tendon is stretched, e.g., by flexion of the knee for the patellar tendon or dorsiflexion of the foot for the Achilles tendon (Figs. 26-6 and 26-7).[5] There are no reports on the applicability of the use of ultrasound contrast agents to enhance the visibility of the blood supply to the largest tendons. A few attempts have been made to use color Doppler imaging to evaluate and quantitate the excursion velocity of some tendons in the hand.[6-8]

A combination of longitudinal and transverse scans provides a three-dimensional approach to tendon examination. Ultrasound scanners that are capable of three-dimensional reconstruction of sonograms are now commercially available, but no direct benefit of the use of **three-dimensional sonography** in the evaluation of superficial tendons has been reported to date (Fig. 26-8). Improvements in the speed (real time) and quality (resolution) of three-dimensional rendering, as well as in the ease of use of the software needed to navigate through the multitude of planes available, are expected to make the advantages of the method appreciable in routine clinical practice in the near future.

Once mandatory with the use of 5- or 7.5-MHz probes, stand-off pads are no longer needed with the very high-frequency transducers, whose focal zone can be adjusted to the very first millimeters of the scan. However, a thin **stand-off pad** remains useful for evaluating very superficial tendons (e.g., the extensor tendons of the fingers at the dorsum of the hand) or tendons coursing in regions with an uneven surface (e.g., the flexor tendons in the fingers) (Fig. 26-9).[9] Another reason to use a stand-off pad is the need to correlate the sonographic findings with the palpation findings. This is

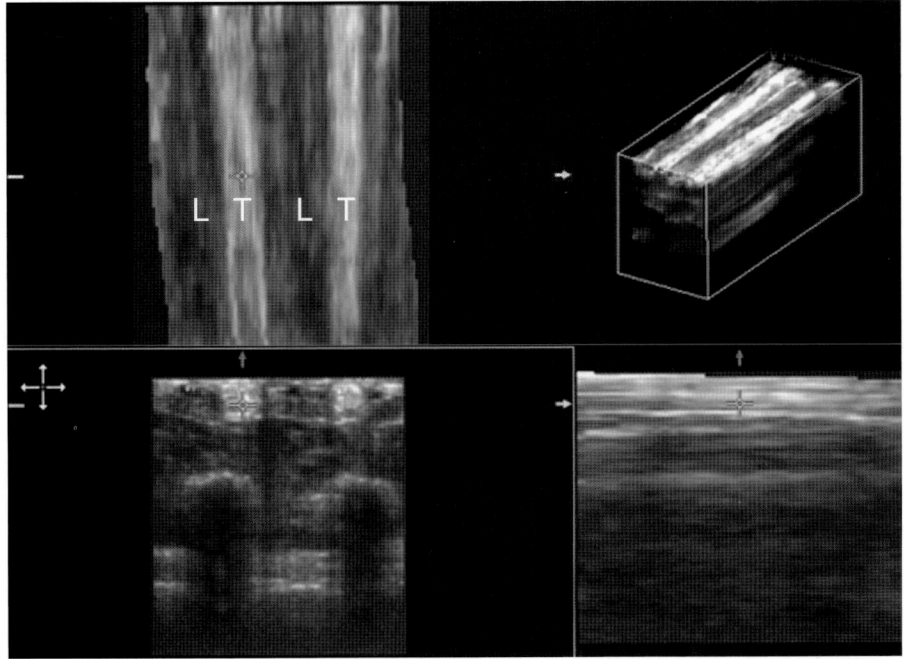

FIGURE 26-8. Three-dimensional sonographic examination of the flexor tendons of the fingers in the palm. *Top left*: Reconstructed coronal sonogram shows the flexor tendons (T) of the third and fourth fingers and the companion lumbrical muscles (L). *Top right*: Volume rendering. *Bottom left*: Transverse sonogram. *Bottom right*: Longitudinal sonogram.

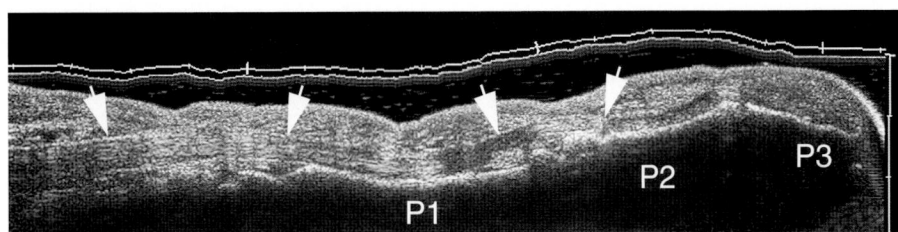

FIGURE 26-9. Normal finger. Longitudinal extended-field-of-view sonogram obtained with a thin stand-off pad shows the normal superficial and deep flexor tendons (*arrows*) coursing along the phalanges. Note that the tendons exhibit normal echogenicity only in the segments that are parallel to the linear-array transducer; the tendons are falsely hypoechoic in the segments that lie oblique to the beam. P1, first phalanx; P2, second phalanx; P3, third phalanx.

accomplished by sliding one or two fingers of one hand between the pad and the skin while keeping the transducer in place over the region of interest with the other hand. This palpation during sonography with a stand-off pad allows the operator to confirm that he or she is focusing on the region of palpable concern and, conversely, to appreciate the firmness of the sonographic abnormality. When a stand-off pad is used, care should be taken to maintain the ultrasound beam strictly perpendicular to the region being examined to avoid artifacts.[10]

When examining tendons, the operator should take full advantage of the real-time capability of sonography by examining the tendon at rest and during active and passive mobilization through **flexion and extension maneuvers**.[10] A valuable reference for the normal anatomy of the region being examined may be obtained by scanning the corresponding area in the contralateral extremity or region, although the possibility of bilateral tendon disorders should be kept in mind.

Another advantage of real-time sonography is its provision of accurate guidance during **interventional procedures**. Aspiration of fluid from or injection of drugs or contrast agent into the fluid-distended synovial sheath of a tendon or an adjacent bursa can be performed safely under ultrasound guidance.[11] Recent research studies have used ultrasound-guided core biopsy of the Achilles tendon under local anesthesia without any complication to correlate sonographic with histopathologic findings.[12]

EXAMINATION TECHNIQUE

Use linear-array transducer.
Use highest frequency available.
Use a stand-off pad only for very superficial structures and for combined palpation and sonography.
Identify and correct anisotropy-related artifacts (false hypoechogenicity) due to improper angle of insonation of the tendon.
Always combine longitudinal and transverse scans.
Check contralateral tendon for reference.
Perform dynamic examination during flexion and extension maneuvers.
Use power Doppler imaging.

NORMAL SONOGRAPHIC APPEARANCE

All normal tendons are echogenic and display a characteristic **fibrillar echotexture** on longitudinal scans (Fig. 26-10).[10] The higher the frequency, the higher the number of visible fibrils. The fine echogenic lines have been shown to correspond to the interfaces between the collagen bundles and the endotenon.[13] No specific sonographic appearance seems to correlate with areas of tendon fragility, the so-called **vulnerable zones**, where ruptures occur most frequently; e.g., the area of the Achilles tendon 2.5 to 6 cm from its insertion into the calcaneus. Although they are easily seen when they are surrounded by hypoechoic muscles, tendons are less well demarcated when they are surrounded by echogenic fat. A key step in the identification of tendons is their mobilization under real-time sonographic monitoring on longitudinal scans. On transverse sonograms, the reflective bundles of fibers give rise to a **finely punctate echogenic pattern** (Fig. 26-11). Transverse scans provide the most accurate measurements of tendon thickness.[10]

Nerves, like tendons, are echogenic with a fibrillar echotexture. However, the hypoechoic bundles of axons are thicker than the bundles of fibrils, and at high frequencies, fewer interfaces are seen within a nerve than within a tendon of the same caliber. On transverse sonograms, this results in a honeycomb pattern for nerves and slightly decreased overall echogenicity compared with tendons (Fig. 26-12).

Sesamoid bones appear as hyper-reflective structures associated with acoustic shadowing (Fig. 26-13). **Synovial sheaths** are not seen at 7.5 MHz, but at frequencies of 15 MHz and higher, they appear as thin, hypoechoic underlining of the tendon (Fig. 26-14). The largest **synovial bursae** (e.g., deep infrapatellar and retrocalcaneal) can be seen on sonograms as collapsed structures that contain only a sliver of fluid and are less than a few millimeters thick (Fig. 26-15).[14]

Optimal display of the echogenic fibrillar texture of a tendon requires that the ultrasound beam be strictly perpendicular to the tendon's axis. The slightest obliquity causes scattering of the beam, which results in an **artifactual hypoechogenicity**[15] that is referred to as the anisotropic property of tendons (Fig. 26-16). Early erroneous descriptions of hypoechoic normal tendons, in particular of the rotator cuff, were due to this artifact. This artifact constantly affects scans obtained with sector transducers—phased-array, mechanical, or curved-array—with which only the midline portion of the scan is free of artifacts and displays the normal echogenicity of a straight tendon lying parallel to the skin (see Fig. 26-16A). When a linear-array transducer is used, the artifact occurs whenever the tendon or a segment of it is not parallel to the transducer's footprint. Rocking the transducer by pressing harder on one end of it usually suffices to bring the footprint of the probe back in a direction parallel to the axis of the tendon. When the artifact is caused by a tendon's curved (concave or convex) course, straightening the tendon through muscle contraction clears the artifact (see Fig. 26-16).

If this is not possible, the alternative is to examine the tendon segment by segment, changing the position of the probe so its footprint is parallel to the segment of the tendon being examined. Another alternative available with linear-array transducers on some high-end scanners is to use the built-in electronic steering of the beam to adjust the direction of the beam to be closer to perpendicular to the concave tendon's axis, e.g., when examining flexor tendons in the fingers (see Fig. 26-16B). When a stand-off pad is used, constant verification that the footprint of the transducer is parallel to the tendon's axis is crucial. Transverse scans are equally affected by the tendon anisotropy artifact, with falsely hypoechoic sections being displayed whenever the transverse scan plane is not perpendicular to the axis of the tendon (see Fig. 26-16G).

Shoulder

Sonography of the shoulder, and especially the rotator cuff, is discussed in Chapter 25.

Elbow

The anterior and lateral aspects of the elbow are best examined with the elbow extended. The common extensor tendon, which includes tendons from the extensor digitorum, extensor digiti minimi, extensor carpi ulnaris, and extensor carpi radialis brevis muscles, inserts into the lateral aspect of the lateral epicondyle (Fig. 26-17). Similarly, a common tendon of origin for the superficial flexor muscles, which include the

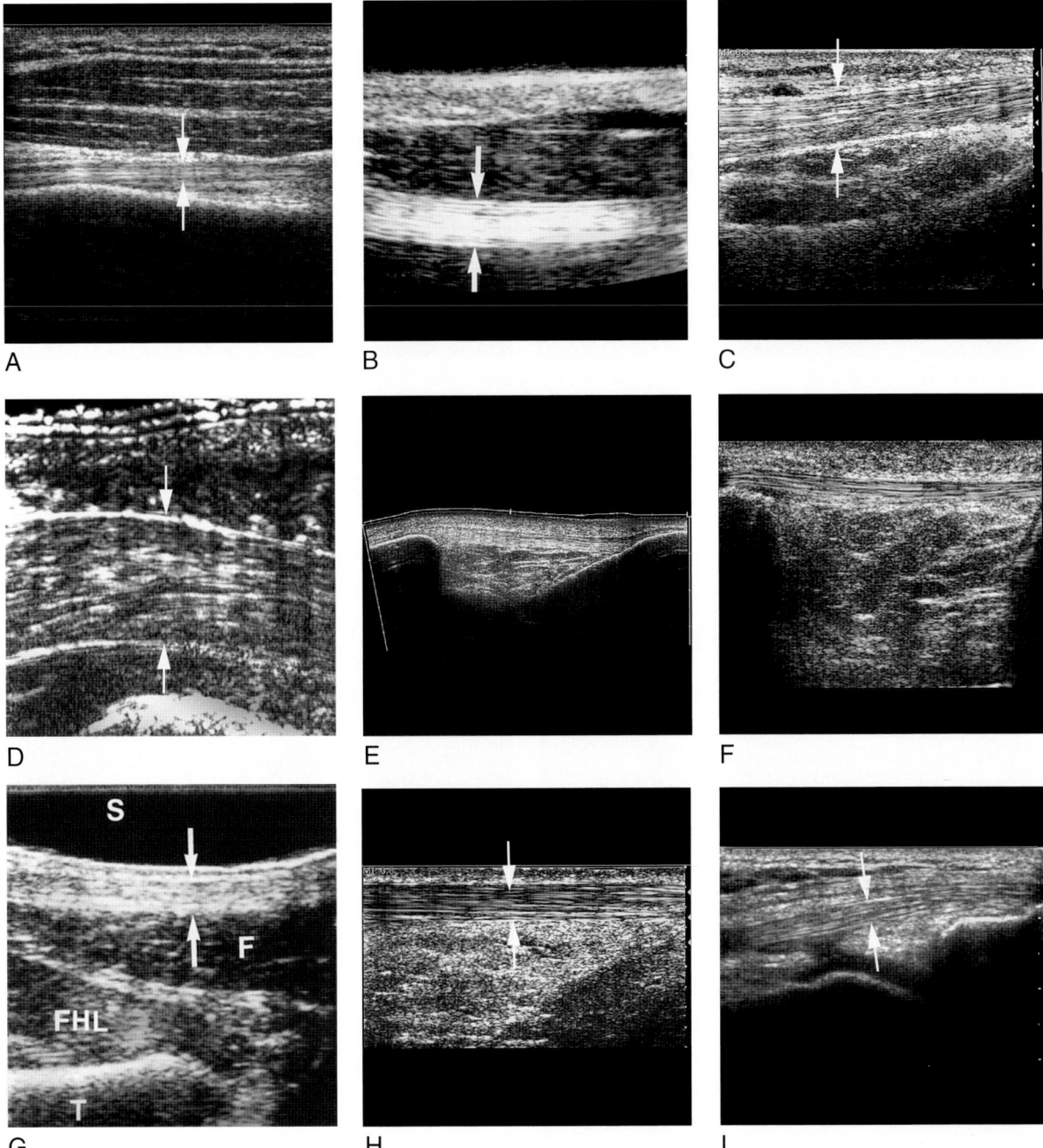

FIGURE 26-10. Spectrum of appearances of normal tendons. All tendons exhibit a fibrillar echotexture with more interfaces being visualized with higher-frequency transducers. Longitudinal views. **A,** Tendon of the long biceps (*arrows*) at the anterior aspect of the shoulder. **B,** Tendon of the flexor pollicis longus (*arrows*) in the thenar area. **C,** Pair of superficial and deep flexor tendons (*arrows*) of the third finger in the palm. **D,** Pair of superficial and deep flexor tendons (*arrows*) of the third finger at the metacarpophalangeal joint obtained with a 20-MHz transducer. Note the higher number of interfaces depicted within the tendons compared with image **C,** which was obtained at 13 MHz. **E,** Patellar tendon scanned at 7.5 MHz. **F,** Patellar tendon scanned at 13 MHz shows more internal interfaces than in image **E. G,** Achilles tendon. Longitudinal scan obtained with a 5-MHz transducer shows the echogenic tendon (*arrows*) with few internal interfaces. F, Kager's fatty triangle; FHL, flexor hallucis longus muscle; S, stand-off pad; T, tibia. **H,** Achilles tendon scanned at 13 MHz. The fibrillar echotexture of the tendon (*arrows*) is much better depicted than in image **G. I,** Tendon of the flexor hallucis longus muscle (*arrows*) in the distal sole of the foot.

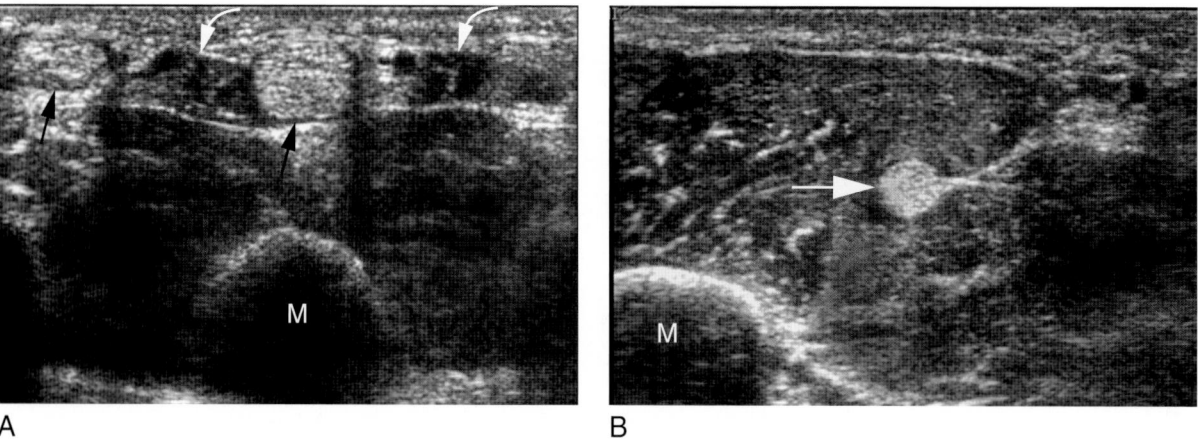

A   B

FIGURE 26-11. Transverse sonograms of normal flexor tendons in the hand. A, Transverse scan of the palm of the hand shows the normal echogenic, rounded superficial and deep flexor tendons of the second and third fingers (*arrows*) adjacent to the hypoechoic lumbrical muscles (*curved arrows*). M, metacarpal bone. **B,** Transverse sonogram of the thenar region shows the echogenic round cross section of the tendon of the flexor pollicis longus muscle (*arrow*) surrounded by the hypoechoic muscles. M, metacarpal bone.

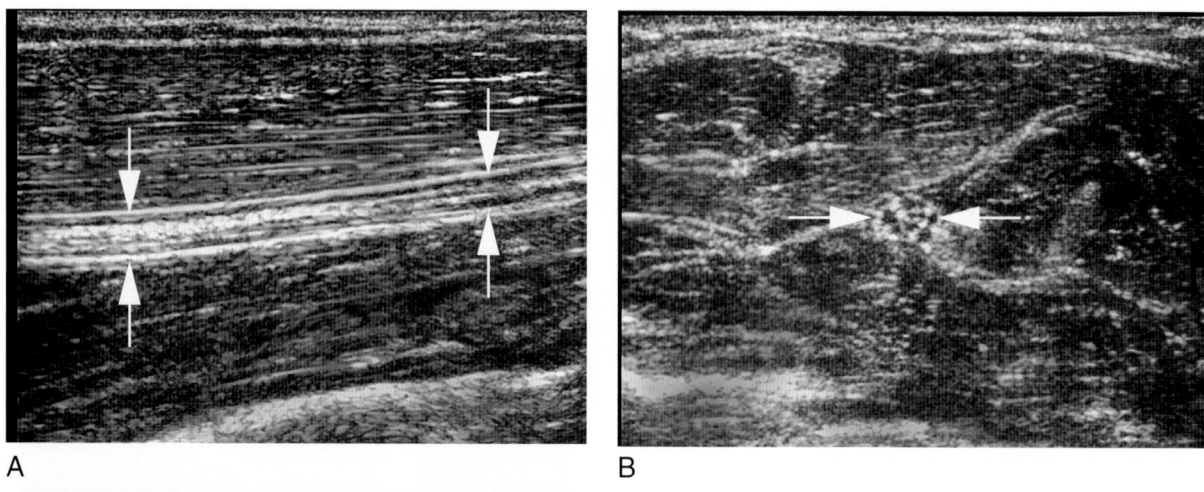

A   B

C

FIGURE 26-12. Normal median nerve. A, Longitudinal sonogram of the volar aspect of the forearm shows the mostly echogenic nerve (*arrows*) between the flexor digitorum superficialis and the flexor digitorum profundus muscles. **B,** Transverse sonogram shows the typical honeycomb pattern (*arrows*) that differentiates nerves from tendons. **C,** Transverse sonogram of the carpal tunnel shows the echogenic cross sections of the flexor tendons (*arrows*) and the cross section of the median nerve (*arrowheads*), which is less echogenic than the tendons.

pronator teres, flexor carpi radialis, palmaris longus, flexor carpi ulnaris, and flexor digitorum superficialis muscles, inserts into the medial epicondyle. At the anterior aspect of the extended elbow, the tendon of the biceps brachii muscle can be visualized as it inserts into the radial tuberosity. Because of the oblique direction of that tendon, it usually appears slightly hypoechoic (Fig. 26-18). The cubital bursa, which is located between the tendon and the radial tuberosity to facilitate the tendon's gliding, is normally not seen.

With the elbow flexed at a 90-degree angle, the tendon of the triceps brachii muscle is readily identifiable on both longitudinal and transverse scans as it inserts into the olecranon (Fig. 26-19).

Hand and Wrist

In the carpal tunnel, the echogenic tendons of the **flexor digitorum profundus (FDP)** and **flexor digitorum superficialis (FDS)** muscles are surrounded by the

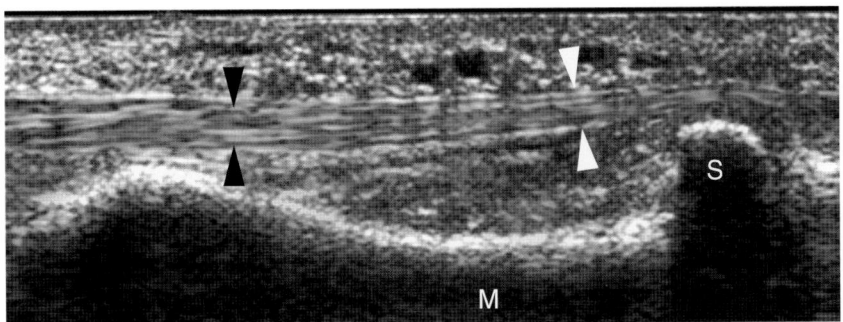

FIGURE 26-13. Normal flexor hallucis tendon. Longitudinal sonogram of the medial aspect of the sole of the foot shows the tendon of the flexor hallucis longus muscle (*arrowheads*) and a sesamoid bone (S). M, first metatarsal bone.

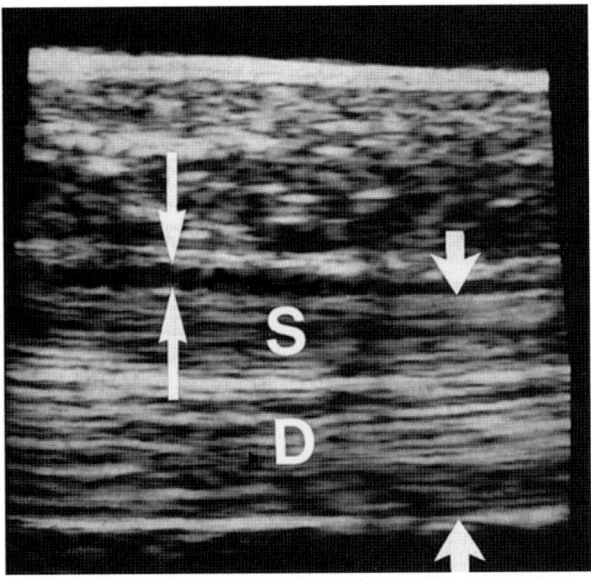

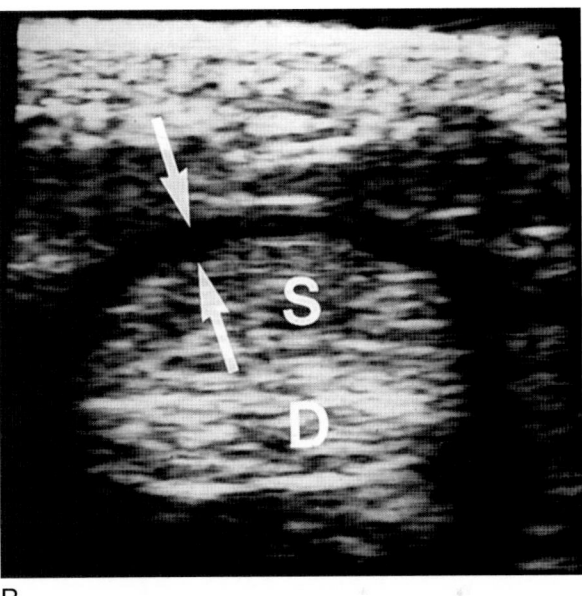

A B

FIGURE 26-14. Synovial sheath of the flexor tendons of the third finger in the palm examined with a 15-MHz transducer. **A**, Longitudinal sonogram shows the echogenic superficial (S) and deep (D) flexor tendons (*short arrows*) with a typical fibrillar texture. Long arrows indicate the synovial sheath. **B**, Transverse scan shows the echogenic cross section of the superficial (S) and deep (D) tendons. The *arrows* point to the synovial sheath.

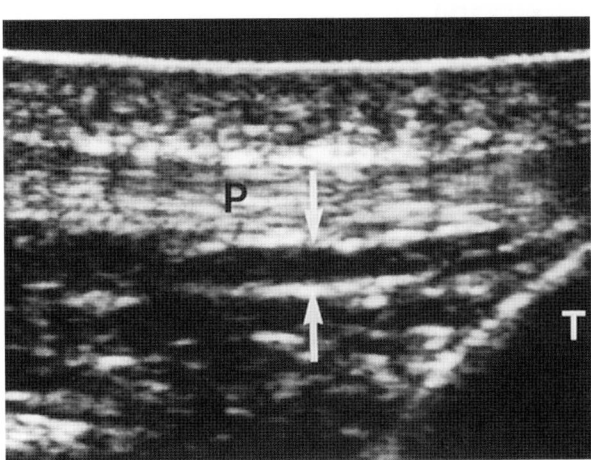

FIGURE 26-15. Normal infrapatellar bursa. Longitudinal scan of the knee shows the deep infrapatellar bursa (*arrows*) posterior to the distal patellar tendon (P). T, tibia.

hypoechoic ulnar bursa and are best seen when the wrist is moderately flexed. The **median nerve** courses outside the ulnar bursa and anterior to the flexor tendons of the second finger (Fig. 26-20A). On transverse scans, the flexor tendons are seen to move dramatically during contraction of the fist. The median nerve is also subject to marked changes in shape at various degrees of flexion of the wrist and fingers as it is displaced by the moving flexor tendons. The median nerve is slightly less echogenic than the tendons. With the use of very high-frequency transducers, the median nerve, like other major peripheral nerve trunks, appears to comprise multiple hypoechoic tubules, with the interfaces between them responsible for the overall echogenicity of the nerve (see Fig. 26-20B).[16]

In the palm, the pairs of FDP and FDS tendons are clearly identified. On longitudinal scans, the play of the tendons of a given finger is appreciated in real-time

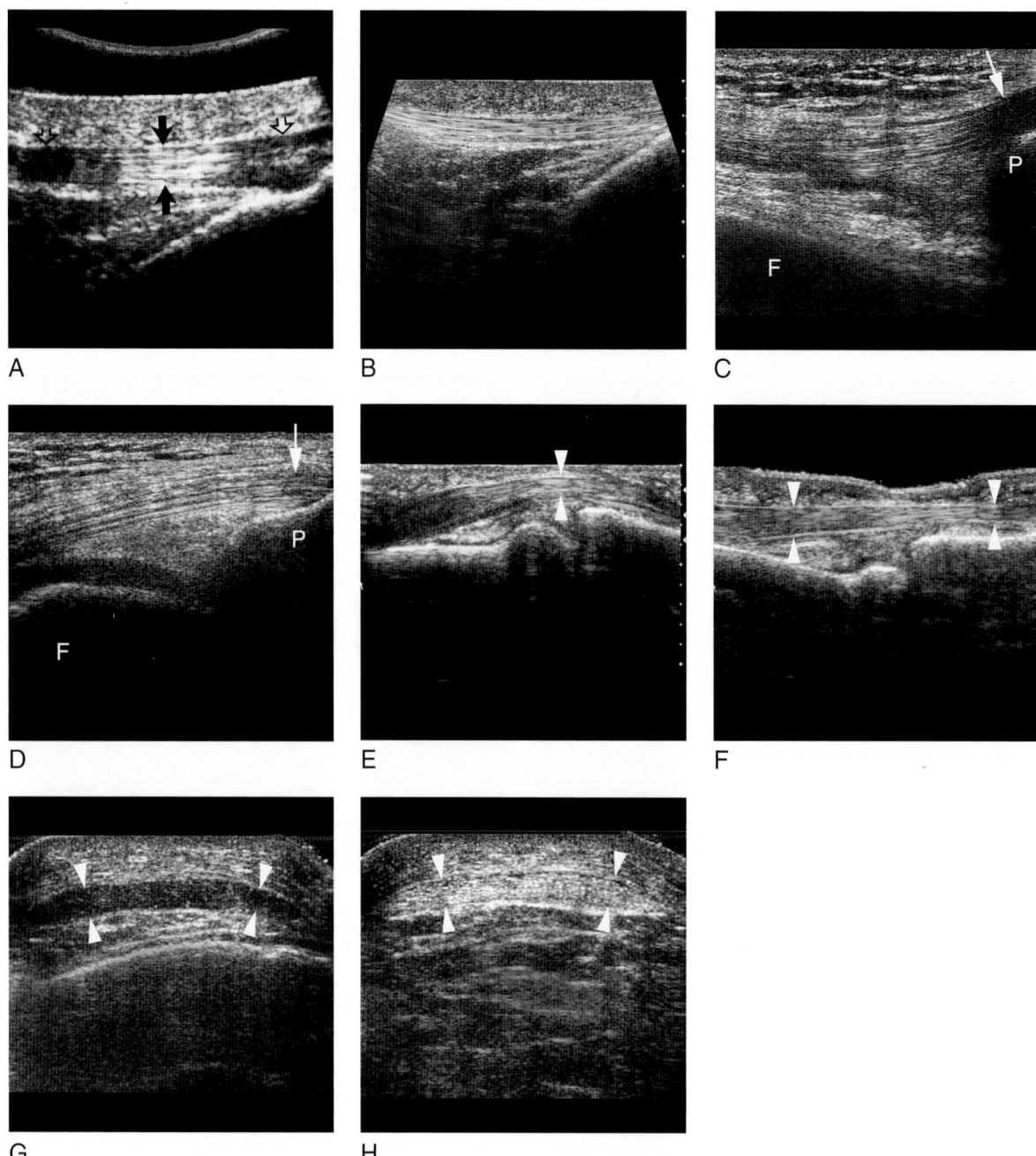

FIGURE 26-16. Spectrum of appearances of false hypoechogenicity due to the anisotropic property of tendons. A, Longitudinal scan of the distal patellar tendon obtained with a 10-MHz curved-array sector transducer. The tendon exhibits normal echogenicity (*arrows*) only in the narrow midportion of the scan, where the beam is perpendicular to the tendon. On either side, the obliquity of the beam is responsible for the artifactual hypoechogenicity (*open arrows*) of the tendon. **B,** Longitudinal sonogram of the patellar tendon obtained using the trapezoidal format (electronic beam steering) of a linear-array transducer. The beam is perpendicular to the tendon fibers along the entire tendon, resulting in the correct display of the tendon's echogenicity. **C, D,** Longitudinal sonograms of the quadriceps tendon. **C,** Sonogram obtained with the knee extended and the quadriceps relaxed shows the false hypoechogenicity of the patellar insertion (*arrow*). **D,** Sonogram obtained with the knee flexed and the quadriceps tendon straightened shows normal echogenicity at the patellar insertion (*arrow*). F, femur; P, patella. **E, F,** Longitudinal sonograms of the flexor tendons of the third finger at the proximal interphalangeal joint. **E,** With the finger fully extended, the flexor tendons are curved and exhibit their normal echogenicity only in the midportion of the scan (*arrowheads*). **F,** Moderate flexion of the joint straightens the tendons, which now display their normal echogenicity along their entire course (*arrowheads*). **G, H,** Transverse sonograms of the patellar tendon. **G,** The scan plane is not strictly perpendicular to the tendon's axis, which results in artifactual hypoechogenicity (*arrowheads*). **H,** When the scan plane is strictly perpendicular to the tendon, normal echogenicity is displayed (*arrowheads*).

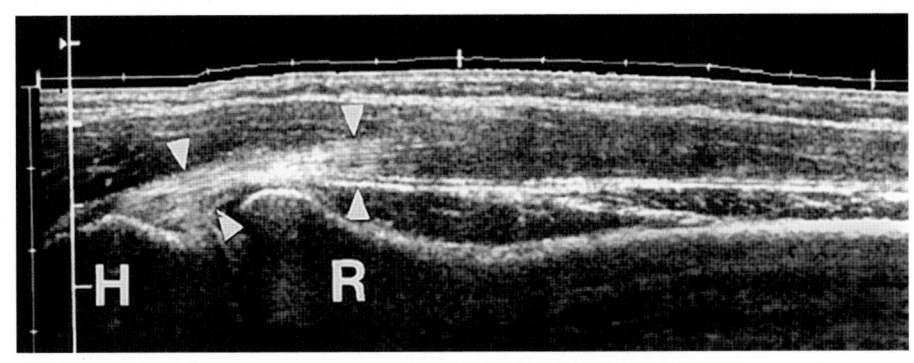

FIGURE 26-17. Normal extensor tendon at elbow. Coronal extended-field-of-view sonogram of the lateral aspect of the elbow shows the normal echogenic common tendon of the extensor muscles of the forearm (*arrowheads*) inserting into the lateral epicondyle. H, humerus; R, radius.

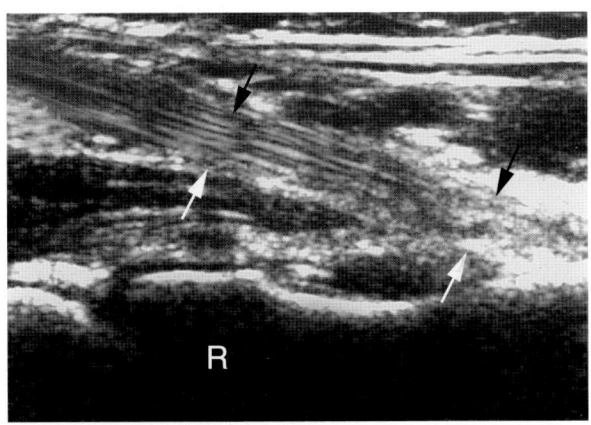

FIGURE 26-18. Normal biceps tendon at elbow. Longitudinal sonogram of the anterior aspect of the extended elbow shows the oblique biceps tendon (*arrows*) inserting into the radial tuberosity. R, radial head.

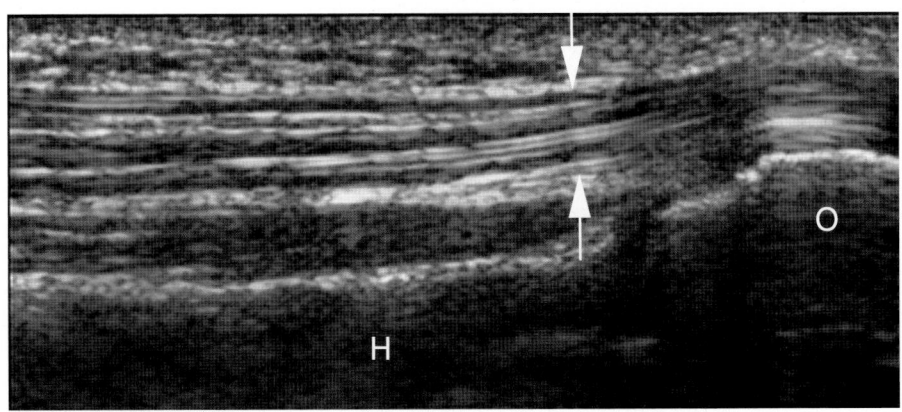

FIGURE 26-19. Normal triceps tendon at elbow. Longitudinal sonogram of the posterior aspect of the flexed elbow shows the tendon of the triceps (*arrows*). H, humerus; O, olecranon.

during flexion and extension of that finger. On transverse scans, the pairs of FDP and FDS tendons appear as rounded echogenic structures adjacent to the corresponding hypoechoic lumbrical muscles (Fig. 26-21). In the fingers, the flexor tendons follow the concavity of the phalanges and therefore are affected by the anisotropy artifact along most of their course, with the exception of the segments that are strictly perpendicular to the ultrasound beam (see Figs. 26-9 and 26-16E, F).[17,18]

Some of the fibrous sheaths (pulleys) that maintain the flexor tendons in place and prevent them from bowstringing during flexion of the finger can be visualized on very high-frequency sagittal sonograms as a barely visible hypoechoic focal thickening of the anterior margin of the flexor tendons (Fig. 26-22). In a cadaver study, sonography demonstrated the A2 (proximal phalanx) pulley in 100% of cases with a mean length of 16 mm and the A4 (middle phalanx) pulley in 67% of cases with a mean length of 6 mm.[19] Transverse sonograms of the fingers at the level of the first phalanx can demonstrate the passage of the rounded FDP tendon, which inserts into the base of the distal phalanx, through the splitting of the FDS tendon, which inserts into the middle phalanx (Fig. 26-23).

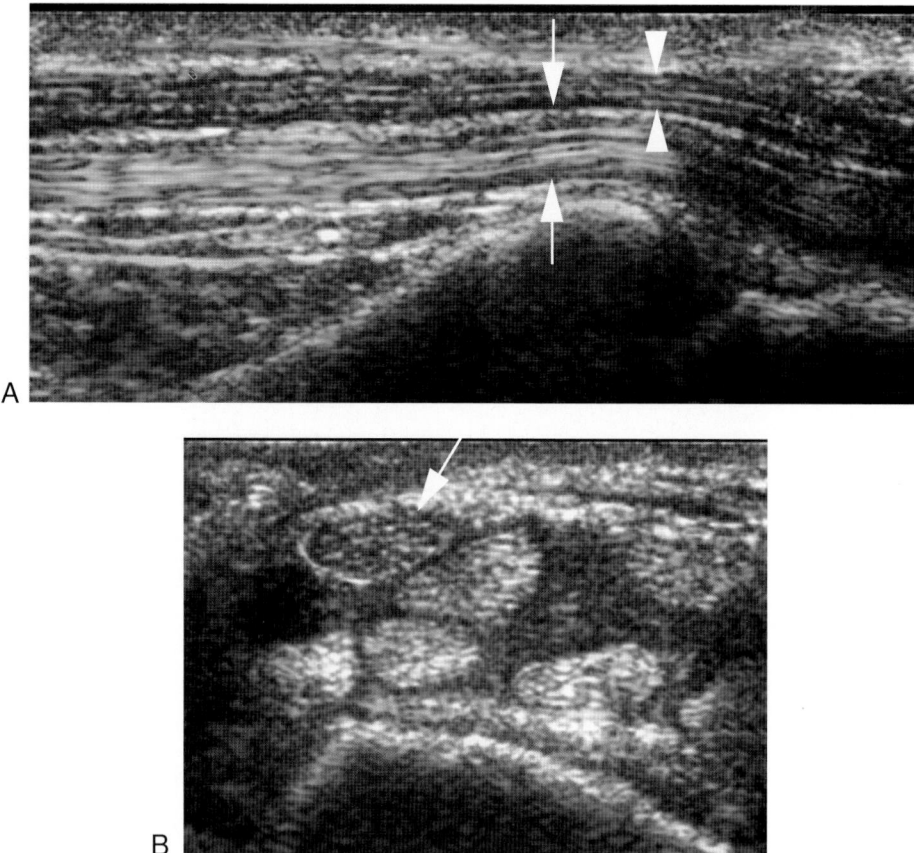

FIGURE 26-20. Flexor tendons of the fingers in the wrist. **A**, Longitudinal sonogram of the volar aspect of the wrist shows the median nerve (*arrowheads*) coursing anterior to the flexor tendons (*arrows*) of the index finger. Note the higher echogenicity of the tendons compared with that of the nerve. **B**, Transverse sonogram of the wrist in moderate flexion shows the echogenic cross sections of the superficial and deep flexor tendons of the fingers in the hypoechoic ulnar bursa. The arrow points to the oval section of the median nerve.

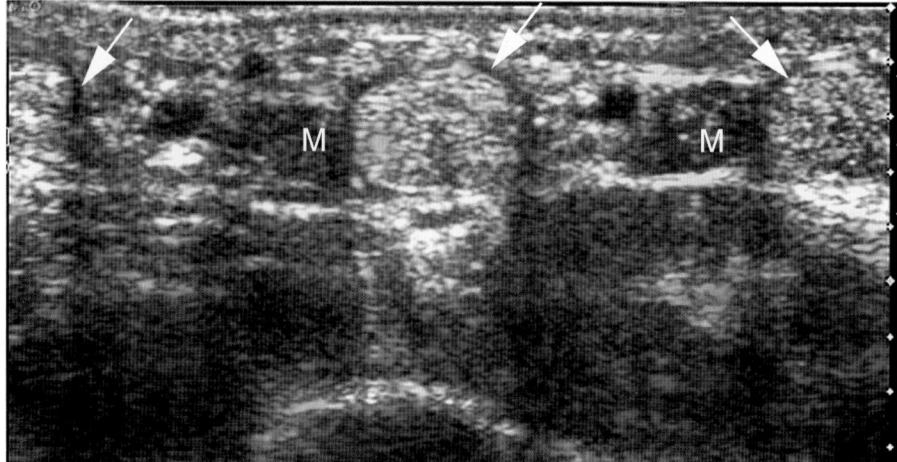

FIGURE 26-21. Normal flexor tendons of fingers. Transverse sonogram of the palm shows the normal echogenic rounded pairs of superficial and deep flexor tendons of the second, third, and fourth fingers (*arrows*) adjacent to the hypoechoic lumbrical muscles (M).

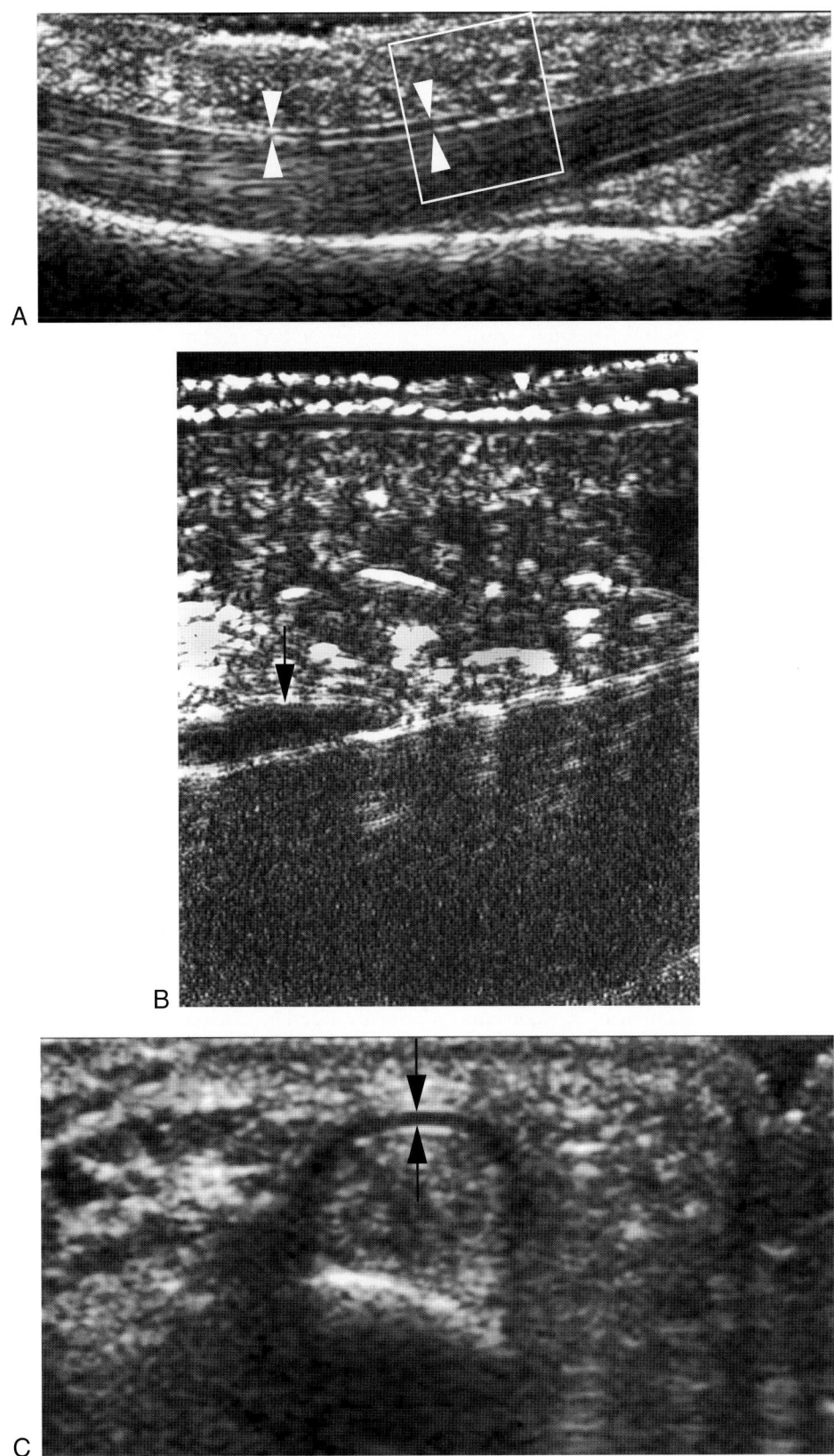

FIGURE 26-22. Tendon pulleys in the first and second phalanges of the third finger. A, Longitudinal sonogram of the first phalanx of the third finger shows the pulley as a very thin (inframillimetric) hypoechoic band of tissue (*arrowheads*) anterior to the flexor tendons. **B**, Longitudinal sonogram of the region indicated with a box on image **A**, obtained at 20 MHz, shows the distal end of the pulley (*arrow*). **C**, Transverse sonogram shows the hypoechoic pulley (*arrows*).

Knee

Sonography is an excellent technique with which to visualize the extensor tendons of the knee.[20,21] Because both the quadriceps and patellar tendons may be slightly concave anteriorly when the knee is extended and the quadriceps relaxed, scans should be obtained during contraction of the quadriceps muscle or with the knee flexed, which straightens the tendons and eliminates the anisotropy-related artifacts (see Fig. 26-16).

The **quadriceps tendon** comprises four tendons (those of the rectus femoris, vastus lateralis, vastus medialis, and vastus intermedius muscles), which are not usually distinguished sonographically as separate structures. The quadriceps tendon lies beneath the subcutaneous fat and anterior to a fat pad and the collapsed suprapatellar bursa (Fig. 26-24). On transverse scans, the quadriceps tendon is oval.

The **patellar tendon** extends from the patella to the tibial tuberosity over a length of 5 to 6 cm (Fig. 26-25A). On transverse sections, the patellar tendon has a convex anterior and a flat posterior surface (see Fig. 26-25B). At its midportion, the tendon is about 4 to 5 mm thick and 20 to 25 mm wide.[21] The subcutaneous prepatellar and infrapatellar bursae are not normally visible, but the deep infrapatellar bursa may appear as a flattened anechoic structure 2 to 3 mm thick (see Fig. 26-15).

Sonography has been used in the evaluation of **collateral ligaments** of the knee and the iliotibial band.[22,23] Normal ligaments are not always easily delineated from the articular capsule and the surrounding subcutaneous fatty tissues. In chronic injury of the medial collateral ligament, sonography can readily demonstrate calcifications within a thickened hypoechoic ligament; this is known as Pellegrini-Stieda disease.[24] A few reports have claimed good results in the evaluation of the **cruciate ligaments**.[25,26] However, sonographic examination of these ligaments is limited by the fact that it is virtually impossible to scan them otherwise than obliquely—which results in an artifactual hypoechoic appearance. It is therefore difficult to evaluate them for anything other than gross rupture. As a rule, the cruciate ligaments are better assessed with MRI.

Foot and Ankle

The **Achilles tendon** is formed by the fusion of the aponeuroses of the soleus and gastrocnemius muscles, and it inserts into the posterior surface of the calcaneus. The Achilles tendon is echogenic and exhibits a characteristic fibrillar texture on longitudinal scans.[27] The termination of the hypoechoic soleus muscle is easily identified anterior to the origin of the tendon (Fig. 26-26). The fatty Kager's triangle, which lies anterior to the distal half of the tendon, is usually echogenic but may show some variation in echogenicity from person to person. More anteriorly lie the hypoechoic flexor hallucis longus muscle and the echogenic posterior surface of the tibia. The small, flattened, hypoechoic retrocalcaneal bursa is sometimes seen in the angle formed by the tendon and the calcaneus. The tendon fibers at the bony insertion have a short, oblique course that causes their artifactual hypoechogenicity (see Fig. 26-26C); this appearance should not be mistaken for the subcutaneous calcaneal bursa, which is not normally seen. A recent sonographic study of the Achilles tendon performed at 10 and 15 MHz revealed the presence of two tendinous portions of different echogenicity representing the portions arising from the soleus and gastrocnemius muscles.[28]

On transverse sonograms, the cross section of the Achilles tendon is grossly elliptical and tapers medially. The tendon plane is remarkable in that instead of being strictly coronal, it is slanted anteriorly and medially (Fig. 26-27). Because of this configuration, there is a risk of overestimating the thickness of the tendon on strictly sagittal scans, and measurements should therefore be taken from transverse scans. At 2 to 3 cm superior to its insertion, the Achilles tendon is 5 to 7 mm thick and 12 to 15 mm wide.[27] A correlation has been found between the tendon's thickness and the subject's height.[29] Results of another study showed that the Achilles tendon is wider in athletes than in control subjects and suggested that long-term physical training results in tendon enlargement.

In the ankle, sonography readily demonstrates the tendons of the peroneus longus and brevis muscles laterally and of the tibialis posterior muscle medially. The tendons of the flexor digitorum longus and flexor hallucis longus muscles can also be identified posterior to the medial malleolus, whereas the tendons of the tibialis anterior, extensor hallucis longus, and extensor digitorum longus muscles are seen at the anterior aspect of the ankle joint. Dynamic examination during specific flexion and extension maneuvers of the ankle and foot helps to identify individual tendons. The ankle tendons are enveloped in synovial sheaths. In a recent study in the ankles of asymptomatic volunteers, a small amount of fluid was found in the posterior tibial and common peroneal tendon sheaths in 71% and 12%, respectively.[30] In the foot, the examination technique and normal sonographic appearance of the flexor and extensor tendons of the toes do not differ significantly from those of the tendons of the fingers.[18]

PATHOLOGY

Tendon disorders result most often from trauma (tears), noninflammatory degenerative conditions now grouped under the term **tendinosis**, and inflammatory conditions (tendinitis and peritendinitis). It is currently

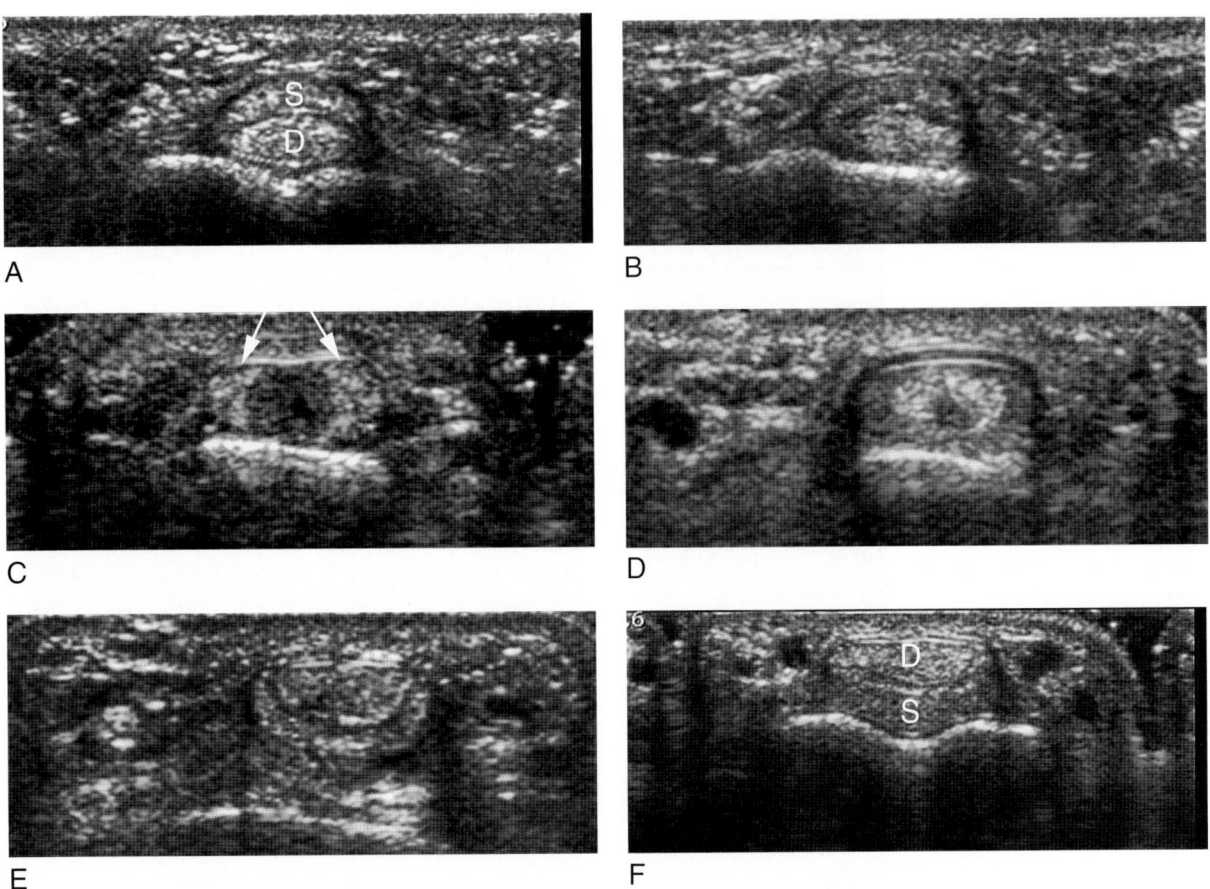

FIGURE 26-23. Relationships between the superficial and deep flexor tendons of fingers. Transverse sonograms at different levels of the first phalanx of the third finger from the base to the proximal interphalangeal joint. **A,** Transverse sonogram at the base of the first phalanx shows the superficial tendon (S) above the deep tendon (D). **B,** The superficial tendon becomes thinner and spreads laterally. **C,** The superficial tendon has split in half (*arrows*), seen on each side of the round, deep tendon, which appears hypoechoic on this scan due to anisotropy. **D,** The two halves of the superficial tendon have reunited behind the deep tendon. **E,** The superficial tendon now has the shape of a cup containing the deep tendon, which is now superficial. **F,** Transverse sonogram obtained at the level of the base of the middle phalanx shows the deep tendon (D) lying anterior to the superficial one (S).

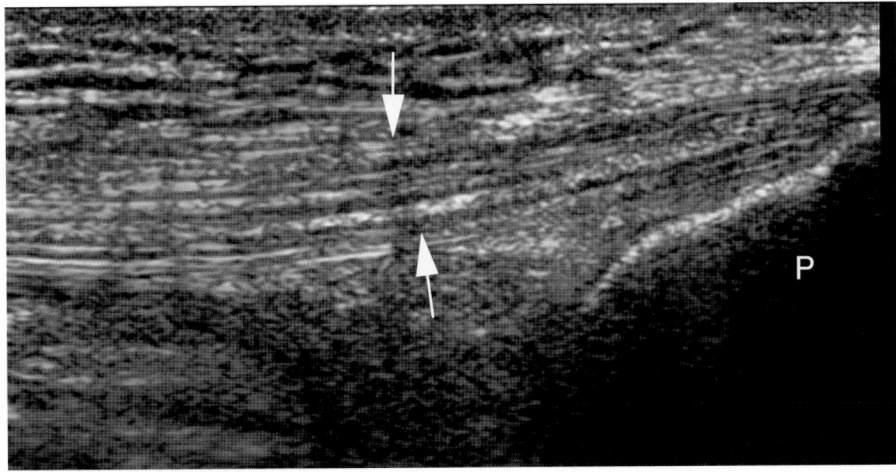

FIGURE 26-24. Normal quadriceps tendon. Longitudinal scan shows the echogenic tendon (*arrows*) surrounded by fat. P, patella.

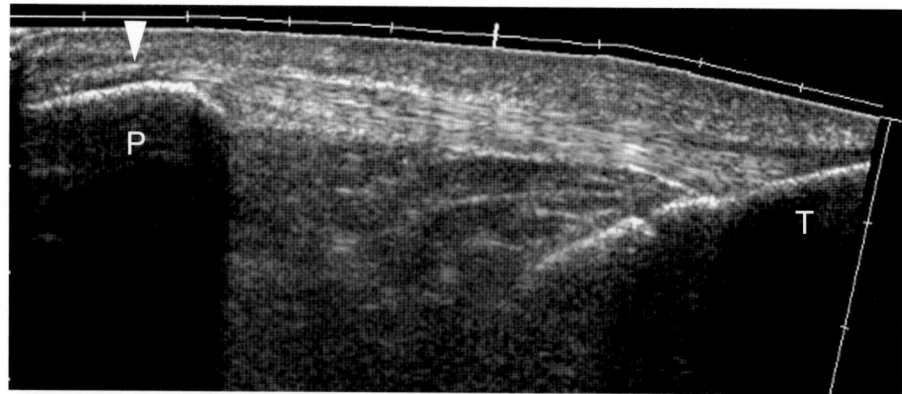

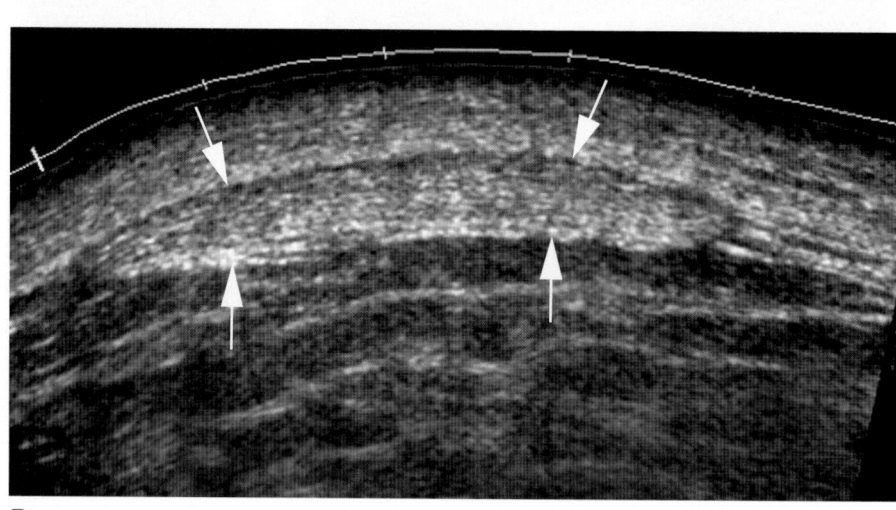

FIGURE 26-25. Normal patellar tendon. A, Longitudinal extended-field-of-view sonogram shows the tendon from its insertion into the patella (P) to its termination into the anterior tibial tuberosity. Note the prepatellar fibers (*arrowhead*). T, tibia. **B,** Transverse sonogram shows the convex anterior and flat posterior surfaces (*arrows*).

SONOGRAPHIC SIGNS OF TENDON TEARS

Discontinuity of fibers (partial or complete)
Focal thinning of the tendon
Hematoma of variable size, usually small
Bone fragment in case of bone avulsion
Nonvisualization of the retracted tendon in case of complete tear

acknowledged that most tendon ruptures represent the final stage of progressive destruction of the fibrils.

Tears

Tears usually occur in tendons that have been rendered fragile by such factors as aging, presence of calcifications, general or local corticosteroid therapy, and underlying systemic diseases (e.g., rheumatoid arthritis, seronegative spondyloarthropathies, lupus erythematosus, diabetes mellitus, and gout).[31-34] In the absence of predisposing factors, biopsy specimens taken from the vicinity of the rupture site often demonstrate degenerative changes, now referred to as tendinosis (see later).

Complete Tears

Tears resulting from direct trauma to the tendons (e.g., lacerations) are rare. The vast majority of **complete tears** result from excessive tension applied to the tendon or from normal tension applied in a movement performed in abnormal conditions. Recent **complete tendon tears** are often correctly diagnosed clinically, but if physical examination is delayed, the diagnosis may be indeterminate because of inflammatory changes. Sonography can show the full-thickness discontinuity of the tendon. The gap between the torn tendon fragments is filled with hypoechoic hemorrhagic fluid (or clot) or granulomatous tissue, depending on the age of the lesion (Fig. 26-28). The gap varies in length, and when the torn fragments are separated by a long distance, the tendon may not be visualized at all. This nonvisualization may occur in complete ruptures of the rotator cuff, biceps brachii tendon, and flexor tendons of the fingers.[35] With the

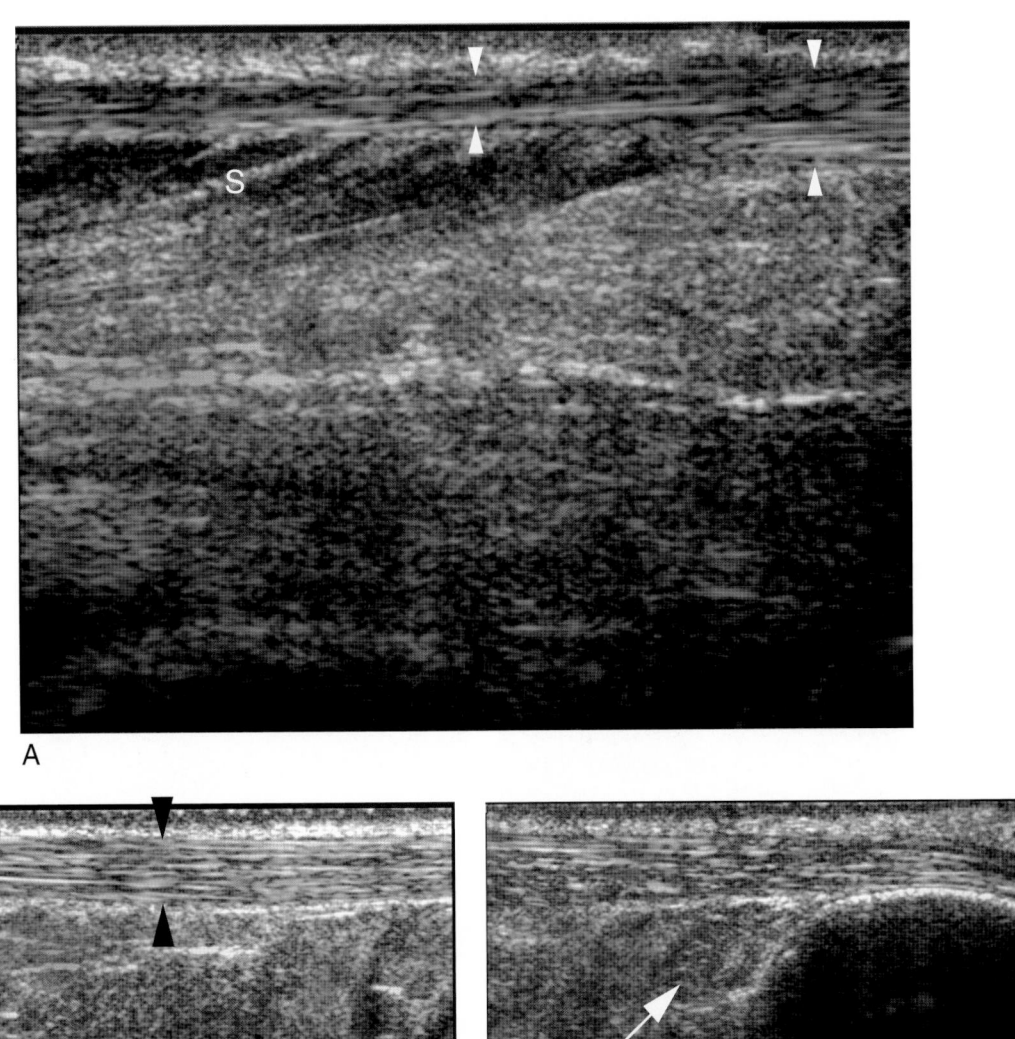

FIGURE 26-26. Normal Achilles tendon. **A**, Longitudinal sonogram of the origin of the tendon (*arrowheads*) shows the termination of the muscular fibers of the soleus muscle (S) that connect to the tendon. **B**, Longitudinal sonogram of the midportion of the tendon (*arrowheads*) shows its typical fibrillar echotexture. **C**, Longitudinal sonogram of the termination of the tendon shows the small retrocalcaneal bursa (*arrow*) with no fluid.

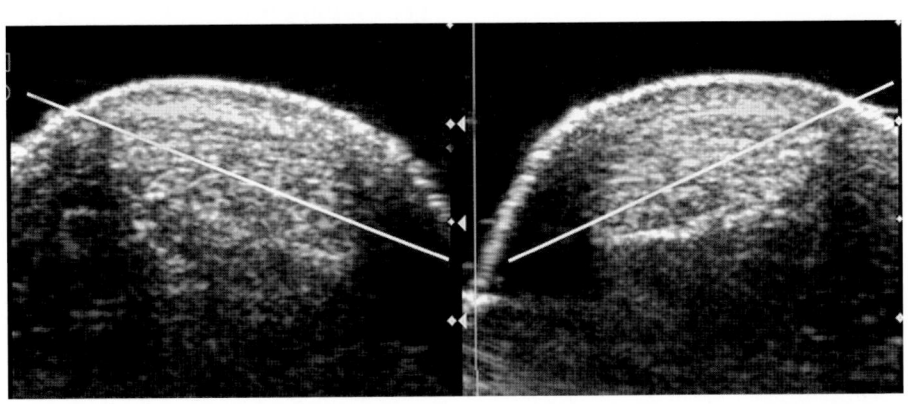

FIGURE 26-27. Both normal Achilles tendons. Transverse sonograms of the same subject show the oblique orientation (*white lines*) of the planes of the left (**A**) and right (**B**) tendons.

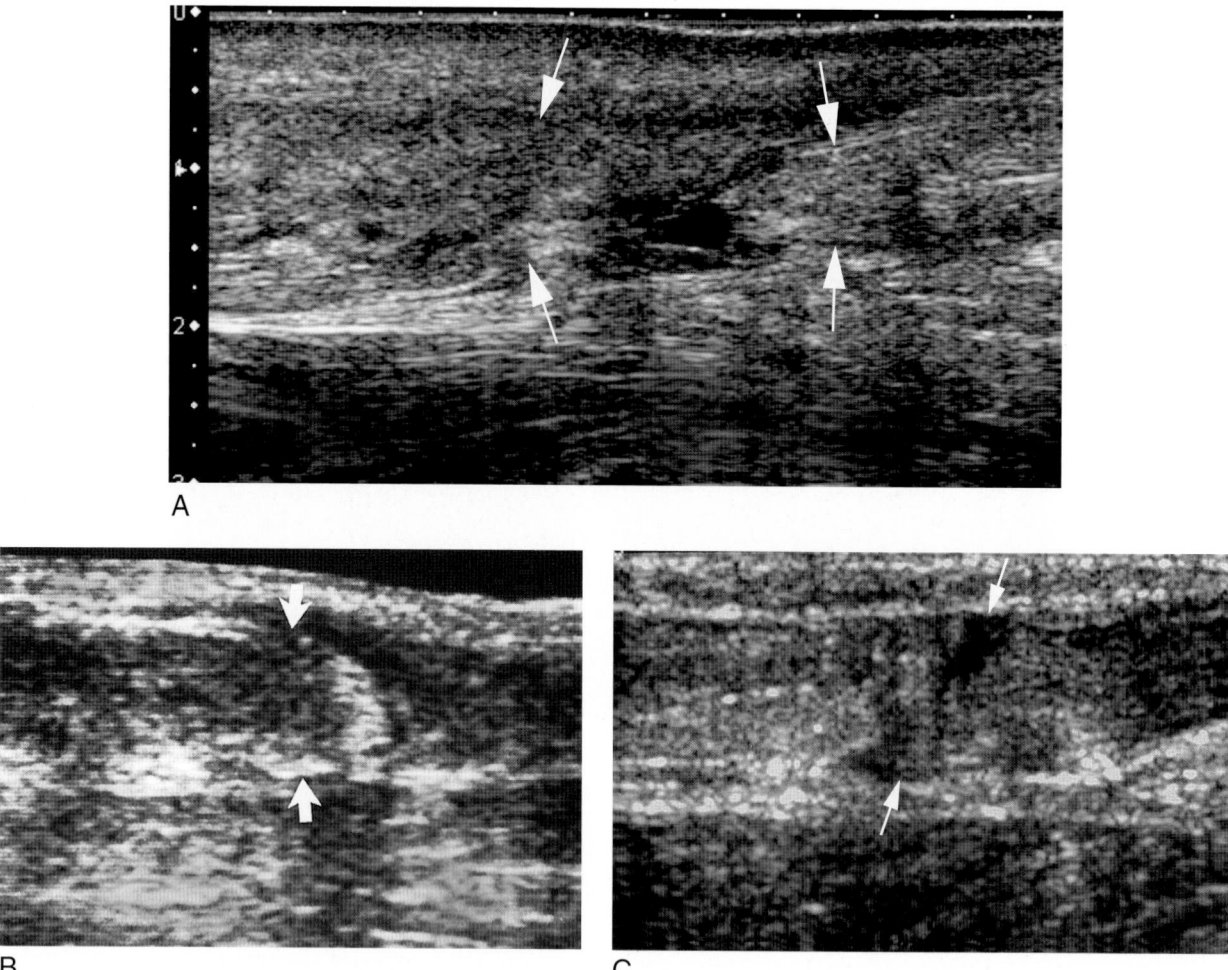

FIGURE 26-28. Complete ruptures involving the middle third of the Achilles tendon. A, Longitudinal sonogram shows the gap between the two ends (*arrows*) of the torn tendon, which is filled with echogenic tissue and a minimal amount of fluid. **B**, Longitudinal sonogram shows the retracted, swollen upper fragment (*arrows*) surrounded by organizing hematoma. **C**, Longitudinal sonogram shows the discontinuity of the tendon fibers (*arrows*).

exception of ruptures of the Achilles tendon, in which a hematoma can develop around the whole tendon, ruptures are usually associated with minimal focal hemorrhage. In the case of avulsion of the tendon from the bone, one or more bone fragments may appear as bright echogenic foci with acoustic shadowing.[36]

Incomplete Tears

Accurate sonographic diagnosis of an incomplete tear is important because early diagnosis and treatment will prevent a subsequent complete rupture. However, **partial tears** are difficult to diagnose clinically and to differentiate from focal areas of tendinosis or tendinitis.

Sonographically, recent partial ruptures appear as focal hypoechoic defects with discontinuity of the fibrillar pattern either within the tendon or at its attachment (Fig. 26-29).[14,37,38] A focal irregularity at the tendon's surface may be the only sign of a small partial

tear. A partial rupture may also appear as only a focal thinning of the tendon, such as may be seen in the rotator cuff. Special mention must be made of **intrasubstance tears or splits**, which often occur in the ankle tendons and appear as longitudinal hypoechoic clefts (see Fig. 26-29C).[39] Subtle sonographic findings may become more apparent on dynamic examination of the tendon during active or passive flexion-extension movements of the associated muscle(s). Three-dimensional evaluation of partial ruptures requires a combination of longitudinal and transverse scans. Indirect signs of tendon rupture include effusion in the tendon sheath or thickening of an adjacent bursa.

A sensitivity of 94% has been reported for sonography in the diagnosis of partial tears of the Achilles tendon.[37] Other studies have reported the superiority of MRI over sonography in the diagnosis of incomplete Achilles tendon tears.[40,41] Although sonography is generally a reliable method for diagnosing complete tears of the

Achilles tendon, it is acknowledged that its use is limited in differentiating between partial ruptures or even micro-ruptures and focal areas of tendinosis.[42] In the knee, when the patellar tendon is partially detached from the patellar apex, longitudinal scans show the discontinuity of the tendon fibers, whereas transverse scans obtained inferior to the patellar apex demonstrate the round defect in the midline of the tendon (see Fig. 26-29B). This may be indistinguishable from classic lesions of tendinosis (e.g., jumper's knee) at the upper insertion of the tendon.

Tendinosis

The recently coined term tendinosis is used to describe degenerative changes in a tendon without clinical or histopathologic signs of inflammation within the tendon or paratenon. Most often, it is associated with painful focal or diffuse nodular thickening of the tendon. Tendinosis has been mainly described in the patellar tendon (jumper's knee) and the Achilles tendon (achillodynia). There is a strong relationship between tendinosis and the repetitive microtrauma of overuse injuries. The normal process of age-related degeneration is probably accelerated with increased stress to or decreased resistance of the tendon; this is particularly obvious in sports-related injuries.

A wide range of histopathologic changes has been described, including degenerative changes (mucoid and hyalin degeneration, fibrinoid necrosis, and microcysts), regeneration (neovascularization and granulation tissue), and microtears, but a constant finding is the absence

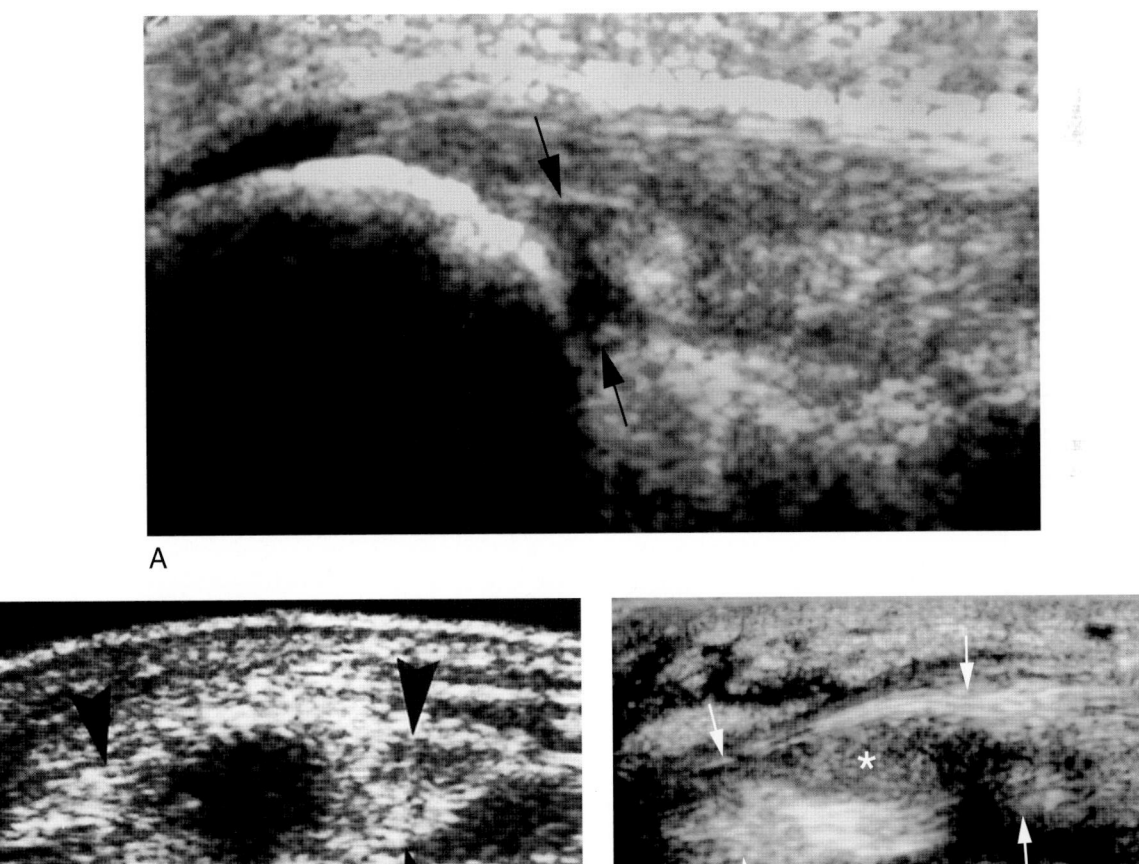

A

B

C

FIGURE 26-29. Partial tendon tears. A, Partial rupture of the patellar tendon at its insertion into the patella. Longitudinal sonogram shows the partial detachment from the patella of the deep fibers of the tendon with a small anechoic hematoma (*arrows*). B, Partial detachment of the superior portion of the patellar tendon. Transverse scan shows a well-defined, round, hypoechoic midline hematoma (*arrow*). The *arrowheads* indicate the tendon's margins. C, Posterior tibial tendon split. Coronal sonogram of the ankle shows the central split (*) separating the tendon's fibers (*arrows*).

of inflammatory cells. However, the clinical distinction between tendinosis and tendinitis is not always possible.

Sonographically, the lesions of tendinosis appear as focal or diffuse areas of markedly decreased echogenicity and tendon enlargement. In the Achilles tendon, the lesions preferentially involve the middle third of the tendon, whereas in the patellar tendon, the lesions are most often located at the upper insertion of the tendon. In both locations, however, the tendon can be diffusely swollen and hypoechoic. Color (power) Doppler imaging shows increased vascularity, usually from the deep surface of the upper patellar tendon and from the deep surface of the distal Achilles tendon (Fig. 26-30). Sonography of the patellar tendon has been shown to detect hypoechoic focal lesions consistent with tendinosis in 14% of asymptomatic athletes with no previous history of jumper's knee.[43] The significance of these abnormalities in asymptomatic athletes remains unclear. In a group of basketball players, it was shown that hypoechoic areas in the patellar tendon can resolve, remain unchanged, or expand without predicting symptoms of jumper's knee.[44] In contrast, in a study of asymptomatic elite soccer players that had revealed the

presence of sonographic abnormalities in 18% of the patellar tendons and 11% of the Achilles tendons, those players with abnormal patellar tendons had a 17% increased risk of developing symptomatic jumper's knee during the 12-month season, whereas those with abnormal Achilles tendons had a 45% increased risk of developing Achilles tendinosis.[45] Early detection of occult tendinosis should prompt adequate treatment to prevent chronic, therapy-resistant symptoms and subsequent tendon ruptures.

Recently, a color Doppler study of Achilles tendinosis has confirmed the presence of vessels not only outside, but also inside the thickened Achilles tendon, mostly in the ventral portion of the tendon; ultrasound-guided sclerosis of these vessels has been attempted in the treatment of painful chronic Achilles tendinosis.[5,46]

Inflammation

Edema associated with inflammation is responsible for the thickening and decreased echogenicity of the tendons, synovial sheath, or paratenon involved. The increased vascularity associated with inflammation can

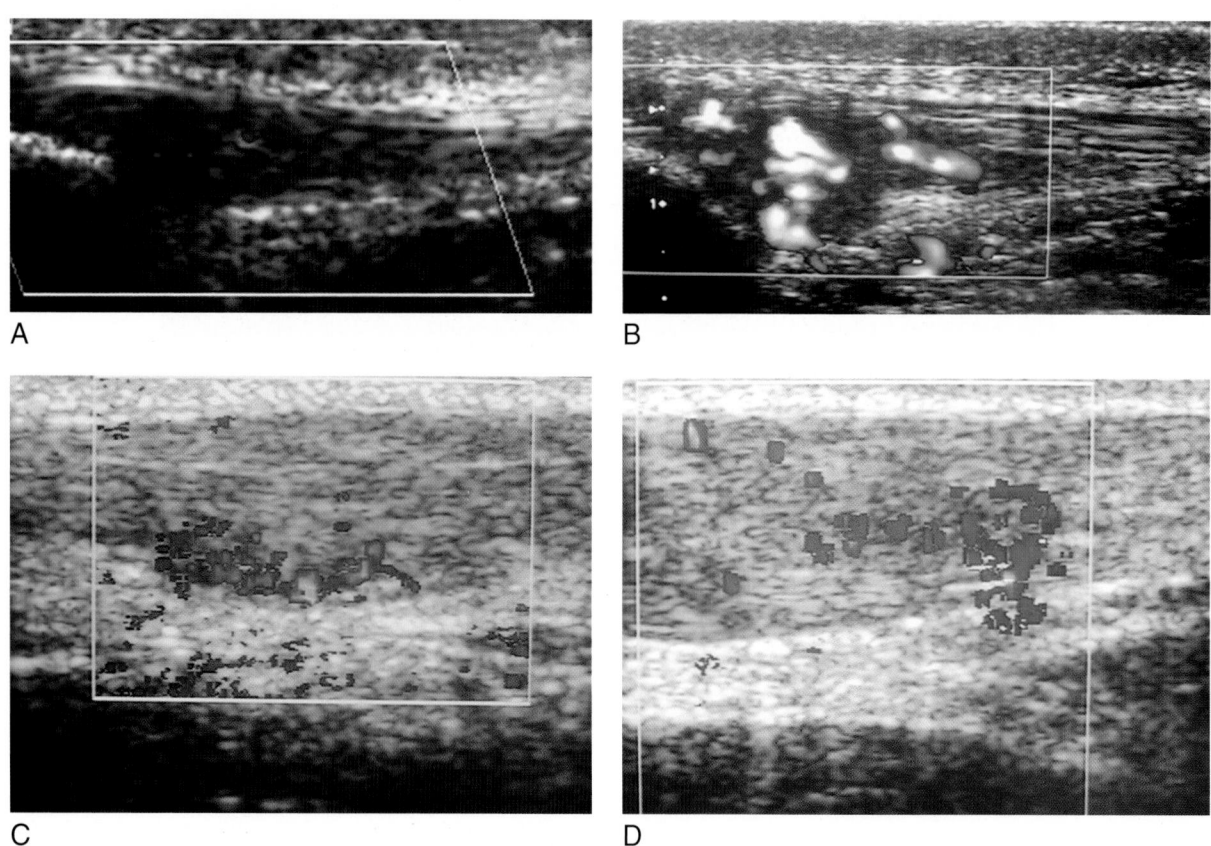

FIGURE 26-30. Tendinosis. A, B, Jumper's knee. Longitudinal color (**A**) and power (**B**) Doppler sonograms show the hypoechoic thickening of the upper third of the patellar tendon with associated hypervascularity. **C** and **D, Achillodynia.** Longitudinal sonograms of the Achilles tendon show thickening and decreased echogenicity of the tendon with a minimal, but unequivocal, increase in vascularity at the deep surface of the tendon.

be depicted with power Doppler imaging.[47,48] When objective quantification of hypervascularity on color Doppler imaging becomes routinely available, it will permit follow-up of patients with inflammatory lesions and documentation of the response to therapy.[49]

Tendinitis

Tendinitis, like tendinosis, can be associated with athletic or occupational activities, but on pathologic examination, there is evidence of acute inflammation, often in addition to preexisting degenerative changes of tendinosis. Tendinitis may affect the whole tendon or only part of it. For example, in the patellar tendon, focal tendinitis, like tendinosis, often involves the upper insertion of the tendon, whereas focal involvement of the distal insertion typically occurs after transposition of the tibial tuberosity.

Sonographically, in **acute tendinitis**, the tendon is thickened and the margins are often ill defined. There is also a diffuse decrease in echogenicity.[21,27] Because improper scanning may result in a falsely hypoechoic tendon, the examination technique used must be flawless. Power Doppler imaging has become critical in documenting the focal or diffuse increase in vascularity (Fig. 26-31). Comparison with sonograms of the unaffected contralateral tendons is often valuable. The presence of flow in a focal area of markedly decreased echogenicity helps confirm the diagnosis of focal tendinitis and rules out an acute partial tear because blood flow is not expected to be present in the blood-filled cavity resulting from the tear. Color Doppler imaging can also be used to monitor a patient's **response to anti-inflammatory therapy**. A decrease in size of the tendon and a return to a normal level of echogenicity and very low vascularity indicate healing.

In **chronic tendinitis**, the margins of the tendon may be deformed and appear bumpy. High-frequency sonography has proved accurate in the detection of minute intratendinous calcifications, which appear as bright foci with or without acoustic shadowing, occasionally with a comet-tail artifact. As a rule, the size and shape of these calcifications are better appreciated on low-kilovoltage radiographs, preferably obtained with the use of a mammographic unit (Fig. 26-32).[50]

SONOGRAPHIC SIGNS OF TENDINITIS

Thickening of the tendon
Decreased echogenicity
Blurred margins
Increased vascularity on color Doppler imaging
Calcifications in chronic tendinitis

Peritendinitis

In peritendinitis, the inflammation takes place in the paratenon, the layer of connective tissue that wraps around the tendon in the absence of a synovial sheath. This condition is frequently found in the Achilles tendon. Sonographically, peritendinitis is characterized by a hypoechoic thickening of the peritenon, with the tendon remaining grossly unaffected. Because gray-scale sonography is often unable to diagnose mild peritendinitis with sufficient reliability,[42] power Doppler imaging is proving very helpful in documenting the increased vascularity associated with this condition (Fig. 26-33).[47]

Tenosynovitis

Tenosynovitis is defined as the inflammation of a tendon sheath. Any tendon surrounded by a synovial sheath—especially tendons in the hand, wrist, and ankle—can be affected. Trauma, including repetitive microtrauma, and pyogenic infection are most commonly responsible for acute tenosynovitis. Cases of tenosynovitis caused by a foreign body retained within a tendon sheath in the hand have been reported.[51] Sonographically, the diagnosis of acute tenosynovitis is made when fluid, even a minimal quantity, is identified in the sheath (Fig. 26-34).[52,53] Internal echoes representing debris can be seen in suppurative tenosynovitis, a serious condition that, if left untreated, can rapidly destroy the tendon.[54]

Chronic tenosynovitis is characterized by a hypoechoic thickening of the synovial sheath, most often with little or no fluid (Fig. 26-35). The thickening of the sheath may impair the movement of tendons in narrow passages. In **de Quervain's tenosynovitis**, the tendons of the abductor pollicis longus and extensor pollicis brevis muscles are constricted by the thickened sheath in the pulley over the radial styloid process. Sonography can demonstrate the hypoechoic thickening of the tendon sheath (see Fig. 26-35C),[18,55,56] and color Doppler imaging may demonstrate increased vascularity in the tissues involved. Sonography can be used to guide the injection of contrast medium into the sheath for **tenography**, a study that silhouettes the sheath wall but cannot demonstrate its thickness.[57] Sonography has also been used to guide injection of steroids into the synovial sheath of the posterior tibial tendon in patients with chronic inflammatory arthropathy.[58]

Rheumatoid arthritis has a predilection for synovial tissues, including tendon sheaths in the distal extremities. Sonography has proved effective in the diagnosis of **rheumatoid tenosynovitis** in the hand.[59,60] The tendon sheath involved by the **pannus** is markedly hypoechoic, and, occasionally, fluid is also present in the sheath, which enhances the visibility of the pannus (Fig. 26-36). Pannus is an inflammatory granulation tissue that arises

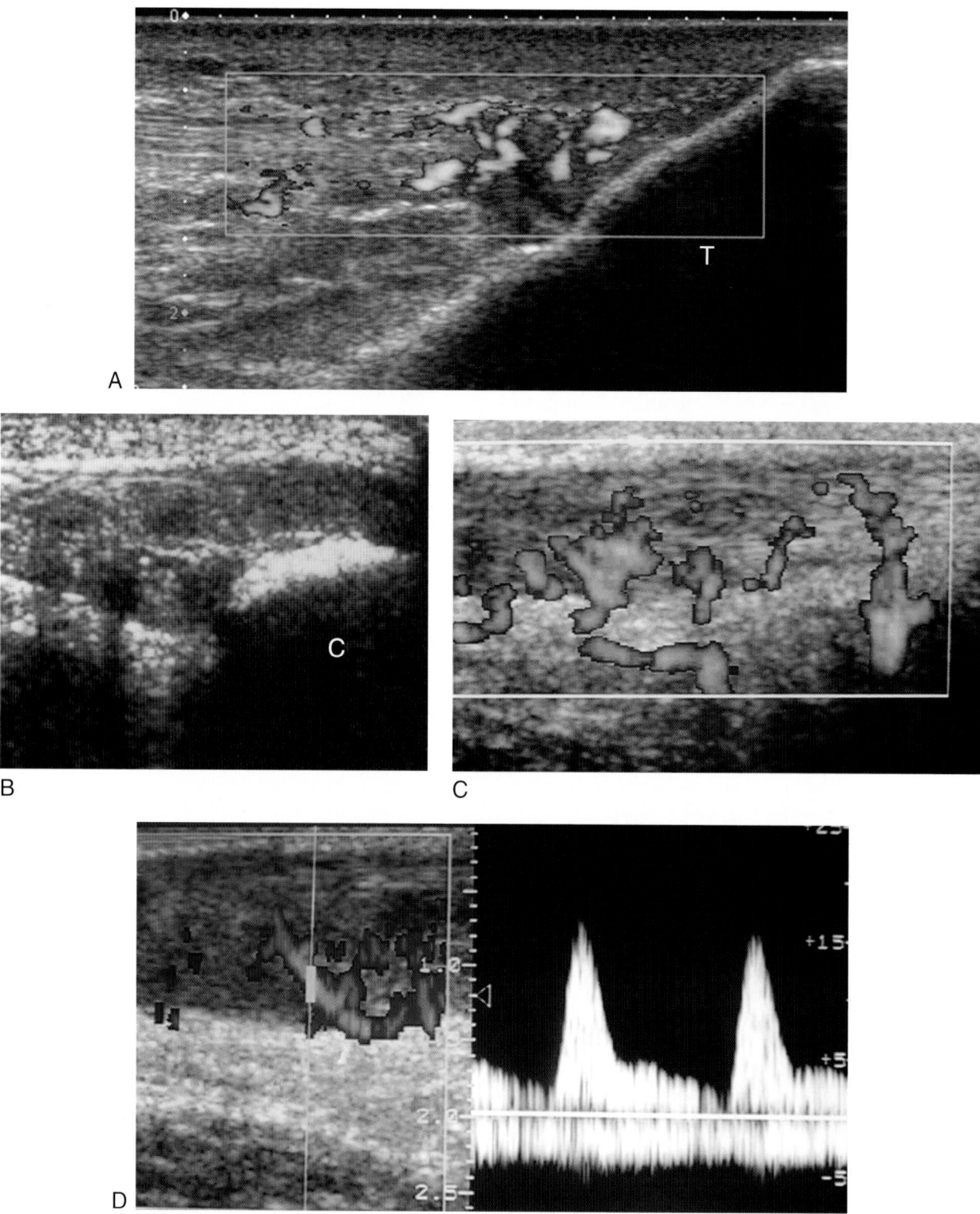

FIGURE 26-31. Tendinitis. A, Tendinitis of the tibial insertion of the patellar tendon. Longitudinal power Doppler sonogram shows the focal area of decreased echogenicity and hypervascularity. T, tibia. **B,** Tendinitis of the distal Achilles tendon. Longitudinal sonogram shows the swelling and decreased echogenicity of the tendon. C, calcaneus. **C, D,** Achilles tendinitis. Longitudinal power and spectral Doppler sonograms show the diffusely swollen and hypoechoic tendons and associated hypervascularity.

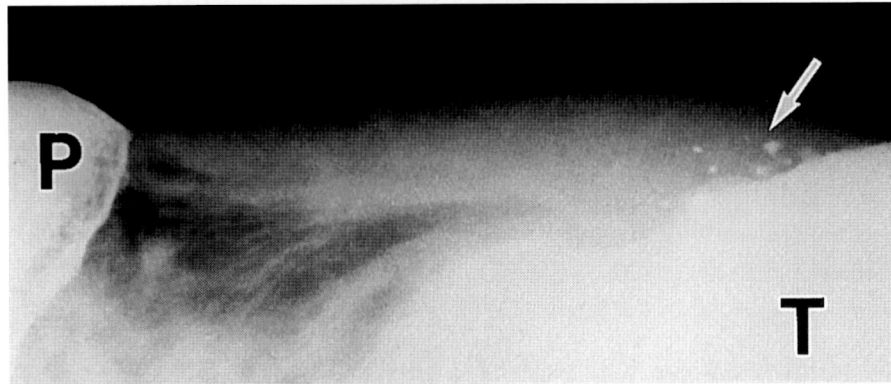

FIGURE 26-32. Chronic calcified patellar tendinitis. A, Longitudinal scan of the lower attachment of the tendon shows a markedly thickened, hypoechoic tendon (*long arrows*) with blurred contours and tiny hyperechoic calcifications (*short arrows*), one with a comet-tail artifact (*arrowhead*). **B,** Lateral low-kilovoltage radiograph obtained with a mammographic unit shows the swollen patellar tendon and the small calcifications (*arrow*). P, patella; T, tibia.

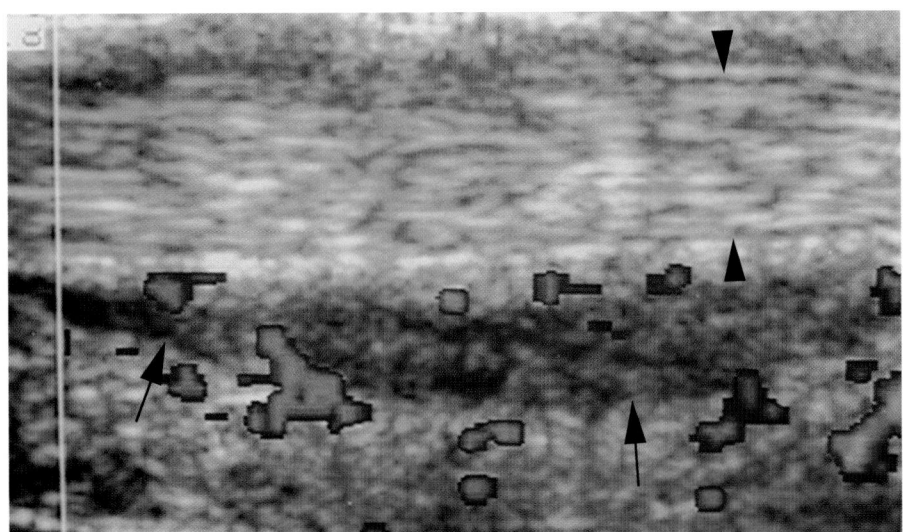

FIGURE 26-33. Peritendinitis of the Achilles tendon. Longitudinal power Doppler sonogram shows the hypoechoic thickening of the paratenon (*arrows*) anterior to the tendon (*arrowheads*) and the associated increased vascularity.

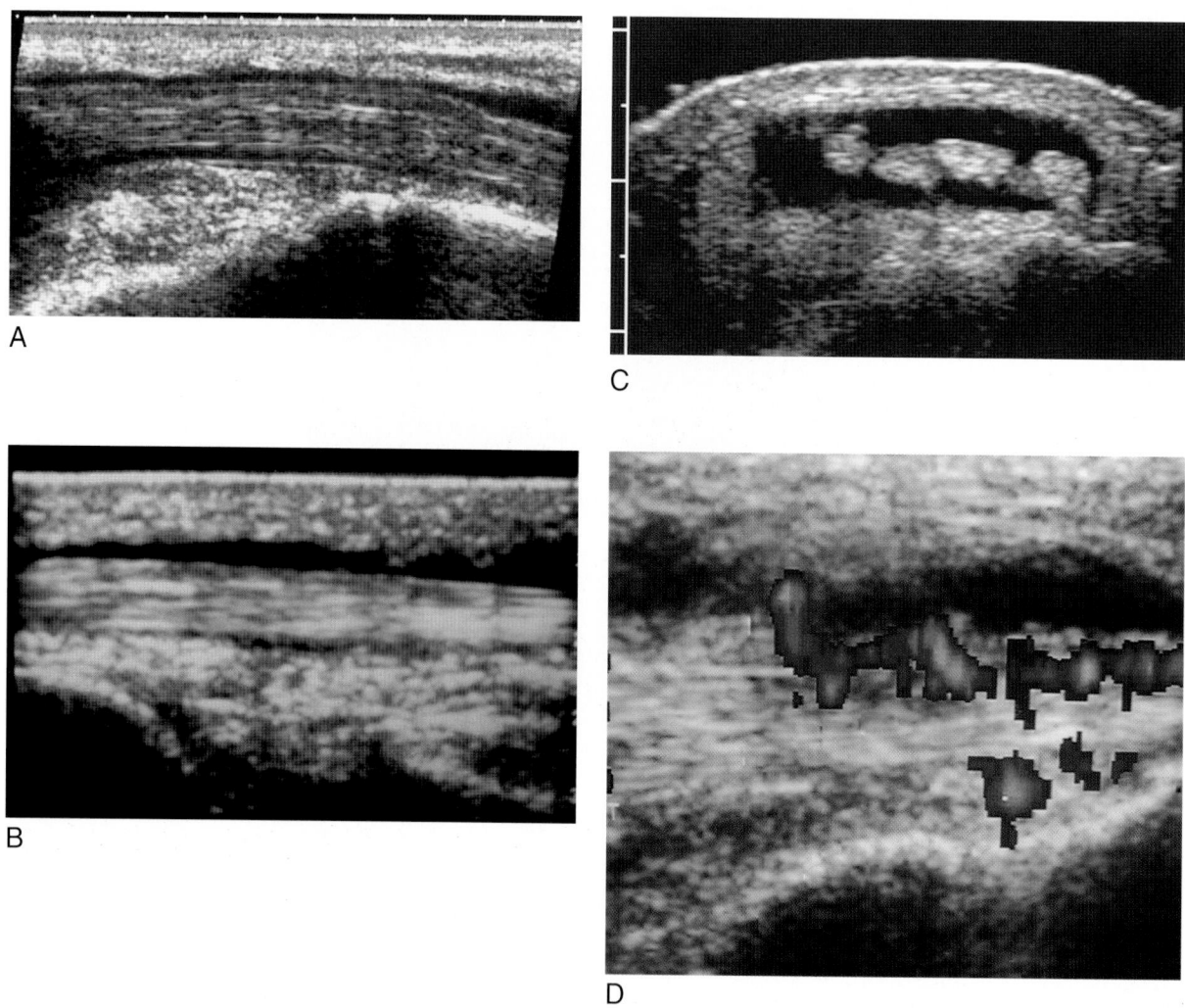

FIGURE 26-34. Acute tenosynovitis. A, Mild tenosynovitis of the posterior tibial tendon at the ankle. Coronal sonogram shows a minimal amount of fluid in the tendon sheath. **B**, Acute tenosynovitis of a flexor digitorum tendon in the hand. **C**, Transverse image of the wrist demonstrates fluid surrounding the flexor tendons. **D**, Tenosynovitis of the peronei tendons. Coronal power Doppler sonogram shows fluid in the synovial sheath and hypervascularity around the tendon.

from the synovial lining. Color Doppler imaging shows significant hypervascularity of the pannus. Sonographic findings of tendon involvement include thickening and inhomogeneity of the tendon whose margins appear jagged.[61] At a later stage, sonography can demonstrate a marked thinning of the tendon or a partial or complete rupture.[62]

Bursitis

Bursitis most often involves the subdeltoid, olecranal, radiohumeral, patellar, and calcaneal bursae. Trauma and, more importantly, repetitive microtrauma are believed to play a major role in bursitis, although no initiating factor can be found in many cases. Prepatellar bursitis is a common finding in subjects who spend extensive periods of time kneeling, such as carpet

layers.[63] It is interesting that transient accumulation of fluid in the subacromial bursa has been demonstrated on sonograms of the shoulder for as long as 16 to 20 hours after handball training.[64] In the early acute stage of bursitis, when the bursa is filled with fluid, sonograms demonstrate a sonolucent, fluid-filled collection with ill-defined margins. In the chronic stage, a complex sonographic appearance with internal echogenic debris results from the presence of granulomatous tissue, precipitated fibrin, and, occasionally, calcification. Power Doppler imaging often shows increased vascularity in the thickened wall of and around the bursa (Fig. 26-37).[65,66] Because the bursa and the adjacent tendon may be involved in the same pathologic process, careful examination of the adjacent tendon is recommended; it has been shown that in 82% of cases of distal-third Achilles tendon tendinosis, retrocalcaneal bursitis was also present.[66]

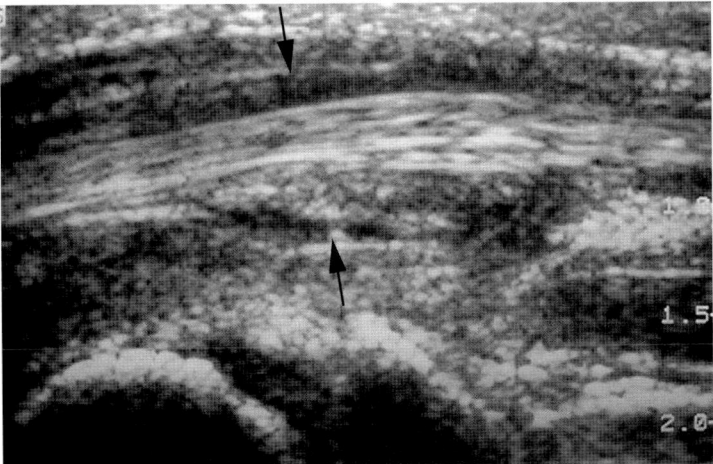

A

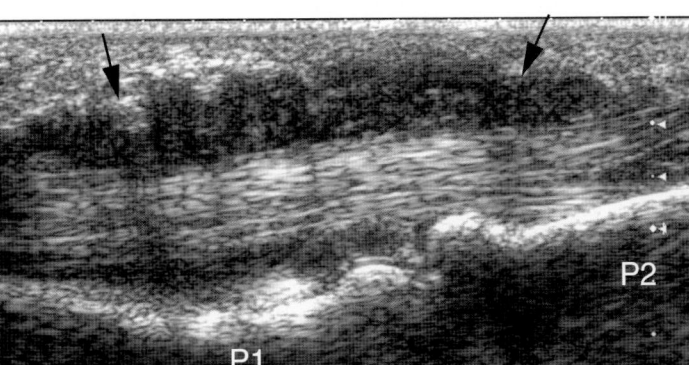

B

P1   P2

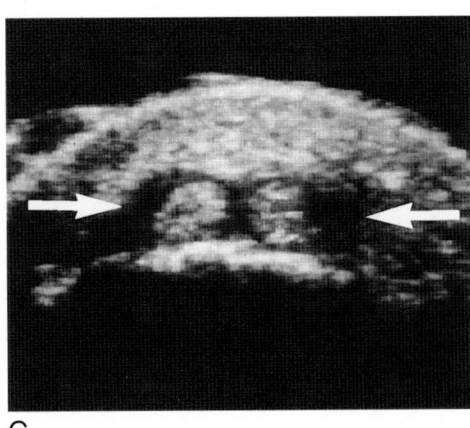

C

FIGURE 26-35. Chronic tenosynovitis. A, Chronic tenosynovitis of the flexor digitorum tendons after surgical treatment of carpal tunnel syndrome. Longitudinal sonogram of the volar aspect of the wrist shows the thickened hypoechoic bursa (*arrows*) and the absence of any substantial amount of fluid. **B,** Chronic posttraumatic tenosynovitis of the flexor digitorum tendons of the index finger. Longitudinal sonogram shows the hypoechoic, thickened synovial sheath (*arrows*), which contains no fluid. Note the grossly intact flexor tendons, with the superficial tendon inserting into the base of the second phalanx. P1, first phalanx; P2, second phalanx. **C,** de Quervain's tenosynovitis. Transverse sonogram of the wrist shows the thickened, hypoechoic synovial sheath (*arrows*) surrounding the tendons of the abductor pollicis longus and extensor pollicis brevis muscles.

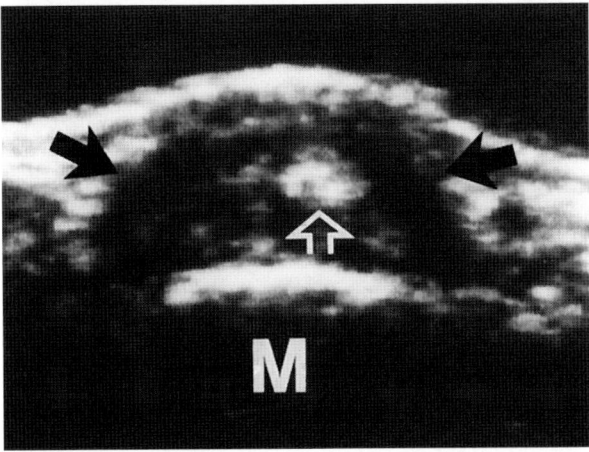

FIGURE 26-36. Rheumatoid tenosynovitis of the extensor tendon of a finger at the dorsum of the hand. Transverse scan shows the hypoechoic pannus (*arrows*) surrounding the tendon (*open arrow*). M, metacarpal bone.

Enthesopathy

Inflammatory **enthesopathy, or enthesitis,** is defined as an inflammation of the insertion of tendons into the bones. This is usually seen in seronegative spondylo-arthropathies, but it can also be occupational, metabolic,

drug induced, infective, or degenerative. Tendons commonly involved include the patellar and Achilles tendons as well as the plantar fascia. Sonographically, the tendon insertion appears swollen and hypoechoic, with calcifications developing in chronic lesions, ranging from fine to bony spurs. Often, there is coexisting bursitis.[67,68]

Nonarticular Osteochondroses

Osgood-Schlatter and Sinding-Larsen-Johansson diseases are both nonarticular osteochondroses of the knee that occur in ossification centers subjected to traction stress. Both conditions occur in adolescents, typically in boys involved in athletic activities. Although the diagnosis is strongly suggested by the clinical history, radiographic studies are often performed to confirm the diagnosis. High-resolution sonography has been used in the evaluation of these two conditions.[69]

Osgood-Schlatter disease is osteochondrosis of the tibial tuberosity. In one study of 70 cases, sonography revealed swelling of the anechoic cartilage in 100% of cases, fragmentation of the echogenic ossification center of the anterior tibial tuberosity in 75% of cases, diffuse thickening of the patellar tendon in 22% of cases, and

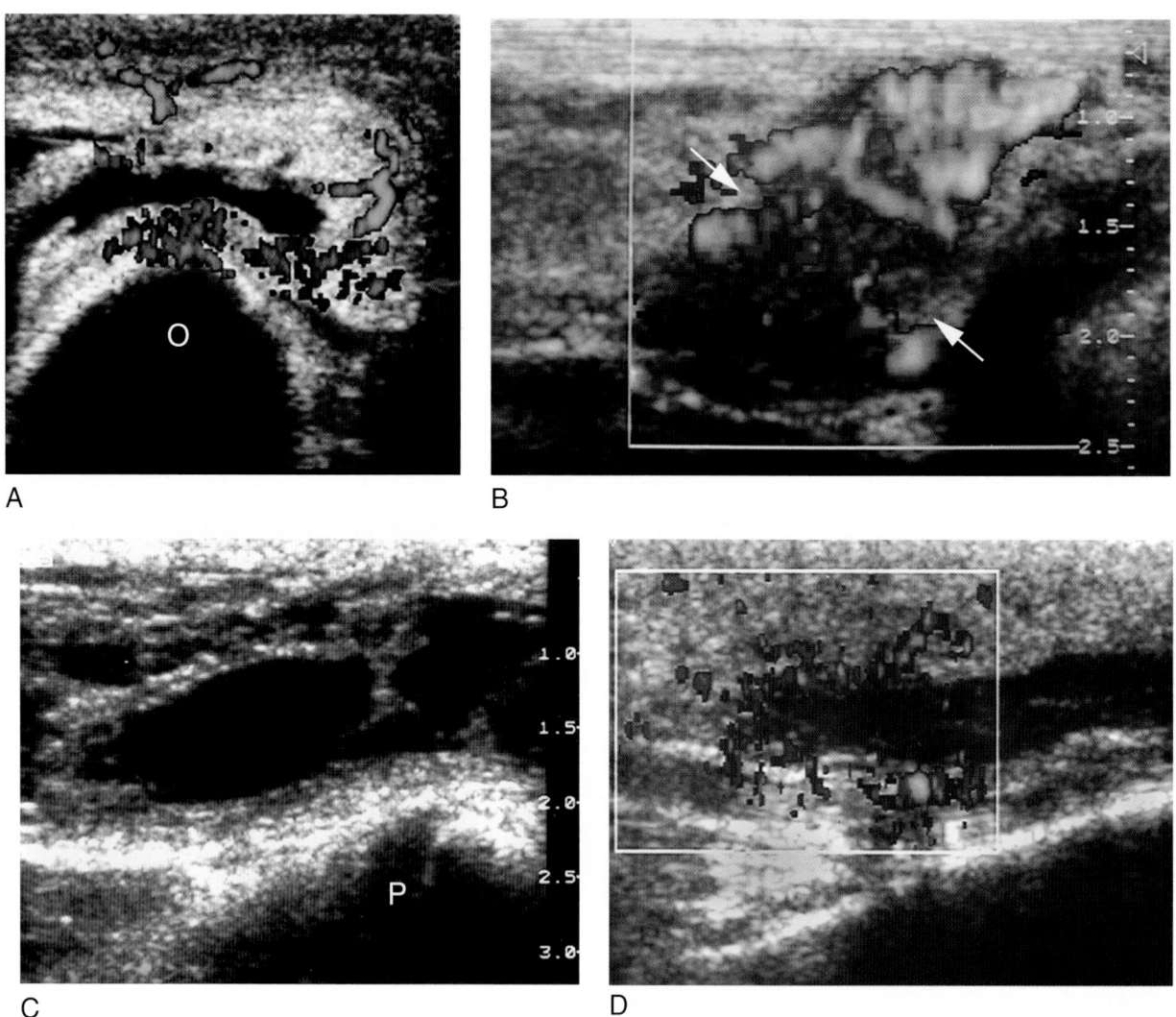

FIGURE 26-37. Bursitis. A, Transverse sonogram of the posterior aspect of the elbow shows the thick-walled, fluid-containing olecranal bursa. Power mode color Doppler sonogram shows the bursa's hypervascularity. O, olecranon. **B,** Longitudinal sonogram of the distal arm with the elbow flexed shows the enlarged, hypervascular subtendinous bursa (*arrows*) of the triceps brachii muscle. **C,** Prepatellar bursitis. Longitudinal sonogram shows the fluid-filled, subcutaneous prepatellar bursa. P, patella. **D,** Bursitis of the subcutaneous infrapatellar bursa. Longitudinal power Doppler sonogram shows the hypervascularity around the distended bursa.

deep infrapatellar bursitis in 17% of cases (Fig. 26-38).[70] A more recent study of 35 children[71] confirmed the findings originally reported by de Flaviis et al.[69]

Sinding-Larsen-Johansson disease is osteochondrosis of the accessory ossification center at the lower pole of the patella. In this rare disease, sonography can demonstrate the fragmented echogenic ossification center and the swollen hypoechoic cartilage and surrounding soft tissues, including the origin of the patellar tendon.[72]

Postoperative Patterns

After surgical repair, tendons appear on sonograms as enlarged, hypoechoic, and heterogeneous with blurred, irregular margins (Fig. 26-39).[14,73,74] The internal linear echoes that constitute the tendon's echotexture are thinner and shorter than in normal tendons. Sonography cannot reliably differentiate recurrent tears and tendinitis from postoperative changes.[75] On postoperative transverse scans, the tendon usually has a rounded cross section. The postoperative pattern may last for several months or even years. Occasionally, sonography can detect bright echogenic foci caused by residual synthetic suture material or calcification. Postoperative Doppler studies may demonstrate residual hypervascularization in tendons (see Fig. 26-39D). Results of a long-term follow-up study of ruptured Achilles tendons, most of them having been repaired surgically, showed that the average thickness of the tendons was 12 mm (range, 7 to 20 mm), compared with 5 mm for the controls, and that 14% of the healed tendons contained calcifications.[76] A study comparing the sonographic appearance after

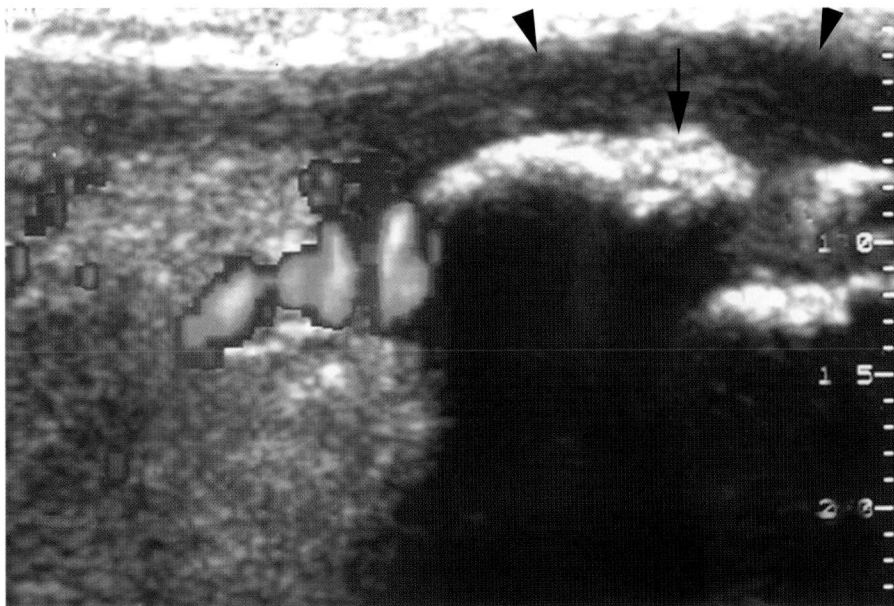

FIGURE 26-38. Osgood-Schlatter disease. Longitudinal power Doppler sonogram shows the swelling of the cartilage (*arrowheads*), fragmentation (*arrow*) of the echogenic ossification center of the anterior tibial tuberosity, and deep infrapatellar bursitis as shown by increased blood flow.

surgical repair of Achilles tendon rupture with that after nonsurgical treatment found no difference except for more limited gliding function of the tendon after surgery. In addition, there was a weak correlation between the sonographic findings and the clinical outcome.[74]

Tumors and Pseudotumors

Benign tumors of tendons or their sheaths include **giant cell tumors** and **osteochondromas**. The giant cell tumor of tendon sheaths is believed to be a circumscribed form of pigmented villonodular synovitis. It preferentially involves the flexor surface of the fingers and is usually found in young and middle-aged women. Local recurrences may occur after incomplete excision. Sonographically, giant cell tumors appear as hypoechoic masses, sometimes with lobulated contours.[18] Malignant tumors are rare. **Synovial sarcomas** may arise from a tendon sheath; they appear as an irregular or lobulated hypoechoic mass that may contain calcifications.

In 95% of patients with **familial hypercholesterolemia**, sonography demonstrates multiple hypoechoic **xanthomas** in the Achilles tendon and can detect early focal xanthomas in tendons that are not yet enlarged.[77] In one group of 30 adults with familial hypercholesterolemia, the mean thickness of the Achilles tendon was 11.1 mm, compared with 4.5 mm in normal subjects and 4.9 mm in a group with nonfamilial hypercholesterolemia.[78] More recently, the use of a cut-off value of 5.8 mm for the thickness of the Achilles tendon has been reported to yield a sensitivity of 75% and a specificity of 85% in the diagnosis of familial hyper-

cholesterolemia.[79] Sonography has also been shown to detect hypoechoic infiltration of the Achilles tendon in 38% of children affected with familial hypercholesterolemia.[80] In contrast, another study showed no significant abnormalities in secondary (nonfamilial) hypercholesterolemia.[81] Sonography can be used to monitor the effect of therapy on the thickness and echotexture of the Achilles tendon.

Intratendinous rheumatoid nodules appear hypoechoic on sonograms.[59] In contrast, various appearances have been reported for **gouty tophi** within or adjacent to tendons. An early report mentioned highly echogenic foci with acoustic shadowing, thus claiming easy differentiation from intratendinous rheumatoid nodules.[82] However, a recent study using color Doppler imaging showed the tophi to be hypoechoic with a peripheral increase of the blood flow.[83] It is likely that the sonographic appearances of gouty tophi parallel the degree of their calcification and associated inflammation. In **dialysis-related amyloidosis**, joint synovial membranes and capsules, as well as tendons (e.g., the supraspinatus tendon) may be thickened—the amount of thickening increasing with the duration of dialysis.[84]

Ganglion cysts most commonly occur in the hand but can develop from any joint or tendon sheath. Sonography demonstrates the oval fluid collection adjacent to the joint space or tendon (Fig. 26-40). Occasionally, chronic cysts have internal echoes, causing the cyst to mimic a hypoechoic solid tumor.

Another type of cyst that occurs adjacent to a joint is the **Baker's cyst**, which is also called a **popliteal cyst**. Baker's cysts are caused by an abnormal distention of the

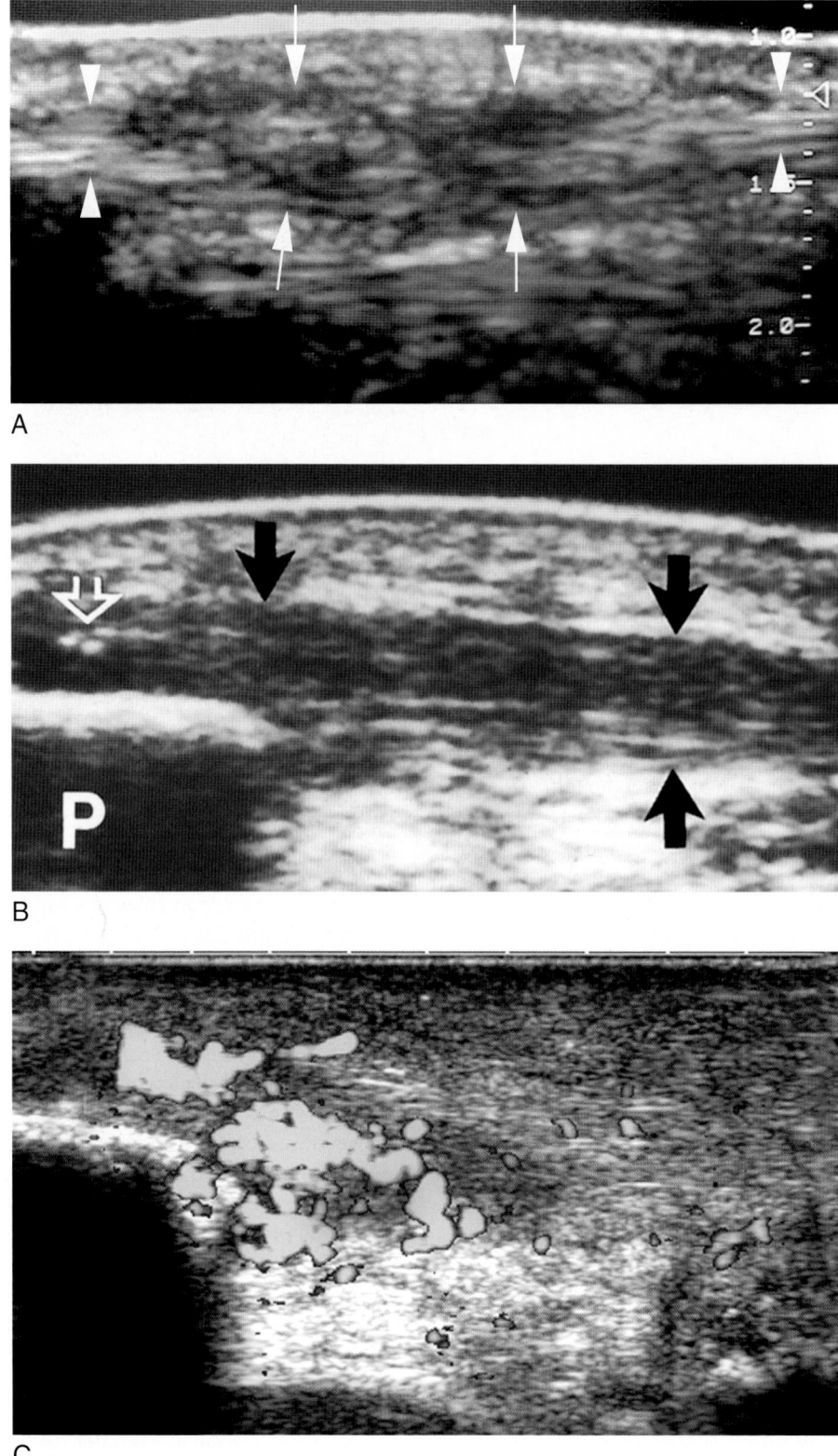

FIGURE 26-39. Postoperative patterns. A, Longitudinal sonogram of the tendon of the palmaris longus muscle after surgical repair of a complete rupture shows the focal hypoechoic thickening of the tendon (*arrows*). The arrowheads point to the normal tendon. **B,** Longitudinal scan of the patellar tendon performed 15 months after surgery for tendinitis shows a diffusely thickened, heterogeneous, hypoechoic tendon (*arrows*) with ill-defined margins and minute calcifications (*open arrow*). P, patella. **C,** Residual chronic postoperative inflammatory changes in the patellar tendon after percutaneous fixation of a fracture of the tibial shaft that consisted of inserting an intramedullary rod through the tendon. Longitudinal power Doppler sonogram shows the residual thickening and hypervascularity of the upper portion of the patellar tendon.

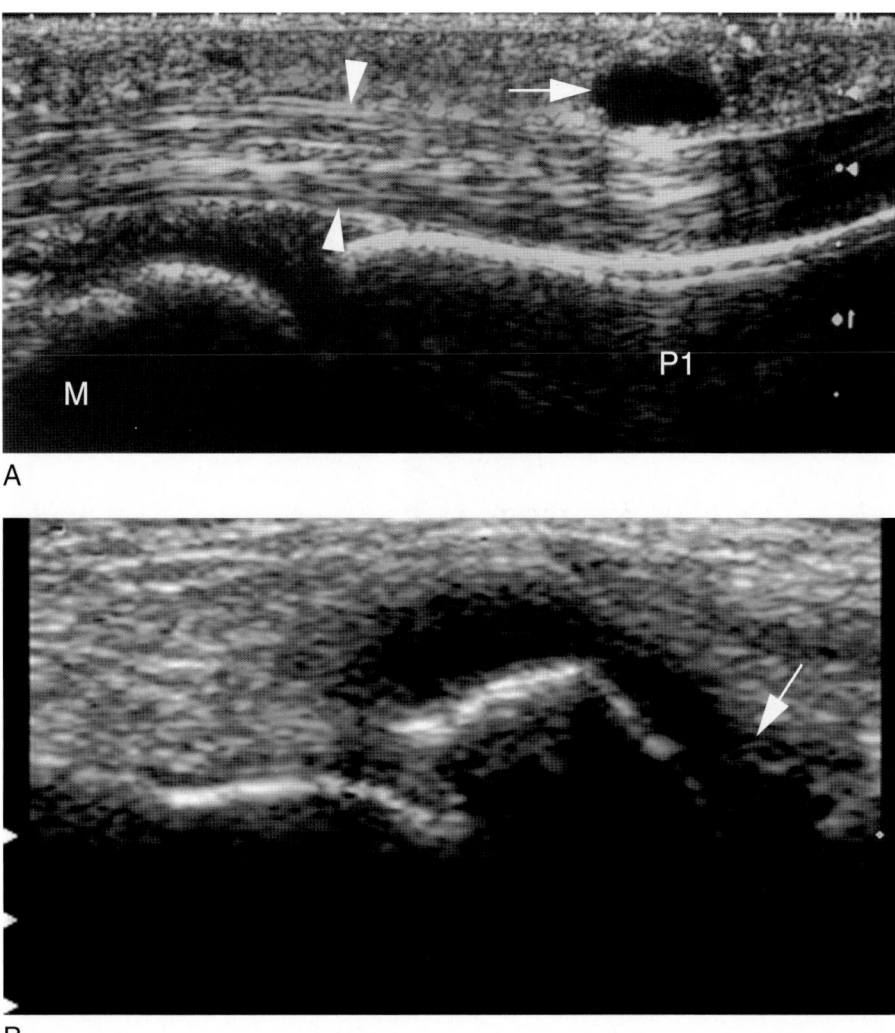

A

B

FIGURE 26-40. Ganglion cysts. A, Longitudinal sonogram of the first phalanx of the third finger shows a well-defined 0.4- × 0.2-cm cyst (*arrow*) anterior to the flexor tendons of the finger (*arrowheads*). Note the distal acoustic enhancement. M, metacarpal bone; P1, first phalanx. **B,** Longitudinal view of the wrist demonstrates a small ganglion cyst dorsal to the wrist bones. Note the small neck (*arrow*) connecting the cyst to the joint.

gastrocnemiosemimembranous bursa, which frequently communicates with the knee joint through a slit-shaped opening at the posteromedial aspect of the joint capsule. They are frequently found in association with pathologic conditions that cause an increase in the intra-articular pressure through overproduction of synovial fluid, capsular sclerosis, or synovial hypertrophy; among these conditions, rheumatoid arthritis is the most common. Baker's cysts appear clinically as popliteal masses that can be asymptomatic or symptomatic. Ruptured cysts or large cysts dissecting into the calf produce a swollen, painful limb that mimics thrombophlebitis. A Baker's cyst typically appears sonographically as a fluid-filled collection.[85-87]

Occasionally, longitudinal scans demonstrate a second anechoic area anterior to the tendon of the gastrocnemius muscle. Transverse scans confirm that both areas represent sections of the same cyst, which surrounds the tendon of the muscle (Fig. 26-41). Internal echoes representing fibrinous strands or debris and synovial thickening can be seen in inflamed or infected cysts. In patients with rheumatoid arthritis, a Baker's cyst may be completely filled with pannus, thus mimicking a solid mass. Color Doppler imaging demonstrates the hypervascularity of the pannus and differentiates it from debris. **Osteochondromatosis** can also develop in a Baker's cyst, giving rise to hyperechoic loose bodies that cast acoustic shadows when calcified.[88] In the case of a recently ruptured cyst, sonography can demonstrate the leak as a subcutaneous fluid collection that extends distally into the lower calf. However, when examination is deferred, the sonographic diagnosis may be more problematic because the leaking fluid has been resorbed, and only an ill-defined residual hypoechoic area remains (Fig. 26-42).[86]

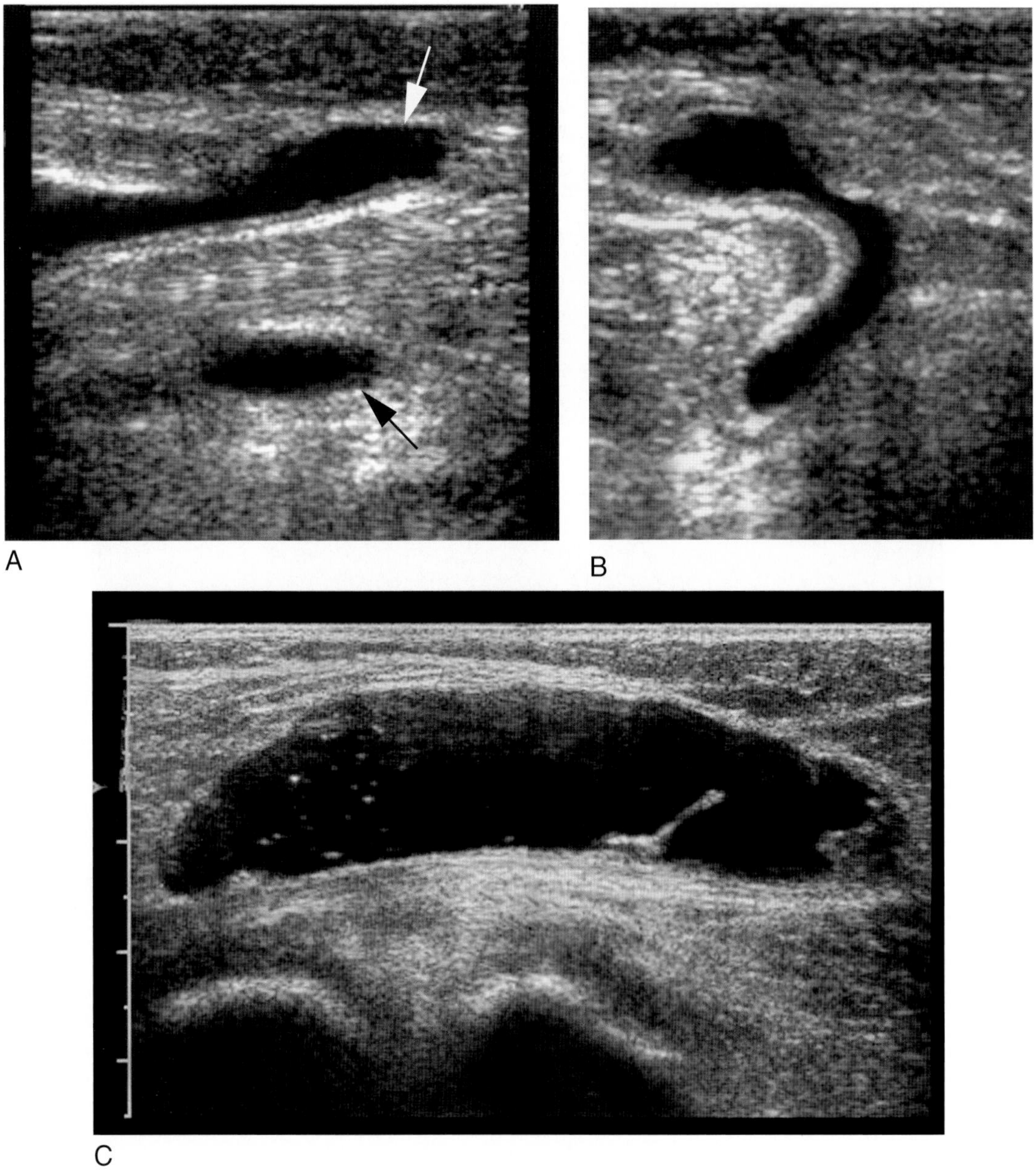

A

B

C

FIGURE 26-41. Baker's cyst. A, Longitudinal sonogram shows two fluid collections (*arrows*) separated by the tendon of the gastrocnemius medialis muscle. **B**, Transverse sonogram shows that the two collections are parts of the same cyst, which wraps around the tendon of the gastrocnemius medialis muscle. **C**, Longitudinal sonogram shows a large popliteal cyst.

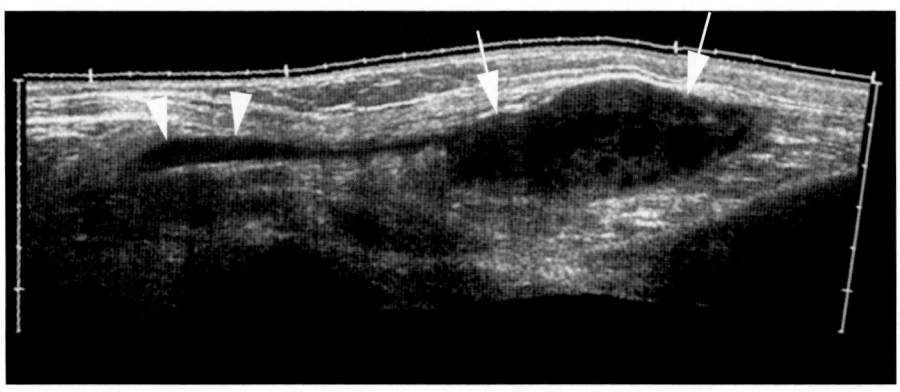

FIGURE 26-42. Ruptured Baker's cyst. Longitudinal extended-field-of-view sonogram of the calf shows a complex mass (*arrows*) that is connected to a small amount of residual fluid in the popliteal fossa (*arrowheads*) representing the ruptured cyst.

SONOGRAPHY VERSUS OTHER IMAGING MODALITIES

For many decades, low-kilovoltage radiography and xeroradiography were the only imaging techniques applicable to tendons. Although they could silhouette tendons, particularly when the tendons were surrounded by fat, these techniques failed to demonstrate their inner structure. However, they are still the best modalities with which to unequivocally document minute calcifications in tendons or bursae.

Tenography is performed by injecting contrast medium into the tendon's synovial sheath. This somewhat neglected imaging technique provides detailed global views of the inner wall of the sheath but cannot appreciate the thickness of the wall as well as sonography.[89,90] Similarly, bursography consists of direct opacification of a bursa. These two techniques are no longer performed, however, because they have been superseded by noninvasive cross-sectional imaging.

Because CT is limited in routine practice to transverse scans of the extremities, it has rarely been used in the evaluation of tendons.[91,92] MRI, on the other hand, because of its excellent contrast and spatial resolution and multiplanar-imaging capability, has emerged as the modality of choice for soft-tissue imaging and has become the standard for imaging tendons in the United States, also to a great extent owing to its operator independence.[93] However, its cost is nearly 10 times that of sonography, often for obtaining similar diagnostic information. High-frequency sonography is currently the only real-time cross-sectional imaging technique, and the dynamic information it provides is unique. Sonograms can be quickly obtained along virtually any orientation, and very high-frequency transducers now provide exquisite spatial and contrast resolution. In fact, in experienced hands, in specific anatomic locations, and for specific pathologic conditions (e.g., ankle tendon tears), high-resolution sonography has been reported to be more accurate than MRI.[94] However, because of the small size of the structures being examined and the possibility of significant technique-related artifacts, tendon sonography is operator dependent, requiring skill, adequate training, and sufficient experience to achieve the best results.

References

Anatomy

1. McMaster PE: Tendon and muscle ruptures. Clinical and experimental studies on the causes and location of subcutaneous ruptures. J Bone Joint Surg 1933;15:705-722.

Instrumentation and Examination Technique

2. Lin EC, Middleton WD, Teefey SA: Extended field of view sonography in musculoskeletal imaging. J Ultrasound Med 1999;18:147-152.

3. Fornage BD, Atkinson EN, Nock LF, et al: US with extended field of view: Phantom-tested accuracy of distance measurements. Radiology 2000;214:579-584.
4. Connolly DJ, Berman L, McNally EG: The use of beam angulation to overcome anisotropy when viewing human tendon with high frequency linear array ultrasound. Br J Radiol 2001;74:183-185.
5. Ohberg L, Lorentzon R, Alfredson H: Neovascularisation in Achilles tendons with painful tendinosis but not in normal tendons: An ultrasonographic investigation. Knee Surg Sports Traumatol Arthrosc 2001;9:233-238.
6. Buyruk HM, Holland WP, Snijders CJ, et al: Tendon excursion measurements with colour Doppler imaging. J Hand Surg [Br] 1998;23:350-353.
7. Sugamoto K, Ochi T: Colour Doppler analysis of tendon and muscle movements. J Hand Surg [Br] 1998;23:237-239.
8. Cigali BS, Buyruk HM, Snijders CJ, et al: Measurement of tendon excursion velocity with colour Doppler imaging: A preliminary study on flexor pollicis longus muscle. Eur J Radiol 1996;23:217-221.
9. Fornage BD, Touche DH, Rifkin MD: Small parts real-time sonography: A new "water-path." J Ultrasound Med 1984;3:355-357.
10. Fornage BD: Ultrasonography of Muscles and Tendons. Examination Technique and Atlas of Normal Anatomy of the Extremities. New York: Springer-Verlag; 1988.
11. Sofka CM, Adler RS: Ultrasound-guided interventions in the foot and ankle. Semin Musculoskelet Radiol 2002;6:163-168.
12. Movin T, Guntner P, Gad A, et al: Ultrasonography-guided percutaneous core biopsy in Achilles tendon disorder. Scand J Med Sci Sports 1997;7:244-248.

Normal Sonographic Appearance

13. Martinoli C, Derchi LE, Pastorino C, et al: Analysis of echotexture of tendons with US. Radiology 1993;186:839-843.
14. Fornage BD, Rifkin MD: Ultrasound examination of tendons. Radiol Clin North Am 1988;26:87-107.
15. Fornage BD: The hypoechoic normal tendon: A pitfall. J Ultrasound Med 1987;6:19-22.
16. Silvestri E, Martinoli C, Derchi LE, et al: Echotexture of peripheral nerves: Correlation between US and histologic findings and criteria to differentiate tendons. Radiology 1995;197:291-296.
17. Fornage BD, Rifkin MD: Ultrasound examination of the hand. Radiology 1986;160:853-854.
18. Fornage BD, Rifkin MD: Ultrasonic examination of the hand and foot. Radiol Clin North Am 1988;26:109-129.
19. Hauger O, Chung CB, Lektrakul N, et al: Pulley system in the fingers: Normal anatomy and simulated lesions in cadavers at MR imaging, CT, and US with and without contrast material distention of the tendon sheath. Radiology 2000;217:201-212.
20. Dillehay GL, Deschler T, Rogers LF, et al: The ultrasonographic characterization of tendons. Invest Radiol 1984;19:338-341.
21. Fornage BD, Rifkin MD, Touche DH, et al: Sonography of the patellar tendon: Preliminary observations. AJR Am J Roentgenol 1984;143:179-182.
22. De Flaviis L, Nessi R, Leonardi M, et al: Dynamic ultrasonography of capsulo-ligamentous knee joint traumas. J Clin Ultrasound 1988;16:487-492.
23. Goh LA, Chhem RK, Wang SC, et al: Iliotibial band thickness: Sonographic measurements in asymptomatic volunteers. J Clin Ultrasound, 2003;31:239-244.

24. Brys P, Velghe B, Geusens E, et al: Ultrasonography of the knee. J Belge Radiol 1996;79:155-159.

25. Röhr E: Die sonographische Darstellung des hinteren Kreuzbandes. Röntgenblatter 1985;38:377-379.

26. Scherer MA, Kraus M, Gerngross H, et al: Importance of ultrasound in postoperative follow-up after reconstruction of the anterior cruciate ligament [in German]. Unfallchirurg 1993;96:47-54.

27. Fornage BD: Achilles tendon: Ultrasound examination. Radiology 1986;159:759-764.

28. Bertolotto M, Perrone R, Martinoli C, et al: High resolution ultrasound anatomy of normal Achilles tendon. Br J Radiol 1995;68:986-991.

29. Koivunen-Niemela T, Parkkola K: Anatomy of the Achilles tendon (tendo calcaneus) with respect to tendon thickness measurements. Surg Radiol Anat 1995;17:263-268.

30. Nazarian LN, Rawool NM, Martin CE, et al: Synovial fluid in the hindfoot and ankle: Detection of amount and distribution with US. Radiology 1995;197:275-278.

Pathology

31. Downey DJ, Simkin PA, Mack LA, et al: Tibialis posterior tendon rupture: A cause of rheumatoid flat foot. Arthritis Rheum 1988;31:441-446.

32. Ismail AM, Balakrishnan R, Rajakumar MK: Rupture of patellar ligament after steroid infiltration. Report of a case. J Bone Joint Surg 1969;51B:503-505.

33. Kricun R, Kricun ME, Arangio GA, et al: Patellar tendon rupture with underlying systemic disease. AJR Am J Roentgenol 1980;135:803-807.

34. Morgan J, McCarty DJ: Tendon ruptures in patients with systemic lupus erythematosus treated with corticosteroids. Arthritis Rheum 1974;17:1033-1036.

35. Souissi M, Giwerc M, Ebelin M, et al: Exploration échographique des tendons fléchisseurs des doigts de la main. Presse Med 1989;18:463-466.

36. Kaempffe FA, Lerner RM: Ultrasound diagnosis of triceps tendon rupture. A report of 2 cases. Clin Orthop 1996;332:138-142.

37. Kalebo P, Allenmark C, Peterson L, et al: Diagnostic value of ultrasonography in partial ruptures of the Achilles tendon. Am J Sports Med 1992;20:378-381.

38. Leekam RN, Salsberg BB, Bogoch E, et al: Sonographic diagnosis of partial Achilles tendon rupture and healing. J Ultrasound Med 1986;5:115-116.

39. Waitches GM, Rockett M, Brage M, et al: Ultrasonographic-surgical correlation of ankle tendon tears. J Ultrasound Med 1998;17:249-256.

40. Weinstabl R: MR and ultrasound study of Achilles tendon injury [in German]. Unfallchirurgie 1992;18:213-217.

41. Neuhold A, Stiskal M, Kainberger F, et al: Degenerative Achilles tendon disease: Assessment by magnetic resonance and ultrasonography. Eur J Radiol 1992;14:213-220.

42. Paavola M, Paakkala T, Kannus P, et al: Ultrasonography in the differential diagnosis of Achilles tendon injuries and related disorders. A comparison between pre-operative ultrasonography and surgical findings. Acta Radiol 1998;39:612-619.

43. Cook JL, Khan KM, Harcourt PR, et al: Patellar tendon ultrasonography in asymptomatic active athletes reveals hypoechoic regions: A study of 320 tendons. Victorian Institute of Sport Tendon Study Group. Clin J Sport Med 1998;8:73-77.

44. Khan KM, Cook JL, Kiss ZS, et al: Patellar tendon ultrasonography and jumper's knee in female basketball players: A longitudinal study. Clin J Sport Med 1997;7:199-206.

45. Fredberg U, Bolvig L: Significance of ultrasonographically detected asymptomatic tendinosis in the patellar and Achilles tendons of elite soccer players: A longitudinal study. Am J Sports Med 2002;30:488-491.

46. Ohberg L, Alfredson H: Ultrasound guided sclerosis of neovessels in painful chronic Achilles tendinosis: Pilot study of a new treatment. Br J Sports Med 2002;36:173-175.

47. Premkumar A, Perry MB, Dwyer AJ, et al: Sonography and MR imaging of posterior tibial tendinopathy. AJR Am J Roentgenol 2002;178:223-232.

48. Richards PJ, Dheer AK, McCall IM: Achilles tendon (TA) size and power Doppler ultrasound (PD) changes compared to MRI: A preliminary observational study. Clin Radiol 2001;56:843-850.

49. Newman JS, Laing TJ, McCarthy CJ, et al: Power Doppler sonography of synovitis: Assessment of therapeutic response—preliminary observations. Radiology 1996;198:582-584.

50. Fornage B, Touche D, Deshayes JL, et al: Diagnostic des calcifications du tendon rotulien. Comparaison échoradiographique. J Radiol 1984;65:355-359.

51. Howden MD: Foreign bodies within finger tendon sheaths demonstrated by ultrasound: Two cases. Clin Radiol 1994;49:419-420.

52. Middleton WD, Reinus WR, Totty WG, et al: Ultrasound of the biceps tendon apparatus. Radiology 1985;157:211-215.

53. Gooding GAW: Tenosynovitis of the wrist. A sonographic demonstration. J Ultrasound Med 1988;7:225-226.

54. Jeffrey RB, Jr, Laing FC, Schechter WP, et al: Acute suppurative tenosynovitis of the hand: Diagnosis with ultrasound. Radiology 1987;162:741-742.

55. Marini M, Boni S, Pingi A, et al: De Quervain's disease: Diagnostic imaging. Chir Organi Mov 1994;79:219-223.

56. Giovagnorio F, Andreoli C, De Cicco ML. Ultrasonographic evaluation of de Quervain disease. J Ultrasound Med 1997;16:685-689.

57. Fornage BD: Ultrasound of the Extremities [in French]. Paris: Vigot; 1991.

58. Brophy DP, Cunnane G, Fitzgerald O, et al: Technical report: Ultrasound guidance for injection of soft tissue lesions around the heel in chronic inflammatory arthritis. Clin Radiol 1995;50:120-122.

59. Fornage BD: Soft-tissue changes in the hand in rheumatoid arthritis: Evaluation with ultrasound. Radiology 1989;173:735-737.

60. Kotob H, Kamel M: Identification and prevalence of rheumatoid nodules in the finger tendons using high frequency ultrasonography. J Rheumatol 1999;26:1264-1268.

61. Grassi W, Tittarelli E, Blasetti P, et al: Finger tendon involvement in rheumatoid arthritis. Evaluation with high-frequency sonography. Arthritis Rheum 1995;38:786-794.

62. Coakley FV, Samanta AK, Finlay DB: Ultrasonography of the tibialis posterior tendon in rheumatoid arthritis. Br J Rheumatol 1994;33:273-277.

63. Myllymaki T, Tikkakoski T, Typpo T, et al: Carpet-layer's knee. An ultrasonographic study. Acta Radiol 1993;34:496-499.

64. Kruger-Franke M, Fischer S, Kugler A, et al: Stress-related clinical and ultrasound changes in shoulder joints of handball players [in German]. Sportverletz Sportschaden 1994;8:166-169.

65. Balint PV, Sturrock RD: Inflamed retrocalcaneal bursa and Achilles tendonitis in psoriatic arthritis demonstrated by ultrasonography. Ann Rheum Dis 2000;59:931-933.

66. Gibbon WW, Cooper JR, Radcliffe GS: Distribution of sonographically detected tendon abnormalities in patients with a clinical diagnosis of chronic Achilles tendinosis. J Clin Ultrasound 2000;28:61-66.

67. Danda D, Shyam Kumar NK, Cherian R, et al: Enthesopathy: Clinical recognition and significance. Natl Med J India 2001;14:90-92.

68. Balint PV, Kane D, Wilson H, et al: Ultrasonography of entheseal insertions in the lower limb in spondyloarthropathy. Ann Rheum Dis 2002;61:905-910.

69. De Flaviis L, Nessi R, Scaglione P, et al: Ultrasonic diagnosis of Osgood-Schlatter and Sinding-Larsen-Johansson diseases of the knee. Skeletal Radiol 1989;18:193-197.

70. Bergami G, Barbuti D, Pezzoli F: Ultrasonographic findings in Osgood-Schlatter disease [in Italian]. Radiol Med (Torino) 1994;88:368-372.

71. Blankstein A, Cohen I, Heim M, et al: Ultrasonography as a diagnostic modality in Osgood-Schlatter disease. A clinical study and review of the literature. Arch Orthop Trauma Surg 2001;121:536-539.

72. Barbuti D, Bergami G, Testa F: Ultrasonographic aspects of Sinding-Larsen-Johansson disease [Italian]. Pediatr Med Chir 1995;17:61-63.

73. Blei CL, Nirschl RP, Grant EG: Achilles tendon: Ultrasonic diagnosis of pathologic conditions. Radiology 1986;159:765-767.

74. Moller M, Kalebo P, Tidebrant G, et al: The ultrasonographic appearance of the ruptured Achilles tendon during healing: A longitudinal evaluation of surgical and nonsurgical treatment, with comparisons to MRI appearance. Knee Surg Sports Traumatol Arthrosc 2002;10:49-56.

75. Karjalainen PT, Ahovuo J, Pihlajamaki HK, et al: Postoperative MR imaging and ultrasonography of surgically repaired Achilles tendon ruptures. Acta Radiol 1996;37:639-646.

76. Bleakney RR, Tallon C, Wong JK, et al: Long-term ultrasonographic features of the Achilles tendon after rupture. Clin J Sport Med 2002;12:273-278.

77. Bude RO, Adler RS, Bassett DR, et al: Heterozygous familial hypercholesterolemia: Detection of xanthomas in the Achilles tendon with US. Radiology 1993;188:567-571.

78. Ebeling T, Farin P, Pyorala K: Ultrasonography in the detection of Achilles tendon xanthomata in heterozygous familial hypercholesterolemia. Atherosclerosis 1992;97:217-228.

79. Descamps OS, Leysen X, Van Leuven F, et al: The use of Achilles tendon ultrasonography for the diagnosis of familial hypercholesterolemia. Atherosclerosis 2001;157:514-518.

80. Koivunen-Niemela T, Viikari J, Niinikoski H, et al: Sonography in the detection of Achilles tendon xanthomata in children with familial hypercholesterolaemia. Acta Paediatr 1994;83:1178-1181.

81. Kainberger F, Seidl G, Traindl O, et al: Ultrasonography of the Achilles tendon in hypercholesterolemia. Acta Radiol 1993;34:408-412.

82. Tiliakos N, Morales AR, Wilson CH, Jr: Use of ultrasound in identifying tophaceous versus rheumatoid nodules [letter]. Arthritis Rheum 1982;25:478-479.

83. Gerster JC, Landry M, Dufresne L, et al: Imaging of tophaceous gout: Computed tomography provides specific images compared with magnetic resonance imaging and ultrasonography. Ann Rheum Dis 2002;61:52-54.

84. Jadoul M, Malghem J, Van de Berg B, et al: Ultrasonographic detection of thickened joint capsules and tendons as marker of dialysis-related amyloidosis: A cross-sectional and longitudinal study. Nephrol Dial Transplant 1993;8:1104-1109.

85. McDonald DG, Leopold GR: Ultrasound B-scanning in the differentiation of Baker's cyst and thrombophlebitis. Br J Radiol 1972;45:729-732.

86. Gompels BM, Darlington LG: Evaluation of popliteal cysts and painful calves with ultrasonography: Comparison with arthrography. Ann Rheum Dis 1982;41:355-359.

87. Strome GM, Bouffard JA, van Holsbeeck M: The knee. In Fornage BD (ed): Musculoskeletal Ultrasound. New York, Churchill Livingstone, 1995, pp 201-219.

88. Moss GD, Dishuk W: Ultrasound diagnosis of osteochondromatosis of the popliteal fossa. J Clin Ultrasound 1984;12:232-233.

Sonography Versus Other Imaging Modalities

89. Engel J, Luboshitz S, Israeli A, et al: Tenography in De Quervain's disease. Hand 1981;13:142-146.

90. Gilula LA, Oloff L, Caputi R, et al: Ankle tenography: A key to unexplained symptomatology. Part II: Diagnosis of chronic tendon disabilities. Radiology 1984;151:581-587.

91. Mourad K, King J, Guggiana P: Computed tomography and ultrasound imaging of jumper's knee: Patellar tendinitis. Clin Radiol 1988;39:162-165.

92. Rosenberg ZS, Feldman F, Singson RD, et al: Ankle tendons: Evaluation with computed tomography. Radiology 1988;166:221-226.

93. Beltran J, Mosure JC: Magnetic resonance imaging of tendons. Crit Rev Diagn Imaging 1990;30:111-182.

94. Rockett MS, Waitches G, Sudakoff G, et al: Use of ultrasonography versus magnetic resonance imaging for tendon abnormalities around the ankle. Foot Ankle Int 1998;19:604-612.

27

THE EXTRACRANIAL CEREBRAL VESSELS

Barbara A. Carroll

Chapter Outline

Stroke secondary to atherosclerotic disease is the third leading cause of death in the United States. Many stroke victims survive the catastrophic event with some degree of neurologic impairment.[1] More than 500,000 new cases of cerebrovascular accidents are reported annually.[2] Ischemia from severe, flow limiting stenosis due to atherosclerotic disease involving the extracranial carotid arteries is implicated in approximately 20% to 30% of strokes.[2] An estimated 80% of strokes are thromboembolic in origin, often with carotid plaque as the embolic source.[3]

Carotid atherosclerotic plaque with resultant stenosis usually involves the internal carotid artery (ICA) within two centimeters of the carotid bifurcation. This location is readily amenable to examination by sonography (US) as well as surgical intervention. Carotid endarterectomy (CEA) was initially proved to be more beneficial than medical therapy in symptomatic patients with greater than 70% carotid stenoses in the North American Symptomatic Carotid Endarterectomy Trial (NASCET) and the European Carotid Surgery Trial (ECST).[4,5]

Subsequent NASCET results for moderate stenoses have shown a net benefit for surgical intervention with narrowings between 50% and 69% diameter. A 15.7% reduction in the 5-year ipsilateral stroke rate was seen in patients treated surgically versus a 22.2% stroke reduction among those treated medically. These results are not as compelling as those for the higher degree stenosis seen in the earlier NASCET trial. The benefit from surgery was greatest among men, in patients with recent stroke, and in patients with hemispheric symptoms. In addition, the NASCET trials dealing with moderate carotid stenoses require a rigorous degree of surgical expertise, such that the risks for disabling stroke or death should not exceed 2% in order to achieve the statistical surgical benefit.[6] The Asymptomatic Carotid Atherosclerosis Study (ACAS) trials published in 1995 report a reduction in ipsilateral stroke in asymptomatic patients with greater than 60% ICA stenoses who undergo CEA.[7] However, these results are less clear cut than the NASCET trials.

Clearly, accurate diagnosis of carotid stenosis is critical to identify those patients who would benefit from surgical treatment. In addition to providing this information, US can assess plaque morphology, such as hemorrhagic plaque, which is known to be an independent risk factor for stroke or transient ischemic attack (TIA).

Over the past 2 decades carotid sonography has largely replaced angiography as the principal screening examination to assess suspected extracranial carotid atherosclerotic disease. Gray-scale, color Doppler, power Doppler, and pulsed Doppler imaging techniques are routinely employed in the evaluation of patients with neurologic symptoms and suspected extracranial cerebral disease.

Ultrasound is an inexpensive, noninvasive, and highly accurate method of diagnosing carotid stenosis. Angiography is an expensive, invasive test not without morbidity, which is why reliance on carotid sonography without preoperative angiography is becoming increasingly common. Magnetic resonance angiography (MRA) and computed tomography (CT) are additional noninvasive screening tools for the identification of carotid bifurcation disease, as well as for clarification of ultrasound findings. Angiography is often now reserved for those patients in whom the US or MRA examination is equivocal or inadequate.

Other carotid ultrasound applications include evaluation of carotid bruits, monitoring progression of known atherosclerotic disease,[8,9] assessment during or after endarterectomy or stent placement,[10] preoperative screening prior to major vascular surgery, and evaluation after detection of retinal cholesterol emboli. Nonatherosclerotic carotid diseases can be evaluated, including follow-up of carotid dissection,[11-15] examination of fibromuscular dysplasia or Takayasu's arteritis, assessment of malignant carotid artery invasion,[16,17] and work-up of pulsatile neck masses and carotid body tumors.[18,19]

CAROTID ARTERY ANATOMY

The first major branch of the aortic arch is the innominate or brachiocephalic artery, which divides into the right subclavian and right common carotid arteries. The second major branch is the left common carotid artery, which is generally separate from the third major branch, the left subclavian artery (Fig. 27-1).

INDICATIONS FOR CAROTID ULTRASOUND

Evaluation of patients with transient ischemic attacks (TIAs)
Evaluation of patients with cerebrovascular accident (CVA)
Evaluation of carotid bruits
Follow-up of known disease
Monitor endarterectomy results/stents, bypass
Preoperative screen prior to major vascular surgery
Evaluation of potential source of retinal emboli
Evaluation of a pulsatile neck mass
Follow-up of carotid dissection

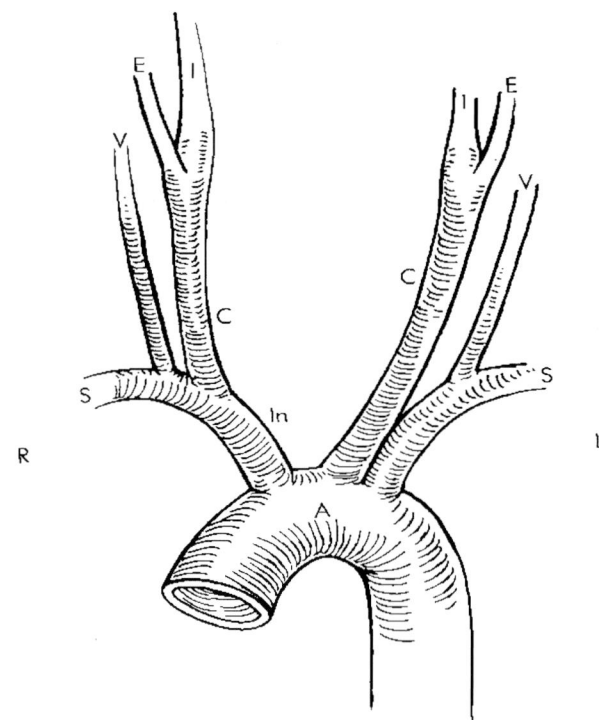

FIGURE 27-1. Branches of the aortic arch and extracranial cerebral arteries. Aortic arch. Common carotid artery (C); external carotid artery (E); innominate artery (In); internal carotid artery (I); left side (L); right side (R); subclavian artery (S); vertebral artery (V).

The common carotid arteries (CCAs) ascend into the neck posterolateral to the thyroid gland and lie deep to the jugular vein and sternocleidomastoid muscle. The CCAs have different proximal configurations with the right originating at the bifurcation of the innominate (brachiocephalic) artery into the common carotid and subclavian arteries. The left CCA usually originates directly from the aortic arch, but often arises with the brachiocephalic trunk. This is known as a bovine arch configuration. The CCA usually has no branches in its cervical region. However, occasionally, it may give off the superior thyroidal artery, vertebral artery, ascending pharyngeal artery, and occipital or inferior thyroid artery. At the carotid bifurcation, the CCA divides into the external carotid artery (ECA) and the internal ICA. The ICA usually has no branching vessels in the neck. The ECA, which supplies the facial musculature, has multiple branches in the neck. The ICA may demonstrate an ampullary region of mild dilation just beyond its origin.

CAROTID ULTRASOUND EXAMINATION

Carotid artery examinations are performed with the patient supine, the neck slightly extended, and the head

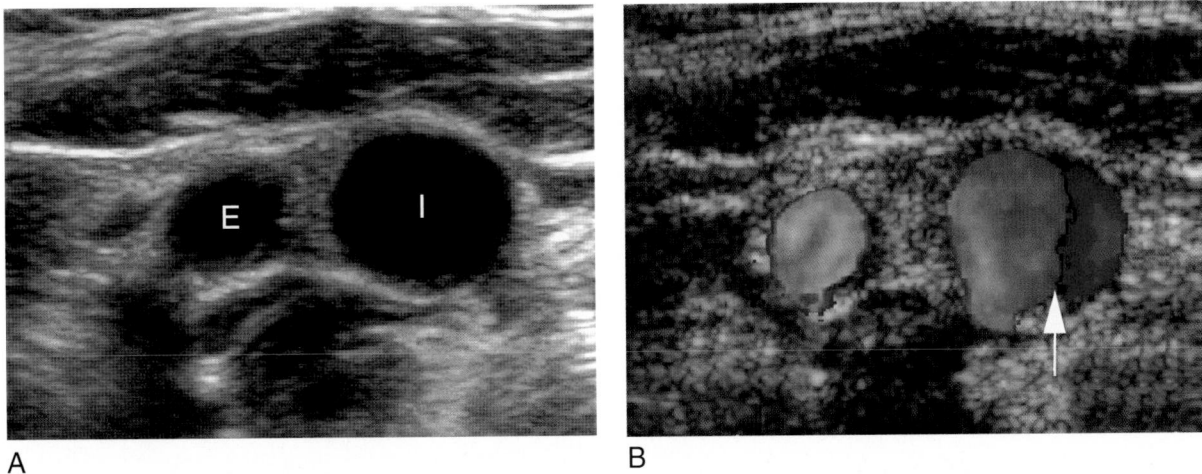

A

B

FIGURE 27-2. Carotid sonographic anatomy. A, Transverse image of left carotid bifurcation. The larger, more lateral vessel is the internal carotid artery (I); external carotid artery (E). **B,** Color Doppler shows normal flow separation (*arrow*) in the proximal internal carotid artery.

turned away from the side being examined. Some operators prefer to perform the examination at the patient's side, and others prefer to sit at the patient's head. The examination sequence also varies with operator preference. This sequence includes the gray-scale examination, Doppler spectral analysis, and Doppler color flow interrogations. Power Doppler imaging may or may not be employed. A 5 to 12 MHz transducer is used for imaging, and a 3 to 7 MHz for Doppler, the choice depending on the patient's body habitus and technical characteristics of the ultrasound machine. Color flow Doppler imaging and power Doppler imaging may be performed with 5 to 10 MHz transducers. In cases of critical stenosis, the Doppler parameters should be optimized to detect very slow flow.

Gray-scale examination begins in the transverse projection. Scans are obtained along the entire course of the cervical carotid artery from the supraclavicular notch cephalad to the angle of the mandible (Fig. 27-2A, B). Inferior angulation of the transducer in the supraclavicular area images the CCA origin. The left CCA origin is deeper and more difficult to image consistently than is the right. The carotid bulb is identified as a mild widening of the CCA near the bifurcation. Transverse views of the carotid bifurcation establish the orientation of the external and internal carotid arteries and help define the optimal longitudinal plane in which to perform Doppler spectral analysis. When the transverse ultrasound images demonstrate occlusive atherosclerotic disease, the percentage of diameter stenosis or area stenosis can be calculated directly using electronic calipers and software analytic algorithms available on most duplex instruments.

After transverse imaging, longitudinal scans of the carotid artery are obtained. The examination plane necessary for optimal longitudinal scans is determined by the course of the vessels demonstrated on the trans-

verse study. In some patients, the optimal longitudinal orientation will be nearly coronal, and in others it will be almost sagittal. In the majority of cases, the optimal longitudinal scan plane will be oblique, somewhere between sagittal and coronal. In approximately 60% of patients, both vessels above the carotid bifurcation and the CCA can be imaged in the same plane (Fig. 27-3); in the remainder, only a single vessel will be imaged in the same plane as the CCA. Images are obtained to display the relationship of both branches of the carotid bifurcation to visualized plaque disease, and the cephalocaudal extent of the plaque is measured. Several anatomic features differentiate the ICA from the ECA. In about 95% of patients, the ICA is posterior and lateral to the ECA. This may vary considerably, however,[10] and the ICA may be medial to the ECA in 3% to 9% of people.

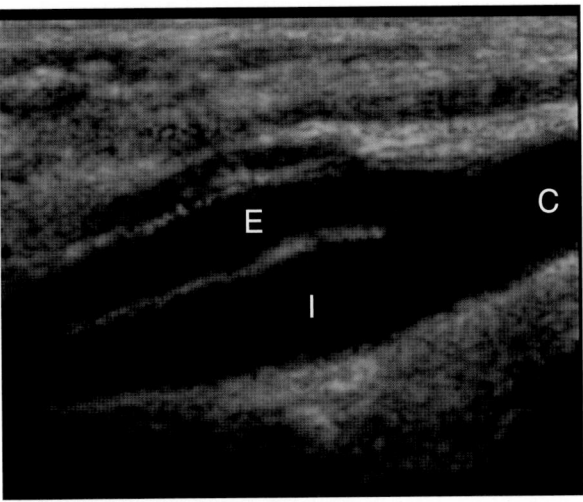

FIGURE 27-3. Carotid bifurcation. Longitudinal image demonstrates common carotid artery (C); external carotid artery (E); and large, posterior internal carotid artery (I).

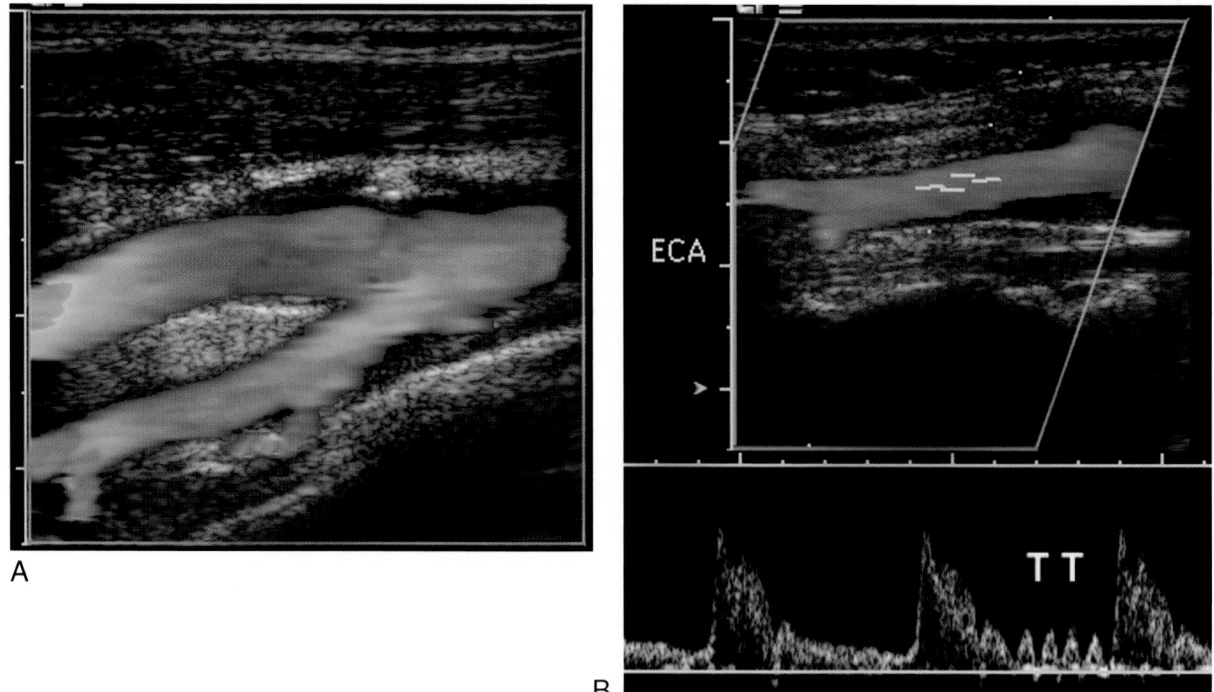

FIGURE 27-4. Normal external carotid artery (ECA). A, Color Doppler of bifurcation demonstrates two small arteries originating from the ECA. **B,** ECA spectral Doppler shows the anticipated serrated flow disturbance from temporal artery tap (TT).

The ICA frequently has an ampullary region of dilation just beyond its origin and is usually larger than the ECA. One reliable distinguishing feature of the ECA is identification of branching vessels (Fig. 27-4A).

The superior thyroidal artery is often seen as the first branch of the ECA after the bifurcation of the CCA. Occasionally an aberrant superior thyroidal artery branch will arise from the distal CCA. The ICA usually has no branches in the neck although, rarely, the ICA gives rise to the ascending pharyngeal, occipital, facial, laryngeal, or meningeal arteries. In some patients, a considerable amount of the ICA will be visible, but in others, only the immediate origin of the vessel will be accessible. Very rarely, the bifurcation may not be visible at all.[19] Rarely the ICA may be hypoplastic or congenitally absent.[20] A useful method to identify the ECA is the tapping of the superficial temporal artery in the preauricular area. The pulsations are transmitted back to the ECA where they cause a "**saw-tooth**" appearance of the spectral waveform (see Fig. 27-4B). Although the temporal tap helps identify the ECA, this tap deflection may be transmitted into the CCA and even the ICA in certain situations.

CAROTID ULTRASOUND INTERPRETATION

Each facet of the carotid sonographic examination is valuable in the final determination of the presence and extent of disease. In most instances, the image and Doppler assessments will agree. However, when there are discrepancies between Doppler and image information, every attempt should be made to discover the source of the disagreement. The more closely the image and Doppler findings correlate, the higher the degree of confidence in the diagnosis. Generally speaking, gray-scale and color/power Doppler images better demonstrate and quantify low-grade stenoses, but high-grade occlusive disease is more accurately defined by Doppler spectral analysis.

Visual Inspection of Gray-Scale Images

Vessel Wall Thickness. Longitudinal views of the layers of the normal carotid wall demonstrate **two nearly parallel echogenic lines,** separated by a hypoechoic to anechoic region (Fig. 27-5). The first echo, bordering the vessel lumen, represents the lumen-intima interface; the second echo is caused by the media-adventitia interface. The media is the anechoic/hypoechoic zone between the echogenic lines. The distance between these lines represents the combined thickness of **the intima and media (I-M complex)**. The far wall of the CCA is measured. Thickening of the I-M complex greater than 0.8 mm is considered abnormal by some and may represent the earliest changes of atherosclerotic disease. However, because thickness of the I-M increases with age, absolute measurements of I-M thickness for any given person may not be a reliable indicator of

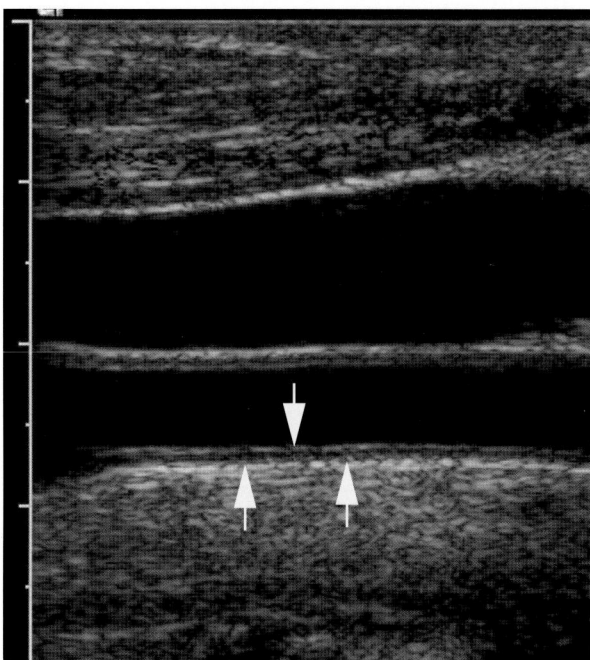

FIGURE 27-5. Normal intima-media (I-M) complex of common carotid artery (CCA). I-M complex (*arrows*) is seen in a left CCA.

atherosclerotic risk factors (Fig. 27-6A, B).[21] Numerous articles support the relationship between I-M thickness (IMT) and increased risk for myocardial infarction or stroke in asymptomatic patient populations.[22-30] A recent reference suggests that IMT may be superior to the coronary artery calcification score for identifying patients at high risk for these cardiovascular events.[25] Assessment of I-M thickness has been advocated as a means of assessing effectiveness of medical interventions

to reduce the progression of I-M thickness or even reverse carotid wall thickening. Whether these measurements have validity for assessment of an individual patient as opposed to large groups of patients remains controversial.

Plaque Characterization. Atheromatous carotid plaques should be carefully evaluated to determine plaque extent, location, surface contour and texture, as well as assessment of luminal stenosis.[31] Embolism is the most common cause of transient ischemic attacks (TIAs) rather than flow-limiting stenosis. Fewer than half of patients with documented TIAs have hemodynamically significant stenosis. It is important to identify low-grade atherosclerotic lesions that may contain hemorrhage or ulceration that can serve as a nidus for emboli that cause both TIAs and stroke.[1] In fact, Polak et al. have shown plaque is an independent risk factor for developing a stroke.[32] Fifty to 70% of patients with hemispheric symptoms demonstrate hemorrhagic or ulcerated plaque. Plaque analysis of CEA specimens has implicated intraplaque hemorrhage as an important factor in the development of neurologic symptoms.[33-39] However, the relationship between sonographic plaque morphology and onset of symptoms is controversial.

Plaque texture is generally classified as being homogeneous or heterogeneous.[9,24,28,31,33-35,40,41] **Homogeneous plaque** has a uniform echo pattern and a smooth surface (Fig. 27-7). The uniform acoustic texture corresponds pathologically to **dense fibrous connective tissue**. **Calcified plaque** produces posterior acoustic shadowing and is common in asymptomatic individuals (Fig. 27-8A, B). **Heterogeneous plaque** has a more complex echo pattern and contains at least one or more focal sonolucent areas (Fig. 27-9A-C). Heterogeneous plaque is characterized pathologically by containing

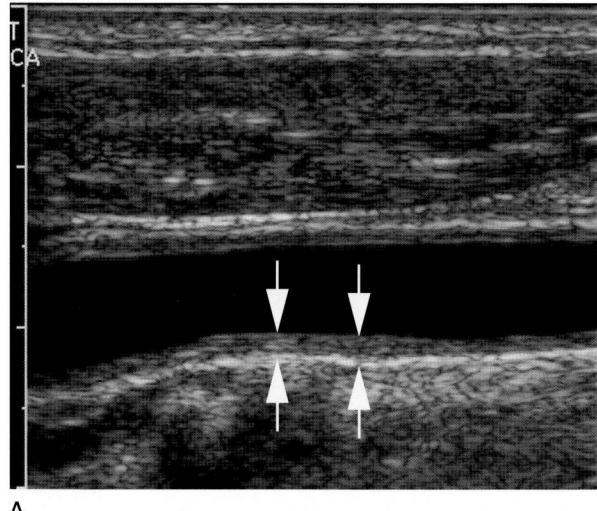

A

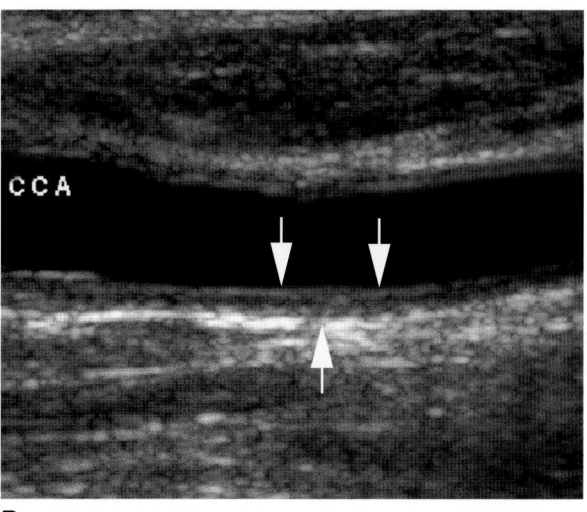

B

FIGURE 27-6. Abnormal intima-media (I-M) complex of common carotic artery. A, Early intima-media hyperplasia with loss of the hypoechoic component of the I-M complex and thickening (*arrows*). **B,** Thickening of the I-M complex with hyperplasia (*arrows*).

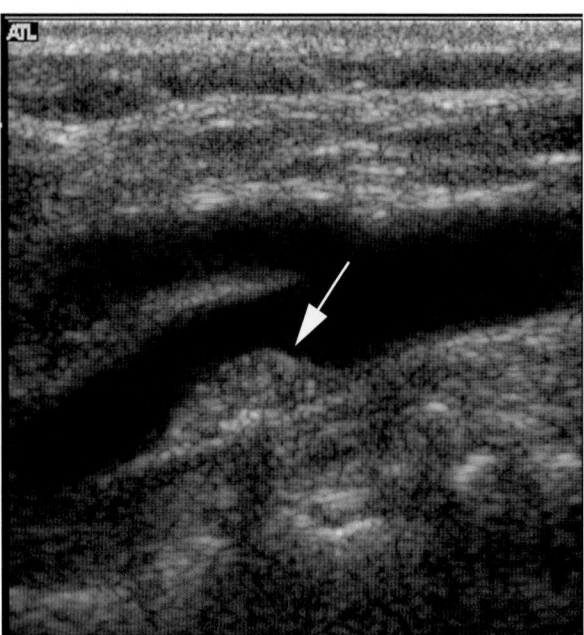

FIGURE 27-7. Homogeneous plaque. Echogenic, homogeneous plaque in a right internal carotid artery (*arrow*).

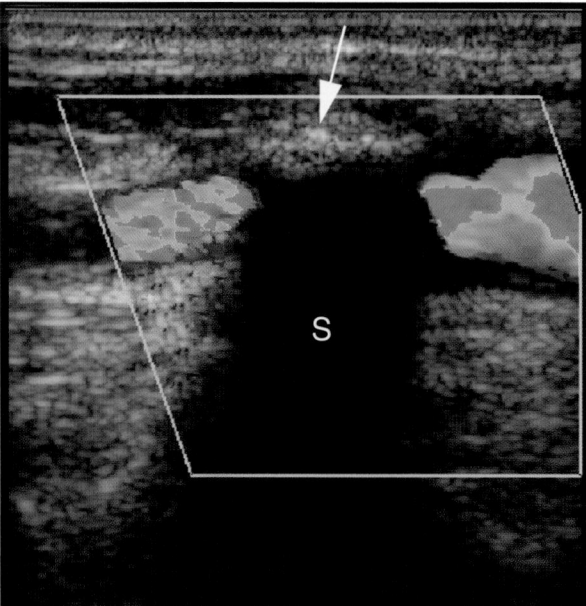

FIGURE 27-8. Calcified plaque. Calcific plaque (*arrow*) produces a shadow (S) which obscures a portion of the left carotid bulb.

intraplaque hemorrhage and/or deposits of lipid, cholesterol, and proteinaceous material.[9] Sonography accurately determines the presence or absence of intraplaque hemorrhage (sensitivity 90% to 94%, specificity 75% to 88%).[33,39,42-44] A "Swiss cheese" plaque appearance with multiple sonolucent areas is characteristic of intraplaque hemorrhage. Virtually all ulcerated plaques are associated with intraplaque hemorrhage. Sonographic findings that suggest **plaque ulceration** include a focal depression or break in the plaque surface, or an anechoic area within the plaque that extends to the plaque surface without an intervening echo between the vessel lumen and the anechoic plaque region. Some sources suggest classifying plaque according to four types (see box). Plaque types 1 and 2 are much more likely to be associated with intraplaque hemorrhage and/or ulceration and are considered unstable and subject to abrupt increase in plaque size following hemorrhage or embolization.[9,42] Types 1 and 2 plaque are typically found in symptomatic patients with greater than 70% diameter stenosis. Types 3 and 4 plaque are generally composed of fibrous tissue and/or calcification. These are generally more benign, stable plaques that are common in asymptomatic older individuals (see Fig. 27-8).

While ultrasound reportedly detects intraplaque hemorrhage reliably, in general, neither angiography nor ultrasound has proved highly accurate in identifying ulcerated plaque. However, recent studies suggest that color Doppler ultrasound and power Doppler ultrasound can improve sonographic identification of plaque ulceration. Color Doppler ultrasound or power Doppler ultrasound or B-flow, a proprietary non-Doppler imaging technique, may demonstrate slow-moving eddies of color within an anechoic region in plaque, which suggests ulceration (Fig. 27-10A, B).[44] The demonstration of these flow vortices was 94% accurate in predicting ulcerative plaque at surgery in one study.[45] Preliminary studies suggest that ultrasound contrast agents may further improve the ability to identify plaque surface characteristics.[46]

A potential pitfall in the diagnosis of plaque ulceration may result from a mirror image duplication artifact producing **pseudoulceration of the carotid artery** (Fig. 27-11A-C). Highly reflective plaque can produce a color Doppler ultrasound ghost artifact simulating ulceration. However, the region of color within the plaque can be recognized as artifactual as the spectral waveform and color shading within the pseudoulceration are of lower amplitude, but otherwise identical to those within the true carotid lumen.[47] Conversely, pulsed Doppler traces from within **ulcer craters** show low velocity damped waveforms (Fig. 27-12A, B). Although the diagnosis of ulceration is controversial, the ability to predict reliably intraplaque hemorrhage, with its associated clinical implications, underscores the importance of ultrasound plaque characterization. The presence of heterogeneous, irregular plaque should be noted because hemorrhagic plaque in a stenosis of less than 50% may be considered a surgical lesion in the appropriate clinical setting.

Evaluation of Stenosis. Measurements of carotid diameter and area stenosis should be made in the transverse plane, perpendicular to the long axis of the vessel using gray-scale imaging, B-flow imaging, or power

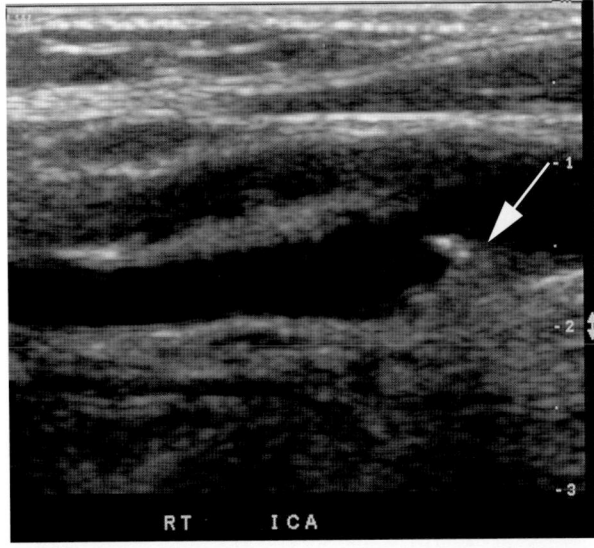

A

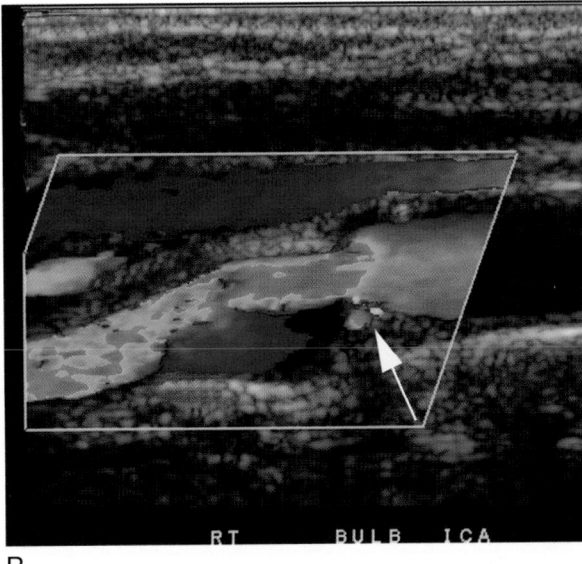

B

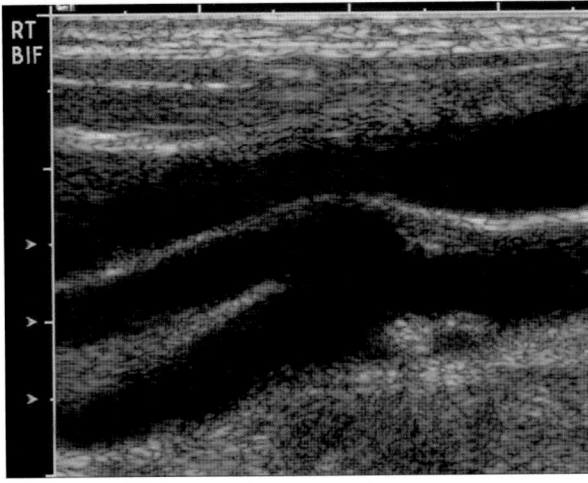

C

FIGURE 27-9. Plaque. A, Longitudinal image shows hypoechoic left internal carotid artery plaque (*arrow*) with possible ulcer crater. **B,** Color Doppler shows low-velocity eddy of flow (*arrow*) in the ulcer. **C,** Heterogeneous plaque in carotid bulb.

ULTRASOUND FEATURES SUGGESTIVE OF PLAQUE MORPHOLOGY

Type 1—Predominantly echolucent plaque, with a thin echogenic cap
Type 2—Substantially echolucent with small areas of echogenicity
Type 3—Predominantly echogenic with small areas of echolucency
Type 4—Uniformly echogenic

US FEATURES SUGGESTIVE OF PLAQUE ULCERATION

Focal depression or break in plaque surface
Anechoic region within plaque extending to vessel lumen
Eddies of color within plaque

Doppler imaging (Fig. 27-13A, B).[31] Measurements made on longitudinal scans may overestimate or underestimate the severity of stenosis by partial "voluming" through an eccentric plaque. Percentage of diameter stenosis and percentage of area stenosis are not always linearly related. Clinical records should state the type of stenosis measured. Asymmetrical stenoses are most appropriately assessed with percentage of area stenosis measurements,[31] although these measurements are often time consuming and technically difficult. The cephalocaudal extent and length of plaques should be noted as should the presence of **tandem plaques**.

As the severity of a stenosis increases, the quality of the real-time image deteriorates.[47,48] Several factors work against successful image assessment of high-grade

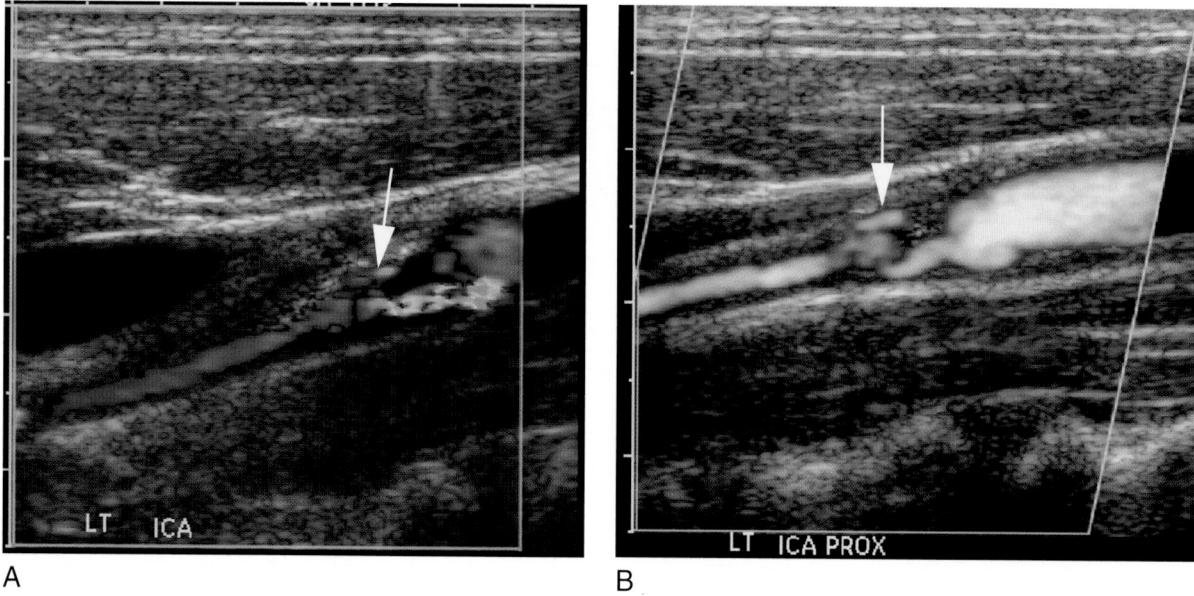

A   B

FIGURE 27-10. Plaque ulceration. Color (**A**) and power (**B**) Doppler longitudinal images show blood flow (*arrow*) into hypoechoic ulcerated plaque.

stenosis. Plaque calcification and irregularity produce shadowing, which obscures the vessel lumen. **Soft plaque** often has acoustic properties similar to flowing blood, producing anechoic plaques or thrombi that are almost invisible on gray-scale images. In the most extreme cases, vessels can show little visible plaque, yet be totally occluded (Fig. 27-14). Color Doppler readily identifies such phenomena. For these reasons, real-time gray-scale ultrasound is best suited for the evaluation of nonrate-limiting lesions, and not for quantifying high-grade stenoses, which are more accurately determined by spectral analysis.[49,50]

Spectral Analysis

Normal Doppler Spectrum. The Doppler spectrum is a quantitative graphic display of the velocities and directions of moving red blood cells present in the Doppler sample volume. Although Doppler assessment of carotid occlusive disease can be performed using frequency data, velocity calculations are preferable. Velocity values are potentially more accurate than frequency shift measurements, because angle theta between the transducer line of sight and the blood flow vector is used to convert a frequency shift to velocity. Frequency shifts vary according to the angle theta and the incident Doppler frequency; velocity measurements take both these factors into account.

The Doppler spectral display represents velocities on the y-axis and time on the x-axis. By convention, flow toward the transducer is displayed above the zero velocity baseline, and flow away from the transducer is below. For ease of spectral analysis, spectra that project

below the baseline are often inverted and placed above the baseline, always keeping in mind the true direction of flow within the vessel. The amplitude of each velocity component (the number of red blood cells with each velocity component) is used to modulate the brightness of the traces. This is also known as a gray-scale velocity plot. In the normal carotid artery, the frequency spectrum is narrow in systole and somewhat wider in early and late diastole. There is usually a black zone between the spectral line and the zero velocity baseline called the **spectral window** (Fig. 27-15).[51,52]

The internal carotid and external carotid branches of the CCA have distinctive spectral waveforms (Fig. 27-16A-C). The **ECA** supplies the high resistance vascular bed of the facial musculature; thus its flow resembles that of other peripheral arterial vessels. Flow velocity rises sharply during systole and falls rapidly in diastole, approaching zero or transiently reversing direction. The **ICA** supplies the low-resistance circulation of the brain and demonstrates flow similar to that in vessels supplying other blood-hungry organs, such as the liver, kidneys, and placenta. The common feature in all low-resistance arterial waveforms is that a large quantity of forward flow continues throughout diastole. The **CCA** waveform is a composite of the internal and external waveforms, but most often the common carotid more closely resembles the internal carotid flow pattern, and diastolic flow is generally above the baseline. Approximately 80% of the blood flowing from the CCA goes through the ICA into the brain, whereas 20% goes through the ECA into the head musculature. The relative decrease in blood flow through the ECA will cause it to have a generally lower amplitude gray-

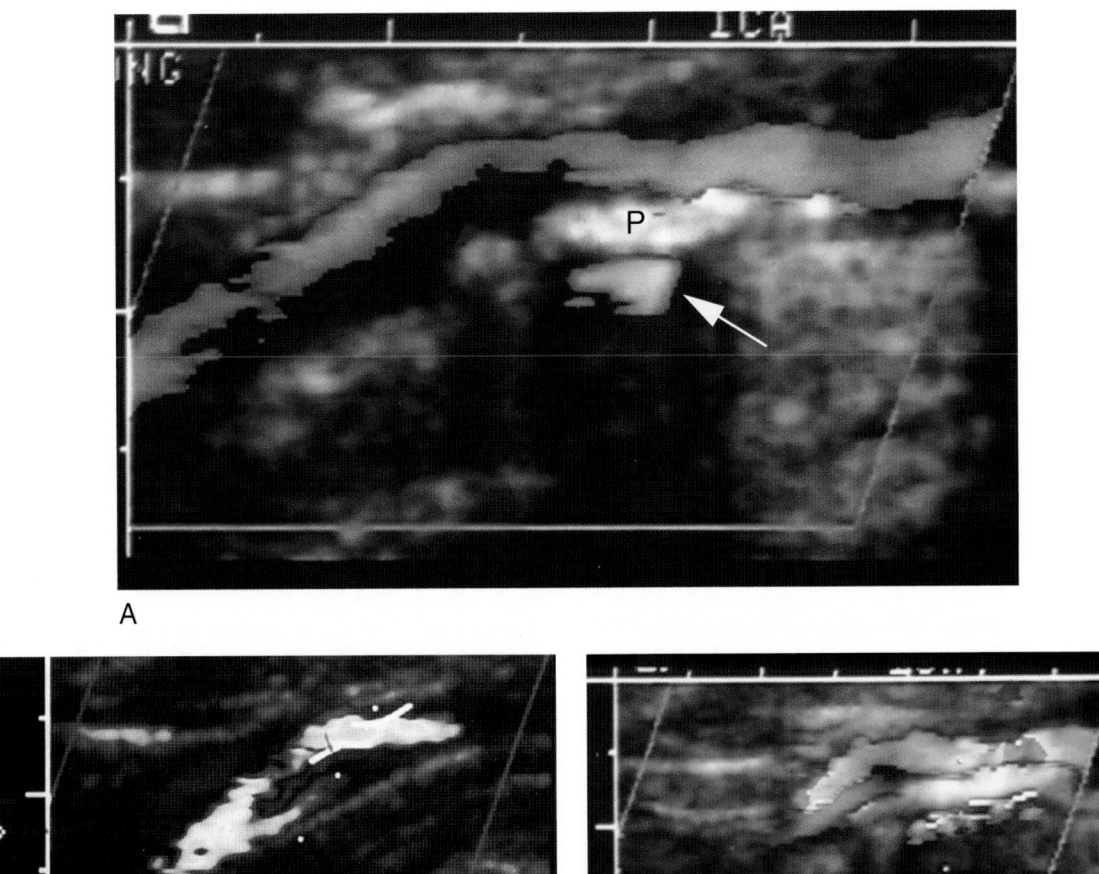

FIGURE 27-11. Plaque pseudoulceration. A, Longitudinal color Doppler image of the proximal left internal carotid artery (ICA) demonstrates an area of pseudoulceration (*arrow*) lying deep to a calcified plaque (P). **B,** Pulsed Doppler traces obtained from the lumen of the ICA demonstrate waveforms consistent with a less than 50% diameter stenosis. **C,** Pulsed Doppler waveforms obtained from the region of the pseudoulcer demonstrate a similar peak systolic velocity. However, the amplitude of the waveform is less than the artery lumen because mirror image artifacts have weaker signals.

scale waveform than that found in either the ICA or the CCA.[10]

Doppler Spectral Examination. Virtually all state-of-the-art US equipment offers color and power Doppler, as well as gray-scale capabilities and pulsed Doppler for the carotid examination. A rapid color Doppler screen allows the detection of abnormal flow patterns, which allows the pulsed Doppler signal volume to be placed in areas that are abnormal, especially those with **high velocity jets**. These high velocity jets are located in the region of and immediately distal to a high-grade stenosis (Fig. 27-17). In cases where both gray-scale and color (power) Doppler images of an entire carotid artery are normal, only representative spectral tracings from the CCA, ICA, and ECA are necessary to complete the examination.

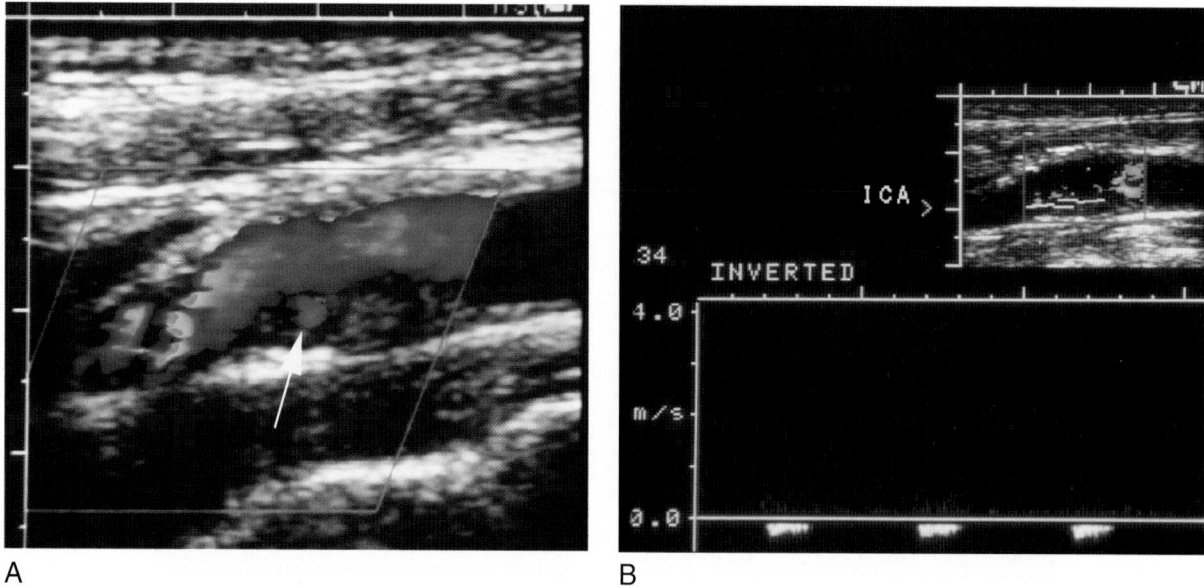

FIGURE 27-12. Plaque ulceration and abnormal flow. A, Longitudinal image of the proximal right internal carotid artery (ICA) demonstrates hypoechoic plaque with an associated area of reversed low velocity eddy flow within an ulcer (*arrow*). **B,** Pulsed Doppler waveforms in this ulcer crater demonstrate the very damped low velocity reversed flow not characteristic of that seen within the main vessel lumen of the ICA.

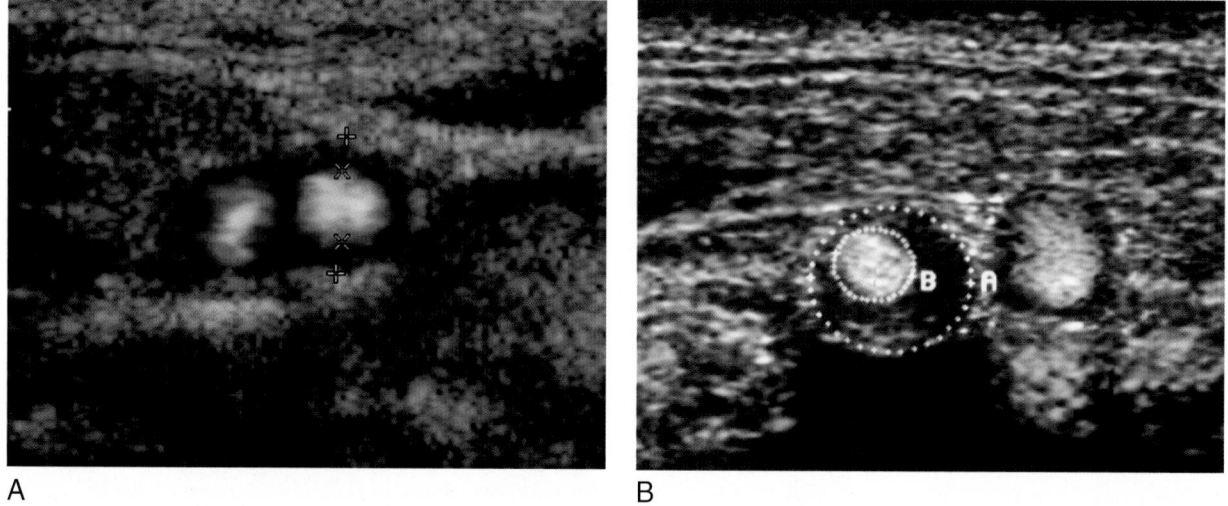

FIGURE 27-13. Measurement of carotid artery diameter. A, Power Doppler transverse image shows a less than 50% diameter stenosis (*cursors*). **B,** Transverse "B-flow" image of the right carotid bifurcation shows a measurement of internal carotid artery (ICA) area stenosis (B). Outer ICA area (A).

A recent publication suggests that a **power Doppler screening examination** could produce an accurate and cost-effective method for patients at risk for carotid disease.[53] Power Doppler imaging used independent of spectral analysis was effectively performed in 89 of 100 patients. The sensitivity for the detection of 40% or greater stenoses using power Doppler was 91% with a 79% specificity. This would be reasonable for a screening test such that those patients with greater than 40% stenoses could be subjected to more expensive spectral analysis. Some believe that the utilization of this less

expensive power Doppler screening could result in a more cost-effective approach to carotid Doppler screening. In addition, carotid power Doppler imaging, as well as carotid B-flow imaging, is ideally suited to utilization in conjunction with vascular contrast agents which may be widely available in the future.

The standard Doppler spectral examination consists of traces obtained from the proximal and distal CCA, the carotid bulb, the proximal ECA, samples in the proximal, middle, and distal ICA, and a representative trace from the vertebral artery. Normal velocities range

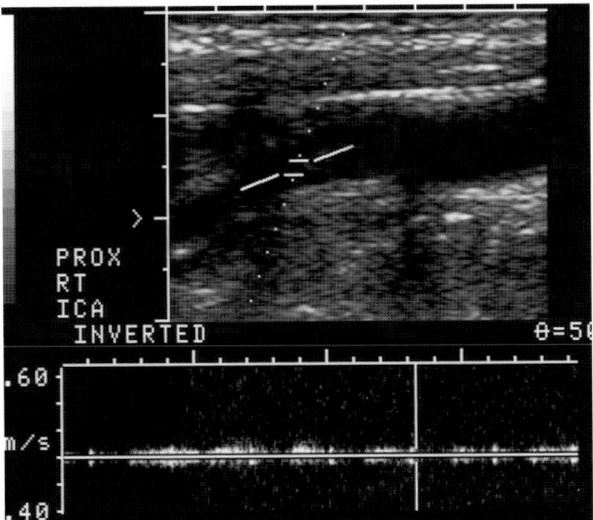

FIGURE 27-14. Sonolucent plaque occludes right internal carotid artery. Image shows no pulsed Doppler flow.

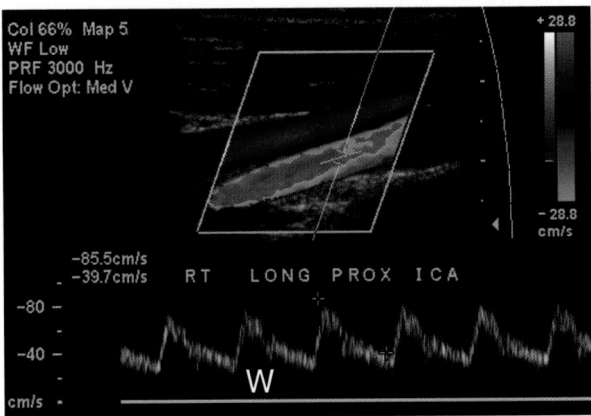

FIGURE 27-15. Normal internal carotid artery (ICA) waveform. Normal, low resistance ICA waveform with clear spectral window (W) indicating absence of spectral broadening.

from higher in the proximal CCA to lower in the distal vessel; normal ICA velocities tend to increase from proximal to distal. In addition, blood flow velocities are obtained immediately proximal to, at, and just beyond regions of maximal visible stenosis and at 1 cm intervals distal to the visualized plaque as far cephalad as possible. Positioning the Doppler angle cursor parallel to the vessel walls determines angle theta, which is used to convert frequency information into velocity values (see Fig. 27-16B). Angle theta is defined as the angle between the Doppler transducer line of sight and the direction of blood flow. The ideal angle theta is 0 degrees, as the cosine of this angle is 1, thus resulting in the greatest possible detectable frequency shift. Because this angle is rarely achievable in the clinical setting, a range of angles from 30 degrees to 60 degrees is considered acceptable for carotid spectral analysis.

Certain schools of US elect a technique in which the Doppler angle is set at 60% and the transducer is "heel and toed" to parallel the carotid artery for Doppler spectral analysis. In our experience, it is frequently not possible to optimize cursor placement in the midportion of the vessel using this technique in tortuous vessels. Therefore, our technique involves selecting the site of spectral analysis and paralleling the wall of the vessel at that point, making certain that the Doppler angle does not exceed 60 degrees. While either technique can be used, results obtained using these different methodologies can result in different velocities. Thus, if the first technique is used, a different set of velocity criteria should be expected than if the second technique is used. This is one of the factors responsible for the differences in velocity spectral criteria utilized in different laboratories (Fig. 27-18A, B). **When angle theta exceeds 60 degrees to 70 degrees, the accuracy of velocity/frequency data declines precipitously to the point where virtually no velocity change is detected at angle theta of 90 degrees.** The entire course of the CCA and ICA should be interrogated with a consistent angle theta maintained throughout the examination, when possible. Generally only the origin of the ECA is evaluated because occlusive plaque is less common here than in the ICA and is rarely clinically significant. A stenosis of the ECA should be noted because it may account for a worrisome cervical bruit when the ICA is normal.[20]

Spectral Broadening. Atheromatous plaque projecting into the arterial lumen disturbs the normal, smooth laminar flow of erythrocytes. The red blood cells move with a wider range of velocities, so the spectral line becomes wider, filling in the normally black spectral window. This phenomenon is termed "**spectral broadening**" (Fig. 27-19). Spectral broadening increases in proportion to the severity of carotid artery stenosis, and a number of schemes have been derived to measure this parameter.[54-56] Some duplex machines allow the operator to measure the spectral spread between the maximal and minimal velocities (bandwidth), and thus quantitate spectral broadening. The validity of these measurements remains to be proved, however, and further correlative studies are needed to document the relationship of quantitative spectral broadening parameters to specific degrees of stenosis.[56] Nevertheless, a visible gestalt of the amount of spectral window obliteration, as well as color Doppler heterogeneity, provides a useful, if not quantitative, predictor of the severity of flow disturbance.

Pitfalls. Pseudospectral broadening can be caused by technical factors, such as **too high a gain setting**. In such instances, the background around the spectral waveform often contains noise. Whenever spectral broadening is suspected, the gain should be lowered to see if the spectral window clears. Similarly, spectral broadening caused by **vessel wall motion** can occur

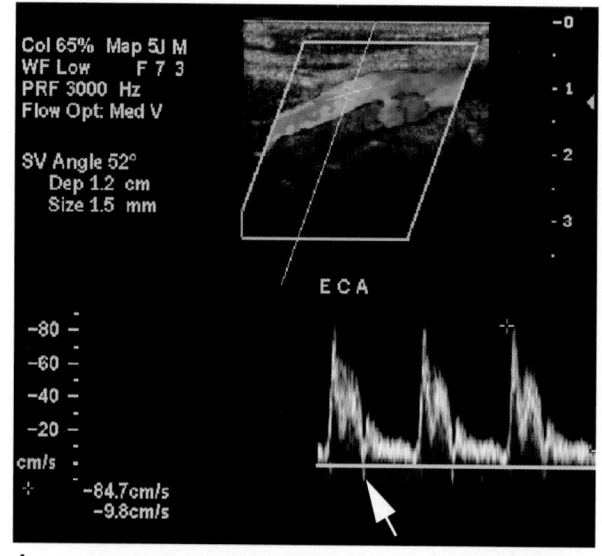

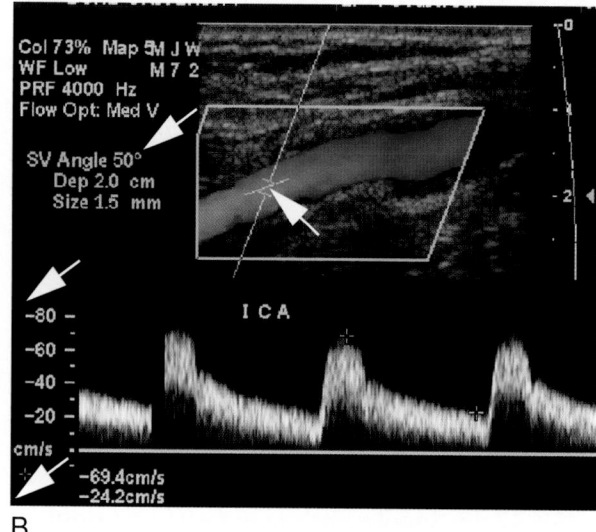

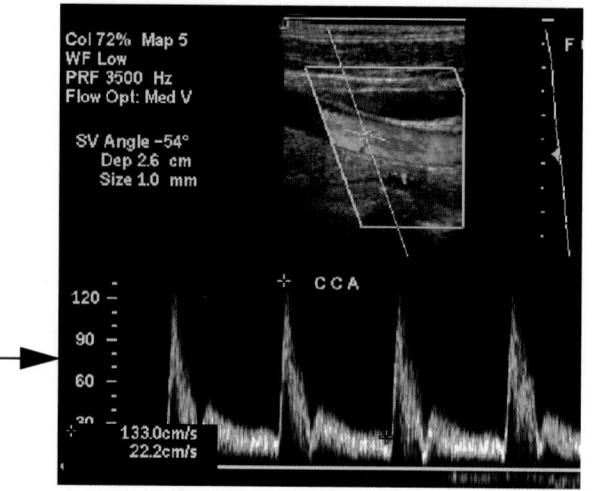

FIGURE 27-16. Normal ECA, ICA, CCA waveforms.
A, Right ECA shows a sharp systolic upstroke and relatively low velocity end-diastolic flow (*arrow*) indicating a vessel supplying high impedance circulation. **B**, ICA shows a larger amount of end-diastolic flow consistent with the low impedance intracerebral circulation. Angle theta (*arrow*) is 50 degrees. **C**, Normal distal CCA waveform is a composite of low resistance ICA and higher resistance CCA waveforms. Note that flow in **C** is toward the transducer (*arrow*) and the Doppler spectrum is plotted above the baseline. In **A** and **B**, flow is directed away from the transducer. Although these spectra have been inverted, the negative velocity signs (*arrows*) remind the operator of the true flow direction. CCA, common carotid artery; ECA, external carotid artery; ICA, internal carotid artery.

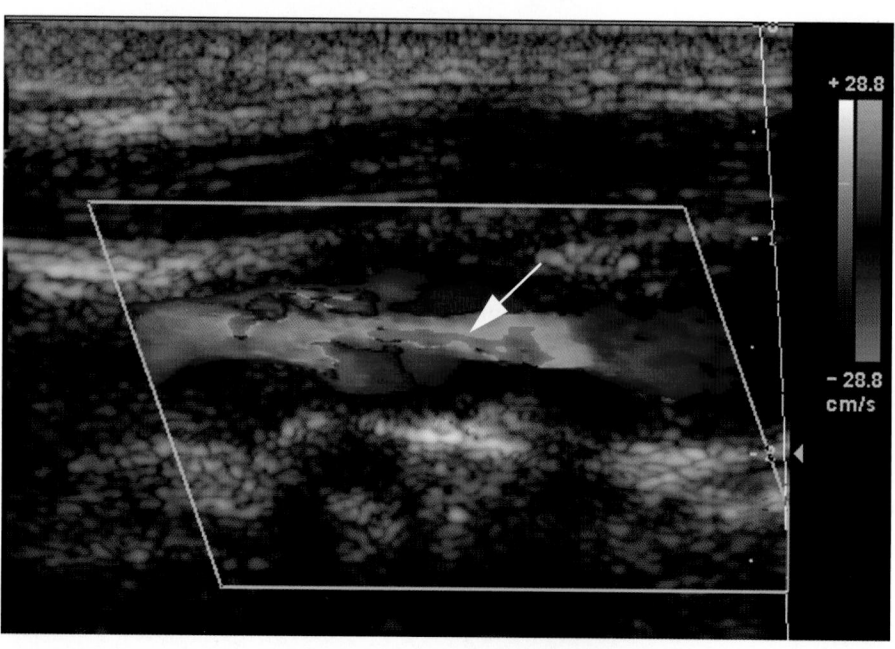

FIGURE 27-17. Color Doppler jet. High velocity jet (*arrow*) or aliasing color demonstrates the area of highest velocity in the area of stenosis.

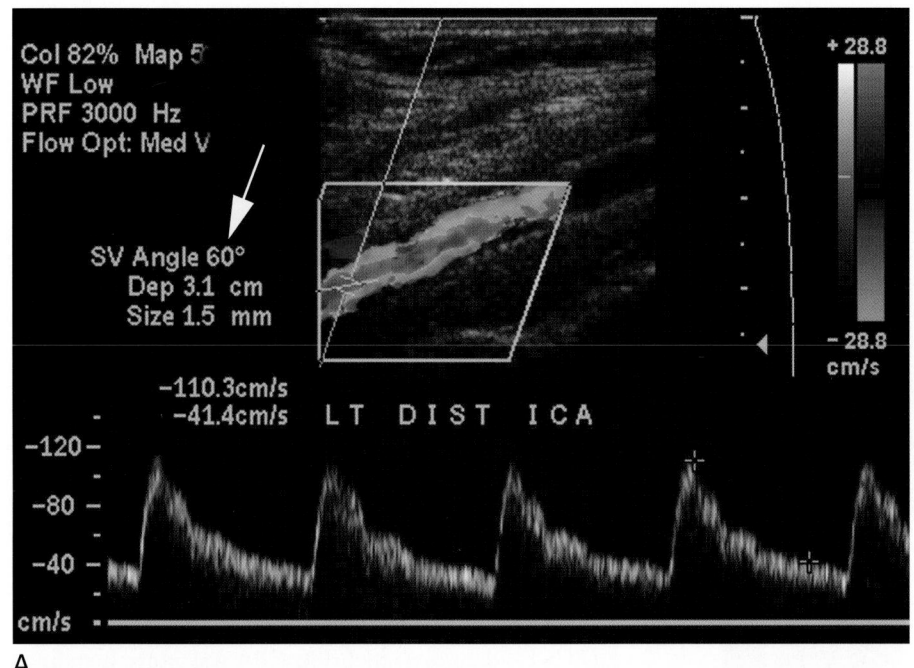

A

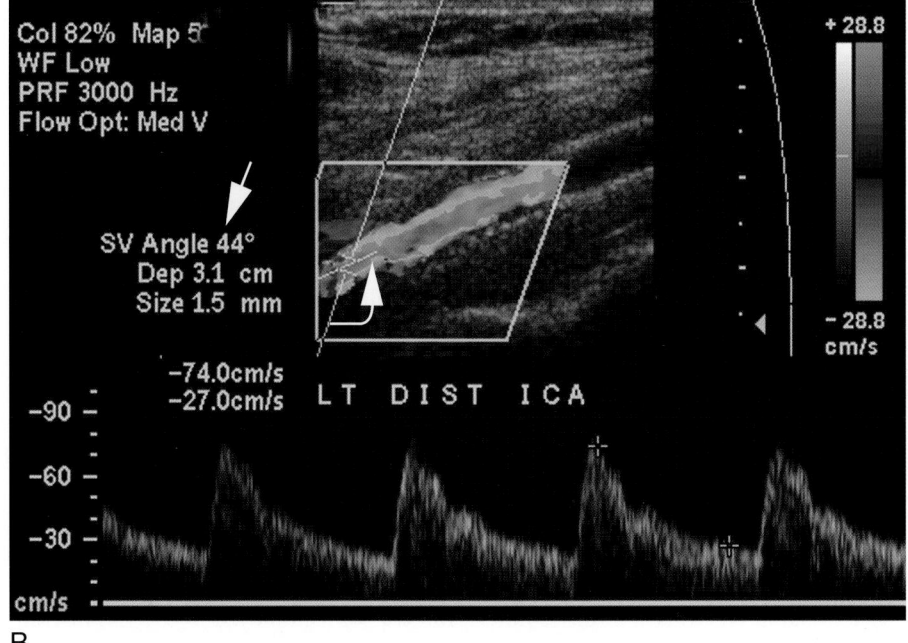

B

FIGURE 27-18. Doppler angle measurement. A, Velocity obtained in the distal ICA with angle theta of 60 degrees is higher than that obtained at 44 degrees (*arrow*) (**B**). However, the sample angle does not parallel the vessel wall at 60 degrees. Note central color aliasing in the region of highest velocity (*curved arrow*).

when the Doppler sample volume is too large or positioned too near the vessel wall. Decreasing the size of the sample volume and placing it midstream should eliminate this potential pitfall.

Altered flow patterns can be found **normally at certain sites** in the carotid system. For instance, it is normal to find flow separation at the **site of branching vessels**, such as where the CCA branches into the ECA and ICA.[57] Flow disturbances also occur at sites where there is an **abrupt change in the vessel diameter**. For instance, flow disturbances and bizarre waveforms due

to flow separation may be encountered in a normal carotid bulb where the CCA terminates in a localized area of dilation as it divides into the ECA and ICA (Fig. 27-20A-C).[10]

The tendency for spectral broadening to occur increases in direct proportion to the velocity of blood flow. For example, it can be observed in normal ECA, vertebral arteries, and in a CCA that is supplying circulation contralateral to an occluded contralateral ICA. **Increased velocity** may also account for the disturbed flow that is sometimes observed in the normal

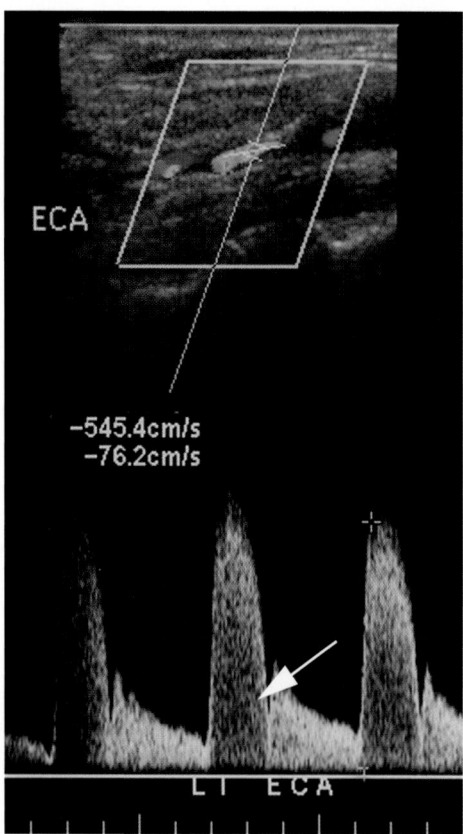

FIGURE 27-19. High-grade external carotid artery stenosis. Elevated velocities and visible narrowing. Spectral broadening is present (*arrow*). Color Doppler spectral broadening is also seen.

extracranial carotid arteries of young athletes with normal cardiac outputs or in patients in pathologic high cardiac output states. It is also seen in arteries supplying **arteriovenous fistulas** and **arteriovenous malformations.**[10,58] Postoperative spectral broadening may persist for months **after CEA** in the absence of significant residual or recurrent disease. This may be due to changes in wall compliance.

Tortuous carotid vessels can demonstrate spectral broadening and asymmetrical high velocity flow jets in the absence of plaque disease. Other nonatheromatous causes of disturbed blood flow in the extracranial carotid arteries include **aneurysms, arterial wall dissections, and fibromuscular dysplasia.**

High Velocity Pulsed Doppler Blood Flow Patterns. Carotid stenoses usually begin to cause velocity changes when they exceed 50% diameter (70% cross-sectional area) (Fig. 27-21A-C).[1] Velocity elevations generally increase as the severity of the stenosis increases. At critical stenoses (>95%), the velocity measurements may actually decrease and the waveform becomes dampened.[50,59] In these cases, correlation with color Doppler or power Doppler imaging is essential to correctly diagnose the severity of the stenosis. Velocity increases are focal and most pronounced in and imme-

diately distal to a stenosis, emphasizing the importance of sampling directly in these regions. As one moves further distal from a stenosis, flow begins to reconstitute and assume a more normal pattern, provided a tandem lesion does not exist distal to the initial site of stenosis. Spectral broadening results in the jets of high velocity flow associated with carotid stenosis; however, correlation with gray-scale and color Doppler images can define other causes of spectral broadening. An awareness of normal flow spectra combined with appropriate Doppler techniques can obviate many potential diagnostic pitfalls.

The degree of carotid stenosis that is considered clinically significant in the symptomatic or asymptomatic patient is in evolution. Initially it was thought that lesions causing 50% diameter stenosis were significant; this perception changed as more information was gathered from two large clinical trials. The **North American Symptomatic Carotid Endarterectomy Trial (NASCET) and the European Carotid Surgery Trial (ECST), demonstrated that CEA was more beneficial than medical therapy in symptomatic patients with 70% to 99% ICA stenosis.**[4,5] Interestingly, the method used to grade stenoses in the ECST study was significantly different than that used in the NASCET trials. The NASCET trials compared the severity of the ICA stenosis on arteriogram with the residual lumen of a presumably more normal distal ICA. The ECST methodology entailed assessment of the severity of stenosis with a "guesstimation" of the lumen of the carotid artery at the level of the stenosis. The ECST assessment is more comparable to the ultrasound visible assessment of the degree of narrowing, whereas velocity tables currently in use have been derived to correspond to the NASCET angiographic determinations for stenosis. The European community trial method for grading carotid artery stenosis tends to give a more severe assessment of narrowing than the NASCET technique.

The initial NASCET trials retrospectively compared velocity data obtained on the Doppler examination with angiographic measurements of stenosis. No standardized ultrasound protocol was employed by the numerous centers involved in the trial. In spite of the lack of uniformity, moderate sensitivity and specificity ranging from 65% to 77% were obtained for grading ICA stenoses using Doppler velocities. If ultrasound technique is standardized and criteria are validated in a given laboratory, peak systolic velocity, as well as peak systolic ratios, have proved to be an accurate method for determining carotid stenosis.[60] A study from the European community surgery trial group compared three different angiographic measurement techniques: the NASCET technique, the ECST technique, and an additional technique comparing measurements of the distal CCA with that of the ICA stenosis. They concluded that the ECST and NASCET techniques

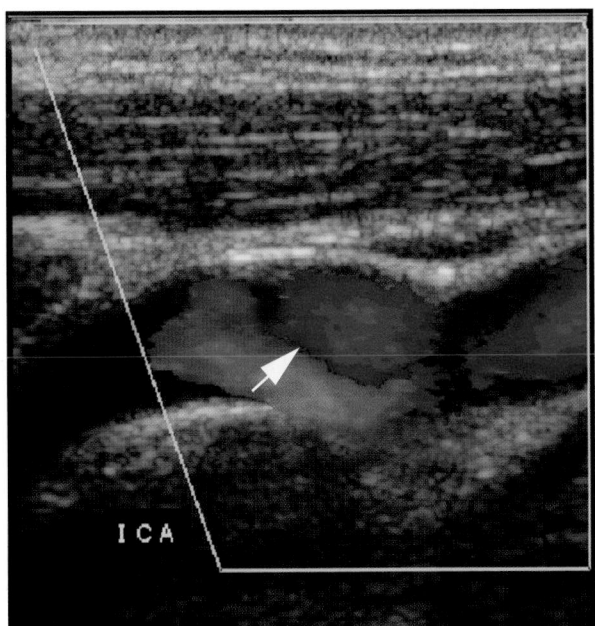

A

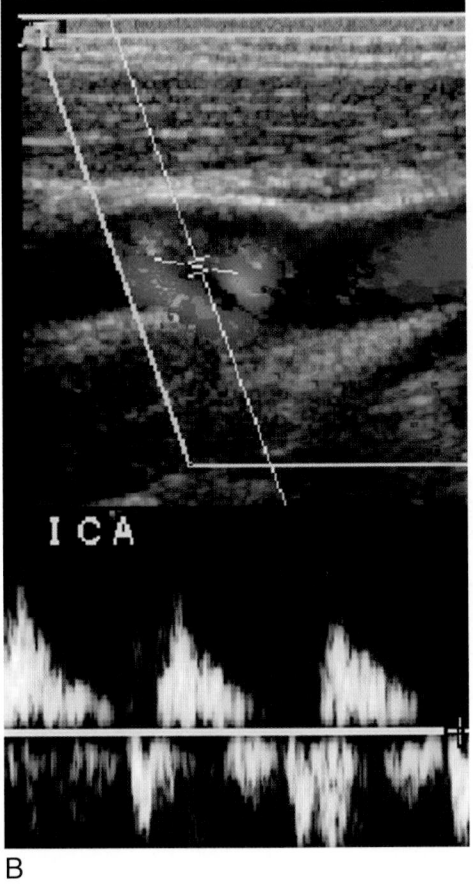

B

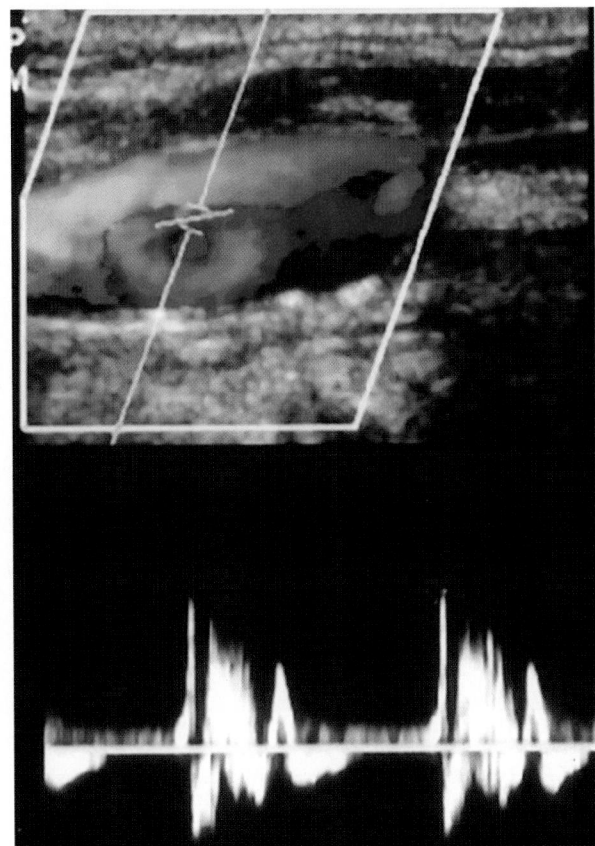

C

FIGURE 27-20. Disturbed flow pattern. A, Longitudinal left bulb image shows color flow separation (*arrow*). **B** and **C,** Two examples of disturbed flow patterns in areas of normal carotid bulb/internal carotid artery flow separation.

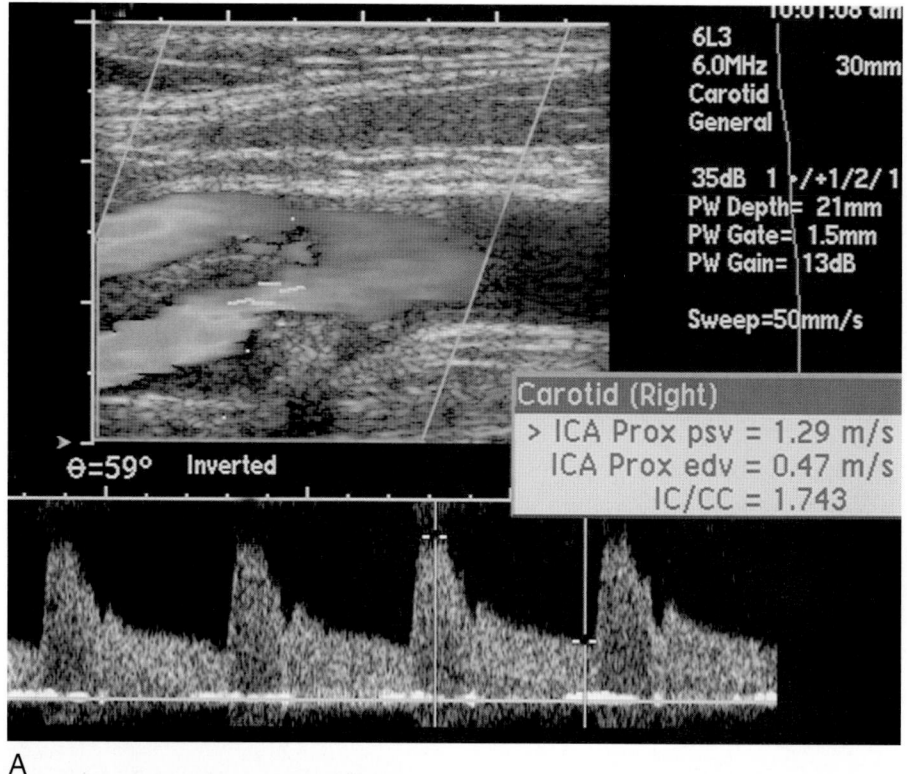

A

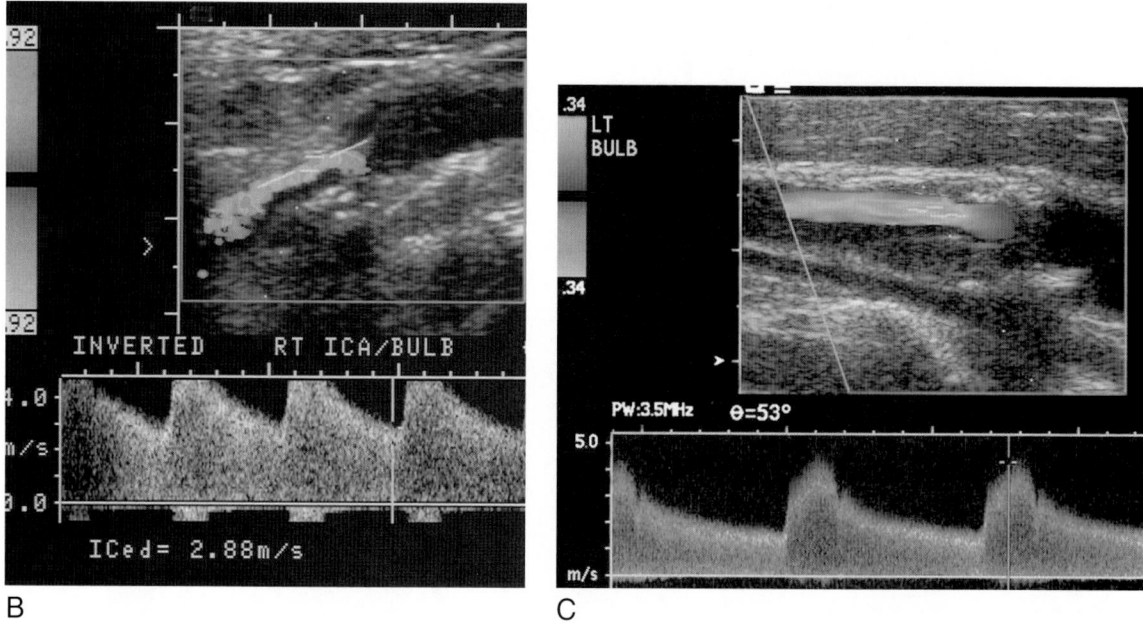

B   C

FIGURE 27-21. ICA Stenosis. A, Internal carotid artery (ICA) stenosis of 50% to 69% diameter shows a peak systolic velocity of 129 cm/sec. **B,** Right ICA demonstrates a visible high-grade stenosis on color Doppler with end-diastolic velocities of greater than 288 cm/sec and peak systolic velocities which alias at greater than 400 cm/sec. This is consistent with a very high-grade stenosis. **C,** Left carotid bulb seen in longitudinal projection with color Doppler demonstrates a high-grade narrowing and spectral broadening with approximately a 400 cm/sec velocity in peak systole and 150 cm/sec in end diastole, consistent with an 80% to 99% stenosis.

were similar in their prognostic value, whereas the CCA/stenosis measurement was the most reproducible of the three techniques. They also concluded that the CCA method, although reproducible, would be invalidated by the presence of CCA disease.[61] Virtually all investigators advocate using the NASCET angiographic measurement technique.

The results of these trials, as well as the more recent ACAS and moderate NASCET studies, have generated reappraisals of the Doppler velocity criteria that most accurately define 70% or greater stenosis and, more recently, greater than 50% diameter stenoses.[62] Attempts have been made to determine the Doppler parameters or combination of parameters that most reliably identify a certain diameter stenosis. Most sources agree that the single best parameter is the peak systolic velocity of the ICA in the region of a stenosis.[59] Using multiple parameters can improve diagnostic confidence, particularly when combined with color and power Doppler imaging.

Degree of stenosis is best assessed using the gray-scale and pulsed Doppler parameters including ICA peak systolic velocity (**PSV**), ICA end-diastolic velocity (**EDV**), CCA PSV, CCA EDV, **peak systolic ICA/CCA ratios,** and **peak end-diastolic ICA/CCA ratios.**[59,60,63] Peak systolic velocity has proved accurate for quantifying high-grade stenoses.[50,60] The relationship of this parameter to the degree of luminal narrowing is well defined and it is easily measured.[64,65] Although Doppler velocities have proved reliable for defining 70% or greater stenosis, Grant showed less favorable results for substenosis classification between 50% and 69% using PSV and ICA/CCA peak systolic velocity ratios.[60] At our institution, a quick rule of thumb is peak systolic ICA velocities less than 125 cm/sec are consistent with less than 50% diameter stenosis; 125 to 250 cm/sec corresponds with 50% to 75% diameter stenosis; greater than 250 cm/sec corresponds with greater than 75% to 80% diameter stenosis.[63] End-diastolic velocity is often useful in distinguishing between degrees of high-grade stenosis.

There are no established criteria for grading ECA stenoses. A good rule of thumb is that if the ECA velocities do not exceed 200 cm/sec, there is not a significant stenosis. However, we usually rely on a visible assessment of the degree of narrowing associated with velocity changes. Occlusive plaque involving the ECA is less common than in the ICA and is rarely clinically significant. Similarly, velocity criteria used to grade CCA stenoses have not been well established. However, if one is able to visualize 2 cm proximal and 2 cm distal to a visible CCA stenosis, a peak-systolic velocity ratio obtained 2 cm proximal to the stenosis versus that in the region of the greatest visible stenosis can be used to grade the percent diameter stenosis in a fashion analogous to that used in peripheral artery studies. A doubling of the peak-systolic velocity across a lesion would correspond to at least a 50% diameter stenosis, and a velocity ratio in excess of 3.5 corresponds to a greater than 75% stenosis. While duplex US remains an accurate method of quantifying ICA stenoses, use of color Doppler and power Doppler has significantly improved diagnostic confidence and reproducibility.[66]

One persistent problem with duplex evaluation of the carotids is that different institutions use peak systolic velocities ranging from 130 cm/sec[67] to 325 cm/sec[62] to diagnose greater than 70% ICA stenosis. Many factors are involved in creating these discrepancies including technique and equipment.[68] This wide range of peak systolic velocities reinforces the need for individual US laboratories to determine which Doppler parameters are most reliable in their own institution.[69] Correlation of the velocity ranges obtained by US with angiographic and surgical results is necessary to achieve accurate, reproducible examinations in a particular US laboratory.[70]

The Society of Radiologists in Ultrasound (SRU) held a consensus conference in October, 2002 to consider Carotid Doppler Ultrasound.[71] The panelists represented multiple medical and surgical specialties. They arrived at a consensus regarding guidelines for performing and interpreting carotid ultrasound examinations and devised a set of criteria that the conference panelists felt were feasible and widely applicable to a broad range of vascular laboratories. Although the consensus conference did not recommend that all established laboratories with internally validated velocity charts alter their practice, it was suggested that physicians establishing new laboratories consider using the consensus criteria; those with pre-existing charts might consider comparing in-house criteria with those provided by the consensus conference. Velocity criteria corresponding to specific degrees of vascular stenosis are listed in Table 27-1A, B. The table used at our institution (Table 27-1B)[71] has a category for 80% to 99% stenoses because our surgeons may be more inclined to operate on asymptomatic greater than 80% stenoses than on less severe stenoses.

Values obtained in the ICA should be obtained at or just distal to the point of maximum visible stenosis and/or at the point of greatest color Doppler spectral abnormality. Values obtained from the CCA should be obtained 2 cm proximal to the widening in the region of the carotid bulb. Because velocities normally decrease from proximal to distal in the CCA and increase from proximal to distal in the ICA, it is important that standardized levels be used routinely for obtaining the ICA/CCA velocity ratio.

Color Doppler Ultrasound

Color Doppler ultrasound displays flow information in real time over the entire image or a selected area. Stationary soft-tissue structures, which lack a detectable phase or frequency shift, are assigned an amplitude value

TABLE 27-1A. SOCIETY OF RADIOLOGISTS IN ULTRASOUND CONSENSUS CONFERENCE ON CAROTID ULTRASOUND OCTOBER 22-23, 2002

	ICA PSV	Plaque	ICA/CCA PSV Ratio	ICA EDV
Normal	<125 cm/sec	None	<2.0	<40 cm/sec
<50%	<125 cm/sec	<50% diameter reduction	<2.0	<40 cm/sec
50%-69%	125-230 cm/sec	≥50% diameter reduction	2.0-4.0	40-100 cm/sec
≥70 to near occlusion	>230 cm/sec	≥50% diameter reduction	>4.0	>100 cm/sec
Near occlusion	May be low or undetectable	Visible	Variable	Variable
Total occlusion	Undetectable	Visible, no detectable lumen	Not applicable	Not applicable

CCA, common carotid artery; EDV, end-diastolic velocity; ICA, internal carotid artery; PSV, peak-systolic velocity.
From Consensus Conference on Carotid Ultrasound, Society of Radiologists in Ultrasound, October 2002, San Francisco. Radiology, 2003; 229:340-346.

TABLE 27-1B. DOPPLER SPECTRAL ANALYSIS

Diameter Stenosis	Peak-Systolic Velocity	ICA/CCA Systolic Ratio	End-Diastolic Ratio
0%-49%	25 cm/sec, <125 cm/sec	<2	<40 cm/sec
50%-69%	125-210 cm/sec	2-3	40-70 cm/sec
70%-79%	>210 cm/sec	>3	70-100 cm/sec
80%-99%*	>280 cm/sec	>3.7	>100 cm/sec
*Near occlusion velocities may be low			
Occlusion	No flow detectable		

CCA, common carotid artery; ICA, internal carotid artery.
From North American Symptomatic Carotid Endarterectomy Trial Collaborators. Beneficial effect of carotid endarterectomy in symptomatic patients with high-grade carotid stenosis. N Engl J Med 1991; 325:445-453; and Consensus Conference on Carotid Ultrasound, Society of Radiologists in Ultrasound, October 2002, San Francisco. Radiology, 2003;229:340-346.

and displayed in a gray-scale format with flowing blood in vessels superimposed in color. The mean Doppler frequency shift produced by red blood cell ensembles pulsing through a selected sample volume is obtained using an autocorrelative method or a time domain processing (speckle motion analysis) method. Color assignments depend on the direction of blood flow relative to the Doppler transducer. Blood flow toward the transducer appears in one color, and flow away from the transducer in another. These color assignments are arbitrary and are generally set up so that arterial flow is depicted as red, and venous flow as blue. Color saturation displays indicate the variable velocity of blood flow. Deeper shades usually indicate low velocities centered around the zero velocity color flow baseline. As velocity increases, the shades become lighter or are assigned a different color hue. Some systems allow selected frequency shifts to be displayed in a contrasting color, such as green. This **green-tag** feature provides a real-time estimation of the presence of high velocity flow.

Setting the color Doppler scale can also be used to create an aliasing artifact corresponding to the highest velocity flow within a vessel (see Fig. 27-18). These **high velocity jets** pinpoint areas for spectral analysis. Color assignments are a function of both the mean frequency shift produced by moving red cell ensembles and the Doppler angle theta. If the vessel is tortuous or diving, angle theta will change along the course of the vessel, resulting in **changing color assignments** that are unrelated to the change in red blood cell velocity. The color assignments will reverse in tortuous vessels as their course changes relative to the Doppler transducer, even though the absolute direction of flow is unchanged. Portions of a vessel that **parallel the Doppler beam** when the angle theta is 90 degrees will have little or no frequency shift detected and no color will be seen.

Optimal Settings for Low Flow Vessel Evaluations. Color Doppler studies should be performed with optimal flow sensitivity and gain settings. Color flow should fill the entire vessel lumen but not spill over into adjacent soft tissues. The pulsed repetition frequency (PRF) and frame rates should be set to allow visualization of flow phenomenon anticipated in a vessel. Frame rates will vary as a function of the width of the area chosen for color Doppler display, as well as for the depth of the region of interest. The greater the color image area, the slower the frame rate will be. The deeper the posterior boundary of the color image, the slower the PRF. Color Doppler sensitivity should be adjusted to detect anticipated velocities, such that if slow flow in a preocclusive carotid lesion is sought, low flow settings with decreased sampling rates are employed. However, the system will then alias at lower velocities because of the decrease in PRF. In addition to **changes in the PRF, optimization of the Doppler angle, gain and power settings, a decrease in the wall filter, an increase in persistence, and an increase in ensemble or dwell time** can be used to optimize low-flow detection.

Flowing blood becomes, in effect, its own contrast medium with color Doppler ultrasound or power Doppler ultrasound outlining the patent vessel lumen. This allows determination of the true course of the vessel, facilitating positioning of the Doppler cursor, and, thus, allowing more reliable velocity determinations. Furthermore, color Doppler ultrasound facilitates Doppler spectral analysis by rapidly identifying areas of flow abnormalities. The highest velocities in the region of and immediately distal to a stenosis are seen as aliasing high velocity jets of color. Color Doppler ultrasound facilitates placing the pulsed Doppler range gate in the region of these most striking color abnormalities for pulsed Doppler spectral analysis. The presence of a stenosis can be determined by color Doppler changes in the vessel lumen, as well as by visible luminal narrowing. Although color Doppler can be used to determine the presence of hypoechoic plaque, color Doppler cannot be used optimally to determine the area of patent lumen in transverse projection because the optimal angle for measuring the area or diameter of narrowing is at 90 degrees to the long axis of the vessel, which is the worst angle for color Doppler imaging. Either gray-scale assessment, power Doppler, or B-flow imaging should be used to assess the diameter/area of the patent carotid (see Fig. 27-13A, B). If a stenosis produces a **bruit or thrill**, the resultant perivascular tissue vibrations may actually be seen as transient speckles of color in the adjacent soft tissues more prominent during systole (Fig. 27-22).[72]

Comparisons of color Doppler ultrasound with conventional duplex sampling techniques and angiography have shown relatively similar accuracy, sensitivity, and specificity.[73] However, color Doppler ultrasound offers many valuable benefits (see box). Color Doppler ultrasound reduces the examination time by pinpointing areas of color Doppler abnormality for pulsed Doppler spectral analysis. Branches of the ECA are readily detected, facilitating differentiation from the ICA. The real-time flow information over a large cross-sectional area provides a global overview of flow abnormalities and allows the course of a vessel to be readily determined. Furthermore, color Doppler improves diagnostic confi-

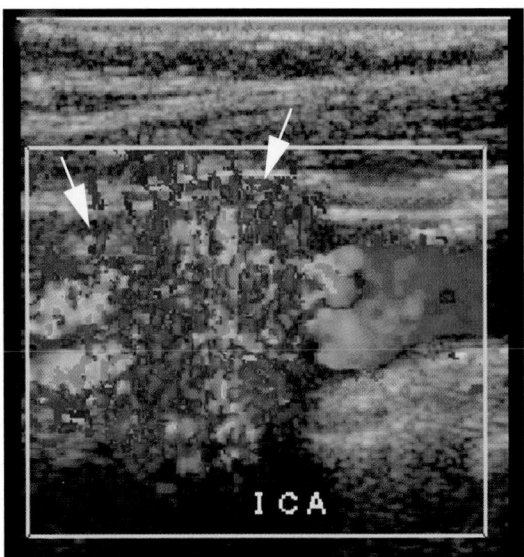

FIGURE 27-22. Color Doppler bruit. Extensive soft tissue color Doppler bruit (*arrows*) surrounds the right carotid bifurcation with a 90% right ICA stenosis.

dence and reproducibility of US studies, thereby avoiding many potential diagnostic pitfalls. The laminar blood flow is disrupted in the region of the carotid bifurcation where there is a **normal transient flow reversal** opposite the origin of the ECA (see Figs. 27-20A-C). Color Doppler displays this normal flow separation as an area of flow reversal located along the outer wall of the carotid bulb, which appears either at early systole or in peak systole and persists for a variable amount of time into the diastolic portion of the cardiac cycle.[74,75] This flow reversal can produce some strikingly bizarre pulsed Doppler waveforms; however, the color Doppler appearance readily discerns the nature of these waveform changes. Furthermore, it has been suggested that the absence of this flow reversal is abnormal and may represent one of the earliest changes of atherosclerotic disease.[74] The flow reversal seen in the region of the carotid bifurcation is clearly different than that seen with color Doppler aliasing. Contiguous saturated areas of red and blue are seen in this low velocity flow separation as compared with the very different contiguous color hues representing the highest color assignments for forward and reversed flow. **Helical flow** in the CCA can be an indirect indication of proximal arterial stenosis, but can occur as a normal variant. Color Doppler graphically displays the eccentric spiraling of flow up the CCA.

Pitfalls of Color Doppler. Color Doppler may help avoid potential diagnostic pitfalls. **Alterations in cardiovascular physiology, tandem lesions, contralateral carotid disease, arrhythmias, postoperative changes,** and **tortuous vessels** can lead to under- or overestimation of the degree of stenosis. In such cases, color Doppler ultrasound can provide direct visualization of the patent lumen in a fashion analogous to angiography.[76] In

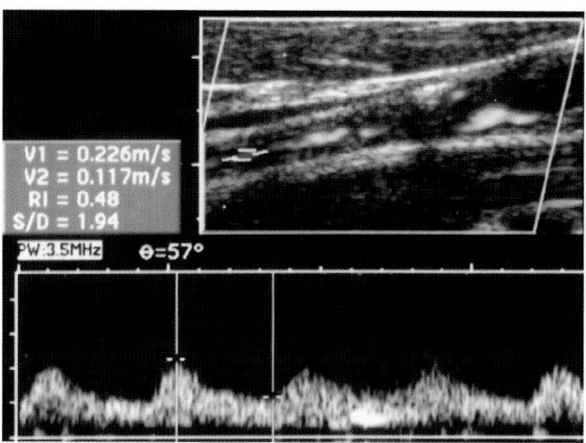

FIGURE 27-23. High-grade "string sign" stenosis of internal carotid artery. Tardus/parvus waveform with low velocity in a long segment.

fact, because angiography images only the vessel lumen, not the vessel wall, color Doppler ultrasound (power Doppler ultrasound) imaging has the potential to evaluate stenoses even more completely than angiography. Because flow patterns are displayed with color Doppler imaging, the local hemodynamic consequences of the lesion are readily discerned. Color Doppler ultrasound/power Doppler ultrasound appears to have particular value in detecting **small residual channels of flow** in areas of high-grade carotid stenoses (Fig. 27-23).[72,73,76-78] Power Doppler ultrasound offers a comparable advantage and has the theoretical potential to be more sensitive for detecting extremely low amplitude, low velocity flow. Finally, color Doppler ultrasound and power Doppler ultrasound have the potential to clarify image Doppler mismatches, further improving diagnostic accuracy and confidence.

Although color Doppler ultrasound offers many advantages, it is angle dependent and prone to artifacts, such as aliasing. The spatial resolution of color Doppler ultrasound is less than that of gray-scale imaging, and the Doppler resolution is inferior to pulsed Doppler

spectral analysis. One cannot equate the color saturation with velocity.[69] The color image is corrected for only one angle, and, thus, changes in color saturation may simply reflect changes in the vessel course and the relative Doppler angle. Color systems generally compute the mean velocity to produce the color pixel in the image. However, the examiner is usually interested in determining the maximum velocity; therefore, pulsed Doppler spectral analysis remains necessary for precise quantification of a hemodynamically significant stenosis.

Power Doppler Ultrasound

The color signal in power Doppler ultrasound is generated from the integrated power Doppler spectrum. The amplitude of the reflected echoes determines the brightness and color tone of the color signal. This amplitude is dependent on the density of red blood cells flowing within the sample volume. Power Doppler ultrasound utilizes a larger dynamic range with a better signal-to-noise ratio than color Doppler ultrasound. Because power Doppler ultrasound does not evaluate frequencies, but rather amplitude or power, artifacts— such as aliasing—do not occur. Power Doppler ultrasound, unlike color Doppler ultrasound, is largely angle independent. These features combine to make power Doppler ultrasound exquisitely sensitive to detecting a residual string of flow in the region of a suspected carotid occlusion.[78]

It is also hypothesized that power Doppler ultrasound has better edge definition than color Doppler ultrasound. The combination of improved edge definition and relative angle-independent flow imaging offer the potential for better visual assessment of the degree of stenosis using power Doppler.[79] Better edge definition may also allow power Doppler ultrasound to more clearly define plaque surface characteristics (see Fig. 27-10B).[80] In spite of the many potential benefits of power Doppler ultrasound, it does not provide velocity or directional flow information.[81] Furthermore, power Doppler is very motion sensitive. The motion sensitivity of power

---

COLOR FLOW DOPPLER IMAGING

ADVANTAGES

Reduction in examination time
Quick identification of areas of stenosis/high velocity, which facilitates spectral analysis to artifacts
Improved diagnostic reproducibility and confidence
Distinguishes occlusion from "string sign"
Simultaneous hemodynamic and anatomic information, velocity, and directional blood flow information
Improved accuracy in quantitating stenoses
Clarifies pulsed Doppler image mismatch

DISADVANTAGES

Angle dependent—prone
Resolution less than gray scale
Less Doppler spectral than pulsed Doppler
Slower frame rates information

POWER DOPPLER ULTRASOUND

ADVANTAGES

No aliasing
Potentially increases accuracy of grading stenoses
Aids in distinguishing preocclusive from occlusive lesions
Potential superior depiction of plaque surface morphology
Increased sensitivity to detecting low-velocity, low-amplitude blood flow
Angle independent

DISADVANTAGES

Does not provide direction or velocity flow information
Very motion sensitive (poor temporal resolution)

CAUSES OF IMAGE DOPPLER MISMATCH

Cardiac arrhythmia
Cardiac valvular disease; cardiomyopathy
Severe aortic stenosis
Hypotension or hypertension
Tandem lesions
Contralateral carotid stenosis
Nonstenotic plaque
Long segment, concentric high-grade stenosis
Carotid dissection
Preocclusive lesion
Tortuous vessels
Calcified plaque; hypoechoic or anechoic plaque
Anatomic variants

Doppler may result in a pseudo-string of flow. If the vibrations of soft tissue at an echogenic interface exceed the clutter filter level, color information may be displayed in areas where there is no blood flow. Pulsed Doppler evaluation of a color power string should always be performed to confirm the presence of real flow.

Pitfalls

Although absolute velocity determinations are valuable in assessing the degree of vascular stenosis, there are times when these measurements are less reliable.[1] Variations in cardiovascular physiology may affect carotid velocity measurements.[82,83] For instance, velocities produced by a stenosis in a **hypertensive patient** may be higher than those in a normotensive individual with a comparable narrowing, especially in the setting of a wide pulsed pressure. On the other hand, a **reduction in cardiac output** will diminish both systolic and diastolic velocities. **Cardiac arrhythmias, aortic valvular lesions,** and **severe cardiomyopathies** can cause significant aberrations in the shape of carotid flow waveforms and alter systolic and diastolic velocity readings (Fig. 27-24A, B). Use of an **aortic balloon pump** (Fig. 27-25) can also distort the Doppler velocity spectrum. These alterations can invalidate the use of standard Doppler parameters to quantify stenoses. **Bradycardia,** for example, produces increased stroke volume, causing systolic velocities to increase, but **prolonged diastolic run-off** causes spuriously decreased end-diastolic values. Patients with **isolated severe or critical aortic stenosis** may demonstrate duplex waveform abnormalities, including prolonged acceleration time, decreased peak velocity, delayed upstroke, and rounded waveforms.[84] However, **mild or moderate aortic stenosis** usually results in little or no sonographic abnormality. **Tortuous or kinked**

carotid arteries represent either congenital or acquired changes in the carotid artery. The clinical significance of these is debatable; however, the **vascular tortuosity** frequently results in eccentric jets of high velocity flow, which may give elevated velocities in the absence of significant stenosis (Fig. 27-26A, B).[85] Conversely, if the carotid bulb is capacious, a large plaque burden may still fail to produce anticipated velocity increases. This is because the relative difference in area between the distal CCA and the residual patent lumen of the large bulb is not sufficient to produce a greater than 50% velocity change. This is referred to by some as **nonstenotic plaque.** (Fig. 27-27A-C). Frequently an **image/Doppler mismatch** alerts the examiner to potential pitfalls.

Color Doppler can be used to overcome diagnostic dilemmas in these situations, particularly when "cine loop" playback capabilities are present. Cine loop allows the computer to store up to 10 seconds of the previous color flow Doppler recording for playback at the real-time rate or frame-by-frame. This allows one to assess filling of all parts of the vessel lumen. **Obstructive lesions** in one carotid can **affect** velocities in the **contralateral vessel.** For instance, severe unilateral ICA stenosis or occlusion may cause shunting of increased flow through the contralateral carotid system. This increased flow artificially increases velocity measurements in the contralateral vessel, particularly in areas of stenosis (Fig. 27-28A, B).[85-88] Conversely, a proximal common carotid or innominate artery stenosis may reduce flow, with consequent reduction of velocity measurements in a stenosis that is distal to the point of obstruction (**tandem lesion**).

Velocity ratios that compare velocity values in the ICA to those in the ipsilateral CCA can help avoid some pitfalls.[50] Of particular value are the peak systolic ratio (PSV in the ICA versus that in the CCA)[56,89] and the end-diastolic ratio (EDV in the ICA/EDV in the CCA).[63] Grant et al. have shown that peak systolic velocity ICA/

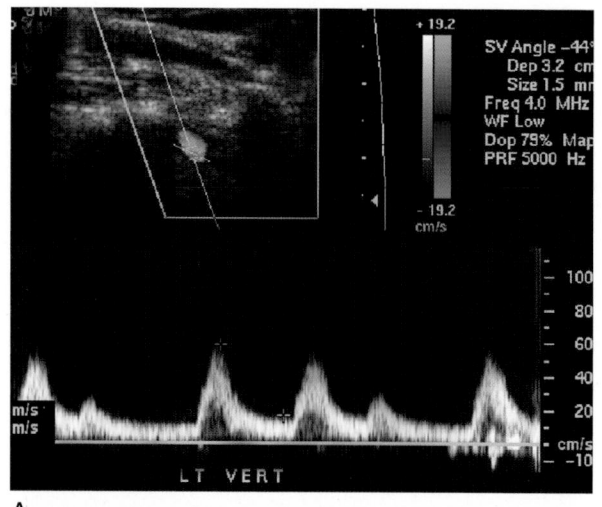

A

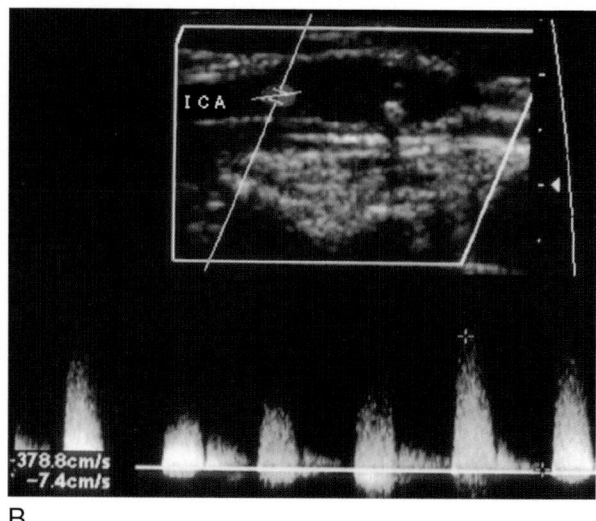

B

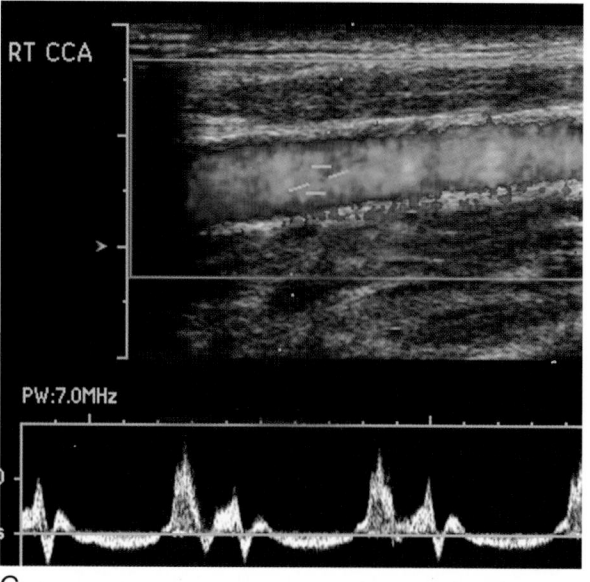

C

FIGURE 27-24. Abnormal Doppler waveforms due to heart disease. A, Patient with aortic valvular disease and atrial fibrillation shows irregular pulsed Doppler rhythm with varying velocities and a delayed upstroke consistent with aortic stenosis. **B,** Pulsed Doppler waveforms in a patient with an 80% to 99% internal carotid artery stenosis and combined aortic stenosis/insufficiency show a striking disparity in peak-systolic and end-diastolic velocities due to severe aortic insufficiency. **C,** Doppler waveform from common carotid artery in a patient with aortic valve insufficiency. Note reversal of flow in diastole.

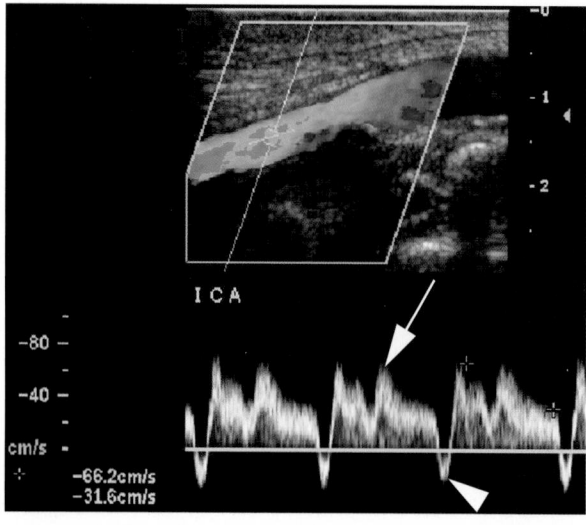

FIGURE 27-25. Abnormal Doppler waveform due to aortic balloon pump. Internal carotid artery pulsed Doppler trace shows the effect on an aortic balloon pump on carotid waveforms. Inflation of the device in systole (*arrow*) produces a second systolic peak, whereas deflation produces flow reversal (*arrowhead*) in end-diastole.

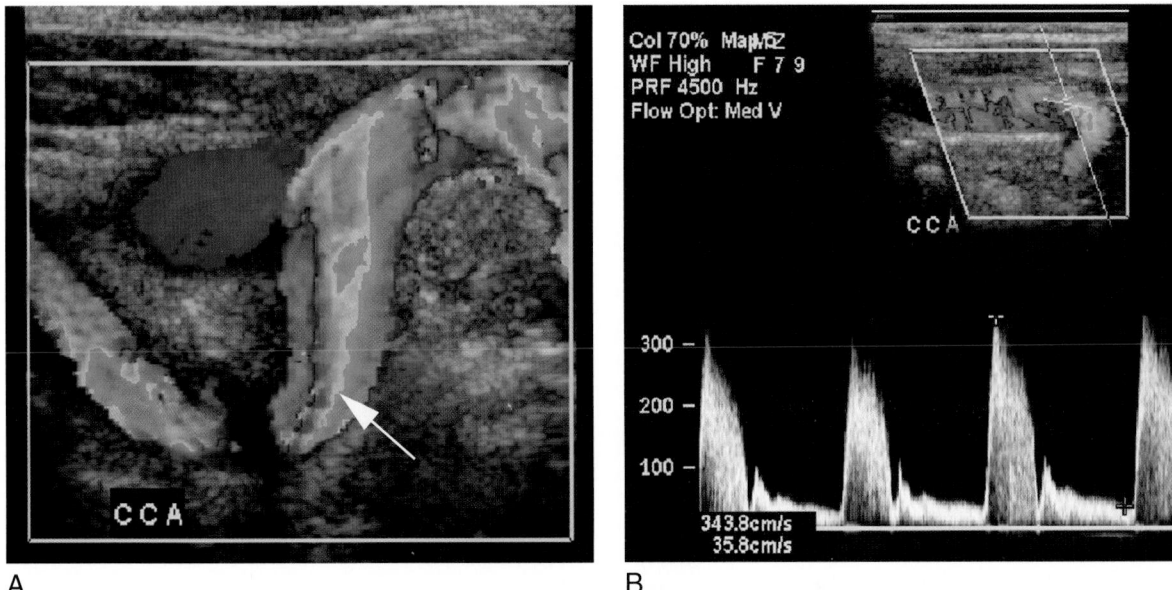

FIGURE 27-26. Abnormal Doppler flow due to tortuous vessel. A, Tortuous common carotid artery (CCA) displays color Doppler eccentric jets of flow (*arrow*). **B,** Spuriously elevated velocity due to an eccentric jet in a **tortuous proximal left CCA** without any visible stenosis.

CCA ratios are comparable in accuracy to peak systolic velocity values for determining the degree of ICA stenosis.[60] Although the peak systolic velocity and peak systolic ICA/CCA velocity ratio have shown relative comparable sensitivities and specificities, there are times when the velocity ratio will more correctly identify the degree of stenosis and the absolute velocity. Velocity ratios should always be employed when unusually high or low common carotid velocities or significant asymmetry of common carotid velocities is detected. Long segment high-grade stenoses frequently will not demonstrate the anticipated degree of ICA velocity elevation. In such situations, the velocity ratio coupled with the gray-scale/color/power Doppler appearance may provide insight into the actual degree of narrowing. As discussed in the previous section on spectral broadening, color flow/power Doppler is invaluable in the avoidance of pitfalls related to spurious Doppler spectral traces.

Although high-grade stenoses usually produce increased velocity in the region of a plaque and distal to it, high-grade intracranial or extracranial occlusive **lesions in tandem may reduce anticipated velocity shifts** and produce an atypical high resistance ICA waveform (Fig. 27-29A-E). Vessels should be examined as far cephalad as possible to avoid missing a distal tandem lesion. Flow immediately distal to stenosis of over 95% frequently demonstrates very low velocity tardus/parvus waveforms as compared to the anticipated high velocities seen in a high-grade stenosis (see Fig. 27-23). **High-grade vascular narrowings**, particularly those of a circumferential nature that occur over a long segment of a vessel, may also produce damped waveforms without a high velocity frequency shift. Although no definite

velocity elevations are present in such a long circumferential narrowing, spectral broadening and disturbed flow distal to such a narrowing are usually apparent. In addition, the fusiform narrowing are usually detected with the real-time image, particularly if color flow Doppler is employed. **Innominate artery occlusions** may result in tardus/parvus waveforms and even carotid steal patterns similar to those noted in the vertebral artery (Fig. 27-30).

Another source of error in pulsed Doppler US analysis is **aliasing**, which is caused by the inability to detect the true peak velocity because the Doppler sampling rate (pulsed repetition frequency, PRF) is too low. A classic visual example of aliasing can be seen in Western films, with the apparent reversal of stage coach wheel spokes when the wagon wheel rotations exceed the film frame rate. The maximal detectable frequency shift can be no greater than half the PRF. With aliasing, the tips of the time velocity spectrum (representing high velocities) are cut off and wrap around to appear below the baseline (Fig. 27-31). If aliasing occurs, **continuous wave probes** used in conjunction with duplex pulsed Doppler can readily demonstrate the true peak velocity shift. Aliasing can also be overcome or decreased by **increasing angle theta** (the angle of Doppler insonation), thereby reducing the detected Doppler shift, or by decreasing the insonating sound beam frequency. **Increasing the PRF** increases the detectable frequency shift, but the PRF increase is limited by the depth of the vessel as well as the center frequency of the transducer.[31,52] One can also **shift the zero baseline** and reassign a larger range of velocities to forward flow to overcome aliasing. It is also valid to **add velocity values above and below the**

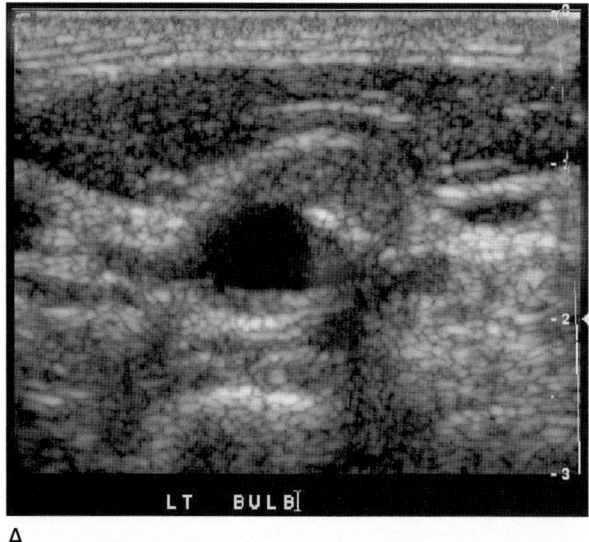

A

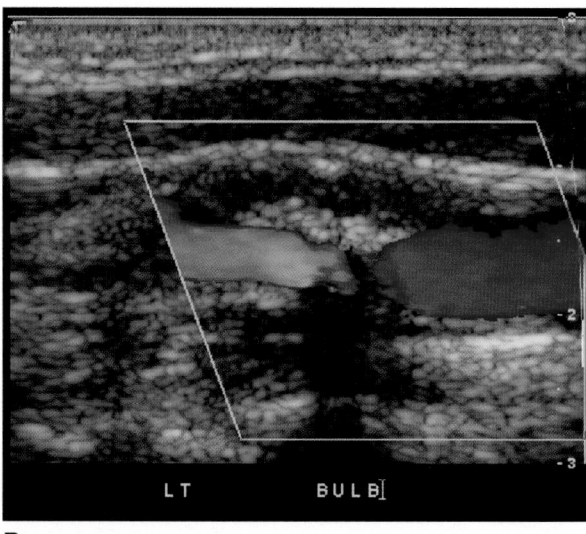

B

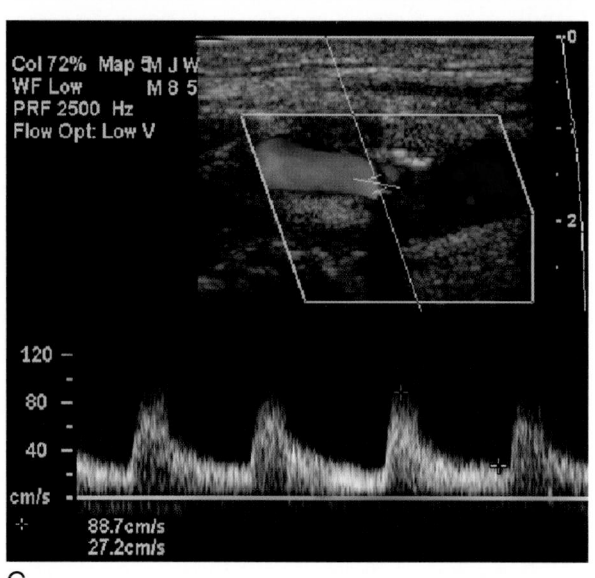

C

FIGURE 27-27. Moderate stenosis carotid bulb.
A, Transverse gray-scale image of the right carotid bulb shows a roughly 50% diameter stenosis. **B,** Color Doppler longitudinal image confirms a moderate stenosis. **C,** On spectral Doppler there are no corresponding increases in systolic velocity (88.7 cm/sec) in the area of apparent narrowing.

baseline to obtain an accurate velocity value, provided multiple wraparounds do not occur, as seen in extremely high velocities. Aliasing may sometimes be useful in color Doppler image interpretation where color flow Doppler aliasing can accent the severity of flow disturbances as well as define the patent lumen.

Internal Carotid Artery Occlusion

Distinguishing between a string sign and a totally occluded carotid has major clinical significance. Grubb et al. have shown that untreated preocclusive lesions carry a roughly 5% per year risk for stroke. Thus, intervention in this patient population is particularly important.[90]

Carotid occlusion is diagnosed when no flow is detected in a vessel. Occasionally transmitted pulsations into an occluded ICA may mimic abnormal flow in a patent vessel. The pulsed Doppler cursor should be

clearly located in the ICA lumen, and arterial pulsatile flow should be identified. Close attention should be paid to the direction of flow and the nature of pulsations. **True center stream sampling** should be documented by transverse scanning, and the sample volume reduced in size as much as possible. Extraneous pulsations should seldom be transmitted to the center of the thrombus.[54]

As a high-grade stenosis approaches occlusion, the high velocity jet is reduced to a mere trickle. It may be difficult to locate the small residual string of flow within a largely occluded lumen using gray-scale imaging alone, particularly if the adjacent plaque or thrombus is anechoic, making the residual lumen invisible during real-time examination, or if there is calcified plaque obscuring visualization.

In critical high-grade stenoses (>95%), standard sensitivity color Doppler settings may fail to demonstrate a

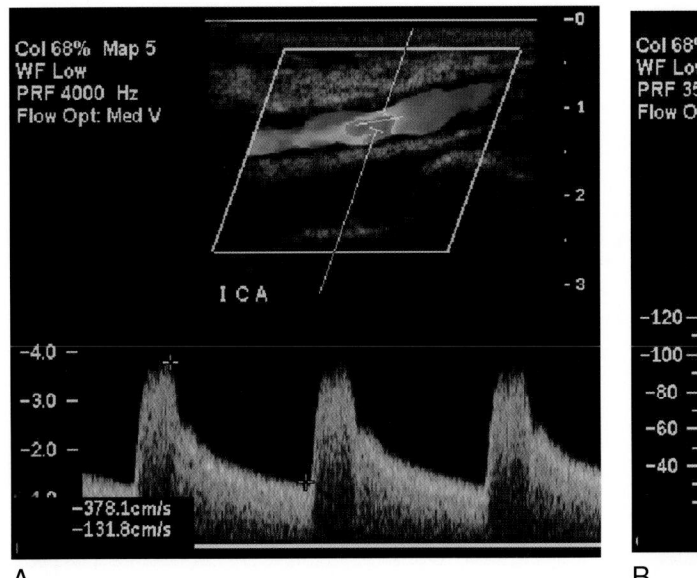

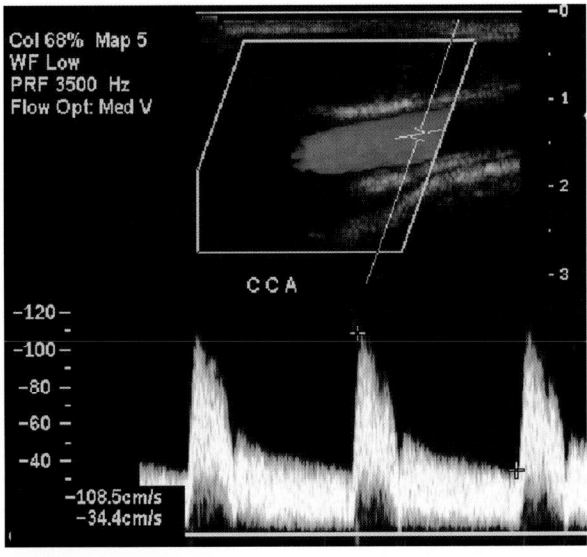

A   B

FIGURE 27-28. Value of ICA/CCA ratio. A, Spuriously increased left ICA velocities in a patient with a less than 50% visible stenosis and a right ICA occlusion (ICA 378). **B,** Left systolic ICA/CCA ratio is also increased 378/109 = 3.5. CCA, common carotid artery; ICA, internal carotid artery.

string of residual flow. Thus, it is always prudent to employ the **slow flow sensitivity settings on color** Doppler to discriminate between critical stenoses and occlusions.[73,76] Alternatively, power Doppler ultrasound (with its increased sensitivity to detecting low amplitude, slow velocity signals) may be utilized to visualize a residual string of blood flow (Fig. 27-32A, B). Color Doppler is 95% to 98% accurate in distinguishing high-grade stenosis from complete occlusion on angiography when appropriate technical parameters are employed.[91-93]

The presence of a high-grade ICA stenosis or occlusion can often be inferred from inspection of the ipsilateral CCA pulsed Doppler waveform or color or power Doppler image (see Fig. 27-30). The pulsed Doppler waveforms in the ipsilateral CCA and ICA proximal to a lesion frequently demonstrate an asymmetrical, high-resistance signal with decreased, absent, or reversed diastolic flow—except when there are ECA collaterals to the **intracranial circulation** (Fig. 27-33A, B). The main intracranial/extracranial collateral pathway exists between the orbital and ophthalmic arteries. Other collateral pathways include the occipital branch of the ECA to the vertebral artery and cervical branches off the arch with the vertebral artery. Similarly, color or power Doppler images may show a flash of color flow in systole, but a conspicuous decrease or absence of color flow in diastole, which is asymmetrical compared to the contralateral side.[91,92] The diagnosis of carotid occlusion versus a string sign is made more accurately with color Doppler and power Doppler than with gray-scale duplex scanning and may obviate the need for angiography to confirm a sonographically diagnosed ICA occlusion.[91,92]

SONOGRAPHIC FINDINGS IN INTERNAL CAROTID ARTERY OCCLUSION

"Internalization" of ipsilateral ECA waveform
Absence of flow within the ICA by color Doppler ultrasound, power Doppler ultrasound, or pulsed Doppler
Reversal of flow within segment of ICA or CCA proximal to occluded segment
Thrombus or plaque completely fills lumen of ICA on gray-scale images, color Doppler ultrasound, or power Doppler ultrasound
Dampened high-resistance waveform within ipsilateral CCA or proximal ICA
Contralateral CCA may demonstrate significantly higher velocities than ipsilateral CCA

Another pitfall in the diagnosis of a totally occluded ICA is **mistaking a patent ECA or one of its branches for the ICA.** The situation is especially confusing when the ECA/ICA collaterals open in response to long-standing ICA disease and the ECA acquires a low resistance waveform (internalization) (Fig. 27-34). One technique that can aid in identifying the ECA is scanning at the origin of the vessel while simultaneously tapping the temporal artery. Percussion of the superficial temporal artery often results in a serrated distortion of the Doppler waveform in the ECA (80% of ECAs percussed in one study) (see Fig. 27-4B).[94] However, this maneuver should be used with caution because the

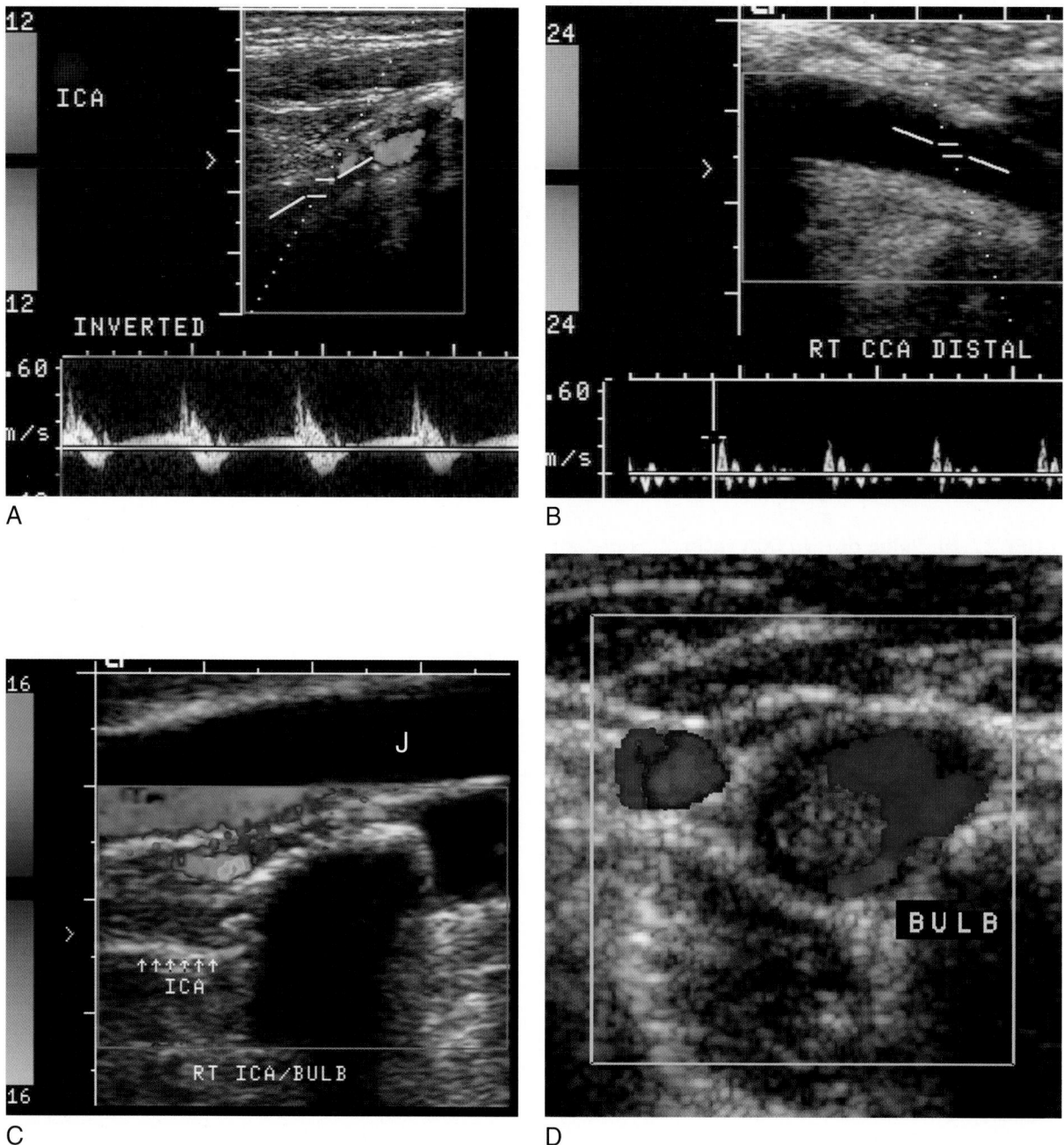

FIGURE 27-29. Abnormal high-resistance waveforms. A, High resistance waveform in a distal ICA due to a high-grade intracranial ICA stenosis. **B,** High resistance, damped flow in a right CCA proximal to an ICA occlusion. **C,** Shows calcified, shadowing plaque proximal to an ICA occlusion. J—jugular vein. **D,** Transverse color Doppler image of the right carotid bulb shows acute thrombus projecting into the lumen with peripheral flow medially. CCA, common carotid artery; ICA, internal carotid artery.

temporal tap can also be seen in the common carotid and internal carotid arteries, although less commonly (54% and 33%, respectively) than in the ECA.[94] Branching vessels are a unique feature of the ECA that can also be used to differentiate this vessel from the ICA. Color Doppler ultrasound can facilitate the identification of such branching vessels (see Fig. 27-4A). Usually, the combination of vessel **size, position, waveform shape, the presence of branches, and the temporal tap response** can correctly **identify** the **ECA**.

Although distal propagation of thrombus almost invariably occurs following an ICA occlusion, CCA occlusions are often localized. Flow may be maintained in the ECA and ICA, but must be reversed in one of the two vessels. Ultrasound is the preferred method for evaluating maintenance of flow around the carotid bifurcation following proximal CCA occlusion. Most commonly, retrograde flow in the ECA will supply antegrade flow in the ipsilateral ICA. Occasionally, the opposite flow pattern will be encountered (Fig. 27-35A-E).[54,95,96]

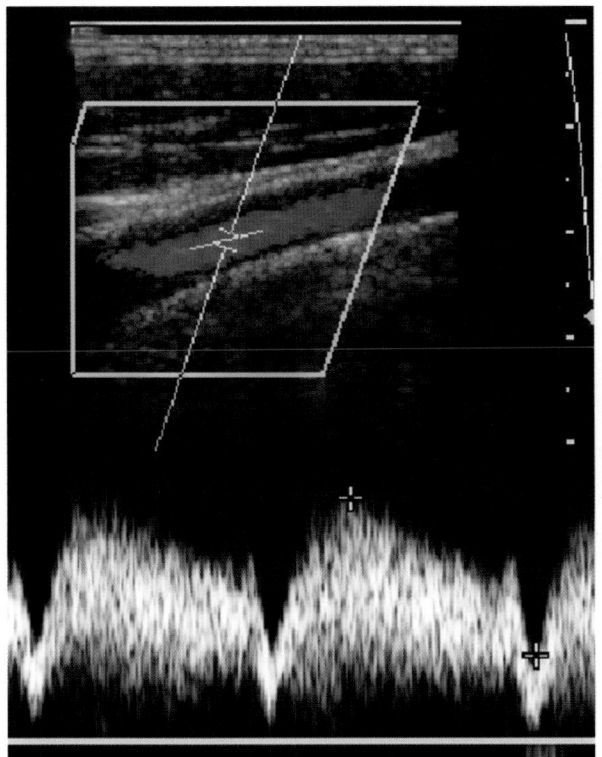

FIGURE 27-30. Abnormal CCA velocity due to innominate artery stenosis. Low right CCA velocities with a pre-steal waveform distal to a severe innominate artery stenosis. CCA, common carotid artery.

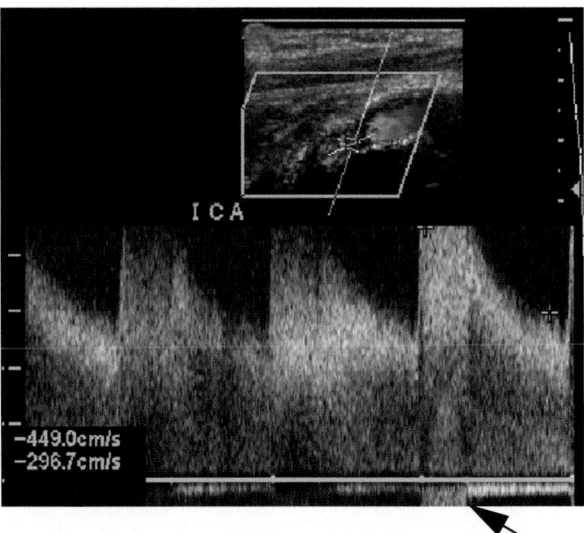

FIGURE 27-31. Aliasing. Aliasing of Doppler waveform in the region of a high-grade (80% to 99%) stenosis. Highest velocities are wrapped around (*arrow*) and displayed below the zero velocity baseline.

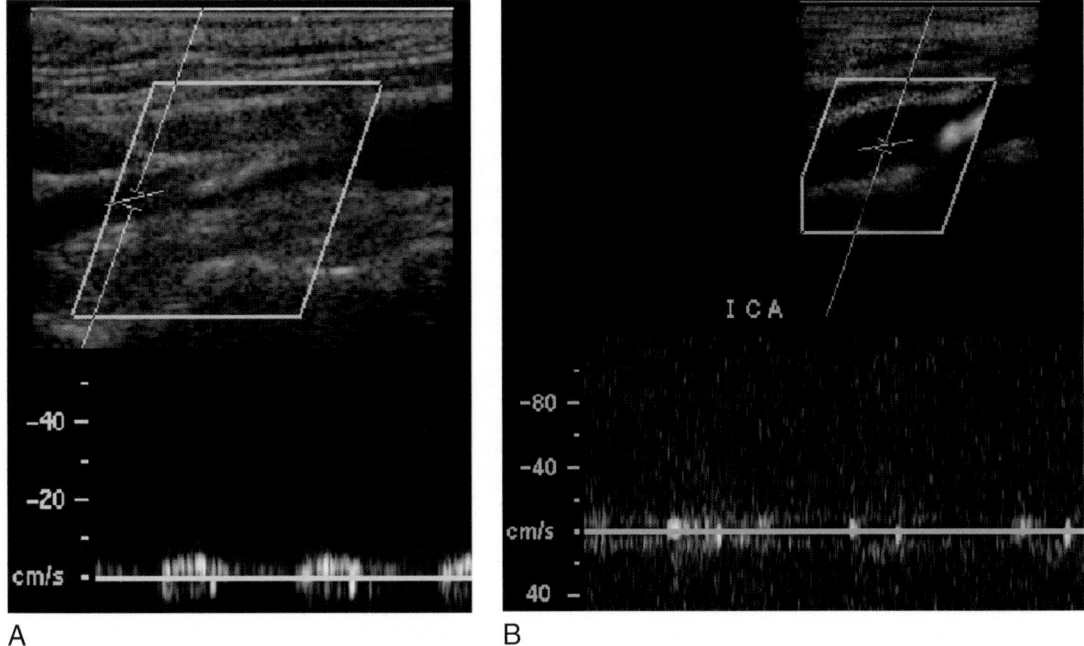

A   B

FIGURE 27-32. Near and total occlusion of ICA. A, A preocclusive trickle of flow in a left ICA. **B,** Hypoechoic plaque with complete ICA occlusion shown on power Doppler. ICA, internal carotid artery.

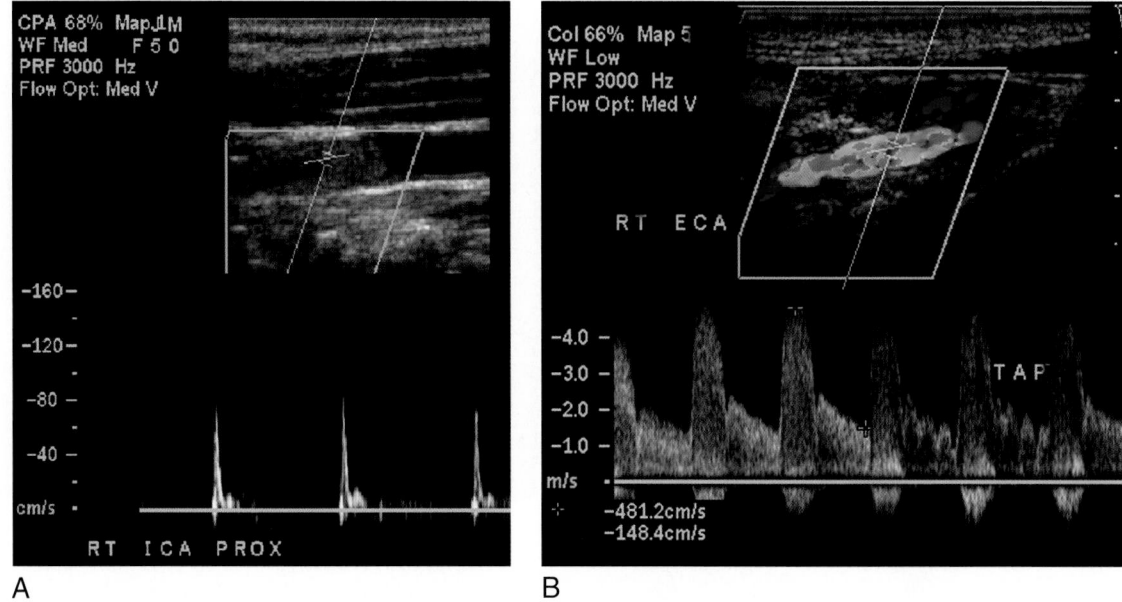

FIGURE 27-33. ICA occlusion. A, Complete left ICA occlusion shows a spiked waveform consistent with an occlusion. **B**, A proximal left ECA trace shows a low-resistance waveform consistent with collaterals to intracranial circulation as well as increased velocity due to an ECA stenosis. ECA, external carotid artery; ICA, internal carotid artery; TAP, temporal artery tap.

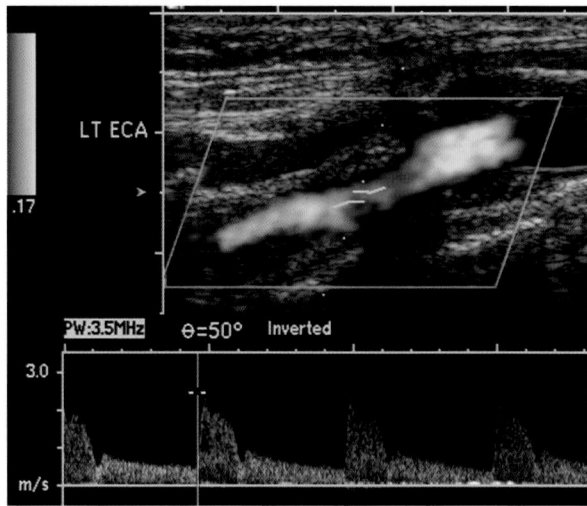

FIGURE 27-34. Long-standing ICA occlusion results in low resistance waveform in ECA.

Preoperative Strategies for Patients with Carotid Artery Disease

The preoperative workup of carotid disease is evolving in response to the results of the NASCET, ECST, and ACAS.[4,5,97] The issue of numbers to be used for a carotid ultrasound examination is predicated on the intent of the examination. Why are we doing the study? How will we use the results? If the examination is a screening test, are we evaluating all patients, symptomatic patients only, and so on? If we intend to select patients for surgery on the basis of ultrasound alone, then a different set of variables is likely to produce the desired outcome. The purpose of a carotid examination and the patient population being screened will impact the selection of velocity thresholds. For example, screening of high-risk, asymptomatic patients might be best performed with high velocity thresholds with increased specificity, whereas symptomatic patients more likely to undergo surgery for optimal treatment would dictate lower thresholds with increased sensitivity.

Although many still consider angiography the standard, there are criticisms of this technique which include significant intraobserver variability, and the fact that angiography may frequently underestimate the degree of stenosis.[98] In fact, comparisons of angiographic and sonographic estimations of carotid stenosis reveal a closer surgical correlation with the ultrasound measurements.[1] Carotid US has proved to be a highly accurate method of detecting high-grade stenoses, as well as differentiating critical stenoses from occlusion, particularly since the advent of color Doppler ultrasound and power Doppler ultrasound. MRA is currently demonstrating comparable accuracy to ultrasound and angiography for the detection and quantification of carotid stenosis. MRA, like ultrasonography, can depict plaque morphology and can additionally evaluate the intracranial circulation. MRA may be helpful in situations where calcified plaque obscures the underlying carotid lumen from insonation.

Many investigators now suggest replacing preoperative angiography with a combination of carotid sonography and MRA. They advocate utilizing angiography

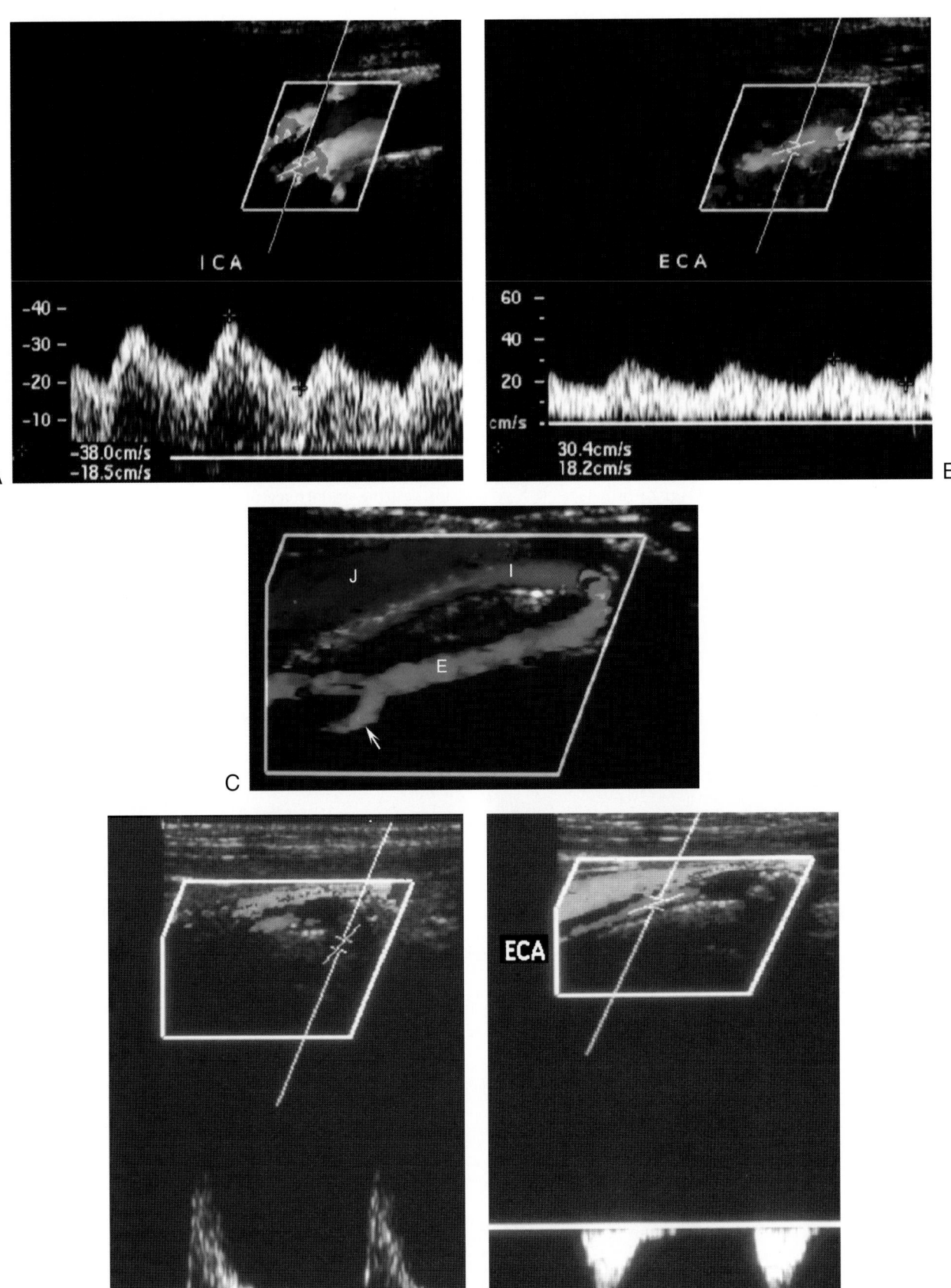

FIGURE 27-35. CCA occlusion causes abnormal ICA waveform. A, Antegrade, tardus/parvus waveform is seen in an ICA distal to a CCA occlusion. **B,** Retrograde ECA flow with a tardus/parvus waveform due to collateral flow from the contralateral ECA to supply the ipsilateral ICA distal to a CCA occlusion is seen. **C,** Color Doppler image shows antegrade ECA flow (E) with an ECA branch (*arrow*) and retrograde ICA flow (I). Internal jugular vein (J). **D,** Spectral Doppler shows high resistance retrograde right ICA flow. **E,** High resistance antegrade flow in the right ECA distal to a CCA occlusion. CCA, common carotid artery; ECA, external carotid artery; ICA, internal carotid artery.

only in cases where MRA and carotid US have discordant results or are inadequate.[99-102] Other studies support the use of carotid US alone prior to endarterectomy.[103-108] Numerous studies show that greater than 90% of surgical candidates can be adequately screened using clinical assessment and US alone. However, in suspected aortic arch proximal vessel disease, or in cases of suspected complete occlusion, some still advocate preoperative angiography.

Randoux et al. report good correlation between CT angiography, MR gadolinium enhanced angiography, and conventional angiography for estimating carotid stenoses.[109] In cases where MR angiography is contraindicated, CT angiography could provide an alternative preoperative noninvasive imaging tool.

Postoperative Ultrasound

The endarterectomized carotid artery demonstrates many characteristic features (Fig. 27-36A-G).[110,111] A discrete wedge between the normal I-M complex and the endarterectomized surface is frequently seen, as are periodically spaced echogenic sutures. The absent I-M complex has also been shown to regrow. While routine surveillance status postendarterectomy is not advocated in asymptomatic patients, one study showed that approximately 6% of patients who underwent endarterectomy had carotid flaps, residual moderate-to-moderately severe stenoses, or an occluded ECA.[112] Two of these patients in their series with postoperative abnormalities on US sustained perioperative stroke. Patients without defects on the postoperative US had no perioperative sequelae or need for redo procedures. Patients with preoperative stenoses greater than 75% have a greater risk for residual stenoses. It appears that utilization of US in the symptomatic postoperative population is useful; the role in the asymptomatic patient population is debatable.[113]

Carotid stenting is largely investigational at this time, and is confined to patients deemed at too high a risk for routine endarterectomy. Carotid **stents** are readily visualized with US allowing one to assess disease before,

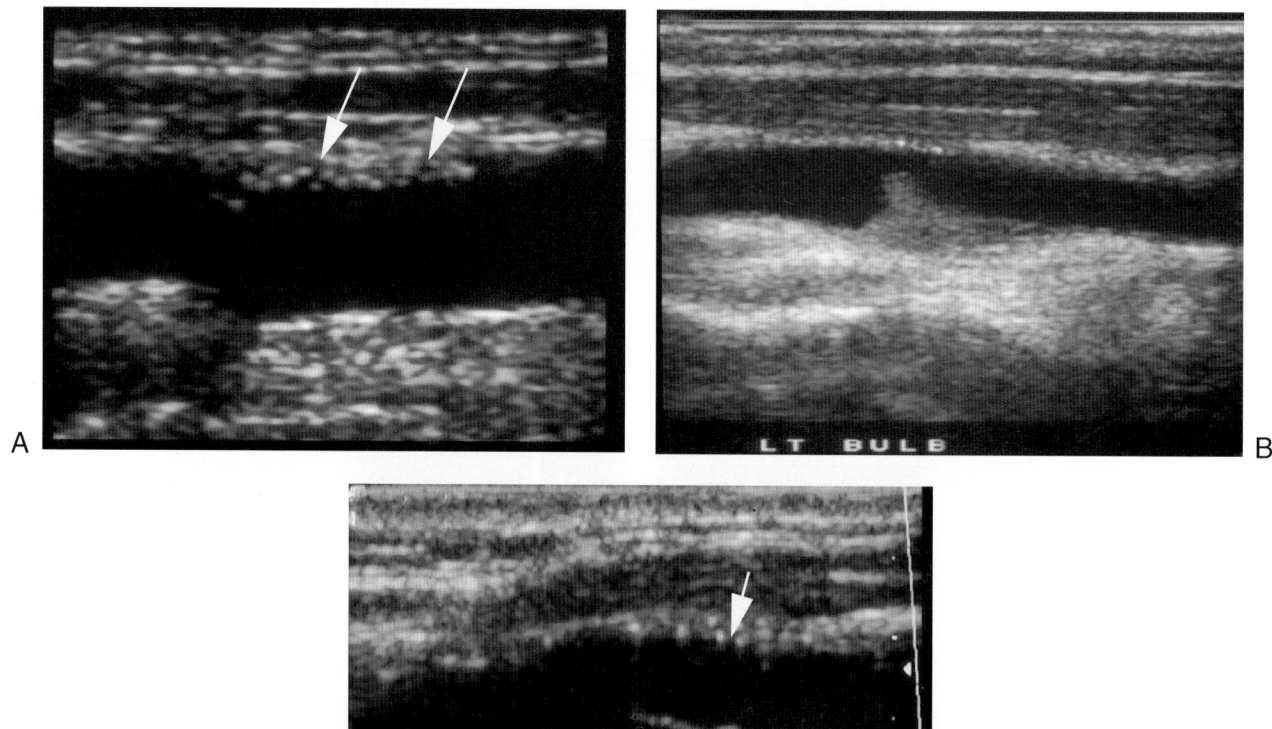

FIGURE 27-36. Postendarterectomy appearances. A, Normal postendarterectomy changes following surgery with a vein patch (*arrows*). **B,** Abnormal wedge of residual/recurrent plaque/thrombus in a newly symptomatic patient status postcarotid endarterectomy. **C,** Postendarterectomy sutures (*arrow*) with a residual intimal flap in lumen.

along, and distal to the stent. US may be helpful in assessing the presence and severity of stenosis, characterizing the carotid bifurcation, assessing anatomic variants and vessel tortuosity, and plaque calcification prior to stent placement (Fig. 27-37A-D).

Velocity criteria employed for grading stenoses in a stent may not be identical for those in the native carotid artery.[114] Some investigators have shown that velocities along the stent are routinely higher than those in a nonstented vessel. Velocity elevations in the range of 125 to 140 cm/sec are fairly common in widely patent stents. In addition, one normally sees an increase in velocity in the distal ICA beyond the deployed stent. The disproportionate velocity elevations along the stent may be due to several factors, including changes in vessel wall compliance and shunting of blood flow away from the ECA. It is also possible that the technique utilized in many of the stent trials, which require strict adherence to the 60° angle theta technique for Doppler interrogation, may result in systematic velocity increases. At present, slight increases in velocity in a stent which appears widely patent on power or color Doppler are unlikely to indicate significant narrowing or warrant further assessment or intervention.

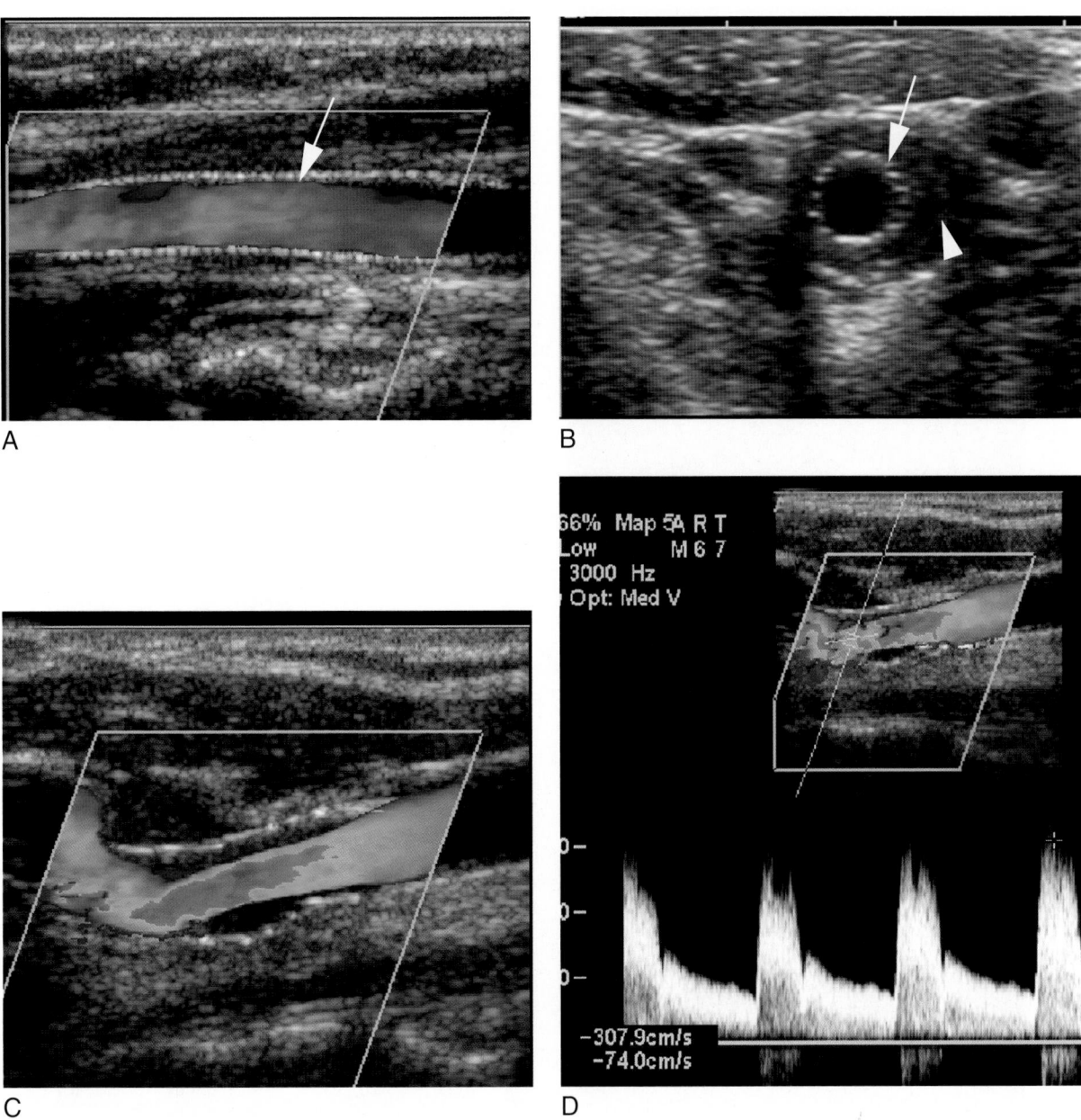

FIGURE 27-37. Carotid stent. A, Normal right carotid stent (*arrow*) shows complete filling on color Doppler examination. **B,** Transverse image of a carotid stent (*arrow*) in the carotid bulb shows residual plaque (*arrowhead*) in the lumen. **C** and **D,** Left carotid stent shows visible narrowing on color Doppler (C) and elevated velocities (D) consistent with a greater than 70% stenosis using standard carotid velocity criteria.

NONATHEROSCLEROTIC CAROTID DISEASE

Nonatherosclerotic carotid disease is far less common than plaque disease. **Fibromuscular dysplasia (FMD),** a noninflammatory process with hypertrophy of muscular and fibrous arterial walls, separated by abnormal zones of fragmentation, involves the mid- and distal ICA more commonly than other carotid segments. A characteristic "string of beads" appearance has been described on angiography. Only a few reports of the ultrasound features of FMD exist.[115,116] Many patients with FMD have nonspecific or no obvious ultrasound abnormalities demonstrated. FMD may be asymptomatic or can result in carotid dissection or subsequent thrombotic embolic events (Fig. 27-38A-C). **Arteritis,** resulting from autoimmune processes, such as Takayasu's arteritis or temporal arteritis, or radiation changes can produce diffuse concentric thickening of carotid walls, which most frequently involves the CCA (Fig. 27-39A-C).[117]

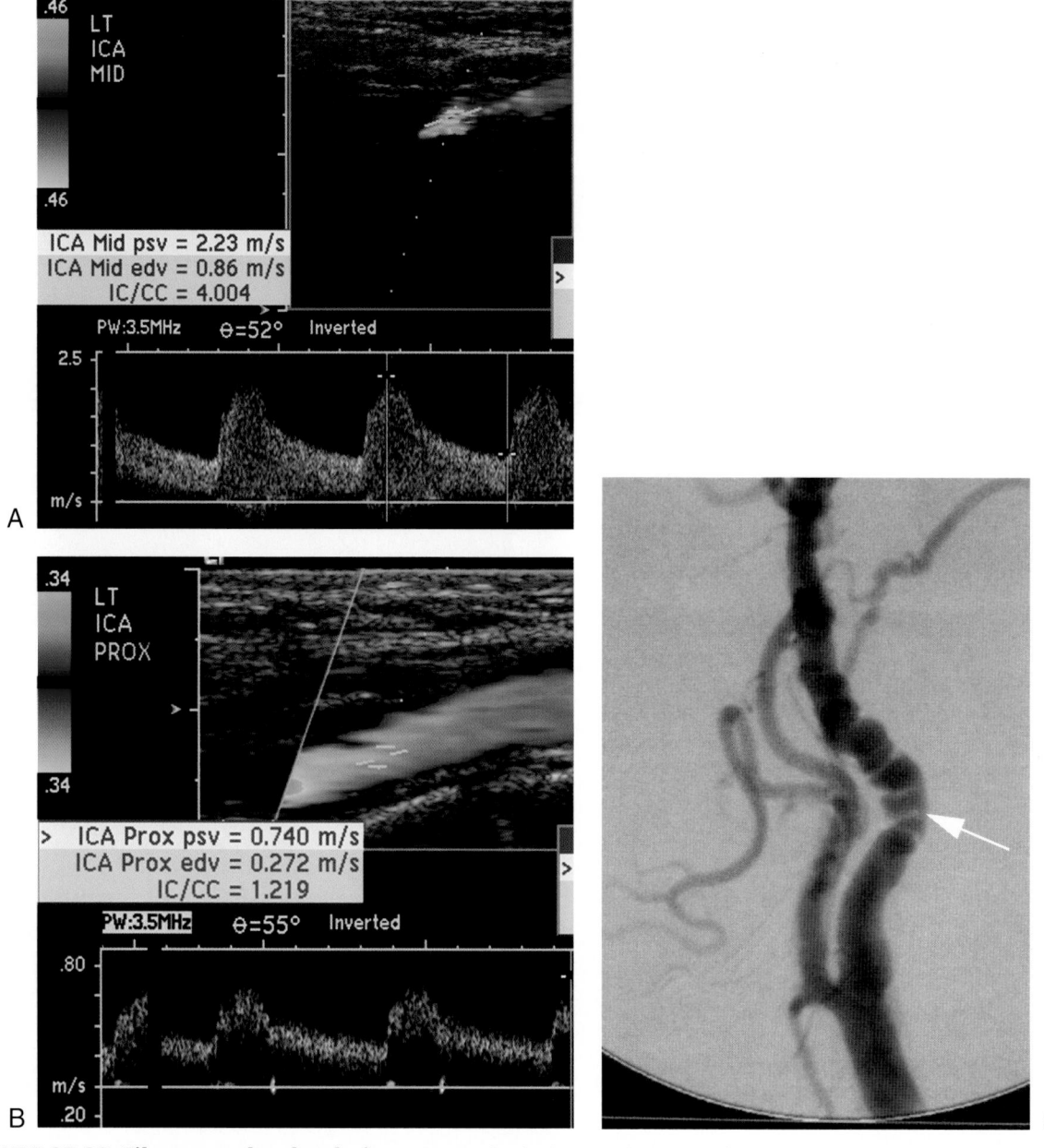

FIGURE 27-38. Fibromuscular dysplasia. A, Longitudinal color Doppler image of the mid- to distal portion of the ICA shows velocity elevation and significant stenosis. **B,** Same patient's proximal portion of the ICA shows no stenosis. **C,** Angiogram demonstrates typical appearance of fibromuscular dysplasia in the mid- and distal ICA. Note the beaded appearance due to focal bands (*arrow*) of thickened tissue that narrow the lumen. ICA, internal carotid artery.

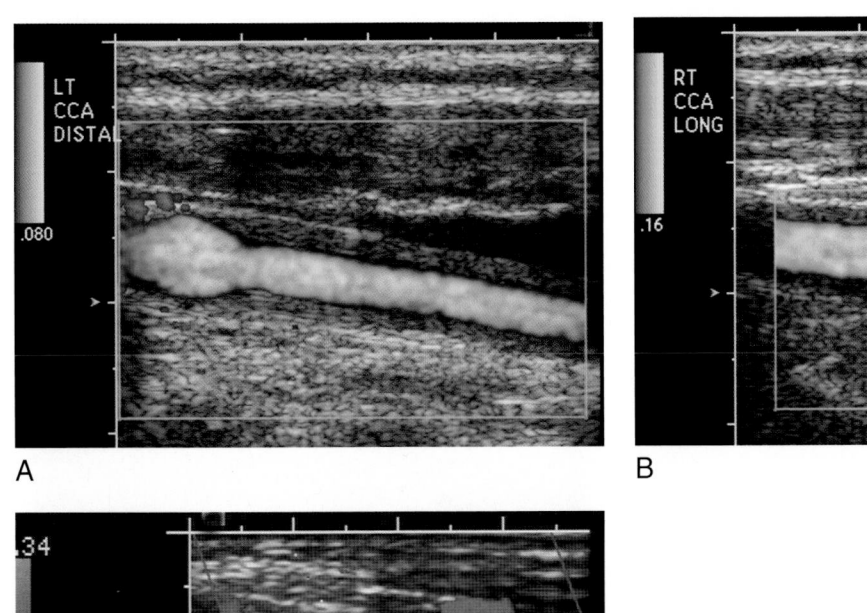

A

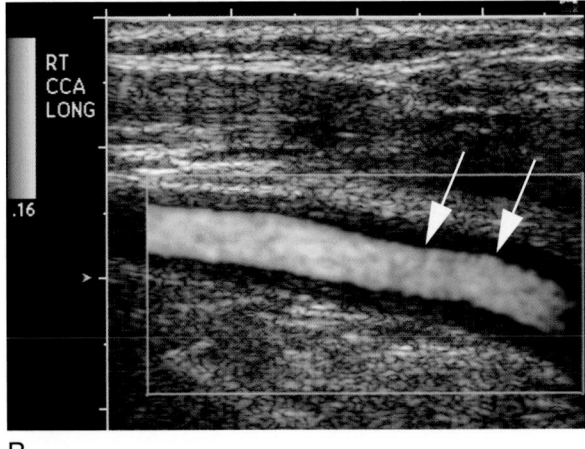

B

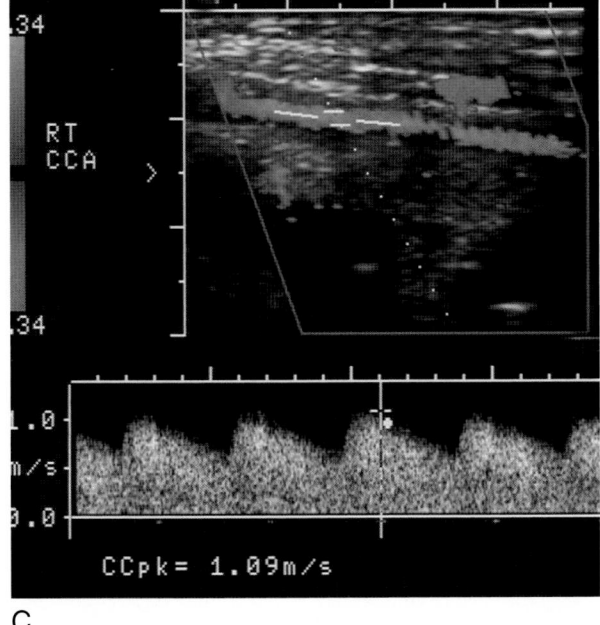

C

FIGURE 27-39. Long segment stenosis CCA due to Takayasu's arteritis. A, Left CCA power Doppler image demonstrates a long segment CCA concentric narrowing due to markedly thickened walls of the artery. **B,** The right CCA power Doppler image of the same patient demonstrates similar concentric narrowing (*arrows*). **C,** The right spectral Doppler waveform shows a mildly tardus/parvus waveform. CCA, common carotid artery.

Cervical trauma can produce carotid **dissections** or aneurysms. Carotid artery dissection results from a tear in the intima, allowing blood to dissect into the wall of the artery producing a false lumen. The false lumen may be blind ended or may re-enter the true lumen. The false lumen may occlude or narrow the true lumen, producing symptoms similar to carotid plaque disease. Dissections may arise spontaneously or secondary to trauma, intrinsic disease with elastic tissue degeneration —such as Marfan's syndrome—or be related to atherosclerotic plaque disease.[15] The US examination of a carotid dissection may reveal a mobile or fixed **echogenic intimal flap**, with or without thrombus formation. There frequently is a striking image-Doppler mismatch with a paucity of gray-scale abnormalities seen in association with marked flow abnormalities (Fig. 27-40A-E).

Color Doppler ultrasound or power Doppler ultrasound may readily clarify the source of this mismatch by demonstrating abrupt tapering of the patent color Doppler-filled lumen to the point of an ICA occlusion, analogous to the findings commonly seen on angiography. Although the ICA is frequently occluded, demonstrating absent flow with a high-resistance waveform in the proximal ipsilateral CCA, flow in the ICA may demonstrate high velocities associated with luminal narrowing secondary to hemorrhage and thrombus in the area of the false lumen. Accordingly, flow velocity waveforms in the CCA may be normal or demonstrate very damped high-resistance waveforms. MRA, another noninvasive imaging test, readily demonstrates mural hematoma confirming the diagnosis of ICA dissection. Although angiography is frequently used to initially diagnose a dissection, ultrasound can be used to follow patients to assess the therapeutic response to anticoagulation. Repeat sonographic evaluation of patients with ICA dissection following anticoagulation

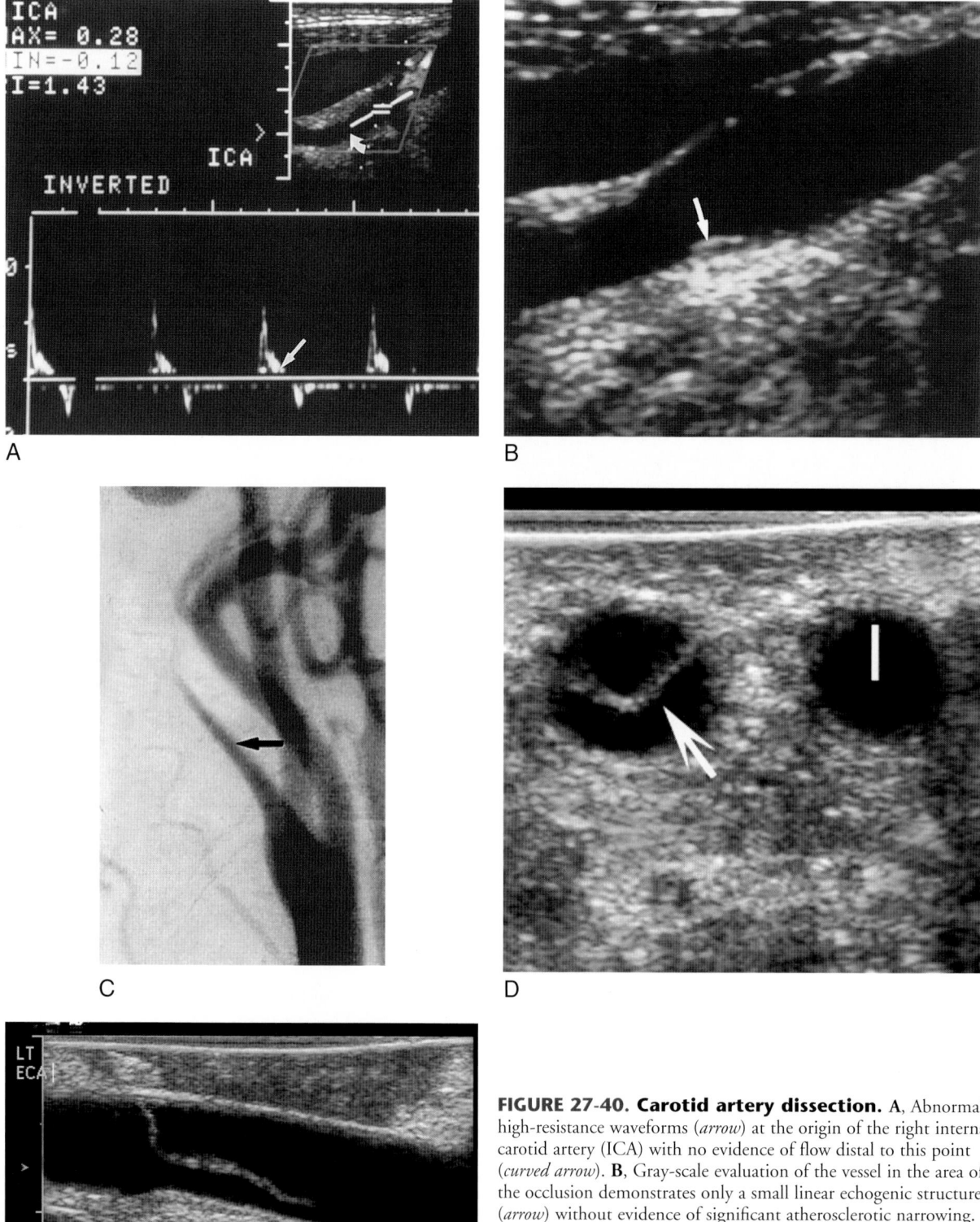

FIGURE 27-40. Carotid artery dissection. **A,** Abnormal high-resistance waveforms (*arrow*) at the origin of the right internal carotid artery (ICA) with no evidence of flow distal to this point (*curved arrow*). **B,** Gray-scale evaluation of the vessel in the area of the occlusion demonstrates only a small linear echogenic structure (*arrow*) without evidence of significant atherosclerotic narrowing. **C,** Subsequent angiogram demonstrates the characteristic tapering to the point of occlusion (*arrow*) associated with carotid artery dissection and thrombotic occlusion. Transverse (**D**) and longitudinal (**E**) images of a different patient show an intimal flap (*arrow*) in an external carotid artery. Internal carotid artery (I).

SONOGRAPHIC FINDINGS IN ICA DISSECTION

ICA

Absent flow/occlusion
Echogenic intimal flap ±thrombus
Hypoechoic thrombus ± luminal narrowing
Normal appearance

CCA

High-resistance waveform
Damped flow
Normal

therapy reveals recanalization of the artery in as many as 70% of cases.[118-120] It is important to consider the diagnosis of dissection as a cause of neurologic symptoms, particularly when the clinical presentation, age, and patient history are atypical for that of atherosclerotic disease or hemorrhagic stroke.

The most common CCA **aneurysm** occurs in the region of the carotid bifurcation. These aneurysms may result from atherosclerosis, infection, trauma, surgery, or infectious etiology, such as syphilis. The normal CCA usually measures no more than 1 cm in diameter.

Carotid body tumors, one of several paragangliomas that involve the head and neck, are usually benign, well-encapsulated masses located at the carotid bifurcation. These tumors may be bilateral, particularly in the familial variant, and are very vascular, often producing an audible bruit. Some of these tumors produce catecholamines, producing sudden changes in blood pressure intra- or postoperatively. Color Doppler ultrasound demonstrates an extremely vascular soft tissue mass at the carotid bifurcation (Fig. 27-41A-D). Color Doppler ultrasound can also be used to monitor embolization or surgical resection of carotid body tumors. A classic nonmass is the **ectatic innominate/proximal CCA** frequently occurring as a pulsatile supraclavicular mass in older women. The request to rule out a carotid aneurysm almost invariably shows the classic normal features of these tortuous vessels (Fig. 27-42). **Extravascular masses,** such as lymph nodes, hematomas, or abscesses, that compress or displace the carotids can be readily distinguished from primary vascular masses, such as aneurysms or pseudoaneurysms (Fig. 27-43). **Post-traumatic pseudoaneurysms** can usually be distinguished from a true carotid aneurysm by demonstrating the characteristic to-and-fro waveforms in the neck of the pseudoaneurysm, as well as the internal variability (yin-yang) characteristic of a pseudoaneurysm (Figs. 27-44A, B).

TRANSCRANIAL DOPPLER SONOGRAPHY

In transcranial Doppler (TCD) US, a low frequency, 2 MHz transducer is used to **evaluate blood flow within the intracranial carotid and vertebrobasilar system and the circle of Willis.** Access is achieved through the orbits, foramen magnum, or, most commonly, the region of temporal calvarial thinning **(transtemporal window).**[121] However, many patients, up to 55% in one series,[122] may not have access for an interpretable TCD examination. Women, particularly African American women, have a thick temporal bone through which it is difficult to insonate the basal cerebral arteries.[122,123] This difficulty limits the feasibility of TCD imaging as a routine part of the noninvasive cerebrovascular work-up.[122]

By using spectral analysis, various parameters, including mean velocity, peak-systolic and end-diastolic velocity, and pulsatility and resistive indices of the blood vessels, are determined. Color (power) Doppler can improve velocity determination by providing better angle theta determination and localizing the course of vessels.[121] TCD has many applications, including evaluation of **intracranial stenoses** and **collateral circulation,** detection and follow-up of **vasoconstriction** from subarachnoid hemorrhage, determination of **brain death,** and identification of **arteriovenous malformation**.[118-121,124] TCD is most reliable in diagnosing stenoses of the middle cerebral artery with sensitivities as high as 91% reported.[122,123] TCD is less reliable for detecting stenoses of the intracranial vertebrobasilar system, anterior and posterior cerebral arteries, and terminal ICA.[122,123] However, TCD is helpful in assessing vertebral artery patency and flow direction when no flow is detected in the extracranial vertebral artery (Fig. 27-45A, B). Diagnosis of an intracranial stenosis is based on an increase in mean velocity of blood flow in the affected vessel compared with the contralateral vessel at the same location.[122,123]

Advantages of TCD US also include its availability to be used to monitor patients in the operating room or angiographic suite for potential cerebrovascular complications.[123] Intraoperative TCD monitoring can be performed with the transducer strapped over the transtemporal window, allowing evaluation of blood flow in the MCA during CEA. **Adequacy of cerebral perfusion** can be assessed while the carotid artery is clamped.[123,124] TCD is also capable of detecting **intraoperative microembolization** ("HITS") which produces high amplitude spikes on the Doppler spectrum.[123,125-127] The technique can be used for the serial evaluation of **vasospasm.** This diagnosis is usually based on serial examinations of the relative increase in blood flow velocity and resistive index changes resulting from a decrease in the lumen of the vessel caused by vasospasm.[123]

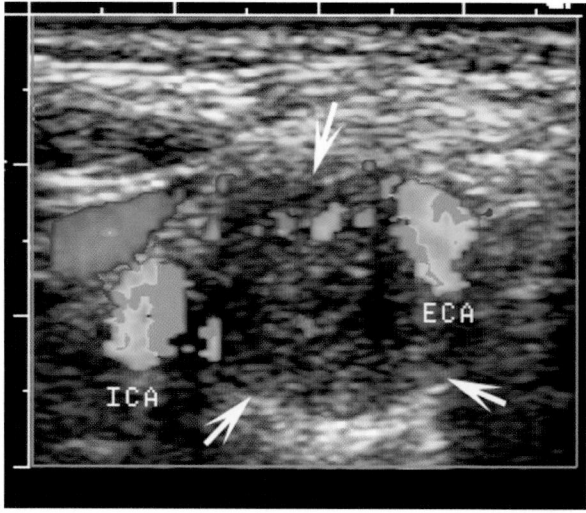

A

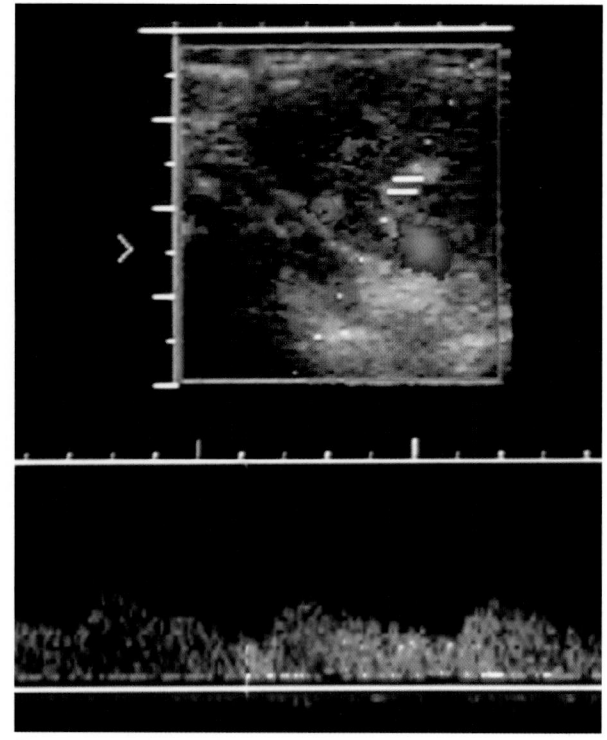

FIGURE 27-41. **Carotid body tumor.** A, Transverse image of the carotid bifurcation shows a mass (*arrows*) splaying the ICA and ECA. **B**, Pulsed Doppler traces of the carotid body tumor show typical A-V shunt (low-resistance) waveform. ECA, external carotid artery; ICA, internal carotid artery.

B

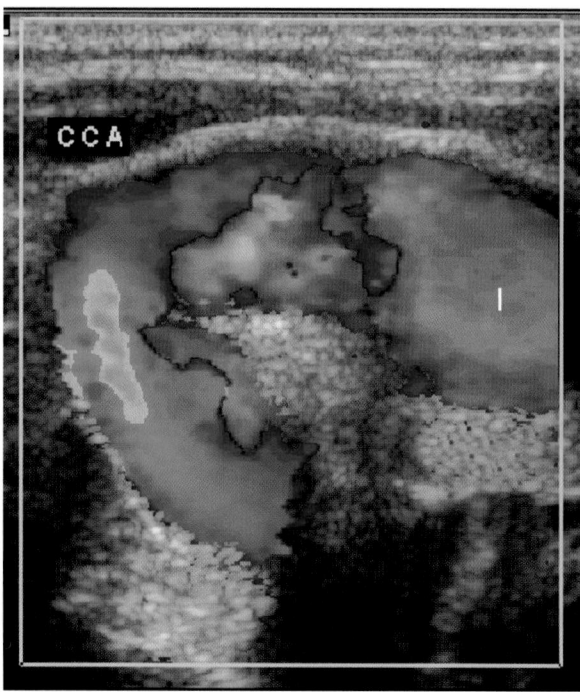

FIGURE 27-42. **Ectatic CCA.** An ectatic proximal CCA as it arises from the innominate (I) artery responsible for a pulsatile right supraclavicular mass. CCA, common carotid artery.

VERTEBRAL ARTERY

The vertebral arteries supply the majority of the posterior brain circulation. Via the circle of Willis, they also provide collateral circulation to other portions of the brain in cases of carotid occlusive disease. Evaluation of the extracranial vertebral artery seems a natural extension of carotid duplex and color Doppler imaging.[128,129] Historically, however, these arteries have not been studied as intensively as the carotids. Symptoms of vertebrobasilar insufficiency also tend to be rather vague and poorly defined, compared with symptoms referable to the carotid circulation. It is often difficult to make an association confidently between a lesion and symptoms. Furthermore, there has been relatively limited interest in surgical correction of vertebral lesions. The anatomic variability, small size, deep course, and limited visualization resulting from overlying transverse processes make the vertebral artery more difficult to examine accurately with ultrasound.[128,130,131] The clinical utility of vertebral duplex scanning remains under investigation. Its role in diagnosing subclavian steal and pre-steal phenomena is well established.[132,133] Less clear cut is the use of vertebral duplex scanning in evaluating vertebral artery stenosis, dissection, or aneurysm.

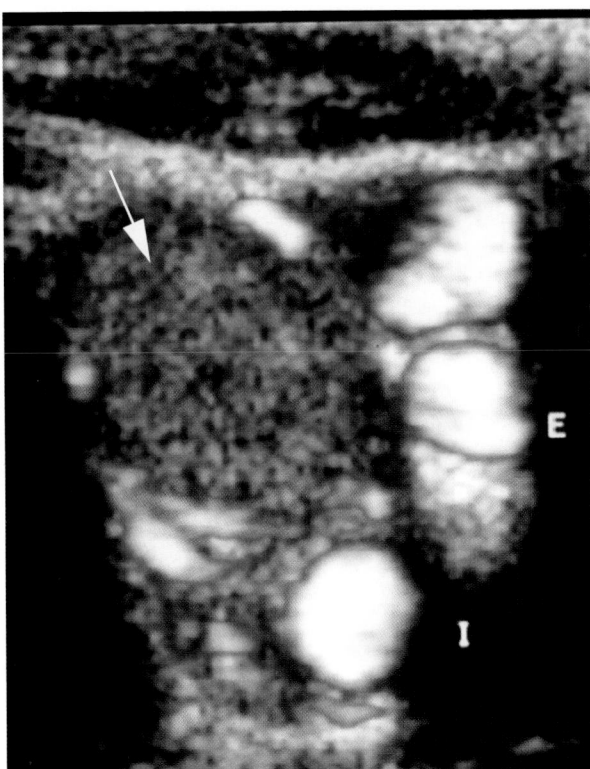

FIGURE 27-43. Pathologic lymph node near carotid bifurcation. A power Doppler image shows a malignant lymph node (*arrow*) lateral to the carotid bifurcation.

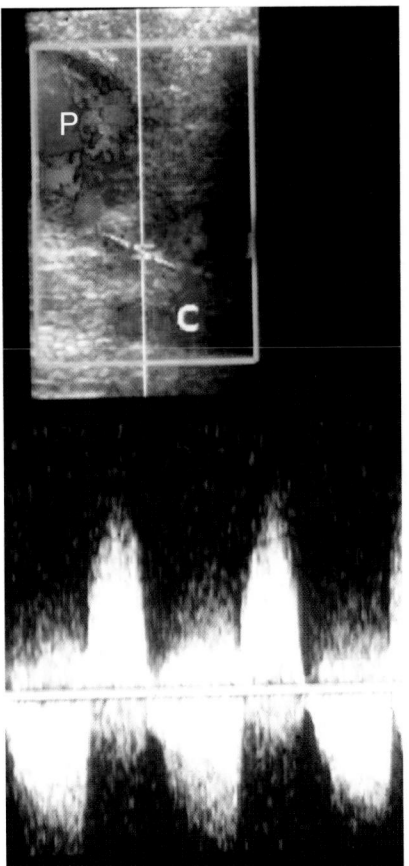

FIGURE 27-44. Pseudoaneurysm of CCA. A transverse image of the left distal CCA (c) demonstrates a characteristic to-and-fro waveform in the neck of the large pseudoaneurysm (P) which resulted from an attempted central venous line placement. CCA, common carotid artery.

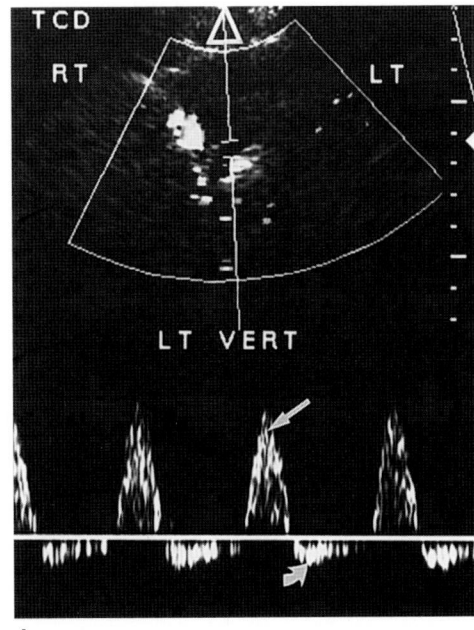

FIGURE 27-45. Transcranial Doppler imaging.
A, Transcranial duplex scan of the posterior fossa in a patient with an incomplete left subclavian steal syndrome demonstrates retrograde systolic flow (*arrow*) and antegrade diastolic flow (*curved arrow*). The scan is obtained in a transverse projection from the region of the foramen magnum (*open arrowhead*). **B**, Color flow Doppler image obtained in the same patient demonstrates that there is not only retrograde flow within the left vertebral artery, but within the basilar artery (*arrow*) as well.

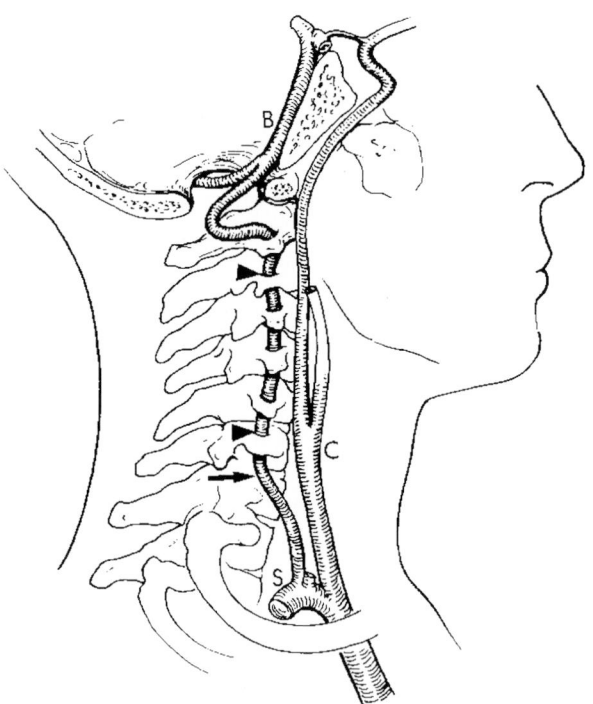

FIGURE 27-46. Vertebral artery course. Vertebral artery (*arrow*) lateral diagram shows its course through the cervical spine transverse foramina (*arrowheads*) en route to joining the contralateral vertebral artery to form the basilar artery (B). Carotid artery (C); subclavian artery (S).

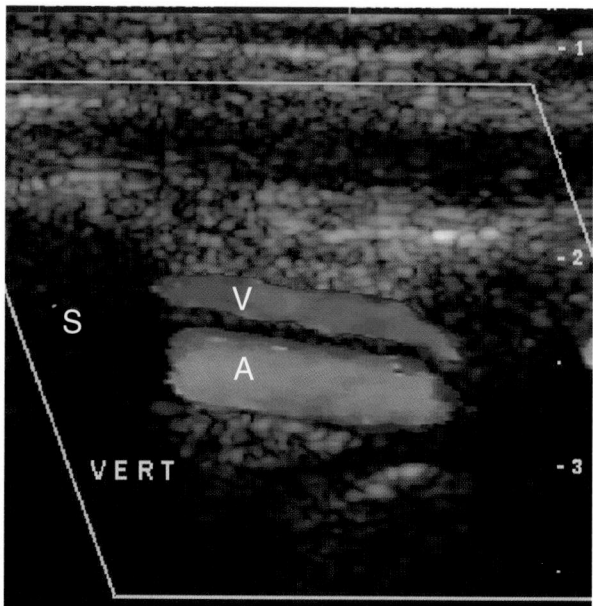

FIGURE 27-47. Normal vertebral artery (A) and vein (V). Longitudinal color Doppler shows the vertebral artery and vein running between the transverse processes of C2 to C6, which are identified by their periodic acoustic shadowing (S).

Anatomy

The vertebral artery is usually the first branch off the subclavian artery (Fig. 27-46). Variation in the origin of the vertebral arteries is common, however. In 6% to 8% of cases, the left vertebral artery arises directly from the aortic arch proximal to the left subclavian artery. In 90% of people, the proximal vertebral artery ascends superomedially, passing anterior to the transverse process of C7, and enters the transverse foramen at the C6 level. The remainder of vertebral arteries enter into the transverse foramina at the C5 or C7 level and, rarely, at the C4 level. Size of vertebral arteries is variable, with the left larger than the right in 42% of cases, the two vertebral arteries equal in size in 26% of cases, and the right larger than the left in 32% of cases.[134] One vertebral artery may even be congenitally absent. Usually the vertebral arteries join at their confluence to form the basilar artery. Rarely the vertebral artery may terminate in a posterior inferior cerebellar artery.

Technique and Normal Examination

Vertebral artery visualization with Doppler flow analysis can be obtained in 92% to 98% of vessels (Fig. 27-47).[130,135] Color Doppler facilitates rapid detection of vertebral arteries, but does not significantly improve this detection rate.[131] Vertebral artery duplex

examinations are performed by first locating the CCA in the longitudinal plane. The direction of flow in the CCA and jugular vein is determined. A gradual sweep of the transducer laterally demonstrates the vertebral artery and vein running between the transverse processes of C2 to C6, which are identified by their periodic acoustic shadowing. Transverse scanning with color Doppler allows the examiner to visualize the carotid artery and jugular vein at the same time and use them as references to determine the direction of flow in the vertebral artery.[130] Angling the transducer caudad allows visualization of the vertebral artery origin in 60% to 70% of the arteries, 80% on the right hand side and 50% on the left. This discrepancy may relate to the fact that the left vertebral artery origin is deeper and that it arises directly from the aortic arch 6% to 8% of the time.[130,136]

The presence and direction of flow should be established. Visible plaque disease should be assessed. The vertebral artery supplies blood to the brain and usually has a low-resistance flow pattern similar to that of the CCA, with continuous flow in systole and diastole; however, wide variability in waveform shape has been noted in angiographically normal vessels.[137] Because the vessel is small, flow tends to demonstrate a broader spectrum. The clear spectral window seen in the normal carotid system is often filled in the vertebral artery (Fig. 27-48).[54]

The **vertebral vein** (often a plexus of veins) runs parallel and adjacent to the vertebral artery. Care must be taken not to mistake its flow for that of the adjacent artery,

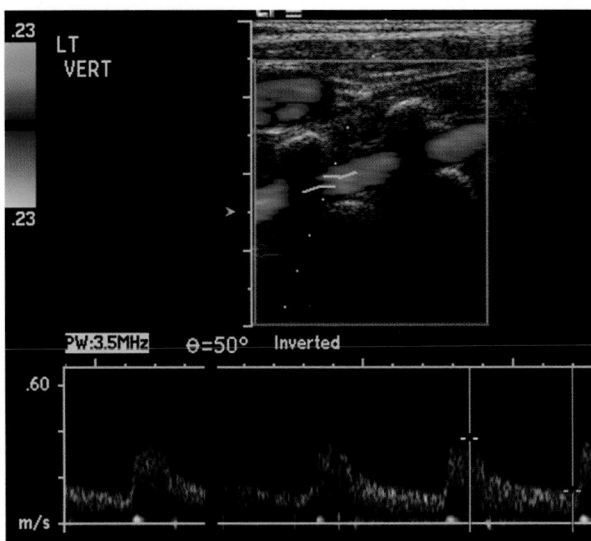

FIGURE 27-48. Normal vertebral artery waveform. Normal low-resistance waveform of the vertebral artery with filling of the spectral window.

particularly if the venous flow is pulsatile. Comparison with jugular venous flow during respiration should readily distinguish between vertebral artery and vein. At times, the ascending cervical branch of the thyrocervical trunk can be mistaken for the vertebral artery. This can be avoided by looking for landmark transverse processes that accompany the vertebral artery and also by paying careful attention to the waveform of the visualized vessel. The ascending cervical branch has a high impedance waveform pattern similar to that of the ECA.[132]

Transcranial Doppler sonographic examination of the vertebrobasilar artery system can be performed as an adjunct to the extracranial evaluation. The examination is conducted with a 2-MHz transducer with the patient sitting, using a suboccipital midline nuchal approach, or with the patient supine, using a retromastoidal approach. Color or power Doppler facilitates transcranial imaging of the vertebrobasilar system.[138]

Subclavian Steal

The **subclavian steal phenomenon** occurs when there is **high-grade stenosis** or **occlusion** of the **proximal subclavian or innominate** arteries with patent vertebral arteries bilaterally. The artery of the ischemic limb "steals" blood from the vertebrobasilar circulation via retrograde vertebral artery flow, which may result in symptoms of vertebrobasilar insufficiency (Fig. 27-49). Symptoms are usually most pronounced during exercise of the upper extremity but can be produced by changes in head position. However, there is often poor correlation between vertebrobasilar symptoms and the subclavian steal phenomenon. Usually flow within the basilar artery

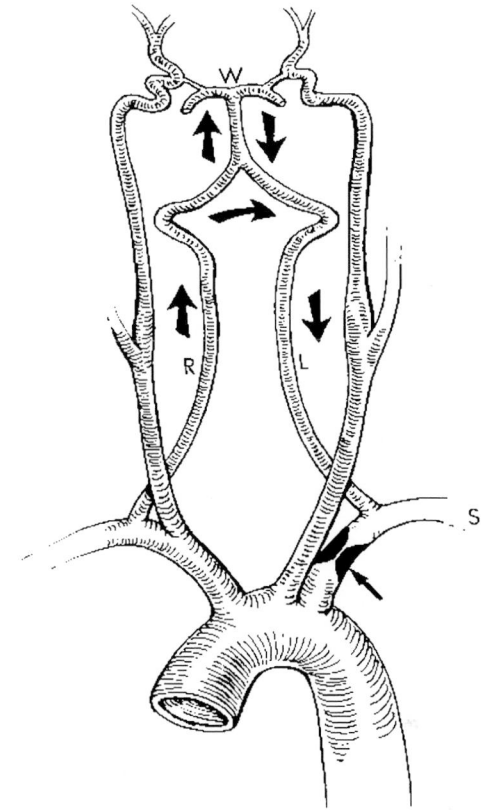

FIGURE 27-49. Hemodynamic pattern in subclavian steal syndrome diagram. Proximal left subclavian artery occlusive lesion (*small arrow*) decreases flow to the distal subclavian artery (S). This produces retrograde flow (*large arrows*) down the left vertebral artery (L) and stealing from the right vertebral artery (R) and other intracranial vessels via the circle of Willis (W).

is unaffected unless there is severe stenosis of the vertebral artery supplying the steal.[138] Additionally, surgical or angioplastic restoration of blood flow may not result in relief of symptoms.[139] The subclavian steal syndrome is most commonly **caused** by **atherosclerotic** disease, although traumatic, embolic, surgical, congenital, and neoplastic factors have also been implicated. Although the proximal subclavian stenosis or occlusion may be difficult to image, particularly on the left, the vertebral artery waveform abnormalities correlate with the severity of the subclavian disease.

Doppler evaluation of the vertebral artery reveals four distinct abnormal waveforms that correlate with subclavian or vertebral artery pathology on angiography. These include the complete subclavian steal, partial or incomplete steal, pre-steal phenomenon, and tardusparvus vertebral artery waveforms.[140] In a **complete subclavian steal**, there is complete reversal of flow within the vertebral artery (Fig. 27-50A, B). **Incomplete or partial steals** demonstrate transient reversal of vertebral flow during systole (Fig. 27-51A, B).[138,140] Incomplete steal suggests high-grade stenosis of the

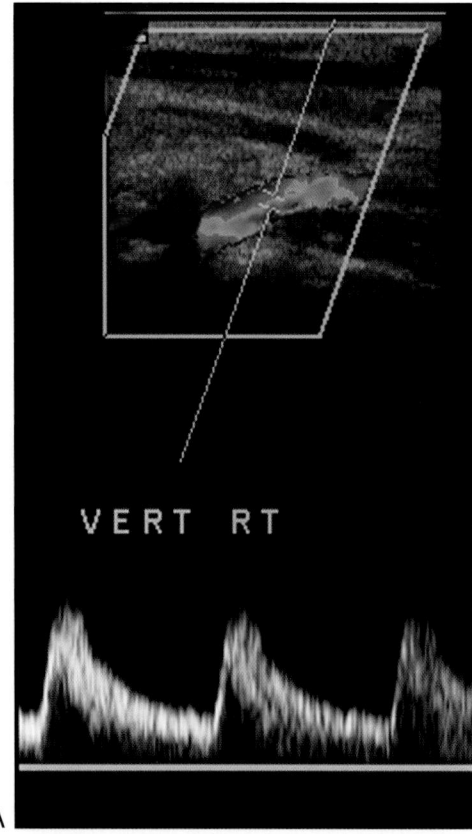

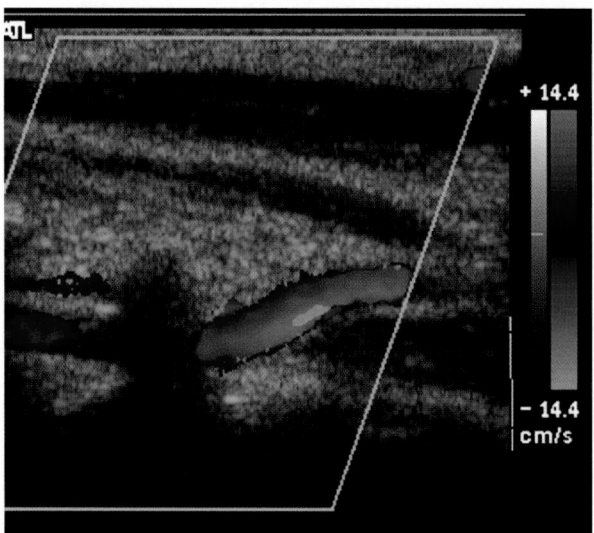

FIGURE 27-50. Vertebral artery flow. A, Subclavian steal causes reversed flow in vertebral artery. Complete vertebral artery flow reversal due to a right subclavian artery occlusion. Flow in this vertebral artery is toward the transducer. **B,** Slightly aberrant vertebral artery with color flow reversal.

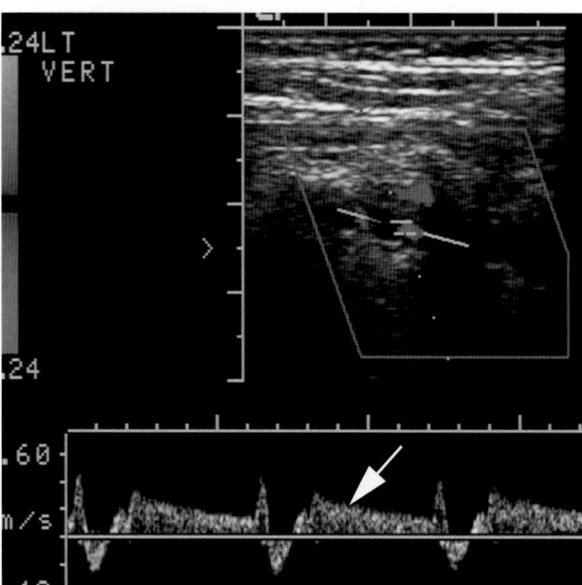

FIGURE 27-51. Incomplete subclavian steal. Flow in early systole is antegrade, flow in peak systole is retrograde, and flow in late systole and diastole (*arrow*) is again antegrade.

subclavian or innominate artery rather than occlusion. Provocative maneuvers, such as exercising the arm for 5 minutes or 5-minute inflation of a sphygmomanometer on the arm to induce rebound hyperemia on the side of the subclavian or innominate lesion can enhance the

sonographic findings and may convert an incomplete steal to a complete steal.[88,108]

The **pre-steal or "bunny" waveform** shows antegrade flow, but with a striking deceleration of velocity in peak systole to a level less than end-diastolic velocity. This is seen in patients with proximal subclavian stenosis, which is usually less severe than in cases of partial steal waveform.[140] The bunny waveform can be converted into a partial steal or complete steal waveform by provocative maneuvers, such as the use of a blood pressure cuff. (Fig. 27-52). A damped, **tardus-parvus waveform** can be seen in patients with high-grade proximal vertebral stenosis.[133,140]

With subclavian steal, color Doppler may show two similarly color-encoded vessels between the transverse processes, representing the vertebral artery and vein.[76] Transverse images of the vertebral artery with color Doppler show reversed flow when compared with the CCA. A Doppler spectral waveform must be produced in all such cases to avoid mistaking flow reversal within an artery for flow in a pulsatile vertebral vein.[76,132]

Stenosis and Occlusion

Diagnosis of **vertebral artery stenosis** is more difficult than diagnosis of flow reversal. Most hemodynamically significant stenoses occur at the origin, which is situated deep in the upper thorax and can be seen in only

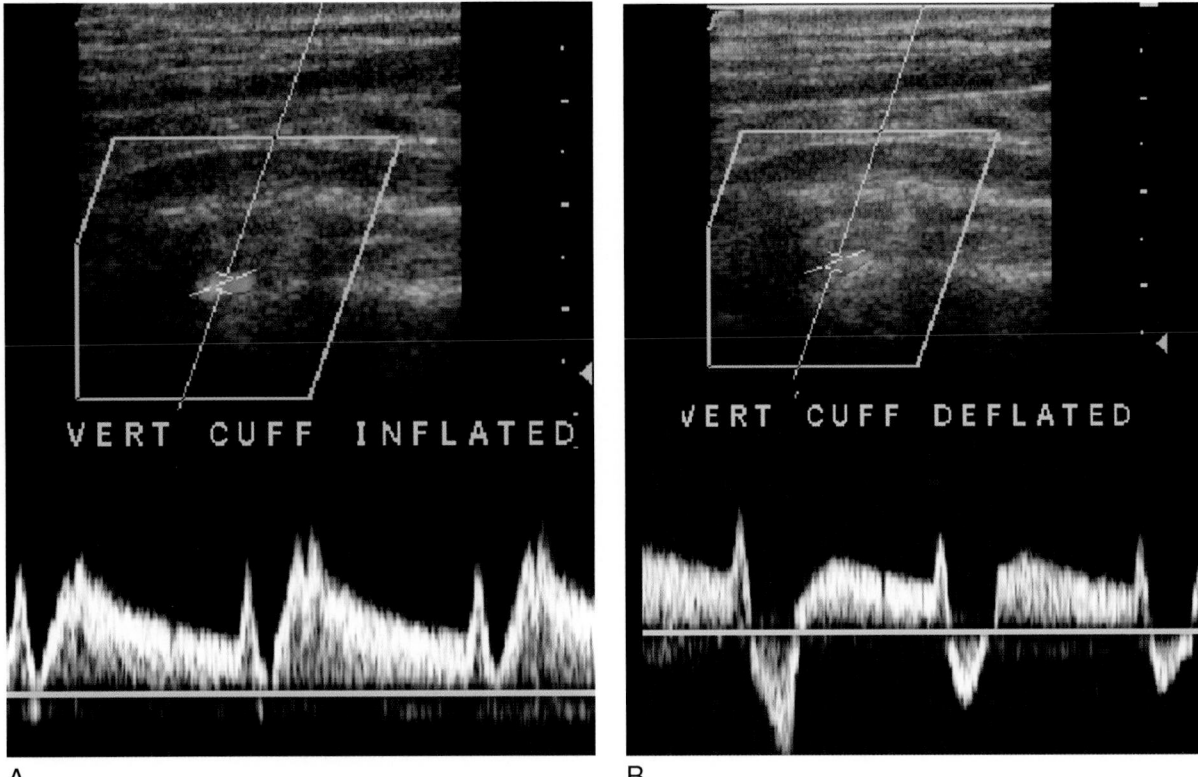

FIGURE 27-52. Incomplete subclavian steal and provocative maneuver. A, Pre-steal left vertebral artery waveform. Flow decelerates in peak systole, but does not reverse. **B,** Post-provocative maneuver, there is reversal of flow in peak systole in response to a decrease in peripheral arterial pressure.

ABNORMAL VERTEBRAL ARTERY WAVEFORMS

COMPLETE SUBCLAVIAN STEAL

Reversal of flow within the vertebral artery ipsilateral to the stenotic or occluded subclavian or innominate artery

INCOMPLETE OR PARTIAL SUBCLAVIAN STEAL

Transient reversal of vertebral artery flow during systole
May be converted into a complete steal using provocative maneuvers
Suggests stenotic, not occlusive, lesion

PRE-STEAL PHENOMENON

"Bunny" waveform: systolic deceleration less than diastolic flow
May be converted into partial steal by provocative maneuvers
Seen with proximal subclavian stenosis

TARDUS-PARVUS OR DAMPED WAVEFORM

Seen with vertebral artery stenosis

approximately 60% to 70% of patients.[130,135,136] Even if the vertebral artery origin off the subclavian is visualized, optimal adjustments of the Doppler angle for accurate velocity measurements may be difficult because of the deep location and vessel tortuosity. No accurate reproducible criteria for evaluating vertebral artery stenosis exist. As flow is normally turbulent within the vertebral artery, spectral broadening cannot be used as an indicator of stenosis. Velocity measurements are not reliable as criteria for stenosis because of the wide normal variation in vertebral artery diameter. Although velocities greater than 100 cm/sec often indicate stenosis, they can occur in angiographically normal vessels. For instance, high flow velocity may be present in a vertebral artery that is serving as a major collateral pathway for cerebral circulation in cases of carotid occlusion (Fig. 27-53).[21,141,142] Thus, only a **focal increase in velocity of at least 50%, visible stenosis on gray-scale or color Doppler, or a striking tardus-parvus vertebral artery waveform** is likely to indicate significant vertebral stenosis. Variability of resistivity indices in normal and abnormal vertebral arteries precludes the use of this parameter as an indicator of vertebral disease.[137]

Diagnosis of **vertebral artery occlusion** is also difficult. Often, inability to detect arterial flow is due to a small or congenitally absent vertebral artery or a

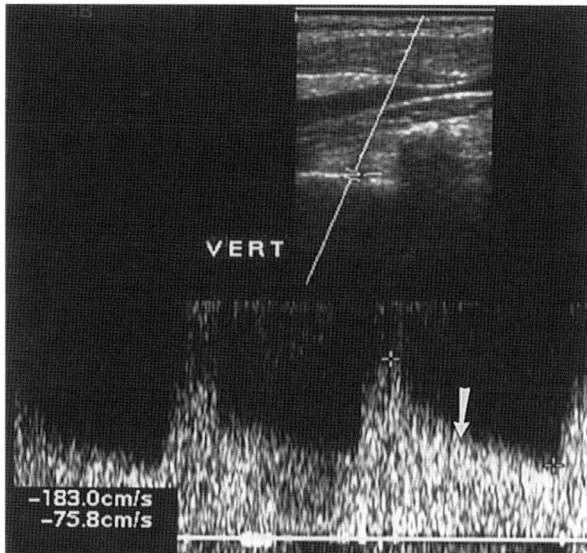

FIGURE 27-53. Increased flow velocity in the vertebral artery. Pulsed Doppler spectral trace from a left vertebral artery demonstrates strikingly high velocities and disturbed flow (*arrow*). While this degree of velocity elevation and flow disturbance could be associated with a focal stenosis, in this case there was increased velocity throughout the vertebral artery due to bilateral internal carotid artery occlusion and increased collateral flow into the vertebral artery.

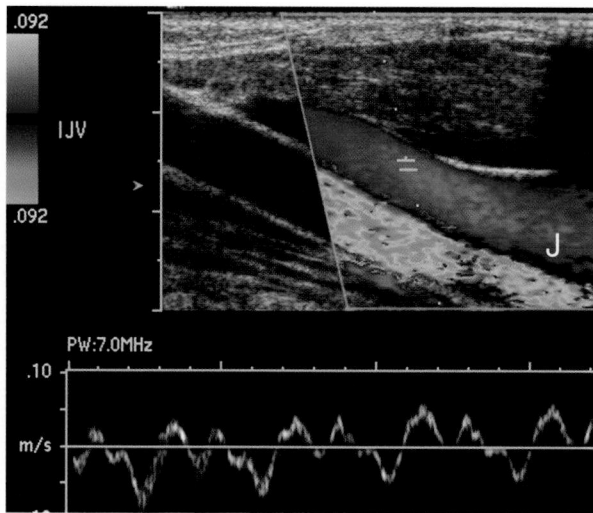

FIGURE 27-54. Normal jugular vein. Complex venous pulsations in the jugular vein (J) reflect the cycle of events in the right atrium.

technically difficult examination. Differentiation of severe stenosis from occlusion is difficult for the same reasons. Markedly damped blood flow velocity in high-grade stenoses and a decreased number of red blood cells traversing the area evaluated may result in a Doppler signal with amplitude too low to be detected.[131] Power Doppler imaging may prove useful in this situation. Visualization of only a vertebral vein is very suggestive of vertebral artery occlusion or congenital absence.

INTERNAL JUGULAR VEIN

The internal jugular veins are the major vessels responsible for return of venous blood from the brain. The most common clinical indication for duplex and color flow US of the internal jugular vein is the evaluation of suspected **jugular venous thrombosis**.[143-150] Thrombus formation may be related to central venous catheter placement. Other indications include diagnosis of **jugular venous ectasia**[149-152] and guidance for **internal jugular or subclavian vein cannulation**,[153-157] particularly in difficult situations where vascular anatomy is distorted.

Technique

The normal internal jugular vein is easily visualized. The vein is scanned with the neck extended and the head turned to the contralateral side. Longitudinal and trans-

verse scans are obtained with light transducer pressure on the neck to avoid collapsing the vein. A coronal view from the supraclavicular fossa is used to image the lower segment of the internal jugular vein and medial segment of the subclavian vein as they join to form the brachiocephalic vein.

The jugular vein lies lateral and anterior to the CCA, lateral to the thyroid gland, and deep to the sternocleidomastoid muscle. The vessel has sharply echogenic walls and a hypoechoic or anechoic lumen. Normally a valve can be visualized in its distal portion.[146,148,158] The right internal jugular vein is usually larger than the left.[153]

Real-time US demonstrates **venous pulsations related to right heart contractions**, as well as changes in venous diameter that vary with changes in intrathoracic pressure. Doppler examination graphically depicts these flow patterns (Fig. 27-54). On inspiration, negative intrathoracic pressure causes flow toward the heart and the jugular veins to decrease in diameter. During expiration and during Valsalva's maneuver, increased intrathoracic pressure causes a decrease in the blood return and the veins enlarge; little or no flow is noted. Walls of the normal jugular vein collapse completely when moderate transducer pressure is applied. Sudden sniffing reduces intrathoracic pressure, causing momentary collapse of the vein on real-time US, accompanied by a brief increase in venous flow toward the heart as shown by Doppler.[145,147,149]

Thrombosis

Clinical features of jugular venous thrombosis (JVT) include a tender, ill-defined, nonspecific neck mass or swelling. The correct diagnosis may not be immediately obvious.[146] Thrombosis of the internal jugular vein can be completely asymptomatic because of the deep position of the vein and the presence of abundant collateral circulation.[149] This condition was previously diagnosed by venography, an invasive procedure prompted only by a high index of suspicion. With the introduction of noninvasive techniques, such as ultrasound, computed tomography (CT),[159] and magnetic resonance angiography (MRA),[160] JVT is being identified more frequently. Internal jugular thrombosis most commonly results from complications of **central venous catheterization**.[144,148,149] Other causes include **intravenous drug abuse, mediastinal tumor, hypercoagulable states, neck surgery,** and **local inflammation/adenopathy**.[146] Some cases are idiopathic or spontaneous.[147] Possible complications of JVT include suppurative thrombophlebitis, clot propagation, and pulmonary embolism.[146,150]

Real-time examination reveals an enlarged noncompressible vein, which may contain visible echogenic intraluminal thrombus. **Acute thrombus** may be anechoic and indistinguishable from flowing blood; however, characteristic lack of compressibility and absent Doppler or color Doppler flow in the region of a thrombus quickly leads to the correct diagnosis. In addition, there is visible loss of vein response to respiratory maneuvers and venous pulsation. Spectral and color flow Doppler interrogations reveal absent flow (Fig. 27-55A, B). Collateral veins may be identified, particularly in cases of chronic internal jugular vein thrombosis. Central liquefaction or other heterogeneity of the thrombus also suggests chronicity. **Chronic thrombi** may be difficult to visualize, as they tend to organize and are difficult to separate from echogenic perivascular fatty tissue.[148] Absence of cardiorespiratory plasticity in a patent jugular or subclavian vein can indicate a more central nonocclusive thrombus (Fig. 27-56A-D). Confirmation of bilateral loss of venous pulsations strongly supports a more central thrombus which can be documented by venography or MRA.

Thrombus that is related to catheter insertion is often demonstrated at the tip of the catheter, although it may be seen anywhere along the course of the vein. The catheter can be visualized as two parallel echogenic lines

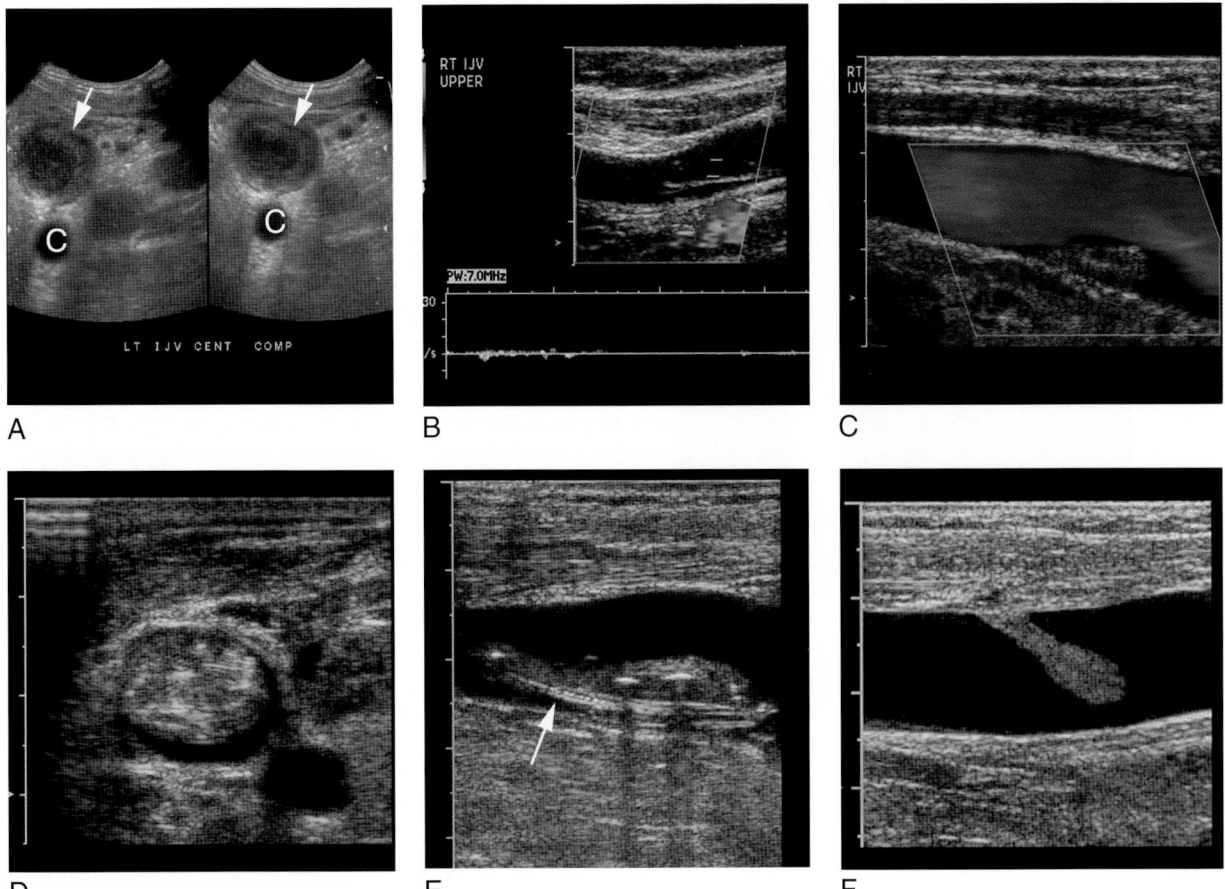

FIGURE 27-55. Internal jugular vein thrombosis—Spectrum of appearances. A, Transverse image of an acute left internal jugular vein thrombus (*arrow*). The vein is distended and noncompressible. Common carotid artery (C). **B,** Longitudinal image of a different patient demonstrates hypoechoic thrombus and no Doppler signal. **C,** Longitudinal color Doppler image shows a small amount of thrombus arising from the posterior wall of the internal jugular vein (IJV). **D,** Transverse image shows echogenic thrombus indicating chronic thrombus in IJV. **E,** Longitudinal image demonstrates thrombus around jugular vein catheter. **F,** Longitudinal images show thrombus arising from anterior wall. This thrombus is probably due to previous catheter placement in this region.

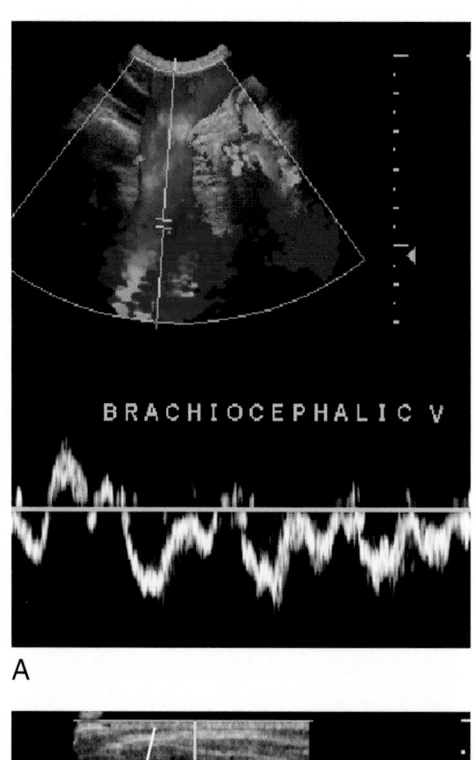

A

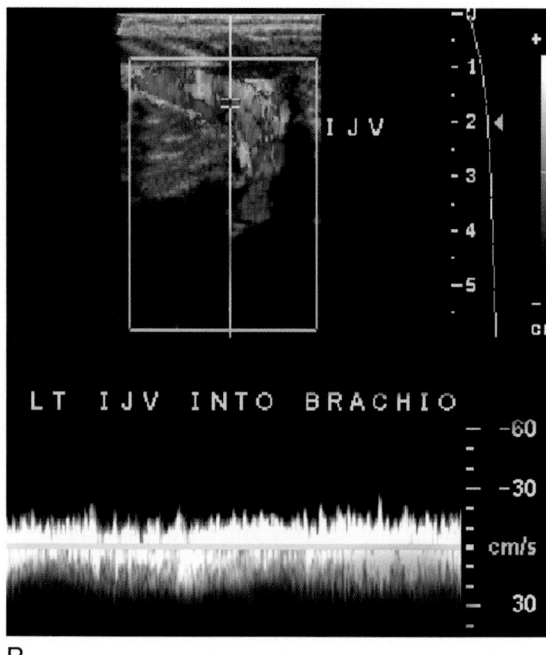

B

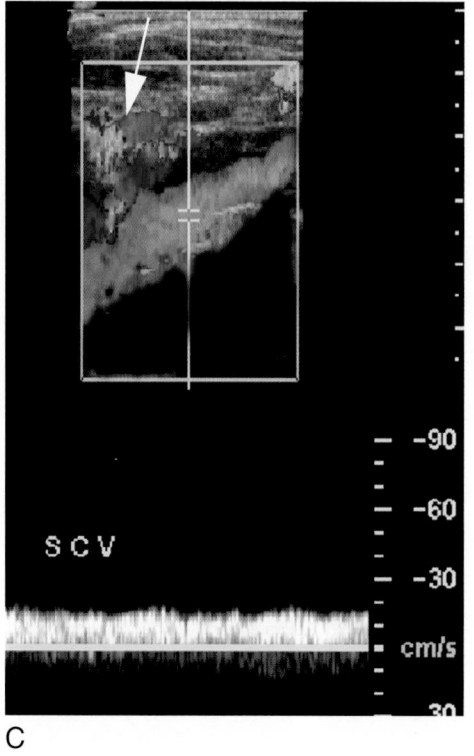

C

FIGURE 27-56. A, Normal and abnormal brachiocephalic vein waveforms. There is normal cardiorespiratory change in the venous waveforms of the brachiocephalic vein implying a patent superior vena cava. **B,** Patient with a near occlusive left central brachiocephalic vein stenosis due to a prior central venous catheter shows reversed nonpulsatile flow in the internal jugular vein on pulsed Doppler waveform. **C,** Left subclavian vein shows centrally directed, but monophasic, flow toward an area of central collaterals (*arrow*) in this patient with a malfunctioning left A-V dialysis fistula.

separated by an anechoic region. Flow is not commonly demonstrated in the catheter, even if the catheter itself is patent.

Sonography has proved to be a reliable means of diagnosing jugular and subclavian vein thrombosis and has the advantage over CT and MRI of being inexpensive, portable, nonionizing, and requiring no intravenous contrast. Sonography has limited access and cannot image all portions of the jugular and subclavian veins, especially those located behind the mandible or below the clavicle. Knowledge of the full extent of thrombus is not frequently a critical factor in treatment planning, however.[146,150] Serial sonographic examination to evaluate response to therapy after the initial assessment can be performed safely and inexpensively. Sonography can also document venous patency prior to vascular line placement, facilitating safer and more successful catheter insertion.

Acknowledgment

Thanks to Susan Murray for her assistance with manuscript preparation.

References

1. Carroll BA: Carotid sonography. Radiology 1991; 178:303-313.
2. Executive Committee for the Asymptomatic Carotid Atherosclerotic Study. Endarterectomy for asymptomatic carotid artery stenosis. JAMA 1995;273(18):1421-1428.
3. Fontenelle LJ, Simper SC, Hanson TL: Carotid duplex scan versus angiography in evaluation of carotid artery disease. Am Surg 1994;60:864-868.
4. North American Symptomatic Carotid Endarterectomy Trial Collaborators: Beneficial effect of carotid endarterectomy in symptomatic patients with high-grade carotid stenosis. N Engl J Med 1991;325:445-453.
5. European Carotid Surgery Trialists' Collaborative Group: MRC European Carotid Surgery Trial: Interim results for symptomatic patients with severe (70-99%) and mild (0-29%) carotid stenosis. Lancet 1991;337:1235-1243.
6. Barnett HJM, Taylor DW, Eliasziw M, et al: Benefit of carotid endarterectomy in patients with symptomatic moderate or severe stenosis. N Engl J Med 1998;339:1415-1425.
7. Executive Committee for the Asymptomatic Carotid Atherosclerosis Study: Endarterectomy for asymptomatic carotid artery stenosis. JAMA 1995;273:1421-1428.
8. Derdeyn CP, Powers WJ, Moran CJ, et al: Role of Doppler US in screening for carotid atherosclerotic disease. Radiology 1995;197:635-643.
9. Merritt CRB, Bluth EI: The future of carotid sonography. AJR 1992;158:37-39.
10. Taylor KJW: Clinical applications of carotid Doppler ultrasound. In Taylor KJW, Burns PN, Wells PNT (eds): Clinical Applications of Doppler Ultrasound. New York, Raven Press, 1988, pp 120-161.
11. Bluth EI, Shyn PB, Sullivan MA, et al: Doppler color flow imaging of carotid artery dissection. J Ultrasound Med 1989;8:149-153.
12. Hennerici M, Steinke W, Rautenberg W: High-resistance Doppler flow pattern in extracranial carotid dissection. Arch Neurol 1989;46:670-672.
13. Rothrock JF, Lim V, Press G, et al: Serial magnetic resonance and carotid duplex examinations in the management of carotid dissection. Neurology 1989;39:686-692.
14. O'Leary DH, Polak JF, Kronmal RA, et al: Carotid-artery intima and media thickness as a risk factor for myocardial infarction and stroke in older adults. N Engl J Med 1999;340:14-22.
15. Sidhu PS, Jonker ND, Khaw KT, et al: Spontaneous dissections of the internal carotid artery: Appearance on colour Doppler ultrasound. Br J Radiol 1997;70:50-57.
16. Gritzmann N, Grasl MCH, Helmer M, et al: Invasion of the carotid artery and jugular vein by lymph node metastases: Detection with sonography. AJR 1990; 154:411-414.
17. Gooding GAW, Langman AW, Dillon WP, et al: Malignant carotid artery invasion: Sonographic detection. Radiology 1989;171:435-438.
18. Steinke W, Hennerici M, Aulich A: Doppler color flow imaging of carotid body tumors. Stroke 1989; 20:1574-1577.
19. Grant EG, Wong W, Tessler F, et al: Cerebrovascular ultrasound imaging. Radiol Clin North Am 1988;26:1111-1130.
20. Ide C, De Coene B, Maileux P, et al: Hypoplasia of the internal carotid artery: A noninvasive diagnosis. Eur Radiol 2000;10:1865-1870.

Examination Performance and Interpretation
21. Polak JF, O'Leary DH, Kronmal RA, et al: Sonographic evaluation of carotid artery atherosclerosis in the elderly: Relationship of disease severity to stroke and transient ischemic attack. Radiology 1993;188:363-370.
22. Veller MG, Fisher CM, Nicolaides AN, et al: Measurement of the ultrasonic intima-media complex thickness in normal subjects. J Vasc Surg 1993;17:719-725.
23. Bort ML, Mulder PGH, Hofman A, et al: Reproducibility of carotid vessel wall thickness measurements. The Rotterdam Study. J Clin Epidemiol 1994;47(8):921-930.
24. Csányi A, Egervári A: Simple clinical method of average intima-media thickness measurement in the common carotid artery. VASA 1996;25:242-248.
25. O'Leary DH, Polak JF, Kronmal RA, et al: Carotid-artery intima and media thickness as a risk factor for myocardial infarction and stroke in older adults. N Engl J Med 1999;340:14-22.
26. Bots ML, Hoes AW, Koudstall PJ, et al: Common carotid intima-media thickness and risk of stroke and myocardial infarction: The Rotterdam study. Circulation 1997;96:1432-1443.
27. Kanters SD, Algra A, van Leeuwen MS, et al: Reproducibility of in vivo carotid intima-media thickness measurements: A review. Stroke 1997;28:665-671.
28. Dwyer JH, Sun P, Kwong-Fu H, et al: Automated intima-media thickness: The Los Angeles atherosclerosis study. Ultrasound Med Biol 1998;24:981-987.
29. Aminbakhsh A, Frohlich J, Mancini GBJ: Detection of early atherosclerosis with B mode carotid ultrasonography: Assessment of a new quantitative approach. Clin Invest Med 1999;22:265-274.
30. Greenland P, Abrams J, Aurigemma GP, et al: Prevention Conference V: Noninvasive tests of atherosclerotic burden. Circulation 2000;101:111-116.
31. Bluth EI, Stavros AT, Marich KW, et al: Carotid duplex sonography: A multicenter recommendation for standardized imaging and Doppler criteria. Radiographics 1988;8:487-506.
32. Polak JF, Shemanski L, O'Leary DH, et al: Hypoechoic plaque at US of the carotid artery: An independent risk factor for incident stroke in adults aged 65 years or older. Radiology 1998;208:649-654.
33. Langsfield M, Gray-Weale AC, Lusby RJ: The role of plaque morphology and diameter reduction in the development of new symptoms in asymptomatic carotid arteries. J Vasc Surg 1989;9:548-557.
34. Leahy AL, McCollum PT, Feeley TM, et al: Duplex ultrasonography and selection of patients for carotid endarterectomy: Plaque morphology or luminal narrowing? J Vasc Surg 1988;8:558-562.
35. Reilly LM, Lusby RJ, Hughes L, et al: Carotid plaque histology using real-time ultrasonography: Clinical and therapeutic implications. Am J Surg 1983;146:188-193.
36. Persson AV, Robichaux WT, Silverman M: The natural history of carotid plaque development. Arch Surg 1983;118:1048-1052.
37. Lusby RJ, Ferrell LD, Ehrenfield WK, et al: Carotid plaque hemorrhage: Its role in production of cerebral ischemia. Arch Surg 1982;117:1479-1488.

38. Edwards JH, Kricheff II, Gorstein F, et al: Atherosclerotic subintimal hematoma of the carotid artery. Radiology 1979;133:123-129.

39. Imparato AM, Riles TS, Gorstein F: The carotid bifurcation plaque: Pathologic findings associated with cerebral ischemia. Stroke 1979;10:238-245.

40. Gerovlakas G, Ramaswami G, Nicolaides A, et al: Characterization of symptomatic and asymptomatic carotid plaques using high-resolution real-time ultrasonography. Br J Surg 1993;80(10):1274-1276.

41. Holdsworth RJ, McCollum PT, Bryce JS, et al: Symptoms, stenosis and carotid plaque morphology. Is plaque morphology relevant? Eur J Vasc Endovasc Surg 1995;9:80-85.

42. Sterpetti AV, Schultz RD, Feldhaus RJ, et al: Ultrasonographic features of carotid plaque and the risk of subsequent neurologic deficits. Surgery 1988;104:652-660.

43. Weinberger J, Marks SJ, Gaul JJ, et al: Atherosclerotic plaque at the carotid artery bifurcation: Correlation of ultrasonographic imaging with morphology. J Ultrasound Med 1987;6:363-366.

44. Stahl JA, Middleton WD: Pseudoulceration of the carotid artery. J Ultrasound Med 1992;11:355-358.

45. Ballard JL, Deiparine MK, Bergan JJ, et al: Cost-effective evaluation and treatment for carotid disease. Arch Surg 1997;132:268-271.

46. Furst H, Hartl WH, Jansen I, et al: Color-flow Doppler sonography in the identification of ulcerative plaques in patients with high-grade carotid artery stenosis. AJNR 1992;13:1581-1587.

47. Abildgaard A, Egge TS, Kløw NE, et al: Use of sonicated albumin (Infoson) to enhance arterial spectral and color Doppler imaging. Cardiovasc Intervent Radiol 1996;19:265-271.

48. Comerota AJ, Cranley JJ, Cook SE: Real-time B-mode carotid imaging in diagnosis of cerebrovascular disease. Surgery 1981;89:718-729.

49. Zwiebel WJ, Austin CW, Sackett JF, et al: Correlation of high-resolution, B-mode and continuous-wave Doppler sonography with arteriography in the diagnosis of carotid stenosis. Radiology 1983;149:523-532.

50. Jacobs NM, Grant EG, Schellinger D, et al: Duplex carotid sonography: Criteria for stenosis, accuracy, and pitfalls. Radiology 1985;154:385-391.

51. Taylor KJW, Holland S: Doppler ultrasound: Part I. Basic principles, instrumentation, and pitfalls. Radiology 1990;174:297-307.

52. Carroll BA, von Ramm OT: Fundamentals of current Doppler technology. Ultrasound Quarterly 1988;6:275-298.

53. Bluth EI, Sunshine JH, Lyons JB, et al: Power Doppler imaging: Initial evaluation as a screening examination for carotid artery stenosis. Radiology 2000;21:791-800.

54. Kassam M, Johnston KW, Cobbold RSC: Quantitative estimation of spectral broadening for the diagnosis of carotid arterial disease: Method and in vitro results. Ultrasound Med Biol 1985;11:425-433.

55. Douville Y, Johnston KW, Kassam M: Determination of the hemodynamic factors which influence the carotid Doppler spectral broadening. Ultrasound Med Biol 1985;11:417-423.

56. Garth KE, Carroll BA, Sommer FG, et al: Duplex ultrasound scanning of the carotid arteries with velocity spectrum analysis. Radiology 1983;147:823-827.

57. Phillips DJ, Greene FM, Langlois Y, et al: Flow velocity patterns in the carotid bifurcations of young, presumed normal subjects. Ultrasound Med Biol 1983;9:39-49.

58. Lichtman JB, Kibble MB: Detection of intracranial arteriovenous malformation by Doppler ultrasound of the extracranial carotid circulation. J Ultrasound Med 1987;6:609-612.

59. Robinson ML, Sacks D, Perlmutter GS, et al: Diagnostic criteria for carotid duplex sonography. AJR 1988;151:1045-1049.

60. Grant EG, Deurinckx AJ, El Saden SM, et al: Ability to use duplex US to quantify internal carotid arterial stenoses: fact or fiction? Radiology 2000;214:247-252.

61. Rothwell PM, Gibson RJ, Slattery J, et al: Prognostic value and reproducibility of measurements of carotid stenosis: A comparison of three methods on 1001 angiograms. Stroke 1994;25:2440-2444.

62. Moneta GL, Edwards JM, Chitwood RW, et al: Correlation of North American Symptomatic Carotid Endarterectomy Trial (NASCET) angiographic definition of 70% to 99% internal carotid artery stenosis with duplex scanning. J Vasc Surg 1993;17:152-159.

63. Friedman SG, Hainline B, Feinberg AW, et al: Use of diastolic velocity ratios to predict significant carotid artery stenosis. Stroke 1988;19:910-912.

64. Kohler TR, Langlois Y, Roederer GO, et al: Variability in measurement of specific parameters for carotid duplex examination. Ultrasound Med Biol 1987;13:637-642.

65. Hunink MGM, Polak JF, Barlan MM, et al: Detection and quantification of carotid artery stenosis: Efficacy of various Doppler velocity parameters. AJR 1993;160:619-625.

66. Horrow MM, Stassi J, Shurman A, et al: The limitations of carotid sonography: Interpretive and technology related errors. AJR 2000;174:189-194.

67. Faught WE, Mattos MA, van Bemmelen, et al: Color-flow duplex scanning of carotid arteries: New velocity criteria based on receiver operator characteristic analysis for threshold stenoses used in the symptomatic and asymptomatic carotid trials. J Vasc Surg 1994;19:818-828.

68. Kuntz KM, Polak JF, Whittemore AD, et al: Duplex ultrasound criteria for the identification of carotid stenosis should be laboratory specific. Stroke 1997;28:597-602.

69. Kuntz KM, Polak JF, Whitemore AD, et al: Duplex ultrasound criteria for the identification of carotid stenosis should be laboratory specific. Stroke 1997;28:597-602.

70. Alexandrov AV, Vital D, Brodie DS, et al: Grading carotid stenosis with ultrasound: An interlaboratory comparison. Stroke 1997;28:1208-1210.

71. Consensus Conference on Carotid Ultrasound, Society of Radiologists in Ultrasound, October 2002, San Francisco. Radiology, 2003;229:340-346.

72. Middleton WD, Erickson S, Melson GL: Perivascular color artifact: Pathologic significance and appearance on color Doppler ultrasound images. Radiology 1989;171:647-652.

73. Erickson SJ, Mewissen MW, Foley WD, et al: Stenosis of the internal carotid artery: Assessment using color Doppler imaging compared with angiography. AJR 1989;152:1299-1305.

74. Middleton WD, Foley WD, Lawson TL: Flow reversal in the normal carotid bifurcation: Color Doppler flow imaging analysis. Radiology 1988;167:207-210.

75. Zierler RE, Phillips DJ, Beach KW, et al: Noninvasive assessment of normal carotid bifurcation hemodynamics with color-flow ultrasound imaging. Ultrasound Med Biol 1987;13:471-476.

76. Erickson SJ, Middleton WD, Mewissen MW, et al: Color Doppler evaluation of arterial stenoses and occlusions involving the neck and thoracic inlet. Radiographics 1989;9:389-406.

77. Middleton WD, Foley WD, Lawson TL: Color-flow Doppler imaging of carotid artery abnormalities. AJR 1988;150:419-425.

78. Branas CC, Weingarten MS, Czeredarczuk M, et al: Examination of carotid arteries with quantitative color Doppler flow imaging. J Ultrasound Med 1994; 13:121-127.

79. Steinke W, Ries S, Artemis N, et al: Power Doppler imaging of carotid artery stenosis: Comparison with color Doppler flow imaging and angiography. Stroke 1997;28:1981-1987.

80. Bluth EI, Althans LE, et al: Comparison of plaque characterization with grayscale imaging and 3-D power Doppler imaging: Can more be learned about intraplaque hemorrhage? JEMU 1999;20:11-15.

81. Griewing B, Morgenstern C, Driesner F, et al: Cerebrovascular disease assessed by color-flow and power Doppler ultrasonography. Stroke 1996;27:95-100.

82. Zbornikova V, Lassvik C: Duplex scanning in presumably normal persons of different ages. Ultrasound Med Biol 1986;12:371-378.

83. Spencer EB, Sheafor DH, Hertzberg BS, et al: Nonstenotic internal carotid arteries: Effects of age and blood pressure at the time of scanning on Doppler US velocity measurements. Radiology 2001;220:174-178.

84. O'Boyle MK, Vibhaker NI, Chung J, et al: Duplex sonography of the carotid arteries in patients with isolated aortic stenosis: Imaging findings and relation to severity of stenosis. AJR 1996;166:197-202.

85. Macchi C, Gulisano M, Giannelli F, et al: Kinking of the human internal carotid artery: A statistical study in 100 healthy subjects by echocolor Doppler. J Cardiovasc Surg 1997;38:629-637.

86. Busuttil SJ, Franklin DP, Youkey JR, et al: Carotid duplex overestimation of stenosis due to severe contralateral disease. Am J Surg 1996;172:144-148.

87. AbuRahma AF, Richmond BK, Robinson PA, et al: Effect of contralateral severe stenosis or carotid occlusion on duplex criteria of ipsilateral stenoses: Comparative study of various duplex parameters. J Vasc Surg 1995; 22:751-762.

88. van Everdingen KJ, van der Gront J, Kappelle LJ: Overestimation of a stenosis in the internal carotid artery by duplex sonography caused by an increase in volume flow. J Vasc Surg 1998;27:479-485.

89. Blackshear WM, Phillips DJ, Chikos PM, et al: Carotid artery velocity patterns in normal and stenotic vessels. Stroke 1980;11:67-71.

90. Grubb RL, Jr, Derdeyn CP, Fritsch SM, et al: Importance or hemodynamic factors in the prognosis of symptomatic carotid occlusion. JAMA 1998;280:1055.

91. Berman SS, Devine JJ, Erdoes LS, et al: Distinguishing carotid artery pseudo-occlusion with color-flow Doppler. Stroke 1995;26:434-438.

92. Görtter M, Niethammer R, Widder B: Differentiating subtotal carotid artery stenoses from occlusions by colour-coded duplex sonography. J Neurol 1994; 241:301-305.

93. AbuRahma AF, Pollack JA, Robinson PA, et al: The reliability of color duplex ultrasound in diagnosing total carotid artery occlusion. Am J Surg 1997;174:185-187.

94. Kliewer MA, Freed KS, Hertzberg BS, et al: Temporal artery tap: Usefulness and limitations in carotid sonography. Radiology 1996;201:481-484.

95. Bebry AJ, Hines GL: Total occlusion of the common carotid artery with a patent internal carotid artery; report of a case. J Vasc Surg 1989;10:469-470.

96. Blackshear WM, Phillips DJ, Bodily KC, et al: Ultrasonic demonstration of external and internal carotid patency with common carotid occlusion: A preliminary report. Stroke 1980;11:249-252.

97. Lee DH, Gao FQ, Rankin RN, et al: Duplex and color Doppler flow sonography of occlusion and near occlusion of the carotid artery. Am J Neuroradiol 1996;17:1267.

98. Alexandrov AV, Bladin CF, Maggisano R, et al: Measuring carotid stenosis—time for a reappraisal. Stroke 1993;24(9):1292-1296.

99. Polak JF, Kalina P, Donaldson MC, et al: Carotid endarterectomy: Preoperative evaluation of candidates with combined Doppler sonography and MR angiography. Radiology 1993;186:333-338.

100. Johnston DC, Goldstein LB: Clinical carotid endarterectomy decision making: Noninvasive vascular imaging versus angiography. Neurology 2001;56:1009-1015.

101. Johnston D, Goldstein LB: Clinical carotid endarterectomy decision making: Noninvasive vascular imaging versus angiography. Neurol 2001; 56:1009-1015.

102. Kuntz KM, Skillman JJ, Whittemore AD, et al: Carotid endarterectomy in asymptomatic patients—Is contrast angiography necessary? A morbidity analysis. J Vasc Surg 1995;22:706-716.

103. Mattos MA, Hodgson KJ, Faught WE, et al: Carotid endarterectomy without angiography: Is color-flow duplex scanning sufficient? Surgery 1994;116:776-783.

104. Cartier R, Cartier P, Fontaine A: Carotid endarterectomy without angiography. The reliability of Doppler ultrasonography and duplex scanning in preoperative assessment. CJS 1993;36(5):411-415.

105. Fontenelle LJ, Simper SC, Hanson TL: Carotid duplex scan versus angiography in evaluation of carotid artery disease. Am Surg 1994;60(11):864-868.

106. Thusay MM, Khoury M, Greene K: Carotid endarterectomy based on duplex ultrasound in patients with and without hemispheric symptoms. Am Surg 2001;67:1-6.

107. Welch HJ, Murphy MC, Raftery KB, et al: Carotid duplex with contralateral disease: The influence of vertebral artery blood flow. Ann Vasc Surg 2000;14:82-88.

108. Chen JC, Salvian AJ, Taylor DC, et al: Can duplex ultrasonography select appropriate patients for carotid endarterectomy? Eur J Vasc Endovasc Surg 1997; 14:451-456.

109. Randoux B, Marro B, Koskas F, et al: Carotid artery stenosis: Prospective comparison of CT, three-dimensional gadolinium-enhanced MR, and conventional angiography. Radiology 2001;220:179-185.

110. Johnson BL, Gupta AK, Bandyk DF, et al: Anatomic patterns of carotid endarterectomy healing. Am J Surg 1996;172:188-190.

111. Kagawa R, Okada Y, Shima T, et al: B-mode ultrasonographic investigations of morphological changes in endarterectomized carotid artery. Surg Neurol 2001;55:50-57.

112. Jackson MR, D'Addio VJ, Gillespie DL, et al: The fate of residual defects following carotid endarterectomy detected by early postoperative duplex ultrasound. Am J Surg 1996;172:184-187.

113. Rocotta KK, DeWeese KA: Is routine carotid ultrasound surveillance after carotid endarterectomy worthwhile? Am J Surg 1996;172:140-143.

114. Robbin ML, Lockhart ME, Weber TM, et al: Carotid artery stents: Early and intermediate follow-up with Doppler US. Radiology 1997;205:749-756.

Nonatherosclerotic Carotid Disease

115. Furie DM, Tien RD: Fibromuscular dysplasia of arteries of the head and neck: Imaging findings. AJR 1994; 162:1205-1209.

116. Kliewer MA, Carroll BA: Ultrasound case of the day. Radiographics 1991;11:504-505.

117. Maeda H, Handa N, Matsumoto M, et al: Carotid lesions detected by B-mode ultrasonography in Takayasu's arteritis: "Macaroni sign" as an indicator of the disease. Ultrasound Med Biol 1991;17(7):695-701.

118. Sturzenegger M: Spontaneous internal carotid artery dissection: Early diagnosis and management in 44 patients. J Neurol 1995;242:231-238.

119. Sturzenegger M, Mattle HP, Rivoir A, et al: Ultrasound findings in carotid artery dissection: Analysis of 43 patients. Neurology 1995;45:691-698.

120. Steinke W, Rautenberg W. Schwartz A, et al: Noninvasive monitoring of internal carotid artery dissection. Stroke 1994;25(5):998-1005.

Transcranial Doppler Sonography

121. Lupetin AR, Davis DA, Beckman J, et al: Transcranial Doppler sonography. Part 1. Principles, technique and normal appearance. Radiographics 1995;15(1):179-191.

122. Comerota AJ, Katz ML, Hosking JD, et al: Is transcranial Doppler a worthwhile addition to screening tests for cerebrovascular disease? J Vasc Surg 1995;21:90-97.

123. Rorick MB, Nichols FT, Adams RJ: Transcranial Doppler correlation with angiography in detection of intracranial stenosis. Stroke 1994;25:1931-1934.

124. Lupetin AR, Davis DA, Beckman, et al: Transcranial Doppler sonography. Part 2. Evaluation of intracranial and extracranial abnormalities and procedural monitoring. Radiographics 1995;15:193-209.

125. Lin SU, Ryu SJ, Chu NS: Carotid Doppler and transcranial color coded sonography in evaluation of carotid-cavernous sinus fistulas. J Ultrasound Med 1994;13:557-564.

126. Mast H, Mohr JP, Thompson JLP, et al: Transcranial Doppler ultrasonography in cerebral arteriovenous malformation. Stroke 1995;26:1024-1027.

127. Gaunt ME, Martin PJ, Smith JL, et al: Clinical relevance of intraoperative embolization detected by transcranial Doppler sonography during carotid endarterectomy: A prospective study of 100 patients. Br J Surg 1994; 81:1435-1439.

Vertebral Artery

128. Bendick PJ, Glover JL: Hemodynamic evaluation of vertebral arteries by duplex ultrasound. Surg Clin North Am 1990;70:235-244.

129. Lewis BD, James EM, Welch TJ: Current applications of duplex and color Doppler ultrasound imaging: Carotid and peripheral vascular system. Mayo Clin Proc 1989;64:1147-1157.

130. Visona A, Lusiani L, Castellani V, et al: The echo-Doppler (duplex) system for the detection of vertebral artery occlusive disease: Comparison with angiography. J Ultrasound Med 1986;5:247-250.

131. Davis PC, Nilsen B, Braun IF, et al: A prospective comparison of duplex sonography vs angiography of the vertebral arteries. AJNR 1986;7:1059-1064.

132. Bluth EI, Merritt CRB, Sullivan MA, et al: Usefulness of duplex ultrasound in evaluating vertebral arteries. J Ultrasound Med 1989;8:229-235.

133. Walker DW, Acker JD, Cole CA: Subclavian steal syndrome detected with duplex pulsed Doppler sonography. AJNR 1982;3:615-618.

134. Elias DA, Weinberg PE: Angiography of the posterior fossa. In Taveras JM, Ferrucci JT (eds): Radiology: Diagnosis-Imaging-Intervention. Philadelphia: J.B. Lippincott, 1989, pp 3, 6-7.

135. Bendick PJ, Jackson VP: Evaluation of the vertebral arteries with duplex sonography. J Vasc Surg 1986; 3:523-530.

136. Ackerstaff RGA, Grosveld WJHM, Eikelboom BC, et al: Ultrasonic duplex scanning of the prevertebral segment of the vertebral artery in patients with cerebral atherosclerosis. Eur J Vasc Surg 1988;2:387-393.

137. Carroll BA, Holder CA: Vertebral artery duplex sonography (abstract). J Ultrasound Med 1990;9:S27-28.

138. de Bray JM, Zenglein JP, Laroche JP, et al: Effect of subclavian syndrome on the basilar artery. Acta Neurol Scand 1994;90:174-178.

139. Thomassen L, Aarli JA: Subclavian steal phenomenon. Acta Neurol Scand 1994;90:241-244.

140. Kliewer MA, Hertzberg BS, Kim DH, et al: Vertebral artery Doppler waveform changes indicating subclavian steal physiology. AJR 2000;174:815-819.

141. Nicolau C, Gilabert R, García A, et al: Effect of internal carotid artery occlusion on vertebral artery blood flow. J Ultrasound Med 2001;20:105-111.

142. Welch HJ, Murphy MC, Raftery KB, et al: Carotid duplex with contralateral disease: The influence of vertebral artery blood flow. Ann Vasc Surg 2000;14:82-88.

Internal Jugular Vein

143. Williams CE, Lamb GHR, Roberts D, et al: Venous thrombosis in the neck: The role of real-time ultrasound. Eur J Radiol 1989;9:32-36.

144. Hubsch PJ, Stiglbauer RL, Schwaighofer BW, et al: Internal jugular and subclavian vein thrombosis caused by central venous catheters: Evaluation using Doppler blood flow imaging. J Ultrasound Med 1988;7:629-636.

145. Gaitini D, Kaftori JK, Pery M, et al: High-resolution real-time ultrasonography: Diagnosis and follow-up of jugular and subclavian vein thrombosis. J Ultrasound Med 1988;7:621-627.

146. Albertyn LE, Alcock MK: Diagnosis of internal jugular vein thrombosis. Radiology 1987;162:505-508.

147. Falk RL, Smith DF: Thrombosis of upper extremity thoracic inlet veins: Diagnosis with duplex Doppler sonography. AJR 1987;149:677-682.

148. Weissleder R, Elizondo G, Stark DD: Sonographic diagnosis of subclavian and internal jugular vein thrombosis. J Ultrasound Med 1987;6:577-587.

149. De Witte BR, Lameris JS: Real-time ultrasound diagnosis of internal jugular vein thrombosis. J Clin Ultrasound 1986;14:712-717.

150. Wing V, Scheible W: Sonography of jugular vein thrombosis. AJR 1983;140:333-336.

151. Gribbin C, Raghavendra BN, Ginsburg HB: Ultrasound diagnosis of jugular venous ectasia. NY State J Med 1989;9:532-533.

152. Hughes PL, Qureshi SA, Galloway RW: Jugular venous aneurysm in children. Br J Radiol 1988;61:1082-1084.

153. Jasinski RW, Rubin JM: Computed tomography and ultrasonographic findings in jugular vein ectasia. J Ultrasound Med 1984;3:417-420.

154. Stevens RK, Fried AM, Hood TR: Ultrasonic diagnosis of jugular venous aneurysm. J Clin Ultrasound 1982; 10:85-87.

155. Lee W, Leduc L, Cotton DB: Ultrasonographic guidance for central venous access during pregnancy. Am J Obstet Gynecol 1989;161:1012-1013.

156. Bond DM, Nolan R: Real-time ultrasound imaging aids jugular venipuncture. Anesth Analg 1989;68:700-701.

157. Machi J, Takeda J, Kakegawa T: Safe jugular and subclavian venipuncture under ultrasonographic guidance. Am J Surg 1987;153:321-323.

158. Dresser LP, McKinney WM: Anatomic and pathophysiologic studies of the human internal jugular valve. Am J Surg 1987;154:220-224.

159. Patel S, Brennan J: Diagnosis of internal jugular vein thrombosis by computed tomography. J Comput Assist Tomogr 1981;5:197-200.

160. Braun IF, Hoffman JC, Malko JA, et al: Jugular venous thrombosis: Magnetic resonance imaging. Radiology 1985;157:357-360.

28

THE PERIPHERAL ARTERIES

Joseph F. Polak

Chapter Outline

$\mathcal{T}$he arteries of the upper and lower extremities are easily accessible to sonographic imaging. Lying in soft tissues of depths of a few centimeters, these vessels are more consistently imaged than the abdominal and thoracic vessels. There are enough imaging windows available so that the transducer can be placed over the artery of interest without the presence of overlying bone. Transducers with imaging frequencies above 5 MHz can normally be used because the arteries lie in close proximity to the skin, typically at depths of 6 cm or less.

Real-time gray-scale imaging is useful for evaluating the presence of atherosclerotic plaque or confirming the presence of extravascular masses. Gray-scale imaging is, however, limited (Fig. 28-1). Color Doppler flow imaging makes it possible to rapidly survey the area of interest, to determine whether or not there are vascular structures, and to characterize their blood flow patterns (see Fig. 28-1). The addition of Doppler waveform analysis to gray-scale imaging is called duplex sonography, a powerful diagnostic tool for confirming the importance of atherosclerotic lesions, differentiating significant arterial stenoses from occlusions, and assessing the nature of perivascular masses, differentiating hematoma from pseudoaneurysm. When compared to duplex sonography, color flow imaging can more rapidly survey arterial segments and detect the presence of arterial stenoses and occlusions. Color flow imaging decreases the length of the peripheral arterial examination as compared to gray-scale and spectral Doppler (duplex) sonography alone[1] and improves diagnostic accuracy.[2] As such, the evaluation of the peripheral arteries requires the use of color Doppler images. Power Doppler imaging, a more sensitive derivative of color Doppler imaging, can further improve the diagnostic performance of Doppler sonography in specific clinical situations.

When compared to angiography, the sonographic approaches discussed in this chapter have the advantage of being noninvasive, relatively inexpensive, and well suited for serial examinations. They also permit the evaluation of soft tissue structures contiguous to the arteries. Computed tomographic angiography (CTA) is a more expensive technology than Doppler sonography and requires the administration of contrast material. Improvements in CTA, with the introduction of multidetector devices, have shortened imaging times, improved resolution, and made this imaging technique competitive with arteriography. Magnetic resonance

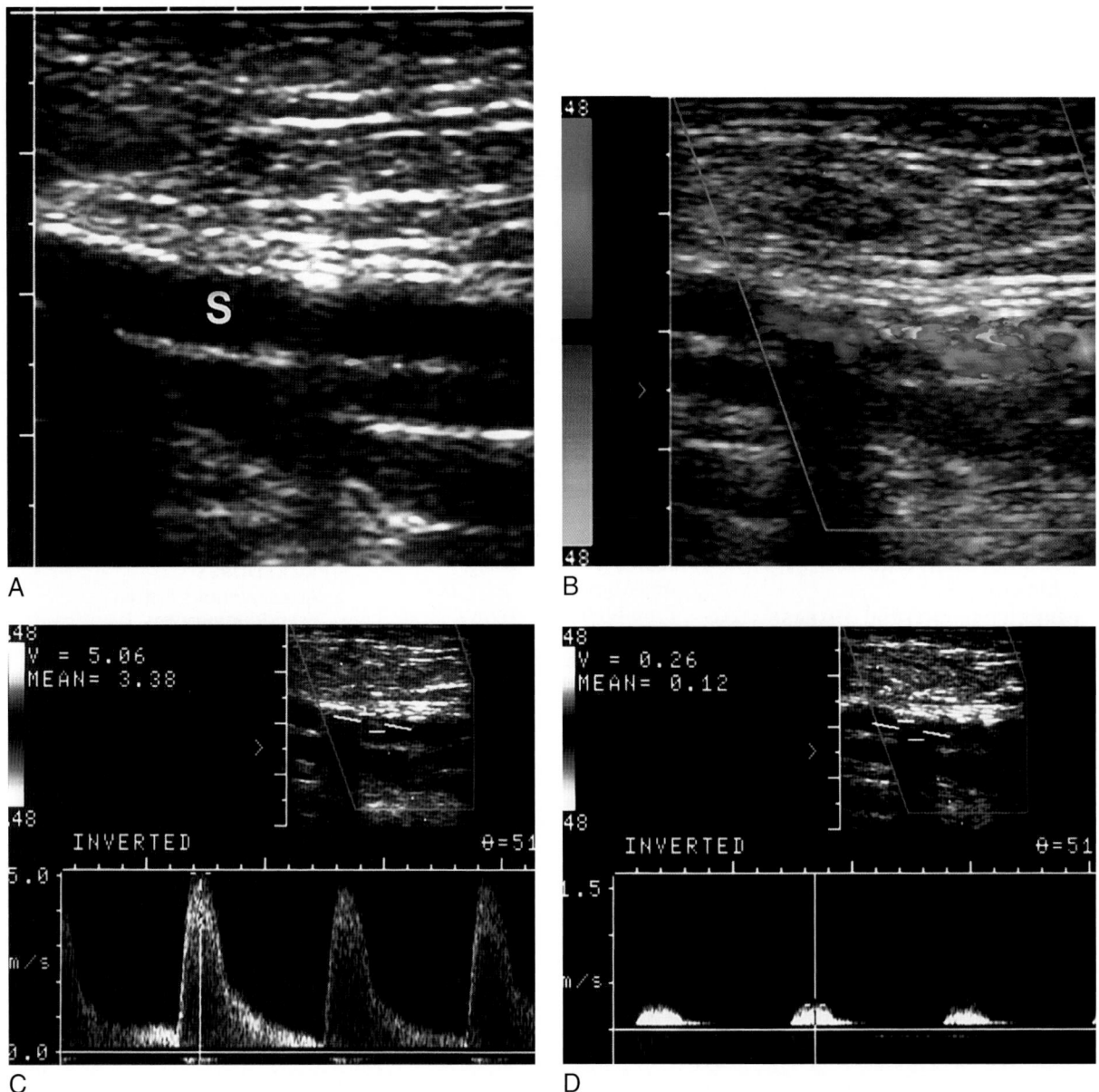

FIGURE 28-1. Comparison of gray-scale and Doppler examinations of arterial stenosis. A, This gray-scale image does not appear to show any significant lesion in the proximal superficial femoral artery (S). **B,** This color flow image shows that the site of stenosis causes an alteration in the color signals from the artery. There is narrowing of the lumen delineated by the color flow signals and aliasing of the color Doppler signals at the site of maximal stenosis. Abnormalities in the color flow signals extend at least 1 cm downstream from the lesion. **C,** Pulsed Doppler sonography shows a marked elevation in the blood flow velocities, indicating a stenosis at the level of a sonolucent lesion not seen on the gray-scale image. **D,** Spectral Doppler image immediately proximal to this site shows dampening of the systolic peak and a high-resistance waveform. The blood flow velocity is decreased to 26 cm/sec. The normal velocities should be approximately 90 to 110 cm/sec in the common femoral arteries.

angiography (MRA) can be used to detect the presence of arterial stenoses and occlusions. Like CTA, MRA can also be used to evaluate the soft tissues for the presence of nonvascular pathologies. However, unlike CTA, this requires additional imaging sequences and increases imaging times. CTA and MRA are less operator dependent than Doppler sonography and, in given clinical situations, more accurate and more reproducible than sonography. Whether MRA and CTA will prove

more cost effective than sonography for evaluating the peripheral arterial system is still under investigation.

INSTRUMENTATION

Real-time Gray-scale Imaging

The diameter of the peripheral arteries that is clinically relevant varies from 1 to 6 mm. Accurate visualization of the arterial wall requires high-resolution transducers, more than 3.5 MHz, in order to visualize different lesions. A broad frequency range of 5 to 10 MHz is preferred because it offers overall good resolution while permitting good depth penetration even in the thigh. For detailed visualization of smaller diameter arteries, higher frequencies of 7 MHz to 12 MHz can be used. At these high frequencies, transducers have poor depth penetration but may be useful for evaluating bypass grafts and the ulnar and radial arteries and smaller arteries of the hand.

The linear phased array transducer is ideal for imaging the extremity arteries. The transducer has sufficient length to permit rapid coverage of long arterial segments by holding it parallel to the artery or graft long axis and by sliding it in a series of nonoverlapping increments. A smaller footprint curved array or sector transducer can be useful for imaging of the iliac arteries and of the more centrally located portions of the subclavian arteries.

Doppler Sonography

Simultaneous display of Doppler spectral information and of the gray-scale image, duplex sonography,[3] is the basic requisite for the evaluation of the peripheral arteries and of arterial bypass grafts. Careful real-time control is needed to position the Doppler sample gate and to accurately detect sites of maximal blood flow velocity in arteries and bypass grafts. The best Doppler transducer frequencies can vary between 3 to 10 MHz, tending to be lower than the simultaneously acquired gray-scale image. Selection of a Doppler transducer frequency of approximately 5 MHz sacrifices some sensitivity for detecting slowly moving blood but decreases the likelihood that the system will alias at sites of rapidly moving blood, such as stenoses or arteriovenous (A-V) fistulas.

Color Doppler imaging is an essential component of a peripheral arterial sonographic examination. The simultaneous display of moving blood superimposed on a gray-scale image[4] makes it possible to rapidly survey the flow patterns within long sections of the peripheral arteries and bypass grafts. In general, an efficient approach to peripheral vascular sonography relies on color flow Doppler sonography to rapidly identify zones of flow disturbances and then on duplex sonography with Doppler spectral analysis to characterize the type of flow abnormality present.[1,5] The color Doppler image displays only the mean frequency shift caused by moving structures. The pixel size (resolution) is also coarser than the corresponding pixel size of gray-scale image. This may cause some ambiguity in alignment of the two separate images and can cause the color Doppler information to overlap beyond the wall of the arteries. Most manufacturers use lower transducer frequencies for the color flow image than for the gray-scale component

of the image. This approach increases the depth penetration of the color flow image without compromising image resolution.

Power Doppler imaging is a variant of color flow imaging that displays a summation of the Doppler signals caused by moving blood. Advantages of power Doppler over color Doppler flow imaging are that the blood flow information does not alias, the signal strengths are much less angle dependent, and slowly moving blood is more easily detected. A disadvantage is the loss of information pertaining to the direction of blood flow, although this option remains in some ultrasound devices.

BLOOD FLOW PATTERNS

Normal Arteries

The normal pattern of arterial blood flow in the extremity is different from that seen in the carotid arteries. At rest, the muscles of the extremities cause a high peripheral (distal) resistance and relatively low diastolic blood flow (Fig. 28-2). The typical blood flow profile is a **triphasic pattern** (Fig. 28-3). This consists of a strong forward component of blood flow during systole, followed by a short reversal of blood flow during early diastole, and then by low-amplitude forward blood flow during diastole. The magnitude of the forward component of blood flow during diastole is variable, disappearing with vasoconstriction due to cold and increasing with warmth or following exercise.

Stenotic Arteries

The high-resistance pattern seen in normal peripheral arteries at rest is transformed into a low-resistance pattern when a significant arterial lesion is located proximal to the artery segment where the Doppler signals are sampled. This low-resistance pattern resembles that of the internal carotid artery. It is thought to reflect the opening of collateral arterial branches and the loss of normal resting arteriolar tone in response to muscle ischemia. It is typically seen distal to an occluded artery segment but can be seen distal to severe stenotic lesion(s).

A localized increase in velocity occurs at the site of a stenosis proper. This increase in blood flow velocity causes a shift in the Doppler frequency sampled at the stenosis. The Doppler frequency shift and increase in estimated blood flow velocity are proportional to the lumen diameter narrowing at the stenosis.[6-8] This can be shown as an increase in the peak systolic velocity on the Doppler spectral display, by an increase in color saturation, or even aliasing on the color Doppler map (see Fig. 28-1). The pattern of blood flow distal to the stenosis is nonlaminar and shows a large variation in both direction and amplitude; this zone of disturbed

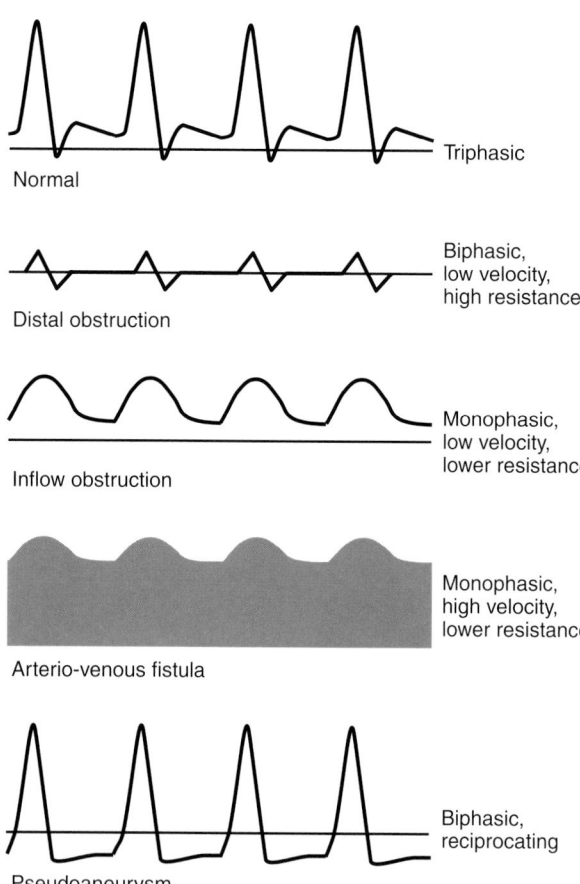

Normal — Triphasic

Distal obstruction — Biphasic, low velocity, high resistance

Inflow obstruction — Monophasic, low velocity, lower resistance

Arterio-venous fistula — Monophasic, high velocity, lower resistance

Pseudoaneurysm — Biphasic, reciprocating

FIGURE 28-2. Normal and abnormal Doppler arterial waveforms. The normal Doppler spectrum of flowing blood in the lower extremity arteries typically has a triphasic pattern: (1) forward flow during systole; (2) a short period of flow reversal in early diastole; and (3) a variable amplitude of low velocity blood flow during the remainder of diastole. Arterial Doppler signals are altered depending on the pathologic change. The four other patterns are examples of common arterial pathologies.

flow is maintained over a distance of slightly more than one centimeter (see Fig. 28-1). In certain cases, the zone of blood flow disturbance can be very small. This zone of disturbed blood flow is captured by the Doppler waveform as a broadening of the spectral window and by color Doppler imaging as increased variance of the color Doppler signals in the vessel.

Arteriovenous Fistulas

Arteriovenous fistulas can either be **congenital or iatrogenic.** Congenital A-V fistulas occur in various forms: abnormal communications between arteries and large distended venous channels or primary venous anomalies. The abnormalities more easily identified with Doppler ultrasound are usually quite obvious clinically and tend to be located close to the skin surface of the involved extremity. These are normally visualized as distended venous channels into which feed single or multiple arterial branches. Smaller, nondistended veins that are not dilated may still contain increased blood flow signals due to the fistula.

Iatrogenic communications often arise following selective arterial or venous catheterization or other forms of penetrating trauma. The communication can be visualized as a jet of blood, with the involved vein being distended when compared to the other side (Fig. 28-4). Blood flow signals in the recipient vein also show an arterial-like appearance, and the feeding artery can have increased diastolic blood flow (see Fig. 28-4). The jet of blood has high velocity signals and, on impact against the opposite vein wall, can cause a perivascular vibration that can be seen as an artifact on color Doppler imaging.[9] An important differential diagnosis is compression of a

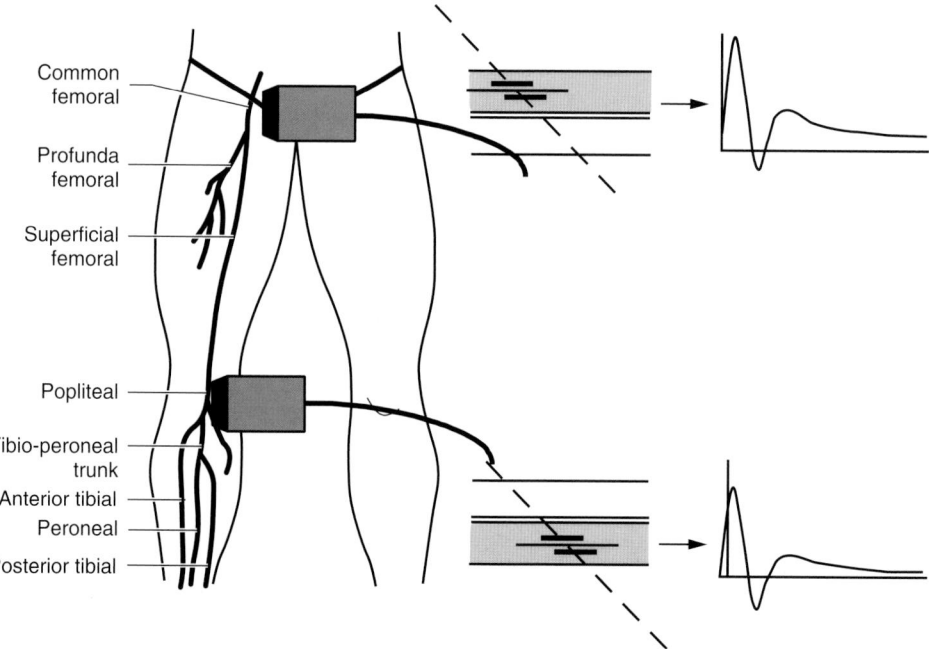

FIGURE 28-3. Normal arterial waveforms. Doppler waveforms at the common femoral and popliteal arteries show triphasic patterns.

Common femoral
Profunda femoral
Superficial femoral
Popliteal
Tibio-peroneal trunk
Anterior tibial
Peroneal
Posterior tibial

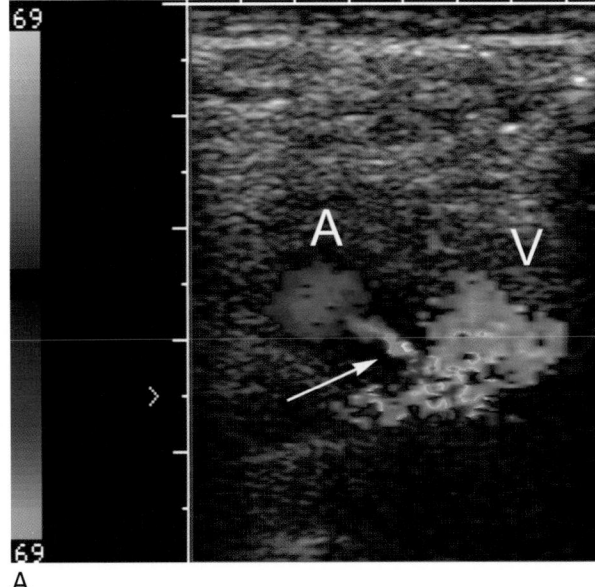

A

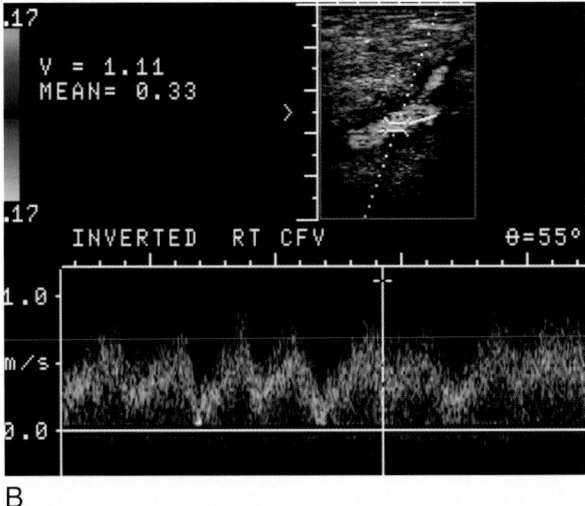

B

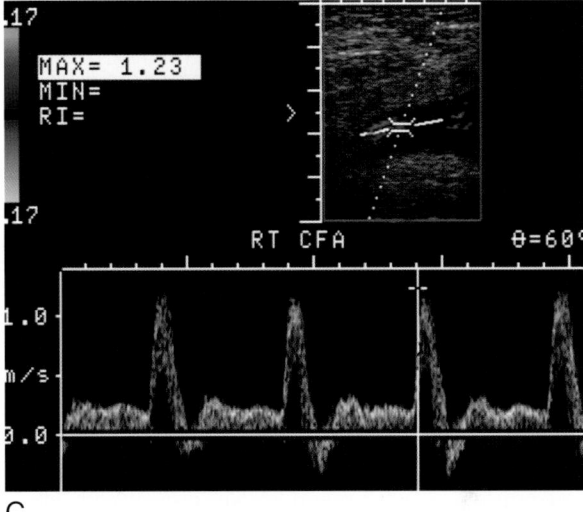

C

FIGURE 28-4. Arteriovenous (A-V) fistula of femoral vessels following angiogram. A, This color flow image shows a high velocity jet (*arrow*) from the common femoral artery (A) into the distended common femoral vein (V). **B**, The arterial type signals sampled in the common femoral vein are consistent with an A-V fistula. **C**, The CFA sampled above the fistula shows a relative increase in blood flow during diastole, and this is indirect evidence of the fistula located downstream. CFA, common femoral artery.

vein by a hematoma. Compression of the vein causes a stenosis that increases blood flow velocity signals in the vein and mimics the high-velocity signals of a fistula (Fig. 28-5).

Masses

The differential diagnosis of perivascular masses is facilitated by the use of color flow imaging, with some diagnostic specificity being offered by Doppler waveform analysis. Blood flow signals within a mass contiguous to an artery suggest the diagnosis of **pseudoaneurysm**, which is a complication that sometimes develops following arterial catheterization or penetrating trauma. The communication tends to have a wide neck if the aneurysm arises at the anastomosis of a synthetic or autologous vein graft.[10] With an iatrogenic pseudoaneurysm of the native artery, a small diameter channel communicates to a larger contained collection of blood. Color Doppler imaging shows blood flow signals in the pseudoaneurysm

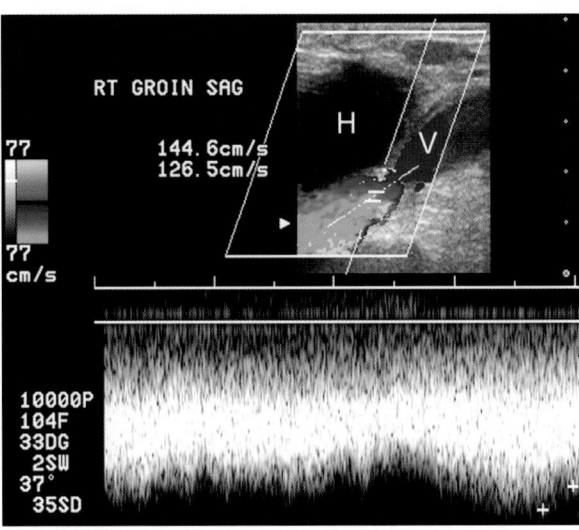

FIGURE 28-5. Hematoma compresses common femoral vein. Extrinsic compression of the common femoral vein (V), a large hematoma (H) causes an increase in blood flow velocity.

cavity. A typical swirling motion or color "yin-yang" sign is typically seen within the collection itself.[11,12] The Doppler waveform sampled in the communicating neck has a very typical appearance: the channel contains a backward-forward or a **to-and-fro blood flow pattern.**[13] The to-and-fro pattern of blood flow shows rapid inflow into the cavity in systole and a slower, lower amplitude exit of blood during diastole (Fig. 28-6).

Hyperplastic or malignant lymph nodes (Fig. 28-7) can show both venous and arterial signals radiating from the hilum of the node. These nodes can be mistaken for pseudoaneurysms.[14,15] Points to consider in the differential diagnosis are detection of arterial and venous signals where the communicating channel should be and the absence of a to-and-fro pattern of blood flow. **Arterial aneurysms** are easily recognized by their typical location within the confines of the arterial wall. Although fusiform aneurysms obey this rule, it may be quite difficult to differentiate a saccular aneurysm from a pseudoaneurysm.[16]

PERIPHERAL ARTERIAL DISEASE

Incidence and Clinical Importance

Peripheral vascular disease is at least as prevalent as coronary artery disease or cerebrovascular disease.[17] Atherosclerosis is a generalized process, wherein the clinical presentation and the development of symptoms depend on the arterial bed and the target organ. Patients with coronary artery disease and carotid artery disease can present in a catastrophic and very noticeable fashion as myocardial infarction and stroke, respectively. This is very different from peripheral arterial disease. Many patients suffer for years from peripheral arterial disease before seeking medical assistance.[18] This is a reflection of the development of collateral arterial channels bypassing the diseased arterial segment as it progressively narrows. The collaterals are often sufficient to maintain perfusion to the lower extremity. The balance between blood supply and oxygen demand is maintained as long as the patient does not exercise or ambulate too vigorously. In general, these patients can go on for years, decreasing their levels of activity as their disease progresses. Disabling claudication is, therefore, more likely to be a presenting symptom in the younger patient with high levels of daily activity.

The patient may also seek medical assistance because of the development of chronic changes of arterial insufficiency and poor wound healing. Acute embolic events originating from a more proximal arterial lesion, either from ulcerated plaques or popliteal aneurysms, can cause acute ischemia, extensive tissue loss, and lead to amputation unless an intervention is performed.

The widespread use of arterial bypass operations has modified the natural history of peripheral arterial disease. The high patency rates of both arterial bypass surgery and similar patency rates for angioplasty have made it possible for patients who would previously have had amputations to remain asymptomatic[19,20] until other causes of mortality intercede. Acute cardiovascular events, myocardial infarction, or sudden death are common causes of mortality in these patients who already have generalized atherosclerosis.

Gray-scale and spectral Doppler (duplex) sonography is well accepted as the primary noninvasive modality for detecting evidence of lower extremity bypass graft dysfunction. It can also be used to evaluate the success of peripheral angioplasty, atherectomy, and stent placement.[21-24] Doppler imaging of the leg arteries to determine the extent and nature of arterial lesions has become practical with the aid of color Doppler flow imaging. Although duplex sonography can be used to determine the presence of significant arterial lesions, the task of evaluating the whole leg is labor and time intensive. It takes 30 to 60 minutes to map the arterial tree of each leg using Duplex ultrasound.[25] With color Doppler mapping, this task can be accomplished in 15 to 20 minutes.[1] Color Doppler imaging also improves the accuracy of Doppler ultrasound as a diagnostic test for detecting and grading the severity of arterial disease.[2,23]

Lower Extremity

Normal Anatomy and Doppler Flow Patterns. The deep arteries of the leg travel with an accompanying vein. The **common femoral artery** starts at the level of the inguinal ligament and continues for 4 to 6 cm until it branches into the **superficial and deep femoral arteries** (profunda femoris) (see Fig. 28-3). The deep femoral artery quickly branches to supply the region of the femoral head and the deep muscles of the thigh. With peripheral arterial disease, collateral pathways often form between this deep femoral artery and the lower portions of the superficial femoral or the popliteal arteries. The superficial femoral artery continues along the medial aspect of the thigh at a depth of 4 to 8 cm until it reaches the adductor canal. At the boundary of the adductor canal, the superficial femoral artery continues as the **popliteal artery**. The popliteal artery crosses posterior to the knee, sending off small geniculate branches and terminating as two major branches: the **anterior tibial artery** and the **tibioperoneal trunk**. The anterior tibial artery courses in the anterior compartment of the lower leg after crossing through the interosseous membrane. It finally crosses the ankle joint as the **dorsalis pedis artery**. The tibioperoneal trunk gives rise to the **posterior tibial** and the **peroneal arteries** that supply the calf muscles. The posterior tibial artery is more superficial than the peroneal artery and can be followed down to its typical location behind the medial malleolus.

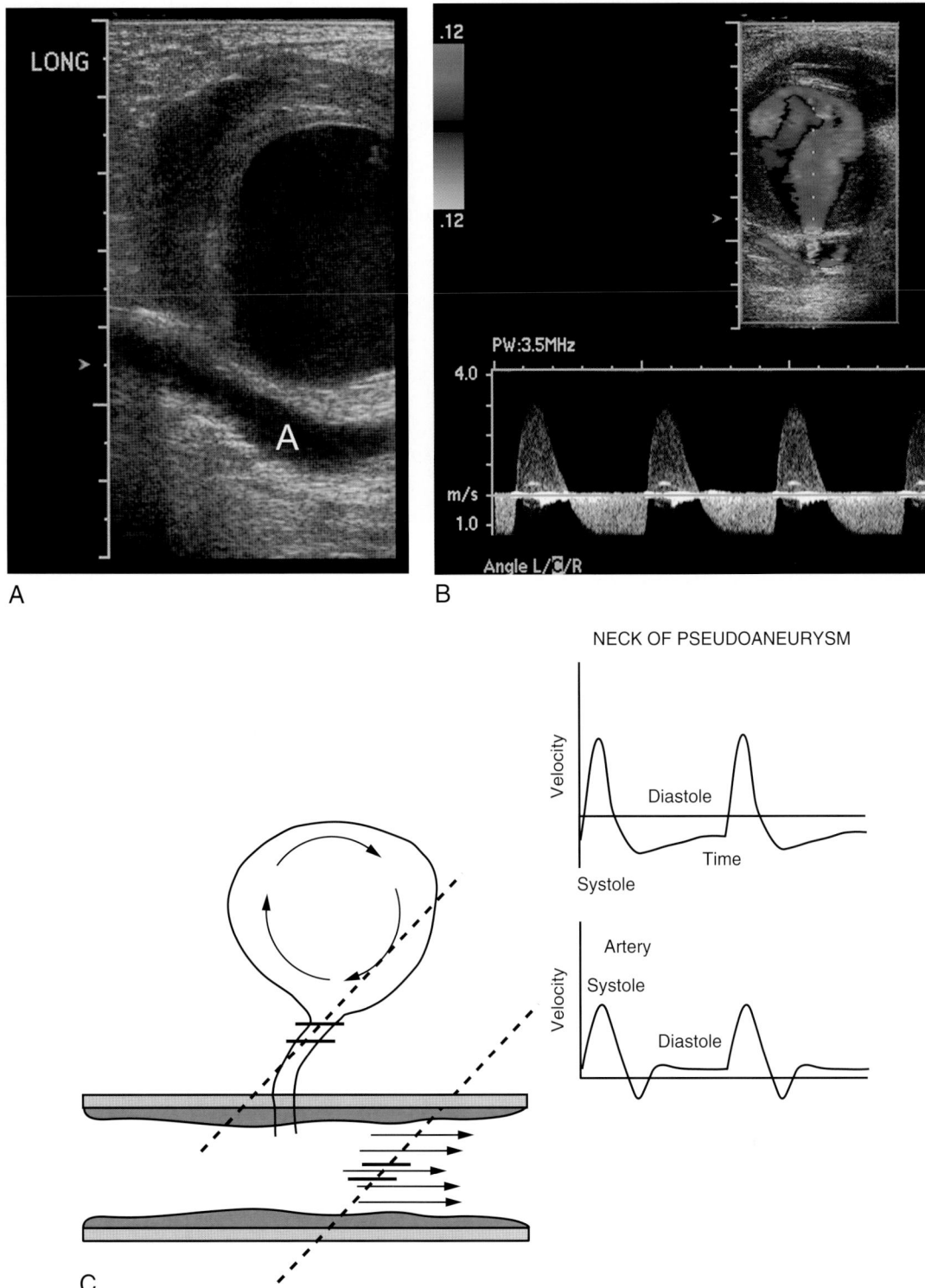

FIGURE 28-6. Femoral artery pseudoaneurysm. A, Longitudinal image of the common femoral artery (A) shows a large perivascular fluid collection. **B,** Color Doppler image shows the yin-yang pattern caused by the swirling of blood in the pseudoaneurysm cavity. Note the thin neck of communication between artery and the perivascular collection. The spectral tracing shows the classic to-and-fro waveform of a pseudoaneurysm. **C,** Diagram showing blood flow as it enters the pseudoaneurysm during systole (to) when blood pressure is higher in the artery than in the cavity. Blood exits during diastole (fro) because the (pressure) energy that has been stored in the soft tissues surrounding the collection is now greater than diastolic pressure.

Continued

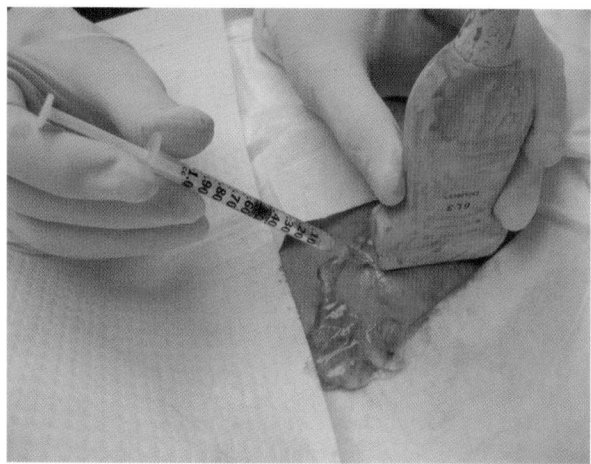

D

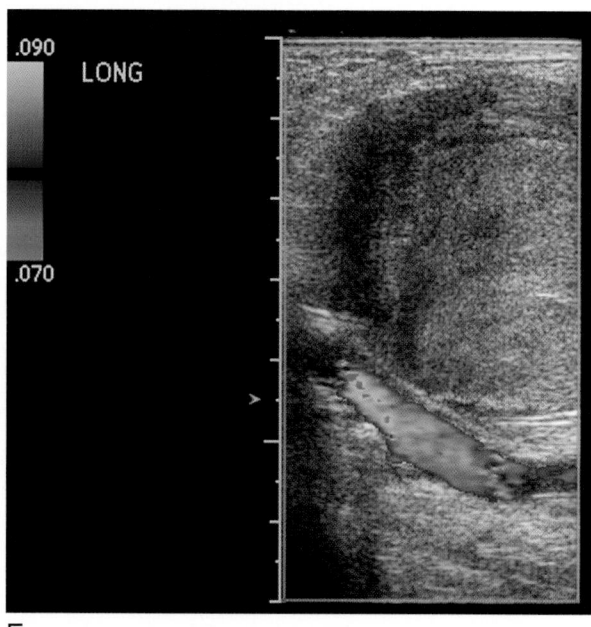

E

FIGURE 28-6, *cont'd*. Femoral artery pseudoaneurysm. D, Ultrasound-guided injection of thrombin to thrombose pseudoaneurysm. A 25 gauge needle is attached to the 1 mL syringe containing the thrombin. **E,** Longitudinal color Doppler image 2 minutes after the injection of thrombin shows that the lumen of the pseudoaneurysm has filled with echoes representing clot and there is no blood flow within it on Doppler examination.

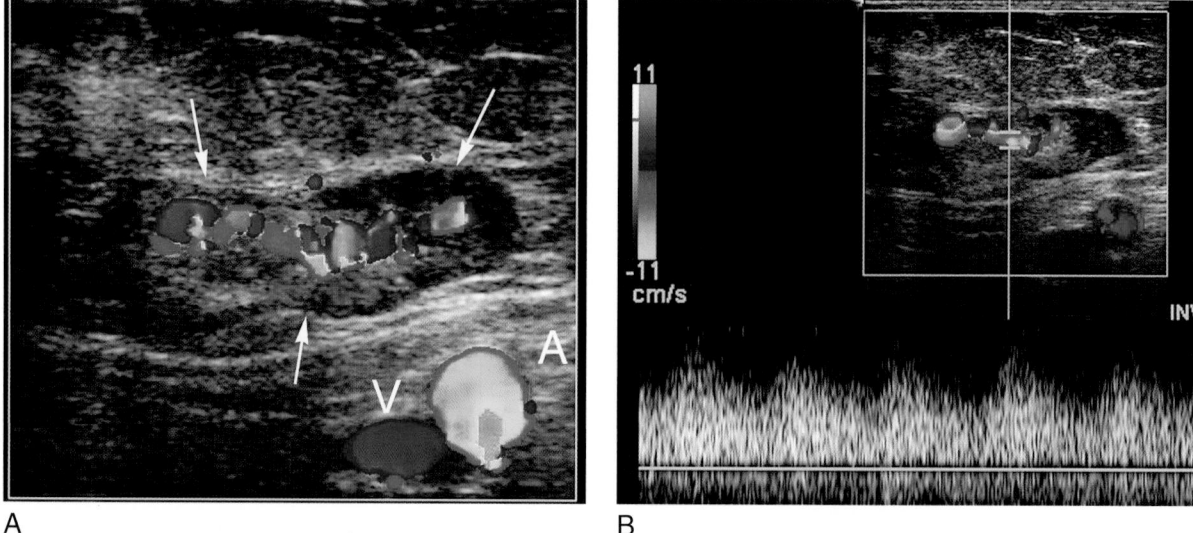

A

B

FIGURE 28-7. Groin lymph node with Doppler signal. A, Color Doppler signals in the soft tissues of the groin are complex. Careful examination shows that these signals are from the center of a structure that is a hyperplastic lymph node (*arrows*) (A, femoral artery; V, femoral vein). **B,** Doppler waveforms from the center of this mass confirm the presence of a mainly arterial waveform and not the to-and-fro of a pseudoaneurysm.

The blood flow pattern in all of these branches is triphasic (see Fig. 28-2). There is an early systolic acceleration in velocity, followed by a brief period of low-amplitude flow reversal before returning to antegrade diastolic flow of low velocity. This pattern can be more pulsatile in the deep femoral (profunda femoris) artery. Peak-systolic velocities vary with the level of the artery, typically at 100 cm/sec at the common femoral artery down to 70 cm/sec at the popliteal artery. The tibioperoneal arteries have peak-systolic velocities of 40 to 50 cm/sec. The response to either **exercise** or **transient ischemia** is a loss of the triphasic pattern and the development of a monophasic pattern with antegrade blood flow with loss of early diastolic blood flow reversal (Fig. 28-8). Although a **monophasic pattern** can be seen in lower extremity disease or following exercise,

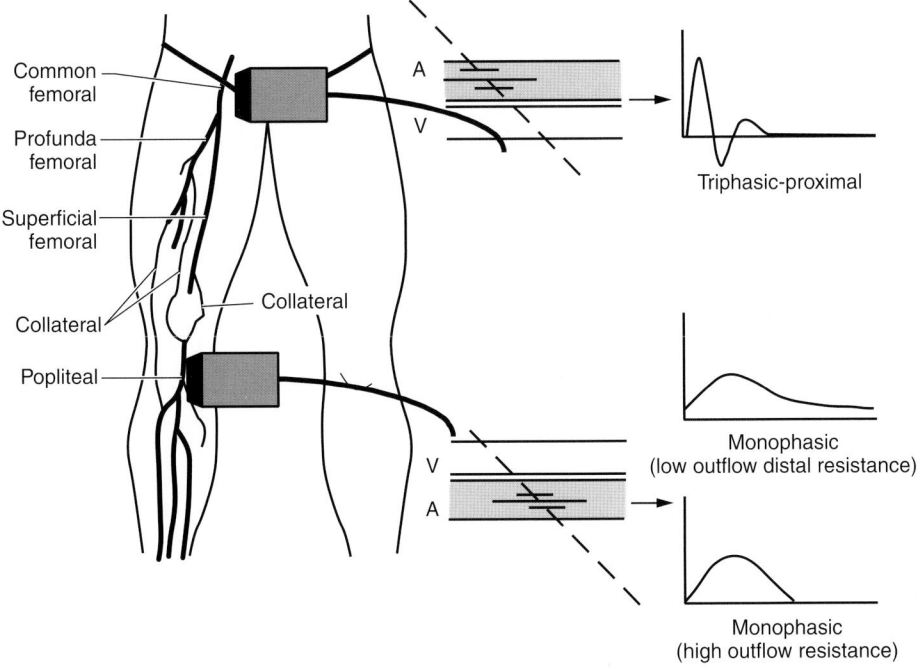

FIGURE 28-8. Significant arterial disease alters the Doppler waveform sampled distal to the lesion. Sampling is taking place distal to an occlusion. The Doppler waveform sampled proximal to a high-grade stenosis may be normal or can show loss of the early and then late components of diastolic flow. The distal waveform is monophasic, most often with a relatively strong diastolic component to the waveform.

peak systolic velocity will be decreased in the ischemic limb of a patient with arterial disease, whereas it is increased in a healthy individual following exercise.

Aneurysms: Diagnostic Criteria. Aneurysms develop as the structural integrity of the arterial wall weakens. A bulge or **focal enlargement of 20%** of the expected vessel diameter constitutes a simple functional definition of an aneurysm. Focal enlargement of the artery is more likely to occur at the level of the popliteal or distal superficial femoral artery (Fig. 28-9). They are often bilateral and can remain asymptomatic for long periods of time. Ultrasound imaging has become a standard in itself for confirming this suspected diagnosis.[26,27] Although ultrasound can visualize the progressive thrombosis that fills in the aneurysm lumen to the level of the dilated wall, the lumen can appear normal at angiography. Ultrasound can be used to follow these aneurysms, as is done for abdominal aneurysm. There are unfortunately no strict size criteria that can be used to determine the suitability for operation. Empirically, a peripheral artery aneurysm of 2 cm or greater usually requires surgical repair.[28] The development of symptoms suggestive of distal embolization by the thrombus accumulating in the lumen is an absolute indication for surgical intervention, regardless of the size of the aneurysm.[28] Aneurysms will typically occlude with time due to accumulating thrombus (see Fig. 28-9). Doppler techniques are useful in confirming the continued patency or occlusion of the lumen within the aneurysm.

Aneurysms: Diagnostic Accuracy. Direct pathologic verification of aneurysms diagnosed by ultrasound has shown that the technique is sensitive and specific and, furthermore, superior to contrast angiography. The accu-

racy of Doppler techniques for confirming patency or occlusion of the lumen at the level of the aneurysm has yet to be reported, but it is accepted as a standard.

Stenosis and Occlusions: Diagnostic Criteria. The effects of peripheral arterial lesions are detectable by a change in the blood flow pattern seen on the arterial Doppler waveform (Table 28-1). At the lesion, peak systolic velocity increases (Figs. 28-1 and 28-10), and early diastolic velocity reversal disappears. Distal to a moderately severe arterial lesion, the early diastolic blood flow reversal decreases and ultimately disappears as the lesion becomes more severe, and peak-systolic blood flow velocity decreases. The diastolic portion of the waveform increases in significance with respect to the decreasing peak systolic blood flow. On occasion, a high-resistance, monophasic pattern with absent diastolic blood flow can be seen, probably due to peripheral vasoconstriction (Fig. 28-11). The low-resistance pattern distal to the lesion is accentuated as the severity of the lesion increases. With severe lesions, the blood flow pattern is mainly that of forward flow with an end-diastolic velocity approaching in amplitude the severely depressed peak systolic velocity. One explanation for the development of this pattern is progressive dilation of the arterioles within the distant vascular bed due to the release of metabolites caused by local ischemia. Another is the development of many small collateral branches that diminish the effective resistance of the distal arterial bed. This pattern is present in most cases of severe-enough proximal lesions but may not be seen when sampling within an artery segment proximal to tandem lesions, such as distal high-grade focal lesions or occlusions. Signals in the artery proximal to a high-grade

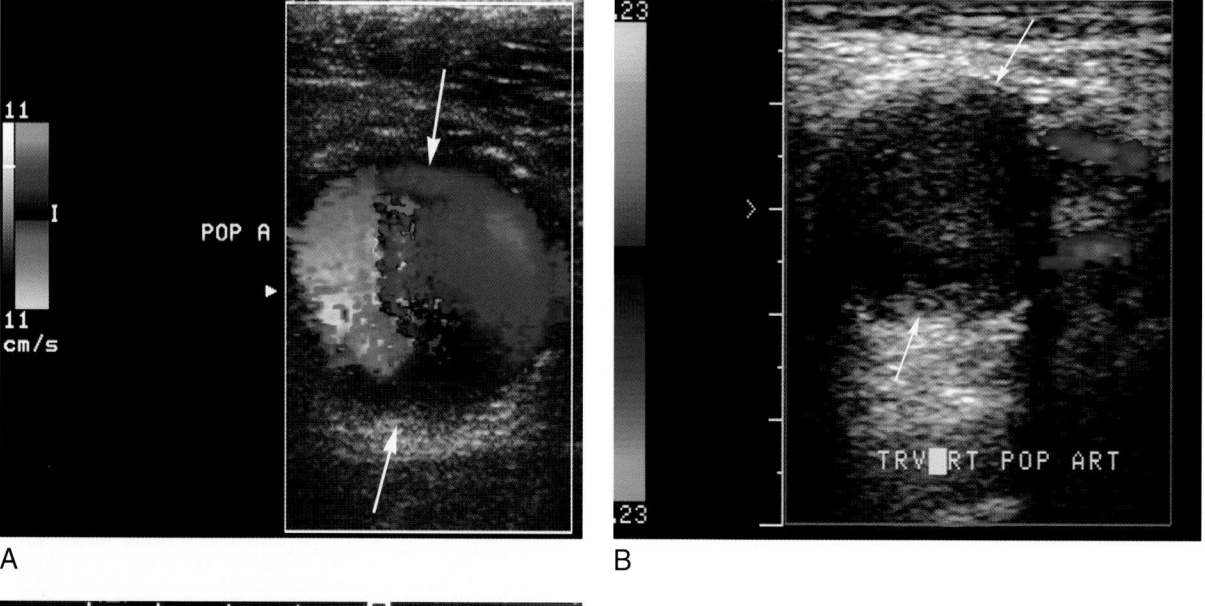

A

B

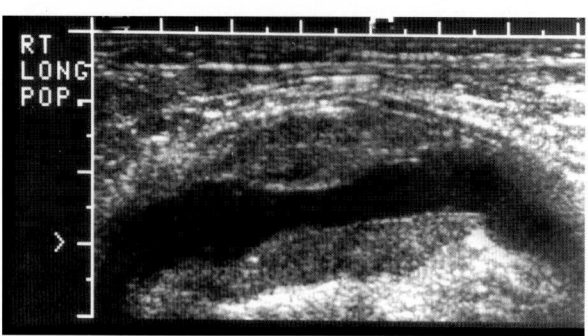

C

FIGURE 28-9. Popliteal artery aneurysm. A, Transverse image of the popliteal space demonstrates a large aneurysm (*arrows*) with swirling blood flow pattern. **B,** Transverse image of the popliteal space of another patient shows a thrombosed popliteal artery (*arrows*), displacing the contiguous duplicated popliteal veins. **C,** Longitudinal gray-scale image of a different patient shows a fusiform aneurysm with a large amount of thrombus seen in the anterior and posterior walls.

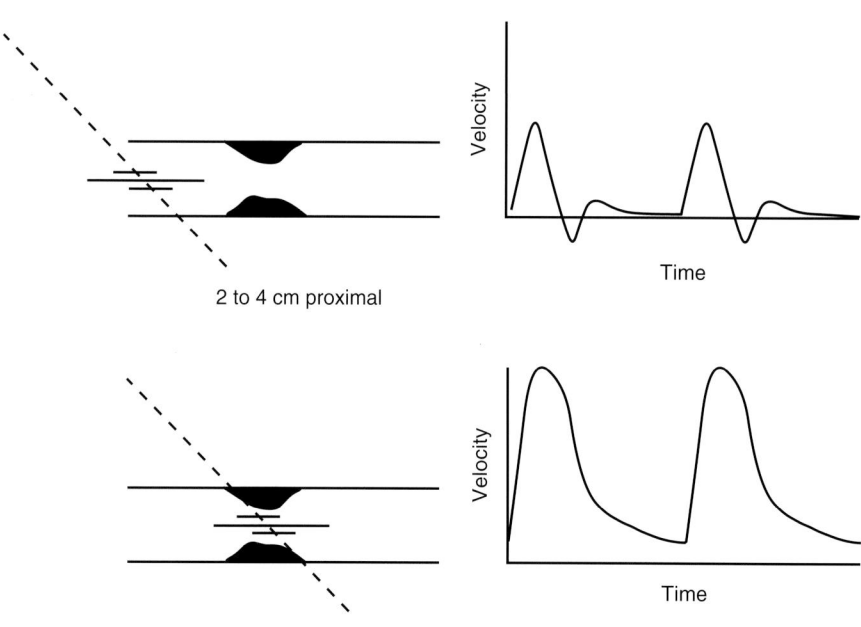

2 to 4 cm proximal

At the stenosis

FIGURE 28-10. Blood flow velocity alterations occur with stenosis of at least 50%. Proximal to the lesion, the flow pattern is normal. At the stenosis, the peak systolic velocity increases in proportion to the degree of stenosis. Alterations in the diastolic portion of the Doppler waveform sampled at the lesion are dependent on the state of the distal arteries and on lesion severity and geometry: diastolic flow may increase dramatically or be almost absent.

TABLE 28-1. STENOSIS DETECTION AND CHARACTERIZATION: FINDINGS AND CORRELATES

Findings	Correlates
Increased peak-systolic velocity >200 cm/sec	Stenosis of at least 50% diameter; near 50% in the proximal femoral artery but closer to 75% in the popliteal arteries
Increased peak-systolic velocity ratio (2 or more)	Normalize to closest arterial segment (stenosis of 50% or more)
Decreased peak-systolic velocity with biphasic (high resistance) or monophasic (high resistance) pattern	Sampling just proximal to high-grade stenosis or occlusion
Absent flow signals (false positive for occlusion, false negative for stenosis)	Calcification
	Poor penetration and poor sensitivity of Doppler
	Sub-total occlusion
Increased flow signals (false positive for stenosis)	Popliteal artery, source not clear but may be due to extrinsic compression
	Kinks
	Sampling in collateral

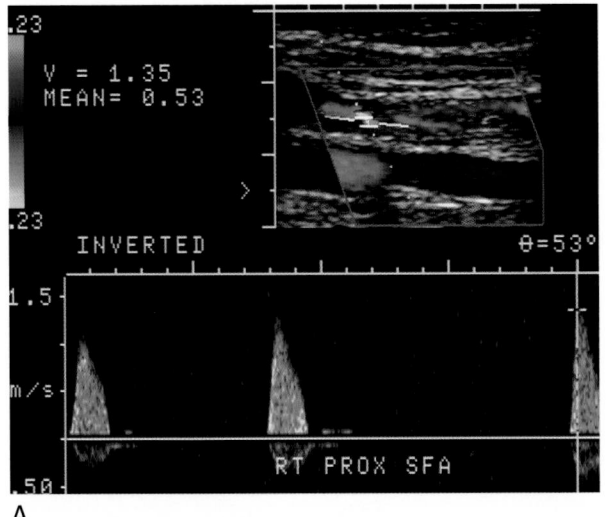

A

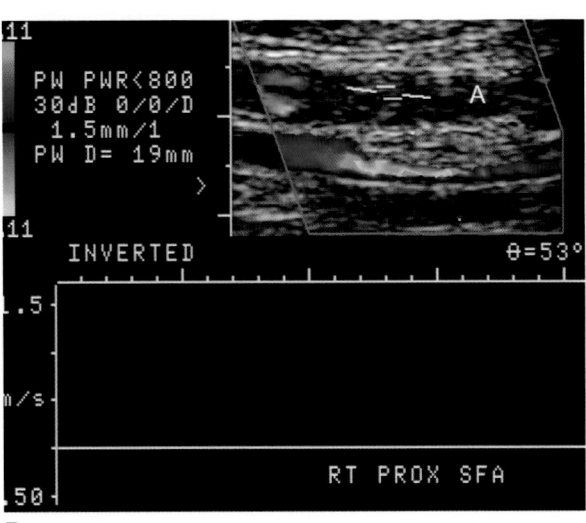

B

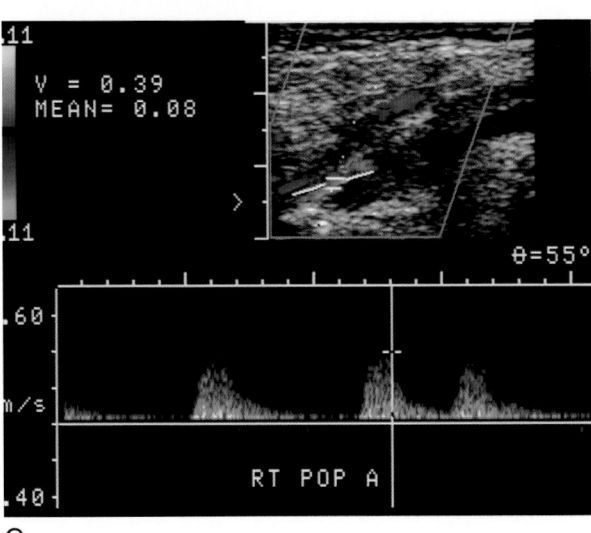

C

FIGURE 28-11. Doppler waveforms above, at, and below occlusion of superficial femoral artery (SFA). **A,** This color flow image shows aliasing of color flow signals in the proximal SFA at point of severe stenosis. Distal to this, there is loss of signal in the artery due to occlusion. Flow is present in area of stenosis due to collateral vessels not seen in this image. **B,** The Doppler waveform sampled more distally confirms the absence of blood flow signals, indicating occlusion of the SFA (A). **C,** Downstream from the SFA occlusion, the popliteal artery signals are monophasic. Diastolic blood flow is low, probably due to peripheral vasoconstriction. There is blood flow in this popliteal artery due to collateral blood supply not shown on this image.

lesion can show a high-resistance pattern (see Fig. 28-11). With absent collaterals, forward blood flow can sometimes be maintained only during systole. A slow rise, low amplitude, low-resistance pattern seen distal to segmental occlusions is called the **tardus-parvus waveform.** Although seen in most arterial segments distal to occlusions, the low-resistance blood flow pattern can be absent when there is peripheral vasoconstriction (Table 28-2 and see Fig. 28-11).

Focal areas where the measured peak systolic velocity more than doubles from a contiguous and normal segment have been shown to correspond to lesions of **greater than 50% narrowing** in the lumen diameter of the artery.[29] The velocity measured at the stenosis is divided by the velocity measured proximal to the stenosis. Because the peak-systolic velocity is less sensitive to the effects of vasodilation or vasoconstriction, it is the preferred Doppler velocity parameter used to grade the severity of lower extremity arterial stenoses. It is possible to use end-diastolic velocities (for example, 80 cm/sec or more) or peak-systolic velocities (>200 and >300 cm/sec) as indicators of stenosis severity. However, end-diastolic velocity estimates are more variable than peak-systolic measurements because they change as a function of peripheral vasodilation.

Stenoses and Occlusions: Diagnostic Accuracy and Applications. The original paper by Kohler et al. reported that Doppler sonography had a diagnostic sensitivity of 82% and a specificity of 92% for detecting segmental arterial lesions of the femoropopliteal arteries.[25] These authors did, however, remark on the fact that selective sampling had to be performed along the full course of the femoral and popliteal arteries.

Because these segments normally measure 30 to 40 cm, it is not surprising that such a survey took from 1 to 2 hours to perform, especially if the iliac arteries were to be evaluated.

Color Doppler sonography has been shown to reduce the time needed to examine the carotid artery for sites of suspected stenosis by 40% when compared to spectral Doppler alone.[5] A similar effect has been shown when color Doppler imaging is used to detect lower extremity arterial lesions. The diagnostic accuracy of the examination is also improved with color Doppler imaging as compared to duplex sonography.[2,30] With color-assisted Doppler sonography, the examination time is reduced to 30 minutes.[1] Many authors have reported on the accuracy of color flow imaging of the peripheral arteries. Accuracy is close to 98% for distinguishing occlusions from nonoccluded segments. Accuracy for the detection of stenoses is better than 85% for the femoropopliteal arteries,[1,31-33] with a few groups including an evaluation of the iliac arteries[25,30,31] and run-off arteries.[34] The evaluation of the run-off arteries is not as accurate as for the femoropopliteal system, especially for the peroneal artery.[35,36] However, selection of possible segments of the tibial arteries that might be suitable as the distal anastomosis of bypass grafts is possible.[37,38] It is possible to forgo other forms of imaging and rely exclusively on Doppler ultrasound before lower extremity bypass grafting.[39,40]

Color Doppler imaging has been shown to be effective in triaging patients with symptoms of lower extremity arterial disease and to decrease the need for diagnostic arteriography in more than one half of patients presenting for clinical evaluation.[41] Doppler sonography can also be used to triage patients likely to need peripheral

---

TABLE 28-2. ARTERIAL OCCLUSIONS: FINDINGS AND CORRELATES

Findings	Correlates
Absence of color Doppler or pulsed Doppler signals	Absence of flow
Echogenic material in artery	Thrombosis associated with occlusion; thrombus typically extends between two largest contiguous collaterals
Large collateral branches seen during color flow imaging	Indicate high likelihood of more distal occlusion or high-grade stenosis
Low amplitude and persistent antegrade flow during systole and diastole	Sampling site is likely distal to occlusion or high-grade stenosis
Low amplitude systolic signals in occluded segment (false negative)	Signals due to motion of thrombus in occluded segment
Flow signals detected at level of occlusion (false negative)	Inadvertent sampling of collateral branch parallel to occluded segment
Failure to detect signals in patent arterial segment (false positive)	Poor sensitivity of Doppler either due to depth or poor adjustment
	Calcification
	Subtotal occlusion with flow diverted away from the stenosis by collaterals

angioplasty and, therefore, better manage more expensive imaging resources such as arteriography.[23,42-44] There are no large studies comparing the efficacy of color Doppler imaging to other technologies, such as magnetic resonance angiography or computed tomographic angiography.

Color Doppler imaging and duplex sonography are extremely well suited for the evaluation of sites having undergone percutaneous interventions, such as angioplasty, atherectomy, or stent placement (Fig. 28-12). An original report indicated that one measurement, made a few days after angioplasty, was predictive of lesion recurrence.[45] Subsequent studies have failed to confirm this observation,[46,47] but they have shown that Doppler sonography can be used to detect recurrence of stenosis or occlusion at the site of a previous intervention. For example, the results following atherectomy have shown a higher incidence of reocclusion than indicated by patients' symptoms,[48] that atherectomy was not as efficient as angioplasty, and that lesion recurrences were higher following atherectomy.[48] There are questions as to whether repeat imaging at the site of previous intervention is needed because a repeat intervention might not be done if the patient remains asymptomatic.[49] It does appear, however, that serial monitoring of sites of angioplasty and stent placement can predict technical success and lesion recurrence.[50,51] There are no data to indicate a benefit of reintervention at the site of lesions detected by Doppler sonography.[22]

Upper Extremity

Normal Anatomy and Doppler Flow Patterns. The arteries of the upper extremity are accompanied by veins: typically, only one vein at the level of the subclavian vein, occasionally duplicated at the level of the axillary

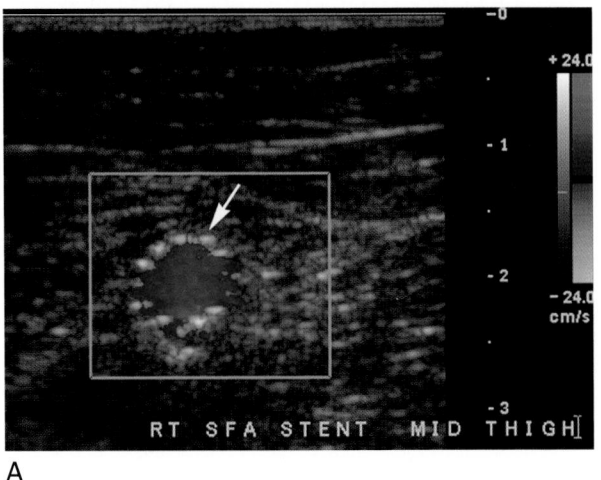

A

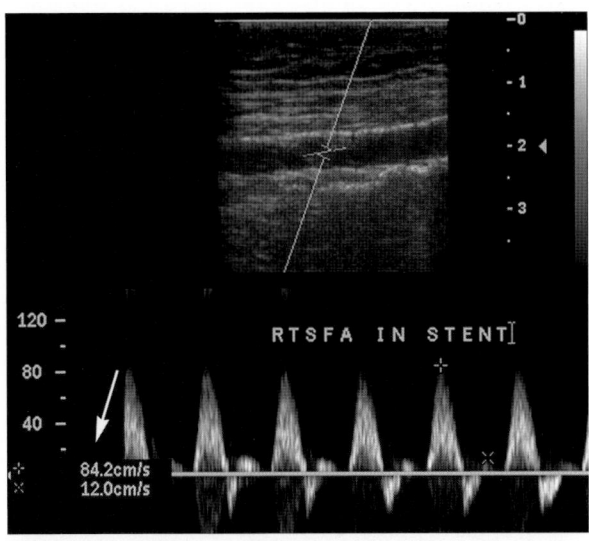

B

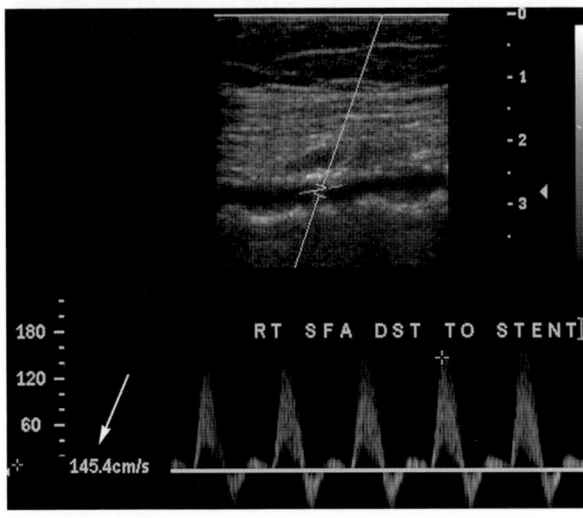

C

FIGURE 28-12. Arterial stent. A, Transverse image of an indwelling stent seen as bright echoes (*arrow*) in the wall of the mid-superficial femoral artery. **B,** The Doppler waveform in the stent is within normal limits at 84 cm/sec (*arrow*). **C,** Distal to the stent, the blood flow velocities are mildly elevated at 145 cm/sec (*arrow*).

veins, always duplicated at the level of the brachial veins and more distally. The junction of the **subclavian artery** with either the **right brachiocephalic** (innominate) or the **left brachiocephalic artery** can be identified using an imaging window superior to the sternoclavicular joint. The artery is located superficial to the vein when the transducer is placed in the supraclavicular fossa. Near the junction of the mid- and proximal third of the clavicle, it is necessary to use a window with the transducer placed on the chest, below the clavicle. The artery now lies deep to the subclavian vein. The origin of the **axillary artery** is lateral to the first rib, normally near the junction of the cephalic and the axillary vein. The axillary artery can be followed as it courses medially over the proximal humerus where it becomes the **brachial artery**. In most subjects, the artery can be followed to the antecubital fossa where it trifurcates into the radial, ulnar, and interosseous branches. The **radial and ulnar arteries** can normally be imaged to the level of the wrist. It is also possible to visualize the smaller digital branches. The normal flow pattern is triphasic and similar to the pattern seen in the leg.

Pathophysiology and Diagnostic Accuracy. Most clinical interest in the noninvasive evaluation of the upper extremity arterial branches is directed to the confirmation of pseudoaneurysms, the detection of focal stenosis due to the thoracic outlet syndrome, the confirmation of native arterial occlusion secondary to emboli or trauma (Fig. 28-13), the detection of complications following cardiac catheterization, the evaluation of dialysis shunts, and preoperative evaluation of the radial artery patency.

There are few reports of subjects with **thoracic outlet syndrome** in the literature. It is possible to induce stenosis in the artery by positioning the arm in the orientation that normally elicits symptoms, most often with the arm abducted. There is an association between the thoracic outlet syndrome and distal arterial embolization. The mechanism is thought to be due to mechanical forces predisposing the artery to develop an aneurysm. Thrombus then forms in the aneurysm and can embolize into the digital arteries. The extent of these acute or chronic occlusions must be mapped to assess the feasibility of possible bypass surgery before subjecting the patient to angiography. Proximal stenoses and occlusions associated with vasculitis can also be confirmed. Following cardiac catheterization, suspected occlusions can be rapidly confirmed. Large hematomas can be readily evaluated, and the possibility of underlying pseudoaneurysms due to jeopardized arteriotomy sutures can be confirmed or excluded.

The radial artery is occasionally used as an access site for cardiac catheterization. **Pseudoaneurysms** (Fig. 28-14) can develop following cardiac catheterization.[52] The radial artery can also be harvested and serve as a donor conduit for coronary bypass surgery. Confirmation of the integrity of the palmar arch of the hand (dominant ulnar artery) is a prerequisite before harvest of the radial artery. This can be tested with Doppler ultrasound, imaging of the distal radial artery, and confirming reversal of blood flow on compression of the more proximal radial artery.[53,54] Ulnar blood flow should increase when the radial artery is compressed and occluded.[54]

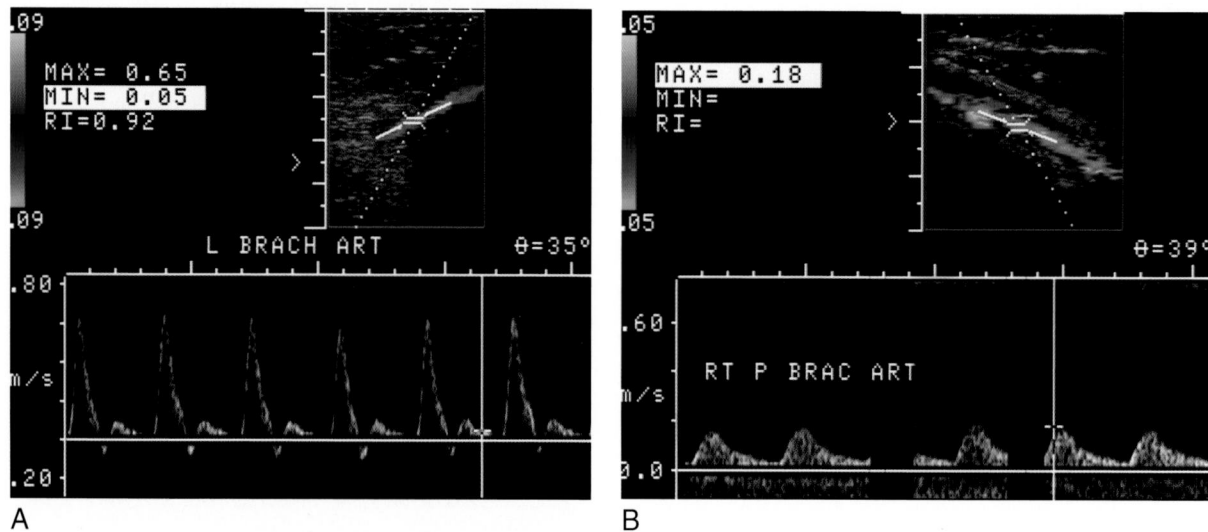

FIGURE 28-13. Normal and abnormal waveforms in the brachial arteries. A, Normal left side resembles the triphasic waveform seen in lower extremity arteries. **B,** Abnormal right side waveform of brachial artery is obtained distal to a subclavian artery occlusion. The Doppler waveform shows a low amplitude (parvus) waveform with a slow systolic rise (tardus). This waveform is typical of what is seen distal to an arterial occlusion.

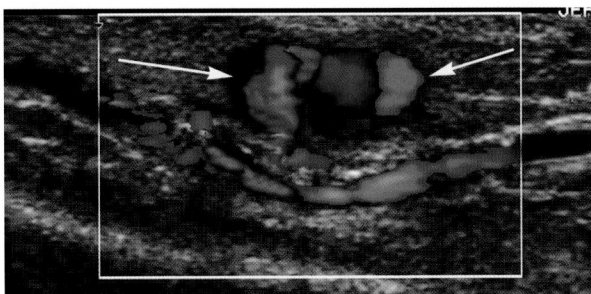

FIGURE 28-14. Radial artery pseudoaneurysm.
Pseudoaneurysm (*arrows*) arising in the radial artery following cardiac catheterization.

VASCULAR AND PERIVASCULAR MASSES AND COMPLICATIONS

Doppler sonography and color flow imaging have the ability to document the presence or absence of blood flow within masses located in close proximity to vessels or vascular prostheses. The presence of blood flow within a perivascular mass can be diagnostic of a pseudoaneurysm that requires treatment, and the absence of blood flow allows a more conservative approach. In the case of a suspected hematoma, serial follow-up examinations can be used to document resolution of the process. In the case of a suspected abscess, a needle aspiration can be performed without fear of uncontrolled hemorrhage.

Synthetic Vascular Bypass Grafts

The complications likely to affect the function of synthetic lower extremity bypass grafts are varied.[10,55] They are a function of the **type of bypass graft utilized** and of the **time since operative placement** (Fig. 28-15). In the first and second years following operation, graft failure can occur secondary to technical errors or to the development of fibrointimal lesions at the anastomoses. Later failures can be due to the progression of atherosclerotic lesions in the native vessels proximal and distal to the graft. The late complication of an anastomotic pseudoaneurysm occurs on average 5 to 10 years following graft placement and preferentially affects the femoral anastomosis of aortofemoral grafts.[5,56] Infections can occur at any time following graft placement and can be associated with the development of an anastomotic pseudoaneurysm. With time, atherosclerotic changes and fibrointimal hyperplastic lesions mixed in with areas of chronic thrombus deposition can also develop in the synthetic graft conduit.

Masses (Hematoma vs. Anastomotic Pseudoaneurysm)

Although the diagnostic accuracy of duplex sonography is above 95% for making the diagnosis of **pseudoaneu-**

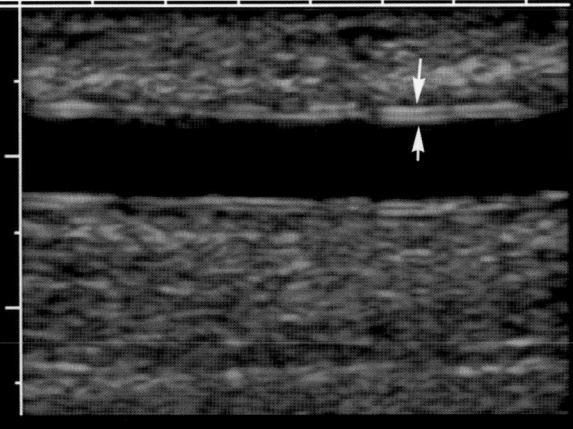

FIGURE 28-15. Synthetic graft. Gray-scale appearance of a synthetic PTFE (polytetrafluoroethylene) lower extremity bypass graft (*arrows*).

rysms at the anastomoses of bypass grafts, no specific waveform patterns have been described.[57,58] The addition of color Doppler imaging can reveal an almost classic appearance of swirling motion of blood in the perivascular mass (Fig. 28-16).[10] This sign is not specific to an anastomotic pseudoaneurysm because saccular aneurysms share similar flow patterns. The differential diagnosis is normally made when careful real-time imaging confirms that the mass is situated beyond the normal lumen of the vessel. The **to-and-fro sign** seen in native pseudoaneurysms is obtained from Doppler spectral analysis of the signal sampled in the communicating channel between the perivascular collection and the native vessel. This neck often does not exist or is very broad, abutting the artery rather than extending as a thin structure for a length of a few centimeters. Typically, anastomotic pseudoaneurysms do not have any distinct communicating channels.

Care must be taken to differentiate perivascular pulsations transmitted within a **hematoma** from flowing blood. Adjustment of the flow sensitivity of the imaging device to minimize this artifact in the normal artery proximal or distal to the site of abnormality can help eliminate this error. Setting the color velocity scale (peak repetition frequency) to a high value can eliminate this artifact, and it should not hamper the detection of the communicating channel.

Occlusions and Perianastomotic Stenoses

The absence of Doppler signals within a bypass graft is diagnostic of an **occlusion**. An **anastomotic stenosis** will typically cause a marked increase in the Doppler velocity signals sampled at the anastomosis or beyond. There is, however, a normal tendency for turbulent flow to develop as the graft tapers to the anastomosis.

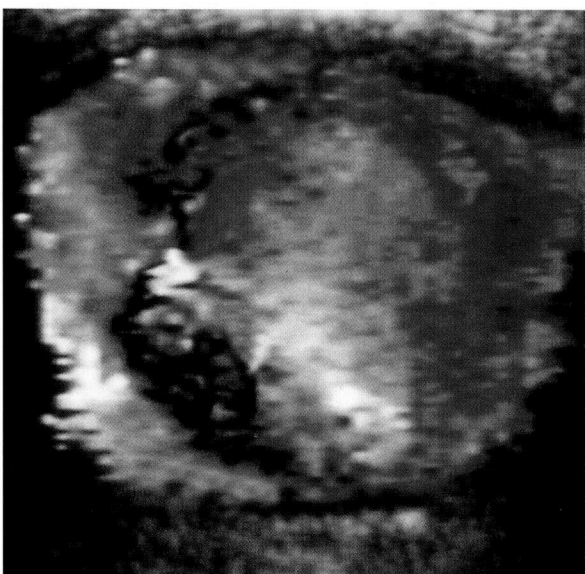

FIGURE 28-16. Anastomotic aneurysm of femoral artery. Transverse image of a large anastomotic aneurysm at the distal anastomosis of an aortobifemoral bypass graft has within it a typical swirling pattern of blood flow.

Increases in velocity due to the geometry of the anastomotic connection are common and can cause up to a 100% increase in velocity without being indicative of a pathologic lesion. There are no studies addressing the actual incidence and significance of this finding. Serial monitoring of these sites of disturbed flow may be used with the premise that an increase in velocity over a few months is indicative of a developing stenosis.[59]

AUTOLOGOUS VEIN GRAFTS

Two types of venous bypass grafts are currently used for arterial revascularization: the reversed vein and the in-situ vein grafts. The **reversed vein** is a segment of native superficial vein that has been harvested from its normal anatomic location, reversed, and then anastomosed to the native artery segments proximal and distal to the diseased segments. The **in situ** technique typically uses the greater saphenous vein, although the lesser saphenous vein can be used for popliteal-to-distal tibioperoneal bypass surgery. The vein is left in its native bed. The valves are lysed and the side branches, perforating veins that normally communicate to the deep venous system, are ligated. The proximal and distal portions are mobilized and anastomosed to the selected arterial segments.

Three different mechanisms are responsible for **bypass graft failure.** Early failures are seen within 1 month of surgery and are normally ascribed to technical errors. These include poor suture line placement, the opening of unsuspected venous channels in the in situ grafts, poor selection of anastomotic sites, and poorly lysed vein valves. During the first 2 years following

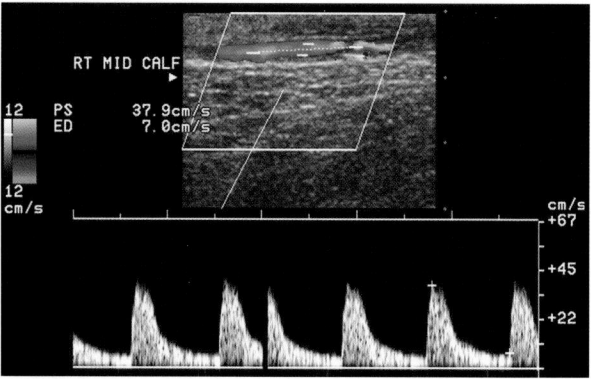

FIGURE 28-17. Abnormal flow velocity of bypass graft. Depressed velocity (<40 cm/sec) in bypass graft in the calf indicative of a high likelihood for future occlusion. The diastolic velocity is still preserved.

surgery, fibrointimal or fibrotic lesions tend to develop, either at the anastomosis or within the graft conduit, most often at the site of a vein valve. Late failures beyond this 2-year period are thought to be secondary to continued progression of the atherosclerotic process in the native vessels proximal and distal to the anastomoses.

Stenosis

A depressed blood flow velocity within a vein bypass graft indicates a high likelihood of incipient graft occlusion and thrombosis (Fig. 28-17). Bandyk et al. have shown that a peak-systolic velocity below 40 or 45 cm/sec can be used to identify such grafts.[60,61] This diagnostic criterion appropriately identifies only the more severely diseased grafts.[62] It does not identify the sites of stenoses that are likely to continue to progress until they become flow restrictive and finally result in graft thrombosis.[63] The lesions that develop within bypass grafts are most often the result of **fibrointimal hyperplasia**, and their existence must be known before they can be monitored for possible progression of severity. Color Doppler sonography can be used to survey the 30 to 80 cm-long bypass graft in a very efficient fashion. The site of a suspected stenosis can be quickly identified, and Doppler spectral analysis can be used to grade the severity of the stenosis with the use of the peak-systolic velocity ratio (Fig. 28-18). Power Doppler imaging and B-flow imaging (a technique that visualizes moving blood) can also be used to better confirm the presence of any stenotic lesions (see Fig. 28-18). This ratio is calculated by dividing the peak systolic velocity measured at the suspected stenosis by that measured in the portion of the graft 2 to 4 cm proximal (Fig. 28-19). Blood flow velocity ratios of 2 or more correspond to 50% diameter stenosis.[25,64] Blood flow velocity ratios of 3 or more correspond to 75% diameter stenosis.[21,64] So-called critical stenoses have been

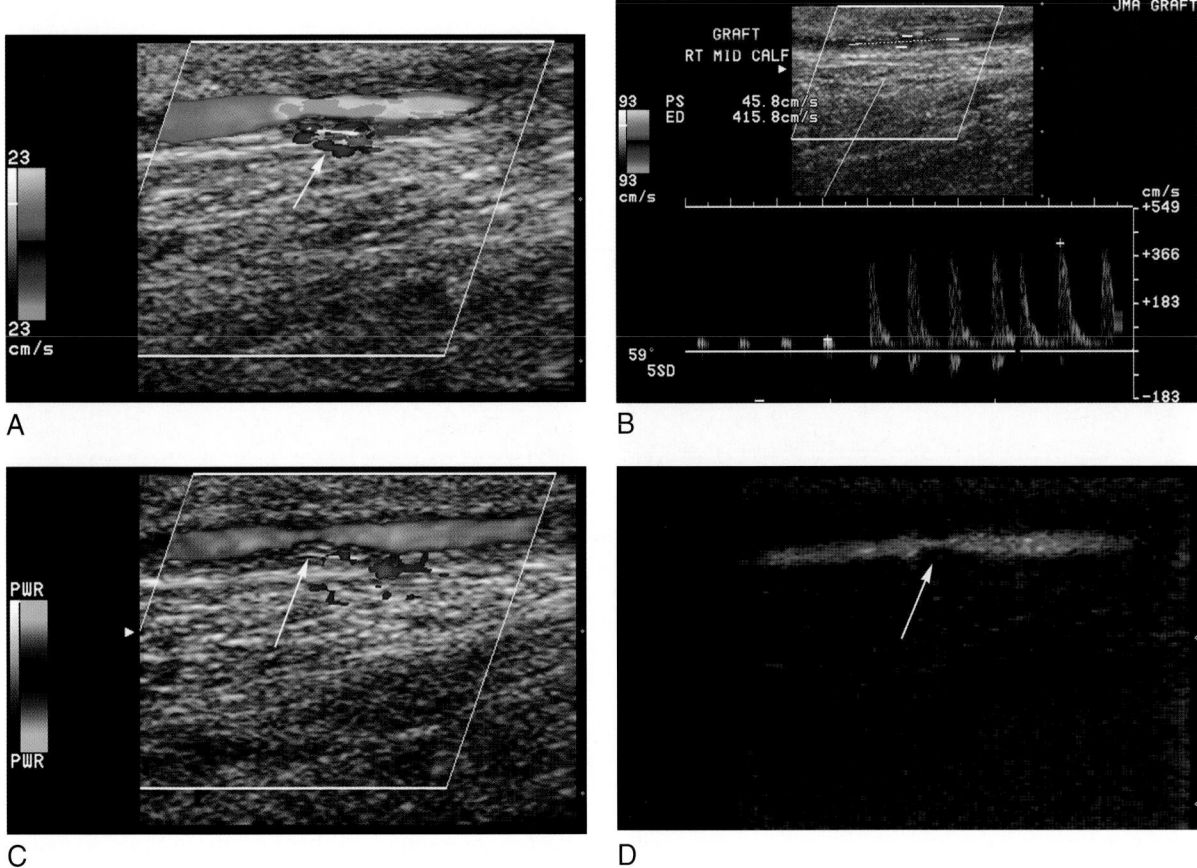

FIGURE 28-18. Focal stenosis of bypass graft in calf. A, Color Doppler image shows a focal site of aliasing with tissue bruit (*arrow*). **B**, The corresponding segment of the bypass graft was then sampled by displacing the Doppler gate along the graft. A significant increase in peak-systolic velocity occurs at the site of aliasing on the color Doppler image. **C**, Power Doppler image confirms the presence of the lesion (*arrow*). **D**, B-flow image also confirms the severity of the stenosis (*arrow*).

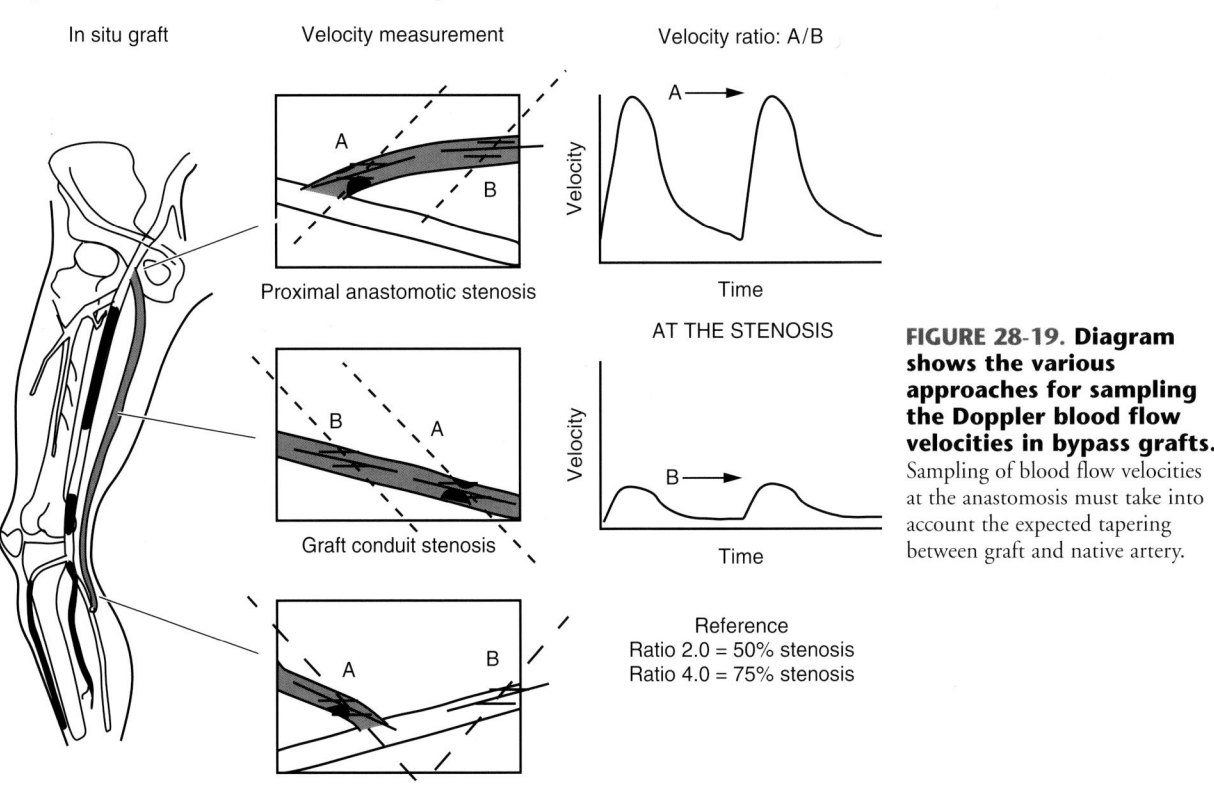

FIGURE 28-19. Diagram shows the various approaches for sampling the Doppler blood flow velocities in bypass grafts. Sampling of blood flow velocities at the anastomosis must take into account the expected tapering between graft and native artery.

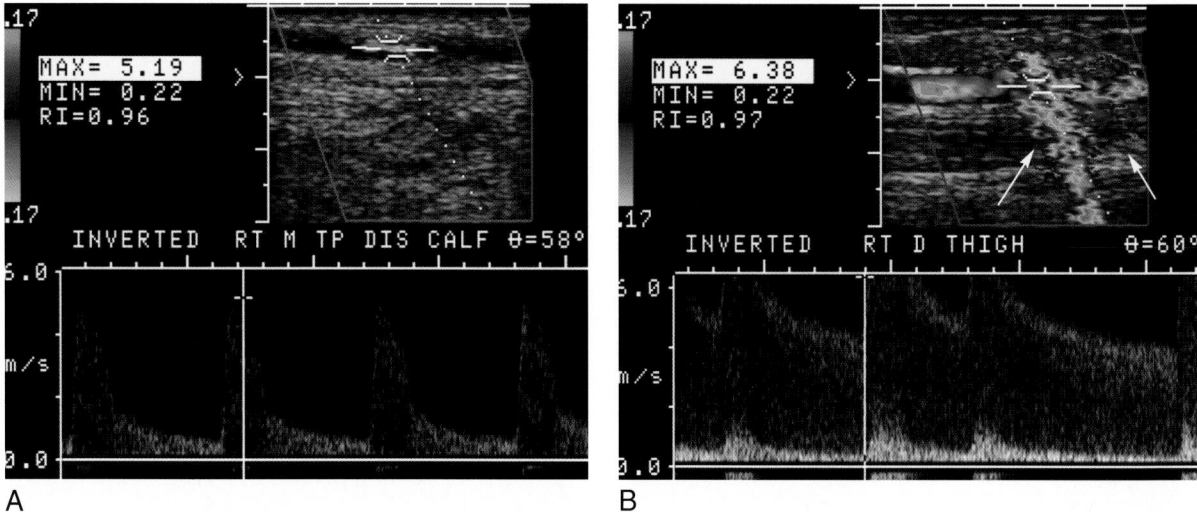

FIGURE 28-20. Bypass graft stenosis and arteriovenous (A-V) fistula causes focal elevation of velocity.
A, Sampling at the site of aliasing of this bypass graft in the calf shows the dramatic increase in blood flow velocity caused by a stenosis.
B, Sampling of same graft in the thigh shows a dramatically different pattern with much more flow in diastole and a perigraft tissue bruit (*arrows*). Although this pattern can be seen with a simple stenosis, in this case, the elevated blood flow velocity was due to a patent A-V fistula arising from the graft at this location.

empirically identified as those causing a velocity increase by a factor of 3.5, 3.7, or even 4.0.[20,65] The blood flow velocity ratio is very accurate for the detection of a stenosis and grading the severity.[66-68]

A potential limitation of the Doppler imaging technique is the presence of tandem lesions where the flow field of one stenosis overlaps the flow field of another situated more distally.[69] It is now recognized that the early lesions develop within 3 months of surgery and are detectable by sonography even before the patient develops any symptoms[70] and that an early examination identifies most of the lesions that will ultimately progress and cause graft thrombosis.[71] An intervention, most often a surgical correction of the developing stenosis, is indicated because it has been shown that these lesions, if left alone, ultimately progress to cause bypass graft occlusion.[70,72] An appropriate peak-systolic velocity ratio cut point for intervention of 4 has been accepted as a threshold defining a critical stenosis and this lesion should be treated.[20] It was recently shown that distal tibial bypass grafts with depressed end diastolic blood flow velocities detected intraoperatively are a high risk for subsequent graft failure.[73]

Arteriovenous Fistula

Persistent arteriovenous communication through nonligated perforating veins occurs with the in situ technique. Arteriovenous fistulas can easily be missed at operation or immediately postoperatively because a good percentage open in the few weeks following surgery. Color Doppler imaging is a simple and elegant way of documenting their presence. The imaging findings can,

however, mimic those of a stenosis (Fig. 28-20). Intraoperative sonography is used to detect fistulas in need of being ligated.[60] Postoperative detection of sites of arteriovenous communication between the in situ graft and the deeper native veins can be done by Doppler ultrasound alone. Ultrasound is typically used as the only guide for surgical correction, without the need for angiography.[74]

DIALYSIS ACCESS GRAFTS AND FISTULAS

The utility of sonography in the evaluation of dialysis A-V fistulas or hemodialysis access grafts (Fig. 28-21) is controversial.[75,76] The native artery-to-vein anastomosis is the favored approach for insuring hemodialysis access and is typically created between the radial artery and a superficial vein (Brescia-Cimino). Its creation requires careful technique, and graft maturation can take weeks or months. Ultrasound offers preoperative information on the status of the native arteries and veins that increases the technical success rate of fistula creation.[77] The alternative type of dialysis access are interposition grafts. They are inserted in the forearm and are either **synthetic PTFE** (polytetrafluoroethylene) or **autologous vein**. Problems common to both types of dialysis access grafts include the development of **microaneurysms, larger aneurysms,** or **stenoses**. Color flow imaging can readily detect perigraft masses or pseudoaneurysm with a high accuracy. Color Doppler imaging and duplex sonography can be used to detect stenoses: the accuracy of the technique is estimated at 86% with a sensitivity of 92% and specificity of 84%.[75] The loss in specificity

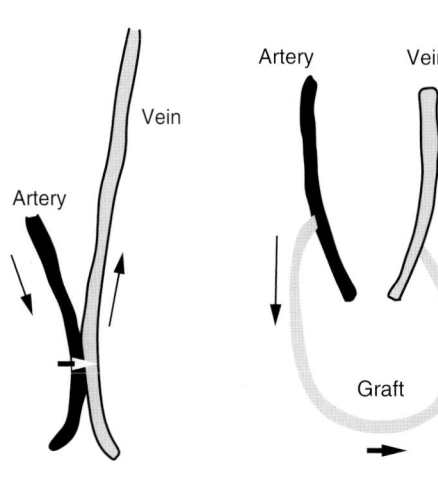

Brescia-Cimino
arterio-venous fistula

Interposition graft
(loop)

Interposition graft
(straight)

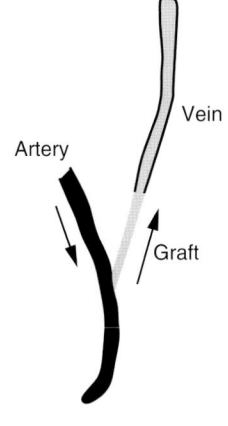

FIGURE 28-21. Dialysis fistula types. Brescia-Cimino arteriovenous fistulas are created by direct suturing (side-to-side) of an artery to a vein. The interposition grafts are created with synthetic PTFE (polytetrafluoroethylene) or biologic analogs for material bridging the artery to a suitable superficial vein.

is explained by turbulent flow patterns set up by a very tortuous course of the outflow vein and the high baseline velocities seen in the outflow vein. The diagnostic accuracy is improved in straight segment grafts to the efferent veins, where the sensitivity increases to 95% for a specificity of 97%.[75] The addition of color Doppler did not seem to improve diagnostic accuracy.[78]

Diagnostic criteria applicable to Doppler ultrasound of hemodialysis access graft stenosis have been reported.[79-81] Peak-systolic velocities in well functioning dialysis access grafts are typically between 100 cm/sec and 200 cm/sec (Fig. 28-22), tending to be higher in the first 6 months after graft placement or shunt creation.[81] Superimposed stenosis can, therefore, be difficult to detect given the high baseline velocities. A blood flow velocity elevation of 100% (velocity ratios of 2 or more) is considered to be consistent with the presence of a significant stenosis. Color Doppler, power Doppler, and gray-scale images are also useful for confirming the presence of an anatomic lesion.[80] Stenotic lesions tend to develop on the venous side of the access fistula in more than 80% of cases.[82] Occasionally, the stenosis can be at the level of the subclavian vein, specifically in individuals who have had hemodialysis catheters inserted in the subclavian vein.[83] Following percutaneous interventions, Doppler ultrasound can be used to monitor development of recurrent stenosis. Low blood flow states of 50 cm/sec or less are also indicative of a high-grade stenosis in the graft conduit or outflow vein.

COMPLICATIONS OF INVASIVE PROCEDURES

The use of duplex or color Doppler sonography for the screening of patients who have had invasive procedures and in whom the diagnosis of A-V fistula or pseudo-

aneurysm is suspected has dramatically increased. The findings on the sonographic examination are commonly taken at face value, without the need for preoperative angiography.

Arteriovenous Fistula

Fistulous communications between vessels following cardiac catheterization or other angiographic procedures can be quickly detected using color Doppler imaging.[84,85] An area of **turbulence** is normally seen within either the common femoral or profunda femoral vein with **arterialized signals** shown on the Doppler spectrum (see Fig. 28-4 and Fig. 28-23). The actual **fistulous communication** can be seen on the color map although it may be difficult to localize with duplex sonography alone. The turbulence associated with the fistula can be confused with turbulent signals due to extrinsic compression of the vein by a hematoma (see Fig. 28-5), also a commonly seen complication following catheterization. Visualization of the communicating channel should therefore be done with a high color velocity setting (high color PRF). An indirect sign of the fistula is dilation of the vein and a poor response to the Valsalva maneuver (Fig. 28-24). Blood flow signals in a vein recipient of a large A-V fistula communication will not decrease during the Valsalva maneuver. With small A-V communications, the venous velocity signals can easily decrease or disappear during the Valsalva maneuver (see Fig. 28-23). Complete abolition of the flow signals during the Valsalva maneuver suggests that the fistula is small and likely to spontaneously occlude over the next few weeks. **Transcutaneus therapy** aimed at achieving closure of the fistula has been described using ultrasound monitoring and by applying pressure over the fistula for periods of 20 to 60 minutes.[86] Success rates of transcutaneous repair attempts are 30% or lower.[86]

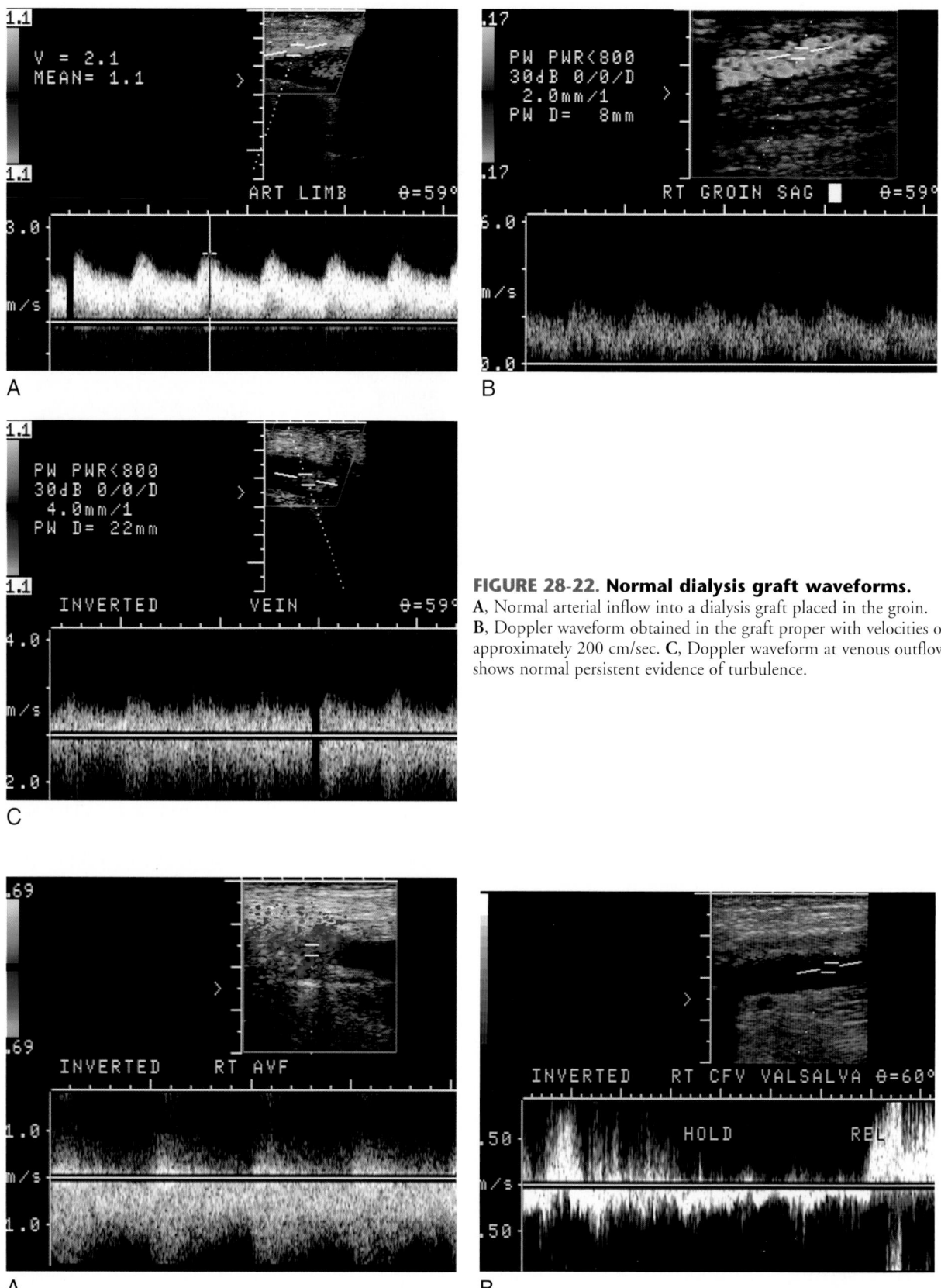

FIGURE 28-22. Normal dialysis graft waveforms.
A, Normal arterial inflow into a dialysis graft placed in the groin.
B, Doppler waveform obtained in the graft proper with velocities of
approximately 200 cm/sec. **C**, Doppler waveform at venous outflow
shows normal persistent evidence of turbulence.

FIGURE 28-23. Waveform in femoral vein suggests small arteriovenous (A-V) fistula. A, Soft tissue bruit is the
only evidence of an A-V fistula. **B**, Sampling of the Doppler waveform in the nearby native common femoral vein shows a partial
response (decreasing blood flow velocity) during a Valsalva maneuver (HOLD) and return to normal after maneuver (REL). This
suggests that the A-V fistula is a small one.

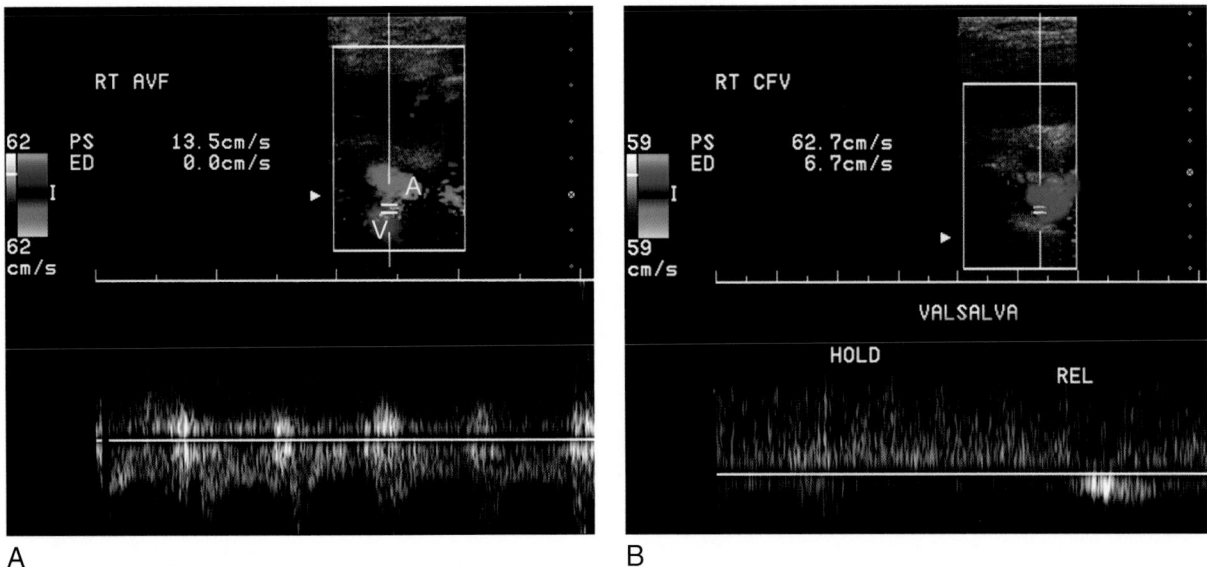

FIGURE 28-24. Waveform in femoral vein suggests large arteriovenous (A-V) fistula. A, This deep-lying A-V fistula is detected by color Doppler imaging (A, common femoral artery; V, common femoral vein). **B,** The poor response (lack of velocity change) to the Valsalva maneuver suggests that the A-V fistula is a relatively large one.

Pseudoaneurysms

This type of complication can develop after **penetrating trauma** or **arterial catheterization**. The direct communication between the pseudoaneurysm and arterial lumen should be detectable by color flow imaging. Often, a high velocity scale (PRF) is needed because blood flow velocities can be very high. The duplex sonographic finding of a to-and-fro sign is typically detected in the communicating channel of the pseudoaneurysm (see Fig. 28-6). Pseudoaneurysms can have multiple compartments as well as be solitary.

Once considered a relative medical emergency, the management of pseudoaneurysms has significantly been affected by the wide use of sonography. The natural history of pseudoaneurysms has been shown to often be benign with spontaneous closure when patients are kept at bed rest.[87]

Fellmeth et al. first described the use of **transcutaneous compression therapy** of pseudoaneurysms following catheterization.[86] They described a simple protocol of applying pressure with the ultrasound probe over the neck of the pseudoaneurysm. The probe was kept along the long axis of the artery as flow into the cavity was obliterated: a sequence of up to three transcutaneous pressure applications, each lasting 20 minutes, was used. Transcutaneous therapy was successful in more than 80% of cases. These authors remarked on the need for good analgesia in their patients, commented on the increased difficulty of performing these repairs when the patient is anticoagulated, and indicated potential complications such as arterial or venous thrombosis. Subsequent reports have confirmed the high success rates of the procedure,[88,89] even in patients undergoing

anticoagulation.[90] Other reports have described a greater likelihood of success for smaller pseudoaneurysms and those with longer communicating channels.[91,92] Pseudoaneurysms arising from other arteries, the axillary[93] or the brachial[94] as examples, have also been successfully treated by transcutaneous compression repair.

An alternative form of therapy has almost completely replaced ultrasound-guided compression repair. **Ultrasound-guided injection of thrombin**[95-97] consists of ultrasound-guided placement of a needle in the cavity of the pseudoaneurysm and injection of up to 1000 units of thrombin (see Fig. 28-6D).[98-100] The basic protocol of using a high concentration of thrombin has been modified to the use of a dilute solution of 1000 units in 10 or 20 mL of saline and then slow injection under ultrasound monitoring. The average dose of thrombin can be decreased to 192 units,[101] thereby reducing the risk of inadvertent injection in the native arteries. As compared to compression ultrasound, the technique is more efficient and has higher success rates[100] than compression repair. It is also successfully applied to patients who are anticoagulated.[102] Even after therapy, a persistent communicating channel can exist (Fig. 28-25).

A very interesting facet of the epidemiology of pseudoaneurysms is the apparent increase in disease incidence seen in the last decade. Kresowik et al. reported incidence rates almost 10 times the 0.5% rate reported in the last few decades.[103] Plausible explanations for this increase in disease incidence were the use of more aggressive anticoagulation and of larger-sized catheters during angioplasty and stent placement procedures. The length of time taken to ensure hemostasis after femoral artery catheterization and removal of the catheter

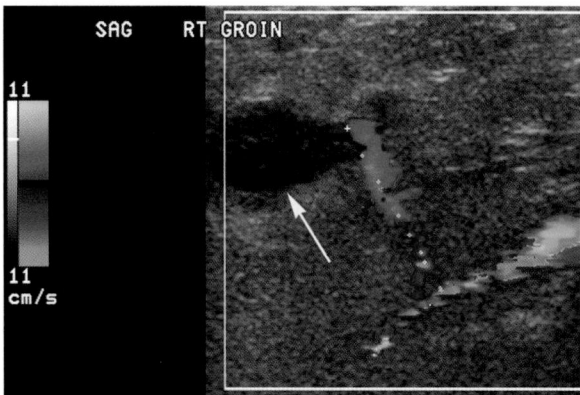

FIGURE 28-25. Persistent neck of pseudoaneurysm. Despite successful thrombosis of the pseudoaneurysm cavity (*arrow*), the small communicating neck remains open. In most patients, this will occlude spontaneously over the next few hours or days.

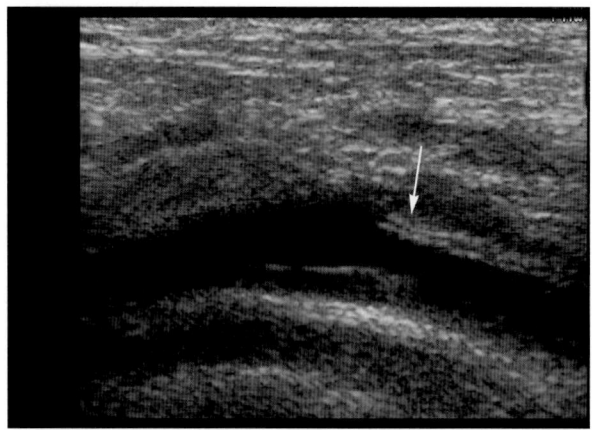

FIGURE 28-26. Arterial closure device causes stenosis of common femoral artery (CFA). A, Closure device (*arrow*) apposed to the near wall of the CFA. **B,** Partial downward displacement of this device causes a stenosis and a corresponding increase in blood flow velocity.

remains the most important predictor of subsequent pseudoaneurysm formation.[104]

The use of **closure devices** that seal the arterial entry site seems to have decreased the overall incidence of pseudoaneurysm formation.[52] However, when pseudoaneurysms occur, they tend to be large and easily identified by ultrasound imaging.[105] Another device, the Angio-Seal, can cause a stenosis (Fig. 28-26) or even arterial occlusion due to inadvertent displacement of the intra-arterial component of the closure device.[106] The key component of some of these devices is an intravascularly placed collagen plug. This plug can migrate and fall into the lumen of the artery.

CONCLUSION

Doppler sonography of the peripheral arterial system is a cost-effective tool for the work-up of many vascular pathologies. Doppler sonography is its own standard for the diagnosis of aneurysms, A-V fistulas, and pseudoaneurysms. These diagnostic tasks are facilitated by the use of color flow imaging. Color flow Doppler imaging with gray-scale and spectral (duplex) sonography can be used to survey and study changes in flow dynamics over long segments of the peripheral arteries. The integration of this diagnostic modality as the main follow-up mechanism for patients having undergone peripheral arterial bypass operations is now well accepted. The near future will see whether Doppler sonography will be shown to be a cost-effective approach for the survey of native arterial disease, detecting lesions, and helping to triage patients to surgery or to other therapeutic options such as angioplasty, atherectomy, or stent placement.

References

1. Polak JF, Karmel MI, Mannick JA, et al: Determination of the extent of lower-extremity peripheral arterial disease with color-assisted duplex sonography: Comparison with angiography. AJR 1990;155:1085-1089.
2. DeVries S, Hunink M, Polak J: Summary receiver operating characteristic curves as a technique for meta-analysis for the diagnostic performance of duplex ultrasonography in peripheral arterial disease. Acad Radiol 1996;3:361-369.
3. Barber FE, Baker DW, Nation AWC, et al: Ultrasonic duplex-scanner. IEEE Trans Biomed Engin 1974; 21:109-113.
4. Kasai C, Namekawa K, Koyano A, et al: Real-time two-dimensional blood flow imaging using an autocorrelation technique. IEEE Trans Sonics Ultrasound 1985;S32:458-463.
5. Polak JF, Dobkin GR, O'Leary DH, et al: Internal carotid artery stenosis: Accuracy and reproducibility of color-Doppler-assisted duplex imaging. Radiology 1989;173:793-798.
6. Spencer MP, Reid JM: Quantitation of carotid stenosis with continuous-wave (C-W) Doppler ultrasound. Stroke 1979;10:326-330.

7. Reneman R, Spencer M: Local Doppler audio spectra in normal and stenosed carotid arteries in man. Ultrasound Med Biol 1979;5:1-11.

8. Ojha M, Johnston K, Cobbold R, et al: Potential limitations of center-line pulsed Doppler recordings: An in-vitro flow visualization study. J Vasc Surg 1989;9:515-520.

9. Middleton WD, Erickson S, Melson GL: Perivascular color artifact: Pathologic significance and appearance on color Doppler US images. Radiology 1989;171:647-652.

10. Polak JF, Donaldson MC, Whittemore AD, et al: Pulsatile masses surrounding vascular prostheses: Real-time US color flow imaging. Radiology 1989;170:363-366.

11. Wilkinson DL, Polak JF, Grass CJ, et al: Pseudoaneurysm of the vertebral artery: Appearance on color-flow Doppler sonography. AJR 1988;151:1051-1052.

12. Mitchell DG: Color Doppler imaging: Principles, limitations, and artifacts. Radiology 1990;177:1-10.

13. Abu-Yousef MM, Wiese JA, Shamma AR: The "to-and-fro" sign: Duplex Doppler evidence of femoral artery pseudoaneurysm. AJR 1988;150:632-634.

14. Morton MJ, Charboneau JW, Banks PM: Inguinal lymphadenopathy simulating a false aneurysm on color-flow Doppler sonography. AJR 1988;151:115-116.

15. Bjork L, Leven H: Intra-arterial DSA and duplex-Doppler ultrasonography in detection of vascularized inguinal lymph node. Acta Radiol 1990;31:106-107.

16. Musto R, Roach M: Flow studies in glass models of aortic aneurysms. Can J Surg 1980;23:452-455.

17. Newman AB, Siscovick DS, Manolio TA, et al: Ankle-arm index as a marker of atherosclerosis in the Cardiovascular Health Study. Circulation 1993;88:837-845.

18. Cronenwett JL, Warner KG, Zelenock GB, et al: Intermittent claudication. Current results of nonoperative management. Arch Surg 1984;119:430-436.

19. Teo NB, Mamode N, Murtagh A, et al: Effectiveness of surveillance of infrainguinal grafts. Eur J Surg 2001;167:605-609.

20. Mills JL, Sr, Wixon CL, James DC, et al: The natural history of intermediate and critical vein graft stenosis: Recommendations for continued surveillance or repair. J Vasc Surg 2001;33:273-278.

21. Dougherty MJ, Calligaro KD, DeLaurentis DA: The natural history of "failing" arterial bypass grafts in a duplex surveillance protocol. Ann Vasc Surg 1998;12:255-259.

22. Back MR, Novotney M, Roth SM, et al: Utility of duplex surveillance following iliac artery angioplasty and primary stenting. J Endovasc Ther 2001;8:629-637.

23. Koelemay MJ, Legemate DA, De Vos H, et al: Duplex scanning allows selective use of arteriography in the management of patients with severe lower leg arterial disease. J Vasc Surg 2001;34:661-667.

24. Katsamouris AN, Giannoukas AD, Tsetis D, et al: Can ultrasound replace arteriography in the management of chronic arterial occlusive disease of the lower limb? Eur J Vasc Endovasc Surg 2001;21:155-159.

25. Kohler TR, Nance DR, Cramer MM, et al: Duplex scanning for diagnosis of aortoiliac and femoropopliteal disease: A prospective study. Circulation 1987;76:1074-1080.

26. Gooding GA, Effeney DJ: Ultrasound of femoral artery aneurysms. AJR 1980;134:477-480.

27. MacGowan SW, Saif MF, O'Neil G, et al: Ultrasound examination in the diagnosis of popliteal artery aneurysms. Br J Surg 1985;72:528-529.

28. Shortell CK, DeWeese JA, Ouriel K, et al: Popliteal artery aneurysms: A 25-year surgical experience. J Vasc Surg 1991;14:771-779.

29. Jager KA, Phillips DJ, Martin RL, et al: Noninvasive mapping of lower limb arterial lesions. Ultrasound Med Biol 1985;11:515-521.

30. Cossman DV, Ellison JE, Wagner WH, et al: Comparison of contrast arteriography to arterial mapping with color-flow duplex imaging in the lower extremities. J Vasc Surg 1989;10:522-529.

31. Mulligan SA, Matsuda T, Lanzer P, et al: Peripheral arterial occlusive disease: Prospective comparison of MR angiography and color duplex US with conventional angiography. Radiology 1991;178:695-700.

32. Fletcher FP, Kershaw LZ, Chan A, et al: Noninvasive imaging of the superficial femoral artery using ultrasound duplex scanning. J Cardiovasc Surg 1990;31:364-367.

33. Whelan FF, Barry MH, Moir JD: Color flow Doppler ultrasonography: Comparison with peripheral arteriography for the investigation of peripheral arterial disease. J Clin Ultrasound 1992;20:369-374.

34. Moneta GL, Yeager RA, Antonovic R, et al: Accuracy of lower extremity arterial duplex mapping. J Vasc Surg 1992;15:275-284.

35. Moneta GL, Yeager RA, Lee RW, et al: Noninvasive localization of arterial occlusive disease: A comparison of segmental pressures and arterial duplex mapping. J Vasc Surg 1993;17:578-582.

36. Karacagil S, Lofberg A, Granbo A, et al: Value of duplex scanning in evaluation of crural and foot arteries in limbs with severe lower limb ischemia. A prospective comparison with angiography. Eur J Vasc Endovasc Surg 1996;12:300-303.

37. Koelemay MJ, Legemate DA, De Vos H, et al: Can cruropedal colour duplex scanning and pulse generated run-off replace angiography in candidates for distal bypass surgery? Eur J Vasc Endovasc Surg 1998;16:13-18.

38. Wain RA, Berdejo GL, Delvalle WN, et al: Can duplex scan arterial mapping replace contrast arteriography as the test of choice before infrainguinal revascularization? Journal of Vascular Surgery 1999;29:100-107.

39. Ascher E, Mazzariol F, Hingorani A, et al: The use of duplex ultrasound arterial mapping as an alternative to conventional arteriography for primary and secondary infrapopliteal bypasses. Am J Surg 1999;178:162-165.

40. Mazzariol F, Ascher E, Salles-Cunha SX, et al: Values and limitations of duplex ultrasonography as the sole imaging method of preoperative evaluation for popliteal and infrapopliteal bypasses. Ann Vasc Surg 1999;13:1-10.

41. Elsman BH, Legemate DA, Van der Heijden FH, et al: Impact of ultrasonographic duplex scanning on therapeutic decision making in lower limb arterial disease. Br J Surg 1995;82:630-633.

42. Collier P, Wilcox G, Brooks D, et al: Improved patient selection for angioplasty utilizing color Doppler imaging. Am J Surg 1990;160:171-174.

43. Edwards JM, Goldwell DM, Goldman ML, et al: The role of duplex scanning in the selection of patients for transluminal angioplasty. J Vasc Surg 1991;13:69-74.

44. Polak JF, Karmel MI, Meyerovitz MF: Accuracy of color Doppler flow mapping for evaluation of the severity of femoropopliteal arterial disease: A prospective study. JVIR 1991;2:471-479.

45. Mewissen MW, Kinney EV, Bandyk DF, et al: The role of duplex scanning versus angiography in predicting outcome after balloon angioplasty in the femoropopliteal artery. J Vasc Surg 1992;15:860-866.

46. Sacks D, Robinson ML, Summers TA, et al: The value of duplex sonography after peripheral artery angioplasty

in predicting subacute stenosis. AJR 1994;
162:179-183.

47. Katzenschlager R, Ahmadi A, Minar E, et al: Color duplex ultrasound guided transluminal angioplasty of the femoropopliteal artery: Initial and 6-months results. Radiology 1996;199:331-334.

48. Vroegindeweij D, Tielbeek A, Buth J, et al: Directional atherectomy versus balloon angioplasty in segmental femoropopliteal artery disease: Two-year follow-up with color-flow duplex scanning. J Vasc Surg 1995;21:255-268.

49. Tielbeek A, Rietjens E, Buth J, et al: The value of duplex surveillance after endovascular intervention for femoropopliteal obstructive disease. Eur J Vasc Endovasc Surg 1996;12:145-150.

50. Spijkerboer A, Nass P, De Valois J, et al: Iliac artery stenoses after percutaneous transluminal angioplasty: Follow-up with duplex ultrasonography. J Vasc Surg 1996;23:691-697.

51. Damaraju S, Cuasay L, Le D, et al: Predictors of primary patency failure in Wallstent self-expanding endovascular prostheses for iliofemoral occlusive disease. Tex Heart Inst J 1997;24:173-178.

52. Dangas G, Mehran R, Kokolis S, et al: Vascular complications after percutaneous coronary interventions following hemostasis with manual compression versus arteriotomy closure devices. J Am Coll Cardiol 2001;38:638-641.

53. Kochi K, Sueda T, Orihashi K, et al: New noninvasive test alternative to Allen's test: Snuff-box technique. J Thorac Cardiovasc Surg 1999;118:756-758.

54. Yokoyama N, Takeshita S, Ochiai M, et al: Direct assessment of palmar circulation before transradial coronary intervention by color Doppler ultrasonography. Am J Cardiol 2000;86:218-221.

55. Hedgcock MW, Eisenberg RL, Gooding GA: Complications relating to vascular prosthetic grafts. J Can Assoc Radiol 1980;31:137-142.

56. Nichols WK, Stanton M, Silver D, et al: Anastomotic aneurysms following lower extremity revascularization. Surgery 1980;88:366-374.

57. Helvie MA, Rubin JM, Silver TM, et al: The distinction between femoral artery pseudoaneurysms and other causes of groin masses: Value of duplex Doppler sonography. AJR 1988;150:1177-1180.

58. Coughlin BF, Paushter DM: Peripheral pseudoaneurysms: Evaluation with duplex US. Radiology 1988;168:339-342.

59. Sanchez LA, Suggs WD, Veith FJ, et al: Is surveillance to detect failing polytetrafluoroethylene bypasses worthwhile? Twelve-year experience with 91 grafts. J Vasc Surg 1993;18:981-990.

60. Bandyk DF, Jorgensen RA, Towne JB: Intraoperative assessment of in situ saphenous vein arterial bypass grafts using pulsed Doppler spectral analysis. Arch Surg 1986;121:292-299.

61. Bandyk DF, Cato RF, Towne JB: A low flow velocity predicts failure of femoropopliteal and femorotibial bypass grafts. Surgery 1985;98:799-809.

62. Mills JL, Harris EJ, Taylor LM, Jr, et al: The importance of routine surveillance of distal bypass grafts with duplex scanning: A study of 379 reversed vein grafts. J Vasc Surg 1990;12:379-389.

63. Grigg MJ, Nicolaides AN, Wolfe JH: Detection and grading of femorodistal vein grafts stenoses: Duplex velocity measurements compared with angiography. J Vasc Surg 1988;8:661-666.

64. Hunink MGM, Polak JF: Response to commentary on accuracy of color Doppler flow mapping for evaluation of

the severity of femoropopliteal arterial disease: A prospective study. JVIR 1991;2:477-478.

65. Ranke C, Creutzig A, Alexander K: Duplex scanning of the peripheral arteries: Correlation of the peak velocity ratio with angiographic diameter reduction. Ultrasound Med Biol 1992;18:433-440.

66. Londrey GL, Hodgson KJ, Spadone DP, et al: Initial experience with color-flow duplex scanning of infrainguinal bypass grafts. J Vasc Surg 1990; 12:284-290.

67. Polak JF, Donaldson MC, Dobkin GR, et al: Early detection of saphenous vein arterial bypass graft stenosis by color-assisted duplex sonography: A prospective study. AJR 1990;154:857-861.

68. Buth J, Disselhoff B, Sommeling C, et al: Color-flow duplex criteria for grading stenosis in infrainguinal vein grafts. J Vasc Surg 1991;14:716-728.

69. Leng GC, Whyman MR, Donnan PT, et al: Accuracy and reproducibility of duplex ultrasonography in grading femoropopliteal stenoses. J Vasc Surg 1993;17:510-517.

70. Mills JL, Bandyk DF, Gathan V, et al: The origin of infrainguinal vein graft stenosis: A prospective study based on duplex surveillance. J Vasc Surg 1995;1:16-25.

71. Ihnat DM, Mills JL, Dawson DL, et al: The correlation of early flow disturbances with the development of infrainguinal graft stenosis: A 10-year study of 341 autogenous vein grafts. J Vasc Surg 1999;30:8-15.

72. Idu MM, Blankestein JD, De Gier P, et al: Impact of a color-flow duplex surveillance program on infrainguinal vein graft patency: A five-year experience. J Vasc Surg 1993;17:42-53.

73. Rzucidlo EM, Walsh DB, Powell RJ, et al: Prediction of early graft failure with intraoperative completion duplex ultrasound scan. J Vasc Surg 2002;36:975-981.

74. Bostrom A, Karacagil S, Jonsson ML, et al: Repeat surgery without preoperative angiography in limbs with patent infrainguinal bypass grafts. Vasc Endovascular Surg 2002;36:343-350.

75. Tordoir JH, De Bruin HG, Hoeneveld H, et al: Duplex ultrasound scanning in the assessment of arteriovenous fistulas created for hemodialysis access: Comparison with digital subtraction angiography. J Vasc Surg 1989; 10:122-128.

76. Scheible W, Skram C, Leopold GR: High resolution real-time sonography of hemodialysis vascular access complications. AJR 1980;134:1173-1176.

77. Mihmanli I, Besirli K, Kurugoglu S, et al: Cephalic vein and hemodialysis fistula: Surgeon's observation versus color Doppler ultrasonographic findings. J Ultrasound Med 2001;20:217-222.

78. Middleton WD, Picus DD, Marx MV, et al: Color Doppler sonography of hemodialysis vascular access: Comparison with angiography. AJR 1989; 152:633-639.

79. Koksoy C, Kuzu A, Erden I, et al: Predictive value of color Doppler sonography in detecting failure of vascular access grafts. Br J Surg 1995;82:50-52.

80. Dousset V, Grenier N, Douws C, et al: Hemodialysis grafts: Color Doppler flow imaging correlated with digital subtraction angiography and functional status. Radiology 1991;181:89-94.

81. Villemarette P, Hower J: Evaluation of functional longevity of dialysis access grafts using color flow Doppler imaging. J Vasc Tech 1992;16:183-188.

82. Kanterman RY, Vesely TM, Pilgram TK, et al: Dialysis access grafts: Anatomic location of venous stenosis and results of angioplasty. Radiology 1995;195:135-139.

83. Schwab SJ, Quarles LD, Middleton JP, et al: Haemodialysis-associated subclavian vein stenosis. Kidney Int 1988;33:1156-1159.

84. Altin RS, Flicker S, Naidech HJ: Pseudoaneurysm and arteriovenous fistula after femoral artery catheterization: Association with low femoral punctures. AJR 1989;152:629-631.

85. Roubidoux MA, Hertzberg BS, Carroll BA, et al: Color flow and image-directed Doppler ultrasound evaluation of iatrogenic arteriovenous fistulas in the groin. JCU 1990;18:463-469.

86. Fellmeth BD, Roberts AC, Bookstein JJ, et al: Postangiographic femoral artery injuries: Nonsurgical repair with US-guided compression. Radiology 1991;178:671-675.

87. Kotval PS, Khoury A, Shah PM, et al: Doppler sonographic demonstration of the progressive spontaneous thrombosis of pseudoaneurysms. J Ultrasound Med 1990;9:185-190.

88. Fellmeth BD, Baron SB, Brown PR, et al: Repair of postcatheterization femoral pseudoaneurysms by color flow ultrasound guided compression. Am Heart J 1992;123:547-551.

89. Cox GS, Young JR, Gray BR, et al: Ultrasound-guided compression repair of postcatheterization pseudoaneurysms: Results of treatment in one hundred cases. J Vasc Surg 1994;19:683-686.

90. Dean S, Olin J, Piedmonte M, et al: Ultrasound-guided compression closure of postcatheterization pseudoaneurysms during concurrent anticoagulation: A review of seventy-seven patients. J Vasc Surg 1996;23:28-35.

91. DiPrete DA, Cronan JJ: Compression ultrasonography: Treatment for acute femoral artery pseudoaneurysms in selected cases. J Ultrasound Med 1992;11:489-492.

92. Paulson EK, Hertzberg BS, Paine SS, et al: Femoral artery pseudoaneurysms: Value of color Doppler sonography in predicting which ones will thrombose without treatment. AJR 1992;159:1077-1081.

93. Rooker KT, Morgan CA, Haseman MK, et al: Color flow guided repair of axillary artery pseudoaneurysm. J Ultrasound Med 1992;11:625-626.

94. Skibo L, Polak JF: Compression repair of a postcatheterization pseudoaneurysm of the brachial artery under sonographic guidance. AJR 1993;160:383-384.

95. Walker TG, Geller SC, Brewster DC: Transcatheter occlusion of a profunda femoral artery pseudoaneurysm using thrombin. AJR 1987;149:185-186.

96. Liau CS, Ho FM, Chen MF, et al: Treatment of iatrogenic femoral artery pseudoaneurysm with percutaneous thrombin injection. J Vasc Surg 1997;26:18-23.

97. Kang SS, Labropoulos N, Mansour MA, et al: Percutaneous ultrasound guided thrombin injection: A new method for treating postcatheterization femoral pseudoaneurysms. J Vasc Surg 1998;27:1032-1038.

98. Lennox AF, Griffin MB, Cheshire NJ, et al: Treatment of an iatrogenic femoral artery pseudoaneurysm with percutaneous duplex-guided injection of thrombin. Circulation 1999;100:39-41.

99. Mohler ER, 3rd, Mitchell ME, Carpenter JP, et al: Therapeutic thrombin injection of pseudoaneurysms: A multicenter experience. Vasc Med 2001;6:241-244.

100. Paulson EK, Sheafor DH, Kliewer MA, et al: Treatment of iatrogenic femoral arterial pseudoaneurysms: Comparison of US-guided thrombin injection with compression repair. Radiology 2000;215:403-408.

101. Reeder SB, Widlus DM, Lazinger M: Low-dose thrombin injection to treat iatrogenic femoral artery pseudoaneurysms. AJR 2001;177:595-598.

102. Brophy DP, Sheiman RG, Amatulle P, et al: Iatrogenic femoral pseudoaneurysms: Thrombin injection after failed US-guided compression. Radiology 2000;214:278-282.

103. Kresowik TF, Khoury MD, Miller BV, et al: A prospective study of the incidence and natural history of femoral vascular complications after percutaneous transluminal coronary angioplasty. J Vasc Surg 1991;13:328-335.

104. Katzenschlager R, Ugurluoglu A, Ahmadi A, et al: The incidence of pseudoaneurysm after diagnostic and therapeutic angiography. Radiology 1995;195:463-466.

105. Sprouse LR, 2nd, Botta DM, Jr, Hamilton IN, Jr: The management of peripheral vascular complications associated with the use of percutaneous suture-mediated closure devices. J Vasc Surg 2001;33:688-693.

106. Kirchhof C, Schickel S, Schmidt-Lucke C, et al: Local vascular complications after use of the hemostatic puncture closure device Angio-Seal. Vasa 2002;31:101-106.

The Peripheral Veins

Bradley D. Lewis

Chapter Outline

$\mathcal{T}$he clinical evaluation of the peripheral venous system is notoriously difficult and inaccurate. Accordingly, numerous imaging and nonimaging methods have been developed to aid clinicians with this diagnostic problem. These methods can be divided into three main categories.

METHODS

Noninvasive, Nonimaging, Physiologic Methods

Noninvasive, nonimaging, physiologic methods rely on altered venous flow hemodynamics to indirectly infer the presence of venous disease. Examples include plethysmographic techniques and continuous wave Doppler ultrasonography. In general, these techniques are highly operator dependent, subjective, lacking in specificity, and they fail to define the anatomy. However, they are inexpensive and may serve as useful screening functions in the hands of competent, experienced clinicians.

Invasive Imaging Methods—Venography

Venography displays the anatomy of the venous system and is the historical standard of venous imaging against which all other techniques are measured. However, its high relative cost, invasive nature, and low but finite risk of contrast reaction and postvenographic phlebitis have led to reluctance to use it. It also lacks the ability to give physiologic information.

Noninvasive Imaging Methods— Ultrasound

Real-time imaging with B-mode ultrasound and the addition of duplex Doppler and color flow Doppler sonography provides objective anatomic information similar to that of venography as well as physiologic information of venous hemodynamics.

The relatively low cost, noninvasive nature, widespread availability, portability, and proven high accuracy of ultrasound have led to its primary role in the diagnosis of venous thrombosis. Sonography has also assumed a role in the evaluation of venous incompetence, preoperative vein mapping, and evaluation of the venous system for patency before the placement of venous catheters.

The peripheral venous system is amenable to evaluation by other imaging techniques as well. Computed tomography (CT) continues to evolve with the availability of multidetector helical and, to a lesser extent, electron-beam CT. The reduced imaging times of these techniques allow vascular imaging, which is directed primarily at the arterial system but also allows exquisite depiction of the venous system. A strategy of adding pelvic and lower extremity venous evaluation to patients undergoing spiral CT to rule out pulmonary embolism has been successfully employed.[1,2] Magnetic resonance imaging (MRI) and magnetic resonance angiography (MRA) also continue to evolve and have shown promise in imaging the peripheral venous system. However, with the high accuracy, portability, availability, and cost of ultrasound, it is unlikely that CT or MRI will supplant ultrasound as the primary screening examination. In most centers, sonography is the primary imaging technique for lower extremity venous evaluation; MRI and CT serve a secondary role, usually in the search of pelvic, abdominal, or thoracic DVT. Venography is reserved for unusual problem-solving situations.

INSTRUMENTATION

Gray-Scale Imaging

The relatively superficial location and lack of overlying bowel and skeletal structures allow high-resolution imaging of most of the peripheral veins, with few exceptions. This superficial location favors the use of higher-frequency transducers. In most patients, a 5 MHz, linear, phased array transducer optimizes gray-scale imaging of the femoropopliteal and subclavian veins. In large patients or in instances in which the iliac veins or the inferior vena cava must be evaluated to determine the proximal extent of a thrombus, a 3.5-MHz transducer may be necessary to obtain adequate depth of penetration. Higher-frequency, 7.5-MHz transducers optimize visualization of superficial veins, such as the greater and lesser saphenous, brachial, and distal calf veins. As in all areas of sonography, the highest-frequency transducer that gives adequate depth of penetration should be used to optimize spatial resolution.

Doppler Sonography

Doppler sonographic techniques include both quantitative duplex spectral analysis and qualitative color flow Doppler sonography. Both techniques have a pivotal role in identifying and objectively quantifying disease states in the peripheral veins and give sonography the ability to detect altered venous hemodynamics. It is this coupling of anatomic and physiologic information that makes sonography such a powerful tool in the evaluation of vascular disease. The same linear, phased array transducers are coupled with Doppler ultrasound, which typically has a lower frequency. Many phased array transducers have the ability to steer the Doppler beam at angles independent of the imaging beam. Thus, shallower Doppler angles can be used, decreasing error

caused by poor Doppler angles. These considerations are even more critical in arterial evaluation. Color flow Doppler sonography is the simultaneous display of flow information in color superimposed on the gray-scale image. This qualitative information demonstrates relative blood velocity, areas of flow disturbance, and direction of blood flow. Color flow Doppler ultrasound has simplified and decreased examination times in many vascular sonographic studies. This technique permits rapid screening of long segments of the venous system and can provide critical information, especially in segments that are not amenable to compression, such as the subclavian veins or the leg veins in very large or obese persons. Power Doppler or Doppler Energy allows angle-independent color sonographic imaging and improves detection of very slow flow. It may have some advantages over standard color Doppler imaging in demonstrating small veins or veins with slow flow, such as calf veins.

LOWER EXTREMITY VEINS

Anatomy

The venous system of the lower extremities is divided into superficial and deep systems. The **superficial system** consists of the greater and lesser saphenous veins and their branches. The **greater saphenous vein** arises from the medial aspect of the common femoral vein in the proximal thigh, inferior to the inguinal ligament but superior to the bifurcation of the common femoral vein (Fig. 29-1). The greater saphenous vein then extends inferiorly to the level of the foot in the subcutaneous tissues of the medial thigh and leg. The normal greater saphenous vein typically is a single vein that is 1 to 3 mm in diameter at the level of the ankle and 3 to 5 mm in diameter at the saphenofemoral junction. These measurements assume importance when this vessel is evaluated before it is harvested for use as an autologous vein graft.

The **lesser saphenous vein** has a variable insertion into the posterior aspect of the proximal or mid-popliteal vein. The lesser saphenous vein then travels in the subcutaneous tissues of the dorsal calf to the ankle. The lesser saphenous vein is normally 1 to 2 mm in diameter distally and 2 to 4 mm in diameter at its junction with the popliteal vein and is also suitable for autologous graft material in many patients. Both the lesser and greater saphenous veins can become abnormally enlarged or varicose when superficial venous incompetence is present. An international forum of vascular specialists recommended changing the nomenclature of the superficial vein. The newly proposed terminology uses great (vs. greater) saphenous vein and small (vs. lesser) saphenous vein in an effort to achieve a common international standard.[3] It is not known if these new terms will become commonly used in North America.

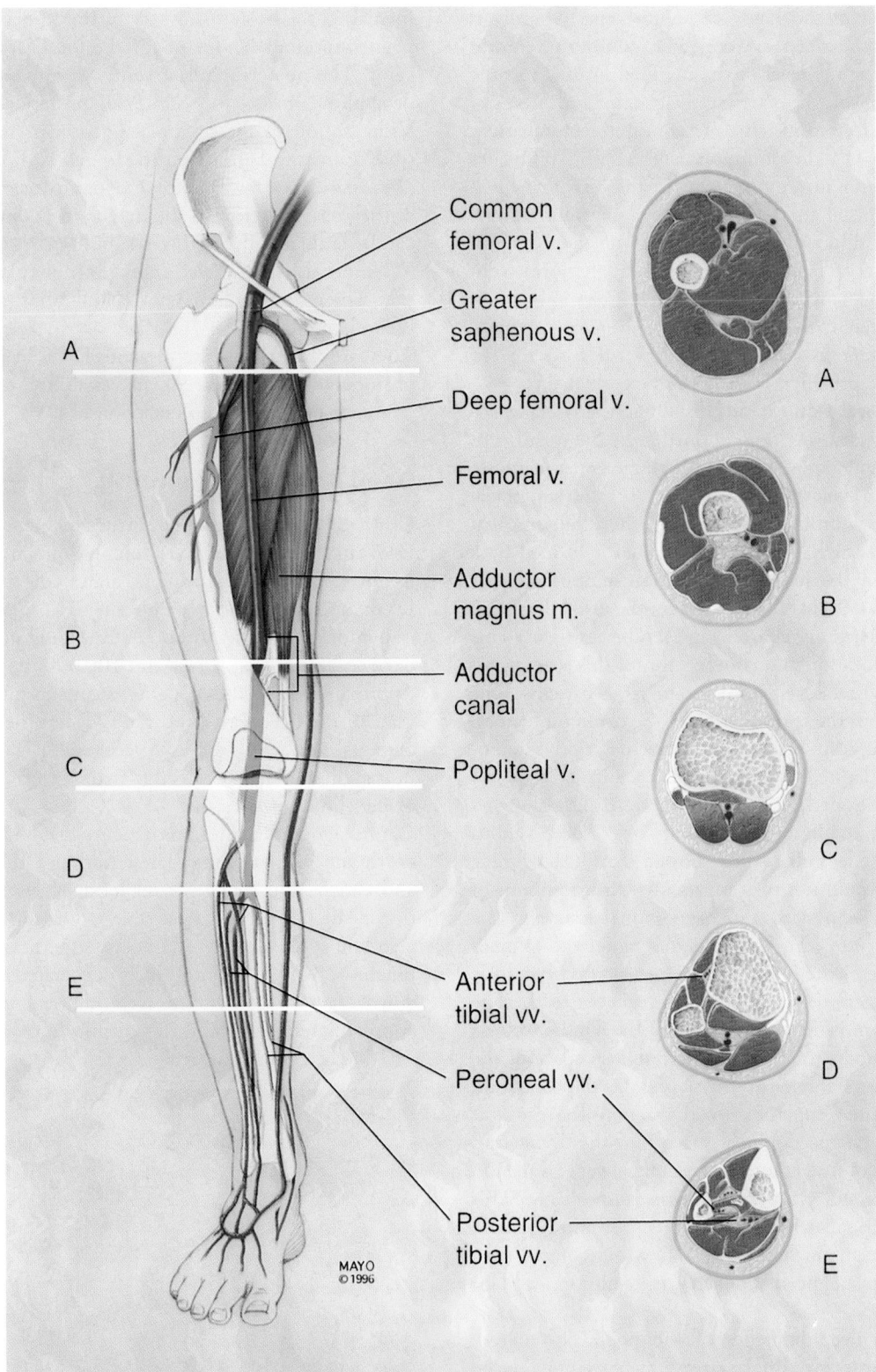

FIGURE 29-1. Anatomy of the lower extremity veins.

Evaluation of the lower extremity veins typically is directed at the **deep system**. The **common femoral vein** begins at the level of the inguinal ligament as the continuation of the external iliac vein and lies just medial and deep to the adjacent common femoral artery (see Fig. 29-1). The common femoral vein bifurcates into the deep and femoral veins in the proximal thigh 6 to 8 cm distal to the inguinal ligament and several centimeters distal to the bifurcation of the common femoral artery. The **deep (profunda) femoral vein** continues to lie medial to its respective artery as it travels deep and laterally to drain the musculature of the thigh. The deep femoral vein typically bifurcates extensively, and only the proximal portion can be evaluated.

The **femoral vein** extends distally in the fascial space deep to the sartorius muscle, medial to the quadriceps muscle group, and lateral to the adductor muscle group. The femoral vein remains medial to the superficial femoral artery until it passes through the adductor canal in the distal thigh. The adductor canal is formed by a separation in the tendinous insertion of the adductor magnus muscle. This canal is deep in the distal thigh and consists of dense aponeurotic and tendinous tissue. This makes visualization and compression of this segment of the distal femoral vein difficult in large patients. The femoral vein is the continuation of the common femoral vein and is a deep vein, but its classic descriptive anatomic nomenclature "superficial" is unfortunate. Studies of family practitioners and general internists have shown a poor understanding of the anatomy of the deep venous system of the leg. One study showed that 76% of these physicians would not treat a patient with thrombosis of the femoral vein with anticoagulation because it is a "superficial" vein.[4] This suggests that radiologists should limit the use of the term *superficial femoral vein* and use the more generic term *femoral vein* instead. The **popliteal vein** is the continuation of the femoral vein as it exits the adductor canal in the popliteal space of the posterior distal thigh. At this level, the popliteal vein lies immediately superficial to the popliteal artery as it passes through the popliteal space into the upper calf. Duplication of the femoral and popliteal veins is seen in up to 20% and 35% of patients, respectively. This anatomic variant is important to keep in mind because acute deep vein thrombosis (DVT) in one branch of a paired system can be overlooked during ultrasound (US) examination.

The first deep branches of the popliteal vein are the paired **anterior tibial veins**, which accompany the corresponding artery into the anterior compartment of the calf. These veins continue distally along the anterior surface of the interosseous membrane to the dorsal aspect of the foot. Shortly after the origin of the anterior tibial veins, the tibioperoneal venous trunk bifurcates into paired peroneal and posterior tibial veins. The **peroneal veins** lie adjacent to the peroneal artery and medial to the posterior aspect of the fibula. The fibula is an important landmark for the localization of these veins. The **posterior tibial veins** accompany the artery deep in the musculature of the calf, posterior to the tibia. Visualization of the proximal portion of the posterior tibial veins can be difficult in the calves of muscular or obese patients. However, these veins are easier to identify as they pass posterior to the medial malleolus and often can be evaluated in a retrograde fashion.

Numerous deep veins drain the musculature of the calf. These gastrocnemial and soleal veins do not have accompanying arteries and they vary in size and extent. They are a common site of acute DVT in high-risk or postoperative patients. Their variability often makes complete evaluation and detection of DVT suboptimal.

Deep Venous Thrombosis

Clinical Significance. The true incidence of acute DVT and its major complication, pulmonary embolism, is not known. In the United States, the incidence of DVT and pulmonary embolism is 70 per 100,000 individuals. As many as 600,000 persons suffer pulmonary embolism (Fig. 29-2) and 100,000 die as a result.[5] Approximately 200,000 patients are hospitalized each year for the treatment of acute DVT, but the majority of patients with DVT are asymptomatic.[6,7] The difficulty in making the diagnosis is due mainly to the inaccuracy of the clinical evaluation.

The signs and symptoms of acute DVT include **pain, erythema,** and **swelling**. These findings are nonspecific and can be caused by several local or systemic conditions. The presence of a palpable "cord," or thrombosed vein, most commonly is due to superficial thrombophlebitis, which is not usually associated with DVT. These factors contribute to a clinical accuracy of approximately 50% for the diagnosis of acute DVT

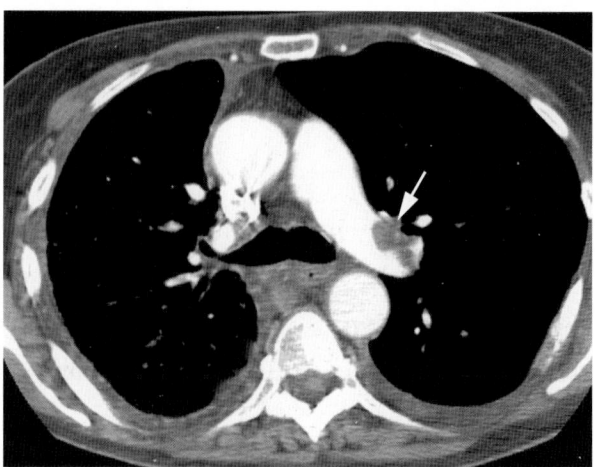

FIGURE 29-2. Acute pulmonary embolism CT.
Contrast-enhanced CT scan of the chest demonstrates an acute pulmonary embolism in the left pulmonary artery (*arrow*).

in symptomatic patients.[7-9] In fact, most hospitalized patients at high risk for developing acute venous thrombosis are asymptomatic.[7] In our vascular laboratory, only 11% of patients referred for suspected acute DVT in 2001 had positive findings on sonographic examination. Because acute DVT is a difficult clinical diagnosis to make and if untreated may have severe complications, including pulmonary embolism and postphlebitic syndrome, an accurate noninvasive method is required to establish the diagnosis. Numerous studies and extensive clinical experience have proved that sonography is an ideal technique for this purpose.

Examination. Evaluation of the deep venous system of the leg in patients with suspected acute DVT relies primarily on gray-scale imaging and venous compression in the transverse plane with color flow Doppler sonography frequently added. A 5-MHz linear array transducer is suitable for most patients. With mild pressure applied to the leg by the transducer, a normal vein will collapse completely and the vein walls will coapt (Fig. 29-3). The degree of pressure required varies, depending on the depth and location of the vein, but it is always less than that required to compress the adjacent artery.

The patient is examined in the supine position. The leg is abducted and rotated externally, with slight flexion of the knee. The standard examination begins with the proximal common femoral vein immediately distal to the inguinal ligament. The veins are visualized in the transverse plane and compressed in a stepwise fashion every 2 to 3 cm through the level of the distal femoral vein in the adductor canal. The proximal deep femoral vein and greater saphenous vein are also visible in this plane and can be evaluated in most patients. The popliteal vein is evaluated best with the patient prone

and the foot resting on a pad to maintain slight knee flexion. The left lateral decubitus position also provides adequate visualization. In these positions, transverse compression sonography can be carried out through the popliteal trifurcation. Many modifications or additions to this standard compression ultrasound examination can be used.

Examination Modifications. The pelvic venous system is poorly visualized because of its depth and overlying bowel gas. However, duplex spectral analysis of the common femoral vein while the patient performs the **Valsalva maneuver** can provide indirect evidence of proximal patency of the pelvic veins. In normal subjects, there is constant antegrade venous flow with slight superimposed variation with each respiratory phase. During the Valsalva maneuver, there is a short period of flow reversal, followed by no flow because of increased intraabdominal pressure. With release of the Valsalva maneuver, there is an abrupt increase in forward venous flow, which quickly returns to baseline (Fig. 29-4A). Patients with complete obstruction of the common or external iliac vein will have decreased or absent flow and loss of variation with respiration. There is no change in this spectral pattern with the Valsalva maneuver (see Fig. 29-4B). Sluggish venous flow may also be appreciated at standard real-time imaging because echogenic red blood cell rouleaux become visible. The Valsalva maneuver provides indirect physiologic evidence of venous patency from the level of the common femoral vein through the inferior vena cava.

False-negative examinations may occur with this indirect portion of the examination because of partial, nonoccluding thrombus in the iliac veins and patients with well-developed pelvic venous collaterals. Both of these conditions may result in a normal response to the

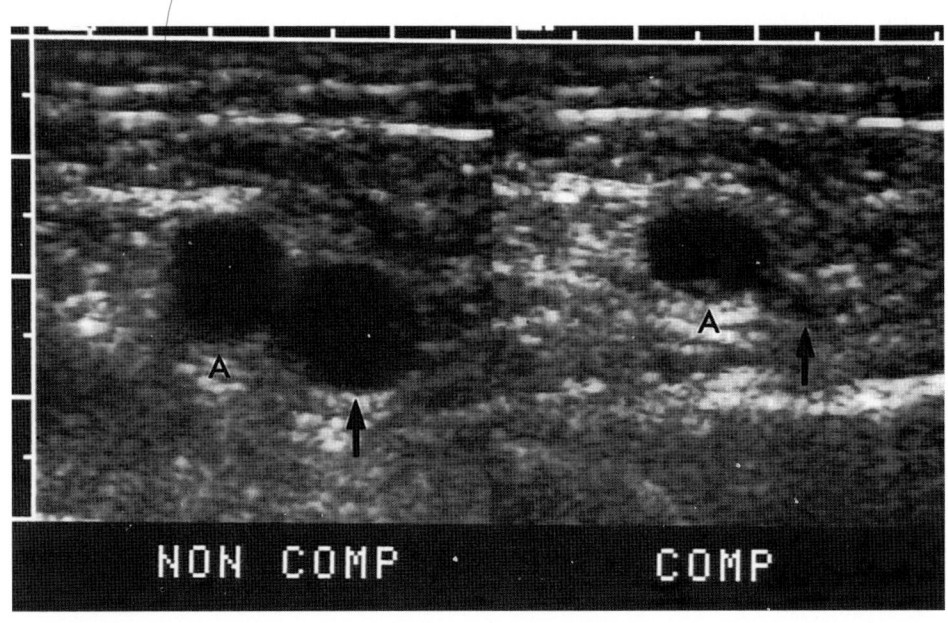

FIGURE 29-3. Normal venous compression ultrasonography. Transverse image of the right common femoral artery (**A**) and vein (*arrows*) before noncompression (NON COMP) and after compression (COMP) with the ultrasonographic transducer. The normal vein collapses completely with compression.

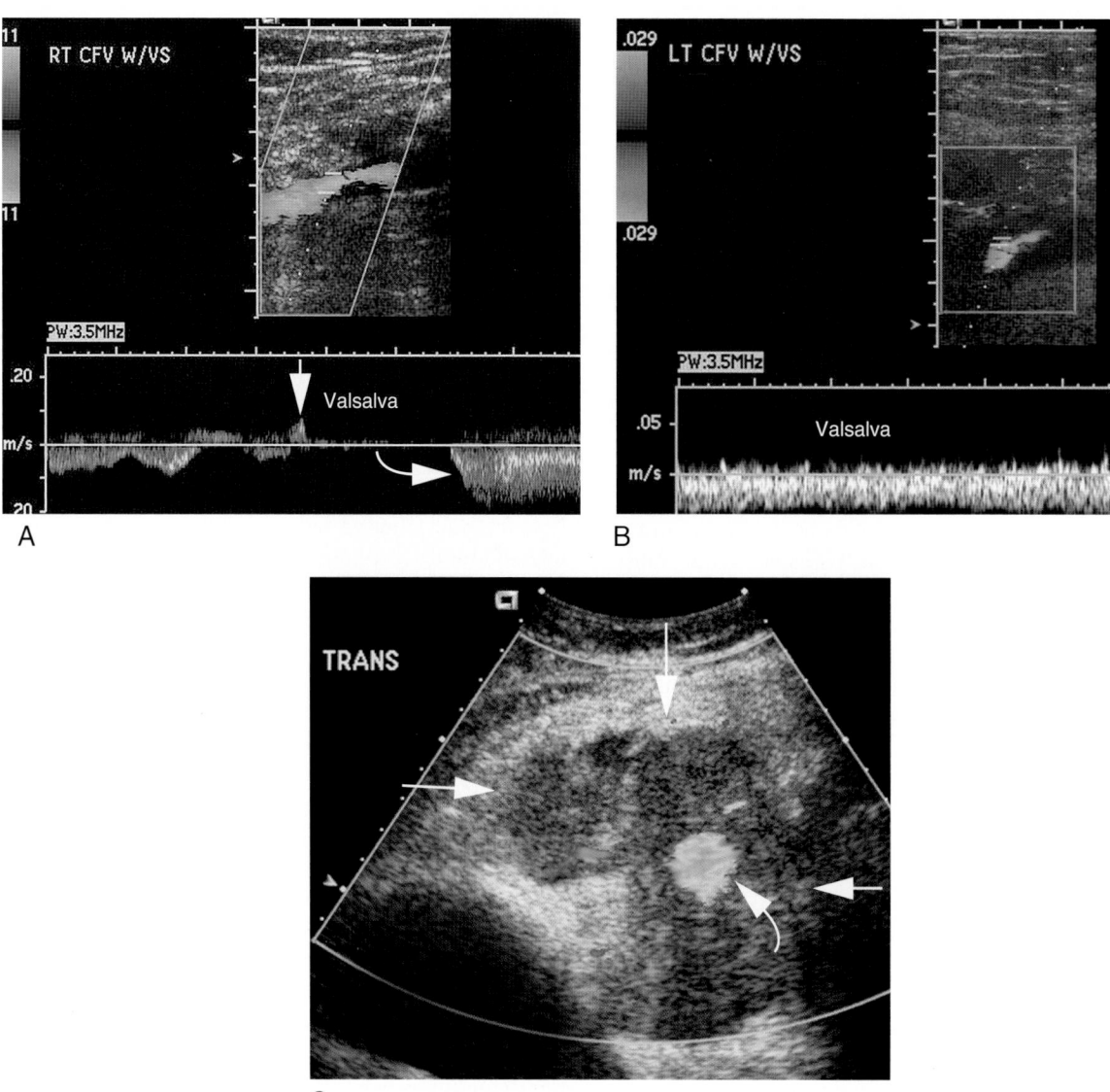

FIGURE 29-4. Iliac vein occlusion with Valsalva's maneuver. A, Normal response. Longitudinal image of the right common femoral vein (CFV) with duplex spectral analysis shows a normal response to Valsalva's maneuver. At the start of Valsalva's maneuver, there is a short period of flow reversal (*straight arrow*), followed by no flow throughout Valsalva's maneuver. With release of Valsalva's maneuver, normal flow returns (*curved arrow*). **B, Abnormal response**. Duplex spectral analysis shows no response to Valsalva's maneuver. **C, Malignant adenopathy** (*arrows*) encasing the external iliac artery (*curved arrow*). The external iliac vein is occluded by the adenopathy.

Valsalva maneuver. In patients with an abnormal Valsalva maneuver or a clinical suspicion of pelvic DVT, dedicated pelvic venous ultrasound can be of value. In thinner patients, the iliac veins may be visualized directly. A 3.5-MHz transducer with color flow Doppler capability may provide adequate visualization. Performing the US examination after an overnight fast decreases bowel gas and can improve visualization of the pelvic veins. If the pelvic veins are poorly seen on US examination and there is a high suspicion of pelvic vein DVT or extrinsic compression, contrast-enhanced CT is usually performed as the next diagnostic examination.

The addition of **color flow Doppler sonography** is a useful modification of the standard compression examination. In normal veins, color should fill the vessel lumen from wall to wall with little or no color aliasing outside the vessel lumen. Venous flow augmentation by squeezing the calf is often necessary to produce complete color filling. Color flow Doppler ultrasound can be helpful in evaluating venous segments that are poorly seen because of the patient's size or the deep location of the segment.[10] Color flow Doppler ultrasound may have some advantages over standard compression techniques in patients with chronic DVT as well.[10,11]

Evaluation of the calf veins is an additional modification of the standard examination that is aided by color flow Doppler techniques,[7-9] but the clinical value and cost-effectiveness of this evaluation are controversial. In some medical centers, the lower leg is not evaluated because it is rare for the isolated calf DVT to cause significant pulmonary emboli.[14] In other medical centers, the calf is evaluated routinely in patients with localized symptoms below the knee due to the 20% incidence of proximal clot propagation, the increased incidence of postphlebitic syndrome, and significant venous insufficiency after untreated calf thrombus. Given these local practice preferences, it is possible to evaluate the tibial and peroneal veins of the calf in many patients with a sensitivity of 92.5% and a specificity of 98.7%.[11-13,15]

Patients can be positioned so they are prone, in the left lateral decubitus position, or in the sitting position. Tilting the examination table into a **reverse Trendelenburg position** or having the patient sit improves visualization by distending the calf veins and decreases the indeterminate examination rate. The paired posterior tibial and peroneal veins are imaged with the transducer placed over the posterior calf. Compression ultrasound in the transverse plane and color Doppler sonography with augmentation of venous flow can be used to confirm venous patency. The anterior tibial veins can be evaluated from an anterior approach. Because thrombus isolated to these veins is rare, anterior examination is not necessary if the peroneal and posterior tibial veins are well seen and normal.[11] The deep veins of the gastrocnemius and soleus muscles do not have an accompanying artery and have variable anatomy. As such, they are not routinely included in the calf vein examination at most centers. However, compression US evaluation of the muscular veins has been shown to be an accurate technique with a sensitivity and specificity similar to that of the posterior tibial and peroneal veins.[16] In centers where calf DVT is treated with anticoagulation, the muscular calf veins should be included as part of the ultrasound examination.

Finally, a modification of the standard examination has been proposed that would greatly abbreviate the examination.[17] A limited venous compression sonographic examination of only the common femoral and popliteal veins in **symptomatic patients** would result in significant time savings, with a minimal decrease in sensitivity. It has been argued that this can be justified because of the relative rarity of isolated femoral vein or iliac vein thrombosis; because calf vein thrombosis is clinically less important; and because there will be potential cost savings from a shortened examination. Frederick et al.[18] recently reported a 4.6% incidence of isolated thrombosis of the femoral vein. It is doubtful that the cost savings of limited compression ultrasound will justify this reduced accuracy. Complete compression ultrasound from the proximal common femoral vein through the distal popliteal vein remains the standard of care.

Findings. The gray-scale compression sonographic findings of acute DVT are based on direct visualization of the thrombus and lack of venous compressibility (Fig. 29-5B). Visualization of thrombus is variable, depending on the extent, age, and echogenicity of the clot. Unfortunately, some acute thrombi may be anechoic, and gray-scale imaging alone can be misleading. Therefore, **the lack of complete venous compression** is the hallmark finding of DVT. **Venous distention** by thrombus can be seen acutely in patients but is less common as the clot ages and becomes organized. **Changes in vein caliber with respiration and the Valsalva maneuver are lost** in patients with DVT. Because this finding is present only in the proximal thigh, it is not usually helpful below the bifurcation of the common femoral vein.

Color flow Doppler ultrasound depiction of DVT relies on identifying either a persistent filling defect or thrombus in the color column of the vessel lumen (see Fig. 29-5) or the absence of flow. Color flow sonography depicts the degree of venous obstruction and any residual patent lumen. It is most helpful in deep segments of the thigh, pelvic, and calf veins.

Accuracy. The accuracy and clinical utility of sonographic assessment of DVT have been studied extensively. The patient population is of critical importance and should be considered in two broad groups: symptomatic and asymptomatic patients. In **symptomatic** patients, studies comparing venography with compression ultrasonography have shown an average sensitivity of 95% and specificity of 98%.[19] Studies of **asymptomatic**, high-risk, or postoperative patients have shown poorer results. Pooled results of six studies showed an average sensitivity of 59% and specificity of 98% in an asymptomatic population.[20] The small size, nonocclusive nature, and higher prevalence of isolated calf thrombi in this group of patients undoubtedly account for the lower sensitivity, because these are more difficult to diagnose with ultrasound as compared with venography. Given these results, the ideal patient for sonographic evaluation has symptoms that extend above the knee.

Chronic Deep Vein Thrombosis. The ability to characterize DVT as acute or chronic is a difficult clinical and imaging problem. Serial studies of patients with acute DVT show that up to 53% of these patients have persistent abnormal findings with compression ultrasound done from 6 to 24 months later.[21,22] These patients may present with postphlebitic syndrome and have symptoms that mimic those of acute DVT. Anticoagulation therapy is not indicated for these patients. Venography has been the standard imaging method for distinguishing between acute and chronic DVT. However, cost consideration and invasiveness have relegated venography to a problem-solving role in most medical centers. Although ultrasound may be able to help in some cases, currently the role of ultrasound in the diagnosis of chronic DVT is unproven.

As an acute thrombus ages, it undergoes fibroelastic organization, with clot retraction, chronic occlusion, or

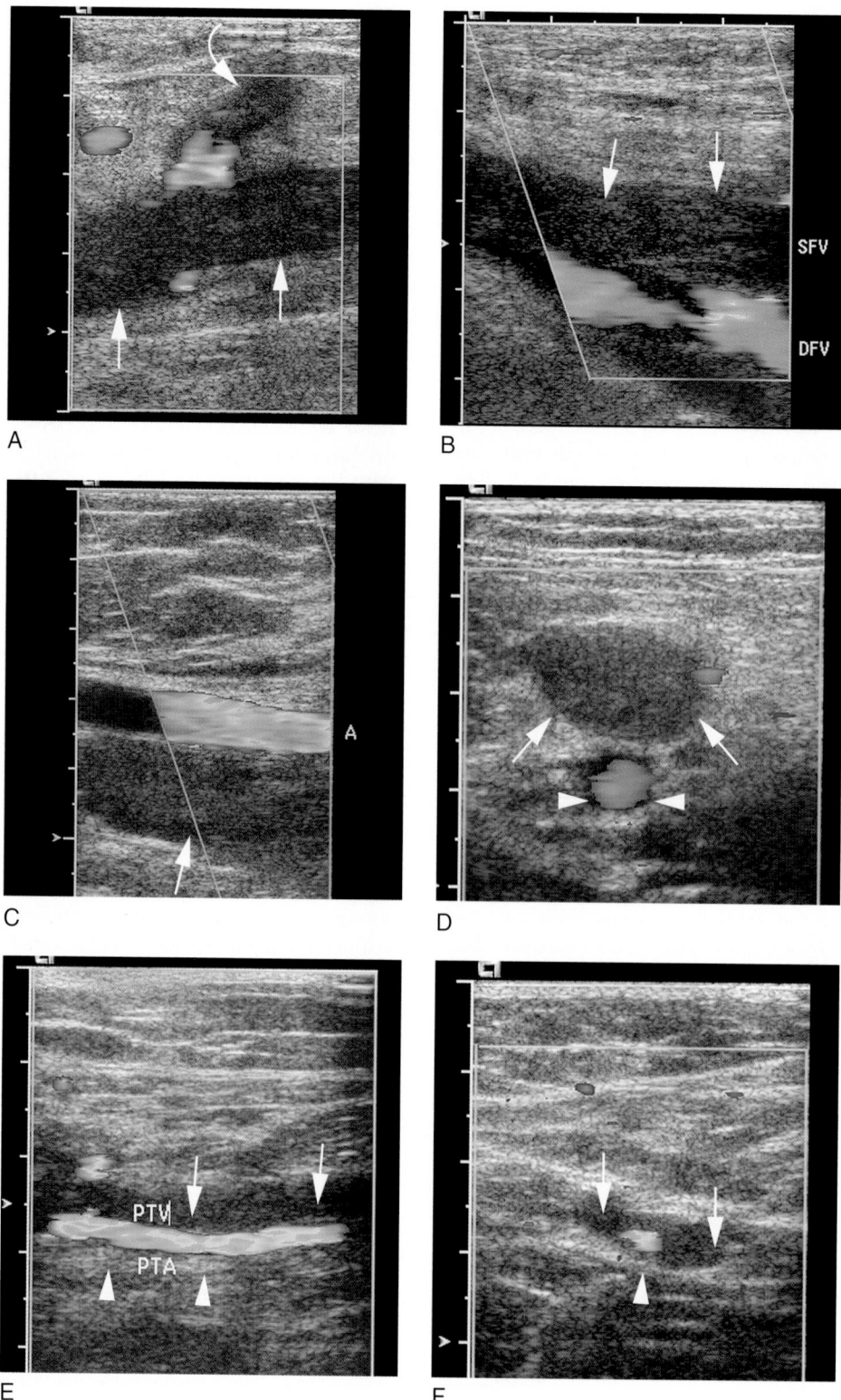

FIGURE 29-5. Appearances of acute deep vein thrombosis (DVT). Acute, hypoechoic thrombus filling and distending various lower deep veins. **A,** Longitudinal image of acute DVT of the CFV (*straight arrows*) and greater saphenous vein (*curved arrow*) at the level of the saphenofemoral junction. **B,** Longitudinal image of thrombus (*arrows*) in the proximal femoral vein (SFV). Note patent proximal deep femoral vein (DFV). **C,** Longitudinal image of the distal SFV showing distention by occlusive thrombus (*arrow*). **D,** Transverse compression image of acute DVT in right popliteal vein (*arrows*). The vein does not compress. Popliteal artery is patent (*arrowheads*). **E,** Longitudinal and **F,** transverse images of acute DVT in paired posterior tibial veins (*arrows*). Posterior tibial artery is patent (*arrowheads*).

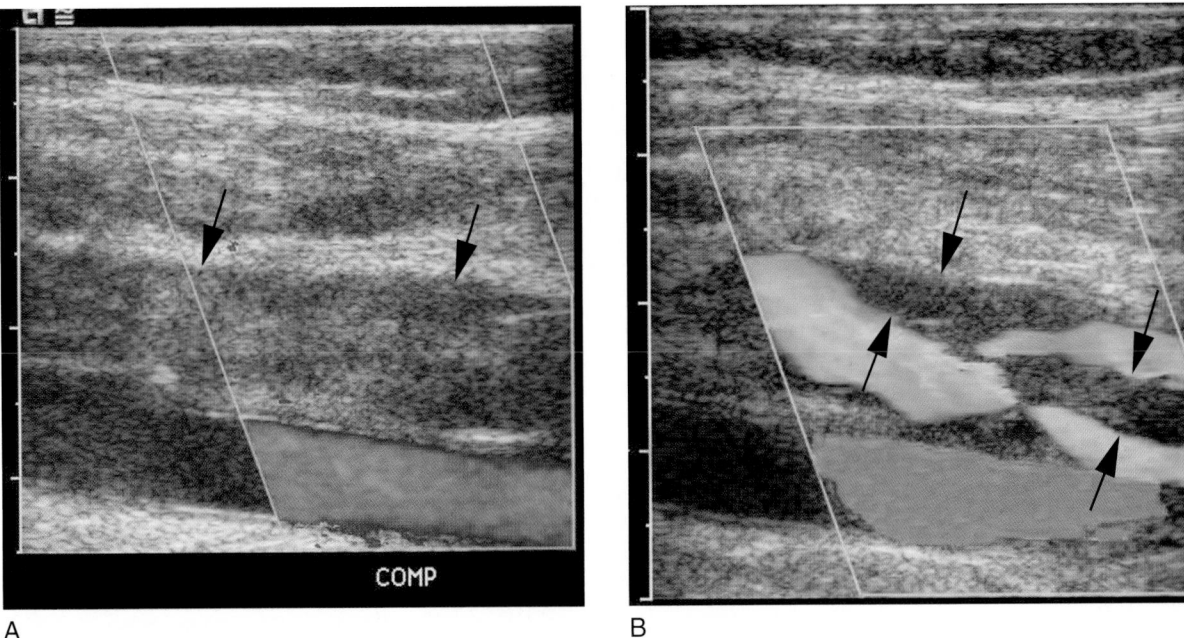

A   B

FIGURE 29-6. Evolution of acute DVT to chronic DVT. A, Longitudinal color Doppler image shows **acute thrombus** of the left popliteal vein (*arrows*). **B,** Color Doppler image after 2 months on anticoagulation therapy shows **partial recannulization** of the popliteal vein with retracted chronic DVT remaining (*arrows*).

wall thickening of the involved segment (Fig. 29-6). These changes lead to poor visualization of the clot and incomplete venous compression. Although compression sonography has little role in the diagnosis of chronic DVT, several authors have suggested that color flow Doppler ultrasound may have a role in some patients to differentiate acute DVT from chronic changes.[10,11] Findings suggestive of chronic DVT at color flow Doppler imaging include irregular echogenic vein walls, thickening of the vein walls due to retracted thrombus, calcified retracted thrombus, decreased diameter of the vein lumina (venous lumina), atretic venous segments, well-developed collateral veins, associated deep venous insufficiency, and absence of distended veins containing hypoechoic or isoechoic thrombus (Fig. 29-7). Although these findings may be suggestive of chronic DVT and should be familiar to practicing radiologists, the accuracy and role of color flow Doppler ultrasound in patients with chronic DVT are not proven. Some centers use US to follow all patients with acute DVT until complete resolution or until changes of chronic DVT have stabilized. These patients then have baseline US studies that permit new or superimposed acute DVT to be more readily identified.

Superficial Venous Thrombosis. Superficial venous thrombosis (SVT) or superficial thrombophlebitis refers to thrombus located in the greater or lesser saphenous veins or in superficial varicosities. SVT does not have the same clinical implications as DVT and is usually treated symptomatically with heat and aspirin. The exception is when SVT extends proximally to within 2 cm of the deep system (Fig. 29-8). Patients with SVT will have progression into the deep system in 11% of cases. Nearly all patients with proximal SVT involving the greater saphenous vein will progress if not anticoagulated.[23] Thus, most centers anticoagulate patients with SVT involving the greater or lesser saphenous vein if it extends to within 2 cm of the saphenofemoral or saphenopopliteal junction.

Venous Insufficiency

Pathophysiology. In many patients, venous insufficiency is caused by venous valvular damage following DVT. The fibroelastic organization and retraction present in the organizing thrombus secondarily involve any adjacent venous valve. This leads to deep venous insufficiency, which develops in approximately one half of the patients with acute DVT.[24] With venous insufficiency, there is direct transmission of the hydrostatic pressure of the standing column of fluid in the venous system to the distal leg. Clinically, this leads to leg swelling, chronic skin and pigmentation changes, woody induration, and finally, nonhealing venous stasis ulcers.

Superficial venous insufficiency leads to distended **subcutaneous varicosities** but has a much better prognosis. Perforating veins communicate from the superficial to the deep system and may also become incompetent, typically because of long-standing deep venous insufficiency.

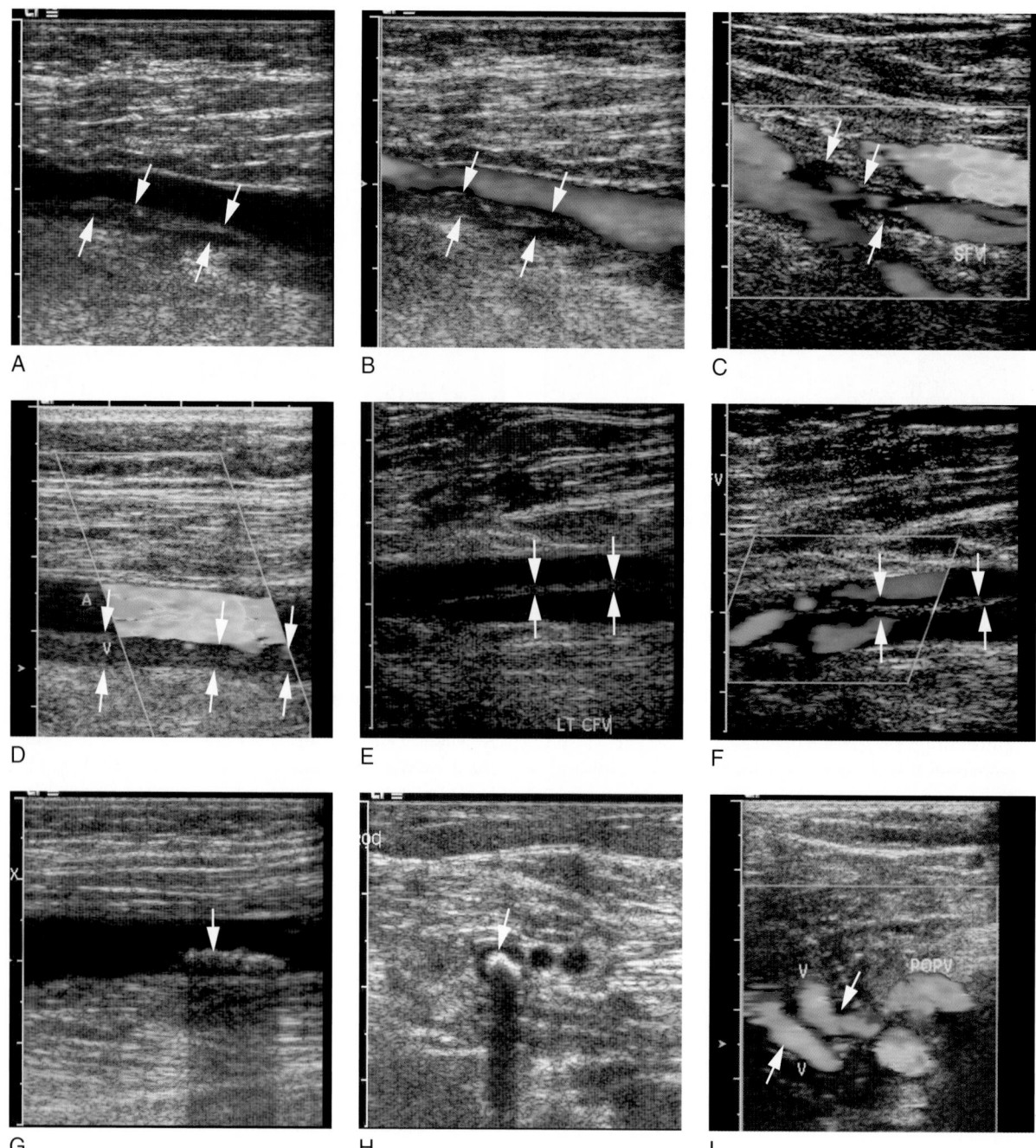

FIGURE 29-7. Chronic deep vein thrombosis (DVT). A and **B, Chronic retracted thrombus** (*arrows*) along the wall of the femoral vein. **C, Irregular wall thickening** (*arrows*) of proximal femoral vein and distal common femoral vein. **D, Atretic, chronically occluded** femoral vein (*arrows*). **E** and **F, Venous webs** (*arrows*) in the common femoral vein. **G,** Longitudinal image of SFV demonstrates chronic calcific thrombus (*arrow*). **H,** Transverse image of muscular vein of the calf demonstrates chronic **calcific thrombus** (*arrow*). **I,** Transverse image of popliteal space shows several **collateral veins** (*arrows*) near the popliteal vein and artery.

Examination. The examination is performed with the patient in an upright or semi-upright position, with the body's weight supported by the contralateral leg. This positioning is necessary to create the hydrostatic pressure needed to reproduce venous insufficiency. Duplex spectral analysis is obtained at several levels of the deep and superficial venous system during provocative maneuvers. Duplex Doppler tracings in the common femoral vein and proximal greater saphenous vein are obtained during Valsalva's maneuver. Several spectral tracings are obtained in the deep and superficial venous system to the level of the popliteal and saphenous veins at the knee. Reverse augmentation by squeezing the thigh above or standard distal venous augmentation by

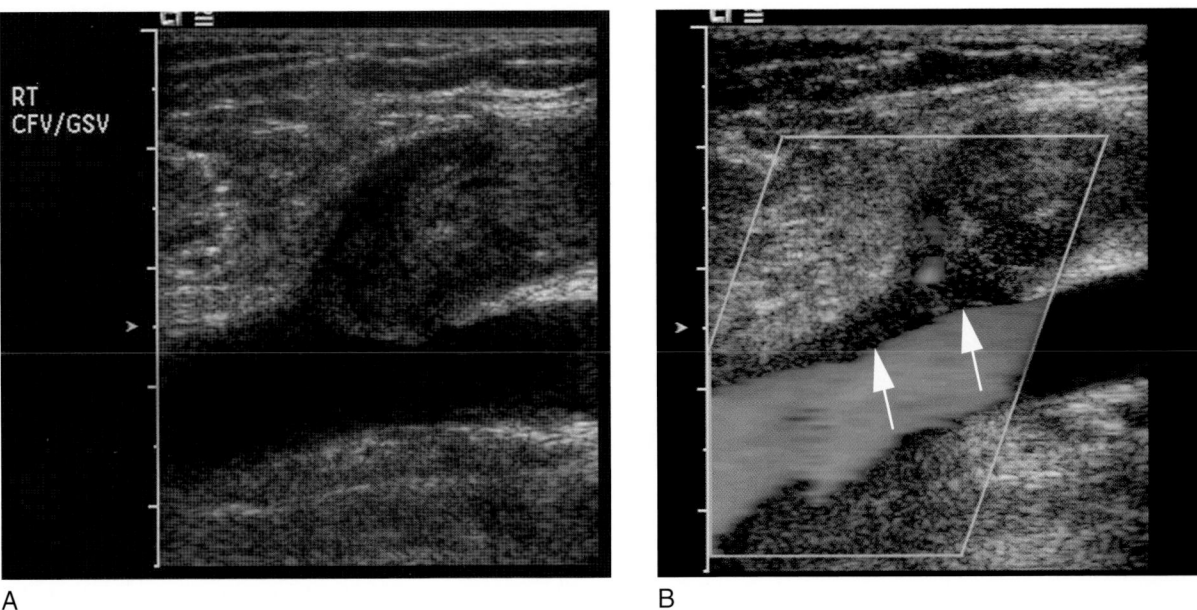

FIGURE 29-8. Superficial thrombophlebitis. A and **B,** Longitudinal gray-scale and color Doppler image of the right greater saphenous vein and saphenofemoral junction. Echogenic thrombus extends from the greater saphenous vein along the anterior wall of the common femoral vein (*arrows*).

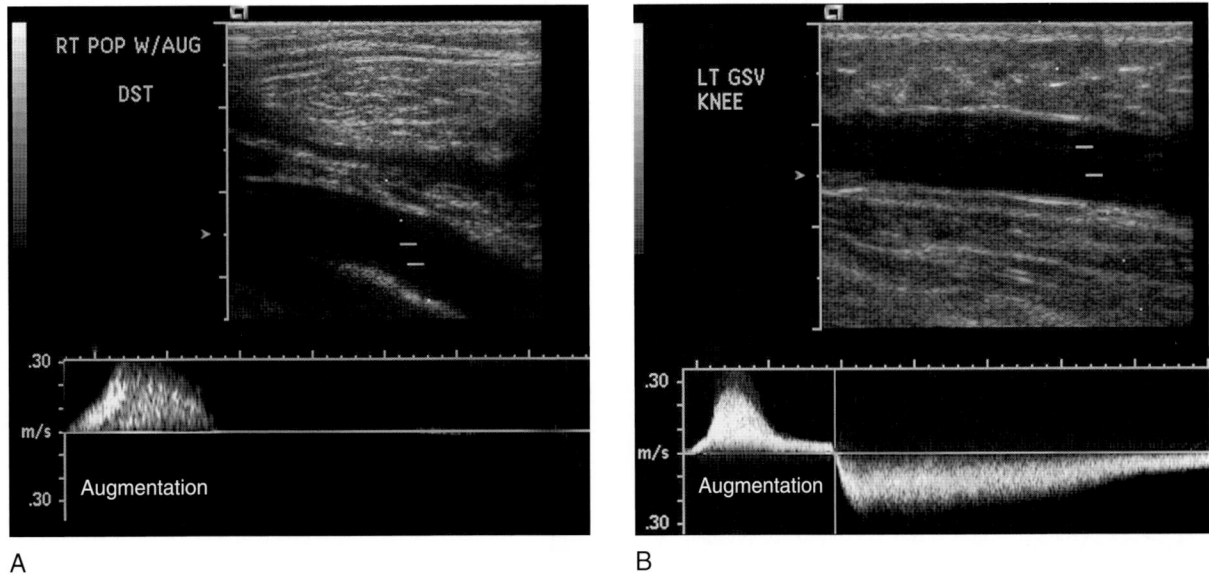

FIGURE 29-9. Venous insufficiency. A, Duplex spectral analysis of the popliteal vein shows a normal waveform with distal augmentation. Note no reversal of flow following distal augmentation. **B,** Duplex spectral analysis of the greater saphenous vein in another patient shows **prolonged (>7 sec) reflux after distal augmentation**, consistent with severe superficial venous insufficiency.

squeezing the calf can be used to assess for insufficiency. Because distal augmentation is more reproducible, it is easier for a single examiner to perform.

Findings. After brisk distal augmentation, the flow in normal veins is antegrade, with a very short period of flow reversal as returning blood closes the first competent venous valve (Fig. 29-9A). Distal augmentation can be performed manually or with automated devices that inflate every 5 to 10 seconds. The automated devices provide a more reproducible calf compression and increase the ease of the examination. Insufficient veins have a greater degree of reversed flow for a longer period of time (see Fig. 29-9B). Quantification schemes have been proposed by evaluating peak flow during venous reflux and measuring the length of time that reflux occurs. These quantification schemes are somewhat subjective and need to be validated in each vascular laboratory.

Venous Mapping

Vein Harvest for Autologous Grafts. Ultrasound mapping and marking are helpful in many patients before a vein is harvested as autologous graft material for peripheral arterial bypass graft. Any superficial vein can be used, but the greater saphenous vein is the most suitable for graft purposes. The examination is performed with the patient in the supine or reverse Trendelenburg position. A tourniquet or blood pressure cuff that is inflated to 50 mm Hg and placed around the proximal thigh can be used to increase venous distention and to aid in mapping. The greater saphenous vein is identified and marked from the level of the sapheno-femoral junction to as far distally as possible. All major branch points should also be marked to aid the surgeon. A superficial vein typically needs to be larger than 3 mm in diameter, but not varicose, to be suitable graft material. The lesser saphenous vein, cephalic vein, and basilic vein are secondary choices and can be used if the greater saphenous vein has already been harvested or is inadequate.

Insufficient Perforating Vein Marking. Newer surgical techniques of subfascial endoscopic ligation of insufficient perforating veins are being used in some medical centers to treat chronic venous stasis changes and nonhealing venous ulcers. These techniques are aided by accurate localization and marking of insufficient venous perforators. The majority of perforating veins are located below the knee in the medical calf. In an upright patient, distended perforating veins are visible as they pass from the subcutaneous tissues through the superficial fascia into the deep muscles of the calf.

These are easily visible on standard gray-scale imaging, and insufficiency can be documented with duplex spectral analysis and flow augmentation (Fig. 29-10). Competent perforating veins are much smaller in caliber and often are difficult or impossible to visualize.

UPPER EXTREMITY VEINS

Anatomy

Venous return from the arm is primarily through the superficial cephalic and basilic veins. The **cephalic vein** travels in the subcutaneous fat of the lateral aspect of the arm. The cephalic vein joins with the deep venous system at the superior aspect of the axillary or distal subclavian vein (Fig. 29-11). The **basilic vein** is located superficially in the medial aspect of the arm. At the level of the teres major muscle, it joins with the paired deep brachial veins. The **brachial veins** are smaller, deeper, and adjacent to the brachial artery. The level where the brachial and basilic veins join, at the teres major muscle, defines the lateral aspect of the axillary vein. The **axillary vein** is adjacent and superficial to the axillary artery as it passes from the teres major muscle to the first rib through the axilla.

As the axillary vein crosses the first rib, it becomes the lateral portion of the subclavian vein. The subclavian vein is inferior and superficial to the adjacent artery as it passes medially deep to the clavicle. The medial portion of the subclavian vein receives the smaller external jugular vein and the larger internal jugular vein in the base of the neck to form the brachiocephalic (innominate) vein. The internal jugular vein extends from the jugular

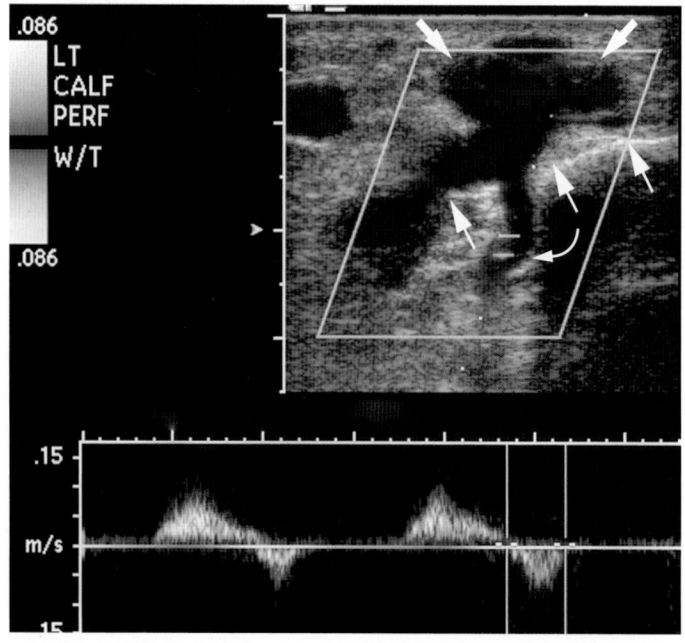

FIGURE 29-10. Incompetent perforating vein. Transverse image and spectral analysis of a dilated perforating vein (*curved arrow*) passing through the fascial plane (*thin arrows*) between the subcutaneous fat and musculature into a superficial varicosity (*thick arrows*). Duplex spectral analysis shows reversed flow in the perforating vein indicating incompetence.

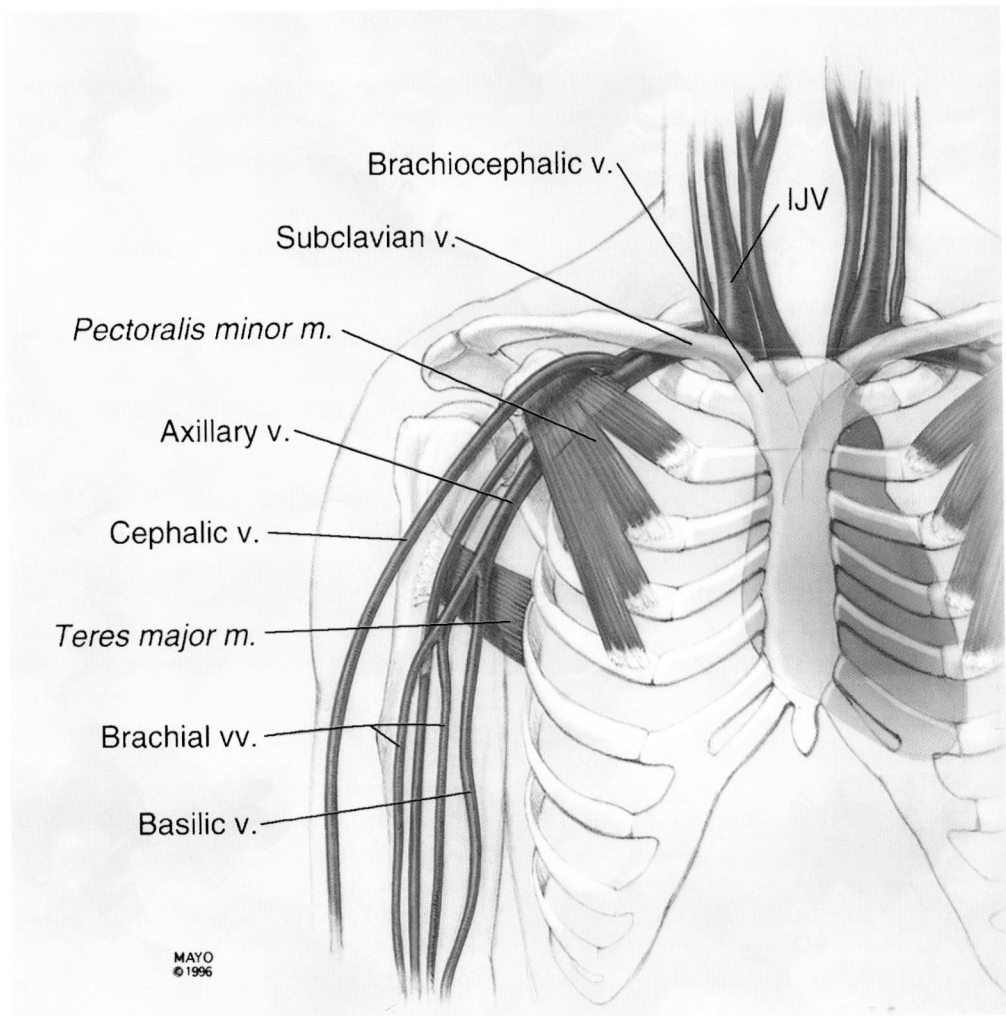

FIGURE 29-11. Anatomy of the upper extremity veins. IJV, internal jugular vein.

foramen in the base of the skull to the confluence with the subclavian vein. The internal jugular vein travels in the carotid sheath and is superficial and lateral to the common carotid artery in the anterior neck. The left and right internal jugular veins are often unequal in size. The brachiocephalic vein is formed by the confluence of the subclavian and internal jugular veins. The right brachiocephalic vein travels along the superficial aspect of the superior right mediastinum. The left brachiocephalic vein is longer and passes from the left superior mediastinum to the right, just deep to the sternum. The right and left brachiocephalic veins join to form the superior vena cava.

Clinical Background

The most common indication for ultrasound evaluation of upper extremity veins is to identify venous thrombosis. The cause and clinical significance of acute DVT of the upper extremity veins differ from those of acute

DVT in the legs. Most cases of arm DVT are thought to be due to the presence of a **central venous catheter** or **pacemaker lead**. Of patients with central catheters, 26% to 67% develop thrombosis, although the majority are asymptomatic.[25,26] **Radiation therapy, effort-induced thrombosis,** and **malignant obstruction** are causes of venous obstruction that are more common in the thorax and arm than in the leg. Although the cause of upper extremity DVT differs from that of the lower extremity, the pathophysiology of its evolution is similar.

The sequelae of upper extremity thrombosis are less severe than those of lower extremity thrombosis. Only 10% to 12% of patients with arm DVT develop pulmonary emboli, and the majority of these are insignificant.[27-29] The development and manifestations of venous stasis and venous insufficiency due to deep venous thrombosis are less common and less severe than in the leg. Chronic swelling, skin changes, and nonhealing venous ulcers are rare in the arm. This is due to two major factors: first, multiple extensive collateral venous pathways usually develop in the arm and upper thorax after an episode of thrombosis or venous obstruction; second, the arm veins are not exposed to the high hydrostatic pressure that leg veins have. Chronic occlusion related to intravenous catheter use and venous thrombosis has made obtaining suitable central venous access difficult in many hospitalized and chronically ill patients. Sonography is ideal for identifying suitable sites for venous access. In difficult cases, direct real-time ultrasonic guidance can be used for placement of venous catheters.

Venous Thrombosis

Examination. Evaluation of the venous system of the upper thorax and arm typically extends from the superior aspect of the brachiocephalic veins through the axillary or brachial veins. The internal jugular veins are also studied. The patient is positioned supine, with the arm to be examined slightly abducted and rotated externally. The patient's head is turned slightly to the opposite side. The highest-frequency transducer that still provides adequate depth of penetration is used. Typically, a 7.5-MHz linear array transducer is used for the internal jugular vein and the arm veins through the axillary vein. A 5-MHz linear array transducer with color Doppler ultrasound capability is often necessary to visualize the subclavian vein.

Evaluation of the venous system of the upper thorax and arm presents several technical challenges different from the lower extremity. First, the overlying skeletal structures and the lung make direct visualization and examination of the inferior brachiocephalic veins and superior vena cava impossible. Second, the clavicle precludes compression ultrasound of the subclavian vein. Third, the typical development of large venous collateral pathways in patients with venous obstruction can be confusing or lead to false-negative sonographic examination results if they are not recognized as collateral pathways. For these reasons, color flow Doppler sonography, attention to detail, and knowledge of the normal anatomic relationships are crucial.

The internal jugular vein is examined initially with compression sonography in the transverse plane and is followed inferiorly to its junction with the subclavian and upper brachiocephalic veins. An inferiorly angled, coronal, supraclavicular approach with color flow Doppler sonography is necessary to evaluate the superior brachiocephalic vein and the medial portion of the subclavian vein. Duplex Doppler sonographic analysis of the inferior internal jugular vein, superior brachiocephalic vein, and medial subclavian vein is helpful to assess transmitted cardiac pulsatility and respiratory phasicity. Because of the proximity to the heart, duplex Doppler spectral tracings in these sites will show greater transmitted pulsatility than in the leg veins. Loss of this pulsatility may be due to a more central venous obstruction (Fig. 29-12). Comparison of these Doppler ultrasound waveforms with those from the contralateral arm is often helpful to confirm the presence or absence of venous obstruction. Response to Valsalva's maneuver or a brisk inspiratory sniff can also be observed and may also help evaluate venous patency. If the patient sniffs, the internal jugular vein or subclavian vein will decrease in diameter, and spectral analysis will show an increase in blood velocity. Patients with central brachiocephalic vein or superior vena cava obstruction lose this response.

The **subclavian vein** is difficult to visualize completely. A coronal, supraclavicular, inferiorly angled approach is used medially, and a coronal, infraclavicular, superiorly angled approach is used laterally. The venous segment deep to the clavicle often is imaged incompletely. Because of the overlying clavicle, color flow Doppler sonography is necessary to confirm complete venous patency. The examiner should also confirm the normal inferior superficial relationship of the vein with the adjacent artery. This will avoid the pitfall of confusing well-developed collateral vessels for a patent subclavian vein in patients with chronic venous occlusion. The axillary and upper arm veins can also be evaluated with transverse compression or color flow Doppler ultrasound. The extent of the examination into the arm depends on the clinical indication, but typically it is continued through the bifurcation of the axillary vein.

Findings. The normal and abnormal findings in the upper extremity veins mirror those seen in the lower extremity veins. Patients with venous thrombosis have incomplete collapse of the vein with compression. Thrombus or an intraluminal filling defect is visible in the color column of the vein with color flow Doppler ultrasound (Fig. 29-13). Absent or decreased cardiac pulsatility with duplex spectral analysis and abnormal response to an inspiratory sniff are also helpful. Abundant, well-developed collateral vessels are common because of long-standing venous occlusion.

Accuracy. The accuracy of ultrasound versus venography in patients with acute DVT of the upper extremity has not been studied as extensively as in the lower extremity. The available literature shows sensitivity ranging from 78% to 100% and specificities of 92% to 100%.[30-32] The lower accuracy in the upper extremity compared with that in the lower extremity is a result of the greater number of technical challenges facing the examiner.

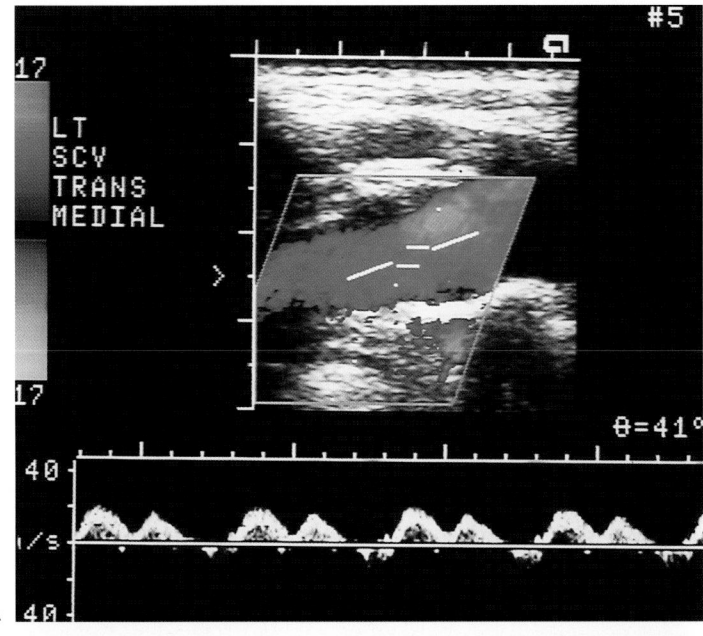

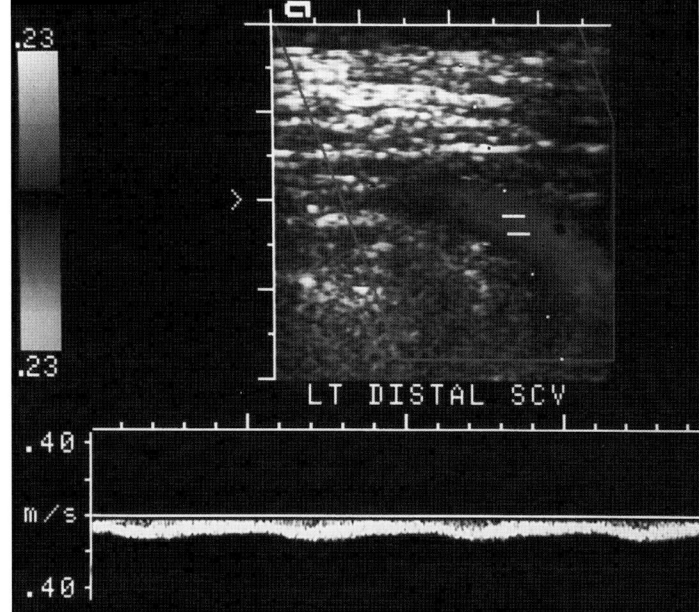

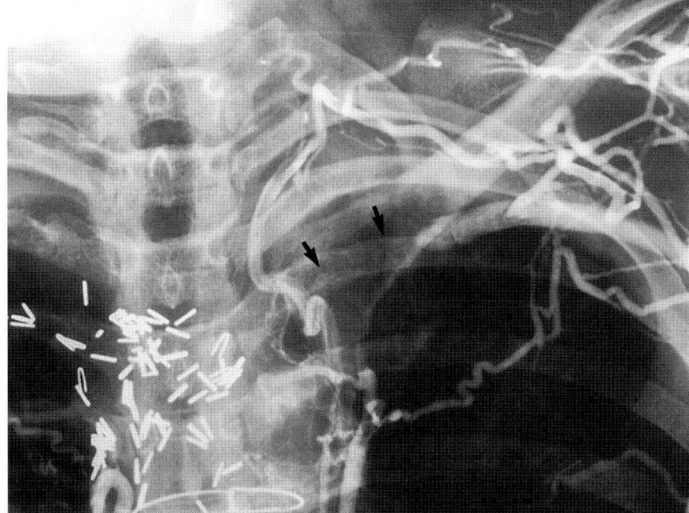

FIGURE 29-12. Comparison of normal and obstructed subclavian veins. A, Normal **subclavian vein (SCV),** transverse color flow Doppler ultrasonography and spectral analysis. There is complete color filling and normal transmitted cardiac pulsations. **B, Loss of the transmitted cardiac pulsations.** Transverse image of the left subclavian vein in another patient. Doppler shows the SCV is patent but has reversed flow direction. **C, Subclavian vein occlusion** (*arrows*) with numerous collateral vessels on venogram.

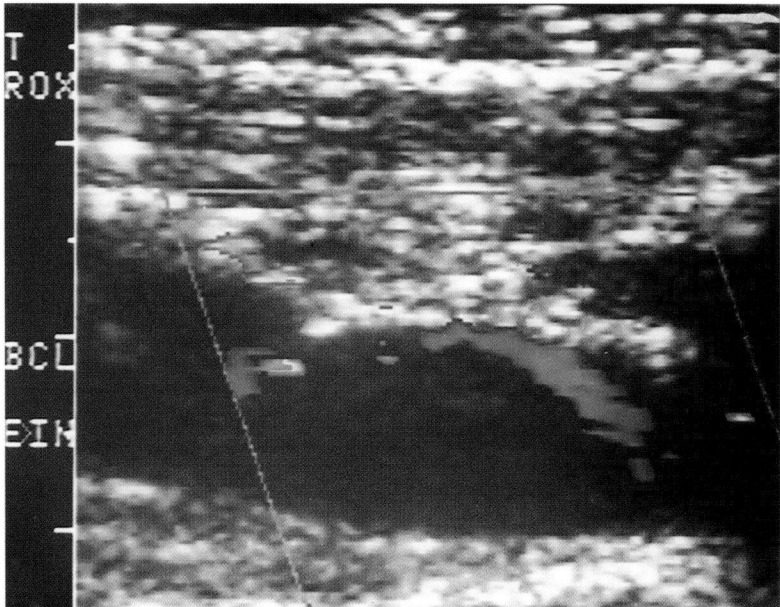

FIGURE 29-13. Acute subclavian vein thrombosis. Transverse color flow Doppler ultrasonogram of the subclavian vein shows extensive hypoechoic thrombus with minimal peripheral flow remaining.

References

Lower Extremity Veins

1. Loud PA, Katz, DS et al: Combined CT venography and pulmonary angiography in suspected thromboembolic disease: Diagnostic accuracy for deep venous evaluation. AJR 2000;174:61-65.
2. Cham MD, Yankelevitz DF, Shaham D, et al: Deep venous thrombosis: Detection by using indirect CT venography. Radiology 2000;216:744-751.
3. Caggiati A, Bergan JJ, Gloviczki P, et al: Nomenclature of the veins of the lower limbs: An international interdisciplinary consensus statement. J Vasc Surg 2002; 36(2):416-422.
4. Bundens WP, Bergan JJ, Halasz NA, et al: The femoral vein. A potentially lethal misnomer. JAMA 1995; 274:1296-1298.
5. Anderson FA, Wheeler HB, Goldberg RJ, et al: A population-based perspective of the hospital incidence and case-fatality rates of deep vein thrombosis and pulmonary embolism. Arch Intern Med 1991;151:933-938.
6. Sandler DA, Martin JF: Autopsy proven pulmonary embolism in hospital patients: Are we detecting enough deep vein thrombosis? J R Soc Med 1989;82:203-205.
7. Salzman EW: Venous thrombosis made easy (editorial). N Engl J Med 1986;314:847-848.
8. Haeger K: Problems of acute deep venous thrombosis. I. The interpretation of signs and symptoms. Angiology 1969;20:219-223.
9. Barnes RW, Wu KK, Hoak JC: Fallibility of the clinical diagnosis of venous thrombosis. JAMA 1975;234:605-607.
10. Lewis BD, James EM, Welch TJ, et al: Diagnosis of acute deep venous thrombosis of the lower extremities: Prospective evaluation of color Doppler flow imaging versus venography. Radiology 1994;192:651-655.
11. Rose SC, Zwiebel WJ, Nelson BD, et al: Symptomatic lower extremity deep venous thrombosis: Accuracy, limitations, and role of color duplex flow imaging in diagnosis. Radiology 1990;175:639-644.
12. Polak JF, Culter SS, O'Leary DH: Deep veins of the calf: Assessment with color Doppler flow imaging. Radiology 1989;171:481-485.
13. Atri M, Herba MJ, Reinhold C, et al: Accuracy of sonography in the evaluation of calf deep vein thrombosis in both postoperative surveillance and symptomatic patients. AJR 1996;166:1361-1367.
14. Gottlieb RH, Widjaja J, Mehra S, Robinette WB: Clinically important pulmonary emboli: Does calf vein US alter outcomes? Radiology 1999;211:25-29.
15. Gottlieb RH, Widjaja J, Tian L, et al: Calf sonography for detecting deep venous thrombosis in symptomatic patients: Experience and review of the literature. J Clin Ultrasound 1999;27:415-420.
16. Krunes U, Teubner K, Knipp H, Holzapfel R: Thrombosis of the muscular calf veins—reference to a syndrome which receives little attention. Vasa 1998;27:172-175.
17. Pezzullo JA, Perkins AB, Cronan JJ: Symptomatic deep vein thrombosis: Diagnosis with limited compression US. Radiology 1996;198:67-70.
18. Frederick MG, Hertzberg BS, Kliewer MA, et al: Can the US examination for lower extremity deep venous thrombosis be abbreviated? A prospective study of 755 examinations. Radiology 1996;199:45-47.
19. Cronan JJ: Venous thromboembolic disease: The role of US. Radiology 1993;186:619-630.
20. Weinmann EE, Salzman EW: Deep-vein thrombosis. N Engl J Med 1994;331:1630-1641.
21. Cronan JJ, Leen V: Recurrent deep venous thrombosis: Limitations of US. Radiology 1989;170:739-742.
22. Baxter GM, Duffy P, MacKechnie S: Colour Doppler ultrasound of the post-phlebitic limb: Sounding cautionary note. Clin Radiol 1991;43:301-304.
23. Chengelis DL, Bendick PJ, Glover JL, et al: Progression of superficial venous thrombosis to deep vein thrombosis. J Vasc Surg 1996;24:745-749.
24. Van Haarst EP, Liasis N, van Ramshorst, Moll FL: The development of valvular incompetence after deep vein thrombosis: A 7 year follow-up study with duplex scanning. Eur J Vasc Endovasc Surg 1996;12:295-299.

Upper Extremity Veins

25. Bonnet F, Loriferne JF, Texier JP, et al: Evaluation of Doppler examination for diagnosis of catheter-related deep vein thrombosis. Intensive Care Med 1989;15:238-240.

26. McDonough JJ, Altemeier WA: Subclavian venous thrombosis secondary to indwelling catheters. Surg Gynecol Obstet 1971;133:397-400.

27. Horattas MC, Wright DJ, Fenton Ah, et al: Changing concepts of deep venous thrombosis of the upper extremity—report of a series and review of the literature. Surgery 1988;104:561-567.

28. Becker DM, Philbrick JT, Walker FB, 4th: Axillary and subclavian venous thrombosis. Prognosis and treatment. Arch Intern Med 1991;151:1934-1943.

29. Monreal M, Lafox E, Ruiz J, et al: Upper-extremity deep venous thrombosis and pulmonary embolism. A prospective study. Chest 1991;99:280-283.

30. Knudson GJ, Wiedmeyer DA, Erickson SJ, et al: Color Doppler sonographic imaging in the assessment of upper-extremity deep venous thrombosis. AJR 1990;154:399-403.

31. Baxter GM, Kincaid W, Jeffrey RF, et al: Comparison of colour Doppler ultrasound with venography in the diagnosis of axillary and subclavian vein thrombosis. Br J Radiol 1991;64:777-781.

32. Morton MJ, James EM, Welch TJ, et al: Duplex and color Doppler imaging in the evaluation of upper extremity and thoracic inlet deep venous thrombosis (exhibit). AJR 1994;162(suppl):192.

Index

i

F

O

DATE DUE
DATE DE RETOUR

AUG 1 5 2011	

CARR McLEAN   38-296